PDR NURSE'S HANDBOOK

FIRST EDITION • 1996

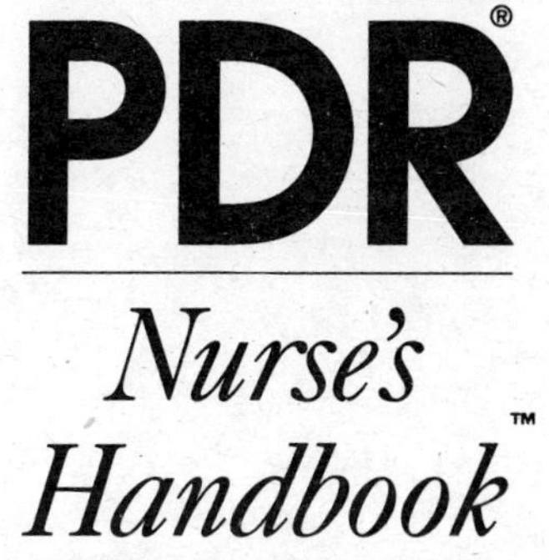

Nurse's Handbook™

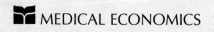
MEDICAL ECONOMICS

PDR NURSE'S HANDBOOK

FIRST EDITION • 1996

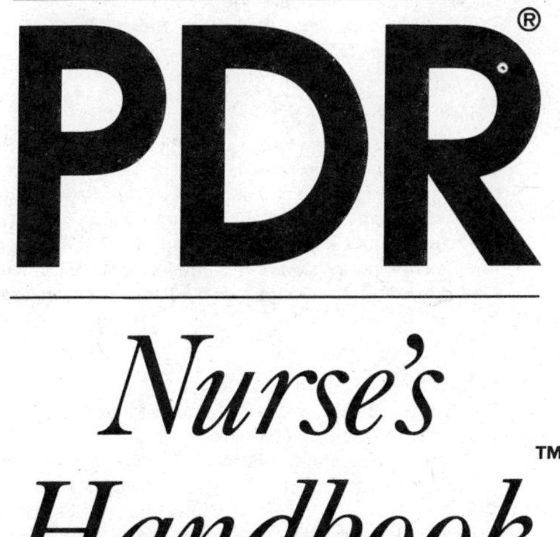

Nurse's Handbook™

MEDICAL ECONOMICS
MONTVALE, NEW JERSEY

PUBLISHING STAFF

President and Chief Operating Officer, Drug Information Services Group: Thomas F. Rice
Director of Product Management: Stephen B. Greenberg
Associate Product Manager: Howard N. Kanter
Director, Professional Support Services: Mukesh Mehta, RPh
Drug Information Specialist: Thomas Fleming, RPh
Director of Database and Systems Development: Robert Charleston
Database Administrator: Tom Y. Gong
Production Manager: Kimberly Hiller-Vivas
Director of Corporate Communications: Gregory J. Thomas
Art Director: Richard A. Weinstock
Electronic Publishing Designer: Kevin J. Leckner
Digital Photography: Shawn W. Cahill, Frank J. McElroy, III
Direct Marketing Manager: Robert W. Chapman

DEVELOPMENT STAFF

Publisher: Diane McOscar
Administrative Editor: Patricia Casey
Developmental Editor: Marjorie A. Bruce
Production Coordinator: Barbara A. Bullock
Art and Design Coordinator: Timothy J. Conners
Editorial Assistant: Tonjia Herman

ISBN: 1-56363-157-1

Manufactured in the United States of America

10 9 8 7 6 5 4 3 2 1

The monographs in this inaugural edition of the *PDR Nurse's Handbook* are the work of two distinguished authors: George R. Spratto, Ph.D., Dean of the School of Pharmacy at West Virginia University, Morgantown, West Virginia, and Adrienne L. Woods, M.S.N., R.N., N.P., Family Nurse Practitioner, Primary Care, at the Department of Veterans Affairs Medical and Regional Office Center, Wilmington, Delaware.

Notice to the Reader

The publisher and the authors do not warrant or guarantee any of the products described herein or perform any independent analysis in connection with any of the product information contained herein. The publisher and the authors do not assume and expressly disclaim any obligation to obtain and include information other than that provided by drug manufacturers.

The reader is expressly warned to consider and adopt all safety precautions that might be indicated by the activities described herein and to avoid all potential hazards. By following the instructions contained herein the reader willingly assumes all risks in connection with such instructions.

The publisher and the authors make no representations or warranties of any kind, including but not limited to the warranties of fitness for particular purpose or merchantability nor are any such representations implied with respect to the material set forth herein, and the publisher and the authors take no responsibility with respect to such material. The publisher and the authors shall not be liable for any special, consequential, or exemplary damages resulting, in whole or in part, from the reader's use of, or reliance upon, this material.

The authors and publisher have made a conscientious effort to ensure that the drug information and recommended dosages in this book are accurate and in accord with accepted standards at the time of publication. However, pharmacology and therapeutics are rapidly changing sciences, so readers are advised, before administering any drug, to check the package insert provided by the manufacturer for the recommended dose, for any additional contraindications for administration, and for any added warnings and precautions. This recommendation is especially important for new, infrequently used, or highly toxic drugs.

Acknowledgments

George Spratto wishes to extend appreciation to his colleagues at West Virginia University for their support and constant encouragement. Greatest appreciation and love go to his wife, Lynne, and sons, Chris and Gregg, who were consistently enthusiastic and supportive throughout the project.

Adrienne Woods would like to thank her colleagues and coworkers at Wilmington College and the Department of Veterans Affairs. She extends special thanks to her husband, Howard, for his love and encouragement and for always being here to pick up all the loose ends, and to her little ones, Katy and Nate, for enduring hectic schedules and missed events.

Appreciation is also expressed to Joyce L. Kee, Associate Professor Emerita, College of Nursing, University of Delaware, Newark, Delaware. Professor Kee revised Appendix 5, "Commonly Use Laboratory Test Values."

Preface

For decades, PDR has been a standard fixture at nursing stations throughout the land. But—until now—it has lacked the one key element that nurses look for first: a thorough discussion of each medication's unique nursing considerations.

With publication of this first edition of the *PDR® Nurse's Handbook™*, however, all that has changed. At last the vital drug information in PDR is available in convenient handbook format designed especially for nurses, complete with the nursing considerations that today's practitioners demand.

The handbook has been organized with all your needs in mind. Medications are organized by therapeutic category, beginning with the category's general characteristics and continuing with individual monographs on specific drugs. A detailed guide to monographs can be found in the "Using the Handbook" section that follows.

Other handy features include:

- Dosage guidelines are labeled by intended use.
- Boldface italics highlight life-threatening side effects.
- Symptoms of overdose, if any, are conveniently listed at the end of the Side Effects section.
- Treatment of overdose, when applicable, is described at the end of the Administration/Storage section.
- Precautions for special populations can be found in an instant in the Special Concerns section.
- Nursing considerations are presented in a nursing process format, with assessment, intervention, teaching, and evaluation guidelines all clearly labeled.

The *PDR® Nurse's Handbook™* is the latest volume in a growing library of medical references from the publishers of PDR. The collection also includes:

- *Physicians' Desk Reference*
- *PDR Guide to Drug Interactions•Side Effects•Indications™*
- *PDR For Nonprescription Drugs®*
- *PDR For Ophthalmology®*
- *PDR® Generics™*
- *PDR® Medical Dictionary™*
- *PDR Supplements*

PDR has also introduced an advanced new *PDR Electronic Library™* on CD-ROM. This Windows-compatible disc provides users with a complete database of PDR prescribing information, electronically searchable for instant retrieval. A standard subscription includes PDR's sophisticated prescription-screening program and an exhaustive file of chemical structures, illustrations, and full-color product photographs. Optional enhancements include the complete contents of *The Merck Manual* and *Stedman's Medical Dictionary,* as well as a handy file of patient handouts drawn from PDR's consumer handbook, *The PDR® Family Guide to Prescription Drugs®*. The disc is available for use on individual PC and PC networks.

For facilities with large, mainframe-based information systems, PDR information is also available as a preformated text file on magnetic tape. For drug interaction information drawn from the peer-reviewed medical literature, there's the new *PDR® Drug REAX™* system, available for Windows-based PCs. And for personal use—on rounds or on the go—there's *Pocket PDR™*, a unique handheld electronic database of prescribing information that literally fits in your pocket. For more information on this or any other member of the PDR family of products, please call, toll-free, 1-800-232-7379 or fax 201-573-4956.

IMPORTANT DRUG INFORMATION NOTICE

The drugs listed below are now off the market. The information of their deactive status was received after the printing deadline. Disregard the individual monographs for these drugs: *Acetophenazine Maleate, Amphetamine Sulfate, Ampicillin with Probenecid, Bisacodyl Tannex, Calcitonin - Human, Lypressin, Methantheline Bromide, Streptomycin Sulfate, Thyrotropin, and Triprolidine Hydrochloride.*

USING THE HANDBOOK

An understanding of the format of the Handbook will help you reference information quickly. The Guide is organized by chapters for therapeutic drug classifications, as listed in the table of contents.

Each chapter begins with a listing of the drugs included in the classification. A separate description of each drug is included within the chapter. Following the listing is information relating to the classification as a whole. This information is contained in the following categories:

- General Statement
- Action/Kinetics
- Uses
- Contraindications
- Special Concerns
- Side Effects
- Drug Interactions
- Laboratory Test Interferences
- Dosage
- Nursing Considerations

Note that information will not be available for every category. These categories are also used for the individual drug entries and will be described below with regard to the specific drugs. (The general statement appears only at the beginning of certain chapters. It provides information about the class of drug and/or what might be specific or unusual about a particular group of drugs. In addition, information may be presented about certain conditions for which the drugs are indicated.

The information at the beginning of each chapter provides an overview of the therapeutic class of drugs. As time permits, it is helpful to review this information for a broad-based understanding of the therapeutic class and the general therapeutic action of the drugs contained in the classification.

The individual drug entries follow a similar format in each chapter. All items listed below may not appear in each drug entry but are represented where appropriate and when information is available. A typical entry may contain the following:

— COMBINATION DRUG HEADING indicates when two or more drugs are combined in the same product

— GENERIC NAME OF DRUG

— PHONETIC PRONUNCIATION of generic name

— FDA PREGNANCY CATEGORY to which drug is assigned; see Appendix 3 for the definition of these categories

— TRADE NAME(S) by which the drug is marketed; a maple leaf indicates that the trade name is available only in Canada

— DRUG SCHEDULE If the drug is controlled by the U. S. Controlled Substances Act, the appropriate schedule is listed. See Appendix 2 for the definition of the five schedules as well as a listing of drugs with their schedules in both the United States and Canada

— Rx = prescription drug; OTC = nonprescription, over-the-counter drug

— HOW SUPPLIED organized by drug form (such as tablet, capsule, IV fluid, etc.), this section gives the strengths in which the drug is available from manufacturers (for drugs marketed in the United States); for example, a specific drug may be available in tablets only for oral use, in the following strengths: 25, 50, 100, and 200 mg tablets

— CONTENT (for combination drugs) is the generic name and amount of each drug in the combination product

— ACTION/KINETICS The action portion describes the mechanism(s) by which a drug achieves its therapeutic effect; not all mechanisms of action are known. The kinetics portion provides information about the rate of drug absorption, distribution, minimum effective serum or plasma level, biologic half-life, duration of action, metabolism and excretion.

The time it takes for half the drug to be excreted or removed from the blood, t½, is important in determining how often a drug is to be administered and how long to assess for side effects. Therapeutic serum or plasma levels indicate the desired concentration, in serum or plasma, for the drug to exert its beneficial effect and is helpful in predicting the possible onset of side effects, as well as achievement of the desired drug effects.

— USES are the therapeutic applications for the drug. Investigational uses are also listed for selected drugs when available.

— DOSAGE provides adult and pediatric doses as well as the dosage forms in which the drug is available. The dosage form or route of administration is clearly shown and is often followed by the disease state (in italics) for which the particular dosage is recommended. The listed dosage is to be considered as a general prescribing guideline; the exact amount of the drug to be given is determined by the provider. However, one should always question orders or prescriptions when dosages differ markedly from the accepted norm.

— ADMINISTRATION/STORAGE provides guidelines to the practitioner in preparing medications for administration, administering the medication, and proper storage and disposal of the medication.

— TREATMENT OF OVERDOSE for selected drugs is included at the end of the Administration/Storage section as described above.

— CONTRAINDICATIONS notes disease states or conditions for which the drug should not be used. The safe use of many of the newer pharmacologic agents during pregnancy, lactation, or childhood has not been established and therefore should generally not be used.

— SPECIAL CONCERNS cover considerations for use with pediatric, geriatric, pregnant, or lactating clients. Situations and disease states when the drug should be used with caution are also listed.

— LABORATORY TEST INTERFERENCES indicates the effect of the drug on laboratory test values for the client. Some of the interferences are caused by the therapeutic or toxic effects of the drugs; others result from interference with the testing method itself. Interferences are described as false positive (+), or increased (↑), values and as false negative (-), or decreased (↓), values. Many of the laboratory test interferences are addressed under *Nursing Considerations*.

— SIDE EFFECTS include potential drug-related undesired or bothersome effects, organized by body system or organ affected. Nearly all potential side effects are listed. In any given clinical situation, a client may show no side effects, one or two side effects, or several side effects. Life-threatening side effects are identified by bold italic print.

— SYMPTOMS OF OVERDOSE includes a listing of the symptoms that may be observed following an overdose of the drug. This information follows the side effects section (as described above).

— DRUG INTERACTIONS lists the results of drugs interacting with one another, usually an increase or decrease in the effect of the drug is evident. Drug interactions may result from a number of different mechanisms (e.g., additive or inhibitory effects, interference with degradation of drug, increased rate of elimination, decreased absorption from the GI tract, and receptor site competition or displacement from plasma protein binding sites).

Any side effects that accompany the administration of a specific drug may be increased as a result of a drug interaction.

Drug interactions are often listed for classes of drugs. Therefore drug interactions are likely to occur for all drugs in the class.

— NURSING CONSIDERATIONS are guidelines to help the practitioner in applying the nursing process to pharmacotherapeutics to ensure safe practice.

- Assessment: Guidelines to assist the practitioner in what to identify and assess before, during, and after drug therapy.
- Interventions: Guidelines for appropriate nursing actions related to the recipient of therapy and to the specific drug being administered.
- Client/Family Teaching: Guidelines to promote education, understanding, and compliance with drug therapy.
- Evaluate: Identifies outcome criteria to determine effectiveness of drug therapy and anticipated client response to therapy.

— ADDITIONAL CONTRAINDICATIONS, ADDITIONAL SIDE EFFECTS, or ADDITIONAL NURSING CONSIDERATIONS provide information relevant to a specific drug but not necessarily to the class overall and serves to reinforce certain areas of importance.

— INDEX is extensively cross-referenced (multiple trade names and the generic name for each drug are paired); information is coded as follows:

- **boldface** = generic drug name
- *italics* = therapeutic drug class
- regular type = trade name
- CAPITALS = combination drugs

VISUAL IDENTIFICATION GUIDE

Use this section to quickly verify the identity of a capsule, tablet, or other solid oral medication. More than 200 leading products are shown in actual size and color, organized alphabetically by generic name. Each product is labeled with its brand name, if applicable, as well as its strength and the name of its supplier.

Table of Contents

Common Sound-Alike Drug Names

The following is a list of common sound-alike and similarly spelled drug names. Generic names are lowercase; trade names are capitalized. The pharmacologic classification/use appears in parentheses next to each drug name.

acetazolamide (diuretic)	acetohexamide (oral antidiabetic)
albuterol (sympathomimetic)	atenolol (beta blocker)
Aldomet (antihypertensive)	Aldoril (antihypertensive)
alprazolam (antianxiety agent)	lorazepam (antianxiety agent)
amiodarone (antiarrhythmic)	amrinone (inotropic agent)
amitriptyline (antidepressant)	nortriptyline (antidepressant)
Apresazide (antihypertensive)	Apresoline (antihypertensive)
Arlidin (peripheral vasodilator)	Aralen (antimalarial)
Atarax (antianxiety agent)	Ativan (antianxiety agent)
atenolol (beta blocker)	timolol (beta blocker)
bacitracin (antibacterial)	Bactroban (anti-infective—topical)
calciferol (vitamin D_2)	calcitriol (vitamin D)
Catapres (antihypertensive)	Combipres (antihypertensive)
cefotaxime (cephalosporin)	cefoxitin (cephalosporin)
chlorpromazine (antipsychotic)	chlorpropamide (oral antidiabetic)
chlorpromazine (antipsychotic)	promethazine (antihistamine)
clonidine (antihypertensive)	Klonopin (anticonvulsant)
Darvocet-N (analgesic)	Darvon-N (analgesic)
desipramine (antidepressant)	diphenhydramine (antihistamine)
digitoxin (cardiac glycoside)	digoxin (cardiac glycoside)
diphenhydramine (antihistamine)	dimenhydrinate (antihistamine)
enalapril (ACE inhibitor)	Anafranil (antidepressant)
enalapril (ACE inhibitor)	Eldepryl (antiparkinson agent)
Eryc (erythromycin base)	Ery-Tab (erythromycin base)
Fioricet (analgesic)	Fiorinal (analgesic)
flurbiprofen (NSAID)	fenoprofen (NSAID)
folinic acid (leucovorin calcium)	folic acid (vitamin B complex)
Gantrisin (sulfonamide)	Gantanol (sulfonamide)
glipizide (oral hypoglycemic)	glyburide (oral hypoglycemic)
Hycodan (cough preparation)	Hycomine (cough preparation)
hydralazine (antihypertensive)	hydroxyzine (antianxiety agent)
hydromorphone (narcotic analgesic)	morphine (narcotic analgesic)
Hydropres (antihypertensive)	Diupres (antihypertensive)
Hytone (topical corticosteroid)	Vytone (topical corticosteroid)
imipramine (antidepressant)	norpramin (antidepressant)
Inderal (beta blocker)	Inderide (antihypertensive)

Indocin (NSAID)	Minocin (antibiotic)
Lioresal (muscle relaxant)	lisinopril (ACE inhibitor)
Lithotabs (lithium carbonate)	Lithobid (lithium carbonate)
Norlutate (progestin)	Norlutin (progestin)
Norvasc (calcium channel blocker)	Navane (antipsychotic)
Orinase (oral hypoglycemic)	Ornade (upper respiratory product)
Percocet (narcotic analgesic)	Percodan (narcotic analgesic)
Platinol (antineoplastic)	Paraplatin (antineoplastic)
prednisolone (corticosteroid)	prednisone (corticosteroid)
Prilosec (inhibitor of gastric acid secretion)	Prozac (antidepressant)
quinidine (antiarrhythmic)	clonidine (antihypertensive)
quinidine (antiarrhythmic)	Quinamm (antimalarial)
quinine (antimalarial)	quinidine (antiarrhythmic)
Regroton (antihypertensive)	Hygroton (diuretic)
Rifamate (antitubercular drug)	rifampin (antitubercular drug)
Seldane (antihistamine)	Feldene (NSAID)
terbutaline (sympathomimetic)	tolbutamide (oral hypoglycemic)
tolazamide (oral hypoglycemic)	tolbutamide (oral hypoglycemic)
Trimox (amoxicillin product)	Diamox (carbonic anhydrase inhibitor)
Vasosulf (sulfonamide decongestant)	Velosef (cephalosporin)
Xanax (antianxiety agent)	Zantac (H_2 histamine blocker)
Zebeta (beta blocker)	DiaBeta (oral hypoglycemic)
Zosyn (anti-infective)	Zofran (antiemetic)

NOTE: Generic names are lowercase; trade names are capitalized.

Anti-Infective Drugs

CHAPTER ONE

Anti-Infectives — General Information

See also the following chapters:

Antibiotics: Aminoglycosides
Antibiotics: Cephalosporins
Antibiotics: Chloramphenicol
Antibiotics: Clindamycin and Lincomycin
Antibiotics: Fluoroquinolones
Antibiotics: Macrolides (including Erythromycins)
Antibiotics: Penicillins
Antibiotics: Sulfonamides
Antibiotics: Tetracyclines
Antibiotics: Miscellaneous
Amebicides, Trichomonacides, and Antiprotozoals
Anthelmintics
Antifungal Drugs
Antimalarial Drugs
Antitubercular Drugs
Leprostatics
Urinary Anti-Infectives and Analgesics
Antiviral Agents

General Statement: The beginning of modern medicine is generally related to two events: the proof by Pasteur that many diseases are caused by microorganisms and the discovery of effective anti-infective drugs. The first of these drugs were the sulfonamides (1938), followed by penicillin during the early 1940s. Since then, dozens of anti-infectives have been added to the list. Moreover, significant progress has been made in the development of antiviral drugs.

Unfortunately, the advent of the anti-infectives has not been a pure panacea. Some of the bacteria and other microorganisms have adapted to the anti-infectives, and there has been a gradual emergence of bacteria resistant to certain anti-infectives, especially the antibiotics. Fortunately, most resistant strains can be eradicated by new and/or different antibiotics, antibiotic combinations, or higher dosages. Nevertheless, awareness of the problem has prompted somewhat greater scrutiny by the physician as to when and how to prescribe antibiotics.

The following general guidelines apply to the use of most anti-infective drugs:

1. Anti-infective drugs can be divided into those that are *bacteriostatic;* that is, arrest the multiplication and further development of the infectious agent, or *bactericidal;* that is, eradicate all living microorganisms. Both time of administration and

length of therapy may be affected by this difference.

2. Some anti-infectives halt the growth of or eradicate many different microorganisms and are termed *broad-spectrum antibiotics*. Others affect only certain specific organisms and are termed *narrow-spectrum antibiotics*.

3. Some of the anti-infectives elicit a hypersensitivity reaction in some persons. Penicillins cause more severe and more frequent hypersensitivity reactions than any other drug.

4. Because of differences in susceptibility of infectious agents to anti-infectives, the sensitivity of the microorganism to the drug ordered should be determined before treatment is initiated. Several sensitivity tests are commonly used for this purpose. The most widely used test—the Kirby-Bauer or disk-diffusion test—gives qualitative results; there are also various quantitative tests aimed at determining the minimal inhibitory concentration (MIC).

5. Certain anti-infective agents have marked side effects, some of the more serious of which are neurotoxicity, including ototoxicity, and nephrotoxicity. Care must be taken not to administer two anti-infectives with similar side effects concomitantly, or to administer these drugs to clients in whom the side effects might be damaging (e.g., a nephrotoxic drug to a client suffering from kidney disease). The choice of anti-infective also depends on its distribution in the body (i.e., whether it passes the blood-brain barrier).

6. Another difficulty associated with anti-infective therapy is that these drugs can eradicate the normal intestinal flora necessary for proper digestion, synthesis of vitamin K, and control of fungi that may gain access to the GI tract (superinfection).

Action/Kinetics: The mechanism of action of the anti-infectives varies. The following modes of action have been identified.* Note the considerable overlap among these mechanisms:

1. Inhibition of synthesis of or activation of enzymes that disrupt bacterial cell walls leading to loss of viability and possibly cell lysis (e.g., penicillins, cephalosporins, cycloserine, bacitracin, vancomycin, miconazole, ketoconazole, clotrimazole).

2. Direct effect on the microbial cell membrane to affect permeability and leading to leakage of intracellular components (e.g., polymyxin, colistimethate, nystatin, amphotericin).

3. Effect on the function of bacterial ribosomes to cause a reversible inhibition of protein synthesis (e.g., chloramphenicol, tetracyclines, erythromycin, clindamycin).

4. Bind to the 30S ribosomal subunit that alters protein synthesis and leads to cell death (e.g., aminoglycosides).

5. Effect on nucleic acid metabolism, inhibits DNA-dependent RNA polymerase (e.g., rifampin), or inhibition of DNA supercoiling and DNA synthesis (e.g., quinolones).

6. Antimetabolites that block specific metabolic steps essential to the life of the microorganism (e.g., trimethoprim, sulfonamides).

7. Bind to viral enzymes that are essential for DNA synthesis leading to a halt of viral replication (e.g., acyclovir, ganciclovir, vidarabine, zidovudine).

Uses: Antibiotics as a group are effective against most bacterial pathogens, as well as against some of the rickettsias and a few of the larger viruses. They are ineffective against viruses that cause influenza, hepatitis, and the common cold. Other anti-infectives are effective against a number of parasites including helminths, the malarial parasite, fungi, trichomonas, and others.

The choice of the anti-infective depends on the nature of the illness

*Sande, M.A., Kapusnik-Uner, J.E., Mandel, G.L.: Antimicrobial agents. In *Goodman and Gilman's The Pharmacological Basis of Therapeutics,* 8th ed. Edited by Gilman, A.G., Rall, T.W., Nies, A.S., Taylor, P. New York, Pergamon Press, 1990, p. 1019.

to be treated, the sensitivity of the infecting agent, and the client's previous experience with the drug. Hypersensitivity and allergic reactions may preclude the use of the agent of choice.

In addition to their use in acute infections, anti-infectives may be given prophylactically in the following instances:

1. To protect persons exposed to a known specific organism
2. To prevent secondary bacterial infections in acutely ill clients suffering from infections unresponsive to antibiotics
3. To reduce risk of infection in clients suffering from various chronic illnesses
4. To inhibit spread of infection from a clearly defined focus, as after accidents or surgery
5. To "sterilize" the bowel or other areas of the body in preparation for extensive surgery

Instead of using a single agent, the physician may sometimes prefer to prescribe a combination of anti-infective agents.

Contraindications: Hypersensitivity or allergic reaction to certain anti-infectives is common and may preclude the use of a particular agent.

Side Effects: The antibiotics and anti-infective agents have few direct toxic effects. Kidney and liver damage, deafness, and blood dyscrasias are occasionally observed.

The following undesirable manifestations, however, occur frequently:

1. Antibiotic therapy often suppresses the normal flora of the body, which in turn keeps certain pathogenic microorganisms, such as *Candida albicans, Proteus,* or *Pseudomonas,* from causing infections. If the flora is altered, *superinfections* (monilial vaginitis, enteritis, UTIs), which necessitate the discontinuation of therapy or the use of other antibiotics, can result.
2. Incomplete eradication of an infectious organism. Casual use of anti-infectives favors the emergence of *resistant* strains insensitive to a particular drug. Resistant strains often are either mutants of the original infectious agents that have developed a slightly different metabolic pathway and can exist despite the antibiotic, or are variants that have developed the ability to release a chemical substance—for instance, the enzyme penicillinase—which can destroy the antibiotic.

To minimize the chances for the development of resistant strains, anti-infectives are usually given for a prescribed length of time after acute symptoms have subsided. Casual use of antibiotics is discouraged for the same reasons.

Laboratory Tests: The bacteriologic sensitivity of the infectious organism to the anti-infective (especially the antibiotic) should be tested by the lab before initiation of therapy and during treatment.

GENERAL NURSING CONSIDERATIONS FOR ALL ANTI-INFECTIVES

Administration/Storage

1. Check expiration date on container.
2. Check for recommended method of storage for the drug and store accordingly.
3. Clearly mark the date and time of reconstitution, your initials, and the strength of solutions of all drugs. Note the length of time that the drug may be stored after dilution and store under appropriate conditions.
4. Complete the administration of anti-infective agents by IVPB (or as ordered) before the drug loses potency.
5. *Treatment of Overdose:* Discontinue the drug and treat symptomatically. Supportive measures should be instituted as needed. Hemodialysis may be used although its effectiveness is questionable, depending on the drug and the status of the client (i.e., more effective in impaired renal function).

Assessment

1. Document indications for therapy, type and onset of symptoms, and lo-

cation and source of infection (if known).
2. Determine if client has experienced any unusual reaction or problems associated with any anti-infectives (usually penicillin) or related drug therapy.
3. Ensure that diagnostic cultures have been done before administering empiric therapy. Use correct procedure for obtaining, storing, and transporting specimen to the lab.

Interventions

1. Conspicuously mark in red on the client's chart, medication record, care plan, pharmacy record, and bed the fact that the client has an allergy and to what. Inform client not to take that drug again unless the physician gives approval after reviewing the history of past allergic reactions to this medication.
2. Once drug therapy is initiated, ask the client about any unusual reactions or problems with the medication. Review with the client possible side effects such as hives, rashes, difficulty breathing, etc. If any of these occur, they may indicate a hypersensitivity or allergic response and the drug should be discontinued and the physician notified immediately.
3. Monitor VS and I&O and ensure adequate hydration.
4. If the anti-infective is mainly excreted by the kidneys, anticipate reduced dosage in clients with renal dysfunction. Nephrotoxic drugs are usually contraindicated in persons with renal dysfunction because toxic levels of the drugs are rapidly attained when renal function is impaired.
5. Verify orders when two or more anti-infectives are ordered for the same client, especially if the drugs have similar side effects, such as nephrotoxicity and/or neurotoxicity.
6. Assess client for therapeutic response, such as reduction of fever, increased appetite, and increased sense of well-being.
7. Assess client for superinfections, particularly of fungal origin, characterized by black furred tongue, nausea, and/or diarrhea.
8. *Prevent superinfections by*
• Limiting client's exposure to persons suffering from an active infectious process
• Rotating the site of IV administration q 72 hr and by changing IV tubing q 24–48 hr
• Providing and emphasizing need for good hygiene
• Instructing care provider to wash own hands carefully before and after contact with the client
9. Have the order for an anti-infective (administered in the hospital) evaluated at least q 5–7 days for renewal, revision, or cancellation.
10. Schedule drug administration throughout 24-hr period to maintain appropriate drug levels. A drug administration schedule is determined by the half-life ($t^{1/2}$) of the drug, the severity of the infection, evidence of organ dysfunction, and the client's need for sleep.
11. Obtain and monitor serum drug levels (peak and trough) throughout therapy to ensure that client is receiving the appropriate dose.

Client/Family Teaching

1. Use anti-infectives only under medical supervision.
2. Do not share medications with friends or family members.
3. Teach the proper method for taking medication and time intervals at which to take the prescribed anti-infective.
4. Provide a printed list of adverse side effects. Report S&S of allergic reactions and superinfections.
5. Prevent recurrence by completing recommended course of therapy, even though client may feel well. Advise clients that incomplete therapy may render them unresponsive to the antibiotic with the next infection.
6. Discard any drug remaining after course of therapy is completed.
7. Instruct client to take antipyretics as prescribed on a regular basis (q 4 hr) for fever reduction.
8. Advise clients with diabetes to perform finger sticks as opposed to

urine testing for a more reliable reflection of blood sugars.

9. Instruct client to seek medical attention if symptoms persist or new S&S appear as medication may require adjustment or change.

10. Advise clients not to stop taking medication if they feel better. Entire prescription should be taken unless otherwise directed. This ensures that the organism is eradicated and diminishes the emergence of drug-resistant bacterial strains.

Evaluate

- Prevention or resolution of infection
- ↓ Fever
- ↓ WBCs
- Negative lab culture results
- ↑ Appetite
- Reports of symptomatic improvement
- Laboratory evidence of therapeutic serum drug levels
- Freedom from complications of drug therapy

CHAPTER TWO

Antibiotics: Aminoglycosides

See also the following individual entries:

Amikacin Sulfate
Gentamicin Sulfate
Kanamycin Sulfate
Neomycin Sulfate
Paromomycin Sulfate
Streptomycin Sulfate
Tobramycin Sulfate

General Statement: The aminoglycosides are broad-spectrum antibiotics, primarily used for the treatment of serious gram-negative infections caused by *Pseudomonas, Escherichia coli, Proteus, Klebsiella,* and *Enterobacter.* Aminoglycoside antibiotics are distributed in the extracellular fluid and cross the placental barrier, but not the blood-brain barrier. Penetration of the CSF is increased when the meninges are inflamed.

The aminoglycosides are excreted, largely unchanged, in the urine. This makes the drugs suitable for UTIs. Concomitant administration of bicarbonate (alkalinization of urine) improves the treatment of such infections. Considerable cross-allergenicity occurs among the aminoglycosides. These drugs are powerful antibiotics and can induce serious side effects. They should not be used for minor infections. Except for streptomycin, resistance of the organisms to aminoglycosides develops slowly. Whenever possible, the sensitivity of the infectious agent should be determined before instituting therapy.

Action/Kinetics: Believed to inhibit protein synthesis by binding irreversibly to ribosomes (30S subunit), thereby interfering with an initiation complex between messenger RNA and the 30S subunit. This leads to production of nonfunctional proteins; polyribosomes are split apart and are unable to synthesize protein. The aminoglycosides are usually bactericidal as a result of disruption of the bacterial cytoplasmic membrane.

The aminoglycosides are poorly absorbed from the GI tract and are therefore usually administered parenterally, the only occasional exceptions being some enteric infections of the GI tract and prior to surgery. They are also absorbed from the peritoneum, bronchial tree, wounds, denuded skin, and joints.

The aminoglycosides are rapidly absorbed after IM injection. **Peak plasma levels:** Usually attained ½–2 hr after IM administration. Measurable levels persist for 8–12 hr after a single administration. **t½:** 2–3 hr. This value increases sharply in clients with impaired kidney function. Ranges of t½ from 24 to 110 hr have been observed. Excreted mainly unchanged in urine.

Uses: Gram-negative bacteria causing bone and joint infections, septicemia (including neonatal sepsis), skin and soft tissue infections (including those from burns), respiratory tract infections, postoperative infections, intra-abdominal infections (including peritonitis), UTIs. In combination with clindamycin for mixed aerobic-anaerobic infections. Also, see individual drugs.

They should be used for gram-positive bacteria only when other less toxic drugs are either ineffective or contraindicated. Their use in CNS *Pseudomonas* infections such as meningitis or ventriculitis is questionable.

Contraindications: Hypersensitivity to aminoglycosides, long-term therapy (except streptomycin for tuberculosis). Use with extreme caution in clients with impaired renal function or preexisting hearing impairment. Safe use in pregnancy and during lactation not established.

Special Concerns: Premature infants, neonates, and older clients receiving aminoglycosides should be assessed closely as they are particularly sensitive to their toxic effects.

Side Effects: *Ototoxicity:* Both auditory and vestibular damage have been noted. The risk of ototoxicity and vestibular impairment is increased in clients with poor renal function and in the elderly. Auditory symptoms include tinnitus and hearing impairment, while vestibular symptoms include dizziness, nystagmus, vertigo, and ataxia.

Renal Impairment: This may be characterized by cylindruria, oliguria, proteinuria, azotemia, hematuria, increase or decrease in frequency of urination; increased BUN, NPN, or creatinine; and increased thirst. *Neurotoxicity:* Neuromuscular blockade, headache, tremor, lethargy, paresthesia, peripheral neuritis (numbness, tingling, or burning of face/mouth), arachnoiditis, encephalopathy, acute organic brain syndrome. CNS depression, characterized by stupor, flaccidity, and rarely, ***coma, and respiratory depression in infants.*** Optic neuritis with blurred vision or loss of vision. *GI:* N&V, diarrhea, increased salivation, anorexia, weight loss. *Allergic:* Rash, urticaria, pruritus, burning, fever, stomatitis, eosinophilia. Rarely, ***agranulocytosis and anaphylaxis.*** Cross-allergy among aminoglycosides has been observed. *Miscellaneous:* Joint pain, ***laryngeal edema, pulmonary fibrosis,*** superinfection.

Symptoms of Overdose: Extension of side effects.

Drug Interactions

Bumetanide / ↑ Risk of ototoxicity
Capreomycin / ↑ Muscle relaxation
Cephalosporins / ↑ Risk of renal toxicity
Ciprofloxacin HCl / Additive antibacterial activity
Cisplatin / Additive renal toxicity
Colistimethate / ↑ Muscle relaxation
Digoxin / Possible ↑ or ↓ effect of digoxin
Ethacrynic acid / ↑ Risk of ototoxicity
Furosemide / ↑ Risk of ototoxicity
Methoxyflurane / ↑ Risk of renal toxicity
Penicillins / ↓ Effect of aminoglycosides
Polymyxins / ↑ Muscle relaxation
Skeletal muscle relaxants (surgical) / ↑ Muscle relaxation
Vancomycin / Additive ototoxicity and renal toxicity
Vitamin A / ↓ Effect of vitamin A due to ↓ absorption from GI tract

Laboratory Test Interferences: ↑ BUN, BSP retention, creatinine, AST, ALT, bilirubin. ↓ Cholesterol values.

NURSING CONSIDERATIONS

See also *General Nursing Considerations for All Anti-Infectives,* Chapter 1.

Administration/Storage

1. Check expiration date.
2. Warn client if the particular drug being administered stings or causes a burning sensation.
3. During IM administration
• Inject drug deep into muscle mass to minimize transient pain.
• Use a Z track method for thin, elderly clients.
• Rotate and document injection sites.
4. With IV administration
• Dilute with the appropriate compatible solution.
• Infuse at the rate ordered to prevent excessive serum concentrations.
5. Administer for only 7–10 days and avoid repeating course of therapy unless a serious infection is present

that does not respond to other antibiotics.
6. Administer around the clock to maintain therapeutic drug levels.
7. *Treatment of Overdose:* Undertake hemodialysis (preferred) or peritoneal dialysis.

Assessment

1. Assess for any history of adverse reactions and hypersensitivity to anti-infective medications.
2. Weigh client prior to administering medication to ensure correct calculation of dosage.
3. Determine baseline renal, auditory, and vestibular function and assess regularly during drug administration.
4. Assess client for the presence and possibly source(s) of infection. Document VS (evidence of fever), culture and lab reports, and wound appearance when applicable.
5. Ensure that appropriate culture studies have been performed before initiating drug therapy.

Interventions

1. Monitor VS and I&O and ensure adequate fluid intake to prevent renal tubule irritation.
2. During therapy, monitor serum drug levels and if levels are elevated, withhold drug and report (e.g., blood levels exceeding 30 mcg/mL of amikacin are considered toxic.)
3. Protect client with vestibular dysfunction by supervising ambulation and providing side rails if necessary. Flag chart and bedside with (potential for) fall hazard.
4. Monitor for signs of ototoxicity; pretreatment audiograms may be helpful, as hearing loss is a dose-related side effect of drug therapy most commonly associated with amikacin, kanamycin, neomycin, or paromomycin. Also, assess for tinnitus, dizziness, and loss of balance, as these are signs of vestibular injury and are more commonly seen with gentamicin and streptomycin. Continue to monitor for ototoxicity, because the onset of deafness may occur several weeks after the aminoglycoside has been discontinued.
5. Do not administer concurrently or sequentially with a topical or systemic nephrotoxic or ototoxic drug (e.g., potent diuretics such as ethacrynic acid or furosemide) unless physician determines that the benefits outweigh the risks.
6. Observe for neuromuscular blockade with muscular weakness leading to apnea, when an aminoglycoside is administered with a muscle relaxant or after anesthesia. Have calcium gluconate or neostigmine available to reverse blockade.
7. Note the presence of cells or casts in the urine, oliguria, proteinuria, lowered specific gravity, or increasing BUN, or creatinine, all of which are indicators of altered renal function.

Client/Family Teaching

1. Review goals of therapy and appropriate prescribed method of administration.
2. Explain the importance of taking medications at the prescribed time intervals, around the clock, until the prescription is finished.
3. Stress the importance of following a well-balanced diet and consuming at least 2 L/day of fluids.
4. Review symptoms of superinfection (black, furry tongue; loose, foul-smelling stools; vaginal itching) and advise to report immediately.
5. Stress that any alterations in hearing, vision, and/or ambulation should also be reported.
6. Discuss the potential side effects for the select drug(s) and stress the importance of reporting these as therapy may need to be discontinued.

Evaluate

- A positive clinical response as evidenced by negative lab culture reports
- Clinical evidence of resolution of infection such as ↓ WBCs, ↓ fever, and reports of symptomatic improvement
- Laboratory confirmation that serum drug levels are within desired therapeutic range

---

Amikacin sulfate

(am-ih-**KAY**-sin)
Pregnancy Category: D
Amikin **(Rx)**

See also *Anti-Infectives,* Chapter 1, and *Aminoglycosides,* Chapter 2.
How Supplied: *Injection:* 50 mg/mL, 250 mg/mL
Action/Kinetics: Amikacin is derived from kanamycin. Its spectrum is somewhat broader than that of other aminoglycosides, including *Serratia* and *Acinetobacter* species, as well as certain staphylococci and streptococci. Amikacin is effective against both penicillinase- and non-penicillinase-producing organisms. **Peak therapeutic serum levels: IM,** 16–32 mcg/mL. **t½:** 2–3 hr. **Toxic serum levels:** >35 mcg/mL (peak measured after 1 hr) and >10 mcg/mL (trough measured before next dose).
Uses: Short-term treatment of gram-negative bacterial infections including *Pseudomonas, Escherichia coli, Proteus, Providencia, Klebsiella, Enterobacter, Serratia,* and *Acinetobacter.* May also be used in infections due to gentamicin or tobramycin resistant strains of *Providencia rettgeri, P. stuartii, Serratia marcescens,* and *Pseudomonas aeruginosa.*

Infections include bacterial septicemia (including neonatal sepsis); serious infections of the respiratory tract, bones, joints, skin, soft tissue, and CNS (including meningitis); intra-abdominal infections (including peritonitis); burns; postoperative infections (including postvascular surgery). Also, serious complicated and recurrent infections of the urinary tract. May be used as initial therapy in certain situations in the treatment of known or suspected staphylococcal disease. *Investigational:* Intrathecal or intraventricular use. As part of multiple drug regimen for *Mycobacterium avium* complex (commonly seen in AIDS clients).

Dosage

• **IM (preferred) and IV**

Adults, children, and older infants: 15 mg/kg/day in two to three equally divided doses q 8–12 hr for 7–10 days; **maximum daily dose:** 15 mg/kg.

Uncomplicated UTIs.

250 mg b.i.d.; **newborns:** loading dose of 10 mg/kg followed by 7.5 mg/kg q 12 hr.

Use in neonates.

Initial: Loading dose of 10 mg/kg; **then,** 7.5 mg/kg q 12 hr. Lower doses may be safer during the first 2 weeks of life.

Intrathecal or intraventricular use.

8 mg/24 hr.

As part of multiple drug regimen for M. avium complex.

15 mg/kg/day IV in divided doses q 8–12 hr.

In clients with impaired renal function.

Normal loading dose of 7.5 mg/kg; **then** administration should be monitored by serum level of amikacin (35 mcg/mL maximum) or creatinine clearance rates. Duration of treatment: **Usual:** 7–10 days.

Administration/Storage (for IV Administration)

1. Add 500-mg vial to 200 mL of sterile diluent, such as NSS or D5W.
2. Administer over a 30- to 60-min period for adults.
3. Administer to infants in the amount of prescribed fluid. The IV administration to infants should be over 1–2 hr.
4. Store colorless liquid at room temperature for no longer than 2 years.
5. Potency is not affected if the solution turns a light yellow.

Special Concerns: Use with caution in premature infants and neonates.

NURSING CONSIDERATIONS

See also *Nursing Considerations* for *Aminoglycosides,* p. 7.

Assessment

1. Obtain audiometric assessment with high dosage or prolonged use.
2. Note any vestibular dysfunction and monitor for eighth cranial nerve impairment R/T elevated peak drug levels.

Evaluate

• Resolution of infection

• Therapeutic serum drug levels (peak 30–35 mcg/mL; trough<10 mcg/mL)

Gentamicin sulfate

(jen-tah-**MY**-sin)
Pregnancy Category: C
Alcomicin ♣, Diogent ♣, Garamycin, Garamycin Intrathecal, Garamycin IV Piggyback, Garamycin Ophthalmic Ointment, Garamycin Ophthalmic Solution, Garamycin Pediatric, Garatec ♣, Genoptic Ophthalmic Liquifilm, Genoptic S.O.P. Ophthalmic, Gentacidin Ophthalmic, Gentafair, Gentak Ophthalmic, Gentamicin, Gentamicin Ophthalmic, Gentamicin Sulfate IV Piggyback, Gentrasul Ophthalmic, G-myticin Topical, Jenamicin, Ocugram ♣, Pediatric Gentamicin Sulfate, PMS Gentamicin Sulfate ♣, R.O.-Gentycin ♣ **(Rx)**

See also *Aminoglycosides,* Chapter 2.

How Supplied: *Cream:* 0.1%; *Injection:* 2 mg/mL, 10 mg/mL, 40 mg/mL; *Ointment:* 1%; *Ophthalmic ointment:* 3 mg/g; *Ophthalmic Solution:* 3 mg/mL

Action/Kinetics: Therapeutic serum levels: IM, 4–8 mcg/mL. **Toxic serum levels:** >12 mcg/mL (peak) and >2 mcg/mL (trough). Prolonged serum levels above 12 mcg/mL should be avoided. **t½:** 2 hr. The drug can be used concurrently with carbenicillin for the treatment of serious *Pseudomonas* infections. However, the drugs should not be mixed in the same flask because carbenicillin will inactivate gentamicin.

Uses: *Systemic:* Serious infections caused by *Pseudomonas aeruginosa, Proteus, Klebsiella, Enterobacter, Serratia, Citrobacter,* and *Staphylococcus.* Infections include bacterial neonatal sepsis, bacterial septicemia, and serious infections of the skin, bone, soft tissue (including burns), urinary tract, GI tract (including peritonitis), and CNS (including meningitis). Should be considered as initial therapy in suspected or confirmed gram-negative infections. In combination with carbenicillin for treating life-threatening infections due to *P. aeruginosa.* In combination with penicillin for treating endocarditis caused by group D streptococci. In combination with penicillin for treating suspected bacterial sepsis or staphylococcal pneumonia in the neonate. Intrathecal administration is used in combination with systemic gentamicin for treating meningitis, ventriculitis, or other serious CNS infections due to *Pseudomonas. Investigational:* Pelvic inflammatory disease.

Ophthalmic: Ophthalmic infections due to *Staphylococcus, S. aureus, Streptococcus pneumoniae,* beta-hemolytic streptococci, *Corynebacterium* species, *Streptococcus pyogenes, Escherichia coli, Haemophilus influenzae, H. aegyptius, H. ducreyi, Klebsiella pneumoniae, Neisseria gonorrhoeae, Proteus* species, *Acinetobacter calcoaceticus, Enterobacter aerogenes, P. aeruginosa, Serratia marcescens, Moraxella lacunata.*

Topical: Prevention of infections following minor cuts, wounds, burns, and skin abrasions. Treatment of superficial infections of the skin.

Dosage

• **IM (usual), IV**

Adults with normal renal function.

Infections.

1 mg/kg q 8 hr, up to 5 mg/kg/day in life-threatening infections; **children:** 2–2.5 mg/kg q 8 hr; **infants and neonates:** 2.5 mg/kg q 8 hr; **premature infants or neonates less than 1 week of age:** 2.5 mg/kg q 12 hr. Therapy may be required for 7–10 days.

Prevention of bacterial endocarditis, dental or respiratory tract procedures.

Adults: 1.5 mg/kg gentamicin (not to exceed 80 mg) plus 1 g ampicillin, each IM or IV, 30–60 min before the procedure; one additional dose of each can be given 8 hr later (alternative: penicillin V, 1 g PO, 6 hr after initial dose).

Prophylaxis of bacterial endocarditis in GI or GU tract procedures or surgery.

Adults: 1.5 mg/kg gentamicin (not to exceed 80 mg) plus 2 g ampicillin, each IM or IV, 30–60 min before procedure; dose should be repeated 8 hr later. **Children:** 2 mg/kg gentamicin plus penicillin G, 30,000 units/kg, or ampicillin, 50 mg/kg in same dosage interval as for adults. Pediatric dosage should not exceed single or 24-hr adult doses.

NOTE: In clients allergic to penicillin, vancomycin, 1 g IV given slowly over 1 hr, may be substituted; the dose of vancomycin should be repeated 8–12 hr later. **Adults with impaired renal function:** To calculate interval (hr) between doses, multiply serum creatinine level (mg/100 mL) by 8.

• **IV**

Septicemia.

Initially: 1–2 mg/kg infused over 30–60 min; **then,** maintenance doses may be administered.

• **Intrathecal**

Meningitis.

Use only the intrathecal preparation. Adults, usual: 4–8 mg/day; **children and infants 3 months and older:** 1–2 mg/day

Pelvic inflammatory disease.

Initial: 2 mg/kg IV; **then,** 1.5 mg/kg t.i.d. plus clindamycin, 500 mg IV q.i.d. Continue for at least 4 days and at least 48 hr after client improves. Continue clindamycin, 450 mg PO q.i.d. for 10–14 days.

• **Ophthalmic solution (0.3%)**

Acute infections.

Initially: 1–2 gtt in conjunctival sac q 15–30 min; **then,** as infection improves, reduce frequency.

Moderate infections.

1–2 gtt in conjunctival sac 4–6 times/day.

Trachoma.

2 gtt in each eye b.i.d.–q.i.d.; treatment should be continued for up to 1–2 months.

• **Ophthalmic ointment (0.3%):** Depending on the severity of infection, ½-in. ribbon from q 3–4 hr to 2–3 times/day.

• **Topical Cream/Ointment (0.1%)**

Apply 1–5 times/day to affected area. The area may be covered with a sterile bandage.

Administration/Storage

1. For intermittent IV administration, the adult dose should be diluted in 50–200 mL of sterile 5% dextrose in water or isotonic saline and administered over a 30–120-min period. The volume should be less for infants and children.

2. Gentamicin should not be mixed with other drugs for parenteral use.

3. For parenteral use, the duration of treatment is 7–10 days, although a longer course of therapy may be required for severe or complicated infections.

4. When used intrathecally, the usual site is the lumbar area.

5. With topical administration:

• Remove the crusts of impetigo contagiosa before applying ointment to permit maximum contact between antibiotic and infection.

• Apply ointment gently and cover with gauze dressing if desirable or as ordered.

• Avoid direct exposure to sunlight as photosensitivity reaction may occur.

• Avoid further contamination of infected skin.

Contraindications: Ophthalmic use to treat dendritic keratitis, vaccinia, varicella, mycobacterial infections of the eye, fungal diseases of the eye, use with steroids after uncomplicated removal of a corneal foreign body.

Special Concerns: Use with caution in premature infants and neonates. Ophthalmic ointments may retard corneal epithelial healing.

Additional Side Effects: Muscle twitching, numbness, ***seizures,*** increased BP, alopecia, purpura, pseudotumor cerebri. Photosensitivity when used topically. *After ophthalmic use:* Transient irritation, burning, stinging, itching, inflammation, angioneurotic edema, urticaria, vesicular and maculopapular dermatitis, mydriasis, conjunctival paresthesia.

Additional Drug Interactions: With carbenicillin or ticarcillin, gentamicin may result in increased effect when used for *Pseudomonas* infections.

NURSING CONSIDERATIONS

See also *Nursing Considerations* for *Aminoglycosides,* Chapter 2.

Assessment

1. Document indications for therapy and type and onset of symptoms.
2. Obtain renal function studies and appropriate specimen for lab C&S.
3. With eye disorders, determine that opthalmologic assessments and cultures have been performed before administering solution.
4. Assess for tinnitus, vertigo, or hearing losses during therapy. Persistently increased gentamycin levels have been associated with 8th CN dysfunction.

Evaluate

- Resolution of infection
- During systemic administration, therapeutic peak serum drug levels (4–8 mcg/mL); (trough<2 mg/mL)

Kanamycin sulfate

(kan-ah-**MY**-sin)
Pregnancy Category: D
Kantrex, Klebcil **(Rx)**

See also *Anti-Infectives,* Chapter 1, and *Aminoglycosides,* Chapter 2.

How Supplied: *Capsule:* 500 mg; *Injection:* 1 g/3 mL, 75 mg/2 mL, 500 mg/2 mL

Action/Kinetics: The activity of kanamycin resembles that of neomycin and streptomycin. **Peak therapeutic serum levels: IM,** 15–40 mcg/mL. **t½:** 2–3 hr. **Toxic serum levels:** >35 mcg/mL (peak) and >10 mcg/mL (trough).

Uses: Parenteral: As initial therapy for infections due to *Escherichia coli, Proteus, Enterobacter aerogenes, Klebsiella pneumoniae, Serratia marcescens,* and *Acinetobacter.* May be combined with a penicillin or cephalosporin before knowing results of susceptibility tests. *Investigational:* As part of a multiple-drug regimen for *Mycobacterium avium* complex in AIDS clients.

PO: As an adjunct to mechanical cleansing of large bowel for suppression of intestinal bacteria; hepatic coma.

Dosage

- **Capsules**

Intestinal bacteria suppression.

1 g every hour for 4 hr; **then,** 1 g q 6 hr for 36–72 hr.

Hepatic coma.

8–12 g/day in divided doses.

- **IM, IV**

Adults and children: 15 mg/kg/day in two to three equal doses. Maximum daily dose should not exceed 1.5 g regardless of route of administration.

For calculating dosage interval (in hr) in clients with impaired renal function, multiply serum creatinine (mg/100 mL) by 9.

- **IM**

Tuberculosis.

Adults: 15 mg/kg/day. Not recommended for use in children.

- **Intraperitoneal**

500 mg diluted in 20 mL sterile distilled water.

- **Inhalation**

250 mg in saline—nebulize b.i.d.–q.i.d.

Irrigation of abscess cavities, pleural space, ventricular cavities.

0.25% solution.

Administration

1. Do not mix with any other medication in IV bottle/bag. Reconstitute 500 mg with 100–200 mL of dextrose or saline solution and infuse over 30–60 min. Administer IV slowly and at concentrations not exceeding 2.5 mg/mL.
2. Unopened vials may change color, but this does not affect potency of drug. Consult pharmacist if unsure of altered vials.
3. Do not mix with other drugs in same syringe for IM injection.
4. Inject deep into large muscle mass to minimize pain and local irritation. Rotate sites of injection. Local irritation may occur with large doses.
5. IV administration is rarely used

and must not be used for clients with renal impairment.
6. Drug should not be administered for more than 12–14 days.
Special Concerns: Use with caution in premature infants and neonates.
Additional Side Effects: Sprue-like syndrome with steatorrhea, malabsorption, and electrolyte imbalance.
Additional Drug Interaction: Procainamide ↑ muscle relaxation.

NURSING CONSIDERATIONS

See also *General Nursing Considerations for All Anti-Infectives,* Chapter 1, and *Aminoglycosides,* Chapter 2.
Client/Family Teaching
1. Consume 2–3 L of fluid/day.
2. Report any symptoms of hearing loss as this is frequently related to elevated peak drug levels.
Evaluate
- Resolution of infection
- Suppression of intestinal bacteria
- During systemic administration, therapeutic drug levels (peak 15–40 mcg/mL; trough 5–10 mcg/mL)

Neomycin sulfate

(nee-oh-**MY**-sin)
Mycifradin Sulfate, Myciguent, Neobiotic **(Rx)**

See also *Anti-Infectives,* Chapter 1, and *Aminoglycosides,* Chapter 2.
How Supplied: *Cream:* 5 mg/g; *Ointment:* 5 mg/g; *Solution:* 125 mg/5 mL; *Tablet:* 500 mg
Action/Kinetics: Peak plasma levels: PO, 1–4 hr; **Therapeutic serum level:** 5–10 mcg/mL. **t½:** 2–3 hr.
Uses: PO: Hepatic coma, sterilization of gut prior to surgery, inhibition of ammonia-forming bacteria in GI tract in hepatic encephalopathy. Therapy of intestinal infections due to pathogenic strains of *Escherichia coli,* primarily in children. *Investigational:* Hypercholesterolemia.

Topical: Used for itching, burning, inflamed skin conditions that are threatened, or complicated, by a secondary bacterial infection.

Dosage
- **Oral solution**

Preoperatively in colorectal surgery.
1 g each of neomycin and erythromycin base for a total of three doses: the first two doses 1 hr apart the afternoon before surgery and the third dose at bedtime the night before surgery.

Hepatic coma, adjunct.
Adults, 4–12 g/day in divided doses for 5–6 days; **children:** 50–100 mg/kg/day in divided doses for 5–6 days.
- **Topical Cream, Ointment**

Neomycin alone or in combination with other antibiotics (bacitracin or gramicidin) and/or an anti-inflammatory agent (corticosteroid). Apply ointment (0.5%) or cream (0.5%) 1–5 times/day to affected area. If necessary, a bandage may be used to cover the area.
Administration/Storage
1. The recommended procedure should be specifically followed to prepare the GI tract for surgery.
2. Have available neostigmine to counteract renal failure, respiratory depression and arrest, side effects that may occur when neomycin is administered intraperitoneally.
Additional Contraindications: Intestinal obstruction (PO). Topical products should not be used in or around the eyes.
Special Concerns: Safe use during pregnancy has not been determined. Due to the possibility of toxicity, some experts do not recommend the parenteral use of neomycin for any purpose. Use with caution in clients with extensive burns, trophic ulceration, or other conditions where significant systemic absorption is possible.
Additional Side Effects: Ototoxicity, nephrotoxicity. Sprue-like syndrome with steatorrhea, malabsorption, and electrolyte imbalance. Skin rashes after topical or parenteral administration. Chronic use in allergic contact dermatitis and chronic der-

matoses increases the risk of sensitization.

Additional Drug Interactions

Digoxin / ↓ Effect of digoxin due to ↓ absorption from GI tract

Penicillin V / ↓ Effect of penicillin due to ↓ absorption from GI tract

Procainamide / ↑ Muscle relaxation produced by neomycin

NURSING CONSIDERATIONS

See also *Nursing Considerations* for *Aminoglycosides,* Chapter 2.

Assessment

1. Document indications for therapy and type and onset of symptoms.
2. Describe findings of abdominal assessment.
3. Obtain appropriate baseline lab studies.

Interventions

1. Monitor I&O and serum electrolyte levels. Encourage fluid intake of 2–3 L/day unless contraindicated.
2. Anticipate a slight laxative effect produced by oral neomycin. Withhold and report in case of suspected intestinal obstruction.
3. Anticipate a low-residue diet for preoperative disinfection and, unless contraindicated, a laxative immediately preceding PO administration of neomycin sulfate.
4. Clean the affected area before applying neomycin topical ointment or solution.

Evaluate

- Improved levels of consciousness in hepatic coma
- Resolution or prevention of infection to skin wounds
- Evidence of effective bowel sterilization before intestinal surgery
- Laboratory evidence of negative culture reports
- Therapeutic serum drug levels (5–10 mcg/mL)

Paromomycin sulfate

(pair-oh-moh-**MY**-sin)
Humatin **(Rx)**

See also *Aminoglycosides,* Chapter 2.

How Supplied: *Capsule:* 250 mg

Action/Kinetics: Paromomycin is obtained from *Streptomyces rimosus forma paromomycina.* Its spectrum of activity resembles that of neomycin and kanamycin. The drug is poorly absorbed from the GI tract and is ineffective against systemic infections when given PO.

Uses: Inhibition of ammonia-forming bacteria in GI tract in hepatic encephalopathy, intestinal amebiasis, preoperative suppression of intestinal flora. Hepatic coma. *Investigational:* Anthelmintic, to treat *Dientamoeba fragilis, Diphyllobothrium latum, Taenia saginata, T. solium, Dipylidium caninum,* and *Hymenolepis nana.*

Dosage

- **Capsules**

Hepatic coma.

Adults: 4 g/day in divided doses for 5–6 days.

Intestinal amebiasis.

Adults and children: 25–35 mg/kg/day administered in three doses with meals for 5–10 days.

D. fragilis infections.

25–30 mg/kg/day in three divided doses for 1 week.

H. nana infections.

45 mg/kg/day for 5–7 days.

D. latum, T. saginata, T. solium, D. caninum infections.

Adults: 1 g/ q 15 min for a total of four doses; **pediatric:** 11 mg/kg/15 min for four doses.

Administration/Storage: Do not administer parenterally and do not administer concurrently with penicillin.

Contraindication: Intestinal obstruction.

Special Concerns: Use during pregnancy only if benefits outweigh risks. To be used with caution in the presence of GI ulceration because of possible systemic absorption.

Additional Side Effects: Diarrhea or loose stools. Heartburn, emesis, and pruritus ani. Superinfections, especially by monilia.

Drug Interaction: Penicillin is inhibited by paromomycin.

NURSING CONSIDERATIONS

See also *Nursing Considerations* for *Aminoglycosides,* p. 7.

Client/Family Teaching

1. Take before or after meals.
2. Report any persistent diarrhea, dehydration, and general weakness because drug therapy may need to be interrupted if symptoms are excessive.

Evaluate: Desired suppression of intestinal flora.

Streptomycin sulfate

(strep-toe-**MY**-sin)
Pregnancy Category: D
(Rx)

See also *Aminoglycosides,* Chapter 2.

How Supplied: *Injection:* 400 mg/mL

Action/Kinetics: Like other aminoglycoside antibiotics, streptomycin is distributed rapidly throughout most tissues and body fluids, including necrotic tubercular lesions. **Therapeutic serum levels: IM,** 20–30 mcg/mL. **t½:** 2–3 hr. **Toxic serum levels:** >50 mcg/mL (peak).

Uses: With other drugs to treat *Mycobacterium tuberculosis* infections. Used in the following infections when less potentially hazardous drugs are either ineffective or contraindicated: UTIs due to *Escherichia coli, Proteus, Enterobacter aerogenes, Klebsiella pneumoniae,* and *Enterococcus faecalis.* With penicillin to treat endocardial infections due to *Streptoccus viridans* and *E. faecalis.* With other drugs to treat bacteremia. With another agent to treat respiratory, endocardial, and meningeal infections due to *H. influenzae.* Infections due to *Brucella, Haemophilus ducreyi* (chancroid), *Francisella tularensis* (tularemia), *Pasturella pestis* (plague), and granuloma inguinale. *Investigational:* As part of multiple-drug regimen to treat *Mycobacterium avium* complex in AIDS clients.

Dosage

- **IM only**

Tuberculosis (adjunct).

The usual regimen for treating drug-susceptible tuberculosis has been 2 months of isoniazid, rifampin, and pyrazinamide, followed by 4 months of isoniazid and rifampin. When streptomycin is added to the drug regimen, the following doses are recommended. **Adults:** 15 mg/kg/day (maximum of 1 g/day), 25–30 mg/kg twice weekly (maximum of 1.5 g), or 25–30 mg/kg thrice weekly (maximum of 1.5 g). The total period of drug treatment is a minimum of 1 year. **Pediatric:** 20–40 mg/kg/day (not to exceed 1 g/day), 25–30 mg/kg twice weekly (maximum of 1.5 g), or 25–30 mg/kg thrice weekly (maximum of 1.5 g). Older, debilitated clients should receive lower dosages.

Bacterial endocarditis due to penicillin-sensitive alpha-hemolytic and nonhemolytic streptococci (with penicillin).

1 g b.i.d. for 1 week; **then,** 0.5 g b.i.d. for second week.

Enterococcal endocarditis (with penicillin).

1 g b.i.d. for 2 weeks; **then,** 0.5 g b.i.d. for 4 weeks. **Plague:** 1 g q 12 hr for at least 10 days.

Tularemia.

0.25–0.5 g q 6 hr for 7–10 days or until client is afebrile for 5–7 days.

Moderate to severe fulminating infections.

Adults: 1–2 g in divided doses q 6–12 hr, depending on severity of infections; **pediatric:** 20–40 mg/kg/day in divided doses q 6–12 hr.

Less severe infections.

Adults: 1–2 g/day.

Mycobacterium avium *complex in AIDS clients.*

11–13 mg/kg/day IV or 15 mg/kg/day IM used with three to five agents as part of a multiple-drug regimen.

Administration/Storage

1. Protect hands when preparing

drug. Wear gloves if drug is prepared often because it is irritating.
2. In a dry form, the drug is stable for at least 2 years at room temperature.
3. Aqueous solutions prepared without preservatives are stable for at least 1 week at room temperature and for at least 3 months under refrigeration.
4. Use only solutions prepared freshly from dry powder for intrathecal, subarachnoid, and intrapleural administration because commercially prepared solutions contain preservatives harmful to tissues of the CNS and pleural cavity.
5. Commercially prepared, ready-to-inject solutions are for IM use only. These solutions are prepared with phenol and are stable at room temperature for prolonged periods of time.
6. When injection into the subarachnoid space is required for treatment of meningitis, only solutions made freshly from the dry powder should be used. Commercial solutions may contain preservatives toxic to the CNS.
7. Administer deep into muscle mass to minimize pain and local irritation.
8. Solutions may darken after exposure to light, but this does not necessarily cause a loss in potency. Check with pharmacist if unsure of potency.
9. *Treatment of Overdose/Toxicity:* Hemodialysis (preferred) or peritoneal dialysis.

Additional Contraindications: Hypersensitivity, contact dermatitis, and exfoliative dermatitis. Do not give to clients with myasthenia gravis.

Special Concerns: Use during pregnancy only if benefits clearly outweigh risks.

Additional Laboratory Test Interference: False urine glucose determinations with Benedict's solution and Clinitest.

NURSING CONSIDERATIONS

See also *Nursing Considerations* for *Aminoglycosides,* Chapter 2.

Assessment

1. Document indications for therapy, onset of symptoms, and any other agents used previously.
2. Ensure that appropriate lab studies, culture specimens, PPD skin testing, and CXR have been performed.
3. Determine if pregnant; drug may cause deafness in newborn.

Client/Family Teaching

1. Solution is malodorous; inform client that this is normal.
2. Report any persistent or bothersome side effects as well as lack of response to drug therapy.
3. Increase fluid intake to 2–3 L/day. Report any evidence of altered urine output or weight gain.
4. Report any evidence of hearing loss, vestibular dysfunction, or loss of balance. High peak streptomycin levels may precipitate eighth cranial nerve dysfunction.

Evaluate

- Laboratory evidence of negative culture reports
- Resolution of infection and reports of symptomatic improvement
- Therapeutic serum drug levels

Tobramycin sulfate

(toe-brah-**MY**-sin)
Pregnancy Category: D
Nebcin, Tobrex Ophthalmic Ointment, Tobrex Ophthalmic Solution
(Rx)

See also *Aminoglycosides,* Chapter 2.

How Supplied: *Injection:* 10 mg/mL, 40 mg/mL; *Powder for injection:* 60 mg, 80 mg, 1.2 g

Action/Kinetics: This aminoglycoside is similar to gentamicin and can be used concurrently with carbenicillin. **Therapeutic serum levels: IM,** 4–8 mcg/mL. **t½:** 2–2.5 hr. **Toxic serum levels:** >12 mcg/mL (peak) and >2 mcg/mL (trough).

Uses: Systemic: Complicated and recurrent UTIs due to *Pseudomonas aeruginosa, Proteus, Escherichia coli, Klebsiella, Enterobacter, Serratia, Staphylococcus aureus, Citrobacter,* and *Providencia.* Lower respiratory tract infections due to *P. aeruginosa, Klebsiella, Enterobacter, E. coli, Serratia,* and *S. aureus.* Intra-abdominal infections (including peritonitis) due to *E. coli, Klebsiella,* and *Enterobacter*. Septicemia in neonates, children, and adults due to *P. aeruginosa, E. coli,* and *Klebsiella*. Skin, bone, and skin structure infections due to *P. aeruginosa, Proteus, E. coli, Klebsiella, Enterobacter,* and *S. aureus*. Serious CNS infections, including meningitis. Can be used with penicillins or cephalosporins in serious infections when results of susceptibility testing are not yet known.

Ophthalmic: Treat superficial ocular infections due to *Staphylococcus, S. aureus, Streptococcus, S. pneumoniae,* beta-hemolytic streptococci, *Corynebacterium, E. coli, Haemophilus aegyptius, H. ducreyi, H. influenzae, Klebsiella pneumoniae, Neisseria, Proteus, Acinetobacter calcoaceticus, Enterobacter, Enterobacter aerogenes, Serratia marcescens, Moraxella, Pseudomonas aeruginosa,* and *Vibrio*.

Dosage

- **IM, IV**

Non-life-threatening serious infections.

Adults: 3 mg/kg/day in three equally divided doses q 8 hr.

Life-threatening infections.

Up to 5 mg/kg/day in three or four equal doses. **Pediatric:** Either 2–2.5 mg/kg q 8 hr or 1.5–1.9 mg/kg q 6 hr; **neonates 1 week of age or less:** up to 4 mg/kg/day in two equal doses q 12 hr.

Impaired renal function.

Initially: 1 mg/kg; **then,** maintenance dose calculated according to information supplied by manufacturer.

- **Ophthalmic Ointment**

Acute infections.

0.5-in. ribbon q 3–4 hr until improvement is noted.

Mild to moderate infections.

0.5-in. ribbon b.i.d.–t.i.d.

- **Ophthalmic Solution**

Acute infections.

Initial: 1–2 gtt q 15–30 min until improvement noted; **then,** reduce dosage gradually.

Moderate infections.

1–2 gtt 2–6 times/day.

Administration/Storage

1. Prepare IV solution by diluting calculated dose of tobramycin with 50–100 mL of dextrose or saline solution and infuse over 30–60 min.
2. Use proportionately less diluent for children than for adults.
3. Do not mix with other drugs for parenteral administration.
4. Store drug at room temperature—no longer than 2 years.
5. Discard solution of drug containing up to 1 mg/mL after 24 hr at room temperature.

Contraindications: Ophthalmically to treat dendritic keratitis, vaccinia, varicella, fungal or mycobacterial eye infections, after removal of a corneal foreign body. Lactation.

Special Concerns: Use with caution in premature infants and neonates. Ophthalmic ointment may retard corneal epithelial healing.

Additional Side Effects: *Symptoms of overdose when used ophthalmically:* Edema, lid itching, punctate keratitis, erythema, lacrimation.

Additional Drug Interactions: With carbenicillin or ticarcillin, tobramycin may have an increased effect when used for *Pseudomonas* infections.

NURSING CONSIDERATIONS

See also *Nursing Considerations* for *Aminoglycosides,* Chapter 2.

Client/Family Teaching

1. Provide a printed list of side effects that require reporting should they occur.
2. Drink plenty of fluids (2–3 L/day) during parenteral drug therapy.
3. With eye infections, review the appropriate method for instillation and observe client technique. Advise to avoid wearing contact lenses until infection is cleared and provider approves.
4. Advise to report if symptoms do not improve or if they worsen after 3 days of therapy.

Evaluate

- Laboratory evidence of negative culture reports

- Resolution of ophthalmic infection
- Therapeutic serum drug levels (4–8 mcg/mL) with systemic therapy

CHAPTER THREE

Antibiotics: Cephalosporins

See also the following individual entries:

Cefaclor
Cefadroxil Monohydrate
Cefamandole Nafate
Cefazolin Sodium
Cefixime Oral
Cefmetazole Sodium
Cefonicid Sodium
Cefoperazone Sodium
Cefotaxime Sodium
Cefotetan Disodium
Cefoxitin Sodium
Cefpodoxime Proxetil
Cefprozil
Ceftazidime
Ceftizoxime Sodium
Ceftriaxone Sodium
Cefuroxime Axetil
Cefuroxime Sodium
Cephalexin Hydrochloride Monohydrate
Cephalexin Monohydrate
Cephalothin Sodium
Cephapirin Sodium
Cephradine
Loracarbef

General Statement: The cephalosporins are semisynthetic antibiotics resembling the penicillins both chemically and pharmacologically. Some cephalosporins are rapidly absorbed from the GI tract and quickly reach effective concentrations in the urinary, GI, and respiratory tracts except in clients with pernicious anemia or obstructive jaundice. The drugs are eliminated rapidly in clients with normal renal function.

The cephalosporins are broad-spectrum antibiotics classified as first-, second-, and third-generation drugs. The difference among generations is based on antibacterial spectra; third-generation cephalosporins have more activity against gram-negative organisms and resistant organisms and less activity against gram-positive organisms than first-generation drugs. Third-generation cephalosporins are also stable against beta-lactamases. Cephalosporins can be destroyed by cephalosporinase. Also, the cost increases from first- to third-generation cephalosporins.

Action/Kinetics: The cephalosporins interfere with a final step in the formation of the bacterial cell wall (inhibition of mucopeptide biosynthesis), resulting in unstable cell membranes that undergo lysis (same mechanism of actions as penicillins). Also, cell division and growth are inhibited. The cephalosporins are most effective against young, rapidly dividing organisms and are considered bactericidal. The **t½** ranges from 69 to 132 min, and serum protein binding ranges from 5% to 86%. Cephalosporins are widely distributed to most tissues and fluids. First- and second-generation drugs do not enter the CSF well but third-generation drugs enter inflamed meninges readily. The cephalosporins are rapidly excreted by the kidneys.

Uses: Cephalosporins are effective against infections of the biliary tract, GI tract, GU system, bones, joints, upper and lower respiratory tract, skin, and skin structures. Also, gynecologic infections, meningitis, osteomyelitis, endocarditis, intra-abdominal infections, peritonitis, otitis media, gonorrhea, septicemia, and prophylaxis prior to surgery. A listing of the organisms against which cephalosporins are effective follows.

First-Generation Cephalosporins. Gram-positive cocci including *Staphylococcus aureus, S. epidermidis, S. pyogenes, Streptococcus pneumoniae, S. viridans,* group A and B streptococci, and anaerobic streptococci. Activity against gram-negative bacteria includes *Escherichia coli, Haemophilus influenzae, Klebsiella,* and *Proteus mirabilis*. Drugs include cefadroxil, cefazolin, cephalexin, cephalothin, cephapirin, cephradine.

Second-Generation Cephalosporins. Spectrum similar to that of first-generation cephalosporins. Also active against certain gram-negative bacteria and anaerobes including *Providencia rettgeri, Bacteroides* species, *Peptococcus,* and *Peptostreptococcus* species. Selected second-generation cephalosporins are effective against the following genera: *Citrobacter, Enterobacter, Providencia, Clostridium,* and *Fusobacterium,* as well as *Morganella morganii, Neisseria gonorrhoeae,* and *Proteus vulgaris*. Second-generation drugs include cefaclor, cefamandole, cefmetazole, cefonicid, cefotetan, cefoxitin, cefpodoxime, cefprozil, cefuroxime, and loracarbef.

Third-Generation Cephalosporins. Less active against gram-positive cocci. Spectrum similar to first- and second-generation cephalosporins. Most are also active against the following gram-negative and anaerobic species: *Acinetobacter, Citrobacter, Enterobacter, Providencia, Salmonella, Serratia, Shigella, Bacteroides, Clostridium, Fusobacterium, Peptococcus,* and *Peptostreptococcus*. Most are effective against *M. morganii, N. gonorrhoeae, Neisseria meningitidis, P. vulgaris, Pseudomonas aeruginosa,* and *Bacteroides fragilis*. Selected third-generation cephalosporins are effective against *Haemophilus parainfluenzae, Moraxella catarrhalis, Salmonella thypi, Clostridium difficile,* and *Eubacterium* species. Third-generation drugs include cefixime, cefoperoxazone, cefotaxime, ceftazidime, ceftizoxime, ceftriaxone.

Contraindications: Hypersensitivity to cephalosporins.

Special Concerns: Safe use in pregnancy and lactation has not been established. Use with caution in the presence of impaired renal or hepatic function or together with other nephrotoxic drugs. Creatinine clearances should be performed on all clients with impaired renal function who receive cephalosporins. Use with caution in clients over 50 years of age. Clients hypersensitive to penicillin may occasionally cross-react to cephalosporins.

Side Effects: *GI:* N&V, diarrhea, abdominal cramps or pain, dyspepsia, glossitis, heartburn, sore mouth or tongue, dysgeusia, anorexia, flatulence, cholestasis. Pseudomembranous colitis. *Allergic:* Urticaria, rashes (maculopapular, morbilliform, or erythematous), pruritus (including anal and genital areas), fever, chills, erythema, ***angioedema,*** serum sickness, joint pain, exfoliative dermatitis, chest tightness, myalgia, erythema multiforme, edema, itching, numbness, chills, ***Stevens-Johnson syndrome, anaphylaxis.*** *NOTE:* Cross-allergy may be manifested between cephalosporins and penicillins. *Hematologic:* Leukopenia, leukocytosis, lymphocytosis, neutropenia (transient), eosinophilia, thrombocytopenia, thrombocythemia, ***agranulocytosis,*** granulocytopenia, bone marrow depression, ***hemolytic anemia,*** pancytopenia, decreased platelet function, ***aplastic anemia,*** hypoprothrombinemia (may lead to bleeding), thrombocytosis (transient). *CNS:* Headache, malaise, fatigue, vertigo, dizziness, lethargy, confusion, paresthesia, precipitation of ***seizures*** (especially in clients with impaired renal function). *Hepatic:* Hepatomegaly, hepatitis. Intrathecal use may result in hallucinations, nystagmus, or ***seizures.*** *Miscellaneous:* Superinfection including oral candidiasis and enterococcal infections, hypotension, sweating, flushing, dyspnea, interstitial pneumonitis.

IV or IM use may result in local swelling, inflammation, cellulitis, paresthesia, burning, phlebitis, thrombophlebitis. IM use may also cause pain and induration, tenderness, increased temperature. Sterile abscesses have been observed following SC use. Nephrotoxicity (↑ BUN with and without ↑ serum creatinine) may occur in clients over 50 and in young children.

Symptoms of Overdose: Parenteral use of large doses of cephalosporins may cause seizures, especially in clients with impaired renal function.

Drug Interactions

Aminoglycosides / ↑ Risk of renal toxicity with certain cephalosporins
Anticoagulants / Certain cephalosporins ↑ PT
Bacteriostatic agents / ↓ Effect of cephalosporins
Bumetanide / ↑ Risk of renal toxicity
Colistimethate / ↑ Risk of renal toxicity
Colistin / ↑ Risk of renal toxicity
Ethacrynic acid / ↑ Risk of renal toxicity
Furosemide / ↑ Risk of renal toxicity
Polymyxin B / ↑ Risk of renal toxicity
Probenecid / ↑ Effect of cephalosporins by ↓ excretion by kidneys
Vancomycin / ↑ Risk of renal toxicity

Laboratory Test Interferences: False + for urinary glucose with Benedict's solution, Fehling's solution, or Clinitest tablets. Enzyme tests (Clinistix, Tes-Tape) are unaffected. False + Coombs' test and urinary 17-ketosteroids.

↑ AST, ALT, total bilirubin, GGTP, LDH, alkaline phosphatase.

Dosage

See individual drugs.

NURSING CONSIDERATIONS

See also *General Nursing Considerations for All Anti-Infectives,* Chapter 1.

Administration/Storage

1. Parenteral solutions infused too rapidly may cause pain and irritation; infuse over 30 min unless otherwise indicated and assess site frequently.
2. Therapy should be continued for at least 2–3 days after symptoms of infection have disappeared.
3. For group A beta-hemolytic streptococcal infections, therapy should be continued for at least 10 days to prevent the development of glomerulonephritis or rheumatic fever.
4. *Treatment of Overdose:* If seizures occur, discontinue the drug immediately and give anticonvulsant drugs. Hemodialysis may also be effective.

Assessment

1. Assess client with a history of hypersensitivity reaction to penicillin for cross-sensitivity to cephalosporins. Cephalosporins are sensitizing and may elicit a hypersensitivity reaction. Do not administer if client history of anaphylaxis to penicillin.
2. Assess client's financial status. Many in this group of antibiotics are quite expensive and clients on fixed incomes with limited health benefits may be unable to afford the prescription expense.
3. Document indications for therapy and symptoms of infection and ensure that appropriate cultures have been performed prior to initiating drug therapy.
4. Obtain baseline CBC, serum glucose, electrolytes, and liver and renal function studies.

Interventions

1. The cephalosporins all have similar sounding and similarly spelled names. Use care when transcribing orders for administration of these drugs and request clarification as needed.
2. Pseudomembranous colitis may

occur in clients receiving cephalosporins. If diarrhea develops, note any fever and report immediately. Continue to monitor VS, I&O, and for lab evidence of electrolyte imbalance.
3. Review liver and renal function studies and anticipate lower doses for clients with renal impairment. For dialysis clients, administer after treatment.
4. Drug may cause a false positive Coombs' test. Document appropriately and instruct client.
5. Persistent temperature elevations may be indicative of drug-induced fever.

Client/Family Teaching

1. Emphasize that oral medications should be taken on an empty stomach but, if GI upset occurs, the drug may be administered with meals.
2. Report any symptoms that may necessitate drug withdrawal such as vaginal itching or drainage, fever, or diarrhea.
3. Explain that yogurt or buttermilk (4 oz) may be prescribed daily for diarrhea related to intestinal superinfections.
4. Advise to report signs of superinfection (black furry tongue, vaginal itching or discharge, and loose, foul-smelling stools). Nystatin may be ordered for secondary infections.
5. Stress the importance of taking medication as ordered and of reporting side effects so that appropriate therapy may be initiated.
6. Advise that any abnormal bleeding or bruising should be reported immediately.
7. Explain that medication may cause a false positive Coombs' test. This would be of concern if client is being cross-matched for blood transfusions or in newborns whose mothers have taken cephalosporins during pregnancy.
8. Avoid alcohol and alcohol-containing products, as a disulfiram-type reaction may occur with some of the cephalasporins.

Evaluate

- Evidence (presence/absence) of pretreatment symptoms and review of C&S results to determine effectiveness of treatment
- Clinical evidence of resolution of infection, such as ↓ WBCs, ↓ temperature, improved appetite
- Reports of symptomatic improvement

Cefaclor

(**SEF**-ah-klor)
Pregnancy Category: B
Ceclor **(Rx)**

See also *Anti-Infectives,* Chapter 1, and *Cephalosporins,* Chapter 3.

How Supplied: *Capsule:* 250 mg, 500 mg; *Powder for Reconstitution:* 125 mg/5 mL, 187 mg/5 mL, 250 mg/5 mL, 375 mg/5 mL

Action/Kinetics: Peak serum levels: 5–15 mcg/mL after 1 hr. **t½: PO,** 36–54 min. Well absorbed from GI tract. From 60% to 85% excreted in urine within 8 hr.

Uses: Otitis media due to *Streptococcus pneumoniae, Hemophilus influenzae, Streptococcus pyogenes,* and staphylococci. Upper respiratory tract infections (including pharyngitis and tonsillitis) caused by *S. pyogenes.* Lower respiratory tract infections (including pneumonia) due to *S. pneumoniae, H. influenzae,* and *S. pyogenes.* Skin and skin structure infections due to *Staphylococcus aureus* and *S. pyogenes.* Urinary tract infections (including pyelonephritis and cystitis) caused by *Escherichia coli, Proteus mirabilis, Klebsiella,* and coagulase-negative staphylococci. *Investigational:* Acute uncomplicated urinary tract infections in select populations using a dose of 2 g.

Dosage

- **Capsules, Oral Suspension**

Adults: 250 mg q 8 hr. Dose may be doubled in more severe infections or those caused by less susceptible organisms. Total daily dose should not exceed 4 g. **Children:** 20 mg/kg/day in divided doses q 8 hr. Dose may be doubled in more serious infections, otitis media, or for infections caused by less susceptible organisms. For otitis media and pharyngitis, the total daily dose may be divided and given q 12 hr. Total daily dose should not exceed 1 g.

Administration/Storage

1. The suspension should be refrigerated after reconstitution and discarded after 2 weeks.
2. The total daily dose for otitis media and pharyngitis can be divided and given q 12 hr.

Special Concerns: Safety for use in infants less than 1 month of age has not been established.

Additional Side Effects: Cholestatic jaundice, lymphocytosis.

NURSING CONSIDERATIONS

See also *General Nursing Considerations* for *All Anti-Infectives,* Chapter 1, and *Cephalosporins,* Chapter 3.

Evaluate: Resolution of infection and reports of symptomatic improvement.

Cefadroxil monohydrate

(sef-ah-**DROX**-ill)
Pregnancy Category: B
Duricef, Ultracef **(Rx)**

See also *Anti-Infectives,* Chapter 1, and *Cephalosporins,* Chapter 3.

How Supplied: *Capsule:* 500 mg; *Powder for Reconstitution:* 125 mg/5 mL, 250 mg/5 mL, 500 mg/5 mL; *Tablet:* 1 g

Action/Kinetics: Peak serum levels: PO, 15–33 mcg/mL after 90 min. **t½: PO,** 70–80 min. Ninety percent of drug is excreted unchanged in urine within 24 hr.

Uses: Pharyngitis, tonsillitis. Infections of the urinary tract, skin, and skin structures.

Dosage

• **Capsules, Oral Suspension, Tablets**

Pharyngitis, tonsillitis, skin and skin structure infections.

Adults: 1 g/day in single or two divided doses.

UTIs.

Adults: 1–2 g/day in single or two divided doses. **Children:** 30 mg/kg/day in divided doses q 12 hr.

For clients with creatinine clearance rates below 50 mL/min.

Initial: 1 g; **maintenance,** 500 mg at following dosage intervals: q 36 hr for creatinine clearance rates of 0–10 mL/min; q 24 hr for creatinine clearance rates of 10–25 mL/min; q 12 hr for creatinine clearance rates of 25–50 mL/min.

Administration/Storage

1. Cefadroxil can be given without regard to meals.
2. The suspension should be shaken well before using.
3. For beta-hemolytic streptococcal infections, treatment should be continued for 10 days.

Special Concerns: Safe use in children not established. Creatinine clearance determinations must be carried out in clients with renal impairment.

NURSING CONSIDERATIONS

See also *General Nursing Considerations* for *All Anti-Infectives,* Chapter 1, and *Cephalosporins,* Chapter 3.

Evaluate

• Reports of symptomatic improvement
• Negative laboratory culture reports

Cefamandole nafate

(sef-ah-**MAN**-dole)
Pregnancy Category: B
Mandol **(Rx)**

See also *Anti-Infectives,* Chapter 1, and *Cephalosporins,* Chapter 3.

How Supplied: *Powder for injection:* 1 g, 2 g, 10 g

Action/Kinetics: Cefamandole nafate has a particularly broad spectrum of activity. **Peak serum levels: IM,** 12–36 mcg/mL after 30–120 min. **t½: IM,** 60 min; **IV,** 30 min. From 65% to 85% excreted unchanged in urine.

Uses: Infections of the urinary tract, lower respiratory tract, bones, joints, skin, and skin structures. Mixed infections of the respiratory tract, skin, and in pelvic inflammatory disease. Peritonitis, septicemia, prophylaxis in surgery. Also, with aminoglycosides in gram-positive or gram-negative sepsis.

Dosage

- **IV or deep IM injection only**

In gluteus or lateral thigh to minimize pain.

Infections.

Adults, usual: 0.5–1 g q 4–8 hr. **Infants and children:** 50–100 mg/kg/day in equally divided doses q 4–8 hr.

Severe infections.

Adults: Up to 2 g q 4 hr. **Infants and children:** Up to 150 mg/kg/day (not to exceed adult dose) divided as above.

Preoperative.

Adults, initial: 1–2 g 30–60 min prior to surgery; **then,** 1–2 g q 6 hr for 1–2 days (3 days for prosthetic arthroplasty). For cesarean section, the first dose should be given just prior to surgery or just after the cord has been clamped. **Pediatric (3 months and older):** 50–100 mg/kg/day in divided doses, using same schedule as for adults.

Impaired renal function.

Initial: 1–2 g; then a maintenance dosage is given, depending on creatinine clearance, according to schedule provided by manufacturer.

Administration/Storage

1. Review package insert for details on how to reconstitute drug.
2. Reconstituted solutions of cefamandole nafate are stable for 24 hr at room temperature and for 96 hr when stored in the refrigerator. Cefamandole solutions reconstituted with dextrose or sodium chloride are stable for 6 months when frozen immediately after reconstitution.
3. For direct IV administration, dilute 1 g in 10 mL of solution and administer over 3–5 min. May be further diluted and administered over 15–30 min.
4. Peripheral IV site *must* be changed every 2–3 days to prevent phlebitis.
5. Carbon dioxide gas forms when reconstituted solutions are kept at room temperature. This gas does not affect the activity of the antibiotic and may be dissipated or used to aid in the withdrawal of the contents of the vial.
6. Use separate IV fluid containers and separate injection sites for each drug when cefamandole is administered concomitantly with another antibiotic such as an aminoglycoside.
7. Follow manufacturer guidelines for dosage with impaired renal function.

Special Concerns: Safety and effectiveness have not been determined in infants less than 1 month of age.

Additional Side Effects: Hypoprothrombinemia leading to bleeding and/or bruising; cholestatic jaundice, decreased creatinine clearance in clients with prior renal impairment.

Additional Drug Interaction: Concomitant use with ethanol produces a disulfiram-type reaction and hypotension.

NURSING CONSIDERATIONS

See also *General Nursing Considerations* for *All Anti-Infectives,* Chapter 1, and *Cephalosporins,* Chapter 3.

Client/Family Teaching

1. Avoid alcohol and any medications or OTC products containing alcohol as a disulfiram-type reaction may occur.
2. Report any evidence of increased bruising or bleeding.
3. Any yellow discoloration of skin, eyes, or stool should be reported immediately.

Evaluate: Resolution of infection.

Cefazolin sodium

(sef-**AYZ**-oh-lin)

Pregnancy Category: B

Ancef, Kefzol, Zolicef **(Rx)**

See also *Anti-Infectives,* Chapter 1, and *Cephalosporins,* Chapter 3.

How Supplied: *Injection:* 1 g/50 mL, 500 mg/50 mL; *Powder for injection:* 500 mg, 1 g, 5 g, 10 g
Action/Kinetics: Peak serum concentration: IM 17–76 mcg/mL after 1 hr. **t½: IM, IV:** 90–130 min. From 80% to 100% excreted unchanged in urine.
Uses: Infections of the urinary tract, biliary tract, respiratory tract, bones, joints, soft tissue, and skin. Endocarditis, septicemia, prophylaxis in surgery.

Dosage
- **IM, IV only**

Mild infections due to gram-positive cocci.
Adults: 250–500 mg q 8 hr.
Mild to moderate infections.
Children over 1 month: 25–50 mg/kg/day in three to four doses.
Moderate to severe infections.
Adults: 0.5–1 g q 6–8 hr.
Acute, uncomplicated UTIs.
Adults: 1 g q 12 hr. *For severe infections,* up to 100 mg/kg/day may be used.
Endocarditis, septicemia.
Adults: 1–1.5 g q 6 hr (rarely, up to 12 g/day).
Pneumococcal pneumonia.
Adults: 0.5 g q 12 hr.
Preoperative.
Adults: 1 g 30–60 min prior to surgery.
During surgery.
Adults: 0.5–1 g.
Postoperative.
Adults: 0.5–1 g q 6–8 hr for 24 hr (may be given up to 5 days, especially in open heart surgery or prosthetic arthroplasty).
Impaired renal function.
Initial: 0.5 g; **then,** maintenance doses are given, depending on creatinine clearance, according to schedule provided by manufacturer.
Administration/Storage
1. Dissolve the solute by shaking vial.
2. For direct IV administration, dilute dose in 10 mL of sterile water and infuse over 3–5 min. For intermittent use, further dilute 500 mg–1 g in 50–100 mL NSS or D5%/W and administer over 30–60 min. Assess carefully for phlebitis.
3. Discard reconstituted solution after 24 hr at room temperature and after 96 hr when refrigerated.
4. Note any evidence of renal dysfunction and follow manufacturer guidelines for dosage.
Special Concerns: Safety in infants under 1 month of age has not been determined.
Additional Side Effects: When high doses are used in renal failure clients: extreme confusion, ***tonic-clonic seizures,*** mild hemiparesis.

NURSING CONSIDERATIONS

See also *General Nursing Considerations* for *All Anti-Infectives,* Chapter 1, and *Cephalosporins,* Chapter 3.
Evaluate
- Resolution of infection
- Negative posttreatment C&S reports

Cefixime oral

(seh-**FIX**-eem)
Pregnancy Category: B
Suprax **(Rx)**

See also *Anti-Infectives,* Chapter 1, and *Cephalosporins,* Chapter 3.
How Supplied: *Powder for Reconstitution:* 100 mg/5 mL; *Tablet:* 200 mg, 400 mg
Action/Kinetics: Stable in the presence of beta-lactamase enzymes. **Peak serum levels:** 2–6 hr. **t½:** averages 3–4 hr. About 50% excreted unchanged in the urine and approximately 10% in the bile. In addition to the microorganisms listed under *Uses* for cephalosporins, cefixime is effective against *Moraxella catarrhalis, Streptococcus agalactiae, Haemophilus parainfluenzae, Pasteurella multocida, Salmonella* species, and *Shigella* species. The following microorganisms are resistant to cefixime: most strains of *Bacteroides fragilis* and clostridia, *Pseudomonas* species, strains of group *D. streptococci* including enterococci, *Listeria*

monocytogenes, and most strains of staphylococci and *Enterobacter.*
Uses: Uncomplicated UTIs caused by *E. coli* and *P. mirabilis.* Otitis media due to *H. influenzae* (beta- lactamase positive and negative strains), *Moraxella catarrhalis,* and *S. pyogenes.* Pharyngitis and tonsillitis caused by *S. pyogenes.* Acute bronchitis and acute exacerbations of chronic bronchitis caused by *S. pneumoniae* and *H. influenzae* (beta-lactamase positive and negative strains). Uncomplicated cervical or urethral gonorrhea due to *N. gonorrhoeae* (both penicillinase- and non-penicillinase-producing strains).

Dosage

• **Oral Suspension, Tablets**
Adults: Either 400 mg once daily or 200 mg q 12 hr. **Children:** Either 8 mg/kg once daily or 4 mg/kg q 12 hr. Clients on renal dialysis or in whom creatinine clearance is 21–60 mL/min, the dose should be 75% of the standard dose (i.e., 300 mg/day). If the creatinine clearance is less than 20 mL/min, the dose should be 50% of the standard dose (i.e., 200 mg/day).

Uncomplicated gonorrhea.
One 400-mg tablet.

Administration/Storage
1. Therapy should be at least 10 days when treating *S. pyogenes.*
2. Children older than 12 years or weighing more than 50 kg should be given the adult dose.
3. Otitis media should be treated using the suspension as higher blood levels are achieved compared with the tablet given at the same dose.
4. Once reconstituted, the suspension should be kept at room temperature where it maintains potency for 14 days.

Special Concerns: Safe use in infants less than 6 months old has not been established.
Additional Side Effects: *GI:* Flatulence. *Hepatic:* Elevated alkaline phosphatase levels. *Renal:* Transient increases in BUN or creatinine.
Additional Laboratory Test Interference: False + test for ketones using nitroprusside test.

NURSING CONSIDERATIONS

See also *Nursing Considerations* for *Cephalosporins,* Chapter 3.

Assessment
1. Take a drug history, noting any prior sensitivity to cephalosporins or penicillins.
2. Assess client financial status and health care coverage because prescription cost may be prohibitive.

Interventions
1. Anticipate reduced dose with impaired renal function.
2. Use the suspension in children and when treating otitis media.
3. Cefixime may alter results of urine glucose and ketone testing; finger sticks may provide more accurate blood sugar recordings during drug therapy.

Client/Family Teaching
1. Cefixime may cause GI upset; report any bothersome side effects, especially persistent diarrhea.
2. Therapy requires only once-a-day dosing and should be taken at the same time each day.
3. Consult physician if child's condition does not improve after 48–72 hr of therapy or if condition deteriorates.
4. Return as scheduled to assess response to therapy.

Evaluate: Resolution of infection and reports of symptomatic improvement.

Cefmetazole sodium

(sef-**MET**-ah-zole)
Pregnancy Category: B
Zefazone **(Rx)**

See also *Anti-Infectives,* Chapter 1, and *Cephalosporins,* Chapter 3.
How Supplied: *Injection:* 1 g/50 mL, 2 g/50 mL; *Powder for injection:* 1 g, 2 g
Uses: Urinary tract, lower respiratory tract, skin and skin structure, and intra-abdominal infections. Preoperatively to decrease incidence of post-

operative infections following cesarean section, cholecystectomy (high risk), colorectal surgery, abdominal or vaginal hysterectomy.

Dosage

- **IV**

Infections.

2 g q 6–12 hr for 5–14 days.

Prophylaxis, abdominal hysterectomy or high-risk cholecystectomy.

1 g 30–90 min prior to surgery and again 8 and 16 hr following surgery.

Prophylaxis, vaginal hysterectomy.

2 g 30–90 min prior to surgery or 1 g 30–90 min prior to surgery and again 8 and 16 hr following surgery.

Prophylaxis, cesarean section.

2 g in a single dose after clamping cord or 1 g after clamping cord and again 8 and 16 hr later.

Prophylaxis, colorectal surgery.

2 g 30–90 min prior to surgery or 2 g 30–60 min prior to surgery and again 8 and 26 hr following surgery.

Administration/Storage

1. The drug should be reconstituted with sterile water for injection, bacteriostatic water for injection, or 0.9% sodium chloride injection.
2. After reconstitution, the drug is stable for 24 hr at room temperature, for 7 days if refrigerated, and for 6 weeks if frozen.
3. If necessary, the reconstituted solution may be further diluted to concentrations of 1–20 mg/mL with 0.9% sodium chloride injection, 5% dextrose injection, or lactated Ringer's injection. Infuse over 15–30 min. Such solutions are stable as described above.
4. Thawed solutions should not be refrozen.
5. Any unused solutions or frozen material should be discarded.

NURSING CONSIDERATIONS

See also *Nursing Considerations* for *Cephalosporins,* Chapter 3.

Assessment

1. Document indications for therapy and the recommended administration frequency and dosage.
2. Obtain baseline renal function studies and anticipate reduced dose and frequency of administration of cefmetazole with impaired renal function.

Evaluate

- Resolution of existing infection
- Infection prophylaxis during surgery

Cefonicid sodium

(seh-**FON**-ih-sid)
Pregnancy Category: B
Monocid **(Rx)**

See also *Anti-Infectives,* Chapter 1, and *Cephalosporins,* Chapter 3.

How Supplied: *Powder for injection:* 1 g, 10 g

Uses: Infections of the lower respiratory tract, urinary tract, bones, joints, skin, and skin structures. Septicemia. Prophylaxis in surgery, especially colorectal surgery, vaginal hysterectomy, cholecystectomy, prosthetic arthroplasty, open heart surgery, cesarean section after the cord has been clamped.

Dosage

- **IV, Deep IM**

Uncomplicated UTIs.

Adults: 0.5 g once daily.

Mild to moderate infections.

Adults: 1 g once daily.

Severe or life-threatening infections.

Adults: 2 g once daily.

Prophylaxis in surgery.

Adults: 1 g 1 hr prior to surgery; dosage may be repeated for 2 more days if required.

In renal impairment.

Initial: 7.5 mg/kg given **IV or IM; then,** follow schedule provided by manufacturer.

Administration/Storage

1. If 2 g is required IM, give half the dose in different large muscle masses.
2. For IV bolus, give cefonicid slowly over 3–5 min either through IV tubing or directly, assess for phle-

bitis, and change peripheral site every 48–72 hr.
3. For IV infusion, reconstitute in 50–100 mL of appropriate diluent and infuse over 30 min (see package insert). Solutions are stable for 24 hr at room temperature and 72 hr if refrigerated.
4. Anticipate reduced dose with renal dysfunction.

NURSING CONSIDERATIONS

See also *Nursing Considerations* for *Cephalosporins,* Chapter 3.

Evaluate

- Resolution of existing infection
- Infection prophylaxis during surgery

Cefoperazone sodium

(sef-oh-**PER**-ah-zohn)
Pregnancy Category: B
Cefobid **(Rx)**

See also *Anti-Infectives,* Chapter 1, and *Cephalosporins,* Chapter 3.

How Supplied: *Powder for injection:* 1 g, 2 g, 10 g

Action/Kinetics: Peak serum levels: 73–153 mcg/mL. **t½:** 102–156 min. Approximately 30% excreted unchanged in the urine.

Uses: Infections of skin, skin structures, urinary tract, and respiratory tract. Intra-abdominal infections including peritonitis. Bacterial septicemia, pelvic inflammatory disease, endometritis, other infections of the female genital tract.

Dosage

- **IM, IV**

Adults, usual: 2–4 g/day in divided doses q 12 hr (up to 12–16 g/day has been used in severe infections or for less sensitive organisms).

NOTE: This drug is significantly excreted in the bile; thus, the daily dose should not exceed 4 g in hepatic disease or biliary obstruction.

Administration/Storage

1. Dilute each gram in 20–40 mL of solution and infuse over 15–30 min.
2. Following reconstitution, the solution should be allowed to stand for dissipation of any foaming and to determine if complete solubilization has occurred. Vigorous shaking may be necessary to dissolve higher concentrations.
3. Reconstituted drug may be frozen; however, after thawing, any unused portion should be discarded.
4. The unreconstituted powder should be protected from light and stored in the refrigerator.
5. If used for neonates, cefoperazone should not be reconstituted with diluents containing benzyl alcohol.

Special Concerns: Use with caution in hepatic disease or biliary obstruction. Safety and effectiveness have not been determined in children.

Additional Side Effects: Hypoprothrombinemia resulting in bleeding and/or bruising.

Additional Drug Interaction: Concomitant use with ethanol may cause an Antabuse-like reaction.

NURSING CONSIDERATIONS

See also *Nursing Considerations* for *Cephalosporins,* Chapter 3.

Assessment

1. Complete a nursing history and assess for bruising, hematuria, black stools, or other evidence of bleeding.
2. Obtain baseline coagulation studies and monitor during therapy as drug may cause hypoprothrombinemia.
3. Assess need for prophylactic vitamin K administration (usually 10 mg/week).
4. If client is receiving treatment for skin lesions, inspect lesions closely, noting size, location, and extent of involvement.
5. Assess for any evidence/history of excessive use of alcohol.
6. Determine if client has liver or biliary disease as dose should be reduced.

Client/Family Teaching

1. Avoid alcohol and any medications containing alcohol for 72 hr after the last dose as an Antabuse-like reaction may occur.

2. Explain the importance of reporting any evidence of bruising or bleeding immediately.

Evaluate

- ↓ Size and number of skin lesions with evidence of wound healing
- Resolution of infection

Cefotaxime sodium

(sef-oh-**TAX**-eem)
Pregnancy Category: B
Claforan **(Rx)**

See also *Anti-Infectives,* Chapter 1, and *Cephalosporins,* Chapter 3.

How Supplied: *Injection:* 1 g/50 mL, 2 g/50 mL; *Powder for injection:* 500 mg, 1 g, 2 g, 10 g

Action/Kinetics: Treatment should be continued for a minimum of 10 days for group A beta-hemolytic streptococcal infections to minimize the risk of glomerulonephritis or rheumatic fever. The IV route is preferable for clients with severe or life-threatening infections; for clients after surgery; or for those manifesting malnutrition, trauma, malignancy, heart failure, or diabetes, especially if shock is present or possible. **t½:** 1 hr. From 20% to 36% is excreted unchanged in the urine.

Uses: Infections of the GU tract, lower respiratory tract (including pneumonia), skin, skin structures, bones, joints, and CNS (including ventriculitis and meningitis). Intra-abdominal infections (including peritonitis), gynecologic infections (including endometritis, pelvic cellulitis, pelvic inflammatory disease), septicemia, bacteremia, and prophylaxis in surgery. Used with aminoglycosides for gram-positive or gram-negative sepsis where the causative agent has not been identified.

Dosage

- **IV, IM**

Uncomplicated infections.

Adults: 1 g q 12 hr.

Moderate to severe infections.

Adults: 1–2 g q 8 hr.

Septicemia.

Adults, IV: 2 g q 6–8 hr.

Life-threatening infections.

Adults, IV: 2 g q 4 hr up to 12 g/day.

Gonorrhea.

Adults, IM: single dose of 1 g.

Preoperative prophylaxis.

Adults: 1 g 30–90 min prior to surgery.

Cesarean section.

IV: 1 g when the umbilical cord is clamped; **then,** give 1 g 6 and 12 hr after the first dose.

Pediatric, 1 month to 12 years, IM, IV: 50–180 mg/kg/day in four to six divided doses; **1–4 weeks, IV:** 50 mg/kg q 8 hr; **0–1 week, IV:** 50 mg/kg q 12 hr. *NOTE:* Use adult dose in children 50 kg or over.

Administration/Storage

1. Cefotaxime should not be mixed with aminoglycosides for continuous IV infusion. If they are to be given to the same client, each should be given separately.
2. Cefotaxime is maximally stable at a pH of 5–7; solutions should not be prepared with diluents having a pH greater than 7.5 (e.g., sodium bicarbonate injection).
3. Dry cefotaxime should be stored below 30°C (86°F) and should be protected from excess heat and light to prevent darkening.
4. Add recommended amount of diluent, shake to dissolve, and observe for particles or discoloration of solution. Do not administer if particles are present or if solution is discolored. The normal color of solution ranges from light yellow to amber.
5. For IM use, reconstitute with sterile water for injection or bacteriostatic water for injection. Inject deeply into large muscle. Divide doses of 2 g and administer into different sites.
6. For direct IV administration, 1 or 2 g cefotaxime should be mixed with 10 mL sterile water for injection and administered over 3–5 min. For intermittent administration, further dilute in 50–100 mL of solution and infuse over 30 min.

7. Discontinue IV administration of other solutions during administration of cefotaxime.
8. After reconstitution, the drug remains stable for 24 hr at room temperature, 5 days refrigerated, and 13 weeks frozen. Thaw frozen samples at room temperature before use. Do not refreeze unused portions.
9. Anticipate reduced dosage in clients with impaired renal function.

NURSING CONSIDERATIONS

See also *Nursing Considerations* for *Cephalosporins,* Chapter 3.

Assessment

1. For clients receiving therapy for joint infections, carefully assess the extent of their ROM and freedom of movement.
2. In clients with gynecologic infections, determine how long symptoms have been evident and how extensive the infection is prior to treatment.
3. Obtain appropriate laboratory studies prior to initiating therapy. Review culture results to determine any organism resistance to this drug.

Interventions

1. Maintain careful documentation of the type and extent of infection and subjective complaints.
2. Monitor and record I&O.
3. Inspect site of injections for pain and redness. IM administration of these medications may cause thrombophlebitis.

Client/Family Teaching

1. Review the drugs being prescribed, their side effects, and the expected outcome of therapy.
2. Reinforce the need to complete the course of therapy as prescribed despite feeling better.
3. Review the appropriate technique for administration and proper storage.
4. Record I&O and report any reduction in urinary output.
5. Persistent diarrhea should also be reported.
6. Avoid alcohol in any form as a disulfiram-type reaction may occur.

Evaluate

- Resolution of infection and reports of symptomatic improvement
- Negative laboratory culture reports

Cefotetan disodium

(sef-oh-**TEE**-tan)
Pregnancy Category: B
Cefotan **(Rx)**

See also *Anti-Infectives,* Chapter 1, and *Cephalosporins,* Chapter 3.

How Supplied: *Injection:* 1 g/50 mL, 2 g/50 mL; *Powder for injection:* 1 g, 2 g, 10 g

Action/Kinetics: Administered parenterally only. **t½:** 3–4.6 hr. From 50% to 80% is excreted unchanged in the urine.

Uses: Infections of the urinary tract, lower respiratory tract, skin and skin structures, bones, and joints. Also gynecologic and intra-abdominal infections. Prophylaxis of postoperative infections (e.g., due to abdominal or vaginal hysterectomy, transurethral surgery, GI or biliary tract surgery, cesarean section).

Dosage

- **IV or IM**

Usual infections.

Adults: 1–2 g q 12 hr for 5–10 days.

UTIs.

Adults: Either 0.5 g q 12 hr, or 1–2 g q 12–24 hr.

Severe infections.

Adults, IV: 2 g q 12 hr.

Life-threatening infections.

Adults, IV: 3 g q 12 hr.

Prophylaxis of postoperative infection.

Adults, IV: 1–2 g 30–60 min prior to surgery.

Administration/Storage

1. Cefotetan disodium must be administered parenterally, because it is not absorbed from the GI tract.
2. IM injections should be made well within a large muscle (e.g., the gluteus maximus).
3. The IV route is preferred for clients with bacterial septicemia, bacteremia, or other severe or life-threatening infections. The IV route is also

preferred for poor-risk clients as the result of malnutrition, surgery, diabetes, trauma, heart failure, malignancy, or if shock is present or impending.
4. Direct IV administration may be completed over 3–5 min following reconstitution (1 g in 10 mL of sterile water for injection). May further dilute in 50–100 mL D5%/W or NSS and infuse over 30–60 min.
5. For IM use, reconstitute with sterile water for injection, NSS, bacteriostatic water for injection, or 0.5%–1% lidocaine HCl.
6. Reconstituted solutions maintain potency for 24 hr at room temperature, for 96 hr if refrigerated, and for 1 week if frozen.
7. Cefotetan should not be mixed with solutions containing aminoglycosides.
8. Dosage should be reduced in impaired renal function and depends on creatinine clearance.
Special Concerns: Safety and effectiveness have not been determined in children.
Additional Side Effects: Concomitant use with ethanol produces a disulfiram-type reaction and hypotension.
Additional Laboratory Test Interference: The drug may affect measurement of creatinine levels by the Jaffe reaction.

NURSING CONSIDERATIONS

See also *Nursing Considerations* for *Cephalosporins,* Chapter 3.

Assessment
1. Obtain a complete nursing history and assess for bruising, hematuria, black stools, or other evidence of bleeding.
2. Assess for any evidence or history of excessive use of alcohol.
3. Obtain baseline coagulation studies and monitor during therapy as drug may cause hypoprothrombinemia.
4. Assess need for prophylactic vitamin K administration (usually 10 mg/week).

Client/Family Teaching
1. Avoid alcohol ingestion during and for 72 hr after cefotetan disodium therapy.
2. Report any side effects, such as diarrhea, bruising/bleeding, or decreased urine output.

Evaluate
- Resolution of infection with reports of symptomatic improvement
- Infection prophylaxis during surgery

Cefoxitin sodium

(seh-**FOX**-ih-tin)
Pregnancy Category: B
Mefoxin **(Rx)**

See also *Anti-Infectives,* Chapter 1, and *Cephalosporins,* Chapter 3.
How Supplied: *Injection:* 1 g/50 mL, 2 g/50 mL; *Powder for injection:* 1 g, 2 g, 10 g
Action/Kinetics: Broad-spectrum cephalosporin that is penicillinase- and cephalosporinase-resistant and is stable in the presence of beta-lactamases. **Peak serum concentration: IM,** 20–30 min. **t½: IM, IV,** 41–65 min; 85% of drug excreted unchanged in urine after 6 hr.
Uses: Infections of the urinary tract (including gonorrhea), bones, joints, lower respiratory tract (including lung abscesses and pneumonia), skin, and skin structures. Intra-abdominal infections (including intra-abdominal abscesses and peritonitis), gynecologic infections (including pelvic inflammatory disease, pelvic cellulitis, and endometritis), septicemia, and prophylaxis in surgery. *NOTE:* Many gram-negative infections resistant to certain cephalosporins and penicillins respond to cefoxitin.

Dosage
- **IM, IV**

Uncomplicated infections (cutaneous, pneumonia, urinary tract).
Adults, IV, IM: 1 g q 6–8 hr.
Severe infections.
Adults, IV: 1 g q 4 hr or 2 g q 6–8 hr.
Gas gangrene.
Adults, IV: 2 g q 4 hr or 3 g q 6 hr.

Gonorrhea.
Adults: 2 g IM with 1 g probenecid PO.

Prophylaxis in surgery.
Adults, IV, IM: 2 g 30–60 min before surgery followed by 2 g q 6 hr after first dose for 24 hr only (72 hr for prosthetic arthroplasty).

Cesarean section, prophylaxis.
2 g **IV** when cord is clamped; **then,** give two additional doses IV or IM 4 and 8 hr later. Subsequent doses may be given q 6 hr for no more than 1 day.

Transurethral prostatectomy, prophylaxis.
1 g before surgery; **then,** 1 g q 8 hr for up to 5 days.

Impaired renal function.
Initial: 1–2 g; **then,** follow maintenance schedule provided by manufacturer.

Infections.
Children over 3 months: 80–160 mg/kg/day in four to six divided doses. Total daily dosage should not exceed 12 g.

Prophylaxis.
Children: 30–40 mg/kg q 6 hr.

Administration/Storage

1. Do not mix with other antibiotics during administration.
2. Reconstituted solutions are stable for 24 hr at room temperature, 1 week in the refrigerator, and 26 weeks when frozen.
3. Store drug vials below 30°C (86°F).
4. Reconstituted solutions are white to light amber. Color does not affect potency. Consult pharmacist if unsure of drug potency.
5. For IM injections, lidocaine hydrochloride 0.05% (without epinephrine) may be used as diluent, by physician's order, to reduce pain at injection site.
6. For direct IV administration dilute 1 g in 10 mL sterile water and infuse over 3–5 min. For intermittent administration, further dilute in 50–100 mL of solution and infuse over 15–30 min.
7. Do not administer cefoxitin rapidly, because it is irritating to veins.

Additional Side Effects: Higher doses have caused increased incidence of eosinophilia and increased AST levels in children over 3 months of age.

Additional Laboratory Test Interference: High concentrations may interfere with the measurement of creatinine by the Jaffe method.

NURSING CONSIDERATIONS

See also *Nursing Considerations* for *Cephalosporins,* Chapter 3.

Interventions

1. Monitor I&O, withhold medication, and report any significant reduction in urinary output.
2. Assess infusion site for pain and redness as medication can cause thrombophlebitis.

Evaluate: Resolution of infection and reports of symptomatic relief.

Cefpodoxime proxetil

(sef-poh-**DOX**-eem)
Pregnancy Category: B
Vantin **(Rx)**

See also *Anti-Infectives,* Chapter 1, and *Cephalosporins,* Chapter 3.

How Supplied: *Granule for Reconstitution:* 50 mg/5 mL, 100 mg/5 mL; *Tablet:* 100 mg, 200 mg

Action/Kinetics: From 29% to 33% is recovered unchanged from the urine.

Uses: Acute, community-acquired pneumonia due to *Streptococcus pneumoniae* or *Hemophilus influenzae* (only non-beta-lactamase-producing strains). Acute otitis media caused by *S. pneumoniae, H. influenzae* (including beta-lactamase-producing strains), and *Moraxella catarrhalis.* Pharyngitis or tonsillitis due to *Streptococcus pyogenes.* Acute, uncomplicated urethral and cervical gonorrhea caused by *Neisseria gonorrhoeae* (including penicillinase-producing strains). Acute, uncomplicated anorectal infections in women due to *N. gonorrhoeae* (including penicillinase-producing strains). Uncomplicated skin and skin structure infections due to

Staphylococcus aureus (including penicillinase-producing strains) or *S. pyogenes*. Uncomplicated UTIs (cystitis) due to *Escherichia coli, Klebsiella pneumoniae, Proteus mirabilis,* or *Staphyloccus saprophyticus*. Acute bacterial exacerbation of chronic bronchitis caused by *S. pneumoniae,* non-beta-lactamase-producing *H. influenzae,* or *M. catarrhalis*.

Dosage

- **Tablets, Suspension**

Acute community-acquired pneumonia.

Adults and children over 13 years: 200 mg q 12 hr for 14 days.

Acute bacterial exacerbations of chronic bronchitis.

Adults and children over 13 years: 200 mg/12 hr for 10 days.

Uncomplicated gonorrhea (men and women) and rectal gonococcal infections (women).

Adults and children over 13 years: Single dose of 200 mg.

Skin and skin structure infections.

Adults and children over 13 years: 400 mg q 12 hr for 7–14 days.

Pharyngitis, tonsillitis.

Adults and children over 13 years: 100 mg q 12 hr for 10 days. **Children, 6 months–12 years:** 5 mg/kg (maximum of 100 mg/dose) q 12 hr (maximum daily dose: 200 mg) for 10 days.

Uncomplicated UTIs.

Adults and children over 13 years: 100 mg q 12 hr for 7 days.

Acute otitis media.

Children, 6 months–12 years: 5 mg/kg (maximum of 200 mg/dose) q 12 hr (maximum daily dose: 400 mg) for 10 days.

Administration/Storage

1. Dosage adjustment is not required in clients with cirrhosis.
2. In severe renal impairment (creatinine clearance less than 30 mL/min), the dosing interval should be increased to q 24 hr. If the client is maintained on hemodialysis, a dosage frequency of 3 times/week after hemodialysis should be used.
3. If only the serum creatinine level is available, the following formula can be used to estimate creatinine clearance (mL/min): males: weight (kg) × (140 - age)/72 × serum creatinine (mg/100 mL); females: 0.85 × male value.
4. The suspension is prepared by adding 58 mL of distilled water to the 50 mg/mL product or 57 mL of distilled water to the 100 mg/5 mL product. After tapping the bottle gently to loosen the powder, add 25 mL of water and shake vigorously for 15 sec to wet the powder. The remainder of the water is then added and the bottle is shaken vigorously for 3 min or until all particles are suspended.
5. After reconstitution, the suspension is stored in the refrigerator and any unused portion should be discarded after 14 days.
6. The reconstituted suspension should be shaken well before using.

NURSING CONSIDERATIONS

See also *General Nursing Considerations* for *All Anti-Infectives,* Chapter 1, and *Cephalosporins,* Chapter 3.

Assessment

1. Determine any previous sensitivity reactions to cephalosporins or penicillins as cross-sensitivity can occur.
2. Document source of infection and ensure that baseline cultures have been performed.
3. Note any history or evidence of renal dysfunction.
4. Obtain a serologic test for syphilis in clients being treated for gonorrhea.

Interventions

1. Closely monitor VS and I&O.
2. Discontinue drug therapy and report if seizures occur.
3. Clients with persistent diarrhea should be evaluated for other causes, such as *C. difficile*.

Client/Family Teaching

1. Take with food to enhance absorption and to diminish GI upset.
2. Report any persistent N&V or diar-

rhea as drug or dosage may require adjustment.
3. Advise clients receiving treatment for gonorrhea to have partner tested and treated and to use barrier contraception to prevent reinfections. Explain that drug is not effective against syphilis and that all partners should be tested so that appropriate treatment may be provided.

Evaluate

- Resolution of infection
- Negative culture reports
- Reports of symptomatic improvement

Cefprozil

(**SEF**-proh-zill)
Pregnancy Category: B
Cefzil **(Rx)**

See also *Anti-Infectives,* Chapter 1, and *Cephalosporins,* Chapter 3.

How Supplied: *Powder for Reconstitution:* 125 mg/5 mL, 250 mg/5 mL; *Tablet:* 250 mg, 500 mg

Action/Kinetics: Sixty percent is recovered in the urine unchanged.

Uses: Pharyngitis and tonsillitis due to *Streptococcus pyogenes.* Otitis media caused by *Streptococcus pneumoniae, Haemophilus influenzae,* and *Moraxella catarrhalis.* Uncomplicated skin and skin structure infections due to *Staphylococcus aureus* (including penicillinase-producing strains) and *S. pyogenes.* Secondary bacterial infection of acute bronchitis and acute bacterial exacerbation of chronic bronchitis due to *S. pneumoniae, H. influenzae* (beta-lactamase positive and negative strains), and *M. catarrhalis.*

Dosage

- **Suspension, Tablets**

Pharyngitis, tonsillitis.

Adults and children over 13 years of age: 500 mg q 24 hr for at least 10 days (especially for *S. pyogenes* infections). **Children, 2–12 years of age:** 7.5 mg/kg q 12 hr for at least 10 days (especially for *S. pyogenes* infections).

Secondary bacterial infections of acute bronchitis and acute bacterial exacerbation of chronic bronchitis.

Adults and children over 13 years of age: 500 mg q 12 hr for 10 days.

Uncomplicated skin and skin structure infections.

Adults and children over 13 years of age: Either 250 mg q 12 hr, 500 mg q 24 hr, or 500 mg q 12 hr (all for a duration of 10 days).

Otitis media.

Infants and children 6 months–12 years: 15 mg/kg q 12 hr for 10 days.

Administration/Storage

1. In clients with impaired renal function (creatinine clearance of 0–30 mL/min), the dose should be 50% of the standard use given at standard intervals.
2. After reconstitution, store the suspension in a refrigerator and discard any unused portion after 14 days.

NURSING CONSIDERATIONS

See also *General Nursing Considerations* for *All Anti-Infectives,* Chapter 1, and *Cephalosporins,* Chapter 3.

Interventions

1. Monitor VS and I&O.
2. Anticipate reduced dose with impaired renal function.

Evaluate: Reports of symptomatic improvement.

Ceftazidime

(sef-**TAY**-zih-deem)
Pregnancy Category: B
Fortaz, Tazicef, Tazidime **(Rx)**

See also *Anti-Infectives,* Chapter 1, and *Cephalosporins,* Chapter 3.

How Supplied: *Powder for injection:* 500 mg, 1 g, 2 g, 6 g, 10 g

Action/Kinetics: Only for IM or IV use. **t½:** 2–3 hr. From 80% to 90% is excreted unchanged in the urine.

Uses: Bacterial septicemia. Infections of the lower respiratory tract, skin and skin structures, bones and joints, CNS (including meningitis), and urinary tract. Also, intra-abdominal (including peritonitis) and gynecologic infections (including endometritis, pelvic cellulitis). Use with aminoglycosides, clindamycin, or vancomycin in severe or life-threatening infections or in the immunocompromised client.

Dosage

- **IM, IV**

Usual infections.

Adults: 1 g q 8–12 hr.

UTIs, uncomplicated.

Adults, IM, IV: 0.25 g q 12 hr.

UTIs, complicated.

Adults, IM, IV: 0.5 g q 8–12 hr.

Uncomplicated pneumonia, skin and skin structure infections.

Adults, IM, IV: 0.5–1 g q 8 hr.

Bone and joint infections.

Adults, IV: 2 g q 12 hr.

Serious gynecologic or intra-abdominal infections, meningitis, severe or life-threatening infections (especially in immunocompromised clients).

Adults, IV: 2 g q 8 hr.

Pseudomonal lung infections in cystic fibrosis clients.

IV: 30–50 mg/kg q 8 hr, not to exceed 6 g/day. **Neonates, 0–4 weeks, IV:** 30 mg/kg q 12 hr. **Infants and children, 1 month–12 years, IV:** 30–50 mg/kg q 8 hr not to exceed 6 g/day.

Administration/Storage

1. Ceftazidime must be administered parenterally, because it is not absorbed from the GI tract.
2. If administering IM, use large muscle mass and inject deeply.
3. The IV route is preferred for clients with bacterial septicemia, peritonitis, bacterial meningitis, or other severe or life-threatening infections. Also, IV should be used for clients considered to be poor risks due to malnutrition, surgery, diabetes, trauma, heart failure, malignancy, or if shock is present or imminent.
4. For direct IV administration, reconstitute 1 g in 10 mL sterile water for injection and administer over 3–5 min.
5. For intermittent administration, further dilute in 50–100 mL of solution and administer over 30–60 min. It is compatible with 0.9% sodium chloride injection, Ringer's injection, lactated Ringer's injection, 5% or 10% dextrose injection, M/6 sodium lactate injection, 5% dextrose and 0.225%, 0.45%, or 0.9% sodium chloride injection, 10% invert sugar in water for injection. Sodium bicarbonate injection should not be used for reconstitution; however, a sodium carbonate formulation should be used for children less than 12.
6. For use as an IV infusion, the 1- or 2-g infusion pack is reconstituted with 100 mL sterile water for injection (or a compatible IV solution).
7. For IM administration, reconstitute in sterile water for injection, bacteriostatic water for injection, or 0.5%–1% lidocaine HCl injection.
8. Ceftazidime should not be added to solutions containing aminoglycosides.
9. Dosage must be reduced in clients with impaired renal function (see package insert).

Special Concerns: A sodium carbonate formulation should be used if the drug is indicated for children less than 12 years of age.

NURSING CONSIDERATIONS

See also *Nursing Considerations* for *Cephalosporins,* Chapter 3.

Evaluate

- Resolution of infection
- Negative laboratory culture reports

Ceftizoxime sodium

(sef-tih-**ZOX**-eem)

Pregnancy Category: B

Cefizox **(Rx)**

See also *Anti-Infectives,* Chapter 1, and *Cephalosporins,* Chapter 3.

How Supplied: *Injection:* 1 g/50 mL, 2 g/50 mL; *Powder for injection:* 500 mg, 1 g, 2 g, 10 g

Action/Kinetics: t½: Approximately 1–2 hr. Approximately 80% excreted unchanged in the urine.

Uses: Infections of the urinary tract, lower respiratory tract, skin, skin structures, bones, and joints. Intra-abdominal infections, septicemia, meningitis (caused by *Haemophilus influenzae* or *Streptococcus pneumoniae)*, gonorrhea (including uncomplicated cervical and urethral gonorrhea caused by *Neisseria*). Pelvic inflammatory disease caused by *Neisseria gonorrhoeae, Escherichia coli,* or *Streptococcus agalactiae*.

Dosage

- **IM, IV**

Uncomplicated urinary tract and other infections.

Adults: 0.5 g q 12 hr.

Severe or resistant infections.

Adults: 1 g q 8 hr or 2 g q 8–12 hr.

Life-threatening infections.

Adults: Up to 3–4 g q 8 hr.

Pelvic inflammatory disease.

2 g q 8 hr IV (doses up to 2 g q 4 hr have been used).

- **IV**

Uncomplicated gonorrhea.

Adults: 1 g as a single dose **IM. Pediatric, over 6 months:** 50 mg/kg q 6–8 hr up to 200 mg/kg/day (not to exceed the maximum adult dose).

Impaired renal function.

Initial, IM, IV: 0.5–1 g; **then,** use maintenance schedule in package insert.

Administration/Storage

1. For IM doses of 2 g, divide the dose equally and give in different large muscle masses.
2. For direct IV administration, reconstitute 1 g in 10 mL sterile water and give slowly over 3–5 min.
3. For intermittent administration, further dilute in 50–100 mL of D5%/W or NSS and infuse over 30 min.
4. Reconstituted solutions are stable at room temperature for 8 hr and, if refrigerated, for 48 hr.

Additional Side Effects: Transient increased levels of eosinophils, AST, ALT, and CPK have been seen in children over 6 months of age.

NURSING CONSIDERATIONS

See also *Nursing Considerations* for *Cephalosporins*, Chapter 3.

Evaluate

- Negative C&S reports
- Resolution of S&S of infection

Ceftriaxone sodium

(sef-try-**AX**-ohn)
Pregnancy Category: B
Rocephin **(Rx)**

See also *Anti-Infectives*, Chapter 1, and *Cephalosporins*, Chapter 3.

How Supplied: *Injection:* 1 g/50 mL, 2 g/50 mL; *Powder for injection:* 250 mg, 500 mg, 1 g, 2 g, 10 g

Action/Kinetics: $t^{1/2}$**:** Approximately 6–8 hr. Significantly protein bound. One-third to two-thirds excreted unchanged in the urine.

Uses: Infections of the lower respiratory tract, urinary tract, skin, skin structures, bones, joints, abdomen. Also, uncomplicated gonorrhea (cervical, urethral, rectal) including both penicillinase- and non-penicillinase-producing strains of *Neisseria gonorrhoeae* and pharyngeal gonorrhea caused by non-penicillinase-producing strains of *N. gonorrhoeae*. Pelvic inflammatory disease, pediatric meningitis, prophylaxis of infections in surgery, bacterial septicemia. *Investigational:* Neurologic complications, arthritis, and carditis associated with Lyme disease (infection caused by *Borrelia burgdorferi)* in clients refractory to penicillin G.

Dosage

- **IV, IM**

General infections.

Adults, usual: 1–2 g/day in single or divided doses q 12 hr, not to exceed 4 g/day. Therapy is maintained for 4–14 days, depending on the infection. **Pediatric:** *Other than meningitis:* 50–75 mg/kg/day not to exceed total daily dose of 2 g given in divided doses q 12 hr.

Meningitis.

Pediatric: 100 mg/kg/day, not to exceed total daily dose of 4 g given once daily or in equally divided doses q 12 hr for 7–14 days.

Prophylaxis of infection in surgery.

1 g 30–120 min prior to surgery.

Uncomplicated gonorrhea.

Adults, IM: 125 mg as a single dose plus doxycycline.

Pharyngeal gonorrhea due to non-penicillinase-producing strains of N. gonorrhoeae.

250 mg as a single IM dose.

Gonococcal infections in children.

Less than 45 kg: 125 mg given once. **Infants:** 25–50 mg/kg/day not to exceed 125 mg IV or IM in a single daily dose for 7 days.

Gonococcal infection during pregnancy.

Adults: 250 mg as a single IM dose plus erythromycin.

Disseminated gonococcal infection.

Adults: 1 g IM or IV q 24 hr.

Gonococcal meningitis or endocarditis.

Adults: 1–2 g IV q 12 hr for 10–14 days (meningitis) or 4 weeks (endocarditis).

Gonococcal ophthalmia.

Adults and children over 20 kg: 1 g given as a single IM dose.

Acute pelvic inflammatory disease.

250 mg IM plus doxycycline or tetracycline.

Lyme disease.

IV: 2–4 g/day for 14 days. Dosage adjustment is not required for renal or hepatic impairment; however, monitor blood levels in dialysis clients.

Administration/Storage

1. IM injections should be deep into the body of a large muscle.
2. IV infusions should contain concentrations of 10–40 mg/mL. Reconstitute 500 mg in 4.8 mL of sterile water, NSS, or D5%/W. Then further dilute in 50–100 mL D5%/W or NSS and infuse over 30–60 min.
3. The drug should not be mixed with other antibiotics.
4. Stability of solutions for IM or IV use varies depending on the diluent used; the package insert should be checked carefully.
5. Dosage should be maintained for at least 2 days after symptoms of infection have disappeared (usual course of therapy is 4–14 days, although complicated infections may require longer therapy).
6. Dosage should be continued for at least 10 days when treating *Streptococcus pyogenes* infections.

Additional Side Effects: Increase in serum creatinine, presence of casts in the urine, alteration of PTs (rare).

NURSING CONSIDERATIONS

See also *Nursing Considerations* for *Cephalosporins,* Chapter 3.

Assessment

1. Note if client has any history of GI disease, especially colitis, because drug should be used cautiously in this setting.
2. Obtain baseline coagulation studies and monitor as drug may alter PTs. May administer vitamin K (10 mg/week) prophylactically if bleeding occurs.
3. Document indications for therapy and include pretreatment findings.

Evaluate

- Resolution of S&S of infection
- Negative laboratory culture reports

Cefuroxime axetil

(sef-your-**OX**-eem)
Pregnancy Category: B
Ceftin **(Rx)**

Cefuroxime sodium

(sef-your-**OX**-eem)
Pregnancy Category: B
Kefurox, Zinacef **(Rx)**

See also *Anti-Infectives,* Chapter 1, and *Cephalosporins,* Chapter 3.

How Supplied: Cefuroxime axetil: *Powder for Reconstitution:* 125 mg/5 mL; *Tablet:* 125 mg, 250 mg, 500 mg

Cefuroxime sodium: *Injection:* 750 mg/50 mL, 1.5 g/50 mL; *Powder for injection:* 750 mg, 1.5 g, 7.5 g

Action/Kinetics: Cefuroxime axetil is used PO, whereas cefuroxime sodium is used either IM or IV. **IM, IV: t½:** 1–2 hr; 66%–100% is excreted unchanged in the urine.

Uses: PO (axetil). Pharyngitis, tonsillitis, otitis media, bronchitis, UTIs, skin and skin structure infections, uncomplicated gonorrhea (urethral and endocervical) caused by non-penicillinase-producing strains of *Neisseria gonorrhoeae*. The suspension is indicated for children from 3 months to 12 years to treat pharyngitis, tonsillitis, acute bacterial otitis media, and impetigo.

IM, IV (sodium). Infections of the urinary tract, lower respiratory tract (including pneumonia), skin and skin structures, bones, and joints. Septicemia, meningitis, uncomplicated and disseminated gonococcal infections due to penicillinase- or non-penicillinase-producing strains of *N. gonorrhoeae* in men and women. Mixed infections in which several organisms have been identified. Prophylaxis of postoperative infections in surgical procedures such as vaginal hysterectomy.

Dosage

• **Tablets (Cefuroxime axetil)**

Infections.

Adults and children over 12 years: 250 mg q 12 hr, up to 500 mg q 12 hr for severe infections or infections due to less susceptible organisms.

Uncomplicated UTIs.

Adults: 125–250 mg q 12 hr. **Infants and children less than 12 years:** 125 mg b.i.d.

Otitis media.

Less than 2 years: 125 mg b.i.d.; **over 2 years:** 250 mg b.i.d.

• **Suspension (Cefuroxime axetil)**

Pharyngitis, tonsillitis.

Children, 3 months to 12 years: 20 mg/kg/day in 2 divided doses, not to exceed 500 mg total dose/ day.

Acute otitis media, impetigo.

Children, 3 months to 12 years: 30 mg/kg/day in 2 divided doses, not to exceed 1,000 mg total dose/ day.

• **IM, IV (Cefuroxime sodium)**

Uncomplicated infections, including urinary tract, pneumonia, disseminated gonococcal, skin and skin structure.

Adults: 0.75 g q 8 hr. **Pediatric, over 3 months:** 50–100 mg/kg/day in divided doses q 6–8 hr (not to exceed adult dose for severe infections).

Severe, complicated, or life-threatening infections; bone and joint infections.

Adults: 1.5 g q 6–8 hr. **Pediatric, over 3 months:** *bone and joint infections,* **IV:** 150 mg/kg/day in divided doses q 8 hr (not to exceed adult dose).

Bacterial meningitis.

Adults: Up to 3 g q 8 hr. **Pediatric, over 3 months: initial, IV,** 200–240 mg/kg/day in divided doses q 6–8 hr; **then,** after clinical improvement, 100 mg/kg/day.

Gonorrhea (uncomplicated).

1.5 g as a single IM dose.

Prophylaxis in surgery.

Adults, IV: 1.5 g 30–60 min before surgery; if procedure is of long duration, **IM, IV,** 0.75 g q 8 hr.

Open heart surgery, prophylaxis.

IV: 1.5 g when anesthesia is initiated; **then,** 1.5 g q 12 hr for a total of 6 g.

Administration/Storage

1. Use IV route for severe or life-threatening infections such as septicemia or in poor-risk clients, especially in presence of shock.
2. For direct IV, reconstitute 750 mg with 8 mL sterile water and give over 3–5 min. For intermittent IV administration, further dilute in 100 mL of dextrose or saline solution and infuse over 30 min.
3. Cefuroxime sodium should not be added to solutions of aminoglycosides; if both drugs are required, each should be given separately to the client.

4. For IM use, inject deep into a large muscle mass.
5. Prior to reconstitution, protect the drug from light. The powder and reconstituted drug may darken without affecting potency.
6. Cefuroxime axetil for PO use is available in tablet and suspension forms.
7. To reconstitute the suspension, loosen the powder by shaking the bottle. Add the appropriate amount of water (depending on bottle size). Invert the bottle and shake vigorously.
8. The suspension must be given with food.
9. Therapy should be continued for at least 10 days in infections due to *Streptococcus pyogenes*.
10. Dosage in adults and children should be reduced in impaired renal function.

Additional Side Effects: Decrease in H&H.

Additional Laboratory Test Interference: False – reaction in the ferricyanide test for blood glucose.

NURSING CONSIDERATIONS

See also *Nursing Considerations* for *Cephalosporins,* Chapter 3.

Assessment

1. Assess for any clinical and laboratory evidence of anemia and renal dysfunction.
2. Document indications for therapy and note baseline assessments.

Client/Family Teaching

1. Take tablets with food to enhance the absorption of the PO medication.
2. Report any signs of anemia (SOB, dizziness, pale skin, etc.) immediately.
3. Crushed cefuroxime axetil tablets have a distinctive bitter taste even when hidden in foods. If unable to tolerate taste, report so alternative drug therapy may be instituted.

Evaluate

- Resolution of S&S of infection
- Normal H&H
- Infection prophylaxis during surgery

Cephalexin hydrochloride monohydrate

(sef-ah-**LEX**-in)
Pregnancy Category: B
Keftab **(Rx)**

Cephalexin monohydrate

(sef-ah-**LEX**-in)
Pregnancy Category: B
Apo-Cephalex ✱, Keflet, Keflex, Novo-Lexin ✱, Nu-Cephalex ✱ **(Rx)**

See also *Anti-Infectives,* Chapter 1, and *Cephalosporins,* Chapter 3.

How Supplied: Cephalexin hydrochloride monohydrate: *Tablet:* 500 mg.
Cephalexin monohydrate: *Capsule:* 250 mg, 500 mg; *Powder for Reconstitution:* 125 mg/5 mL, 250 mg/5 mL; *Tablet:* 250 mg, 500 mg

Action/Kinetics: Peak serum levels: PO, 9–39 mcg/mL after 1 hr. **t½, PO:** 30–72 min. Absorption delayed in children. The HCl monohydrate does not require conversion in the stomach before absorption. Ninety percent of drug excreted unchanged in urine within 8 hr.

Uses: Respiratory tract infections caused by *Streptococcus pneumoniae* and group A β-hemolytic streptococci. Otitis media due to *S. pneumoniae, Hemophilus influenzae, Moraxella catarrhalis* (use monohydrate only), staphylococci, and streptococci. Genitourinary tract infections (including prostatitis) due to *Escherichia coli, Proteus mirabilis,* and *Klebsiella.* Bone infections caused by *P. mirabilis* and staphylococci. Skin and skin structure infections due to staphylococci and streptococci.

Dosage

• Capsules, Oral Suspension, Tablets

General infections.

Adults, usual: 250 mg q 6 hr up to 4 g/day. **Pediatric:** *Monohydrate,*

25–50 mg/kg/day in four equally divided doses.

Infections of skin and skin structures, streptococcal pharyngitis, uncomplicated cystitis, over 15 years.
Adults: 500 mg q 12 hr. For streptococcal pharyngitis in children over 1 year and for skin and skin structure infections, the total daily dose should be divided and given q 12 hr.

Otitis media.
Pediatric: 75–100 mg/kg/day in four divided doses.

Administration/Storage

1. After reconstitution, the drug should be refrigerated and the unused portion discarded after 14 days.
2. If the total daily dose is more than 4 g, parenteral drug therapy should be undertaken.
3. Treatment should be continued for at least 10 days for beta-hemolytic streptococcal infections.
4. Dosage may have to be reduced in clients with impaired renal function or increased for severe infections. Action of drug can be prolonged by the concurrent administration of PO probenecid.

Special Concerns: Safety and effectiveness of the HCl monohydrate have not been determined in children.

Additional Side Effects: Nephrotoxicity, cholestatic jaundice.

NURSING CONSIDERATIONS

See also *Nursing Considerations* for *Cephalosporins,* Chapter 3.

Client/Family Teaching

1. Advise to take with meals if GI upset is evident.
2. Take 2–3 L/day of fluids to prevent dehydration.
3. Report any changes in elimination patterns, or a yellow discoloration of the skin or eyes.

Evaluate

- Resolution of infection
- Reports of symptomatic improvement

Cephalothin sodium

(sef-**AL**-oh-thin)
Pregnancy Category: B
Keflin ✱, Keflin Neutral **(Rx)**

See also *Anti-Infectives,* Chapter 1, and *Cephalosporins,* Chapter 3.

How Supplied: *Injection:* 1 g/50 mL, 2 g/50 mL; *Powder for injection:* 1 g, 2 g

Action/Kinetics: Poorly absorbed from GI tract; must be given parenterally. **Peak serum levels: IM,** 6–21 mcg/mL after 30 min. **t½, IM, IV:** 30–60 min. Fifty-five percent to 90% excreted unchanged in urine. Its low nephrotoxicity, ototoxicity, and neurotoxicity make the drug suitable for clients with impaired renal function.

Uses: Infections of the GU tract, GI tract, respiratory tract, skin, soft tissues, bones, and joints. Meningitis, septicemia (including endocarditis), and prophylaxis in surgery.

Dosage

- **Deep IM, IV**

General infections.
Adults, usual: 0.5–1 g q 4–6 hr. **Pediatric:** 80–160 mg/kg/day in divided doses.

UTIs, uncomplicated pneumonia, furunculosis with cellulitis.
Adults: 0.5 g q 6 hr (for severe infections increase the dose to 1 g or give 0.5 g q 4 hr).

Life-threatening infections.
Adults: 2 g q 4 hr (up to 12 g/day for bacteremia, septicemia).

Preoperative and during surgery.
Adults: 1–2 g 30–60 min prior to surgery and during surgery. **Pediatric:** *Prophylaxis in surgery:* 20–30 mg/kg using adult schedule.

Postoperative.
Adults: 1–2 g q 6 hr for 24 hr.

Impaired renal function.
Initial: 1–2 g; **then,** use manufacturer's guidelines for maintenance doses.

Administration/Storage

1. Dilute according to directions on package insert. For direct IV administration, dilute 1 g in 10 mL of solution and infuse over 3–5 min. For intermittent IV administration further dilute 1 g in 50 mL of dextrose or saline solution and infuse over 15–30 min.
2. Discard reconstituted solution after 12 hr at room temperature and after 96 hr when refrigerated.

3. Dissolve precipitate by warming vial in hand and shaking. Do not overheat.
4. For prolonged IV infusion, the medication should be replaced with a freshly prepared solution every 24 hr to ensure stability.
5. For direct IV administration, add a small needle into larger veins.
6. Alter dose and follow manufacturer's guidelines for clients with impaired renal function.

Additional Side Effects: Nephrotoxicity, severe phlebitis, hemolytic anemia, increased PT.

Laboratory Test Interferences: Large doses may produce false + results in urinary protein tests that use sulfosalicylic acid.

NURSING CONSIDERATIONS

See also *Nursing Considerations* for *Cephalosporins,* Chapter 3.

Assessment

1. Monitor PT and assess for bleeding. May administer vitamin K (10 mg/week) if bleeding occurs.
2. Monitor I&O and assess renal function studies.

Evaluate

- Resolution of infection
- Infection prophylaxis during surgery

Cephapirin sodium

(sef-ah-**PIE**-rin)
Pregnancy Category: B
Cefadyl **(Rx)**

See also *Anti-Infectives,* Chapter 1, and *Cephalosporins,* Chapter 3.

How Supplied: *Powder for injection:* 1 g

Action/Kinetics: Peak serum levels: IM, 9.4 mcg/mL after 30 min. **t½, IM, IV:** 21–47 min. Virtually entirely excreted in the urine within 6 hr, with 41%–60% excreted unchanged.

Uses: Infections of the respiratory tract, urinary tract, skin, and skin structures. Septicemia, endocarditis, osteomyelitis, prophylaxis in surgery.

Dosage

- **IM, IV only**

General infections.

Adults: 0.5–1 g q 4–6 hr up to 12 g/day for serious or life-threatening infections.

Preoperatively.

Adults: 1–2 g 30–60 min before surgery.

During surgery.

Adults: 1–2 g.

Postoperatively.

Adults: 1–2 g q 6 hr for 24 hr. **Pediatric, over 3 months:** 40–80 mg/kg/day in four equally divided doses.

In clients with impaired renal function, a dose of 7.5–15 mg/kg q 12 hr may be adequate.

Administration/Storage

1. For direct IV administration reconstitute 1 g in 10 mL of solution and infuse over 3–5 min. For intermittent infusions, further dilute in 50–100 mL of solution and infuse over 15–20 min.
2. Discard after 12 hr when kept at room temperature and after 10 days when refrigerated at 4°C (39°F).
3. Concurrent administration with probenecid may inhibit excretion of cephapirin.
4. Anticipate reduced dose with impaired renal function.

Special Concerns: Before use in children less than 3 months, assess benefits versus risks.

Additional Side Effect: Increase in serum bilirubin.

NURSING CONSIDERATIONS

See also *Nursing Considerations* for *Cephalosporins,* Chapter 3.

Evaluate

- Resolution of infection
- Infection prophylaxis in surgery

Cephradine

(**SEF**-rah-deen)
Pregnancy Category: B
Anspor, Velosef **(Rx)**

See also *Anti-Infectives,* Chapter 1, and *Cephalosporins,* Chapter 3.

How Supplied: *Capsule:* 250 mg, 500 mg; *Powder for Reconstitution:* 125 mg/5 mL, 250 mg/5 mL

Action/Kinetics: Similar to that of cephalexin. Rapidly absorbed from GI tract or IM injection site (30 min–2 hr); 60%–90% excreted after 6 hr. **Peak serum levels: PO,** 8–24 mcg/mL after 30–60 min; **IM,** 5.6–13.6 mcg/mL after 1–2 hr. **t½:** 42–120 min; 80%–95% excreted in urine unchanged.

Uses: Infections of the respiratory tract (including lobar pneumonia, tonsillitis, pharyngitis), urinary tract (including prostatitis and enterococcal infections), skin, skin structures, and bone. Otitis media, septicemia, prophylaxis in surgery, following cesarean section to prevent infection. In severe infections, therapy is usually initiated parenterally.

Dosage

- **Capsules, Oral Suspension**

Skin and skin structures, respiratory tract infections.

Adults, usual: 250 mg q 6 hr or 500 mg q 12 hr.

Lobar pneumonia.

Adults: 500 mg q 6 hr or 1 g q 12 hr.

Uncomplicated UTIs.

Adults, usual: 500 mg q 12 hr.

More serious infections and prostatitis.

500 mg q 6 hr or 1 g q 12 hr (severe, chronic infections may require up to 1 g q 6 hr).

Pediatric, over 9 months: 25–50 mg/kg/day in equally divided doses q 6–12 hr (75–100 mg/kg/day for otitis media).

- **Deep IM, IV**

General infections.

Adults: 2–4 g/day in equally divided doses q.i.d.

Surgical prophylaxis.

Adults: 1 g 30–90 min before surgery; **then,** 1 g q 4–6 hr for one to two doses (or up to 24 hr postoperatively).

Cesarean section, prophylaxis.

IV: 1 g when the umbilical cord is clamped; **then,** give two additional 1-g doses **IV or IM** 6 and 12 hr after the initial dose. **Pediatric, over 1 year:** 50–100 mg/kg/day in equally divided doses q.i.d.

Administration/Storage

1. Dilute according to directions on package insert.
2. For direct IV administration dilute 1 g in 10 mL of D5%/W or NSS and infuse over 3–5 min. For intermittent infusions further reconstitute in 50–100 mL of dextrose or saline solution and infuse over 30–60 min. Discontinue other IV solutions during IV administration of cephalosporins.
3. Do not mix with lactated Ringer's solution.
4. Discard reconstituted solution after 10 hr at room temperature and after 48 hr when refrigerated at 5°C.
5. A slightly yellow solution may be retained for use; if unsure of solution potency, consult with pharmacist.
6. Be especially careful to inject into muscle, because sterile abscesses from accidental SC injection have occurred.
7. Before and after reconstitution, protect from excessive heat and light.
8. To ensure stability, replace medication infusion solution during prolonged IV administration q 10 hr.
9. Administer PO medication without regard to meals.
10. Reduce dose in clients with impaired renal function.
11. Rotate and document injection sites carefully.

Special Concerns: Safe use during pregnancy has not been established. Safe use of the parenteral form in infants under 1 month of age and the PO form in children less than 9 months of age have not been established.

Additional Laboratory Test Interferences: False + reactions using sulfosalicylic acid for urinary protein tests. High concentrations may interfere with measurement of creatinine by the Jaffe method.

NURSING CONSIDERATIONS

See also *Nursing Considerations* for *Cephalosporins,* Chapter 3.

Evaluate
- Resolution of S&S of infection
- Infection prophylaxis in surgery
- Negative laboratory culture reports

Loracarbef

(**lor**-ah-**KAR**-bef)
Pregnancy Category: B
Lorabid **(Rx)**

See also *Anti-Infectives,* Chapter 1.

How Supplied: *Capsule:* 200 mg, 400 mg; *Powder for reconstitution:* 100 mg/5 mL, 200 mg/5 mL

Action/Kinetics: Loracarbef is related chemically to the cephalosporin antibiotics. The drug acts by inhibiting cell wall synthesis; it is stable in the presence of certain bacterial beta-lactamases. **Average peak plasma levels:** 8 mcg/mL following a single 200-mg dose in a fasting subject after 90 min and 14 mcg/mL following a single 400-mg dose in a fasting subject after 90 min. Following doses of 7.5 mg/kg and 15 mg/kg of the oral suspension to children, average peak plasma levels were 13 and 19 mcg/mL, respectively, within 40–60 min. **Elimination t½:** 1 hr (increased to 5.6 hr in clients with a creatinine clearance from 10 to 50 mL/min/1.73 m^2 and to 32 hr in clients with a creatinine clearance of less than 10 mL/min/1.73 m^2). The drug is not metabolized in humans.

Uses: Secondary bacterial infections of acute bronchitis caused by *Streptococcus pneumoniae, Haemophilus influenzae,* or *Morazella catarrhalis* (including beta-lactamase-producing strains of both organisms). Acute bacterial exacerbations of chronic bronchitis caused by *S. pneumoniae, H. influenzae,* or *M. catarrhalis* (including beta-lactamase-producing strains of both organisms). Pneumonia caused by *S. pneumoniae* or *H. influenzae* (only non-beta-lactamase-producing strains). Otitis media caused by *S. pneumoniae, Streptococcus pyogenes, H. influenzae,* or *M. catarrhalis* (including beta-lactamase-producing strains of both organisms). Acute maxillary sinusitis caused by *S. pneumoniae, H. influenzae* (only non-beta-lactamase-producing strains), or *M. catarrhalis* (including beta-lactamase-producing strains). Pharyngitis and tonsillitis caused by *S. pyogenes.* Uncomplicated skin and skin structure infections caused by *Staphylococcus aureus* (including penicillinase-producing strains) or *S. pyogenes.* Uncomplicated UTIs caused by *Escherichia coli* or *Staphylococcus saprophyticus.* Uncomplicated pyelonephritis caused by *E. coli.*

Dosage

- **Capsules, Oral Suspension**

Secondary bacterial infection of acute bronchitis.

Adults 13 years of age and older: 200–400 mg q 12 hr for 7 days.

Acute bacterial exacerbation of chronic bronchitis.

Adults 13 years of age and older: 400 mg q 12 hr for 7 days.

Pneumonia.

Adults 13 years of age and older: 400 q 12 hr for 14 days.

Pharyngitis, tonsillitis.

Adults 13 years of age and older: 200 mg q 12 hr for 10 days. **Infants and children, 6 months–12 years:** 15 mg/kg/day in divided doses q 12 hr for 10 days.

Sinusitis.

Adults 13 years of age and older: 400 mg q 12 hr for 10 days.

Acute otitis media.

Infants and children, 6 months–12 years: 30 mg/kg/day in divided doses q 12 hr for 10 days. The suspension should be used as it is more rapidly absorbed than the capsules, resulting in higher peak plasma levels when given at the same dose.

Skin and skin structure infections (impetigo).

Infants and children, 6 months–12 years: 15 mg/kg/day in divided doses q 12 hr for 7 days.

Administration/Storage

1. Should be taken at least 1 hr before or at least 2 hr after meals.
2. The manufacturer provides a chart to assist with establishing the dosage regimen for pediatric clients.
3. Clients with creatinine clearance levels of 10–49 mL/min may be given one-half the recommended dose at the usual dosage interval. Clients with creatinine clearance less than 10 mL/min may be treated with the recommended dose given every 3–5 days. Clients on hemodialysis should receive another dose following dialysis.
4. The oral suspension is reconstituted by adding 30 mL water to the 50-mL bottle or 60 mL water to the 100-mL bottle. After mixing, the suspension may be kept at room temperature for 14 days without significant loss of potency. The bottle should be kept tightly closed. After 14 days any unused portion should be discarded.
5. *Treatment of Overdose:* Hemodialysis may be effective in increasing the elimination of loracarbef from plasma from clients with chronic renal failure.

Contraindication: Hypersensitivity to loracarbef or cephalosporin-class antibiotics.

Special Concerns: Use during labor and delivery only if clearly needed. Pseudomembranous colitis is possible with most antibacterial agents. Use with caution and at reduced dosage in clients with impaired renal function, in those with a history of colitis, in clients receiving concurrent treatment with potent diuretics, during lactation, and in clients with known penicillin allergies. Safety and efficacy in children less than 6 months of age have not been determined.

Side Effects: The incidence of certain side effects is different in the pediatric population compared with the adult population. *GI:* Diarrhea, N&V, abdominal pain, anorexia, pseudomembranous colitis. *Hypersensitivity:* Skin rashes, urticaria, pruritus, erythema multiforme. *CNS:* Headache, somnolence, nervousness, insomnia, dizziness. *Hematologic:* Transient thrombocytopenia, leukopenia, eosinophilia. *Miscellaneous:* Vasodilation, vaginitis, vaginal moniliasis, rhinitis.

Symptoms of Overdose: N&V, epigastric distress, diarrhea.

Drug Interactions

Diuretics, potent / ↑ Risk of renal dysfunction

Probenecid / ↓ Renal excretion resulting in ↑ plasma levels of loracarbef

NURSING CONSIDERATIONS

See also *General Nursing Considerations* for *All Anti-Infectives,* Chapter 1.

Assessment

1. Note any history or evidence of sensitivity to cephalosporins and penicillin derivatives.
2. Obtain baseline cultures and renal function studies.
3. List drugs currently prescribed to ensure that none interact unfavorably.

Client/Family Teaching

1. Take only as directed 1 hr before or 2 hr after meals.
2. Provide a printed list of drug side effects stressing those that require immediate reporting.
3. Report persistent diarrhea, which may be secondary to pseudomembranous colitis; this requires medical intervention.

Evaluate

- Negative lab C&S reports with resolution of infection
- Relief of ear pain and/or sore throat
- Improved breathing patterns
- Evidence of wound healing

CHAPTER FOUR

Antibiotics: Chloramphenicol

See the following individual entries:

Chloramphenicol
Chloramphenicol Ophthalmic
Chloramphenicol Sodium Succinate

Chloramphenicol

(klor-am-**FEN**-ih-kohl)
Chloromycetin (Cream, Kapseals, and Otic), Mychel, PMS-Chloramphenicol **(Rx)**

Chloramphenicol ophthalmic

(klor-am-**FEN**-ih-kohl)
AK Chlor, Chloromycetin Ophthalmic, Chloroptic Ophthalmic, Chloroptic S.O.P. Ophthalmic, Ophtho-Chloram ✦, Sopamycetin ✦ **(Rx)**

Chloramphenicol sodium succinate

(klor-am-**FEN**-ih-kohl)
Chloromycetin Sodium Succinate, Mychel-S **(Rx)**

See also *Anti-Infectives,* Chapter 1.

How Supplied: Chloramphenicol: *Capsule:* 250 mg
Chloramphenicol ophthalmic: *Ointment:* 1%; *Powder for reconstitution:* 25 mg; *Solution:* 0.5%
Chloramphenicol sodium succinate: *Powder for injection:* 1 g

General Statement: This antibiotic was originally isolated from *Streptomyces venezuellae* and is now produced synthetically. The antibiotic can be extremely toxic (due to protein synthesis inhibition in rapidly proliferating cells, as in bone marrow) and should not be used for trivial infections.

Action/Kinetics: Chloramphenicol interferes with or inhibits protein synthesis in bacteria by binding to 50S ribosomal subunits. Therapeutic serum concentrations: *peak,* 10–20 mcg/mL; *trough:* 5–10 mcg/mL (less for neonates). **Peak serum concentration: IM,** 2 hr. **t½:** 4 hr. Drug is metabolized in the liver; 75%–90% of drug excreted in urine within 24 hr, as parent drug (8%–12%) and inactive metabolites. The drug is mostly bacteriostatic. Chloramphenicol is well absorbed from the GI tract and is distributed to all parts of the body, including CSF, pleural, and ascitic fluids; saliva; milk; and aqueous and vitreous humors.

Uses: *Not to be used for trivial infections, prophylaxis of bacterial infections, or to treat colds, flu, or throat infections.* **Systemic Use.** Treatment of choice for typhoid fever but not for typhoid carrier state. Serious infections caused by *Salmonella, Rickettsia, Chlamydia,* and lymphogranuloma-psittacosis group. Meningitis due to *Haemophilus influenzae.* Brain abscesses due to *Bacteroides fragilis.* Cystic fibrosis anti-infective. Meningococcal or pneumococcal meningitis. **Topical Use.** Otitis externa. Prophylaxis of infection in minor cuts, wounds, skin abrasions, burns; promote healing in superficial infections of the skin. **Ophthalmic Use.** Superficial ocular infections due to *Staphylococcus aureus; Streptococcus* species, including *S. pneumoniae; Escherichia coli, H. influenzae, H.*

aegyptius, H. ducreyi, Klebsiella species, *Neisseria* species, *Enterobacter* species, *Moraxella lacunata, Pseudomonas aeruginosa,* and *Vibrio* species. Chloramphenicol should be used only for serious ocular infections for which less dangerous drugs are either contraindicated or ineffective.

Dosage

- **Capsules, Oral Suspension, IV: Chloramphenicol, chloramphenicol palmitate**

Adults: 50 mg/kg/day in four equally divided doses q 6 hr. Can be increased to 100 mg/kg/day in severe infections, but dosage should be reduced as soon as possible. **Neonates and children with immature metabolic function:** 25 mg/kg once daily in divided doses q 12 hr. **Neonates, less than 2 kg:** 25 mg/kg once daily. **Neonates, over 2 kg, over 7 days of age:** 50 mg/kg/day q 12 hr in divided doses. **Neonates, over 2 kg, from birth to 7 days of age:** 50 mg/kg once daily. **Children:** 50–75 mg/kg/day in divided doses q 6 hr (50–100 mg/kg/day in divided doses q 6 hr for meningitis). *NOTE:* Carefully follow dosage for premature and newborn infants less than 2 weeks of age because blood levels differ significantly from those of other age groups.

- **Chloramphenicol sodium succinate–IV only**

Same dosage as chloramphenicol (see above). Switch to **PO** as soon as possible.

- **Chloramphenicol Ophthalmic Ointment 1%**

0.5-in. ribbon placed in lower conjunctival sac q 3–4 hr for acute infections and b.i.d.–t.i.d. for mild to moderate infections.

- **Chloramphenicol Ophthalmic Solution 0.5%**

1–2 gtt in lower conjunctival sac 2–6 times/day (or more for acute infections).

- **Chloramphenicol Otic Solution 0.5%**

2–3 gtt in ear t.i.d.

- **Chloramphenicol Topical Cream 1%**

Apply 1–4 times/day.

Administration/Storage

1. Administer IV as a 10% solution over at least a 60-sec interval. Reconstitute 1 g in 10 mL of water for injection or 5% dextrose injection. May further dilute in 50–100 mL of dextrose or saline solution and infuse over 30–60 min.
2. When used for skin infections, a sterile bandage may be used if necessary.

Contraindications: Hypersensitivity to chloramphenicol; pregnancy, especially near term and during labor; lactation. Avoid simultaneous administration of other drugs that may depress bone marrow. Ophthalmically in the presence of dendritic keratitis, vaccinia, varicella, mycobacterial or fungal eye infections, or following removal of a corneal foreign body. Topical products should not be used near or in the eye.

Special Concerns: Use with caution in clients with intermittent porphyria or G6PD deficiency. To avoid gray syndrome, use with caution and in reduced doses in premature and full-term infants. Ophthalmic ointments may retard corneal epithelial healing.

Side Effects: *Hematologic* (most serious): ***Aplastic anemia, hypoplastic anemia,*** thrombocytopenia, granulocytopenia, ***hemolytic anemia,*** pancytopenia, hemoglobinuria (paroxysmal nocturnal). *Hematologic studies should be undertaken before and every 2 days during therapy. GI:* N&V, diarrhea, glossitis, stomatitis, unpleasant taste, enterocolitis, pruritus ani. *Allergic:* Fever, angioedema, macular and vesicular rashes, urticaria, hemorrhages of the skin, intestine, bladder, mouth. ***Anaphylaxis.*** *CNS:* Headache, delirium, confusion, mental depression. *Neurologic:* Optic neuritis, peripheral neuritis. *Following topical use:* Burning, itching, irritation, redness of skin. Hypersensitive clients may exhibit ***angioneurotic edema,*** urticaria, vesicular and maculopapular dermatoses. *Miscellaneous:*

Superinfection. Jaundice (rare). Herxheimer-like reactions when used for typhoid fever (may be due to release of bacterial endotoxins). ***Gray syndrome in infants:*** Rapid respiration, ashen gray color, failure to feed, abdominal distention with or without vomiting, progressive pallid cyanosis, vasomotor collapse, death. Can be reversed when drug is discontinued. *NOTE: Neonates should be observed closely, since the drug accumulates in the bloodstream and the infant is thus subject to greater hazards of toxicity.*

Drug Interactions

Acetaminophen / ↑ Effect of chloramphenicol due to ↑ serum levels
Anticoagulants, oral / ↑ Effect of anticoagulants due to ↓ breakdown by liver
Antidiabetics, oral / ↑ Effect of antidiabetics due to ↓ breakdown by liver
Barbiturates / ↑ Effect of barbiturates due to ↓ breakdown by liver; also, ↓ serum levels of chloramphenicol
Chymotrypsin / Chloramphenicol will inhibit chymotrypsin
Cyclophosphamide / Delayed or ↓ activation of cyclophosphamide
Iron preparations / ↑ Serum iron levels
Penicillins / Either ↑ or ↓ effect when combined to treat certain microorganisms
Phenytoin / ↑ Effect of phenytoin due to ↓ breakdown by liver; also, chloramphenicol levels may be ↑ or ↓
Rifampin / ↓ Effect of chloramphenicol due to ↑ breakdown by liver
Vitamin B_{12} / ↓ Response to vitamin B_{12} when treating pernicious anemia

NURSING CONSIDERATIONS

See also *General Nursing Considerations for All Anti-Infectives,* Chapter 1.

Assessment

1. Note any history of hypersensitivity to chloramphenicol.
2. If client is a nursing mother, transmission of the drug to breast milk can result in the infant receiving the drug as well. Infants have underdeveloped capacity to metabolize chloramphenicol.
3. Take a complete nursing history. Clients who are diabetic and taking oral hypoglycemic agents may have to use insulin during treatment with chloramphenicol.
4. Chloramphenicol may produce a false positive reaction with Fehling's or Benedict's solutions, both of which contain copper sulfate. In diabetic clients, use Lab-Stix to test the urine or, if available, do finger sticks for enhanced accuracy of glucose determinations.
5. If client is concomitantly receiving drugs that cause bone marrow depression, use of chloramphenicol is contraindicated.
6. Be certain that baseline hematologic studies are completed before drug treatment begins.
7. Arrange for hematologic studies to be conducted q 2 days to detect early signs of bone marrow depression. This may also develop weeks to months following drug therapy.
8. Anticipate reduced dosage in clients with impaired renal function and in newborn infants.
9. Document indications for therapy and note pretreatment findings.

Interventions

1. Become familiar with drugs that enhance the effects of chloramphenicol and monitor closely for evidence of severe toxicity in clients on concurrent therapy.
2. Client should receive the drug only as necessary; avoid repeated courses of therapy with chloramphenicol because the drug is highly toxic.
3. Monitor client for the development of any of the following:
- *Bone marrow depression* characterized by weakness, fatigue, sore throat, and bleeding; discontinuation of the drug may be indicated.

• *Optic neuritis* characterized by bilaterally reduced visual acuity, an indication to discontinue the drug immediately.
• *Peripheral neuritis* characterized by pain and disturbance of sensation, both of which are indications to discontinue the drug immediately.
• Development of *gray syndrome* in premature and newborn infants, characterized by rapid respiration, failure to feed, abdominal distention with or without vomiting, loose green stools, progressive cyanosis, and vasomotor collapse. Withhold drug and report if evident.
4. Assess for toxic and irritative effects, such as N&V, unpleasant taste, diarrhea, and perineal irritation following PO administration. Differentiation of drug-induced diarrhea from that caused by a superinfection is critical and may be accomplished by assessment and analysis of all presenting symptoms.

Client/Family Teaching

1. Chloramphenicol should be taken 1 hr before or 2 hr after meals; however, if GI upset occurs, it can be taken with food.
2. The drug should be taken at regularly spaced intervals *around the clock* to be most effective.
3. Avoid the use of alcohol during therapy.
4. Do not take salicylates or NSAIDs without approval.
5. Review the signs of hypersensitivity, such as itching and rash, and stress the importance of reporting.
6. Report the development of sore throat or any unusual fatigue, bruising, or bleeding immediately because drug may need to be discontinued.
7. Ophthalmic solutions may cause blurred vision immediately after instillation; this should clear.
8. During IV administration client may experience a bitter taste, but this should subside after several minutes.

Evaluate

• Resolution of infection
• Therapeutic serum drug levels (peak 10–20 mcg/mL; trough 5–10 mcg/mL)

CHAPTER FIVE

Antibiotics: Clindamycin and Lincomycin

See the following individual entries:

Clindamycin Hydrochloride Hydrate
Clindamycin Palmitate Hydrochloride
Clindamycin Phosphate
Lincomycin Hydrochloride

Clindamycin hydrochloride hydrate

(klin-dah-**MY**-sin)
Cleocin Hydrochloride, Dalacin C ✱
(Rx)

Clindamycin palmitate hydrochloride

(klin-dah-**MY**-sin)
Cleocin Pediatric, Dalacin C Palmitate ✱ **(Rx)**

Clindamycin phosphate

(klin-dah-**MY**-sin)
Pregnancy Category: B (vaginal cream; topical gel, lotion, solution)
Cleocin Vaginal Cream, Cleocin Phosphate, Cleocin T, Dalacin C Phosphate ✱, Dalacin T Topical ✱
(Rx)

See also *Anti-Infectives,* Chapter 1.

How Supplied: Clindamycin hydrochloride hydrate: *Capsule:* 75 mg, 150 mg, 300 mg
Clindamycin palmitate hydrochloride: *Granule for reconstitution: 75 mg/5 mL*
Clindamycin phosphate: *Vaginal cream:* 2%; *Gel:* 1%; *Injection:* 150 mg/mL, 300 mg/50 mL, 600 mg/50 mL, 900 mg/50 mL; *Lotion:* 1%; *Solution:* 1%; *Swab:* 1%

General Statement: Clindamycin is a semisynthetic antibiotic. Its spectrum resembles that of the erythromycins and includes a variety of gram-positive organisms, particularly staphylococci, streptococci, and pneumococci, and some gram-negative organisms. Should not be used for trivial infections.

Action/Kinetics: Suppresses protein synthesis by microorganism by binding to ribosomes (50S subunit) and preventing peptide bond formation. Is both bacteriostatic and bactericidal. **Peak serum concentration: PO,** 4 mcg/mL after 300 mg; **IM,** 4.9 mcg/mL after 300 mg; **IV,** 14.7 mcg/mL after 300 mg. **t½:** 2.4–3 hr. In serious infections the rate of IV administration is adjusted to maintain appropriate serum drug concentrations: 4–6 mcg/mL.

Uses: Systemic. Serious respiratory tract infections (e.g., empyema, lung abscess, pneumonia) caused by staphylococci, streptococci, and pneumococci. Serious skin and soft tissue infections, septicemia, intra-abdominal infections, pelvic inflammatory disease, female genital tract infections. May be the drug of choice for *Bacteroides fragilis.* In combination with aminoglycosides for mixed aerobic and anaerobic bacterial infections. Staphylococci-induced acute hematogenous osteomyelitis.

Adjunct to surgery for chronic bone/joint infections. *Investigational:* Alternative to sulfonamides in combination with pyrimethamine in the acute treatment of CNS toxoplasmosis in AIDS clients. In combination with primaquine to treat *Pneumocystis carinii* pneumonia. Chlamydial infections in women. Bacterial vaginosis due to *Gardnerella vaginalis*. **Topical Use.** Used topically for inflammatory acne vulgaris. Vaginally to treat bacterial vaginosis.

Dosage

• PO only: Capsules, Oral Solution

Adults: Clindamycin HCl, Clindamycin palmitate HCl: 150–450 mg q 6 hr, depending on severity of infection. **Pediatric: Clindamycin HCl hydrate:** 8–20 mg/kg/day divided into three to four equal doses; clindamycin palmitate HCl: 8–25 mg/kg/day divided into three to four equal doses. **Children less than 10 kg:** Minimum recommended dose is 37.5 mg t.i.d.

• IV

Clindamycin phosphate. Adults: 0.6–2.7 g/day in two to four equal doses depending on severity of infection.

Life-threatening infections.

4.8 g. **Pediatric over 1 month:** 15–40 mg/kg/day in three to four equal doses depending on severity of infections.

Severe infections.

No less than 300 mg/day, regardless of body weight.

Acute pelvic inflammatory disease.

IV: 600 mg q.i.d. plus gentamicin, 2 mg/kg IV; **then,** gentamicin, 1.5 mg/kg t.i.d. IV. IV therapy should be continued for 2 days after client improves. The 10–14-day treatment cycle should be completed using clindamycin, **PO:** 450 mg q.i.d.

• Topical Gel, Lotion, or Solution

Apply thin film b.i.d. to affected areas.

• Vaginal cream (2%)

One applicatorful (containing about 100 mg clindamycin phosphate), preferably at bedtime, for 7 consecutive days.

Administration/Storage

1. Give parenteral clindamycin only to hospitalized clients.
2. Dilute IV injections to maximum concentration of 12 mg/mL, with no more than 1,200 mg administered in 1 hr.
3. Single IM injections greater than 600 mg are not advisable. Inject deeply into muscle to prevent induration, pain, and sterile abscesses.
4. Do not refrigerate; otherwise, solution may become thickened.
5. Administer IV over a period of 20–60 min, depending on dose and therapeutic serum concentration to be attained.
6. Dosage should be reduced in severe renal impairment.

Contraindications: Hypersensitivity to either clindamycin or lincomycin. Not for use in treating viral and minor bacterial infections. Use in clients with a history of regional enteritis, ulcerative colitis, or antibiotic-associated colitis.

Special Concerns: Safe use during pregnancy has not been established. Use with caution in infants up to 1 month of age. Use with caution in clients with GI disease, liver or renal disease, history of allergy or asthma. Safety and efficacy of topical products have not been established in children.

Laboratory Test Interferences: ↓ Levels of AST, ALT, NPN, alkaline phosphatase, bilirubin, BSP retention, and ↓ platelet count.

Side Effects: *GI:* N&V, diarrhea, abdominal pain, tenesmus, flatulence, bloating, anorexia, weight loss, esophagitis. Nonspecific colitis, pseudomembranous colitis (may be severe). *Allergic:* Morbilliform rash (most common). Also, maculopapular rash, urticaria, pruritus, fever, hypotension. Rarely, polyarteritis, anaphylaxis, erythema multiforme. *Hematologic:* Leukopenia, neutropenia, eosinophilia, thrombocytopenia, ***agranulocytosis.*** *Miscellaneous:* Superinfection. Also sore throat, fatigue, urinary frequency, headache.

Following IV use: Thrombophlebitis, erythema, pain, swelling. *Following IM use:* Pain, induration, sterile abscesses.

Following topical use: Erythema, irritation, dryness, peeling, itching, burning, oiliness of skin.

Following vaginal use: Cervicitis, vaginitis, vulvar irritation, urticaria, rash. *NOTE:* The injection contains benzyl alcohol, which has been associated with ***a fatal "gasping syndrome"*** in infants.

Drug Interactions

Antiperistaltic antidiarrheals (opiates, Lomotil) / ↑ Diarrhea due to ↓ removal of toxins from colon

Ciprofloxacin HCl / Additive antibacterial activity

Erythromycin / Cross-interference → ↓ effect of both drugs

Kaolin (e.g., Kaopectate) / ↓ Effect due to ↓ absorption from GI tract

Neuromuscular blocking agents / ↑ Effect of blocking agents

NURSING CONSIDERATIONS

See also *General Nursing Considerations* for *All Anti-Infectives,* Chapter 1.

Assessment

1. Take a complete nursing history. Document indications for therapy and type and onset of symptoms.
2. Auscultate lungs and note extensiveness of respiratory tract infections.
3. Document presence of serious skin and soft tissue infections, septicemia, and female genital tract infections.
4. List any client complaints indicative of pelvic inflammatory disease or intra-abdominal infections.
5. Note any history of liver or renal disease, allergies, or history of GI problems.
6. Obtain baseline liver and renal function studies.

Interventions

1. Be prepared to manage pseudomembranous colitis, which can occur 2–9 days or several weeks after initiation of therapy. Provide fluids, electrolytes, protein supplements, systemic corticosteroids, and oral antibiotics as prescribed.
2. Do not administer, and caution client against using, antiperistaltic agents if diarrhea occurs because these can prolong or aggravate the condition.
3. Do not administer kaolin concomitantly because this will reduce absorption of antibiotic. If kaolin is required, administer 3 hr before antibiotic.
4. Do not use any acne or topical mercury preparations containing a peeling agent in an area affected by medication because severe irritation may occur.
5. Administer on an empty stomach to ensure optimum absorption. Drug should be administered only as long as necessary.
6. During IV administration observe for hypotension and keep client in bed for 30 min following therapy. Advise that a bitter taste may also be evident.
7. Observe for drug interactions caused by concurrent administration of neuromuscular blocking agents. Be alert to hypotension, bronchospasms, cardiac disturbances, hyperthermia, and respiratory depression.
8. Observe closely for:
   - Skin rash because this is the most frequently reported side effect
   - Clients with renal and/or hepatic impairment and newborns for organ dysfunction
   - GI disturbances, such as abdominal pain, diarrhea, anorexia, N&V, bloody or tarry stools, and excessive flatulence. Discontinuation of drug may be indicated.

Client/Family Teaching

1. Take PO medication with a full glass of water to prevent esophageal ulceration.
2. If client has slight GI disturbance, the drug may be taken with food because food does not significantly affect the rate of absorption.

3. Report any side effects such as persistent vomiting, diarrhea, fever, or abdominal pain and cramping.
4. Review symptoms of colitis that may be severe and should be reported immediately, especially when working with the frail elderly.
5. The vaginal cream contains mineral oil, which may weaken latex or rubber products, such as condoms or vaginal contraceptive diaphragms. Use of such products is not recommended for 72 hr following treatment.
6. Clients should not engage in intercourse when using the vaginal cream as this may enhance irritation.

Evaluate

- Resolution of infection
- Reports of symptomatic improvement
- Negative laboratory culture reports
- Therapeutic serum drug concentrations with IV therapy (4–6 mcg/mL)

Lincomycin hydrochloride

(link-oh-**MY**-sin)
Lincocin **(Rx)**

See also *Anti-Infectives,* Chapter 1.

How Supplied: *Capsule:* 500 mg; *Injection:* 300 mg/mL

Action/Kinetics: Lincomycin is isolated from *Streptomyces lincolnensis.* Its spectrum resembles that of the erythromycins and includes a variety of gram-positive organisms, in particular staphylococci, streptococci, and pneumococci, and some gram-negative organisms. Lincomycin suppresses protein synthesis by microorganisms by binding to ribosomes (50S subunit), which is essential for transmittal of genetic information. It is both bacteriostatic and bactericidal. Lincomycin is absorbed rapidly from the GI tract and is widely distributed. **Peak serum levels: PO,** 2.6 mcg/mL after 500 mg; **IM,** 9.5 mcg/mL after 600 mg; **IV,** 19 mcg/mL after 600 mg. **t½:** 4.4–6.4 hr. This drug should not be used for trivial infections.

Uses: Not a first-choice drug but useful for clients allergic to penicillin. Used for serious respiratory tract, skin, and soft tissue infections due to staphylococci, streptococci, or pneumococci. Septicemia. In conjunction with diphtheria antitoxin in the treatment of diphtheria.

Dosage

- **Capsules**

  Infections.

Adults: 500 mg t.i.d.–q.i.d.; **children over 1 month of age:** 30–60 mg/kg/day in three to four divided doses, depending on severity of infection.

- **IM**

  Infections.

Adults: 600 mg q 12–24 hr; **children over 1 month of age:** 10 mg/kg q 12–24 hr, depending on severity of infection.

- **IV**

  Infections.

Adults: 0.6–1.0 g q 8–12 hr up to 8 g/day, depending on severity of infection; **children over 1 month of age:** 10–20 mg/kg/day, depending on severity of infection.

NOTE: In impaired renal function, reduce dosage by 70%–75%.

- **Subconjunctival Injection**

0.75 mg/0.25 mL.

Administration/Storage

1. Prepare drug for administration as directed on package insert.
2. Administer slowly IM to minimize pain.
3. For IV use, carefully follow concentration and recommended rate for administration to prevent severe cardiopulmonary reactions.
4. Injection contains benzyl alcohol.

Contraindication: Hypersensitivity to drugs. Use in infants up to 1 month of age.

Special Concerns: Safe use during pregnancy has not been established. Use with caution in clients with GI disease, liver or renal disease, or a history of allergy or asthma. Not for use in treating viral and minor bacterial infections.

Laboratory Test Interferences: ↓ Levels of AST, ALT, NPN, alkaline phosphatase, bilirubin, BSP retention, and ↓ platelet count.

Side Effects: *GI:* N&V, diarrhea, abdominal pain, tenesmus, flatulence, bloating, anorexia, weight loss, esophagitis. Nonspecific colitis, pseudomembranous colitis (may be severe). *Allergic:* Morbilliform rash (most common). Also, maculopapular rash, urticaria, pruritus, fever, hypotension. Rarely, polyarteritis, ***anaphylaxis,*** erythema multiforme. *Hematologic:* Leukopenia, neutropenia, eosinophilia, thrombocytopenia, ***agranulocytosis.*** *Miscellaneous:* Superinfection.

Following IV use: Thrombophlebitis, erythema, pain, swelling. IV lincomycin may cause hypotension, syncope, and ***cardiac arrest*** (rare). *Following IM use:* Pain, induration, sterile abscesses. *Following topical use:* Erythema, irritation, dryness, peeling, itching, burning, oiliness. Also, sore throat, fatigue, urinary frequency, headache.

NOTE: The injection contains benzyl alcohol, which has been associated with a fatal gasping syndrome in infants.

Drug Interactions

Antiperistaltic antidiarrheals (opiates, Lomotil) / ↑ Diarrhea due to ↓ removal of toxins from colon

Erythromycin / Cross-interference → ↓ effect of both drugs

Kaolin (e.g., Kaopectate) / ↓ Effect due to ↓ absorption from GI tract

Neuromuscular blocking agents / ↑ Effect of blocking agents

NURSING CONSIDERATIONS

See also *General Nursing Considerations for All Anti-Infectives,* Chapter 1.

Interventions

1. Be prepared to manage colitis, which can occur 2–9 days to several weeks after initiation of therapy, by providing fluids, electrolytes, protein supplements, systemic corticosteroids, and vancomycin.
2. Do not administer, and caution client against using, antiperistaltic agents if diarrhea occurs, because these agents can prolong or aggravate condition.
3. Do not use any acne or topical mercury preparations containing a peeling agent in an area affected by medication because severe irritation can occur.
4. Do not administer kaolin concomitantly with lincomycin because kaolin will reduce absorption of the antibiotic. If kaolin is required, administer 3 hr before antibiotic.
5. Observe for adverse drug interactions caused by concurrent administration of neuromuscular blocking agents. Be alert to hypotension, bronchospasms, cardiac disturbances, hyperthermia, and respiratory depression.
6. Assess for transient flushing and sensations of warmth and cardiac disturbances, which may accompany IV infusions. Monitor pulse rate before, during, and after infusion until rate is stable at levels normal for client.
7. CBC and liver function tests should be done periodically during long-term therapy.

Client/Family Teaching

1. Instruct client to take lincomycin on an empty stomach between meals and not with a sugar substitute.
2. Administer on an empty stomach to ensure optimum absorption. GI disturbances, including abdominal pain, diarrhea, anorexia, N&V, bloody or tarry stools, and excessive flatulence, should be reported as drug may need to be discontinued.

Evaluate

- Negative lab culture reports
- Resolution of infection

CHAPTER SIX

Antibiotics: Fluoroquinolones

See also the following individual entries:

Ciprofloxacin Hydrochloride
Enoxacin
Lomefloxacin Hydrochloride
Norfloxacin
Ofloxacin

Action/Kinetics: These antibiotics are synthetic, broad-spectrum antibacterial agents. The fluorine molecule confers increased activity against gram-negative organisms as well as broadens the spectrum against gram-positive organisms. These drugs act as bactericidal agents by interfering with DNA gyrase, an enzyme needed for the synthesis of bacterial DNA. Food may delay the absorption of ciprofloxacin, lomefloxacin, and norfloxacin. Both ciprofloxacin and ofloxacin may be given IV; all fluoroquinolones may be given PO.

Uses: See individual drugs; these drugs are used for a large number of gram-positive and gram-negative infections. Generally ciprofloxacin and ofloxacin are used for lower respiratory tract infections, skin and skin structure infections, and UTI. In addition ofloxacin is used for STDs and ciprofloxacin is used for bone and joint infections and infectious diarrhea. Enoxacin and norfloxacin are approved only for complicated and uncomplicated UTIs and uncomplicated urethral and cervical gonorrhea caused by *Neisseria gonorrhoeae*. Lomefloxacin has been approved for use in lower respiratory tract infections and both uncomplicated and complicated UTI.

Specific diseases for which these drugs are used include bronchitis, pneumonia (including *Legionella* and *Mycoplasma*), prostatitis, osteomyelitis, traveler's diarrhea, gonorrheal cervicitis or urethritis, prophylaxis in urological surgery, pelvic inflammatory disease, otitis media, septic arthritis, sinusitis, bacterial meningitis, bacteremia (both pseudomonal and staphylococcal), and endocarditis.

Contraindications: Hypersensitivity to the quinolone group of antibiotics, including cinoxacin and nalidixic acid. Lactation. Use in children less than 18 years of age.

Special Concerns: Lower doses are necessary in impaired renal function. Evidence suggests there may be differences in CNS toxicity between the various fluoroquinolones.

Side Effects: See individual drugs. The following side effects are common to each of the fluoroquinolone antibiotics. *GI:* N&V, diarrhea, abdominal pain or discomfort, dry or painful mouth, heartburn, dyspepsia, flatulence, constipation, pseudomembranous colitis. *CNS:* Headache, dizziness, malaise, lethargy, fatigue, drowsiness, somnolence, depression, insomnia, ***seizures,*** paresthesia. *Dermatologic:* Rash, photosensitivity, pruritus (except for ciprofloxacin). *Hypersensitivity reactions:* Facial or ***pharyngeal edema,*** dyspnea, urticaria, itching, tingling, loss of consciousness, ***CV collapse.*** *Other:* Visual disturbances and ophthalmologic abnormalities, hearing loss, superinfection, phototoxicity, eosinophilia, crystalluria. Fluoroquinolones, except norfloxacin, may also cause vaginitis, syncope, chills, and edema.

Symptoms of Overdose: Extension of side effects.

Drug Interactions

Antacids / ↓ Serum levels of fluoroquinolones due to ↓ absorption from the GI tract
Anticoagulants / ↑ Effect of anticoagulant
Antineoplastic agents / ↓ Serum levels of fluoroquinolones
Cimetidine / ↓ Elimination of fluoroquinolones
Cyclosporine / ↑ Risk of nephrotoxicity
Didanosine / ↓ Serum levels of fluoroquinolones due to ↓ absorption from the GI tract
Iron salts / ↓ Serum levels of fluoroquinolones due to ↓ absorption from the GI tract
Probenecid / ↑ Serum levels of fluoroquinolones due to ↓ renal clearance
Sucralfate / ↓ Serum levels of fluoroquinolones due to ↓ absorption from the GI tract
Theophylline / ↑ Plasma levels and ↑ toxicity of theophylline due to ↓ clearance
Zinc salts / ↓ Serum levels of fluoroquinolones due to ↓ absorption from the GI tract

Laboratory Test Interferences: ↑ ALT, AST. See also individual drugs.

Dosage

See individual drugs.

NURSING CONSIDERATIONS

See also *General Nursing Considerations for All Anti-Infectives,* Chapter 1.

Administration/Storage

1. Clients should drink liberal amounts of fluids.
2. Products containing iron or zinc and antacids containing magnesium or aluminum should not be taken simultaneously or within 4 hr before or 2 hr after dosing with fluoroquinolones.
3. Enoxacin and norfloxacin should be taken 1 hr before or 2 hr after meals; ciprofloxacin and lomefloxacin may be taken without regard to meals. Ofloxacin should not be taken with food.
4. *Treatment of Overdose:* For acute overdose, vomiting should be induced or gastric lavage performed. The client should be carefully observed and, if necessary, symptomatic and supportive treatment given. Hydration should be maintained.

Assessment

1. Document indications for therapy and type and onset of symptoms.
2. Note any previous experiences with antibiotics in this class and document results.
3. Determine that baseline CBC, liver and renal function studies, and lab cultures have been performed.
4. List medications client currently prescribed noting any that may interact unfavorably.

Interventions

1. Monitor VS and I&O, and encourage increased intake of fluids.
2. Observe client closely for any evidence of adverse effects as hypersensitivity reactions may be observed even following the first dose. The drug should be discontinued at the first sign of skin rash or other allergic manifestations.
3. If phototoxicity occurs, excessive sunlight or artificial ultraviolet light should be avoided.
4. During prolonged or chronic administration of fluoroquinolones, periodic assessment of renal, hepatic, and hematopoietic function should be performed.
5. In clients receiving anticoagulants and theophyllines, monitor closely as quinolones can cause increased drug levels with toxic drug effects, including increased bleeding or seizures.

Client/Family Teaching

1. Take only as directed and preferably not with meals, as food may delay absorption (enoxacin, norfloxacin, ofloxacin).
2. Encourage adequate fluid intake (>2 L/day).

3. Advise client not to take any mineral supplements or antacids containing magnesium or aluminum concomitantly.
4. Do not perform hazardous tasks until drug effects are realized as dizziness may be experienced.
5. Describe symptoms of a hypersensitivity reaction and stress the importance of immediate reporting; instruct client to discontinue drug therapy in this event.
6. Review list of drug side effects noting those that require immediate reporting and also advise client to report any other persistent, bothersome symptoms. The most frequently reported side effects include N&V and diarrhea.
7. Review symptoms of superinfection (furry tongue, vaginal or rectal itching, diarrhea) and advise client to report if evident.
8. Wear protective clothing and sunscreens. Avoid excessive sunlight or artificial ultraviolet light; if phototoxicity occurs, discontinue the drug and report. Photosensitivity reactions may occur up to several weeks after stopping fluoroquinolone therapy.

Evaluate

- Reports of symptomatic improvement
- Clinical evidence of resolution of infection (↓ WBCs, ↓ temperature, ↑ appetite)
- Laboratory evidence of negative culture reports

Ciprofloxacin hydrochloride

(sip-row-**FLOX**-ah-sin)
Pregnancy Category: C
Ciloxan Ophthalmic, Cipro, Cipro I.V.
(Rx)

See also *Fluoroquinolones,* Chapter 6.

How Supplied: *Injection:* 10 mg/mL, 200 mg/100 mL, 400 mg/200 mL; *Ophthalmic solution:* 0.3%; *Tablet:* 250 mg, 500 mg, 750 mg

Action/Kinetics: Ciprofloxacin is effective against both gram-positive and gram-negative organisms. Rapidly and well absorbed following PO administration. Food delays absorption of the drug. **Maximum serum levels:** 1–2 hr. **t½:** 4 hr for PO use and 5–6 hr for IV use. Peak serum levels above 5 mcg/mL should be avoided. About 40%–50% of a PO dose and 50%–70% of an IV dose is excreted unchanged in the urine.

Uses: Systemic. UTIs caused by *Escherichia coli, Enterobacter cloacae, Citrobacter diversus, Citrobacter freundii, Klebsiella pneumoniae, Proteus mirabilis, Providencia rettgeri, Pseudomonas aeruginosa, Morganella morganii, Serratia marcescens, Serratia epidermidis,* and *Streptococcus faecalis. H. ducreyi* (chancroid) and gonococcal infections. Uncomplicated gonorrhea.

Lower respiratory tract infections caused by *E. coli, E. cloacae, K. pneumoniae, P. mirabilis, P. aeruginosa,* and *Haemophilus influenzae, parainfluenzae,* and *pneumoniae.*

Bone and joint infections due to *E. cloacae, P. aeruginosa,* and *S. marcescens.*

Skin and skin structure infections caused by *E. coli, E. cloacae, Citrobacter freundii, M. morganii, P. aeruginosa, P. mirabilis, Proteus vulgaris, Providencia stuartii, Staphylococcus pyogenes, Staphylococcus epidermidis,* and penicillinase- and non-penicillinase-producing strains of *Staphylococcus aureus.*

Infectious diarrhea caused by enterotoxigenic strains of *E. coli.* Also, *Campylobacter jejuni, Shigella flexneri,* and *Shigella sonnei.* Typhoid fever.

Investigational: Clients, over 14 years of age, with cystic fibrosis who have pulmonary exacerbations due to susceptible microorganisms. Malignant external otitis. In combination with rifampin and other tuberculostatics for tuberculosis.

Ophthalmic. Superficial ocular infections due to *Staphylococcus* species (including *S. aureus*), *Streptococcus* species (including *S. pneumoniae, S. pyogenes*), *E. coli, Hemophilus ducreyi, H. influenzae, K. pneumoniae, Neisseria gonorrhoeae,*

Proteus species, *Acinetobacter calcoaceticus, Enterobacter aerogenes, P. aeruginosa, S. marcescens, Chlamydia trachomatis,* and *Vibrio* species.

Dosage

• **Tablets**

UTIs.

250 mg (mild) to 500 mg (severe/complicated) q 12 hr for 7–14 days.

Chancroid

500 mg b.i.d. for 3 days.

Gonococcal infections, uncomplicated

500 mg in a single dose given with doxycycline.

Gonococcal infections, disseminated

500 mg b.i.d. to complete a full week of therapy after an initial regimen of ceftriaxone 1 g IM or IV q 24 hr for 24–48 hr after improvement begins.

Infectious diarrhea.

500 mg q 12 hr for 5–7 days.

Skin, skin structures, respiratory tract, bone and joint infections.

500 mg (mild) to 750 mg (severe or complicated) q 12 hr for 7–14 days. Treatment may be required for 4–6 weeks in bone and joint infections.

Cystic fibrosis, malignant external otitis.

750 mg b.i.d.

NOTE: Dose must be reduced in clients with a creatinine clearance less than 50 mL/min.

• **IV Infusion**

UTIs.

200 mg (mild) to 400 mg (severe or complicated) q 12 hr for 7–14 days.

Skin, skin structures, respiratory tract, bone and joint infections.

400 mg (for mild to moderate infections) q 12 hr for 7–14 days.

• **Ophthalmic Solution**

Acute infections.

Initial, 1–2 gtt q 15–30 min; **then,** reduce dosage as infection improves.

Moderate infections.

1–2 gtt 4–6 (or more) times/day.

Administration/Storage

1. Although food delays the absorption of the drug, it may be taken with or without meals. The recommended time for dosing is 2 hr after a meal.
2. Clients on theophylline or probenecid require close observation and potential medication adjustments.
3. Do not administer to children.
4. Following instillation of the ophthalmic solution, light finger pressure should be applied to the lacrimal sac for 1 min.
5. The IV solution dose should be reconstituted to 0.5–2 mg/mL and then given over a period of 60 min. To minimize discomfort and irritation, slowly infuse a dilute solution into a large vein.
6. The IV product can be diluted with 0.9% sodium chloride injection or 5% dextrose injection. Such dilutions are stable up to 14 days at refrigerated or room temperatures and should not be frozen.

Contraindications: Hypersensitivity to quinolones. Use in children. During lactation, consideration should be given either to discontinuing nursing or the drug. Ophthalmic use in the presence of dendritis keratitis, varicella, vaccinia, mycobacterial and fungal eye infections, and after removal of foreign bodies from the cornea.

Special Concerns: Safety and effectiveness of ophthalmic, PO, or IV use has not been determined in children.

Laboratory Test Interferences: ↑ ALT, AST, alkaline phosphatase, serum bilirubin, LDH, serum creatinine, BUN, serum gamma-glutamyltransferase, serum amylase, uric acid, blood monocytes, potassium, PT, triglycerides, cholesterol. ↓ H&H. Either ↑ or ↓ blood glucose, platelets.

Additional Side Effects

See also *Side Effects* for *Fluoroquinolones,* Chapter 6.

GI: N&V, abdominal pain/discomfort, diarrhea, dry/painful mouth, dyspepsia, heartburn, constipation, flatulence, pseudomembranous colitis, oral candidiasis, ***intestinal perforation,*** anorexia, GI bleeding, bad taste in mouth. *CNS:* Headache, dizziness, fatigue, lethargy, malaise, drowsiness, restlessness, insomnia, nightmares, hallucinations, tremor, lightheadedness, irritability, confusion, ataxia, mania, weakness, psychotic reactions, depression, depersonalization, seizures. *GU:* Nephritis, hematuria, cylindruria, renal failure, urinary retention, polyuria, vaginitis, urethral bleeding, acidosis, renal calculi, interstitial nephritis, vaginal candidiasis. *Skin:* Urticaria, photosensitivity, hypersensitivity, flushing, erythema nodosum, cutaneous candidiasis, hyperpigmentation, rash, paresthesia, edema (of lips, neck, face, conjunctivae, hands), angioedema, toxic epidermal necrolysis, exfoliative dermatitis, ***Stevens-Johnson syndrome.*** *Ophthalmic:* Blurred or disturbed vision, double vision, eye pain, nystagmus. *CV:* Hypertension, syncope, angina pectoris, palpitations, atrial flutter, ***MI, cerebral thrombosis,*** ventricular ectopy, ***cardiopulmonary arrest,*** postural hypotension. *Respiratory:* Dyspnea, ***bronchospasm, pulmonary embolism, edema of larynx or lungs,*** hemoptysis, hiccoughs, epistaxis. *Hematologic:* Eosinophilia, pancytopenia, leukopenia, anemia, leukocytosis, ***agranulocytosis,*** bleeding diathesis. *Miscellaneous:* Superinfections; fever; chills; tinnitus; joint pain or stiffness; back, neck or chest pain; flare-up of gout; flushing; worsening of myasthenia gravis; ***hepatic necrosis;*** cholestatic jaundice; hearing loss, dysphasia.

After ophthalmic use: Irritation, burning, itching, angioneurotic edema, urticaria, maculopapular and vesicular dermatitis, crusting of lid margins, conjunctival hyperemia, bad taste in mouth, corneal staining, keratitis, keratopathy, allergic reactions, photophobia, decreased vision, tearing, lid edema. Also, a white, crystalline precipitate in the superficial part of corneal defect (onset within 1–7 days after initiating therapy; lasts about 2 weeks and does not affect continued use of the medication).

Additional Drug Interactions
Azlocillin / ↓ Excretion of ciprofloxacin → possible ↑ effect
Caffeine / ↓ Excretion of caffeine → ↑ pharmacologic effects
Cyclosporine / ↑ Nephrotoxic effect of cyclosporine
Hydantoins / ↓ Phenytoin serum levels

NURSING CONSIDERATIONS

See also *Nursing Considerations* for *Fluoroquinolones,* Chapter 6.

Assessment

1. Determine age. Not for use in children under 18 as irreversible collagen destruction has been noted.
2. Note medications currently prescribed. Fatal reactions have been reported in clients receiving concurrent administration of IV ciprofloxacin and theophylline.

Client/Family Teaching

1. Take medication 2 hr after meals because food may delay absorption.
2. Avoid ingestion of antacids containing magnesium or aluminum within 2 hr of taking drug because antacids may also interfere with absorption.
3. Stress the importance of drinking increased amounts of fluids (2–3 L/day) and keeping the urine acidic to minimize the risk of crystalluria.
4. The medication may cause dizziness; use caution in any activity that requires mental alertness or coordination.
5. Report any persistent GI symptoms such as diarrhea, vomiting, or abdominal pain.
6. Provide a printed list of side effects stressing those that should be reported immediately.

Evaluate:

- Improvement in symptoms of infection as evidenced by ↓ fever, ↓ WBCs, ↑ appetite
- Negative laboratory culture reports

Enoxacin

(ee-**NOX**-ah-sin)

Pregnancy Category: C
Penetrex **(Rx)**

See also *Fluoroquinolones,* Chapter 6.
How Supplied: *Tablet:* 200 mg, 400 mg
Action/Kinetics: Peak plasma levels: 0.83 mcg/mL 1–3 hr after a 200-mg dose and 2 mcg/mL 1–3 hr after a 400-mg dose. Mean peak plasma levels are 50% higher in geriatric clients than in young adults. The drug diffuses into the cervix, fallopian tubes, and myometrium at levels 1–2 times those seen in plasma and into kidney and prostate at levels 2–4 times those seen in plasma. **t½:** 3–6 hr. The drug inhibits certain isozymes of the cytochrome P-450 hepatic microsomal enzyme system, resulting in alterations of metabolism of some drugs. More than 40% is excreted unchanged through the urine.
Uses: To treat uncomplicated urethral or cervical gonorrhea due to *Neisseria gonorrhoeae.* To treat uncomplicated UTIs due *Escherichia coli, Staphylococcus epidermidis,* or *S. saprophyticus;* for complicated UTIs due to *E. coli, Klebsiella pneumoniae, Proteus mirabilis, Pseudomonas aeruginosa, S. epidermidis,* or *Enterobacter cloacae.* Not effective for syphilis.

Dosage

- **Tablets**

Uncomplicated gonorrhea.
Adults: 400 mg for one dose.
Uncomplicated UTIs, cystitis.
Adults: 200 mg q 12 hr for 7 days.
Complicated UTIs.
Adults: 400 mg q 12 hr for 14 days.
Administration/Storage
1. Should be taken 1 hr before or 2 hr after meals.
2. The dose should be adjusted in clients with a creatinine clearance of 30 mL (or less)/min/1.73 m^2. After a normal initial dose, a 12-hr interval and one-half the recommended dose should be used.
Contraindication: Lactation.
Special Concerns: Safety and efficacy have not been determined in children less than 18 years of age. Dosage adjustment is not required in elderly clients with normal renal function. Enoxacin is not efficiently removed by hemodialysis or peritoneal dialysis.
Laboratory Test Interferences: ↑ ALT, AST, alkaline phosphatase, bilirubin. Proteinuria, albuminuria.
Additional Side Effects: *GI:* Anorexia, bloody stools, gastritis, stomatitis. *CNS:* Confusion, nervousness, anxiety, tremor, agitation, myoclonus, depersonalization, hypertonia. *Dermatologic:* Toxic epidermal necrolysis, ***Stevens-Johnson syndrome,*** urticaria, hyperhidrosis, mycotic infection, erythema multiforme. *CV:* Palpitations, tachycardia, vasodilation. *Respiratory:* Dyspnea, cough, epistaxis. *GU:* Vaginal moniliasis, urinary incontinence, renal failure. *Hematologic:* Eosinophilia, leukopenia, increased or decreased platelets, decreased hemoglobin, leukocytosis. *Miscellaneous:* Glucosuria, pyuria, increased or decreased potassium, asthenia, back or chest pain, myalgia, arthralgia, purpura, vertigo, unusual taste, tinnitus, conjunctivitis.
Additional Drug Interactions
Bismuth subsalicylate / Bioavailability of enoxacin is ↓ when bismuth subsalicylate is given within 1 hr; should not use together
Digosin / ↓ Serum digoxin levels

NURSING CONSIDERATIONS

See also *General Nursing Considerations for All Anti-Infectives,* Chapter 1, and for *Fluoroquinolones,* Chapter 6.
Assessment
1. Identify source of infection and determine that appropriate cultures have been performed.
2. Obtain baseline CBC and liver and renal function studies.
3. Anticipate reduced dosage with renal dysfunction.
Client/Family Teaching
1. Take only as directed; 1 hr before or 2 hr after meals.
2. Advise clients with STDs that partners should be informed and tested so

that appropriate treatment can be instituted.
3. Provide a printed list of drug side effects and stress those that require immediate attention.

Evaluate

- Negative urethral or cervical cultures for *N. gonorrhoeae*
- Resolution of infection
- Relief of pain and burning R/T UTI

Lomefloxacin hydrochloride

(**loh**-meh-**FLOX**-ah-sin)
Pregnancy Category: C
Maxaquin **(Rx)**

See also *Fluoroquinolones*, Chapter 6.

How Supplied: *Tablet:* 400 mg

Action/Kinetics: Mean peak plasma levels: 4.2 mcg/mL after a 400-mg dose. The rate and extent of absorption is decreased if taken with food. **t½:** 8 hr. The drug is metabolized in the liver with 65% excreted unchanged through the urine and 10% excreted unchanged in the feces.

Uses: Acute bacterial exacerbation of chronic bronchitis caused by *Haemophilus influenzae* or *Morazella catarrhalis*. Uncomplicated UTIs due to *Escherichia coli*, *Klebsiella pneumoniae, Proteus mirabilis,* or *Staphylococcus saprophyticus*. Complicated UTIs due to *E. coli, K. pneumoniae, P. mirabilis, Pseudomonas aeruginosa, Citrobacter diversus,* or *Enterobacter cloacae*. Preoperatively to decrease the incidence of UTIs 3–5 days after surgery in clients undergoing transurethral procedures. *NOTE:* Not to be used for the empiric treatment of acute bacterial exacerbation of chronic bronchitis if the probable cause is *Streptococcus pneumoniae*.

Dosage

- **Tablets**

Acute bacterial exacerbation of chronic bronchitis. Cystitis. Complicated UTIs.

Adults: 400 mg once daily for 10 days.

Prophylaxis of infection before surgery for transurethral procedures.
Single 400-mg dose 2–6 hr before surgery.

Uncomplicated gonococcal infections.
400 mg as a single dose (as an alternative to ciprofloxacin or ofloxacin).

Administration/Storage

1. Can be taken without regard for meals.
2. Dosage modification is required for clients with creatinine clearance less than 40 mL/min/1.73 m^2 and more than 10 mL/min/1.73 m^2. Following an initial loading dose of 40 mg, daily maintenance doses of 200 mg should be given for the duration of treatment. Lomefloxacin levels should be performed to determine any necessary alteration in the next dosing interval. This same regimen should be followed for clients on hemodialysis.

Contraindications: Use in minor urologic procedures for which prophylaxis is not indicated (e.g., simply cystoscopy, retrograde pyelography). Use for the empiric treatment of acute bacterial exacerbation of chronic bronchitis due to *S. pneumoniae*. Lactation.

Special Concerns: Plasma clearance is reduced in the elderly. Safety and efficacy have not been determined in children less than 18 years of age. Serious hypersensitivity reactions that are occasionally fatal have occurred, even with the first dose. No dosage adjustment is needed for elderly clients with normal renal function. Lomefloxacin is not efficiently removed from the body by hemodialysis or peritoneal dialysis.

Laboratory Test Interferences: ↑ ALT, AST, alkaline phosphatase, bilirubin, BUN, gamma-glutamyltransferase. ↑ or ↓ Potassium. Abnormalities of urine specific gravity or serum electrolytes.

Additional Side Effects: *CNS:* Confusion, tremor, vertigo, nervousness, anxiety, hyperkinesia, anorexia, agitation, increased appetite, depersonalization, paranoia, ***coma.*** *GI:* GI inflammation or bleeding, dysphagia, tongue discoloration, bad taste in mouth. *GU:* Dysuria, hematuria, micturition disorder, anuria, strangury, leukorrhea, intermenstrual bleeding perineal pain, vaginal moniliasis, orchitis, epididymitis, proteinuria, albuminuria. *Hypersensitivity Reactions:* Urticaria, itching, pharyngeal or facial edema, ***CV collapse,*** tingling, loss of consciousness, dyspnea. *CV:* Hypotension, tachycardia, bradycardia, extrasystoles, cyanosis, ***arrhythmia, cardiac failure,*** angina pectoris, ***MI, pulmonary embolism, cardiomyopathy,*** phlebitis, cerebrovascular disorder. *Respiratory:* Dyspnea, respiratory infection, epistaxis, ***bronchospasm,*** cough, increased sputum, respiratory disorder, stridor. *Hematologic:* Eosinophilia, leukopenia, increase or decrease in platelets, increase in ESR, lymphocytopenia, decreased hemoglobin, anemia, bleeding, increased PT, increase in monocytes. *Dermatologic:* Urticaria, eczema, skin exfoliation, skin disorder. *Ophthalmologic:* Conjunctivitis, eye pain. *Otic:* Earache, tinnitus. *Musculoskeletal:* Back or chest pain, asthenia, leg cramps, arthralgia, myalgia. *Miscellaneous:* Increase or decrease in blood glucose, flushing, increased sweating, facial edema, influenza-like symptoms, decreased heat tolerance, purpura, lymphadenopathy, increased fibrinolysis, thirst, gout, hypoglycemia, phototoxicity.

NURSING CONSIDERATIONS

See also *General Nursing Considerations for All Anti-Infectives,* Chapter 1, and *Fluoroquinolones,* Chapter 6.

Assessment

1. Document indications for drug therapy and type and onset of symptoms.
2. Obtain baseline cultures and renal function studies. Modify dosage in clients with renal dysfunction.

Evaluate

- UTI prophylaxis during transurethral procedures
- Reports of symptomatic relief (↓ frequency and burning with UTIs)
- Improved breathing patterns with lower respiratory tract infections
- Negative lab culture reports

Norfloxacin

(nor-**FLOX**-ah-sin)

Pregnancy Category: C

Chibroxin, Noroxin Ophthalmic Solution ✱ **(Rx)**

See also *Anti-Infectives,* Chapter 1, and *Fluoroquinolones,* Chapter 6.

How Supplied: *Ophthalmic solution:* 0.3%; *Tablet:* 400 mg

Action/Kinetics: Norfloxacin manifests activity against gram-positive and gram-negative organisms by inhibiting bacterial DNA synthesis. It is not effective against obligate anaerobes. **Peak plasma levels:** 1.4–1.6 mcg/mL after 1–2 hr following a dose of 400 mg and 2.5 mcg/mL 1–2 hr after a dose of 800 mg. **t½:** 3–4.5 hr. Food decreases the absorption of norfloxacin. Approximately 30% excreted unchanged in the urine and 30% through the feces.

Uses: **Systemic:** Uncomplicated UTIs caused by *Escherichia coli, Klebsiella pneumoniae, Enterobacter cloacae, Proteus mirabilis, P. vulgaris, Pseudomonas aeruginosa, Citrobacter freundii, Staphylococcus aureus, S. epidermidis, Enterococcus faecalis, Enterobacter aerogenes, S. saprophyticus,* and *S. agalactiae.* Complicated UTIs caused by *Enterococcus faecalis, E. coli, K. pneumoniae, P. mirabilis, P. aeruginosa,* or *Serratia marcescens.* Urethral gonorrhea and endocervical gonococcal infections due to penicillinase- or non- penicillinase-producing *Neisseria gonorrhoeae.* Prostatitis.

Ophthalmic: Superficial ocular infections involving the cornea or conjunctiva due to *Staphylococcus, S. aureus, Streptococcus pneumoniae, E. coli, Haemophilus aegyptius, H. influenzae, Klebsiella pneumoniae, Neisseria gonorrhoeae, Proteus* species, *Enterobacter aerogenes, Serratia marcescens, Pseudomonas aeruginosa,* and *Vibrio* species.

Dosage

- **Tablets**

Uncomplicated UTIs due to E. coli, K. pneumoniae, or P. mirabilis.
400 mg q 12 hr for 3 days.

Uncomplicated UTIs due to other organisms.
400 mg q 12 hr for 7–10 days.

Complicated UTIs.
400 mg q 12 hr for 10–21 days. Maximum dose for UTIs should not exceed 800 mg/day.

Uncomplicated gonorrhea.
800 mg as a single dose.

Impaired renal function, with creatinine clearance equal to or less than 30 mL/min/1.73 m².
400 mg/day for 7–10 days.

- **Ophthalmic solution**

Acute infections.
Initially, 1–2 gtt q 15–30 min; **then,** reduce frequency as infection is controlled.

Moderate infections.
1–2 gtt 4–6 times/day.

Administration/Storage: Food decreases the absorption of norfloxacin; therefore, the drug should be taken 1 hr before or 2 hr after meals

Contraindications: Hypersensitivity to nalidixic acid, cinoxacin, or norfloxacin. Lactation, infants, and children. Ophthalmic use for dendritic keratitis, vaccinia, varicella, mycobacterial infections of the eye, fungal disease of the eye, and use with steroid combinations after uncomplicated removal of a corneal foreign body.

Special Concerns: Use with caution in clients with a history of seizures and in impaired renal function. Geriatric clients eliminate norfloxacin more slowly.

Laboratory Test Interferences: ↑ AST, ALT, alkaline phosphatase, BUN, serum creatinine, and LDH.

Side Effects: See also *Side Effects for Fluoroquinolones,* Chapter 6.

GI: Nausea, vomiting, diarrhea, abdominal pain or discomfort, dry/painful mouth, dyspepsia, flatulence, constipation, pseudomembranous colitis, stomatitis. *CNS:* Headache, dizziness, fatigue, malaise, drowsiness, depression, insomnia, confusion, psychoses. *Hematologic:* Decreased hematocrit, eosinophilia, leukopenia, neutropenia, either increased or decreased platelets. *Dermatologic:* Photosensitivity, rash, pruritus, exfoliative dermatitis, ***toxic epidermal necrolysis,*** erythema, erythema multiforme, ***Stevens-Johnson syndrome.*** *Other:* Paresthesia, hypersensitivity, fever, visual disturbances, hearing loss, crystalluria, cylindruria, candiduria, myoclonus (rare), hepatitis, pancreatitis, arthralgia.

Following ophthalmic use: Conjunctival hyperemia, photophobia, chemosis, bitter taste in mouth.

Additional Drug Interaction: Nitrofurantoin ↓ antibacterial effect of norfloxacin.

NURSING CONSIDERATIONS

See also *Nursing Considerations for Fluoroquinolones,* Chapter 6.

Assessment

1. Document indications for therapy and type and onset of symptoms.
2. Note any history of seizure disorder or impaired renal function and anticipate reduced dosage with impaired renal function.
3. Obtain baseline CBC and appropriate cultures prior to initiating therapy.
4. Determine if client is pregnant. The drug is not for use in pregnant women or in children.

Client/Family Teaching

1. The medication should be taken 1 hr before or 2 hr after meals, with a glass of water.
2. Advise taking at evenly spaced intervals, generally every 12 hr.
3. Antacids should not be taken with or for 2 hr after a dose of norfloxacin.
4. To prevent crystalluria, clients should be well hydrated. Encourage fluid intake of 2–3 L/day unless contraindicated.
5. Use caution if operating equipment or driving a motor vehicle because the drug may cause dizziness.
6. Advise females of childbearing age to practice contraception during drug therapy.
7. Avoid prolonged sun exposure and wear sunglasses, protective

clothing, and a sunscreen to prevent photosensitivity reactions.

Evaluate

- Negative lab culture reports
- Reports of symptomatic improvement (with UTI: ↓ dysuria, hematuria, and frequency; with ophthalmic use: ↓ itching, burning, and discharge).

Ofloxacin

(oh-**FLOX**-ah-zeen)
Pregnancy Category: C
Floxin, Floxin I.V., Ocuflox **(Rx)**

See also *Anti-Infectives,* Chapter 1 and *Fluoroquinolones,* Chapter 6.

How Supplied: *Injection:* 4 mg/mL, 20 mg/mL, 40 mg/mL; *Ophthalmic solution:* 0.3%; *Tablet:* 200 mg, 300 mg, 400 mg

Action/Kinetics: Ofloxacin has activity against a wide range of gram-positive and gram-negative aerobic and anaerobic bacteria. The production of penicillinase should have no effect on the activity of ofloxacin. The drug is widely distributed to body fluids. **Maximum serum levels:** 1–2 hr. **t½, first phase:** 5–7 hr; **second phase:** 20–25 hr. **Peak serum levels at steady state, after PO doses:** 1.5 mcg/mL after 200-mg doses, 2.4 mcg/mL after 300-mg doses, and 2.9 mcg/mL after 400-mg doses. **Peak serum levels after IV doses:** 2.7 mcg/mL after 200-mg dose and 4 mcg/mL after 400-mg dose. Between 70% and 80% is excreted unchanged in the urine.

Uses: Systemic: Pneumonia or acute bacterial exacerbations of chronic bronchitis due to *Haemophilus influenzae* or *Streptococcus pneumoniae*. Not a drug of first choice in the treatment of presumed or confirmed pneumococcal pneumonia. Not effective for syphilis.

Acute, uncomplicated urethral and cervical gonorrhea due to *Neisseria gonorrhoeae;* nongonococcal urethritis, and cervicitis due to *Chlamydia trachomatis*. Mixed infections of the urethra and cervix due to *N. gonorrhoeae* and *C. trachomatis*.

Mild to moderate skin and skin structure infections due to *Staphylococcus aureus, Streptococcus pyogenes,* or *Proteus mirabilis*.

Uncomplicated cystitis due to *Citrobacter diversus, Enterobacter aerogenes, E. coli, Klebsiella pneumoniae, Proteus mirabilis,* or *Pseudomonas aeruginosa*. Complicated UTIs due to *Escherichia coli, K. pneumoniae, P. mirabilis, C. diversus,* or *P. aeruginosa*. Prostatitis due to *E. coli*.

IV therapy is indicated when the client is unable to take PO medication.

Ophthalmic: Treatment of conjunctivitis caused by *S. aureus, Staphylococcus epidermidis, S. pneumoniae, Enterobacter cloacae, H. influenzae, P. mirabilis,* and *P. aeruginosa*.

Dosage

- **Tablets, IV**

Pneumonia, exacerbation of chronic bronchitis.

400 mg q 12 hr for 10 days.

Acute uncomplicated gonorrhea.

One 400-mg dose. The Centers for Disease Control also recommend adding doxycycline.

Cervicitis/urethritis due to C. trachomatis or N. gonorrhoeae.

300 mg q 12 hr for 7 days.

Mild to moderate skin and skin structure infections.

400 mg q 12 hr for 10 days.

Cystitis due to E. coli or K. pneumoniae.

200 mg q 12 hr for 3 days.

Cystitis due to other organisms.

200 mg q 12 hr for 7 days.

Complicated UTIs.

200 mg q 12 hr for 10 days.

Prostatitis.

300 mg q 12 hr for 6 weeks.

Chlamydia.

300 mg PO b.i.d. for 7 days.

Epididymitis.

300 mg PO b.i.d. for 10 days.

Pelvic inflammatory disease, outpatient.

400 mg PO b.i.d. for 14 days plus clindamycin or metronidazole.

NOTE: The dose should be adjusted in clients with a creatinine clearance of 50 mL/min or less. If the creatinine clearance is 10–50 mL/min, the dosage interval should be q 24 hr, and if creatinine clearance is less than 10 mL/min, the dose should be half the recommended dose given q 24 hr.

• **Ophthalmic Solution (0.3%)**
Conjunctivitis.

Initial: 1–2 gtt in the affected eye(s) q 2–4 hr for the first 2 days; **then,** 1–2 gtt q.i.d. for five additional days.

Administration/Storage

1. The drug should not be taken with food.
2. The drug should be stored in tightly closed containers at a temperature below 30°C (86°F).
3. The ophthalmic solution should not be injected subconjunctivally and it should not be introduced directly into the anterior chamber of the eye.
4. Care should be taken so that the ophthalmic applicator tip does not get contaminated with material from the eye, fingers, or other sources.
5. For IV use, give slowly over a period of time not less than 60 min; not to be given by rapid or bolus IV infusion.
6. The IV product must be diluted prior to use to a final concentration of 4 mg/mL. The following solutions may be used for dilution: 0.9% sodium chloride; 5% dextrose; 5% dextrose and 0.9% sodium chloride; 5% dextrose in lactated Ringer's; 5% sodium bicarbonate; Plasma-Lyte 56 in 5% dextrose; 5% dextrose, 0.45% sodium chloride, and 0.15% KCl; sodium lactate (M/6); water for injection. Infuse slowly, over 1 hr.
7. Oflaxacin in premixed bottles or flexible containers does not have to be diluted further as it is already premixed in 5% dextrose. The premixed product should be stored at 25°C or less (77°F).
8. The drug should be protected from excessive heat, freezing, and light.

Contraindications: Hypersensitivity to quinolone antibacterial agents. Use during lactation. Use for syphilis (ineffective). Ophthalmic use in dendritic keratitis, vaccinia, varicella, mycobacterial infections of the eye, fungal diseases of the eye, and with steroid combinations after uncomplicated removal of a corneal foreign body.

Special Concerns: Safety and effectiveness of the systemic forms have not been established in children, adolescents under the age of 18 years, pregnant women, and lactating women. Safety and effectiveness of the ophthalmic form have not been established in children less than 1 year of age. Use with caution in clients with known or suspected CNS disorders such as severe cerebral atherosclerosis, epilepsy, or factors that predispose to seizures. The effectiveness of the IV dosage form in treating severe infections has not been determined.

Laboratory Test Interferences: ↑ ALT, AST.

Side Effects: See also *Side Effects* for *Fluroquinolones,* Chapter 6.

*GI:*Nausea, diarrhea, vomiting, abdominal pain or discomfort, dry or painful mouth, dyspepsia, flatulence, constipation, pseudomembranous colitis, dysgeusia, decreased appetite. *CNS:* Headache, dizziness, fatigue, malaise, somnolence, depression, insomnia, seizures, sleep disorders, nervousness, anxiety, cognitive change, dream abnormality, euphoria, hallucinations, vertigo. *CV:* Chest pain, edema, hypertension, palpitations, vasodilation. *Hypersensitivity reactions:* Dyspnea, ***anaphylaxis.*** *GU:* External genital pruritus in women, vaginitis, vaginal discharge; burning, irritation, pain, and rash of the female genitalia; glucosuria, proteinuria, hematuria, pyuria, dysmenorrhea, menorrhagia, metrorrhagia, urinary frequency or pain. *Respiratory:* Cough, rhinorrhea. *Dermatologic:* Diaphoresis, vasculitis, photosensitivity, rash, pruritus. *Hematologic:* Leukocytosis, lymphocytopenia, eosinophilia. *Musculoskeletal:* Asthenia, extremity pain, arthralgia, myalgia, possibility of osteochondrosis. *Miscellaneous:* Chills, malaise, syncope, hyperglycemia or hypoglycemia, whole body pain, thirst, weight loss, photophobia, trunk pain, paresthesia, visual disturbances, hypersensitivity, hearing loss, fever.

After ophthalmic use: Transient ocular burning or discomfort, stinging, redness, itching, photophobia, tearing, and dryness.

NURSING CONSIDERATIONS

See also *Nursing Considerations* for *Fluoroquinolones,* Chapter 6.

Assessment

1. Note any client history of hypersensitivity to quinolone derivatives.
2. Document indications for therapy and type and onset of symptoms.
3. Determine that baseline CBC and liver and renal function studies as well as necessary cultures have been performed prior to administering drug.
4. Assess client and history carefully and document any evidence of CNS disorders.

Interventions

1. Anticipate reduced dosage with altered renal function. Review other prescribed agents; probenecid may block tubular excretion.
2. Perform C&S studies throughout therapy to assess for any evidence of bacterial resistance.
3. Observe client with CNS disorders closely. Document and report any evidence of CNS effects such as tremors, restlessness, confusion, and hallucinations as drug therapy may need to be discontinued.

Client/Family Teaching

1. Do not take with food. Take oral medication 1 hr before or 3 hr after meals.
2. Do not take any vitamins, iron or mineral combinations, or aluminum- or magnesium-based antacids for 2 hr before or 2 hr after ingestion of ofloxacin.
3. Do not perform activities that require mental alertness until drug effects are realized as drug may cause drowsiness and lightheadedness.
4. Review appropriate method for eye administration and have client demonstrate technique.
5. Advise that after ophthalmic use client may experience burning, stinging, itching, or tearing but this should subside.
6. Drink 2–3 L/day of fluids to assist in drug elimination.
7. Most common side effects include N&V and diarrhea. Provide a printed list of drug side effects stressing those that require immediate reporting.
8. Avoid direct sunlight as a photosensitivity reaction may occur. If exposure is necessary, wear sunglasses, protective clothing, and sunscreens.
9. Clients with diabetes should monitor their blood sugars closely during drug therapy as extreme variations may occur.

Evaluate

- Negative culture reports
- Reports of symptomatic improvement

CHAPTER SEVEN

Antibiotics: Macrolides (Including Erythromycins)

See also the following individual entries:

Azithromycin
Clarithromycin
Erythromycin Base
Erythromycin Estolate
Erythromycin Ethylsuccinate
Erythromycin Lactobionate
Erythromycin Stearate

Action/Kinetics: The erythromycins are produced by strains of *Streptomyces erythraeus* and have bacteriostatic and bactericidal activity (at high concentrations or if microorganism is particularly susceptible). The erythromycins are considered to be macrolide antibiotics.

The erythromycins inhibit protein synthesis of microorganisms by binding reversibly to a ribosomal subunit (50S), thus interfering with the transmission of genetic information and inhibiting protein synthesis. The drugs are effective only against rapidly multiplying organisms. The erythromycins are absorbed from the upper part of the small intestine. Erythromycins for PO use are manufactured in enteric-coated or film-coated forms to prevent destruction by gastric acid. Erythromycin is approximately 70% bound to plasma proteins and achieves concentrations in body tissues about 40% of those in the plasma. Erythromycin diffuses into body tissues; peritoneal, pleural, ascitic, and amniotic fluids; saliva; through the placental circulation; and across the mucous membrane of the tracheobronchial tree. It diffuses poorly into spinal fluid, although penetration is increased in meningitis. Alkalinization of the urine (to pH 8.5) increases the gram-negative antibacterial action. **Peak serum levels: PO,** 1–4 hr. **t½:** 1.5–2 hr, *but prolonged in clients with renal impairment.* The drug is partially metabolized by the liver and primarily excreted in bile. Erythromycins are also excreted in breast milk. The strength of erythromycin products is based on erythromycin base equivalents. Many erythromycins are available in ointments and solutions for ophthalmic, otic, and dermatologic use.

Uses

1. Upper respiratory tract infections due to *Streptococcus pyogenes* (group a beta-hemolytic streptococci), *Streptococcus pneumoniae,* and *Haemophilus influenzae* (combined with sulfonamides).
2. Mild to moderate lower respiratory tract infections due to *S. pyogenes* and *S. pneumoniae.* Respiratory tract infections due to *Mycoplasma pneumoniae.*
3. Pertussis (whooping cough) caused by *Bordetella pertussis;* may also be used as prophylaxis of pertussis in exposed individuals.
4. Mild to moderate skin and skin structure infections due to *S. pyogenes* and *Staphylococcus aureus.*
5. As an adjunct to antitoxin in diphtheria (caused by *Corynebacterium diphtheriae*), to prevent carriers, and to eradicate the organism in carriers.
6. Intestinal amebiasis due to *Enta-*

moeba histolytica (PO erythromycin only).
7. Acute pelvic inflammatory disease due to *Neisseria gonorrhoeae.*
8. Erythrasma due to *Corynebacterium minutissimum.*
9. *Chlamydia trachomatis* infections causing urogenital infections during pregnancy, conjunctivitis in the newborn, or pneumonia during infancy. Also, uncomplicated chlamydial infections of the urethra, endocervix, or rectum in adults (when tetracyclines are contraindicated or not tolerated).
10. Nongonococcal urethritis caused by *Ureaplasma urealyticum* when tetracyclines are contraindicated or not tolerated.
11. Legionnaires' disease due to *Legionella pneumophilia.*
12. As an alternative to penicillin (in penicillin-sensitive clients) to treat primary syphilis caused by *Treponema pallidum.*
13. Prophylaxis of initial or recurrent attacks of rheumatic fever in clients allergic to penicillin or sulfonamides.
14. Infections due to *Listeria monocytogenes.*
15. Bacterial endocarditis due to alpha-hemolytic streptococci, Viridans group, in clients allergic to penicillins.

Investigational: Infections due to *N. gonorrhoeae,* including uncomplicated urethral, rectal, or endocervical infections and disseminated gonococcal infections (including use in pregnancy). Severe or prolonged diarrhea due to *Campylobacter jejuni.* Genital, inguinal, or anorectal infections due to *Lymphogranuloma venereum.* Chancroid due to *Haemophilus ducreyi.* Primary, secondary, or early latent syphilis due to *T. pallidum.* Erythromycin base used with PO neomycin prior to elective colorectal surgery to reduce wound complications. As an alternative to penicillin to treat anthrax, Vincent's gingivitis, erysipeloid, actinomycosis, tetanus, with a sulfonamide to treat *Nocardia* infections, infections due to *Eikenella corrodens,* and *Borrelia* infections (including early Lyme disease).

Contraindications: Hypersensitivity to erythromycin; in utero syphilis.

Special Concerns: Use with caution in liver disease and during lactation. Use may result in bacterial and fungal overgrowth (i.e., superinfection).

Side Effects: Erythromycins have a low incidence of side effects (except for the estolate salt). *GI* (most common): N&V, diarrhea, cramping, abdominal pain, stomatitis, anorexia, melena, heartburn, pruritus ani, pseudomembranous colitis. *Allergic:* Skin rashes with or without pruritus, bullous fixed eruptions, urticaria, eczema, ***anaphylaxis*** (rare). *CNS:* Fear, confusion, altered thinking, uncontrollable crying or hysterical laughter, feeling of impending loss of consciousness. *CV:* Rarely, ventricular arrhythmias, including ***ventricular tachycardia and torsades de pointes in clients with prolonged QT intervals.*** *Miscellaneous:* Superinfection, hepatotoxicity, ototoxicity. *Following topical use:* Itching, burning, irritation, or stinging of skin. Dry, scaly skin.

IV use may result in venous irritation and thrombophlebitis; IM use produces pain at the injection site, with development of necrosis or sterile abscesses.

Symptoms of Overdose: N&V, diarrhea, epigastric distress, acute pancreatitis (mild), hearing loss (with or without tinnitus and vertigo).

Drug Interactions

Alfentanil / ↓ Excretion of alfentanil → ↑ effect
Anticoagulants / ↑ Anticoagulant effect → possible hemorrhage
Astemizole / Serious CV side effects, including torsades de pointes and other ventricular arrhythmias (including QT interval prolongation), cardiac arrest, and death
Bromocriptine / ↑ Serum levels of bromocriptine → ↑ pharmacologic and toxic effects
Carbamazepine / ↑ Effect (and tox-

icity requiring hospitalization and resuscitation) of carbamazepine due to ↓ breakdown by liver
Cyclosporine / ↑ Effect of cyclosporine due to ↓ excretion (possibly with renal toxicity)
Digoxin / Erythromycin ↑ bioavailability of digoxin
Disopyramide / ↑ Plasma levels of disopyramide → arrhythmias and ↑ QTc intervals
Ergot alkaloids / Acute ergotism manifested by peripheral ischemia
Lincosamides / Drugs antagonize each other
Methylprednisolone / ↑ Effect of methylprednisolone due to ↓ breakdown by liver
Penicillin / Erythromycins either ↓ or ↑ effect of penicillins
Sodium bicarbonate / ↑ Effect of erythromycin in urine due to alkalinization
Terfenadine / Serious CV side effects, including torsades de pointes and other ventricular arrhythmias (including QT interval prolongation), cardiac arrest, and death
Theophyllines / ↑ Effect of theophylline due to ↓ breakdown in liver; ↓ erythromycin levels may also occur
Triazolam / ↑ Bioavailability of triazolam → ↑ CNS depression
Laboratory Test Interferences: False + or ↑ values of urinary catecholamines, urinary steroids, and AST and ALT.

Dosage

PO and IM (painful); some preparations can be given IV. See individual drugs.

NURSING CONSIDERATIONS

See also *General Nursing Considerations for All Anti-Infectives,* Chapter 1.
Administration/Storage
1. Inject deep into muscle mass. Injections are painful and irritating.
2. *Treatment of Overdose:* Induce vomiting. General supportive measures. Allergic reactions should be controlled with conventional therapy.
Assessment
1. Note if client is allergic to any other antibiotics or to other allergens.
2. Document indications for therapy, type and onset of symptoms, other agents used, and the outcome.
3. Ensure that appropriate cultures have been performed prior to initiating therapy.
4. Determine that baseline hematologic profile and liver and renal function studies have been performed, if prolonged therapy is anticipated.
5. Assess for skin reactions when using erythromycin ointment. Plan to discontinue therapy and report if reactions are evident.
6. When using ophthalmic solutions, assess for mild reaction which, although usually transient, should be reported.
7. If also prescribed oral anticoagulants, digoxin, and theophyllines, monitor closely because erythromycins can inhibit cytochrome P-450 and enhance effects of these drugs.
Interventions
1. Do not administer with or immediately prior to ingestion of fruit juice or other acidic drinks because acidity may decrease activity of drug. However, adequate water (up to 8 oz) should be consumed with each dose.
2. Do not routinely administer PO medication with meals because food decreases the absorption of most erythromycins. However, provider may order medication to be given with food to reduce GI irritation.
3. Instill otic solutions at room temperature. Gently pull pinna of ear down and back for children under 3 years of age; pull pinna of ear up and back for clients over 3 years of age.
4. Observe for evidence of impaired liver function, especially among the elderly. Review appropriate lab data.
5. Note any evidence of hearing loss, which is usually temporary.
Client/Family Teaching
1. May take with food to diminish GI upset. Advise to take only as directed and to complete the entire course of therapy, despite feeling better.
2. If tablets are not coated, advise to take them 2 hr after meals. Do not take erythromycins with juices. Ex-

plain that stomach acid destroys the erythromycin base thus it must be administered with an enteric coating.
3. Doses of erythromycins should be evenly spaced throughout a 24-hr period.
4. Question clients to ensure they are eating a balanced diet and that fluid intake is adequate (>2 L/day).
5. If nausea is intolerable, notify provider so the prescription can be changed to coated tablets that can be taken with meals.
6. Review symptoms of superinfection, such as furry tongue, vaginal itching, rectal itching, or diarrhea and advise to report.
7. Stress that any evidence of rash, yellow discoloration of skin or eyes, or any irritation of the mouth or tongue should be reported.
8. Advise clients with diabetic gastric paresis that erythromycin may increase GI motility.
9. With topical use, remind client to clean affected area before applying ointment.
10. Advise to instill otic solutions at room temperature. Demonstrate the appropriate method for administration and have client/family return demonstrate.

Evaluate

- Clinical evidence of resolution of infection (negative lab culture reports, ↓ temperature, evidence of wound healing, ↓ WBCs, improved appetite)
- Reports of symptomatic improvement

Azithromycin

(az-**zith**-roh-**MY**-sin)
Pregnancy Category: B
Zithromax **(Rx)**

See also *Macrolides,* Chapter 7.
How Supplied: *Capsule:* 250 mg
Action/Kinetics: Azithromycin is an azalide antibiotic (subclass of macrolides) derived from erythromycin. The drug acts by binding to the 50S ribosomal subunit of susceptible organisms, thus interfering with microbial protein synthesis. It is rapidly absorbed and distributed widely throughout the body. Food decreases the absorption of azithromycin. **$t^{1/2}$, terminal:** 68 hr. A loading dose will achieve steady-state levels more quickly. The major route of elimination is biliary excretion of unchanged drug with a small amount being excreted through the kidneys.
Uses: Mild to moderate infections in clients 16 years of age or older as described below. Acute bacterial exacerbations of COPD due to *Hemophilus influenzae, Moraxella catarrhalis,* or *Streptococcus pneumoniae.* Community-acquired pneumonia due to *S. pneumoniae* or *H. influenzae* in clients who can take outpatient PO therapy. As an alternative to first-line therapy to treat streptococcal pharyngitis or tonsillitis due to *Streptococcus pyogenes.* Uncomplicated skin and skin structure infections due to *Staphylococcus aureus, Staphyloccus pyogenes,* or *Streptococcus agalactiae.* Nongonococcal urethritis and cervicitis due to *Chlamydia trachomatis.*

Dosage

- **Capsules**

Upper and lower respiratory tract infections due to COPD, pneumonia, pharyngitis/tonsillitis; uncomplicated skin and skin structure infections.
Adults and children over 16 years of age: 500 mg as a single dose on day 1 followed by 250 mg once daily on days 2–5 for a total dose of 1.5 g.

Nongonococcal urethritis and cervicitis due to C. trachomatis, *chancroid, chlamydia.*
1 g given as a single dose.
Administration/Storage: The drug should be given at least 1 hr prior to a meal or at least 2 hr after a meal.
Contraindications: Hypersensitivity to azithromycin, any macrolide antibiotic, or erythromycin. In clients who are not eligible for outpatient PO therapy (e.g., known or suspect-

ed bacteremia, immunodeficiency, functional asplenia, nosocomially acquired infections, geriatric or debilitated clients).

Special Concerns: Use with caution in clients with impaired hepatic or renal function and during lactation. Safety and effectiveness have not been determined in children less than 16 years of age.Recommended doses should not be relied upon to treat gonorrhea or syphilis.

Laboratory Test Interferences: ↑ Serum CPK, potassium, ALT, GGT, AST, serum alkaline phosphatase, bilirubin, BUN, creatinine, blood glucose, LDH, and phosphate.

Side Effects: *GI:* N&V, diarrhea, loose stools, abdominal pain, dyspepsia, flatulence, melena, cholestatic jaundice, pseudomembranous colitis. *CNS:* Dizziness, headache, somnolence, fatigue, vertigo. *CV:* Chest pain, palpitations, ***ventricular arrhythmias (including ventricular tachycardia and torsades de pointes in clients with prolonged QT intervals observed with other macrolides).*** *GU:* Monilia, nephritis, vaginitis. *Allergic:* Angioedema, photosensitivity, rash. *Hematologic:* Leukopenia, neutropenia, decreased platelet count.

Drug Interactions: See also *Drug Interactions* for *Macrolides,* Chapter 7.

Aluminum- and magnesium-containing antacids will decrease the peak serum levels of azithromycin but not the total amount absorbed.

NURSING CONSIDERATIONS

See also *Nursing Considerations* for *Macrolides,* Chapter 7.

Assessment

1. Determine any history of sensitivity to erythromycins.
2. Note any previous experience with macrolide antibiotics and results.
3. Obtain baseline liver and renal function studies.
4. Determine if client is currently prescribed warfarin or theophylline. Azithromycin may cause an increase in serum concentrations of these drugs so levels should be monitored throughout therapy.
5. Obtain documentation that clients with sexually transmitted cervicitis or urethritis are tested for gonorrhea and syphilis at the time of diagnosis. Ensure that appropriate drug therapy is instituted if necessary.

Client/Family Teaching

1. Do not administer with meals because food decreases absorption.
2. Avoid ingesting aluminum- or magnesium-containing antacids simultaneously with azithromycin.
3. Notify provider if N&V or diarrhea is excessive.
4. With STDs advise client to encourage sexual partner to seek medical evaluation and treatment to prevent reinfections and stress that condoms should be used during intercourse throughout therapy.

Evaluate

- Resolution of S&S of infection
- Laboratory confirmation of negative culture reports

Clarithromycin

(klah-**rith**-roh-**MY**-sin)
Pregnancy Category: C
Biaxin **(Rx)**

See also *Macrolides,* Chapter 7.

How Supplied: *Granule for Reconstitution:* 125 mg/5 mL, 250 mg/5 mL; *Tablet:* 250 mg, 500 mg

Action/Kinetics: Clarithromycin is a macrolide antibiotic that acts by binding to the 50S ribosomal subunit of susceptible organisms, thus interfering with or inhibiting microbial protein synthesis. The drug is rapidly absorbed from the GI tract although food slightly delays the onset of absorption as well as the formation of the active metabolite but does not affect the extent of the bioavailability. **Peak serum levels:** 2 hr when fasting. **Steady-state peak serum levels:** 1 mcg/mL within 2–3 days after 250 mg q 12 hr and 2–3 mcg/mL after 500 mg q 12 hr. Clarithromycin and 14-OH clarithromycin (active metabolite) are readily distributed to body tissues and fluids. **t½, elimination:** 3–7 hr (depending on the dose) for clarithromycin and 5–6 hr for 14-OH clarithromycin. Up to 30% of a dose is excreted unchanged in the urine.

Uses: Mild to moderate infections caused by susceptible strains of the following: Pharyngitis/tonsillitis due to *Streptococcus pyogenes* and acute maxillary sinusitis due to *Saccharomyces pneumoniae*. Acute otitis media in children. Acute bacterial exacerbation of chronic bronchitis due to *Haemophilus influenzae, Moraxella catarrhalis,* or *S. pneumoniae*. Pneumonia due to *Mycoplasma pneumoniae* or *S. pneumoniae*. Uncomplicated skin and skin structure infections due to *Staphylococcus aureus* or *S. pyogenes*. The active metabolite, 14-OH clarithromycin, has significant activity (twice the parent compound) against *H. influenzae*. Disseminated mycobacterial infections due to *Mycobacterium avium* (commonly seen in AIDS clients) and *M. intracellulare*.

Dosage

- **Tablets, Oral Suspension**

Pharyngitis, tonsillitis.

250 mg q 12 hr for 10 days.

Lower respiratory tract infections.

250–500 mg q 12 hr for 7–14 days.

Acute exacerbation of chronic bronchitis due to S. pneumoniae or M. catarrhalis; pneumonia due to S. pneumoniae or M. pneumoniae; skin and skin structure infections.

250 mg q 12 hr for 7–14 days.

Acute maxillary sinusitis, acute exacerbation of chronic bronchitis due to H. influenzae.

500 mg q 12 hr for 7–14 days.

Disseminated M. avium complex.

Adults: 0.5 g b.i.d.; **children:** 7.5 mg/kg b.i.d. up to 500 mg b.i.d.

Administration/Storage

1. The drug may be given with or without meals.
2. Decreased doses or prolonging the dosing interval should be considered in clients with severe renal impairment with or without coexisting impaired hepatic function.
3. Drug may cause a bitter taste.
4. The reconstituted suspension should be shaken well before each use; it should be used within 14 days and should not be refrigerated.

Contraindications: Hypersensitivity to clarithromycin, other macrolide antibiotics, or erythromycin.

Special Concerns: Use with caution in severe renal impairment with or without concomitant hepatic impairment and during lactation. Safety and effectiveness in children less than 12 years of age have not been determined.

Laboratory Test Interferences: ↑ ALT, AST, GGT, alkaline phosphatase, LDH, total bilirubin, BUN, serum creatinine.

Side Effects: *GI:* Diarrhea, nausea, abnormal taste, dyspepsia, abdominal discomfort or pain, pseudomembranous colitis. *CNS:* Headache. *Hematologic:* Decreased WBC count, elevated PT.

Drug Interactions

See also Drug Interactions for *Macrolides,* Chapter 7.

Carbamazepine / ↑ Blood levels of carbamazepine

Theophylline / ↑ Serum levels of theophylline

NURSING CONSIDERATIONS

See also *Nursing Considerations* for *Macrolides,* Chapter 7.

Assessment

1. Note any sensitivity to erythromycin or any of the macrolide antibiotics.
2. Obtain baseline liver and renal function studies.
3. Determine that appropriate laboratory cultures are done prior to initiation of drug therapy.
4. List drugs client currently prescribed noting any potential interactions.
5. Document indications for therapy and note type and onset of symptoms.

Interventions: Monitor I&O and observe client for any evidence of persistent diarrhea. Report if evident as an antibiotic-associated colitis may be precipitated by C. difficile and require alternative management.

Evaluate

- Clinical evidence and reports of symptomatic improvement
- Laboratory evidence of negative culture reports

Erythromycin base

(eh-**rih**-throw-**MY**-sin)
Pregnancy Category: B
Capsules/Tablets: Apo-Erythro Base ✱, Apo-Erythro-EC ✱, Diomycin ✱, E-Base Caplets, E-Base Tablets, E-Mycin, Erybid ✱, Eryc, Ery-Tab, Erythromid ✱, Erythromycin Base Film-Tabs, Novo-Rythro EnCap ✱, PCE ✱, PCE Dispertab, PMS-Erythromycin, Robimycin Robitabs. **Gel, topical:** Erygel. **Ointment, topical:** Akne-mycin. **Ointment, ophthalmic:** AK-Mycin, Ilotycin Ophthalmic. **Pledgets:** Erycette, T-Stat. **Solution, topical:** Akne-mycin, A/T/S, EryDerm, Erymax, ETS, Mythromycin, Staticin, T-Stat **(Rx)**

See also *Macrolides,* Chapter 7, and *Anti-Infective Agents,* Chapter 1.

How Supplied: *Enteric Coated Capsule:* 250 mg; *Enteric Coated Tablet:* 250 mg, 333 mg, 500 mg; *Gel/Jelly:* 2%; *Ointment:* 2%; *Ophthalmic ointment:* 5 mg/g; *Pad:* 2%; *Solution:* 1.5%, 2%; *Swab:* 2%; *Tablet:* 250 mg, 500 mg; *Tablet, Coated Particles:* 333 mg, 500 mg

Uses: See *Macrolides,* Chapter 7. *Ophthalmic solution:* Treatment of ocular infections (along with PO therapy) due to *Streptococcus pneumoniae, Staphylococcus aureus, S. pyogenes, Corynebacterium* species, *Haemophilus influenzae,* and *Bacteroides* infections. Also prophylaxis of ocular infections due to *Neisseria gonorrhoeae* and *Chlamydia trachomatis. Topical solution:* Acne vulgaris. *Topical ointment:* Prophylaxis of infection in minor skin abrasions; treatment of superficial infections of the skin. Acne vulgaris.

Dosage

- **Delayed-Release Capsules, Enteric-Coated Tablets, Delayed-Release Tablets, Film-Coated Tablets, Suspension**

Respiratory tract infections due to Mycoplasma pneumoniae.
500 mg q 6 hr for 5–10 days (up to 3 weeks for severe infections).

Upper respiratory tract infections (mild to moderate) due to S. pyogenes *and* S. pneumoniae.
250–500 mg q.i.d. (or 20–50 mg/kg/day in divided doses) for 10 days.

Upper respiratory tract infections due to H. influenzae.
Erythromycin ethylsuccinate, 50 mg/kg/day, plus sulfisoxazole, 150 mg/kg/day, given together for 10 days.

Lower respiratory tract infections (mild to moderate) due to S. pyogenes *and* S. pneumoniae.
250–500 mg q.i.d. (or 20–50 mg/kg/day in divided doses) for 10 days.

Intestinal amebiasis due to Entamoeba histolytica.
Adults: 250 mg q.i.d. for 10–14 days; **pediatric:** 30–50 mg/kg/day in divided doses for 10–14 days.

Legionnaire's disease.
500–1,000 mg q.i.d. for 3 weeks (or 1–4 g/day in divided doses).

Bordetella pertussis.
500 mg q.i.d. for 10 days (or 40–50 mg/kg/day in divided doses for 5–14 days).

Infections due to Corynebacterium diphtheriae.
500 mg q.i.d. for 10 days.

Erythrasma.
250 mg t.i.d. for 3 weeks.

Primary syphilis.
20 g in divided doses over 10 days.

Chlamydial infections.
Infants: 50 mg/kg/day in four divided doses for 14 (conjunctivitis) to 21 (pneumonia) days; **adults:** 500 mg q.i.d. for 7 days or 250 mg q.i.d. for 14 days for urogenital infections.

Mild to moderate skin and skin structure infections due to S. pyogenes *and* S. aureus.
250–500 mg q 6 hr (or 50 mg/kg/day in divided doses—to a maximum of 4 g/day) for 10 days.

Listeria monocytogenes infections.
500 mg q 12 hr (or 250 mg q 6 hr), up to maximum of 4 g/day.

Pelvic inflammatory disease, acute N. gonorrhoeae.
Erythromycin lactobionate, 500 mg IV q 6 hr for 3 days; **then,** 250 mg erythromycin base q 6 hr for 7 days.

Alternatively for pelvic inflammatory disease, 500 mg PO q.i.d. for 10–14 days.

Prophylaxis of initial or recurrent rheumatic fever.
250 mg b.i.d.

Bacterial endocarditis due to alpha-hemolytic streptococcus.
Adults: 1 g 2 hr prior to the procedure; **then,** 500 mg 6 hr after the initial dose. **Pediatric,** 20 mg/kg 2 hr prior to the procedure; **then,** 10 mg/kg 6 hr after the initial dose.

Pneumonia of infancy, conjunctivitis of the newborn, and urogenital infections during pregnancy due to C. trachomatis.
500 mg q.i.d. for 7 days (or 250 mg q.i.d. for 14 days).

Nongonococcal urethritis due to Ureaplasma urealyticum.
500 mg q.i.d. for at least 7 days.

Erythrasma due to Corynebacterium minutissimum.
250 mg t.i.d. for 21 days.

• **Ophthalmic Ointment**

Mild to moderate infections.
0.5-in. ribbon b.i.d.–t.i.d.

Acute infections.
0.5 in. q 3–4 hr until improvement is noted.

Prophylaxis of neonatal gonococcal or chlamydial conjunctivitis.
0.2–0.4 in. into each conjunctival sac.

• **Topical Solution**

Apply morning and evening to affected areas.

• **Topical Ointment (2%)**

Apply 1–5 times/day to affected area.

Administration/Storage

1. The ophthalmic ointment should not be washed from the eyes.
2. Before applying the topical solution, the affected areas should be washed, rinsed, and dried.
3. A sterile bandage may be used with the topical ointment.
4. Food does not affect oral absorption.

Additional Contraindications: Ophthalmic use in dendritic keratitis, vaccinia, varicella, myobacterial infections of the eye, fungal diseases of the eye. Use with steroid combinations following uncomplicated removal of a corneal foreign body.

NURSING CONSIDERATIONS

See also *Nursing Considerations* for *Macrolides,* Chapter 7.

Assessment

1. Document indications for therapy and describe symptoms and onset.
2. Determine that cultures, CBC, and appropriate diagnostic studies have been performed prior to initiating therapy.

Evaluate

- Negative C&S results
- Reports of symptomatic relief
- Desired infection prophylaxis

Erythromycin estolate

(eh-**rih**-throw-**MY**-sin)
Pregnancy Category: B
Ilosone **(Rx)**

See also *Macrolides,* Chapter 7.

How Supplied: *Capsule:* 250 mg; *Suspension:* 125 mg/5 mL, 250 mg/5 mL; *Tablet:* 500 mg

Action/Kinetics: Most active form of erythromycin, with relatively long-lasting activity.

Uses: See *Macrolides,* Chapter 7.

Dosage

• **Capsules, Suspension, Tablets**

See *Erythromycin base,* p. 72. Similar blood levels are achieved using erythromycin base, estolate, or stearate.

Administration/Storage

1. Shake oral suspension well before pouring.
2. Do not store suspension longer than 2 weeks at room temperature.
3. Chewable tablets must be chewed or crushed.

Additional Contraindications: Cholestatic jaundice or preexisting liver dysfunction. Not recommended for treatment of chronic disorders such as acne or furunculosis or for prophylaxis of rheumatic fever.

Additional Side Effect: Hepatotoxicity.

NURSING CONSIDERATIONS

See also *Nursing Considerations* for *Macrolides,* Chapter 7.

Assessment

1. Document indications for therapy and onset of symptoms.
2. Note any evidence of liver dysfunction.

Evaluate: Resolution of infection.

Erythromycin ethylsuccinate

(eh-**rih**-throw-**MY**-sin)
Pregnancy Category: B
Apo-Erythro-ES, E.E.S. 200 and 400, E.E.S. Granules, EryPed, EryPed 200, EryPed 400, EryPed Drops **(Rx)**

See also *Macrolides,* Chapter 7.

How Supplied: *Chew Tablet:* 200 mg; *Granule for Reconstitution:* 100 mg/2.5 mL, 200 mg/5 mL, 400 mg/5 mL; *Suspension:* 200 mg/5 mL, 400 mg/5 mL; *Tablet:* 400 mg

Uses: See *Macrolides,* Chapter7.

Dosage

• Oral Suspension, Tablets, Chewable Tablets

See *Erythromycin base,* p. 72. *NOTE:* 400 mg of erythromycin ethylsuccinate will achieve the same blood levels of erythromycin as 250 mg of the base, estolate, or stearate forms.

Hemophilus influenzae infections.

Erythromycin ethylsuccinate, 50 mg/kg/day with sulfisoxazole, 150 mg/kg/day, both for a total of 10 days.

Administration/Storage

1. Refrigerate aqueous suspension, and store for maximum of 1 week.
2. Chewable tablets must be chewed or crushed.

Additional Contraindication: Preexisting liver disease.

NURSING CONSIDERATIONS

See also *Nursing Considerations* for *Macrolides,* Chapter 7.

Evaluate: Resolution of infection.

Erythromycin lactobionate

(eh-**rih**-throw-**MY**-sin)
Pregnancy Category: B
Erythrocin Lactobionate IV **(Rx)**

See also *Macrolides,* Chapter 7.

How Supplied: *Powder for injection:* 500 mg, 1 g

Uses: For seriously ill or vomiting clients with infections caused by susceptible organisms; acute pelvic inflammatory disease due to gonorrhea. Legionnaire's disease.

Dosage

• IV

Adults and children: 15–20 mg/kg/day up to 4 g/day in severe infections.

Acute pelvic inflammatory disease caused by gonorrhea.

500 mg q 6 hr for 3 days followed by 250 mg erythromycin stearate, **PO,** q 6 hr for 7 days.

Legionnaire's disease.

1–4 g/day in divided doses. Change to PO therapy as soon as possible.

Administration/Storage

1. Sterile water for injection is the preferred diluent. However, 5% dextrose injection or 5% dextrose and lactated Ringer's injection may also be used provided that they are first buffered with 4% sodium bicarbonate injection.
2. For intermittent IV administration, solution may be further diluted in 100 to 250 mL of D5/W or NSS and infused over 20–60 min.
3. The initial reconstituted solution is stable for 2 weeks if refrigerated or for 24 hr at room temperature. However, the final diluted solution should be given within 8 hr. The reconstituted piggyback vial should be used within 24 hr if stored in the refrigerator or 8 hr if stored at room temperature.
4. If the reconstituted solution is frozen, it can be stored for 30 days. Once thawed, it should be used within 8 hr. A thawed solution should not be refrozen.

Additional Side Effect: Transient deafness.

Additional Drug Interaction: Some physicians recommend that no drugs be added to IV solutions of erythromycin lactobionate.

NURSING CONSIDERATIONS

See also *Nursing Considerations* for *Macrolides,* Chapter 7.

Assessment

1. Document indications for therapy, noting type and onset of symptoms.
2. Obtain baseline CBC and C&S studies.
3. Assess for any hearing deficits.

Evaluate

- Resolution of infection
- Negative C&S reports

Erythromycin stearate

(eh-**rih**-throw-**MY**-sin)
Pregnancy Category: B
Apo-Erythro-S ✱, Eramycin, Erythrocin Stearate, Wyamycin S **(Rx)**

See also *Macrolides,* Chapter 7.

How Supplied: *Tablet:* 250 mg, 500 mg

Uses: See *Macrolides,* Chapter 7.

Dosage

- **Tablets, film coated**

See *Erythromycin base,* p. 72. Similar blood levels are achieved using erythromycin base, estolate, or stearate forms.

Additional Side Effects: Drug causes more allergic reactions (e.g., skin rash and urticaria) than other erythromycins. Hepatotoxicity.

NURSING CONSIDERATIONS

See also *Nursing Considerations* for *Macrolides,* Chapter 7.

Client/Family Teaching

1. Do not administer with meals because food decreases absorption.
2. Report any evidence of allergic reaction such as rash or itching.

Evaluate: Resolution of infection.

CHAPTER EIGHT

Antibiotics: Penicillins

See also the following individual entries:

- Amoxicillin
- Amoxicillin and Potassium Clavulanate
- Ampicillin Oral
- Ampicillin with Probenecid
- Ampicillin Sodium Parenteral
- Ampicillin Sodium/Sulbactam Sodium
- Bacampicillin Hydrochloride
- Carbenicillin Indanyl Sodium
- Cloxacillin Sodium
- Dicloxacillin Sodium
- Methicillin Sodium
- Mezlocillin Sodium
- Nafcillin Sodium
- Oxacillin Sodium
- Penicillin G Benzathine, Parenteral
- Penicillin G, Benzathine and Procaine Combined
- Penicillin G Potassium for Injection
- Penicillin G Sodium for Injection
- Penicillin G Procaine Suspension, Sterile
- Penicillin V Potassium
- Piperacillin Sodium
- Piperacillin and Tazobactam Sodium
- Ticarcillin Disodium
- Ticarcillin Disodium and Clavulanate Potassium

Action/Kinetics: The bactericidal action of penicillins depends on their ability to bind penicillin-binding proteins (PBP-1 and PBP-3) in the cytoplasmic membranes of bacteria, thus inhibiting cell wall synthesis. Some penicillins act by acylation of membrane-bound transpeptidase enzymes, thereby preventing cross-linkage of peptidoglycan chains, which are necessary for bacterial cell wall strength and rigidity. Cell division and growth are inhibited and often lysis and elongation of susceptible bacteria occur. Penicillin is most effective against young, rapidly dividing organisms and has little effect on mature resting cells. Depending on the concentration of the drug at the site of infection and the susceptibility of the infectious microorganism, penicillin is either bacteriostatic or bactericidal. Penicillins are distributed throughout most of the body and pass the placental barrier. They also pass into synovial, pleural, pericardial, peritoneal, ascitic, and spinal fluids. Although normal meninges and the eyes are relatively impermeable to penicillins, they are better absorbed by inflamed meninges and eyes. **Peak serum levels, after PO:** 1 hr. **t½:** 30–110 min; protein binding: 20%–98% (see individual agents). The renal, cardiac, and hematopoietic functions, as well as the electrolyte balance, of clients receiving penicillin should be monitored at regular intervals. Excreted largely unchanged by the urine as a result of glomerular filtration and active tubular secretion.

Uses: See individual drugs. Depending on the penicillin, these drugs are effective against one or more of the following organisms. **Gram-positive organisms:** *Bacillus anthracis,* beta-hemolytic streptococci, *Corynebacterium diphtheriae, Listeria monocytogenes,* staphylococci, *Staphylococcus aureus,* streptococci, *Streptococcus faecalis, S. pneumoniae,* and *S. viridans.* **Gram-negative organisms:** *Acinetobacter* species, *Citrobacter* species, *Enterobacter* species, *Escherichia coli, Haemophi-*

lus influenzae, Klebsiella species, *Moraxella catarrhalis, Morganella morganii, Neisseria gonorrhoeae, Neisseria meningitidis, Proteus mirabilis, Proteus vulgaris, Providencia* species, *Providencia rettgeri, Providencia stuartii, Pseudomonas aeruginosa, Salmonella* species, *Serratia* species, *Shigella* species, and *Streptobacillus moniliformis*. **Anaerobic organisms:** *Actinomyces bovis, Bacteroides* species, *Clostridium* species, *Eubacterium* species, *Fusobacterium* species, *Peptococcus* species, *Peptostreptococcus* species, *Treponema pallidum, Veillonella* species.

Contraindications: Hypersensitivity to penicillins, imipenem, and cephalosporins. PO use of penicillins during the acute stages of empyema, bacteremia, pneumonia, meningitis, pericarditis, and purulent or septic arthritis.

Special Concerns: Use of penicillins during lactation may lead to sensitization, diarrhea, candidiasis, and skin rash in the infant. Use with caution in clients with a history of asthma, hay fever, or urticaria. Clients with cystic fibrosis have a higher incidence of side effects with broad spectrum penicillins. Safety and effectiveness of carbenicillin, piperacillin, and the beta-lactamase inhibitor/penicillin combinations (e.g., amoxicillin/potassium clavulanate, ticarcillin/ potassium clavulanate) have not been determined in children less than 12 years of age. The incidence of resistant strains of staphylococci to penicillinase-resistant penicillins is increasing. Use of prolonged therapy may lead to superinfection (i.e., bacterial or fungal overgrowth of nonsusceptible organisms).

Side Effects: Penicillins are potent sensitizing agents; it is estimated that up to 10% of the US population is allergic to the antibiotic. Hypersensitivity reactions are reported to be on the increase in pediatric populations. Sensitivity reactions may be immediate (within 20 min) or delayed (as long as several days or weeks after initiation of therapy). *Allergic:* Skin rashes (including maculopapular and exanthematous), exfoliative dermatitis, erythema multiforme (rarely, ***Stevens-Johnson syndrome***), hives, pruritus, wheezing, ***anaphylaxis,*** fever, eosinophilia, ***angioedema,*** serum sickness, ***laryngeal edema, laryngospasm, prostration, angioneurotic edema, bronchospasm, hypotension, vascular collapse, death.*** *GI:* Diarrhea (may be severe), abdominal cramps or pain, N&V, bloating, flatulence, increased thirst, bitter/unpleasant taste, glossitis, gastritis, stomatitis, dry mouth, sore mouth or tongue, furry tongue, black "hairy" tongue, bloody diarrhea, rectal bleeding, enterocolitis, pseudomembranous colitis. *CNS:* Dizziness, insomnia, hyperactivity, fatigue, prolonged muscle relaxation. Neurotoxicity including lethargy, neuromuscular irritability, ***seizures,*** hallucinations following large IV doses (especially in clients with renal failure). *Hematologic:* Thrombocytopenia, leukopenia, ***agranulocytosis,*** anemia, thrombocytopenic purpura, ***hemolytic anemia,*** granulocytopenia, neutropenia, bone marrow depression. *Renal:* Oliguria, hematuria, hyaline casts, proteinuria, pyuria (all symptoms of interstitial nephritis), nephropathy. Electrolyte imbalance following IV use. *Miscellaneous:* Hepatotoxicity (cholestatic jaundice), superinfection, swelling of face and ankles, anorexia, hyperthermia, transient hepatitis, vaginitis, itchy eyes. IM injection may cause pain and induration at the injection site, ecchymosis, and hematomas. IV use may cause vein irritation, deep vein thrombosis, and thrombophlebitis. For **emergency treatment** of severe allergic or anaphylactic reactions, administer epinephrine (0.3–0.5 mL of a 1:1,000 solution SC or IM, or 0.2–0.3 mL diluted in 10 mL saline, given slowly by IV). Corticosteroids should be on hand. In those instances where penicillin is the drug of choice, the physician may decide to use it even though the client is allergic, adding a medication to the regimen to control the allergic response.

Symptoms of Overdose: Neuromuscular hyperexcitability, convulsive seizures. Massive IV doses may cause agitation, asterixis, hallucinations, confusion, stupor, multifocal myoclonus, seizures, coma, hyperkalemia, and encephalopathy.

Drug Interactions

Aminoglycosides / Penicillins ↓ effect of aminoglycosides
Antacids / ↓ Effect of penicillins due to ↓ absorption from GI tract
Antibiotics, Chloramphenicol, Erythromycins, Tetracyclines / ↓ Effect of penicillins
Anticoagulants / Penicillins may potentiate pharmacologic effect
Aspirin / ↑ Effect of penicillins by ↓ plasma protein binding
Chloramphenicol / Either ↑ or ↓ effects
Erythromycins / Either ↑ or ↓ effects
Heparin / ↑ Risk of bleeding following parenteral penicillins
Oral contraceptives / ↓ Effect of oral contraceptives
Phenylbutazone / ↑ Effect of penicillins by ↓ plasma protein binding
Probenecid / ↑ Effect of penicillins by ↓ excretion
Tetracyclines / ↓ Effect of penicillins

Laboratory Test Interferences: ↓ Hematocrit, hemoglobin, WBC lymphocytes, serum potassium, albumin, total proteins, uric acid. ↑ Basophils, lymphocytes, monocytes, platelets, serum alkaline phosphatase, serum sodium. ↑ AST, ALT, bilirubin, LDH following semisynthetic penicillins.

Dosage

Penicillins are available in a variety of dosage forms for PO, parenteral, inhalation, and intrathecal administration. Dosages for individual drugs are given in drug entries. Long-acting preparations are frequently used. PO doses must be higher than IM or SC doses because a large fraction of penicillin given PO may be destroyed in the stomach.

NURSING CONSIDERATIONS

See also *General Nursing Considerations for All Anti-Infectives,* Chapter 1.

Administration/Storage

1. IM and IV administration of penicillin causes a great deal of local irritation. These antibiotics should thus be injected slowly.
2. IM injections are made deeply into the gluteal muscle. IV injections are usually made through the tubing of an IV infusion.

Assessment

1. Assess rigorously for allergic reactions because the incidence is higher with penicillin therapy than with other antibiotics. If a reaction occurs, the drug must be discontinued immediately. Epinephrine, oxygen, antihistamines, and corticosteroids must be immediately available.
2. Anticipate that allergic reactions are more likely to occur in clients with a history of asthma, hay fever, urticaria, or allergy to cephalosporins.

Interventions

1. Detain client in an ambulatory care site for at least 20 min after administering a penicillin injection to assess for the onset of anaphylaxis. Be prepared for prompt treatment of anaphylactic reaction.
2. Do not administer long-acting types of penicillin IV, because these types are only for IM use. They may cause emboli or CNS or cardiac pathology if administered IV.
3. Do not massage repository (long-acting) penicillin products after injection, because rate of absorption should not be increased.
4. Prevent rapid administration of IV penicillin because this method may cause local irritation and may precipitate convulsions. With some agents, high-dose therapy may precipitate aplastic anemia.
5. The elderly may be more sensitive to the effects of penicillin than are younger people. Therefore, care should be exerted when calculating the dose based on client weight and height.

6. Most penicillins are excreted in breast milk and should be prescribed cautiously to nursing mothers.

Client/Family Teaching

1. Review the drugs prescribed, the method and frequency of administration, their side effects, and the expected outcome of therapy.
2. Address the S&S of allergic reactions, i.e., rashes, fever, joint swelling, angioneurotic edema, intense itching, and respiratory distress (during therapy and in some cases 7–12 days after therapy). Instruct client to stop the medication when noted and to call someone for help immediately.
3. Oral penicillins may cause GI upset (N&V and diarrhea). Take oral penicillin with a glass of water 1 hr before or 2 hr after meals to minimize binding to foods.
4. Explain when to return for repository penicillin injections to complete treatment.
5. Instruct clients to complete the entire prescribed course of therapy, even though they may feel well. Incomplete therapy will predispose the individual to a lack of response due to the development of resistant bacterial strains. A person with alpha-hemolytic *Streptococcus* infection must continue with penicillin therapy for a minimum of 10 days, and preferably 14 days, to prevent development of rheumatic fever or glomerulonephritis.
6. Review S&S of superinfections (furry tongue, vaginal or rectal itching, diarrhea) and instruct client to report if evident.
7. Notify provider if symptoms do not improve or get worse after 24–48 hr of drug therapy.

Evaluate

- Knowledge and understanding of illness and evidence of compliance with prescribed medication therapy
- Reports of symptomatic improvement
- Clinical evidence of resolution of symptoms of infection such as ↓ fever, ↓ WBCs, ↑ appetite, and negative lab culture reports

Amoxicillin (amoxycillin)

(ah-mox-ih-**SILL**-in)

Amoxil, Amoxil Pediatric Drops, APO-Amoxi ✤, Biomox, Novamoxin ✤, Nu-Amoxi ✤, Polymox, Polymox Drops, Trimox 125, 250, and 500, Wymox **(Rx)**

See also *Anti-Infectives,* Chapter 1, and *Penicillins,* Chapter 8.

How Supplied: *Capsule:* 250 mg, 500 mg; *Chew tablet:* 125 mg, 250 mg; *Powder for reconstitution:* 50 mg/mL, 125 mg/5 mL, 250 mg/5 mL

Action/Kinetics: Semisynthetic broad-spectrum penicillin closely related to ampicillin. Destroyed by penicillinase, acid stable, and better absorbed than ampicillin. From 50% to 80% of a PO dose is absorbed from the GI tract. **Peak serum levels: PO:** 4–11 mcg/mL after 1–2 hr. **t½:** 60 min. Mostly excreted unchanged in urine.

Uses: Gram-positive streptococcal infections including *Streptococcus faecalis, S. pneumoniae,* and non-penicillinase-producing staphylococci. Gram-negative infections due to *Hemophilus influenzae, Proteus mirabilis, Escherichia coli,* and *Neisseria gonorrhoeae.*

Dosage

• **Capsules, Oral Suspension, Chewable Tablets**

Susceptible infections of ear, nose, throat, GU tract, skin and soft tissues, lower respiratory tract.

Adults: 250–500 mg q 8 hr; **pediatric under 20 kg:** 20–40 (or more) mg/kg/day in three equal doses. The pediatric dose should not exceed the maximum adult dose.

Prophylaxis of bacterial endocarditis.

3 g 60 min prior to procedure (dental, oral, or upper respiratory tract) and 1.5 g 6 hr later. Alternatively, ampicillin, 1–2 g (50 mg/kg for children) plus gentamicin, 1.5 mg/kg (2 mg/kg for children) not to exceed 80 mg, both either IM or IV 30 min before procedure followed by amoxicillin, 1.5 g (25 mg/kg for children) 6 hr after initial dose. Amoxicillin may be

given as an alternate procedure for GU or GI procedures at a dose of 3 g 1 hr before procedure followed by 1.5 g 6 hr after the initial dose.

Gonococcal infections.
3 g with probenecid, 1 g, given as a single dose. In addition, tetracycline, 0.5 mg, q.i.d. for 7 days.

Gonococcal infection in pregnancy.
3 g with probenecid, 1 g, given as a single dose. In addition, erythromycin base, 0.5 g q.i.d. for 7 days.

Disseminated gonococcal infections.
3 g with probenecid, 1 g, given as a single dose; **then,** 0.5 g q.i.d. for 7 days.

Acute pelvic inflammatory disease.
3 g with probenecid, 1 g, given as a single dose. In addition, doxycycline, 100 mg b.i.d. for 10–14 days.

Sexually transmitted epididymo-orchitis.
3 g with probenecid, 1 g, given as a single dose. In addition, tetracycline, 0.5 g q.i.d. for 10 days.

Bacterial vaginosis.
0.5 g q.i.d. for 7 days.

Chlamydia trachomatis during pregnancy (as an alternative to erythromycin).
0.5 g t.i.d. for 7 days.

Administration/Storage
1. Dry powder is stable at room temperature for 18–30 months. Reconstituted suspension is stable for 1 week at room temperature and for 2 weeks at 2°C–8°C.
2. Chewable tablets are available for pediatric use. These may be administered with food.

Special Concern: Safe use during pregnancy has not been established.

NURSING CONSIDERATIONS

See also *Nursing Considerations* for *Penicillins,* Chapter 8.

Evaluate
- Resolution of infection
- Therapeutic peak serum drug levels (4–11 mcg/mL)

—COMBINATION DRUG—

Amoxicillin and Potassium clavulanate

(ah-mox-ih-**SILL**-in, poh-**TASS**-ee-um klav-you-**LAN**-ayt)
Pregnancy Category: B
Augmentin '125', '250', and '500', Clavulin ✱ **(Rx)**

See also *Anti-Infectives,* Chapter 1, and *Penicillins,* Chapter 8.

How Supplied: See Content.

Content: Each "250" tablet contains: 250 mg amoxicillin, 125 mg potassium clavulanate. Each "500" tablet contains: 500 mg amoxicillin, 125 mg potassium clavulanate.
Each "125" chewable tablet contains: 125 mg amoxicillin, 31.25 mg potassium clavulanate. Each "250" chewable tablet contains: 250 mg amoxicillin, 62.5 mg potassium clavulanate.
"125" powder for oral suspension contains: 125 mg amoxicillin and 31.25 mg potassium clavulanate/5 mL. "250" powder for oral suspension contains: 250 mg amoxicillin and 62.5 potassium clavulanate/5 mL.

Action/Kinetics: *For details, see amoxicillin.* Potassium clavulanate inactivates lactamase enzymes, which are responsible for resistance to penicillins. Thus, this preparation is effective against microorganisms that have manifested resistance to amoxicillin. For potassium clavulanate: **Peak serum levels:** 1–2 hr. **t½:** 1 hr. *NOTE:* Both the "250" and "500" tablets contain 125 mg potassium clavulanate.

Uses: For beta-lactamase-producing strains of the following organisms: *Hemophilus influenzae* causing lower respiratory tract infections, otitis media, and sinusitis; *Staphylococcus aureus, Escherichia coli,* and *Klebsiella,* causing skin and skin structure infections; *E. coli, Klebsiella,* and *Enterobacter,* causing UTI.

Dosage
- **Oral Suspension, Chewable**

Tablets, Tablets

Susceptible infections.

Adults, usual: One "250" tablet q 8 hr; **children less than 40 kg:** 20 mg/kg/day in divided doses q 8 hr.

Respiratory tract and severe infections.

Adults: one "500" tablet q 8 hr; **children, less than 40 kg:** 40 mg/kg/day in divided doses q 8 hr (this dose is also used in children for otitis media, lower respiratory tract infections, or sinusitis).

Chancroid.

Adults: One "500" tablet t.i.d. for 7 days (alternative to erythromycin).

Disseminated gonococcal infections.

Following therapy with an appropriate cephalosporin, uncomplicated disease therapy may be completed with 1 "500" mg tablet t.i.d. for 1 week.

Administration/Storage

1. Both the "250" and "500" tablets contain 125 mg clavulanic acid; therefore, two "250" tablets are not the same as one "500" tablet.
2. The reconstituted suspension should be refrigerated and discarded after 10 days.

NURSING CONSIDERATIONS

See also *Nursing Considerations* for *Penicillins,* Chapter 8.

Evaluate

- Resolution of infecting organism
- Reports of symptomatic improvement
- Healing of venereal ulcers

Ampicillin oral

(am-pih-**SILL**-in)
Pregnancy Category: B
Ampicin ✱, APO-Ampi ✱, D-Amp, Novo-Ampicillin ✱, Nu-Ampi ✱, Omnipen, Penbritin ✱, Polycillin, Polycillin Pediatric Drops, Principen, Totacillin **(Rx)**

—COMBINATION DRUG—

Ampicillin with Probenecid

(am-pih-**SILL**-in, proh-**BEN**-ih-sid)
Ampicin-PRB ✱, Polycillin-PRB, Probampacin **(Rx)**

Ampicillin sodium, parenteral

(am-pih-**SILL**-in)
Pregnancy Category: B
Ampicin ✱, Omnipen-N, Penbritin ✱, Polycillin-N, Totacillin-N **(Rx)**

See also *Anti-Infectives,* Chapter 1, and *Penicillins,* Chapter 8.

How Supplied: Ampicillin oral: *Capsule:* 250 mg, 500 mg; *Powder for reconstitution:* 125 mg/5 mL, 250 mg/5 mL.

Ampicillin with Probenecid: See Content.

Ampicillin sodium parenteral: *Powder for injection:* 125 mg, 250 mg, 500 mg, 1 g, 2 g, 10 g

Content: Ampicillin with Probenecid: Powder for oral suspension: 3.5 g ampicillin and 1 g probenecid/bottle

Action/Kinetics: Synthetic, broad-spectrum antibiotic suitable for gram-negative bacteria. Acid resistant, destroyed by penicillinase. Absorbed more slowly than other penicillins. From 30% to 60% of PO dose absorbed from GI tract. **Peak serum levels: PO:** 1.8–2.9 mcg/mL after 2 hr; **IM,** 4.5–7 mcg/mL. **t½:** 80 min—range 50–110 min. Partially inactivated in liver; 25%–85% excreted unchanged in urine.

Uses: Infections of respiratory, GI, and GU tracts caused by *Shigella, Salmonella, Escherichia coli, Hemophilus influenzae, Proteus* strains, *Neisseria gonorrhoeae, N. meningitidis,* and *Enterococcus.* Also, otitis media in children, bronchitis, rat-bite fever, and whooping cough. Penicillin G-sensitive staphylococci, streptococci, pneumococci.

Dosage

- **Ampicillin: Capsules, Oral Suspension; Ampicillin sodium: IV, IM**

Respiratory tract and soft tissue infections.

PO: 20 kg or more: 250 mg q 6 hr; **less than 20 kg:** 50 mg/kg/day in equally divided doses q 6–8 hr. **IV, IM: 40 kg or more:** 250–500 mg q 6 hr; **less than 40 kg:** 25–50 mg/kg/day in equally divided doses q 6–8 hr.

Disseminated gonococcal infections.

PO: 1 g q 6 hr.

Bacterial meningitis.

Adults: A total of 8–12 g/day given in divided doses q 3–4 hr. **Pediatric:** 100–200 mg/kg/day in divided doses q 3–4 hr.

Bacterial endocarditis prophylaxis (dental, oral, or upper respiratory tract procedures; GI or GU tract surgery or instrumentation).

Adult, IM, IV: 1–2 g (use 2 g for GI or GU tract surgery) plus gentamicin, 1.5 mg/kg (not to exceed 80 mg) IM or IV, given 30 min before procedure followed by amoxicillin, 1.5 g, 6 hr after initial dose; or, repeat parenteral dose 8 hr after initial dose. **Pediatric:** Ampicillin, 50 mg/kg with gentamicin, 2 mg/kg 30 min prior to procedure followed by amoxicillin, 25 mg/kg, after 6 hr or a parenteral dose of ampicillin is given after 8 hr.

Septicemia.

Adults/children: 150–200 mg/kg, IV for first 3 days, then IM q 3–4 hr.

• **Ampicillin with Probenecid: Oral Suspension**

Urethral, endocervical, or rectal infections due to N. gonorrhoeae.

Adults: 3.5 g ampicillin and 1 g probenecid as a single dose.

Prophylaxis of infection in rape victims.

3.5 g with 1 g probenecid.

Administration/Storage

1. After reconstitution for IM or direct IV administration, the solution of sodium ampicillin **must be used within the hour**.
2. For IM use, dilute only with sterile water for injection or bacteriostatic water for injection.
3. For IVPB, ampicillin may be reconstituted with sodium chloride injection.
4. IV injections of reconstituted sodium ampicillin should be given slowly; 2 mL should be given over a period of at least 3–5 min.
5. For administration by IV drip, check compatibility and length of time that drug retains potency in a particular solution.
6. If the creatinine clearance is less than 10 mL/min, the dosing interval should be increased to 12 hr.

Additional Drug Interactions

Allopurinol / ↑ Incidence of skin rashes

Ampicillin / ↓ Effect of oral contraceptives

NURSING CONSIDERATIONS

See also *Nursing Considerations* for *Penicillins,* Chapter 8.

Interventions

1. Obtain and monitor liver and renal function studies.
2. When administering IM, tell the client that it will be painful. Rotate and document injection sites.
3. Monitor urinary output and serum potassium levels especially in the elderly.
4. Observe skin closely for rashes because they occur more often with this drug than with other penicillins.
5. If clients develop a skin rash, have them tested for mononucleosis because this may be the cause of the rash.
6. Observe for an "Ampicillin rash" which may develop. It is a dull red, itchy, macular or macropapular rash and is generally benign.

Client/Family Teaching

1. Take the medication 1 hr before or 2 hr after meals.
2. Teach the person administering the drug the appropriate method for administration and storage.
3. Take the drug for the prescribed number of days even if the symptoms subside.
4. Review side effects that may occur and advise to report and refrain from taking the drug until medically cleared.
5. Ampicillin chewable tablets should not be swallowed whole.

6. Do not save any of the drug for future use or share with family members or friends who may seem to have the same type of infection.
7. Drug may decrease effectiveness of oral contraceptives. Advise client to practice alternative method of contraception during this period.

Evaluate

- Resolution of S&S of infection
- Reports of symptomatic improvement
- Negative laboratory culture reports (note any evidence of resistance to drug therapy)

—COMBINATION DRUG—

Ampicillin sodium/Sulbactam sodium

(am-pih-**SILL**-in/sull-**BACK**-tam)
Pregnancy Category: B
Unasyn **(Rx)**

See also *Anti-Infectives,* Chapter 1, and *Penicillins,* Chapter 8.

How Supplied: See Content

Content: Powder for injection: 1 g ampicillin sodium and 0.5 g sulbactam sodium; 2 g ampicillin sodium and 1 g sulbactam sodium.

Action/Kinetics: For details, see *Ampicillin oral.* Sulbactam is present in this product because it irreversibly inhibits beta-lactamases, thus ensuring activity of ampicillin against beta-lactamase-producing microorganisms. Thus, sulbactam broadens the antibiotic spectrum of ampicillin to those bacteria normally resistant to it. **Peak serum levels, after IV infusion:** 15 min. **$t^1/_2$, both drugs:** about 1 hr. From 75%–85% of both drugs is excreted unchanged in the urine within 8 hr after administration.

Uses: To treat infections caused by beta-lactamase-producing strains of the following: (a) skin and skin structure infections caused by *Staphylococcus aureus, Escherichia coli, Klebsiella* species (including *K. pneumoniae*), *Proteus mirabilis, Bacteroides fragilis, Enterobacter* species, and *Acinetobacter calcoaceticus;* (b) intra-abdominal infections caused by *E. coli, Klebsiella* species (including *K. pneumoniae*), *Bacteroides* (including *B. fragilis* and *Enterobacter*) (c) gynecologic infections caused by *E. coli* and *Bacteroides* (including *B. fragilis*). *NOTE:* Mixed infections caused by ampicillin-susceptible organisms and beta-lactamase-producing organisms are susceptible to this product; thus, additional antibiotics do not have to be used.

Dosage

- **IV, IM**

Adults: 1 g ampicillin/0.5 g sulbactam to 2 g ampicillin/1 g sulbactam q 6 hr, not to exceed 4 g sulbactam daily. Doses must be decreased in renal impairment.

Administration/Storage

1. For IV use, drug can be given by slow injection over 10–15 min or, if mixed with 50–100 mL of diluent, can be given over 15–30 min.
2. For IV use, the drug can be reconstituted with any of the following: 5% dextrose injection, 5% dextrose injection in 0.45% saline, 10% invert sugar, lactated Ringer's injection, 0.9% sodium chloride injection, M/6 sodium lactate injection, or sterile water for injection.
3. For IM use, the drug can be reconstituted with sterile water for injection or 0.5% or 2% lidocaine HCl injection.
4. After reconstitution, solutions should stand so that any foaming will dissipate and the vial can be inspected visually to ensure dissolution.
5. Solutions for IM administration must be used within 1 hr after preparation.
6. If aminoglycosides are prescribed concomitantly, administer each separately (1 hr apart) because ampicillin will inactivate aminoglycosides.
7. *Treatment of Overdose:* Both ampicillin and sulbactam may be removed by hemodialysis.

Special Concerns: Safety and efficacy in children less than 12 years of age have not been established.

Laboratory Test Interferences: ↑ AST, ALT, alkaline phosphatase, LDH, creatinine, BUN; also, ↑ basophils, eosinophils, lymphocytes, monocytes, platelets. ↓ Serum albumin and total proteins, H&H, RBCs, WBCs, and platelets. Presence of RBCs and hyaline casts in urine.

Side Effects: *At site of injection:* Pain and thrombophlebitis. *GI:* Diarrhea, N&V, flatulence, abdominal distention, glossitis. *CNS:* Fatigue, malaise, headache. *GU:* Dysuria, urinary retention. *Miscellaneous:* Itching, chest pain, edema, facial swelling, erythema, chills, tightness in throat, epistaxis, substernal pain, mucosal bleeding, candidiasis.

Symptoms of Overdose: ***Neurologic symptoms, including convulsions.***

NURSING CONSIDERATIONS

See also *Nursing Considerations* for *Penicillins, Ampicillin,* Chapter 8.

Interventions

1. Anticipate reduced doses in clients with impaired renal function.
2. IM injections are extremely painful; follow manufacturer's recommendations for IM reconstitution and tell the client to expect some discomfort.
3. If clients develop a skin rash, have them tested for mononucleosis because this may be the cause of the rash.

Evaluate

- Resolution of infection
- Reports of symptomatic improvement

Bacampicillin hydrochloride

(bah-kam-pih-**SILL**-in)
Pregnancy Category: B
Penglobe ♣, Spectrobid **(Rx)**

See also *Anti-Infectives,* Chapter 1, and *Penicillins,* Chapter 8.

How Supplied: *Tablet:* 400 mg

Action/Kinetics: Bacampicillin is a semisynthetic, acid-resistant penicillin that is hydrolyzed to the active ampicillin in the GI tract. Food does not affect absorption of the drug. The drug is 98% absorbed from the GI tract and is approximately 20% plasma protein bound. **Peak serum levels:** Obtained in 0.9 hr are approximately 3 times those seen with equivalent doses of ampicillin. Seventy-five percent is excreted in the urine as active ampicillin within 8 hr.

Uses: Upper and lower respiratory tract infections caused by beta-hemolytic streptococcus, *Staphylococcus pyogenes,* pneumococci, non-penicillinase-producing staphylococci, and *Haemophilus influenzae.* UTIs caused by *Escherichia coli, Proteus mirabilis,* and enterococci. Skin infections caused by streptococci and susceptible staphylococci. Acute uncomplicated urogenital infections caused by *Neisseria gonorrhoeae.*

Dosage

- **Oral Suspension, Tablets**

Upper respiratory tract infections, otitis media, UTIs, skin and skin structure infections.

Adults (25 kg or more), 400 mg q 12 hr; **pediatric:** 25 mg/kg/day in equally divided doses q 12 hr. Dose may be doubled in cases of lower respiratory tract infections, severe infections, or in treating less susceptible organisms.

Gonorrhea.

Males and females: 1.6 g with 1 g probenecid as a single dose. No pediatric dosage has been established.

Contraindications: History of penicillin allergy. Concomitant use with disulfiram (Antabuse).

Laboratory Test Interferences: False + reaction to Clinitest, Benedict's solution, and Fehling's solution. ↑ AST.

Drug Interaction: Bacampicillin should not be used concomitantly with disulfiram.

NURSING CONSIDERATIONS

See also *General Nursing Considerations* for *Penicillins,* Chapter 8.

Client/Family Teaching

1. Take on an empty stomach unless otherwise prescribed.

2. Warn client not to start disulfiram therapy while taking bacampicillin.
3. Advise clients with diabetes to perform finger sticks to enhance accuracy of blood sugar determinations and replacement needs.
4. Advise clients also on allopurinol therapy to report any evidence of a skin rash.

Evaluate

- Negative C&S results
- Resolution of infection and reports of improvement

Carbenicillin indanyl sodium

(kar-ben-ih-**SILL**-in)
Pregnancy Category: B
Geocillin, Geopen Oral ✱ **(Rx)**

See also *Anti-Infectives,* Chapter 1, and *Penicillins,* Chapter 8.
How Supplied: *Tablet:* 382 mg
Action/Kinetics: The drug is acid stable. **Peak serum levels: PO:** 6.5 mcg/mL after 1 hr. **t½:** 60 min. Rapidly excreted unchanged in urine.
Uses: Upper and lower UTIs or bacteriuria due to *Escherichia coli, Proteus vulgaris and P. mirabilis, Morganella morganii, Providencia rettgeri, Enterobacter, Pseudomonas,* and enterococci. Prostatitis due to *E. coli, Streptococcus faecalis* (enterococci), *P. mirabilis,* and *Enterobacter* species.

Dosage

- **Tablets**

UTIs due to E. coli, Proteus, Enterobacter.
382–764 mg q.i.d.
UTIs due to Pseudomonas *and enterococci.*
764 mg q.i.d.
Prostatitis due to E. coli, P. mirabilis, Enterobacter, *and enterococci.*
764 mg q.i.d.

Administration/Storage

1. Protect from moisture.
2. Store at temperature of 30°C or less.

Additional Contraindication: Pregnancy.
Special Concerns: Safe use in children not established. Use with caution in clients with impaired renal function.
Additional Side Effect: Neurotoxicity in clients with impaired renal function.
Additional Drug Interaction: When used in combination with gentamicin or tobramycin for *Pseudomonas* infections, effect of carbenicillin may be enhanced.

NURSING CONSIDERATIONS

See also *General Nursing Considerations* for *All Anti-Infectives,* Chapter 1, and *Penicillins,* Chapter 8.

Interventions

1. Provide frequent mouth care to minimize nausea and unpleasant aftertaste.
2. Monitor renal function studies and assess client with impaired renal function for evidence of neurotoxicity, manifested by hallucinations, impaired sensorium, muscular irritability, and seizures.
3. Monitor CBC and assess for any hemorrhagic manifestations, such as ecchymosis, petechiae, and frank bleeding of gums and/or rectum.

Evaluate

- Negative laboratory C&S results
- Resolution of infection and reports of symptomatic improvement

Cloxacillin sodium

(klox-ah-**SILL**-in)
Apo-Cloxi ✱, Cloxapen, Novo-Cloxin ✱, Nu-CLoxi ✱, Orbenin ✱, Tegopen **(Rx)**

See also *Anti-Infectives,* Chapter 1, and *Penicillins,* Chapter 8.
How Supplied: *Capsule:* 250 mg, 500 mg; *Powder for Reconstitution:* 125 mg/5 mL
Action/Kinetics: Resistant to penicillinase and is acid stable. **Peak plasma levels:** 7–15 mcg/mL after 30–60 min. **t½:** 30 min. Protein binding: 88%–96%. Well absorbed from GI tract. Mostly excreted in urine, but some excreted in bile.
Uses: Infections caused by penicillinase-producing staphylococci, in-

cluding pneumococci, group A beta-hemolytic streptococci, and penicillin G-sensitive staphylococci.

Dosage

- **Capsules, Oral Solution**

Skin and soft tissue infections, mild to moderate upper respiratory tract infections.

Adults and children over 20 kg: 250 mg q 6 hr; **pediatric, less than 20 kg:** 50 mg/kg/day in divided doses q 6 hr.

Lower respiratory tract infections or disseminated infections.

Adults and children over 20 kg: 0.5 g q 6 hr; **pediatric, less than 20 kg:** 100 (or more) mg/kg/day in divided doses q 6 hr. Alternatively, a dose of 50–100 mg/kg/day (up to a maximum of 4 g/day) divided q 6 hr may be used for infants and children.

Administration/Storage

1. Add amount of water stated on label in two portions; shake well after each addition.
2. Shake well before pouring each dose.
3. Refrigerate reconstituted solution and discard unused portion after 14 days.
4. Administer 1 hr before or 2 hr after meals because food interferes with absorption of drug.

NURSING CONSIDERATIONS

See also *Nursing Considerations* for *Penicillins,* Chapter 8.

Client/Family Teaching

1. Review appropriate guidelines for administration; include frequency and amount.
2. Advise to take only as directed.
3. Stress importance of taking for the full prescribed time despite feeling better.

Evaluate

- Eradication of infection and reports of symptomatic improvement
- ↓ Fever, ↓ WBCs, ↑ appetite, and negative laboratory culture reports

Dicloxacillin sodium

(dye-klox-ah-**SILL**-in)

Dycill, Dynapen, Pathocil **(Rx)**

See also *Anti-Infectives,* Chapter 1, and *Penicillins,* Chapter 8.

How Supplied: *Capsule:* 125 mg, 250 mg, 500 mg; *Powder for reconstitution:* 62.5 mg/5 mL

Action/Kinetics: This drug is penicillinase-resistant and acid-resistant. **Peak serum levels: IM, PO,** 4–20 mcg/mL after 1 hr. **t½:** 40 min. Chiefly excreted in urine.

Uses: Resistant staphylococcal infections. To initiate therapy in any suspected staphylococcal infection. Infections due to *Streptococcus pneumoniae.*

Dosage

- **Capsules, Oral Suspension**

Skin and soft tissue infections, mild to moderate upper respiratory tract infections.

Adults and children over 40 kg: 125 mg q 6 hr; **pediatric:** 12.5 mg/kg/day in four equal doses given q 6 hr.

Lower respiratory tract infections or disseminated infections.

Adults and children over 40 kg: 250 mg q 6 hr, up to a maximum of 4 g/day; **pediatric:** 12–25 mg/kg/day in four equal doses given q 6 hr. Dosage not established for the newborn.

Administration/Storage

1. To prepare PO suspension, shake container to loosen powder, measure water for reconstitution as indicated on label, add half of the water, and immediately shake vigorously because usual handling may cause lumps. Add the remainder of the water and again shake vigorously.
2. Shake well before pouring each dose.
3. The reconstituted PO solution is stable for 7 days at room temperature, 10 days if refrigerated, and 21 days if frozen.
4. Give at least 1 hr before meals or no sooner than 2–3 hr after a meal with a full glass of water.

Contraindication: Treatment of meningitis.

NURSING CONSIDERATIONS

See also *General Nursing Considerations for All Anti- Infectives,* Chapter 1, and *Penicillins,* Chapter 8.

Evaluate

- Reports of symptomatic relief
- Negative laboratory culture reports

Methicillin sodium

(meth-ih-**SILL**-in)
Staphcillin **(Rx)**

See also *Anti-Infectives,* Chapter 1, and *Penicillins,* Chapter 8.

How Supplied: *Powder for injection:* 1 g, 4 g, 10 g

Action/Kinetics: This drug is a semisynthetic, penicillinase-resistant salt suitable for soft tissue, penicillin G-resistant, and resistant staphylococcal infections. **Peak plasma levels: IM,** 10–20 mcg/mL after 30–60 min; **IV,** 15 min. **t½:** 30 min. Excreted chiefly in the urine.

Additional Uses: Infections by penicillinase-producing staphylococci, osteomyelitis, septicemia, enterocolitis, bacterial endocarditis.

Dosage

- **IM, continuous IV infusion**

General infections.

Adults: 4–12 g/day, depending on the infection, in divided doses q 4–6 hr. (*NOTE:* If creatinine clearance is less than 10 mL/min, the dose should not exceed 2 g q 12 hr.) **Pediatric:** 100–300 mg/kg/day in divided doses q 4–6 hr. **Infants over 7 days of age and weighing more than 2 kg:** 100 mg/kg/day in divided doses q 6 hr. **Infants more than 7 days of age and weighing less than 2 kg or less than 7 days of age and weighing more than 2 kg:** 75 mg/kg/day in divided doses q 8 hr. **Infants under 7 days of age and weighing less than 2 kg:** 50 mg/kg/day in divided doses q 12 hr.

Meningitis.

Infants over 7 days of age and weighing more than 2 kg: 150–200 mg/kg/day. **Infants more than 7 days of age and weighing less than 2 kg or less than 7 days and weighing more than 2 kg:** 150 mg/kg/day. **Infants under 7 days of age and weighing less than 2 kg:** 100 mg/kg/day.

Administration/Storage

1. Do not use dextrose solutions for diluting methicillin because their low acidity may destroy the antibiotic.
2. Inject medication slowly. Methicillin injections are particularly painful.
3. Inject deeply into gluteal muscle. Use caution to avoid sciatic nerve injury.
4. To prevent sterile abscesses at injection site, include 0.2–0.3 mL of air in syringe before starting injection so that when the needle is withdrawn the irritating solution will not leak into tissue.
5. If used IV, care should be taken as thrombophlebitis can occur, especially in geriatric clients.
6. Check for redness or edema at site of injection and for pain along the course of the vein into which the drug is administered. Methicillin is a vesicant.
7. Methicillin is sensitive to heat when dissolved. Therefore, solutions for IM administration must be used within 24 hr if standing at room temperature or within 4 days if refrigerated. Solutions for IV use must be used within 8 hr.
8. For IV administration, dilute 1 mL (500 mg) with 20–25 mL of sterile water for injection or sodium chloride injection USP and administer at a rate of 10 mL/min. May further dilute and administer IVPB over 30 min.
9. Do not mix methicillin with any other drug in the same syringe or IV solution.

Special Concerns: Use with caution in clients with renal failure. Safe use in neonates has not been established. Periodic renal function tests are indicated for long-term therapy.

NURSING CONSIDERATIONS

See also *General Nursing Considerations for All Anti-Infectives,* Chapter 1 and for *Penicillins,* Chapter 8.

Assessment

1. Document indications for therapy and type and onset of symptoms.
2. Ensure that blood cultures and CBC are taken prior to start of therapy and weekly during therapy. Many strains of methicillin-resistant staphylococci have been identified. It has been recommended that these clients be isolated until appropriate antibiotic therapy can be instituted to prevent major institutional outbreaks.
3. Obtain CBC and liver and renal function studies.

Interventions

1. Monitor I&O. Note any evidence of hematuria or casts in the urine.
2. Observe for any evidence of pallor, ecchymosis, or bleeding tendencies (drug enhances anticoagulants); monitor CBC.
3. Observe for fever, nausea, and other signs of hepatotoxicity, especially with prolonged therapy.
4. Drug contains sodium; calculate accordingly for clients on strict sodium restrictions.

Evaluate

- Negative lab C&S reports and no evidence of organism resistance
- Eradication of infection and evidence of ↓ fever, ↓ WBC
- Reports of symptomatic improvement

Mezlocillin sodium

(mez-low-**SILL**-in)
Pregnancy Category: B
Mezlin **(Rx)**

See also *Anti-Infectives,* Chapter 1, and *Penicillins,* Chapter 8.

How Supplied: *Powder for injection:* 1 g, 2 g, 3 g, 4 g, 20 g

Action/Kinetics: Mezlocillin is a broad-spectrum (gram-negative and gram-positive organisms, including aerobic and anaerobic strains) antibiotic used parenterally. **Therapeutic serum levels:** 35–45 mcg/mL. **t½: IV,** 55 min. Excreted mostly unchanged by the kidneys. Penetration to CSF is poor unless meninges are inflamed.

Uses: Septicemia and infections of the lower respiratory tract, urinary tract, abdomen, skin, and female genital tract caused by *Klebsiella, Proteus, Pseudomonas, Escherichia coli, Bacteroides, Peptococcus, Streptococcus faecalis* (enterococcus), *Peptostreptococcus,* and *Enterobacter.* Also, *Neisseria gonorrhoeae* infections of the urinary tract and female genital system. Infections caused by *Streptococcus pneumoniae* and group A beta-hemolytic streptococcus.

Dosage

- **IV, IM**

Serious infections.

Adults: 200–300 mg/kg/day in four to six divided doses; **usual:** 3 g q 4 hr or 4 g q 6 hr. **Infants and children, 1 month–12 years:** 50 mg/kg q 4 hr given **IM** or **IV** over 30 min; **infants more than 2 kg and less than 1 week of age or less than 2 kg and less than 1 week of age:** 75 mg/kg q 12 hr; **infants less than 2 kg and more than 1 week of age:** 75 mg/kg q 8 hr; **infants more than 2 kg and more than 1 week of age:** 75 mg/kg q 6 hr.

Life-threatening infections.

Adults: Up to 350 mg/kg/day, not to exceed 24 g/day.

Gonococcal urethritis.

Adults: Single dose of 1–2 g with probenecid, 1 g.

Prophylaxis of postoperative infection.

Adults: 4 g 30–90 min prior to start of surgery; **then,** 4 g, IV, 6 and 12 hr later.

Prophylaxis of infection in clients undergoing cesarean section.

First dose: 4 g IV when cord is clamped; **second and third doses:** 4 g IV 4 and 8 hr after the first dose.

Administration/Storage

1. When given by IV infusion (including piggyback), administration of other drugs should be discontinued during administration of mezlocillin.
2. Drug is very irritating to veins. Direct IV administration should be slow to prevent phlebitis; 1 g over 3–5

min. May further dilute in 50–100 mL of dextrose or saline solution and administer over 30 min.
3. For pediatric IV administration, infuse over 30 min.
4. Vials and infusion bottles should be stored at temperatures below 30°C (86°F).
5. The powder and reconstituted solution may darken slightly, but potency is not affected.
6. IM doses should not exceed 2 g/injection. Mezlocillin should be continued for at least 2 days after symptoms of infection have disappeared.
7. For group A beta-hemolytic streptococcus, therapy should continue for at least 10 days.

Laboratory Test Interferences: ↑ AST, ALT, serum alkaline phosphatase, serum bilirubin, serum creatinine, and/or BUN. ↓ Serum potassium.

Additional Side Effects: Bleeding abnormalities. Decreased hemoglobin or hematocrit values.

NURSING CONSIDERATIONS

See also *Nursing Considerations* for *Penicillins,* Chapter 8.

Assessment

1. Note any sensitivity to penicillin or cephalosporins.
2. Obtain appropriate specimens for culture prior to initiating therapy.
3. Obtain baseline CBC, PT, PTT, electrolytes, and renal function studies and monitor during therapy.
4. Anticipate reduced dosage in clients with impaired renal function.

Client/Family Teaching

1. Immediately report any evidence of increased bruising and/or bleeding.
2. Advise that symptoms of drug-induced anemia may be manifested by fatigue, pallor, weakness, vertigo, headache, dyspnea, and palpitations and to report if evident.

Evaluate

- Negative culture reports
- Reports of symptomatic improvement
- Serum drug levels within therapeutic range (35–45 mcg/mL)

Nafcillin sodium

(naf-**SILL**-in)
Nafcil, Nallpen, Unipen **(Rx)**

See also *Anti-Infectives,* Chapter 1, and *Penicillins,* Chapter 8.

How Supplied: *Capsule:* 250 mg; *Injection:* 1 g/50 mL, 2 g/50 mL; *Powder for injection:* 500 mg, 1 g, 2 g, 10 g

Action/Kinetics: Nafcillin is penicillinase-resistant and acid stable. Used for resistant staphylococcal infections. Parenteral therapy is recommended initially for severe infections. **Peak plasma levels: PO,** 7 mcg/mL after 30–60 min; **IM,** 14–20 mcg/mL after 30–60 min. **t1/2:** 60 min. Significantly bound to plasma proteins.

Uses: Infections by penicillinase-producing staphylococci; also certain pneumococci and streptococci. As initial therapy if staphylococcal infection is suspected (i.e., until results of culture have been obtained).

Dosage

• IV

Adults: 0.5–1 g q 4 hr.

• IM

Adults: 0.5 g q 4–6 hr. **Children and infants:** 25 mg/kg b.i.d. **Neonates:** 10 mg/kg b.i.d. Or, for neonates weighing less than 2,000 g and less than 7 days of age, a dose of 25 mg/kg b.i.d. can be given; for neonates weighing less than 2,000 g but older than 7 days, a dose of 75 mg/kg/day divided q 6 hr.

• Capsules, Oral Solution, Tablets

Mild to moderate infections.

Adults: 250–500 mg q 4–6 hr.

Severe infections.

Adults: Up to 1 g q 4–6 hr.

Pneumonia/scarlet fever.

Children: 25 mg/kg/day in four divided doses.

Staphylococcal infections.
Children: 50 mg/kg/day in four divided doses. **Neonates:** 10 mg/kg t.i.d.–q.i.d.

Streptococcal pharyngitis.
Children: 250 mg t.i.d.

NOTE: IV administration is not recommended for neonates or infants.

Administration/Storage

1. Reconstitute for PO use by adding powder to bottle of diluent. Replace cap tightly. Then *shake* thoroughly until all powder is in solution. Check carefully for undissolved powder at the bottom of bottle. Solution must be stored in refrigerator and unused portion discarded after 1 week.
2. Reconstitute for parenteral use by adding required amount of sterile water. Shake vigorously. Date, time, and initial bottle. Refrigerate after reconstitution and discard unused portion after 48 hr.
3. For direct IV administration, dissolve powder in 15–30 mL of sterile water for injection or isotonic sodium chloride solution and inject over 5–10-min period into the tubing of flowing IV infusion. For IV drip, dissolve the required amount in 100–150 mL of isotonic sodium chloride injection and administer by IV drip over a period of 30–90 min.
4. IV use should be reserved for therapy of 24–48 hr duration due to the possibility of thrombophlebitis, especially in geriatric clients. Reduce rate of flow and report any pain, redness, or edema at site of IV administration.
5. Do not administer IV to newborn infants.
6. Administer IM by deep intragluteal injection.
7. Serum levels after PO administration are low and unpredictable.

Additional Side Effects: Sterile abscesses and thrombophlebitis occur frequently, especially in the elderly.

NURSING CONSIDERATIONS

See also *Nursing Considerations* for *Penicillins,* Chapter 8.

Client/Family Teaching

1. Take 1 hr before or 2 hr after meals with a full glass of water. Report any GI distress.
2. Report any unusual side effects or worsening of condition.

Evaluate

- Laboratory evidence of ↓ number of colonies of the infecting organism
- ↓ WBC, ↓ temperature, and reports of symptomatic improvement

Oxacillin sodium

(ox-ah-**SILL**-in)
Bactocill, Prostaphlin **(Rx)**

See also *Anti-Infectives,* Chapter 1, and *Penicillins,* Chapter 8.

How Supplied: *Capsule:* 250 mg, 500 mg; *Injection:* 1 g/50 mL, 2 g/50 mL; *Powder for injection:* 500 mg, 1 g, 2 g, 4 g, 10 g; *Powder for reconstitution:* 250 mg/5 mL

Action/Kinetics: This is a penicillinase-resistant, acid-stable drug used for resistant staphylococcal infections. **Peak plasma levels: PO,** 1.6–10 mcg after 30–60 min; **IM,** 5–11 mcg/mL after 30 min. **$t^1/_2$:** 30 min.

Uses: Infections caused by penicillinase-producing staphylococci; also certain pneumococci and streptococci.

Dosage

- **Capsules, Oral Solution**

Mild to moderate infections of the upper respiratory tract, skin, soft tissue.
Adults and children (over 20 kg): 500 mg q 4–6 hr for at least 5 days. **Children less than 20 kg:** 50 mg/kg/day in equally divided doses q 6 hr for at least 5 days.

Septicemia, deep-seated infections.
Parenteral therapy (see below) followed by PO therapy. **Adults:** 1 g q 4–6 hr; **children:** 100 mg/kg/day in equally divided doses q 4–6 hr.

- **IM, IV**

General infections.
Adults and children over 40 kg: 250–500 mg q 4–6 hr. **Children less than 40 kg:** 50 mg/kg/day in equally divided doses q 6 hr.

Severe infections of the lower respiratory tract or disseminated infections. **Adults and children over 40 kg:** Up to 1 g q 4–6 hr. **Children less than 40 kg:** Up to 100 mg/kg/day. **Neonates and premature infants, less than 2,000 g:** 50 mg/kg/day divided q 12 hr if less than 7 days of age and 100 mg/kg/day divided q 8 hr if more than 7 days of age. **Neonates and premature infants, more than 2,000 g:** 75 mg/kg/day divided q 8 hr if less than 7 days of age and 150 mg/kg/day divided q 6 hr if more than 7 days of age. Maximum daily dose: **Adults,** 12 g; **children,** 100–300 mg/kg.

Administration/Storage

1. Administer IM by deep intragluteal injection, rotate injection sites, and observe for pain and swelling at IM injection site.
2. Reconstitution: Add sterile water for injection or sodium chloride injection in amount indicated on vial. Shake until solution is clear. For parenteral use, reconstituted solution may be kept for 3 days at room temperature or 1 week in refrigerator. Discard outdated solutions.
3. IV administration (two methods):
• For rapid, direct administration, add an equal amount of sterile water or isotonic saline to reconstituted dosage (usually 250–500-mg vial with 5 mL of solution) and administer over a period of 10 min.
• For IV infusion, add reconstituted solution to either dextrose, saline, or invert sugar solution for a concentration of 0.5–40 mg/mL and administer over a 6-hr period, during which time drug remains potent.
• Observe for pain, redness, and edema at the site of IV injection and along the course of the vein.
4. Treatment of osteomyelitis may require several months of intensive PO therapy.

NURSING CONSIDERATIONS

See also *Nursing Considerations* for *Penicillins,* Chapter 8.

Evaluate

• Clinical evidence and reports of improvement in S&S of infection
• Negative lab culture reports

Penicillin G benzathine, parenteral

(pen-ih-**SILL**-in, **BEN**-zah-theen)
Pregnancy Category: B
Bicillin ✱, Bicillin L-A, Megacillin Suspension ✱, Permapen **(Rx)**

See also *Anti-Infectives,* Chapter 1, and *Penicillins,* Chapter 8.

How Supplied: *Injection:* 300,000 U/mL, 600,000 U/mL

Action/Kinetics: Penicillin G is neither penicillinase resistant nor acid stable. The product is a long-acting (repository) form of penicillin in an aqueous vehicle; it is administered as a sterile suspension. **Peak plasma levels: IM** 0.03–0.05 unit/mL.

Uses: Most gram-positive (streptococci, staphylococci, pneumococci) and some gram-negative (gonococci, meningococci) organisms. Syphilis. Prophylaxis of glomerulonephritis and rheumatic fever. Surgical infections, secondary infections following tooth extraction, tonsillectomy.

Dosage

• **Parenteral Suspension (IM only)**

Upper respiratory tract infections, erysipeloid, yaws.

Adults: 1,200,000 units as a single dose; **older children:** 900,000 units as a single dose; **children under 27 kg:** 300,000–600,000 units as a single dose; **neonates:** 50,000 units/kg as a single dose.

Early syphilis.

Adults: 2,400,000 units as a single dose.

Late syphilis.

Adults: 2,400,000 units/ q 7 days for 3 weeks.

Neurosyphilis.

Adults: Penicillin G, 12,000,000–24,000,000 units IV/day for 10–14 days followed by penicillin G benzathine, 2,400,000 units IM q week for 3 weeks.

Congenital syphilis, older children.
50,000 units/kg IM (up to adult dose of 2,400,000 units).

Prophylaxis of rheumatic fever.
Adults and children over 27.3 kg: 1,200,000 units/ q 4 weeks; **children and infants less than 27.3 kg:** 50,000 units/kg as a single dose.

Administration/Storage
1. Shake multiple-dose vial vigorously before withdrawing the desired dose because medication tends to clump on standing. Check that all medication is dissolved and that no residue is present at bottom of bottle.
2. Use a 20-gauge needle and do not allow medication to remain in the syringe and needle for long periods of time before administration because the needle may become plugged and the syringe "frozen."
3. Inject slowly and steadily into the muscle and *do not massage* injection site.
4. For adults, use the upper outer quadrant of the buttock; for infants and small children, the midlateral aspect of the thigh should be used. Benzathine penicillin should not be administered in the gluteal region in children less than 2 years of age.
5. *Do not administer IV.* Before injection of medication, aspirate needle to ascertain that needle is not in a vein.
6. Rotate and chart site of injections.
7. Divide between two injection sites if dose is large or available muscle mass is small.

NURSING CONSIDERATIONS

See also *Nursing Considerations* for *Penicillins,* Chapter 8.

Client/Family Teaching
1. Explain the importance of returning for repository penicillin injections.
2. Determine need for sexual counseling or referral in clients being treated for venereal disease. Stress the importance of the sexual partner also undergoing treatment.

Evaluate
- Effective prophylaxis of poststreptococcal rheumatic fever
- Resolution of symptoms of infection
- Negative serologic tests for syphilis

COMBINATION DRUG

Penicillin G benzathine and Procaine combined

(pen-ih-**SILL**-in, **BEN**-zah-theen, **PROH**-kain)
Pregnancy Category: B
Bicillin C-R, Bicillin C-R 900/300 **(Rx)**

See also *Anti-Infectives,* Chapter 1, and *Penicillins,* Chapter 8.

How Supplied: See Content

Content: Injection, 300,000 units/mL contains: 150,000 units penicillin G benzathine and 150,000 units penicillin G procaine; 600,000 units/dose contains: 300,000 units penicillin G benzathine and 300,000 units penicillin G procaine; 1,200,000 units/dose contains: 600,000 units penicillin G benzathine and 600,000 units penicillin G procaine; 2,400,000 units/dose contains: 1,200,000 units penicillin G benzathine and 1,200,000 units penicillin G procaine.
Injection, 900/300 per dose contains: 900,000 units penicillin G benzathine and 300,000 units penicillin G procaine.

Uses: Streptococcal infections (A, C, G, H, L, and M) without bacteremia, of the upper respiratory tract, skin, and soft tissues. Scarlet fever, erysipelas, pneumococcal infections, and otitis media.

Dosage
- **IM Only**

Streptococcal infections.
Adults and children over 27 kg: 2,400,000 units, given at a single session using multiple injection sites or, alternatively, in divided doses on days 1 and 3; **children 13.5–27 kg:** 900,000–1,200,000 units; **infants and children under 13.5 kg:** 600,000 units.

Pneumococcal infections, except meningitis.
Adults: 1,200,000 units; **pediatric:**

600,000 units. Give q 2–3 days until temperature is normal for 48 hr.

Administration/Storage

1. For adults, administer by deep IM injection in the upper outer quadrant of the buttock. For infants and children, use the midlateral aspect of the thigh.

2. Injection sites should be rotated for repeated doses.

Contraindications: Use to treat syphilis, gonorrhea, yaws, bejel, and pinta.

NURSING CONSIDERATIONS

See also *Nursing Considerations* for *Penicillins,* Chapter 8.

Evaluate: Resolution of infection.

Penicillin G potassium for injection

(pen-ih-**SILL**-in)
Pregnancy Category: B
Pfizerpen **(Rx)**

Penicillin G (Aqueous) sodium for injection

(pen-ih-**SILL**-in)
Pregnancy Category: B
(Rx)

See also *Anti-Infectives,* Chapter 1, and *Penicillins,* Chapter 8.

How Supplied: Penicillin G potassium for injection: *Injection:* 1 million U/50 mL, 2 million U/50 mL, 3 million U/50 mL; *Powder for injection:* 1 million U, 5 million U, 10 million U, 20 million U

Penicillin G (Aqueous) sodium for injection: *Powder for injection:* 5 million U

Action/Kinetics: The low cost of penicillin G still makes it the first choice for treatment of many infections. Rapid onset makes it especially suitable for fulminating infections. Penicillin G is neither penicillinase resistant nor acid stable. **Peak plasma levels: IM or SC,** 6–20 units/mL after 15–30 min **t½:** 30 min.

Uses: Streptococci of groups A, C, G, H, L, and M are sensitive to penicillin G. High serum levels are effective against streptococci of the D group.

Dosage

- **Penicillin G Potassium and Sodium Injections (IM, continuous IV infusion)**

Streptococcal infections.

Adults: 300,000–30 million units/day, depending on the use. **Pediatric:** 100,000–250,000 units/kg/day (given in divided doses q 4 hr). **Infants over 7 days of age weighing more than 2 kg:** 100,000 units/kg/day (given in divided doses q 6 hr). **Infants over 7 days of age weighing less than 2 kg:** 75,000 units/day (given in divided doses q 8 hr). **Infants less than 7 days of age weighing more than 2 kg:** 50,000 units/kg/day (given in divided doses q 8 hr). **Infants less than 7 days of age weighing less than 2 kg:** 50,000 units/kg/day (given in divided doses q 12 hr).

Meningitis.

Infants over 7 days of age weighing more than 2 kg: 200,000 units/kg. **Infants over 7 days of age weighing less than 2 kg:** 150,000 units/kg. **Infants less than 7 days of age weighing more than 2 kg:** 150,000 units/kg. **Infants less than 7 days of age weighing less than 2 kg:** 100,000 units/kg/day for 14 days.

Gram-negative bacillary bacteremia.

20 million or more units daily.

Anthrax.

A minimum of 5 million units/day (up to 12–20 million units have been used).

Clostridial infections.

20 million units/day used with an antitoxin.

Actinomycosis, cervicofacial.

1–6 million units/day; *thoracic and abdominal disease:* **initial,** 12–20 million units/day IV for 6 weeks followed by penicillin V, PO, 500 mg q.i.d. for 2–3 months.

Rat-bite fever, Haverhill fever.
12–20 million units/day for 3–4 weeks.

Endocarditis due to Listeria.
15–20 million units/day for 4 weeks (in adults).

Endocarditis due to Erysipelothrix rhusiopathiae.
12–20 million units/day for 4–6 weeks.

Meningitis due to Listeria.
15–20 million units/day for 2 weeks (in adults).

Pasteurella infections causing bacteremia and meningitis.
4–6 million units/day for 2 weeks.

Severe fusospirochetal infections of the oropharynx, lower respiratory tract, and genital area.
5–10 million units/day.

Pneumococcal infections causing empyema.
5–24 million units/day in divided doses q 4–6 hr.

Pneumococcal infections causing meningitis.
20–24 million units/day for 14 days.

Pneumococcal infections causing endocarditis, pericarditis, peritonitis, suppurative arthritis, osteomyelitis, mastoiditis.
12–20 million units/day for 2–4 weeks.

Adjunct with antitoxic to prevent diphtheria.
2–3 million units/day in divided doses for 10–12 days.

Meningococcal meningitis.
20–30 million units/day by continuous IV drip for 14 days (or until there is no fever for 7 days) or 200,000–300,000 units/kg/day q 2–4 hr in divided doses for a total of 24 doses.

Neurosyphilis.
12–24 million units/day for 10–14 days (can be followed by benzathine penicillin G, 2.4 million units IM weekly for 3 weeks).

Congenital syphilis in newborns.
50,000 units/kg/day (IV) in divided doses q 8–12 hr for 10–14 days; *in infants after newborn period:* 50,000 units/kg/ q 4–6 hr for 10–14 days.

Gonococcal infections in infants.
100,000 units/kg/day in two equal doses.

• **Oral Solution, Tablets**

General use.
Adults: 200,000–500,000 units/ q 6–8 hr; **pediatric under 12 years of age:** 25,000–90,000 units/kg/day in three to six divided doses. *NOTE:* 250 mg Penicillin G potassium, PO, is equivalent to 400,000 units.

Upper respiratory tract infections due to streptococci.
200,000–250,000 units/ q 6–8 hr for 10 days (for severe infections, use 400,000–500,000 units/ q 8 hr for 10 days or 800,000 units/ q 12 hr).

Infections of the respiratory tract due to pneumococci.
400,000–500,000 units/ q 6 hr until client has no fever for 48 hr.

Infections of the skin and skin structures due to staphylococci.
200,000–500,000 units/ q 6–8 hr until cured.

Infections of the oropharynx due to fusospirochetes.
400,000–500,000 units/ q 6–8 hr.

Prophylaxis of rheumatic fever and/or chorea.
200,000–250,000 units b.i.d. chronically.

Administration/Storage

1. IM administration is preferred; discomfort is minimized by using solutions of up to 100,000 units/mL.
2. Use sterile water, isotonic saline USP, or 5% D5W and mix with recommended volume for desired strength.
3. Loosen powder by shaking bottle before adding diluent.
4. Hold vial horizontally and rotate slowly while directing the stream of the diluent against the wall of the vial.
5. Shake vigorously after addition of diluent.
6. Solutions may be stored at room temperature for 24 hr or in refrigerator for 1 week. Discard remaining solution.
7. Use 1%–2% lidocaine solution as diluent for IM (if ordered by physician) to lessen pain at injection site. Do not use procaine as diluent for aqueous penicillin.
8. The PO products should be taken

at least 1 hr before or 2 hr after meals.

9. Note the drugs that should *not* be mixed with penicillin during IV administration: aminophylline, amphotericin B, ascorbic acid, chlorpheniramine, chlorpromazine, gentamicin, heparin, hydroxyzine, lincomycin, metaraminol, novobiocin, oxytetracycline, phenylephrine, phenytoin, polymyxin B, prochlorperazine, promazine, promethazine, sodium bicarbonate, sodium salts of barbiturates, sulfadiazine, tetracycline, tromethamine, vancomycin, vitamin B complex.

10. For intermittent IV administration (q 6 hr) drug may be reconstituted with 100 mL of dextrose or saline solution and infused over 1 hr.

11. Electrolyte contents: Penicillin G Sodium (1 mg =1,600 units) contains 2 mEq sodium/1 million units; Penicillin G Potassium (1 mg =1,600 units) contains 1.7 mEq potassium and 0.3 mEq sodium/1 million units.

Additional Side Effects: Rapid IV administration may cause hyperkalemia and cardiac arrhythmias. Renal damage occurs rarely.

NURSING CONSIDERATIONS

See also *Nursing Considerations* for *Penicillins,* Chapter 8.

Assessment

1. Document indications for therapy and type and onset of symptoms.
2. List other agents prescribed and the outcome.
3. Ensure that appropriate cultures have been obtained before initiating therapy.

Interventions

1. Order drug by specifying sodium or potassium salt.
2. Monitor I&O. Dehydration decreases excretion of the drug and may raise the blood level of penicillin G to dangerously high levels that can cause kidney damage.
3. Assess client for GI disturbances, which may lead to dehydration.
4. Very high doses (>20 million units) may cause seizures or platelet dysfunction, especially in clients with impaired renal function.

Evaluate

- Clinical evidence and reports of symptomatic improvement
- Negative lab culture reports
- Prophylaxis of rheumatic fever or chorea

Penicillin G Procaine Suspension, Sterile

(pen-ih-**SILL**-in, **PROH**-caine)
Pregnancy Category: B
Ayercillin ✦, Crysticillin 300 A.S. and 600 A.S., Pfizerpen-AS, Wycillin **(Rx)**

See also *Anti-Infectives,* Chapter 1, and *Penicillins,* Chapter 8.

How Supplied: *Injection:* 600,000 U/mL

Action/Kinetics: Long-acting (repository) form in aqueous or oily vehicle. Destroyed by penicillinase. Because of slow onset, a soluble penicillin is often administered concomitantly for fulminating infections.

Uses: Penicillin-sensitive staphylococci, pneumococci, streptococci, and bacterial endocarditis (for *Streptococcus viridans* and *S. bovis* infections). Gonorrhea, all stages of syphilis. *Prophylaxis:* Rheumatic fever, pre- and postsurgery. Diphtheria, anthrax, fusospirochetosis (Vincent's infection), erysipeloid, rat-bite fever.

Dosage

- **IM Only**

Pneumococccal, staphylococcal, streptococcal infections; erysipeloid, rat-bite fever, anthrax, fusospirochetosis.

Adults, usual: 600,000–1,200,000 units/day for 10–14 days. **Newborns, usual:** 50,000 units/kg/day in a single dose.

Bacterial endocarditis.

Adults: 1,200,000 units penicillin G procaine q.i.d. for 2–4 weeks with streptomycin, 500 mg b.i.d. for the first 14 days.

Diphtheria carrier state.

300,000 units/day for 10 days.

Diphtheria, adjunct with antitoxin.

300,000–600,000 units/day.

Gonococcal infections.

4.8 million units divided into at least two doses and given with 1 g PO probenecid (given 30 min before the injections).

Neurosyphilis.

2.4 million units/day for 10 days (given at two sites) with probenecid 500 mg PO q.i.d.; **then,** benzathine penicillin G, 2.4 million units/week for 3 weeks.

Congenital syphilis in infants, symptomatic and asymptomatic.

50,000 units/kg/day for 10–14 days.

Syphilis: primary, secondary, latent with negative spinal fluid.

Adults and children over 12 years: 600,000 units/day for 8 days (total of 4.8 million units).

Administration/Storage

1. Note on package whether medication is to be refrigerated, since some brands require this to maintain stability.
2. Shake multiple-dose vial thoroughly to ensure uniform suspension before injection. If the medication is clumped at the bottom of the vial, it must be shaken until clump dissolves.
3. Use a 20-gauge needle and aspirate immediately after withdrawing medication from the vial; otherwise needle may become clogged and syringe may "freeze."
4. Administer into two sites if dose is large or available muscle mass is small.
5. Aspirate to check that the needle is not in a vein.
6. Inject deep into muscle at a slow rate.
7. Do not massage after injection.
8. Rotate and chart injection sites.
9. Drug is for IM use only.

NURSING CONSIDERATIONS

See also *Nursing Considerations* for *Penicillins,* Chapter 8.

Assessment

1. Document indications for therapy, onset of symptoms, and any other treatments prescribed.
2. Obtain appropriate pretreatment lab specimens for C&S analysis.

Client/Family Teaching

1. Observe for wheal or other skin reactions at site of injection that may indicate a reaction to procaine as well as to penicillin and report.
2. Determine need for sexual counseling/referral in clients being treated for venereal disease. Stress importance of the partner also undergoing treatment.
3. Clients with a history of rheumatic fever or congenital heart disease need to understand the importance of using antibiotic prophylaxis prior to any invasive medical or dental procedure.

Evaluate: Laboratory confirmation of successful treatment of underlying pathogenic agent.

Penicillin V potassium (Phenoxymethyl penicillin potassium)

(pen-ih-**SILL**-in)

Pregnancy Category: B

Apo-Pen-VK ✦, Beepen-VK, Betapen-VK, Ledercillin VK, Nadopen-V ✦, Novo-Pen-VK ✦, Nu-Pen-VK ✦, Penicillin VK, Pen-V, Pen-Vee K, PVF K ✦, Robicillin VK, V-Cillin K, Veetids 125, 250, and 500 **(Rx)**

See also *Anti-Infectives,* Chapter 1, and *Penicillins,* Chapter 8.

How Supplied: *Powder for reconstitution:* 125 mg/5 mL, 250 mg/5 mL; *Tablet:* 250 mg, 500 mg

Action/Kinetics: These preparations are related closely to penicillin G. They are not penicillinase resistant but are acid stable and resist inactivation by gastric secretions. They are well absorbed from the GI tract and are not affected by foods. **Peak plasma levels:** Penicillin V, **PO:** 2.7 mcg/mL after 30–60 min; penicillin V potassium, **PO:** 1–9 mcg/mL after 30–60 min. **t½:** 30 min.

Periodic blood counts and renal function tests are indicated during long-term usage.

Uses: Penicillin-sensitive staphylococci, pneumococci, streptococci, gonococci. Vincent's infection of the oropharynx. Lyme disease. *Prophylaxis:* Rheumatic fever, chorea, bacterial endocarditis, pre- and post-surgery. Should *not* be used as prophylaxis for GU instrumentation or surgery, sigmoidoscopy, or childbirth or during the acute stage of severe pneumonia, bacteremia, arthritis, empyema, pericarditis, and meningitis. Penicillin G, IV, should be used for treating neurologic complications due to Lyme disease.

Dosage

- **Oral Solution, Tablets**

Streptococcal infections.

Adults and children over 12 years: 125–250 mg/ q 6–8 hr for 10 days. **Children, usual:** 25–50 mg/ kg/day in divided doses q 6–8 hr.

Pneumococcal or staphylococcal infections, fusospirochetosis of oropharynx.

Adults and children over 12 years: 250–500 mg/ q 6–8 hr.

Prophylaxis of rheumatic fever/chorea.

125–250 mg b.i.d.

Prophylaxis of bacterial endocarditis.

Adults and children over 27 kg: 2 g 30–60 min prior to procedure; **then,** 1 g/ q 6 hr. **Pediatric:** 1 g 30–60 min prior to procedure; **then,** 500 mg/ q 6 hr.

Anaerobic infections.

250 mg q.i.d. See also *Penicillin G, Procaine, Aqueous, Sterile,* p. 95

Prophylaxis of septicemia caused by Staphylococcus pneumoniae in children with sickle cell anemia.

125 mg b.i.d.

Streptococcal pharyngitis in children.

250 mg b.i.d. for 10 days.

Streptococcal otitis media and sinusitis.

250–500 mg/ q 6 hr for 14 days.

Lyme disease.

250–500 mg q.i.d. for 10–20 days (for children less than 2 years of age, 50 mg/kg/day in four divided doses for 10–20 days).

NOTE: 250 mg penicillin V is equivalent to 400,000 units.

Administration/Storage

1. Administer without regard to meals. Blood levels may be slightly higher when administered on an empty stomach, however.
2. Do not administer at the same time as neomycin because malabsorption of penicillin V may occur.

Special Concerns: More and more strains of staphylococci are resistant to penicillin V, necessitating culture and sensitivity studies.

Additional Drug Interactions

Contraceptives, oral / ↓ Effectiveness of oral contraceptives
Neomycin, oral / ↓ Absorption of penicillin V

NURSING CONSIDERATIONS

See also *Nursing Considerations* for *Penicillins,* Chapter 8.

Client/Family Teaching

1. Clients with a history of rheumatic fever or congenital heart disease need to understand the importance of using antibiotic prophylaxis prior to any invasive medical or dental procedure.
2. Review appropriate dose, frequency of administration, and length of therapy prescribed.
3. Advise parents to report if throat and/or ear symptoms do not improve after 48 hr of therapy as child may need to be reevaluated and therapy altered.
4. Explain that with oral administration if a reaction is going to occur, you usually see it after the second dose. Advise client/parent to seek medical intervention immediately if respiratory distress or skin wheals appear.
5. Women of childbearing age should use an additional nonhormonal form of birth control if taking oral contraceptives because their effectiveness may be diminished.
6. Report for all scheduled follow-up exams and lab studies (especially CBC and renal function during long-term therapy).

Evaluate
• Reports of symptomatic improvement
• Negative lab C&S reports
• Endocarditis and/or rheumatic fever prophylaxis during invasive medical and/or dental procedures

Piperacillin sodium

(pie-**PER**-ah-sill-in)
Pregnancy Category: B
Pipracil **(Rx)**

See also *Anti-Infectives,* Chapter 1 and *Penicillins,* Chapter 8.

How Supplied: *Powder for injection:* 2g, 3g, 4g, 40g

Action/Kinetics: Piperacillin is a semisynthetic, broad-spectrum penicillin for parenteral use. It is not penicillinase resistant. The drug penetrates CSF in the presence of inflamed meninges. **Peak serum level:** 244 mcg/mL. **t½:** 36–72 min. Excreted unchanged in urine and bile.

Uses: Intra-abdominal infections, gynecologic infections, septicemia, skin and skin structure infections, bone and joint infections, UTIs, lower respiratory tract infections, gonococcal infections, streptococcal infections. Mixed infections prior to the identification of the causative organisms. Prophylaxis in surgery including GI, biliary, hysterectomy, cesarean section.

Aminoglycosides have been used with piperacillin sodium, especially in clients with impaired host defenses.

Dosage

• **IM, IV**

Serious infections.

IV: 3–4 g/ q 4–6 hr (12–18 g/day) as a 20–30-min infusion.

Complicated UTIs.

IV: 8–16 g/day (125–200 mg/kg/day) in divided doses q 6–8 hr.

Uncomplicated UTIs and most community-acquired pneumonias.

IM, IV: 6–8 g/day (100–125 mg/kg/day) in divided doses q 6–12 hr.

Uncomplicated gonorrhea infections.

2 g **IM** with 1 g probenecid **PO** 30 min before injection (both given as single dose).

Prophylaxis in surgery.

First dose: IV, 2 g prior to surgery; **second dose:** 2 g either during surgery (abdominal) or 4–6 hr after surgery (hysterectomy, cesarean); **third dose:** 2 g at an interval depending on use. Dosage should be decreased in renal impairment.

Dosages have not been established in infants and children under 12 years of age although the following doses have been suggested: **Neonates,** 100 mg/kg/ q 12 hr; **children,** 200–300 mg/kg/day (up to a maximum of 24 g/day) divided q 4–6 hr.

For cystic fibrosis.

350–500 mg/kg/day divided q 4–6 hr.

Administration/Storage

1. No more than 2 g should be administered IM at any one site.
2. For IM administration, use upper, outer quadrant of gluteus or well-developed deltoid muscle. Do not use lower or mid-third of upper arm.
3. For IV administration reconstitute each gram with at least 5 mL diluent, such as sterile or bacteriostatic water for injection, sodium chloride for injection, or bacteriostatic sodium chloride for injection. Shake until dissolved.
4. Inject IV slowly over a period of 3–5 min to avoid vein irritation.
5. Administer by intermittent IV infusion in at least 50 mL of dextrose or saline solutions over a period of 20–30 min.
6. After reconstitution, solution may be stored at room temperature for 24 hr, refrigerated for 1 week, or frozen for 1 month.

Laboratory Test Interferences: Positive Coombs' test; ↑ (especially in infants) AST, ALT, LDH, bilirubin.

Additional Side Effect: Rarely, prolonged muscle relaxation.

NURSING CONSIDERATIONS

See also *Nursing Considerations* for *Penicillins,* Chapter 8.

Assessment

1. Document indications for therapy and type and onset of symptoms.

2. Ensure that appropriate pretreatment cultures have been sent.
3. Obtain baseline electrolytes, hematologic, liver, and renal function studies and monitor throughout therapy.
4. Assess for diarrhea or any other evidence of superinfection.

Evaluate
- Infection prophylaxis during surgery
- Clinical evidence and reports of symptomatic improvement
- Negative lab C&S reports

—COMBINATION DRUG—

Piperacillin sodium and Tazobactam sodium

(pie-**PER**-ah-**sill**-in, tay-zoh-**BAC**-tam)
Pregnancy Category: B
Zosyn **(Rx)**

See also *Piperacillin sodium,* and *Penicillins,* Chapter 8.

How Supplied: See Content.

Content: *Powder for injection:* 2 g piperacillin with 0.25 g tazobactam sodium; 3 g piperacillin with 0.372 g tazobactam sodium; 4 g piperacillin with 0.5 g tazobactam sodium.

Action/Kinetics: This product is a combination of piperacillin sodium and tazobactam sodium, a beta-lactamase inhibitor. Tazobactam inhibits beta- lactamases, thus ensuring activity of piperacillin against beta- lactamase-producing microorganisms. Thus, tazobactam broadens the antibiotic spectrum of piperacillin to those bacteria normally resistant to it. **Peak plasma levels:** Attained immediately after completion of an IV infusion. **t½, piperacillin and tazobactam:** 0.7–1.2 hr. Both drugs are eliminated through the kidney with piperacillin excreted unchanged and tazobactam excreted both unchanged and as inactive metabolites. The t½ of both drugs is increased in clients with renal impairment and in hepatic cirrhosis (dose adjustment not required).

Uses: Appendicitis complicated by rupture or abscess and peritonitis caused by piperacillin-resistant, beta-lactamase-producing strains of *Escherichia coli, Bacteroides fragilis, B. ovatus, B. thetaiotaomicron,* and *B. vulgatus*. Uncomplicated and complicated skin and skin structure infections (including cellulitis, cutaneous abscesses, and ischemic/diabetic foot infections) caused by piperacillin-resistant, beta-lactamase-producing strains of *Staphylococcus aureus*. Postpartum endometritis or pelvic inflammatory disease caused by piperacillin-resistant, beta-lactamase-producing strains of *E. coli*. Community-acquired pneumonia of moderate severity caused by piperacillin-resistant, beta-lactamase-producing strains of *Haemophilus influenzae*.

Infections caused by piperacillin-susceptible organisms for which piperacillin is effective may also be treated with this combination. The treatment of mixed infections caused by piperacillin-susceptible organisms and piperacillin-resistant, beta-lactamase-producing organisms susceptible to this combination do not require addition of another antibiotic.

Dosage

- **IV infusion**

Susceptible infections.

Adults: 12 g/day piperacillin and 1.5 g/day tazobactam, given as 3.375 g (i.e., 3 g piperacillin and 0.375 g tazobactam) q 6 hr for 7–10 days. In clients with renal insufficiency, the IV dose is adjusted depending on the extent of impaired function. If creatinine clearance is 20–40 mL/min, the dose is 8 g/day piperacillin and 1 g/day tazobactam in divided doses of 2.25 g q 6 hr. If the creatinine clearance is less than 20 mL/min, the dose is 6 g/day piperacillin and 0.75 g/day tazobactam in divided doses of 2.25 g q 8 hr.

Administration/Storage

1. For IV administration or by infusion, the powder for injection is reconstituted with 5 mL suitable diluent/g piper-

acillin. IV diluents that can be used include 0.9% sodium chloride for injection, sterile water for injection, dextran 6% in saline, dextrose 5%, potassium chloride 40 mEq, bacteriostatic saline/parabens, bacteriostatic water/parabens, bacteriostatic saline/benzyl alcohol, bacteriostatic water/benzyl alcohol. **Lactated Ringer's is not compatible.**
2. After the diluent is added, the vial is shaken well until the powder is dissolved. It may be further diluted to the desired final volume with the diluent.
3. If intermittent IV infusion is used, the 5 mL diluent/g piperacillin is further diluted to a volume of at least 50 mL. The infusion is given over a period of 30 min. During the infusion, the primary infusion solution should be discontinued.
4. If concomitant therapy with aminoglycosides is indicated, piperacillin/tazobactam and the aminoglycoside are given separately, as penicillin can inactivate the aminoglycoside if they are mixed.
5. Single-dose vials should be used immediately after reconstitution. Any unused drug should be discarded after 24 hr if stored at room temperature or after 48 hr if stored in the refrigerator at 2°C–8°C (36°F–46°F).
6. After reconstitution, piperacillin/tazobactam is stable in glass and plastic syringes, IV bags, and tubing. The drug is stable in IV bags for up to 24 hr at room temperature and up to 1 week in the refrigerator. The drug is stable in an ambulatory IV infusion pump for 24 hr at room temperature.

Contraindications: Hypersensitivity to penicillins, cephalosporins, or beta-lactamase inhibitors.

Special Concerns: Use with caution during lactation. Safety and efficacy have not been determined in children less than 12 years of age.

Laboratory Test Interferences: ↓ H&H. Transient ↑ AST, ALT, alkaline phosphatase, and bilirubin. ↑ Serum creatinine, BUN. Prolonged PT and PTT. Positive direct Coomb's test. Proteinuria, hematuria, pyuria, abnormalities in electrolytes (↑ and ↓ sodium, potassium, calcium), hyperglycemia, ↓ total protein or albumin.

Side Effects: See *Penicillins,* Chapter 8. The highest incidence of side effects include the following. *GI:* Diarrhea, constipation, N&V, dyspepsia, stool changes, abdominal pain. *CNS:* Headache, insomnia, fever, agitation, dizziness, anxiety. *Dermatologic:* Rash, including maculopapular, bullous, urticarial, and eczematoid; pruritus. *Hematologic:* Thrombocytopenia, eosinophilia, leukopenia, neutropenia. *Miscellaneous:* Pain, moniliasis, hypertension, chest pain, edema, rhinitis, dyspnea.

Drug Interactions
Heparin / Possible ↑ effect of heparin
Oral anticoagulants / Possible ↑ effect of oral anticoagulants
Tobramycin / ↓ Area under the curve, renal clearance, and urinary recovery of tobramycin
Vecuronium / Prolongation of the neuromuscular blockade of vecuronium

NURSING CONSIDERATIONS

See also *Nursing Considerations* for *Piperacillin,* and *Penicillins,* Chapter 8.

Assessment
1. Document indications for therapy and type, location, and onset of symptoms.
2. Determine any sensitivity to penicillins, cephalosporins, beta-lactamase inhibitors, or other allergens.
3. List drugs prescribed to ensure none interact unfavorably. Use of heparin and oral anticoagulants may require dosage adjustments.
4. Obtain baseline electrolytes, urinalysis, hematologic and coagulation profile, and liver and renal function studies and monitor throughout therapy.
5. Anticipate reduced dosage with renal impairment.

Evaluate: Clinical and lab evidence of resolution of infecting organism.

Ticarcillin disodium

(tie-kar-**SILL**-in)
Pregnancy Category: B
Ticar **(Rx)**

See also *Anti-Infectives,* Chapter 1, and *Penicillins,* Chapter 8.

How Supplied: *Powder for injection:* 1 g, 3 g, 20 g, 30 g

Action/Kinetics: This drug is a parenteral, semisynthetic antibiotic with an antibacterial spectrum of activity resembling that of carbenicillin. Primarily suitable for treatment of gram-negative organisms but also effective for mixed infections. Combined therapy with gentamicin or tobramycin is sometimes indicated for treatment of *Pseudomonas* infections. *The drugs should not be mixed during administration because of gradual mutual inactivation.* **Peak plasma levels: IM,** 25–35 mcg/mL after 1 hr; **IV,** 15 min. **t½:** 70 min. Elimination complete after 6 hr.

Uses: Bacterial septicemia, skin and soft tissue infections, acute and chronic respiratory tract infections caused by susceptible strains of *Pseudomonas aeruginosa, Proteus, Escherichia coli,* and other gram-negative organisms. GU tract infections caused by above organisms and by *Enterobacter* and *Streptococcus faecalis.* Anaerobic bacteria causing empyema, anaerobic pneumonitis, lung abscess, bacterial septicemia, peritonitis, intra-abdominal abscess, skin and soft tissue infections, salpingitis, endometritis, pelvic inflammatory disease, pelvic abscess. Ticarcillin may be used in infections in which protective mechanisms are impaired such as during use of oncolytic or immunosuppressive drugs or in clients with acute leukemia. Clients seriously ill should receive higher doses such as in serious urinary tract and systemic infections.

Dosage

- **IV infusion, direct IV, IM**

Bacterial septicemia, intra-abdominal infections, skin and soft tissue infections, infections of the female genital system and pelvis, respiratory tract infections.

Adults: 200–300 mg/kg/day by IV infusion in divided doses q 3, 4, or 6 hr, depending on the severity of the infection; **pediatric, less than 40 kg,** 200–300 mg/kg/day by IV infusion q 4 or 6 hr (daily dose should not exceed the adult dose).

UTIs, uncomplicated.

Adults: 1 g IM or direct IV q 6 hr; **pediatric, less than 40 kg,** 50–100 mg/kg/day IM or direct IV in divided doses q 6 or 8 hr.

UTIs, complicated.

Adults: 150–200 mg/kg/day by IV infusion in divided doses q 4 or 6 hr (usual dose is 3 g q.i.d. for a 70-kg client).

Neonates with sepsis due to *Pseudomonas, Proteus,* or *E. coli.*

Less than 7 days of age and less than 2 kg, 75 mg/kg q 12 hr; **more than 7 days of age and less than 2 kg,** 75 mg/kg q 8 hr; **less than 7 days of age and more than 2 kg,** 75 mg/kg q 8 hr; **more than 7 days of age and more than 2 kg,** 100 mg/kg q 8 hr. Can be given IM or by IV infusion over 10–20 min.

Clients with renal insufficiency should receive a loading dose of 3 g **IV,** and subsequent doses, as indicated by creatinine clearance.

Administration/Storage

1. Discard unused reconstituted solutions after 24 hr when stored at room temperature and after 72 hr when refrigerated.
2. For IM use, reconstitute each gram with 2 mL sterile water for injection, sodium chloride injection, or 1% lidocaine HCl (without epinephrine) to prevent pain and induration. The reconstituted solution should be used quickly and should be injected well into a large muscle.
3. For IV use, reconstitute each gram with 4 mL of the desired solution. Administer slowly to prevent vein irritation and phlebitis. A dilution of 1 g/20 mL (or more) will decrease the chance of vein irritation.

4. For an IV infusion, use 50 or 100 mL *ADD-Vantage* container of either 5% dextrose in water or sodium chloride injection and give by intermittent infusion over 30–120 min in equally divided doses.
5. Do not administer more than 2 g of the drug in each IM site.
6. Children weighing over 40 kg should receive the adult dose.
7. Ticarcillin should not be mixed together with amikacin, gentamicin, or tobramycin due to the gradual inactivation of these aminoglycosides.
8. Anticipate reduced dosage with liver or renal dysfunction.

Additional Contraindication: Pregnancy.

Special Concerns: Use with caution in presence of impaired renal function and for clients on restricted salt diets.

Laboratory Test Interferences: ↑ Alkaline phosphatase, AST, ALT.

Additional Side Effects: Neurotoxicity and neuromuscular excitability, especially in clients with impaired renal function.

Additional Drug Interactions: Effect of carbenicillin may be enhanced when used in combination with gentamicin or tobramycin for *Pseudomonas* infections.

NURSING CONSIDERATIONS

See also *Nursing Considerations* for *Penicillins,* Chapter 8.

Assessment

1. Document indications for therapy and type and onset of symptoms.
2. Ensure that appropriate specimens have been sent for culture.
3. Obtain bleeding times and liver and renal function studies, and monitor during therapy.

Interventions

1. Monitor client on high doses of drug for signs of electrolyte imbalance (especially sodium and potassium levels).
2. Note sodium content of drug (usually 4.75 mEq Na/g) and calculate accordingly for clients on strict sodium restrictions.

Client/Family Teaching

1. Report any symptoms of bleeding abnormalities, such as petechiae, ecchymosis, or frank bleeding.
2. Observe for edema, weight gain, or respiratory distress and report. This may be precipitated by drug's large sodium content.
3. Provide a printed list of drug side effects that should be reported if evident.

Evaluate

- Laboratory evidence of negative culture reports
- Clinical evidence and reports of symptomatic improvement

—COMBINATION DRUG—

Ticarcillin disodium and Clavulanate potassium

(tie-kar-**SILL**-in, klav-you-**LAN**-ate poe-**TASS**-ee-um)
Pregnancy Category: B
Timentin **(Rx)**

See also *Ticarcillin,* and *Penicillins,* Chapter 8.

How Supplied: See Content

Content: Powder for injection contains: 3 g ticarcillin disodium and 0.1 g clavulanate potassium. Solution contains: 3 g ticarcillin disodium and 0.1 g clavulanate potassium.

Action/Kinetics: This preparation contains clavulanic acid, which protects the breakdown of ticarcillin by beta-lactamase enzymes, thus ensuring appropriate blood levels of ticarcillin.

Uses: Complicated and uncomplicated UTIs; infections of the bones and joints, lower respiratory tract, skin and skin structures; gynecologic infections, bacterial septicemia. In combination with an aminoglycoside for certain *Pseudomonas aeruginosa* infections.

Dosage

- **IV Infusion**

Systemic and UTIs.

Adults more than 60 kg: 3.1 g (containing 0.1 g clavulanic acid) q 4–6 hr for 10–14 days. **Adults less**

than 60 kg: 200–300 mg ticarcillin/kg/day in divided doses q 4–6 hr for 10–14 days.

Gynecologic infections.

Adults more than 60 kg, moderate infections: 200 mg/kg/day in divided doses q 6 hr; **severe infections:** 300 mg/kg/day in divided doses q 4 hr.

In renal insufficiency.

Initially, loading dose of 3.1 g ticarcillin and 0.1 g clavulanic acid; **then,** dose based on creatinine clearance (see package insert).

Administration/Storage

1. To attain the appropriate dilution for 3.1 g ticarcillin and 0.1 g clavulanic acid, dilute with 13 mL of either sodium chloride injection or sterile water for injection. Further dilutions, if necessary, can be undertaken with 5% dextrose injection, lactated Ringer's injection, or sodium chloride injection.
2. The drugs should be administered over a period of 30 min, either through a Y-type IV infusion or by direct infusion.
3. This product is incompatible with sodium bicarbonate.
4. Dilutions with sodium chloride injection or lactated Ringer's injection may be stored at room temperature for 24 hr or refrigerated for 7 days. Dilutions with 5% dextrose injection are stable at room temperature for 12 hr or for 3 days if refrigerated.
5. If used with another anti-infective agent (e.g., an aminoglycoside), each drug should be given separately.

NURSING CONSIDERATIONS

See also *Nursing Considerations* for *Ticarillin disodium* and *Penicillins,* Chapter 8.

Evaluate: Resolution of infection and reports of symptomatic improvement.

CHAPTER NINE

Antibiotics: Sulfonamides

See also the following individual entries:

- Mafenide Acetate
- Pediazole
- Sulfacetamide Sodium
- Sulfadiazine
- Sulfamethizole
- Sulfamethoxazole
- Sulfamethoxazole and Phenazopyridine
- Sulfasalazine
- Sulfisoxazole
- Sulfisoxazole Acetyl
- Sulfisoxazole Diolamine
- Sulfisoxazole and Phenazopyridine
- Trimethoprim and Sulfamethoxazole

Action/Kinetics: Sulfonamides are structurally related to PABA and, as such, competitively inhibit the enzyme dihydropteroate synthetase, which is responsible for incorporating PABA into dihydrofolic acid. Thus, the synthesis of dihydrofolic acid is inhibited, resulting in a decrease in tetrahydrofolic acid, which is required for synthesis of DNA, purines, and thymidine. Thus, sulfonamides halt multiplication of bacteria (bacteriostatic) but do not kill fully formed microorganisms. Resistance to sulfonamides has occurred with increasing frequency.

The various sulfonamides are absorbed and excreted at widely differing rates. This has an important bearing on their therapeutic use. For instance, agents that are poorly absorbed from the GI tract are particularly indicated for intestinal infections because they remain localized in the intestine for a long time.

Sulfonamides are absorbed into the bloodstream and distributed throughout all tissues, including the CSF, where concentrations attain 50%–80% of those found in the blood. The sulfonamides are metabolized in the liver and primarily excreted by the kidneys. Small amounts are found in the feces, bile, breast milk, and other secretions.

It is always desirable to determine the susceptibility of the pathogen before, or soon after, initiation of therapy.

Sulfonamides have the advantage of being relatively inexpensive.

Uses: PO, Parenteral. The range of usefulness of the sulfonamides has been greatly reduced by the emergence of resistant strains of bacteria and the development of more effective antibiotics.

Acute, nonobstructive UTIs caused by *Escherichia coli, Klebsiella, Enterobacter, Staphylococcus aureus, Proteus mirabilis, Proteus vulgaris*. Drug of choice for nocardiosis. Elimination of meningococci from the nasopharynx in asymptomatic *Neisseria meningitidis* carriers when organism is sulfonamide-sensitive group A strain. As an alternative to penicillin for prophylaxis of rheumatic fever. As an alternative to tetracyclines for chlamydial infections or for trachoma and inclusion conjunctivitis or lymphogranuloma venereum. In conjunction with pyrimethamine for toxoplasmosis. In combination with quinine sulfate and pyrimethamine for chloroquine-resistant *Plasmodium falciparum*. In combination with penicillin or erythromycin for otitis media. Chancroid. In conjunction with streptomycin for meningitis caused by *Haemophilus influenzae*.

Ophthalmic. Conjunctivitis, corneal ulcer, and other superficial ocular infections due to susceptible organisms. Adjunct to systemic sulfonamides to treat trachoma.

Vaginal. Triple sulfa is used to treat *Gardnerella vaginalis* vaginitis and sulfanilamide is used to treat *Candida albicans* vulvovaginitis only.

Contraindications: Except for hypersensitivity reactions to sulfonamides and chemically related drugs (e.g., thiazides, sulfonylureas, loop diuretics, carbonic anhydrase inhibitors, local anesthetics, PABA-containing sunscreens), there are few absolute contraindications. Sulfonamides, however, are potentially dangerous drugs and cause a 5% overall incidence of major and minor side effects.

Sulfonamides may cause mental retardation and never should be administered during the third term of pregnancy, to nursing mothers, or to infants under 2 months of age, except for the treatment of congenital toxoplasmosis (a serious parasitic disease that can cause brain inflammation) or in life-threatening situations. Porphyria. Group A beta-hemolytic streptococcal infections.

Special Concerns: Sulfonamides should be used with caution, and in reduced dosage, in clients with impaired liver or renal function, intestinal or urinary tract obstructions, blood dyscrasias, allergies, asthma, and hereditary G6PD deficiency. Use with caution if exposed to sunlight or ultraviolet light as photosensitivity may occur. Superinfection is a possibility. Ophthalmic products should be used with caution in clients with dry eye. Safety and efficacy of ophthalmic use in children have not been determined.

Side Effects: Systemic. *GI:* N&V, diarrhea, abdominal pain, glossitis, stomatitis, anorexia, pseudomembranous enterocolitis, pancreatitis. *Allergic:* Rash, pruritus, photosensitivity, erythema nodosum or multiforme, generalized skin eruptions, ***Stevens-Johnson syndrome,*** conjunctivitis, rhinitis, balanitis. Serum sickness, urticaria, pruritus, exfoliative dermatitis, ***anaphylaxis, toxic epidermal necrolysis*** with or without corneal damage, periorbital edema, conjunctival and scleral injection, allergic myocarditis, decreased pulmonary function, disseminated lupus erythematosus, periarteritis nodosa, arteritis. *CNS:* Headaches, dizziness, mental depression, ***seizures,*** hallucinations, vertigo, insomnia, apathy, ataxia, confusion, psychoses, drowsiness, restlessness. *Renal:* Renal damage due to precipitation of sulfonamide or its acetyl derivative in the tubules (manifested by crystalluria, hematuria, oliguria); nephrotic syndrome. *Hematologic:* Acute hemolytic anemia especially in G6PD deficiency, ***aplastic anemia,*** leukopenia, ***agranulocytosis,*** thrombocytopenia, methemoglobinemia, purpura megaloblastic anemia, hypoprothrombinemia, Heinz body anemia. *Miscellaneous:* Jaundice, hepatitis, hepatocellular necrosis, tinnitus, hypoglycemia, arthralgia, acidosis, superinfection, hearing loss, transverse myelitis, drug fever, pyrexia, alopecia, arthralgia, myalgia, periarteritis nodosum.

By killing the intestinal flora, the sulfonamides also reduce the bacterial synthesis of vitamin K. This may result in ***hemorrhage.*** Administration of vitamin K to clients on long-term sulfonamide therapy is recommended.

Ophthalmic Use. Headache, browache. Blurred vision, eye irritation, itching, transient epithelial keratitis, reactive hyperemia, conjunctival edema, burning and transient stinging. Rarely, ***Stevens-Johnson syndrome,*** exfoliative dermatitis, ***toxic epidermal necrolysis,*** photosensitivity, fever, skin rash, GI disturbances, and bone marrow depression.

Symptoms of Overdose: N&V, anorexia, colic, dizziness, drowsiness, headache, unconsciousness, toxic fever. More serious manifestations include ***acute hemolytic anemia, agranulocytosis,*** acidosis, maculopapular dermatitis, hepatic jaundice, sensitivity reactions, toxic neuritis, ***death*** (several days after the first dose).

Drug Interactions

Anesthetics, local / ↓ Effect of sulfonamides
Antacids / ↓ Effect of sulfonamides due to ↓ absorption from GI tract
Anticoagulants, oral / ↑ Effect of anticoagulants due to ↓ plasma protein binding
Antidiabetics, oral / ↑ Hypoglycemic effect due to ↓ plasma protein binding
Cyclosporine / ↓ Effect of cyclosporine and ↑ nephrotoxicity
Methenamine / ↑ Chance of sulfonamide crystalluria due to acid urine
Methotrexate / ↑ Effect of methotrexate due to ↓ plasma protein binding and ↓ renal tubular excretion → bone marrow suppression
Oxacillin / ↓ Effect of oxacillin due to ↓ absorption from GI tract
Paraldehyde / ↑ Chance of sulfonamide crystalluria
Phenylbutazone / ↑ Effect of sulfonamides by ↑ blood levels
Phenytoin / ↑ Effect of phenytoin due to ↓ breakdown in liver
Probenecid / ↑ Effect of sulfonamides by ↓ in plasma protein binding
Salicylates / ↑ Effect of sulfonamides by ↑ blood levels
Silver products / Incompatible with ophthalmic products

Laboratory Test Interferences: False + or ↑ liver function tests (amino acids, bilirubin, BSP), renal function (BUN, NPN, creatinine clearance), blood counts, PT, Coombs' test. False + or ↑ urine glucose (copper reduction methods, such as Benedict's solution or Clinitest), protein, urobilinogen.

Dosage

See individual drugs.

Sulfonamides are usually given PO. Dosage is adjusted individually. An initial loading dose is usually recommended. Short-acting compounds must be given q 4–6 hr.

Topical application of sulfonamides is rarely ordered today, except for mafenide acetate, which is used as a 10% ointment to treat burn infections.

Creams of triple sulfa or sulfanilamide are used for vaginitis. Systemic absorption is possible when used intravaginally.

When sulfonamides are given as adjuncts to GI surgery, medication is usually started 3–5 days before surgery and is given for 1–2 weeks postoperatively after peristalsis has resumed.

NURSING CONSIDERATIONS

See also *General Nursing Considerations for All Anti-Infectives,* Chapter 1.

Administration/Storage

1. Ophthalmic solutions should not be used if they have darkened or contain a precipitate.
2. Care must be taken to avoid contamination of ophthalmic products.
3. Vaginal applicators and inserts should be used with caution after the seventh month of pregnancy, although use may be contraindicated in pregnancy.
4. The medication should be inserted high into the vagina using the applicator provided with the product.
5. *Treatment of Overdose:* Immediately discontinue the drug.

- Induce emesis or perform gastric lavage, especially if large doses were taken.
- To hasten excretion, alkalinize the urine and force fluids (if kidney function is normal). If there is renal blockage due to sulfonamide crystals, catheterization of the ureters may be needed.
- In the event of agranulocytosis, antibiotic therapy is needed to combat infection.
- To treat severe anemia or thrombocytopenia, blood or platelet transfusions are required.

Assessment

1. Obtain a thorough nursing and drug history.
2. Note if the client has ever received sulfonamide therapy and the response.
3. Document indications for therapy and type and onset of symptoms. List other agents prescribed and the outcome.
4. Question clients concerning any conditions that may preclude drug therapy, such as intestinal problems, urinary tract obstructions, G6PD deficiency (may precipitate hemolysis), or allergies.
5. Determine if the client is pregnant so that another type of medication, not harmful to a developing fetus, may be used.
6. Document symptoms of infection. Ensure that appropriate liver and renal function studies as well as C&S data have been performed prior to initiating therapy.
7. Obtain baseline CBC, blood sugar levels, and bleeding times, and monitor throughout drug therapy.
8. For ophthalmic use, the provider should be contacted if improvement is not seen within 5–7 days, if the condition worsens, or if pain, redness, itching, or swelling of the eye occurs.

Interventions

1. During drug therapy, assess clients for any of the following reactions that may require withdrawal of the drug:
- Skin rashes, abdominal pain, reports of anorexia, irritation of the mouth or tingling of the extremities
- Blood dyscrasias (characterized by sore throat, fever, pallor, purpura, jaundice, or weakness)
- Serum sickness (characterized by eruptions of purpuric spots and pain in limbs and joints). Serum sickness may develop 7–10 days after initiation of therapy.
- Early symptoms of Stevens-Johnson syndrome (characterized by high fever, severe headaches, stomatitis, conjunctivitis, rhinitis, urethritis, and balanitis [inflammation of the tip of the penis])
- Jaundice, which may indicate hepatic involvement, with onset 3–5 days after initiation of therapy
- Renal involvement (characterized by renal colic, oliguria, anuria, hematuria, and proteinuria)
- Ecchymosis and hemorrhage (caused by decreased synthesis of vitamin K by intestinal bacteria)
- Hemolytic anemia especially in the elderly
- Behavioral changes or acute mental disturbances

2. Monitor I&O and record. Encourage adequate fluid intake to prevent crystalluria. Observe urinalysis for evidence of crystals. Minimum output of urine should be 1.5 L/day. Test urine pH to determine excess acidity. Administration of a particularly insoluble sulfonamide may require alkalinization of urine. The drug of choice for this purpose is sodium bicarbonate.
3. If administering long-acting sulfonamides, adequate fluid intake must be maintained for 24–48 hr after the drug has been discontinued.

Client/Family Teaching

1. Provide a printed list of drug side effects and advise which to report immediately.
2. Take drug on time and as prescribed and remain under medical supervision during course of therapy despite feeling better.
3. Certain sulfonamides may color urine orange-red or brown. This should not be cause for alarm but should be reported.
4. Take medication with 6–8 oz (180–240 mL) of water and maintain adequate fluid intake for 24–48 hr after discontinuing drug.
5. Drug may cause N&V and loss of appetite. Explain how to monitor I&O and instruct client to maintain a record during the course of therapy. Unless contraindicated, encourage client to consume greater than 2.5 L/day of fluids.

6. Demonstrate how to test urine pH daily and advise when to report changes in acidity because additional drug therapy may be necessary.
7. Discourage the use of vitamin C while on therapy since it may make the urine more acidic and contribute to crystal formation.
8. If clients are also taking anticoagulants, instruct them to be particularly alert to evidence of an increase in bleeding tendencies (bruising, cuts that bleed for a longer time than usual, etc.) and to report.
9. Avoid prolonged exposure to sunlight because drug may cause a photosensitivity reaction. Wear protective clothing, sunglasses, and sunscreen when exposure is necessary.
10. Report any changes in vision or hearing.
11. Do not perform activities that require mental alertness until drug effects realized.
12. Vaginal intercourse should be avoided when vaginal sulfonamide products are being used.
13. Report for lab studies as scheduled.

Evaluate

• Knowledge and understanding of illness and evidence of compliance with prescribed therapy
• Negative lab C&S results (note any evidence of organism resistance to sulfonamide at this time)
• Clinical evidence of resolution of infection and reports of symptomatic improvement

Mafenide acetate

(**MAH**-fen-eyed)
Pregnancy Category: C
Sulfamylon **(Rx)**

See also *Sulfonamides,* Chapter 9.

How Supplied: *Cream:* 85 mg/g

Action/Kinetics: Mafenide is active against many gram-positive and gram-negative organisms. It is active in the presence of serum and pus. When applied topically, it diffuses through devascularized areas, is absorbed, and is rapidly metabolized.

Uses: Topical application to prevent infections in second- and third-degree burns.

Dosage

• **Cream**

1/16-in.-thick film applied over entire surface of burn with gloves once or twice daily until healing is progressing satisfactorily or until site is ready for grafting.

Administration/Storage

1. Mafenide, unlike other sulfonamides, is not inhibited by pus or body fluids.
2. Daily bathing should be undertaken to assist in debridement.
3. Continue mafenide therapy until healing is progressing well or until the burn site is ready for grafting. The drug should not be withdrawn if there is still the possibility of infections.
4. Avoid exposure to excessive heat.

Contraindication: Not to be used for already established infections.

Special Concerns: Use with caution during lactation and in those with acute renal failure. Use not recommended in infants less than 1 month of age.

Side Effects: *Allergic:* Rash, itching, swelling, hives, blisters, facial edema, erythema, eosinophilia. *Dermatologic:*Pain or burning (common) on application; excoriation of new skin, bleeding (rare). *Respiratory:*Hyperventilation or tachypnea, decrease in arterial pCO_2. *Metabolic:*Acidosis, increase in serum chloride. *Miscellaneous:* ***Fatal hemolytic anemia with disseminated intravascular coagulation,*** diarrhea.

NURSING CONSIDERATIONS

See also *General Nursing Considerations for All Anti-Infectives,* Chapter 1, and for *Sulfonamides,* Chapter 9.

Client/Family Teaching

1. Demonstrate the appropriate method for administration/application.
2. Mafenide cream should be applied aseptically to a cleansed, debrided, burn site using a gloved hand.
3. Burns treated with mafenide are to be covered only with a thin dressing.
4. The drug causes pain on application; use analgesics as prescribed.

5. Report at once any unusual reactions including rashes, bruising, bleeding, swelling, or breathing difficulty.

Evaluate: Evidence of readiness for grafting at burn site and freedom from infection.

—COMBINATION DRUG—

Pediazole

(**PEE**-dee-ah-zohl)

Pregnancy Category: C

(Rx)

How Supplied: See Content

Content: This product is available as granules that, when reconstituted, provide an oral suspension.

Antibacterial, antibiotic: Erythromycin ethylsuccinate, 200 mg/5 mL erythromycin activity. *Antibacterial, sulfonamide:* Sulfisoxazole, 600 mg/5 mL. See also information on individual components.

Use: Acute otitis media in children caused by *Haemophilus influenzae.*

Contraindications: Pregnancy at term and in children less than 2 months of age. Use with caution during other times of pregnancy.

Dosage

- **Oral Suspension**

Usual: Equivalent of 50 mg/kg/day of erythromycin and 150 mg/kg/day of sulfisoxazole, up to a maximum of 6 g/day. **Over 45 kg:** 10 mL/ q 6 hr; **24 kg:** 7.5 mL/ q 6 hr; **16 kg:** 5 mL/ q 6 hr; **8 kg:** 2.5 mL/ q 6 hr; **less than 8 kg:** Calculate dose according to body weight.

Administration/Storage

1. The reconstituted suspension should be refrigerated and used within 14 days.
2. Therapy should be continued for 10 days.
3. May be taken without regard to meals.

NURSING CONSIDERATIONS

See also *General Nursing Considerations for All Anti-Infectives,* Chapter 1, and *Sulfonamides,* Chapter 9.

Client/Family Teaching

1. Review the appropriate method, dosage, and frequency for administration.
2. Remind parent to keep medication refrigerated and to shake well before using.
3. Stress the importance of giving every 6 hr RTC for 10 days for drug to be effective.
4. Schedule to return in 2 weeks for follow-up ear check to ensure that infection has responded to therapy.

Evaluate

- Resolution of infection
- Reports of symptomatic improvement

Sulfacetamide sodium

(sul-fah-**SEAT**-ah-myd)

AK-Sulf, Bleph-10, Cetamide, Diosulf ✦, Isopto-Cetamide, I-Sulfacet, Ocu-Sul-10, Ocu-Sul-15, Ocu-Sul-30, Ocu-sulf-10, Ophthacet, Ophtho-Sulf ✦, PMS-Sulfacetamide Sodium ✦, Sebizon, Sodium Sulamyd, Spectro-Sulf, Steri-Units Sulfacetamide, Sulf-10, Sulfacetamide Minims ✦, Sulfair, Sulfair 10, Sulfair 15, Sulfair Forte, Sulfamide, Sulfex 10% ✦, Sulten-10 **(Rx)**

See also *Sulfonamides,* Chapter 9.

How Supplied: *Lotion:* 10%; *Ophthalmic Ointment:* 10%; *Ophthalmic Solution:* 10%, 15%, 30%

Uses: Topically for ophthalmic infections including trachoma, seborrheic dermatitis, dandruff, and cutaneous bacterial infections.

Dosage

- **Ophthalmic Solution**

1–3 gtt of 10%, 15%, or 30% solution in conjunctival sac q 2–3 hr.

- **Ophthalmic Ointment (10%)**

Apply 1–4 times/day and at bedtime in conjunctival sac.

For cutaneous infections.

Apply locally (10%) to affected area b.i.d.–q.i.d.

- **Lotion**

Seborrheic dermatitis.

Apply 1–2 times/day (for mild cases, apply overnight).

Cutaneous bacterial infections. Apply b.i.d.–q.i.d. until infection clears.

Administration/Storage: *Treatment of Overdose:* Client should ingest large amounts of fluid. Mannitol infusions may help if oliguria is present. Administration of bicarbonate may prevent crystallization in the kidney.

Special Concerns: Safe use during pregnancy and lactation or in children less than 12 years of age has not been established. Use with caution in clients with dry eye syndrome.

Side Effects: *Topical:* Itching, redness, swelling, irritation.

Symptoms of Overdose: If taken PO, N&V, hematuria, crystalluria, and ***renal shutdown*** (due to precipitation of sulfa crystals) may occur.

Drug Interactions: Preparations containing silver are incompatible with sulfacetamide sodium.

NURSING CONSIDERATIONS

See also *General Nursing Considerations for All Anti-Infectives,* Chapter 1, and for *Sulfonamides,* Chapter 9.

Assessment

1. Document indications for therapy, onset of symptoms, and a description of the area requiring treatment.
2. List other agents prescribed, duration of therapy, and the outcome.
3. Note any allergy to sulfa drugs.

Client/Family Teaching

1. Stress that medication is for topical use only.
2. When used for seborrheic dermatitis of the scalp, medication should be applied at bedtime and allowed to remain overnight. The hair and scalp may be washed the following morning, if desired. Hair should be washed at least once a week. The medication should be applied for 8–10 consecutive nights.
3. If hair and scalp are oily or if there is debris, shampoo scalp before application.
4. Ophthalmic products may cause sensitivity to bright light; this can be minimized by wearing sunglasses.
5. Report any purulent eye drainage as this inactivates sulfacetamide.
6. If client is prescribed additional eye drops, advise to wait 5 min after sulfacetamide instillation.
7. Do not wear contact lenses until infection is resolved.

Evaluate

- Resolution of infection
- Reports of symptomatic improvement

Sulfadiazine

(sul-fah-**DYE**-ah-zeen)
Microsulfon **(Rx)**

See also *Sulfonamides,* Chapter 9.

How Supplied: *Tablet:* 500 mg

Action/Kinetics: Short-acting, and often combined with other anti-infectives.

Uses: Urinary tract infections, bacillary dysentery, rheumatic fever prophylaxis. Adjunct with pyrimethamine in toxoplasmosis in selected immunocompromised clients (e.g., those with AIDS, neoplastic disease, or congenital immune compromise).

Dosage

- **Tablets**

UTIs, bacillary dysentery.

Adults, initial: 2–4 g; **maintenance:** 4–8 g/day in four to six divided doses; **infants over 2 months, initial:** 75 mg/kg/day (2 g/m^2); **maintenance:** 120–150 mg/kg/day (4 g/m^2/day) in four to six divided doses, not to exceed 6 g/day.

Rheumatic fever prophylaxis.

Under 30 kg: 0.5 g/day; **over 30 kg:** 1 g/day.

As adjunct with pyrimethamine in congenital toxoplasmosis.

Infants less than 2 months, initial: 75–100 mg/kg; **maintenance:** 100–150 mg/kg/day in four divided doses.

Special Concerns: Safe use during pregnancy has not been established. Should not be used in infants less than 2 months of age unless combined with pyrimethamine to treat congenital toxoplasmosis.

NURSING CONSIDERATIONS

See also *General Nursing Considerations For All Anti-Infectives,* Chapter 1, and for *Sulfonamides,* Chapter 9.

Assessment

1. Document indications for therapy and anticipated time frame for therapy.
2. Ensure that appropriate lab culture studies have been performed.

Evaluate

- Negative culture reports
- Rheumatic fever prophylaxis during invasive procedures

Sulfamethizole

(sul-fah-**METH**-ih-zohl)
Thiosulfil Forte **(Rx)**

See also *Sulfonamides,* Chapter 9.
How Supplied: *Tablet:* 500 mg
Use: Urinary tract infections.
Special Concerns: Safe use during pregnancy has not been established.
Additional Drug Interactions: Sulfamethizole ↑ effects of tolbutamide, phenytoin, and chlorpropamide due to ↓ breakdown by liver.

Dosage

- **Tablets**

Adults, 0.5–1 g t.i.d.–q.i.d.; **infants over 2 months:** 30–45 mg/kg/day in four divided doses.

NURSING CONSIDERATIONS

See also *General Nursing Considerations for All Anti-Infectives,* Chapter 1, and for *Sulfonamides,* Chapter 9.

Evaluate

- Negative urine culture results
- Reports of symptomatic improvement

Sulfamethoxazole

(sul-fah-meth-**OX**-ah-zohl)
Pregnancy Category: C
Apo-Sulfamethoxazole ✦, Gantanol, Urobak **(Rx)**

See also *Sulfonamides,* Chapter 9.
How Supplied: *Tablet:* 500 mg
Action/Kinetics: **t½:** 8.6 hr. Sulfamethoxazole is also a component of Bactrim, Bactrim DS, Septra, and Septra DS.

Dosage

- **Oral Suspension, Tablets**

Mild to moderate infections.

Adults, initially: 2 g; **then,** 1 g in morning and evening.

Severe infections.

Adults, initially: 2 g; **then,** 1 g t.i.d. **Infants over 2 months, initial:** 50–60 mg/kg; **then,** 25–30 mg/kg in morning and evening, not to exceed 75 mg/kg/day.

Lymphogranuloma venereum.

1 g b.i.d. for 2 weeks.

Uses: Urinary and upper respiratory tract infections; lymphogranuloma venereum.
Special Concerns: May be an increased risk of severe side effects in elderly clients.

NURSING CONSIDERATIONS

See also *General Nursing Considerations for All Anti-Infectives,* Chapter 1, and for *Sulfonamides,* Chapter 9.

Client/Family Teaching

1. Drug may cause dizziness; assess response prior to any activity requiring mental alertness.
2. Advise the use of sunglasses, sunscreens, and protective clothing during sun exposure as a photosensitivity reaction may occur.

Evaluate

- Resolution of infection
- Reports of symptomatic improvement

COMBINATION DRUG

Sulfamethoxazole and Phenazopyridine

(sul-fah-meth-**OX**-ah-zohl, fen-ay-zoh-**PEER**-ih-deen)
Pregnancy Category: C
Azo Gantanol, Azo Sulfamethoxazole **(Rx)**

How Supplied: See Content
Content: *Sulfonamide:* Sulfamethoxazole, 500 mg. *Urinary analgesic:* Phenazopyridine, 100 mg. See also *Sulfamethoxazole,* Chapter 9, and *Phenazopyridine,* Chapter 18.

Uses: Acute, painful phase of uncomplicated UTIs due to susceptible strains of *Escherichia coli, Enterobacter, Klebsiella, Proteus mirabilis, Proteus vulgaris,* and *Staphylococcus aureus.*

Dosage

- **Tablets**

Adults and children over 12 years of age, initially: 2 g sulfamethoxazole and 400 mg phenazopyridine (4 tablets); **then,** 1 g sulfamethoxazole and 200 mg phenazopyridine (2 tablets) q 12 hr for 2 days.

Administration/Storage

1. Dose should be decreased in clients with impaired renal function.
2. Treatment should not exceed 2 days.

Contraindications: Pregnancy at term, during lactation. Use in children less than 12 years of age. Glomerulonephritis, severe hepatitis, uremia, and pyelonephritis of pregnancy with GI disturbances.

Special Concerns: Use with caution in impaired hepatic or renal function and in severe allergy or bronchial asthma.

NURSING CONSIDERATIONS

See also *General Nursing Considerations for All Anti-Infectives,* Chapter 1, and for *Sulfamethoxazole,* Chapter 9.

Client/Family Teaching

1. If GI upset occurs, the drug may be taken with or after meals.
2. Fluid intake must be adequate for urine output to be at least 1.2–1.5 L/day to prevent crystalluria and stone formation. Maintain record of I&O.

Evaluate

- Resolution of infection
- ↓ GU pain and discomfort

Sulfasalazine

(sul-fah-**SAL**-ah-zeen)
Pregnancy Category: B
Azulfidine, Azulfidine EN-Tabs, PMS Sulfasalazine ✸, PMS Sulfasalazine E.C. ✸, Salazopyrin ✸, Salazopyrin-EN Tabs ✸, SAS Enteric-500 ✸, SAS-500 ✸ **(Rx)**

See also *Sulfonamides,* Chapter 9.

How Supplied: *Enteric Coated Tablet:* 500 mg; *Tablet:* 500 mg

Action/Kinetics: About one-third of the dose of sulfasalazine is absorbed from the small intestine while two-thirds passes to the colon, where it is split to 5-aminosalicylic acid and sulfapyridine. The drug does not affect the microflora.

Use: Ulcerative colitis.

Dosage

- **Oral Suspension, Enteric-Coated Tablets, Tablets**

Adults: initial, 3–4 g/day in divided doses (1–2 g/day may decrease side effects); **maintenance:** 500 mg q.i.d. **Pediatric, initial:** 40–60 mg/kg/day in four to six equally divided doses; **maintenance:** 20–30 mg/kg/day in four divided doses.

For desensitization to sulfasalazine.

Reinstitute at level of 50–250 mg/day; **then,** give double dose q 4–7 days until desired therapeutic level reached. Use oral suspension.

Additional Contraindications: Children below 2 years, persons with marked sulfonamide and salicylate hypersensitivity.

Side Effects: Anorexia, vomiting, nausea.

Additional Drug Interactions

Digoxin / Sulfasalazine ↓ effect due to ↓ absorption from GI tract
Ferrous sulfate / Ferrous sulfate ↓ blood levels of sulfasalazine

NURSING CONSIDERATIONS

See also *General Nursing Considerations for All Anti-Infectives,* Chapter 1, and for *Sulfonamides,* Chapter 9.

Assessment

1. Note indications for therapy. Document frequency, quantity, and consistency of stool production as well as characteristics of abdominal pain.
2. Obtain baseline CBC and urinalysis. Send a stool specimen for analysis.

Client/Family Teaching

1. Take with food to reduce GI upset.
2. Stress the importance of taking medication exactly as ordered be-

cause intermittent therapy (2 weeks on, 2 weeks off) is generally recommended.
3. Drug may discolor urine or skin a yellow-orange color.
4. Take at least 2–3 L/day of water to decrease incidence of crystalluria and stone formation.
5. Avoid prolonged exposure to sunlight because drug may increase sensitivity. Wear protective clothing, sunglasses, and sunscreen if exposure is necessary.

Evaluate
- ↓ Frequency of loose stools and control of associated abdominal pain
- ↓ Colon inflammation

Sulfisoxazole
(sul-fih-**SOX**-ah-zohl)
Pregnancy Category: C
Gantrisin, Novo-Soxazole ✱ **(Rx)**

Sulfisoxazole acetyl
(sul-fih-**SOX**-ah-zohl)
Pregnancy Category: C
Gantrisin, Lipo Gantrisin **(Rx)**

Sulfisoxazole diolamine
(sul-fih-**SOX**-ah-zohl)
Pregnancy Category: C
Gantrisin Diolamine **(Rx)**

See also *Sulfonamides,* Chapter 9.
How Supplied: Sulfisoxazole: *Tablet:* 500 mg.
Sulfisoxazole acetyl: *Suspension:* 500 mg/5 mL
Sulfisoxazole diolamine: *Ophthalmic Solution:* 4%
Action/Kinetics: t½: 5.9 hr. Lipo Gantrisin contains sulfisoxazole acetyl in a homogenized vegetable oil mixture.
Uses: Urinary tract and topical infections. Conjunctivitis, corneal ulcer, and other superficial ocular infections due to *Escherichia coli, Haemophilus aegyptius, Chlamydia trachomatis,* and other susceptible infections. Ophthalmically as an adjunct with systemic sulfonamides to treat trachoma.

Dosage
- **Oral Suspension, Extended-Release Tablets**

Adults, initial: 2–4 g; **maintenance:** 1 g b.i.d.–t.i.d. depending on severity of the infection. **Infants over 2 months, initial:** 50–60 mg/kg/day; **maintenance:** 25–30 mg/kg in the morning and evening, not to exceed 75 mg/kg/day. Alternative dose: 50–60 mg/kg/day divided q 12 hr, not to exceed 3 g/day.
- **IM, IV (slow injection or drip), SC**

Initially, 50 mg/kg; **then,** 100 mg/kg in two to four divided doses.
- **Ophthalmic Solution (4%)**

Conjunctivitis or corneal ulcer.
1–2 gtt into conjunctival sac q 1–3 hr, depending on the severity of the infection.
Trachoma.
2 gtt q 2 hr with concomitant systemic therapy.

Administration/Storage
1. For SC administration, dilute commercial solution containing 400 mg/mL with sterile water for injection, to obtain solution containing 50 mg/mL.
2. Ophthalmic use may cause sensitivity to bright light (can be minimized by wearing sunglasses.
3. For ophthalmic use, the provider should be notified if improvement is not seen after 7–8 days, if the condition worsens, or if pain, increased redness, itching, or swelling of the eye occurs.

Special Concerns: Safety and efficacy of the ophthalmic products have not been established in children. Use with caution in clients with severe dry eye.
Additional Side Effects: *Following ophthalmic use:* Blurred vision, itching, local irritation, epithelial keratitis, reactive hyperemia, conjunctival edema, burning, headache or browache, transient stinging.
Additional Drug Interaction: Sulfisoxazole may ↑ effects of thiopental due to ↓ plasma protein binding.

NURSING CONSIDERATIONS

See also *General Nursing Considerations for All Anti-Infectives,* Chapter 1, and for *Sulfonamides,* Chapter 9.

Evaluate

- Negative culture results
- Reports of symptomatic improvement

—COMBINATION DRUG—

Sulfisoxazole and Phenazopyridine

(sul-fih-**SOX**-ah-zohl, fen-**ay**-zoh-**PEER**-ih-deen)

Pregnancy Category: C

Azo-Cheragan, Azo Gantrisin, Axo-Sulfisoxazole, Azo-Truxazole, Sul-Azo

(Rx)

How Supplied: See Content

Content: Each of the products contains sulfisoxazole (antibacterial), 500 mg and phenazopyridine (urinary analgesic), 50 mg. Also, see information on individual components.

Uses: For the first 2 days in treating uncomplicated UTIs due to *Escherichia coli, Enterobacter, Klebsiella, Proteus mirabilis, Proteus vulgaris,* and *Staphylococcus aureus*. Sulfisoxazole can be used alone after the first 2 days.

Dosage

- **Tablets**

Adults, initial: 4–6 tablets; **then,** 2 tablets q.i.d. for 2 days.

Contraindications: Pregnancy at term, during lactation, and in children less than 12 years of age. Glomerulonephritis, severe hepatitis, uremia, and pyelonephritis of pregnancy with GI disturbances.

Special Concerns: Use with caution in impaired hepatic or renal function and in severe allergy or bronchial asthma.

NURSING CONSIDERATIONS

See *General Nursing Considerations for All Anti-Infectives,* Chapter 1, and for *Sulfonamides,* Chapter 9.

Evaluate: Resolution of infection with reports of symptomatic relief.

Trimethoprim and Sulfamethoxazole

(try-**METH**-oh-prim, sul-fah-meh-**THOX**-ah-zohl)

Pregnancy Category: C

Apo-Sulfatrim ✦, Bactrim, Bactrim DS, Bactrim IV, Bactrim Pediatric, Bactrim Roche ✦, Cotrim, Cotrim D.S., Cotrim Pediatric, Novo-Trimel ✦, Novo-Trimel DS ✦, Nu-Cotrimix ✦, Roubac ✦, Septra, Septra DS, Septra IV, Sulfatrim

(Rx)

See also *Sulfonamides,* Chapter 9.

How Supplied: See Content

Content: These products contain the antibacterial agents sulfamethoxazole and trimethoprim. See also *Sulfamethoxazole,* Chapter 9. **Oral Suspension:** Sulfamethoxazole, 200 mg and trimethoprim, 40 mg/5 mL.

Tablets: Sulfamethoxazole, 400 mg and trimethoprim, 80 mg/tablet.

Double Strength (DS) Tablets: Sulfamethoxazole, 800 mg and trimethoprim, 160 mg/tablet.

Concentrate for injection: Sulfamethoxazole, 80 mg and trimethoprim, 16 mg/mL.

Uses: PO, Parenteral: UTIs due to *Escherichia coli, Klebsiella, Enterobacter, Pseudomonas mirabilis* and *vulgaris,* and *Morganella morganii.* Enteritis due to *Shigella flexneri* or *S. sonnei. Pneumocystis carinii* pneumonitis in children and adults. **PO:** Acute otitis media in children due to *Haemophilus influenzae* or *Streptococcus pneumoniae*. Traveler's diarrhea in adults due to *E. coli. Prophylaxis of P. carinii* pneumonia in immunocompromised clients (including those with AIDS). Acute exacerbations of chronic bronchitis in adults due to *H. influenzae* or *S. pneumoniae. Investigational:* Cholera, salmonella, nocardiosis, prophylaxis of recurrent UTIs in women, prophylaxis of neutropenic clients with *P. carinii* infections or leukemia clients to decrease incidence of gram-negative rod bacteremia. Treatment of acute and chronic prostatitis. Decrease chance of urinary and blood bacterial infections in renal transplant clients.

Dosage

• Oral Suspension, Double-Strength Tablets, Tablets

UTIs, shigellosis, bronchitis, acute otitis media.

Adults: 1 DS tablet, 2 tablets, or 4 teaspoonfuls of suspension q 12 hr for 10–14 days. **Pediatric:** Total daily dose of 8 mg/kg trimethoprim and 40 mg/kg sulfamethoxazole divided equally and given q 12 hr for 10–14 days (*NOTE:* For shigellosis, give adult or pediatric dose for 5 days.) For clients with impaired renal function the following dosage is recommended: creatinine clearance of 15–30 mL/min: one-half the usual regimen and for creatinine clearance less than 15 mL/min: use is not recommended.

Chancroid.

1 DS tablet b.i.d. for at least 7 days (alternate therapy: 4 DS tablets in a single dose).

Pharyngeal gonococcal infection due to penicillinase-producing Neisseria gonorrhoeae.

720 mg trimethoprim and 3,600 mg sulfamethoxazole once daily for 5 days.

Prophylaxis of P. carinii *pneumonia.*

Adults: 160 mg trimethoprim and 800 mg sulfamethoxazole q 24 hr. **Children:** 150 mg/m^2 of trimethoprim and 750 mg/m^2 sulfamethoxazole daily in equally divided doses b.i.d. on three consecutive days per week. The total daily dose should not exceed 320 mg trimethoprim and 1,600 mg sulamethoxazole.

Treatment of P. carinii *pneumonia.*

Adults and children: Total daily dose of 15–20 mg/kg trimethoprim and 100 mg/kg sulfamethoxazole divided equally and given q 6 hr for 14–21 days.

Prophylaxis of P. carinii *pneumonia in immunocompromised clients.*

1 DS tablet daily.

Traveler's diarrhea.

Adults, 1 DS tablet q 12 hr for 5 days.

Prostatitis, acute bacterial.

1 DS tablet b.i.d. until client is afebrile for 48 hr; treatment may be required for up to 30 days.

Prostatitis, chronic bacterial.

1 DS tablet b.i.d. for 4–6 weeks.

• IV

UTIs, shigellosis, acute otitis media.

Adults and children: 8–10 mg/kg/day (based on trimethoprim) in two to four divided doses q 6, 8, or 12 hr for up to 14 days for severe UTIs or 5 days for shigellosis.

Treatment of P. carinii *pneumonia.*

Adults and children: 15–20 mg/kg/day (based on trimethoprim) in 3–4 divided doses q 6–8 hr for up to 14 days.

Administration/Storage

1. The IV infusion must be administered over a period of 60–90 min.
2. Each 5-mL vial must be diluted to 125 mL with D5W and used within 6 hr. If the amount of fluid should be restricted, each 5 mL can be diluted up to 75 mL with D5W and used within 2 hr. The diluted solution should not be refrigerated.
3. The IV infusion should not be mixed with any other drugs or solutions.
4. If the diluted IV infusion is cloudy or precipitates after mixing, it should be discarded and a new solution prepared.

Additional Contraindications: Infants under 2 months of age. During pregnancy at term. Megaloblastic anemia due to folate deficiency. Lactation.

Special Concerns: Use with caution in impaired liver or kidney function. AIDS clients may not tolerate or respond to this product. Use with caution in clients with possible folate deficiency.

Laboratory Test Interferences: Jaffe alkaline picrate reaction overestimation of creatinine by 10%.

Additional Drug Interactions

Cyclosporine / ↓ Effect of cyclosporine; ↑ risk of nephrotoxicity
Dapsone / ↑ Effect of both dapsone and trimethoprim
Methotrexate / ↑ Risk of methotrexate toxicity due to displacement from plasma protein binding sites
Phenytoin / ↑ Effect of phenytoin due to ↓ hepatic clearance
Sulfonylureas / ↑Hypoglycemic effect of sulfonylureas
Thiazide diuretics / ↑ Risk of thrombocytopenia with purpura in geriatric clients
Warfarin / ↑ PT
Zidovudine↑Serum levels of AZT due to ↓ renal clearance

NURSING CONSIDERATIONS

See also *General Nursing Considerations for All Anti-Infectives,* Chapter 1, and for *Sulfonamides,* Chapter 9.

Assessment

1. Obtain baseline lab data to evaluate liver and renal functions. Anticipate reduced dose with renal dysfunction.
2. Assess for anemia (leukopenia and granulocytopenia) because megaloblastic anemia due to folate deficiency is a contraindication as drug inhibits ability to produce folinic acid.
3. Simultaneous administration of folinic acid (6–8 mg/day) may prevent antifolate drug effects.
4. Document, when known, in clients infected with AIDS virus as they may be intolerant to this product.

Client/Family Teaching

1. Take only as directed; do not share medications.
2. Report any symptoms of drug fever, vasculitis, N&V, or CNS disturbances immediately.

Evaluate

- Resolution of infection
- Negative culture results
- Prophylaxis of *P. carinii* pneumonia

CHAPTER TEN

Antibiotics: Tetracyclines

See also the following individual entries:

Doxycycline Calcium
Doxycycline Hyclate
Doxycycline Monohydrate
Tetracycline
Tetracycline Hydrochloride

Action/Kinetics: The tetracyclines inhibit protein synthesis by microorganisms by binding to a crucial ribosomal subunit (50S), thereby interfering with protein synthesis. The drugs block the binding of aminoacyl transfer RNA to the messenger RNA complex. Cell wall synthesis is not inhibited. The drugs are mostly bacteriostatic and are effective only against multiplying bacteria. Tetracyclines are well absorbed from the stomach and upper small intestine. They are well distributed throughout all tissues and fluids and diffuse through noninflamed meninges and the placental barrier. They become deposited in the fetal skeleton and calcifying teeth. **t½:** 7–18.6 hr (see individual agents) and is increased in the presence of renal impairment. The drugs bind to serum protein (range: 20%–93%; see individual agents). The drugs are concentrated in the liver in the bile and are excreted mostly unchanged in the urine and feces.

Uses: Used mainly for infections caused by *Rickettsia, Chlamydia,* and *Mycoplasma*. Due to development of resistance, tetracyclines are usually not used for infections by common gram-negative or gram-positive organisms.

Tetracyclines are the drugs of choice for rickettsial infections such as Rocky Mountain spotted fever, endemic typhus, and others. They are also the drugs of choice for psittacosis, lymphogranuloma venereum, and urethritis due to *Mycoplasma hominis* and *Ureaplasma urealyticum*. Epididymo-orchitis due to *Chlamydia trachomatis* and/or *Neisseria gonorrhoeae*. Atypical pneumonia caused by *Mycoplasma pneumoniae*. Adjunct in the treatment of trachoma.

Tetracyclines are the drugs of choice for gram-negative bacteria causing bartonellosis, brucellosis, granuloma inguinale, cholera. They are used as alternatives for the treatment of plague, tularemia, chancroid, or *Campylobacter fetus* infections. Prophylaxis of plague after exposure. Infections caused by *Acinetobacter, Bacteroides, Enterobacter aerogenes, Escherichia coli, Shigella*. Respiratory and/or urinary tract infections caused by *Haemophilus influenzae* or *Klebsiella pneumoniae*.

As an alternative to penicillin for uncomplicated gonorrhea or disseminated gonococcal infections, especially with penicillin allergy. Acute pelvic inflammatory disease. Tetracyclines are also useful as an alternative to penicillin for early syphilis.

Although not generally used for gram-positive infections, tetracyclines may be beneficial in anthrax, *Listeria* infections, and actinomycosis. They have also been used in conjunction with quinine sulfate for chloroquine-resistant *Plasmodium falciparum* malaria and as an intracavitary injection to control pleural or pericardial effusions caused by metastatic carcinoma. As an adjunct to amebicides in acute intestinal amebiasis. Used PO to treat uncomplicated endocervical, rectal, or urethral *Chlamydia* infections.

Topical uses include skin granulomas caused by *Mycobacterium marinum;* ophthalmic bacterial infections causing blepharitis, conjunctivitis, or keratitis; and as an adjunct in the treatment of ophthalmic chlamydial infections such as trachoma or inclusion conjunctivitis. Tetracyclines are used as an alternative to silver nitrate for prophylaxis of neonatal gonococcal ophthalmia. Vaginitis. Severe acne.

Contraindications: Hypersensitivity; avoid drug during tooth development stage (last trimester of pregnancy, neonatal period, during breast-feeding, and during childhood up to 8 years) because tetracyclines interfere with enamel formation and dental pigmentation. Never administer intrathecally.

Special Concerns: Use with caution and at reduced dosage in clients with impaired kidney function.

Side Effects: *GI* (most common): N&V, thirst, diarrhea, anorexia, sore throat, flatulence, epigastric distress, bulky loose stools. Less commonly, stomatitis, dysphagia, black hairy tongue, glossitis, or inflammatory lesions of the anogenital area. Rarely, pseudomembranous colitis. PO dosage forms may cause esophageal ulcers, especially in clients with esophageal obstructive element or hiatal hernia. *Allergic* (rare): Urticaria, pericarditis, polyarthralgia, fever, rash, pulmonary infiltrates with eosinophilia, ***angioneurotic edema,*** worsening of SLE, ***anaphylaxis,*** purpura. *Skin:* Photosensitivity, maculopapular and erythematous rashes, exfoliative dermatitis (rare), onycholysis, discoloration of nails. *CNS:* Dizziness, lightheadedness, unsteadiness, paresthesias. *Hematologic:* Eosinophilia, ***hemolytic anemia,*** neutropenia, thrombocytopenia, thrombocytopenic purpura. *Hepatic:* Fatty liver, increases in liver enzymes; rarely, hepatotoxicity, hepatitis, hepatic cholestasis. *Miscellaneous:* Candidal superinfections including oral and vaginal candidiasis, discoloration of infants' and children's teeth, bone lesions, delayed bone growth, abnormal pigmentation of the conjunctiva, pseudotumor cerebri in adults and bulging fontanels in infants.

IV administration may cause thrombophlebitis; IM injections are painful and may cause induration at the injection site.

The administration of deteriorated tetracyclines may result in Fanconi-like syndrome characterized by N&V, acidosis, proteinuria, glycosuria, aminoaciduria, polydipsia, polyuria, hypokalemia.

Drug Interactions

Aluminum salts / ↓ Effect of tetracyclines due to ↓ absorption from GI tract

Antacids, oral / ↓ Effect of tetracyclines due to ↓ absorption from GI tract

Anticoagulants, oral / IV tetracyclines ↑ hypoprothrombinemia

Bismuth salts / ↓ Effect of tetracyclines due to ↓ absorption from GI tract

Bumetanide / ↑ Risk of kidney toxicity

Calcium salts / ↓ Effect of tetracyclines due to ↓ absorption from GI tract

Cimetidine / ↓ Effect of tetracyclines due to ↓ absorption from GI tract

Contraceptives, oral / ↓ Effect of oral contraceptives

Digoxin / Tetracyclines ↑ bioavailability of digoxin

Diuretics, thiazide / ↑ Risk of kidney toxicity

Ethacrynic acid / ↑ Risk of kidney toxicity

Furosemide / ↑ Risk of kidney toxicity

Insulin / Tetracyclines may ↓ insulin requirement

Iron preparations / ↓ Effect of tetracyclines due to ↓ absorption from GI tract

Lithium / Either ↑ or ↓ levels of lithium
Magnesium salts / ↓ Effect of tetracyclines due to ↓ absorption from GI tract
Methoxyflurane / ↑ Risk of kidney toxicity
Penicillins / Tetracyclines may mask bactericidal effect of penicillins
Sodium bicarbonate / ↓ Effect of tetracyclines due to ↓ absorption from GI tract
Zinc salts / ↓ Effect of tetracyclines due to ↓ absorption from GI tract
Laboratory Test Interferences: False + or ↑ urinary catecholamines and urinary protein (degraded); ↑ coagulation time. False – or ↓ urinary urobilinogen, glucose tests (see *Nursing Considerations*). Prolonged use or high doses may change liver function tests and WBC counts.

Dosage

See individual drugs.

NURSING CONSIDERATIONS

See also *General Nursing Considerations for All Anti-Infectives,* Chapter 1.

Administration/Storage

1. Do not use outdated or deteriorated drugs because a Fanconi-like syndrome may occur (see *Side Effects*).
2. Discard unused capsules to prevent use of deteriorated medication.
3. Administer IM into large muscle mass to avoid extravasation into subcutaneous or fatty tissue.
4. Administer on an empty stomach at least 1 hr before or 2 hr after meals. Withhold antacids, iron salts, dairy foods, and other foods high in calcium for at least 2 hr after PO administration. Do not administer milk with tetracyclines.

Assessment

1. Determine any drug allergens or sensitivity. Be aware that IM form contains procaine HCl.
2. Document indications for therapy and type and onset of symptoms. List other agents prescribed and the outcome.
3. Assess for and note any evidence of impaired kidney function.
4. Determine if client has any history of colitis or other bowel problems.
5. If the client is pregnant, determine the trimester.
6. Note symptoms of infection and ensure that baseline lab studies have been performed, including CBC, BUN, creatinine, C&S, etc.
7. Document baseline VS and weights.

Interventions

1. If client experiences gastric distress following administration of medication, suggest that they be permitted to have a light meal with the medication to reduce distress. An alternative would be to reduce the individual dose of the medication but increase the frequency of administration.
2. Monitor VS and I&O. Maintain adequate I&O because renal dysfunction may result in drug accumulation, leading to toxicity. Assess client with impaired kidney function for increased BUN, acidosis, anorexia, N&V, weight loss, and dehydration. Continue assessment after cessation of therapy because symptoms may appear latently.
3. To prevent or treat pruritus ani instruct and assist client to cleanse the anal area with water several times a day and/or after each bowel movement. Observe for symptoms of enterocolitis, such as diarrhea, pyrexia, abdominal distention, and scanty urine. These symptoms may necessitate discontinuing drug and substituting another antibiotic.
4. If GI disturbances occur, avoid antacids that contain calcium, magnesium, or aluminum.
5. Assess client on IV therapy for N&V, chills, fever, and hypertension resulting from too rapid administration or an excessively high dose. Slow rate of IV infusion and report if symptoms occur.
6. Observe infant for bulging fonta-

nelle, which may be caused by a too rapid rate of IV infusion. Slow IV infusion rate and report.
7. Side effects such as sore throat, dysphagia, fever, dizziness, hoarseness, and inflammation of mucous membranes of the body may be candidal superinfections and should be reported.
8. Assess client with impaired hepatic or renal function for altered level of consciousness or other CNS disturbances, as drug may cause hepatic and renal toxicity.
9. Observe for onycholysis (loosening or detachment of the nail from the nail bed) or discoloration and take appropriate precautions.

Client/Family Teaching

1. Take on a full stomach to enhance absorption. Do not lay down after administration as this may precipitate erosive esophagitis.
2. Do not take tetracyclines with milk, cheese, ice cream, yogurt, or other foods containing calcium. If dose is taken with meals, avoid these foods for 2 hr after administration.
3. Zinc tablets or vitamin preparations containing zinc may interfere with absorption of tetracyclines. Identify food sources high in zinc that should be avoided (oysters, fresh and raw; cooked lobster, dry oat flakes, steamed crabs, veal, liver, etc.)
4. Avoid direct or artificial sunlight, which can cause a severe sunburn-like reaction, and report erythema if it occurs. Wear protective clothing, sunglasses, and a sunscreen if exposure is necessary and for up to 3 weeks following therapy.
5. Tetracyclines interfere with formation of tooth enamel and dental pigmentation from pregnancy through age 8.
6. Explain how to prevent or treat pruritus ani by cleansing the anal area with water several times a day and/or after each bowel movement.
7. Advise females of childbearing age to use an alternative method of birth control, as drug may interfere with oral contraceptives. It may also cause an overgrowth vaginal infection so call if symptoms become evident.
8. Advise client to take only as directed and to complete full prescription unless otherwise indicated. Remind client to discard any leftover medications to prevent adverse effects from the consumption of deteriorated drugs.

Evaluate

- Knowledge and understanding of illness and evidence of compliance with prescribed therapy
- Resolution of infection (↓ temperature, ↓ WBCs, ↑ appetite)
- Reports of symptomatic improvement
- Negative C&S reports and no evidence of organism resistance to drug therapy

Doxycycline calcium

(dox-ih-**SYE**-kleen)
Pregnancy Category: D
Vibramycin **(Rx)**

Doxycycline hyclate

(dox-ih-**SYE**-kleen)
Pregnancy Category: D
Apo-Doxy ✱, Doryx, Doxy 100 and 200, Doxy-Caps, Doxycin ✱, Doxychel Hyclate, Novo-Doxylin ✱, Vibramycin, Vibramycin IV, Vibra-Tabs, Vivox **(Rx)**

Doxycycline monohydrate

(dox-ih-**SYE**-kleen)
Pregnancy Category: D
Monodox, Vibramycin **(Rx)**

See also *Anti-Infectives,* Chapter 1, and *Tetracyclines,* Chapter 10.

How Supplied: Doxycycline calcium: *Syrup:* 50 mg/5 mL.
Doxycyline hyclate: *Capsule:* 50 mg, 100 mg; *Enteric Coated Capsule:* 100 mg; *Powder for injection:* 100 mg, 200 mg; *Tablet:* 100 mg.
Doxycycline monohydrate: *Capsule:* 50 mg, 100 mg; *Powder for Reconstitution:* 25 mg/5 mL

Action/Kinetics: More slowly absorbed, and thus more persistent, than other tetracyclines. Preferred for clients with impaired renal function for treating infections outside the urinary tract. From 80% to 95% is bound to serum proteins. **t½:** 14.5–22 hr; 30%–40% excreted unchanged in urine.

Additional Uses: Orally for uncomplicated gonococcal infections in adults (except anorectal infections in males); acute epididymo-orchitis caused by *Neisseria gonorrhoeae* and *Chlamydia trachomatis;* gonococcal arthritis-dermatitis syndrome; nongonococcal urethritis caused by *C. trachomatis* and *Ureaplasma urealyticum.* Prophylaxis of malaria due to *Plasmodium falciparum* in short-term travelers (< 4 months) to areas with chloroquine- or pyrimethamine-sulfadoxine-resistant strains.

Dosage

• Capsules, Delayed-Release Capsules, Oral Suspension, Tablets, IV

Infections.

Adult: First day, 100 mg q 12 hr; **maintenance:** 100–200 mg/day, depending on severity of infection. **Children, over 8 years (45 kg or less): First day,** 4.4 mg/kg in 1–2 doses; **then,** 2.2–4.4 mg/kg/day in divided doses depending on severity of infection. Children over 45 kg should receive the adult dose.

Acute gonorrhea.

200 mg at once given PO; **then,** 100 mg at bedtime on first day, followed by 100 mg b.i.d. for 3 days. Alternatively, 300 mg immediately followed in 1 hr with 300 mg.

Syphilis (primary/secondary).

300 mg/day in divided PO doses for 10 days.

C. trachomatis *infections.*

100 mg b.i.d. PO for minimum of 7 days.

Prophylaxis of "traveler's diarrhea."

100 mg/day given PO.

Prophylaxis of malaria.

Adults: 100 mg PO once daily; **children, over 8 years of age:** 2 mg/kg/day up to 100 mg/day.

• IV

Endometritis, parametritis, peritonitis, salpingitis.

100 mg b.i.d. with 2 g cefoxitin, IV, q.i.d. continued for at least 4 days or 2 days after improvement observed. This is followed by doxycycline, PO, 100 mg b.i.d. for 10–14 days of total therapy.

NOTE: The Centers for Disease Control have established treatment schedules for STDs.

Administration/Storage

1. Powder for suspension has expiration date of 12 months from date of issue.
2. Solution stable for 2 weeks when stored in refrigerator.
3. Follow directions on vial for dilution. Concentrations should be no lower than 0.1 mg/mL and no higher than 1.0 mg/mL.
4. During infusion protect solution from light.
5. Complete administration of solutions diluted with NaCl injection, D5W, Ringer's injection, and 10% invert sugar within 12 hr.
6. Complete administration of solutions diluted with lactated Ringer's injection or 5% dextrose in lactated Ringer's injection within 6 hr.
7. Prophylaxis for malaria can begin 1–2 days before travel begins, during travel, and for 4 weeks after leaving the malarious area.

Contraindications: Prophylaxis of malaria in pregnant individuals and in children less than 8 years old. Use during the last half of pregnancy and in children up to 8 years of age (tetracycline may cause permanent discoloration of the teeth). Lactation.

Special Concern: Safety for IV use in children less than 8 years of age has not been established.

Additional Drug Interaction: Carbamazepine, phenytoin, and barbiturates ↓ effect of doxycycline by ↑ breakdown of doxycycline by the liver.

NURSING CONSIDERATIONS

See also *General Nursing Considera-*

tions for All Anti-Infectives, Chapter 1, and for *Tetracyclines,* Chapter 10.

Client/Family Teaching

1. May take with food. To prevent esophageal ulceration take with a full glass of water.
2. Avoid direct exposure to sunlight and wear protective clothing and sunscreens when exposure is necessary.
3. With STDs advise that partner be tested and treated. Use condoms until medically cleared.

Evaluate

- Resolution of infection and reports of symptomatic improvement
- Negative laboratory culture reports

Tetracycline

(teh-trah-**SYE**-kleen)

Pregnancy Category: D

Achromycin Ophthalmic Ointment, Achromycin Ophthalmic Suspension, Actisite Periodontal Fiber **(Rx)**

Tetracycline hydrochloride

(teh-trah-**SYE**-kleen)

Pregnancy Category: D

Achromycin IM and IV, Achromycin Ophthalmic Ointment, Achromycin Topical Ointment, Achromycin V, Ala-Tet, Apo-Tetra ✱, Nor-Tet, Novo-Tetra ✱, Nu-Tetra ✱, Panmycin, Robitet, Robicaps, Sumycin 250 and 500, Sumycin Syrup, Teline, Teline-500, Tetracap, Tetracyn ✱, Tetralan-250 and -500, Tetralan Syrup, Tetram **(Rx)**

See also *General Information* on *Tetracyclines,* Chapter 10.

How Supplied: Tetracycline: *Syrup:* 125 mg/5 mL

Tetracycline hydrochloride: *Capsule:* 100 mg, 250 mg, 500 mg; *Ointment:* 3%; *Ophthalmic ointment:* 1%; *Solution:* 2.2 mg/mL; *Tablet:* 250 mg, 500 mg

Action/Kinetics: t½: 7–11 hr. From 40% to 70% excreted unchanged in urine; 65% bound to serum proteins. Dosage is always expressed as the hydrochloride salt.

Additional Uses: Ophthalmic: Superficial ophthalmic infections due to *Staphylococcus aureus, Streptococcus, Streptococcus pneumoniae, Escherichia coli, Neisseria,* and *Bacteroides*. Prophylaxis of *Neisseria gonorrhoeae* in newborns. With oral therapy for treatment of *Chlamydia trachomatis*. **Topical:** Acne vulgaris, prophylaxis or treatment of infection following skin abrasions, minor cuts, wounds, or burns. **Tetracycline fiber:** Adult periodontitis. *Investigational:* Pleural sclerosing agent in malignant pleural effusions (administered by chest tube); in combination with gentamicin for *Vibrio vulnificus* infections due to wound infection after trauma or by eating contaminated seafood. Mouthwash (use suspension) to treat nonspecific mouth ulcerations, canker sores, aphthous ulcers. Possible drug of choice for stage I Lyme disease.

Dosage

- **Capsules, Tablets**

Mild to moderate infections.

Adults, usual: 500 mg b.i.d. or 250 mg q.i.d.

Severe infections.

Adult: 500 mg q.i.d. **Children over 8 years:** 25–50 mg/kg/day in four equal doses.

Brucellosis.

500 mg q.i.d. for 3 weeks with 1 g streptomycin IM b.i.d. for first week and once daily the second week.

Syphilis.

Total of 30–40 g over 10–15 days.

Gonorrhea.

Initially, 1.5 g; **then,** 500 mg q 6 hr until 9 g has been given.

Gonorrhea sensitive to penicillin.

Initially, 1.5 g; **then,** 500 mg q 6 hr for 4 days (total: 9 g).

GU or rectal Chlamydia trachomatis infections.

500 mg q.i.d. for minimum of 7 days.

Severe acne.

Initially, 1 g/day; **then,** 125–500 mg/day (long-term).

NOTE: The Centers for Disease Control have established treatment schedules for STDs.

- **Ophthalmic Suspension**

Acute infections.
Initially: 1–2 gtt q 15–30 min; **then,** as infection improves, decrease frequency.
Moderate infections.
1–2 gtt q 4 hr.
Trachoma.
2 gtt in each eye b.i.d.–q.i.d. for up to 2 or more months (PO tetracycline may be given concomitantly).
• **Ophthalmic Ointment**
Acute infections.
½ in. q 3–4 hr until improvement noted.
Mild to moderate infections.
½ in. b.i.d.–t.i.d.
• **Topical**
Acne.
Apply topical solution to affected areas in the morning and at night, making sure that skin is completely wet after each application.
Infections.
Apply OTC ointment (3%) to affected areas 1–4 times/day. A sterile bandage may be used.
• **Tetracycline fiber**
Adult periodontitis.
The fiber should be placed into the periodontal pocket until the pocket is filled (amount of fiber will vary with pocket depth and contour) ensuring that the fiber is in contact with the base of the pocket. The fiber should remain in place for 10 days, after which it is to be removed. The effectiveness of subsequent therapy with the fiber has not been assessed.

Administration/Storage

1. To reconstitute solutions for IV use, vials containing 250 or 500 mg should be diluted with 5 or 10 mL, respectively, of sterile water for injection. Further dilution (100–1,000 mL) can be done with sodium chloride injection, 5% dextrose injection, 5% dextrose and sodium chloride, Ringer's injection, and lactated Ringer's injection.
2. Except for Ringer's and lactated Ringer's injections, calcium-containing solutions should not be used to dilute tetracycline HCl.
3. For IM administration, inject into a large muscle mass.
4. The tetracycline fiber product consists of a monofilament of ethylene/vinyl acetate copolymer evenly dispersed with tetracycline. The fiber provides for continuous release of tetracycline for 10 days. The fiber releases about 2 mcg/cm/hr of tetracycline.
5. Clients should avoid actions that may dislodge the fiber; i.e., they should not chew hard, crusty, or sticky foods; should not brush or floss near any treated areas; should not engage in hygienic practices that might dislodge the fiber; should not probe the treated area with tongue or fingers.
6. The dentist should be contacted immediately if the fiber is dislodged or falls out before the next scheduled visit or if pain or swelling occur.

Contraindications: The topical ointment should not be used in or around the eyes. Ophthalmic products should not be used to treat fungal diseases of the eye, dendritic keratitis, vaccinia, varicella, mycobacterial eye infections, or following removal of a corneal foreign body.

Special Concerns: The tetracycline fiber should be used with caution in clients with a history of oral candidiasis. Use of the fiber in chronic abscesses has not been evaluated. Safety and efficacy of the fiber have not been determined in children.

Additional Side Effects: Temporary blurring of vision or stinging following administration. Dermatitis and photosensitivity following ophthalmic use. *Use of the tetracycline fiber:* Oral candidiasis, glossitis, staining of the tongue, severe gingival hyperplasia, minor throat irritation, pain following placement in an abscessed area, throbbing pain, hypersensitivity reactions.

NURSING CONSIDERATIONS

See also *Nursing Considerations* for *Tetracyclines,* Chapter 10, and *Gener-*

al Nursing Considerations for All Anti-Infectives, Chapter 1.

Assessment

1. Document indications for therapy, type and onset of symptoms, and any other agents or treatments prescribed.
2. Determine that appropriate cultures and/or diagnostic studies have been performed prior to starting therapy.
3. With long-term therapy, obtain baseline CBC and liver and renal function studies and monitor periodically.

Client/Family Teaching

1. Take PO form 1 hr before or 2 hr after meals.
2. Avoid dairy products, antacids, or iron preparations for 2 hr of ingestion of medication.
3. Drug may cause photosensitivity reaction. Avoid exposure to sunlight and wear protective clothing and sunscreen when exposure is necessary.
4. Transient blurring of vision or stinging may occur when tetracycline is instilled into the eye.
5. The topical ointment may stain clothing.
6. Drug may cause increased yellow-brown discoloration and softening of teeth and bones. *Not* advised for children under 8 years of age.
7. With PO application for gum disease, review proper care of site(s), foods to avoid, and proper cleaning while avoiding floss or pics for the entire length of therapy. Review symptoms that require immediate reporting (pain, abnormal discharge, fever, swelling, expulsion of fiber) and stress the importance of returning as scheduled for removal and follow-up.

Evaluate

- Resolution of infection and reports of symptomatic improvement
- Evidence of ↓ acne lesions
- Radiologic evidence of resolution of effusion with desired pleural sclerosing.

CHAPTER ELEVEN

Antibiotics: Miscellaneous

See the following individual entries:

Aztreonam for Injection
Bacitracin Intramuscular
Bacitracin Ointment
Bacitracin Ophthalmic Ointment
Imipenem-Cilastatin Sodium
Mupirocin
Pentamidine Isethionate
Polymyxin B Sulfate, Sterile Ophthalmic
Spectinomycin Hydrochloride
Trimetrexate Glucuronate
Vancomycin Hydrochloride

Aztreonam for injection

(as-**TREE**-oh-nam)
Pregnancy Category: B
Azactam for Injection **(Rx)**

See also *Anti-Infectives,* Chapter 1.
How Supplied: *Injection:* 1 g/50 mL, 2 g/50 mL; *Powder for injection:* 500 mg, 1 g, 2 g
Action/Kinetics: Aztreonam belongs to a class of antibiotics called *monobactams.* It is a synthetic drug that is bactericidal against gram-negative aerobic pathogens. The drug acts by inhibiting cell wall synthesis due to a high affinity of the drug for penicillin binding protein 3; this results in cell lysis and death. Widely distributed to all body fluids. **Time to peak serum levels:** 0.6–1.3 hr. **t½:** 1.5–2 hr. The t½ is prolonged in clients with impaired renal function. Approximately 60%–75% excreted unchanged in the urine within 8 hr.
Uses: Complicated and uncomplicated urinary tract infections (including pyelonephritis and cystitis) due to *E. coli, Klebsiella pneumoniae, Proteus mirabilis, Pseudomonas aeruginosa, Enterobacter cloacae, Klebsiella oxytoca, Citrobacter* species, and *Serratia marcescens.* Lower respiratory tract infections (including bronchitis and pneumonia) due to *E. coli, K. pneumoniae, P. aeruginosa, Hemophilus influenzae, P. mirabilis, Enterobacter* species, and *S. marcescens.* Septicemia due to *E. coli, K. pneumoniae, P. aeruginosa, P. mirabilis, S. marcescens* and *Enterobacter* species. Skin and skin structure infections (including postoperative wounds, ulcers, and burns) caused by *E. coli, P. mirabilis, S. marcescens, Enterobacter* species, *P. aeruginosa, K. pneumoniae,* and *Citrobacter* species. Intra-abdominal infections (including peritonitis) due to *E. coli, K. pneumoniae, Enterobacter* species, *P. aeruginosa, Citrobacter* species, and *Serratia* species. Gynecologic infections (including endometritis and pelvic cellulitis) due to *E. coli, K. pneumoniae, P. mirabilis,* and *Enterobacter* species. As an adjunct to surgery to manage infections caused by susceptible organisms. As an alternative to spectinomycin in clients with acute uncomplicated gonorrhea who are resistant to penicillin. Concomitant initial therapy with other anti-infective drugs and aztreonam in seriously ill clients is recommended before the causative organism is known and who are at risk for an infection due to gram-positive aerobic pathogens.

Dosage

- **IM, IV**

Urinary tract infections.
Adults: 0.5–1 g q 8–12 hr, not to exceed 8 g/day. **Children:** 30 mg/kg q 6–8 hr.

Moderate to severe systemic infections.
1–2 g q 8–12 hr, not to exceed 8 g/day.

Severe systemic or life-threatening infections.
2 g q 6–8 hr, not to exceed 8 g/day.

P. aeruginosa *infections in children.*
50 mg/kg q 4–6 hr.

NOTE: Dose must be reduced in clients with impaired renal function.

Administration/Storage

1. The IV route should be used for doses greater than 1 g or in clients with septicemia.
2. Therapy should be continued for at least 48 hr after the client becomes asymptomatic or until laboratory tests indicate that the infection has been eradicated.
3. For use as a bolus, the 15-mL vial should be diluted with 6–10 mL sterile water for injection. For IM use, the 15-mL vial should be diluted with at least 3 mL of either sterile water for injection, sodium chloride injection, bacteriostatic water for injection, or bacteriostatic sodium chloride injection. Final dilution should not exceed 20 mg/mL.
4. An IV bolus injected slowly over 3–5 min may be used to initiate therapy. IV infusion should be given over 20–60 min.
5. For IM use, the drug should be given in a large muscle mass.
6. Aztreonam is incompatible with cephradine, nafcillin sodium, and metronidazole. Data for other drugs are not available and therefore use of other admixtures is not recommended.
7. *Treatment of Overdose:* Hemodialysis or peritoneal dialysis to reduce serum levels.

Contraindication: Allergy to aztreonam. Lactation.

Special Concerns: Safety and effectiveness have not been determined in children and infants. Use with caution in clients allergic to penicillins or cephalosporins and in those with impaired hepatic or renal function.

Laboratory Test Interferences: ↑ AST, ALT, alkaline phosphatase, serum creatinine, PT, PTT. Positive Coombs' test.

Side Effects: *GI:* N&V, diarrhea, abdominal cramps, mouth ulcers, numb tongue, halitosis, *Clostridium difficile*-associated diarrhea or GI bleeding. *CNS:* Confusion, ***seizures,*** vertigo, paresthesia, insomnia, dizziness. *Hematologic:* Anemia, neutropenia, thrombocytopenia, leukocytosis, thrombocytosis, pancytopenia. *Dermatologic:* Rash, purpura, erythema multiforme, urticaria, petechiae, pruritus, diaphoresis, exfoliative dermatitis. *CV:* Hypotension, transient ECG changes, flushing. *Following parenteral use:* Phlebitis and thrombophlebitis after IV use; discomfort and swelling at the injection site after IM use. *Miscellaneous:* ***Anaphylaxis,*** hypersensitivity reactions, headache, weakness, fever, malaise, hepatitis, jaundice, muscle aches, tinnitus, diplopia, nasal congestion, altered taste, sneezing, vaginal candidiasis, vaginitis, breast tenderness, chest pain, eosinophilia.

Drug Interactions: Antibiotics that increase levels of beta-lactamase (e.g., cefoxitin, imipenem) may inhibit the activity of aztreonam.

NURSING CONSIDERATIONS

See also *General Nursing Considerations For All Anti-Infectives,* Chapter 1.

Assessment

1. Obtain baseline CBC and liver and renal function studies and monitor throughout therapy.
2. Monitor renal function if used with an aminoglycoside (especially if high doses are used or if therapy is prolonged).
3. Anticipate reduced dosage in clients with impaired renal function (see package insert).
4. Note any allergy to penicillins or cephalosporins.

Client/Family Teaching

1. Reassure client that during therapy

a slightly itchy, red rash and nasal congestion may occur.
2. Advise that a taste alteration may be experienced during IV therapy and to report if eating is impaired.

Evaluate

- Resolution of infecting organism
- Reports of symptomatic improvement

Bacitracin intramuscular

(bass-ih-**TRAY**-sin)
Bacitin ✤, Bacitracin Sterile **(Rx)**

Bacitracin ointment

(bass-ih-**TRAY**-sin)
Baciguent **(OTC)**

Bacitracin ophthalmic ointment

(bass-ih-**TRAY**-sin)
AK-Tracin, Bacitracin Ophthalmic Ointment **(Rx)**

See also *Anti-Infectives,* Chapter 1.
How Supplied: Bacitracin ointment: *Ointment:* 500 U/g
Bacitracin ophthalmic ointment: *Ointment:* 500 U/g
Action/Kinetics: This antibiotic is produced by *Bacillus subtilis.* The drug interferes with synthesis of cell wall, preventing incorporation of amino acids and nucleotides. Bacitracin is bactericidal, bacteriostatic, and active against protoplasts. It is not absorbed from the GI tract. When given parenterally, drug is well distributed in pleural and ascitic fluids.

Bacitracin has high nephrotoxicity. Its systemic use is restricted to infants (see *Uses*). Renal function must be carefully evaluated prior to, and daily, during use. **Peak plasma levels: IM,** 0.2–2 mcg/mL after 2 hr. From 10% to 40% is excreted in the urine after IM administration.
Uses: Bacitracin is used locally during surgery for cranial and neurosurgical infections caused by susceptible organisms.

As an ointment (preferred) or solution, bacitracin is prescribed for superficial pyoderma-like impetigo and infectious eczematoid dermatitis, for secondary infected dermatoses (atopic dermatitis, contact dermatitis), and for superficial infections of the eye, ear, nose, and throat by susceptible organisms. Ophthalmically, the drug is effective against species of *Staphylococcus, S. aureus, Streptococcus, S. pneumoniae, S. pyogenes, Corynebacterium, Neisseria, N. gonorrhoeae,* and alpha-hemolytic streptococci (viridans group).

Parenteral use is limited to the treatment of staphylococcal pneumonia and staphylococcus-induced empyema in infants.

Dosage

- **IM only**

Infants, 2.5 kg and below: 900 units/kg/day in two to three divided doses; **infants over 2.5 kg:** 1,000 units/kg/day in two to three divided doses.

- **Ophthalmic ointment (500 units/g)**

Acute infections.
½ in. in lower conjunctival sac q 3–4 hr until improvement occurs. Treatment should be reduced before the drug is discontinued.

Mild to moderate infections.
½ in. b.i.d.–t.i.d.

- **Topical ointment (500 units/g)**

Apply 1–5 times/day to affected area.
Administration/Storage: Do not mix bacitracin with glycerin or other polyalcohols that cause drug to deteriorate. Bacitracin unguentin base is anhydrous, consisting of liquid and white petrolatum.
Contraindications: Hypersensitivity or toxic reaction to bacitracin. Pregnancy. Epithelial herpes simplex keratitis, vaccinia, varicella, mycobacterial eye infections, fungal diseases of the eye. Topical antibiotics should not be used in deep-seated ocular infections or in those that are likely to become systemic.
Special Concerns: Ophthalmic ointments may retard corneal epithelial healing. Prolonged or repeated use

may result in bacterial or fungal overgrowth of nonsusceptible organisms leading to a secondary infection.

Side Effects: ***Nephrotoxicity due to tubular and glomerular necrosis, renal failure;*** toxic reactions; N&V.

Drug Interactions

Aminoglycosides / Additive nephrotoxicity and neuromuscular blocking activity

Anesthetics / ↑ Neuromuscular blockade → possible muscle paralysis

Neuromuscular blocking agents / Additive neuromuscular blockade → possible muscle paralysis

NURSING CONSIDERATIONS

See also *General Nursing Considerations* for *All Anti-Infectives,* Chapter 1.

Assessment

1. Document indications for therapy, type, and onset of symptoms.
2. List any previous experiences with this type of infection (especially of ocular origin), agents used, and the outcome.
3. Recurrent ophthalmic infections should be cultured and carefully assessed by an ophthalmologist.

Interventions

1. Monitor and maintain adequate I&O with parenteral use of drug.
2. Withhold drug and report when output is inadequate. Monitor renal function studies.
3. Test pH of urine daily; pH should be kept at 6 or greater to decrease renal irritation.
4. Have sodium bicarbonate or other alkali available to administer if urine pH drops below 6.
5. Do not administer concurrently or sequentially with a topical or systemic nephrotoxic drug.
6. Cleanse area before applying bacitracin as a wet dressing or ointment.

Evaluate

- Resolution of S&S of infection
- Restoration of skin integrity
- Negative laboratory C&S reports

—COMBINATION DRUG—

Imipenem-Cilastatin sodium

(em-ee-**PEN**-em, sigh-lah-**STAT**-in)

Pregnancy Category: C

Primaxin I.M., Primaxin I.V. **(Rx)**

See also *Anti-Infectives,* Chapter 1.

How Supplied: See Content

Content: Powder for IV injection contains: 250 mg imipenem, 250 mg cilastatin sodium; 500 mg imipenem, 500 mg cilastatin sodium.

Powder for IM injection contains: 500 mg imipenem, 500 mg cilastatin sodium; 750 mg imipenem, 750 mg cilastatin sodium.

Action/Kinetics: Imipenem, an antibiotic, inhibits cell wall synthesis and is thus bactericidal against a wide range of gram-positive and gram-negative organisms. It is stable in the presence of beta-lactamases. Addition of cilastatin prevents the metabolism of imipenem in the kidneys by dehydropeptidase I, thus ensuring high levels of the imipenem in the urinary tract. **t½, after IV:** 1 hr for each component. **Peak plasma levels, after 20 min IV infusion:** 15–25 mcg/mL for the 250-mg dose, 31–49 mcg/mL for the 500-mg dose, and 56–88 mcg/mL for the 1-g dose. **Peak plasma levels, after IM:** 10–12 mcg/mL within 2 hr. Compared with IV administration, imipenem is approximately 75% bioavailable after IM use with cilastatin being 95% bioavailable. **t½, imipenem:** 2–3 hr. About 70% of imipenem and cilastin is recovered in the urine within 10 hr of administration.

Uses: IV. To treat the following serious infections: lower respiratory tract, urinary tract, gynecologic, skin and skin structures, bone and joint, endocarditis, intra-abdominal, bacterial septicemia, and infections caused by more than one agent. Infections resistant to aminoglycosides, cephalosporins, or penicillins have responded to imipenem. Bacterial eradication may not be achieved in clients with cystic fibrosis, chronic pulmonary disease, and lower respiratory tract infections caused by *Pseudomonas aeruginosa*.

IM. This route of administration is not intended for severe or life-threatening infections (including endocarditis, or bacterial sepsis). Lower respiratory tract infections, intra-abdominal infections, skin and skin structure infections, gynecologic infections.

Dosage

- **IV**

Fully susceptible gram-positive organisms, gram-negative organisms, anaerobes.

Mild: 250 mg q 6 hr; *moderate:* 500 mg q 6 hr or q 8 hr; *severe/life-threatening:* 500 mg q 6 hr.

Urinary tract infections due to fully susceptible organisms.

Uncomplicated: 250 mg q 6 hr; *complicated:* 500 mg q 6 hr.

Moderately susceptible organisms (especially some strains of P. aeruginosa.

Mild: 500 mg q 6 hr; *moderate,* 500 mg q 6 hr–1 g q 6 hr; *severe/life-threatening,* 1 g q 6–8 hr.

Urinary tract infections due to moderately susceptible organisms.

Uncomplicated: 250 mg q 6 hr; *complicated:* 500 mg q 6 hr.

The total daily dose should not exceed 50 mg/kg or 4 g, whichever is lower.

- **IM**

Lower respiratory tract, skin and skin structure, or gynecologic infections: mild to moderate.

500 or 750 mg q 12 hr depending on severity.

Intra-abdominal infections: mild to moderate.

750 mg q 12 hr. The total daily dose should not exceed 1.5 g.

Administration/Storage

1. Reconstitute each vial with 10 mL of diluent and swirl; further dilute in at least 100 mL of dextrose or saline solution.
2. The initial dose should be based on the type and severity of infection. Doses between 250 and 500 mg should be given by IV infusion over 20–30 min; doses of 1 g should be given by IV infusion over 40–60 min. If nausea develops, the infusion rate should be decreased.
3. The following solutions can be used as diluents: 0.9% sodium chloride injection, 5% or 10% dextrose injection, 5% dextrose injection with 0.02% sodium bicarbonate solution, 5% dextrose and 0.9% sodium chloride injection, 5% dextrose injection with either 0.225% or 0.45% saline solution, Normosol-M in D5W, 5% dextrose with 0.15% potassium chloride solution, mannitol (2.5%, 5%, or 10%).
4. Reconstituted IV solutions vary from colorless to yellow while reconstituted IM solutions vary from white to light tan in color. Variations in color do not affect the potency.
5. Imipenem-cilastatin should not be physically mixed with other antibiotics; however, the drug may be administered with other antibiotics, if necessary.
6. Most reconstituted IV solutions can be stored at room temperature for 4 hr and, if refrigerated, for 24 hr. The exception is imipenem-cilastatin reconstituted with 0.9% sodium chloride solution, which is stable at room temperature for 10 hr and, if refrigerated, for 48 hr. Reconstituted IM solutions should be used within 1 hr of preparation.
7. When used IM, the dose should be given in a large muscle mass with a 21-gauge 2-in. needle.
8. IM use should be continued for at least 2 days after S&S of infection are absent. Safety and effectiveness have not been established for use for more than 14 days.
9. Dosage should be reduced in clients with a creatinine clearance of 70 mL/min/1.73 m^2 or less. Check package insert for specific dosage information.

Contraindications: In clients allergic to local anesthetics of the amide type. IM use in clients with heart block (due to the use of lidocaine HCl diluent) or severe shock.

Special Concerns: Use with caution in pregnancy and lactation. Due to cross sensitivity, use with caution in clients with penicillin allergy. Safety and effectiveness have not

been determined in children less than 12 years of age.
Laboratory Test Interferences: ↑ AST, ALT, alkaline phosphatase, LDH, bilirubin, potassium, chloride, BUN, creatinine. ↓ Serum sodium. Positive Coombs' test and abnormal PT. Presence of protein, RBCs, WBCs, casts, bilirubin, or urobilinogen in the urine.
Side Effects: *GI:* ***Pseudomembranous colitis,*** nausea, diarrhea, vomiting, abdominal pain, heartburn, increased salivation, ***hemorrhagic colitis,*** gastroenteritis, glossitis, pharyngeal pain, tongue papillar hypertrophy. *CNS:* Fever, confusion, ***seizures,*** dizziness, sleepiness, myoclonus, headache, vertigo, paresthesia, encephalopathy, tremor, psychic disturbances. *CV:* Hypotension, tachycardia, palpitations. *Dermatologic:* Rash, urticaria, pruritus, flushing, cyanosis, facial edema, erythema multiforme, skin texture changes, ***toxic epidermal necrolysis.*** *CV:* Hypotension, palpitations, tachycardia. *Respiratory:* Chest discomport, dyspnea, hyperventilation. *GU:* Pruritus vulvae, anuria/oliguria, acute renal failure. *Miscellaneous:* Candidiasis, superinfection, tinnitus, polyuria, increased sweating, polyarthralgia, muscle weakness, transient hearing loss in clients with existing hearing impairment, taste perversion, hepatitis, thrombocytopenia, leukopenia, thoracic spine pain.

The following side effects may occur at the injection site: Thrombophlebitis, phlebitis, pain, erythema, vein induration, infused vein infection.
Drug Interactions: Use of ganciclovir with imipenem-cilastatin may result in generalized seizures.

NURSING CONSIDERATIONS

See also *General Nursing Considerations for All Anti-Infectives,* Chapter 1.

Evaluate

- Resolution of infection
- Reports of symptomatic improvement

Mupirocin

(myou-**PEER**-oh-sin)
Pregnancy Category: B
Bactroban **(Rx)**

How Supplied: *Ointment:* 2%
Action/Kinetics: Mupirocin exerts its antibacterial action by binding to bacterial isoleucyl transfer RNA synthetase, which results in inhibition of protein synthesis by the organism. The drug is not absorbed into the systemic circulation. Serum present in exudative wounds decreases the antibacterial activity. Mupirocin is metabolized to the inactive monic acid in the skin and is then removed by normal skin desquamation. There is no cross resistance with other antibiotics such as chloramphenicol, erythromycin, gentamicin, lincomycin, methicillin, neomycin, novobiocin, penicillin, streptomycin, or tetracyclines.
Uses: Topically to treat impetigo due to *Staphylococcus aureus, Streptococcus pyogenes,* and beta-hemolytic streptococcus.

Dosage

- **Topical Ointment**

A small amount of ointment is applied to the affected area t.i.d.
Administration/Storage: A gauze dressing may be used if desired.
Contraindications: Ophthalmic use. Lactation.
Special Concerns: Superinfection may result from chronic use.
Side Effects: Superinfection, rash, burning, stinging, pain, nausea, tenderness, erythema, swelling, dry skin, contact dermatitis, and increased exudate.

NURSING CONSIDERATIONS

Client/Family Teaching

1. Demonstrate the appropriate technique for applying topical medications. Review hygienic measures and stress the importance of hand washing to prevent spread of infection.
2. Report any symptoms of chemical irritation or hypersensitivity such as increased rash, itching, or pain at the site.

3. Report if no improvement is noted after 3–5 days of therapy.
4. Notify school nurse to ensure appropriate screening is performed when treating school-aged children.

Evaluate

- Evidence of healing in skin lesions
- Reports of symptomatic improvement

Pentamidine isethionate

(pen-**TAM**-ih-deen)

Pregnancy Category: C

NebuPent, Pentacarinate ✱, Pentam **(Rx)**

Classification: Antibiotic, miscellaneous (antiprotozoal)

Action/Kinetics: The drug inhibits synthesis of DNA, RNA, phospholipids, and proteins, thereby interfering with cell metabolism. It may interfere also with folate transformation. About one-third of the dose may be excreted unchanged in the urine. Plasma levels following inhalation are significantly lower than after a comparable IV dose.

Uses: Parenteral. Pneumonia caused by *Pneumocystis carinii*. **Inhalation.** Prophylaxis of *P. carinii* in high-risk HIV-infected clients defined by one or both of the following: (a) a history of one or more cases of pneumonia caused by *P. carinii* and/or (b) a peripheral CD4+ lymphocyte count less than 200/mm^3. *Investigational:* Trypanosomiasis, visceral leishmaniasis.

Dosage

- **IV, Deep IM**

Adults and children: 4 mg/kg/day for 14 days. Dosage should be reduced in renal disease.

- **Aerosol**

Prevention of P. carinii pneumonia. 300 mg/ q 4 weeks given via the Respirgard II nebulizer.

Administration/Storage

1. To prepare IM solution, dissolve one vial in 3 mL of sterile water for injection.
2. To prepare IV solution, dissolve one vial in 3–5 mL of sterile water for injection or 5% dextrose injection. The drug is then further diluted in 50–250 mL of 5% dextrose solution. This solution then can be infused slowly over 60 min.
3. IV solutions in concentrations of 1 and 2.5 mg/mL in 5% dextrose injection are stable for 48 hr at room temperature.
4. The dose using the nebulizer should be delivered until the chamber is empty (30–45 min). The suggested flow rate is 5–7 L/min from a 40–50-psi (pounds per square inch) air or oxygen source.
5. Reconstitution for use in the nebulizer is accomplished by dissolving the contents of the vial in 6 mL sterile water for injection. Saline solution cannot be used because it causes the drug to precipitate.
6. When used for nebulization, pentamidine should not be mixed with any other drug.
7. The solution for nebulization is stable at room temperature for 48 hr if protected from light.

Contraindications: Clients manifesting anaphylaxis to inhaled or parenteral pentamidine.

Special Concerns: Use with caution in clients with hepatic or kidney disease, hypertension or hypotension, hyperglycemia or hypoglycemia, hypocalcemia, leukopenia, thrombocytopenia, anemia, ventricular tachycardia, pancreatitis, Stevens-Johnson syndrome.

Side Effects: Parenteral. *CV:* Hypotension, ***ventricular tachycardia,*** phlebitis. *GI:* Nausea, anorexia, bad taste in mouth. *Hematologic:* Leukopenia, thrombocytopenia, anemia. *Electrolytes/glucose:* Hypoglycemia, hypocalcemia, hyperkalemia. *CNS:* Dizziness without hypotension, confusion, hallucinations. *Miscellaneous:* Acute renal failure, ***Stevens-Johnson syndrome,*** elevated serum creatinine, elevated liver function tests, pain or induration at IM injection site, sterile abscess at injection site, rash, neuralgia.

Inhalation. Most frequent include the following. *GI:* Decreased appetite, N&V, metallic taste, diarrhea, abdominal pain. *CNS:* Fatigue, dizziness, headache. *Respiratory:* SOB, cough, pharyngitis, chest pain, chest congestion, ***bronchospasm,*** pneumothorax. *Miscellaneous:* Rash, night sweats, chills, myalgia, headache, anemia, edema.

NURSING CONSIDERATIONS

See also *General Nursing Considerations for All Anti-Infectives,* Chapter 1.

Assessment

1. Document indications for therapy and assess extent of infection.
2. Determine history of kidney disease, hypertension, and past blood disorders. Ensure that appropriate baseline lab studies have been performed (cultures, CBC, electrolytes, blood sugar, calcium, liver and renal function) and monitor throughout therapy.
3. Note results of tuberculosis screening tests.
4. Auscultate lung sounds and document respiratory assessment findings.

Interventions

1. Observe for symptoms of hypoglycemia, hypocalcemia, and/or hyperkalemia.
2. During IV therapy monitor BP frequently (q 15 min during therapy and q 2 hr following therapy until stable).
3. Monitor and record VS and I&O.
4. Obtain apical pulse and auscultate for any evidence of arrhythmia if client not monitored.
5. During administration of aerosolized pentamidine, appropriate precautions should be followed to protect the health care worker. Wear:
   - Eye protection with side shields
   - Disposable gowns
   - Respiratory protective equipment such as an organic dust-mist respirator unless client is under hood stalls or in a ventilated booth
   - Gloves
   - Administer with the Respirgard II nebulizer
   - Document worker exposure(s) and report any persistent or unusual symptoms
6. Follow appropriate institutional guidelines and Occupational Safety and Health Association (OSHA) standards for administration of drug.
7. Incorporate Universal Precautions to protect immunocompromised clients.

Client/Family Teaching

1. Advise client to report any adverse effects such as bruising, hematuria, blood in stools, or other evidence of bleeding.
2. Avoid aspirin-containing compounds, alcohol, IM injections, or rectal thermometers.
3. Advise to use a soft toothbrush, electric razor, and night light to prevent injury and falls.
4. Be alert for S&S of hypoglycemia (which may be severe) and report immediately after consuming juice with sugar.
5. Report early signs of Stevens-Johnson syndrome (characterized by high fever, severe headaches, stomatitis, conjunctivitis, rhinitis, urethritis, and balanitis), all of which may necessitate the discontinuation of drug therapy.
6. Intake of fluids should be increased to 2–3 L/day during drug therapy.
7. Rise from a prone position slowly and dangle legs before standing as drug may cause dizziness and postural hypotension.
8. During inhalation, advise that a metallic taste may be experienced.
9. Stress the importance of completing the prescribed course of therapy.

Evaluate

- (Parenterally) radiographic evidence and reports of improvement in symptoms of *P. carinii* pneumonia
- (Inhalation) evidence of prophylaxis of *P. carinii* pneumonia in HIV-infected at-risk individuals

Polymyxin B sulfate, sterile ophthalmic

(pol-ee-**MIX**-in)
(Rx)

See also *Anti-Infectives,* Chapter 1.
How Supplied: *Powder for injection:* 500,000 U
Action/Kinetics: Polymyxin B sulfate is derived from the spore-forming soil bacterium *Bacillus polymyxa.* It is bactericidal against most gram-negative organisms and rapidly inactivated by alkali, strong acid, and certain metal ions. Polymyxin increases the permeability of the plasma cell membrane of the bacterium (i.e., similar to detergents), causing leakage of essential metabolites and ultimately inactivation. **Peak serum levels: IM,** 2 hr. **t½:** 4.3–6 hr. Longer in presence of renal impairment. Sixty percent of drug excreted in urine. It is virtually unabsorbed from the GI tract except in newborn infants. After parenteral administration, polymyxin B seems to remain in the plasma.
Uses: Systemic. Acute infections of the urinary tract and meninges, septicemia caused by *Pseudomonas aeruginosa.* Meningeal infections caused by *Haemophilus influenzae,* UTIs caused by *Escherichia coli,* bacteremia caused by *Enterobacter aerogenes* or *Klebsiella pneumoniae.* Combined with neomycin for irrigation of the urinary bladder to prevent bacteriuria and bacteremia from indwelling catheters.

Ophthalmic. Conjunctival and corneal infections (e.g., conjunctivitis, keratitis, keratoconjunctivitis, corneal ulcers, blepharitis, blepharoconjunctivitis, acute meibomianitis, dacryocystitis) due to *E. coli, H. influenzae, K. pneumoniae, E. aerogenes,* and *P. aeruginosa.* Used alone or in combination for ear infections.

Dosage

- **IV**

Infections.
Adults and children: 15,000–25,000 units/kg/day (maximum) in divided doses q 12 hr. **Infants,** up to 40,000 units/kg/day.

- **IM**

Not usually recommended due to pain at injection site.
Infections.
Adults and children: 25,000–30,000 units/kg/day in divided doses q 4–6 hr. **Infants,** up to 40,000 units/kg/day.

Both IV and IM doses should be reduced in renal impairment.

- **Intrathecal**

Meningitis.
Adults and children over 2 years: 50,000 units/day for 3–4 days; **then,** 50,000 units every other day until 2 weeks after cultures are negative; **children under 2 years,** 20,000 units/day for 3–4 days or 25,000 units once every other day; dosage of 25,000 units should be continued every other day for 2 weeks after cultures are negative.

- **Ophthalmic Solution**

1–2 gtt 2–6 times/day, depending on the infection. Treatment may be necessary for 1–2 months or longer.
Administration/Storage
1. Store and dilute as directed on package insert.
2. Pain on IM injection can be lessened by reducing drug concentration as much as possible. It is preferable to give drug more frequently in more dilute doses. If ordered, procaine hydrochloride (2 mL of a 0.5%–1.0% solution per 5 units of dry powder) may be used for mixing the drug for IM injection.
3. For IV administration, reconstitute 500,000 units with 300–500 mL of D5W and infuse over 60–90 min.
4. *Never use preparations containing procaine hydrochloride for IV or intrathecal use.*
Contraindications: Hypersensitivity. Polymyxin B sulfate is a potentially toxic drug to be reserved for the treatment of severe, resistant infections in hospitalized clients. The drug is not indicated for clients with severely im-

paired renal function or nitrogen retention. Ophthalmic use in dendritic keratitis, vaccinia, varicella, mycobacterial infections of the eye, fungal diseases of the eye, use with steroid combinations after uncomplicated removal of a foreign body from the cornea.
Special Concern: Safe use during pregnancy has not been established.
Laboratory Test Interferences: False + or ↑ levels of urea nitrogen and creatinine. Casts and RBCs in urine.
Side Effects: *Nephrotoxic:* Albuminuria, cylindruria, azotemia, hematuria, proteinuria, leukocyturia, electrolyte loss. *Neurologic:* Dizziness, flushing of face, mental confusion, irritability, nystagmus, muscle weakness, drowsiness, paresthesias, blurred vision, slurred speech, ataxia, ***coma, seizures. Neuromuscular blockade may lead to respiratory paralysis.*** *GI:* N&V, diarrhea, abdominal cramps. *Miscellaneous:* Fever, urticaria, skin exanthemata, eosinophilia, ***anaphylaxis.***

Following intrathecal use: Meningeal irritation with fever, stiff neck, headache, increase in leukocytes and protein in the CSF. Nerve-root irritation may result in neuritic pain and urine retention. *Following IM use:* Irritation, severe pain. *Following IV use:* Thrombophlebitis. *Following ophthalmic use:* Burning, stinging, irritation, inflammation, angioneurotic edema, itching, urticaria, vesicular and maculopapular dermatitis.

Drug Interactions

Aminoglycoside antibiotics / Additive nephrotoxic effects
Cephalosporins / ↑ Risk of renal toxicity
Phenothiazines / ↑ Risk of respiratory depression
Skeletal muscle relaxants (surgical) / Additive muscle relaxation

NURSING CONSIDERATIONS

See also *General Nursing Considerations for All Anti-Infectives,* Chapter 1.

Assessment

1. Determine kidney function and urinary output. Note any evidence of urinary tract problems or edema.
2. Assess respiratory function and note any history of problems.
3. Ensure that appropriate specimens have been obtained for C&S prior to initiating therapy.

Interventions

1. Note any muscle weakness, an early sign of muscle paralysis related to neuromuscular blockade. Assess closely for evidence of respiratory paralysis and withhold drug. Neuromuscular blockade may respond to calcium chloride. Have emergency equipment readily available.
2. Monitor I&O. Anticipate reduced dose in clients with impaired renal function; observe for nephrotoxicity, characterized by albuminuria, urinary casts, nitrogen retention, and hematuria. Advise a fluid intake of at least 2 L/day.
3. Use safety precautions and supervise ambulatory or bedridden clients with neurologic disturbances.
4. Anticipate a prolonged regimen of topical application of polymyxin B solution because drug is not toxic when used in wet dressings, and the provider may wish to prevent emergence of resistant strains.

Client/Family Teaching

1. Avoid hazardous tasks until drug effects realized because drug may cause dizziness, vertigo, and ataxia.
2. Report any neurologic disturbances, demonstrated by dizziness, blurred vision, irritability, circumoral and peripheral numbness and tingling, weakness, and ataxia. Advise that these symptoms usually disappear within 24–48 hr after the drug is discontinued and are associated with high serum drug levels.

Evaluate

- Negative lab culture reports
- Resolution of infection and reports of symptomatic improvement

Spectinomycin hydrochloride

(speck-tin-oh-**MY**-sin)
Trobicin **(Rx)**

See also *Anti-Infectives,* Chapter 1.
How Supplied: *Powder for injection:* 2 g
Action/Kinetics: Spectinomycin is produced by *Streptomyces spectabilis.*

It inhibits bacterial protein synthesis by binding to ribosomes (30S subunit), thereby interfering with transmission of genetic information crucial to life of microorganism. Spectinomycin is mainly bacteriostatic. It is only given IM. **Peak plasma concentration:** 100 mcg/mL (2-g dose) after 1 hr and 160 mcg/mL (4-g dose) after 2 hr. **t½:** 1.2–2.8 hr. Not significantly bound to protein. Excreted in urine.
Uses: Acute gonorrheal proctitis and urethritis in males and acute gonorrheal cervicitis and proctitis in females due to susceptible strains of *Neisseria gonorrhoeae.* It is ineffective against syphilis and thus is a poor drug to choose when mixed infections are present. The drug is also ineffective against pharyngeal infections.

Dosage

- **IM only**

Gonorrheal urethritis in males, proctitis, and cervicitis.
2 g. In geographic areas where antibiotic resistance is known to be prevalent, give 4 g divided between two gluteal injection sites.

Alternative regimen for urethral, endocervical, or rectal gonococcal infections in clients who cannot take ceftriaxone.
Adults and children weighing more than 45 kg: Spectinomycin, 2 g, as a single dose followed by doxycycline. **Children weighing less than 45 kg:** 40 mg/kg given IM once.

Gonococcal infections in pregnancy where client is allergic to beta-lactams.
2 g followed by erythromycin.

Disseminated gonococcal infection where client is allergic to beta-lactams.
2 g q 12 hr.

Administration/Storage
1. Powder is stable for 3 years.
2. Use reconstituted solution within 24 hr.
3. Inject deeply into the upper, outer quadrant of the gluteus muscle.
4. Injections may be divided between two sites for clients requiring 4 g. Rotate and document injection sites.

Contraindication: Sensitivity to drug.
Special Concerns: Safe use during pregnancy, in infants, and in children has not been established.
Side Effects: A single dose of spectinomycin has caused soreness at the site of injection, urticaria, dizziness, nausea, chills, fever, and insomnia. Multiple doses have caused a decrease in H&H and creatinine clearance and an increase in alkaline phosphatase, BUN, and ALT.

NURSING CONSIDERATIONS

See also *General Nursing Considerations for All Anti-Infectives,* Chapter 1.

Client/Family Teaching
1. Advise clients who are suspected to have syphilis to return for serologic tests monthly for at least 3 months.
2. Refer clients for counseling and encourage treatment of sexual partners.
3. Advise to abstain from sex until infection is resolved. Review safe sex practices to prevent reinfections.

Evaluate
- Laboratory confirmation of negative culture reports
- Clinical evidence and reports of improvement in symptoms of gonorrheal urethritis, cervicitis, and/or proctitis

Trimetrexate Glucuronate

(**try**-meh-**TREX**-ayt gloo-**KYOU**-roh-nayt)
Pregnancy Category: D
NeuTrexin **(Rx)**

See also *Anti-Infectives,* Chapter 1.
How Supplied: *Powder for injection:* 25 mg
Action/Kinetics: Trimetrexate inhibits the enzyme dihydrofolate reductase that results in interference with thymidylate biosynthesis and inhibition of folate-dependent formyl-

transferases. This leads to inhibition of purine synthesis and disruption of DNA, RNA, and protein synthesis and ultimately cell death. Trimetrexate must be given together with leucovorin to prevent serious or life-threatening complications, including bone marrow suppression, oral and GI mucosal ulceration, and renal and hepatic dysfunction. **t½:** 11 hr. The drug is highly bound to plasma protein and is metabolized by the liver. The metabolites also appear to have an inhibitory effect on dihydrofolate reductase.

Uses: As alternative therapy with concurrent leucovorin for the treatment of moderate to severe *Pneumocystis carinii* pneumonia (PCP) in immunocompromised clients. Treatment is indicated in clients with AIDS who are intolerant of or refractory to trimethoprim-sulfamethoxazole (TMP/SMZ) therapy or in whom this combination is contraindicated. *Investigational:* Treatment of non-small-cell lung, prostate, or colorectal cancer.

Dosage

• **IV infusion**

Pneumocystis carinii *pneumonia.*

Adults: 45 mg/m² once daily by IV infusion over 60–90 min. Leucovorin is given IV at a dose of 20 mg/m² over 5–10 min q 6 hr for a total daily dose of 80 mg/m². Leucovorin may also be given orally in four doses of 20 mg/m² spaced equally throughout the day (the oral dose should be rounded up to the next higher 25-mg increment). Doses of trimetrexate and leucovorin are modified depending on hematologic toxicity. If neutrophils are between 750 and 1,000/mm³ and platelets between 50,000 and 75,000/mm³, the dose of trimetrexate remains at 45 mg/m² once daily but the dose of leucovorin is increased to 40 mg/m² q 6 hr. If neutrophils are between 500 and 749/mm³ and platelets between 25,000 and 49,999, the dose of trimetrexate is reduced to 22 mg/m² once daily and the dose of leucovorin is 40 mg/m² q 6 hr. If neutrophils are less than 500/mm³ and platelets are less than 25,000/mm³, trimetrexate is discontinued for 9 days with leucovorin still given at a dose of 40 mg/m² q 6 hr; from days 10 to 21, trimetrexate should be interrupted up to 96 hr.

Administration/Storage

1. Leucovorin therapy must be given for 72 hr after the last dose of trimetrexate.
2. The recommended course of therapy is 21 days for trimetrexate and 24 days for leucovorin.
3. The lyophilized powder is reconstituted with 2 mL of 5% dextrose injection or sterile water for injection to yield a concentration of 12.5 mg/mL. The reconstituted product appears as a pale greenish-yellow solution. The solution should not be used if it is cloudy or a precipitate is observed. The solution should be filtered before dilution.
4. The powder should not be reconstituted with solutions containing either chloride ion or leucovorin as precipitation occurs immediately.
5. The reconstituted solution may be further diluted with 5% dextrose injection to yield a final concentration of from 0.25 to 2 mg/mL.
6. Before and after administering trimetrexate, the IV line must be flushed thoroughly with at least 10 mL of 5% dextrose injection.
7. Trimetrexate and leucovorin solutions must be given separately.
8. If trimetrexate comes in contact with the skin or mucosa, the areas should be immediately and thoroughly washed with soap and water.
9. After reconstitution, the solution is stable under refrigeration or at room temperature for at least 24 hr. The reconstituted solution should not be frozen. Any unused portion should be discarded after 24 hr.
10. *Treatment of Overdose:* Discontinue trimetrexate and administer leucovorin at a dose of 40 mg/m² q 6 hr for 3 days.

Contraindications: Hypersensitivity to trimetrexate, leucovorin, or methotrexate. Use during lactation.

Special Concerns: Use with caution in clients with impaired hematologic, renal, or hepatic function. Safety and efficacy have not been determined for clients less than 18 years of age for use in treating histologically confirmed PCP.

Side Effects: *GI:* N&V. *Hematologic:* Neutropenia, thrombocytopenia, anemia. *Hepatic:* Hepatic toxicity manifested by increased ALT, AST, alkaline phosphatase, and bilirubin. *Renal:* Increased serum creatinine. *Electrolytes:* Hyponatremia, hypocalcemia.

Symptoms of Overdose: Primarily hematologic.

Drug Interactions: Since trimetrexate is metabolized by the P-450 enzyme system in the liver, drugs that stimulate or inhibit this enzyme system may cause drug interactions that may alter plasma levels of trimetrexate (e.g., erythromycin, rifabutin, rifampin).

Acetaminophen / May alter the levels of trimetrexate metabolites
Cimetidine / May ↓ metabolism of trimetrexate
Clotrimazole / ↓ Metabolism of trimetrexate
Ketoconazole / ↓ Metabolism of trimetrexate
Miconazole / ↓ Metabolism of trimetrexate

NURSING CONSIDERATIONS

See also *Nursing Considerations* for *All Anti-Infectives,* Chapter 1.

Assessment

1. Document indications for therapy, any other agents prescribed, and the outcome.
2. Note if client is intolerant or refractory to trimethoprim-sulfamethoxazole.
3. List drugs currently prescribed to ensure none interact unfavorably.
4. Determine any hypersensitivity to leucovorin, methotrexate, or trimetrexate.
5. Obtain baseline hematologic profile and liver and renal function studies. During therapy, obtain these values twice a week to assess hematologic, renal, and hepatic function.

Interventions

1. Drug is to be administered concurrently with leucovorin to avoid its hematologic, hepatic, renal, and GI toxicities.
2. Clients who require concomitant therapy with myelosuppressive, nephrotoxic, or hepatotoxic drugs should be carefully monitored.
3. To allow for use of full therapeutic doses of trimetrexate, anticipate that zidovudine therapy should be discontinued during trimetrexate therapy.
4. Observe client carefully and report any changes. It may be difficult to distinguish side effects caused by trimetrexate from symptoms due to underlying medical conditions.
5. Trimetrexate should be discontinued under the following circumstances:
   - Serum transaminase or alkaline phosphatase increases to more than 5 times the upper limit of the normal range
   - Serum creatinine increases to 2.5 mg/dL
   - Mucosal toxicity becomes so severe it interferes with oral intake
   - Body temperature increases to more than 40.5°C (105°F) when taken orally

Client/Family Teaching

1. Explain the reasons for drug therapy and the anticipated results.
2. Advise clients receiving trimetrexate that they must be followed closely by the provider. This would involve frequent lab work and follow-up visits.
3. Review the potential drug-related side effects and those situations that would warrant discontinuation of drug therapy.
4. Identify appropriate support groups that would assist client and family to understand and cope with the disease.

Evaluate: Resolution of PCP in immunocompromised clients.

Vancomycin hydrochloride

(van-koh-**MY**-sin)
Pregnancy Category: C
Lyphocin, Vancocin, Vancocin CP ✱, Vancoled **(Rx)**

See also *Anti-Infectives,* Chapter 1.
How Supplied: *Capsule:* 125 mg, 250 mg; *Powder for injection:* 500 mg, 1 g, 5 g, 10 g; *Powder for reconstitution:* 250 mg/5 mL, 500 mg/6 mL
Action/Kinetics: This antibiotic, derived from *Streptomyces orientalis,* diffuses in pleural, pericardial, ascitic, and synovial fluids after parenteral administration. It appears to bind to bacterial cell wall, arresting its synthesis and lysing the cytoplasmic membrane by a mechanism that is different from that of penicillins and cephalosporins. Vancomycin may also change the permeability of the cytoplasmic membranes of bacteria, thus inhibiting RNA synthesis. The drug is bactericidal for most organisms and bacteriostatic for enterococci. It is poorly absorbed from the GI tract. **Peak plasma levels, IV:** 33 mcg/mL 5 min after 0.5-g dosage. **t½, after PO:** 4–8 hr for adults and 2–3 hr for children; **t½, after IV:** 4–11 hr for adults and ranging from 2–3 hr in children to 6–10 hr for newborns. The half-life is increased markedly in the presence of renal impairment (240 hr has been noted). Primarily excreted in urine unchanged. Auditory and renal function tests are indicated before and during therapy.
Uses: PO. Antibiotic-induced pseudomembranous colitis due to *Clostridium difficile.* Staphylococcal enterocolitis. Severe or progressive antibiotic-induced diarrhea caused by *C. difficile* that is not responsive to the causative antibiotic being discontinued; also for debilitated clients.

IV. Severe staphylococcal infections in clients who have not responded to penicillins or cephalosporins, who cannot receive these drugs, or who have resistant infections. Infections include lower respiratory tract infections, bone infections, endocarditis, septicemia, and skin and skin structure infections. Alone or in combination with aminoglycosides to treat endocarditis caused by *Streptococcus viridans* or *S. bovis.* Must combine with an aminoglycoside to treat endocarditis due to *Streptococcus faecalis.* Used with rifampin, an aminoglycoside (or both) to treat early onset prosthetic valve endocarditis caused by *Staphylococcus epidermidis* or other diphtheroids. Prophylaxis of bacterial endocarditis in pencillin-allergic clients who have congenital heart disease or rheumatic or other acquired or valvular heart disease if such clients are undergoing dental or surgical procedures of the upper respiratory tract. The parenteral dosage form may be given PO to treat pseudomembranous colitis or staphylococcal enterocolitis due to *C. difficile.*

Dosage

• **Capsules, Oral Solution**
Adults: 0.5–2 g/day in three to four divided doses for 7–10 days. Alternatively, 125 mg t.i.d.–q.i.d. for *C. difficile* may be as effective as the 500-mg dosage. **Children:** 40 mg/kg/day in three to four divided doses for 7–10 days, not to exceed 2 g/day. **Neonates:** 10 mg/kg/day in divided doses.

• **IV**

Severe staphylococcal infections.
Adults: 500 mg q 6 hr or 1 g q 12 hr. **Children:** 10 mg/kg/6 hr. **Infants and neonates, initial:** 15 mg/kg for one dose; **then,** 10 mg/kg q 12 hr for neonates in the first week of life and q 8 hr thereafter up to 1 month of age.

Prophylaxis of bacterial endocarditis in dental, oral, or upper respiratory tract procedures in penicillin-allergic clients.
Adults: 1 g vancomycin over 1 hr plus 1.5 mg/kg gentamicin (IV or IM), not to exceed 80 mg, 1 hr before the procedure. May repeat once, 8 hr after the initial dose. **Children:** 20 mg/kg vancomycin plus 2 mg/kg gentamicin (IV or IM), not to exceed 80 mg, 1 hr before the procedure.

May repeat once, 8 hr after the initial dose.

Administration/Storage

1. Dosage must be reduced in clients with renal disease; see package insert for procedure.
2. The oral solution is prepared by adding 115 mL distilled water to the 10-g container. The appropriate dose of oral solution may be mixed with 1 oz of water or flavored syrup to improve the taste. The diluted drug may also be given by NGT.
3. The parenteral form may be administered PO by diluting the 1-g vial with 20 mL distilled or deionized water (each 5 mL contains about 250 mg vancomycin).
4. For IV use, dilute each 500-mg vial with 10 mL of sterile water. This may be further diluted in 200 mL of dextrose or saline solution and infused over 60 min.
5. Intermittent infusion is the preferred route, but continuous IV drip may be used.
6. Avoid rapid IV administration because this may result in hypotension, nausea, warmth, and generalized tingling. Administer over 1 hr in at least 200 mL of NSS or D5W.
7. Avoid extravasation during injections as this may cause tissue necrosis.
8. Reduce risk of thrombophlebitis by rotating injection sites or adding additional diluent.
9. Aqueous solution is stable for 2 weeks.
10. Once rubber stopper is punctured, ampule should be refrigerated to maintain stability.

Contraindications: Hypersensitivity to drug. Minor infections. Lactation.

Special Concerns: Use with extreme caution in the presence of impaired renal function or previous hearing loss. Geriatric clients are at a greater risk of developing ototoxicity.

Side Effects: Ototoxicity (may lead to deafness), nephrotoxicity (may lead to uremia). *Red-neck syndrome:* Chills, erythema of neck and back, fever, paresthesias. *Dermatologic:* Urticaria, macular rashes. *Allergic:* Drug fever, hypersensitivity, ***anaphylaxis.*** *Miscellaneous:* Nausea, tinnitus, eosinophilia, neutropenia (reversible), hypotension (due to rapid administration). Thrombophlebitis at site of injection. Deafness may progress after drug is discontinued.

Drug Interactions

Aminoglycosides / ↑ Risk of nephrotoxicity
Anesthetics / Risk of erythema and histamine-like flushing in children
Muscle relaxants, nondepolarizing / ↑ Neuromuscular blockade

NURSING CONSIDERATIONS

See also *General Nursing Considerations for All Anti-Infectives,* Chapter 1.

Assessment

1. Document indications for therapy and type and onset of symptoms.
2. Determine that baseline renal and auditory functions (including 8th cranial nerve function) have been assessed.
3. Anticipate reduced dose with renal dysfunction.
4. Ensure that baseline lab C&S tests have been performed.

Interventions

1. Monitor and record weight, VS, and I&O; ensure adequate hydration.
2. Assess and report any evidence of adverse drug effects, such as:
• Ototoxicity, demonstrated by tinnitus, progressive hearing loss, dizziness, and/or nystagmus
• Nephrotoxicity, demonstrated by albuminuria, hematuria, anuria, casts, edema, and uremia
3. During IV drug administration ensure that peak and trough drug levels are performed at the prescribed dosing interval, usually 30 min prior to scheduled IV dose (trough) and 1 hr following IV dose (peak) to accurately assess serum levels.

Evaluate

• Laboratory evidence of negative culture reports
• Serum drug levels within therapeutic range (trough 1–5 mcg/mL; peak 20– 50 mcg/mL)

CHAPTER TWELVE

Amebicides, Trichomonacides, and Antiprotozoals

See also the following individual entries:

Atovaquone
Eflornithine Hydrochloride
Erythromycins - See Chapter 7
Gentian Violet
Metronidazole
Paromomycin Sulfate - See Chapter 2
Tetracyclines - See Chapter 10

General Statement: Amebiasis is a widely distributed disease caused by the protozoan *Entamoeba histolytica*. The disease has a high incidence in areas with low standards of hygiene. In the United States, the average rate of infestation is generally 1%–10% of the population; however, in certain southern localities, the incidence is as high as 40% of the population.

E. histolytica has two forms: (1) an active motile form known as the trophozoite form, and (2) a cystic form that is resistant to destruction and is responsible for the transmission of the disease.

The overt manifestations of amebiasis vary. Some clients manifest violent acute dysentery (characterized by sudden development of severe diarrhea, cramps, and passage of bloody, mucoid stools); others have few overt symptoms or are even completely asymptomatic.

Diagnosis is made on the basis of microscopic examination of fresh, or at least moist, stools by a trained examiner. More than one sample of stool must be negative before amebiasis can be ruled out.

Amoebae often migrate from the GI tract to other parts of the body (extraintestinal amebiasis). The spleen, lungs, or liver are frequently affected. The amoebae colonize in these organs and form abscesses that may rupture and thereby serve as infectious foci.

At present, no one drug can cure both intestinal and extraintestinal amebic infestations; physicians prefer to use a combination of therapeutic agents. Often the more effective but toxic agents are used initially for a short period of time, while long-term eradication or prophylaxis is carried out with less toxic agents.

Since many of the agents used in the treatment of amebiasis are also used for trichomoniasis, nursing considerations for both amebicides and trichomonacides are listed below.

Infestation with the parasite *Trichomonas vaginalis* causes vaginitis, characterized by an irritating, profuse, creamy, or frothy vaginal discharge associated with severe itching and burning. Diagnosis is made by demonstrating the presence of the trichomonad microscopically in the vaginal secretion.

Vaginitis caused by *T. vaginalis* is treated by various locally applied antitrichomonal agents—often effective amebicides—and also by the oral administration of metronidazole. This drug is usually prescribed for both sexual partners to prevent reinfection. Acid douches (vinegar or lactic acid) are a helpful adjunct to treatment.

Eradication of the infectious agent—which frequently becomes resistant—should be ascertained for 3 months after treatment has ceased. The examination usually is made after menstruation, since trichomonal infections often flare up during menstruation.

The incidence of infections by another protozoan organism, *Giardia lamblia,* is increasing in North America. The organism is transmitted in the feces. Infections are characterized by mucous diarrhea, abdominal pain, and weight loss. Drugs of choice are metronidazole and quinacrine.

NURSING CONSIDERATIONS

See also *General Nursing Considerations for All Anti-Infectives,* Chapter 1.

AMEBICIDES

Assessment

1. Document type and onset of symptoms. Assist client to identify causative factors/conditions and possible exposures.
2. Determine that lab studies (i.e., CBC, electrolytes, nutrition profile) and appropriate cultures have been performed.
3. Closely assess clients on therapy for acute dysentery or extraintestinal amebiasis because the agents of choice are highly toxic.

Interventions

1. Anticipate that clients frequently are on combination-drug therapy for amebiasis; observe for toxic reactions to compounds.
2. Be prepared to give intensive supportive nursing care to clients having acute dysentery; assist in the effort to control diarrhea, maintain fluid and electrolyte balance, skin integrity, comfort, and prevent complications caused by malnutrition. The client's activity may have to be curtailed during the acute phase of the disease.
3. Administer drugs only for the period of time ordered and allow for rest periods between courses of therapy. Advise clients against self-medication.

Client/Family Teaching

1. Carriers must continue with drug therapy; stress the benefit to themselves, their families, and their coworkers.
2. Emphasize the necessity for thorough washing of hands, especially in factories, schools, and other institutions where disease is easily spread. Advise daily disinfecting of toilets.
3. Explain the need for food handlers to be particularly conscientious about washing hands after toileting. Emphasize the need to use soap, water, and clean towels.
4. Client and carriers need to have regular stool examinations to check for recurrence.
5. Instruct clients with certain infestations to have well water tested, as this may be one source of contamination.
6. Stress that client and carriers need to report for follow-up visits to ensure eradication of organisms.

TRICHOMONACIDES

Client/Family Teaching

1. Review the prescribed method for administration.
2. If the prescribed method of administration is insufflation or vaginal suppository, instruct client in self-administration and be available to answer any questions or concerns.
3. Review the proper methods for douching and stress the importance of good feminine hygiene.
4. Advise to wear a sanitary napkin to prevent clothing or bed linen from becoming stained by the medication in vaginal suppositories, especially if they contain iodine (which does stain). Stress that the sanitary pad must be changed frequently and immediately upon staining because it may serve as a growth medium for the infecting organisms.
5. Stress that the sexual partner may be an asymptomatic carrier and may also require therapy to prevent reinfection of the woman.

6. Instruct to use condoms during sexual intercourse while undergoing treatment to prevent reinfections.

Evaluate

• Negative lab culture reports and resolution of symptoms of infection
• Clinical and laboratory confirmation of successful eradication and prophylaxis of amebiasis and trichomoniasis

Atovaquone

(ah-**TOV**-ah-kwohn)
Pregnancy Category: C
Mepron **(Rx)**

How Supplied: *Suspension:* 750 mg/5 mL; *Tablet:* 250 mg

Action/Kinetics: The mechanism of action of atovaquone against *Pneumocystis carinii* is not known. However, in *Plasmodium,* the drug appears to act by inhibiting electron transport resulting in inhibition of nucleic acid and ATP synthesis. The bioavailability of the drug is increased when taken with food. Plasma levels in AIDS clients are about one-third to one-half the levels achieved in asymptomatic HIV-infected volunteers. **t½:** 2.2 days in AIDS clients; the long half-life is believed to be due to enterohepatic cycling and eventually fecal elimination. The drug is not metabolized in the liver and is not excreted appreciably through the urine.

Uses: Acute oral treatment of mild to moderate *P. carinii* in clients who are intolerant to trimethoprim-sulfamethoxazole. The drug has not been evaluated as an agent for prophylaxis of *P. carinii.* Atovaquone is not effective for concurrent pulmonary diseases such as bacterial, viral, or fungal pneumonia or in mycobacterial diseases.

Dosage

• **Tablets**

Adults: 750 mg (three 250-mg tablets) given with food t.i.d. for 21 days (total daily dose: 2,250 mg).

Administration/Storage

1. The drug should be taken with meals as food significantly enhances the absorption of the drug. Failure to give the drug with food may result in lower plasma levels and may limit the response to therapy.
2. The drug should be dispensed in a well-closed container and stored at 15°C –25°C (59°F –77°F).

Contraindications: Hypersensitivity to atovaquone or any components of the formulation.

Special Concerns: Use with caution during lactation and in elderly clients. There are no efficacy studies in children. GI disorders may limit absorption of atovaquone.

Laboratory Test Interferences: ↑ ALT, AST, alkaline phosphatase, amylase, creatinine.

Side Effects: Since many clients taking atovaquone have complications of HIV disease, it is often difficult to distinguish side effects caused by atovaquone from symptoms caused by the underlying medical condition. *Dermatologic:* Rash (including maculopapular), pruritus. *GI:* Nausea, diarrhea, vomiting, abdominal pain, constipation, dyspepsia, taste perversion. *CNS:* Headache, fever, insomnia, dizziness, anxiety, anorexia. *Respiratory:* Cough, sinusitis, rhinitis. *Hematologic:* Anemia, neutropenia. *Miscellaneous:* Asthenia, oral monilia, pain, sweating, hypoglycemia, hyperglycemia, hypotension, hyponatremia, hyperkalemia.

Drug Interactions: Since atovaquone is highly bound to plasma proteins (>99.9%), caution should be exercised when giving the drug with other highly plasma protein-bound drugs with narrow therapeutic indices as competition for binding may occur.

NURSING CONSIDERATIONS

Assessment

1. Document any previous therapy for *P. carinii,* the agents used, and the response.
2. Assess baseline pulmonary status, CBC, and pulmonary culture results.
3. Clients with acute *P. carinii* must be carefully evaluated/screened for other related pulmonary diseases of viral, bacterial, or fungal origin and treated with additional drugs as appropriate.

Client/Family Teaching

1. Take only as directed and with meals to enhance absorption.
2. Provide a printed list of drug side effects and identify those that require immediate reporting.
3. Emphasize that this is not a cure but alleviates symptoms of *P. carinii.*
4. Do not exceed prescribed dose and do not share medication.
5. Review criteria and precautions for safe sex, stressing that the risk of transmission of HIV to others is not reduced.
6. Identify appropriate support groups and individuals to assist the client/family to understand and cope with the disease.

Evaluate: Relief of symptoms R/T *Pneumocystis carinii.*

Eflornithine hydrochloride

(ee-**FLOR**-nih-theen)
Pregnancy Category: C
Ornidyl **(Rx)**

See also *Anti-Infectives,* Chapter 1.

How Supplied: *Injection:* 200 mg/mL

Action/Kinetics: Eflornithine inhibits the enzyme ornithine decarboxylase; this enzyme decarboxylates ornithine, which is a necessary step in the biosynthesis of polyamines such as putrescine, sperimidine, and spermine. These polyamines are thought to play an important function in cell division and differentiation. The drug crosses the blood-brain barrier. **$t^{1}/_{2}$, terminal elimination:** 3 hr. Approximately 80% of an IV dose is excreted unchanged in the urine within 1 day.

Uses: Treatment of the meningoencephalitic stage of African trypanosomal infections (sleeping sickness) due to *Trypanosoma brucei gambiense.*

Dosage

• **Injection Concentrate (must be diluted before use)**

Sleeping sickness.

Adults: 100 mg/kg q 6 hr by IV infusion for 14 days.

Administration/Storage

1. The concentrate must be diluted with sterile water for injection before being infused.
2. To prepare the infusion, withdraw the entire contents of each 100-mL vial using strict aseptic technique. Inject 25 mL into each of four IV diluent bags, each bag containing 100 mL sterile water. This results in an eflornithine concentration of 40 mg/mL.
3. The infusion should be given over a minimum of 45 consecutive minutes.
4. The diluted drug must be used within 24 hr of preparation and should be stored at 4°C (39°F). The undiluted vial may be stored at room temperature, preferably below 30°C (86°F).
5. Other drugs should not be given during IV infusion of eflornithine.
6. The dose should be reduced in clients with impaired renal function depending on the serum creatinine level.

Contraindication: Use during lactation.

Special Concerns: Safety and effectiveness have not been determined in children. Use with caution in clients with impaired renal function. Clients should be carefully monitored for 24 months to ensure that therapy is reinstituted if relapses occur.

Side Effects: *Hematologic:* Anemia (over 50% of clients), leukopenia (over one-third of clients), thrombocytopenia, eosinophilia. *GI:* Diarrhea, vomiting, anorexia, abdominal pain. *CNS:* ***Seizures,*** headache, dizziness. *Miscellaneous:* Alopecia, hearing impairment, asthenia, facial edema.

NURSING CONSIDERATIONS

See also *General Nursing Considerations for All Anti-Infectives,* Chapter 1.

Assessment

1. Document dates and location of suspected exposure.
2. Obtain baseline CBC, platelets, and liver and renal function studies.

3. Perform baseline audiogram and assess hearing periodically throughout eflornithine therapy.

Interventions

1. Observe closely for seizure activity resulting from drug therapy and incorporate appropriate precautions.
2. Monitor hematologic studies throughout therapy, documenting any evidence of anemia, myelosuppression, leukopenia, or thrombocytopenia as the dosage may require modification or interruption if severe.
3. At the conclusion of therapy stress the importance of medical follow-up for 24 months to evaluate for relapses, as therapy then must be reinstituted.

Evaluate: Positive clinical response based on appropriate lab culture results.

Gentian Violet

(**JEN**-shun **VYE**-oh-let)
Pregnancy Category: C
Genapax **(Rx)**

How Supplied: *Solution:* 1%, 2%

Action/Kinetics: This traditional rosaniline dye is effective against some gram-positive bacteria, many fungi (yeasts and dermatophytes), and many strains of *Candida*. Treatment should continue until symptoms subside and cultures are negative.

Uses: Topically for treatment of cutaneous and mucocutaneous *Candida albicans* infections such as thrush, intertriginous and paronychial candidiasis. Secondary agent to treat vulvovaginal candidiasis.

Dosage

- **Topical solution**

Apply 1% or 2% solution to affected areas b.i.d.–t.i.d. for 3 days.

- **Vaginal**

One tampon (5 mg) inserted for 3–4 hr once or twice daily for 12 consecutive days. An additional tampon may be used overnight in resistant cases.

Administration/Storage

1. Tampon should be inserted high into vagina. During last trimester of pregnancy, the suppository should be inserted partially into vagina, preferably by hand.
2. The solution should not be used in or around the eyes.

Contraindications: Hypersensitivity to gentian violet, presence of other vaginal infections, extensive vaginal excoriation, and ulceration. Ulcerative lesions of the face.

Special Concerns: Use with caution in clients suspected of having diabetes mellitus because vaginal infections often are the first symptoms of this disease.

Side Effects: *Topical:* Irritation, hypersensitivity, ulceration of mucous membranes, permanent staining if applied to granulation tissue. *GI:* Following use for oral candidiasis, esophagitis, laryngitis, tracheitis, laryngeal obstruction. *Vaginal:* Vaginal burning, pain, itching, or other signs of irritation. Use of tampons has been associated with toxic shock syndrome.

NURSING CONSIDERATIONS

Assessment

1. Document indications for therapy and type and onset of symptoms, and their location.
2. Inspect area for application to ensure it is not ulcerated or excoriated.

Client/Family Teaching

1. Review the appropriate method for administration.
2. Stress the importance of good skin care and proper hygiene to prevent further infection.
3. Keep exposed areas as dry as possible.
4. Wear clean panties with a cotton crotch.
5. Protect skin and clothing from dye as it will stain.
6. Male partner should wear a condom to prevent reinfection.

Evaluate

- Negative lab culture results
- Improved skin lesions with evidence of healing
- Reports of symptomatic improvement

Metronidazole

(meh-troh-**NYE**-dah-zohl)
Pregnancy Category: B
Apo-Metronidazole ✱, Femazole, Flagyl, Flagyl I.V., Flagyl I.V. RTU, Metric 21, MetroGel, MetroGel-Vaginal, Metro I.V., Metryl, Metryl-500, Metryl I.V., Novo-Nidazol ✱, Protostat, Satric, Satric 500, Trikacide ✱ **(Rx)**

See also *Anti-Infectives,* Chapter 1.
How Supplied: *Capsule:* 375 mg; *Gel/jelly:* 0.75%; *Injection:* 500 mg/100 mL; *Tablet:* 250 mg, 500 mg
Action/Kinetics: Effective against anaerobic bacteria and protozoa. Specifically inhibits growth of trichomonae and amoebae by binding to DNA, resulting in loss of helical structure, strand breakage, inhibition of nucleic acid synthesis, and cell death. Well absorbed from GI tract and widely distributed in body tissues. **Peak serum concentration: PO,** 6–40 mcg/mL, depending on the dose, after 1–2 hr. **t½: PO,** 6–12 hr average: 8 hr. Eliminated primarily in urine (20% unchanged), which may be red-brown in color following either PO or IV use.
Uses: Systemic. Amebiasis. Symptomatic and asymptomatic trichomoniasis; to treat asymptomatic partner. Amebic dysentery and amebic liver abscess. To reduce postoperative anaerobic infection following colorectal surgery, elective hysterectomy, and emergency appendectomy. Anaerobic bacterial infections of the abdomen, female genital system, skin or skin structures, bones and joints, lower respiratory tract, and CNS. Also, septicemia, endocarditis, hepatic encephalopathy. PO for Crohn's disease and pseudomembranous colitis. *Investigational:* giardiasis, *Gardnerella vaginalis.*

Topical. Inflammatory papules, pustules, and erythema of rosacea.

Vaginal. Bacterial vaginosis.

Dosage

• **Capsules, Tablets**

Amebiasis: Acute amebic dysentery or amebic liver abscess.

Adult: 500–750 mg t.i.d. for 5–10 days; **pediatric:** 35–50 mg/kg/day in three divided doses for 10 days.

Trichomoniasis, female.

250 mg t.i.d. for 7 days, 2 g given on 1 day in single or divided doses, or 375 mg b.i.d. for 7 days. **Pediatric:** 5 mg/kg t.i.d. for 7 days. An interval of 4–6 weeks should elapse between courses of therapy. *NOTE:* Pregnant women should not be treated during the first trimester. *Male:* Individualize dosage; usual, 250 mg t.i.d. for 7 days.

Giardiasis.

250 mg t.i.d. for 7 days.

G. vaginalis.

500 mg b.i.d. for 7 days.

• **IV**

Anaerobic bacterial infections.

Adults, initially: 15 mg/kg infused over 1 hr; **then,** after 6 hr, 7.5 mg/kg q 6 hr for 7–10 days (daily dose should not exceed 4 g). Treatment may be necessary for 2–3 weeks, although PO therapy should be initiated as soon as possible.

Prophylaxis of anaerobic infection during surgery.

Adults: 15 mg/kg given over a 30–60-min period, with completion 1 hr prior to surgery and 7.5 mg/kg infused over 30–60 min 6 and 12 hr after the initial dose.

• **Topical**

Rosacea.

After washing, apply a thin film and rub in well in the morning and evening for 9 weeks.

• **Vaginal (0.75%)**

One applicatorful (5 g) in the morning and evening for 5 days.

Administration/Storage

1. If used IV, drug should not be given by IV bolus. Administer each single dose over a period of 1 hr.
2. Syringes with aluminum needles or hubs should not be used.
3. If a primary IV fluid setup is used, discontinue the primary solution during infusion of metronidazole.
4. The order of mixing to prepare the powder for injection is important:

• Reconstitute.
• Dilute in IV solutions (in glass or plastic containers).
• Neutralize pH with sodium bicarbonate solution. Neutralized solutions should not be refrigerated.
5. Premixed, ready to use Flagyl usually comes 5 mg/mL (500 mg Metronidazole in 100 mL of solution) in plastic bags.
6. For topical use, therapeutic results should be seen within 3 weeks with continuing improvement through 9 weeks of therapy.
7. Cosmetics may be used after application of topical metronidazole.
8. IV metronidazole has a high sodium content.
9. *Treatment of Overdose:* Supportive treatment.

Contraindications: Blood dyscrasias; active organic disease of the CNS. Not recommended for trichomoniasis during the first trimester of pregnancy. During lactation. For topical use: hypersensitivity to parabens or other ingredients of the formulation.

Special Concerns: Safety and efficacy have not been established in children. Clients should not drink alcohol during use.

Side Effects: Systemic Use. *GI:* Nausea, dry mouth, metallic taste, vomiting, diarrhea, abdominal discomfort, constipation. *CNS:* Headache, dizziness, vertigo, incoordination, ataxia, confusion, irritability, depression, weakness, insomnia, syncope, seizures, peripheral neuropathy including paresthesias. *Hematologic:* Leukopenia, ***bone marrow aplasia.*** *GU:* Burning, dysuria, cystitis, polyuria, incontinence, dryness of vagina or vulva, dyspareunia, decreased libido. *Allergic:* Urticaria, pruritus, erythematous rash, flushing, nasal congestion, fever, joint pain. *Miscellaneous:* Furry tongue, glossitis, stomatitis (due to overgrowth of *Candida*.) ECG abnormalities, thrombophlebitis.

Topical Use: Watery eyes if gel applied too closely to this area; transient redness; mild burning, dryness, and skin irritation.

Vaginal Use: Symptomatic candida vaginitis, N&V.

Symptoms of Overdose: Ataxia, N&V, peripheral neuropathy, ***seizures*** up to 5–7 days.

Drug Interactions
Barbiturates / Possible therapeutic failure of metronidazole
Cimetidine / ↑ Serum levels of metronidazole due to ↓ clearance
Disulfiram / Concurrent use may cause confusion or acute psychosis
Ethanol / Possible disulfiram-like reaction, including flushing, palpitations, tachycardia, and N&V
Hydantoins / ↑ Effect of hydantoins due to ↓ clearance
Lithium / ↑ Lithium toxicity
Warfarin / ↑ Anticoagulant effect

NURSING CONSIDERATIONS

See also *General Nursing Considerations for All Anti-Infectives,* Chapter 1.

Client/Family Teaching
1. Take with food or milk to reduce GI upset.
2. Report any symptoms of CNS toxicity immediately, such as ataxia or tremor, that may necessitate withdrawal of drug.
3. Do not perform tasks that require mental alertness until drug effects are realized as dizziness may occur.
4. During treatment for trichomoniasis, explain the necessity for the male partner to have therapy also, since organisms may be located in the male urogenital tract.
5. Clients should not engage in intercourse while using the vaginal gel. With all other therapy, sexual partners should use a condom to prevent reinfection.
6. The drug may turn urine brown; do not be alarmed.
7. Avoid alcohol because a disulfiram-like reaction may occur. Symptoms include abdominal cramps, vomiting, flushing, and headache.

Evaluate
• Resolution of infection and reports of symptomatic improvement
• Negative lab culture reports

CHAPTER THIRTEEN

Anthelmintics

See also the following individual entries:

Mebendazole
Oxamniquine
Piperazine Citrate
Praziquantel
Pyrantel Pamoate
Thiabendazole

General Statement: Helminthiasis, or infestation of the body by parasites, is a common affliction. Helminths (worms) may infect the intestinal lumen or the worm also may migrate to a particular tissue. Treatment of helminth infections is complicated by the fact that a worm may have one or more morphologic stages. Thus, it is important to ensure that therapy rids the body of eggs and larvae, as well as worms. Also, a client may be infected by more than one type of worm. Factors such as availability and cost of the drug, toxicity, ease of administration, and how long it takes to complete therapy also have a significant impact on successful treatment of helminths. Accurate diagnosis is extremely important before treatment is started because its success depends on selecting the drug best suited for the eradication of a specific infestation. Parasites that infest only the intestinal tract can be eradicated by locally acting drugs. Other parasites enter tissues and must be treated by drugs that are absorbed from the GI tract.

Since many parasitic infestations are transmitted by persons sharing bathroom facilities, the physician may wish to examine all members of the household for parasitic infestation. Treatment is often accompanied or followed by repeated laboratory examinations to determine whether the parasite has been eradicated.

Helminths can be divided into three groups: cestodes (flatworms, tapeworms), nematodes (roundworms), and trematodes (flukes). The following is a brief description of the more common helminths and the drug of choice to treat infections by that particular helminth.

CESTODES (FLATWORMS, TAPEWORMS): The more common tapeworms are the beef tapeworm (*Taenia saginata*), pork tapeworm (*T. solium*), dwarf tapeworm (*Hymenolepis nana*), and fish tapeworm (*Diphyllobothrium latum*). The tapeworm consists of a scolex or head that hooks into a segment of intestine. The body is that of a segmented flatworm, sections of which are found in the stools. Tapeworm infestations are difficult to eradicate but have few side effects. **Drug treatment:** Niclosamine and praziquantel.

NEMATODES: 1. **Filaria (filariasis).** Infections due to *Wuchereria bancrofti, Brugia malayi,* and *B. timori* are transmitted by mosquitoes. These parasites are tiny roundworms that migrate into the lymphatic system and bloodstream. Living and dead worms can obstruct the lymphatic system, causing elephantiasis. Mosquito control is the best means of combating this infestation.

Other filarial infections include *Loa loa,* transmitted by the bite of a horsefly, and *Onchocerca volvulus* (onchocerciasis, river blindness), which is transmitted by the bite of a blackfly. **Drug treatment:** Diethylcarbamazine. Suramin sodium (available from Centers for Disease Control) is used to treat onchocerciasis.

2. **Hookworm (uncinariasis).** Intestinal infection caused by *Ancylostoma duodenale* or *Necator americanus,* these infections cause debilitation resulting in iron-deficiency anemia, characterized by fatigue, lassitude, and apathy. **Drug treatment:** Mebendazole or pyrantel pamoate.

3. **Pinworm (enterobiasis).** These intestinal infestations are common in school-age children. Complications are rare, although heavy infestations may cause abdominal pain, weight loss, and insomnia. **Drug treatment:** Mebendazole, piperazine, pyrantel pamoate, pyrvinium pamoate, thiabendazole.

4. **Roundworm (ascariasis).** Caused by *Ascaris lumbricoides,* this infection can cause obstruction of the respiratory and GI tracts. **Drug treatment:** Mebendazole, pyrantel pamoate.

5. **Trichinosis.** Caused by *Trichinella spiralis,* these parasites are transmitted by the consumption of raw or inadequately cooked pork. The infection is serious; larvae burrow into the bloodstream and form cysts in skeletal muscle. **Drug treatment:** Corticosteroids to control the inflammation caused by systemic infestation; mebendazole, thiabendazole.

6. **Threadworm (strongyloidiasis).** This parasite (*Strongyloides stercoralis*) infests the upper GI tract. Heavy infestations can result in malabsorption syndrome, diarrhea, and general discomfort. **Drug treatment:** Thiabendazole.

7. **Whipworm (trichuriasis).** This threadlike parasite (*Trichuris trichiura*) lodges in the mucosa of the cecum. **Drug treatment:** Mebendazole.

TREMATODES: Schistosomiasis (blood flukes or bilharziasis) can be transmitted by contaminated water supplies. The organisms are *Schistosoma mansoni, S. japonicum, S. haematobium,* and *S. mekongi.* The infection is difficult to eradicate. **Drug treatment:** Praziquantel, oxamniquine (*S. mansoni* only).

Side Effects: Since the anthelmintics do not belong to any one chemical group, their side effects are related to specific compounds. However, N&V, cramps, and diarrhea are common to most.

NURSING CONSIDERATIONS

See also *General Nursing Considerations for All Anti-Infectives,* Chapter 1.

Assessment

1. Document indications for therapy and type and onset of symptoms. Assist client to identify causative factors and possible exposure(s).
2. List other agents prescribed and the outcome.
3. Obtain appropiate specimens for microscopic examination.
4. Determine if pregnant and note any evidence of GI ulcers.

Client/Family Teaching

1. Provide written instructions regarding prescribed diet, cathartics, enemas, medications, and follow-up tests when treatment is to be carried out at home.
2. Review these instructions to be sure they are understood by the person responsible for the client's treatment and care. *Good hygienic practices reduce the incidence of helminthiasis.*
3. Advise parent to notify school or institution that child is undergoing therapy. Identify any close contacts that should also be treated.
4. Emphasize the need for follow-up examinations to check the results of treatment.
5. Specific practices are as follows:

PINWORMS

1. Advise that therapy generally consists of a single dose with meals and is repeated in 2 weeks.
2. Instruct responsible family member how to prevent infestation with pinworms by:

• Washing hands with soap and water before and after contact with infected person and when changing their clothes or bed linens

• Washing hands frequently during the day, after toileting, and before meals
• Keeping nails short
• Washing ova from anal area in the morning as these may cause itching
• Applying antipruritic ointment to anal area to reduce scratching, which transfers pinworms. Scratching causes pinworms to attach to the fingers, which when placed in the mouth causes reinfection
• Changing clothes daily and checking for evidence of eggs or worms
• Wearing tight underpants
• Wearing gloves to prepare food
• Washing linens in hot water
• Not sharing washcloths and towels
• Disinfecting toilet daily
• For several days after therapy, wet mop or vacuum bedroom floor; do not sweep
• Wash bed linens and night clothes after therapy and do not shake

3. Explain that the eggs are not visible but contaminate everything they come in contact with (i.e., food, hands, clothes, linens, rugs). Eggs floating in the air can be swallowed and cause infestation. This is very contagious and easily transmissable and all family members may need to be examined for pinworms.
4. After the end of the treatment course, swab the perianal area each morning with transparent tape and return to provider. Advise that a cure is considered when no further eggs are found on microscopic examination for 7 consecutive days.

ROUNDWORMS, HOOKWORMS, WHIPWORMS:

1. Two to 3 weeks after therapy, stools should undergo microscopic examination to determine fecal egg count.
2. Record stool color and consistency and examine for any evidence of expulsed worm.
3. After administration of medication, cathartics, and enema, examine the results of the enema for the head of the worm.
4. Advise responsible family member:

• Stools must go to the laboratory warm and be examined daily until no further roundworm ova are found
• Wash hands with soap and water frequently during the day, after toileting, and before eating
• Wash all fruits and vegetables before eating; cook meats and vegetables thoroughly
• Wear shoes, do not defecate outside, use a bathroom, and double flush to ensure proper disposal

TREMATODES:

1. Advise that dizziness, drowsiness, N&V, headache, diarrhea, and pruritis may occur 3 hr after a dose of medication and last for several hours.
2. Report any low-grade fever, discoloration of urine, or seizure activity.
3. Advise clients with prior seizure disorder that they should be hospitalized for treatment.

Evaluate

• Knowledge and understanding of illness, how acquired, prevention of transmission, and compliance with prescribed therapy
• Successful treatment evidenced by expulsion of worm(s)
• Three consecutive negative stool exams, perianal swabs, and/or cultures
• Causes for repeated infestation and the need for further treatment

Mebendazole

(meh-**BEN**-dah-zohl)
Pregnancy Category: C
Vermox **(Rx)**

See also *Anthelmintics,* Chapter 13.

How Supplied: *Chew Tablet:* 100 mg

Action/Kinetics: Mebendazole exerts its anthelmintic effect by blocking the glucose uptake of the organisms, thereby reducing their energy until death results. It also inhibits the formation of microtubules in the helminth. **Peak plasma levels:** 2–4 hr.

Poorly absorbed from the GI tract. Excreted in feces.

Uses: Whipworm, pinworm, roundworm, common and American hookworm infections; in single or mixed infections.

Dosage

- **Tablets, Chewable**

Whipworm, roundworm, and hookworm.

Adults and children: 1 tablet morning and evening on 3 consecutive days.

Pinworms.

1 tablet, one time. All treatments can be repeated after 3 weeks.

Contraindication: Hypersensitivity to mebendazole.

Special Concerns: Use with caution in children under 2 years of age and during lactation.

Side Effects: Transient abdominal pain and diarrhea.

Drug Interactions: Carbamazepine and hydantoin may ↓ effect due to ↓ plasma levels of mebendazole.

NURSING CONSIDERATIONS

See also *Nursing Considerations* for *Anthelmintics,* Chapter 13.

Client/Family Teaching

1. Tablet may be chewed, crushed, and/or mixed with food.
2. No prior fasting, purging, or other procedures are required.
3. With pinworms, advise that condition may be highly contagious. Stress careful handwashing with soap and water before and after eating and toileting.
4. Advise school nurse of treatment.
5. Do not share washcloths and towels. Wear tight underpants and change daily.
6. Review the appropriate method for handling linens and clothing (no shaking or sharing, wash in hot water).
7. Clean toilet seats and vacuum or wetmop bedroom floors daily.
8. Wash all fruits and vegetables thoroughly.
9. Thoroughly cook all meats and vegetables.

Evaluate

- Negative stool specimens and/or negative perianal swabs
- Destruction of causative organism
- Reports of symptomatic improvement

Oxamniquine

(ox-**AM**-nih-kwin)
Pregnancy Category: C
Vansil **(Rx)**

How Supplied: *Capsule:* 250 mg

Action/Kinetics: *Schistosoma mansoni* is a trematode parasite found in Egypt, elsewhere in Africa, South America, and the West Indies, including Puerto Rico. The agent is found in water and is transmitted by snails. The drug causes the worms to shift from the mesenteric veins to the liver, where they are destroyed. Oxamniquine is more effective against male than against female schistosomes, but females cease laying eggs following treatment; thus, the infection eventually subsides due to decreased reproduction. **Peak plasma concentration:** 1–1.5 hr. **t½:** 1–2.5 hr. The drug is well absorbed after PO administration. Inactive metabolites are excreted in urine.

Uses: All stages of *S. mansoni* infections (acute and chronic), including involvement of the liver and spleen. *Investigational:* With praziquantel to treat neurocysticercosis (single dose only).

Dosage

- **Capsules**

Adults: 12–15 mg/kg as single PO dose. **30–40 kg:** 500 mg; **41–60 kg:** 750 mg; **61–80 kg:** 1,000 mg; **81–100 kg:** 1,250 mg. **Children (under 30 kg):** 10 mg/kg followed in 2–8 hr with a second 10-mg/kg dose.

Special Concerns: Use during pregnancy and lactation only when potential benefits outweigh risks.

Side Effects: Well tolerated. *CNS:* Transient drowsiness and dizziness, headaches. ***Convulsions (mostly in epileptics);*** therefore, closely monitor clients with history of convulsive disorders. *GI:* N&V, abdominal pain, anorexia. *Dermatologic:* Urticaria.

NURSING CONSIDERATIONS

See also *Nursing Considerations* for *Anthelmintics,* Chapter 13.

Client/Family Teaching

1. Do not drive a car or operate hazardous machinery because drug may cause dizziness and/or drowsiness.
2. Administer after food to minimize GI distress.
3. Report any evidence of seizures or CNS symptoms.
4. May discolor urine orange/red; report so that hematuria may be ruled out.
5. Advise that cough, pulmonary infiltrates, elevated liver enzymes, and urticaria have been associated with death of parasites and not drug toxicity. These symptoms may occur several days to 1 month following treatment.

Evaluate: Laboratory evidence of eradication of S. mansoni parasitic infection

Piperazine citrate

(pie-**PER**-ah-zeen)

(Rx)

See also *Anthelmintics,* Chapter 13.

Action/Kinetics: The drug is believed to paralyze the muscles of parasites; this dislodges the parasites and promotes their elimination by peristalsis. The drug has little effect on larvae in tissues. The drug is readily absorbed from the GI tract, is partially metabolized by the liver, and the remainder is excreted in urine. Rate of elimination differs among clients although it is excreted nearly unchanged in the urine within 24 hr.

Uses: Pinworm (oxyuriasis) and roundworm (ascariasis) infestations. Particularly recommended for pediatric use.

Dosage

- **Syrup, Tablets**

  Pinworms.

Adults and children: 65 mg/kg/day as a single dose for 7 days up to a maximum daily dose of 2.5 g.

Roundworms.

Adults: one dose of 3.5 g/day for 2 consecutive days; **pediatric:** one dose of 75 mg/kg/day for 2 consecutive days, not to exceed 3.5 g/day. For severe infections, repeat therapy after 1 week.

Contraindications: Impaired liver or kidney function, seizure disorders, hypersensitivity. Lactation.

Special Concerns: Safe use during pregnancy has not been established. Due to neurotoxicity, prolonged, repeated, or excessive use in children should be avoided.

Laboratory Test Interference: False – or ↓ uric acid values.

Side Effects: Piperazine has low toxicity. *GI:* N&V, diarrhea, cramps. *CNS:* Tremors, headache, vertigo, decreased reflexes, paresthesias, ***seizures,*** ataxia, chorea, memory decrement. *Ophthalmologic:* Nystagmus, blurred vision, cataracts, strabismus. *Allergic:* Urticaria, fever, skin reactions, purpura, lacrimation, rhinorrhea, arthralgia, ***bronchospasm,*** cough. *Miscellaneous:* Muscle weakness.

Drug Interactions: Concomitant administration of piperazine and phenothiazines may result in an increase in extrapyramidal effects (including violent convulsions) caused by phenothiazines.

NURSING CONSIDERATIONS

See also *Nursing Considerations* for *Anthelmintics,* Chapter 13.

Assessment

1. Note any evidence of impaired hepatic or renal function.
2. Document any history of seizure disorder or chronic neurologic disease as drug is contraindicated.
3. Determine previous treatments and length of therapy as excessive drug therapy should be avoided in children due to neurotoxic effects.
4. Use cautiously with severe malnutrition or anemia.

Client/Family Teaching

1. The drug should be taken on an empty stomach. Take before breakfast or in two divided doses.

2. Report any adverse drug effects immediately.
3. Strict hygiene is required to prevent reinfection.
4. Keep pleasant-tasting medication out of reach of children.
5. Explain that drug causes paralysis of ascariasis parasite and they are expelled live by peristalsis. Instruct to flush 2–3 times to ensure that contents are completely removed.

Evaluate

- Eradication of infecting parasite
- Negative stool examinations and perianal swabs
- Cause(s) for repeated infestation and/or reinfection (assess need for further treatment)

Praziquantel

(pray-zih-**KWON**-tell)
Pregnancy Category: B
Biltricide, Cysticide **(Rx)**

How Supplied: *Tablet:* 600 mg
Action/Kinetics: Praziquantel causes increased cell permeability in the helminth, resulting in a loss of intracellular calcium with massive contractions, and paralysis of musculature with breakdown of the integrity of the organism. Thus, phagocytes can attack the parasite and death follows. **Maximum serum levels:** 1–3 hr. **t½:** 0.8–1.5 hr. Levels in the CSF are approximately 14%–20% of the total amount of the drug in the plasma. Significant first-pass effect. Excreted primarily in the urine.
Uses: Schistosomal infections due to *Schistosoma japonicum, S. mansoni, S. mekongi,* and *S. hematobium*. Liver flukes (*Chonorchis sinensis, Opisthorchis viverrini). Investigational:* Neurocysticercosis, other tissue flukes, and intestinal cestodes.

Dosage

- **Tablets**

Schistosomiasis.
Three doses of 20 mg/kg with an interval between doses not less than 4 hr or more than 6 hr.

Chonorchiasis and opisthorchiasis.
Three doses of 25 mg/kg as a 1-day treatment.

Administration/Storage: *Treatment of Overdose:* Administer a fast-acting laxative.
Contraindications: Ocular cysticercosis. Lactation.
Special Concerns: Safety in children less than 4 years of age not established.
Side Effects: *GI:* Nausea, abdominal discomfort. *CNS:* Malaise, headache, dizziness, drowsiness. *Miscellaneous:* Fever, urticaria (rare). *NOTE:* These side effects may also be due to the helminth infection itself.

Symptoms of Overdose: Extension of side effects.

NURSING CONSIDERATIONS

See also *Nursing Considerations* for *Anthelmintics,* Chapter 13.

Assessment

1. Determine if the schistosomiasis or fluke infection is accompanied by cerebral cysticercosis; if so, the client should be hospitalized for treatment.
2. Note any liver dysfunction as a reduced dosage may be indicated.

Client/Family Teaching

1. The tablets should be taken as directed, during meals with liquids. The tablets should not be chewed as their bitter taste can cause retching and vomiting.
2. Due to dizziness and drowsiness, caution should be exercised while driving or performing tasks requiring alertness.
3. Do not nurse baby on treatment day and for 3 days following treatment.

Evaluate

- Eradication of parasitic infestation
- Negative culture reports

Pyrantel pamoate

(pie-**RAN**-tell)
Antiminth, Combantrin ✦, Reese's Pinworm **(Rx)**

See also *Anthelmintics,* Chapter 13.
How Supplied: *Suspension:* 144 mg/30 mL, 720 mg/5 mL; *Tablet:* 180 mg
Action/Kinetics: The anthelmintic effect is attributed to the neuromuscu-

lar blocking effect of this agent, which paralyzes the helminth, allowing it to be expelled through the feces. It is poorly absorbed from GI tract. **Peak plasma levels:** 0.05–0.13 mcg/mL after 1–3 hr. Partially metabolized in liver. Fifty percent is excreted unchanged in feces and less than 15% excreted unchanged in urine.
Uses: Pinworm (enterobiasis) and roundworm (ascariasis) infestations. Multiple helminth infections.

Dosage

- **Liquid Oral Suspension**

Adults and children: one dose of 11 mg/kg (maximum). **Maximum total dose:** 1.0 g.
Contraindications: Pregnancy. Hepatic disease.
Special Concerns: Use with caution in presence of liver dysfunction. Safe use in children less than 2 years of age has not been established.
Side Effects: *GI* (most frequent): Anorexia, N&V, cramps, diarrhea. *Hepatic:* Transient elevation of AST. *CNS:* Headache, dizziness, drowsiness, insomnia. *Miscellaneous:* Skin rashes.
Drug Interaction: Use with piperazine for ascariasis results in antagonism of the effect of both drugs.

NURSING CONSIDERATIONS

See also *Nursing Considerations* for *Anthelmintics,* Chapter 13.
Client/Family Teaching
1. Drug may be taken without regard to food intake.
2. Caution that drug may cause dizziness or drowsiness and not to engage in activities that require mental alertness.
3. Purging is not necessary prior to or during treatment.
4. Drug may be taken with milk or fruit juice.
5. Provide a printed list of drug side effects, stressing those that require immediate reporting.
6. When treating pinworms, review with client/family the appropriate precautions R/T transmission (see *Anthelmintics,* Chapter 13.)

Evaluate
- Resolution of infection
- Negative consecutive stool examinations and perianal swabs

Thiabendazole

(thigh-ah-**BEN**-dah-zohl)
Pregnancy Category: C
Mintezol, Minzolum **(Rx)**

See also *Anthelmintics,* Chapter 13.
How Supplied: *Chew Tablet:* 500 mg; *Suspension:* 500 mg/5 mL
Action/Kinetics: The drug interferes with the enzyme fumarate reductase, which is specific to several helminths. It is readily absorbed from the GI tract. **Peak plasma levels:** 1–2 hr. **t½:** 0.9–2 hr. Most of the drug is excreted within 24 hr, mainly through the urine.
Uses: Primarily for threadworm infections, cutaneous larva migrans, visceral larva migrans when these infections occur alone or if pinworm is also present. Use in the following infections only if specific therapy is not available or cannot be used or if a second drug is desirable: hookworm, whipworm, large roundworm. To reduce symptoms of trichinosis during the invasive phase.

Dosage

- **Oral Suspension, Chewable Tablets**

Over 68 kg: 1.5 g/dose; **less than 68 kg:** 22 mg/kg/dose.
Administration/Storage
1. For strongyloidiasis, cutaneous larva migrans, hookworm, whipworm, or roundworm; two doses daily are given for 2 days. For trichinelliasis, give two doses daily for 2–4 days. For pinworm, give two doses for 1 day, repeat after 7–14 days.
2. *Treatment of Overdose:* Induce vomiting or perform gastric lavage. Treat symptoms.

Contraindications: Lactation. Use in mixed infections with ascaris as it may cause worms to migrate.
Special Concerns: Safety and efficacy not established in children less than 13.6 kg. Use with caution in clients with hepatic disease or impaired hepatic function.
Side Effects: *GI:* N&V, anorexia, diarrhea, epigastric distress. *CNS:* Dizziness, drowsiness, headache, irritability, ***seizures.*** *Allergic:* Pruritus, angioedema, flushing of face, chills, fever, skin rashes, ***Stevens-Johnson syndrome, anaphylaxis,*** lymphadenopathy. *Hepatic:* Jaundice, cholestasis, liver damage, transient increase in AST. *GU:* Crystalluria, hematuria, enuresis, foul odor of urine. *Miscellaneous:* Tinnitus, blurred vision, hypotension, collapse, hyperglycemia, leukopenia, perianal rash.

Symptoms of Overdose: Psychic changes, transient vision changes.
Drug Interaction: ↑ Serum levels of xanthines due to ↓ breakdown by liver.

NURSING CONSIDERATIONS

See also *Nursing Considerations* for *Anthelmintics,* Chapter 13.
Assessment: Document indications for therapy, onset of symptoms, and attempt to identify how and when acquired.
Client/Family Teaching
1. Administer the drug after meals; chew tablets thoroughly.
2. CNS disturbances (including muscular weakness and loss of mental alertness) may be caused by the drug and should be reported.
3. Do not operate hazardous machinery after taking the medication, as drug may cause dizziness and drowsiness.
4. May notice an odor to the urine 24 hr following ingestion; this is normal.
5. Report any evidence of rash, fever, or itching immediately.

Evaluate
- Negative consecutive stool cultures
- Eradication of infestation

CHAPTER FOURTEEN

Antifungal Drugs

See the following individual entries:

Amphotericin B
Butoconazole Nitrate
Ciclopirox Olamine
Clotrimazole
Econazole Nitrate
Fluconazole
Flucytosine
Griseofulvin Microsize
Griseofulvin Ultramicrosize
Itraconazole
Ketoconazole
Miconazole
Naftifine Hydrochloride
Natamycin
Nystatin
Oxiconazole Nitrate
Sulconazole Nitrate
Terbinafine Hydrochloride
Terconazole Nitrate
Tioconazole
Tolnaftate

Amphotericin B

(am-foe-**TER**-ih-sin)
Pregnancy Category: B
Fungizone, Fungizone IV **(Rx)**

See also *Anti-Infectives,* Chapter 1.
How Supplied: *Cream:* 3%; *Lotion:* 3%; *Powder for injection:* 50 mg
Action/Kinetics: This antibiotic is produced by *Streptomyces nodosus;* it is fungistatic or fungicidal depending on the concentration of the drug in body fluids and the susceptibility of the fungus. Amphotericin B binds to specific chemical structures—sterols—of the fungal cellular membrane, increasing cellular permeability and promoting loss of potassium and other substances. Amphotericin B is used either IV or topically. It is highly bound to serum protein (90%) **Peak plasma levels:** 0.5–2 mcg/mL. $t^1/_2$**, initial:** 24 hr; **second phase:** 15 days. Slowly excreted by kidneys.
Uses: The drug is toxic and should be used only for clients under close medical supervision with progressive or potentially fatal fungal infections. *Systemic:* Disseminated North American blastomycosis, cryptococcosis, and other systemic fungal infections, including coccidioidomycosis, histoplasmosis, mucormycosis, sporotrichosis, aspergillosis, disseminated candidiasis, and monilial overgrowth resulting from oral antibiotic therapy. Secondary therapy to treat American mucocutaneous leishmaniasis. *Topical:* Cutaneous and mucocutaneous infections of *Candida (Monilia)* infections.

Dosage

- **Slow IV infusion**

Antifungal. **Initial:** 0.25 mg/kg/day. May be increased gradually by 0.1–0.2 mg/kg/day, up to a maximum dose of 1.5 mg/kg/day to 1.5 mg/kg every other day. A test dose (1 mg) should be given first to assess client tolerance. Depending on use, treatment may be required for several months.

- **Intrathecal**

Antifungal. **Initial:** 0.025–0.1 mg (of the base) q 48–72 hr; **then,** the dose may be increased to 0.5 mg, as tolerated, to a maximum total dose of 15 mg.

- **Continuous Bladder Irritation**

Antifungal. 50 mg (of the base) in 1,000 mL sterile water/day given at a rate of 50 mL/hr via a three-way catheter for 5–10 days.

- **Topical (Lotion, Cream, Ointment—Each 3%)**

Apply liberally to affected areas b.i.d.–q.i.d. Depending on the type of lesion, up to 4 weeks of therapy may be necessary.

Administration/Storage

1. Follow directions on vial for dilution. Use only distilled water without a bacteriostatic agent or 5% dextrose as diluent to avoid precipitation of drug.
2. Strict aseptic technique must be used in preparation because there is no bacteriostatic agent in the medication.
3. Use a sterile 20-gauge needle every time entrance is made into the vial.
4. Do not use saline solution or distilled water with bacteriostatic agent as a diluent because a precipitate may result. Use sterile water with continuous bladder irrigation.
5. Do not use the initial concentrate if any precipitate is present.
6. An in-line membrane filter with a pore diameter of 1 μm may be used. Since preparation is a colloidal suspension, anything smaller may remove the medication.
7. Protect from light during administration and storage.
8. Minimize local inflammation and danger of thrombophlebitis by administering the solution below the recommended dilution of 0.1 mg.
9. Initiate therapy in the most distal veins. When administered peripherally, changing sites with each dose may decrease phlebitis.
10. Have on hand 200–400 units of heparin sodium, since it may be ordered for the infusion to prevent thrombophlebitis.
11. Administer IV infusion for 6 hr (usually diluted in 500 mL D5W) with an infusion pump and preferably in a central line.
12. After reconstitution, amphotericin may be stored for 24 hr in a dark room or in a refrigerator for 1 week without significant loss of potency.
13. Use dilutions of 0.1 mg/mL immediately after preparation.
14. Rub creams and lotions into lesion.
15. The cream may cause drying and slight skin discoloration; the lotion and ointment may cause staining of nail lesions, but not skin.

Contraindications: Hypersensitivity to drug. Use to treat common forms of fungal diseases showing only positive skin or serologic tests.

Special Concerns: The bone marrow depressant effects may result in increased incidence of microbial infection, delayed healing, and gingival bleeding. Although used in children, safety and efficacy have not been determined.

Laboratory Test Interferences: ↑ AST, ALT, alkaline phosphatase, creatinine, BUN, NPN, BSP retention values.

Side Effects: After topical use. Irritation, pruritus, dry skin. Redness, itching, or burning especially in skin folds. **After IV use.** *GI:* N&V, diarrhea, dyspepsia, anorexia, abdominal cramps, epigastric pain, melena, hemorrhagic gastroenteritis. *CNS:* Fever, chills, headache, malaise, vertigo; rarely, ***seizures,*** peripheral neuropathy, and other neurologic symptoms. *CV:* Thrombophlebitis, phlebitis. Rarely, arrhythmias, hyper- or hypotension, ***ventricular fibrillation, cardiac arrest.*** *Renal:* Anuria, oliguria, azotemia, hypokalemia, renal tubular acidosis, nephrocalcinosis, hyposthenuria. *Hematologic:* Normochromic, normocytic anemia. Rarely, ***coagulation defects,*** thrombocytopenia, leukopenia, agranulocytosis, eosinophilia, leukocytosis. *Dermatologic:* Maculopapular rash, pruritus. *Miscellaneous:* Muscle and joint pain, generalized pain, weight loss, tinnitus, blurred or double vision, hearing loss, hepatic failure, dyspnea, flushing, anaphylaxis. **After intrathecal use:** Blurred vision, changes in vision, difficulty in urination, numbness, tingling, pain, or weakness.

Drug Interactions

Aminoglycosides / Additive nephrotoxicity and/or ototoxicity
Corticosteroids, Corticotropin / ↑ Potassium depletion caused by amphotericin B
Cyclosporine / ↑ Nephrotoxic effects of cyclosporine
Digitalis glycosides / ↑ Potassium depletion caused by amphotericin B; ↑ incidence of digitalis toxicity

Flucytosine / Synergistic antifungal effect
Miconazole / Amphotericin B ↓ effect of miconazole
Rifampin / Synergistic antifungal effect
Skeletal muscle relaxants, surgical (e.g., succinylcholine, *d*-tubocurarine) / ↑ Muscle relaxation
Tetracyclines / Synergistic antifungal effect

NURSING CONSIDERATIONS

See also *General Nursing Considerations For All Anti-Infectives,* Chapter 1.

Assessment

1. Assess for any history of adverse effects and hypersensitivity to any anti-infectives or drugs in the antifungal category.
2. During the nursing and drug history, assess mental status and note client age.
3. Ensure that baseline CBC, liver and renal function, and laboratory cultures have been performed.
4. Assess and describe characteristics of lesions requiring therapy.

Interventions

1. Determine that a 1-mg test dose has been administered (1 mg in 20 mL D5W over 20–30 min) to assess client's tolerance to amphotericin.
2. Ascertain if client is to be premedicated with antipyretics, antihistamines, corticosteroids, and/or antiemetic drugs to reduce side effects. Rashes, fevers, and chills may occur frequently with this therapy.
3. Infuse IV slowly, monitor VS frequently (every 15–30 min during first dose), and interrupt if client develops any adverse effects.
4. Monitor I&O. Report a reduction in blood sediment or cloudiness in the urine.
5. Weigh client twice weekly and assess for possible malnutrition or dehydration.
6. Anticipate hypokalemia in clients concomitantly taking digoxin. Observe for toxicity, muscle weakness and monitor serum digoxin levels.
7. Intrathecal administration of amphotericin may cause inflammation of the spinal roots; assess for sensory loss or foot drop in these clients.

Client/Family Teaching

1. GI effects may be reduced by administering an antihistamine or antiemetic before drug therapy and by administering the drug before mealtime. If diarrhea develops, try small frequent meals.
2. Report any incidents of anorexia, nausea, vomiting, headache, or chills.
3. Stress the importance of reporting any decrease in I&O and extreme weight loss. Advise adequate hydration (2½ L/day) to prevent nephrotoxic effects.
4. Amphotericin therapy usually requires long-term treatments (6–10 weeks) to ensure an adequate response and to prevent any relapse.
5. Neurologic symptoms such as tinnitus, blurred vision, or vertigo should be reported immediately.
6. Review guidelines for therapy with creams and lotions:
   - Drug does not stain skin when it is rubbed into lesion.
   - Any discoloration of fabric caused by cream or lotion may be removed by washing with soap and water.
   - Any discoloration of clothing caused by ointment may be removed with a standard cleaning fluid.
   - Report any increased itching, burning, or rash at site of local application.
   - Do not apply an occlusive dressing as this may promote yeast growth.

Evaluate

- Clinical and laboratory evidence of successful resolution of fungal infection
- Reports of symptomatic improvement

Butoconazole nitrate

(byou-toe-**KON**-ah-zohl)
Pregnancy Category: C
Femstat **(Rx)**

How Supplied: *Vaginal cream:* 2%
Action/Kinetics: By permeating chitin in the fungal cell wall, butoconazole increases membrane permeability to intracellular substances,

leading to reduced osmotic resistance and viability of the fungus. Approximately 5.5% of drug is absorbed following vaginal administration; plasma. **t½:** 21–24 hr.

Uses: Vulvovaginal fungal infections caused by *Candida* species.

Dosage

- **Vaginal cream (2%)**

During pregnancy, second and third trimesters only.

One full applicator (about 5 g) of the cream intravaginally at bedtime for 6 days.

Nonpregnant.

One full applicator (about 5 g) intravaginally at bedtime for 3 days (if necessary, may be used for up to 6 days). *NOTE:* Vaginal infections may also be treated by one dose of butoconazole.

Administration/Storage

1. During pregnancy, use of a vaginal applicator may be contraindicated.
2. If there is no response, studies should be repeated to confirm the diagnosis before reinstituting antifungal therapy.
3. Not to be stored above 40°C (104°F).

Contraindications: Use during first trimester of pregnancy.

Special Concerns: Pediatric dosage has not been established. Use with caution during lactation.

Side Effects: *GU:* Vaginal burning, vulvar burning or itching, discharge; soreness, swelling, and itching of the fingers.

NURSING CONSIDERATIONS

Assessment

1. Document symptoms requiring treatment and length of time experienced.
2. Determine if client is pregnant.
3. Obtain appropriate pretreatment lab studies.

Client/Family Teaching

1. Instruct in the appropriate technique for medication administration.
2. Administer as prescribed and continue during menstrual cycle.
3. Insert cream high into the vagina.
4. Report if irritation or burning occurs.
5. The use of sanitary napkins may prevent soiling and staining of undergarments and clothing.
6. To prevent reinfection, the sexual partner should use a condom during intercourse and also seek treatment if symptomatic.
7. If the client is having recurrent vaginal infections and has been exposed to HIV, the provider should be consulted to determine the cause of symptoms. If the symptoms return within 2 months, the client could be pregnant or there could be a serious underlying medical cause (e.g., diabetes, HIV infection).

Evaluate

- Eradication of fungal infection
- Reports of symptomatic improvement

Ciclopirox olamine

(sye-kloh-**PEER**-ox)

Pregnancy Category: B

Loprox **(Rx)**

How Supplied: *Cream:* 1%; *Lotion:* 1%

Action/Kinetics: This broad-spectrum fungicide is effective against dermatophytes, yeast, *Malassezia furfur, Trichophyton rubrum, T. mentagrophytes, Epidermophyton floccosum, Microsporum canis,* and *Candida albicans*. At lower concentrations the drug blocks the transport of amino acids into the cell, whereas at higher concentrations the cell membrane of the fungus is altered so that intracellular material leaks out. The drug may also inhibit synthesis of RNA, DNA, and protein in growing fungal cells. A small amount of drug is absorbed through the skin; it also penetrates to the sebaceous glands and dermis as well as into the hair.

Uses: Tinea pedis, tinea corporis, tinea cruris, tinea versicolor, candidiasis.

Dosage

- **Topical cream (1%)**

Massage gently into the affected area and surrounding skin morning and

evening. If no improvement after 4 weeks, diagnosis should be reevaluated.
Contraindication: Use in or around the eyes.
Special Concerns: Safety and efficacy in lactation and in children under 10 years of age not established.
Side Effects: *Dermatologic:* Irritation, redness, burning, pain, skin sensitivity, pruritus at application site.

NURSING CONSIDERATIONS

Assessment

1. Document indications for therapy and type and onset of symptoms.
2. If drug is used for suspected *M. furfur* infection, assist with establishing the diagnosis by describing lesions and obtaining scrapings because a technique for culture of organism does not exist.

Client/Family Teaching

1. Cleanse skin with soap and water and dry thoroughly.
2. Occlusive dressings or wrappings should not be used. Adult incontinence pads/diapers are an occlusive dressing and should not be used during therapy.
3. Even if symptoms have improved, the drug should be used for the full prescribed time.
4. Shoes and socks should be changed at least once daily. Shoes should be well-fitted and ventilated.
5. Report if the area of application shows evidence of blistering, burning, itching, oozing, redness, or swelling.

Evaluate

- Resolution of infection and desired wound healing
- Reports of symptomatic improvement

Clotrimazole

(kloh-**TRY**-mah-zohl)
Pregnancy Category: C (systemic use); B (topical/vaginal use)
Canesten ✦, Canestin 1 ✦, Canestin 3 ✦, Clotrimaderm ✦, FemCare, Gyne-Lotrimin, Lotrimin, Lotrimin AF, Mycelex, Mycelex-7, Mycelex-G, Mycelex OTC, Myclo ✦, Neo-Zol **(OTC) (Rx)**

See also *Anti-Infectives,* Chapter 1.
How Supplied: *Kit; Lotion:* 1%; *Lozenge/Troche:* 10 mg; *Solution:* 1%; *Topical cream:* 1%; *Vaginal cream:* 1%; *Vaginal tablet:* 100 mg, 500 mg
Action/Kinetics: Depending on concentration, this drug may be fungistatic or fungicidal. The drug acts by inhibiting the biosynthesis of sterols, resulting in damage to the cell wall and subsequent loss of essential intracellular elements due to altered permeability. Clotrimazole may also inhibit oxidative and peroxidative enzyme activity and inhibit the biosynthesis of triglycerides and phospholipids by fungi. When used for *Candida albicans,* the drug inhibits transformation of blastophores into the invasive mycelial form. It is poorly absorbed from the GI tract and metabolized in the liver to inactive compounds that are excreted through the feces. **Duration:** up to 3 hr.
Uses: Broad-spectrum antifungal effective against *Malassezia furfur, Trichophyton rubrum, Trichophyton mentagrophytes, Epidermophyton floccosum, Microsporum canis, C. albicans. Oral troche:* Oropharyngeal candidiasis. Reduce incidence of oropharyngeal candidiasis in clients who are immunocompromised due to chemotherapy, radiotherapy, or steroid therapy used for leukemia, solid tumors, or kidney transplant. *Topical OTC products:* Topically to treat tinea pedis, tinea cruris, and tinea corporis. *Topical prescription products:* Same as OTC plus candidiasis and tinea versicolor. *Vaginal products:* Vulvovaginal candidiasis.

Dosage

- **Troche**

Treatment.
One troche (10 mg) 5 times/day for 14 consecutive days.
Prophylaxis.
One troche t.i.d. for duration of che-

motherapy or until maintenance doses of steroids are instituted.

• **Topical Cream, Lotion, Solution (each 1%)**

Massage into affected skin and surrounding areas b.i.d. in morning and evening for 7 consecutive days. Diagnosis should be reevaluated if no improvement occurs in 4 weeks.

• **Vaginal tablets**

One 100-mg tablet/day at bedtime for 7 days. One 500-mg tablet can be inserted once at bedtime.

• **Vaginal cream (1%)**

5 g (one full applicator)/day at bedtime for 7 consecutive days.

Administration/Storage

1. Mycelex-G vaginal cream can be stored at 2°C–30°C (36°F–86°F). Mycelex-G, 100-mg vaginal tablets should not be stored above 35°C (95°F); the 500-mg vaginal tablets should be stored below 30°C (86°F).
2. The troche should be slowly dissolved in the mouth.
3. Topical products should not come in contact with the eyes.

Contraindications: Hypersensitivity. First trimester of pregnancy.

Special Concerns: Use with caution during lactation. Safety and effectiveness for PO use in children less than 3 years of age has not been determined.

Side Effects: *Skin:* Irritation including rash, stinging, pruritus, urticaria, erythema, peeling, blistering, edema. *Vaginal:* Lower abdominal cramps; urinary frequency; bloating; vaginal irritation, itching or burning; dyspareunia. *Hepatic:* Abnormal liver function tests. *GI:* N&V following use of troche.

NURSING CONSIDERATIONS

See also *General Nursing Considerations for All Anti-Infectives,* Chapter 1.

Client/Family Teaching

1. Review goals of therapy and appropriate method for administration.
2. Unless otherwise directed, apply only after cleaning the affected area.
3. When treating vaginal infections, the client should not engage in intercourse; or, to prevent infection, the partner should wear a condom.
4. To prevent staining of clothes, a sanitary napkin should be used with vaginal tablets or cream.
5. If exposed to HIV and recurrent vaginal yeast infections occur, the client should seek prompt medical intervention to determine the cause of the symptoms.

Evaluate

• Eradication of fungal infection
• Reports of symptomatic improvement

Econazole nitrate

(ee-**KON**-ah-zohl)
Pregnancy Category: C
Ecostatin ✱, Spectazole **(Rx)**

How Supplied: *Cream:* 1%

Action/Kinetics: This drug may be fungistatic or fungicidal, depending on concentration. The drug inhibits the synthesis of sterols that damages the cell membrane and increases the permeability, resulting in a loss of essential intracellular elements. It may also inhibit biosynthesis of triglycerides and phospholipids and inhibit oxidative and peroxidative enzyme activity. Effective concentrations are found in the stratum corneum, epidermis, and the dermis. Systemic absorption is low.

Uses: Broad-spectrum fungicide effective against *Microsporum audouinii, M. canis, M. gypseum, Epidermophyton floccosum, Trichophyton mentagrophytes, T. rubrum, T. tonsurans, Candida albicans, Malassezia furfur,* and some gram-positive bacteria. Used to treat tinea cruris, tinea corporis, tinea pedis, tinea versicolor, cutaneous candidiasis.

Dosage

• **Topical cream (1%)**

Tinea cruris, tinea corporis, tinea pedis, tinea versicolor.

Apply sufficient cream to cover the affected areas once daily.

Cutaneous candidiasis.

Apply b.i.d. in the morning and evening. If no improvement is noted after recommended treatment period, diagnosis should be reevaluated.

Contraindications: Hypersensitivity. Ophthalmic use.

Special Concerns: Use with caution in pregnancy and lactation.
Side Effects: *Topical:* Burning, erythema, itching, stinging.

NURSING CONSIDERATIONS

See also *General Nursing Considerations for All Anti-Infectives,* Chapter 1.
Client/Family Teaching
1. Review goals of therapy and the appropriate method for application.
2. The skin should be cleansed with soap and water and dried thoroughly. Cream should be applied as directed after cleaning the affected area.
3. For athlete's foot, the shoes and socks should be changed at least once daily. Shoes should be well-fitted and ventilated.
4. To reduce chance of reinfection, tinea pedis should be treated for 1 month and tinea cruris, tinea corporis, and candidal infections should be treated for 2 weeks.
5. The drug should be used for the full prescribed time even though symptoms may have improved.
6. Report if the condition worsens or symptoms of burning, itching, redness, and stinging occur.
Evaluate
- Resolution of fungal infection
- Reports of symptomatic improvement

Fluconazole

(flew-**KON**-ah-zohl)
Pregnancy Category: C
Diflucan **(Rx)**

How Supplied: *Injection:* 2 mg/mL, 200 mg/100 mL, 400 mg/200 mL; *Powder for Reconstitution:* 10 mg/mL, 40 mg/mL; *Tablet:* 50 mg, 100 mg, 150 mg, 200 mg
Action/Kinetics: Fluconazole inhibits the enzyme cytochrome P-450, which is essential to survival of fungal cells. Inhibition of the enzyme results in a decrease in cell wall integrity and extrusion of intracellular material. Fluconazole apparently does not affect the cytochrome P-450 enzyme in animals or humans. **Peak plasma levels:** 1–2 hr. **t½:** 30 hr, which allows for once daily dosing. The drug penetrates all body fluids at steady state. Bioavailability is not affected by agents that increase gastric pH. Eighty percent of the drug is excreted unchanged by the kidneys.
Uses: Oropharyngeal and esophageal candidiasis. Serious systemic candidal infection (including UTIs, peritonitis, and pneumonia). Cryptococcal meningitis. Maintenance therapy to prevent cryptococcal meningitis in AIDS clients. Vaginal candidiasis. To decrease the incidence of candidiasis in clients undergoing a bone marrow transplant who receive cytotoxic chemotherapy or radiation therapy.

Dosage

- **Tablets, Oral Suspension, IV**

Vaginal candidiasis.
150 mg as a single oral dose.

Oropharyngeal or esophageal candidiasis.
Adults, First day: 200 mg; **then,** 100 mg/day for a minimum of 14 days (for oropharyngeal candidiasis) or 21 days (for esophageal candidiasis). Up to 400 mg/day may be required for esophageal candidiasis.

Candidal UTI and peritonitis.
50–200 mg/day.

Systemic candidiasis (e.g., candidemia, disseminated candidiasis, and pneumonia)
Optimal dosage and duration have not been determined although doses up to 400 mg/day have been used.

Acute cryptococcal meningitis.
Adults, First day: 400 mg; **then,** 200 mg/day (up to 400 mg may be required) for 10–12 weeks after CSF culture is negative.

Maintenance to prevent relapse of cryptococcal meningitis.
Adults: 200 mg once daily. **Pediatric:** 3–6 mg/kg/day.

Prevention of candidiasis in bone marrow transplant.
400 mg once daily. In clients expected to have severe granulocytopenia

(less than 500 neutrophils/mm^3), fluconazole should be started several days before the anticipated onset of neutropenia and continued for 7 days after the neutrophil count rises about 1,000 cells/mm^3. In clients with renal impairment, an initial loading dose of 50–400 mg can be given; daily dose is based then on creatinine clearance.

Administration/Storage

1. The daily dose is the same for oral and IV administration.
2. Usually, a loading dose of twice the daily dose is recommended for the first day of therapy in order to obtain plasma levels close to the steady state by the second day of therapy.
3. The IV solution should not be used if it is cloudy or precipitated or the seal is not intact.
4. The rate of IV infusion of fluconazole should not exceed 200 mg/hr as a continuous infusion.
5. Supplementary medication should not be added to the IV bag.
6. Due to a long half-life, once daily dosing (either IV or PO) is possible.
7. To prevent relapse, maintenance therapy is usually required in clients with AIDS, cryptococcal meningitis, or recurrent oropharyngeal candidiasis.

Contraindication: Hypersensitivity to fluconazole.

Special Concerns: Use with caution if client shows hypersensitivity to other azoles. Care should be used when fluconazole is prescribed during lactation. The effectiveness of the drug has not been adequately assessed in children.

Laboratory Test Interferences: ↑ AST, serum transaminase (especially if used with isoniazid, oral hypoglycemic agents, phenytoin, rifampin, valproic acid).

Side Effects: Following single doses. *GI:* Nausea, abdominal pain, diarrhea, dyspepsia, taste perversion. *CNS:* Headache, dizziness. *Other:* Angioedema, ***anaphylaxis (rare).***

Following multiple doses. Side effects are more frequently reported in HIV-infected clients than in non-HIV-infected clients. *GI:* N&V, abdominal pain, diarrhea, ***serious hepatic reactions***. *CNS:* Headache, ***seizures.*** *Dermatologic:* Skin rash, exfoliative skin disorders (including ***Stevens-Johnson syndrome,*** and toxic epidermal necrolysis), alopecia. *Hematologic:* Leukopenia, thrombocytopenia. *Other:* Hypercholesterolemia, hypertriglyceridemia, hypokalemia.

Drug Interactions

Cimetidine / ↓ Plasma levels of fluconazole

Cyclosporine / Fluconazole may ↑ cyclosporine levels in renal transplant clients with or without impaired renal function

Hydrochlorothiazide / ↑ Plasma levels of fluconazole due to ↓ renal clearance

Glipizide / ↑ Plasma levels of glipizide due to ↓ breakdown by the liver

Glyburide / ↑ Plasma levels of glyburide due to ↓ breakdown by the liver

Phenytoin / Fluconazole ↑ plasma levels of phenytoin

Rifampin / ↓ Plasma levels of fluconazole due to ↑ breakdown by the liver

Theophylline / ↑ Plasma levels of theophylline

Tolbutamide / ↑ Plasma levels of tolbutamide due to ↓ breakdown by the liver

Warfarin / ↑ PT

Zidovudine / ↑ Plasma levels of AZT

NURSING CONSIDERATIONS

See also *General Nursing Considerations for All Anti-Infectives,* Chapter 1.

Assessment

1. Take a thorough nursing and drug history. Note any history of hypersensitivity to azoles or similar class of drugs.
2. Determine if client is HIV infected (if possible) because this may place client at an increased risk for possible side effects.
3. Obtain baseline liver and renal function studies. Clients who develop abnormal liver function tests should

be closely monitored for the development of more serious liver toxicity.
4. Determine that baseline cultures have been obtained prior to initiating therapy.

Client/Family Teaching
1. Review goals of therapy and appropriate method and schedule for medication administration.
2. Stress the importance of reporting any rash or persistent side effects (especially in immunocompromised clients), as drug may need to be discontinued.
3. Report for all scheduled lab studies to carefully assess drug response.

Evaluate
- Elimination of pathogenic fungi
- Candida prophylaxis in transplant recipients
- Reports of symptomatic improvement

Flucytosine

(flew-**SYE**-toe-seen)
Pregnancy Category: C
Ancobon, Ancotil ✱ **(Rx)**

How Supplied: *Capsule:* 250 mg, 500 mg

Action/Kinetics: Flucytosine is indicated only for serious systemic fungal infections. The drug is less toxic than amphotericin B. Liver, renal system, and hematopoietic system must be monitored closely.

Flucytosine appears to penetrate the fungal cell membrane and then, after metabolism, to act as an antimetabolite interfering with nucleic acid and protein synthesis. It is well absorbed from the GI tract and is distributed to the joints, aqueous humor, peritoneal and other body fluids and tissues. **Peak plasma concentration:** 2–6 hr. **Therapeutic serum concentration:** 20–25 mcg/mL. **t½:** 2–5 hr, higher in presence of impaired renal function. Eighty percent to 90% of the drug is excreted unchanged in urine.

Uses: Serious systemic infections by susceptible strains of *Candida* (e.g., endocarditis, septicemia, UTIs) or *Cryptococcus* (pulmonary or UTIs, meningitis, septicemia).

Dosage
- **Capsules**

Adult and children: 50–150 mg/kg/day in four divided doses. Clients with renal impairment receive lower dosages.

Administration/Storage
1. Reduce or avoid nausea by administering capsules a few at a time over a 15-min period.
2. *Treatment of Overdose:* Prompt induction of vomiting or gastric lavage. Adequate fluid intake (by IV if necessary). Monitor blood, liver, and kidney parameters frequently. Hemodialysis will quickly decrease serum levels.

Contraindications: Hypersensitivity to drug. Lactation.

Special Concerns: Safety and effectiveness have not been determined in children. Use with extreme caution in clients with kidney disease or history of bone marrow depression. The bone marrow depressant effects may cause an increased incidence of microbial infection, gingival bleeding, and delayed healing.

Side Effects: *GI:* N&V, diarrhea, abdominal pain, dry mouth, anorexia, duodenal ulcer, GI hemorrhage, ulcerative colitis. *Hematologic:* Anemia, leukopenia, thrombocytopenia, ***aplastic anemia, agranulocytosis,*** pancytopenia, eosinophilia. *CNS:* Headache, vertigo, confusion, sedation, hallucinations, paresthesia, parkinsonism, psychosis, pyrexia. *Hepatic:* Hepatic dysfunction, jaundice, elevation of hepatic enzymes, increase in bilirubin. *GU:* Increase in BUN and creatinine, azotemia, crystalluria, renal failure. *Respiratory:* Chest pain, dyspnea, ***respiratory arrest.*** *Dermatologic:* Pruritus, rash, urticaria, photosensitivity. *Other:* Ataxia, hearing loss, peripheral neuropathy, weakness, hypoglycemia, fatigue, ***cardiac arrest,*** hypokalemia.

Symptoms of Overdose (serum levels greater than 100 mcg/mL): N&V, diarrhea, leukopenia, thrombocytopenia, hepatitis.

Drug Interactions

Amphotericin B / ↑ Effect and toxicity of flucytosine due to kidney impairment

Cytosine / Inactivates antifungal effect of flucytosine

NURSING CONSIDERATIONS

See also *General Nursing Considerations for All Anti-Infectives,* Chapter 1.

Assessment

1. Obtain baseline CBC and liver and renal function studies and monitor throughout therapy.
2. Before administering first dose, check that cultures have been taken.
3. Anticipate reduced dose with impaired renal function.

Client/Family Teaching

1. Report as scheduled so that weekly cultures are taken to determine that strains have not become resistant. A strain is considered resistant if the MIC value is greater than 100.
2. Report any reduction in urine output as well as any blood, sediment, or cloudiness in the urine.
3. Stress that any side effects that interfere with dosing should be reported.

Evaluate: Resolution of fungal infection.

Griseofulvin microsize

(griz-ee-oh-**FULL**-vin)
Pregnancy Category: C
Fulvicin-U/F, Grifulvin V, Grisactin, Grisactin 250, Grisactin 500, Grisovin-FP ✱ **(Rx)**

Griseofulvin ultramicrosize

(griz-ee-oh-**FULL**-vin)
Pregnancy Category: C
Fulvicin-P/G, Grisactin Ultra, Gris-PEG **(Rx)**

See also *Anti-Infectives,* Chapter 1.

How Supplied: Griseofulvin microsize: *Capsule:* 250 mg; *Suspension:* 125 mg/5 mL; *Tablet:* 250 mg, 500 mg.

Griseofulvin ultramicrosize: *125 mg; 165 mg; 250 mg; 330 mg*

Action/Kinetics: Griseofulvin is a natural antibiotic derived from a species of *Penicillium.* It is believed to interfere with cell division (metaphase) or DNA replication. When taken systemically, the drug is deposited in the newly formed skin and nails, which are then resistant to reinfection by the tinea. Griseofulvin is absorbed from the duodenum. **Peak plasma concentration:** 0.37–2 mcg/mL after 4 hr. **t1/2:** 9–24 hr. Levels may be increased by giving the drug with a high-fat diet. The GI absorption of the ultramicrosize products is about 1.5 times that of the microsize products; however, there is no evidence this causes any difference in the safety and effectiveness of the drug compared with the microsize form.

Uses: Tinea (ringworm) infections of skin (including athlete's foot), scalp, groin, and nails. The drug is effective against tinea corporis, tinea pedis, tinea barbae, tinea unguium, tinea cruris, tinea capitis due to *Trichophyton* species, *Microsporum audouinii, M. canis, M. gypseum,* and *Epidermophyton floccosum.* It is the only PO drug effective against dermatophytid (tinea ringworm) infections. The drug is not effective against *Candida.* Susceptibility of the infectious agent should be established before treatment is begun.

Dosage

- **Capsules, Oral Suspension, Tablets**

Tinea corporis, cruris, or capitis.

Adults: 0.5 g griseofulvin microsize daily in a single dose or divided dose (or 330–375 mg ultramicrosize).

Tinea pedis or unguium.

Adults: 0.75–1 g/day of griseofulvin microsize (or 660–750 mg ultramicrosize). After response, decrease dose of microsize to 0.5 g/day. **Pediatric, 13.6–22.7 kg:** 125–250 mg griseofulvin microsize daily (or 82.5–165 mg ultramicrosize); **pediatric, over 22.7 kg:** 250–500 mg microsize daily (or 165–330 mg ultramicrosize). *NOTE:* Dose has not been determined in children less than 2 years of age.

Administration/Storage

1. Treatment must be of sufficient duration to eradicate the infecting organism. For example, treatment for tinea capitis should be from 4 to 6 weeks; 2–4 weeks for tinea corporis; 4–8 weeks for tinea pedis; and 4–6 months (fingernails) and 6–18 months (toe nails) for tinea unguium.
2. With prolonged therapy, evaluate liver, renal, and hematologic function.

Contraindications: Pregnancy. Porphyria or history thereof, hepatocellular failure, and hypersensitivity to drug. Exposure to artificial light or sunlight. Use for infections due to bacteria, candidiasis, actinomycosis, sporotrichosis, tinea versicolor, histoplasmosis, chromoblastomycosis, coccidioidomycosis, cryptococcosis, and North American blastomycosis.

Special Concerns: Cross sensitivity with penicillin is possible.

Laboratory Test Interferences: ↑ ALT, AST, alkaline phosphatase, BUN, and creatinine level values.

Side Effects: *Hypersensitivity:* Rashes, urticaria, ***angioneurotic edema,*** allergic reactions. *GI:* N&V, diarrhea, epigastric pain, ***GI bleeding.*** *CNS:* Dizziness, headache, confusion, mental fatigue, insomnia. *Miscellaneous:* Oral thrush, acute intermittent porphyria, paresthesias of extremities after long-term therapy, proteinuria, leukopenia, photosensitivity, worsening of lupus erythematosus, menstrual irregularities, hepatic toxicity, granulocytopenia.

Drug Interactions

Alcohol, ethyl / Tachycardia and flushing

Anticoagulants, oral / ↓ Effect of anticoagulants due to ↑ breakdown in liver

Barbiturates / ↓ Effect of griseofulvin due to ↓ absorption from GI tract

Cyclosporine / ↓ Plasma levels of cyclosporine → ↓ pharmacologic effect

Oral contraceptives / ↓ Effect of contraceptives → breakthrough bleeding, pregnancy, or amenorrhea

Salicylates / ↓ Serum salicylate levels

NURSING CONSIDERATIONS

See also *General Nursing Considerations for All Anti-Infectives,* Chapter 1.

Client/Family Teaching

1. Eat a high-fat diet because fat enhances the absorption of griseofulvin from the intestines. Refer to a dietitian as necessary for assistance with diet and meal planning. Suggest ice cream, bread and butter, fried chicken, etc.
2. Take all medication as prescribed to prevent any recurrence of infection. If the course of therapy is interrupted or not completed, therapy may have to be started over again.
3. Practice appropriate hygiene to prevent reinfection.
4. Avoid exposure to intense natural and artificial light because photosensitivity reactions may occur. Wear protective clothing, sunglasses, and a sunscreen if exposure is necessary.
5. Report any fever, sore throat, and malaise, (all symptoms of leukopenia).
6. Advise client to practice a nonhormonal form of birth control.
7. Advise client that to be considered cured, repeated cultures and scrapings of affected sites must be negative.
8. Persistent N&V and diarrhea and any mental confusion should be immediately reported.

Evaluate

- Improvement in pretreatment symptoms
- Negative culture and scraping results

Itraconazole

(**ih**-trah-**KON**-ah-zohl)

Pregnancy Category: C

Sporanox **(Rx)**

How Supplied: *Capsule:* 100 mg

Action/Kinetics: The drug is believed to inhibit cytochrome P-450-dependent synthesis of ergosterol, which is a necessary component of fungal cell membranes. The drug concentrates in fatty tissues, omentum, liver, kidney, and skin. **t½, at steady-state:** 64 hr. Extensively metabolized by the liver; the major metabolite is hydroxyitraconazole, which also has antifungal activity. Metabolites are excreted in both the urine and feces.

Uses: Treatment of blastomycosis (pulmonary and extrapulmonary) and histoplasmosis (including chronic cavitary pulmonary disease and disseminated, nonmeningeal histoplasmosis) in both immunocompromised and nonimmunocompromised clients. To treat aspergillus infections in clients intolerant or refractory to amphotericin B. The drug is effective against *Blastomyces dermatitidis, Histoplasma capsulatum* and *H. duboisii, Aspergillus flavus* and *A. fumigatis,* and *Cryptococcus neoformans.* In vitro activity has also been found for a number of other organisms. *Investigational:* (1) Superficial mycoses including dermatophytoses (tinea capitis, tinea corporis, tinea cruris, tinea pedis, and tinea manuum), pityriasis versicolor, candidiasis (vaginal, oral, chronic mucocutaneous), onychomycosis, and sebopsoriasis. (2) Systemic mycoses including dimorphic infections (paracoccidioidomycosis, coccidioidomycosis), cryptococcal infections (meningitis, disseminated), and candidiasis. (3) Miscellaneous mycoses including fungal keratitis, alternariosis, leishmaniasis (cutaneous), subcutaneous mycoses (chromomycosis, sporotrichosis), and zygomycosis.

Dosage

- **Capsules**

Blastomycosis or histoplasmosis.

Adults: 200 mg once daily. If there is no improvement or the disease is progressive, the dose may be increased in 100-mg increments to a maximum of 400 mg/day. **Children, 3–16 years of age:** 100 mg/day (for systemic fungal infections).

Aspergilliosis.

200–400 mg daily.

Life-threatening infections.

Adults: A loading dose of 200 mg t.i.d. for the first 3 days should be given.

Unlabeled Uses.

Adults: 50–400 mg/day for 1 day to more than 6 months, depending on the condition and the response.

Administration/Storage

1. The drug should be taken with food to ensure maximal absorption.
2. Daily doses greater than 200 mg should be given in two divided doses.
3. Treatment should be continued for a minimum of 3 months and until symptoms and lab tests indicate the active fungal infection has subsided. Recurrence of active infection may occur if there is an inadequate period of treatment.
4. *Treatment of Overdose:* Use supportive measures, including gastric lavage and sodium bicarbonate. Dialysis will not remove itraconazole.

Contraindications: Concomitant use of astemizole or terfenadine. Hypersensitivity to the drug or its excipients. Lactation.

Special Concerns: Safety and efficacy have not been determined in children although pediatric clients have been treated for systemic fungal infections.

Side Effects: *GI:* N&V, diarrhea, abdominal pain, anorexia, flatulence. *CNS:* Headache, dizziness, insomnia, decreased libido, somnolence, depression. *Dermatologic:* Rash (occurs more frequently in immunocompromised clients also taking immunosuppressant drugs), pruritus. *Miscellaneous:* Edema, fatigue, fever, malaise, hypertension, abnormal hepatic function, hypokalemia, albuminuria, tinnitus, impotence, adrenal insufficiency, gynecomastia, breast pain in males.

Symptoms of Overdose: Extension of side effects.

Drug Interactions

Astemizole / ↑ Astemizole levels → serious CV toxicity including ven-

tricular tachycardia, torsades de pointes, and death.
Cyclosporine / ↑ Cyclosporine levels (dose of cyclosporine should be ↓ by 50% if itraconazole doses are much greater than 100 mg/day)
Digoxin / ↑ Digoxin levels
H_2 Antagonists / ↓ Plasma levels of itraconazole
Isoniazid / ↓ Plasma levels of itraconazole
Phenytoin / ↓ Plasma levels of itraconazole; also, metabolism of phenytoin may be altered
Rifampin / ↓ Plasma levels of itraconazole
Sulfonylureas / ↑ Risk of hypoglycemia
Terfenadine / ↑ Terfenadine levels → serious CV toxicity including ventricular tachycardia, torsades de pointes, and death
Warfarin / ↑ Anticoagulant effect of warfarin

NURSING CONSIDERATIONS

Assessment

1. List drugs currently prescribed to prevent any unfavorable interactions.
2. Obtain baseline CBC, electrolytes, fungal cultures, and liver and renal function studies.
3. Drug is not intended for pregnant or nursing mothers.

Interventions

1. Monitor hepatic enzyme test values in clients with preexisting abnormal liver function.
2. The response rate of histoplasmosis in HIV-infected clients is similar to non-HIV-infected clients, although the clinical course of histoplasmosis in HIV-infected clients is more severe and usually requires maintenance therapy to prevent relapse.
3. Absorption may be decreased in HIV-infected clients with hypochlorhydria.

Client/Family Teaching

1. Take with food to enhance absorption.
2. Take only as directed; usually for 3 months. Noncompliance or inadequate periods of treatment may lead to a recurrence of active infection.
3. Report any S&S that may suggest liver dysfunction. These may include anorexia, unusual fatigue, N&V, diarrhea, jaundice, dark urine, and pale stool.
4. Symptoms that may indicate reactivation of histoplasmosis, such as weight loss, chest pain, SOB, fever, rales, pain, etc., should be reported immediately.
5. Advise that S&S of blastomycosis include SOB, rales, hemoptysis, chest pain, fever, cough, skin lesions, rashes, and weight loss and require immediate attention.

Evaluate: Eradication of infecting organisms and reports of symptomatic relief.

Ketoconazole

(kee-toe-**KON**-ah-zohl)
Pregnancy Category: C
Nizoral (Rx; 1% shampoo is OTC)

How Supplied: *Cream:* 2%; *Shampoo:* 2%; *Tablet:* 200 mg

Action/Kinetics: Ketoconazole inhibits synthesis of sterols (e.g., ergosterol), damaging the cell membrane and resulting in loss of essential intracellular material. It also inhibits biosynthesis of triglycerides and phospholipids and inhibits oxidative and peroxidative enzyme activity. When used to treat *Candida albicans,* it inhibits transformation of blastospores into the invasive mycelial form. Use in Cushing's syndrome is due to its ability to inhibit adrenal steroidogenesis. **Peak plasma levels:** 3.5 mcg/mL after 1–2 hr after a 200-mg dose. **t½** [biphasic]: first, 2 hr; second, 8 hr. Requires acidity for dissolution. Metabolized in liver to inactive metabolites and most excreted through feces.

Uses: PO. Candidiasis, chronic mucocutaneous candidiasis, candiduria, histoplasmosis, chromomycosis, oral thrush, blastomycosis, coccidioidomycosis, paracoccidioidomycosis. Recalcitrant cutaneous dermatophyte infections not responding to other therapy. **Cream.** Tinea pedis. Tinea corporis and tinea cruris due to *Trichophyton rubrum, T. mentagrophytes,* and *Epidermophyton floccosum.* Tinea versicolor caused by *Microsporum furfur;* cutaneous candidiasis caused by *Candida* species; seborrheic dermatitis. **Shampoo.** To reduce scaling due to dandruff. *Investigational:* Onychomycosis due to *Candida* and *Trichophyton.* High doses to treat CNS fungal infections. Advanced prostate cancer, Cushing's syndrome.

Dosage

- **Tablets**

Fungal infections.

Adults: 200–400 mg once daily. **Pediatric, over 2 years:** 3.3–6.6 mg/kg once daily.

CNS fungal infections.

Adults: 800–1,200 mg/day.

Advanced prostate cancer.

400 mg q 8 hr.

Cushing's syndrome.

800–1,200 mg/day.

- **Topical cream (2%)**

Tinea corporis, tinea cruris, tinea versicolor, tinea pedis, cutaneous candidiasis.

Cover the affected and immediate surrounding areas once daily (twice daily for more resistant cases). Duration of treatment is usually 2 weeks.

Seborrheic dermatitis.

Apply to affected area b.i.d. for 4 weeks or until symptoms clear.

- **Shampoo (1%, 2%)**

Use twice a week for 4 weeks with at least 3 days between each shampooing. **Then,** use as required to maintain control.

Administration/Storage

1. Ketoconazole should be given a minimum of 2 hr before administration of drugs that increase gastric pH (such as antacids, anticholinergics, or H_2 blockers). If antacids are needed, delay administration by 2 hr.
2. To decrease GI upset, take tablets with food.
3. The shampoo should be applied in sufficient quantities to cover the entire scalp for 1 min. Rinse with warm water and repeat, leaving the shampoo on the scalp for 3 min. After the second washing, rinse thoroughly and dry hair with towel or warm air flow.
4. The minimum treatment for candidiasis (using tablets) is 1–2 weeks and for other systemic mycoses is 6 months.

Contraindications: Hypersensitivity, fungal meningitis. Topical product not for ophthalmic use. Use during lactation.

Special Concerns: Use tablets with caution in children less than 2 years of age. The safety and effectiveness of the shampoo and cream have not been determined in children. Use with caution during lactation.

Laboratory Test Interferences: Transient ↑ serum liver enzymes. ↓ Serum testosterone.

Side Effects: *GI:* N&V, abdominal pain, diarrhea. *CNS:* Headache, dizziness, somnolence, fever, chills. *Hematologic:* Thrombocytopenia, leukopenia, ***hemolytic anemia.*** *Miscellaneous:* Hepatotoxicity, photophobia, pruritus, gynecomastia, impotence, bulging fontanelles, urticaria, decreased serum testosterone levels, anaphylaxis (rare). *Topical cream:* Stinging, irritation, pruritus. *Shampoo:* Increased hair loss, irritation, abnormal hair texture, itching, oiliness or dryness of the scalp and hair, scalp pustules.

Drug Interactions

Antacids / ↓ Absorption of ketoconazole due to ↑ pH induced by these drugs

Anticoagulants / ↓ Effect of anticoagulants

Anticholinergics / ↓ Absorption of ketoconazole due to ↑ pH induced by these drugs

Astemizole / ↑ Plasma levels of astemizole → serious CV effects

Corticosteroids / ↑ Risk of corticosteroid toxicity due to ↑ bioavailability

Cyclosporine / ↑ Levels of cyclosporine (may be used therapeutically to decrease the dose of cyclosporine)

Histamine H_2 antagonists / ↓ Ab-

sorption of ketoconazole due to ↑ pH induced by these drugs
Isoniazid / ↓ Bioavailability of ketoconazole
Rifampin / ↓ Serum levels of both drugs
Terfenadine / ↑ Plasma levels of terfenadine → serious CV effects
Theophyllines / ↓ Serum levels of theophylline

NURSING CONSIDERATIONS

See also *General Nursing Considerations for All Anti-Infectives,* Chapter 1.

Client/Family Teaching

1. Review the appropriate method for drug administration.
2. Report persistent fever, pain, or diarrhea.
3. If clients have achlorhydria, instruct them to dissolve each tablet in 4 mL aqueous solution of 0.2 N HCl and to use a straw (glass or plastic) to take this solution to avoid contact with their teeth. This is followed by drinking a glass of tap water.
4. Use caution when driving or when performing hazardous tasks because drug can cause headaches, dizziness, and drowsiness.
5. Avoid alcohol or alcohol-containing products.
6. Wear sunglasses, sunscreen, and protective clothing and avoid sun exposure to prevent a photosensitivity reaction.
7. During long-term therapy, report for periodic liver function evaluation.

Evaluate

- Eradication of fungal infections
- Reports of symptomatic improvement

Miconazole

(my-**KON**-ah-zohl)
Pregnancy Category: C
Systemic: Monistat I.V. **Topical:** Micatin, Monistat-Derm. **Vaginal:** Monistat ✦, Monistat 3, Monistat 5 ✦, Monistat 7 (Rx and OTC)

See also *Anti-Infectives,* Chapter 1.
How Supplied: *Injection:* 10 mg/mL

Action/Kinetics: Miconazole may be fungistatic or fungicidal, depending on the concentration. It is a broad-spectrum fungicide that alters the permeability of the fungal membrane by inhibiting synthesis of sterols; thus, essential intracellular materials are lost. The drug also inhibits biosynthesis of triglycerides and phospholipids and also inhibits oxidative and peroxidative enzyme activity. **Peak blood levels:** 1 mcg/mL. The drug is eliminated in three phases; **t½ of each phase:** 0.4, 2.1, and 24 hr. More than 90% of miconazole is bound to serum proteins. Excretion of the drug is unaltered in clients with renal insufficiency, including those on hemodialysis.

Uses: Systemic. Fungal infections caused by coccidioidomycosis, candidiasis, cryptococcosis, paracoccidioidomycosis, chronic mucocutaneous candidiasis, pseudoallescheriosis. When used for the treatment of either fungal meningitis or urinary bladder infection, IV infusion must be supplemented with intrathecal administration or bladder irrigation of the drug. **Topical, Vaginal:** Tinea pedis, tinea cruris, tinea corporis caused by *Trichophyton rubrum, T. mentagrophytes,* and *Epidermophyton floccosum* (both OTC and Rx). Moniliasis and tinea versicolor (Rx only).

Dosage

- **IV infusion**

Candidiasis.

Adults: 600–1,800 mg/day for 1 to more than 20 weeks.

Coccidioidomycosis.

Adults: 1,800–3,600 mg for 3 to more than 20 weeks.

Cryptococcosis.

Adults: 1,200–2,400 mg/day for 3 to more than 12 weeks.

Paracoccidioidomycosis.

Adults: 200–1,200 mg/day for 2 to more than 16 weeks.

Pseudoallescheriosis.

Adults: 600–3,000 mg/day for 5 to more than 20 weeks. **Pediatric, less than 1 year of age:** 15–30 mg/

kg/day; **1–12 years of age:** 20–40 mg/kg/day, not to exceed 15 mg/kg/dose.

• **Intrathecal**

20 mg/dose of the undiluted solution as an adjunct to **IV** therapy.

• **Bladder instillation**

200 mg of diluted solution as adjunct in treatment of fungal infections of urinary bladder.

• **Topical, Aerosol Powder, Aerosol Solution, Cream, Lotion, Powder**

Apply to cover affected areas in morning and evening (once daily for tinea versicolor) for 7 days.

• **Vaginal**

Monistat 3.

One suppository daily at bedtime for 7 days (100-mg suppositories) or 3 consecutive days (200-mg suppositories).

Monistat 7.

One applicator full of cream or one suppository at bedtime daily for 7 days. Course may be repeated after presence of other pathogens has been ruled out.

Administration/Storage

1. For IV infusion, the drug should be diluted in at least 200 mL of either 0.9% sodium chloride or 5% dextrose solution and administered over a period of 30–60 min. Discard if solution darkens.
2. The IV dose may be divided over three infusions daily.
3. The lotion is preferred for intertriginous areas.
4. To reduce recurrence of symptoms, tinea cruris, tinea corporis, and candida should be treated for 2 weeks; tinea pedis should be treated for 1 month.
5. For intrathecal use, the drug is given as the undiluted solution (20 mg/dose) as an adjunct to IV treatment for fungal meningitis. Doses are alternated between lumbar, cervical, and cisternal punctures every 3–7 days; document sites.
6. The vaginal products should be refrigerated below 15°C–30°C (59°F–86°F).

Contraindications: Hypersensitivity. Use of topical products in or around the eyes.

Special Concerns: Safe use in children less than 1 year of age has not been established.

Side Effects: Following systemic use. *GI:* N&V, diarrhea, anorexia. *Hematologic:* Thrombocytopenia, aggregation of erythrocytes, rouleaux formation on blood smears. Transient decrease in hematocrit. *Dermatologic:* Pruritus, rash, flushing, phlebitis at injection site. *CV:* Transient tachycardia or arrhythmias following rapid injection of undiluted drug. *Miscellaneous:* Fever, chills, drowsiness, transient decrease in serum sodium values. Hyperlipemia due to the vehicle (polyethylene glycol 40 and castor oil). **Following topical use:** Vulvovaginal burning, pelvic cramps, hives, skin rash, headache, itching, irritation, maceration, and allergic contact dermatitis.

Drug Interactions

Amphotericin B / ↓ Activity of miconazole of each drug

Coumarin anticoagulants / Miconazole ↑ anticoagulant effect

NURSING CONSIDERATIONS

See also *General Nursing Considerations for All Anti-Infectives,* Chapter 1.

Assessment

1. Determine any previous client experience with this drug and document any evidence of sensitivity and response obtained.
2. Obtain baseline CBC, electrolytes, and liver function studies and monitor throughout therapy.
3. Obtain appropriate pretreatment lab studies and cultures, as IV therapy may be required for periods ranging from 1 to more than 20 weeks, depending on the organism.

Client/Family Teaching

1. Demonstrate appropriate technique for medication administration and instruct client to take/use medication only as directed.
2. Use sanitary pads to protect clothing and linens when using cream or suppositories.
3. When used for vaginal infections,

refrain from intercourse or have sexual partner use a condom to prevent reinfection.
4. When used vaginally, miconazole treatment should be continued during menses.
5. Persistent N&V, diarrhea, dizziness, and pruritus should be reported.
6. If exposed to HIV and recurrent vaginal yeast infections occur, the client should seek prompt medical intervention to determine the cause of the symptoms.

Evaluate

- Negative lab culture results
- Reports of resolution of vaginitis evidenced by ↓ in itching and burning and ↓ discharge

Naftifine hydrochloride

(**NAF**-tih-feen)
Pregnancy Category: B
Naftin **(Rx)**

See also *Anti-Infectives,* Chapter 1.
How Supplied: *Cream:* 1%; *Gel/jelly:* 1%
Action/Kinetics: Naftifine is a synthetic antifungal agent with a broad spectrum of activity. The drug is thought to inhibit squalene 2,3-epoxidase, which is responsible for synthesis of sterols. The decreased levels of sterols (especially ergosterol) and the accumulation of squalene in cells result in fungicidal activity. Although used topically, approximately 6% of the drug is absorbed. Naftifine and its metabolites are excreted via the feces and urine. **t½:** 2–3 days.
Uses: To treat tinea cruris, tinea pedis, and tinea corporis caused by *Candida albicans, Epidermophyton floccosum, Microsporum canis, M. audouinii, M. gypseum, Trichophyton rubrum, T. mentagrophytes,* and *T. tonsurans.*

Dosage

- **Topical Cream (1%), Topical Gel (1%)**

Massage into affected area and surrounding skin once daily if using the cream and twice daily (morning and evening) if using the gel.
Contraindication: Ophthalmic use.
Special Concerns: Consideration should be given to discontinuing nursing while using naftifine and for several days after the last application. Safety and efficacy in children have not been determined.
Side Effects: *Topical cream:* Burning, stinging, dryness, itching, local irritation, erythema. *Topical gel:* Burning, stinging, itching, rash, tenderness, erythema.

NURSING CONSIDERATIONS

Client/Family Teaching

1. Demonstrate the appropriate technique for topical application.
2. Wash hands before and after applying medication.
3. Use care to avoid contact with the eyes, nose, mouth, or other mucous membranes.
4. Occlusive dressings, diapers, or wrappings should not be used. Area should not be covered unless specifically ordered.
5. Beneficial effects are usually observed within 1 week; treatment should be continued as prescribed for 1–2 weeks after symptoms have decreased.
6. Medication is for external use only.
7. Report any excessive itching or burning.
8. Advise that the client should be reevaluated if beneficial effects are not evident after 4 weeks of treatment.

Evaluate

- Negative lab culture results for pathogenic fungi
- Reports of symptomatic improvement

Natamycin

(nah-tah-**MY**-sin)
Natacyn **(Rx)**

See also *Anti-Infectives,* Chapter 1.

How Supplied: *Suspension:* 5%
Action/Kinetics: Natamycin is an antifungal antibiotic derived from *Streptomyces natalensis*. The drug, which is fungicidal, binds to the fungal cell membrane, resulting in alteration of permeability and loss of essential intracellular materials. After topical administration, the drug reaches therapeutic levels in the corneal stroma but not in the intraocular fluid. It is not absorbed systemically.
Uses: For ophthalmic use only. Drug of choice for *Fusarium solanae* keratitis. For treatment of fungal blepharitis, conjunctivitis, and keratitis caused by susceptible organisms. It is active against a variety of yeasts and filamentous fungi including *Candida, Aspergillus, Cephalosporium, Fusarium,* and *Penicillium*. Before initiating therapy, determine the susceptibility of the infectious organism to drug in smears and cultures of corneal scrapings. Effectiveness of natamycin for use as single agent in fungal endophthalmitis not established.

Dosage

• **Ophthalmic Suspension (5%)**
Fungal keratitis.
Initially, 1 gtt in conjunctival sac q 1–2 hr; can be reduced usually, after 3–4 days to 1 gtt 6–8 times/day. Continue therapy for 14–21 days, during which dosage can be reduced gradually at 4–7-day intervals.
Fungal blepharitis/conjunctivitis.
1 gtt 4–6 times/day.

Administration/Storage
1. Store natamycin at room temperature or in refrigerator avoiding exposure to light and excessive heat.
2. Shake well before using.
3. Avoid contamination of dropper.
4. Discontinue drug if toxicity is suspected.
5. Review therapy if no improvement noted after 7–10 days.

Contraindication: Hypersensitivity to drug.
Special Concerns: Safe use during pregnancy not established. Effectiveness as a single agent to treat fungal endophthalmitis has not been established.
Side Effects: Eye irritation, occasional allergies.

NURSING CONSIDERATIONS

See also *General Nursing Considerations for All Anti-Infectives,* Chapter 1.
Client/Family Teaching
1. Stress the importance of close medical supervision (initially report twice weekly) to regulate dosage.
2. Demonstrate proper administration technique and observe self-administration.
3. Continue therapy for 14–21 days as ordered, even though condition may appear to be under control.

Evaluate
• Laboratory evidence of negative lab culture reports
• Ophthalmic and symptomatic improvement

Nystatin
(nye-**STAT**-in)
Pregnancy Category: C (A for vaginal use)
Tablets: Mycostatin, Nilstat. **Oral Suspension:** Mycostatin, Nadostine ✱, Nilstat, Nystex, PMS Nystatin ✱. **Troches:** Mycostatin Pastilles. **Vaginal Tablets:** Mycostatin, Nadostine ✱, **Topical:** Mycostatin, Nadostine ✱, Nilstat, Nyaderm ✱, Nystex **(Rx)**

See also *Anti-Infectives,* Chapter 1.
How Supplied: *Capsule:* 500,000 U, 1 million U; *Cream:* 100,000 U/gm; *Lozenge/troche:* 200,000 U; *Ointment:* 100,000 U/gm; *Powder:* 100,000 U/gm; *Suspension:* 100,000 U/mL; *Tablet:* 100,000 U, 500,000 U
Action/Kinetics: This natural antifungal antibiotic is derived from *Streptomyces noursei* and is both fungistatic and fungicidal against all species of *Candida*. Nystatin binds to fungal cell membranes (sterols), resulting in altered cellular permeability and leakage of potassium and other essential intracellular components. Nystatin is poorly absorbed from the GI tract; unabsorbed nystatin is excreted in the feces.
Uses: *Candida* infections of the skin, mucous membranes, GI tract, vagina, and mouth (thrush). The drug is too toxic for systemic infec-

tions although it can be given PO for intestinal moniliasis infections as it is not absorbed from the GI tract.

Dosage

• **Lozenge, Oral Suspension, Tablets**

Intestinal candidiasis.

Tablets, 500,000–1,000,000 units t.i.d.; continue treatment for 48 hr after cure to prevent relapse.

Oral candidiasis.

Oral Suspension, adults and children: 400,000–600,000 units q.i.d. (½ dose in each side of mouth, held as long as possible before swallowing); **infants:** 200,000 units q.i.d. (same procedure as with adults); **premature or low birth weight infants:** 100,000 units q.i.d. **Lozenge, adults and children:** 200,000–400,000 units 4–5 times/day, up to 14 days. *NOTE:* Lozenges should not be chewed or swallowed.

• **Vaginal Tablets**

100,000 units (1 tablet) inserted in vagina once each day for 2 weeks.

• **Topical Cream, Ointment, Powder (100,000 units/g each)**

Apply to affected areas b.i.d.–t.i.d., or as indicated, until healing is complete.

Administration/Storage

1. A powder for extemporaneous compounding of the oral suspension is available. To reconstitute, add ⅛ tsp of the powder (about 500,000 units) to approximately ½–1 cup water and stir well. This product is administered immediately after mixing.
2. Protect drug from heat, light, moisture, and air.
3. The suspension can be stored for 7 days at room temperature or for 10 days in the refrigerator without loss of potency.
4. For *Candida* infections of the feet, the powder can be freely dusted on the feet as well as in socks and shoes.
5. The cream is generally used in *Candida* infections involving intertriginous areas; however, moist lesions should be treated with powder.
6. Vaginal tablets should be refrigerated.

Contraindication: Use for systemic mycoses. Use of topical products in or around the eyes.

Special Concerns: Occlusive dressings should not be used when treating candidiasis. Lozenges should not be used in children less than 5 years of age.

Side Effects: Nystatin has few toxic effects. *GI:* Epigastric distress, N&V, diarrhea. *Other:* Rarely, irritation.

NURSING CONSIDERATIONS

See also *General Nursing Considerations for All Anti-Infectives,* Chapter 1.

Interventions

1. Anticipate that vaginal tablets may be continued in the gravid client for 3–6 weeks before term to reduce incidence of thrush in the newborn.
2. Do not mix oral suspension in foods because the medication will be inactivated.
3. Apply cream or ointment to mycotic lesions with a swab or wear gloves to avoid direct contact with hands as contact dermatitis may ensue.
4. Drop 1 mL of oral suspension in each side of mouth or apply with a swab to treat oral moniliasis. Instruct client to swish around and keep medication in the mouth as long as possible before swallowing.
5. Do not use mouthwash in clients with oral candidiasis as this may alter normal flora and promote infections.
6. Vaginal tablets may be administered PO for candidiasis. These should be sucked on as a lozenge and not chewed or swallowed.
7. For pediatric use, 250,000 units of cherry flavor nystatin has been given frozen in the form of popsicles.
8. Insert vaginal tablets high in vagina with an applicator.

Client/Family Teaching

1. Provide written guidelines and review the appropriate method and technique for administration (according to the area being treated).

2. Continue using vaginal tablets even when menstruating because the treatment should be continued for 2 weeks. Avoid tampons.
3. To prevent reinfection, avoid intercourse during therapy or use condoms. Advise partner to seek treatment if symptomatic.
4. Provide a printed list of drug side effects. Advise to report any bothersome or persistent symptoms.
5. Discontinue drug and report if vaginal tablets cause irritation, redness, or swelling.
6. Drug may stain; sanitary pads may help protect clothing and linens.

Evaluate

- Negative culture results
- Improvement in skin and mucous membrane irritation with less associated discomfort

Oxiconazole nitrate

(ox-ee-**KON**-ah-zohl)
Pregnancy Category: B
Oxistat **(Rx)**

See also *Anti-Infectives,* Chapter 1.

How Supplied: *Cream:* 1%; *Lotion:* 1%

Action/Kinetics: Oxiconazole acts by inhibiting ergosterol synthesis, which is required for cytoplasmic membrane integrity of fungi. It is active against a broad range of organisms including many strains of *Trichophyton rubrum* and *T. mentagrophytes.* Systemic absorption of the drug is low.

Uses: Topical treatment of tinea pedis (athlete's foot), tinea cruris (jock itch), and tinea corporis (ringworm) due to *T. rubrum, T. mentagrophytes,* and *Epidermophyton floccosum.*

Dosage

- **Cream (1%), Lotion (1%)**

Apply 1% cream or lotion to cover affected areas once daily in the evening. To prevent recurrence, treatment should continue for 2 weeks for tinea corporis and tinea cruris and for 1 month for tinea pedis.

Contraindications: Ophthalmic or vaginal use.

Special Concerns: Use with caution during lactation.

Side Effects: *Dermatologic:* Pruritus, burning, stinging, irritation, erythema, fissuring, maceration, contact dermatitis, scaling, tingling, pain, dyshidrotic eczema, folliculitis, papules, rash, nodules.

NURSING CONSIDERATIONS

Assessment

1. Assess and describe area of involvement, noting presentation and onset of symptoms.
2. The diagnosis should be reviewed if the client shows no clinical response after the designated treatment period (tinea corporis and tinea cruris require 2 weeks of therapy; tinea pedis requires 1 month of therapy to prevent recurrence).

Client/Family Teaching

1. Demonstrate how to apply the medication and instruct client/family to use only as directed.
2. Report any itching and/or burning associated with therapy because treatment should be discontinued if symptoms suggesting sensitivity or chemical irritation appear.
3. Stress the importance of following prescribed therapy as some infections may require 2 weeks to a month of daily treatments to ensure there is no recurrence.
4. Oxiconazole is intended for external use only and should not be introduced into the eye.

Evaluate

- Resolution of fungal infection
- Reports of symptomatic improvement

Sulconazole nitrate

(sul-**KON**-ah-zohl)
Pregnancy Category: C
Exelderm **(Rx)**

How Supplied: *Cream:* 1%; *Solution:* 1%

Action/Kinetics: This broad-spectrum antifungal and antiyeast agent inhibits growth of *Trichophyton mentagrophytes, Epidermophyton floccosum, Microsporum canis,* and *Malassezia furfur* as well as certain gram-positive bacteria.

Uses: Treatment of tinea cruris (jock itch), tinea corporis (ringworm), and tinea versicolor. Efficacy has not been demonstrated for tinea pedis (athlete's foot).

Dosage

- **Cream, Solution (1% each)**

A small amount of the cream or solution is gently massaged into the affected area and surrounding skin once or twice daily.

Contraindication: Ophthalmic use.
Special Concerns: Use with caution during lactation. Safety and efficacy have not been demonstrated in children.
Side Effects: *Dermatologic:* Burning, itching, stinging, redness.

NURSING CONSIDERATIONS

Client/Family Teaching

1. Demonstrate how to apply medication and advise to use only as directed.
2. Drug is for external use only.
3. Contact with the eyes should be avoided.
4. Relief of symptoms usually occurs within a few days of initiating treatment, with clinical improvement occurring within 1 week. Report if symptoms do not improve after 4–6 weeks as an alternate diagnosis should be considered.
5. To reduce the chance of recurrent tinea cruris, tinea corporis, and tinea versicolor, client should be treated for 3 weeks. Clients with tinea pedis should be treated for 4 weeks.

Evaluate

- ↓ Skin irritation
- Reports of symptomatic improvement

Terbinafine hydrochloride

(ter-**BIN**-ah-feen)
Pregnancy Category: B
Lamisil **(Rx)**

How Supplied: *Cream:* 1%
Action/Kinetics: Terbinafine inhibits squalene epoxidase, a key enzyme in the sterol biosynthesis in fungi. This results in ergosterol deficiency and a corresponding accumulation of squalene leading to fungal cell death. Systemic absorption is highly variable. Approximately 75% of cutaneously absorbed drug is excreted in the urine, mostly as metabolites.
Uses: Interdigital tinea pedis (athletes's foot), tinea cruris (jock itch), or tinea corporis (ringworm) due to *Epidermophyton floccosum, Trichophyton mentagrophytes,* or *T. rubrum. Investigational:* Cutaneous candidiasis and tinea versicolor.

Dosage

- **Cream**

Interdigital tinea pedis.

Apply to cover the affected and immediately surrounding areas b.i.d. until symptoms are significantly improved. Drug therapy should be maintained for a minimum of 1 week and should not exceed 4 weeks.

Tinea cruris or tinea corporis.

Apply to cover the affected and immediately surrounding areas 1–2 times/day until symptoms are significantly improved. Drug therapy should be maintained for a minimum of 1 week and should not exceed 4 weeks.

Administration/Storage

1. Contact with eyes, nose, mouth, or other mucous membranes should be avoided.
2. Occlusive dressings should be avoided.
3. Many clients treated for 1–2 weeks continue to improve during the 2–4 weeks after drug therapy has been completed. Thus, clients should not be considered therapeutic failures until they have been observed for a period of 2–4 weeks off therapy.

Contraindications: Oral, ophthalmic, or intravaginal use. Lactation.
Special Concerns: Safety and efficacy have not been determined in children less than 12 years of age.
Side Effects: *Dermatologic:* Irritation, burning, itching, dryness.

NURSING CONSIDERATIONS

Assessment

1. Describe clinical presentation and note onset of symptoms.
2. Document that infected tissue scrapings (culture or microscopic examination in KOH solution) confirm diagnosis.

Client/Family Teaching

1. Stress importance of using exactly as prescribed. Review appropriate method for application; drug is for topical dermatologic use only.
2. Advise client to avoid contact with mouth, nose, eyes, and other mucous membranes and not to cover treated areas with an occlusive dressing.
3. Symptoms of increased irritation or possible sensitization such as redness, itching, burning, blistering, swelling, or oozing should be reported to the provider.
4. Stress the importance of reporting if irritation or sensitivity develop, as treatment should be discontinued and alternative therapy instituted.
5. Remind client to use the medication for the prescribed time frame.
6. Explain that continued improvement in skin condition may be noted for 2–4 weeks following the completion of drug therapy.

Evaluate

- Symptomatic relief with improvement in dermatologic condition
- Laboratory evidence of negative mycologic results (culture or KOH preparation)

Terconazole nitrate

(ter-**KON**-ah-zohl)

Pregnancy Category: C

Terazol ✱, Terazol 3, Terazol 7 **(Rx)**

How Supplied: *Vaginal cream:* 0.4%, 0.8%; *Vaginal suppository:* 80 mg

Action/Kinetics: Terconazole, a triazole derivative, is thought to exert its antifungal activity by disrupting cell membrane permeability leading to loss of essential intracellular materials. The drug also inhibits synthesis of triglycerides and phospholipids as well as inhibiting oxidative and peroxidative enzyme activity. When used for *Candida,* terconazole inhibits transformation of blastospores into the invasive mycelial form.

Uses: Vulvovaginitis caused by *Candida*. Ineffective in infections due to *Trichomonas* or *Haemophilus vaginalis*.

Dosage

- **Vaginal Cream (0.4%, 0.8%)**

One applicator full (5 g) intravaginally, once daily at bedtime for 7 consecutive days for the 0.4% cream and for 3 consecutive days for the 0.8% cream.

- **Vaginal Suppository**

One 80-mg suppository once daily at bedtime for 3 consecutive days.

Special Concerns: During lactation, consider discontinuing nursing or the drug. Safety and efficacy have not been established in children.

Side Effects: *GU:* Vulvovaginal burning, irritation, or itching; dysmenorrhea, pain of the female genitalia. *Miscellaneous:* Headache (most common), body pain, photosensitivity, abdominal pain, chills, fever.

NURSING CONSIDERATIONS

Assessment

1. Obtain a thorough nursing history because recurrent candidiasis may be caused by oral contraceptives, antibiotics, or diabetes whereas intractable candidiasis may be the result of undetected diabetes mellitus or reinfection.
2. Prior to a second course of therapy, the diagnosis should be confirmed to rule out other pathogens associated with vulvovaginitis.

Client/Family Teaching

1. Demonstrate the appropriate method for administration and cleansing (the cream should be inserted high into the vagina). Sitz baths and vaginal douches may also be ordered with this therapy.
2. Discontinue use and report if any burning, irritation, or pain occurs.
3. Medication may stain clothes; use sanitary napkins during therapy and change frequently because damp

sanitary napkins may harbor infecting organisms.
4. To avoid reinfection, the client should refrain from sexual intercourse, or the partner should be advised to use a condom as medication may also irritate partner.
5. Continue to take medication for prescribed time frame even if symptoms subside.
6. The drug should continue to be used during menses to ensure a full course of therapy. Effectiveness is not altered by menstruation.

Evaluate

- Resolution of fungal infections
- Reports of symptomatic improvement

Tioconazole

(tie-oh-**KON**-ah-zohl)
Pregnancy Category: C
Gyno-Trosyd ✦, Trosyd ✦, Vagistat-1 **(Rx)**

How Supplied: *Ointment:* 6.5%
Action/Kinetics: The antifungal activity of tioconazole is thought to be due to alteration of the permeability of the cell membrane of the fungus, causing leakage of essential intracellular compounds. The systemic absorption of the drug in nonpregnant clients is negligible.
Uses: *Candida albicans* infections of the vulva and vagina. Also effective against *Torulopsis glabrata.*

Dosage

- **Vaginal Ointment, 6.5%**

One applicator full (about 4.6 g) should be inserted intravaginally at bedtime for 3 days. If needed, the treatment period can be extended to 6 days.
Contraindication: Use of a vaginal applicator during pregnancy may be contraindicated.
Special Concerns: Safety and effectiveness have not been determined during lactation or in children.
Side Effects: *GU:* Burning, itching, irritation, vulvar edema and swelling, discharge, vaginal pain, dysuria, dyspareunia, nocturia, desquamation, dryness of vaginal secretions.

NURSING CONSIDERATIONS

Assessment

1. Obtain a thorough nursing history. Clients who do not respond to treatment may have unrecognized diabetes mellitus.
2. Any persistent resistant infection may be due to reinfection; therefore the sources of infection should be carefully evaluated.
3. Obtain appropriate lab studies as indicated, prior to initiating therapy.

Client/Family Teaching

1. Demonstrate the appropriate method for administration (the cream should be inserted high into the vagina).
2. Use the medication just prior to bedtime.
3. Report if any burning, irritation, or pain occurs.
4. Medication may stain clothes; use sanitary napkins during therapy and change frequently because damp sanitary napkins may harbor infecting organisms.
5. To avoid reinfection, the client should refrain from sexual intercourse, or the partner should be advised to use a condom.
6. Continue to take medication for prescribed time frame even if symptoms subside.
7. The drug should continue to be used during menses to ensure a full course of therapy. Effectiveness is not altered by menstruation.

Evaluate

- Resolution of fungal infection
- Reports of symptomatic improvement

Tolnaftate

(toll-**NAF**-tayt)
Aftate for Athlete's Foot, Aftate for Jock Itch, Genaspor, NP-27, Pitrex ✦, Quinsana Plus, Tinactin, Tinactin for Jock Itch, Ting, Zeasorb-AF **(OTC)**

See also *Anti-Infectives,* Chapter 1.

How Supplied: *Cream:* 1%; *Powder:* 1%; *Solution:* 1%; *Spray:* 1%
Action/Kinetics: The exact mechanism is not known although the drug is thought to stunt mycelial growth causing a fungicidal effect.
Uses: Tinea pedis, tinea cruris, tinea corporis, and tinea versicolor. Fungal infections of moist skin areas.

Dosage

• **Topical: Aerosol Powder, Aerosol Solution, Cream, Gel, Powder, Solution. Spray Solution**
Apply b.i.d. for 2–3 weeks although treatment for 4–6 weeks may be necessary in some instances.
Contraindications: Scalp and nail infections. *Avoid getting into eyes.*
Special Concerns: Should not be used in children less than 2 years of age.
Side Effect: Mild skin irritation.

NURSING CONSIDERATIONS

See also *General Nursing Considerations for All Anti-Infectives,* Chapter 1.
Assessment
1. Carefully inspect the source of infection and document because the choice of vehicle is important for effective therapy.
• Powders are used in mild conditions as adjunctive therapy.
• For primary therapy and prophylaxis, creams, liquids, or ointments are used, especially if the area is moist.
• Liquids and solutions are used if the area is hairy.
2. Obtain appropriate lab data because concomitant therapy should be used if bacterial or *Candida* infections are also present.
Client/Family Teaching
1. Demonstrate and observe client demonstrate the appropriate technique for medication administration.
2. Stress that the skin should be thoroughly cleaned and dried before the medication is applied.
3. Use care when administering and do not inadvertently rub medication into the eye.
4. Report any bothersome side effects; local relief of symptoms should be evident within the first 24–48 hr of therapy.
5. Continue to use as directed, despite improvement of symptoms.
6. Discontinue use if improvement is not noted within 10 days and report.
Evaluate
• Reports of symptomatic relief with evidence of skin healing
• Eradication of fungal infection

CHAPTER FIFTEEN

Antimalarial Drugs

See also the following drug classes and individual drugs:

4-Aminoquinolines

Chloroquine Hydrochloride
Chloroquine Phosphate
Hydroxychloroquine Sulfate

Miscellaneous

Mefloquine Hydrochloride
Primaquine Phosphate
Quinine Sulfate
Sulfadoxine and Pyrimethamine

4-AMINOQUINOLINES

See also the following individual entries:

Chloroquine Hydrochloride
Chloroquine Phosphate
Hydroxychloroquine Sulfate

Action/Kinetics: Several mechanisms have been proposed for the action of 4-aminoquinolines. These include (a) an active chloroquine-concentrating mechanism in the acid vesicles of the parasite causing inhibition of growth, (b) release of aggregates of ferriprotoporphyrin IX from erythrocytes in the parasite causing membrane damage and erythrocyte or parasite lysis, (c) interference with hemoglobin digestion by the parasite, and (d) interference with synthesis of nucleoprotein by the parasite. The drugs are active against the erythrocytic forms of *Plasmodium vivax* and *P. malariae* as well as most strains of *P. falciparum*. The aminoquinolines are rapidly and almost completely absorbed from the GI tract and are widely distributed throughout the body. **Peak serum levels:** 1–6 hr. These agents are excreted extremely slowly, and the presence of some drug has been demonstrated in the bloodstream weeks and even months after the drug has been discontinued. Up to 70% may be excreted unchanged. Urinary excretion is increased by acidifying the urine; excretion is slowed by alkalinization.

Uses: Treatment or prophylaxis of acute attacks of malaria caused by *Plasmodium falciparum, P. vivax, P. ovale,* and *P. malariae*. Will cause a radical cure of vivax and malariae malaria if combined with primaquine. The drugs are effective only against the erythrocytic stages and therefore will not prevent infections. However, the drugs will completely cure infection due to sensitive strains of falciparum malaria.

Extraintestinal amebiasis caused by *Entamoeba histolytica*. Discoid or lupus erythematosus, scleroderma, pemphigus, lichen planus, polymyositis, sarcoidosis, porphyria cutanea tarda.

Contraindications: Hypersensitivity. Changes in retinal or visual field. Lactation. Use in psoriasis or porphyria only if benefits clearly outweigh risks. Not to be used concomitantly with gold or phenylbutazone or in clients receiving drugs that depress blood-forming elements of bone marrow.

Special Concerns: To be used with extreme caution in the presence of hepatic, severe GI, neurologic, and blood disorders. Infants and children are sensitive to the effects of 4-aminoquinolines. Certain strains of *P. falciparum* are resistant to 4-aminoquinolines.

Side Effects: *GI:* N&V, diarrhea,

cramps, anorexia, epigastric distress, stomatitis, dry mouth. *CNS:* Headache, fatigue, nervousness, anxiety, irritability, agitation, apathy, confusion, personality changes, depression, psychoses, ***seizures.*** *CV:* Hypotension, ECG changes (inversion or depression of T wave, widening of QRS complex). *Dermatologic:* Pruritus, changes in pigment of skin and mucous membranes, dermatoses, bleaching of hair. *Hematologic:* Neutropenia, ***aplastic anemia,*** thrombocytopenia, ***agranulocytosis.*** *Ocular:* Retinopathy that may be permanent and may lead to blindness. Blurred vision, difficulty in focusing or in accommodation; chronic use may lead to corneal deposits or keratopathy. *Miscellaneous:* Peripheral neuritis, ototoxicity, neuromyopathy manifested by muscle weakness.

Symptoms of Overdose: Headache, drowsiness, visual disturbances, ***CV collapse, seizures followed by sudden and early respiratory and cardiac arrest.*** Infants and children have manifested respiratory depression, ***CV collapse, shock, seizures, and death following overdoses of parenteral chloroquine.*** ECG changes include nodal rhythm, atrial standstill, prolonged intraventricular conduction, and bradycardia, which lead to ***ventricular fibrillation or arrest.***

Drug Interactions

Acidifying agents, urinary (ammonium chloride, etc.) / ↑ Urinary excretion of antimalarial and thus ↓ its effectiveness

Alkalinizing agents, urinary (bicarbonate, etc.) / ↓ Excretion of antimalarial and thus ↑ amount of drug in system

Antipsoriatics / 4-Aminoquinolines inhibit antipsoriatic drugs

MAO inhibitors / ↑ Toxicity of 4-aminoquinolines due to ↓ breakdown in liver

Laboratory Test Interference: Colors urine brown.

Dosage

See individual drug entries.

NURSING CONSIDERATIONS

See also *General Nursing Considerations for All Anti-Infectives,* Chapter 1.

Administration/Storage

1. Store in amber-colored containers.
2. *Treatment of Overdose:* Undertake gastric lavage or emesis followed by activated charcoal. Seizures should be controlled prior to gastric lavage. Seizures due to anoxia can be treated by oxygen, mechanical ventilation, or vasopressors (in shock with hypotension). Tracheostomy or tracheal intubation may be required. Forced fluids and acidification of the urine may hasten excretion. Peritoneal dialysis and exchange transfusions may also help.

Assessment

1. Identify indications for drug therapy: prophylaxis or acute therapy.
2. Determine that pretreatment lab studies and cultures have been performed.
3. Assist client to identify source of infections and exposure.
4. Assess for retinopathy manifested by visual disturbances. Retinal changes are not reversible. Regular ophthalmologic examinations are mandatory during prolonged therapy.
5. Note any evidence of hepatic, neurologic, or blood disorders and assess lab parameters.

Interventions

1. Observe for acute toxicity, which may occur in accidental overdosage in children or in suicidal clients. Symptoms of acute toxicity develop within 30 min of ingestion. Death may occur within 2 hr.
2. Observe closely for drug interactions, adverse side effects, and drug-resistant organisms. Symptoms of acute toxicity for may include headache, drowsiness, visual disturbances, CV collapse, convulsions, and cardiac arrest.
3. Monitor and record VS, I&O, and state of consciousness at frequent intervals.
4. With some therapies, anticipate that fluids will have to be forced and ammonium chloride administered

for weeks to months to acidify urine and promote renal excretion of the drug.
5. Check toxic effects of other drugs being used because the combination with chloroquine may intensify toxic effects.
6. When used for suppressive therapy, administer the drug on the same day each week. Give immediately before or after meals to minimize gastric irritation (e.g., hydroxychloroquine).
7. Administer with the evening meal when managing discoid lupus erythematosus.
8. Evaluate ophthalmologic examination findings to determine if any retinal damage has occurred.

Client/Family Teaching

1. Review the prescribed method for administration and time intervals at which to take the medication.
2. Provide a printed list of the S&S of drug toxicity. Instruct client to report any persistent or bothersome side effects.
3. Stress the importance of reporting for scheduled medical visits and lab studies.
4. Explain and ensure that adequate fluid intake as well as the medications prescribed to acidify urine are taken as ordered.
5. Advise that some drugs may discolor urine brown and not to be alarmed.
6. Keep medications in child-proof containers and warn to keep out of children's reach.

Evaluate

- Knowledge and understanding of illness and compliance with prescribed therapy
- Malaria prophylaxis when traveling to an endemic area
- Clinical evidence of elimination of causative organism
- Reports of symptomatic improvement
- Freedom from complications or adverse drug effects

Chloroquine hydrochloride

(**KLOR**-oh-kwin)

Aralen HCl **(Rx)**

Chloroquine phosphate

(**KLOR**-oh-kwin)

Aralen Phosphate, Novo-Chloroquine ✱ **(Rx)**

See also *Antimalarial Drugs, 4-Aminoquinolines,* Chapter 15.

How Supplied: Chloroquine hydrochloride: *Injection:* 50 mg/mL

Chloroquine phosphate: *Tablet:* 250 mg, 500 mg

Dosage

- **Tablets**

Acute malarial attack.

Adults, initial: 1 g; **then,** 500 mg after 6–8 hr and 500 mg/day for next 2 days. **Children:** Total dose of 41.7 mg/kg given over a 3-day period as follows, **initial:** 16.7 mg/kg (not to exceed a single dose of 1 g); **then,** 8.3 mg/kg (not to exceed a single dose of 500 mg) given 6, 24, and 48 hr after the first dose.

Suppression (prophylaxis) of malaria.

Adults: 500 mg/week (on same day each week). If therapy has not been initiated 14 days before exposure, an initial loading dose of 1 g may be given in 500-mg doses 6 hr apart. **Children:** 8.3 mg/kg (not to exceed the adult dose) per week (on same day each week). If therapy has not been initiated 14 days before exposure, an initial loading dose of 16.7 mg/kg may be given in two divided doses 6 hr apart.

Amebiasis.

Adults: 250 mg q.i.d. for 2 days; **then,** 250 mg b.i.d. for 2–3 weeks (combine with an intestinal amebicide). **Children:** 10 mg/kg (not to exceed 500 mg) daily for 3 weeks.

- **IM**

Acute malarial attack.

Adults, initial: 200–250 mg; repeat dosage in 6 hr if necessary. Total daily dose in first 24 hr should not exceed 1 g. Begin PO therapy as soon as possible. **IM, SC. Children and infants:** 6.25 mg/kg repeated in 6 hr; dose should not exceed 12.5 mg/kg/day.

Amebiasis.

Adults: 200–250 mg/day for 10–12 days. Begin PO therapy as soon as possible. **Children:** 7.5 mg/kg/day for 10–12 days.

- **IV infusion**

Acute malarial attack.

Adults, initial: 16.6 mg/kg over 8 hr; **then,** 8.3 mg/kg q 6–8 hr by continuous infusion.

Special Concern: Use during pregnancy only if benefits outweigh risks.

Additional Side Effects: Chloroquine may exacerbate psoriasis and precipitate an acute attack.

Drug Interactions

Cimetidine / ↓ Oral clearance rate and metabolism of chloroquine
Kaolin / ↓ Effect of chloroquine due to ↓ absorption from GI tract
Magnesium trisilicate / ↓ Effect of chloroquine due to ↓ absorption from GI tract

NURSING CONSIDERATIONS

See also *Nursing Considerations* for *Antimalarial Drugs, 4-Aminoquinolines,* Chapter 15.

Assessment

1. Determine if client has a history of psoriasis because drug may exacerbate condition and precipitate an acute attack.
2. Note drugs client currently prescribed to assess the possibility of any unfavorable drug interactions.
3. Document indications for therapy and onset of symptoms.

Client/Family Teaching

1. Take only as directed and complete prescribed full course of therapy.
2. Avoid activities that require mental alertness until drug effects realized as drug may cause dizziness.
3. Avoid direct sun exposure. When exposure necessary, wear protective clothing, sunglasses, and sunscreens.
4. Urine may be discolored dark yellow or reddish brown.
5. Review appropriate methods for protection against mosquitoes, i.e., wear long pants and long-sleeved shirts, apply repellents, and use netting or screens as indicated.
6. Avoid ingestion of alcohol in any form.

Evaluate

- Reports of symptomatic improvement
- Negative laboratory culture reports
- Effective malarial prophylaxis

Hydroxychloroquine sulfate

(hy-drox-ee-**KLOR**-oh-kwin)
Plaquenil Sulfate **(Rx)**

See also *Antimalarial Drugs, 4-Aminoquinolines,* Chapter 15.

How Supplied: *Tablet:* 200 mg

Action/Kinetics: Hydroxychloroquine is not a drug of choice for rheumatoid arthritis and should be discontinued after 6 months if no beneficial effects are noted. **Peak plasma levels:** 1–3 hr. Unchanged drug is excreted in the urine. Excretion may be enhanced by acidifying the urine and decreased by alkalizing the urine.

Uses: Antimalarial, antirheumatic, discoid and lupus erythematosus. Not used as a first line of therapy.

Dosage

- **Tablets**

Acute malarial attack.

Adults, initial: 800 mg; **then,** 400 mg after 6–8 hr and 400 mg/day for next 2 days. **Children:** A total of 32 mg/kg given over a 3-day period as follows: **initial:** 12.9 mg/kg (not to exceed a single dose of 800 mg); **then,** 6.4 mg/kg (not to exceed a single dose of 400 mg) 6, 24, and 48 hr after the first dose.

Suppression of malaria.

Adults: 400 mg q 7 days. If therapy has not been initiated 14 days prior to exposure, an initial loading dose of 800 mg may be given in two divided doses 6 hr apart. **Children:** 6.4 mg/kg (not to exceed the adult dose) q 7 days. If therapy has not been initiated 14 days prior to exposure, an initial loading dose of 12.9 mg/kg may be given in two doses 6 hr apart.

Rheumatoid arthritis.

Adults: 400–600 mg/day taken with milk or meals; **maintenance** (usually after 4–12 weeks): 200–400 mg/day. (*NOTE:* Several months may be required for a beneficial effect to be seen.)

Lupus erythematosus.

Adults, usual: 400 mg once or twice daily; **prolonged maintenance:** 200–400 mg/day.

Additional Contraindications: Long-term therapy in children, ophthalmologic changes due to 4-aminoquinolines.

Special Concerns: Use with caution in alcoholism or liver disease.

Additional Side Effects: The appearances of skin eruptions or of misty vision and visual halos are indications for withdrawal. Clients on long-term therapy should be examined thoroughly at regular intervals for knee and ankle reflexes and hematopoietic studies.

Drug Interactions

Digoxin / Hydroxychloroquine ↑ serum digoxin levels

Gold salts / Dermatitis and ↑ risk of severe skin reactions

Phenylbutazone / Dermatitis and ↑ risk of severe skin reactions

NURSING CONSIDERATIONS

See also *Nursing Considerations* for *Antimalarial Drugs, 4-Aminoquinolines,* Chapter 15, and *General Nursing Considerations for All Anti-Infectives,* Chapter 1.

Assessment

1. Document indications for therapy and onset of symptoms.
2. Note condition of skin and record strength of ankle and knee reflexes.
3. Determine if client has any history of liver disease or alcohol abuse.
4. Ensure that baseline CBC, liver function studies, and ophthalmic exams are noted and evaluated every 3 months.

Client/Family Teaching

1. Any skin eruptions or muscular weakness should be reported because this is an indication to stop drug therapy.
2. Stress the importance of reporting for regular ophthalmic exams and of reporting any visual disturbances because the drug may need to be discontinued. Retinopathy has been found to be dose related.
3. Advise client that when the drug is given for rheumatoid arthritis:
   - GI irritation may be reduced by administering drug with meal or glass of milk.
   - Corticosteroids and salicylates or NSAIDs may be used concomitantly and should be continued at the anti-inflammatory dose for several weeks into initial therapy.
   - Report all side effects and anticipate that excessive side effects may necessitate a reduction of therapy. After 5–10 days of reduced dosage, under medical supervision, drug may gradually be increased again to the desired level.
   - Dosage will be reduced when the desired response is attained so that drug will again be effective in case of flare-up.
   - Stress that benefits may not occur until 6–12 months after therapy has been initiated.
4. When the drug is given for lupus erythematosus, administer dose with the evening meal.
5. Suppressive antimalarial therapy should be initiated 2 weeks prior to exposure and should be continued for 6–8 weeks after leaving the endemic area. If therapy is not started prior to exposure, the initial loading dose should be doubled and given in two doses 6 hr apart.

Evaluate

- Termination of acute malarial attack and suppression of malarial symptoms
- Reports of improvement in joint pain and mobility with ↓swelling

MISCELLANEOUS

See the following individual entries:
Mefloquine Hydrochloride
Primaquine Phosphate
Quinine Sulfate
Sulfadoxine and Pyrimethamine

Mefloquine hydrochloride

(meh-**FLOH**-kwin)
Pregnancy Category: C
Lariam **(Rx)**

How Supplied: *Tablet:* 250 mg
Action/Kinetics: Although the precise mechanism of action is not known, mefloquine is related chemically to quinine and acts as a blood schizonticide. It may increase intravesicular pH in acid vesicles of parasite. Mefloquine is a mixture of enantiomeric molecules that results in differences in the rates of release, absorption, distribution, metabolism, elimination, and activity of the drug. **t½:** 13–24 days (average 3 weeks). The drug is 98% bound to plasma proteins and is concentrated in blood erythrocytes (i.e., the target cells in treatment of malaria).
Uses: Mild to moderate acute malaria caused by mefloquine-susceptible strains of *Plasmodium falciparum* (both chloroquine susceptible and resistant strains) or *P. vivax*. Data are not available regarding effectiveness in treating *P. ovale* or *P. malariae*. Also, prophylaxis of *P. falciparum* and *P. vivax* infections, including prophylaxis of chloroquine-resistant strains of *P. falciparum*. *NOTE:* Clients with acute *P. vivax* malaria are at a high risk for relapse as mefloquine does not eliminate the exoerythrocytic (hepatic) parasites. Thus, these clients should also be treated with primaquine.

Dosage

• **Tablets**

Mild to moderate malaria caused by susceptible strains of P. falciparum *or* P. vivax.
1,250 mg (5 tablets) as a single dose with at least 8 oz of water.

Prophylaxis of malaria.
250 mg (1 tablet) once a week for 4 weeks; **then,** 1 tablet every other week. **Pediatric, 15–19 kg:** ¼ tablet (62.5 mg) weekly; **20–30 kg:** ½ tablet (125 mg) weekly; **31–45 kg:** ¾ tablet (187.5 mg) weekly; **over 45 kg:** 1 tablet (250 mg) weekly.

Administration
1. For prophylaxis, therapy with mefloquine should be initiated 1 week prior to travel to an endemic area and should be continued for 4 additional weeks after return from an endemic area.
2. *Treatment of Overdose:* Induce vomiting and administer fluid therapy to treat vomiting and diarrhea.

Contraindications: Hypersensitivity to mefloquine or related compounds.
Special Concerns: Use with caution during lactation. Safety and effectiveness have not been determined in children.
Laboratory Test Interferences: When used for prophylaxis: Transient ↑ transaminases, leukocytosis, thrombocytopenia. **When used for treatment of acute malaria:** ↓ Hematocrit, transient ↑ transaminases, leukocytosis, thrombocytopenia.
Side Effects: *NOTE:* At the doses used, it is difficult to distinguish side effects due to the drug from symptoms attributable to the disease itself. **When used for treatment of acute malaria.** *GI:* N&V, diarrhea, abdominal pain, loss of appetite. *CNS:* Dizziness, fever, headache, fatigue, emotional problems, ***seizures.*** *Miscellaneous:* Myalgia, chills, skin rash, tinnitus, bradycardia, hair loss. **When used for prophylaxis of malaria.** *CNS:* Dizziness, syncope, encephalopathy of unknown etiology. *Miscellaneous:* Vomiting, extrasystoles. **Postmarketing surveillance.** *CNS:* Vertigo, psychoses, confusion, anxiety, depression, hallucinations. *Miscellaneous:* Visual disturbances.

Symptoms of Overdose: Cardiotoxic effects, vomiting, diarrhea.

Drug Interactions
Beta-adrenergic blocking agents / ECG abnormalities or cardiac arrest

Chloroquine / ↑ Risk of seizures
Quinidine / ↑ Risk of ECG abnormalities or cardiac arrest
Quinine / ↑ Risk of seizures, ECG abnormalities, or cardiac arrest
Valproic acid / Loss of seizure control and ↓ blood levels of valproic acid

NURSING CONSIDERATIONS

See also *General Nursing Considerations for All Anti-Infectives,* Chapter 1.

Assessment

1. Note lab confirmation of causative organism.
2. Determine liver function and monitor closely during long-term drug therapy.

Interventions

1. If the client has a life-threatening *P. falciparum* infection, treatment should be initiated with an IV antimalarial drug. This can be followed by mefloquine, PO, to complete therapy.
2. To reduce the potential of cardiotoxic effects, vomiting should be induced in cases of overdose.
3. Periodic ophthalmic examinations are recommended.

Client/Family Teaching

1. Do not take the drug on an empty stomach; take with at least 8 oz of water.
2. Provide a printed list of side effects and stress those that require immediate reporting.
3. Advise client to report any early evidence of visual disturbance, stressing the importance of periodic ophthalmic examinations during therapy.

Evaluate

- Control and prevention of acute attacks of malaria (in clients with drug-sensitive malarial parasites)
- Negative lab culture reports

Primaquine phosphate

(PRIM-ah-kwin)
(Rx)

How Supplied: *Tablet:* 26.3 mg
Action/Kinetics: Mechanism of action not known, but the drug binds to and may alter the properties of DNA leading to decreased protein synthesis. Both the gametocyte and exoerythrocyte forms are inhibited. Well absorbed from GI tract. **Peak plasma levels:** 2 hr. Poorly distributed in body tissues. **t½ elimination:** 4 hr.
Uses: Primaquine produces a radical cure of vivax malaria by eliminating both exoerythrocytic and erythrocytic forms (thus preventing relapse). Primaquine also is active against the sexual forms (gametocytes) of plasmodia resulting in disruption of transmission of the disease by eliminating the reservoir from which the mosquito carrier is infected. Also used following termination of chloroquine phosphate suppression therapy where vivax malaria is endemic.

Dosage

- **Tablets**

Acute attack of vivax malaria, clients with parasitized RBCs.

15 mg (base) daily for 14 days together with chloroquine phosphate (to destroy erythrocytic parasites).

Suppression of malaria.

Adults, 26.3 mg (15 mg base) daily for 14 days or 78.9 mg once a week for 8 weeks; **children:** 0.68 mg/kg/day (0.5 mg/kg base) for 14 days.

Administration/Storage

1. Store in tightly closed containers.
2. For suppression therapy, initiate during the last 2 weeks of or after suppressive therapy with chloroquine or a similar drug.
3. *Treatment of Overdose:* Treat symptoms.

Contraindications: Very active forms of vivax and falciparum malaria. Use during pregnancy only if benefits outweigh risks. Concomitant use with quinacrine. In clients with rheumatoid arthritis or lupus erythematosus who are acutely ill or who have a tendency to develop granulocytopenia. Concomitant use with other bone marrow depressants or hemolytic drugs.
Special Concern: Use during pregnancy only when benefits outweigh risks.

Side Effects: *GI:* Abdominal cramps, epigastric distress, N&V. *Hematologic:* Methemoglobinemia. Blacks and members of certain Mediterranean ethnic groups (Sardinians, Sephardic Jews, Greeks, Iranians) manifest a high incidence of G6PD deficiency and as a result have a low tolerance for primaquine. These individuals manifest ***marked hemolytic anemia*** following primaquine administration. *Miscellaneous:* Headache, pruritus, interference with visual accommodation, ***cardiac arrhythmias,*** hypertension.

Symptoms of Overdose: Abdominal cramps, burning and epigastric distress, cyanosis, methemoglobinemia, anemia, leukocytosis or leukopenia, CNS and CV disturbances. Granulocytopenia and ***acute hemolytic anemia*** in sensitive clients.

Drug Interactions

Bone marrow depressants, hemolytic drugs / Additive side effects

Quinacrine / Quinacrine interferes with metabolic degradation of primaquine and thus enhances its toxic side reactions. **Do not give primaquine** to clients who are receiving or have received quinacrine within the past 3 months.

NURSING CONSIDERATIONS

See also *General Nursing Considerations for All Anti-Infectives,* Chapter 1, and *Antimalarial Drugs, 4-Aminoquinolines,* Chapter 15.

Assessment

1. Note any history of rheumatoid arthritis or lupus erythematosus.
2. List other medications currently prescribed to ensure no unfavorable interactions.
3. Determine if pregnant. Do not give during first trimester and preferably not until after delivery.
4. Ensure that baseline hematologic profile and cultures have been performed.

Interventions

1. Monitor for indications to withdraw drug: dark urine that indicates hemolysis and a marked fall in hemoglobin or erythrocyte count.
2. Assess dark-skinned clients closely. Because of a possible inborn deficiency of G6PD, these clients are particularly susceptible to hemolytic anemia while on primaquine.

Client/Family Teaching

1. Take medication immediately before or after meals or with antacids to minimize gastric irritation.
2. For suppressive therapy, take drug on same day each week.
3. Monitor color of urine and report immediately any darkening or brown color.
4. Stress the importance of completing a full course of therapy for effective results.
5. Review symptoms of overdose (GI, CNS, and CV disturbances) and advise client to report if evident.

Evaluate

- Termination of acute malarial attacks and suppression of malarial symptoms
- Negative lab culture reports

Quinine sulfate

(**KWYE**-nine)
Pregnancy Category: X
Formula Q, Legatrim, M-KYA, Novo-Quinine ✱, Quinamm, Quiphile, Q-vel **(Rx)**

How Supplied: *Capsule:* 180 mg, 200 mg, 260 mg, 324 mg, 325 mg; *Tablet:* 260 mg, 325 mg

Action/Kinetics: This drug is a natural alkaloid obtained from the bark of the cinchona tree. In addition to its antimalarial properties, it has antipyretic, analgesic, and oxytocic properties similar to those of the salicylates. It relieves muscle spasms and is used as a diagnostic agent for myasthenia gravis. Quinine has been used increasingly in the last several years since resistant forms of vivax and falciparum were observed in Southeast Asia. No resistant forms of the parasite have been found for quinine.

The precise antimalarial mechanism of action is not known; quinine does affect DNA replication. The drug may also act to raise intracellular pH. The drug eradicates the

erythrocytic stages of plasmodia. Quinine also increases the refractory period of skeletal muscle and decreases the excitability of the motor end-plate region, making it useful for nocturnal leg cramps. Quinine is rapidly and completely absorbed from the GI tract and is widely distributed in body tissues. **Peak plasma levels:** 1–3 hr **t½:.** 4–5 hr. The drug is highly bound to protein (70%–85%) and about 5% is excreted unchanged in urine. Small amounts of the drug are found in saliva, bile, feces, and gastric juice. Acidifying the urine increases the rate of excretion.
Uses: In combination with pyrimethamine and a sulfonamide or a tetracycline for resistant forms of *Plasmodium falciparum*. Chloroquine sensitive stains of *P. falciparum, P. malariae, P. ovale,* and *P. vivax*. Due to lack of effectiveness, the drug is no longer recommended for nocturnal leg cramps.

Dosage

- **Capsules, Tablets**

Chloroquine-resistant malaria.
Adults: 650 mg/8 hr for at least 3 days (7 days in Southeast Asia) along with pyrimethamine, 25 mg b.i.d. for the first 3 days and sulfadiazine, 2 g/day for the first 5 days. There are two alternative regimens: (1) quinine, 650 mg/8 hr for at least 3 days (7 days in Southeast Asia) along with a tetracycline, 250 mg/6 hr for 10 days or (2) quinine, 650 mg/8 hr for 3 days with sulfadoxine, 1.5 g and pyrimethamine, 75 mg as a single dose.

Chloroquine-sensitive malaria.
Adults: 600 mg/8 hr for 5–7 days. **Pediatric:** 10 mg/kg q 8 hr for 5–7 days.

Administration/Storage

1. The parenteral form is available from the Centers for Disease Control if client unable to take orally.
2. *Treatment of Overdose:*
- Induce vomiting or undertake gastric lavage.
- Maintain BP and renal function.
- If necessary, provide artificial respiration.
- Sedatives, oxygen, and other supportive measures may be required.
- Give IV fluids to maintain fluid and electrolyte balance.
- Treat angioedema or asthma with epinephrine, corticosteroids, and antihistamines.
- Urinary acidification will hasten excretion; however, in the presence of hemoglobinuria, acidification of the urine will increase renal blockade.

Contraindications: Clients with tinnitus. G6PD deficiency, optic neuritis, history of blackwater fever, and thrombocytopenia purpura associated with previous use of quinine. Pregnancy (category X) as the drug is oxytocic and may cause congenital malformations.
Special Concerns: Use with caution in clients with cardiac arrhythmias and during lactation.
Side Effects: Use of quinine may result in a syndrome referred to as *cinchonism*. Mild cinchonism is characterized by tinnitus, headache, nausea, slight visual disturbances. Larger doses, however, may cause severe CNS, CV, GI, or dermatologic effects.

Allergic: Flushing, rashes, fever, facial edema, pruritus, dyspnea, tinnitus, gastric upset. *GI:* N&V, gastric pain. *Ophthalmologic:* Blurred vision, photophobia, diplopia, night blindness, decreased visual fields, impaired color perception. *CNS:* Headache, confusion, restlessness, vertigo, syncope, fever. *Hematologic:* Thrombocytopenia, hypoprothrombinemia. *CV:* Symptoms of angina, ventricular tachycardia, conduction disturbances. *Miscellaneous:* Sweating.

Symptoms of Overdose: Dizziness, intestinal cramping, skin rash, tinnitus. With higher doses, symptoms include apprehension, confusion, fever, headache, vomiting, and seizures.

Drug Interactions

Acetazolamide / ↑ Effect of quinine due to ↓ rate of elimination

Aluminum-containing antacids / Absorption of quinine ↓ or delayed
Anticoagulants, oral / Additive hypoprothrombinemia due to ↓ synthesis of vitamin K–dependent clotting factors
Cimetidine / ↑ Effect of quinine due to ↓ rate of excretion
Digoxin / Quinine ↑ effect of digoxin
Heparin / Effect ↓ by quinine
Mefloquine / ↑ Risk of ECG abnormalities or cardiac arrest. **Do not use together.**
Pyrimethamine / ↑ Effect of quinine due to ↓ plasma protein binding
Skeletal muscle relaxants (surgical) / ↑ Respiratory depression and apnea
Sodium bicarbonate / ↑ Effect of quinine due to ↓ rate of elimination

NURSING CONSIDERATIONS

See also *General Nursing Considerations For All Anti-Infectives,* Chapter 1.

Assessment

1. Note any history or evidence of cardiac arrhythmias.
2. Obtain baseline CBC and ophthalmic exam and monitor throughout drug therapy.

Client/Family Teaching

1. Do not take medication with antacids. Take with or immediately after meals to reduce GI upset.
2. Drug may cause dizziness or blurred vision. Do not drive a car or operate machinery until drug effects are realized.
3. If also taking cimetidine or digoxin, report any side effects immediately because dosage may need to be adjusted.
4. If female and of childbearing age, advise to use birth control because drug may harm fetus.
5. Report any ringing of the ears, blurring of vision, and headache, which may be followed by digestive disturbances, impairment of hearing and sight, confusion, and delirium. This may indicate intolerance or overdosage and requires immediate medical intervention.

Evaluate

• Termination of acute malarial attack and control of symptoms of malaria

—COMBINATION DRUG—

Sulfadoxine and Pyrimethamine

(sul-fah-**DOX**-een, pie-rih-**METH**-ah-meen)
Pregnancy Category: C
Fansidar **(Rx)**

See also *Sulfonamides,* Chapter 9.
How Supplied: See Content
Content: Each tablet contains: 500 mg sulfadoxine, 25 mg pyrimethamine.
Action/Kinetics: Sulfadoxine competes with para-aminobenzoic acid for biosynthesis of folic acid, whereas pyrimethamine inhibits the formation of tetrahydrofolate from dihydrofolate. These reactions are necessary for one-carbon transfer reactions in the synthesis of nucleic acids. Well absorbed following PO use and is widely distributed throughout the body. Each tablet contains sulfadoxine, 500 mg, and pyrimethamine, 25 mg. **Peak plasma levels:** sulfadoxine, 2.5–6 hr; pyrimethamine, 1.5–8 hr. Both drugs are long-acting with a **t½** of 170 hr for sulfadoxine and 110 hr for pyrimethamine. Both drugs are excreted through the urine with about 20%–30% of pyrimethamine excreted unchanged.
Uses: Prophylaxis and treatment of falciparum malaria, especially chloroquine-resistant strains. *Investigational:* Prophylaxis of *Pneumocystis carinii* pneumonia in AIDS clients (second-line agents).

Dosage

• **Tablets**

Acute malaria (in combination with quinine).

Adults: 2–3 tablets as a single dose. **Pediatric, 9–14 years of age:** 2 tablets as a single dose; **4–8 years of age:** 1 tablet as a single dose; **under 4 years of age:** ½ tablet as a single dose.

Prophylaxis of malaria.

Adults: 1 tablet/week or 2 tablets biweekly; **Pediatric, 9–14 years of age:** weekly, 3/4 tablet; biweekly, 1 1/2 tablets. **4–8 years of age:** weekly, 1/2 tablet; biweekly, 1 tablet. **Under 4 years of age:** weekly, 1/4 tablet; biweekly, 1/2 tablet.

Administration

1. High intake of fluid should occur to prevent precipitation in the urine.
2. For prophylaxis, therapy should be initiated 1–2 days before the person enters the endemic area; therapy should continue during stay and for 4–6 weeks after leaving. Primaquine should be given.
3. If folic acid deficiency occurs, leucovorin can be given in a dose of 5–15 mg/day IM for 3 or more days.

Contraindications: Megaloblastic anemia. Infants less than 2 months old. Pregnancy (near term) and lactation. Significant liver parenchymal disease, renal insufficiency, in presence of blood dyscrasias.

Special Concerns: Use with caution in severe allergy, folate deficiency, bronchial asthma, and clients with G6PD deficiency. Fatalities have resulted due to Stevens-Johnson syndrome and toxic epidermal necrolysis.

Side Effects: See *Sulfonamides,* Chapter 9. ***Stevens-Johnson syndrome, toxic epidermal necrolysis.***

Drug Interactions: Sulfonamides, including trimethoprim/sulfamethoxazole, will ↑ risk of folic acid deficiency if used with sulfadoxine, pyrimethamine, and methotrexate.

NURSING CONSIDERATIONS

See also *Nursing Considerations for All Anti-Infectives,* Chapter 1.

Assessment

1. Document indications for therapy and type and onset of symptoms and/or contact with endemic area.
2. Determine any history or evidence of G6PD deficiency.
3. Note any severe allergic conditions such as asthma, bronchitis, or severe nutritional disorders, as drug should be used cautiously in this setting.
4. Review CBC and assess lab values for evidence of liver or renal dysfunction.

Client/Family Teaching

1. Report immediately if fever, sore throat, purpura, jaundice, pallor, or glossitis is observed.
2. The drug should be discontinued immediately if erythema, rash, pruritus, orogenital lesions, or pharyngitis is noted.
3. Adequate fluids should be taken (2–3 L/day) to prevent crystalluria and stone formation.
4. Contraceptive measures should be used to prevent pregnancy while on this medication.
5. Breast-feeding should not be undertaken while on this medication.
6. Report for lab studies as scheduled because blood counts and urinalysis should be performed periodically if chronic therapy is required.

Evaluate: Prevention of acute malarial attacks and ↓ severity of malarial symptoms.

CHAPTER SIXTEEN

Antitubercular Drugs

See the following individual entries:

Cycloserine
Ethambutol Hydrochloride
Isoniazid
Rifabutin
Rifampin
Rifampin and Isoniazid

Cycloserine

(sye-kloh-**SEE**-reen)
Pregnancy Category: C
Seromycin **(Rx)**

How Supplied: *Capsule:* 25 mg
Action/Kinetics: This drug is produced by a strain of *Streptomyces orchidaceus* or *Garyphalus lavendulae*. It acts by inhibiting cell wall synthesis by interfering with the incorporation of the amino acid alanine. The drug is well absorbed from the GI tract and widely distributed in body tissues. **Time to peak plasma levels:** 3–8 hr. Cerebrospinal levels are similar to those in plasma. **t½:** 10 hr. From 60% to 70% is excreted unchanged in urine.
Uses: With other drugs to treat active pulmonary and extrapulmonary tuberculosis only when primary therapy cannot be used. Has been used to treat UTIs when other therapy has failed or if the organism has demonstrated sensitivity.

Dosage

• **Capsules**

Adults, initially: 250 mg q 12 hr for first 2 weeks; **then,** 0.5–1 g/day in divided doses based on blood levels. Dosage should not exceed 1 g/day. **Pediatric:** 10–20 mg/kg/day, not to exceed 0.75–1 g/day. *NOTE:* Pyridoxine, 200–300 mg/day may prevent neurotoxic effects.
Administration/Storage: *Treatment of Overdose:* Supportive therapy. Charcoal may be more effective than emesis or gastric lavage. Hemodialysis may be used for life-threatening toxicity. Pyridoxine may treat neurotoxic effects.
Contraindications: Hypersensitivity to cycloserine, epilepsy, depression, severe anxiety, psychosis, severe renal insufficiency, and alcoholism. Lactation.
Special Concerns: Safe use during pregnancy and in children has not been established.
Side Effects: *CNS:* Drowsiness, headache, mental confusion, tremors, vertigo, loss of memory, psychoses (possibly with ***suicidal tendencies)***, character changes, hyperirritability, aggression, increased reflexes, ***seizures,*** paresthesias, paresis, coma. Neurotoxic effects depend on blood levels of cycloserine. Hence, frequent determinations of cycloserine blood levels are indicated, especially during the initial period of therapy. *Other:* Sudden development of CHF, skin rashes, increased transaminase.

Symptoms of Overdose: CNS depression, including drowsiness, mental confusion, headache, vertigo, paresthesias, dysarthrias, hyperirritability, psychosis, paresis, ***seizures,*** and ***coma.***

Drug Interactions

Ethanol / ↑ Risk of epileptic episodes
Isoniazid / ↑ Risk of cycloserine CNS side effects (especially dizziness)

NURSING CONSIDERATIONS

See also *General Nursing Considerations for All Anti-Infectives,* Chapter 1.

Assessment
1. Obtain a thorough nursing and drug history.
2. Note any evidence of depression, anxiety, seizures, or excessive use of alcohol.
3. Obtain baseline parameters and monitor liver and renal function studies throughout therapy.

Interventions
1. Monitor I&O and observe for any sudden development of CHF in clients receiving high doses of cycloserine.
2. Report any psychotic or neurologic reactions that will necessitate withdrawing the drug, at least for a short period of time.
3. Monitor serum cycloserine levels throughout therapy (less than 25–30 mcg/mL).

Client/Family Teaching
1. Drug causes drowsiness and dizziness; caution against performing tasks that require mental alertness and advise to report if symptoms persist.
2. Consume 2–3 L/day of fluids.
3. Avoid alcohol.
4. Report any SOB or skin rashes.
5. Overt behavior changes, especially suicide ideations, require immediate reporting.

Evaluate
- Resolution of infection
- Negative sputum cultures for acid-fast bacilli
- Improved CXR and pulmonary function parameters

Ethambutol hydrochloride

(eh-**THAM**-byou-tohl)
Myambutol **(Rx)**

How Supplied: *Tablet:* 100 mg, 400 mg

Action/Kinetics: Tuberculostatic. Inhibits the synthesis of metabolites resulting in impairment of cell metabolism, arrest of multiplication, and ultimately cell death. The drug is active against *Mycobacterium tuberculosis,* but not against fungi, other bacteria, or viruses. Readily absorbed after PO administration. Widely distributed in body tissues except CSF. **Peak plasma concentration:** 2–5 mcg/mL after 2–4 hr. **t½:** 3–4 hr. About 65% of metabolized and unchanged drug excreted in urine and 20%–25% unchanged drug excreted in feces. Drug accumulates in clients with renal insufficiency.

Uses: Pulmonary tuberculosis in combination with other tuberculostatic drugs.

Dosage

- **Tablets**

Adults, initial treatment: 15 mg/kg/day until maximal improvement noted; **for retreatment:** 25 mg/kg/day as a single dose with at least one other tuberculostatic drug; **after 60 days:** 15 mg/kg/day.

Administration/Storage: Ethambutol should only be used in conjunction with at least one other antituberculosis drug.

Contraindications: Hypersensitivity to ethambutol, preexisting optic neuritis, and in children under 13 years of age.

Special Concerns: Should be used with caution and in reduced dosage in clients with gout and impaired renal function and in pregnant women.

Side Effects: *Ophthalmologic:* Optic neuritis, decreased visual acuity, loss of color (green) discrimination, temporary loss of vision or blurred vision. *GI:* N&V, anorexia, abdominal pain. *CNS:* Fever, headache, dizziness, confusion, disorientation, malaise, hallucinations. *Allergic:* Pruritus, dermatitis, ***anaphylaxis.*** *Miscellaneous:* Peripheral neuropathy (numbness, tingling), precipitation of gout, thrombocytopenia, joint pain, toxic epidermal necrolysis. Renal damage. Also ***anaphylactic shock,*** peripheral neuritis (rare), hyperuricemia, and decreased liver function. Adverse symptoms usually appear during the early months of therapy and disappear thereafter. Periodic renal and hepatic function tests as well as uric acid determinations are recommended.

Drug Interactions: Aluminum may delay and decrease the absorption of ethambutol.

NURSING CONSIDERATIONS

See also *General Nursing Considerations for All Anti-Infectives,* Chapter 1.

Assessment

1. Note indications for therapy, other treatments prescribed, and the outcomes.
2. Ascertain that client has had a visual acuity test before ethambutol therapy. Document no preexisting visual problems (especially if dose exceeds 15 mg/kg/day).
3. Obtain baseline CBC and liver and renal function studies and monitor throughout therapy.

Client/Family Teaching

1. Take as prescribed to prevent any relapses or complications.
2. Consume 2–3 L/day of fluids to ensure adequate hydration.
3. Avoid aluminum-based antacids because these may interfere with drug absorption.
4. Stress importance of vision testing every 2–4 weeks while on therapy and to report any vision changes.
5. Reassure client that adverse ocular side effects generally disappear within several weeks to several months after therapy has been discontinued.
6. Women of childbearing age should practice birth control during therapy. If pregnancy is suspected, discontinue drug and report immediately.

Evaluate

- Negative sputum cultures for acid-fast bacilli
- Resolution of infection (↓ fever, ↓ WBC, ↓ sputum production and improved CXR)

Isoniazid (INH, Isonicotinic acid hydrazide)

(eye-so-**NYE**-ah-zid)

Pregnancy Category: C

Laniazid, Laniazid C.T., Nydrazid Injection, PMS Isoniazid ✱ **(Rx)**

How Supplied: *Injection:* 100 mg/mL; *Syrup:* 50 mg/5 mL; *Tablet:* 100 mg, 300 mg

General Statement: Isoniazid is the most effective tuberculostatic agent. The metabolism of isoniazid is genetically determined and involves the level of a hepatic enzyme. Clients on isoniazid fall into two groups, depending on the manner in which they metabolize isoniazid. As a rule, 50% of whites and blacks inactivate the drug slowly, whereas the majority of American Indians, Eskimos, Japanese, and Chinese are rapid acetylators (inactivators).

1. **Slow acetylators:** These clients show earlier, favorable response but have more toxic reactions (e.g., neuropathies because of higher blood levels of drug).
2. **Rapid acetylators:** These clients have possible poor clinical response due to rapid inactivation, which is 5–6 times faster than slow acetylators. This group requires an increased daily dose of the drug. They are more likely to develop hepatitis.

Action/Kinetics: Isoniazid probably interferes with lipid and nucleic acid metabolism of growing bacteria, resulting in alteration of the bacterial wall. The drug is tuberculostatic. It is readily absorbed after PO and parenteral (IM) administration and is widely distributed in body tissues, including cerebrospinal, pleural, and ascitic fluids. **Peak plasma concentration: PO,** 1–2 hr. **t½, fast acetylators:** 0.5–6 hr; **t½, slow acetylators:** 2–5 hr. These values are increased in association with liver and kidney impairment. Drug is metabolized in liver and excreted primarily in urine.

Uses: Tuberculosis caused by human, bovine, and BCG strains of *Mycobacterium tuberculosis.* The drug should not be used as the sole tuberculostatic agent. Prophylaxis of tuberculosis. *Investigational:* To improve severe tremor in clients with multiple sclerosis.

Dosage

- **Syrup, Tablets**

Active tuberculosis.

Adults: 5 mg/kg/day (up to 300 mg/day) as a single dose; **children and infants:** 10–20 mg/kg/day (up to 300 mg total) in a single dose.

Prophylaxis.

Adults: 300 mg/day in a single dose; **children and infants:** 10 mg/kg/day (up to 300 mg total) in a single dose.

• **IM**

Active tuberculosis.

Adults: 5 mg/kg (up to 300 mg) once daily. **Pediatric:** 10–20 mg/kg (up to 300 mg) once daily.

Prophylaxis.

Adults/adolescents: 300 mg/day. **Pediatric:** 10 mg/kg/day.

NOTE: Pyridoxine, 6–50 mg/day, is recommended in the malnourished and those prone to neuropathy (e.g., alcoholics, diabetics).

Administration/Storage

1. Store in dark, tightly closed containers.
2. Solutions for IM injection may crystallize at low temperature and should be allowed to warm to room temperature if precipitation is evident.
3. Anticipate a slight local irritation at the site of injection. Rotate and document injection sites.
4. Isoniazid should be administered with pyridoxine, 10–50 mg/day, in malnourished, alcoholic, or diabetic clients to prevent symptoms of peripheral neuropathy.
5. *Treatment of Overdose:* Maintain respiration and undertake gastric lavage (within first 2–3 hr providing seizures are not present). To control seizures, give diazepam or a short-acting IV barbiturate followed by pyridoxine (1 mg IV/1 mg isoniazid ingested). Sodium bicarbonate, IV, to correct metabolic acidosis. Forced osmotic diuresis; monitor fluid I&O. For severe cases, hemodialysis or peritoneal dialysis should be considered.

Contraindications: Severe hypersensitivity to isoniazid or in clients with previous isoniazid-associated hepatic injury or side effects.

Special Concerns: Severe, and sometimes fatal, hepatitis may occur even after several months of therapy; incidence is age-related and current alcohol use increases the risk. Extreme caution should be exercised in clients with convulsive disorders, in whom the drug should be administered only when the client is adequately controlled by anticonvulsant medication. Also, use with caution for the treatment of renal tuberculosis and, in the lowest dose possible, in clients with impaired renal function and in alcoholics.

Laboratory Test Interferences: Altered liver function tests. False + or ↑ potassium, AST, ALT, urine glucose (Benedict's test, Clinitest).

Side Effects: *Neurologic:* Peripheral neuropathy characterized by symmetrical numbness and tingling of extremities (dose-related). Rarely, toxic encephalopathy, optic neuritis, optic atrophy, ***seizures,*** impaired memory, toxic psychosis. *GI:* N&V, epigastric distress, xerostomia. *Hypersensitivity:* Fever, skin rashes and eruptions, vasculitis, lymphadenopathy. *Hepatic:* Liver dysfunction, jaundice, bilirubinemia, bilirubinuria, ***serious and sometimes fatal hepatitis (especially in clients over 50 years of age).*** Increases in serum AST and ALT. *Hematologic:* ***Agranulocytosis,*** eosinophilia, thrombocytopenia, ***hemolytic, sideroblastic, or aplastic anemia.*** *Metabolic/Endocrine:* Metabolic acidosis, pyridoxine deficiency, pellagra, hyperglycemia, gynecomastia. *Miscellaneous:* Tinnitus, urinary retention, rheumatic syndrome, lupus-like syndrome, arthralgia.

NOTE: Pyridoxine, 10–50 mg/day, may be given concomitantly with isoniazid to decrease CNS side effects. Ophthalmologic and liver function tests are recommended periodically.

Symptoms of Overdose: N&V, dizziness, blurred vision, slurred speech, visual hallucinations within 30–180 min. Severe overdosage may cause respiratory distress, ***CNS depression (coma can occur), severe seizures,*** metabolic acidosis, acetonuria, hyperglycemia.

Drug Interactions

Aluminum salts / ↓ Effect of isoniazid due to ↓ absorption from GI tract
Anticoagulants, oral / ↓ Anticoagulant effect
Atropine / ↑ Side effects of isoniazid
Benzodiazepines / ↑ Effect of benzodiazepines that undergo oxidative metabolism (e.g., diazepam, triazolam)
Carbamazepine / ↑ Risk of both carbamazepine and isoniazid toxicity
Cycloserine / ↑ Risk of cycloserine CNS side effects
Disulfiram / ↑ Risk of acute behavioral and coordination changes
Enflurane / Isoniazid may produce high levels of hydrazine, which increases defluorination of enflurane
Ethanol / ↑ Chance of isoniazid-induced hepatitis
Halothane / ↑ Risk of hepatotoxicity and hepatic encephalopathy
Hydantoins (phenytoin) / ↑ Effect of hydantoins due to ↓ breakdown in liver
Ketoconazole / ↓ Serum levels of ketoconazole → ↓ effect
Meperidine / ↑ Risk of hypotension or CNS depression
PAS / ↑ Effect of isoniazid by ↑ blood levels
Rifampin / Additive liver toxicity

NURSING CONSIDERATIONS

See also *General Nursing Considerations for All Anti-Infectives,* Chapter 1.

Assessment

1. Document indications for therapy and type and onset of symptoms.
2. Determine any other agents used previously for these symptoms and the outcome.
3. Obtaine baseline lab studies, CXR, and sputum cultures. Monitor liver and renal function studies and anticipate reduced dose with renal dysfunction.
4. Perform a thorough pulmonary assessment and describe the characteristics of any sputum produced.

Interventions

1. If CNS stimulation is marked, withhold drug and report.
2. Assess clients with diabetes closely because it is more difficult to control when isoniazid is administered.
3. Monitor I&O to ascertain that renal output is adequate to prevent systemic accumulation of the drug.
4. Provide client with only a 1-month supply of the drug because client should be examined and evaluated monthly while on isoniazid.

Client/Family Teaching

1. Take drug on an empty stomach 1 hr before or 2 hr after meals.
2. Consume 2–3 L/day of fluids to ensure adequate hydration.
3. Explain that pyridoxine is given to prevent neurotoxic effects of isoniazid.
4. Avoid alcohol while on drug therapy.
5. Withhold drug and report fatigue, weakness, malaise, and anorexia immediately because these may be S&S of hepatitis.
6. Stress the importance of taking drugs as ordered and of reporting for monthly follow-up and lab studies and ophthalmic assessments.

Evaluate

- Negative sputum cultures for acid-fast bacilli
- Prevention of neurotoxic drug side effects
- Reports of symptomatic improvement (↓ fever, ↓ secretions, ↑ appetite)

Rifabutin

(**rif**-ah-**BYOU**-tin)
Pregnancy Category: B
Mycobutin **(Rx)**

How Supplied: *Capsule:* 150 mg
Action/Kinetics: Rifabutin is an antimycobacterial drug derived from rifamycin. It inhibits DNA-dependent RNA polymerase in susceptible strains of *Escherichia coli* and *Bacil-*

lus subtilis. The drug is rapidly absorbed from the GI tract. **Peak plasma levels after a single dose:** 3.3 hr. **Mean terminal t½:** 45 hr. About 85% is bound to plasma proteins. High-fat meals slow the rate, but not the extent, of absorption. About 30% of a dose is excreted in the feces and 53% excreted in the urine, primarily as metabolites. The 25-O-desacetyl metabolite is equal in activity to rifabutin.

Use: Prevention of disseminated *Mycobacterium avium* complex (MAC) disease in clients with advanced HIV infection.

Dosage

- **Capsules**

Prophylaxis of MAC disease in clients with advanced HIV infection.

Adults: 300 mg/day.

Administration/Storage

1. The drug can be given at doses of 150 mg b.i.d. with food if clients experience N&V or other GI upset.
2. Urine, feces, saliva, sputum, perspiration, tears, and skin may be colored brown-orange. Soft contact lenses may be permanently stained.
3. *Treatment of Overdose:* Gastric lavage followed by instillation into the stomach of an activated charcoal slurry.

Contraindications: Hypersensitivity to rifabutin or other rifamycins (e.g., rifampin). Use in clients with active tuberculosis. Lactation.

Special Concerns: Safety and efficacy have not been determined in children, although the drug has been used in HIV-positive children.

Laboratory Test Interferences: ↑ AST, ALT, alkaline phosphatase.

Side Effects: *GI:* Anorexia, abdominal pain, diarrhea, dyspepsia, eructation, flatulence, N&V, taste perversion. *Respiratory:* Chest pain, chest pressure or pain with dyspnea. *CNS:* Insomnia, ***seizures,*** paresthesia, aphasia, confusion. *Musculoskeletal:* Asthenia, myalgia, arthralgia, myositis. *Body as a whole:* Fever, headache, generalized pain, flu-like syndrome. *Dermatologic:* Rash, skin discoloration. *Hematologic:* Neutropenia, leukopenia, anemia, eosinophilia, thrombocytopenia. *Miscellaneous:* Discolored urine, nonspecific T wave changes on ECG, hepatitis, hemolysis, uveitis.

Symptoms of Overdose: Worsening of side effects.

Drug Interactions: Rifabutin has liver enzyme-inducing properties and may be expected to have similar interactions as does rifampin. However, rifabutin is a less potent enzyme inducer than rifampin.

AZT / ↓ Steady-state plasma levels of AZT after repeated rifabutin dosing

Oral contraceptives / Rifabutin may ↓ the effectiveness of oral contraceptives

NURSING CONSIDERATIONS

See also *General Nursing Considerations for All Anti-Infectives,* Chapter 1.

Assessment

1. Document onset of HIV and symptoms necessitating therapy.
2. Obtain baseline CBC.
3. Ensure that CXR, PPD, and sputum cultures have been performed to rule out active tuberculosis. Clients who develop active tuberculosis during therapy must be covered with appropriate antituberculosis medications.

Client/Family Teaching

1. Review the S&S of both MAC and tuberculosis and instruct client to call provider if new symptoms develop that are consistent with either disease.
2. Any S&S of muscle or eye pain, irritation, or inflammation should be promptly reported.
3. All secretions, skin, and mucous membranes may become discolored orange-brown.
4. Advise that soft contact lens may become permanently discolored.
5. Practice nonhormonal form of birth control if sexually active.

Evaluate: Prevention of disseminated MAC disease in clients with advanced HIV.

Rifampin

(rih-**FAM**-pin)

Pregnancy Category: C

Rifadin, Rimactane, Rofact ✱ **(Rx)**

How Supplied: *Capsule:* 150 mg, 300 mg; *Powder for injection:* 600 mg

Action/Kinetics: Semisynthetic antibiotic derived from *Streptomyces mediterranei*. Rifampin suppresses RNA synthesis by binding to the beta subunit of DNA-dependent RNA polymerase. This prevents attachment of the enzyme to DNA and blockade of RNA transcription. The drug is both bacteriostatic and bactericidal and is most active against rapidly replicating organisms. The drug is well absorbed from the GI tract and is widely distributed in body tissues. **Peak plasma concentration:** 4–32 mcg/mL after 2–4 hr. **t½:** 1.5–5 hr; (higher in clients with hepatic impairment). In normal clients t½ decreases with usage. The drug is metabolized in liver; 60% is excreted in feces.

Uses: All types of tuberculosis. Must be used in conjunction with at least one other tuberculostatic drug (such as isoniazid, ethambutol, pyrazinamide) but is the drug of choice for retreatment. Also for treatment of asymptomatic meningococcal carriers to eliminate *Neisseria meningitidis*. *Investigational:* Used in combination for infections due to *Staphylococcus aureus* and *S. epidermidis* (endocarditis, osteomyelitis, prostatitis); Legionnaire's disease; in combination with dapsone for leprosy; prophylaxis of meningitis due to *Haemophilus influenzae* and gram-negative bacteremia in infants.

Dosage

- **Capsules, IV**

Pulmonary tuberculosis.

Adults: Single dose of 600 mg/day; **children over 5 years:** 10–20 mg/kg/day, not to exceed 600 mg/day.

Meningococcal carriers.

Adults: 600 mg b.i.d. for 2 days; **children:** 10–20 mg/kg q 12 hr for four doses. Dosage should not exceed 600 mg/day.

Administration/Storage

1. Administer capsules once daily 1 hr before or 2 hr after meals to ensure maximum absorption.
2. Check to be sure that there is a desiccant in the bottle containing capsules of rifampin because these are relatively moisture sensitive.
3. If administered concomitantly with PAS, drugs should be given 8–12 hr apart because the acid interferes with the absorption of rifampin.
4. When used for tuberculosis, therapy should continue for 6–9 months.
5. Reconstitute 600-mg vial using 10 mL of sterile water for injection. Gently swirl vial to dissolve. The resultant solution contains 60 mg/mL rifampin; it is stable at room temperature for 24 hr.
6. Add the volume of reconstituted solution needed to 500 mL of D5W and infuse over 3 hr or it may be added to 100 mL D5W and infused over 30 min. Sterile saline may be used when dextrose is contraindicated; however, the stability of rifampin is slightly less.
7. The dilution solution must be used within 4 hr or drug may precipitate from solution.
8. Injectable solution appears dark reddish brown.
9. A PO suspension (10 mg/mL) may be prepared as follows: The contents of either four 300-mg rifampin capsules or eight 150-mg capsules are emptied into a 4-oz amber glass bottle. To this is added 20 mL of simple syrup; shake vigorously. Add 100 mL of simple syrup and shake again. The suspension is stable for 4 weeks when stored at room temperature or in the refrigerator.
10. *Treatment of Overdose:* Gastric lavage followed by activated charcoal slurry introduced into the stomach. Antiemetics to control N&V. Forced diuresis to enhance excretion. If hepatic function is seriously

impaired, bile drainage may be required. Extracorporeal hemodialysis may be necessary.

Contraindications: Hypersensitivity; not recommended for intermittent therapy.

Special Concerns: Safe use during lactation has not been established. Safety and effectiveness not determined in children less than 5 years of age. Use with extreme caution in clients with hepatic dysfunction.

Laboratory Test Interferences: ↑ AST, ALT, alkaline phosphatase, BUN, bilirubin, uric acid, BSP retention values. False + Coombs' test.

Side Effects: *GI:* N&V, diarrhea, anorexia, gas, pseudomembranous colitis, pancreatitis, sore mouth and tongue, cramps, heartburn, flatulence. *CNS:* Headache, drowsiness, fatigue, ataxia, dizziness, confusion, generalized numbness, fever, difficulty in concentrating. *Hepatic:* Jaundice, hepatitis. Increases in AST, ALT, bilirubin, alkaline phosphatase. *Hematologic:* Thrombocytopenia, eosinophilia, hemolysis, leukopenia, hemolytic anemia. *Allergic:* Flu-like symptoms, dyspnea, wheezing, SOB, purpura, pruritus, urticaria, skin rashes, sore mouth and tongue, conjunctivitis. *Renal:* Hematuria, hemoglobinuria, renal insufficiency, acute renal failure. *Miscellaneous:* Visual disturbances, muscle weakness or pain, arthralgia, decreased BP, osteomalacia, menstrual disturbances, edema of face and extremities, adrenocortical insufficiency, increases in BUN and serum uric acid. *NOTE:* Body fluids and feces may be red-orange.

Symptoms of Overdose: Shortly after ingestion, N&V, and lethargy will occur. Followed by severe hepatic involvement (liver enlargement with tenderness, increased direct and total bilirubin, change in hepatic enzymes) with unconsciousness. Also, brownish red or orange discoloration of urine, saliva, tears, sweat, skin, and feces.

Drug Interactions

Acetaminophen / ↓ Effect of acetaminophen due to ↑ breakdown by liver

Aminophylline / ↓ Effect of aminophylline due to ↑ breakdown by liver

Anticoagulants, oral / ↓ Effect of anticoagulants due to ↑ breakdown by liver

Antidiabetics, oral / ↓ Effect of oral antidiabetic due to ↑ breakdown by liver

Barbiturates / ↓ Effect of barbiturates due to ↑ breakdown by liver

Benzodiazepines / ↓ Effect of benzodiazepines due to ↑ breakdown by liver

Beta-adrenergic blocking agents / ↓ Effect of beta-blocking agents due to ↑ breakdown by liver

Chloramphenicol / ↓ Effect of chloramphenicol due to ↑ breakdown by liver

Clofibrate / ↓ Effect of clofibrate due to ↑ breakdown by liver

Contraceptives, oral / ↓ Effect of oral contraceptives due to ↑ breakdown by liver

Corticosteroids / ↓ Effect of corticosteroids due to ↑ breakdown by liver

Cyclosporine / ↓ Effect of cyclosporine due to ↑ breakdown by liver

Digitoxin / ↓ Effect of digitoxin due to ↑ breakdown by liver

Digoxin / ↓ Serum levels of digoxin

Disopyramide / ↓ Effect of disopyramide due to ↑ breakdown by liver

Estrogens / ↓ Effect of estrogens due to ↑ breakdown by liver

Halothane / ↑ Risk of hepatotoxicity and hepatic encephalopathy

Hydantoins / ↓ Effect of hydantoins due to ↑ breakdown by liver

Isoniazid / ↑ Risk of hepatotoxicity

Ketoconazole / ↓ Effect of either ketoconazole or rifampin

Methadone / ↓ Effect of methadone due to ↑ breakdown by liver

Mexiletine / ↓ Effect of mexiletine due to ↑ breakdown by liver

Quinidine / ↓ Effect of quinidine due to ↑ breakdown by liver

Sulfones / ↓ Effect of sulfones due to ↑ breakdown by liver

Theophylline / ↓ Effect of theophylline due to ↑ breakdown by liver
Tocainide / ↓ Effect of tocainide due to ↑ breakdown by liver
Verapamil / ↓ Effect of verapamil due to ↑ breakdown by liver

NURSING CONSIDERATIONS

See also *General Nursing Considerations for All Anti-Infectives,* Chapter 1.

Assessment

1. Document indications for therapy and type and onset of symptoms.
2. List any previous therapy, the duration, and the outcome.
3. Obtain appropriate baseline lab studies and cultures. Evaluate for impaired renal function, blood dyscrasias, and liver dysfunction.
4. Assess for GI disturbance and auditory nerve impairment; document and report.
5. Obtain baseline CXR; auscultate and document lung sounds and characteristics of sputum. Note PPD skin test results.

Client/Family Teaching

1. Take drug on an empty stomach 1 hr before or 2 hr after meals. Advise to report if GI upset occurs.
2. Explain the importance of taking this medication for months to effectively treat tuberculosis.
3. Advise not to stop taking medication or skip doses without provider consent.
4. Avoid alcohol as this increases the risk of liver toxicity.
5. Symptoms such as headache, drowsiness, confusion, fever, and muscle and joint aches may occur during the first few weeks of therapy; report if symptoms persist or increase in intensity.
6. Rifampin may impart a red-orange color to urine, feces, saliva, sputum, and tears; contact lenses may become *permanently* discolored.
7. Women of childbearing age should practice alternative birth control since oral contraceptives may not be effective. Advise that drug has teratogenic properties.
8. Review drug side effects stressing those which require medical intervention.

Evaluate

- Effectiveness as a combination agent in treating tuberculosis based on radiographic and lab evidence
- Prophylaxis of meningitis due to *H. influenzae* and gram-negative bacteremia in infants

—COMBINATION DRUG—

Rifampin and Isoniazid

(rih-**FAM**-pin, **eye**-soh-**NYE**-ah-zid)
Rifamate, Rimactane/INH Dual Pack
(Rx)

See also *Rifampin, Isoniazid,* Chapter 16.

How Supplied: See Content

Content: Each capsule contains the following antituberculosis drugs: rifampin, 300 mg, and isoniazid, 150 mg.

Uses: Pulmonary tuberculosis following completion of initial therapy. Concomitant treatment with pyridoxine is recommended in malnourished clients, in those predisposed to neuropathy (e.g., alcoholics, diabetics), and in adolescents.

Dosage

- **Capsules**

  Pulmonary tuberculosis.

Adults: Two capsules once daily.

Administration/Storage: The drug should be taken either 1 hr before or 2 hr after a meal.

Contraindications: To treat meningococcal infections or asymptomatic carriers of *Neisseria meningitidis* to eliminate meningococci from the nasopharynx. In those who have previous isoniazid-induced hepatic injury or who have had severe side effects to isoniazid.

Special Concerns: Use with caution in impaired liver function as rifampin and isoniazid can cause liver dysfunction and fatal hepatitis, respectively. Use with caution, if at all, during lactation.

Side Effects: See individual entries for rifampin and isoniazid.

NURSING CONSIDERATIONS

See also *Nursing Considerations* for *Rifampin, Isoniazid,* Chapter 16.

Assessment

1. Document onset of symptoms, source of contact, and any other agents prescribed with the outcome.
2. Note any previous experience with this drug. Renal hypersensitivity has been reported when therapy was resumed after interruption.
3. Note any evidence of alcohol abuse or liver or renal dysfunction.
4. Obtain baseline CBC, CXR, and liver and renal function studies and monitor periodically throughout therapy.

Client/Family Teaching

1. Take exactly as prescribed and do not skip doses or share medications. Caution against intentional or accidental interruption of the daily dosage regimen.
2. Body secretions (urine, feces, tears, sputum, sweat) may become discolored orange-red. Do not wear soft contact lenses as these may become permanently stained.
3. Report any numbness or tingling in hands and feet as this is suggestive of peripheral neuropathy or toxicity. Coadministration of pyridoxine may help prevent CNS toxic effects.
4. Symptoms of fatigue, weakness, malaise, N&V, and anorexia (symptoms of hepatitis) should be reported immediately.
5. Do not use oral birth control methods, as these may be ineffective.
6. Advise that therapy will be continued until bacterial conversion and maximal improvement have been observed.

Evaluate: Successful treatment and resolution of tubercle bacilli.

CHAPTER SEVENTEEN

Leprostatics

See the following individual entries:

Clofazimine
Dapsone

Clofazimine

(kloh-**FAYZ**-ih-meen)
Pregnancy Category: C
Lamprene **(Rx)**

How Supplied: *Capsule:* 50 mg
Action/Kinetics: This drug is thought to exert a bactericidal effect on the mycobacterium; the drug inhibits mycobacterial growth and binds to mycobacterial DNA. Cross-resistance with rifampin or dapsone is not observed. The drug is concentrated in fatty tissues and the reticuloendothelial system. **t½:** 70 days. The drug is excreted in the feces via the bile, as well as in sputum, sweat, and sebum.
Uses: Lepromatous leprosy (including dapsone-resistant leprosy and leprosy complicated by erythema nodosum leprosum). In combination with other drugs to prevent resistance in multibacillary leprosy.

Dosage

- **Capsules**

Leprosy resistant to dapsone.
100 mg/day together with one or more other leprostatic drugs for a period of 3 years; **maintenance:** clofazimine alone, 100 mg/day.

Erythema nodosum leprosum.
Dosage depends on severity of symptoms, but doses greater than 200 mg/day are not recommended. Goal is 100 mg/day.

Administration/Storage
1. Clofazimine should be given with one or more other leprostatic agents to prevent the development of resistance to each drug.
2. *Treatment of Overdose:* Gastric lavage or induction of vomiting. General supportive measures.
Special Concerns: Use with caution in clients with abdominal pain or diarrhea. Use during lactation only if benefits outweigh risks. Safety and efficacy have not been determined in children.
Laboratory Test Interferences: ↑ AST, serum bilirubin, albumin.
Side Effects: *GI:* N&V, diarrhea, abdominal or epigastric pain. Rarely, GI bleeding, intestinal obstruction, anorexia, constipation, liver enlargement. *Dermatologic:* Pink to brownish black pigmentation of skin, ichthyosis, dryness of skin, pruritus, rash. *Ophthalmologic:* Pigmentation of conjunctiva and cornea (due to clofazimine crystals), phototoxicity, decreased vision, eye irritation, burning, itching, or dryness. *CNS:* Headache, dizziness, drowsiness, neuralgia, fatigue, depression. *Miscellaneous:* Jaundice, weight loss, hepatitis, anemia, ***thromboembolism,*** bone pain, edema, cystitis, fever, vascular pain, lymphadenopathy, eosinophilia, hypokalemia. Discoloration of urine, feces, sweat, or sputum.

NURSING CONSIDERATIONS

Client/Family Teaching
1. Take medication as ordered and with food to minimize GI irritation.
2. Report any increased GI distress, depression, and/or unusual side effects immediately.
3. Although reversible, clofazimine will cause pink to brownish black skin discoloration, which may persist after therapy.
4. Do not be alarmed because all body fluids become discolored during therapy.

5. Oil baths and frequent lotion application may minimize itchy, dry skin formation.

Evaluate

- Reports of symptomatic improvement
- ↓ Size and number of skin lesions

Dapsone (DDS, Diphenylsulfone)

(**DAP**-sohn)
Pregnancy Category: C
Avlosulfon ✤ **(Rx)**

How Supplied: *Tablet:* 25 mg, 100 mg

Action/Kinetics: Dapsone is a synthetic agent with both bacteriostatic and bactericidal activity, especially against *Mycobacterium leprae* (Hansen's bacillus). Although the exact mechanism is not known, dapsone is thought to act similarly to sulfonamides in that it interferes with the metabolism of the infectious organism. Widely distributed throughout the body. **Peak plasma levels:** 4–8 hr. Doses of 200 mg/day for 8 days will lead to a plateau plasma level of 0.1–7 mcg/mL. **t½:** About 28 hr. The drug is acetylated in the liver and metabolites are excreted in the urine.

Uses: Lepromatous and tuberculoid types of leprosy, dermatitis herpetiformis, and for prophylaxis of malaria. *Investigational:* Relapsing polychondritis.

Dosage

- **Tablets**

Leprosy.

Adults: 50–100 mg/day. The full dose should be initiated and continued without interruption.

Leprosy, bacteriologically negative tuberculoid and indeterminate type.

Adults: 100 mg/day with rifampin, 600 mg/day for 6 months; **then,** continue dapsone for a minimum of 3 years.

Leprosy, lepromatous and borderline clients.

100 mg/day for at least 10 years.

Dermatitis herpetiformis.

Adults, initial: 50 mg/day; dosage may be increased to 300 mg/day or higher, if necessary. **Maintenance:** Reduce dosage to minimum maintenance dose as soon as possible; maintenance dosage may be reduced or eliminated in clients on a gluten-free diet. Dosage should be correspondingly less in children.

Administration/Storage

1. For tuberculoid and indeterminate clients, dosage should be continued for at least 3 years.
2. For lepromatous clients, full dosage may be necessary for life.
3. Possible resistance to dapsone should be carefully evaluated, especially if lepromatous or borderline lepromatous clients relapse. If there is no response to dapsone therapy within 3–6 months, dapsone resistance can be confirmed.
4. *Treatment of Overdose:* Gastric lavage. In normal and methemoglobin-reductase deficient clients, give methylene blue, 1–2 mg/kg by slow IV (may need to be repeated if methemoglobin reaccumulates). In nonemergencies, methylene blue may be given PO, 3–5 mg/kg/4–6 hr.

Contraindications: Advanced amyloidosis of kidneys. Lactation.

Laboratory Test Interference: Altered liver function tests.

Side Effects: *Hematologic:* ***Hemolytic anemia,*** methemoglobinemia. *GI:* N&V, anorexia, abdominal discomfort. *CNS:* Headache, insomnia, vertigo, paresthesia, psychoses, peripheral neuropathy. *Dermatologic:* Photosensitivity, lupus-like syndrome. *Hypersensitivity:* Severe skin reactions including exfoliative dermatitis, erythema multiforme, urticaria, erythema nodosum, toxic erythema, toxic epidermal necrolysis, morbilliform and scarlatiniform reactions. *Miscellaneous:* Muscle weakness, hypoalbuminemia, albuminuria, nephrotic syndrome, renal papillary necrosis, blurred vision, tinnitus, male infertility, fever, tachycardia, mononucleosis-type syndrome.

A leprosy-reactional state may occur in large numbers of clients during therapy with dapsone. Type 1 occurs soon after therapy is initiated. Clients manifest an enhanced delayed hypersensitivity syndrome, leading to swelling of existing nerve and skin lesions with possible neuritis. However, this is not an indication to discontinue therapy. Steroids, analgesics, and surgical decompression of swollen nerve trunks may be used to reduce symptoms. Type 2 occurs in nearly 50% of clients during the first year of therapy. Symptoms include fever, erythematous skin nodules, joint swelling, neuritis, orchitis, malaise, depression, iritis, or epistaxis. Usually therapy is continued with the use of analgesics, steroids, or clofazimine to suppress the reaction.

Symptoms of Overdose: N&V, hyperexcitability (up to 24 hr after ingestion of an overdose). Methemoglobin-induced depression, ***seizures,*** severe cyanosis, headache, hemolysis.

Drug Interactions

Para-aminobenzoic acid / ↓ Effect of dapsone

Probenecid / ↑ Effect of dapsone due to inhibition of renal excretion

Pyrimethamine / ↑ Risk of hematologic reactions

Rifampin / ↓ Effect of dapsone due to ↑ plasma clearance

NURSING CONSIDERATIONS

See also *General Nursing Considerations for All Anti-Infectives,* Chapter 1.

Assessment

1. Obtain baseline CBC and liver and renal function studies, and monitor throughout therapy.
2. Note indications for therapy and type and onset of symptoms. Document size, extent, and location of lesions.

Interventions

1. Dosage will be increased slowly during initiation period.
2. Check whether client is to receive hematinics.
3. Use strict medical asepsis because client may have leukopenia.
4. Observe clients in whom there are other concurrent chronic conditions particularly closely and anticipate reduction in dosage of sulfones.
5. Assess for symptoms of anemia. Report RBC count below 2,500,000/mm^3 or if it remains low during first 6 weeks of therapy. Also note when WBCs fall below 5,000/mm^3.

Client/Family Teaching

1. Take medication exactly as ordered.
2. Follow diet as prescribed (e.g., gluten-free) and refer to dietitian as needed for additional counseling and instruction.
3. Instruct lactating mothers to report cyanosis of nursing infant because this indicates high sulfone levels, and withdrawal of drug may be indicated.
4. Provide a printed list of drug side effects. Any evidence of psychoses, GI disturbances, lepra reaction, headaches, dizziness, lethargy, severe malaise, tinnitus, paresthesias, deep aches, neuralgic pains, and ocular disturbances should be reported.
5. Report allergic dermatitis, which usually appears before week 10 of therapy. Allergic dermatitis may develop into fatal exfoliative dermatitis.
6. Stress the importance of reporting for scheduled laboratory studies and follow-up visits to evaluate effectiveness of therapy.
7. Identify local support groups that may assist the client to understand and cope with this chronic disease.

Evaluate

- ↓ Size and extent of lesions
- Improvement in inflammation and ulceration of the mucous membranes during the first 3–6 months of therapy. (Lack of response may indicate a need for other therapy.)
- Malaria prophylaxis

CHAPTER EIGHTEEN

Urinary Anti-Infectives and Analgesics

See the following individual entries:

Cinoxacin
Flavoxate Hydrochloride
Methenamine Hippurate
Methenamine Mandelate
Methylene Blue
Nalidixic Acid
Nitrofurantoin Macrocrystals
Oxybutynin Chloride
Phenazopyridine Hydrochloride

Cinoxacin

(sin-**OX**-ah-sin)
Pregnancy Category: B
Cinobac Pulvules **(Rx)**

See also *Anti-Infectives,* Chapter 1.

How Supplied: *Capsule:* 250 mg, 500 mg

Action/Kinetics: Cinoxacin, which is related chemically to nalidixic acid, acts by inhibiting DNA replication, resulting in a bactericidal action. It is rapidly absorbed after PO administration; a 500-mg dose results in a urine concentration of 300 mcg/mL during the first 4-hr period and 100 mcg/mL during the second 4-hr period. Within 24 hr, 97% is excreted in the urine, 60% unchanged. **Mean serum t½:** 1.5 hr. Food decreases peak serum levels by approximately 30% but not the total amount absorbed.

Uses: Initial and recurrent UTIs caused by *Escherichia coli, Proteus mirabilis, P. vulgaris, Klebsiella,* and *Enterobacter* species. Prevents UTIs for up to 5 months in women with a history of UTIs. *NOTE:* Cinoxacin is ineffective against *Pseudomonas,* staphylococci, and enterococci infections. Prophylaxis of UTIs.

Dosage

- **Capsules**

UTIs.

Adults: 1 g/day in two to four divided doses for 7–14 days. *In clients with impaired renal function:* **Initial,** 500 mg; **then,** dosage schedule based on creatinine clearance (see package insert).

Prophylaxis of UTIs in women.

250 mg at bedtime for up to 5 months.

Administration/Storage: *Treatment of Overdose:* Well hydrate the client to prevent crystalluria. Maintain an airway and support ventilation and perfusion. VS, blood gases, and serum electrolytes should be meticulously monitored. Decrease absorption by giving activated charcoal.

Contraindications: Hypersensitivity to cinoxacin or other quinolones. Infants and prepubertal children. Anuric clients. Lactation.

Special Concerns: Use with caution in clients with hepatic or kidney disease. Safety and efficacy in children less than 18 years of age have not been determined.

Laboratory Test Interferences: ↑ BUN, AST, ALT, serum creatinine, and alkaline phosphatase. ↓ Hematocrit/hemoglobin.

Side Effects: *GI:* N&V, anorexia, abdominal cramps and pain, diarrhea, altered sensation of taste. *CNS:* Headache, dizziness, insomnia, drowsiness, confusion, nervousness. *Hypersensitivity:* Rash, pruritus, urticaria, edema, angioedema, eosinophilia, ***anaphylaxis (rare)***, toxic epidermal necrolysis (rare), erythema multiforme, ***Stevens-Johnson syndrome***. *Other:* Tingling sensation, photophobia, perineal burning, tinnitus, thrombocytopenia.

Symptoms of Overdose: Anorexia, N&V, epigastric distress, diarrhea, headache, dizziness, insomnia, photophobia, tinnitus, and a tingling sensation.

Drug Interaction: Probenecid ↓ excretion of cinoxacin → ↓ concentration in the urine.

NURSING CONSIDERATIONS

See also *Nursing Considerations for All Anti-Infectives,* Chapter 1.

Assessment

1. Ascertain that renal and hepatic function tests are completed before initiating therapy.
2. Determine if client is anuric; if so do not administer.

Client/Family Teaching

1. Take exactly as directed.
2. Consume 2–3 L/day of fluids to ensure adequate hydration.
3. Advise that acidic fluids enhance drug action (cranberry, prune juice) and to limit intake of alkaline products (milk, bicarbonate).
4. Photosensitivity reaction may occur; avoid unnecessary sun exposure, use sunscreens, protective clothing, and sunglasses.

Evaluate

- ↓ S&S of UTI (dysuria, frequency)
- Negative urine culture results

Flavoxate hydrochloride

(flay-**VOX**-ayt)
Pregnancy Category: B
Urispas **(Rx)**

How Supplied: *Tablet:* 100 mg

Action/Kinetics: Flavoxate relieves muscle spasms of the urinary tract by acting directly on the smooth muscle; it relaxes the detrusor muscle by cholinergic blockade. The drug has local anesthetic and analgesic effects also. It is well absorbed from GI tract; 10%–30% is excreted in urine.

Uses: Symptomatic relief of urinary tract irritation, dysuria, urgency, nocturia, suprapubic pain, incontinence associated with cystitis, prostatitis, urethritis, urethrocystitis, and other urinary tract disorders. Compatible for use with urinary tract germicides.

Dosage

- **Tablets**

Adults and children over 12 years: 100 or 200 mg t.i.d.–q.i.d. Dose may be reduced when symptoms decrease.

Contraindications: Obstructive disorders of urinary tract, including pyloric or duodenal obstructions, intestinal lesions, ileus, achalasia (absence of gastric acid), and GI hemorrhage.

Special Concerns: Use with caution in glaucoma. Use with caution during lactation. Confusion is more likely to occur in geriatric clients. Safety and effectiveness have not been determined in children less than 12 years of age.

Side Effects: *GI:* N&V, xerostomia. *CNS:* Drowsiness, headache, vertigo, nervousness, mental confusion (especially in the elderly). *CV:* Tachycardia, palpitations. *Hematologic:* Eosinophilia, leukopenia. *Ophthalmologic:* Blurred vision, increased ocular tension, accommodation disturbances. *Other:* Urticaria, skin rashes, fever, dysuria.

NURSING CONSIDERATIONS

See also *Nursing Considerations* for *Cholinergic Blocking Agents,* Chapter 49.

Client/Family Teaching

1. Do not drive a car or operate hazardous machinery because drug may cause drowsiness and blurred vision.
2. Practice good oral hygiene. Relieve dryness of mouth with ice chips or hard candy. Ensure adequate hydration.
3. Avoid strenuous exercise; advise that the body's heat-regulating mechanism may be altered and sweating inhibited.
4. Report any persistent, bothersome, or new symptoms.

Evaluate

- Reports of symptomatic relief in urinary tract symptoms and discomfort
- Normal patterns of urinary elimination

Methenamine hippurate

(meh-**THEEN**-ah-meen)
Pregnancy Category: C
Hip-Rex ✱, Hiprex, Urex **(Rx)**

Methenamine mandelate

(meh-**THEEN**-ah-meen)
Pregnancy Category: C
Mandelamine **(Rx)**

How Supplied: Methenanamine hippurate: *Tablet:* 1 g
Methenamine mandelate: *Tablet:* 0.5 g, 1 g; *Suspension:* 0.5 g/5 mL

Action/Kinetics: This drug is converted in an acid medium into ammonia and formaldehyde (the active principle), which denatures protein. Formaldehyde levels in the urine may be bacteriostatic or bactericidal, depending on the pH; it is most effective when the urine has a pH value of 5.5 or less, which is maintained by using the hippurate or mandelate salt. Readily absorbed from GI tract but up to 60% may be hydrolyzed by gastric acid if tablets are not enteric-coated. To be effective, urinary formaldehyde concentration must be greater than 25 mcg/mL. **Peak levels of formaldehyde:** 2 hr if using hippurate and 3–8 hr if using mandelate (if urinary pH is 5.5 or less) **t¹/₂:** 3–6 hr. Seventy to 90% of drug and metabolites excreted in urine within 24 hr.

Uses: Acute, chronic, and recurrent UTIs by susceptible organisms, especially gram-negative organisms including *Escherichia coli.* As a prophylactic before urinary tract instrumentation. Never used as sole agent in the treatment of acute infections.

Dosage

- **Tablets**

Hippurate: **Adults and children over 12 years:** 1 g b.i.d. in the morning and evening; **children, 6–12 years:** 0.5 g b.i.d.

- **Oral Suspension, Enteric-Coated Tablets**

Mandelate: **Adults:** 1 g q.i.d. after meals and at bedtime; **children 6–12 years:** 0.5 g q.i.d.; **children under 6 years:** 0.25 g/13.6 kg q.i.d.

Administration/Storage: *Treatment of Overdose:*Absorption following overdose may be minimized by inducing vomiting or by gastric lavage, followed by activated charcoal. Fluids should be forced.

Contraindications: Renal insufficiency, severe liver damage, severe dehydration. Concurrent use of sulfonamides as an insoluble precipitate may form with formaldehyde.

Special Concerns: Use with caution in gout (methenamine may cause urate crystals to precipitate in the urine).

Laboratory Test Interference: False + urinary glucose with Benedict's solution. Drug interferes with determination of urinary catecholamines and estriol levels by acid hydrolysis technique (enzymatic techniques not affected). False + catecholamines, hydroxycorticosteroids, vanillylmandelic acid; false – 5-hydroxyindoleacetic acid.

Side Effects: *GI:* N&V, diarrhea, anorexia, cramps, stomatitis. *GU:* Hematuria, albuminuria, crystalluria, dysuria, urinary frequency or urgency, bladder irritation. *Dermatologic:* Skin rashes, urticaria, pruritus, erythematous eruptions. *Other:* Headache, dyspnea, edema, lipoid pneumonitis.

Drug Interactions

Acetazolamide / ↓ Effect of methenamine due to inhibition of conversion to formaldehyde
Sodium bicarbonate / ↓ Effect of methenamine due to inhibition of conversion to formaldehyde
Sulfonamides / ↑ Chance of sulfonamide crystalluria due to acid urine produced by methenamine
Thiazide diuretics / ↓ Effect of me-

thenamine due to ↑ alkalinity of urine produced by thiazides

NURSING CONSIDERATIONS

See also *Nursing Considerations for All Anti-Infectives,* Chapter 1.

Assessment

1. Note any history of gout.
2. List other agents prescribed and ensure that client is not concurrently prescribed sulfonamides.

Interventions

1. An acidic urine should be maintained, especially when treating *Proteus* or *Pseudomonas* infections.
2. Oral methenamine mandelate suspensions have a vegetable oil base; particular care should thus be taken in the elderly or debilitated to prevent lipid pneumonia.
3. Clearly indicate on chart that client is receiving drug because drug will interfere with tests to determine urinary estriol, catecholamines, and HIAA.
4. Urine may become turbid and full of sediment when methenamine mandelate is administered concomitantly with sulfamethizole.
5. Monitor urine sample for any evidence of hematuria and/or albuminuria.

Client/Family Teaching

1. If GI upset occurs, the drug can be taken with food.
2. Maintain an adequate fluid intake of 1.5–2 L/day. Instruct client on how to keep a record of I&O and the appropriate foods to include in the diet.
3. To maintain an acidic urine, alkalizing foods (e.g., milk products) or medication (e.g., acetazolamide, bicarbonate) should not be taken in excess.
4. Advise which foods (such as prunes, plums, and cranberry juice) may help maintain acid urine. Drugs such as ascorbic acid, methionine, ammonium chloride, or sodium diphosphate may additionally be required.
5. Instruct client in the use of Labstix or Nitrazine paper to test that pH of urine is 5.5 or lower.
6. Clients on high dosage of drug should report any evidence of bladder irritation or painful and frequent micturition.
7. Report adverse drug effects such as N&V, skin rash, tinnitus, and muscle cramps as these may require termination of drug therapy.

Evaluate

- Resolution of UTI and reports of symptomatic improvement
- Negative urine C&S results

Methylene blue (Methylthionine blue)

(**METH**-ih-leen)

Urolene Blue **(Rx)**

How Supplied: *Injection:* 10 mg/mL; *Solution:* 2%; *Tablet:* 65 mg

Action/Kinetics: Methylene blue is a dye possessing bacteriostatic activity. High doses oxidize Fe^2 (ferrous ion) of reduced hemoglobin to Fe^3 (ferric ion), resulting in methemoglobinemia (basis for use in cyanide poisoning). Lower doses increase the conversion of methemoglobin to hemoglobin.

Uses: Mild GU tract antiseptic for cystitis and urethritis. Drug-induced or idiopathic methemoglobinemia. Antidote for cyanide poisoning. *Investigational:* Treatment of oxalate and phosphate urinary tract calculi.

Dosage

- **Tablets**

  GU antiseptic.

65–130 mg t.i.d. after meals with a full glass of water.

- **IV**

  Antidote.

1–2 mg/kg slowly over several minutes.

Contraindications: Hypersensitivity to drug. Renal insufficiency. G6PD deficiency because hemolysis may result.

Side Effects: *GI:* N&V, diarrhea. *GU:* Dysuria, bladder irritation, may cause urine or feces to turn blue-green. *Other:* Anemia, fever, cyanosis, CV abnormalities.

NURSING CONSIDERATIONS

Client/Family Teaching: Stress that medication may turn urine and stools a blue-green color and will stain body tissues.

Evaluate
- Resolution of cyanide toxicity
- Evidence of fistula formation

Nalidixic acid

(nah-lih-**DICKS**-ick **AH**-sid)
Pregnancy Category: B
NegGram **(Rx)**

How Supplied: *Suspension:* 250 mg/5 mL; *Tablet:* 250 mg, 500 mg, 1 g

Action/Kinetics: Nalidixic acid is believed to inhibit the DNA synthesis of the microorganism, probably by interfering with DNA polymerization. The drug is either bacteriostatic or bactericidal. Nalidixic acid is rapidly absorbed from the GI tract. **Peak plasma concentration:** 20–40 mcg/mL after 1–2 hr; **peak urine levels:** 150–200 mcg/mL after 3–4 hr. **t½, plasma:** 1.5 hr (increased to 21 hr in anuric clients); **t½, urine:** 6 hr. The drug is metabolized in the liver to hydroxynalidixic acid (comparable activity to nalidixic acid) and inactive compounds which are rapidly excreted. The drug is extensively protein bound.

Sensitivity determinations are recommended before and periodically during prolonged administration of nalidixic acid. Renal and liver function tests are advisable if course of therapy exceeds 2 weeks.

Uses: Acute and chronic UTIs caused by susceptible gram-negative organisms, including *Escherichia coli, Proteus, Enterobacter,* and *Klebsiella.*

Dosage

- **Oral Suspension, Tablets**

Adults: initially, 1 g q.i.d. for 1–2 weeks; **maintenance,** if necessary, 0.5 g q 6 hr. Maximum daily dose: 4 g. **Children, 3 months to 12 years, initial:** 55 mg/kg/day in four equally divided doses; **maintenance:** 33 mg/kg/day.

Administration/Storage

1. Underdosage (less than 4 g/day) initially may lead to emergence of bacterial resistance.
2. *Treatment of overdose:* Gastric lavage if the overdose is identified early. If absorption has occurred, fluid administration is increased with supportive measures. In severe cases, use of anticonvulsants may be necessary.

Contraindications: To be used with caution in clients with liver disease, severely impaired kidney function, epilepsy, and severe cerebral arteriosclerosis. Lactation. Use not recommended for infants less than 3 months of age.

Special Concerns: Use with care in prepubertal children.

Laboratory Test Interferences: False + for urinary glucose with Benedict's solution, Fehling's solution, or Clinitest Reagent tablets. Falsely elevated 17-ketosteroids.

Side Effects: *GI:* N&V, diarrhea, abdominal pain. *CNS:* Drowsiness, headache, dizziness, weakness, vertigo, toxic psychoses, intracranial hypertension, ***seizures (rare)***. Also, increased intracranial pressure with bulging anterior fontanel, papilledema, and headache; sixth cranial nerve palsy in children and infants. *Allergic:* Photosensitivity (e.g., erythema, painful bullae on exposed skin), skin rashes, arthralgia (joint swelling and stiffness), pruritus, urticaria, angioedema, eosinophilia, anaphylaxis (rare). *Hematologic:* Leukopenia, thrombocytopenia, ***hemolytic anemia*** (especially in clients with G6PD deficiency). *Ophthalmic:* Reversible subjective visual disturbances, including overbrightness of lights, difficulty in focusing, changes in color perception, double vision, decreased visual acuity. *Other:* Metabolic acidosis, cholestatic jaundice, cholestasis, paresthesia.

Symptoms of Overdose: Toxic psychoses, convulsions, increased intracranial pressure, nausea, vomiting, lethargy, metabolic acidosis.

Drug Interactions

Antacids, oral / ↓ Effect of nalidixic acid due to ↓ absorption from GI tract
Anticoagulants, oral / ↑ Effect of anticoagulants due to ↓ plasma protein binding

Nitrofurantoin / ↓ Effect of nalidixic acid

NURSING CONSIDERATIONS

See also *Nursing Considerations for All Anti-Infectives,* Chapter 1.

Assessment

1. Note any history of liver or renal dysfunction.
2. Determine that baseline CBC and urine cultures have been performed.
3. Assess for any adverse CNS effects, e.g., seizures, psychosis, severe headaches or evidence of increased ICP. Withhold drug and report if evident.

Client/Family Teaching

1. Take drug 1 hr before meals, on an empty stomach. If GI upset occurs, may be taken with food.
2. Drink at least 2–3 L/day of water during drug therapy.
3. Do not perform tasks that require mental alertness until drug effects realized. Drug may cause drowsiness, confusion, blurred vision, and dizziness.
4. Avoid prolonged exposure to sunlight or ultraviolet light. Wear protective clothing and sunscreen if exposure is necessary. Advise that photosensitivity may remain for 3 months following therapy.

Evaluate

• Negative urine culture reports
• Reports of symptomatic improvement (↓ dysuria, ↓ frequency)

Nitrofurantoin macrocrystals

(**nye**-troh-fyour-**AN**-toyn)
Pregnancy Category: B
Macrobid, Macrodantin **(Rx)**

See also *Anti-Infectives,* Chapter 1.

How Supplied: *Capsule:* 25 mg, 50 mg, 100 mg

Action/Kinetics: Nitrofurantoin interferes with bacterial carbohydrate metabolism by inhibiting acetyl coenzyme A; the drug also interferes with bacterial cell wall synthesis. It is bacteriostatic at low concentrations and bactericidal at high concentrations. Tablets are readily absorbed from the GI tract; bioavailability is increased by food. **$t^1/_2$:** 20 min (60 min in anephric clients). **Urine levels:** 50–250 mcg/mL. If the creatinine clearance is less than 40 mL/min, urine antibacterial levels are inadequate with the subsequent higher blood levels increasing the possibility of toxicity. Antibacterial activity is best in an acid urine. From 30% to 50% excreted unchanged in the urine. Nitrofurantoin macrocrystals (Macrodantin) are available; this preparation maintains effectiveness while decreasing GI distress.

Uses: UTIs due to susceptible strains of *Escherichia coli, Staphylococcus aureus* (not for treatment of pyelonephritis or perinephric abscesses), enterococci, and certain strains of *Enterobacter* and *Klebsiella.*

Dosage

• Capsules, Oral Suspension, Tablets

UTIs.

Adults: 50–100 mg q.i.d., not to exceed 600 mg/day. For cystitis, Macrobid is given in doses of 100 mg b.i.d. for 7 days. **Pediatric, 1 month of age and over:** 5–7 mg/kg/day in four equal doses.

Prophylaxis of UTIs.

Adults: 50–100 mg at bedtime. **Pediatric, 1 month of age and over:** 1 mg/kg/day at bedtime or in two divided doses daily.

Administration/Storage

1. Administer PO medication with meals or milk to promote absorption and reduce gastric irritation.
2. Preferably, administer capsules containing crystals, instead of tablets, because crystals cause less GI intolerance.
3. Store PO medications in amber-colored bottles.
4. The medication should be continued for a minimum of 3 days after obtaining a negative urine culture.
5. *Treatment of overdose:* Induce emesis. High fluid intake to promote urinary excretion. The drug is dialyzable.

Contraindications: Anuria, oliguria, and clients with impaired renal function (creatinine clearance below

40 mL/min); pregnant women, especially near term; infants less than 1 month of age; and nursing mothers.
Special Concerns: To be used with extreme caution in clients with anemia, diabetes, electrolyte imbalance, avitaminosis B, or a debilitating disease. Safety during lactation has not been established.
Laboratory Test Interferences: ↑ AST, ALT, serum phosphorus. ↓ Hemoglobin.
Side Effects: Nitrofurantoin is a potentially toxic drug with many side effects. *GI:* N&V, anorexia, diarrhea, abdominal pain, parotitis, pancreatitis. *CNS:* Headache, dizziness, vertigo, drowsiness, nystagmus, confusion, depression, euphoria, psychotic reactions (rare). *Hematologic:* Leukopenia, thrombocytopenia, eosinophilia, megaloblastic anemia, ***agranulocytosis,*** granulocytopenia, ***hemolytic anemia (especially in clients with G6PD deficiency).*** *Allergic:* Drug fever, skin rashes, pruritus, urticaria, angioedema, exfoliative dermatitis, erythema multiforme ***(rarely, Stevens-Johnson syndrome), anaphylaxis,*** arthralgia, myalgia, chills, sialadenitis, asthma symptoms in susceptible clients; maculopapular, erythematous, or eczematous eruption. *Pulmonary:* Sudden onset of dyspnea, cough, chest pain, fever and chills; pulmonary infiltration with consolidation or pleural effusion on x-ray, elevated sedimentation rate, eosinophilia. *After subacute or chronic use:* dyspnea, nonproductive cough, malaise, interstitial pneumonitis. Permanent impairment of pulmonary function with chronic therapy. A lupus-like syndrome associated with pulmonary reactions. *Hepatic:* Hepatitis, cholestatic jaundice, chronic active hepatitis, hepatic necrosis (rare). *CV:* Benign intracranial hypertension, changes in ECG, collapse, cyanosis. *Miscellaneous:* Peripheral neuropathy, asthenia, alopecia, superinfections of the GU tract, muscle pain.

Drug Interactions

Acetazolamide / ↓ Effect of nitrofurantoin due to ↑ alkalinity of urine produced by acetazolamide
Antacids, oral / ↓ Effect of nitrofurantoin due to ↓ absorption from GI tract
Anticholinergic drugs / ↑ Effect of nitrofurantoin due to ↑ absorption from stomach
Magnesium trisilicate / ↓ Absorption of nitrofurantoin from GI tract
Nalidixic acid / Nitrofurantoin ↓ effect of nalidixic acid
Probenecid / High doses ↓ secretion of nitrofurantoin → toxicity
Sodium bicarbonate / ↓ Effect of nitrofurantoin due to ↑ alkalinity of urine produced by sodium bicarbonate

NURSING CONSIDERATIONS

See also *General Nursing Considerations for All Anti-Infectives,* Chapter 1.

Interventions

1. Ensure that appropriate pretreatment lab studies have been performed (CBC, urine C&S, liver and renal functions; also CXR and pulmonary function tests with chronic therapy).
2. Observe client for acute or delayed onset anaphylactic reaction and have emergency equipment readily available.
3. Clearly label chart to show that client is on drug because it may alter certain lab determinations.
4. Monitor for recurrent UTI symptoms and report because urinary superinfections may occur.
5. Blacks and ethnic groups of Mediterranean and Near Eastern origin should be assessed for symptoms of anemia.

Client/Family Teaching

1. Take with food to minimize GI upset and enhance absorption.
2. Take as prescribed and complete the full course of therapy.
3. Increase fluid intake, drink at least 2 quarts of water a day, unless contraindicated. Acidic foods (prunes, cranberry juice, plums) enhance drug action whereas alkaline foods (milk products) minimize drug action.
4. Acid urine enhances antibacterial activity. Teach how to monitor urine pH as needed. Drug may turn urine a dark yellow or brown color.
5. Report any persistent or bothersome side effects. Symptoms of respir-

atory dysfunction require immediate intervention.

6. Immediately report any numbness and tingling in the extremities or flu-like symptoms. These side effects are indications for drug withdrawal because the condition may worsen and become irreversible.

7. Report persistent N&V and diarrhea as these may be symptoms of a GI superinfection.

Evaluate

• Negative urine cultures results

• Resolution of infection and reports of symptomatic improvement (↓ dysuria, ↓ frequency)

Oxybutynin chloride

(ox-ee-**BYOU**-tih-nin)
Pregnancy Category: B
Ditropan **(Rx)**

How Supplied: *Syrup:* 5 mg/5 mL; *Tablet:* 5 mg

Action/Kinetics: Oxybutynin causes increased vesicle capacity and delay of initial urgency to void by exerting a direct antispasmodic effect. Has no effect at either the neuromuscular junction or autonomic ganglia. Has 4–10 times the antispasmodic effect of atropine but only one-fifth the anticholinergic activity. **Onset:** 30–60 min; **Time to peak effect:** 3–6 hr; **duration:** 6–10 hr. Eliminated through the urine.

Use: Neurogenic bladder disease characterized by urinary retention, urinary overflow, incontinence, nocturia, urinary frequency or urgency, reflex neurogenic bladder.

Dosage

• **Syrup, Tablets**

Adults: 5 mg b.i.d.–t.i.d.; maximum dosage, 20 mg/day. **Children, over 5 years:** 5 mg b.i.d.–t.i.d.; maximum dosage, 15 mg/day.

Administration/Storage

1. Store in tight containers at 15°C–30°C (59°F–86°F).

2. *Treatment of Overdose:* Stomach lavage, physostigmine (0.5–2 mg IV; repeat as necessary up to maximum of 5 mg). Supportive therapy, if necessary. Counteract excitement with sodium thiopental (2%) or chloral hydrate (100–200 mL of 2% solution) rectally. Artificial respiration may be necessary if respiratory muscles become paralyzed.

Contraindications: Glaucoma (angle closure), GI obstruction, paralytic ileus, intestinal atony, megacolon, severe colitis, myasthenia gravis, obstructive urinary tract disease, acute hemorrhage.

Special Concerns: *Use with caution when increased cholinergic effect is undesirable and in the elderly.* Safe use in children less than 5 years of age has not been determined. Use with caution in geriatric clients; in clients with autonomic neuropathy, renal, or hepatic disease; and in clients with hiatal hernia with reflex esophagitis. Heat stroke and fever (due to decreased sweating) may occur if given at high environmental temperatures.

Side Effects: *GI:* N&V, constipation, bloated feeling, decreased GI motility. *CNS:* Drowsiness, insomnia, weakness, dizziness, restlessness, hallucinations. *EENT:* Dry mouth, blurred vision, dilation of pupil, cycloplegia, increased ocular tension. *CV:* Tachycardia, palpitations, vasodilation. *Miscellaneous:* Decreased sweating, urinary hesitancy and retention, impotence, suppression of lactation, ***severe allergic reactions,*** drug idiosyncrasies, urticaria, and other dermal manifestations. *NOTE:* The drug may aggravate symptoms of prostatic hypertrophy, hypertension, coronary heart disease, CHF, hyperthyroidism, cardiac arrhythmias, and tachycardia.

Symptoms of Overdose: Intense CNS disturbances (restlessness, psychoses), circulatory changes (flushing, hypotension) and failure, respiratory failure, paralysis, coma.

NURSING CONSIDERATIONS

See also *Nursing Considerations* for *Cholinergic Blocking Agents,* Chapter 49.

Assessment

1. Document indications for therapy and type and onset of symptoms.

2. Review conditions that may be ag-

gravated by oxybutynin and determine if present.

Client/Family Teaching

1. Review prescription and instruct to take only as directed.
2. Provide a printed list of side effects, stressing those that require immediate reporting.
3. Use caution driving a car or in operating dangerous machinery because drug may cause drowsiness and blurred vision.
4. Withhold medication and report if diarrhea occurs (especially in clients with an ileostomy or colostomy) because diarrhea may be an early symptom of intestinal obstruction.
5. Consume 2–3 L/day of fluids to ensure adequate hydration and to relieve symptoms of dry mouth.
6. Vegetables, fruit, fiber, and fluids should be consumed in adequate quantities to prevent constipation.
7. Wear sunglasses, sunscreens, and protective clothing during sunlight exposure as drug may cause a photosensitivity reaction.
8. Avoid overexposure to heat and acknowledge the body's need for increased fluids in hot weather because sweating is inhibited by the drug and heat stroke may occur.
9. Report any loss of effect as dosage may require adjustment.
10. Clients with neurogenic bladder should return as scheduled for cystometry and to evaluate response to therapy to determine the need for continuation of medication.

Evaluate

- Reports of relief of spasms and associated GU pain
- Normal urinary elimination patterns
- Evidence of positive cystometry findings

Phenazopyridine hydrochloride (Phenylazodiaminopyridine HCl)

(fen-**AY**-zoh-**PEER**-ih-deen)
Pregnancy Category: B

Azo-Standard, Baridium, Eridium, Geridium, Phenazo ✱, Phenazodine, Prodium, Pyrazodine, Pyridiate, Pyridin, Pyridium, Urodine, Urogesic, Viridium **(OTC) (Rx)**

How Supplied: *Tablet:* 95 mg, 100 mg, 200 mg

Action/Kinetics: Phenazopyridine HCl is an azo dye with local analgesic and anesthetic effects on the urinary tract. Sixty-five percent excreted unchanged or as metabolites within 24 hr.

Uses: Relief of pain, urgency or frequency, and burning in chronic UTIs or irritation, including cystitis, urethritis and pyelitis, trauma, surgery, or urinary tract instrumentation. May also be used as an adjunct to antibacterial therapy. The underlying cause of the irritation must be determined.

Dosage

- **Tablets**

Adults: 200 mg t.i.d. with or after meals. **Pediatric, 6–12 years:** 4 mg/kg t.i.d. with food.

Administration/Storage: *Treatment of Overdose:* Methylene blue, 1–2 mg/kg IV or 100–200 mg PO of ascorbic acid to treat methemoglobinemia.

Contraindications: Renal insufficiency. Use in children less than 12 years of age. Chronic use to treat undiagnosed pain of the urinary tract.

Side Effects: *GI:* Nausea. *Hematologic:* Methemoglobinemia, ***hemolytic anemia*** (especially in clients with G6PD deficiency). *Dermatologic:* Yellowish tinge of the skin or sclerae may indicate accumulation of drug due to renal insufficiency. *Miscellaneous:* Renal and hepatic toxicity, headache, pruritus, rash.

Symptoms of Overdose: Methemoglobinemia following massive overdoses. Hemolysis due to G6PD deficiency.

Laboratory Test Interferences: Ehrlich's test for urine urobilinogen, phenolsulfonphthalein excretion test for kidney function, urine bilirubin, Clinistix or Tes-Tape, colorimetric laboratory test procedures (e.g., urine ketone tests, urine protein tests, urine steroid determinations).

NURSING CONSIDERATIONS

Assessment

1. Document indications for therapy and type and onset of symptoms.
2. Note any history of liver and/or renal dysfunction.

Client/Family Teaching

1. Take medication with or after meals to prevent GI upset.
2. Should be used for only 2 days when taken together with an antibacterial agent for UTIs.
3. Monitor I&O; consume 2–3 L/day of fluids.
4. In clients with diabetes, finger sticks should be performed to evaluate blood sugar levels.
5. Drug turns urine orange-red; may stain fabrics. Wear a sanitary napkin to avoid staining garments. A 0.25% sodium dithionate or sodium hydrosulfite solution, available from a pharmacy, will remove these stains.
6. Provide a printed list of side effects that indicate toxicity (e.g., yellowing of skin) and advise to report if evident.

Evaluate: Reports of relief of pain and discomfort upon urination in client with UTI.

CHAPTER NINETEEN

Antiviral Agents

See also the following individual entries:

Acyclovir (Acycloguanosine)
Amantadine Hydrochloride
Didanosine (ddI, Dideoxyinosine)
Famciclovir
Foscarnet Sodium
Ganciclovir Sodium (DHPG)
Idoxuridine (IDU)
Ribavirin
Rimantadine Hydrochloride
Stavudine
Trifluridine
Vidarabine
Zalcitabine (Dideoxycytidine, ddC)
Zidovudine (Azidothymidine, AZT)

General Statement: Viruses are among the simplest living organisms in that they are comprised of one or more strands of a linear or helical nucleic acid core, which consists of either DNA or RNA, but not both. Viruses may possess an outer protein or lipoprotein envelope. Classification of viruses is undertaken by the type of nucleic acid present with subclassification based on the cellular site of viral multiplication or some morphologic characteristic.

To maintain their growth and reproduce, viruses must enter living cells; i.e., they use many of the biochemical mechanisms and products of the host cell to survive. Thus, it is difficult to find a drug that is specific for the virus and that does not interfere with the function of the host cell. However, there are enzymes and replicative mechanisms that are unique to viruses and, in recent years, an increasing number of drugs with specific antiviral activity have been developed. Since a mature virus can survive outside the host cell and maintain its infective properties, agents with antiviral activity have been targeted at viral replication. To replicate, the virus must enter the host cell and direct the cell to make new viral particles.

As knowledge of viral replication increased, various stages were identified at which viral replication could thus be affected. These are as follows:

1. Attachment to and penetration of susceptible cells. The virus enters the host cell by a phagocytosis-like mechanism; it is then encapsulated by the host cell cytoplasm. Gamma globulin interferes with entry of the virus particle into a cell, probably by blocking penetration.
2. Uncoating. The protein coat of the virus is dissolved by viral enzymes, thus liberating free viral DNA or RNA. Amantadine inhibits the uncoating of certain viruses after they have entered susceptible cells, thus inhibiting the replication of these viruses.
3. Synthesis of viral components. The genome (total genetic component) of the virus is duplicated and viral proteins are synthesized in the appropriate sequence. Most of the currently approved antiviral drugs act to inhibit the synthesis of RNA and DNA. For example, nucleic acid synthesis is inhibited by acyclovir, didanosine (ddI), famciclovir, foscarnet, ganciclovir, idoxuridine, interferons, ribavirin, stavudine, and vidarabine.
4. Assembly of the viral particle. The viral components are assembled to form the mature virus particle. The vi-

ral genome may or may not be encapsulated by viral protein. Both puromycin and 5-fluoro-2'-deoxyuridine can inhibit assembly of intact viral particles.
5. Release of the virus from the host cell. Viral release may be rapid and result in lysis and death of the host cell or it may be slow and result in cell survival. At the present time, there are no approved drugs that act on this phase of viral replication.

Since replication of certain viruses reaches a maximum at about the time clinical symptoms of the disease are seen, drugs that block viral replication must often be given before the onset of the disease (i.e., prophylactically). Amantadine is a drug that must be given prophylactically against influenza A. On the other hand, with other viruses, replication continues for a period of time after symptoms of the disease are seen. In these infections, inhibition of viral replication will promote healing. Examples are drugs that inhibit DNA replication.

NURSING CONSIDERATIONS

See *General Nursing Considerations For All Anti-Infectives,* Chapter 1.

Assessment

1. Document indications for therapy, type and onset of symptoms, and exposure characteristics if known.
2. Determine which pretreatment baseline lab data should be documented, based on indications for therapy.
3. List other agents and route prescribed to ensure none interact unfavorably.
4. Note underlying medical conditions that may preclude drug therapy with these agents.

Client/Family Teaching

1. Review the appropiate method and frequency for drug administration. Provide written guidelines to promote client understanding and compliance.
2. Stress the importance of taking exactly as directed and counsel not to share medications.
3. Review the anticipated benefits of therapy and identify the associated side effects of prescribed agent(s).
4. Address specific measures necessary to decrease or halt the spread of the disease.
5. Stress the importance of maintaining adequate nutrition and advise to consume 2–3 L/day of fluids during therapy.
6. Report the development of any rashes or unusual symptoms associated with drug therapy.
7. If symptoms do not improve or worsen after specified time frame, report to provider.
8. Stress the importance of close medical supervision and follow-up during drug therapy.

Evaluate

- Prophylaxis of viral infections
- Reduction in length and severity of symptoms of viral infections

Acyclovir (Acycloguanosine)

(ay-**SYE**-kloh-veer, ay-**SYE**-kloh-**GWON**-oh-seen)
Pregnancy Category: C
Zovirax **(Rx)**

How Supplied: *Capsule:* 200 mg; *Ointment:* 5%; *Powder for injection:* 500 mg, 1000 mg; *Suspension:* 200 mg/5 mL; *Tablet:* 400 mg, 800 mg
Action/Kinetics: Acyclovir is converted by HSV-infected cells to acyclovir triphosphate, which interferes with HSV DNA polymerase, thereby inhibiting DNA replication. Systemic absorption is slow from the GI tract (although therapeutic levels are reached) and following topical administration. Food does not affect absorption. **Peak levels after PO:** 1.5–2 hr. The drug is widely distributed in tissues and body fluids. **t½, PO:** 3.3 hr. Metabolites and unchanged drug (up to 85%) are excreted through the kidney. Dosage should be reduced in clients with impaired renal function. It has been found that clients who take acyclovir (600–800 mg/day) along with zidovudine had a significantly prolonged

survival rate compared with clients taking only acyclovir.

Uses: PO. Initial and recurrent genital herpes in immunocompromised and nonimmunocompromised clients. Prophylaxis of frequently recurrent genital herpes infections in nonimmunocompromised clients. Treatment of chickenpox in children ranging from 2 to 18 years of age. Acute treatment of herpes zoster (shingles).

Parenteral. Initial therapy for severe genital herpes in clients who are not immunocompromised; initial and recurrent mucosal and cutaneous HSV-1 and HSV-2 infections in immunocompromised individuals. Varicella zoster infections (shingles) in immunocompromised clients. HSE in clients over 6 months of age. Severe initial cases of genital herpes in clients who are not immunocompromised.

Topical. Acyclovir decreases healing time and duration of viral shedding in initial herpes genitalis. Also used for limited non-life-threatening mucocutaneous HSV infections in immunocompromised clients. The drug does not seem to be beneficial in recurrent herpes genitalis or in herpes labialis in nonimmunocompromised clients.

Investigational: Cytomegalovirus and HSV infection following bone marrow or renal transplantation; herpes simplex ocular infections; herpes simplex proctitis; herpes simplex whitlow; herpes zoster encephalitis; disseminated primary eczema herpeticum; herpes simplex–associated erythema multiforme; infectious mononucleosis; and varicella pneumonia.

Dosage

- **Capsules, Suspension, Tablets**

Initial genital herpes.

200 mg q 4 hr (while awake) for a total of 5 capsules/day for 10 days.

Chronic genital herpes.

400 mg b.i.d., 200 mg t.i.d., or 200 mg 5 times/day for up to 12 months.

Intermittent therapy for genital herpes.

200 mg q 4 hr (while awake) for a total of 5 capsules/day for 5 days.

Herpes zoster, acute treatment.

800 mg q 4 hr 5 times/day for 7–10 days.

Chickenpox.

20 mg/kg (of the suspension) q.i.d. for 5 days. A single dose should not exceed 800 mg.

- **IV infusion**

Mucosal and cutaneous herpes simplex in immunocompromised clients.

Adults: 5 mg/kg infused at a constant rate over 1 hr, q 8 hr (15 mg/kg/day) for 7 days. **Children less than 12 years of age:** 250 mg/m^2 infused at a constant rate over 1 hr, q 8 hr for 7 days.

Varicella-zoster infections (shingles) in immunocompromised clients.

Adults: 10 mg/kg infused at a constant rate over 1 hr, q 8 hr for 7 days. **Children less than 12 years of age:** 500 mg/m^2 infused at a constant rate over at least 1 hr, q 8 hr for 7 days.

Herpes simplex encephalitis.

Adults: 10 mg/kg infused at a constant rate over at least 1 hr, q 8 hr for 10 days. **Children less than 12 years of age:** 500 mg/m^2 infused at a constant rate over at least 1 hr, q 8 hr for 10 days.

- **Topical (5% ointment)**

Adults and children: Lesion should be covered with sufficient amount of ointment (0.5-in. ribbon/4 in.^{2} of surface area) q 3 hr, 6 times/day for 7 days.

Administration/Storage

1. The IV solution is prepared by dissolving the contents of the 500- or 1000-mg vial in 10 or 20 mL sterile water for injection, respectively (final concentration of 50 mg/mL). Infusion concentrations of 7 mg/mL or lower are recommended; thus, the calculated dose must be added to an appropriate IV solution at the correct volume. Reconstituted solution should be used within 12 hr. Bacteriostatic water containing benzyl alco-

hol or parabens should not be used as it will cause a precipitate.
2. IV infusion should be accompanied by adequate hydration to prevent precipitation in renal tubules.
3. The drug is for IV infusion only administered over 1 hr; it should not be administered by rapid or bolus IV, IM, or SC injections.
4. If refrigerated, reconstituted solution may show a precipitate, which dissolves at room temperature.
5. Store ointment in a dry place at room temperature.
6. To prevent spread of infection to other body sites, use a finger cot or rubber glove when applying the cream.
7. Do not exceed recommended dose.
8. Medication should not be shared with others.
9. Both the PO and parenteral dose and/or dosing interval should be adjusted in acute or chronic renal impairment.
10. The suspension may be used to treat varicella zoster infections.
11. *Treatment of Overdose:* Hemodialysis (peritoneal dialysis is less effective).

Contraindications: Hypersensitivity to formulation. Use in the eye. Use to prevent recurrent HSV infections.

Special Concerns: Use with caution during lactation. Use with caution with concomitant intrathecal methotrexate or interferon. Safety and efficacy of PO form not established in children less than 2 years of age. Prolonged or repeated doses in immunocompromised clients may result in emergence of resistant viruses.

Side Effects: PO. *Short-term treatment of herpes simplex. GI:* N&V, diarrhea, anorexia, sore throat, taste of drug. *CNS:* Headache, dizziness, fatigue. *Miscellaneous:* Edema, skin rashes, leg pain, inguinal adenopathy.

Long-term treatment of herpes simplex. GI: N&V, diarrhea, sore throat. *CNS:* Headache, vertigo, insomnia, fatigue, fever, depression, irritability. *Other:* Arthralgia, rashes, palpitations, superficial thrombophlebitis, muscle cramps, menstrual abnormalities, acne, lymphadenopathy, alopecia.

Treatment of herpes zoster. GI: N&V, diarrhea, constipation. *CNS:* Headache, malaise.

Treatment of chickenpox. GI: Diarrhea, constipation, abdominal pain, flatulence. *Dermatologic:* Rash.

Parenteral. *At injection site:* Phlebitis, inflammation. *CNS:* Encephalopathic changes, including lethargy, obtundation, tremors, agitation, confusion, hallucination, ***seizures, coma***, jitters, headache. *Miscellaneous:* Skin rashes, urticaria, sweating, hypotension, nausea, thrombocytosis.

Topical. Transient burning, stinging, pain. Pruritus, rash, vulvitis. *NOTE:* All of these effects have also been reported with the use of a placebo preparation.

Symptoms of Overdose: Increased BUN and serum creatinine, ***renal failure following parenteral overdose.***

Drug Interactions
Probenecid / ↑ Bioavailability and half-life of acyclovir → ↑ effect
Zidovudine / Severe lethargy and drowsiness

NURSING CONSIDERATIONS

See also *General Nursing Considerations for Antiviral Agents,* Chapter 19.

Assessment
1. Ensure that appropriate laboratory studies (CBC, electrolytes, liver and renal functions) have been performed.
2. Document indications for therapy and carefully assess all skin lesions.
3. With chickenpox or herpes zoster, institute appropriate precautions for all susceptible individuals (e.g., pregnant women, immunocompromised clients, and those who have not had chickenpox [may check titer if unknown]).

Client/Family Teaching
1. Apply acyclovir ointment in the amount directed with a finger cot or rubber glove to prevent transmission of infection.
2. Cover all lesions with topical acyclovir as ordered, but do not exceed

the frequency or length of time of recommended treatment.
3. Report any burning, stinging, itching, and rash if they occur when applying acyclovir.
4. Complete all examinations and tests to rule out possible presence of other sexually transmitted diseases.
5. Return for medical supervision if HSV recurs because acyclovir is ineffective for treatment of reinfection. Stress that it is not a cure, it is only used to help manage symptoms.
6. Acyclovir will not prevent transmission of disease to others or prevent reinfection.
7. Use condoms for sexual intercourse to prevent reinfections while undergoing treatment. Advise abstinence during acute outbreaks (lesions present) and condoms at other times during sexual intercourse.
8. The total dose and dosage schedule differ depending on whether the infection is initial or chronic and whether intermittent therapy regimen is being used. Therefore, following prescribed dosage, dosage combinations (i.e., with AZT) and duration of treatment are extremely important.
9. Consume 2–3 L/day of fluids, especially during parenteral therapy, to prevent renal toxicity and crystalluria.
10. Instruct females to have an annual Pap test and explain that an increased risk of cervical cancer has been associated with genital herpes.

Evaluate

- Reports of less severe and less frequent herpes outbreaks
- Crusting and healing of herpetic lesions

Amantadine hydrochloride

(ah-**MAN**-tah-deen)
Pregnancy Category: C
Symadine, Symmetrel **(Rx)**

How Supplied: *Capsule:* 100 mg; *Syrup:* 50 mg/5 mL

Action/Kinetics: As an antiviral agent, amantadine is believed to prevent penetration of the virus into cells, possibly by inhibiting uncoating of the RNA virus. Amantadine may also prevent the release of infectious viral nucleic acid into the host cell. The drug reduces symptoms of viral infections if given within 24–48 hr after onset of illness. For the treatment of parkinsonism, amantadine may increase the release of dopamine from dopaminergic nerve terminals in the substantia nigra of parkinson clients, resulting in an increase in dopamine levels in dopaminergic synapses. Well absorbed from GI tract. **Onset:** 48 hr. **Peak serum concentration:** 0.2 mcg/mL after 1–4 hr. **t½:** range of 9–37 hr, longer in presence of renal impairment. Ninety percent excreted unchanged in urine.

Uses: Influenza A viral infections of the respiratory tract (prophylaxis and treatment of high-risk clients with immunodeficiency, CV, metabolic, neuromuscular, or pulmonary disease). Symptomatic treatment of idiopathic parkinsonism and parkinsonism syndrome resulting from encephalitis, carbon monoxide intoxication, drugs, or cerebral arteriosclerosis. The drug decreases extrapyramidal symptoms, including akinesia, rigidity, tremors, excessive salivation, gait disturbances, and total functional disability. Favorable results have been obtained in about 50% of the clients. Improvements can last for up to 30 months, although some clients report that the effect of the drug wears off in 1–3 months. A rest period or an increased dosage may reestablish effectiveness. For parkinsonism, amantadine hydrochloride is usually used concomitantly with other agents, such as levodopa and anticholinergic agents.

Dosage

- **Capsules, Syrup**

Antiviral.

Adults: 200 mg/day as a single or divided dose. **Children, 1–9 years:**

4.4–8.8 mg/kg/day up to a maximum of 150 mg/day in one or two divided doses (use syrup); **9–12 years:** 100 mg b.i.d.

Prophylactic treatment.
Institute before or immediately after exposure and continue for 10–21 days if used concurrently with vaccine or for 90 days without vaccine.

Symptomatic management.
Initiate as soon as possible and continue for 24–48 hr after disappearance of symptoms. Dose should be decreased in renal impairment (see package insert). Dose should be reduced to 100 mg/day for persons with active seizure disorders due to the increased risk of seizure frequency using daily doses of 200 mg.

Parkinsonism.
When used as sole agent, usual dose is 100 mg b.i.d.; may be necessary to increase up to 400 mg/day in divided doses. When used with other antiparkinson drugs: 100 mg 1–2 times/day.

Drug-induced extrapyramidal symptoms.
100 mg b.i.d. (up to 300 mg/day may be required in some). Dosage should be reduced in clients with impaired renal function.

Administration/Storage
1. Protect capsules from moisture.
2. Therapy should be started for viral illness as soon as possible after symptoms begin and for 24–48 hr after symptoms disappear.
3. *Treatment of Overdose:* Gastric lavage or induction of emesis followed by supportive measures. Ensure that client is well hydrated; give IV fluids if necessary. To treat CNS toxicity, IV physostigmine, 1–2 mg given q 1–2 hr in adults or 0.5 mg at 5–10-min intervals (maximum of 2 mg/hr) in children. Sedatives and anticonvulsants may be given if needed; antiarrhythmics and vasopressors may also be required.

Contraindication: Hypersensitivity to drug.

Special Concerns: Administer with caution to clients with liver and renal disease, history of epilepsy, CHF, peripheral edema, orthostatic hypotension, recurrent eczematoid dermatitis, or severe psychosis, in clients taking CNS stimulant drugs, to those exposed to rubella, and to nursing mothers. Safe use in lactating mothers and in children less than 1 year has not been established.

Side Effects: *GI:* N&V, constipation, anorexia, xerostomia. *CNS:* Depression, psychosis, ***convulsions,*** hallucinations, lightheadedness, confusion, ataxia, irritability, anxiety, headache, dizziness, fatigue, insomnia. *CV:* ***CHF,*** orthostatic hypotension, peripheral edema. *Miscellaneous:* Urinary retention, leukopenia, neutropenia, mottling of skin of the extremities due to poor peripheral circulation (livedo reticularis), skin rashes, visual problems, slurred speech, oculogyric episodes, dyspnea, weakness, eczematoid dermatitis.

Symptoms of Overdose: Anorexia, N&V, CNS effects.

Drug Interactions
Anticholinergics / Additive anticholinergic effects (including hallucinations, confusion), especially with trihexyphenidyl and benztropine
CNS stimulants / May ↑ CNS and psychic effects of amantadine; use cautiously together
Hydrochlorothiazide/triamterene combination / ↓ Urinary excretion of amantadine → ↑ plasma levels
Levodopa / Potentiated by amantadine

NURSING CONSIDERATIONS

See also *General Nursing Considerations For Antiviral Agents,* Chapter 19.

Assessment
1. Obtain a thorough nursing history and note any evidence of seizures, CHF, and renal insufficiency.
2. With active seizure disorder drug dosage must be reduced to prevent breakthrough seizures.
3. With Parkinson's disease, following loss of effectiveness of the drug, benefits may be regained by increasing the dosage or discontinuing the drug for several weeks and then reinstituting it.

Interventions
1. Observe for an increase in seizure

activity and take appropriate precautions. Ensure that dosage is reduced to 100 mg/day.
2. Assess clients with a history of CHF or peripheral edema for increased edema and/or respiratory distress and report promptly.
3. Monitor I&O. Observe clients with renal impairment for crystalluria, oliguria, and increased BUN or creatinine levels.
4. Monitor CNS status and immediately report any mental status changes.

Client/Family Teaching

1. Administer last daily dose several hours before retiring to prevent insomnia.
2. Do not drive a car or work in a situation where alertness is important because medication can affect vision, concentration, and coordination.
3. Rise slowly from a prone position because orthostatic hypotension may occur.
4. Lie down if dizzy or weak to relieve symptoms of orthostatic hypotension.
5. Report diffuse patchy discoloration or mottling of the skin. Discoloration lessens when legs are elevated and usually fades completely within weeks after discontinuing drug.
6. Report any exposure to rubella because drug may increase susceptibility to disease.
7. Susceptible individuals (elderly, immunocompromised) should avoid crowds during "flu" season.
8. Psychologic changes such as confusion, nervousness, or depression should be reported as well as any persistent, bothersome, or new symptoms.
9. Avoid alcohol or any other unprescribed OTC products.
10. Clients with parkinsonism should not stop drug abruptly.
11. Clients with seizure disorders should be advised to report any early signs or symptoms of seizure activity as dosage may require adjustment.

Evaluate

- ↓ Drug-induced extrapyramidal symptoms
- Improved motor control
- Improvement in symptoms of influenza A viral infections

Didanosine (ddI, dideoxyinosine)

(die-**DAN**-oh-seen)
Pregnancy Category: B
Videx **(Rx)**

See also *Antiviral Agents,* Chapter 19.

How Supplied: *Chew Tablet:* 25 mg, 50 mg, 100 mg, 150 mg; *Powder for reconstitution:* 100 mg, 167 mg, 250 mg, 2 g, 4 g

Action/Kinetics: Didanosine is a nucleoside analog of deoxyadenosine. After entering the cell, it is converted to the active dideoxyadenosine triphosphate (ddATP) by cellular enzymes. Due to the chemical structure of ddATP, its incorporation into viral DNA leads to chain termination and therefore inhibition of viral replication. ddATP also inhibits viral replication by interfering with the HIV–RNA-dependent DNA polymerase by competing with the natural nucleoside triphosphate for binding to the active site of the enzyme. Didanosine has shown in vitro antiviral activity in a variety of HIV-infected T cell and monocyte/macrophage cell cultures. Didanosine is broken down quickly at acidic pH; therefore, PO products contain buffering agents to increase the pH of the stomach. Food will decrease the rate of absorption of the drug. **t½, elimination:** 1.6 hr for adults and 0.8 hr for children. The drug is metabolized in the liver and excreted mainly through the urine.

Uses: Advanced HIV infection in adult and pediatric (over 6 months of age) clients who are intolerant of AZT therapy or who have demonstrated decreased effectiveness of AZT therapy. Use in adults with HIV infection who have received prolonged AZT therapy. AZT should be considered as initial therapy for the treatment of advanced HIV infection, unless contraindicated, since this drug prolongs survival and decreases the incidence of opportunistic infections.

Dosage

• **Chewable/Dispersible Buffered Tablets, Buffered Powder for Oral Solution, Powder for Pediatric Oral Solution**

Adults, initial, weight over 60 kg: 200 mg q 12 hr (with 250 mg buffered powder q 12 hr). **Weight less than 60 kg:** 125 mg q 12 hr (with 167 mg buffered powder q 12 hr). **Pediatric, BSA 1.1–1.4 m²:** Two 50-mg tablets q 12 hr or 125 mg of the pediatric powder q 12 hr; **BSA 0.8–1.0 m²:** One 50- and one 25-mg tablet q 12 hr or 94 mg of the pediatric powder q 12 hr. **BSA 0.5–0.7 m²:** Two 25-mg tablets q 12 hr or 62 mg of the pediatric powder q 12 hr. **BSA less than 0.4 m²:** One 25-mg tablet q 12 hr or 31 mg of the pediatric powder q 12 hr.

Administration/Storage

1. Didanosine should be administered on an empty stomach.
2. To prevent gastric acid degradation, adult and pediatric (over 1 year) clients should take a 2-tablet dose. Pediatric clients under 12 months of age should receive a 1-tablet dose.
3. Tablets should not be swallowed whole. Tablets may be chewed or crushed thoroughly before taking or tablets may be dispersed in at least 1 oz of drinking water (stir thoroughly and drink immediately).
4. To prepare the buffered powder for PO solution, the contents should be mixed with 4 oz of drinking water; the powder should *not* be mixed with fruit juice or other acid-containing beverages. The mixture should be stirred until the powder dissolves completely (about 2–3 min). The entire solution should be consumed immediately.
5. To prepare the powder for pediatric oral solution, the dry powder must be mixed with purified water to an initial concentration of 20 mg/mL. The resulting solution is then mixed with antacid to a final concentration of 10 mg/mL. This admixture must be shaken thoroughly prior to use and may be stored in a tightly closed container in the refrigerator for up to 30 days.
6. *Treatment of Overdose:* There are no antidotes; treatment should be symptomatic.

Contraindication: Lactation.

Special Concerns: Administer with caution in clients with renal and hepatic impairment and in those on sodium-restricted diets. Clients may continue to develop opportunistic infections and other complications of HIV infection and should thus remain under close observation.

Laboratory Test Interferences: ↑ AST, ALT, alkaline phosphatase, bilirubin, uric acid, amylase.

Side Effects: Commonly pancreatitis and peripheral neuropathy (manifested by distal numbness, tingling, or pain in the feet or hands). Neuropathy occurs more frequently in clients with a history of neuropathy or neurotoxic drug therapy.

In adults. *GI:* Diarrhea, abdominal pain, N&V, anorexia, dry mouth, ileus, colitis, constipation, eructation, flatulence, gastroenteritis, ***GI hemorrhage,*** oral moniliasis, stomatitis, mouth sores, sialadenitis, ***stomach ulcer hemorrhage,*** melena, oral thrush, liver abnormalities. *CNS:* Headache, ***tonic-clonic seizures,*** abnormal thinking, anxiety, nervousness, twitching, confusion, depression, acute brain syndrome, amnesia, aphasia, ataxia, dizziness, hyperesthesia, hypertonia, incoordination, ***intracranial hemorrhage,*** paralysis, paranoid reaction, psychosis, insomnia, sleep disorders, speech disorders, tremor. *Hematologic:* Leukopenia, granulocytopenia, thrombocytopenia, microcytic anemia, ***hemorrhage,*** ecchymosis, petechiae. *Dermatologic:* Rash, pruritus, herpes simplex, skin disorder, sweating, eczema, impetigo, excoriation, erythema. *Musculoskeletal:* Asthenia, myopathy, arthralgia, arthritis, myalgia, muscle atrophy, decreased strength, hemiparesis, neck rigidity, joint disorder, leg cramps. *CV:* Chest pain, hypertension, hypotension, migraine, palpitation, peripheral vascular disorder, syncope, vasodilation, arrhythmias. *Body as a whole:* Chills, fever, infection, allergic reaction, pain, abscess, cellulitis, cyst, dehydration, malaise, flu syndrome, numbness of hands and feet, weight loss, alopecia. *Respiratory:* Pneumonia, dyspnea, asthma, bronchitis, increased cough, rhinitis, rhinorrhea, epistaxis, laryngitis, decreased lung function, pharyngitis, hypoventilation, sinusitis, rhonchi, rales, congestion, interstitial pneumonia, respiratory disorders. *Ophthalmic:* Blurred vision, conjunctivitis, diplopia, dry eye, glaucoma, retinitis, photophobia, strabismus. *Otic:* Ear disorder, otitis (externa and media), ear pain. *GU:* Impotency, kidney calculus, kidney failure, abnormal kidney function, nocturia, urinary frequency, vaginal hemorrhage. *Miscellaneous:* Peripheral edema, sarcoma, hernia, hypokalemia, lymphoma-like reaction.

In children. *GI:* Diarrhea, N&V, liver abnormalities, abdominal pain, stomatitis, mouth sores, pancreatitis, anorexia, increase in appetite, constipation, oral thrush, melena, dry mouth. *CNS:* Headache, nervousness, insomnia, dizziness, poor coordination, lethargy, neurologic symptoms, ***seizures.*** *Hematologic:* Ecchymosis, ***hemorrhage,*** petechaie, leukopenia, granulocytopenia, thrombocytopenia, anemia. *Dermatologic:* Rash, pruritus, skin disorder, eczema, sweating, impetigo, excoriation, erythema. *Musculoskeletal:* Arthritis, myalgia, muscle atrophy, decreased strength. *Body as a whole:* Chills, fever, asthenia, pain, malaise, failure to thrive, weight loss, flu syndrome, alopecia, dehydration. *CV:* Vasodilation, arrhythmia. *Respiratory:* Cough, rhinitis, dyspnea, asthma, rhinorrhea, epistaxis, pharyngitis, hypoventilation, sinusitis, rhonchi, rales, congestion, pneumonia. *Ophthalmic:* Photophobia, strabismus, visual impairment. *Otic:* Ear pain, otitis. *Miscellaneous:* Urinary frequency, diabetes mellitus, diabetes insipidus, liver abnormalities.

Symptoms of Overdose: Pancreatitis, peripheral neuropathy, diarrhea, hyperuricemia, hepatic dysfunction.

Drug Interactions

Ketoconazole / ↓ Absorption of ketoconazole due to gastric pH change caused by buffering agents in didanosine

Pentamidine (IV) / ↑ Risk of pancreatitis

Quinolone antibiotics / ↓ Plasma levels of quinolone antibiotics

Ranitidine / ↓ Absorption of ranitidine due to gastric pH change caused by buffering agents in didanosine

Tetracyclines / ↓ Absorption of tetracyclines from the stomach due to the buffering agents in didanosine

NURSING CONSIDERATIONS

Assessment

1. Document all previous experience with AZT therapy and the outcome listing reasons for transfer to didanosine.
2. Obtain baseline CBC, CD_4 counts, and liver and renal function studies and monitor throughout therapy.
3. Note baseline VS and weight.

Interventions

1. Anticipate reduced dose with liver and renal impairment. Monitor I&O and laboratory parameters.
2. Assess clients on sodium-restricted diets as sodium content is more in the single-dose packet than in the two-tablet dose.
3. Observe for evidence of diarrhea and/or hyperuricemia as drug dosage may require adjustment. Encourage to drink plenty of fluids.
4. Any changes in vision should be documented and evaluated with an ophthalmic examination.

Client/Family Teaching

1. Food decreases the rate of drug absorption so take on an empty stomach.
2. Tablets should be chewed or

crushed; follow administration guidelines carefully.
3. Advise clients to report any symptoms of neuropathy (numbness, burning, or tingling in the hands or feet) as drug should be discontinued until symptoms subside. Client may tolerate a reduced dose of didanosine once these symptoms have been resolved.
4. Report any symptoms of abdominal pain and N&V immediately as these may be clinical signs of pancreatitis. The drug should be stopped immediately and the client evaluated with dosing resumed only after pancreatitis has been ruled out.
5. Advise client to avoid alcohol and any other drugs that may exacerbate the toxicity of didanosine.
6. Remind client and family that didanosine is not a cure, but it alleviates the symptoms of HIV infections. Stress that clients may continue to acquire opportunistic infections.
7. Stress that didanosine therapy has *not* been shown to reduce the risk of transmission of HIV to others through sexual contact or blood contamination and that appropriate precautions should continue to be taken.
8. Provide referrals to local support groups that may assist client/family to understand and cope with disease.

Evaluate: Control and successful management of symptoms of AIDS, ARC, and opportunistic infections in clients with HIV who are intolerant to or have clinically deteriorated during therapy with AZT.

Famciclovir

(fam-**SY**-kloh-veer)
Pregnancy Category: B
Famvir **(Rx)**

See also *Antiviral Agents,* Chapter 19.

How Supplied: *Tablet:* 500 mg

Action/Kinetics: Famciclovir undergoes rapid biotransformation to the active compound penciclovir. The drug inhibits viral DNA synthesis and therefore replication in HSV types 1 (HSV-1) and 2 (HSV-2) and varicella-zoster virus. Penciclovir is further metabolized to inactive compounds that are excreted through the urine. **t½:** 2 hr following IV administration and 2.3 hr following PO use. The half-life was increased in clients with renal insufficiency.

Use: Management of acute herpes zoster (shingles).

Dosage

- **Tablets**

Herpes zoster infections.

500 mg q 8 hr for 7 days. Dosage reduction is recommended in clients with impaired renal function: for creatinine clearance of 40–50 mL/min, the dose should be 500 mg q 12 hr, and for creatinine clearance of 20–39 mL/min, the dose should be 500 mg q 24 hr (data are not available for dosing in clients with a creatinine clearance less than 20 mL/min).

Administration/Storage

1. Therapy should be initiated as soon as herpes zoster is diagnosed.
2. Drug therapy is most useful if started within the first 48 hr of appearance of rash.
3. The effect of famciclovir appears to be more pronounced in clients greater than 50 years of age.

Contraindications: Use during lactation.

Special Concerns: Safety and efficacy have not been determined in children less than 18 years of age.

Side Effects: *GI:*N&V, diarrhea, constipation, anorexia, abdominal pain. *CNS:*Headache, dizziness, paresthesia, somnolence. *Body as a whole:* Fatigue, fever, pain, rigors. *Musculoskeletal:* Back pain, arthralgia. *Respiratory:* Pharyngitis, sinusitis. *Dermatologic:* Pruritus; signs, symptoms, and complications of zoster-related signs.

Drug Interactions

Digoxin / ↑Levels of digoxin
Probenecid / Probenecid↑plasma levels of penciclovir
Theophylline / ↑Levels of penciclovir

NURSING CONSIDERATIONS

See also *Nursing Considerations* for *Antiviral Agents,* Chapter 19.

Assessment
1. Document location and onset of symptoms, frequency of recurrence, and extent of lesions.
2. Therapy should be initiated as soon as diagnosis is confirmed.
3. Obtain baseline CBC and renal function studies. Anticipate reduced dosage with renal dysfunction.

Client/Family Teaching
1. Review the appropriate method, frequency, and amount of drug to consume and the duration of therapy.
2. Identify side effects frequently associated with therapy (diarrhea, nausea, headaches, fatigue) and advise to report if intolerable.
3. Remind clients that they are extremely contagious when lesions are open and draining and should avoid any exposure or contact unless it can be confirmed that the person(s) have had the chickenpox and are not pregnant.

Evaluate
- Resolution of lesions with relief of pain
- ↓Duration of postherpetic neuralgia

Foscarnet sodium

(fos-**KAR**-net)
Pregnancy Category: C
Foscavir **(Rx)**

See also *Antiviral Agents* Chapter 19.
How Supplied: *Injection:* 24 mg/mL
Action/Kinetics: Foscarnet inhibits replication of all known herpes viruses. The drug acts by selective inhibition at the pyrophosphate binding site on virus-specific DNA polymerases and reverse transcriptases at levels that do not affect cellular DNA polymerases. It is active against herpes simplex virus mutants deficient in thymidine kinase. CMV strains resistant to ganciclovir may be sensitive to foscarnet; viral reactivation of CMV occurs after termination of foscarnet therapy. The latent state of any of the human herpes viruses is not sensitive to foscarnet. The drug is believed to accumulate in human bone and has variable penetration into the CSF. Approximately 80%–90% of IV foscarnet is excreted unchanged through the urine.
Use: Treatment of CMV retinitis in clients with AIDS.

Dosage
- **IV infusion**

Individualized. Induction: 60 mg/kg for clients with normal renal function given IV at a constant rate over a minimum of 1 hr q 8 hr for 2–3 weeks, depending on the response. **Maintenance:** 90–120 mg/kg/day (depending on renal function) given as an IV infusion over 2 hr. Most clients should be started on the 90-mg/kg/day dose.

Administration/Storage
1. To avoid local irritation, foscarnet should be infused only into veins with adequate blood flow to allow rapid dilution and distribution.
2. The rate of infusion must be no more than 1 mg/kg/min using controlled IV infusion either by a central venous line or a peripheral vein.
3. If using a central venous catheter for infusion, the standard 24-mg/mL solution may be used without dilution. However, if a peripheral vein catheter is used, the 24-mg/mL solution should be diluted to 12 mg/mL with 5% dextrose in water or with NSS to avoid vein irritation. Diluted solutions should be used within 24 hr of first entry into a sealed bottle.
4. The potential for renal impairment may be minimized by hydrating the client during administration of the drug to establish and maintain diuresis.
5. The dose must be adjusted in renal impairment using the dosing guide provided with the drug.
6. No other drug or supplement should be given through the same catheter as foscarnet. Foscarnet is incompatible with 30% dextrose, amphotericin B, and calcium-containing solutions (e.g., Ringer's lactate and TPN). Other incompatibilities include acyclovir sodium, diazepam, digoxin, ganciclovir, leucovorin,

midazolam, pentamidine, phenytoin, prochlorperazine, trimethoprim/sulfamethoxazole, and vancomycin. A precipitate can result if foscarnet is given at the same time as divalent cations.

7. *Treatment of Overdose:* Monitor the client for S&S of electrolyte imbalance and renal impairment. Symptomatic treatment. Hemodialysis and hydration may be of some benefit.

Special Concerns: Use with caution during lactation and in clients with impaired renal function (the effects of the drug have not been determined in clients with a creatinine clearance less than 50 mL/min or serum creatinine more than 2.8 mg/dL). Safety and effectiveness in children have not been determined. Transient changes in electrolytes may increase the risk of cardiac disturbances and seizures. Safety and effectiveness have not been determined for the treatment of other CMV infections such as pneumonitis or gastroenteritis, for congenital or neonatal CMV disease, and in nonimmunocompromised clients. Use with caution with drugs that alter serum calcium levels as foscarnet decreases serum levels of ionized calcium. Side effects such as renal impairment, electrolyte abnormalities, and seizures may contribute to client death.

Laboratory Test Interferences: ↑ Alkaline phosphatase, AST, ALT, LDH, BUN, creatine phosphokinase, serum creatinine. ↓ Creatinine clearance. Abnormal X-ray. Abnormal A-G ratio.

Side Effects: *GU:* Renal impairment (most common), albuminuria, dysuria, polyuria, urinary retention, urethral disorder, UTIs, ***acute renal failure,*** nocturia, hematuria, glomerulonephritis, urinary frequency, toxic nephropathy, nephrosis, urinary incontinence, pyelonephritis, renal tubular disorders, urethral irritation, uremia, perineal pain in women, penile inflammation. *Metabolic/Electrolyte:* Hypocalcemia, hypokalemia, hypomagnesemia, hypophosphatemia, hyperphosphatemia, hyponatremia, hypercalcemia, acidosis, thirst, decreased weight, dehydration, glycosuria, diabetes mellitus, abnormal glucose tolerance, hypochloremia, hypervolemia, hypoproteinemia. *Hematologic:* Anemia (one-third of clients), granulocytopenia, neutropenia, leukopenia, thrombocytopenia, platelet abnormalities, thrombosis, WBC abnormalities, lymphadenopathy, coagulation disorders, decreased coagulation factors, decreased prothrombin, hypochromic anemia, pancytopenia, hemolysis, leukocytosis, cervical lymphadenopathy, lymphopenia. *Body as a whole:* Fever, fatigue, asthenia, pain, infection, rigors, malaise, sepsis, death, back or chest pain, cachexia, flu-like symptoms, edema, bacterial or fungal infections, abscess, moniliasis, leg edema, peripheral edema, hypothermia, syncope, substernal chest pain, ascites, ***malignant hyperpyrexia,*** herpes simplex, viral infections, toxoplasmosis. *CNS:* Headache, dizziness, ***seizures (including tonic-clonic),*** tremor, ataxia, dementia, stupor, meningitis, aphasia, abnormal coordination, EEG abnormalities, vertigo, coma, encephalopathy, dyskinesia, extrapyramidal disorders, hemiparesis, paraplegia, speech disorders, tetany, cerebral edema, depression, confusion, anxiety, insomnia, somnolence, amnesia, aggressive reaction, nervousness, agitation, hallucinations, impaired concentration, emotional liability, psychosis, ***suicide attempt,*** delirium, sleep disorders, personality disorders. *Peripheral nervous system:* Hypesthesia, neuropathy, sensory disturbances, generalized spasms, abnormal gait, hyperesthesia, hypertonia, hyperkinesia, vocal cord paralysis, hyporeflexia, hyperreflexia, neuralgia, neuritis, peripheral neuropathy. *Musculoskeletal:* Arthralgia, myalgia, involuntary muscle contractions, leg cramps, arthrosis, synovitis, torticollis. *GI:* N&V, diarrhea, anorexia, abdominal pain, dry mouth, dysphagia, dyspepsia, rectal hemorrhage, constipation, melena, flatulence, pancreatitis, ulcerative stomatitis, enteritis, glossitis, enterocolitis, proctitis, stomatitis, tenesmus, pseudomembranous colitis, gastroenteritis, oral leukoplakia, oral hemorrhage, rectal disorders, colitis, duodenal ulcer, hematemesis, paralytic ileus, ulcerative proctitis, tongue ulceration, esophageal ulceration. *Hepatic:* Abnormal hepatic function, cholecystitis, cholelithiasis, hepatitis, hepatosplenomegaly, cholestatic hepatitis, jaundice. *CV:* Hypertension, palpitations, sinus tachycardia, first degree AV block, nonspecific ST-T segment changes, hypotension, flushing, cerebrovascular disorder, ***cardiomyopathy, cardiac failure, cardiac arrest,*** bradycardia, arrhythmias, extrasystole, atrial fibrillation, phlebitis, superficial thrombophlebitis of arm, mesenteric vein thrombophlebitis. *Respiratory:* Cough, dyspnea, pneumonia, sinusitis, rhinitis, pharyngitis, respiratory insufficiency, pulmonary infiltration, ***pulmonary embolism,*** pneumothorax, hemoptysis, stridor, bronchospasm, laryngitis, bronchitis, respiratory depression, pleural effusion, ***pulmonary hemorrhage,*** pneumonitis. *Ophthalmic:* Visual field defects, nystagmus, periorbital edema, eye pain, conjunctivitis, diplopia, blindness, retinal detachment, mydriasis, photophobia. *Ear:* Deafness, earache, tinnitus, otitis. *Dermatologic:* Increased sweating, rash, skin ulceration, pruritus, seborrhea, erythematous rash, maculopapular rash, facial edema, skin discoloration, acne, alopecia, dermatitis, anal pruritus, genital pruritus, aggravated psoriasis, psoriaform rash, skin disorders, dry skin, urticaria, skin hypertrophy, verruca. *Miscellaneous:* Epistaxis, taste perversions, pain or inflammation at injection site, lymphoma-like disorder, sarcoma, ***malignant lymphoma,*** ADH disorders, decreased gonadotropins, gynecomastia.

Symptoms of Overdose: Extensions of the above side effects. Of most concern are development of ***seizures,*** renal function impairment, paresthesias in limbs or periorally, and electrolyte disturbances especially involving calcium and phosphate.

Drug Interactions
Aminoglycosides / ↓ Elimination of foscarnet → ↑ risk of renal impairment
Amphotericin / ↓ Elimination of foscarnet → ↑ risk of renal impairment
AZT / ↑ Risk of anemia
Pentamidine, IV / ↓ Elimination of foscarnet → ↑ risk of renal impairment; also, pentamidine causes hypocalcemia

NURSING CONSIDERATIONS

Assessment

1. Document indications for therapy and the onset of symptoms.
2. Determine confirmation of the diagnosis of CMV retinitis by indirect ophthalmoscopy.
3. Note any history of cardiac or neurologic dysfunction.
4. Ensure that appropriate lab cultures have been performed before instituting therapy.
5. Obtain baseline CBC, serum electrolytes, calcium, phosphorus, magnesium, and liver and renal function studies.

Interventions

1. Due to the possibility of decreased renal function, creatinine clearance should be determined at baseline, 2–3 times/week during induction therapy, and at least once every 1–2 weeks during maintenance therapy. This is especially true in geriatric clients who commonly have decreased glomerular filtration rates.
2. Monitor I&O and VS. Ensure that client is well hydrated.
3. Monitor appropriate lab values and observe clients for the possibility of chelation of divalent metal ions, which will alter serum levels of electrolytes. Thus, levels of electrolytes, calcium, magnesium, and creatinine should be monitored closely.
4. Observe for any evidence of seizure activity and use seizure precautions.
5. Follow dilution and administration guidelines carefully. Ideally, product should be prepared daily,

under a biologic hood, by the pharmacist.

Client/Family Teaching

1. Remind clients that foscarnet is not a cure for CMV retinitis and that they may continue to experience progression of the condition during or following treatment.
2. Review long list of drug side effects, stressing those that require immediate medical attention.
3. Stress the importance of reporting for regularly scheduled ophthalmic examinations.
4. Report any evidence of numbness of the extremities, paresthesias, or perioral tingling as these are symptoms of hypocalcemia. Stop the infusion and seek appropriate medical intervention to correct the imbalance before resuming the infusion.

Evaluate: Ophthalmic evidence of successful treatment of CMV retinitis in clients with AIDS.

Ganciclovir sodium (DHPG)

(gan-**SYE**-kloh-veer)
Pregnancy Category: C
Cytovene **(Rx)**

See also *Antiviral Agents,* Chapter 19.

How Supplied: *Capsule:* 250 mg; *Powder for injection:* 500 mg

Action/Kinetics: Upon entry into viral cells infected by CMV, ganciclovir is converted to ganciclovir triphosphate by the CMV. Ganciclovir triphosphate inhibits viral DNA synthesis by competitive inhibition of viral DNA polymerases and direct incorporation into viral DNA; this results in eventual termination of viral DNA elongation. Ganciclovir is active against CMV, herpes simplex virus-1 and -2, Epstein-Barr virus, and varicella zoster virus. **t½:** Approximately 2.9 hr. The drug is believed to cross the blood-brain barrier. Most of the drug is excreted unchanged through the urine. Renal impairment increases the t½ of the drug.

Uses: Immunocompromised clients with CMV retinitis, including AIDS clients. Diagnosis may be confirmed by culture of CMV from the blood, urine, or throat; note that a negative CMV culture does not rule out CMV retinitis. Prevention of CMV disease in transplant clients at risk; duration of treatment depends on duration and degree of immunosuppression. *Investigational:* Treatment of CMV infections (e.g., gastroenteritis, hepatitis, pneumonitis) in immunocompromised clients.

Dosage

- **IV infusion**

CMV retinitis.

Induction treatment: 5 mg/kg over 1 hr q 12 hr for 14–21 days in clients with normal renal function. **Maintenance:** 5 mg/kg over 1 hr by IV infusion daily for 7 days or 6 mg/kg/day for 5 days each week. Dosage must be reduced in clients with renal impairment.

Prophylaxis of CMV disease in transplant clients.

Initial dose: 5 mg/kg over 1 hr q 12 hr for 7–14 days. **Maintenance:** 5 mg/kg/day on 7 days each week (or 6 mg/kg/day on 5 days each week).

Administration/Storage

1. Doses greater than 6 mg/kg infused over 1 hr may result in increased toxicity.
2. Due to the high pH (9–11) of reconstituted ganciclovir, the drug should not be given by IM or SC injection. The drug should not be given by IV bolus or rapid IV injection.
3. To minimize phlebitis or pain at the injection site, ganciclovir should be given into veins with an adequate blood flow to allow rapid dilution and distribution.
4. The dose should not exceed 1.25 mg/kg/day in clients undergoing hemodialysis.
5. The drug should be reconstituted by injecting 10 mL sterile water for injection followed by shaking. The vial should be discarded if particulate matter or discoloration is noted. Because parabens is incompatible with ganciclovir, bacteriostatic water for injection should not be used for reconstitution.

6. The reconstituted solution is stable for 12 hr at room temperature.
7. IV infusion concentrations greater than 10 mg/mL are not recommended. Further reconstitute ganciclovir with 100 mL of any of the following solutions: 5% dextrose, lactated Ringer's or Ringer's solution, 0.9% sodium chloride. Infuse over 1 hr.
8. Follow guidelines for handling cytotoxic drugs during handling and disposal of drug. Avoid inhalation and contact with skin. Latex gloves and safety glasses should be used when handling drug. Ideally, ganciclovir should be mixed by the pharmacist under a biologic hood.
9. *Treatment of Overdose:* Hydration, hemodialysis.

Contraindications: Hypersensitivity to acyclovir or ganciclovir. Lactation.

Special Concerns: Safety and effectiveness of ganciclovir have not been established for nonimmunocompromised clients, treatment of other CMV infections such as pneumonitis or colitis, or congenital or neonatal CMV disease. Use with caution in impaired renal function and in elderly clients. Use in children only if potential benefits outweigh potential risks. Ganciclovir is not a cure for CMV retinitis and progression of the disease may continue in immunocompromised clients. Treatment with AZT and ganciclovir (e.g., in AIDS clients) will likely not be tolerated and lead to severe granulocytopenia.

Laboratory Test Interferences: ↑ Serum creatinine, BUN. ↓ Blood glucose.

Side Effects: *Hematologic:* Granulocytopenia, thrombocytopenia, neutropenia (may be irreversible), eosinophilia, anemia. *CNS:* Ataxia, ***coma,*** confusion, abnormal dreams or thoughts, dizziness, headache, paresthesia, psychosis, nervousness, somnolence, tremor. *GI:* N&V, diarrhea, anorexia, ***GI hemorrhage,*** abdominal pain. *CV:* Hypertension or hypotension, arrhythmias. *Body as a whole:* Fever (most common), chills, edema, infections, malaise. *Dermatologic:* Rash (most common), alopecia, pruritus, urticaria. *GU:* Hematuria, increased serum creatinine, increased BUN. *Miscellaneous:* Abnormal liver function values; inflammation, pain, or phlebitis at injection site; decreased blood glucose, dyspnea, retinal detachment in CMV retinitis clients.

Symptoms of Overdose: Neutropenia. Possibility of hypersalivation, anorexia, vomiting, bloody diarrhea, inactivity, cytopenia, testicular atrophy, increased BUN and liver function test results.

Drug Interactions
Adriamycin / Additive cytotoxicity in rapidly dividing cells
Amphotericin B / Additive cytotoxicity in rapidly dividing cells; also, ↑ serum creatinine levels
Cyclosporine / ↑ Serum creatinine levels
Dapsone / Additive cytotoxicity in rapidly dividing cells
Flucytosine / Additive cytotoxicity in rapidly dividing cells
Imipenem/Cilastatin combination / Possibility of seizures
Pentamidine / Additive cytotoxicity in rapidly dividing cells
Probenecid / ↑ Effect of ganciclovir due to ↓ renal excretion
Sulfamethoxazole/Trimethoprim combinations / Additive cytotoxicity in rapidly dividing cells
Vinblastine / Additive cytotoxicity in rapidly dividing cells
Vincristine / Additive cytotoxicity in rapidly dividing cells
AZT / ↑ Risk of granulocytopenia

NURSING CONSIDERATIONS

Assessment

1. Document indications for therapy and onset of symptoms.
2. Determine confirmation of CMV retinitis by indirect opthalmoscopy.
3. Assess orientation and mentation levels.
4. Determine that appropriate lab studies have been performed. Note any evidence of hematologic disorders that may preclude drug use.

Interventions

1. Monitor CBC frequently because granulocytopenia and thrombocytopenia are side effects of drug therapy. Ganciclovir should not be administered if neutrophil count drops below 500 cells/mm^3 or the platelet count falls below 25,000/mm^3. Concomitant therapy with AZT may increase neutropenia.
2. Anticipate reduced dose in clients with impaired renal function; monitor renal function studies throughout therapy.
3. Monitor I&O. Ensure that client is adequately hydrated before and during IV therapy with ganciclovir because drug is excreted through the kidneys.
4. Client may experience pain and/or phlebitis at infusion site because pH of *diluted* solution is high (pH 9–11). Follow administration guidelines carefully.
5. Review list of drug interactions as some may induce renal failure and have additive toxicity if given during ganciclovir therapy.

Client/Family Teaching

1. Drug therapy should not be interrupted unless deemed necessary by provider because a relapse may occur.
2. Report any dizziness, confusion, and/or seizures immediately.
3. Stress the importance of reporting for scheduled lab studies because results may require adjustment of dose or even discontinuation of therapy.
4. Stress the importance of regular ophthalmologic examinations because retinitis may progress to blindness (retinal detachment).
5. Ganciclovir may impair fertility.
6. During and for 90 days following drug therapy, women of childbearing age should use safe contraception and men should practice barrier contraception.
7. Report any unusual behavior or altered thought processes.

Evaluate

- Resolution of CMV infection
- CMV prophylaxis in transplant clients
- Ophthalmic evidence demonstrating control of progression of CMV retinitis

Idoxuridine (IDU)

(eye-dox-**YOUR**-ih-deen)
Pregnancy Category: C
Herplex Liquifilm, Herplex-D ✱ **(Rx)**

See also *Antiviral Agents,* Chapter 19.

How Supplied: *Solution:* 0.1%

Action/Kinetics: Idoxuridine, which resembles thymidine, inhibits thymidylic phosphorylase and specific DNA polymerases required for incorporation of thymidine into viral DNA. Idoxuridine, instead of thymidine, is incorporated into viral DNA, resulting in faulty DNA and the inability of the virus to infect tissue or reproduce. Idoxuridine may also be incorporated into mammalian cells. The drug does not penetrate the cornea well. It is rapidly inactivated by nucleotidases or deaminases.

Uses: Herpes simplex keratitis, especially for initial epithelial infections characterized by the presence of thread-like extensions. *NOTE:* Idoxuridine will control infection but will not prevent scarring, loss of vision, or vascularization. Alternative form of therapy must be instituted if no improvement is noted after 7 days or if complete reepithelialization fails to occur after 21 days of therapy.

Dosage

- **Ophthalmic (0.1%) solution.**

Initially: 1 gtt every hour during the day and q 2 hr during the night; **following improvement:** 1 gtt q 2 hr during the day and q 4 hr at night. Continue for 3–5 days after healing is complete. Alternate dosing schedule: 1 gtt q min for 5 min; repeat q 4 hr, day and night.

Administration/Storage

1. Store idoxuridine solution at 2°C–8°C (36°F–46°F) and protect from light.
2. Do not mix with other medications.
3. Store idoxuridine ointment at 2°C–15°C (36°F–59°F).
4. Administer ophthalmic medication as scheduled, even during the night.
5. Do not use drug that was improp-

erly stored because of loss of activity and increased toxic effects.
6. Topical corticosteroids may be used with idoxuridine in the treatment of herpes simplex with corneal edema, stromal lesions, or iritis.
7. To control secondary infections, antibiotics may be used with idoxuridine.
8. Atropine may be used concomitantly with idoxuridine, if appropriate.
9. Improvement is usually observed within 7–8 days; if there is continuous improvement, therapy should be continued for 21 days.
10. Some strains of herpes simplex may be resistant to idoxuridine; if there is no decrease in fluorescein staining after 14 days of use, another form of therapy should be undertaken.

Contraindications: Hypersensitivity; deep ulcerations involving stromal layers of cornea. Lactation. Concomitant use of corticosteroids in herpes simplex keratitis.

Special Concerns: Idoxuridine may be sensitizing, especially with dermal use. Safety and efficacy have not been determined in children.

Side Effects: Localized to eye. Temporary visual haze, irritation, pain, pruritus, inflammation, follicular conjunctivitis with preauricular adenopathy, mild edema of eyelids and cornea, allergic reactions (rare), photosensitivity, corneal clouding and stippling, small punctate defects. *NOTE:* Squamous cell carcinoma has been reported at the site of application.

Symptom of Overdose (frequent administration): Defects on corneal epithelium.

Drug Interaction: Concurrent use of boric acid may cause irritation.

NURSING CONSIDERATIONS

See also *General Nursing Considerations for Antiviral Agents,* Chapter 19.

Client/Family Teaching

1. Review appropriate method for instillation, frequency for administration, and proper storage.
2. Report any symptoms of vision loss.
3. *Do not* apply boric acid to the eye during idoxuridine therapy because boric acid may cause irritation.
4. Reassure that hazy vision following instillation of medication will be of short duration.
5. Wear dark glasses if photophobia occurs.
6. If idoxuridine has been used concurrently with corticosteroids, explain that the idoxuridine will be continued longer than the steroid, to prevent reinfection.
7. Report for scheduled ophthalmic exams to determine drug response and to assess application site.

Evaluate

- Control of ophthalmic infection
- Reepithelialization of herpetic eye lesions

Ribavirin

(rye-bah-**VYE**-rin)
Pregnancy Category: X
Virazole, Virazole (Lyophilized) ✦ **(Rx)**

See also *Antiviral Agents,* Chapter 19.

How Supplied: *Powder for reconstitution:* 6 g

Action/Kinetics: Although the precise mechanism is not known, ribavirin may act as a competitive inhibitor of cellular enzymes that act on guanosine and xanthosine. Ribavirin is distributed to the plasma, respiratory tract, and RBCs and is rapidly taken up by cells. **t½:** 9.5 hr. Eliminated through both the urine and feces.

Uses: Hospitalized pediatric clients (including infants) with severe lower respiratory tract infections (viral pneumonia including bronchiolitis) due to respiratory syncytial virus (RSV). Ribavirin is intended to be used along with standard treatment (including fluid management) for such clients with severe lower respiratory tract infections. *Investigational:* Ribavirin aerosol has been used against influenza A and B.

Oral ribavirin has been used against herpes genitalis, acute and chronic hepatitis, measles, and Lassa fever.

Dosage

• **Aerosol only, to an infant oxygen hood using the Small Particle Aerosol Generator-2 (SPAG-2)**

The concentration administered is 20 mg/mL and the average aerosol concentration for a 12-hr period is 190 mcg/L of air. See *Administration/Storage.*

Administration/Storage

1. Administration of the drug should be carried out for 12–18 hr/day for 3 (minimum)–7 (maximum) days.
2. Treatment is most effective if initiated within the first 3 days of the respiratory syncytial virus, which causes lower respiratory tract infections.
3. Ribavirin aerosol should only be administered using the SPAG-2 aerosol generator.
4. Therapy should *not* be instituted in clients requiring artificial respiration.
5. No other aerosolized medications should be given if ribavirin aerosol is being used.
6. The drug may be solubilized with sterile water (USP) for injection or inhalation in the 100-mL vial. The solution is then transferred to the SPAG-2 reservoir utilizing a sterilized 500-mL wide-mouth Erlenmeyer flask and further diluted to a final volume of 300 mL with sterile water.
7. Solutions in the SPAG-2 reservoir should be replaced daily. Also, if the liquid level is low, it should be discarded before new drug solution is added.
8. Reconstituted solutions of ribavirin may be stored at room temperature for 24 hr.
9. Drug is not to be administered by women of childbearing age. *Post* this advisement so they do not come in contact with the drug.

Contraindications: Infants requiring artificial respiration (the drug may precipitate in the equipment and interfere with appropriate ventilation of the client). Children with mild RSV lower respiratory tract infections who require a shorter hospital stay than required for a full course of ribavirin therapy. Pregnancy or women who may become pregnant during drug therapy (the drug may cause fetal harm and is known to be teratogenic). Lactation.

Special Concerns: Use with caution in adults with asthma or chronic obstructive lung disease (deterioration of respiratory function may occur).

Side Effects: *Pulmonary:* Worsening of respiration, pneumothorax, apnea, bacterial pneumonia, dependence on ventilator. *CV:* Hypotension, ***cardiac arrest,*** manifestations of digitalis toxicity. *Other:* Anemia (with IV or PO ribavirin); conjunctivitis and rash (with the aerosol).

NURSING CONSIDERATIONS

Interventions

1. It is essential that constant monitoring be undertaken for both the fluid and respiratory status of the client.
2. Assess frequently for evidence of respiratory distress; stop therapy and report if distress occurs. Do not leave child unattended and unstimulated in the tent for long periods during therapy.
3. Monitor and record VS and I&O.
4. Anticipate limited use in infants and adults with COPD or asthma.
5. With prolonged therapy (more than 7 days), observe for S&S of anemia; monitor CBC values.

Evaluate

• Auscultatory and radiographic evidence of improved airway exchange
• Clinical and lab evidence of resolution of RSV pneumonia

Rimantadine hydrochloride

(rih-**MAN**-tih-deen)
Pregnancy Category: C
Flumadine **(Rx)**

See also *Antiviral Agents,* and *Amantadine,* Chapter 19.

How Supplied: *Syrup:* 50 mg/5 mL; *Tablet:* 100 mg

Action/Kinetics: Rimantadine is thought to act early in the viral replication cycle, possibly by inhibiting the uncoating of the virus. It has been suggested that a virus protein specified by the virion M_2 gene plays an important role in the inhibition of the influenza A virus by rimantadine. The drug has little or no activity against influenza B virus. Plasma trough levels following 100 mg b.i.d. for 10 days range from 118 to 468 ng/mL; however, levels are higher in clients over the age of 70 years. The drug is metabolized in the liver, and both unchanged drug (25%) and metabolites are excreted through the urine.

Uses: In adults for prophylaxis and treatment of illness caused by strains of influenza A virus. In children for prophylaxis against influenza A virus.

Dosage

- **Syrup, Tablets**

Prophylaxis.

Adults and children over 10 years of age: 100 mg b.i.d. In clients with severe hepatic dysfunction (creatinine clearance less than 10 mL/min) and in elderly nursing home clients, the dose should be reduced to 100 mg/day. **Children, less than 10 years of age:** 5 mg/kg once daily, not to exceed a total dose of 150 mg/day.

Treatment.

Adults: 100 mg b.i.d. In clients with severe hepatic dysfunction and in elderly nursing home clients, reduce the dose to 100 mg/day.

Administration/Storage

1. For treatment of influenza A virus infections, therapy should be initiated as soon as possible, preferably within 48 hr after onset of S&S. Treatment should continue for approximately 7 days from the initial onset of symptoms.
2. *Treatment of Overdose:* Supportive therapy. IV physostigmine at doses of 1–2 mg IV in adults and 0.5 mg in children, not to exceed 2 mg/hr, has been reported to be beneficial in treating overdose for amantadine (a related drug).

Contraindications: Hypersensitivity to amantadine, rimantadine, or other drugs in the adamantine class. Use during lactation.

Special Concerns: Use with caution in clients with renal or hepatic insufficiency. An increased incidence of seizures is possible in clients with a history of epilepsy who have received amantadine. Influenza A virus strains resistant to rimantadine can emerge during treatment and be transmitted, causing symptoms of influenza. Safety and efficacy of rimantadine in the treatment of symptomatic influenza infections in children have not been established. Safety and efficacy for prophylaxis of infections have not been determined in children less than 1 year of age. The incidence of side effects in geriatric clients is higher than other clients.

Side Effects: GI and CNS side effects are the most common. *GI:* N&V, anorexia, dry mouth, abdominal pain, diarrhea, dyspepsia, constipation, dysphagia, stomatitis. *CNS:* Insomnia, dizziness, headache, nervousness, fatigue, asthenia, impairment of concentration, ataxia, somnolence, agitation, depression, gait abnormality, euphoria, hyperkinesia, tremor, hallucinations, confusion, ***convulsions,*** agitation, diaphoresis, hypesthesia. *Respiratory:* Dyspnea, ***bronchospasm,*** cough. *CV:* Pallor, palpitation, hypertension, ***cerebrovascular disorder, cardiac failure,*** pedal edema, heart block, tachycardia, syncope. *Miscellaneous:* Tinnitus, taste loss or change, parosmia, eye pain, rash, nonpuerperal lactation, increased lacrimation, increased frequency of micturition, fever, rigors.

Symptoms of Overdose: Extensions of side effects including the possibility of agitation, hallucinations, ***cardiac arrhythmias, and death.***

Drug Interactions

Acetaminophen / ↓ Peak concentration and area under the curve for rimantadine

Aspirin / ↓ Peak plasma levels and area under the curve for rimantadine

Cimetidine / ↓ Clearance of rimantadine

NURSING CONSIDERATIONS

See also *Nursing Considerations* for *Amantadine,* Chapter 19.

Assessment

1. Document indications for therapy. Determine if client has been vaccinated, or if not, then why not.
2. List other drugs prescribed to ensure none interact unfavorably.
3. Obtain baseline liver and renal function studies to determine any dysfunction.
4. Anticipate reduced dosage with severe hepatic dysfunction and with elderly nursing home clients.
5. Note any history of epilepsy and assess for loss of seizure control.

Client/Family Teaching

1. Instruct to take only as directed and not to share medication with friends or family.
2. Stress that therapy should be initiated as soon as symptoms appear and should be continued for approximately 7 days from the onset of symptoms.
3. Emphasize to clients that early annual vaccination is the method of choice for influenza prophylaxis. The 2–4-week time frame required to develop an antibody response can be managed with rimantadine.

Evaluate: Prevention and management of symptoms of influenza A virus.

Stavudine

(**STAH**-vyou-deen)
Pregnancy Category: C
Zerit

How Supplied: *Capsule:* 15 mg, 20 mg, 30 mg, 40 mg

Action/Kinetics: Stavudine acts to inhibit replication of HIV due to phosphorylation by cellular kinases to stavudine triphosphate, which has antiviral activity. The mechanism for the antiviral activity includes inhibition of HIV reverse transcriptase by competing with the natural substrate deoxythymidine triphosphate and by causing DNA chain termination, thereby inhibiting viral DNA synthesis. Stavudine is rapidly absorbed with peak plasma levels in 1 hr or less after dosing. **t½, terminal:** Approximately 1.2 hr. About 40% of the drug is eliminated through the kidney.

Uses: Treatment of adults with advanced HIV infection who cannot tolerate approved therapies or who have experienced significant clinical or immunologic deterioration while receiving such therapies (or for whom such therapies are contraindicated).

Dosage

- **Capsules**

Advanced HIV infections.

Adults, initial: 40 mg b.i.d. for clients weighing 60 or more kg and 30 mg b.i.d. for clients weighing less than 60 kg. In clients developing peripheral neuropathy, the following dosage schedule may be used if symptoms of neuropathy resolve completely: 20 mg b.i.d. for clients weighing 60 or more kg and 15 mg b.i.d. for clients weighing less than 60 kg.

The following dosage schedule is recommended for clients with impaired renal function: (a) creatinine clearance greater than 50 mL/min: 40 mg q 12 hr for clients weighing 60 or more kg and 30 mg q 12 hr for clients weighing less than 60 kg; (b) creatinine clearance from 26–50 mL/min: 20 mg q 12 hr for clients weighing 60 or more kg and 15 mg q 12 hr for clients weighing less than 60 kg; (c) creatinine clearance from 10–25 mL/min: 20 mg q 24 hr for clients weighing 60 or more kg and 15 mg q 24 hr for clients weighing less than 60 kg. Insufficient data are available to recommend doses for clients with a creatinine clearance less than 10 mL/min or for clients undergoing dialysis.

Administration/Storage: Stavudine may be taken without regard to meals.

Contraindications: Lactation.

Special Concerns: The effect of stavudine on the clinical progression of HIV infection, such as incidence of opportunistic infections or survival, has not been determined.

Laboratory Test Interferences: ↑ AST, ALT.

Side Effects: *Neurologic:* Peripheral neuropathy (common), including numbness, tingling, or pain in feet or hands. *CNS:* Insomnia, anxiety, depression, nervousness, dizziness, confusion, migraine, somnolence, tremor, neuralgia, dementia. *GI:* Diarrhea, N&V, anorexia, dyspepsia, constipation, ulcerative stomatitis, aphthous stomatitis, ***pancreatitis.*** *Body as a whole:* Headache, chills, fever, asthenia, abdominal pain, back pain, malaise, weight loss, allergic reactions, flu syndrome, lymphadenopathy, pelvic pain, ***neoplasms, death.*** *CV:* Chest pain, vasodilation, hypertension, peripheral vascular disorder, syncope. *GU:* Dysuria, genital pain, dysmenorrhea, vaginitis, urinary frequency, hematuria, impotence, urogenital neoplasm. *Respiratory:* Dyspnea, pneumonia, asthma. *Dermatologic:* Rash, sweating, pruritus, maculopapular rash, benign skin neoplasm, urticaria, exfoliative dermatitis. *Ophthalmic:* Conjunctivitis, abnormal vision.

NURSING CONSIDERATIONS

Assessment

1. Document onset of symptoms, date confirmed, and other agents prescribed and symptoms, and note date of intolerance.
2. Obtain baseline CBC, PT, and liver and renal function studies. Anticipate reduced dosage with impaired renal function.

Client/Family Teaching

1. Take exactly as prescribed, do not exceed prescribed dose, and do not share medications.
2. Remind clients/family that the medication is not a cure, but it alleviates/manages the symptoms of HIV infections. Advise that they may continue to acquire illnesses associated with AIDS or ARC, including opportunistic infections, and should remain under close medical supervision when taking stavudine.
3. The risk of transmission of HIV to others through blood or sexual contact is not reduced in individuals on stavudine therapy. Review the criteria and precautions for safe sex and advise not to share needles.
4. Caution to report any symptoms of peripheral neuropathy characterized by numbness and tingling or pain in the hands and/or feet. Stress that drug therapy should be discontinued if these symptoms are evident. Advise that symptoms may temporarily worsen following cessation of drug therapy but, once completely resolved, drug may be reintroduced at a lower dose.
5. Report for all scheduled lab studies and follow-up visits to assess response to therapy and to identify early any adverse drug effects.
6. Provide a list of local support groups that may assist client/family to understand and cope with this disease.

Evaluate: Clinical and immunologic improvement in clients with AIDS and ARC.

Trifluridine

(try-**FLUR**-ih-deen)
Pregnancy Category: C
Viroptic **(Rx)**

See also *Antiviral Agents,* Chapter 19.

How Supplied: *Ophthalmic Solution:* 1%

Action/Kinetics: Trifluridine closely resembles thymidine; the drug inhibits thymidylic phosphorylase and specific DNA polymerases necessary for incorporation of thymidine into viral DNA. Trifluridine, instead of thymidine, is incorporated into viral DNA, resulting in faulty DNA and the ability to infect or reproduce in tissue. Trifluridine is also incorporated into mammalian DNA. **t½:** 12–18 min.

Uses: Primary keratoconjunctivitis and recurrent epithelial keratitis caused by HSV types 1 and 2. Epithelial keratitis resistant to idoxuridine. Is especially indicated for infections resistant to idoxuridine or vidarabine.

Dosage

- **Solution, 1%.**

1 gtt solution q 2 hr onto cornea, up to maximum of 9 gtt/day in each eye during acute stage (presence of corneal ulcer). Following reepithelialization, decrease dosage to 1 gtt/4 hr (or minimum of 5 gtt/day in each eye) for 7 days. Do not use for more than 21 days.

Administration/Storage

1. May be used concomitantly in the eye with antibiotics (chloramphenicol, bacitracin, polymyxin B sulfate, erythromycin, neomycin, gentamicin, tetracycline, sulfacetamide sodium), corticosteroids, anticholinergics, epinephrine HCl, and sodium chloride.
2. Drug is heat-sensitive. Store in refrigerator at 2°C–8°C (35.6°F–46.4°F).

Contraindications: Hypersensitivity or chemical intolerance to drug.

Special Concern: Safe use during pregnancy not established. Use with caution during lactation.

Side Effects: *Ophthalmic:* Local, usually transient; irritation of conjunctiva and cornea, including burning or stinging and edema of eyelids. Increased intraocular pressure. *Other:* Superficial punctate keratopathy, epithelial keratopathy, hypersensitivity reaction, stromal edema, irritation, keratitis sicca, hyperemia.

NURSING CONSIDERATIONS

See also *General Nursing Considerations for Antiviral Agents,* Chapter 19.

Client/Family Teaching

1. Instill drop onto cornea. Apply finger pressure lightly to lacrimal sac for 1 min after instillation.
2. A mild, transient burning sensation may occur on instillation.
3. Report any new or bothersome side effects but do not stop medication without specific instructions as herpetic keratitis may recur.
4. Arrange for regular examination by an ophthalmologist.
5. Improvement usually occurs within 7 days and healing takes place within 14 days. Thereafter, 7 more days of therapy are necessary to prevent recurrence.
6. Report if no improvement is noted within 7 days.
7. Do not administer drug for more than 21 days because toxicity may occur (remaining medication should be discarded after 21 days).
8. Keep medication in the refrigerator.

Evaluate

- Resolution of infection
- Reepithelialization of herpetic eye lesions

Vidarabine

(vye-**DAIR**-ah-been)
Pregnancy Category: C
Vira-A **(Rx)**

See also *Antiviral Agents,* Chapter 19 and *Anti-Infectives,* Chapter 1.

How Supplied: *Ophthalmic ointment:* 3%

Action/Kinetics: Vidarabine is phosphorylated in the cell to arabinosyl adenosine monophosphate (ara-AMP) or the triphosphate (ara-ATP). These compounds cause inhibition of viral DNA polymerase, inhibition of virus-induced ribonucleotide reductase. The drug may also incorporate into the viral DNA molecule leading to chain termination. Vidarabine is rapidly metabolized to ara-HX, which has decreased antiviral activity. **Peak plasma levels:** Vidarabine, 0.2–0.4 mcg/mL; ara-HX, 3–6 mcg/mL. **t½: IV,** vidarabine, 1 hr; ara-HX, 3.3. hr. Drug and metabolites excreted by kidneys. Due to low solubility, very little vidarabine penetrates following ophthalmic use.

Uses: Systemic: Herpes simplex virus encephalitis. Neonatal herpes simplex viral infections including disseminated infection with encephalitis, visceral involvement, and infections of the eyes, mouth, and skin. Herpes zoster in immunocompromised clients.

Topical: Primary keratoconjunctivitis and recurrent epithelial keratitis caused by HSV types 1 and 2. Superficial keratitis caused by HSV that is resistant to idoxuridine. It is more effective than idoxuridine for deep recurrent infections.

Dosage

- **Slow IV Infusion**

Herpes simplex viral encephalitis, neonatal herpes simplex viral infections.

15 mg/kg/day for 10 days.

Herpes zoster.

10 mg/kg/day for 5 days.

- **Ophthalmic Ointment**

½ in. of 3% ointment applied to lower conjunctival sac 5 times/day at 3-hr intervals. Continue therapy for 7 days after complete reepithelialization but at reduced dosage (e.g., b.i.d.).

Administration/Storage

1. To be effective, vidarabine therapy should be initiated as soon as possible, but no later than 72 hr after the appearance of vesicular lesions.
2. Systemic: slowly infuse total daily dose at constant rate over 12–24 hr.
3. A total of 2.2 mL of IV solution is required to dissolve 1 mg of medication. A maximum of 450 mg may be dissolved in 1 L and administered over 12–24 hr. Should be used within 48 hr after dilution. Do not refrigerate solution.
4. Since such a small amount is needed for newborns, 1 mL of the injection should be added to 9 mL of sterile NSS or sterile water for injection to provide a suspension of 20 mg/mL.
5. Any carbohydrate or electrolyte solution is suitable as diluent. Do not use biologic or colloidal fluids.
6. Shake vidarabine vial well before withdrawing dosage. Add to prewarmed (35°C–40°C, 95°F–104°F) infusion solution. Shake mixture until completely clear.
7. For final filtration use an in-line filter (0.45 μm).
8. Dilute just before administration and use within 48 hr.
9. Due to insolubility, the drug may have to be given in a large fluid volume. Care should be exercised in administering such a volume to clients susceptible to fluid overloading or with cerebral edema (e.g., with CNS infections or renal impairment).
10. Topical corticosteroids or antibiotics may be used concomitantly with vidarabine, but benefits and risks must be assessed.
11. Wait 10 min before use of an additional topical ointment.
12. *Treatment of Overdose:* Monitor hematologic as well as liver and kidney function.

Contraindications: Hypersensitivity to drug. Concomitant use of corticosteroids usually contraindicated. Lactation. IM, SC, or IV use by rapid or bolus injection. Ophthalmic use in presence of sterile trophic ulcers.

Special Concerns: *Systemic:* Use with caution in clients susceptible to fluid overload, cerebral edema, or with impaired renal or hepatic function. The drug may be carcinogenic and mutagenic. Early diagnosis and treatment of viral infections are essential. The drug is ineffective against infections due to adenovirus or RNA viruses, bacteria, fungi, or chlamydial infections of the cornea.

Drug Interaction: Allopurinol may interfere with the metabolism of vidarabine.

Laboratory Test Interferences: ↑ Bilirubin, AST.

Side Effects: Systemic. *GI:* N&V, diarrhea, anorexia, hematemesis. *CNS:* Tremor, dizziness, ataxia, confusion, malaise, headache, hallucinations, psychoses, metabolic encephalopathy (may be fatal). *Hematologic:* Decrease in reticulocytes, H&H, WBC count, and platelet count. *Miscellaneous:* Weight loss, rash, pruritus, pain at injection site, neurologic abnormalities in infants. **Topical.** Photophobia, lacrimation, conjunctival injection, foreign body sensation, temporal visual haze, burning, irritation, superficial punctate keratitis, pain, punctal occlusion, sensitivity to bright light.

Symptoms of Overdose: Bone marrow depression with thrombocytopenia and leukopenia. Acute fluid overloading may pose a greater risk than vidarabine itself.

NURSING CONSIDERATIONS

See also *General Nursing Considerations for Antiviral Agents,* Chapter 19.

Assessment

1. Document indications for therapy and type and onset of symptoms. Drug must be initiated within 72 hr of appearance of vesicular lesions to be effective.
2. List other agents prescribed and the outcome.
3. Obtain baseline renal, liver, and hematologic studies and monitor for any evidence of dysfunction precipitated by vidarabine therapy.

Client/Family Teaching

1. Take only as directed and do not share medications.
2. Wash hands before and after applying ointment. If other agents prescribed wait 10 min before instilling.
3. Ophthalmic ointment will cause a temporary haze after application. Avoid hazardous activities until vision clears.
4. Report any new, persistent, or bothersome side effects.
5. Wear sunglasses outside and avoid bright lights because drug may cause photophobic reactions.
6. Do not wear contact lenses until infection clears.
7. Client must remain under close supervision of an ophthalmologist while receiving therapy for ophthalmic problem.

Evaluate

- Resolution of infection
- Negative lab culture results
- Healing of skin lesions
- Reepithelialization of herpetic eye lesions with complete healing of eyes in 1–3 weeks

Zalcitabine (Dideoxycytidine, ddC)

(zal-**SIGH**-tah-been)
Pregnancy Category: C
Hivid **(Rx)**

See also *Antiviral Agents,* Chapter 19, and *Anti-Infectives,* Chapter 1.

How Supplied: *Tablet:* 0.375 mg, 0.75 mg

Action/Kinetics: Zalcitabine is converted in cells to the active metabolite, dideoxycytidine 5'-triphosphate (ddCTP), by cellular enzymes. ddCTP serves as an alternative substrate to deoxycytidine triphosphate for HIV-reverse transcriptase, thereby inhibiting the in vitro replication of HIV-1 and inhibiting viral DNA synthesis. The incorporation of ddCTP into the growing DNA chain leads to premature chain termination. ddCTP serves as a competitive inhibitor of the natural substrate for deoxycytidine triphosphate for the active site of the viral reverse transcriptase, which further inhibits viral DNA synthesis. Food reduces the rate of absorption of the drug. Zalcitabine does not appear to undergo significant metabolism by the liver. **Elimination t½:** 1–3 hr. Approximately 70% of a PO dose is excreted through the kidneys and 10% in the feces. Prolonged elimination (t½ up to 8.5 hr) is observed in clients with impaired renal function.

Uses: In combination with AZT or in advanced HIV infections (CD_4 cell count of 300/mm^3 or less and who have shown significant clinical or immunologic deterioration). Alone for HIV-infected adults with advanced disease who are intolerant to AZT or where the disease has progressed while taking AZT.

Dosage

- **Tablets**

In combination with AZT in advanced HIV infection.

Adults: 0.75 mg given at the same time with 200 mg AZT q 8 hr for a total daily dose of 2.25 mg zalcitabine and 600 mg AZT.

Alone in advanced HIV infection. 2.25 mg/day.

Administration/Storage

1. If the creatinine clearance is 10–40 mL/min, the dose should be reduced to 0.75 mg/12 hr and if creatinine clearance is less than 10 mL/min, the dose should be reduced to 0.75 mg/24 hr.
2. Reduction of dosage is not required for client weights down to 30 kg.

Contraindications: Hypersensitivity to zalcitabine or any components of the product. Use in clients with moderate or severe peripheral neuropathy or with drugs that have the potential to cause peripheral neuropathy (see *Drug Interactions*). Concomitant use with didanosine. Lactation.

Special Concerns: Use with extreme caution in clients with low CD_4 cell counts (<50/mm^3). Use with caution in clients with a history of pancreatitis or known risk factors for the development of pancreatitis. Clients with a creatinine clearance less than 55 mL/min may be at a greater risk for toxicity due to decreased clearance. Safety and efficacy have not been determined in HIV-infected children less than 13 years of age.

Laboratory Test Interferences: ↑ ALT, AST, alkaline phosphatase.

Side Effects: The incidence of certain side effects is dependent on the duration of use and the dose of the drug. *Neurologic:* Peripheral neuropathy (common) characterized by numbness and burning dysesthesia involving the distal extremities; this may be followed by sharp shooting pains or severe continuous burning pain if the drug is not withdrawn. The neuropathy may progress to severe pain requiring narcotic analgesics and may be irreversible. *GI:* ***Fatal pancreatitis*** when given alone or with AZT. Esophageal ulcers, oral ulcers, nausea, dysphagia, anorexia, abdominal pain, vomiting, constipation, ulcerative stomatitis, aphthous stomatitis, diarrhea, dry mouth, dyspepsia, glossitis, ***rectal hemorrhage,*** hemorrhoids, enlarged abdomen, gum disorders, flatulence, anorexia, tongue ulceration, dysphagia, eructation, gastritis, ***GI hemorrhage,*** left quadrant pain, salivary gland enlargement, esophageal pain, esophagitis, rectal ulcers. *Dermatologic:* Rash (including erythematous, maculopapular, follicular), pruritus, night sweats, dermatitis, skin lesions, acne, alopecia, bullous eruptions, increased sweating, urticaria, hot flashes. *CNS:* Headache, dizziness, seizures, ataxia, abnormal coordination, Bell's palsy, dysphonia, hyperkinesia, hypokinesia, migraine, neuralgia, neuritis, stupor, tremor, vertigo, hypertonia, hand tremor, twitching, confusion, impaired concentration, insomnia, agitation, depersonalization, hallucinations, emotional lability, nervousness, anxiety, depression, euphoria, manic reaction, dementia, amnesia, somnolence, abnormal thinking, crying. *Respiratory:* Coughing, dyspnea, flu-like symptoms, cyanosis. *Musculoskeletal:* Myalgia, arthralgia, pain in the feet or arms, arthritis, arthropathy, cold feet, leg cramps, myositis, shoulder pain, wrist pain, cold extremities. *Hepatic:* Exacerbation of hepatic dysfunction, especially in those with preexisting liver disease or with a history of alcohol abuse. Abnormal hepatic function, hepatitis, jaundice, hepatocellular damage. *CV:* ***Cardiomyopathy,*** CHF, hypertension, palpitations, syncope, atrial fibrillation, tachycardia, heart racing, epistaxis. *Hematologic:* Anemia, leukopenia, neutropenia, eosinophilia, thrombocytopenia. *Hypersensitivity:* Urticaria, ***anaphylaxis*** (rare). *Endocrine:* Diabetes mellitus, hyperglycemia, hypocalcemia, impotence. *GU:* Gout, toxic nephropathy, polyuria, renal calculi, ***acute renal failure,*** hyperuricemia, increased frequency of micturition, abnormal renal function, renal cyst. *Ophthalmologic:* Abnormal vision, burning or itching eyes, xerophthalmia, eye pain or abnormality. *Miscellaneous:* Fatigue, pharyngitis, fever, rigors, chest pain, weight decrease, pain, malaise, asthenia, generalized edema, ear blockage, taste perversion, deafness, tinnitus.

Drug Interactions: The following drugs have the potential to cause peripheral neuropathy: chloramphenicol, cisplatin, dapsone, disulfiram, ethionamide, glutethimide, gold, hydralazine, iodoquinol, isoniazid, metronidazole, nitrofurantoin, phenytoin, ribavirin, vincristine. Drugs such as amphotericin, foscarnet, and aminoglycosides may increase the risk of peripheral neuropathy by interfering with the renal clearance of zalcitabine, thus increasing plasma levels.

NURSING CONSIDERATIONS

Assessment

1. Document any history of pancreatitis or associated risk factors. Clients with a history of pancreatitis or elevated serum amylase should be followed closely while on zalcitabine therapy.
2. Baseline serum amylase and triglyceride levels should be performed in clients with a history of pancreatitis, increased amylase, those on parenteral nutrition, or those with a history of drug abuse.
3. Hematology and chemistry profiles should be undertaken before beginning therapy with zalcitabine and AZT and at appropriate intervals thereafter.
4. Obtain baseline liver and renal function studies and monitor closely throughout therapy.
5. Note drugs currently prescribed to prevent any unfavorable interactions.

Interventions

1. In clients exhibiting symptoms of peripheral neuropathy, the drug may be reintroduced at 50% of the initial dose (i.e., 0.375 mg/8 hr) only if all symptoms related to the peripheral neuropathy have improved to mild symptoms. The drug should be permanently discontinued if severe discomfort due to peripheral neuropathy progress for 1 week or longer.
2. Frequent monitoring of hematologic indices is recommended to detect serious anemia or granulocytopenia.
3. In clients manifesting hematologic toxicity, decreases in hemoglobin may occur as early as 2–4 weeks after beginning therapy, whereas granulocytopenia may be seen after 6–8 weeks of therapy.

Client/Family Teaching

1. Take only as directed and with concurrently prescribed AZT every 8 hr round the clock.
2. Reinforce that clients receiving zalcitabine may continue to develop opportunistic infections and other complications of HIV infection and should remain under close medical supervision.
3. Advise women of childbearing age to use an effective contraceptive while taking zalcitabine.
4. Discontinue zalcitabine and report if symptoms of peripheral neuropathy occur, especially if the symptoms are bilateral and progress for more than 72 hr. Explain that the peripheral neuropathy may continue to worsen despite interruption of therapy. If the symptoms improve, then the drug may be reintroduced.
5. Advise client that drug is not a cure but may offer symptomatic improvement.
6. Provide a list of local support groups that may assist client/family to understand and cope with this disease.

Evaluate: Improved CD_4 cell counts, ↓ incidence of opportunistic infection, and improved survival rates in clients with advanced HIV infections.

Zidovudine (Azidothymidine, AZT)

(zye-**DOH**-vyou-deen, ah-**zee**-doh-**THIGH**-mih-deen)

Pregnancy Category: C

Apo-Zidovudine ✦, Novo-AZT ✦, Retrovir **(Rx)**

See also *Antiviral Agents,* Chapter 19, and *Anti-Infectives,* Chapter 1.

How Supplied: *Capsule:* 100 mg; *Injection:* 10 mg/mL; *Syrup:* 50 mg/5 mL

Action/Kinetics: The active form of the drug is AZT triphosphate, which is derived from AZT by cellular enzymes. AZT triphosphate competes with thymidine triphosphate (the natural substrate) for incorporation into growing chains of viral DNA by retroviral reverse transcriptase. Once incorporated, AZT triphosphate causes premature termination of the growth of the DNA chain. Low concentrations of AZT also inhibit the activity of *Shigella, Klebsiella, Salmonella, Enterobacter, Escherichia coli,* and *Citrobacter,* although resistance develops rapidly. The drug is absorbed rapidly from the GI tract and is distributed to both plasma and CSF. **Peak serum levels:** 0.1–1.5 hr. **t½:** approximately 1 hr. The drug is metabolized rapidly by the liver and excreted through the urine.

Uses: Adults manifesting symptoms due to HIV (i.e., AIDS or ARC) and who have confirmed *Pneumocystis carinii* pneumonia or a peripheral blood T_4 helper/inducer lymphocyte count of less than 200/mm^3. To prevent HIV transmission from pregnant women to their fetuses.

NOTE: AZT syrup has been authorized for use in HIV-infected children from 3 months to 12 years of age who have either HIV-associated symptoms or a CD_4 (T_4) cell count of less than 400.

Dosage

• **Capsules, Syrup**

Symptomatic HIV infections.

Adults, initial: 200 mg (two 100-mg capsules or 20 mL syrup) q 4 hr around the clock. After 1 month, the dose may be reduced to 100 mg q 4 hr.

Asymptomatic HIV infections.

Adults: 100 mg q 4 hr while awake (500 mg/day); **Pediatric, 3 months–12 years,** 180 mg/m^2 q 6 hr, not to exceed 200 mg q 6 hr.

Prevent transmission of HIV from mothers to their fetuses.

500 mg/day.

• **IV**

Initially: 1–2 mg/kg infused over 1 hr. The IV dose is given q 4 hr around the clock only until PO therapy can be instituted. Dosage adjustment may be necessary due to hematologic toxicity.

Administration/Storage

1. The nurse and client must be aware that AZT therapy is not a cure for HIV infections, and clients may continue to develop opportunistic infections and other complications due to AIDS or ARC.
2. Blood counts should be performed at least q 2 weeks. If anemia or granulocytopenia is severe, the dose of AZT must be adjusted or discontinued. Epoetin alfa recombinant may be administered with iron to stimulate RBC production. A blood transfusion may also be required.
3. Safety and effectiveness of chronic AZT therapy in adults are not known, especially in clients who have a less advanced form of disease.
4. Capsules and syrup should be protected from light.
5. Drug should not be mixed with blood products or protein solutions.
6. After dilution, the solution is stable at room temperature for 24 hr and if refrigerated (2°C–8°C, 35.6°F–46.4°F) for 48 hr. However, to ensure safety from microbial contamination, the solution should be given within 8 hr if stored at room temperature and 24 hr if refrigerated.
7. When used to prevent maternal-fetal transmission of HIV, AZT should be initiated in pregnant women between 14 and 24 weeks of gestation; also, IV AZT should be given during labor, and newborn infants should receive AZT syrup.

8. *Treatment of Overdose:* Treat symptoms. Hemodialysis will enhance the excretion of the primary metabolite of AZT.

Contraindications: Allergy to AZT or its components. Lactation.

Special Concerns: Use with caution in clients who have a hemoglobin level of less than 9.5 g/dL or a granulocyte count less than 1,000/mm³.

Side Effects: *Hematologic:* Anemia, granulocytopenia. *GI:* N&V, diarrhea, anorexia, GI pain, dyspepsia. *CNS:* Dizziness, headache, malaise, sleepiness, insomnia, paresthesias. *Other:* Myalgia, asthenia, diaphoresis, dyspnea, rash, change in taste perception.

Symptoms of Overdose: N&V. Transient hematologic changes.

Drug Interactions

Acetaminophen / ↑ Risk of granulocytopenia
Adriamycin / ↑ Risk of cytotoxicity, nephrotoxicity, or hematologic toxicity
Amphotericin B / See *Adriamycin*
Dapsone / See *Adriamycin*
Flucytosine / See *Adriamycin*
Interferon / See *Adriamycin*
Pentamidine / See *Adriamycin*
Probenecid / ↓ Biotransformation or renal excretion of AZT
Vinblastine / See *Adriamycin*
Vincristine / See *Adriamycin*

NURSING CONSIDERATIONS

See also *General Nursing Considerations for Antiviral Agents,* Chapter 19.

Client/Family Teaching

1. Stress the importance of taking the medication q 4 hr ATC as ordered; sleep must be interrupted to take medication.
2. Report for all lab studies, especially CBC, because drug causes anemia and additional medications or a blood transfusion may be necessary.
3. Report early S&S of anemia, such as SOB, weakness, lightheadedness, or palpitations, and increased tiredness.
4. Consume 2–3 L/day fluids to ensure adequate hydration. Maintain a record of weights and I&O.
5. Report any symptoms of superinfections (e.g., furry tongue, mouth lesions, vaginal or rectal itching, thrush).
6. Avoid acetaminophen and any other unprescribed drugs that may exacerbate the toxicity of AZT.
7. Remind clients/family that the medication is not a cure, but it alleviates/manages the symptoms of HIV infections.
8. Clients should be advised not to share medication and not to exceed the recommended dose of AZT.
9. The risk of transmission of HIV to others through blood or sexual contact is not reduced in individuals on AZT therapy. Review the criteria and precautions for safe sex and advise not to share needles.
10. Provide a list of local support groups that may assist client/family to understand and cope with this disease.

Evaluate

- Control of symptoms of HIV, AIDS, or ARC
- Reports of symptomatic improvement
- ↑ CD_4 (T_4) lymphocyte counts
- ↓ Risk of maternal transmission of HIV infection to fetus

Antineoplastic Agents

CHAPTER TWENTY

General Information

See also the following chapters:

Antineoplastic Agents: Alkylating Agents
Antineoplastic Agents: Antimetabolites
Antineoplastic Agents: Antibiotics
Antineoplastic Agents: Hormone and Antihormones
Antineoplastic Agents: Natural Products and Miscellaneous Agents

General Statement: Significant progress continues to be made in the drug therapy of neoplastic diseases. Some types of cancer can now be considered "curable" by chemotherapy alone. In many other forms of cancer, especially in cases of suspected metastatic disease, chemotherapy is an important adjunct in treatment. Progress can be attributed, in part, to the more judicious use of an increasing number of combination regimens of antineoplastic agents, the composition and time of administration of which are based on a better understanding of the characteristics of a specified neoplastic disease, on the kinetics of the cell cycle (see *Action/Kinetics*), and on the mechanism of action of the drugs used. Some of the principles underlying successful cancer chemotherapy are reviewed below. Extensive nursing implications to increase the comfort of the client during cancer therapy are provided.

General Impact of Antineoplastic Agents: Many antineoplastic agents slow down the disease process and induce a remission. All antineoplastic agents are cytotoxic (i.e., cell poisons) and therefore interfere with normal as well as neoplastic cells. However, neoplastic cells are much more active and multiply more rapidly than normal cells, and are thus more affected by the antineoplastic agents. Normal tissue cells, such as those of the bone marrow, the GI mucosal epithelium, and hair follicles are naturally active and particularly susceptible to antineoplastic agents. The margin between the dose of antineoplastic drug needed to destroy the neoplastic cells and that needed to cause bone marrow damage, for example, is narrow. Thus, clients who receive antineoplastic agents are closely watched for signs of bone marrow depression, which is characterized by low blood counts (leukocytes, erythrocytes, platelets). Since WBCs or platelets show the effect of an overdose more rapidly than do erythrocytes, the platelet and WBC counts are often used as a guide to dosage. If a blood or marrow test indicates a precipitous fall in the WBC or platelet count, the antineoplastic agent may have to be discontinued or the dosage modified significantly. Drugs are usually withheld when the WBC count falls below 2,000/mm^3 and the platelet count falls below 100,000/mm^3. Sometimes the effect of the antineoplastic drugs on the bone marrow is cumulative, with the depression of WBCs and platelets occurring weeks or months after initiation of therapy. Thus, clients must be followed carefully. Antineoplastic agents should be administered only by people knowledgeable in their management. Facilities must be available for frequent laboratory evaluations, especially total blood counts and bone marrow tests. The toxicity of the antineoplastic agents is manifested in the lining of the GI tract by development of oral ulcers, intestinal bleeding, and diarrhea. Finally, since hair follicles are also rapidly proliferating tissue, alopecia often accompanies the drug treatment of antineoplastic disease. Antineoplastic agents fall into several broad categories: Alkylating Agents, Antimetabolites, Antibiotics, Natural Products and Miscellaneous Agents, Hormonal and Antihormonal Agents, and Radioactive Isotopes. The choice of the chemotherapeutic agent(s) depends both on the type of the tumor and on its site of growth. Although it has been said that cancer is not one disease but many, a simpler major subdivision involves separation into solid tumors and hematologic malignancies. The former are confined to a specific tissue or organ site initially and usually involve surgery and/or irradiation. Chemotherapy is used to eradicate remaining cells or metastases, or when primary treatment is insufficient or impossible. Chemotherapy is usually the major form of therapy in hematologic malignancies (i.e., leukemias, lymphomas); some cures have been achieved, notably in Hodgkin's disease and the leukemias of childhood. General information applying to all antineoplastic agents (*Action, Uses, Contraindications, Side Effects, Administration,* and extensive *Nursing Considerations*) is presented below.

Action: During division, cells go through a definite number of stages during which they are more or less susceptible to various chemotherapeutic agents (see *Action/Kinetics* of various agents). Some agents, notably the alkylating agents, are effective during all stages of the cycle, while others, the antimetabolites, e.g., are effective only during stages of DNA synthesis. The various cell stages are described in Figure 2.

Uses: Most of the drugs discussed in this section are used exclusively for neoplastic disease. A few are used on an experimental basis for some of the rheumatic diseases.

Contraindications: Hypersensitivity to drug. Most antineoplastic agents are contraindicated for a period of 4 weeks after radiation therapy or chemotherapy with similar drugs. Use with caution, and at reduced dosages, in clients with preexisting bone marrow depression, malignant infiltration of bone marrow or kidney, or liver dysfunction. The safe use of these drugs during pregnancy has not been established; they are contraindicated during the first trimester.

Side Effects: *Bone marrow depression* (leukopenia, thrombocytopenia, ***agranulocytosis,*** anemia) *is the major danger of antineoplastic therapy.* ***Bone marrow depression can sometimes be irreversible.*** *It is mandatory that the client have frequent total blood counts and bone marrow examinations. Precipitous falls must be reported to a physician.* Other side effects include: *GI:* N&V (may be severe), anorexia, diarrhea (may be hemorrhagic), stomatitis, enteritis, abdominal cramps, intestinal ulcers. *Hepatic:* Hepatic toxicity including jaundice and changes in liver enzymes. *Dermatologic:* Dermatitis,

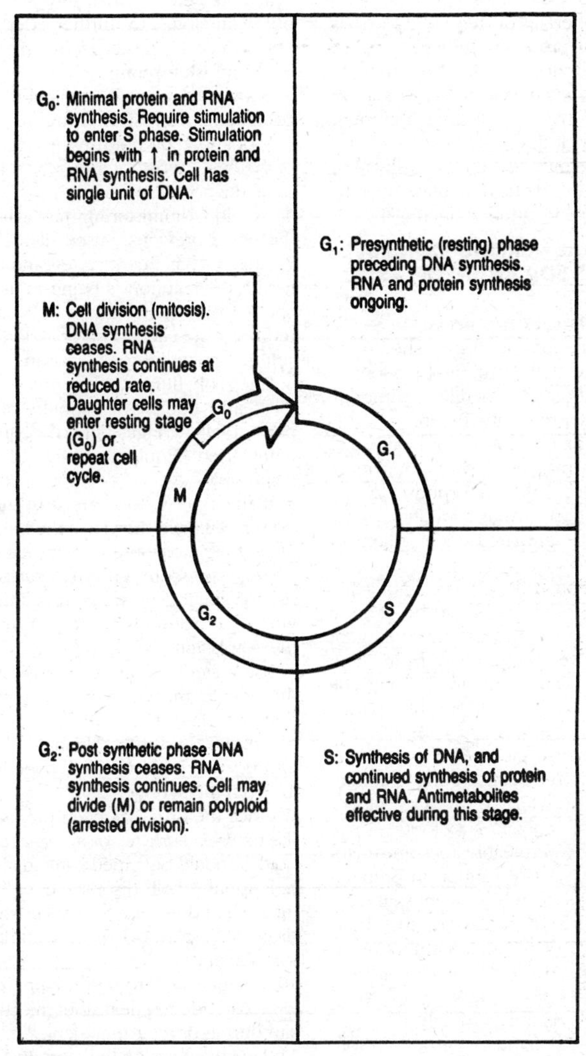

Figure 2 Cell Stages

erythema, various dermatoses including maculopapular rash, alopecia (reversible), pruritus, urticaria, cheilosis. *Immunologic:* Immunosuppression with increased susceptibility to viral, bacterial, or fungal infections. *CNS:* Depression, lethargy, confusion, dizziness, headache, fatigue, malaise, fever, weakness. *GU:* ***Acute renal failure,*** reproductive abnormalities including amenorrhea and azoospermia. *NOTE:* Alkylating agents, in particular, may be both carcinogenic and mutagenic.

GENERAL NURSING CONSIDERATIONS FOR ANTINEOPLASTIC AGENTS

Administration/Storage

1. Antineoplastic drugs should be prepared only by trained personnel; preparation is generally contraindicated by pregnant women.
2. Cytotoxic exposure for health care workers may be through inhalation, ingestion, and absorption during preparation. Antineoplastic drugs should be prepared under a laminar flow (biologic) hood.
• If a laminar flow hood is not available, preparation should be done in a work area away from cooling or heating vents and away from other people. The work area should be covered with a disposable plastic liner.
• Use latex gloves to protect the skin when reconstituting antineoplastic drugs. Do not use gloves made of polyvinyl chloride since these are permeable to some cytotoxic drugs. Use caution in preparation, particularly to prevent skin reactions. Prevent contact of the drugs with skin or mucous membranes. If this occurs, wash the area immediately with copious amounts of water and document accordingly.
• Wash the hands well both before and after removing the gloves used for drug preparation.
• Before beginning preparation the nurse should put on a disposable, nonpermeable surgical gown with a closed front and knit cuffs that completely cover the wrists.
• Wear goggles. Should material accidentally enter the eyes, wash eyes out well with isotonic saline eyewash (or water if isotonic saline is unavailable) and immediately see an ophthalmologist for further care.
3. Use piggyback setup with an electronic infusion pump.
4. Start infusion with a solution not containing the vesicant drug.
5. If possible, do not use the dorsum of the hand, wrist, or antecubital fossa as the site of infusion.
6. Avoid administering medication through a previously used site.
7. After IV has been started and unmedicated solution is being infused, check for blood return and for pain, redness, or edema before starting solution containing medication.
8. Luer-Lok fittings, protective needles, and connectors should be a part of all syringes and IV equipment used. Equipment should be disposable.
• If the drug is to be reconstituted from a vial, vent the vial at the beginning of the procedure. This lowers the internal pressure and reduces the risk of spilling or spraying solution when the needle is withdrawn from the diaphragm.
• Use a sterile alcohol wipe around the needle and vial top when withdrawing the drug.
• Place a sterile alcohol wipe around the needle when expelling air from the syringe.
9. Once the drug has been prepared the external surfaces of syringes and bottles should be wiped with an alcohol sponge. All disposable equipment should be placed in a separate disposable plastic bag and marked for incineration.
10. Instruct client to report pain, redness, or edema near the injection site during or after treatment.
11. Due to effects on the reproductive system, client should be advised to practice some form of reliable contraception.
12. Nurses should wear latex gloves when disposing of vomitus, urine, or feces from clients receiving cytotoxic drug therapy.

13. Maintain a record of all exposure during preparation, administration, cleanup, and spills. Follow appropriate institutional guidelines governing exposures allowed, extravasation, and periodic lab evaluations.

Interventions

1. Establish a team involving the client, family, nurse, physician, pharmacist, social worker, and other health care workers to develop a holistic, therapeutic plan for the client's physical, emotional, social, and spiritual concerns.
2. The entire family may comprise a strong support system for the client and enhance the client's coping abilities. Initially, identify one family member through which the health care team can direct and receive information and have that person function as a liaison for all family members. This should be someone in whom the client has complete confidence and has identified as such. Assess this person's response to the illness, as this impacts on the client's adaptation as well.
3. Whenever possible, ensure that the members of the health team are people who are committed to a long-term relationship with the client. This ensures that there will be consistency in follow-through of care and provides the client with the emotional support that will be necessary for treatment in the long months and possibly years ahead.
4. Use the nursing process format while working with the client and family. Learn from the client and family what they understand from what the physician has explained to them and clarify any misconceptions they may have. Provide written guidelines of the therapy and what to expect.
5. Work closely with the client and family as they experience the effects and problems of chemotherapy associated with cure, remission, or palliation.
6. Determine that informed consent has been obtained.

NURSING CONSIDERATIONS DURING INITIATION OF CHEMOTHERAPY

Assessment

1. Identify indications for therapy, type and onset of symptoms, and any other previous treatments with the outcome.
2. Determine the client's emotional status, and note any history of hypersensitivity to drugs or foods.
3. Assess nutritional status and obtain baseline height, weight, and VS. Drug doses are usually based on BSA (m^2).
4. Perform a complete physical assessment and document findings.
5. Examine the client's mouth for any abnormalities or problems. If indicated, contact the client's dentist to clarify any findings.
6. Determine what experience the client has had concerning surgery, prior radiation therapy, or with chemotherapy.
7. If dealing with someone who has just moved to the area or who is visiting and has experienced problems concerning the illness, contact the health professional with whom the client has been working to ensure continuity of care and to learn of any potential problems.
8. Ensure that the necessary blood work has been completed. This provides important baseline data against which to measure client's progress and should include bone marrow function (CBC with differential), platelets, and renal and liver function.
9. Note the prescribed route of administration: oral, IV, IM, or directly at the tumor site (intracavity, intrapleural, intrathecal, intravesical, intraperitoneal intra-arterial, or topical).
10. Depending on the route of administration, longevity of therapy, frequency of access, venous integrity, and client preference determine if long-term venous access with a venous access device would be more comfortable and benefit the client.

11. Review the client's current pain control regimen. Make sure that pain medication is made available and in quantities necessary to relieve pain.
12. Anticipate premedication with an antiemetic, antihistamine, and possibly an anti-inflammatory agent 30–60 min before initiating therapy (and throughout as needed).

Interventions

1. Place client on careful I&O and record.
2. Instruct client to report any pain, redness, or edema that occurs near the site of injection during or after treatment.
3. If extravasation occurs, stop the infusion and follow the institutional protocol for minimizing the effects. General guidelines for managing an extravasation include:
• Aspirate drug through the cannula with a small syringe (tuberculin size).
• Administer appropriate antidote.
• Remove needle and apply ice or heat (if vinca alkaloids).
• Document and assess site closely.
4. Chart administration of antineoplastic drugs on the medication record and according to the established protocol for the institution.
• Record client's drug protocol on the medication administration record.
• Day 1 is the first day of the first dose.
• Number each day after that in sequence, even though client may not receive drug daily.
• Indicate when the nadir (the time of most severe physiologic depression) is likely to occur so that possible complications, such as infection and bleeding, can be anticipated and treated early. Also note anticipated recovery time, when available.
• When the drug regimen is repeated, the first day of therapy is charted as day 1.
5. Establish appropriate principles to promote client compliance. Keep client and family informed and interpret complicated terminology and therapy; support client and family and help them to understand unconventional emotions and anger.
6. Assist the client and family in locating an appropriate support group to assist them in coping with the client's illness, associated therapy, and emotional turmoil in the family unit.

Client/Family Teaching

1. Stress the importance of complying with all aspects of the therapeutic regimen.
2. Supply information and literature appropriate to the particular type of cancer or illness the client has.
3. Outline the types of side effects the client may be expected to experience and identify a means for coping with these problems.
4. Explain that local cancer support groups in their community may assist them to understand and perhaps begin to cope with their illness.
5. Appropriate literature related to the type and location of cancer may be useful as a guide during treatment. The American Cancer Society provides free, many booklets related to the various types of cancers, chemotherapy, and how to deal with the side effects of treatments. Encourage client to go to the library, local cancer society, and physician with unanswered questions.
6. Identify how and where to contact their health care providers to report any side effects, ask questions, or to request clarification of instructions.
7. Review the drugs to be used and the anticipated results.
8. In the event that antineoplastic agents are prepared and administered in the home, families need to be advised as to the proper disposal of urine, feces, and vomitus.
9. If solutions are prepared in the home and accidents of spilling the drug occur, medical attention must be sought immediately. The health department should be notified. The name of the drug and the type and duration of exposure must be recorded and reported.
10. When the clients are at home, instruct them to maintain accurate I&O records. Provide them with appro-

priate conversion charts as necessary.

Evaluate

• Knowledge and understanding of illness, drug side effects, and goals of therapy
• Any complaints of N&V, pain, anorexia, or diarrhea that may indicate lack of effectiveness of the currently prescribed agents
• Evidence of acute renal failure or hepatic toxicity or changes in liver enzymes
• The presence of and extent of psychologic depression, lethargy, or other signs of possible changes in mental status
• Reports that pain is controlled
• Clinical, lab, and/or radiologic evidence of control or regression of malignant cell proliferation
• Successful administration of chemotherapy with a minimum of adverse side effects
• Desired cure

NURSING CONSIDERATIONS FOR BONE MARROW DEPRESSION (MYELOSUPPRESSION)

LEUKOPENIA

Assessment

1. Check for granulocytopenia or decreased WBCs (normal values: 5,000–10,000/mm^3).
2. Review differential (normal values: neutrophils 60%–70%, lymphocytes 25%–30%, monocytes 2%–6%, eosinophils 1%–3%, basophils 0.25%–0.5%).
3. Note any sudden sharp drop in WBC count or a reduction below 2,000/mm^3, because these findings might necessitate reduction in dosage or withdrawal of the drug.
4. Calculate the nadir (time the blood count reaches its lowest point after chemotherapy) for the prescribed agent (generally 7–14 days). This assists to predict, monitor, and respond to effects of the bone marrow depression.
5. Check temperature q 4 hr and recheck in 1 hr if there is a slight elevation. Report fever above 38°C (100°F) because client has limited resistance to infection resulting from leukopenia and immunosuppression.
6. Assess skin and orifices of body for signs of infection. Early identification is extremely important, since due to reduced or absent granulocytes, local abscesses do not form with pus, but infection becomes systemic as a septicemia.
7. Be aware of any signs of infection. Check the oral cavity for sores or the presence of ulcerated areas. Check urine for odor or particulate matter.
8. Be alert to any client report of increased weakness or fatigue. These symptoms may indicate anemia or electrolyte imbalance.
9. Continually assess for any changes in client morale.

Interventions

1. *Prevent infection by* using strict medical asepsis and frequent handwashing.
2. Provide frequent, meticulous, physical hygiene and maintain a clean environment.
3. Cleanse and dry the rectal area after each bowel movement. Apply ointment if there is irritation; use Tucks and/or Nupercainal for discomfort.
4. Use a gentle antiseptic to wash client who has a tendency to have skin eruptions.
5. Provide mouth care q 4–6 hr, with either NSS or hydrogen peroxide diluted to half strength with water. Follow with a substrate of milk of magnesia. (Make substrate of milk of magnesia by discarding the clear liquid in the top of the bottle and using the thick white liquid that remains to coat the oral mucosa.) Do not use lemon or glycerin, because they tend to reduce the production of saliva and change the pH of the mouth. Mucosal deterioration occurs if mouth care is not provided at least q 6 hr.
6. Be prepared to initiate reverse iso-

lation if WBC count falls below 1,500–2,000/mm^3 by:

• Maintaining client in private room and explaining reasons for this procedure
• Practicing universal precautions; use gloves, masks, and gowns as ordered
• Avoiding indwelling urinary catheters
• Limiting articles brought into room
• Providing private bathroom or bedside commode
• Minimizing unnecessary traffic into and out of room
• Screening visitors for infection before they enter room and limiting visitations
• Avoiding exposure to dust, sprays, contaminated medical equipment
• Advising to avoid deodorants, as these block sebaceous gland secretion
• Keeping fresh fruits and vegetables, cut flowers, and any source of stagnant water (water pitcher, humidifiers, flower vases) away from client
• Reviewing and stressing kitchen hygiene and food safety at home
• Cautioning that dogs, cats, birds, and other animals may carry infection and to avoid
• Assessing orders for requests for administration of granulocyte colony-stimulating factors and ensure availability

7. Prevent nosocomial infections from invasive procedures by:

• Cleansing skin with an antiseptic before procedure
• Changing tubing of IV infusion q 24 hr
• Changing site of IV infusion q 48 hr, if client does not have an implanted venous access device or other designated catheter for long-term use
• Practice strict asepsis with all treatments and dressing changes

THROMBOCYTOPENIA

Assessment

1. Obtain platelet count (normal values: 150,000–400,000/mm^3). Client with a platelet count below 50,000/mm^3 should be monitored closely.
2. Check urine for blood cells.
3. Check stool and gastric contents for occult blood.
4. Inspect skin for petechiae or bruising.
5. Assess all orifices for bleeding.
6. Expect spontaneous hemorrhage if platelets are below 20,000 and anticipate platelet transfusions.
7. Assess BP of hospitalized client b.i.d. and as necessary.

Interventions

1. Prevent bleeding by minimizing SC or IM injections. When injections are necessary, apply pressure for 3–5 min to prevent leakage or hematoma.
2. Report and document any unusual bleeding after injection.
3. Do not apply a BP cuff or other tourniquet for excessive periods of time.
4. Avoid rectal temperatures and test all urine, GI secretions, and stool for occult blood. Prevent constipation.
5. *Assist with the treatment of bleeding*

• Due to epistaxis. Pinch nose for 10 min and apply pressure to upper lip to stop nosebleed; in severe cases, small sponges saturated with neosynephrine ¼% and gently inserted into affected nare, or nasal packing, may be necessary.
• With transfusion (usually ordered if platelet count falls significantly below 150,000/mm^3). Take baseline VS before start of transfusion and then q 15 min after transfusion is started. Monitor VS for at least 2 hr after transfusion is completed. Assess for histoincompatibility, indicated by chills, fever, and urticaria. Stop transfusion, provide supportive care, and follow appropriate institutional protocol for transfusion reaction.

6. Advise the client to use safety measures to *prevent bleeding* from cuts or bruises by:

• Not picking or forcefully blowing their nose, as bleeding may result
• Avoiding contact sports and any activities that may lead to injury
• Reporting any frontal headaches to provider
• Using an electric razor for shaving rather than a blade

• Providing a soft-bristled toothbrush or having client massage gums with fingers or a cotton ball and avoid dental floss to limit irritation
• Avoiding rectal irritation with enemas, suppositories, or thermometers
• Using a water-based lubricant before intercourse
• Consuming plenty of fluids, increasing activity, and taking stool softeners to prevent constipation
• Rearranging furniture so that area for ambulation is unimpeded and also, to prevent bumping into furniture at night when getting out of bed to go to the bathroom
• Having a night light to permit visualization in the event client must get up during the night
• Wearing shoes or slippers when ambulating

ANEMIA

Assessment

1. Check hemoglobin (normal values: men, 13.5–18.0 g/dL blood; women, 11.5–15.5 g/dL blood) and hematocrit (normal values: men, 40%–52%; women, 35%–46%).
2. Assess client for pallor, lethargy, dizziness, increased SOB, or unusual fatigue.

Interventions

1. *Minimize anemia by:*
• Providing a nutritious diet that client can tolerate
• Administering or instructing client to take vitamins and iron supplements as ordered
2. *Assist with treatment of anemia by:*
• Administering diet high in iron that client can tolerate
• Administering vitamins and iron supplements as ordered
• Administering blood transfusions when ordered
• Spacing and scheduling activities to allow for frequent periods of rest
• Positioning to facilitate ventilation; teaching breathing and relaxation techniques and administering oxygen as prescribed
• Controlling room temperature for comfort and providing emotional support

NURSING CONSIDERATIONS FOR GI TOXICITY

NAUSEA AND VOMITING; ANOREXIA

Assessment

1. Expect that N&V may be due to either a CNS effect on the chemoreceptor trigger zone or direct irritation to the GI tract. With radiation therapy, N&V may be attributed to the accumulation of toxic waste products of cell destruction and localized damage to the lining of the throat, stomach, and intestine.
2. Anticipatory N&V is considered a conditioned response of unknown origin prior to chemotherapy, but it does respond to premedication.
3. Determine if the client is refusing food or fluids or just experiencing anorexia.
4. Compare client's nutritional status and weight with the baseline established at the start of therapy and monitor on subsequent visits.
5. Include the family in discussions on nutrition problems as they often supply information the client either forgets to mention or is afraid to talk about.
6. Examine the frequency, character, and amount of vomitus. If the client has been vomiting at home be sure the family member in attendance has been taught to follow this procedure and document accordingly.
7. List antiemetics prescribed and their results.

Interventions

1. *Prevent N&V by:*
• Premedicating with antiemetic as ordered, before administering antineoplastic drug. Usually the antiemetic is ordered to be administered 30–60 min before or just after administration of antineoplastic agent.
• Administering antineoplastic on an empty stomach, with meals, or at bedtime, to minimize N&V and to produce the most therapeutic effect for the client

• Teaching client and/or family how to insert an antiemetic suppository
• Providing ice chips at onset of nausea
• Providing carbonated beverages to counteract nausea
• Encouraging ingestion of dry carbohydrates such as toast and dry crackers before initiating activity
• Waiting for N&V to pass before serving food
• Providing small, nutritious snacks and planning meal schedules to coincide with client's best tolerance time
• Providing nourishing foods that the client likes
• Encouraging intake of a high-protein diet
• Freezing dietary supplements and serving them like ice cream to make them more palatable
• Avoiding foods with overpowering aroma
• Encouraging client to chew foods well
• Providing good oral hygiene both before and after meals
• Encourage the client to eat favorite foods where possible. Such encouragement tends to ensure some nutrition will be provided even though the client feels ill.
• Where possible, encourage clients to eat their meals with others, preferably at a table. Sharing with other clients has been shown to encourage some clients to eat.

2. Antiemetics that have different actions/pharmacokinetics may be administered concurrently in an effort to control severe N&V.

3. *Assist with the treatment of N&V by:*
• Administering antiemetic(s), as ordered, or contacting provider if antiemetic has not been ordered. All vomiting should be reported, because a change in chemotherapeutic regimen or correction of electrolyte balance may be required.
• Altering the timing of other medication doses to after meals
• Offering simple foods: rice, toast, noodles, bananas, scrambled eggs, mashed potatoes, custards, ice cream
• Offering salty foods (pretzels, crackers), as these are usually tolerated
• Avoiding solid and liquid foods at the same meal
• Eliminating any odors in the room and avoiding malodorous foods (e.g., cabbage, sauerkraut, etc.)
• Providing supportive care to keep client as comfortable, clean, and free from odor as possible
• Trying another or concurrent antiemetic agents, if one prescribed is ineffective
• Correcting electrolyte balance and providing hyperalimentation, as necessary
• Screening visitors and calls until client feels able to resume these interactions

4. *Approach anorexia by:*
• Providing small, frequent meals q 2 or 3 hr on schedule
• Maximizing caloric intake by offering nutrient-dense snacks and drinks (yogurt, cheese and crackers, peanut butter and jelly sandwiches, cereal, dried fruit, fruit nectars, and instant breakfast drink mixes)
• Making nutrient-dense supplements with whole milk
• Suggesting a walk or activity before eating to boost appetite
• Concentrating on and obtaining favorite foods

5. *Increase caloric intake and protein consumption by:*
• Adding high-calorie foods such as mayonnaise, butter, and gravy to foods
• Using whole milk in puddings, cream soups, custards
• Making double-strength milk by adding powdered milk to whole milk for gravies, hot cereals, mashed potatoes, eggs, casseroles, baked things, etc.
• Adding whipped cream to frosting and desserts
• Offering milkshakes, nectar, and eggnog when thirsty
• Offering peanut butter on crackers, bagels with cream cheese, trail mix, and nuts and seeds for snacks
• Cutting up meats and cheeses and

adding to salads, soups, scrambled eggs, etc.

BOWEL DYSFUNCTION (DIARRHEA/ABDOMINAL CRAMPING)

Assessment

1. Note frequency and severity of cramping caused by hypermotility.
2. Document frequency, color, consistency, and amount of diarrhea, all of which indicate amount of tissue destruction occurring.
3. Assess for signs of dehydration and acidosis indicating electrolyte imbalance, and maintain careful I&O records.
4. Determine if stool samples have been sent for culture.

Interventions

1. *Prevent diarrhea/abdominal cramping by:*
• Providing small, frequent meals on a schedule
• Identifying any factors that tend to aggravate or increase the incidence
• Increasing the use of constipating foods, such as hard cheeses, in the diet

2. *Assist with the treatment of diarrhea by:*
• Administering an antidiarrheal and narcotic agent (i.e., codeine, tincture of opium, imodium, or lomotil), if ordered, or requesting if antidiarrheal has not been ordered. Diarrhea or abdominal cramping should be reported, because a change in chemotherapeutic regimen or correction of electrolyte balance may be required.
• Increasing fluids to avoid dehydration
• Providing foods to correct sodium and potassium losses, e.g., bananas, potatoes, fish and meat, apricot nectar, tomato juice, and sports drinks with "electrolytes"
• Avoiding high-fiber foods that contain "insoluble fiber," such as wheat bran, brown rice, and popcorn
• Administering bulk-forming agents (i.e., metamucil) as needed
• Offering "soluble-fiber" foods, such as white rice, oatmeal, applesauce, mashed potatoes, and pears
• Avoiding fried foods and greasy foods
• Avoiding excessive sweets, which may aggravate diarrhea (usually due to sorbitol, which is found in many gums and candies)
• Using alumimum-containing antacids when needed
• Avoiding gas-forming foods, such as broccoli, corn, onion, garlic, lentils, and kidney beans
• Considering lactose-free products or Lact-Aid, which facilitates digestion of lactose
• Restricting oral intake to rest the bowel if necessary
• Providing good skin care, especially to the perianal area to prevent skin breakdown. Apply A&D ointment for perianal tenderness. Change client's gown and bed linens frequently; use special mattresses and room deodorizers as needed.

3. *Prevent constipation by:*
• Providing a high-fiber diet
• Administering stool softeners and bulk-forming agents as prescribed
• Promoting increased fluid intake
• Increasing activity levels
• Monitoring frequency, consistency, and amount of stool

4. *Prevent obstruction by:*
• Aggressive GI management in the area of constipation
• Assessing for early S&S such as abdominal pain, N&V, and diminished or absent bowel sounds
• Attempting conservative management, i.e., NPO, NG suction to relieve before referring for surgical intervention (if unsuccessful)

STOMATITIS (MUCOSAL ULCERATION)

Assessment

• Assess for dryness of the mouth, erythema, mouth sore, painful swallowing, and white patchy areas of the oral mucous membranes that indicate developing stomatitis.
• Assessment should be done each time the drug/drugs are adminis-

tered. Expect symptoms 5 days to 2 weeks after starting therapy

Interventions

1. *Prevent stomatitis by:*

• Assessing oral cavity t.i.d. and reporting bleeding gums or burning sensation especially when acid liquids such as fruit juice are ingested

• Setting up a regular schedule for oral preventive care

• Providing good mouth care

• Applying lubricant (Vaseline) to lips at least t.i.d.

2. *Assist with treatment of stomatitis by:*

• Continuing to provide good oral care

• Applying topical viscous anesthetic, such as benzocaine 20%, or a swish and gargle anesthetic dyclonine hydrochloride 0.5%, or a swish, swallow/discard agent such as lidocaine 2% (Xylocaine), before meals or as needed to anesthetize oral mucosa. Client may swallow lidocaine after swishing it around oral cavity but should be encouraged to expectorate it.

• Puncture a vitamin E capsule and apply to painful lesions in an effort to promote healing

• Offering "Magic Mouthwash," which consists of 4 g (approx. 1/8 teaspoon) baking soda, 30mL viscous xylocaine, 30mL benedryl elixir, and 30mL Maalox (optional) in 1 L NSS; advise client to swish and spit out q 1–2 hr as needed

• Providing an allopurinol mouthwash for fluorouracil-related stomatitis

• Offering small, frequent meals of bland foods at medium temperatures

• Administering nystatin solution or clotrimazole troches for fungal infections as prescribed

3. Administer medications (antifungals, antivirals) as prescribed to prevent general infections.

NURSING CONSIDERATIONS FOR NEUROTOXICITY

Assessment

1. Assess for symptoms of minor neuropathies, such as tingling in hands and feet and loss of deep tendon reflexes.

2. Assess for symptoms of serious neuropathies, such as weakness of hands, ataxia, loss of coordination, foot drop, wrist drop, or paralytic ileus.

3. Note what kind of activities the clients liked to do that required using their hands. This could be an important clue when asking clients about changes in sensation or weakness involving the hands.

Interventions

1. *Prevent functional loss due to neurotoxicity by:*

• Reporting symptoms of neuropathies early and discussing findings as the physician may decide to change the medication regimen

• Practicing and teaching seizure precautions

2. *Assist with treatment of neuropathies by:*

• Using appropriate safety measures in caring for client with a functional loss

• Maintaining good body alignment by frequent and anatomically correct repositioning. Determine the need and frequency for ROM exercises.

• Obtaining medical orders for stool softeners and laxatives as needed

NURSING CONSIDERATIONS FOR OTOTOXICITY

Assessment: Assess for hearing difficulties before initiating therapy.

Interventions

1. Instruct client to report tinnitus or alteration in hearing.

2. Perform audiometry testing, if indicated, throughout therapy.

NURSING CONSIDERATIONS FOR HEPATOTOXICITY

Assessment

1. Obtain and assess the following liver function tests:

• Total serum bilirubin (normal values: 0.1–1.0 mg/dL). An elevation may indicate liver disease or an increased rate of RBC hemolysis is present.

• AST (normal values: 8–33 units/L). Elevation is indicative of changes in the liver, skeletal muscles, lungs, pancreas, and heart. Hepatitis produces striking elevations in the AST.

• ALT (normal values: 8–20 units/L).

Elevation may be indicative of conditions leading to hepatic necrosis.
• LDH (normal values: 70–250 units/L). Elevation may be indicative of hepatitis, pulmonary infarction, and CHF.
2. Observe for signs of liver involvement, such as abdominal pain, high fever, diarrhea, and yellowing of skin and sclera.

Interventions

1. Prevent further hepatotoxicity by immediate reporting of elevations in liver function tests and signs of liver involvement, as these are indications for changing medication regimen.
2. Assist with the treatment for hepatotoxicity by providing supportive nursing care to relieve symptoms, such as pain, fever, diarrhea, and symptoms associated with jaundice.

NURSING CONSIDERATIONS FOR RENAL TOXICITY

Assessment

1. Obtain and assess the following renal function tests:
• BUN (normal values: 5–20 mg/dL)
• Serum uric acid (normal values: men, 3.5–7.0 mg/dL; women, 2.4–6.0 mg/dL)
• Creatinine clearance (normal values: women, 0.8–1.7 g/24 hr; men, 1.0–1.9 g/24 hr)
• Quantitative uric acid (normal values: 250–750 mg/day)
2. Observe and document any stomach pain, swelling of feet or lower legs, shakiness, unusual body movement, and stomatitis.

Interventions

1. Record I&O.
2. Limit hyperuricemia by encouraging extra fluid intake to speed excretion of uric acid and to decrease hazard of crystal and urate stone formation.
3. Test pH and assist with alkalinization of urine as ordered.

NURSING CONSIDERATIONS FOR IMMUNOSUPPRESSION

Assessment

1. Assess for the presence of fever, chills, or sore throat.
2. Note any changes in WBC count and differential.

Interventions

1. Assist with treatment of client with immunosuppression by:
• Preventing infection as noted under bone marrow depression for leukopenia
• Advising delay of active immunization for several months after therapy is completed because there may be either a hypo- or hyperactive response
• Avoiding contact with children who have recently taken the oral polio vaccine
• Administering granulocyte colony-stimulating factor when prescribed
2. Review food safety (e.g., storage, handling, washing, cooking meats thoroughly, avoiding raw eggs) and stress the importance of kitchen hygiene for clients preparing meals at home

NURSING CONSIDERATIONS FOR GU ALTERATIONS

Assessment

1. Assess for altered GU function.
2. Determine client understanding that most symptoms, such as amenorrhea, cease after medication is discontinued.
3. Ascertain client's comprehension of risks before initiation of therapy, by asking whether physician has informed client that sterility may be a permanent result of therapy.

Interventions: Prevent teratogenesis by teaching client and partner of childbearing age to use contraceptive measures to avoid pregnancy, both during and for several months after therapy. Drug could have a teratogenic effect on the fetus if the woman were to conceive during this period.

NURSING CONSIDERATIONS FOR ALOPECIA

Client/Family Teaching

1. Advise that hair loss is a normal occurrence with chemotherapy. Explain that the treatment disrupts the mitotic activity of the hair follicle

which weakens the hair shaft which causes it to break off. This includes all hair, i.e., eyebrows, body, and pubic hair.

2. Alopecia may occur within 2–3 weeks after the initial treatment. Assist client to understand, be prepared for, and expect this as normal with this therapy. Advise that people respond differently and that while some may lose hair with a certain agent, others may not.

3. Reinforce that it will grow back but that hair may be of a different texture or color. It should start to grow in again about 8 weeks after therapy is completed.

4. In clients receiving more than 4,500 rad to the cranium, this may be permanent.

5. Several alternatives for managing alopecia include:

- Encouraging client to shop for a wig before hair loss begins
- Wearing a bandana or hat to cover head, and taking special care to protect the bare head from sun exposure
- Shaving head, if hair starts to fall out in large clumps, and using a wig or scarf until scalp hair has grown in again
- Using a wig or scarf while hair is falling out and growing in again
- Wearing a night cap at bedtime. This ensures that hair that falls out during the night will be collected in one place and will not be all over the bed in the morning.
- Encouraging expression of feelings related to changes in self-image

NURSING CONSIDERATIONS FOR ALTERATIONS IN SKIN

Assessment

1. Assess skin turgor and integrity. Document baseline data for comparison.

2. Anticipate and explain to family that some clients have slight changes in skin color during therapy.

Interventions

1. Maintain cleanliness of skin through bathing and frequent linen changes.

2. Prevent dryness and replenish moisture of skin with emollient lotions.

3. Prevent excessive exposure to sun or artificial ultraviolet light, and use a sunscreen and protective clothing when exposure is necessary.

4. Use a special mattress or bed to redistribute weight on bony prominences and to minimize pressure and friction on pressure points.

5. Establish a schedule for repositioning, massaging, and assessing client's skin condition with appropriate documentation.

6. Ensure adequate nutritional intake.

7. Refer for assistance with makeup application as needed.

8. With pruritus, attempt to stop scratching as this may impair skin integrity. Administer antihistamines, corticosteroids, nonirritating moisturizers, and cool compresses as needed.

CHAPTER TWENTY-ONE

Antineoplastic Agents: Alkylating Agents

See also the following individual entries:

Busulfan
Carboplatin for Injection
Carmustine
Chlorambucil
Cisplatin
Cyclophosphamide
Dacarbazine
Ifosfamide
Lomustine
Mechlorethamine Hydrochloride
Mesna
Streptozocin
Thiotepa
Uracil Mustard

Action/Kinetics: Alkylating agents are highly reactive in that under physiologic conditions they donate an alkyl group (carbonium ion) to biologically important macromolecules, such as DNA. These reactions inactivate the molecule, bringing *cell division* to a halt. This cytotoxic activity is not limited to cancerous cells, but affects replication of the other cells of an organism, especially that of rapidly proliferating tissues, such as the bone marrow, intestinal epithelium, and hair follicles.

The toxic effects of the alkylating agents are usually cell-cycle nonspecific. The cytotoxic effect on cell division becomes apparent when the cell enters the S phase and cell division is blocked at the G_2 phase (premitotic phase), resulting in cells having a double complement of DNA.

Resistance of cancer cells to alkylating agents usually develops slowly and gradually. The resistance seems to be the sum total of several minor adaptations and not a reaction to a single one. Such mechanisms include decreased permeability of the cells, increased production of noncancer receptors (nucleophilic substances), and increased efficiency of the DNA repair system.

NURSING CONSIDERATIONS

See *Nursing Considerations* for individual agents and *Nursing Considerations* for *Antineoplastic Agents,* Chapter 20.

Evaluate: Clinical and radiographic evidence of tumor and disease regression or stabilization.

Busulfan

(byou-**SUL**-fan)
Pregnancy Category: D
Myleran (Abbreviation: Bus) **(Rx)**

See also *Antineoplastic Agents,* Chapter 20, and *Alkylating Agents,* above.

How Supplied: *Tablet:* 2 mg

Action/Kinetics: Busulfan is cell cycle-phase nonspecific and acts predominately against cells of the granulocytic type and is thought to act by alkylating cellular thiol groups. Cross-linking of nucleoproteins occurs. Busulfan may cause severe bone marrow depression. Leukocyte count drops during the second or third week. Thus, close medical supervision, including weekly laboratory tests, is mandatory. Resistance may develop and is thought to be due to the altered transport into the cell and/or increased intracellular inactivation. Rapidly absorbed from the GI tract; appears in serum 0.5–2 hr after PO administration. **t½:** 2.5 hr. It is slowly excreted by the kidney.

Increased appetite and sense of well-being may occur a few days after therapy is started. Sometimes administered with allopurinol to prevent symptoms of clinical gout.

Uses: Chronic myelogenous leukemia (granulocytic, myelocytic, myeloid). Less effective in individuals with chronic myelogenous leukemia who lack the Philadelphia (Ph^1) chromosome. Not effective in individuals where the disease is in the "blastic" phase.

Dosage

• **Tablets**

Individualized according to leukocyte count.

Chronic myelocytic leukemia.

Adults, remission, induction, usual dose: 4–8 mg/day until leukocyte count falls below 15,000/mm^3; **maintenance:** 1–3 mg/day. Discontinue therapy if there is a precipitous fall in leukocyte count. **Children, induction:** 0.06–0.12 mg/kg or 1.8–4.6 mg/m^2 daily; **maintenance:** dosage is titrated to maintain a leukocyte count of 20,000/mm^3.

Administration/Storage

1. Busulfan should be taken at the same time each day.
2. Extra fluid intake may be required during therapy.
3. Busulfan should not be administered without supervision and the availability of facilities for weekly CBCs.
4. *Treatment of Overdose:* If ingestion is recent, gastric lavage or induction of vomiting followed by activated charcoal. Hematologic status must be monitored.

Contraindications: Use during lactation only if benefits outweigh risks.

Laboratory Test Interference: ↑ Uric acid in blood and urine.

Additional Side Effects: Pancytopenia (more severe than with other agents), bronchopulmonary dysplasia, ***interstitial pulmonary fibrosis***, cataracts (after prolonged use), hyperpigmentation, adrenal insufficiency-like syndrome, gynecomastia, suppression of ovarian function, amenorrhea, cholestatic jaundice, myasthenia gravis. Cellular dysplasia in the adrenal glands, bone marrow, lymph nodes, liver, pancreas, and thyroid.

Symptoms of Overdose: ***Bone marrow toxicity.***

Drug Interactions: Use with thioguanine may cause esophageal varices with abnormal liver function tests.

NURSING CONSIDERATIONS

See also *Nursing Considerations* for *Antineoplastic Agents,* Chapter 20.

Assessment

1. Note previous experience with drug therapy and determine any resistance.
2. In clients with chronic myelogenous leukemia note presence of Philadelphia (Ph^1) chromosome.
3. Document when disease is in "blastic" phase as drug is not effective.
4. Drug may cause moderate to severe granulocyte suppression. Monitor appropriate weekly hematologic profiles. Nadir: 21 days; recovery: 42–56 days.

Evaluate

• ↑ Appetite and improved sense of well-being

• Maintenance of leukocytes at 20,000/mm^3

• Absence of blasts on peripheral blood smear

• ↓ Spleen size

• In combination with allopurinol, prevention of symptoms of gout

Carboplatin for Injection

(**KAR**-boh-plah-tin)

Pregnancy Category: D

Paraplatin **(Rx)**

See also *Antineoplastic Agents,* Chapter 20, and *Alkylating Agents,* Chapter 21.

How Supplied: *Powder for injection:* 50 mg, 150 mg, 450 mg

Action/Kinetics: Related to cisplatin. Carboplatin acts by producing interstrand DNA cross-links and is thus thought to be cell-cycle nonspecific. **t½, initial:** 1.1–2 hr; **postdistribution:** 2.6–5.9 hr. Carboplatin is not bound to plasma proteins although platinum from carboplatin is irreversibly bound to plasma protein with a slow half-life (5 days). The drug is eliminated unchanged in the urine at a rate related to creatinine clearance. **Uses:** Initial treatment of advanced ovarian cancer in combination with other chemotherapeutic agents. Palliative treatment of recurrent ovarian cancer either initially or previously treated with chemotherapy, including cisplatin. *Investigational:* Small cell lung carcinoma (in combination with etoposide); advanced or recurrent squamous cell tumors of the head and neck (in combination with fluorouracil); seminoma of testicular cancer; advanced endometrial cancer; relapsed or refractory acute leukemia.

Dosage

• **IV**

Ovarian cancer, as a single agent. 360 mg/m² q 4 weeks on day 1. Lower doses are recommended in clients with low creatinine clearances.

In combination with cyclophosphamide.

Carboplatin, 300 mg/m² plus cyclophosphamide, 600 mg/m², both on day 1 q 4 weeks.

Administration/Storage

1. Single intermittent doses of carboplatin should not be repeated until the neutrophil count is at least 2,000/mm³ and the platelet count is 100,000/mm³.
2. The dose may be escalated by no more than 125% of the starting dose if platelet counts are greater than 100,000/mm³ and neutrophil counts are greater than 2,000/mm³. If platelet counts are less than 50,000/mm³ and neutrophil counts are less than 500/mm³, subsequent doses should be 75% of the prior dose.
3. For clients with impaired kidney function, the dose should be adjusted as follows: creatinine clearance of 41–59 mL/min, 250 mg/m² on day 1; creatinine clearance of 16–40 mL/min, 200 mg/m². There is no recommended dose if the creatinine clearance is less than 15 mL/min.
4. Immediately before use, the drug should be reconstituted with either sterile water for injection, 5% dextrose in water, or sodium chloride injection to obtain a final concentration of 10 mg/mL. Carboplatin can be further diluted to concentrations as low as 0.5 mg/mL with 5% dextrose in water or sodium chloride injection. The dose is administered by infusion lasting 15 min or longer.
5. Reconstituted solutions are stable for 8 hr at room temperature. Discard after this period of time because there is no antibacterial preservative in the formulation.
6. Unopened vials should be stored at room temperature, protected from light.
7. Should not be used with needles or IV administration sets containing aluminum.
8. Cisplatin has been confused with carboplatin. Signs should be placed in the storage areas warning of the name mix-ups. Products should not be referred to as "platinum."
9. *Treatment of Overdose:* Monitor bone marrow and liver function tests. Treat symptomatically.

Additional Contraindications: History of severe allergy to mannitol or platinum compounds (including cisplatin). Severe bone marrow depression, significant bleeding, lactation.

Laboratory Test Interferences: ↑ Alkaline phosphatase, AST, total bilirubin.

Additional Side Effects: ***Bone marrow suppression*** may be severe. Vomiting is a frequent side effect. *Neurologic:*Central neurotoxicity, peripheral neuropathies (more common in ages 65 and over), ototoxicity. *GU:* Nephrotoxicity (including increased BUN and serum creatinine). *Electrolytes:* Loss of calcium, magnesium, potassium, sodium. *Allergic:* Rash, urticaria, pruritus, erythema; ***bronchospasm*** and hypotension (rare). *Miscellaneous:* Pain, alopecia, asthenia. CV, respiratory, mucosal side effects, ***anaphylaxis.***

Symptoms of Overdose: ***Bone marrow suppression, hepatic toxicity.***

Drug Interactions: Carboplatin can react with aluminum (e.g., needles, IV administration sets) causing formation of a precipitate and loss of potency.

NURSING CONSIDERATIONS

See also *Nursing Considerations* for *Antineoplastic Agents,* Chapter 20.

Assessment

1. Note any evidence of kidney impairment.
2. Determine if client has a history of allergic responses to mannitol or platinum compounds.
3. Document and assess any evidence of neurologic disorders as a means of determining if those that may occur at a later date are drug related or exacerbations of a prior condition.
4. Obtain CBC and assess closely for drug-induced anemia, a frequent side effect of carboplatin therapy.
5. Ascertain that alkaline phosphatase, AST, and total bilirubin have been done. These results serve as baseline data against which to measure client reactions to the drug therapy.

Interventions

1. Premedicate client with antiemetics because vomiting is a frequent side effect of drug therapy.
2. Drug dose is based on CBC and creatinine clearance results; monitor carefully. Anticipate reduced dose with impaired liver and/or renal function.
3. If the client has evidence of kidney impairment, give 1–2 L of fluids before starting therapy. This may be given over a period of time. Have diuretics available should the client begin to show signs of overhydration.

Client/Family Teaching

1. Warn that N&V may be experienced.
2. Report if a rash, pruritus, redness of the skin, or bronchospasm develops.
3. Maintain adequate fluid intake. Favorite fluids may be given, especially those with potassium and calcium, since these electrolytes may be lost in excess as a result of therapy.
4. Report any sore throat, fever, fatigue, or mouth sores. This may be an indication of bone marrow depression, which can be severe with this drug therapy.

Evaluate: Evidence of ↓ size and spread of tumor and stabilization of malignant disease.

Carmustine

(kar-**MUS**-teen)

Pregnancy Category: D

BiCNU (Abbreviation: BCNU) **(Rx)**

See also *Antineoplastic Agents,* Chapter 20, and *Alkylating Agents,* Chapter 21.

How Supplied: *Powder for injection:* 100 mg

Action/Kinetics: Carmustine acts by alkylating DNA and RNA as well as by inhibiting several enzymes by carbamoylation of amino acids in proteins. It is cell-cycle nonspecific. The drug is not cross-resistant with other alkylating agents. Drug rapidly cleared from plasma and metabolized. Crosses blood-brain barrier (concentration in CSF at least 50% greater than in plasma). **t½:** 15–30 min. Thirty percent excreted in urine after 24 hr, 60%–70% after 96 hr.

Uses: Alone or in combination with other antineoplastic agents for palliative treatment of primary (e.g., brainstem glioma, astrocytoma, glioblastoma, ependymoma) and metastatic brain tumors, multiple myeloma (in combination with prednisone). Advanced Hodgkin's disease and non-Hodgkin's lymphomas (not the drug of choice). *Investigational:* GI cancer, malignant melanoma, mycosis fungoids.

Dosage

- **IV**

In previously untreated clients. 150–200 mg/m^2 q 6–8 weeks as a single or divided dose (on consecutive days). Alternate dosing schedule: 75–100 mg/m^2 on 2 successive days q 6 weeks or 40 mg/m^2 on 5 successive days q 6 weeks. Subsequent dosage should be reduced if platelet levels are less than 100,000/mm^3 and leukocyte levels are less than 4,000/mm^3.

Administration/Storage

1. Discard vials in which powder has become an oily liquid.
2. Store unopened vials at 2°C–8°C (36°F–46°F) and protect from light. Store diluted solutions at 4°C (39°F) and protect from light.
3. Reconstitute powder with absolute ethyl alcohol (provided); then add sterile water. For injection, these dilutions are stable for 24 hr when stored as noted above.
4. Stock solutions diluted to 500 mL with 0.9% sodium chloride for injection or with 5% dextrose for injection are stable for 48 hr when stored as noted above.
5. Administer by IV over 1–2-hr period; faster injection may produce intense pain and burning at site of injection.
6. Check for extravasation if client complains of burning or pain at site of injection. Discomfort may be due to alcohol diluent. If there is no extravasation, and client complains of burning at site of injection, reduce rate of flow.
7. Slow rate of IV infusion and report if client demonstrates intense flushing of skin and/or redness of conjunctiva.
8. Contact of reconstituted carmustine with skin may result in hyperpigmentation (transient). If contact occurs, the skin or mucosa should be washed thoroughly with soap and water.
9. *Do not use vial for multiple doses* because there is no preservative in vial.

Special Concerns: Not recommended for use during lactation. Delayed bone marrow toxicity may be observed. Safety and effectiveness have not been established in children.

Additional Side Effects: *GI:* N&V within 2 hr after administration, lasting 4–6 hr. *GU:* Renal failure, azotemia, decrease in kidney size. *Hepatic:* Reversible increases in alkaline phosphatase, bilirubin, and transaminase. *Other:* Rapid IV administration may produce transitory intense flushing of skin and conjunctiva (onset: after 2 hr; duration: 4 hr). ***Pulmonary fibrosis,*** ocular toxicity including retinal hemorrhage.

Drug Interactions

Cimetidine / Additive bone marrow suppression
Digoxin / ↓ Serum levels of digoxin → ↓ effect
Phenytoin / ↓ Serum levels of phenytoin → ↓ effect

NURSING CONSIDERATIONS

See also *Nursing Considerations* for *Antineoplastic Agents,* Chapter 20.

Assessment

1. Obtain baseline CBC and monitor for at least 6 weeks after a dose of carmustine because delayed bone marrow toxicity may develop. Drug causes granulocyte and bone marrow suppression. Nadir: 21 days; recovery: 35–42 days.
2. Determine if baseline ophthalmic examination is needed.

Client/Family Teaching

1. Report any S&S of fever or infection; increased SOB, abnormal bruising or bleeding.
2. Avoid vaccinations.
3. Avoid smoking as this enhances pulmonary toxicity.
4. May experience hair loss.
5. If mouth sores develop, advise provider so a special mouthwash can be prescribed.

Evaluate

- ↓ Extent and size of metastatic tumor process
- Platelet counts > 100,000/mm^3 and leukocyte counts > 4,000/mm^3

Chlorambucil

(klor-**AM**-byou-sill)
Pregnancy Category: D
Leukeran (Abbreviation: CHL) **(Rx)**

See also *Antineoplastic Agents,* Chapter 20, and *Alkylating Agents,* Chapter 21.

How Supplied: *Tablet:* 2 mg

Action/Kinetics: Chlorambucil is cell-cycle nonspecific although it is also cytotoxic to nonproliferating cells. The drug forms an unstable ethylenimmonium ion which binds (alkylates) with intracellular substances such as nucleic acids. The cytotoxic effect is due to cross-linking of strands of DNA and RNA and inhibition of protein synthesis. The drug also has immunosuppressant activity. Is rapidly absorbed from the GI tract. **Peak plasma levels:** 1 hr. Plasma **t½:** about 60 min. Chlorambucil is 99% bound to plasma proteins, especially albumin. Is extensively metabolized by the liver and at least one metabolite is active. Sixty percent of the drug is excreted through the urine 24 hr after drug administration, and 40% is bound to tissues, including fat.

Uses: Palliation in chronic lymphocytic leukemia, malignant lymphomas (including lymphosarcoma), giant follicular lymphomas, and Hodgkin's disease. *Investigational:* Ovarian and testicular cancer, hairy cell leukemia, polycythemia vera, in combination with prednisone for nephrotic syndrome in adults and children unresponsive to other therapy.

Dosage

- **Tablets**

Leukemia, lymphomas.

Individualized according to response of client. **Adults, children, initial dose:** 0.1–0.2 mg/kg body weight (or 4–10 mg) daily in single or divided doses for 3–6 weeks; **maintenance:** 0.03–0.1 mg/kg/day depending on blood counts.

Alternative for chronic lymphocytic leukemia.

Initial: 0.4 mg/kg; **then,** repeat this dose every 2 weeks increasing by 0.1 mg/kg until either toxicity or control of condition is observed.

Nephrotic syndrome, immunosuppressant.

Adults, children: 0.1–0.2 mg/kg body weight daily for 8–12 weeks.

Special Concerns: Use during lactation only if benefits outweigh risks. Safety and efficacy have not been established in children. The drug is carcinogenic in humans and may be both mutagenic and teratogenic in humans. It also affects fertility.

Administration/Storage: *Treatment of Overdose:* General supportive measures. Blood should be carefully monitored; blood transfusions may be required.

Laboratory Test Interference: ↑ Uric acid levels in serum and urine.

Additional Side Effects: *Hepatic:* Hepatotoxicity with jaundice. *Pulmonary:* ***Pulmonary fibrosis,*** bronchopulmonary dysplasia. *CNS:* Children with nephrotic syndrome have an increased risk of seizures. *Miscellaneous:* Keratitis, drug fever, sterile cystitis, interstitial pneumonia, peripheral neuropathy. Cross-sensitivity (skin rashes) may occur with other alkylating agents.

Symptoms of Overdose: Pancytopenia (reversible), ataxia, agitated behavior, ***clonic-tonic seizures.***

NURSING CONSIDERATIONS

See also *Nursing Considerations* for *Antineoplastic Agents,* Chapter 20.

Assessment

1. Document indications for therapy, noting pretreatment laboratory and physical assessment findings.
2. Drug may cause severe granulocyte and lymphocyte suppression. Nadir: 21 days; recovery: 42–56 days.

Client/Family Teaching

1. The drug should be taken 1 hr before breakfast or 2 hr after the evening meal.
2. Monitor and record intake; consume 2–3 L/day of fluids.
3. Provide a printed list of adverse side effects. Advise that skin rash may be a result of cross-sensitivity with oth-

er alkylating agents and should be reported if present.

4. Stress that drug is carcinogenic and may also be mutagenic and teratogenic. Explain what this means and the associated risks of this form of drug therapy. Stress the importance of practicing birth control during therapy.

Evaluate

• Positive tumor response as evidenced by ↓ tumor size and spread and suppression of malignant cell proliferation

• Desired immunosuppressant activity

Cisplatin

(sis-**PLAH**-tin)

Platinol, Platinol-AQ (Abbreviation: CDDP) **(Rx)**

See also *Antineoplastic Agents,* Chapter 20.

How Supplied: *Injection:* 1 mg/mL; *Powder for injection:* 10 mg, 50 mg

Action/Kinetics: Cisplatin, a heavy metal inorganic coordination complex, acts similarly to alklyating agents in that it produces interstrand and intrastrand crosslinks in DNA. The drug is cell-cycle nonspecific. **t½: Initial,** 25–49 min; **postdistribution,** 58–73 hr. Incomplete urinary excretion (only 27%–43% after 5 days). Drug concentrates in liver, kidneys, large and small intestines, with low penetration of CNS. The drug is over 90% bound to plasma protein.

Uses: Treatment of metastatic testicular (in combination with bleomycin and vinblastine) and ovarian (in combination with doxorubicin) tumors in clients with prior radiotherapy or surgery. Advanced bladder cancer unresponsive to other treatment. *Investigational:* Cancer of the adrenal cortex, head and neck, breast, cervix, endometrium, stomach, lung, prostate. Neuroblastoma. Germ cell tumors of the ovary and in children. Osteosarcoma.

Dosage

• **IV**

Metastatic testicular tumors, remission induction.

Usual dosage: cisplatin, 20 mg/m²/day for 5 days q 3 weeks for three courses; bleomycin sulfate, **IV (rapid infusion):** 30 units/week (on day 2 of each week) for 12 consecutive weeks; vinblastine sulfate, **IV,** 0.15–0.2 mg/kg twice weekly (days 1 and 2) q 3 weeks for four courses (i.e., eight doses total).

Metastatic ovarian tumor, as single agent.

100 mg/m² q 4 weeks.

In combination with doxorubicin hydrochloride, cisplatin: 50 mg/m²/3 weeks (on day 1); doxorubicin hydrochloride: 50 mg/m² once every 3 weeks (on day 1). The drugs are given sequentially.

Advanced bladder cancer.

50–70 mg/m² q 3–4 weeks as a single agent.

NOTE: Repeat courses should not be administered until (1) serum creatinine is below 1.5 mg/dL and/or the BUN is below 25 mg/dL; (2) platelets are equal to or greater than 100,000/mm³ and leukocyte count is equal to or greater than 4,000/mm³; and (3) auditory activity is within the normal range.

Administration/Storage

1. Store unopened vials of dry powder in refrigerator at 2°C–8°C to maintain stability for 2 years.

2. Reconstitute 10- and 50-mg vials with 10 or 50 mL of sterile water for injection as instructed on package insert.

3. Add dosage recommended from reconstituted vial to 2 L of 5% dextrose in one-half or one-third NSS containing 37.5 g mannitol. Infuse over a period of 6–8 hr. Furosemide is ordered by some practitioners instead of mannitol.

4. Do not refrigerate reconstituted vials because a precipitate will form. Reconstituted solution is stable at room temperature for 20 hr.

5. Use of a 0.45-μm filter is advised.
6. Before administration of cisplatin, hydrate client with 1–2 L of fluid by IV route over a period of 8–12 hr.
7. Do *not* use any equipment with aluminum for preparing or administering because a black precipitate will form and loss of potency will occur.
8. Platinol-AQ is a sterile, multidose vial without preservatives. Unopened containers should be stored at 15°C–25°C, protected from light. Once opened, the solution is stable for 28 days protected from light or for 7 days under fluorescent room light.
9. Cisplatin has been confused with carboplatin. Signs should be placed in the storage areas warning of the name mix-ups. Products should not be referred to as "platinum."
10. Have emergency equipment readily available to treat any occurrence of an anaphylactic reaction to cisplatin.

Additional Contraindications: Preexisting renal impairment, bone marrow suppression, hearing impairment, and allergic reactions to platinum. Lactation.

Special Concern: Safe use during pregnancy has not been established; use is generally not recommended.

Laboratory Test Interferences: ↑ Plasma iron levels. Nephrotoxicity results in ↑ serum uric acid, BUN, and creatinine and ↓ creatinine clearance.

Additional Side Effects: *Renal:* Severe cumulative renal toxicity, including renal tubular damage and renal insufficiency. *Electrolytes:* Low levels of calcium, magnesium, potassium, phosphate, and sodium. *Neurologic:* Seizures, taste loss, peripheral neuropathies. Neurotoxicity may occur 4–7 months after prolonged therapy. *Otic:* Ototoxicity characterized by tinnitus, especially in children. *Ophthalmologic:* Papilledema, cerebral blindness, optic neuritis. High doses have resulted in blurred vision and altered color perception. *Miscellaneous:* ***Anaphylactic reactions,*** hyperuricemia.

Additional Drug Interactions
Aminoglycosides / Cumulative nephrotoxity
Anticonvulsants / Plasma levels of anticonvulsants may become subtherapeutic
Loop diuretics / Additive ototoxicity
Phenytoin / ↓ Effect of phenytoin due to ↓ plasma levels

NURSING CONSIDERATIONS

See also *Nursing Considerations* for *Antineoplastic Agents,* Chapter 20.

Assessment
1. Document indications for therapy and anticipated results.
2. Identify any previous treatments and the outcome.
3. Ascertain that baseline renal tests are performed before therapy is instituted because cisplatin may cause severe cumulative renal toxicity.
4. Anticipate that additional doses of cisplatin will not be administered until the client's renal function has returned to baseline value and usually not more frequently than every 3–4weeks.
5. Recommend audiometry testing before initiating therapy and before administering subsequent doses, to ascertain that client's hearing has not been affected.
6. Obtain baseline CBC and assess for mild granulocyte suppression. Nadir: 14 days; recovery: 21 days.

Interventions
1. *During therapy monitor client closely for:*
• Facial edema, bronchoconstriction, tachycardia, and shock.
• Tremors that may progress to seizures due to hypomagnesemia.
• Tetany, confusion, or signs of hypocalcemia associated with hypomagnesemia; monitor calcium and magnesium levels.
2. Hydrate well and monitor I&O for 24 hr after treatment.
3. Be alert to complaints of ringing in ears, difficulty in hearing, edema of lower extremities, and decreased urination and report.

Client/Family Teaching

1. Report any numbness, tingling, swelling, or joint pain.
2. Avoid vaccinations.
3. Use birth control. Drug may also cause infertility.
4. Avoid alcohol and salicylates as these may increase gastric bleeding.

Evaluate: Evidence of ↓ tumor size and spread and suppression of malignant cell proliferation.

Cyclophosphamide

(sye-kloh-**FOS**-fah-myd)
Pregnancy Category: D
Cytoxan, Cytoxan Lyophilized, Neosar, Procytox ✱ (Abbreviation: CYC)
(Rx)

See, also *Antineoplastic Agents,* Chapter 20, and *Alkylating Agents,* Chapter 21.

How Supplied: *Powder for injection:* 100 mg, 200 mg, 500 mg, 1 g, 2 g; *Tablet:* 25 mg, 50 mg

Action/Kinetics: Cyclophosphamide is metabolized in the liver to both active antineoplastic alkylating agents and inactive metabolites. The active metabolites alkylate nucleic acids, thus interfering with the growth of neoplastic and normal tissues. The cytotoxic action is due to cross-linking of strands of DNA and RNA and inhibition of protein synthesis. The drug also possesses immunosuppressive activity. **t½:** 3–12 hr, but remnants of drug and/or metabolites detectable in serum after 72 hr; in children, the **t½** averages 4.1 hr. Metabolites are excreted through the urine with up to 20% of cyclophosphamide excreted unchanged. Cyclophosphamide is also excreted in milk.

Uses: Often used in combination with other antineoplastic drugs. Multiple myeloma. Malignant lymphomas: Hodgkin's disease, follicular lymphoma, lymphocytic lymphosarcoma, reticulum cell sarcoma, lymphoblastic lymphosarcoma, Burkitt's lymphoma. Mycosis fungoides. Leukemias: Chronic lymphocytic and granulocytic leukemia, acute myelogenous and monocytic leukemia, acute lymphoblastic leukemia in children. Neuroblastoma, adenocarcinoma of ovary, retinoblastoma. Carcinoma of breast. *Investigational:* Rheumatic diseases including rheumatoid arthritis and lupus erythematosus, multiple sclerosis, polyarteritis nodosa, Ewing's sarcoma, osteosarcoma, soft tissue sarcomas, prophylaxis of rejection in organ transplants. Also, cancer of the cervix, lung, endometrium, bladder, prostate and testes; Wilms' tumor.

Dosage

- **IV**

Malignancies.

Adults, loading dose: 40–50 mg/kg in divided doses over 2–5 days. *Alternative therapy:* 10–15 mg/kg q 7–10 days, 3–5 mg/kg twice weekly, or 1.5–3 mg/kg/day. **Children, induction:** 2–8 mg/kg (or 60–250 mg/m^2/day in divided doses for 6 or more days); **maintenance:** 10–15 mg/kg q 7–10 days or 30 mg/kg q 3–4 weeks (or when bone marrow recovery occurs).

- **Oral Solution, Tablets**

Malignancies.

Adults: 1–5 mg/kg depending on client tolerance. **Maintenance** (various schedules): **PO:** 1–5 mg/kg/day. **Children, induction:** 2–8 mg/kg (or 60–250 mg/m^2 in divided doses for 6 or more days); **maintenance:** 2–5 mg/kg (or 50–150 mg/m^2) twice a week. Attempt to maintain leukocyte count at 3,000–4,000/mm^3. Dosage should be adjusted for kidney or liver disease.

Nephrotic syndrome in children.

2.5–3 mg/kg/day for 60–90 days.

Administration/Storage

1. IV/IM: Dissolve 100 mg cyclophosphamide in 5 mL sterile water for injection or bacteriostatic water.
2. Solutions may be given IV, IM, intraperitoneally, or intrapleurally. Also, they may be infused IV with 5% dextrose injection, 5% dextrose and 0.9% sodium chloride injection, 5% dextrose and Ringer's injection,

lactated Ringer's injection, 0.45% sodium chloride injection, or 1/6M sodium lactate injection.
3. The reconstituted solution may be stored at room temperature for 24 hr and for 6 days if refrigerated at 2°C–8°C (36°F–46°F).
4. An oral solution may be prepared by dissolving injectable cyclophosphamide in aromatic elixir.
5. PO: Administer preferably on empty stomach. Give with meals in case of GI disturbance.
6. Fluid intake should be increased before, during, and for 24 hr after cyclophosphamide administration.
7. The initial loading dose may need to be reduced by one-third to one-half in clients who have previously received cytotoxic drugs or radiation therapy.
8. *Treatment of Overdose:* General supportive measures. Dialysis.

Contraindications: Lactation. Severe bone marrow depression.

Special Concerns: Use with caution in clients with thrombocytopenia, leukopenia, previous radiation therapy, bone marrow infiltration of tumor cells, previous therapy causing cytotoxicity, and impaired liver and kidney function. May interfere with wound healing.

Laboratory Test Interferences: ↑ Uric acid in blood and urine; false + Pap test; ↓ serum pseudocholinesterase. Suppression of certain skin tests.

Additional Side Effects: Acute hemorrhagic cystitis. ***Bone marrow depression appears frequently during days 9–14 of therapy.*** Alopecia occurs more frequently than with other drugs. ***Secondary neoplasia (especially of urinary bladder), pulmonary fibrosis, cardiotoxicity,*** darkening of skin or fingernails. Interference with oogenesis and spermatogenesis.

Drug Interactions
Allopurinol / ↑ Chance of bone marrow toxicity
Anticoagulants / ↑ Effect of anticoagulants
Chloramphenicol / ↓ Metabolism of cyclophosphamide to active metabolites → ↓ pharmacologic effect
Doxorubicin / ↑ Cardiotoxicity due to doxorubicin
Insulin / ↑ Hypoglycemia
Phenobarbital / ↑ Rate of metabolism of cyclophosphamide in liver
Succinylcholine / ↑ Succinylcholine-induced apnea due to ↓ breakdown in plasma
Thiazide diuretics / ↑ Chance of leukopenia

NURSING CONSIDERATIONS

See also *Nursing Considerations* for *Antineoplastic Agents,* Chapter 20.

Assessment
1. Note any client history of prior radiation therapy and/or chemotherapy because this is an indication for dose reduction of cyclophosphamide.
2. Assess skin condition and integrity. Document evidence of breakdown as drug may interfere with wound healing.
3. Review drugs currently prescribed to determine if any may interact unfavorably.
4. Obtain baseline CBC as drug may cause moderate granulocyte suppression. Nadir: 14 days; recovery: 17–21 days.

Interventions
1. Administer the drug in the morning so that kidneys can eliminate the drug before bedtime. Encourage frequent voiding.
2. Keep client well hydrated to help prevent hemorrhagic cystitis due to excessive concentration of drug in urine.
3. Observe for any evidence of dysuria and hematuria. Monitor urinalysis and specific gravity of urine to assess for syndrome of inappropriate antidiuretic hormone (SIADH).
4. Monitor for cardiotoxicity; client complaints of SOB, presence of pulmonary crackles, or tachycardia.
5. Observe for increased coughing or SOB. Obtain periodic CXR and pulmonary function tests.
6. See *Nursing Considerations* for *Neuromuscular Blocking Agents,* Chapter 53, if client is also receiving succinylcholine because apnea may be induced.

7. May suppress skin test response for *Candida*, mumps, trichophyton, and purified protein derivative.

Client/Family Teaching

1. Take medication on an empty stomach unless otherwise ordered.
2. Increase consumption of fluids during and for 24 hr after cyclophosphamide therapy.
3. May discolor skin and nails.
4. Report any unusual bruising, bleeding, or fever.
5. Avoid vaccinations during therapy.
6. Reassure client with alopecia that hair should grow back when drug is stopped or when a maintenance dosage is given.
7. Advise women that drug may cause a false positive Pap test.
8. May also cause sterility and menstrual irregularities.
9. Contraception should be practiced by both men and women during therapy.
10. Advise diabetic client that S&S of hypoglycemia may be precipitated by drug interactions with insulin. Instruct to monitor sugars closely and to consult with provider for possible insulin dosage adjustment.
11. Report any evidence of injury or delayed healing of wounds.

Evaluate

- Improved hematologic parameters
- ↓ Tumor size and spread
- Suppression of malignant cell proliferation

Dacarbazine

(dah-**KAR**-bah-zeen)
Pregnancy Category: C
DTIC ✱, DTIC-Dome, Imidazole Carboxamide (Abbreviation: DTIC) **(Rx)**

See also *Antineoplastic Agents,* Chapter 20, and *Alkylating Agents,* Chapter 21.

How Supplied: *Powder for injection:* 100 mg, 200 mg

Action/Kinetics: The drug is thought to act by three mechanisms, including: alkylation by an activated carbonium ion, antimetabolite to inhibit DNA synthesis, and by combining with protein sulfhydryl groups. The drug is cell-cycle nonspecific. **t½, biphasic, initial,** 19 min; **terminal,** 5 hr. Drug probably localizes in liver. Limited amounts (14% of plasma level) enter CSF. Approximately 40% of drug excreted in urine unchanged within 6 hr. Dacarbazine is secreted through the kidney tubules rather than filtered through the glomeruli.

Uses: Metastatic malignant melanoma. Hodgkin's disease (with other agents).

Dosage

- **IV only**

Malignant melanoma.

2–4.5 mg/kg/day for 10 days; may be repeated at 4-week intervals; or 250 mg/m²/day for 5 days; may be repeated at 3-week intervals.

Hodgkin's disease.

150 mg/m²/day for 5 days; or 375 mg/m² on day 1, with other drugs repeated q 15 days.

Administration/Storage

1. To minimize adverse GI effects, antiemetics, fasting, and limited fluid intake (4–6 hr preceding treatment) have been suggested.
2. Extreme care should be taken to avoid extravasation.
3. Reconstitute with sterile water for injection to 10 mg/mL. Drug can be given by IV push over 1-min period. May be further diluted in 250 mL of D5%/W or NSS and administered (preferred) over 15–30 min.
4. Protect dry vials from light and store at 2°C–8°C.
5. Reconstituted solutions are stable for up to 72 hr at 4°C or for 8 hr at 20°C. More dilute solutions for IV infusions are stable for 24 hr when stored at 2°C–8°C.
6. *Treatment of Overdose:* Monitor blood cell counts; supportive treatment.

Contraindication: Use during lactation.

Special Concerns: Dosage has not been established in children.

Additional Side Effects: ***Especially serious (fatal) hematologic toxicity.*** More than 90% of clients develop N&V and anorexia 1 hr after initial administration, which persists for 12–48 hr. Rarely, diarrhea, stomatitis, and intractable nausea. Also, flu-like syndrome, severe pain along injected vein, facial flushing, alopecia, photosensitivity. Elevation of AST, ALT, and other enzymes, CNS symptoms.

NURSING CONSIDERATIONS

See also *Nursing Considerations* for *Antineoplastic Agents,* Chapter 20.

Interventions

1. Ascertain how fluid status is to be handled (have client fast for 4–6 hr before treatment to reduce emesis or allow client to have fluids up to 1 hr before administration to minimize dehydration following treatment).
2. Anticipate antiemetic administration before and throughout therapy. Report N&V because these side effects may last for 1–12 hr after injection.
3. Have phenobarbital and/or prochlorperazine available for palliation of vomiting following administration of dacarbazine.
4. Clients may develop flu-like symptoms with fever, aches, fatigue, usually starting 7–10 days after dose of drug. Administer antipyretics and analgesics as needed.
5. Monitor client and laboratory studies closely for evidence of bone marrow depression, liver toxicity, or hypersensitivity reaction. Anticipitate mild granulocyte toxicity. Nadir: 10 days; recovery: 21 days.

Client/Family Teaching

1. Reassure client that after the first 1–2 days of dacarbazine therapy, vomiting should cease because tolerance develops to the drug.
2. Report any flu-like symptoms (fever, myalgia, and malaise) that may occur. Usually occurs 1 week after treatment and may persist for 1–3 weeks. Acetaminophen may assist to relieve symptoms.
3. Avoid prolonged exposure to sun or ultraviolet light, as photosensitivity reaction may occur. Wear protective clothing, sunscreens, and sunglasses as needed.
4. Prepare client for hair loss.
5. Practice contraception during and for several months following therapy.

Evaluate

- ↓ Tumor size and spread
- Suppression of malignant cell proliferation

Ifosfamide

(eye-**FOS**-fah-myd)
Pregnancy Category: D
Ifex **(Rx)**

See also *Antineoplastic Agents,* Chapter 20, and *Alkylating Agents,* Chapter 21.

How Supplied: *Powder for injection:* 1 g, 3 g

Action/Kinetics: Ifosfamide, a synthetic analog of cyclophosphamide, must be converted in the liver to active metabolites. The alkylated metabolites of ifosfamide then interact with DNA. **t½:** 7 hr. Excreted in the urine both as unchanged drug and metabolites.

Uses: As third-line therapy, in combination with other antineoplastic drugs, for germ cell testicular cancer. Ifosfamide should always be given with mesna (p. 842) to prevent ifosfamide-induced hemorrhagic cystitis. *Investigational:* Cancer of the breast, lung, pancreas, ovary, and stomach. Also for sarcomas, acute leukemias (except AML), malignant lymphomas.

Dosage

- **IV**

Testicular cancer.

1.2 g/m²/day for 5 consecutive days. Treatment may be repeated q 3 weeks or if platelet counts are at least 100,000/mm³ and WBCs are at least 4,000/mm³.

Administration/Storage

1. To prevent bladder toxicity, ifosfamide should be given with at least 2 L/day of PO or IV fluid as well as with mesna.
2. Dosage should be administered slowly over 30 min.
3. The drug is reconstituted by adding either sterile water for injection or

bacteriostatic water for injection for a final concentration of 50 mg/mL. Solutions may be further diluted to achieve concentrations from 0.6 to 20 mg/mL by adding 5% dextrose injection, 0.9% sodium chloride injection, sterile water for injection, or lactated Ringer's injection. Infuse over 30 min.
4. Reconstituted solutions (50 mg/mL) are stable for 1 week at 30°C (86°F) or 3 weeks at 5°C (41°F).
5. Dilutions of ifosfamide not prepared with bacteriostatic water for injection should be refrigerated and used within 6 hr.

Contraindications: Severe bone marrow depression. Lactation.

Special Concerns: Use with caution in clients with compromised bone marrow reserve, impaired renal function, and during lactation. Safety and efficacy have not been established in children. May interfere with wound healing.

Laboratory Test Interferences: ↑ Liver enzymes, bilirubin.

Additional Side Effects: *GU:* ***Hemorrhagic cystitis,*** hematuria, dysuria, urinary frequency. *CNS:* Confusion, depressive psychosis, somnolence, hallucinations. Less frequently: dizziness, disorientation, cranial nerve dysfunction, ***seizures, coma.*** *GI:* Salivation, stomatitis. *Miscellaneous:* Alopecia, infection, liver dysfunction, phlebitis, fever of unknown origin, dermatitis, fatigue, hypertension, hypotension, polyneuropathy, pulmonary symptoms, ***cardiotoxicity,*** interference with normal wound healing.

NURSING CONSIDERATIONS

See also *Nursing Considerations* for *Antineoplastic Agents,* Chapter 20.

Interventions

1. Anticipate concomitant administration with mesna to minimize occurrence of hemorrhagic cystitis.
2. Monitor I&O; promote high fluid intake during therapy.
3. Obtain and send urine for analysis prior to each dose of ifosfamide.
4. Monitor CBC and platelets closely; obtain WBC and platelet parameters prior to each drug administration.
5. Note the presence of marked leukopenia and protect the client from possible infection. Immunosuppression may activate latent infections such as herpes.
6. Check client's mouth for furry patches on the tongue or oral membranes and report if evident.

Client/Family Teaching

1. Reinforce that hair loss and N&V are frequent side effects of drug therapy.
2. Stress that normal wound healing may be impaired during drug therapy. Report any injury or interference with normal wound healing.
3. Report any confusion, hallucinations, or marked drowsiness because these symptoms may necessitate discontinuation of drug therapy.
4. Warn there may be hyperpigmentation of their skin and mucous membranes.
5. Advise female clients to practice contraceptive measures during the treatment and for at least 4 months after treatments have ceased.
6. If the treatment is to last 6 months, the client should be told that infertility may result.
7. Consume 2 L of fluids per day. Report the presence of frothy dark urine, jaundice, or light colored stools. These are signs of hepatotoxicity and adjustments may be needed in the dosage of drug or therapy may need to be changed.
8. Explain that joint or flank pain may be caused by the increase in uric acid that results from the rapid cytolysis of tumor and RBCs.
9. Review symptoms of neurotoxicity and advise client to report if evident. During outpatient treatment it is particularly important to elicit the support of the family in making observations and evaluations and encouraging them to keep a record of events and the times of their occurrence.
10. Do not take any salicylates or alcohol.

11. Avoid crowds, vaccinations, and persons with known infections.

Evaluate

• Evidence of ↓ tumor size and spread

• Designated hematologic parameters (platelet counts at least 100,000/mm^3 and WBCs at least 4,000/mm^3 in order to continue the therapy)

Lomustine

(loh-**MUS**-teen)

Pregnancy Category: D

CeeNu (Abbreviation: CCNU) **(Rx)**

See also *Antineoplastic Agents,* Chapter 20, and *Alkylating Agents,* Chapter 21.

How Supplied: *Capsule:* 10 mg, 40 mg, 100 mg

Action/Kinetics: Lomustine is an alkylating agent with cross-reactivity to carmustine. The drug interferes with the function of DNA and RNA and is cell-cycle nonspecific. Lomustine also inhibits protein synthesis by inhibiting necessary enzyme reactions. Rapidly absorbed from the GI tract; crosses the blood-brain barrier resulting in concentrations higher than in plasma. **Peak plasma level:** 1–6 hr; **t½:** biphasic; **initial,** 6 hr; **postdistribution:** 1–2 days. From 15% to 20% of drug remains in body after 5 days. Fifty percent of drug excreted within 12 hr through the kidney, 75% within 4 days. Small amounts are excreted through the lungs and feces. Metabolites present in milk.

Uses: Used alone or in combination with other drugs. Primary and metastatic brain tumors. Secondary therapy in disseminated Hodgkin's disease (in combination with other antineoplastics). *Investigational:* Cancer of the lung, breast, kidney; multiple myeloma; malignant melanoma.

Dosage

• Capsules

Adults and children, initial: 100–130 mg/m^2 as a single dose q 6 weeks. If bone marrow function is reduced, decrease dose to 100 mg/m^2 q 6 weeks. Subsequent dosage based on blood counts of clients (platelet count above 100,000/mm^3 and leukocyte count above 4,000/mm^3). Blood tests should be undertaken weekly, and repeat therapy should not be undertaken before 6 weeks.

Administration/Storage

1. Store below 40°C.
2. Lomustine may be given alone or in combination with other drugs, surgery, or radiotherapy.
3. Nadir: 3–7 weeks.

Contraindication: Use during lactation.

Laboratory Test Interference: Elevated liver function tests (reversible).

Additional Side Effects: High incidence of N&V 3–6 hr after administration and lasting for 24 hr. Renal and pulmonary toxicity. Dysarthria. ***Delayed bone marrow suppression*** may occur due to cumulative bone marrow toxicity. ***Thrombocytopenia and leukopenia may lead to bleeding and overwhelming infections.***

NURSING CONSIDERATIONS

See also *Nursing Considerations* for *Antineoplastic Agents,* Chapter 20.

Client/Family Teaching

1. Inform client that medication comes in capsules of three strengths and a combination of capsules will make up the correct dose; this combination should be taken at one time.
2. Client may have N&V up to 36 hr after treatment; this period may be followed by 2–3 days of anorexia. Take antiemetics as prescribed.
3. GI distress may be reduced by the administration of antiemetics before drug administration or by taking the drug after fasting.
4. Report feelings of depression caused by prolonged N&V so that various antiemetics can be tried and to ensure that psychological support is available as needed.
5. Any abnormal bruising or bleeding, sore throat or flu symptoms should be reported.
6. Explain that intervals of 6 weeks are

necessary between doses for optimum effect with minimal toxicity but that hematologic profiles should be assessed weekly.
Evaluate: Control or remission of metastatic processes.

Mechlorethamine hydrochloride (Nitrogen mustard)

(meh-klor-**ETH**-ah-meen)
Pregnancy Category: D
Mustargen **(Rx)**

See also *Antineoplastic Agents,* Chapter 20, and *Alkylating Agents,* Chapter 21.
How Supplied: *Powder for injection:* 10 mg
Action/Kinetics: Mechlorethamine is cell-cycle nonspecific. It acts by forming an unstable ethylenimmonium ion, which then alkylates or binds with various compounds, including nucleic acids. The cytotoxic activity is due to cross-linking of DNA and RNA strands and protein synthesis. When used for intracavitary tumors, the drug exerts both an inflammatory reaction and sclerosis on serous membranes, which causes adherence of the drug to serosal surfaces. It reacts rapidly with tissues and within minutes after administration the active drug is no longer present. Metabolites are excreted through the urine.
Uses: IV: Bronchogenic carcinoma; chronic lymphocytic and chronic myelocytic leukemia; palliative treatment of stages III and IV of Hodgkin's disease, polycythemia vera, mycosis fungoides. **Intracavitary:** Intrapericardially, intraperitoneally, or intrapleurally for treatment of metastatic carcinoma resulting in effusion. *Investigational:* **Topical:** Cutaneous mycosis fungoides.

Dosage

• **IV**
Adults, children: a total dose of 0.4 mg/kg per course of therapy given as a single dose or in two to four divided doses over 2–4 days. Depending on blood cell count, a second course may be given after 3 weeks.
• **Intracavitary**
0.4 mg/kg.
• **Intrapericardial**
0.2 mg/kg.
• **Topical Ointment, Solution**
Apply to entire skin surface once daily until 6–12 months after a complete response is obtained; **then,** use once to several times a week for up to 3 years.

Administration/Storage
1. Because drug is highly irritating, any contact with skin should be avoided; plastic or rubber gloves should be worn during preparation.
2. Drug is best administered through tubing of a rapidly flowing IV saline infusion.
3. Prepare solution immediately before administration because it decomposes on standing.
4. Medication is available in a rubber-stoppered vial to which 10 mL of either sterile water for injection or sodium chloride injection should be added to give a concentration of 1 mg/mL over 3–5 min.
5. Insert the needle and keep it inserted until the medication is dissolved and the required dose withdrawn. Carefully discard the vial with the remaining solution so that no one will come in contact with it.
6. For intracavitary administration, may be further diluted in 100 mL of NSS; turn client every 60 sec for 5 min to the following positions: prone, supine, right side, left side, and knee-chest. Lack of effect often results from failure to move the client often enough. Remaining fluid may be removed after 24–36 hr.
7. An aqueous solution of equal parts of 5% sodium thiosulfate and 5% sodium bicarbonate should be used to clean glassware, tubings, and other articles after drug administration. Soak for 45 min.
8. Monitor IV closely because extravasation causes swelling, erythema, induration, and sloughing.

9. In case of extravasation, remove IV, assist in infusion of area with isotonic sodium thiosulfate (4.14% solution of USP salt), and apply cold compresses. If sodium thiosulfate is not available, use isotonic sodium chloride solution or 1% lidocaine. Apply ice for 6–12 hr.

Contraindications: Use during lactation. During infectious disease.

Special Concerns: Extravasation into SC areas causes painful inflammation and induration. Use in children has been limited although the drug has been used in MOPP (mechlorethamine, Oncovin, procarbazine, prednisone) therapy.

Additional Side Effects: High incidence of N&V. Amyloidosis, hyperuricemia, petechiae, SC hemorrhages, tinnitus, deafness, herpes zoster, or temporary amenorrhea. Extravasation into SC tissue causes painful inflammation.

Drug Interaction: Amphotericin B: combination increases possibility of blood dyscrasias.

NURSING CONSIDERATIONS

See also *Nursing Considerations* for *Antineoplastic Agents,* Chapter 20.

Assessment

1. Document indications for therapy and route of administration. Note any agents used previously.
2. Monitor hematologic profile. Drug may cause granulocyte and platelet suppression. Nadir: 7–14 days; recovery 21 days.

Interventions

1. Administer phenothiazine and/or a sedative as ordered (30–45 min prior to medication and RTC as needed) to control severe N&V that usually occur 1–3 hr after administration of nitrogen mustard.
2. Administer in late afternoon or early evening, and follow with a sedative (sleeping pill) at an appropriate time to control any adverse symptoms and to induce sleep.
3. If mechlorethamine comes in contact with the eye, irrigate with copious amounts of saline solution and consult with an ophthalmologist.
4. Irrigate skin with water for 15 min and then with 2% solution of sodium thiosulfate in the event of accidental contact.
5. Monitor for symptoms of dehydration, anemia, infection, and gout.
6. Coadministration of allopurinol may decrease uric acid levels.

Client/Family Teaching

1. Advise client that hair loss may occur.
2. Avoid vaccinia and protect from any exposure to infections or infected persons.
3. Drug may cause irreversible gonadal suppression.
4. Practice birth control during and for 4 months following therapy.

Evaluate

- Evidence of ↓ tumor size and spread
- Laboratory evidence of improved hematologic parameters
- Radiographic evidence of resolution of effusion

Mesna

(**MEZ**-nah)

Pregnancy Category: B

Mesnex, Uromitexan ✱ **(Rx)**

How Supplied: *Injection:* 100 mg/mL

Action/Kinetics: Ifosfamide is metabolized to products that cause hemorrhagic cystitis. In the kidney, mesna reacts chemically with these ifosfamide metabolites to cause their detoxification. Following IV use, mesna is rapidly oxidized to mesna disulfide (dimesna), which is eliminated by the kidneys. **t½ in blood, mesna:** 0.36 hr; **dimesna:** 1.17 hr.

Uses: Prophylactically to reduce the incidence of hemorrhagic cystitis caused by ifosfamide. *Investigational:* Reduce incidence of hemorrhagic cystitis caused by cyclophosphamide.

Dosage

- **IV bolus.**

Prophylaxis of ifosfamide-induced hemorrhagic cystitis.

Dosage of mesna equal to 20% of the ifosfamide dose given at the time of ifosfamide and at 4 and 8 hr after each dose of ifosfamide. Thus, the total daily dose of mesna is 60% of the ifosfamide dose (e.g., an ifosfamide dose of 1.2 g/m^2 would mean doses of mesna would be 240 mg/m^2 at the time the ifosfamide dose was given, 240 mg/m^2 after 4 hr, and 240 mg/m^2 after 8 hr). This dosage should be given on each day that ifosfamide is administered.

Administration/Storage

1. If the dosage of ifosfamide is increased or decreased, the dosage of mesna should be adjusted accordingly.
2. The drug can be reconstituted to a final concentration of 20 mg mesna/mL fluid by adding either 5% dextrose injection, 5% dextrose and sodium chloride injection, 0.9% sodium chloride injection, or lactated Ringer's injection.
3. Diluted solutions are stable for 24 hr at 25°C (77°F). However, when mesna is exposed to oxygen, dimesna is formed; thus, a new ampule should be used for each administration.
4. Mesna is not compatible with cisplatin.

Contraindication: Hypersensitivity to thiol compounds.

Special Concerns: Use with caution during lactation.

Laboratory Test Interference: False + test for urinary ketones.

Side Effects: Since mesna is used with ifosfamide and other antineoplastic agents, it is difficult to identify those side effects due to mesna. The following symptoms are believed possible. *GI:* N&V, diarrhea, bad taste in mouth.

NURSING CONSIDERATIONS

Interventions

1. Drug must be administered with each dose of ifosfamide and at 4- and 8-hr intervals following the initial dose to be effective against drug-induced hemorrhagic cystitis.
2. Obtain a morning urine specimen for analysis each day before ifosfamide therapy.

Client/Family Teaching

1. May experience a bad taste in the mouth during drug therapy; use hard candy to mask taste.
2. N&V and diarrhea are frequent side effects of drug therapy; report if persistent or bothersome.

Evaluate: Prevention of ifosfamide-induced hemorrhagic cystitis.

Streptozocin

(strep-toe-**ZOH**-sin)
Pregnancy Category: C
Zanosar **(Rx)**

See also *Antineoplastic Agents,* Chapter 20, and *Alkylating Agents,* Chapter 21.

How Supplied: *Powder for injection:* 1 g

Action/Kinetics: Streptozocin is cell-cycle nonspecific although it does inhibit progression out of the G_2 phase of cell division. The drug forms methylcarbonium ions that alkylate or bind with intracellular substances such as nucleic acids. It is also cytotoxic by virtue of cross-linking of DNA strands resulting in inhibition of DNA synthesis. It may also cause hyperglycemia. Streptozocin does not penetrate the blood-brain barrier well, although within 2 hr after administration, metabolites do and produce levels similar to those in plasma. **t½, unchanged drug, initial,** 35 min. **t½, metabolites, initial:** 6 min; **intermediate:** 3.5 hr; **terminal:** 40 hr. Unchanged drug and metabolites excreted in urine.

Uses: Metastatic islet cell pancreatic carcinomas (functional and nonfunctional) in clients with symptomatic or progressive metastases. *Investigational:* Malignant carcinoid tumors.

Dosage

• **IV**

Daily schedule: 500 mg/m^2 for 5 consecutive days q 6 weeks (until maximum benefit is achieved or toxicity occurs). Dose should not be increased. *Weekly schedule:* **Initial:** 1,000 mg/m^2/week for 2 weeks; **then,** if no response or no toxicity, dose can be increased, not to exceed a single dose of 1,500 mg/m². Response should be seen in 17–35 days.

Administration/Storage

1. Drug should be reconstituted with 50–100 mL dextrose injection or 0.9% sodium chloride injection and administered slowly over 1–2 hr. Reconstituted solution is pale gold in color.
2. No preservatives are found in the product; thus, total storage time for reconstituted drug is 12 hr. The ampule is not considered to be multiple dose.
3. Caution should be observed (wear gloves) in handling the drug.
4. Drug is a vesicant. Infiltration may result in tissue ulceration and necrosis.

Contraindication: Use during lactation.

Special Concerns: Dosage has not been determined for children.

Additional Side Effects: Renal toxicity (up to two-thirds of clients) manifested by anuria, azotemia, glycosuria, hypophosphatemia, and renal tubular acidosis. ***Toxicity is dose-related and cumulative and may be fatal.*** Glucose intolerance (reversible) or insulin shock with hypoglycemia, depression.

NURSING CONSIDERATIONS

See also *Nursing Considerations* for *Antineoplastic Agents,* Chapter 20.

Interventions

1. Premedicate with antiemetic as drug may cause severe N&V.
2. Monitor I&O and weight. Encourage 3 L/day of fluids to reduce the risk of renal damage. Note if urine output decreases as streptozocin can cause anuria.
3. Perform finger sticks at least once a day and observe for symptoms of hypoglycemia.
4. Monitor serum blood sugar, CBC, uric acid, and liver and renal function studies during and following therapy. Drug may cause lymphocyte and platelet suppression. Nadir: 10 days; recovery: 14–17 days.

Evaluate: ↓ Tumor size and spread and suppression of malignant cell proliferation.

Thiotepa

(thigh-oh-**TEP**-ah)
(Abbreviation: Thio) **(Rx)**

See also *Antineoplastic Agents,* Chapter 20, and *Alkylating Agents,* Chapter 21.

How Supplied: *Powder for injection:* 15 mg

Action/Kinetics: Thiotepa is cell-cycle nonspecific; it is thought to act by causing the release of ethylenimmonium ions that bind or alkylate various intracellular substances such as nucleic acids. The drug is cytotoxic by virtue of cross-linking of DNA and RNA strands as well as by inhibition of protein synthesis. It is cleared rapidly from the plasma following IV use. Thiotepa may be significantly absorbed through the bladder mucosa. Approximately 85% is excreted through the urine, mainly as metabolites.

Uses: Adenocarcinoma of the breast or ovary. Control of serious effusions of pleural, pericardial, and peritoneal cavities. Superficial papillary carcinoma of the urinary bladder. Hodgkin's and non-Hodgkin's disease, lymphosarcoma, bronchogenic carcinoma. *Investigational:* Prevention of pterygium recurrences after surgery.

Dosage

- **IV (may be rapid)**

0.3–0.4 mg/kg at 1–4-week intervals or 0.2 mg/kg for 4–5 days q 2–4 weeks.

- **Intratumor or Intracavitary Administration**

0.6–0.8 mg/kg q 1–4 weeks; **maintenance (intratumor):** 0.07–0.8 mg/kg at 1–4-week intervals, depending on condition of client.

Carcinoma of bladder.

30–60 mg in 30–60 mL distilled water instilled into the bladder and retained for 2 hr. Give once a week for 4 weeks. May be repeated monthly, if necessary.

Administration/Storage
1. Reconstitute with sterile water for injection (usually 1.5 mL to give a concentration of 5 mg/0.5 mL). The reconstituted solution can then be mixed with sodium chloride injection, dextrose injection, dextrose and sodium chloride injection, Ringer's injection, or lactated Ringer's injection (i.e., if a large volume is needed for intracavitary use, IV drip, or perfusion).
2. Minimize pain on injection and retard rate of absorption by simultaneous administration of local anesthetics. Drug may be mixed with procaine HCl 2% or epinephrine HCl 1:1,000, or both, upon order of the physician.
3. Store vials in the refrigerator. Reconstituted solutions may be stored for 5 days in the refrigerator without substantial loss of potency.
4. Since thiotepa is not a vesicant, it may be injected quickly and directly into the vein with the desired volume of sterile water. Usual amount of diluent is 1.5 mL.
5. Do not use NSS as a diluent.
6. Discard solutions grossly opaque or with precipitate.
7. When used for bladder carcinoma, the client is dehydrated for 8–12 hr prior to each dose.
8. When used for intracavitary purposes, administer through the same tube used to remove fluid from the cavity.
9. *Treatment of Overdose:* To treat hematopoietic toxicity, transfusions of whole blood, platelets, or leukocytes have been used.

Contraindications: Use during lactation. Pregnancy. Renal, hepatic, or bone marrow damage. Acute leukemia. Use with other alkylating agents due to increased toxicity.
Special Concerns: Thiotepa is both carcinogenic and mutagenic.
Additional Side Effects: Anorexia or decreased spermatogenesis. Significant toxicity to the hematopoietic system.

Symptoms of Overdose: ***Hematopoietic toxicity.***
Drug Interaction: Thiotepa increases the pharmacologic and toxic effect of succinylcholine due to a decrease in breakdown by the liver.

NURSING CONSIDERATIONS

See also *Nursing Considerations* for *Antineoplastic Agents,* Chapter 20.
Assessment
1. Document indications for therapy, onset of symptoms, and any other agents used for this condition.
2. Obtain baseline lab studies (e.g., hematologic profile) as drug causes platelet and granulocyte suppression. Nadir: 21 days; recovery: 40–50 days.

Interventions
1. Encourage clients who receive drug as bladder instillations to retain fluid for 2 hr. They should be NPO for 6 hr to ensure drug retention. Observe for hematuria and dysuria.
2. Reposition client with a bladder instillation q 15 min to ensure maximum bladder area contact.
3. Stress importance of practicing contraception because drug is carcinogenic and mutagenic.

Evaluate: Control of tumor size and malignant cell proliferation.

Uracil mustard
(**YOUR**-ah-sill)
(Rx)

See also *Antineoplastic Agents,* Chapter 20, and *Alkylating Agents,* Chapter 21.
How Supplied: *Capsule:* 1 mg
Action/Kinetics: Uracil mustard is a bifunctional alkylating agent and is cell-cycle nonspecific. It is not a vesicant. The drug forms unstable ethylenimmonium ions that bind or alkylate various intracellular substances. The drug cross-links with DNA and interferes with the function of DNA and RNA. The drug is excreted through the kidneys.

Uses: Chronic lymphocytic leukemia, non-Hodgkin's lymphomas (of the lymphocytic or histiocytic type), chronic myelogenous leukemia. Palliative therapy for polycythemia vera and mycosis fungoides.

Dosage

- **Capsules**

Adults: 0.15 mg/kg once weekly for 4 weeks. **Pediatric:** 0.30 mg/kg once weekly for 4 weeks. If a response is obtained, the weekly dose should be continued until relapse is noted.

Administration/Storage

1. Uracil mustard should not be administered until 2–3 weeks after the maximum effect of other cytotoxic drugs or X-ray therapy has been determined.
2. Uracil capsules contain tartrazine; note any sensitivity to compound.
3. Complete blood counts should be done once or twice weekly during therapy and 1 month thereafter. Nadir: 2–3 weeks.
4. Effect of drug sometimes takes 3 months to become apparent, and drug should be given that long unless precluded by a toxicity reaction.

Contraindications: Pregnancy and lactation. Leukopenia, thrombocytopenia, aplastic anemia.

Laboratory Test Interference: ↑ Serum uric acid levels.

Additional Side Effects: During therapy significant decreases in leukocyte and platelet counts occur. Also, hepatotoxicity, amenorrhea, azoospermia.

NURSING CONSIDERATIONS

See also *Nursing Considerations* for *Antineoplastic Agents,* Chapter 20.

Client/Family Teaching

1. Encourage intake of 2–3 L/day of fluids during therapy to prevent hyperuricemia. Allopurinol may be prescribed to decrease uric acid formation.
2. Warn client not to have immunizations with vaccines containing live virus during therapy with uracil mustard because vaccinia may result as a complication of immunosuppression.
3. Encourage continuation with therapy because beneficial effect may take as long as 3 months to appear.

Evaluate: Control of proliferation of malignant cells and hematologic stabilization.

CHAPTER TWENTY-TWO

Antineoplastic Agents: Antimetabolites

See the following individual entries:

Cladribine Injection
Cytarabine
Floxuridine
Fludarabine Phosphate
Fluorouracil
Hydroxyurea
Idarubicin Hydrochloride
Levamisole Hydrochloride
Mercaptopurine
Methotrexate
Methotrexate Sodium
Teniposide
Thioguanine

Cladribine injection

(**KLAD**-rih-bean)
Pregnancy Category: D
Leustatin **(Rx)**

See also *Antineoplastic Agents,* Chapter 20.

How Supplied: *Injection:* 1 mg/mL

Action/Kinetics: Cladribine is toxic to both actively dividing and quiescent lymphocytes and monocytes by inhibiting both DNA synthesis and repair. Specifically, the drug results in accumulation of 2-chloro-2'-deoxy-beta-D-adenosine monophosphate (2-CdAMP), which is subsequently converted to the active triphosphate deoxynucleotide (2-CdATP). Cells with high deoxycytidine kinase and low deoxynucleotidase activities (as in lymphocytes and monocytes) will be selectively killed by cladribine as toxic deoxynucleotides accumulate intracellularly. **t½:** 5.4 hr. The drug is excreted mainly through the urine.

Uses: To treat hairy cell leukemia as defined by clinically significant anemia, neutropenia, thrombocytopenia, or disease-related symptoms. *Investigational:* Advanced cutaneous T-cell lymphomas; chronic lymphocytic leukemia; non-Hodgkin's lymphomas; acute myeloid leukemia; autoimmune hemolytic anemia; mycosis fungoides or the Sezary syndrome.

Dosage

- **IV infusion**

  Hairy cell leukemia.

A single course given by continuous infusion for 7 consecutive days at a dose of 0.09 mg/kg/day.

Administration/Storage

1. If neurotoxicity or renal toxicity occur, drug therapy should be delayed or discontinued.
2. Aseptic technique and proper environmental precautions must be observed as the drug product does not contain any antimicrobial preservative.
3. To prepare a single daily dose, 0.09 mg/kg or 0.09 mL/kg of cladribine is added to an infusion bag containing 500 mL of 0.9% sodium chloride injection. The use of 5% dextrose is not recommended due to increased degradation of the drug. Admixtures of cladribine are stable for at least 24 hr at room temperature under normal room fluorescent light in Baxter Viaflex PVC infusion containers.
4. To prepare the 7-day infusion, the drug should be mixed only with bacteriostatic 0.9% sodium chloride injection (benzyl alcohol preserved). To minimize the risk of microbial contamination, both the cladribine

and diluent should be passed through a sterile 0.22-µm disposable hydrophilic syringe filter as each solution is being introduced into the infusion reservoir. The calculated dose of cladribine (0.09 mg/kg or mL/kg for 7 days) is first added to the infusion reservoir through the sterile filter; then, a calculated amount of bacteriostatic 0.9% sodium chloride injection is run through the filter to bring the total volume of the solution to 100 mL. After completing the preparation of the solution, the line should be clamped and the filter disconnected and discarded. Air bubbles should be aseptically aspirated from the reservoir as necessary using the syringe and a dry second sterile filter assembly. Admixtures for the 7-day infusion are stable in Pharmacia Deltic medication cassettes.

5. Adherence to the recommended diluents and infusion systems is advised due to limited availability of compatibility data.

6. Solutions containing cladribine should not be mixed with other IV drugs or additives or infused simultaneously in a common IV line.

7. Unopened vials should be refrigerated, protected from light, at 2°C–8°C (36°F–46°F). Although freezing does not affect the solution, a precipitate may form at low temperatures. The drug may be resolubilized by allowing the solution to warm naturally to room temperature and by shaking vigorously. The solution is not to be heated or microwaved. Once thawed, the solution should not be refrozen.

8. Once diluted, solutions containing cladribine should be injected promptly or stored in the refrigerator for no more than 8 hr prior to administration.

9. Vials of cladribine are for single use only; any unused portion should be discarded in an appropriate manner.

10. *Treatment of Overdose:* Discontinue infusion of the drug. Institute appropriate supportive measures as there is no antidote for cladribine.

Contraindication: Use during lactation.

Special Concerns: Use with caution in clients with known or suspected renal or hepatic insufficiency. Benzyl alcohol, a constituent of the 7-day infusion solution, has been associated with a fatal "gasping syndrome" in premature infants. Although used in children, safety and efficacy have not been established.

Side Effects: *Hematologic:* Neutropenia, anemia, thrombocytopenia, prolonged depression of CD_4 counts, prolonged bone marrow hypocellularity. *Body as a whole:* Fever, infections (including septicemia, pneumonia), fatigue, chills, asthenia, diaphoresis, malaise, trunk pain. *GI:* Nausea, decreased appetite, vomiting, diarrhea, constipation, abdominal pain. *CV:* Edema, tachycardia, purpura, petechiae, epistaxis. *CNS:* Headache, dizziness, insomnia. *Dermatologic:* Rashes, reactions at injection site, pruritus, pain, erythema. *Respiratory:* Abnormal breath sounds, cough, abnormal chest sounds, SOB. *Musculoskeletal:* Myalgia, arthralgia. *Following IV injection:* Redness, swelling pain, thrombosis, phlebitis.

Symptoms of Overdose: Irreversible neurologic toxicity (paraparesis/quadriparesis), ***acute nephrotoxicity, severe bone marrow suppression.***

NURSING CONSIDERATIONS

See also *Nursing Considerations* for *Antineoplastic Agents,* Chapter 20.

Assessment

1. Document onset of symptoms and note any other previous therapies.

2. Obtain baseline hematologic profile and liver and renal function studies. Drug causes myelosuppression; monitor hematologic profile for 4–8 weeks after treatment.

3. Reconstituted infusion solution contains benzyl alcohol. Do not use with premature infants.

4. Determine that client is infection free prior to administering drug. Assess appropriate laboratory data and radiologic studies.

Interventions

1. Fevers during the first 1–2 months following therapy should be evaluated carefully (e.g., lab studies, X rays) to determine need for treatment with antibiotics.
2. Monitor VS, I&O, and neurologic status.
3. High dose drug therapy may precipitate acute nephrotoxity and delayed neurotoxity (from demyelination).
4. Anticipate that with large tumor burdens, allopurinol may be prescribed to empirically treat hyperuricemia and tumor lysis syndrome.
5. Clients with preexisting hepatic or renal disease warrant close observation.
6. Monitor hematologic profile closely; anticipate that blood transfusions may be required, and to a lesser extent platelet transfusions, due to cladribine's severe myelosuppressive effects.

Client/Family Teaching

1. Explain the recommended dosing which requires a continuous infusion for 7 consecutive days.
2. Instruct client to report any evidence of abnormal bleeding, pain, or fever.
3. Advise that nausea may be relieved with chlorpromazine if evident and to call for a prescription.
4. Fever and fatigue are common side effects but should be reported if prolonged or debilitating. Schedule activities accordingly and include frequent rest periods.
5. Advise women of childbearing age to practice a safe form of contraception as drug is teratogenic.
6. Explain that bone marrow aspiration and biopsy will be repeated after treatment to confirm pharmacologic response.

Evaluate

- Normalization of hematologic profile (i.e., Hb > 12 g/dL; Plts > 100,000; ANC > 1,500 x 10^6/L)
- Absence of hairy cells in peripheral blood and bone marrow
- Inhibition of pathologic and clinical disease progression

Cytarabine (ARA-C, Cytosine arabinoside)

(sye-**TAIR**-ah-been)
Pregnancy Category: D
Cytosar ✱, Cytosar-U **(Rx)**

See also *Antineoplastic Agents,* Chapter 20.

How Supplied: *Liquid:* 120 mg/mL; *Powder for injection:* 100 mg, 500 mg, 1 g, 2 g

Action/Kinetics: Cytarabine is thought to act by inhibiting DNA polymerase as well as by being incorporated into both DNA and RNA. The drug is cell-phase specific, acting in the S phase and also blocking the progression of cells from the G_1 phase to the S phase. Cytarabine may also decrease the immune response. After PO administration, cytarabine is rapidly broken down by the GI mucosa and liver, resulting in systemic availability of less than 20%. **t½ after IV:** distribution, 10 min; elimination, 1–3 hr. The drug is metabolized in the liver to uracil arabinoside, which is excreted in the urine. Crosses blood-brain barrier. Eighty percent eliminated in urine in 24 hr.

Uses: Induction and maintenance of remission in acute myelocytic leukemia in adults and children, acute lymphocytic leukemia, chronic myelocytic leukemia, erythroleukemia, and meningeal leukemia. In combination with other drugs for non-Hodgkin's lymphoma in children. *Investigational:* Hodgkin's lymphomas, myelodysplastic syndrome.

Dosage

NOTE: Cytarabine is frequently used in combination with other drugs; thus, dosage varies and must be carefully checked.

- **IV infusion**

Acute myelocytic leukemia, acute lymphocytic leukemia.

100–200 mg/m^2 as a continuous infusion over 24 hr or in divided doses (by rapid injection) for 5–10 days; repeat q 2 weeks.

Acute nonlymphocytic leukemia (in combination with other drugs). 100 mg/m^2/day by continuous IV infusion (days 1–7) or 100 mg/m^2 q 12 hr (days 1–7).

Refractory acute leukemia.

IV: 3 g/m^2 q 12 hr for 4–12 doses; repeat at 2–3-wk intervals.

• **Intrathecal**

Meningeal leukemia.

Usual: 30 mg/m^2 q 4 days with hydrocortisone sodium succinate and methotrexate, each at a dose of 15 mg/m^2, until CSF findings are normal, followed by one additional dose.

NOTE: The drug should be discontinued if platelet level falls to 50,000/mm^3 or less or polymorphonuclear granulocyte level falls to 1,000/mm^3 or less.

Administration/Storage

1. Cytarabine may be given SC, IV infusion, or IV injection. It is ineffective PO.
2. The 100-mg vial of cytarabine should be reconstituted with 5 mL bacteriostatic water for injection with benzyl alcohol (0.9%) with the resultant solution containing 20 mg/mL. The 500-mg vial should be reconstituted with 10 mL of bacteriostatic water for injection with benzyl alcohol (0.9%) with the resultant solution containing 50 mg/mL cytarabine. Benzyl alcohol should not be used for reconstitution if the drug will be used intrathecally; rather, 0.9% saline or Elliott's B solution should be used.
3. To administer direct IV, reconstitute 100 mg and administer over 1–3 min. May be further diluted into 100 mL of D5%/W or NSS and infused over 30 min.
4. Reconstituted solution should be stored at room temperature and used within 48 hr.
5. Discard hazy solution.
6. Assess closely during drug administration for evidence of anaphylactic reaction. Have appropriate resuscitative drugs and equipment readily available.
7. *Treatment of Overdose:* General supportive measures.

Contraindications: Use during lactation. Anaphylaxis has occurred causing acute cardiopulmonary arrest. Use with caution in impaired hepatic function.

Special Concerns: Anaphylaxis has occurred, causing acute cardiopulmonary arrest. Use with caution in clients with impaired renal function.

Additional Side Effects: "Cytarabine syndrome" (6–12 hr following drug administration) manifested by bone pain, fever, myalgia, maculopapular rash, conjunctivitis, chest pain, or malaise. Nephrotoxicity, neuritis, skin ulceration, sepsis, acute pancreatitis (in clients previously treated with l-asparaginase), pneumonia, hyperuricemia. Thrombophlebitis at injection site.

The incidence of side effects (N&V for several hours) is higher in clients receiving rapid IV injection than in those receiving drug by IV infusion. Intrathecal administration may result in systemic side effects including N&V, fever, and rarely neurotoxicity and paraplegia.

Symptoms of Overdose: CNS toxicity.

Drug Interaction: Absorption of digoxin may be impaired when cytarabine is used with other antineoplastics.

NURSING CONSIDERATIONS

See also *Nursing Considerations* for *Antineoplastic Agents,* Chapter 20.

Assessment

1. Determine baseline CBC, platelets, and liver function. Note any history of impaired hepatic function.
2. Document any previous therapy for leukemia and the results.
3. Drug may cause severe granulocyte and platelet toxicity. Nadir: 10 days; recovery: 21 days.

Interventions

1. Observe closely 6–12 hr following drug administration for the develop-

ment of "cytarabine syndrome" (see *Additional Side Effects*).
2. Monitor VS and I&O during therapy. Encourage 2–3 L/day of fluids to prevent renal damage from hyperuricemia related to cell lysis. Alkalinization of the urine may enhance uric acid excretion.
3. Obtain written hematologic parameters that would necessitate the interruption of drug therapy.
4. Report any inflammation of the eye, which may require treatment with steroid eye drops.
5. Anticipate that systemic toxicity may result from intrathecal use of cytarabine.

Client/Family Teaching

1. Report any unusual bruising, bleeding, or fever.
2. Avoid vaccinations during therapy.
3. Use birth control during and for at least 4 months following therapy.

Evaluate

- ↓ Tumor size and spread
- Improved hematologic parameters
- Evidence of disease remission

Floxuridine

(flox-**YOUR**-ih-deen)
Pregnancy Category: D
FUDR **(Rx)**

See also *Antineoplastic Agents*, Chapter 20.

How Supplied: *Powder for injection:* 0.5 g

Action/Kinetics: Floxuridine is cell-cycle specific for the S phase of cell division. The drug is rapidly metabolized to fluorouracil (see below). The drug inhibits DNA and RNA synthesis. Crosses blood-brain barrier. **t½:** 5–20 min. From 60% to 80% of fluorouracil is excreted as respiratory CO_2 (8–12 hr); small amount (15%) excreted in urine (1–6 hr).

Uses: Intra-arterially as palliative treatment of GI adenocarcinoma metastatic to the liver (especially in clients incurable by surgery or other treatment). Used in clients with disease limited to an area capable of infusion by a single artery. *Investigational:* Cancer of the breast, ovaries, cervix, bladder, kidney, and prostate.

Dosage

- **Intra-arterial infusion**

0.1–0.6 mg/kg/day by continuous infusion over 24 hr. Infusion is continued until a response or toxicity occurs (usually for 14–21 days with a rest period of 2 weeks between courses of therapy).

Administration/Storage

1. Higher doses (0.4–0.6 mg) are best given by hepatic artery infusion because the liver metabolizes the drug, reducing the possibility of systemic toxicity.
2. The drug should be given until adverse effects are manifested. Resume therapy after adverse effects have subsided. WBC nadir: 1 week. Platelet nadir: 10 days.
3. An infusion pump should be used to overcome pressure in the large arteries and to assure a uniform rate of infusion.
4. Each vial should be reconstituted with 5 mL sterile water to yield a 100-mg/mL concentration. This may be further reconstituted in D5/W or NSS and infused intra-arterially.
5. Reconstituted vials should be stored in the refrigerator at 2°C–8°C (36°F–46°F) for no longer than 2 weeks.

Contraindications: If client is at poor risk, including depressed bone marrow function, nutritionally poor, or potentially serious infections. Lactation. Should not be used during pregnancy unless benefits clearly outweigh risks.

Laboratory Test Interferences: ↑ Excretion of 5-hydroxyindoleacetic acid. ↑ Serum transaminase and bilirubin, LDH, alkaline phosphatase. ↓ Plasma albumin.

Additional Side Effects: Esophagopharyngitis, myocardial ischemia, angina, acute cerebellar syndrome, photophobia, lacrimation, decreased vision. Complications of intra-arterial administration are arterial aneurysm, arterial ischemia, arterial thrombosis, bleeding at catheter site, occluded, displaced, or leaking catheters, embolism, fibromyositis, infection at catheter site, thrombophlebitis.

NURSING CONSIDERATIONS

See also *Nursing Considerations* for *Antineoplastic Agents,* Chapter 20.
Evaluate: Suppression of metastatic processes.

Fludarabine phosphate

(floo-**DAIR**-ah-bean)
Pregnancy Category: D
Fludara **(Rx)**

See also *Antineoplastic Agents,* Chapter 20.
How Supplied: *Powder for injection:* 50 mg
Action/Kinetics: Fludarabine is rapidly dephosphorylated to 2-fluoro-ara-A and then phosphorylated within the cell by the enzyme deoxycytidine kinase to the active 2-fluoro-ara-ATP. This compound inhibits DNA polymerase alpha, ribonucleotide reductase, and DNA primase, resulting in inhibition of DNA synthesis. **t½, 2-fluoro-ara-A:** About 10 hr. Approximately 23% of a dose of fludarabine is excreted in the urine as unchanged 2-fluoro-ara-A.
Uses: Chronic lymphocytic leukemia in individuals who have not responded to at least one standard alkylating agent-containing regimen. *Investigational:* Non-Hodgkin's lymphoma, macroglobulinemic lymphoma, prolymphocytic leukemia or prolymphocytoid variant of chronic lymphocytic leukemia, mycosis fungoides, hairy cell leukemia, Hodgkin's disease.

Dosage

• **IV**

Adults, usual: 25 mg/m² given over a period of 30 min for 5 consecutive days. A 5-day course of therapy should be initiated every 28 days.

Administration/Storage

1. The dose may be decreased or delayed based on the presence of hematologic or neurotoxicity.
2. It is recommended that after a maximal response has been seen three additional cycles be administered; the drug should then be discontinued.
3. The lyophilized product should be reconstituted with 2 mL of sterile water for injection, USP. Each mL of the resulting solution will contain 25 mg fludarabine phosphate with the final pH ranging from 7.2 to 8.2. This may then be diluted in 100 or 125 mL of 5% dextrose injection, USP, or 0.9% sodium chloride, USP and administered over 30 min.
4. Reconstituted fludarabine contains no preservatives; thus, it must be used within 8 hr.
5. If the solution comes in contact with the skin or mucous membranes, wash thoroughly with soap and water. Eyes should be rinsed thoroughly with plain water.
6. The product should be stored under refrigeration at a temperature of 2°C–8°C (36°F–46°F).
7. *Treatment of Overdose:* Discontinue administration of the drug and treat symptoms. The hematologic profile should be monitored.

Contraindication: Lactation.
Special Concerns: Use with caution in clients with renal insufficiency. The safety and effectiveness of fludarabine in children and in previously untreated or nonrefractory chronic lymphocytic leukemia clients have not been established. Fludarabine produces dose-dependent toxic effects. An increased risk of toxicity is possible in geriatric clients, in renal insufficiency, and in bone marrow impairment.
Side Effects: *Hematologic:* Neutropenia, thrombocytopenia, anemia. *Tumor lysis syndrome:* Hyperuricemia, hyperphosphatemia, hypocalcemia, hyperkalemia, hematuria, metabolic acidosis, urate crystalluria, renal failure. Flank pain and hematuria may signal the onset of the syndrome. *GI:* N&V, anorexia, stomatitis,

diarrhea, GI bleeding. *CNS:* Malaise, fatigue, weakness, agitation, confusion, coma. *Neuromuscular:* Peripheral neuropathy, paresthesia, myalgia. *Respiratory:* Pneumonia, dyspnea, cough, interstitial pulmonary infiltrate. *GU:* Dysuria, urinary infection, hematuria. *Miscellaneous:* Edema (common), skin rashes, fever, chills, ***serious opportunistic infections,*** pain, visual disturbances, hearing loss.

Symptoms of Overdose: Irreversible CNS toxicity including delayed blindness, ***coma, and death.*** Severe thrombocytopenia and neutropenia.

NURSING CONSIDERATIONS

See also *Nursing Considerations* for *Antineoplastic Agents,* Chapter 20.

Assessment

1. Document indications for therapy, noting previous agents used and the outcome.
2. Perform a baseline CNS assessment and document. High doses may precipitate neurotoxicity.
3. Obtain baseline hematologic parameters and renal function studies and monitor throughout therapy. Nadir: 5–25 days.

Client/Family Teaching

1. Advise client to report any evidence of flank pain or hematuria as this may preclude a tumor lysis syndrome.
2. Practice barrier birth control during drug therapy.
3. Report any evidence of infection (sore throat, fever) and the development of any abnormal bruising or bleeding.

Evaluate: Hematologic evidence of control of the malignant process.

Fluorouracil (5-Fluorouracil,5-FU)

(flew-roh-**YOUR**-ah-sill)
Pregnancy Category: X
Adrucil, Efudex, Fluoroplex (Abbreviation: 5-FU) **(Rx)**

See also *Antineoplastic Agents,* Chapter 20.

How Supplied: *Cream:* 1%, 5%; *Injection:* 50 mg/mL; *Solution:* 1%, 2%, 5%

Action/Kinetics: Pyrimidine antagonist that inhibits the methylation reaction of deoxyuridylic acid to thymidylic acid. Thus, the synthesis of DNA and, to a lesser extent, RNA is inhibited. The drug is cell-cycle specific for the S phase of cell division. **t½, initial:** 5–20 min; **final:** 20 hr. From 60% to 80% eliminated as respiratory CO_2 (8–12 hr); small amount (15%) excreted unchanged in urine (1–6 hr). Highly toxic; initiate use in hospital. When used topically, the following response occurs:

• Early inflammation: erythema for several days (minimal reaction)
• Severe inflammation: burning, stinging, vesiculation
• Disintegration: erosion, ulceration, necrosis, pain, crusting, reepithelialization
• Healing: within 1–2 weeks with some residual erythema and temporary hyperpigmentation

Uses: Systemic: Palliative management of certain cancers of the rectum, stomach, colon, pancreas, and breast. In combination with levamisole for Dukes' stage C colon cancer after surgical resection. In combination with leucovorin for metastatic colorectal cancer. *Investigational:* Cancer of the bladder, ovaries, prostate, cervix, endometrium, lung, liver, head, and neck. Also, malignant pleural, peritoneal, and pericardial effusions. **Topical (as solution or cream):** Multiple actinic or solar keratoses. Superficial basal cell carcinoma. *Investigational:* Condylomata acuminata (1% solution in 70% ethanol or the 5% cream).

Dosage

• **IV**

Palliative management of selected carcinomas.

Individualize dosage. Initial: 12 mg/kg/day for 4 days, not to exceed 800 mg/day. If no toxicity seen, administer 6 mg/kg on days 6, 8, 10, and

12. Discontinue therapy on day 12 even if there are no toxic symptoms. **Maintenance:** Repeat dose of first course q 30 days or when toxicity from initial course of therapy is gone; or, give 10–15 mg/kg/week as a single dose. Do not exceed 1 g/week. **If client is debilitated or is a poor risk:** 6 mg/kg/day for 3 days; if no toxicity, give 3 mg/kg on days 5, 7, and 9 (daily dose should not exceed 400 mg).

Metastatic colorectal cancer.
Leucovorin, **IV,** 200 mg/m^2/day for 5 days followed by fluorouracil, **IV,** 370 mg/m^2/day for 5 days. Repeat q 28 days to maximize response and to prolong survival.

Dukes' stage C colon cancer after surgical resection.
See *Levamisole HCL,* Chapter 22.

- **Cream, Topical Solution**

Actinic or solar keratoses.
Apply 1%–5% cream or solution to cover lesion 1–2 times/day for 2–6 weeks.

Superficial basal cell carcinoma.
Apply 5% cream or solution to cover lesion b.i.d. for 3–6 weeks (up to 10–12 weeks may be required).

Administration/Storage

IV

1. Store in a cool place (50°F–80°F or 10°C–27°C). Do not freeze. Excessively low temperature causes precipitation.
2. Do not expose the solution to light.
3. Solution may discolor slightly during storage, but potency and safety are not affected.
4. If precipitate forms, resolubilize by heating to 60°C (140°F) with vigorous shaking. Allow to return to room temperature and allow air to settle out before withdrawing and administering medication.
5. Further dilution is not needed, and solution may be injected directly into the vein with a 25-gauge needle over 1–2 min.
6. Drug can be diluted in D5/W or NSS and administered by IV infusion for periods of 30 min–8 hr. This method has been reported to produce less systemic toxicity than rapid injection.
7. The drug should not be mixed with other drugs or IV additives.
8. *Treatment of Overdose:* Monitor hematologically for at least 4 weeks.

TOPICAL

1. Apply with fingertips, nonmetallic applicator, or rubber gloves. Wash hands immediately thereafter.
2. Avoid contact with eyes, nose, and mouth.
3. Limit occlusive dressings to lesions, since they are responsible for an increased incidence of inflammatory reactions in normal skin.
4. Complete healing of keratoses may require 2 months.

Additional Contraindications: **Systemic:** Clients in poor nutritional state, with severe bone marrow depression, severe infection, or recent (4-week-old) surgical intervention. Lactation. To be used with caution in clients with hepatic or liver dysfunction.
Special Concerns: Safety and efficacy of topical products have not been established in children. Occlusive dressings may result in increased inflammation in adjacent normal skin when topical products are used.
Laboratory Test Interferences: ↑ Alkaline phosphatase, LDH, serum bilirubin, and serum transaminase.
Additional Side Effects: Systemic: Esophagopharyngitis, myocardial ischemia, angina, acute cerebellar syndrome, photophobia, lacrimation, decreased vision. Also, arterial thrombosis, arterial ischemia, arterial aneurysm, bleeding or infection at site of catheter, thrombophlebitis, embolism, fibromyositis, abscesses. **Topical:** *Dermatologic:* Pain, pruritus, hyperpigmentation, irritation, inflammation, burning at site of application, scarring, soreness, allergic contact dermatitis, tenderness, scaling, swelling, suppuration, alopecia, photosensitivity, urticaria. *CNS:* Insomnia, irritability. *GI:* Stomatitis, medicinal taste. *Miscellaneous:* Lacri-

mation, telangiectasia, toxic granulation.

Symptoms of Overdose: N&V, diarrhea, GI ulceration, GI bleeding, thrombocytopenia, ***agranulocytosis,*** leukopenia.

Drug Interactions: Leucovorin calcium ↑ toxicity of fluorouracil.

NURSING CONSIDERATIONS

See also *Nursing Considerations* for *Antineoplastic Agents,* Chapter 20.

Interventions

1. Observe for intractable vomiting, stomatitis, and diarrhea, all of which are early signs of toxicity and thus indicate immediate discontinuation of drug.
2. The drug also should be discontinued if WBC and platelet counts are depressed below 3,500/mm^3 and 100,000/mm^3, respectively. Nadir: 10–20 days; recovery: 30 days.
3. Practice reverse isolation techniques when WBC count is below 2,000/mm^3.
4. Protect client and supervise ambulation if symptoms of cerebellar dysfunction occur (altered balance, dizziness, or weakness).
5. Advise that hair loss and mouth lesions may occur but are usually transient.
6. Prevent exposure to strong sunlight and other ultraviolet rays because these rays intensify skin reaction to the drug.

Client/Family Teaching

1. Review and demonstrate appropriate method for topical administration.
2. Explain that affected area may appear much worse before healing takes place in 1–2 months.
3. Advise to drink plenty of fluids (2–3 L/day) during therapy.
4. Instruct both men and women to practice barrier contraception during drug therapy.
5. Avoid exposure to sunlight. If exposure is necessary, wear protective clothing, sunglasses, and sunscreen.
6. Provide a printed list of drug side effects. Stress those that require immediate reporting.
7. Advise that hair loss and mouth sores may appear but are usually transient.

Evaluate

- Relief of pain and ↓ tumor size
- Reepithelialization of malignant skin lesion

Hydroxyurea

(hy-**DROX**-ee-you-**ree**-ah)

Hydrea (Abbreviation: HYD)

See also *Antineoplastic Agents,* Chapter 20.

How Supplied: *Capsule:* 500 mg

Action/Kinetics: Thought to be cell-cycle specific for the S phase of cell division. Believed to interfere with DNA but not synthesis of RNA or protein. Most active in inhibiting incorporation of thymidine into DNA. Rapidly absorbed from GI tract. **Peak serum concentration:** 2 hr. **t½:** 3–4 hr. The drug crosses the blood-brain barrier. Degraded in liver; 80% excreted through the urine with 50% unchanged; also excreted as respiratory CO_2.

Uses: Chronic, resistant, myelocytic leukemia. Carcinoma of the ovary (recurrent, inoperable, or metastatic). Melanoma. With irradiation to treat primary squamous cell carcinoma of the head and neck (but not the lip).

Dosage

- **Capsules**

Solid tumors, intermittent therapy or when used together with irradiation.

Dose individualized. Usual: 80 mg/kg as a single dose every third day. Intermittent dosage offers advantage of reduced toxicity. If effective, maintain client on drug indefinitely unless toxic effects preclude such a regimen.

Solid tumors, continuous therapy.

20–30 mg/kg/day as a single dose.

Resistant chronic myelocytic leukemia.

20–30 mg/kg/day in a single dose or two divided daily doses.

Concomitant therapy with irradiation for carinoma of the head and neck.
80 mg/kg as a single dose every third day.

Administration/Storage

1. Dosage should be calculated on the basis of actual or ideal weight (whichever is less).
2. Therapy should be continued for at least 6 weeks before efficacy is assessed.
3. If the client cannot swallow a capsule, contents may be given in glass of water that should be drunk immediately, even though some material may not dissolve and may float on top of glass.
4. Hydroxyurea should be started at least 7 days before initiation of irradiation; hyroxyurea is continued through irradiation and indefinitely afterward as long as the client can tolerate the dose. The dosage of radiation is not usually adjusted with concomitant usage of hydroxyurea.
5. Excessive heat should be avoided when storing hydroxyurea.

Contraindications: Leukocyte count less than 2,500/mm^3 or thrombocyte count less than 100,000/mm^3. Severe anemia.

Special Concerns: Use during pregnancy only if benefits clearly outweigh risks. Give with caution to clients with marked renal dysfunction. Geriatric clients may be more sensitive to the effects of hydroxyurea necessitating a lower dose. Dosage has not been established in children.

Laboratory Test Interferences: ↑ Uric acid in serum; ↑ BUN and creatinine.

Additional Side Effects: Erythrocyte abnormalities including megaloblastic erythropoiesis. Constipation, redness of the face, maculopapular rash.

NURSING CONSIDERATIONS

See also *Nursing Considerations* for *Antineoplastic Agents,* Chapter 20.

Interventions

1. Observe for exacerbation of postirradiation erythema.
2. Monitor liver and renal function studies during therapy.
3. Monitor hematologic profiles at least weekly. Drug may cause severe granulocyte and platelet suppression. Nadir: 7 days; recovery: 14 days.

Evaluate

- Improved hematologic parameters
- Suppression of malignant cell proliferation
- ↓ Tumor size and spread

Idarubicin hydrochloride

(eye-dah-**ROOB**-ih-sin)
Pregnancy Category: D
Idamycin For Injection **(Rx)**

How Supplied: *Powder for injection:* 5 mg, 10 mg

Action/Kinetics: Idarubicin is an anthracycline that inhibits nucleic acid synthesis and interacts with the enzyme topoisomerase II. It is rapidly taken up into cells due to its significant lipid solubility. **t½ (terminal):** 22 hr when used alone and 20 hr when used with cytarabine. The drug is metabolized in the liver to the active idarubicinol, which is excreted through both the bile and urine. Both idarubicin and idarubicinol are significantly bound (97% and 94%, respectively) to plasma proteins.

Uses: In combination with other drugs (often cytarabine) to treat AML in adults, including French-American-British classifications M1–M7. Comparison with daunorubicin indicates that idarubicin is more effective in inducing complete remissions in clients with AML.

Dosage

- **IV**

Induction therapy in adults: 12 mg/m^2/day for 3 days by slow (10–15 min) IV injection in combination with cytarabine, 100 mg/m^2/day given by continuous infusion for 7 days or as a 25-mg/m^2 IV bolus followed by 200 mg/m^2/day for 5 days by continuous infusion. A second course may be given if there is evidence of leukemia after the first course.

Administration/Storage

1. The 5-mg and 10-mg vials should be reconstituted with 5 mL and 10 mL, respectively, of 0.9% sodium chloride injection to give a final concentration of 1 mg/mL. Diluents containing bacteriostatic agents should not be used.
2. To minimize aerosol formation during reconstitution, the contents of the vial are under negative pressure. Care should be taken to avoid inhalation of any aerosol formed.
3. The drug should be given slowly into a freely flowing IV infusion over 10–15 min.
4. If extravasation is suspected or has occurred, elevate the extremity and apply intermittent ice packs (immediately for ½ hr, then 4 times/day at ½-hr intervals for 3 days) over the affected area.
5. The IV solution of idarubicin should not be mixed with any other drugs.
6. Reconstituted solutions are stable for 7 days if refrigerated and 3 days at room temperature. Unused solution should be discarded.
7. If the drug comes in contact with the skin, the area should be washed thoroughly with soap and water. Goggles, gloves, and protective gowns should be used during preparation and administration of idarubicin.
8. *Treatment of Overdose:* Supportive treatment including antibiotics and platelet transfusions. Treat mucositis.

Contraindications: Lactation. Preexisting bone marrow suppression induced by previous drug therapy or radiotherapy (unless benefit outweighs risk). Administration by the IM or SC routes.

Special Concerns: Safety and effectiveness have not been demonstrated in children. Skin reactions may occur if the powder is not handled properly.

Side Effects: *GI:* N&V, mucositis, diarrhea, abdominal pain, abdominal cramps, ***hemorrhage.*** *Hematologic:* ***Severe myelosuppression.*** *Dermatologic:* Alopecia, generalized rash, urticaria, bullous erythrodermatous rash of the palms and soles, hives at injection site. *CNS:* Headache, ***seizures,*** altered mental status. *CV:* CHF, ***serious arrhythmias including atrial fibrillation, chest pain, MI, cardiomyopathies,*** decrease in LV ejection fraction. *NOTE:* Cardiac toxicity is more common in clients who have received anthracycline drugs previously or who have preexisting cardiac disease. *Miscellaneous:* Altered hepatic and renal function tests, infection (95% of clients), fever, pulmonary allergy, neurologic changes in peripheral nerves.

Symptoms of Overdose: Severe GI toxicity, myelosuppression.

NURSING CONSIDERATIONS

See also *Nursing Considerations* for *Antineoplastic Agents,* Chapter 20.

Assessment

1. Document any preexisting cardiac disease.
2. Note any history of previous radiation therapy or treatment with anthracyclines; document indications for therapy.
3. Obtain baseline CBC, platelets, and liver and renal function studies and monitor throughout therapy.

Interventions

1. Anticipate that the dose should be reduced in clients with impaired hepatic or renal function or if bilirubin levels are 5 mg/dL.
2. Severe myelosuppression is a side effect of drug therapy. Observe closely for early evidence of hemorrhaging and infection.
3. Medicate as needed for nausea and diarrhea, frequent side effects of drug therapy.
4. Evaluate complaints of severe abdominal pain and perform careful abdominal assessments.
5. Document any evidence of SOB or chest pain as drug may cause myocardial toxicity.
6. Monitor I&O, encourage a high fluid intake, and keep the urine

slightly alkaline to prevent the formation of uric acid stones. In clients with gout, administer colchicine or Indocin as needed.

Evaluate

• Presence of leukemia cells (as a second course of therapy may be indicated after hematologic recovery)

• Evidence of a complete remission and improved hematologic parameters

Levamisole hydrochloride

(lee-**VAM**-ih-sohl)

Pregnancy Category: C

Ergamisol **(Rx)**

How Supplied: *Tablet:* 50 mg

Action/Kinetics: Levamisole is used in combination with fluorouracil and is considered to be an immunomodulator. The drug is thought to restore depressed immune function. As such, it stimulates formation of antibodies, stimulates T-cell activation and proliferation, potentiates monocyte and macrophage function (including phagocytosis and chemotaxis), and increases mobility adherence and chemotaxis of neutrophils. Levamisole is rapidly absorbed from the GI tract. **Peak plasma levels:** 0.13 mcg/mL after 1.5–2 hr. **t½:** 3–4 hr. Metabolized by the liver and excreted mainly in the urine.

Use: In combination with fluorouracil to treat clients with Dukes' stage C colon cancer following surgical resection.

Dosage

• Tablets

Adults, initial: Levamisole, 50 mg q 8 hr for 3 days (starting 7–30 days after surgery) given together with fluorouracil, 450 mg/m^2/day by IV push for 5 days (starting 21–34 days after surgery). **Maintenance:** Levamisole, 50 mg q 8 hr for 3 days q 2 weeks for 1 year; fluorouracil, 450 mg/m^2/day by IV push once a week beginning 28 days after the beginning of the 5-day course and continuing for 1 year.

Administration/Storage

1. Levamisole therapy should be started no earlier than 7 and no later than 30 days after surgery; fluorouracil therapy should be initiated no earlier than 21 days and no later than 35 days after surgery. Before fluorouracil therapy is started, the client should be out of the hospital, ambulatory, eating normally, have well-healed wounds, and have recovered from any postoperative complications.

2. If levamisole therapy has been started 7–20 days after surgery, fluorouracil therapy should be started at the same time as the second course of levamisole (i.e., 21–34 days after surgery).

Contraindication: Lactation.

Special Concern: Safety and effectiveness have not been demonstrated in children. Agranulocytosis, caused by levamisole, may be accompanied by a flu-like syndrome, or it may be asymptomatic. Thus, hematologic monitoring is required.

Side Effects: *GI:* Commonly nausea and diarrhea; vomiting, stomatitis, anorexia, abdominal pain, constipation, flatulence, dyspepsia. *Hematologic:* Leukopenia, thrombocytopenia, anemia, granulocytopenia. *Dermatologic:* Commonly, dermatitis and pruritus; alopecia, skin discoloration. *CNS:* Dizziness, headache, inability to concentrate, weakness, memory loss, paresthesia, ataxia, somnolence, depression, insomnia, confusion, nervousness, anxiety, forgetfulness. *Musculoskeletal:* Arthralgia, myalgia. *Ophthalmologic:* Abnormal tearing, conjunctivitis, blurred vision. *Miscellaneous:* Fatigue, fever, rigors, chest pain, edema, taste perversion, altered sense of smell, infection, hyperbilirubinemia, epistaxis.

Drug Interactions

Ethanol / Disulfiram-like reaction when used with levamisole

Phenytoin / ↑ Phenytoin plasma levels

NURSING CONSIDERATIONS

Assessment

1. Document indications for therapy, onset of symptoms, and any previous treatments prescribed.

2. Record pretreatment weight.
3. Obtain baseline CBC with differential, platelets, electrolytes, and liver function studies; monitor throughout therapy.

Interventions

1. Ensure that IV fluorouracil is prescribed for concomitant administration.
2. Observe if client manifests stomatitis or diarrhea after fluorouracil administration because the drug should be discontinued before the full five doses are given.
3. Monitor and carefully evaluate hematologic studies.
• If the WBC is between 2,500 and 3,500/mm^3, the dose of fluorouracil should be deferred until the WBC count is 3,500/mm^3.
• If the WBC count is less than 2,500/mm^3, the dose of fluorouracil should be deferred until the WBC count is 3,500/mm^3 and then reinstituted at a dose reduced by 20%.
• If the WBC count is less than 2,500/mm^3 for more than 10 days even though fluorouracil has not been given, the administration of levamisole should be discontinued.
• Administration of both levamisole and fluorouracil should be deferred until the platelet count is at least 100,000/mm^3.

Client/Family Teaching

1. Provide a printed list of drug side effects that should be reported.
2. Instruct client to report immediately any malaise, confusion, fever, or chills (flu-like symptoms).
3. Avoid alcohol because drug may cause a disulfiram-like effect.
4. Advise female clients of childbearing age to practice safe contraception.
5. Stress the importance of weekly lab studies for CBC and platelets prior to therapy with fluorouracil and every 3-month electrolyte and liver function determinations for 1 year.

Evaluate

• Control of tumor size and spread
• Restoration of immune function and inhibition of malignant cell proliferation

Mercaptopurine (6-Mercaptopurine)

(mer-kap-toe-**PYOUR**-een)
Pregnancy Category: D
Purinethol (Abbreviation: 6-MP) **(Rx)**

See also *Antineoplastic Agents,* Chapter 20.

How Supplied: *Tablet:* 50 mg

Action/Kinetics: Mercaptopurine is cell-cycle specific for the S phase of cell division. The drug is converted to thioinosinic acid by the enzyme hypoxanthine-guanine phosphoribosyltransferase. Thioinosinic acid then inhibits reactions involving inosinic acid. Also, both thioinosinic acid and 6-methylthioinosinate (also formed from mercaptopurine) inhibit RNA synthesis. About 50% absorbed from GI tract. **Plasma t$^1/_2$:** 47 min in adults and 21 min in children. Metabolites are excreted in urine with up to 39% excreted unchanged. Cross-resistance with thioguanine has been observed.

Uses: Acute lymphocytic or myelocytic leukemia. Lymphoblastic leukemia, especially in children. Acute myelogenous and myelomonocytic leukemia. Effectiveness varies depending on use. The drug is not effective for leukemia of the CNS, solid tumors, lymphomas, or chronic lymphatic leukemia. *Investigational:* Inflammatory bowel disease, chronic myelocytic leukemia, polycythemia vera, non-Hodgkin's lymphoma, psoriatic arthritis.

Dosage

• **Tablets**

Highly individualized: 2.5 mg/kg/day. **Adults, usual:** 100–200 mg; **pediatric:** 50 mg. Dosage may be increased to 5 mg/kg/day after 4 weeks if beneficial effects are not noted. Dosage is increased until symptoms of toxicity appear. **Maintenance after remission:** 1.5–2.5 mg/kg/day.

Administration/Storage

1. Since the maximum effect of mercaptopurine on the blood count may be delayed and the blood count may drop for several days after drug has been discontinued, therapy should be discontinued at first sign of abnormally large drop in leukocyte count. Nadir: 14 days.
2. Administer drug in one dose daily at any convenient time.
3. Discourage intake of alcoholic beverages.
4. *Treatment of Overdose:* Induction of emesis if detected soon after ingestion. Supportive measures.

Contraindications: Use in resistance to mercaptopurine or thioguanine. To treat CNS leukemia, chronic lymphatic leukemia, lymphomas (including Hodgkin's disease), solid tumors. Lactation.

Special Concerns: Use with caution in clients with impaired renal function. Use during lactation only if benefits clearly outweigh risks. Severe bone marrow depression (anemia, leukopenia, thrombocytopenia) may occur. There is an increased risk of pancreatitis when used for inflammatory bowel disease.

Additional Side Effects: Hepatotoxicity, oral lesions, drug fever, hyperuricemia. Produces less GI toxicity than folic acid antagonists, and side effects are less frequent in children than in adults. Pancreatitis (when used for inflammatory bowel disease).

Symptoms of Overdose: Immediate symptoms include N&V, diarrhea, and anorexia while delayed symptoms include myelosuppression, gastroenteritis, and liver dysfunction.

Drug Interactions

Allopurinol / ↑ Effect of methotrexate due to ↓ breakdown by liver (reduce dose of methotrexate by 25%–33%)

Trimethoprim–Sulfamethoxazole / ↑ Risk of bone marrow suppression

NURSING CONSIDERATIONS

See also *Nursing Considerations* for *Antineoplastic Agents,* Chapter 20.

Assessment

1. Document indications for therapy, onset of symptoms, and any other treatments prescribed.
2. Obtain liver function studies and hematologic profile. Drug causes granulocyte and platelet suppression. Nadir: 10–14 days; recovery: 21–28 days.

Evaluate

- Improved hematologic parameters
- Suppression of malignant cell proliferation
- Symptoms of disease remission

Methotrexate, Methotrexate sodium

(meth-oh-**TREKS**-ayt)

Pregnancy Category: D (X for pregnant psoriatic or rheumatoid arthritis clients)

Amethopterin, Folex PFS, Rheumatrex Dose Pack (Abbreviation: MTX) **(Rx)**

See also *Antineoplastic Agents,* Chapter 20.

How Supplied: *Injection:* 25 mg/mL; *Powder for injection:* 20 mg, 50 mg, 1 g; *Tablet:* 2.5 mg

Action/Kinetics: Methotrexate is cell-cycle specific for the S phase of cell division. The drug acts by inhibiting dihydrofolate reductase, which prevents reduction of dihydrofolate to tetrahydrofolate; this results in decreased synthesis of purines and consequently DNA. The most sensitive cells are bone marrow, fetal cells, dermal epithelium, urinary bladder, buccal mucosa, intestinal mucosa, and malignant cells. The mechanism of action for use in rheumatoid arthritis is not known although the drug may affect immune function. Variable absorption from GI tract. **Peak serum levels, IM:** 30–60 min; **PO:** 1–2 hr. **t½:** initial, 1 hr; intermediate, 2–3 hr; final, 8–12 hr. Drug may accumulate in the body. Excreted by kidney (55%–92% in 24 hr). Renal function tests are recommended before initiation of therapy; daily leukocyte counts should be taken during therapy.

Uses: Uterine choriocarcinoma (curative), chorioadenoma des truens, hydatidiform mole, acute lymphocytic and lymphoblastic leukemia, lymphosarcoma, and other disseminated neoplasms in children; meningeal leukemia, some beneficial effect in regional chemotherapy of head and neck tumors, breast tumors, and lung cancer. In combination for advanced stage non-Hodgkin's lymphoma. Advanced mycosis fungoides. High doses followed by leucovorin rescue in combination with other drugs for prolonging relapse-free survival in nonmetastatic osteosarcoma in individuals who have had surgical resection or amputation for the primary tumor. Severe, recalcitrant, disabling psoriasis. Rheumatoid arthritis (severe, active, classical or definite) in clients who have had inadequate response to NSAIDs and at least one or more antirheumatic drugs (disease modifying). *Investigational:* Severe corticosteroid-dependent asthma to reduce corticosteroid dosage; adjunct to treat osteosarcoma. Psoriatic arthritis and Reiter's disease.

Dosage

• Tablets (Methotrexate). IM, IV, IA, Intrathecal (Methotrexate sodium)

Choriocarcinoma, and similar trophoblastic diseases.

Dose individualized. PO, IM: 15–30 mg/day for 5 days. May be repeated 3–5 times with 1-week rest period between courses.

Acute lymphatic (lymphoblastic) leukemia.

Initial: 3.3 mg/m² (with 60 mg/m² prednisone daily); **maintenance: PO, IM,** 30 mg/m² 2 times/week or **IV,** 2.5 mg/kg q 14 days.

Meningeal leukemia.

Intrathecal: 12 mg/m² q 2–5 days until cell count returns to normal.

Lymphomas.

PO: 10–25 mg/day for 4–8 days for several courses of treatment with 7–10-day rest periods between courses.

Mycosis fungoides.

PO: 2.5–10 mg/day for several weeks or months; **alternatively, IM:** 50 mg once weekly or 25 mg twice weekly.

Lymphosarcoma.

0.625–2.5 mg/kg/day in combination with other drugs.

Osteosarcoma.

Used in combination with other drugs, including doxorubicin, cisplatin, bleomycin, cyclophosphamide, and dactinomycin. **Usual IV starting dose for methotrexate:** 12 g/m²; dose may be increased to 15 g/m² to achieve a peak serum level of 10^{-3} mol/L at the end of the methotrexate infusion.

Psoriasis.

Adults, usual: PO, IM, IV, 10–25 mg/week, continued until beneficial response observed. Weekly dose should not exceed 50 mg. **Alternate regimens: PO,** 2.5 mg q 12 hr for three doses or q 8 hr for four doses each week (not to exceed 30 mg/week); **or** 2.5 mg **PO** daily for 5 days followed by 2 days of rest (dose should not exceed 6.25 mg/day). Once beneficial effects are noted, reduce dose to lowest possible level with longest rest periods between doses.

Rheumatoid arthritis.

Initial: single PO doses of 7.5 mg/week or divided PO doses of 2.5 mg at 12-hr intervals for three doses given once a week; **then,** adjust dosage to achieve optimum response, not to exceed a total weekly dose of 20 mg. Once response has been reached, the dose should be reduced to the lowest possible effective dose.

Administration/Storage

1. Use only sterile, preservative-free sodium chloride injection to reconstitute powder for intrathecal administration.
2. Prevent inhalation of particles of medication and skin exposure.
3. When used for rheumatoid arthritis, improvement is thought to be maintained for up to 2 years with continuous therapy. When the drug is

discontinued, the arthritis usually worsens within 3–6 weeks.
4. Methotrexate products containing preservatives should not be used intrathecally.
5. Six hours prior to initiation of a methotrexate infusion, the client should be hydrated with 1 L/m^2 of IV fluid. Hydration should be continued at 125 mL/m^2/hr during the methotrexate infusion and for 2 days after the infusion has been completed.
6. The urine should be alkalinized (see *Chapter* 77.) to a pH above 7 during methotrexate infusion.
7. Follow guidelines provided for leucovorin rescue schedule following high doses of methotrexate.
8. *Treatment of Overdose:* Leucovorin, given as soon as possible, may decrease toxic effects. The dose used is 10 mg/m^2 PO or parenterally followed by 10 mg/m^2 PO q 6 hr for 72 hr. Charcoal hemoperfusion will reduce serum levels. In massive overdosage, hydration and urinary alkalinization are needed to prevent precipitation of methotrexate and metabolites in the renal tubules.

Contraindications: Psoriasis clients with kidney or liver disease; blood dyscrasias as hypoplasia, thrombocytopenia, anemia, or leukopenia. Alcoholism, alcoholic liver disease, or other chronic liver disease. Immunodeficiency syndromes. Pregnancy and lactation.

Special Concerns: Use with caution in impaired renal function and elderly clients. Use with extreme caution in the presence of active infection and in debilitated clients. Safety and efficacy have not been established for juvenile rheumatoid arthritis.

Additional Side Effects: ***Severe bone marrow depression.*** Hepatotoxicity, fibrosis, cirrhosis. ***Hemorrhagic enteritis, intestinal ulceration or perforation,*** acne, ecchymosis, hematemesis, melena, increased pigmentation, diabetes, leukoencephalopathy, chronic interstitial obstructive pulmonary disease, acute renal failure. Intrathecal use may result in chemical arachnoiditis, transient paresis, or ***seizures.*** Concomitant exposure to sunlight may aggravate psoriasis.

Drug Interactions
Alcohol, ethyl / Additive hepatotoxicity; combination can result in coma
Aminoglycosides, oral / ↓ Absorption of PO methotrexate
Anticoagulants, oral / Additive hypoprothrombinemia
Chloramphenicol / ↑ Effect of methotrexate by ↓ plasma protein binding
Etretinate / Possible hepatotoxicity if used together for psoriasis
Folic acid–containing vitamin preparations / ↓ Response to methotrexate
Ibuprofen / ↑ Effect of methotrexate by ↓ renal secretion
NSAIDs / Possible fatal interaction
PABA / ↑ Effect of methotrexate by ↓ plasma protein binding
Phenylbutazone / ↑ Effect of methotrexate by ↓ renal secretion
Phenytoin / ↑ Effect of methotrexate by ↓ plasma protein binding
Probenecid / ↑ Effect of methotrexate by ↓ renal clearance
Procarbazine / Possible ↑ nephrotoxicity
Pyrimethamine / ↑ Methotrexate toxicity
Salicylates (aspirin) / ↑ Effect of methotrexate by ↓ plasma protein binding; also, salicylates ↓ renal excretion of methotrexate
Smallpox vaccination / Methotrexate impairs immunologic response to smallpox vaccine
Sulfonamides / ↑ Effect of methotrexate by ↓ plasma protein binding
Tetracyclines / ↑ Effect of methotrexate by ↓ plasma protein binding
Thiopurines / ↑ Plasma levels of thiopurines

NURSING CONSIDERATIONS

See also *Nursing Considerations* for *Antineoplastic Agents,* Chapter 20.

Assessment
1. Determine if client is receiving other organic acids, such as aspirin, phenylbutazone, probenecid, and/or

sulfa drugs, because these agents affect renal clearance of methotrexate and increase thrombocytopenia and GI side effects.
2. Identify indications for therapy. List drugs client currently prescribed to determine if any interact unfavorably with methotrexate.
3. Note any evidence of acute infections.
4. Obtain baseline CBC and renal function studies. Drug causes granulocyte and platelet suppression. Nadir: 10 days; recovery: 14 days.

Interventions

1. Monitor I&O, and encourage fluid intake (2–3 L/day) to facilitate excretion of drug.
2. Assess renal function and report oliguria, since this symptom may indicate the need to discontinue this drug.
3. Have calcium leucovorin—a potent antidote for folic acid antagonists—readily available in case of overdosage. Antidotes are ineffective if not administered within 4 hr of overdosage. Corticosteroids are sometimes given concomitantly with initial dose of methotrexate.

Client/Family Teaching

1. Take tablets at bedtime with an antacid to minimize GI upset.
2. Avoid salicylates and ingestion of alcohol as liver toxicity and bleeding may result.
3. Report oral ulcerations, one of the first signs of toxicity.
4. Avoid vaccinations (especially for smallpox) because the impaired immunologic response may result in vaccinia.
5. Consume 2–3 L/day of fluids to prevent renal damage.
6. Instruct how to test urine pH and advise to report if less than 6.5. Explain that bicarbonate tablets may be prescribed to assist in alkalizing the urine.
7. Allopurinol may be prescribed to reduce uric acid levels.
8. Avoid sun exposure and use sunscreens, sunglasses, and appropriate clothing when necessary.

Evaluate

- Suppression of malignant cell proliferation
- ↓ Size and spread of tumor
- Improved hematologic parameters
- Improvement in skin lesions with severe psoriasis
- Reports of ↓ joint swelling and pain and ↑ mobility

Teniposide (VM-26)

(teh-**NIP**-ah-side)
Pregnancy Category: D
Vumon **(Rx)**

See also *Antineoplastic Agents,* Chapter 20.

How Supplied: *Injection:* 10 mg/mL

Action/Kinetics: Teniposide is a derivative of podophyllotoxin. It acts in the late S or early G_2 phase of the cell cycle, preventing cells from entering mitosis. The drug inhibits type II topoisomerase activity resulting in both single- and double-stranded breaks in DNA and DNA: protein cross-links. The drug is active against sublines of certain murine leukemias that have developed resistance to amsacrine, cisplatin, daunorubicin, doxorubicin, mitoxantrone, or vincristine. **Terminal t½:** 5 hr. Is significantly bound to plasma proteins (over 99%). Teniposide is metabolized in the liver and excreted mainly through the urine (4%–12% unchanged) with small amounts excreted in the feces.

Uses: In combination with other antineoplastic agents for induction therapy in clients with refractory childhood acute lymphoblastic leukemia (ALL). Has also been used for relapsed ALL.

Dosage

- **IV Infusion**

Regimen 1 for childhood ALL clients failing induction therapy with cytarabine.

Teniposide, 165 mg/m², and cytarabine, 300 mg/m² IV twice weekly for eight to nine doses.

Regimen 2 for childhood ALL refractory to vincristine/prednisone-containing regimens.
Teniposide, 250 mg/m², and vincristine, 1.5 mg/m², IV weekly for 4–8 weeks, and prednisone, 40 mg/m² orally for 28 days.

Administration/Storage

1. Teniposide should be given over 30–60 min or longer and is not to be given by rapid IV infusion as hypotension may occur.
2. The IV catheter or needle must be in the proper position and functional prior to infusion. Improper administration may cause extravasation resulting in local tissue necrosis or thrombophlebitis. Also, occlusion of central venous access devices has occurred during 24-hr infusion at concentrations of 0.1–0.2 mg/mL.
3. Teniposide must be diluted with either 5% dextrose injection or 0.9% sodium chloride injection to give a final concentration of 0.1, 0.2, 0.4, or 1 mg/mL.
4. Contact of undiluted teniposide with plastic equipment or devices used to prepare IV infusions may result in softening or cracking and possible drug product leakage. To prevent extraction of plasticizer DEHP, solutions should be prepared and given in non-DEHP-containing LVP containers such as glass or polyolefin plastic bags of containers. The use of polyvinylchloride containers is not recommended.
5. Lipid administration sets or low DEHP-containing nitroglycerin sets will keep exposure to DEHP at low levels and can be used. Diluted solutions are chemically and physically compatible with the recommended IV administration sets and LVP containers for up to 24 hr at ambient room temperature and lighting conditions.
6. Caution must be exercised in handling and preparing the solution as skin reactions may occur with accidental exposure and the drug is cytotoxic. Use of gloves is recommended; if the solution comes in contact with the skin, it should be washed immediately with soap and water. If the drug comes in contact with mucous membranes, they should be flushed thoroughly with water.
7. Heparin solution can cause precipitation of teniposide; thus, flush the administration apparatus thoroughly with 5% dextrose injection or 0.9% sodium chloride injection before and after teniposide administration.
8. Unopened ampules are stable until the date indicated if stored at 2°C–9°C (36°F–46°F) in the original package (protected from light).
9. Solutions containing 1 mg/mL should be given within 4 hr of preparation to reduce the potential for precipitation. Refrigeration of solutions is not recommended.
10. Precipitation of teniposide may occur at the recommended concentrations, especially if the diluted solution is agitated more than is recommended during preparation. Also, storage time should be minimized prior to administration and care should be taken to avoid contact of the diluted solution with other drugs or fluids.
11. Not for use in premature infants as product contains benzyl alcohol.
12. *Treatment of Anaphylaxis or Overdose:*

- Anaphylaxis must be promptly treated with antihistamines, corticosteroids, epinephrine, IV fluids, and other supportive measures. If a client who manifested a hypersensitivity reaction must be retreated, pretreatment with corticosteroids and antihistamines should be undertaken with the client carefully observed during and after the infusion.
- If hypotension occurs, the infusion should be stopped and fluids given. Other supportive therapy should be undertaken as needed.
- Myelosuppression may be treated with supportive care including blood products and antibiotics.

Contraindications: Hypersensitivity to teniposide, etoposide, or the polyoxylethylated castor oil that is present in teniposide products. Lactation.

Special Concerns: Clients with both Down syndrome and leukemia may be especially sensitive to myelosuppressive chemotherapy; thus, initial dosing with teniposide should be reduced. An anaphylactic reaction may occur with the first dose and may be life-threatening (incidence appears to be greater in clients with brain tumors and neuroblastoma). Use with caution in clients with impaired hepatic function. Teniposide contains benzyl alcohol which has been associated with a fatal "gasping" syndrome in premature infants.

Side Effects: *Hematologic:* ***Severe myelosuppression,*** leukopenia, neutropenia, thrombocytopenia, anemia. *Hypersensitivity reactions:* ***Anaphylaxis*** manifested by chills, fever, ***bronchospasm,*** dyspnea, facial flushing, hypertension or hypotension, tachycardia. *CV:* Hypotension. *GI:* Mucositis, N&V, diarrhea. *Dermatologic:* Alopecia (reversible), rash, hepatic dysfunction or toxicity, peripheral neurotoxicity, infection, bleeding, renal dysfunction, metabolic abnormalities.

Symptoms of Overdose: Myelosuppression, hypotension.

Drug Interactions

Antiemetic drugs / Acute CNS depression and hypotension in clients receiving high doses of teniposide and who were pretreated with antiemetics

Methotrexate / ↑ Plasma clearance of methotrexate

Sodium salicylate / ↑ Effect of teniposide due to displacement from plasma protein binding sites

Sulfamethizole / ↑ Effect of teniposide due to displacement from plasma protein binding sites

Tolbutamide / ↑ Effect of teniposide due to displacement from plasma protein binding sites

NURSING CONSIDERATIONS

See also *Nursing Considerations* for *Antineoplastic Agents,* Chapter 20, and *Etoposide,* Chapter 25.

Assessment

1. Note any sensitivity to product derivatives especially polyoxylethylated castor oil.
2. Product contains benzyl alcohol; assess for any client intolerance.
3. Obtain baseline hematologic profile and liver and renal function studies, and assess throughout therapy. Drug may cause granulocyte and platelet suppression. Nadir: 14 days; recovery: 21 days.

Interventions

1. Premedicate with antiemetics. Monitor VS closely during infusion.
2. Anticipate reduced dosage in clients with liver or renal dysfunction or in clients with Down syndrome.
3. Observe for enhanced CNS effects when clients are premedicated with antiemetics.
4. Observe closely for S&S of myelosuppression. Withhold treatment if platelet count is less than 50,000 mm^3 or ANC is less than 500 mm^3 and do not resume treatment until hematologic recovery is evident.
5. If client experiences symptoms of anaphylaxis (chills, fever, tachycardia, dyspnea, or altered BP), interrupt infusion and obtain immediate medical support.

Client/Family Teaching

1. Explain that drug is a "possible carcinogen" and review risk of developing secondary acute nonlymphocytic leukemia with intensive therapy schedules (1–2 times/week during remission).
2. Report promptly if any of the following are noted: fever, chills, rapid heartbeat, or difficulty in breathing.
3. Advise that N&V and hair loss are frequent drug side effects.
4. Stress that drug will cause fetal harm and contraceptive measures must be followed during treatment.

Evaluate: Remission of acute lymphoblastic leukemia in clients with relapsed or refractory ALL.

Thioguanine

(thigh-oh-**GWON**-een)
Pregnancy Category: D

Lanvis ✱, TG, 6-Thioguanine (Abbreviation: 6-TG) **(Rx)**

See also *Antineoplastic Agents,* Chapter 20.

How Supplied: *Tablet:* 40 mg

Action/Kinetics: Purine antagonist that is cell-cycle specific for the S phase of cell division. Thioguanine is converted to 6-thioguanylic acid, which in turn interferes with the synthesis of guanine nucleotides by competing with hypoxanthine and xanthine for the enzyme phosphoribosyltransferase (HGPRTase). Ultimately the synthesis of RNA and DNA is inhibited. Resistance to the drug may result from increased breakdown of 6-thioguanylic acid or loss of HGPRTase activity. Partially absorbed (30%) from GI tract. **t½:** 80 min. Detoxified by liver and excreted in the urine. More effective in children than in adults. Cross-resistance with mercaptopurine. Perform platelet counts weekly; discontinue drug if abnormally large fall in blood count is noted, indicating severe bone marrow depression.

Uses: Acute and nonlymphocytic leukemias (usually in combination with other drugs such as cyclophosphamide, cytarabine, prednisone, vincristine). Chronic myelogenous leukemia (not first-line therapy).

Dosage

• Tablets

Individualized and determined by hematopoietic response. **Adults and pediatric, initial:** 2 mg/kg/day (or 75–100 mg/m²) given at one time. From 2 to 4 weeks may elapse before beneficial results become apparent. Compute dose to nearest multiple of 20 mg. If no response, dosage may be increased to 3 mg/kg/day. **Usual maintenance dose (even during remissions):** 2–3 mg/kg/day (or 100 mg/m²). Dosage of thioguanine does not have to be decreased during administration of allopurinol (to inhibit uric acid production).

Administration/Storage: *Treatment of Overdose:* Induce vomiting if client is seen immediately after an acute overdosage. Treat symptoms. Hematologic toxicity may be treated by platelet transfusions (for bleeding) and granulocyte transfusions. Antibiotics are indicated for sepsis.

Contraindications: Resistance to mercaptopurine or thioguanine.

Special Concerns: Use not recommended during lactation.

Laboratory Test Interference: ↑ Uric acid in blood and urine.

Additional Side Effects: Loss of vibration sense, unsteadiness of gait. ***Hepatotoxicity,*** myelosuppression (common), hyperuricemia. Adults tend to show a more rapid fall in WBC count than children.

Symptoms of Overdose: N&V, hypertension, malaise, and diaphoresis may be seen immediately, which may be followed by myelosuppression and azotemia. ***Severe hematologic toxicity.***

NURSING CONSIDERATIONS

See also *Nursing Considerations* for *Antineoplastic Agents,* Chapter 20.

Interventions

1. Provide assistance to ambulatory clients who may experience loss of vibration sense and thus have unsteady gait (these clients may be unable to rely on canes).
2. Expect hyperuricemia after tumor lysis, which may be reduced with administration of allopurinol, which prevents purine breakdown and excessive uric acid formation.
3. Monitor hematologic profile and liver function tests initially; repeat hematologic profile weekly and liver function tests monthly during course of therapy. Obtain parameters for withholding drug. Note any evidence of anemia and assess for evidence of fatigue or dyspnea. Drug may cause granulocyte and platelet suppression. Nadir: 10 days; recovery: 21 days.

Client/Family Teaching

1. Take tablets on an empty stomach for best results.
2. Encourage increased fluid intake (2–3 L/day) to minimize hyperuricemia and hyperuricosuria.

3. Withhold drug and report if jaundice, ↓ urine output, diarrhea, or extremity swelling occurs.
4. Any sore throat, fever, or flu-like symptoms as well as increased bruising and bleeding tendencies require immediate reporting.
5. Emphasize that contraceptive measures are advised with this drug.

Evaluate

• Suppression of malignant cell proliferation

• Hematologic evidence of a remission of leukemia

CHAPTER TWENTY-THREE

Antineoplastic Agents: Antibiotics

See the following individual entries:

Bleomycin Sulfate
Dactinomycin
Daunorubicin
Doxorubicin Hydrochloride
Mitomycin
Mitotane
Mitoxantrone Hydrochloride
Pentostatin
Plicamycin

Bleomycin sulfate

(blee-oh-**MY**-sin)
Blenoxane (Abbreviation: BLM) **(Rx)**

See also *Antineoplastic Agents,* Chapter 20.

How Supplied: *Powder for injection:* 15 U

Action/Kinetics: Bleomycin is a glycopeptide antibiotic produced by *Streptomyces verticillus.* It is most effective in the G_2 and M phases of cell division although some activity is noted in noncycling cells. The action may be due to binding to DNA, inducing lability of the DNA structure and decreasing synthesis of DNA and to a lesser extent RNA and protein. Drug currently used is mostly a mixture of bleomycin A_2 and B_2. Drug has relatively low bone marrow depressant activity, localizes in certain tissues, and is an important component of some combination regimens. **Peak plasma levels** (after 4–5 days of therapy): 50 ng/mL. **t½, after rapid IV and intrapleural, adults:** 24 min and 4 hr; **children, less than 3 years of age:** 54 min and 3 hr. **t½, continuous IV, adults:** 79 min and 9 hr; **children, less than 3 years of age:** 2.3 hr (terminal phase). Two-thirds excreted in urine as active bleomycin. 60%–70% excreted in the urine unchanged.

Uses: Palliative treatment, either alone or in combination, for Hodgkin's and non-Hodgkin's lymphomas (including lymphosarcoma and reticulum cell sarcoma), testicular carcinomas, and squamous cell carcinomas (especially of the head and neck, larynx, paralarynx, penis, cervix, vulva, and skin). *Investigational:* Soft tissue sarcomas, osteosarcoma, malignant effusions (peritoneal, pleural), ovarian tumors. Also for severe, recalcitrant common warts (verruca vulgaris).

Dosage

- **SC, IM, IV**

Hodgkin's disease.

Initial: 0.25–0.5 units/kg (10–20 units/m² once or twice weekly. **Maintenance:** 1 unit/day or 5 units/week given IM or IV.

Squamous cell carcinoma of head, neck, or cervical.

Initial: 0.25–0.5 units/kg (10–30 units/m² once or twice weekly. **Maintenance:** 30–60 units/day over a period of 1–24 hr given by regional arterial infusion.

Lymphosarcoma, reticulum cell sarcoma, testicular carcinoma.

0.25–0.5 unit/kg (10–20 units/m² once or twice weekly.

- **Intralesional**

Warts.

0.2–0.8 unit (depending on the size) one or more times q 2–4 weeks (up to a maximum total dose of 2 units using a solution of 15 units of sterile bleomycin solution in 15 mL 0.9% saline or water for injection).

Administration/Storage

1. For IM or SC use, the drug should be reconstituted with 1–5 mL sterile

water for injection, 5% dextrose injection, sodium chloride for injection, or bacteriostatic water for injection.
2. Administer IV slowly over 10 min. May be further diluted in 50–100 mL of D5%/W or NSS and infused.
3. Hodgkin's disease and testicular tumors should respond within 2 weeks; squamous cell cancers require at least 3 weeks.
4. Bleomycin is stable for 24 hr at room temperature (14 days if refrigerated) in sodium chloride, 5% dextrose solution, and 5% dextrose containing heparin, 100 or 1,000 units/mL.

Additional Contraindications: Renal or pulmonary diseases. Pregnancy, lactation.

Additional Side Effects: ***Pulmonary fibrosis, especially in older clients.*** Mucocutaneous toxicity and hypersensitivity reactions. In approximately 1% of lymphoma clients, an idiosyncratic reaction manifested by hypotension, fever, chills, mental confusion, and wheezing has been reported.

Additional Drug Interactions: Bleomycin may decrease plasma levels and renal excretion of digoxin.

NURSING CONSIDERATIONS

See also *Nursing Considerations* for *Antineoplastic Agents,* Chapter 20.

Assessment

1. Document indications for therapy and onset and describe symptoms.
2. Determine that baseline pulmonary function studies have been performed. Assess client for basilar rales, cough, dyspnea on exertion, and tachypnea, all of which are dose-related symptoms of pulmonary toxicity.
3. Document to avoid adhesive on the skin as drug accumulates in keratin and may discolor epithelium.
4. Note if client is receiving digoxin. Digoxin levels should be monitored during therapy as levels may be enhanced.
5. Clients with lymphoma may be prescribed two test doses of 2 units each initially to assess for idiosyncratic response.
6. Drug may cause mild granulocyte suppression. Nadir: 10 days; recovery: 14 days.

Client/Family Teaching

1. Review the symptoms of idiosyncratic reaction (see *Additional Side Effects*) that may occur in clients with lymphoma.
2. Explain that fever 3–6 hr after treatment is common and to take prescribed antipyretics to relieve symptoms.
3. Avoid vaccinations.
4. Practice safe, barrier form of contraception.
5. Report any abnormal oral or skin rashes.
6. Advise that smoking may aggravate pulmonary symptoms.

Evaluate:

- Evidence of ↓ tumor size and spread
- Resolution of warts

Dactinomycin

(dack-tin-oh-**MY**-sin)
Pregnancy Category: C
Actinomycin D, Cosmegen **(Rx)**

See also *Antineoplastic Agents,* Chapter 20.

How Supplied: *Powder for injection:* 0.5 mg

Action/Kinetics: Chromopeptide antibiotic produced by *Streptomyces parvullus.* Dactinomycin acts by intercalating into the purine–pyrimidine base pair, thereby inhibiting synthesis of messenger RNA. The activity is cell-cycle nonspecific although the maximum number of cells are destroyed in the G_1 phase. The drug is cleared from the blood within 2 min and concentrated in nucleated cells. **t½:** 36 hr. The drug does not cross the blood-brain barrier and is excreted mainly unchanged.

During therapy, leukocyte counts should be performed daily, and platelet counts q 3 days. Frequent liver and kidney function tests are recommended. Appearance of toxic manifestations may be delayed by several weeks. Irreversible bone marrow depression may occur in clients with preexisting renal, hepatic, or bone marrow impairment. The drug is corrosive to soft tissue.

Uses: In combination with vincristine, surgery, and/or irradiation for treatment of Wilms' tumor (nephroblastoma) and its metastases. In combination with methotrexate to treat metastatic and nonmetastatic choriocarcinoma. In combination with cyclophosphamide, doxorubicin, and vincristine to treat rhabdomyosarcoma. Nonseminomatous testicular carcinoma. With cyclophosphamide and radiotherapy to treat Ewing's sarcoma. In combination with radiotherapy to treat sarcoma botryoides. Endometrial carcinoma. *Investigational:* Ovarian cancer, Kaposi's sarcoma, osteosarcoma, malignant melanoma.

Dosage

• **IV**

Carcinomas.

Adults, usual: 0.5 mg/m²/week for 3 weeks; or, 0.01–0.015 mg/kg/day for a maximum of 5 days q 4–6 weeks. Dose is individualized. **Pediatric:** 10–15 mcg/kg (0.45 mg/m²) daily for 5 days; **alternatively,** a total dose of 2.4 mg/m² over 1 week. Total daily dosage for both adults and children should not exceed 15 mcg/kg over a 5-day period. Course of treatment may be repeated after 3 weeks unless contraindicated due to toxicity. If no toxicity, second course can be given after 3 weeks.

• **Isolation Perfusion**

Ewing's sarcoma/sarcoma botryoides.

0.05 mg/kg for pelvis and lower extremities and 0.035 mg/kg for upper extremities.

Administration/Storage

1. For IV use, dactinomycin is available in a lyophilized dactinomycin-mannitol mixture that turns a gold color upon reconstitution with sterile water. Use only sterile water without a preservative to reconstitute the drug for IV use, as it will precipitate. Solutions should not be exposed to direct sunlight.

2. Any portion of the solution not used for the injection should be discarded.

3. *The drug is extremely corrosive.* It is most safely administered through the tubing of a running IV (e.g., 5% dextrose or sodium chloride). It may be given directly into the vein, but the needle used to draw up the solution should be discarded and another sterile needle attached, before injection, to prevent SC reaction and thrombophlebitis.

4. Extreme care should be exercised in reconstituting and administering dactinomycin so that the dust or vapors are not inhaled or come in contact with skin or mucous membranes. Special care should be exercised to prevent contact with the eyes. Drug should be prepared under a laminar flow hood.

5. For direct IV administration, reconstitute 0.5-mg vial with 1.1 mL of sterile water for injection and infuse at a rate of 500 mcg/min. May be further diluted in 50 mL of D5W or NSS and infused over 10–15 min.

Contraindications: Concurrent infection with chickenpox or herpes zoster (death may result). Lactation. Infants less than 6–12 months of age.

Special Concerns: When used with X-ray therapy, erythema is seen in normal skin and the buccal and pharyngeal mucosa.

Laboratory Test Interference: Interferes with bioassay tests used to determine antibacterial drug levels.

Additional Side Effects: ***Anaphylaxis.*** Due to corrosiveness, extravasation causes severe damage to soft tissues. Hypocalcemia. When combined with radiation, increased severity of skin reactions, GI toxicity, and ***bone marrow depression.***

NURSING CONSIDERATIONS

See also *Nursing Considerations* for *Antineoplastic Agents,* Chapter 20.

Assessment

1. Assess and report if client is pregnant, lactating, or infected with herpes, all of which are contraindications for dactinomycin therapy.
2. Determine baseline CBC and monitor closely throughout therapy for evidence of bone marrow depression. Drug may cause severe granulocyte and platelet toxicity. Nadir: 10 days; recovery 21–28 days.

Interventions

1. Report erythema of the skin, which can lead to desquamation and sloughing, particularly in areas previously affected by radiation. Erythema may be seen in normal skin and the buccal and pharyngeal mucosa.
2. Monitor I&O and provide 2–3 L/day of fluids to prevent dehydration and urate crystal formation. Determine need for allopurinol therapy if unable to maintain adequate PO fluid intake.
3. Report any stomatitis or persistent diarrhea as drug dose may require adjustment.
4. Warn client of the possibility of delayed toxic reactions and stress importance of returning for blood tests.
5. Anticipate that dactinomycin may be administered intermittently if N&V persist even when an antiemetic is given.
6. Anticipate that penicillin will not be used if client contracts an infection because dactinomycin inhibits the action of penicillin.
7. Drug interferes with bioassay test used to measure antibacterial drug levels; monitor client response to antibiotic therapy carefully.

Client/Family Teaching

1. Report any unusual bruising, bleeding, or fever.
2. Avoid vaccinations.
3. Practice contraception during and for 4 weeks following therapy.
4. May experience hair loss 7–10 days after therapy.

Evaluate: Evidence of ↓ tumor size and spread and suppression of malignant cell proliferation.

Daunorubicin

(daw-noh-**ROO**-bih-sin)
Pregnancy Category: D
Cerubidine (Abbreviation: DNR) **(Rx)**

See also *Antineoplastic Agents,* Chapter 20.

How Supplied: *Powder for injection:* 20 mg

Action/Kinetics: Anthracycline antibiotic produced by *Streptomyces coeruleorubidus.* Daunorubicin is most active in the S phase of cell division but is not cell-cycle specific. The drug inhibits synthesis of nucleic acid by inserting into the double helix of DNA. Daunorubicin also possesses immunosuppressive, cytotoxic, and antimitotic activity. Rapidly cleared from the plasma. Metabolized to the active daunorubinicol. **t½:** daunorubicin, 18.5 hr; daunorubinicol, 27 hr. Drug rapidly taken up by heart, kidneys, lung, liver, and spleen. Chiefly excreted in bile (40%) and unchanged in urine (25%). Does not pass blood-brain barrier.

Uses: Acute nonlymphocytic leukemia in adults (myelogenous, erythroid, monocytic). When combined with cytarabine, effectiveness is increased. Acute lymphocytic leukemia in children (increased effectiveness when combined with vincristine and prednisone). *Investigational:* Ewing's sarcoma, chronic myelocytic leukemia, neuroblastoma, non-Hodgkin's lymphomas, Wilms' tumor.

Dosage

• **IV infusion**

Acute nonlymphocytic leukemia.

Adults: Daunorubicin, 45 $mg/m^2/day$ on days 1, 2, and 3 of first course and days 1 and 2 of additional courses; *cytosine arabinoside (Ara-c),* 100 $mg/m^2/day$, by IV infusion, for 7 days during first course and for 5 days during any additional courses of treatment. Some recommend reducing the dose of daunorubicin to 30 mg/m^2 in clients 60 years of age and older. Up to three courses may be required.

Acute lymphocytic leukemia. **Adults:** Daunorubicin, 45 mg/m^2, IV, on days 1, 2, and 3; vincristine, IV, on days 1, 8, and 15; prednisone, PO, 40 mg/m^2/day for days 1–22 and then taper between days 22 and 29; and, L-asparaginase, IV, 500 IU/kg/day on days 22–32.

Acute lymphocytic leukemia. **Children:** Daunorubicin, 25 mg/m^2, and vincristine, 1.5 mg/m^2, each IV, on day 1 every week with prednisone, 40 mg/m^2, PO, daily. Usually four courses will induce remission. *NOTE:* Calculate the dose on the basis of milligrams per kilogram if the child is less than 2 years of age or if the body surface is less than 0.5 m^2.

Acute nonlymphocytic leukemia. **Geriatric clients:** 30 mg/m^2 on days 1, 2, and 3 of the first course and days 1 and 2 of the second course in combination with cytarabine.

Dosage should be reduced in clients with renal or hepatic disease.

Administration/Storage

1. Dilute in vial with 4 mL sterile water for injection USP. Agitate gently until dissolved (solution contains 5 mg daunorubicin/mL). Withdraw desired dose into syringe containing 10–15 mL isotonic saline; inject into tubing of rapidly flowing 5% glucose or NSS IV and administer over 3–5 min. May further dilute in 50 mL of D5%/W or NSS and infuse over 10–15 min (or in 100 mL of solution and infuse over 30–45 min.)
2. *Never administer daunorubicin IM or SC.*
3. Reconstituted solution stable for 24 hr at room temperature; for 48 hr when refrigerated.
4. Protect from sunlight.
5. Do not mix with other drugs or heparin.
6. Extravasation may cause severe local tissue necrosis.

Special Concerns: Not recommended for use during lactation. Use with caution in preexisting heart disease or bone marrow depression, renal or hepatic failure.

Additional Side Effects: ***Myocardial toxicity: Potentially fatal CHF, especially if total dosage exceeds 550 mg/m^2 for adults, 300 mg/m^2 for children more than 2 years of age, and 10 mg/kg for children less than 2 years of age.*** Mucositis (3–7 days after administration), red-colored urine, hyperuricemia. Severe tissue necrosis if extravasation occurs. Cross-resistance with doxorubicin (produced by similar microorganism) and vinca alkaloids. Hyperuricemia may occur due to lysis of leukemic cells; allopurinol should be given as a precaution, before starting antileukemic therapy.

NURSING CONSIDERATIONS

See also *Nursing Considerations* for *Antineoplastic Agents,* Chapter 20.

Assessment

1. Document indications for therapy and clinical findings.
2. Monitor hematologic profile as drug may cause severe granulocyte and platelet toxicity. Nadir: 10 days; recovery: 21– 28 days.
3. Allow for bone marrow recovery before subsequent treatments.
4. Follow appropriate guidelines for dose adjustment in liver dysfunction (e.g., bilirubin 1.2–3.0 mg%, give 75% of dose; bilirubin greater than 3.0 mg%, give 50% of dose).

Interventions

1. Assess client during and after termination of therapy for myocardial toxicity, manifested by changes in baseline ECG, edema, dyspnea, and cyanosis. A 30% decrease in QRS voltage and a reduction in the systolic ejection fraction may be early signals of cardiomyopathy. Clients with a cardiac history who receive doses above 550 mg/m^2 are more susceptible to CHF.
2. Allopurinol should be administered prior to antileukemic therapy as drug may precipitate hyperuricemia.

Client/Family Teaching

1. Review side effects and have client report any S&S of cardiac toxicity (i.e., increased SOB, increased fatigue, and edema).

2. Report if mouth ulcers or pain interferes with eating.
3. Urine may appear red for several days following therapy with daunorubicin; this is not blood.
4. Consume 1.5–2 L/day of fluids. Record I&O and report any altered elimination patterns.
5. Avoid foods high in purines and avoid alcohol.
6. Practice contraception during and for at least 1 month following therapy.
7. Avoid vaccinations.
8. Anticipate hair loss. Hair should grow back in about 5 weeks following therapy.

Evaluate

- Improved hematologic parameters
- Suppression of malignant cell proliferation

Doxorubicin hydrochloride (ADR)

(dox-oh-**ROO**-bih-sin)
Adriamycin PFS, Adriamycin RDF, Rubex **(Rx)**

See also *Antineoplastic Agents,* Chapter 20.

How Supplied: *Injection:* 2 mg/mL; *Powder for injection:* 10 mg, 20 mg, 50mg, 100 mg, 150 mg

Action/Kinetics: Anthracycline antibiotic produced by *Streptomyces peucetius*. Doxorubicin is cell-cycle specific for the S phase of cell division. Its antineoplastic activity may be due to binding to DNA by intercalating between base pairs resulting in inhibition of synthesis of DNA and RNA by template disordering and steric obstruction. The drug is metabolized in the liver to the active adriamycinol as well as inactive metabolites, which are excreted through the bile. **t½, doxorubicin: biphasic, initial:** 0.6 hr; **final,** 16.7 hr.

Uses: Acute lymphoblastic leukemia, acute myeloblastic leukemia, Wilms' tumor, soft tissue and osteogenic sarcomas, neuroblastoma, cancer of the breast, ovaries, lungs, bladder, and thyroid, lymphomas (Hodgkin's and non-Hodgkin's), bronchogenic carcinoma (especially small cell histologic type). *Investigational:* Cancer of the head and neck, cervix, liver, pancreas, prostate, testes, and endometrium.

Dosage

- **IV only**

Adults, highly individualized: 60–75 mg/m² q 21 days, or 25–30 mg/m² for 3 successive days q 3–4 weeks, or 20 mg/m² q week. Total dose should not exceed 550 mg/m² (440 mg/m² in clients with previous chest irradiation or medications increasing cardiotoxicity). **Pediatric:** 30 mg/m² on 3 successive days q 4 weeks. Use reduced dosage in clients with hepatic dysfunction, depending on serum bilirubin level. If bilirubin is 1.2–3 mg/100 mL, give 50% of usual dose; if it is greater than 3 mg/100 mL, give 25% of usual dose.

Administration/Storage

1. Initiate therapy only in hospitalized clients.
2. The drug should be reconstituted with saline to give a final concentration of 2 mg/mL (e.g., dilute 10-mg vial with 5 mL) and administered over 3–5 min. The reconstituted solution is stable for 24 hr at room temperature and 48 hr if stored at 2°C–8°C (36°F–46°F).
3. If the powder or solution comes in contact with the skin or mucous membranes, wash with soap and water thoroughly.
4. *Do not administer SC or IM because severe necrosis of tissue may result.* To minimize danger of extravasation, inject slowly into tubing of free-flowing IV infusion of either 5% dextrose or sodium chloride injection.
5. Monitor IV administration carefully. Stinging, burning, or edema at injection site indicates extravasation. Administration should be stopped and injection site moved to avoid tissue necrosis.

6. Be prepared with an injectable corticosteroid for local infiltration and flood site with NSS. Examine area frequently for ulceration that may necessitate early wide excision followed by plastic surgery.
7. Should not be mixed with heparin, dexamethasone sodium phosphate, or cephalothin because a precipitate may form. Mixing with aminophylline or 5-fluorouracil will result in a change from red to blue-purple indicating decomposition.
8. *Treatment of Overdose:* If the client is myelosuppressed, antibiotics and platelet and granulocyte transfusions may be necessary. Treat symptoms of mucositis.

Additional Contraindications: Lactation. Depressed bone marrow or cardiac disease. IM or SC use.

Special Concerns: Use in pregnancy only if benefits outweigh risks. Use with caution in impaired hepatic function and necrotizing colitis. Cardiotoxicity may be more frequent in children up to 3 years of age.

Additional Side Effects: *Myocardial toxicity:* Potentially fatal ***CHF.*** Mucositis, lacrimation, conjunctivitis. Hyperpigmentation of nail beds. Facial flushing if injection is too rapid. Hyperuricemia, red-colored urine (initially). Extravasation may cause severe cellulitis and tissue necrosis. Drug may reactivate previous cardiac, skin, mucosal, and liver radiation damage. Cross-resistance with daunorubicin. ***Severe myelo-suppression.*** When combined with cytarabine, necrotizing colitis may occur.

Symptoms of Overdose: Mucositis, leukopenia, thrombocytopenia. Increased risk of ***cardiomyopathy*** and subsequent ***CHF*** with chronic overdosage.

Drug Interactions

Barbiturates / ↑ Plasma clearance of doxorubicin

Cyclophosphamide / ↑ Risk of hemorrhagic cystitis

Digoxin / ↓ Digoxin plasma levels and renal excretion

6-Mercaptopurine / ↑ Risk of hepatotoxicity

NURSING CONSIDERATIONS

See also *Nursing Considerations* for *Antineoplastic Agents,* Chapter 20.

Assessment

1. Document indications for therapy and onset of symptoms.
2. Obtain and monitor hematologic profile as drug may cause granulocyte toxicity. Nadir: 14 days; recovery: 21 days.

Interventions

1. Administer antiemetics 30–45 min before therapy and round-the-clock as needed.
2. Observe for cardiac arrhythmias, ST segment depression, sinus tachycardia, and/or respiratory difficulties indicative of cardiac toxicity.
3. Monitor I&O and VS. Observe for late onset (up to 6 months) CHF.
4. Encourage fluid intake of 2–3 L/day. Anticipate allopurinol administration and alkalinization of the urine to decrease urate stone formation.

Client/Family Teaching

1. If medication reactivates previous radiotherapy damage, such as erythema, edema, and desquamation, reassure the client that these symptoms should disappear after 7 days.
2. Consume 2–3 L/day of fluids.
3. Urine will turn red-brown for 1–2 days after initiation of therapy; this is not blood.
4. Nail beds may become very discolored.
5. Alopecia may occur but hair should grow back 2–3 months after discontinuation of therapy.
6. Report any flu-like symptoms immediately because drug causes severe myelosuppression.
7. Avoid vaccinations.
8. Practice contraception during and for 4 months after therapy.
9. Report any mouth ulcers as stomatitis may be evident 5–10 days after the dose and last for 3–7 days. A special mouthwash may be prescribed to decrease symptoms.

Evaluate

- ↓ Tumor size and spread
- Improved hematologic parameters

Mitomycin

(my-toe-**MY**-sin)
Mutamycin (Abbreviation: MTC) **(Rx)**

See also *Antineoplastic Agents,* Chapter 20.

How Supplied: *Powder for injection:* 5 mg, 20 mg, 40 mg

Action/Kinetics: Antibiotic produced by *Streptomyces caespitosus* that inhibits DNA synthesis. At high doses both RNA and protein synthesis are inhibited. Most active during late G_1 and early S stages. Not recommended as a single agent for primary treatment or in place of surgery and/or radiotherapy. **t¹/₂, initial:** 5–15 min; **final:** 50 min. Metabolized in liver; 10% excreted unchanged in urine, more when dose is increased.

Uses: Palliative treatment and adjunct to surgical or radiologic treatment of disseminated adenocarcinoma of the stomach and pancreas. Used in combination with other agents. *Investigational:* Superficial bladder cancer; cancer of the breast, head and neck, lung, cervix; colorectal cancer; biliary cancer; chronic myelocytic leukemia. Ophthalmic solution used as an adjunct to surgical excision to treat primary or recurrent pterygia.

Dosage

- **IV only**

10–20 mg/m² as a single dose via infusion q 6–8 wk. Subsequent courses of treatment are based on hematologic response and should not be repeated until leukocyte count is at least 4,000/mm³ and platelet count is at least 100,000/mm³.

Administration/Storage

1. Drug is toxic, and extravasation is to be avoided. Observe infusion site closely for any evidence of erythema or client complaints of discomfort.
2. Reconstitute 5-, 20-, or 40-mg vial with 10, 40, or 80 mL sterile water for injection, respectively, as indicated on label and administer over 5–10 min. Medication will dissolve if allowed to remain at room temperature.
3. Drug at concentration of 0.5 mg/mL is stable for 14 days under refrigeration or for 7 days at room temperature.
4. Diluted to a concentration of 20–40 mcg/mL, the drug is stable for 3 hr in D5W, for 12 hr in isotonic saline, and for 24 hr in sodium lactate injection.
5. Mitomycin (5–15 mg) and heparin (1,000–10,000 units) in 30 mL of isotonic saline is stable for 48 hr at room temperature.

Contraindications: Pregnancy and lactation. Thrombocytopenia, coagulation disorders, increase in bleeding tendency due to other causes. In clients with a serum creatinine level greater than 1.7 mg/dL.

Special Concerns: Use with extreme caution in presence of impaired renal function.

Additional Side Effects: ***Severe bone marrow depression, especially leukopenia and thrombocytopenia.*** Pulmonary toxicity including dyspnea with nonproductive cough. ***Microangiopathic hemolytic anemia with renal failure and hypertension (hemolytic uremic syndrome),*** especially when used long-term in combination with fluorouracil. Cellulitis. Extravasation causes severe necrosis of surrounding tissue. ***Respiratory distress syndrome in adults, especially when used with other chemotherapy.***

Drug Interactions: Severe bronchospasm and SOB when used with vinca alkaloids.

NURSING CONSIDERATIONS

See also *Nursing Considerations* for *Antineoplastic Agents,* Chapter 20.

Assessment

1. Obtain baseline CBC, PT, PTT, and platelets, and note any evidence of abnormalities. Drug may cause platelet and granulocyte suppression. Nadir: 28 days; recovery: 40–55 days.
2. Assess renal function and do not initiate drug therapy if serum creatinine level is greater than 1.7 mg/dL.
3. Auscultate lung fields and assess pulmonary function. Ensure that

CXR has been performed (pulmonary infiltrates and fibrosis can occur with cumulative doses). Observe closely for early evidence of pulmonary complications, such as dyspnea, nonproductive cough, and abnormal lung sounds and ABGs.
Evaluate: Evidence of ↓ tumor size and spread.

Mitotane (O,P'-DDD)

(**MY**-toe-tayn)
Pregnancy Category: C
Lysodren **(Rx)**

See also *Antineoplastic Agents,* Chapter 20.
How Supplied: *Tablet:* 500 mg
Action/Kinetics: Mitotane directly suppresses activity of adrenal cortex. It also changes the peripheral metabolism of corticosteroids resulting in a decrease in 17-hydroxycorticosteroids. About 40% of drug absorbed from GI tract; detectable in serum for long periods of time (6–9 weeks after administration). Drug, however, mostly stored in adipose tissue. **t^1/$_2$:** After therapy terminated, 18–159 days. Unchanged drug and metabolites are excreted in the bile and eventually the feces. Steroid replacement therapy may have to be instituted (i.e., increased) to correct adrenal insufficiency. Therapy is continued as long as drug seems effective. Beneficial results may not become apparent until after 3 months of therapy.
Use: Inoperable cancer of the adrenal cortex. *Investigational:* Cushing's syndrome.

Dosage

• **Tablets**

Carcinoma of the adrenal cortex.
Adults, initial: 8–10 g/day in three to four equally divided doses (maximum tolerated dose may range from 2 to 16 g/day). Adjust dosage upward or downward according to severity of side effects or lack thereof. **Usual maintenance:** 8–10 g/day. **Pediatric, initial:** 1–2 g/day in divided doses; **then,** dose can be increased gradually to 5–7 g/day.

Cushing's syndrome.
Initial: 3–6 g/day in three to four divided doses; **then,** 0.5 mg 2 times/week to 2 g/day.
Administration/Storage
1. Institute treatment in hospital until stable dosage schedule is achieved.
2. Treatment should be continued for 3 months to determine beneficial effects.
3. To counteract shock or trauma, be prepared to administer steroid medications in high doses, because depressed adrenals may not produce sufficient steroids.
Contraindications: Hypersensitivity to drug. Discontinue temporarily after shock or severe trauma.
Special Concerns: Use with caution in the presence of liver disease other than metastatic lesions. Long-term usage may cause brain damage and functional impairment. Use during lactation only if benefits outweigh risks.
Laboratory Test Interferences: ↓ PBI and urinary 17-hydroxycorticosteroids.
Additional Side Effects: Adrenal insufficiency. *CNS:* Depression, sedation, vertigo, lethargy. *Ophthalmic:* Blurring, diplopia, retinopathy, opacity of lens. *Renal:* Hemorrhagic cystitis, hematuria, proteinuria. *CV:* Flushing, orthostatic hypotension, hypertension. *Miscellaneous:* Hyperpyrexia, skin rashes, aching of body.
Drug Interaction: Mitotane may ↑ rate of metabolism of heparin, requiring an increase of dosage.

NURSING CONSIDERATIONS

See also *Nursing Considerations* for *Antineoplastic Agents,* Chapter 20.
Assessment
1. Note any history of sensitivity to mitotane and document any episodes of shock or severe trauma that would necessitate discontinuation of drug therapy.
2. Assess for evidence of brain damage by performing behavioral and neurologic assessments of client.
Client/Family Teaching
1. Report any symptoms of adrenal insufficiency, such as weakness, in-

creased fatigue, lethargy, and GI effects (including weight loss and anorexia).
2. Stress the importance of wearing identification in case of trauma or shock and carrying a list of drugs currently prescribed.
3. Avoid tasks that require mental alertness until drug effects are realized.
4. Advise that desired effects may not be evident for 3 months.
5. Avoid situations that may cause injury or exposure to infections.

Evaluate

- ↓ Tumor size and spread
- Serum cortisol level within desired range

Mitoxantrone hydrochloride

(my-toe-**ZAN**-trohn)
Pregnancy Category: D
Novantrone **(Rx)**

See also *Antineoplastic Agents,* Chapter 20.

How Supplied: *Injection:* 2 mg/mL

Action/Kinetics: Mitoxantrone is most active in the late S phase of cell division but is not cell-cycle specific. The drug appears to bind to DNA by intercalation between base pairs and a nonintercalative electrostatic interaction; this results in inhibition of DNA and RNA synthesis. Distribution to tissues such as the brain, spinal cord, spinal fluid, and eyes is low. **t½:** Approximately 6 days. Mitoxantrone is highly bound to plasma proteins. The drug is excreted through both the feces (via the bile) and the urine (up to 65% unchanged).

Uses: In combination with other drugs, for the initial treatment of acute nonlymphocytic leukemias, including monocytic, promyelocytic, myelocytic, and acute erythroid leukemias. *Investigational:* Alone or in combination with other drugs to treat breast and liver cancer; non-Hodgkin's lymphomas.

Dosage

- **IV infusion**

Initial therapy for acute nonlymphocytic leukemia, induction.
Mitoxantrone, 12 mg/m²/day on days 1–3 combined with cytosine arabinoside, 100 mg/m² as a continuous 24-hr infusion on days 1–7. If the response is incomplete, a second induction course may be given using the same daily dosage, but giving mitoxantrone for 2 days and cytosine arabinoside for 5 days. *Consolidation therapy, approximately 6 weeks after final induction therapy:* mitoxantrone, 12 mg/m²/day on days 1 and 2 combined with cytosine arabinoside, 100 mg/m² as a continuous 24-hr infusion on days 1–5. A second consolidation course of therapy may be given 4 weeks after the first.

Administration/Storage

1. The drug should not be frozen.
2. The client must be closely monitored for chemical, lab, and hematologic values.
3. Mitoxantrone should not be mixed in the same infusion with other drugs.
4. Mitoxantrone must be diluted prior to use with a minimum of 50 mL of either 5% dextrose injection or 0.9% sodium chloride injection.
5. The diluted solution is given into a freely running IV infusion of either 5% dextrose injection or 0.9% sodium chloride injection over a period of at least 3 min.
6. Maintain infusion on an electronic infusion device.
7. Care should be taken to avoid extravasation at the injection site. Also, the solution should not come in contact with the eyes, mucous membranes, or skin.
8. Hospital procedures for the handling and disposal of antineoplastic drugs should be followed closely.
9. *Treatment of Overdose:* Antibiotic therapy. Monitor hematology.

Contraindications: Preexisting myelosuppression (unless benefits outweigh risks). During lactation. Intrathecal use.

Special Concerns: Safety and efficacy have not been established in children. The drug may be mutagenic.
Laboratory Test Interference: Transient ↑ AST and ALT.
Side Effects: *Hematologic:* Severe myelosuppression, ecchymosis, petechiae. *GI:* N&V, diarrhea, stomatitis, mucositis, abdominal pain, GI bleeding. *CNS:* Headache, seizures. *CV:* CHF, decreases in LV ejection fraction, arrhythmias, tachycardia, chest pain, hypotension. *Respiratory:* Cough, dyspnea. *Miscellaneous:* Conjunctivitis, urticaria, rashes, renal failure, hyperuricemia, alopecia, fever, phlebitis (at infusion site), tissue necrosis (as a result of extravasation), jaundice. In addition, there is an increased risk of pneumonia, urinary tract and fungal infections, and sepsis.

Symptoms of Overdose: Severe leukopenia with infection.

NURSING CONSIDERATIONS

See also *Nursing Considerations* for *Antineoplastic Agents,* Chapter 20.

Assessment

1. Obtain baseline hematologic and chemistry studies and monitor throughout therapy. Drug may cause granulocyte and platelet suppression. Nadir: 10–14 days; recovery: 21 days.
2. Note any history of cardiac disease; perform baseline ECG and assess for symptoms of cardiotoxicity during therapy.
3. Assess liver and renal function and determine uric acid level.

Interventions

1. Monitor VS and observe closely for any adverse side effects.
2. Initiate appropriate precautions for clients with severe myelosuppression.
3. Anticipate N&V, mucositis, and stomatitis as side effects, and initiate appropriate protocol.
4. Monitor uric acid levels and, if elevated, determine the need for allopurinol therapy.

Client/Family Teaching

1. Advise females of childbearing age to practice contraception during drug therapy.
2. Drug may temporarily discolor urine and/or sclera greenish blue for 24 hr after therapy.
3. Provide a printed list of drug side effects, stressing those that require immediate reporting such as persistent diarrhea, N&V, abnormal bruising and bleeding, severe dyspnea, and any evidence of infection.
4. Consume 2–3 L/day of fluids to prevent hyperuricemia.
5. Avoid vaccinia and crowds, especially during flu season.

Evaluate

- Improved hematologic parameters
- Suppression of malignant cell proliferation

Pentostatin (2'-deoxycoformycin; DCF)

(**PEN**-toh-**stah**-tin)
Pregnancy Category: D
Nipent **(Rx)**

How Supplied: *Powder for injection:* 10 mg
Action/Kinetics: Pentostatin is isolated from *Streptomyces antibioticus;* the drug inhibits the enzyme ADA. Inhibition of ADA, especially in the presence of adenosine or deoxyadenosine, results in cellular toxicity (T cells, B cells) due to elevated intracellular levels of dATP; this blocks the synthesis of DNA through inhibition of ribonucleotide reductase. Pentostatin also inhibits RNA synthesis and causes increased DNA damage. **t½, distribution,** 11 min; **terminal,** 5.7 hr. Approximately 90% is excreted in the urine as unchanged pentostatin or metabolites.
Uses: Hairy cell leukemia in adults who are refractory to alpha-interferon; such individuals have progressive disease after a minimum of 3 months of alpha-interferon therapy or no response after a minimum of 6 months of alpha-interferon therapy. During lactation.

Dosage

- **IV Bolus, IV Infusion**

Alpha-interferon-refractory hairy cell leukemia.
4 mg/m² every other week.

Administration/Storage

1. To reconstitute, 5 mL of sterile water for injection is added to the vial; the vial is mixed thoroughly to obtain complete dissolution for a concentration of 2 mg/mL.
2. Pentostatin may be given by IV bolus or diluted in 25–50 mL of 5% dextrose injection or 0.9% sodium chloride injection. Dilution of the entire contents of the reconstituted vial with 25 or 50 mL provides a concentration of diluted pentostatin of 0.33 or 0.18 mg/mL, respectively. Such a dilution does not interact with polyvinylchloride infusion containers or administration sets.
3. Pentostatin vials can be stored in the refrigerator at temperatures of 2°C–8°C (36°F–46°F). Reconstituted vials or reconstituted vials further diluted may be stored at room temperature and ambient light for up to 8 hr.
4. The optimum duration of treatment has not been determined; if major toxicity has not occurred, treatment should continue until a complete response has been achieved. This should be followed by two additional doses and then treatment should be stopped. If, after 12 months, there is only a partial response, treatment should be discontinued.
5. A dose should be withheld if there is severe rash, CNS toxicity, infection, or elevated serum creatinine.
6. Pentostatin should be temporarily withheld if the absolute neutrophil count falls below 200 cells/mm³ during treatment in a client who had an initial neutrophil count greater than 500 cells/mm³. Treatment may be continued when the count returns to pretreatment levels.
7. *Treatment of Overdose:* General supportive measures.

Contraindication: In combination with fludarabine phosphate.

Special Concerns: Treat clients with infection only if the potential benefit outweighs the risk; infection should be treated before pentostatin therapy is initiated or resumed. Safety and effectiveness have not been determined in children.

Laboratory Test Interferences: ↑ Liver function test, BUN, creatinine, LDH, CPK, gamma globulins. Albuminuria, glycosuria, hyponatremia, hypocholesterolemia.

Side Effects: *Hematologic:* Leukopenia, anemia, thrombocytopenia, ecchymosis, lymphadenopathy, petechia, abnormal erythrocytes, leukocytosis, pancytopenia, purpura, splenomegaly, eosinophilia, hematologic disorder, hemolysis, lymphoma-like reaction. *GI:* N&V, anorexia, abdominal pain, diarrhea, constipation, flatulence, stomatitis, colitis, dysphagia, dyspepsia, eructation, gastritis, ***GI hemorrhage,*** gum hemorrhage, intestinal obstruction, leukoplakia, melena, periodontal abscess, proctitis, abnormal stools, esophagitis, gingivitis, mouth disorder. *Hepatic:* Hepatitis, hepatomegaly, ***hepatic failure.*** *CNS:* Headache, anxiety, abnormal thinking, confusion, depression, dizziness, insomnia, nervousness, paresthesia, somnolence, agitation, amnesia, ataxia, abnormal dreams, depersonalization, emotional lability, hyperesthesia, hypesthesia, hypertonia, incoordination, decreased libido, neuropathy, stupor, tremor, vertigo, ***coma, seizures.*** *CV:* Arrhythmia, abnormal ECG, ***hemorrhage,*** thrombophlebitis, aortic stenosis, arterial anomaly, cardiomegaly, CHF, ***cardiac arrest,*** flushing, hypertension, ***MI,*** palpitation, varicose vein, ***shock.*** *Dermatologic:* Rash, skin disorder, eczema, dry skin, herpes simplex, herpes zoster, maculopapular rash, pruritus, seborrhea, skin discoloration, sweating, vesiculobullous rash, acne, alopecia, exfoliative dermatitis, contact dermatitis, fungal dermatitis, benign skin neoplasm, psoriasis, SC nodule, skin hypertrophy, urticaria. *GU:* GU disorder, dysuria, hematuria, fibrocystic breast(s), gynecomastia, hydronephrosis, oliguria, polyuria, pyuria, hydronephrosis, toxic nephropathy, urinary frequency, urinary retention, urinary urgency, UTI, impaired urination, urolithiasis, vaginitis. *Musculoskeletal:* Myalgia, arthralgia, asthenia, facial paralysis, abnormal gait, arthritis, bone pain, osteomyelitis, neck rigidity, pathologic fracture. *Respiratory:* Cough, upper respiratory infection, lung disorder, bronchitis, dyspnea, epistaxis, lung edema, pneumonia, pharyngitis, rhinitis, sinusitis, asthma, atelectasis, hemoptysis, hyperventilation, hypoventilation, increased sputum, laryngitis, larynx edema, lung fibrosis, pleural effusion, pneumothorax, ***pulmonary embolus.*** *Body as a whole:* Fever, infection, fatigue, weight loss or gain, peripheral edema, pain, allergic reaction, chills, sepsis, chest pain, back pain, flu syndrome, malaise, neoplasm, abscess, enlarged abdomen, ascites, acidosis, dehydration, diabetes mellitus, gout, abnormal healing, cellulitis, facial edema, cyst, fibrosis, granuloma, hernia, hemorrhage or inflammation of the injection site, moniliasis, pelvic pain, photosensitivity, ***anaphylaxis,*** mucous membrane disorder, immune system disorder, neck pain. *Ophthalmic:* Abnormal vision, conjunctivitis, eye pain, blepharitis, cataract, diplopia, exophthalmos, lacrimation disorder, optic neuritis, retinal detachment. *Miscellaneous:* Ear pain, deafness, otitis media, parosmia, taste perversion, tinnitus.

Symptoms of Overdose: ***Severe renal, hepatic, pulmonary, and CNS toxicity; death can result.***

Drug Interactions

Fludarabine / Use with pentostatin may cause ↑ risk of fatal pulmonary toxicity

Vidarabine / ↑ Effect of vidarabine, including side effects

NURSING CONSIDERATIONS

See also *Nursing Considerations* for *Antineoplastic Agents,* Chapter 20.

Assessment

1. Note any previous experience with alpha-interferon and describe the response.
2. Obtain baseline hematologic parameters and renal function studies.
3. Question client and note any symptoms of infection prior to initiating therapy.

Client/Family Teaching

1. Advise client to report the development of rashes as these may progress and require discontinuation of drug therapy.
2. Practice effective birth control during drug therapy.
3. Stress the importance of reporting for scheduled lab studies to evaluate hematologic parameters. Advise that periodic bone marrow aspirates and biopsies may be necessary.

Evaluate: Laboratory evidence of improved hematologic parameters (↑ hemoglobin, granulocyte, and platelet counts) in clients with hairy cell leukemia.

Plicamycin (Mithramycin)

(plye-kah-**MY**-sin, mith-rah-**MY**-sin)

Pregnancy Category: X

Mithracin (Abbreviation: MTH) **(Rx)**

See also *Antineoplastic Agents,* Chapter 20.

How Supplied: *Powder for injection:* 2.5 mg

Action/Kinetics: Antibiotic produced by *Streptomyces plicatus, S. argillaceus,* and *S. tanashiensis*. Plicamycin complexes with DNA in the presence of magnesium (or other divalent cations), resulting in inhibition of cellular and enzymatic RNA synthesis. The drug decreases blood calcium by blocking the hypercalcemic effect of vitamin D, acting on osteoclasts, and preventing the action of parathyroid hormone. Plicamycin is cleared rapidly from the blood and is concentrated in the Kupffer cells of the liver, renal tubular cells, and along formed bone surfaces. The drug crosses the blood-

brain barrier. It is excreted through the urine.
Uses: Malignant testicular tumors usually associated with metastases and when radiation or surgery is not an alternative. Hypercalcemia and hypercalciuria associated with advanced malignancy and not responsive to other therapy.

Dosage

- **IV only**

Testicular tumor.

Dose individualized. Usual: 25–30 (maximum) mcg/kg (given over a period of 4–6 hr) daily for 8–10 (maximum) days. A second approach is to use 25–50 mcg/kg on alternate days for an average of eight doses.

Hypercalcemia, hypercalciuria.

Dose individualized: 15–25 mcg/kg (given over a period of 4–6 hr) daily for 3–4 days. Additional courses of therapy may be warranted at weekly intervals if initial course is unsuccessful.

Administration/Storage

1. Store vials of medication in refrigerator at temperatures below 10°C (36°F–46°F). Discard unused portion of drug.
2. Reconstitute fresh for each day of therapy.
3. Drug is unstable in acid solution (pH 5 and below) and in reconstituted solutions (pH 7) and thus deteriorates rapidly.
4. Add 4.9 mL of sterile water to the 2.5-mg vial of plicamycin (or as recommended on the package insert) and shake to dissolve the drug. Final concentration 500 mcg/mL.
5. Add the calculated dosage of the drug to the IV solution ordered (recommended 1 L of D5W) and adjust the rate of flow as ordered (recommended infusion time is 4–6 hr for 1 L).
6. Closely check peripheral IV for extravasation. Stop IV if extravasation occurs; apply moderate heat to disperse drug and to reduce pain and tissue damage. Restart IV at another site.
7. Should be used only for hospitalized clients.
8. *Treatment of Overdose:* Monitor hematologic status, especially clotting factors. Also, closely monitor serum electrolytes and hepatic and renal functions.

Additional Contraindications: Thrombocytopenia, thrombocytopathy, coagulation disorders, and increased tendency to hemorrhage. Impaired bone marrow function. Pregnancy (category: X). Lactation. Do not use for children under 15 years of age.
Special Concerns: Use with caution in impaired liver or kidney function.
Laboratory Test Interferences: ↓ Serum calcium, potassium, and phosphorus. ↑ Serum BUN, creatinine, AST, ALT, alkaline phosphatase, bilirubin, isocitric dehydrogenase, ornithine carbamyltransferase, LDH. ↑ BSP retention.
Additional Side Effects: Severe thrombocytopenia, ***hemorrhagic tendencies.*** Facial flushing. Hepatic and renal toxicity. Extravasation may cause irritation or cellulitis. Electrolyte imbalance including hypocalcemia, hypokalemia, and hypophosphatemia.

Symptoms of Overdose: Hematologic toxicity.

NURSING CONSIDERATIONS

See also *Nursing Considerations* for *Antineoplastic Agents,* Chapter 20.

Assessment

1. Document indications for therapy and any other treatments prescribed.
2. Obtain baseline hematologic profile, calcium, potassium, phosphorus, and hepatic and renal function studies. Monitor and correct electrolytes and minerals throughout therapy.
3. Assess clients for evidence of abnormal bleeding such as epistaxis, hemoptysis, hematemesis, purpura, or ecchymoses. Drug may cause granyu-

locyte and platelet suppression. Nadir: 10–14 days; recovery: 21 days.

Interventions

1. If antiemetic drugs are ordered, administer before or during therapy with mithramycin.
2. Monitor I&O. Correct dehydration and administer 2–3 L/day of fluids during therapy.
3. Rapid IV drug flow precipitates more severe GI side effects; administer slowly over 4–6 hr.
4. Monitor electrolytes; calcium and phosphate may rebound after therapy.

Evaluate

- ↓ Tumor size and spread
- ↓ Serum calcium levels

CHAPTER TWENTY-FOUR

Antineoplastic Agents: Hormone and Antihormones

See the following individual entries:

Diethylstilbestrol Phosphate - See Chapter 68
Estramustine Phosphate Sodium
Flutamide
Goserelin Acetate
Leuprolide Acetate
Megestrol Acetate - See Chapter 68
Tamoxifen
Testolactone
Vinblastine Sulfate
Vincristine Sulfate
Vinorelbine Tartrate

Estramustine phosphate sodium

(es-trah-**MUS**-teen)
Emcyt **(Rx)**

See also *Antineoplastic Agents,* Chapter 20.

How Supplied: *Capsule:* 140 mg

Action/Kinetics: Estramustine is a water-soluble drug that combines estradiol and mechlorethamine (a nitrogen mustard). The estradiol facilitates uptake into cells containing the estrogen receptor while the nitrogen mustard acts as an alkylating agent. Chronic estramustine administration results in plasma levels and effects of estradiol similar to those of conventional estradiol therapy. It is well absorbed from the GI tract and dephosphorylated before reaching the general circulation. Metabolites include estromustine, estrone, and estradiol. **$t^1/_2$:** 20 hr. Major route of excretion is in the feces.

Uses: Palliative treatment of metastatic and/or progressive prostatic carcinoma.

Dosage

- **Capsules**

14 mg/kg/day in three to four divided doses (range: 10–16 mg/kg/day) or 600 mg (base)/m² daily in three divided doses. Treat for 30–90 days before assessing beneficial effects; continue therapy as long as the drug is effective. Some clients have taken doses from 10 to 16 mg/kg/day for more than 3 years.

Administration/Storage

1. Capsules should be stored in the refrigerator at 2°C–8°C (36°F–46°F), although they may be kept at room temperature up to 48 hr without affecting potency.
2. Capsules should be taken with water 1 hr before or 2 hr after meals.
3. *Treatment of Overdose:* Gastric lavage; treat symptoms. Monitor blood counts and liver profiles for at least 6 weeks.

Contraindications: Active thrombophlebitis or thromboembolic disease unless the tumor mass is causing the thromboembolic disorder. Allergy to nitrogen mustard or estrogen.

Special Concerns: Use with caution in presence of cerebrovascular disease, CAD, diabetes, hypertension, CHF, impaired liver or kidney function, and metabolic bone diseases associated with hypercalcemia.

Laboratory Test Interferences: ↑ Bilirubin, AST, LDH. ↓ Glucose tolerance. Abnormal hematologic tests for leukopenia and thrombocytopenia.

Additional Side Effects: *CV: **MI, CV accident,*** thrombosis, CHF, increased BP, thrombophlebitis, leg cramps, edema. *Respiratory: **Pulmonary embolism,*** dyspnea, upper respiratory discharge, hoarseness. *GI:* Flatulence, burning sensation of throat, thirst. *CNS:* Emotional lability, insomnia, anxiety, lethargy, headache. *Dermatologic:* Easy bruising, flushing, peeling of skin or fingertips. *Miscellaneous:* Chest pain, tearing of eyes, breast tenderness or enlargement, decreased glucose tolerance.

Symptoms of Overdose: Extensions of the side effects.

Drug Interaction: Drugs or food containing calcium may ↓ absorption of estramustine phosphate sodium.

NURSING CONSIDERATIONS

See also *Nursing Considerations* for *Antineoplastic Agents,* Chapter 20.

Assessment

1. Note any history of client allergy to nitrogen mustard or estrogen.
2. Assess clients with diabetes for hyperglycemia because glucose tolerance may be decreased. Ask clients about their glucose tests at home and any difficulties or changes they may have noted in their condition such as increased fatigue, weakness, etc.
3. Assess for symptoms of hypercalcemia: insomnia, lethargy, anorexia, N&V, coma, and vascular collapse.
4. Determine that serum calcium levels are routinely done; assess results (normal: 4.5–5.5 mEq/L). The effect of the steroid and osteolytic metastases may result in hypercalcemia.

Interventions

1. Withhold drug and report high serum calcium levels. Encourage high fluid intake to minimize hypercalcemia.
2. For severe hypercalcemia, be prepared to assist with administration of IV fluids, diuretics, corticosteroids, and phosphate supplements.
3. Closely monitor clients who resume therapy after drug-induced hypercalcemia is corrected.

Client/Family Teaching

1. Teach the client and/or family member how to take the BP and instruct to maintain a record. BP elevation occurs in conjunction with this therapy.
2. Consume 2–3 L/day of fluids.
3. Provide a list of symptoms of hypercalcemia that require reporting if evident.
4. Explain to male clients that impotence resulting from previous estrogen therapy may be reversed.
5. Estramustine phosphate sodium may cause genetic mutation. Therefore, contraceptive measures should be practiced to prevent teratogenesis.

Evaluate: ↓ Size and spread of prostatic carcinoma.

Flutamide

(**FLOO**-tah-myd)
Pregnancy Category: D
Euflex ✱, Eulexin **(Rx)**

See also *Antineoplastic Agents,* Chapter 20.

How Supplied: *Capsule:* 125 mg

Action/Kinetics: Flutamide acts either to inhibit uptake of androgen or to inhibit nuclear binding of androgen in target tissues. Thus, the effect of androgen is decreased in androgen-sensitive tissues. Flutamide is rapidly metabolized to active (alpha-hydroxylated derivative) and inactive metabolites in the liver and mainly excreted in the urine. **$t^{1/2}$ of active metabolite:** 6 hr (8 hr in geriatric clients). Ninety-four percent to 96% is bound to plasma proteins.

Uses: In combination with leuprolide acetate (i.e., a luteinizing hormone releasing hormone—LHRH-agonist) to treat stage D_2 metastatic prostatic carcinoma. Treatment must be initiated simultaneously with both drugs for maximum benefit.

Dosage

- **Capsules**

250 mg (2 capsules) t.i.d. q 8 hr for a total daily dose of 750 mg.

Administration/Storage: *Treatment of Overdose:* Induce vomiting if client is alert. Frequently monitor VS and observe client closely.

Contraindication: Use during pregnancy.

Laboratory Test Interferences: ↑ AST, ALT, creatinine, alpha-glutamyl transferase.

Side Effects: Side effects are listed for treatment of flutamide with LHRH-agonist. *GU:* Loss of libido, impotence. *CV:* Hot flashes, hypertension. *GI:* N&V, diarrhea, GI disturbances, anorexia. *CNS:* Confusion, depression, drowsiness, anxiety, nervousness. *Hematologic:* Anemia, leukopenia, thrombocytopenia, ***hemolytic anemia,*** macrocytic anemia. *Hepatic:* Elevated transaminases, bilirubin, or creatinine; hepatitis, cholestatic jaundice, hepatic encephalopathy, ***hepatic necrosis.*** *Dermatologic:* Rash, photosensitivity, irritation at injection site. *Miscellaneous:* Gynecomastia, edema, neuromuscular symptoms, pulmonary symptoms.

Symptoms of Overdose: Breast tenderness, gynecomastia, increases in AST. Also possible are ataxia, anorexia, vomiting, decreased respiration, lacrimation, sedation, hypoactivity, and piloerection.

NURSING CONSIDERATIONS

See also *Nursing Considerations* for *Antineoplastic Agents,* Chapter 20.

Assessment

1. Document indications for therapy, onset of symptoms, and any agents previously used and the outcome.
2. Anticipate concomitant administration with an LHRH-agonist (such as leuprolide acetate).
3. Obtain baseline and periodic CBC and liver function tests during long-term flutamide therapy.

Client/Family Teaching

1. Clients should be informed to take flutamide and the LHRH-agonist (leuprolide) at the same time.
2. Drug therapy should not be interrupted or discontinued without consulting the provider.
3. Hot flashes, impotence, and diarrhea are all potential side effects of drug therapy; report if persistent or bothersome.
4. Review male sexual problems that are drug induced (impotence, decreased libido, gynecomastia). Assist client and partner to understand and identify need for counseling.

Evaluate

- Evidence of a ↓ in size and spread of tumor
- Decreased production of testosterone in prostatic cancer
- Control of metastatic processes

Goserelin acetate

(**GO**-seh-rel-in)
Pregnancy Category: X
Zoladex **(Rx)**

How Supplied: *Implant:* 3.6 mg

Action/Kinetics: Goserelin acetate is a synthetic decapeptide analog of LHRH (or GnRH). The drug is a potent inhibitor of gonadotropin secretion from the pituitary gland. Initially, there is actually an increase in serum luteinizing hormone and FSH. This is followed by a long-term suppression of pituitary gonadotropins with serum levels of testosterone decreasing to those seen in surgically castrated males. When used for endometriosis, the drug controls the secretion of hormones required for the ovary to synthesize estrogen resulting in plasma estrogen levels seen in menopause. **Peak serum levels after SC implantation:** 12–15 days. **Mean peak serum levels:** Approximately 2.5 ng/mL. The drug is available as an implant in a preloaded syringe. For the first 8 days of the treatment cycle, the rate of absorption is slower than for the remainder of the period.

Uses: Palliative treatment of advanced prostatic carcinoma as an alternative to orchiectomy or estrogen administration when these are either unacceptable to the client or not indicated. Endometriosis, including pain relief and reduction of endometriotic lesions. *Investigational:* Advanced breast cancer in premenopausal and postmenopausal women.

Dosage

- **SC Implant**

Prostatic carcinoma, endometriosis.
3.6 mg q 28 days into the upper abdominal wall using sterile technique under the direction of a physician.

Administration/Storage

1. The sterile syringe, in which the drug is contained, should not be removed until immediately before use. The syringe should be examined for damage and to ensure the drug is visible in the translucent chamber.
2. Administration of the drug should be under the supervision of a physician.
3. The area should be cleaned with an alcohol swab; a topical (i.e., ethyl chloride) or a local anesthetic may be used prior to the injection.
4. To administer the drug, the client's skin should be stretched with one hand and the needle gripped with the fingers around the barrel of the syringe. The needle is inserted into the SC fat and should not be aspirated. If a large vessel is penetrated, blood will be seen immediately in the syringe; the needle should be withdrawn and the injection made elsewhere with a new syringe.
5. The direction of the needle is changed so it parallels the abdominal wall. The needle is then pushed in until the barrel hub touches the client's skin and then withdrawn approximately 1 cm to create a space to inject the drug. The plunger is depressed to deliver the drug.
6. The needle is then withdrawn and the area bandaged.
7. To confirm the drug has been delivered, ensure that the tip of the plunger is visible within the tip of the needle.
8. If there is need to remove goserelin surgically, it can be located by ultrasound.
9. The 28-day schedule should be adhered to as closely as possible.
10. The drug should be stored at room temperature not exceeding 25°C (77°F).
11. There is no evidence the drug accumulates in clients with either hepatic and/or renal dysfunction.
12. The duration of treatment for endometriosis is 6 months.

Contraindications: Pregnancy, lactation.

Special Concerns: Safety and effectiveness have not been determined in clients less than 18 years of age. There may be transient worsening of symptoms during the first few weeks of therapy.

Side Effects: *GU:* Sexual dysfunction, decreased erections, lower urinary tract symptoms, renal insufficiency, urinary obstruction, UTI. Impairment of fertility. *CNS:* Lethargy, dizziness, insomnia, anxiety, depression, headache. *GI:* Anorexia, nausea, constipation, diarrhea, vomiting, ulcer formation. *CV:* Edema, CHF, arrhythmias, ***CVA, MI,*** peripheral vascular disorder, hypertension, chest pain. *Miscellaneous:* Hot flashes (common), upper respiratory tract infection, rash, sweating, COPD, worsened pain for the first 30 days, breast swelling/tenderness, fever, chills, anemia, gout, hyperglycemia, weight increase.

NURSING CONSIDERATIONS

See also *Nursing Considerations* for *Antineoplastic Agents,* Chapter 20.

Client/Family Teaching

1. Remind client that the most common adverse side effects (especially hot flashes, decreased erections, and sexual dysfunction) are due to decreased testosterone levels.
2. Goserelin should not be used in women who are likely to become pregnant or who are pregnant. Advise of potential hazards to the fetus in the event of pregnancy and also stress that drug may impair fertility.
3. Advise that there may be initial worsening of symptoms or the occurrence of new symptoms of prostatic cancer. This is the result of transient increases of testosterone.

4. Client may complain of an increase in bone pain and develop spinal cord compression or ureteral obstruction. Client and family should be reassured that these symptoms are usually only temporary but should be reported.
5. Identify appropriate resources and support groups to provide emotional support to client and family.

Evaluate

• Reports of symptom control and ↑ comfort

• Evidence of ↓ tumor size and spread

Leuprolide acetate

(loo-**PROH**-lyd)
Pregnancy Category: X
Lupron, Lupron Depot, Lupron Depot-PED **(Rx)**

See also *Antineoplastic Agents,* Chapter 20.

How Supplied: *Injection:* 5 mg/mL; *Kit:* 5 mg/mL, 7.5 mg, 11.25 mg, 15 mg; *Powder for injection:* 3.75 mg, 7.5 mg

Action/Kinetics: Leuprolide is related to the naturally occurring GnRH. By desensitizing GnRH receptors, gonadotropin secretion is inhibited. Initially, however, LH and FSH levels increase, leading to increases of sex hormones. However, decreases in these hormones will be observed within 2–4 weeks. **t½:** 3 hr. **Peak plasma level following depot injection:** 20 ng/mL after 4 hr and 0.36 ng/mL after 4 weeks.

Uses: Palliative treatment in advanced prostatic cancer when orchiectomy or estrogen treatment are not appropriate. Endometriosis (use depot form). Treat central precocious puberty (use depot-PED form). *Investigational:* Breast, ovarian, and endometrial cancer; leiomyoma uteri; precocious puberty: prostatic hypertrophy; infertility.

Dosage

• **SC**

Advanced prostatic cancer.

1 mg/day, using the syringes provided.

Central precocious puberty.

Initial: 50 mcg/kg/day as a single dose. Dose may increased by 10 mcg/kg/day, which is the maintenance dose.

• **Depot**

Advanced prostatic cancer.

7.5 mg IM q 28–33 days.

Endometriosis.

3.75 mg once a month for at least 6 months. Retreatment is not recommended.

• **Depot-PED**

Central precocious puberty.

Initial: 0.3 mg/kg/4 weeks IM (minimum is 7.5 mg).

Administration/Storage

1. If unrefrigerated, injection should be stored below 30°C (86°F).
2. The injection should be administered using only the syringes provided.
3. Depot may be stored at room temperature. The injection should be refrigerated until used.
4. The depot should be reconstituted only with the diluent provided; after reconstitution, the preparation is stable for 24 hr. However, since there is no preservative, it should be used immediately.
5. When injecting the depot form, needles smaller than 22 gauge should not be used.

Contraindications: Depot form is contraindicated during pregnancy, in women who may become pregnant while receiving the drug, and during lactation. Clients sensitive to benzyl alcohol (found in leuprolide injection). Undiagnosed abnormal vaginal bleeding.

Special Concerns: Safety and efficacy have not been determined in children (except depot-PED). May cause increased bone pain and difficulty in urination during the first few weeks of therapy.

Laboratory Test Interferences: Injection: ↑ BUN, creatinine. **Depot:** ↑ LDH, alkaline phosphatase, AST, uric acid, cholesterol, LDL, triglycerides. ↓ WBC counts and HDL. Misleading results from tests of pituitary gonadotropic and gonadal function up to 4–8 weeks after discontinuing depot therapy.

Side Effects: Injection and Depot. *GI:* N&V, anorexia, diarrhea. *CNS:* Paresthesia, insomnia, pain. *CV:* Peripheral edema, angina, ***cardiac arrhythmias.*** *GU:* Hematuria, urinary frequency or urgency, dysuria, testicular pain. *Respiratory:* Dyspnea, hemoptysis. *Endocrine:* Gynecomastia, breast tenderness, impotency, hot flashes, sweating, decreased testicular size, decreased libido. *Other:* Myalgia, bone pain, dermatitis, asthenia, diabetes, fever, chills, increased calcium.

Injection. *CV:* ***MI, pulmonary emboli,*** hypotension, transient ischemic attack, ***stroke.*** *GI:* Dysphagia, ***GI bleeding,*** rectal polyps, GI disturbance, peptic ulcer, hepatic dysfunction. *CNS:* Anxiety, lethargy, memory disorder, mood swings, numbness, syncope, blackouts. *Musculoskeletal:* Peripheral neuropathy, spinal fracture, spinal paralysis, joint pain, pelvic fibrosis, ankylosing spondylitis. *EENT:* Blurred vision, ophthalmologic disorders, hearing disorder, taste disorders. *Respiratory:* Cough, pneumonia, ***pulmonary fibrosis,*** pleural rub, pulmonary infiltrate. *Dermatologic:* Carcinoma of the skin/ear, ecchymosis, hair loss, itching, dry skin, pigmentation, skin lesion. *GU:* Bladder spasms, incontinence, urinary obstruction, penile swelling, prostate pain. *Miscellaneous:* Fatigue, hypoglycemia, infection, inflammation, temporal bone swelling, increased libido, thyroid enlargement, increased BUN, increased creatinine, decreased WBC, hypoproteinemia.

Depot. *CV:* Syncope, vasodilation. *GI:* Dysphagia, gingivitis. *CNS:* Somnolence, personality disorder. *GU:* Urinary incontinence, cervic disorder. *Dermatologic:* Rash, erythema multiforme, hair growth, skin striae, alopecia. *Miscellaneous:* Hard nodule in throat, changes in bone density, abscess at injection site, body odor, infection, accelerated sexual maturity, epistaxis.

NURSING CONSIDERATIONS

See also *Nursing Considerations* for *Antineoplastic Agents,* Chapter 20.

Client/Family Teaching

1. Review the appropriate method and frequency of administration. Have clients return/demonstrate. Explain drug reconstitution, storage, and proper disposal of syringes and equipment.
2. Stress that hot flashes are a common side effect of drug therapy.
3. Record weight and report gains of 2 lb/day.
4. Provide a printed list of drug side effects. Stress those that require immediate reporting such as weakness, numbness, respiratory difficulty, and impaired urination.
5. Explain altered sexual effects (impotence, ↓ testes size). Assist client and partner to understand and identify appropriate resources for counseling and support.
6. Advise that increased bone pain may be evident at the start of therapy. Analgesics may be prescribed for pain control.

Evaluate

- Regression or control of tumor size and spread
- Improvement in symptoms of endometriosis

Tamoxifen

(tah-**MOX**-ih-fen)
Pregnancy Category: D
Alpha-Tamoxifen ✱, Apo-Tamox ✱, Nolvadex, Nolvadex-D ✱, Novo-Tamoxifen ✱, Tamofen ✱, Tamone ✱
(Rx)

See also *Antineoplastic Agents,* Chapter 20.

How Supplied: *Tablet:* 10 mg

Action/Kinetics: Antiestrogen is believed to compete with estrogen for estrogen-binding sites in target tissue (breast). It also blocks uptake of estradiol. **Steady-state plasma levels (after 10 mg b.i.d. for 3 months):** 120 ng/mL for tamoxifen and 336 ng/mL for N-desmethyl tamoxifen. Steady-state levels for tamoxifen are reached in about 4 weeks and for N-desmethyl tamoxifen in about 8 weeks (**t½ for metabolite:** about 14 days). Metabolized to the equally active N-desmethyltamoxifen. Tamoxifen and metabolites are excreted mainly through the feces. Objective response may be delayed 4–10 weeks with bone metastases.

Uses: Adjuvant treatment of axillary node-negative or node-positive breast cancer in women following total or segmental mastectomy, axillary dissection, and breast irradiation. Metastatic breast cancer in premenopausal women as an alternative to oophorectomy or ovarian irradiation (especially in women with estrogen-positive tumors). Advanced metastatic breast cancer in men. *Investigational:* Mastalgia, gynecomastia (to treat pain and size), prophylaxis of breast cancer in high-risk women, pancreatic carcinoma.

Dosage

• Tablets

10–20 mg b.i.d. (morning and evening). Doses of 10 mg b.i.d.–t.i.d. for 2 years and 10 mg b.i.d. for 5 years have been used. There is no evidence that doses greater than 20 mg daily are more effective.

Contraindication: Lactation.

Special Concerns: Use with caution in clients with leukopenia or thrombocytopenia. Women should not become pregnant while taking tamoxifen.

Laboratory Test Interference: ↑ Serum calcium (transient), thyroid-binding globulin in postmenopausal women, BUN, AST.

Side Effects: *GI:* N&V, distaste for food, anorexia, diarrhea, abdominal cramps. *CV:* Peripheral edema, superficial phlebitis, ***pulmonary embolism, thromboembolic disorders (especially when tamoxifen is combined with other cytotoxic agents).*** *CNS:* Depression, dizziness, lightheadedness, headache, fatigue. *Hepatic:* Rarely, fatty liver, cholestasis, hepatitis, ***hepatic necrosis.*** *GU:* Hot flashes, vaginal bleeding and discharge, menstrual irregularities, pruritus vulvae, ovarian cysts, hyperplasia of the uterus, polyps, uterine carcinoma. *Other:* Skin rash, skin changes, hypercalcemia, musculoskeletal pain, hyperlipidemias, weight gain or loss, increased bone and tumor pain, mild to moderate thrombocytopenia and leukopenia, retinopathy, hair thinning or partial loss, fluid retention, coughing. In men, may be loss of libido and impotency.

Drug Interactions

Anticoagulants / ↑Hypoprothrombinemic effect

Bromocriptine / ↑Serum levels of tamoxifen and N-desmethyl tamoxifen

NURSING CONSIDERATIONS

See also *Nursing Considerations* for *Antineoplastic Agents,* Chapter 20.

Assessment

1. Document indications for therapy, any other therapies prescribed, and the outcome.
2. Obtain baseline hematologic profile and monitor periodically throughout therapy. Drug may cause granulocyte suppression. Nadir: 14 days; recovery: 21 days.
3. Monitor and report high serum calcium levels. The effect of the steroid and osteolytic metastases may result in hypercalcemia. Assess for symptoms of hypercalcemia (insomnia, lethargy, anorexia, N&V, coma, and vascular collapse).
4. Closely monitor clients who resume therapy after drug-induced hypercalcemia is corrected.
5. Be certain that client with increased pain has adequate orders for analgesics and provide as needed.

Client/Family Teaching

1. Provide a printed list of side effects that should be reported; a reduction in dosage may be indicated.
2. Explain to client experiencing increased bone and lumbar pain or local disease flares that these symptoms may be associated with a good (tumor) response to medication. Advise to take prescribed analgesics as needed.

3. Encourage high fluid intake (2–3 L/day) to minimize hypercalcemia.
4. Review benefits of exercise. Perform ROM exercises on bedridden clients and encourage others to exercise to reduce calcium levels, improve circulation, and prevent thrombophlebitis.
5. Perform weights weekly and assess for edema. Report excessive weight gain or evidence of peripheral edema.
6. Advise that drug may cause "hot flashes" and to dress accordingly.
7. Wear protective clothing, sunscreens, and sunglasses to prevent photosensitivity reactions.
8. Practice safe, nonhormonal methods of contraception during drug therapy and for 1 month following therapy.
9. Have regular ophthalmologic examinations if doses of drug are much higher than those usually recommended for antihormonal antineoplastic agents.
10. Continue with regular gynecologic examinations and report promptly any menstrual irregularities, abnormal vaginal bleeding, change in vaginal discharge, or pelvic pain or pressure.

Evaluate

- Suppression of tumor growth and malignant cell proliferation
- Breast cancer prophylaxis in select high-risk women

Testolactone

(tes-toe-**LACK**-tohn)
Pregnancy Category: C
Teslac **(Rx)**

See also *Antineoplastic Agents,* Chapter 20.

How Supplied: *Tablet:* 50 mg

Action/Kinetics: Synthetic steroid related to testosterone. The drug may act to reduce synthesis of estrone from adrenal androstenedione by inhibiting steroid aromatase activity. The drug is well absorbed from the GI tract. It is metabolized in the liver and unchanged drug and metabolites are excreted through the urine. Does not cause virilization.

Uses: Palliative treatment of advanced or disseminated mammary cancer in postmenopausal women or in premenopausal ovariectomized clients. Is effective in only 15% of clients.

Dosage

- **Tablets**

250 mg q.i.d. Therapy usually should be continued for 3 months unless there is active progression of the disease.

Additional Contraindications: Breast cancer in men; premenopausal women with intact ovaries. Lactation.

Special Concerns: Safety and efficacy have not been determined in children.

Laboratory Test Interferences: ↑ Plasma calcium, urinary excretion of creatine (24 hr) and 17-ketosteroids. ↓ Estradiol levels using radioimmunoassays.

Additional Side Effects: *GI:* N&V, glossitis, anorexia. *CNS:* Numbness or tingling of fingers, toes, face. *Miscellaneous:* Inflammation and irritation at injection site; increases BP during parenteral administration. Hypercalcemia. Maculopapular erythema, alopecia, nail growth disturbances. See also *Testosterone,* Chapter 70.

Drug Interactions: Testolactone may ↑ effect of oral anticoagulants.

NURSING CONSIDERATIONS

See also *Nursing Considerations* for *Antineoplastic Agents,* Chapter 20, and *Testosterone,* Chapter 70.

Interventions

1. Anticipate a reduction in dose of anticoagulants if client is on concomitant therapy.
2. The effect of the steroid and osteolytic metastases may result in hypercalcemia. Assess routinely for symptoms of hypercalcemia (insomnia, lethargy, anorexia, N&V). Closely monitor clients who resume therapy after drug-induced hypercalcemia is corrected. Withhold drug and report high serum calcium levels.
3. Monitor BP and report any signifi-

cant increases (e.g. diastolic increase of 20 mm Hg).
4. Encourage high fluid intake (2–3 L/day) to minimize hypercalcemia.
5. Perform ROM exercises on bedridden clients and encourage others to exercise to reduce calcium levels, improve circulation, and prevent thrombophlebitis.
Evaluate: ↓ Tumor size and spread.

Vinblastine sulfate

(vin-**BLAS**-teen)
Pregnancy Category: D
Velban, Velbe ✱ (Abbreviation: VLB)
(Rx)

See also *Antineoplastic Agents,* Chapter 20.
How Supplied: *Injection:* 1 mg/mL; *Powder for injection:* 10 mg
Action/Kinetics: Alkaloid, isolated from the periwinkle plant, is believed to inhibit mitosis (metaphase in cell cycle). Rapidly cleared from plasma but poor penetration to the brain. About 75% bound to serum proteins. Almost completely metabolized in the liver after IV administration. **t½, triphasic:** initial, 3.7 min; intermediate 1.6 hr; final, approximately 25 hr. Metabolites are excreted in the bile with smaller amounts in the urine. No cross-resistance with vincristine.
Uses: Palliative treatment of Hodgkin's disease, lymphocytic leukemia, mycosis fungoides, advanced carcinoma of testis, histiocytic lymphoma, Kaposi's sarcoma, Letterer-Siwe disease, trophoblastic tumors, and breast cancer (especially cancer unresponsive to other drugs or surgery). Usually administered in combination with other drugs. *Investigational:* Cancer of the head and neck, bladder, lung, kidney, chronic myelocytic leukemia, and ovarian germ cell tumors.

Dosage
• IV
Individualized, using WBC count as guide. Vinblastine is administered once every 7 days. **Adults, initial:** 3.7 mg/m^2; **then,** after 7 days, graded doses of 5.5, 7.4, 9.25, and 11.1 mg/m^2 at intervals of 7 days (maximum dose should not exceed 18.5 mg/m^2). **Children, initial:** 2.5 mg/m^2; **then,** after 7 days, graded doses of 3.75, 5.0, 6.25, and 7.5 mg/m^2 at intervals of 7 days (maximum dose should not exceed 12.5 mg/m^2). **Maintenance** doses are calculated based on WBC count—at least 4,000/mm^3.
Administration/Storage
1. Dilute vinblastine with 10 mL of sodium chloride injection.
2. Inject into tubing of flowing IV infusion or directly into vein and administer over 1 min. May be further diluted in 50–100 mL of NSS and infused over 15–30 min.
3. Assess peripheral IV site for patency to prevent extravasation and local irritation and pain. If extravasation occurs, move infusion to another vein. Treat affected area with injection of hyaluronidase and application of moderate heat to decrease local reaction.
4. Remainder of solution may be stored in refrigerator for 30 days.
5. If the drug gets into the eye, immediately wash eye thoroughly with water to prevent irritation and ulceration.
6. To reconstitute, under a laminar flow hood, add 10 mL sodium chloride injection, which is preserved with either benzyl alcohol or phenol for a final concentration of 1 mg/mL.
7. The drug should not be reconstituted with solutions that raise or lower the pH from between 3.5 and 5.
8. *Treatment of Overdose:*
• If ingestion is discovered early enough, oral activated charcoal slurry should be given followed by a cathartic.
• Treat side effects due to inappropriate secretion of ADH.
• Prevent ileus (e.g., enemas, cathartic).
• Administer an anticonvulsant (e.g., phenobarbital), if necessary.

• Monitor the CV system.
• Monitor blood counts daily to determine risk of infection and whether blood transfusions are necessary.

Contraindications: Leukopenia, granulocytopenia. Bacterial infections. Lactation.

Additional Side Effects: Toxicity is dose-related and more pronounced in clients over age 65 or in those suffering from cachexia (profound general ill health) or skin ulceration. *GI:* Ileus, rectal bleeding, ***hemorrhagic enterocolitis,*** vesiculation of the mouth, ***bleeding from a former ulcer.*** *Dermatologic:* Total epilation, skin vesiculation. *Neurologic:* Paresthesias, neuritis, mental depression, loss of deep tendon reflexes, ***seizures.*** Extravasation may result in phlebitis and cellulitis with sloughing.

Symptoms of Overdose: Exaggeration of side effects (see above). Neurotoxicity.

Drug Interactions

Bleomycin sulfate / Combination of bleomycin and vinblastine may produce signs of Raynaud's disease in clients with testicular cancer
Glutamic acid / Inhibits effect of vinblastine
Mitomycin C / Severe bronchospasm with SOB
Phenytoin / ↓ Effect of phenytoin due to ↓ plasma levels
Tryptophan / Inhibits effect of vinblastine

NURSING CONSIDERATIONS

See also *Nursing Considerations* for *Antineoplastic Agents,* Chapter 20.

Assessment

1. Take a thorough drug history, noting indications for therapy.
2. Note any evidence of neuropathies prior to onset of therapy.
3. Obtain baseline hematologic profile. Drug may cause granulocyte and platelet suppression. Nadir: 10 days; recovery: 21 days.

Interventions

1. Administer an antiemetic to control N&V.
2. Monitor I&O. Encourage fluid intake of 2–3 L/day.
3. Observe client for cyanosis and pallor of extremities and for signs of Raynaud's disease if also receiving bleomycin.
4. Check for manifestations of neurotoxicity and report if evident because the dosage of drug may need to be adjusted. Monitor neurologic toxicity by checking client reflexes and strength of hand grip.
5. Observe for symptoms of gout. Assess need for adding allopurinol or for alkalization of urine to decrease uric acid levels.

Client/Family Teaching

1. Report any signs of infection, fever, sore throat, unusual bruising, or bleeding.
2. Instruct women and men undergoing therapy to practice barrier contraception.
3. Avoid vaccinations and exposure to persons with infectious diseases.
4. To prevent constipation, eat a high-fiber diet, increase intake of fluids, remain active, and take stool softeners as prescribed.
5. Wear protective clothing and a sunscreen if exposure to sunlight is necessary.
6. Advise that partial hair loss may occur and assist with planning for cosmetic replacement.
7. Report any evidence of jaw pain, numbness, tingling, and deep tendon loss as well as diminished reflexes (S&S of neurotoxicity) in the lower extremities because this is an indication to discontinue drug therapy.

Evaluate: Control and/or regression of malignant process.

Vincristine sulfate

(vin-**KRIS**-teen)
Pregnancy Category: D
Oncovin, Vincasar PFS, Vincrex (Abbreviation: VCR or LCR) **(Rx)**

See also *Antineoplastic Agents,* Chapter 20.

How Supplied: *Injection:* 1 mg/mL

Action/Kinetics: Vincristine is an alkaloid obtained from periwinkle. Vincristine inhibits mitosis at metaphase. The antineoplastic effect is due to interference with intracellular tubulin function by binding to microtubule and spindle proteins in the S phase. After IV use, drug is distributed within 15–30 min to tissues. Poorly penetrates blood-brain barrier. **t½, triphasic:** initial, 5 min; intermediate, 2.3 hr; final, 85 hr. Approximately 80% is excreted in the feces and up to 20% in the urine. No cross-resistance with vinblastine.

Uses: Frequently used in combination therapy. Acute lymphocytic leukemia in children. Hodgkin's and non-Hodgkin's lymphomas (lymphocytic, mixed-cell, histiocytic, undifferentiated, nodular, and diffuse). Wilms' tumor, neuroblastoma, lymphosarcoma, rhabdomyosarcoma, reticulum cell sarcoma. *Investigational:* Idiopathic thrombocytopenic purpura; cancer of the breast, ovary, cervix, lung, colorectal area; malignant melanoma, osteosarcoma, multiple myeloma, ovarian germ cell tumors, mycosis fungoides, chronic lymphocytic leukemia, chronic myelocytic leukemia. Kaposi's sarcoma.

Dosage

• **IV only (direct, infusion)**

Individualized with extreme care as overdose can be fatal. **Adults, usual, initial:** 0.4–1.4 mg/m² (or 0.01–0.03 mg/kg) 1 time/week; **children:** 1.5–2 mg/m² 1 time/week. **Children less than 10 kg or with body surface area less than 1 m²,** 0.05 mg/kg 1 time/week.

For hepatic insufficiency.

If serum bilirubin is 1.5–3, administer 50% of the dose; if serum bilirubin is more than 3.1 or AST is more than 180, dose should be omitted.

Administration/Storage

1. Dissolve powder in sterile water or isotonic saline injection to a concentration ranging from 0.01 to 1 mg/mL.
2. Medication is injected either directly into a vein or into the tubing of a flowing IV infusion over a period of 1 min.
3. If extravasation occurs, move infusion to another vein. Treat affected area with injection of hyaluronidase and application of moderate heat to decrease local reaction.
4. Store in refrigerator. Dry powder is stable for 6 months. Solutions are stable for 2 weeks under refrigeration.
5. Protect drug from exposure to light.
6. Vincristine should not be mixed with any solution that alters the pH outside the range of 3.5–5.5.
7. Should not be mixed with anything other than NSS or glucose in water.
8. *Treatment of Overdose:*

• Treat side effects due to inappropriate secretion of ADH.
• Use an anticonvulsant (e.g., phenobarbital), if necessary.
• Prevent ileus by use of enemas, cathartics, or decompression of the GI tract.
• Monitor the CV system.
• Monitor blood counts daily to determine risk of infection and whether blood transfusions are necessary.
• Folinic acid, 100 mg IV q 3 hr for 24 hr and then q 6 hr for a minimum of 48 hr, may help with treating the symptoms of overdose.

Contraindications: Clients with demyelinating Charcot-Marie-Tooth syndrome. Lactation. Use during radiation therapy.

Special Concerns: Geriatric clients are more susceptible to the neurotoxic effects. Intrathecal use (may cause death).

Additional Side Effects: *Neurologic:* Paresthesias, depression of deep tendon reflexes, foot drop, ***seizures,*** difficulties in gait. *GI:* ***Intestinal necrosis or perforation.*** Constipation, paralytic ileus. *Renal:* Inappropriate ADH secretion (polyuria or dysuria). Acute uric acid nephropathy. *Ophthalmic:* Blindness, ptosis, diplopia, photophobia. *Miscellaneous:* CNS leukemia, leukopenia or complicating infection, ***bronchospasm,*** SOB. Less bone marrow depression than vinblastine. Significant tissue irritation if leakage occurs during IV use.

Symptoms of Overdose: Exaggeration of side effects.

Drug Interactions

L-Asparaginase / Asparaginase ↓ liver clearance of vincristine

Calcium channel blocking drugs / ↑ Accumulation of vincristine in cells

Digoxin / Vincristine ↓ effect of digoxin

Glutamic acid / Inhibits effect of vincristine

Methotrexate / Combination may cause hypotension

Mitomycin C / Severe bronchospasm and acute SOB

Phenytoin / ↓ Effect of phenytoin due to ↓ plasma levels

NURSING CONSIDERATIONS

See also *Nursing Considerations* for *Antineoplastic Agents,* Chapter 20, and *Vinblastine,* Chapter 24.

Assessment

1. Note indications for therapy. Perform baseline neurologic assessment and monitor for early S&S of neurologic and neuromuscular side effects (e.g., sensory impairment and paresthesias) before neuritic pain and motor difficulties are apparent because neuromuscular manifestations are irreversible.
2. Obtain baseline liver, renal, and hematologic profiles and monitor. Drug may cause granulocyte suppression. Nadir: 10 days; recovery: 21 days.

Interventions

1. Premedicate and regularly administer antiemetic to control N&V.
2. Record I&O, weights, and assess nutritional status.
3. Prevent constipation by increased intake of fluids (2–3 L/day), regular exercise, a high-fiber diet, and stool softeners as needed.
4. Observe for symptoms of gout. Assess need for adding allopurinol or for alkalization of urine to decrease uric acid levels.
5. Be prepared with laxatives and enemas to treat high colon impaction caused by vincristine.
6. Assess for absence of bowel sounds indicative of paralytic ileus, which requires symptomatic care and temporary discontinuation of vincristine therapy.
7. Advise to avoid vaccinations and persons with infectious diseases.
8. Review S&S of neurotoxicity (paresthesias, difficulty walking, and diminished reflexes) and stress importance of reporting.
9. Advise to practice reliable form of birth control during and for 2 months following therapy.

Evaluate: Inhibition of malignant cell proliferation.

Vinorelbine tartrate

Pregnancy Category: D
Navelbine **(Rx)**

How Supplied: Information not available at time of printing.

Action/Kinetics: Vinorelbine is a semisynthetic vinca alkaloid. The antineoplastic effect is thought to be due to inhibition of mitosis at metaphase through the drug's interaction with tubulin. Other possible actions may include interference with (a) amino acid, cyclic AMP, and glutathione metabolism, (b) calmodulin-dependent calcium transport ATPase activity, (c) cellular respiration, and (d) nucleic acid and lipid biosynthesis. Following IV administration, the concentration of vinorelbine in plasma decays in a triphasic manner. The initial rapid decline is due to distribution of the drug to peripheral compartments. The prolonged terminal phase is due to a slow efflux of the drug from peripheral compartments. **Terminal phase t½:** Averages 27.7–43.6 hr. The drug is metabolized by the liver and excreted through the urine and feces.

Uses: Alone or in combination with cisplatin for first-line treatment of ambulatory clients with unresectable, advanced non-small-cell lung cancer. *Investigational:* Breast cancer, cisplatin-resistant ovarian carcinoma, and Hodgkin's disease.

Dosage

• **IV only**

Non-small-cell lung cancer.

Granulocytes (1,500 or more cells/mm³) on the day of treatment: 30 mg/m² weekly given over 6–10 min into the side port of a free-flowing IV closest to the IV bag followed by flushing with at least 75–125 mL of the solution used to dilute the product. May also be given, at the same dose level, with cisplatin, 120 mg/m² on days 1 and 29 and then q 6 weeks. **Granulocytes (1,000–1,499 cells/mm³) on the day of treatment:** 15 mg/m² weekly given over 6–10 min as described previously.

Breast cancer, Hodgkin's disease.

30 mg/m²/week.

Administration/Storage

1. For clients who, during treatment with vinorelbine, have manifested fever or sepsis while granulocytopenic or who had two consecutive weekly doses held due to granulocytopenia, subsequent doses of vinorelbine should be as follows: 22.5 mg/m² for granulocytes equal to or greater than 1,500 cells/mm³ or 11.25 mg/m² for granulocytes from 1,000 to 1,499 cells/mm³.
2. Granulocyte counts should be equal to or greater than 1,000 cells/mm³ prior to giving vinorelbine. Dosage should be based on granulocyte counts on the day of drug treatment.
3. If hyperbilirubinemia develops during treatment, the dose of vinorelbine should be adjusted as follows: 30 mg/m² for a total bilirubin of 2 or less mg/dL, 15 mg/m² for a total bilirubin of 2.1–3 mg/dL, and 7.5 mg/m² for a total bilirubin greater than 3 mg/dL.
4. The drug must be given IV with the IV needle or catheter properly positioned before any drug is given. Leakage into surrounding tissue may cause considerable irritation, local tissue necrosis, or thrombophlebitis. If extravasation occurs, the injection should be stopped immediately and the remaining dose given in another vein. Institutional guidelines should be used to treat extravasation injuries.
5. Due to the toxicity of vinorelbine, caution must be used in handling and preparing the solution. The use of gloves is recommended. If the solution comes in contact with skin or mucosa, the area should be washed immediately with soap and water. If the eye is affected, it should be flushed with water immediately and thoroughly.
6. Vinorelbine must be diluted in either a syringe or IV bag. If an IV bag is used, the dose should be diluted to a concentration between 0.5 and 2 mg/mL using one of the following solutions: 5% dextrose injection, 0.45% or 0.9% sodium chloride injection, 5% dextrose and 0.45% sodium chloride injection, Ringer's injection, and lactated Ringer's injection. When dilution in a syringe is used, the dose should be diluted to a concentration between 1.5 and 3 mg/mL with 5% dextrose injection or 0.9% sodium chloride injection.
7. Diluted vinorelbine solutions may be used for up to 24 hr under normal room light when stored in polypropylene syringes or polyvinyl chloride bags at 5°C–30°C (41°F–96°F). Unopened vials are stable until the expiration date indicated if stored under refrigeration at 2°C–8°C (36°F–46°F). Unopened vials should be protected from light and not frozen. They should not be used if particulate matter is seen.
8. *Treatment of Overdose:* There is no known antidote for vinorelbine. For overdosage, begin general supportive measures together with appropriate blood transfusions and antibiotics, as necessary.

Contraindications: Clients with pretreatment granulocyte counts less than 1,000 cells/mm³. Use during lactation.

Special Concerns: Use with caution in clients with severe hepatic injury or impairment. Use with extreme caution in clients whose bone marrow reserve may have been compromised by chemotherapy or prior to irradiation; also, in those whose bone marrow function is recovering from the effects of previous chemotherapy. Older clients may be more sensitive to the effects of the drug. Safety and efficacy have not been determined in children.

Laboratory Test Interferences: ↑ Total bilirubin, AST. Transient elevations of liver enzymes.

Side Effects: *Hematologic:*Granulocytopenia (may require hospitalization), leukopenia, thrombocytopenia, anemia. *GI:* N&V, constipation, diarrhea, paralytic ileus, anorexia, stomatitis. *CNS:* Mild to severe peripheral neuropathy including paresthesia and hypesthesia, loss of deep tendon reflexes. *CV:* Chest pain, especially in those with a history of CV disease or tumor within the chest; phlebitis. *Respiratory:* SOB (may be severe), dyspnea, interstitial pulmonary changes. *Dermatologic:* Erythema, pain at injection site and vein discoloration, chemical phlebitis along the vein proximal to the site of injection. *Miscellaneous:* Alopecia, asthenia, fatigue, jaw pain, myalgia, arthralgia, rash, hemorrhagic cystitis, syndrome of inappropriate ADH secretion.

Symptoms of Overdose: Bone marrow suppression, peripheral neurotoxicity.

Drug Interactions

Cisplatin / ↑ Incidence of granulocytopenia

Mitomycin / Acute pulmonary reactions

NURSING CONSIDERATIONS

See also *Nursing Considerations* for *Antineoplastic Agents,* Chapter 20.

Assessment

1. Document indications for therapy, other agents and therapies prescribed, and when administered.
2. Obtain baseline CBC with differential initially and before each dose of vinorelbine. Do not administer if granulocyte counts are not at least 1,000 cells/mm^3. Graunlocyte nadir: 7–10 days; Recovery: 7–14 days thereafter.

Client/Family Teaching

1. Report any fever or chills immediately because drug-induced granulocytopenia makes the client much more susceptible to infections.
2. Avoid crowds, persons with infectious diseases, and vaccinations during therapy.
3. Advise women of childbearing age to practice reliable contraception during therapy and for several months thereafter.

Evaluate: Control of malignant cell proliferation.

CHAPTER TWENTY-FIVE

Antineoplastic Agents: Natural Products and Miscellaneous Agents

See the following individual entries:

Aldesleukin
Altretamine
Asparaginase
Etoposide
Interferon Alfa-2A Recombinant
Interferon Alfa-2B Recombinant
Interferon Alfa-N3
Octreotide Acetate
Paclitaxel
Pegaspargase
Procarbazine Hydrochloride
Strontium-89 Chloride

Aldesleukin (Interleukin-2; IL-2)

(al-des-**LOO**-kin)
Pregnancy Category: C
Proleukin **(Rx)**

See also *Antineoplastic Agents,* Chapter 20.

How Supplied: *Powder for injection:* 22 million IU

Action/Kinetics: Aldesleukin, produced by recombinant DNA technology, is a human interleukin-2 (IL-2) product. The recombinant form differs from natural IL-2 in that aldesleukin is not glycosylated, the molecule has no N-terminal alanine, the molecule has serine substituted for cysteine at amino acid position 125, and the aggregation state of aldesleukin may be different from that of native IL-2. However, aldesleukin possesses the biologic activity of human native IL-2. Drug effects include activation of cellular immunity with profound lymphocytosis, eosinophilia, and thrombocytopenia; the production of cytokines, including tumor necrosis factor, IL-1, and gamma interferon; and, inhibition of tumor growth. The exact mechanism of action of aldesleukin is not known. The drug reaches high plasma levels after a short IV infusion and it is rapidly distributed to the extravascular, extracellular space. It is rapidly cleared from the circulation by both glomerular filtration and peritubular extraction; the drug is metabolized in the kidneys with little or no active form excreted through the urine. **t¹/₂, distribution:** 13 min; **t¹/₂, elimination:** 85 min.

Uses: Metastatic renal cell carcinoma in adults 18 years of age and older. *Investigational:* Kaposi's sarcoma in combination with zidovudine, metastatic melanoma in combination with low-dose cyclophosphamide, colorectal cancer and non-Hodgkin's lymphoma often in combination with lymphokine-activated killer cells.

Dosage

- **Intermittent IV infusion**

Metastatic renal cell carcinoma in adults.

Each course of treatment consists of two 5-day treatment cycles separated by a rest period. **Adults:** 600,000 IU/kg (0.037 mg/kg) given q 8 hr by a 15 min IV infusion for a total of 14 doses. Following 9 days of rest, this schedule is repeated for another 14 doses, for a maximum of 28 doses per course. *NOTE:* Due to toxicity clients may not be able to receive all 28 doses (median number of doses given is 20).

Retreatment for metastatic renal cell carcinoma.
Clients should be evaluated for a response about 4 weeks after completion of a course of therapy and again just prior to the start of the next treatment course. Additional courses should be given only if there is evidence of some tumor shrinkage following the last course and retreatment is not contraindicated (See *Contraindications* above). Each treatment course should be separated by at least 7 weeks from the date of hospital discharge.

Administration/Storage

1. Dose modification for toxicity should be undertaken by withholding or interrupting a dose rather than reducing the dose to be given.
2. Therapy should be permanently discontinued for the following toxicities:
• CV: Sustained ventricular tachycardia, uncontrolled or unresponsive cardiac rhythm disturbances, recurrent chest pain with ECG changes indicating angina or MI, pericardial tamponade
• Pulmonary: Intubation required for more than 72 hr
• Renal: Renal dysfunction requiring dialysis for more than 72 hr
• CNS: Coma or toxic psychosis lasting more than 48 hr, seizures that are repetitive or difficult to control
• GI: Bowel ischemia, bowel perforation, GI bleeding requiring surgery
3. The guidelines for held doses and subsequent doses of aldesleukin are detailed in the information provided by the manufacturer and should be consulted carefully.
4. Vials should be reconstituted aseptically with 1.2 mL sterile water for injection. If reconstituted as directed, each milliliter will contain 18 million IU (1.1 mg) of aldesleukin. Such solutions should be clear and colorless to slightly yellow.
5. The vial is for a single use only and any unused portion should be discarded. Drug is not for use with transplant clients, as the risk of allograft rejection may occur.
6. During reconstitution, the sterile water for injection should be directed at the side of the vial. The contents should be swirled gently to avoid foaming. The vial should not be shaken.
7. The reconstituted drug may be diluted in 50 mL of 5% dextrose injection and then infused over 15 min.
8. Plastic bags should be used as this results in more consistent drug delivery. In-line filters should *not* be used when giving aldesleukin.
9. Reconstitution is not to be undertaken using bacteriostatic water for injection or 0.9% sodium chloride injection due to increased aggregation.
10. Dilution with albumin can alter the pharmacology of aldesleukin. Also, aldesleukin should not be mixed with other drugs.
11. After reconstitution, the drug is stable for 48 hr if stored at room temperature or 2°C–8°C (36°F–46°F). The product should be administered within 48 hr of reconstitution, bringing the solution to room temperature before infusing. The product should not be frozen.
12. The undiluted drug is stable for 5 days if refrigerated in 1-mL B-D syringes.
13. The drug is compatible with glass, PVC (preferred), or polypropylene syringes.
14. *Treatment of Overdose:* Side effects will usually reverse if the drug is stopped, especially because the serum half-life is short. Continuing toxicity is treated symptomatically. Life-threatening side effects have been treated by the IV administration of dexamethasone (which may result in loss of the therapeutic effectiveness of aldesleukin).

Contraindications: Hypersensitivity to IL-2 or any components of the product. Abnormal thallium stress test or pulmonary function tests. Organ allografts. Use in either men or women not practicing effective contraception. Lactation.

Retreatment is contraindicated in those who have experienced the following during a previous course of therapy: sustained ventricular tachycardia; uncontrolled or unresponsive cardiac rhythm disturbances; recurrent chest pain with ECG changes that are consistent with angina or MI; intubation required for more than 72 hr; pericardial tamponade; renal dysfunction requiring dialysis for more than 72 hr; coma or toxic psychosis lasting more than 48 hr; seizures that are repetitive or difficult to control; ischemia or perforation of the bowel; and GI bleeding requiring surgery.

Special Concerns: Aldesleukin may worsen symptoms in clients with unrecognized or untreated CNS metastases. Use of medications known to be nephrotoxic or hepatotoxic may further increase toxicity to the kidney and liver caused by aldesleukin. The drug may increase the risk of allograft rejection in transplant clients. Safety and efficacy have not been established in children less than 18 years of age.

Laboratory Test Interferences: ↑ BUN, bilirubin, serum creatinine, transaminase, alkaline phosphatase. See also *Electrolyte and other disturbances* under *Side Effects*.

Side Effects: Side effects are frequent, often serious, and sometimes fatal. Most clients will experience fever, chills, rigors, pruritus, and GI side effects. The frequency and severity of side effects are usually dose-related and schedule-dependent. Incidence of side effects is greater in PS 1 clients than in PS 0 clients. The side effects listed have an incidence of 1% or greater.

Capillary leak syndrome (CLS): Results from extravasation of plasma proteins and fluid into the extracellular space with loss of vascular tone. This results in a drop in mean arterial BP within 2–12 hr after the start of treatment and reduced organ perfusion that may be severe and result in death. CLS causes hypotension, hypoperfusion, and extravasation that leads to edema and effusion. ***CLS may be associated with supraventricular and ventricular arrhythmias, MI,*** angina, respiratory insufficiency requiring intubation, GI bleeding or infarction, renal insufficiency, and changes in mental status.

CV: Hypotension (sometimes requiring vasopressor therapy), sinus tachycardia, ***arrhythmias (atrial, junctional, supraventricular, ventricular)***, bradycardia, PVCs, premature atrial contractions, myocardial ischemia, ***MI, cardiac arrest, CHF,*** myocarditis, endocarditis, gangrene, ***stroke, pericardial effusion, thrombosis.*** *Respiratory:* Pulmonary congestion, dyspnea, pulmonary edema, ***respiratory failure,*** tachypnea, pleural effusion, wheezing, apnea, pneumothorax, hemoptysis. *GI:* N&V, diarrhea, stomatitis, anorexia, ***GI bleeding*** (sometimes requiring surgery), dyspepsia, constipation, ***intestinal perforation,*** intestinal ileus, pancreatitis. *CNS:* Changes in mental status (may be an early indication of bacteremia or early bacterial sepsis), dizziness, sensory dysfunction, disorders of special senses (speech, taste, vision), syncope, motor dysfunction, ***coma, seizure***. *GU:* Oliguria or anuria, proteinuria, hematuria, dysuria, impaired renal function requiring dialysis, urinary retention, urinary frequency. *Hepatic:* Jaundice, ascites, hepatomegaly. *Hematologic:* Anemia, thrombocytopenia, leukopenia, coagulation disorders, leukocytosis, eosinophilia. *Dermatologic:* Pruritus, erythema, rash, dry skin, exfoliative dermatitis, purpura, petechiae, urticaria, alopecia. *Musculoskeletal:* Arthralgia, myalgia, arthritis, muscle spasm. *Electrolyte and other disturbances:* Hypomagnesemia, acidosis, hypocalcemia, hypophosphatemia, hypokalemia, hyperuricemia, hypoalbuminemia, hypoproteinemia, hyponatremia, hyperkalemia, alkalosis, hypoglycemia, hyperglycemia, hypocholesterolemia, hypercalcemia, hypernatremia, hyperphosphatemia. *Miscellaneous:* Fever, chills, pain (abdominal, chest, back), fatigue, malaise, weakness, edema, infection (including the injection site, urinary tract, catheter tip, phlebitis, sepsis), weight gain or weight loss, headache, conjunctivitis, reactions at the injection site, allergic reactions, hypothyroidism.

Symptoms of Overdose: See *Side Effects* above. Administration of more than the recommended dose will cause a more rapid onset of toxicities.

Drug Interactions

Aminoglycosides / ↑ Risk of kidney toxicity
Antihypertensives / Potentiate hypotension seen with aldesleukin
Asparaginase / ↑ Risk of hepatic toxicity
Cardiotoxic agents / ↑ Risk of cardiac toxicity
Corticosteroids / Concomitant use may ↓ the antitumor effectiveness of aldesleukin (although the corticosteroids ↓ side effects of aldesleukin)
Cytotoxic chemotherapy / ↑ Risk of myelotoxicity
Doxorubicin / ↑ Risk of cardiac toxicity
Hepatotoxic drugs / ↑ Risk of liver toxicity
Indomethacin / ↑ Risk of kidney toxicity
Methotrexate / ↑ Risk of hepatic toxicity
Myelotoxic agents / ↑ Risk of myelotoxicity
Nephrotoxic agents / ↑ Risk of kidney toxicity

NURSING CONSIDERATIONS

See also *Nursing Considerations* for *Antineoplastic Agents,* Chapter 20.

Assessment

1. Note any history of liver or renal dysfunction as well as cardiac, pulmonary, or CNS impairment.
2. The following baseline parameters should be determined prior to initiation of therapy and daily during drug use: CBC, including differential and platelet counts, blood chemistries (including electrolytes), renal and hepatic function tests, CXRs. All clients should have baseline pulmonary function tests with ABGs.
3. Clients should be screened with a thallium stress test to document normal ejection fraction and unimpaired wall motion. If minor abnormalities in wall motion of questionable significance are noted, a stress echocardiogram may be useful to exclude significant CAD.
4. Assess carefully for any S&S of infection. Obtain cultures to R/O any potential sources. Preexisting bacterial infections must be treated prior to initiation of aldesleukin therapy as intensive treatment may cause impaired neutrophil function and an increased risk of disseminated infection leading to sepsis and bacterial endocarditis.
5. All clients with indwelling central lines should receive antibiotic prophylaxis against *Saccharomyces aureus*.

Interventions

1. Therapy should be initiated in a closely monitored environment where VS and I&O are assessed often.
2. Cardiac function should be assessed daily by clinical examination and assessment of VS. Clients who have signs or symptoms of chest pain, murmurs, gallops, irregular rhythm, or palpitations should be further assessed with an ECG examination and CPK evaluation. If there is evidence of cardiac ischemia or CHF, a repeat thallium study should be undertaken.
3. Perform daily CV evaluations to identify any early S&S of drug toxicity. Monitor client carefully for symptoms of CLS characterized by hypotension and hypoperfusion, altered mental status and decreased urine output. Mental status changes are usually transient but should be evaluated carefully. Alterations in urinary output may signal renal toxicity.

Client/Family Teaching

1. Report any persistent abdominal pain or discomfort.
2. Review list of potential drug side effects and note those (dyspnea, palpitations, chest pain, or impaired vision) requiring immediate medical intervention.

3. Practice reliable contraceptive methods.
4. Avoid any OTC drugs unless specifically ordered.
Evaluate: Disease regression with evidence of ↓ tumor size and spread.

Altretamine (Hexylmethylmelamine)

(all-**TRET**-ah-meen)
Pregnancy Category: D
Hexalen, Hexastat ✱ **(Rx)**

See also *Antineoplastic Agents,* Chapter 20.
How Supplied: *Capsule:* 50 mg
Action/Kinetics: The mechanism of action of altretamine is unknown although metabolism of the drug is required for cytotoxicity. Altretamine is well absorbed following PO ingestion and undergoes rapid demethylation in the liver, yielding the principal metabolites–pentamethylmelamine and tetramethylmelamine. **Peak plasma levels:** 0.5–3 hr. **t½:** 4.7–10.2 hr. Metabolites of the drug are excreted mainly through the kidney.
Uses: Used alone in the palliative treatment of persistent or recurrent ovarian cancer after first-line cisplatin- or alkylating agent-based combination therapy.

Dosage

- **Capsules**

  Ovarian cancer.

260 mg/m²/day given either for 14 or 21 consecutive days in a 28-day cycle. The total daily dose is given as four divided doses PO after meals and at bedtime.
Contraindications: Preexisting bone marrow depression or severe neurologic toxicity, although the drug has been used safely in clients with preexisting cisplatin neuropathies. Use during lactation.
Special Concerns: Safety and effectiveness have not been determined in children. High daily doses may result in gradual onset of N&V.
Laboratory Test Interferences: ↑ Serum creatinine, BUN, alkaline phosphatase.
Side Effects: *GI:* N&V (most common). *Neurologic:* Peripheral sensory neuropathy, fatigue, anorexia, seizures. *CNS:* Mood disorders, disorders of consciousness, ataxia, dizziness, vertigo. *Hematologic:* Leukopenia, thrombocytopenia, anemia. *Miscellaneous:* ***Hepatic toxicity,*** skin rash, pruritus, alopecia.
Drug Interactions: Use with MAO inhibitors may cause severe orthostatic hypotension, especially in clients over the age of 60 years.

NURSING CONSIDERATIONS

See also *Nursing Considerations* for *Antineoplastic Agents,* Chapter 20.
Assessment
1. Document onset of symptoms and note all previous therapeutic regimens.
2. Document baseline neurologic findings.
3. Obtain hematologic and liver function studies prior to initiating drug therapy.

Interventions
1. Anticipate neurotoxicity as a side effect of drug therapy. A neurologic exam should be performed prior to each course of altretamine.
2. Administering pyridoxine with altretamine may reduce the severity of the neurotoxic effects.
3. Peripheral blood counts should be monitored monthly, prior to the initiation of each course of therapy and as clinically indicated.

Client/Family Teaching
1. Report any adverse symptoms, such as tingling, decreased sensation, dizziness, and N&V. Drug dose may need to be decreased or therapy discontinued.
2. Practice barrier contraception as drug may cause fetal damage.
3. Emphasize the importance of reporting for monthly hematologic studies.

Evaluate: Control of tumor growth and spread.

Asparaginase

(ah-**SPAIR**-ah-jin-ays)
Pregnancy Category: C
Colaspase, Elspar, Kidrolase ✱ (Abbreviation: Lcf-ASP) **(Rx)**

See also *Antineoplastic Agents,* Chapter 20.

How Supplied: *Powder for injection:* 10,000 IU

Action/Kinetics: Drug isolated from *Escherichia coli.* Cell cycle specific (G_1 phase). Neoplastic cells are unable to synthesize sufficient asparagine, an amino acid, to meet their metabolic needs. The supply of asparagine is further decreased by the enzyme asparaginase, which breaks down asparagine to aspartic acid and ammonia. Asparaginase interferes with synthesis of DNA, RNA, and protein and is cell-cycle specific for the G_1 phase of cell division. **Time to peak plasma levels, after IM:** 14–24 hr. **t½, after IV:** 8–30 hr; **after IM:** 39–49 hr. The drug accumulates in plasma and tissue, and a small amount (1%) appears in CSF. Excretion is unknown. More toxic in adults than in children.

Uses: Acute lymphocytic leukemia in children; mostly used in combination with other drugs. Not to be used for maintenance therapy. *Investigational:* Acute myelocytic and myelomonocytic leukemia, chronic lymphocytic leukemia, Hodgkin's and non-Hodgkin's lymphomas, melanosarcoma.

Dosage

• **IV, IM**

When used as sole agent. **Adults and children:** 200 IU/kg/day **IV** for 28 days.

In combination with prednisone and vincristine. Asparaginase: 1,000 IU/kg/day **IV** for 10 days beginning on day 22 of course of therapy; vincristine: 2 mg/m² **IV** once weekly on days 1, 8, and 15 of course of treatment (single dosage should not exceed 2 mg); prednisone: 40 mg/m²/day **PO** in three doses for 15 days; **then,** 20 mg/m² for 2 days, 10 mg/m² for 2 days, 5 mg/m² for 2 days, and 2.5 mg/m² for 2 days, followed by discontinuance of therapy.

Alternative combination regimen. Asparaginase: 6,000 IU/m² **IM** on days 4, 7, 10, 13, 16, 19, 22, 25, and 28 of course of treatment; vincristine: 1.5 mg/m² **IV** weekly on days 1, 8, 15, and 22 of course of treatment (maximum single dose should not exceed 2 mg); prednisone: 40 mg/m²/day **PO** in three divided doses for 28 days, followed by gradual discontinuation over a 2-week period.

Administration/Storage

1. An intradermal skin test (0.1 mL of a 20-IU/mL solution) should be done at least 1 hr before initial administration of drug and when 1 week or more has elapsed between treatments.
2. A desensitization procedure, with increasing amounts of asparaginase, is sometimes carried out in clients hypersensitive to the drug (1 IU, then double dose every 10 min until total dose for day or reaction occurs).
3. Treatment should be initiated only in hospitalized clients.
4. Asparaginase should not be used as the sole induction agent unless a combined regimen is not possible due to toxicity or because the client is refractory.
5. For IV use, reconstitute the 10,000-unit vial with either 5 mL sterile water for injection or sodium chloride injection. The solution may be given by direct IV administration or by infusion. When infused, give over at least 30 min in side of arm; use an infusion of either sodium chloride injection or dextrose injection (5%).
6. When used IM, no more than 2 mL should be given at a single injection site.
7. Reconstitute for IM use by adding 2 mL sodium chloride injection to the 10,000-unit vial. Do not use after 8 hr following reconstitution.
8. The drug should be handled with care because it is a contact irritant.
9. Have emergency equipment readily available during each administration of asparaginase because a severe hypersensitivity reaction is more likely to occur with this drug.

Contraindications: Anaphylactic reactions to asparaginase, acute hemorrhagic pancreatitis. Lactation. Institute retreatment with great care.
Special Concerns: Use with caution in presence of liver dysfunction.
Laboratory Test Interferences: ↑ Blood ammonia, BUN, glucose, uric acid, AST, ALT, alkaline phosphatase, bilirubin (direct and indirect). ↓ Serum calcium albumin, cholesterol, plasma fibrinogen. Interference with interpretation of thyroid function tests.
Side Effects: Hypersensitivity reaction including those with negative skin tests. Hyperglycemia, uricemia, azotemia, acute hemorrhagic pancreatitis, ***fatal hyperthermia.*** Hallucinations, Parkinson-like syndrome (rare).
Drug Interactions
Methotrexate / Asparaginase ↓ effect of methotrexate
Prednisone / Even though used with asparaginase, may cause ↑ toxicity
Vincristine / Even though used with asparaginase, may cause ↑ toxicity; ↑ hyperglycemic effect

NURSING CONSIDERATIONS

See also *General Nursing Considerations* for *Antineoplastic Agents,* Chapter 20.
Assessment
1. Document indications for therapy and baseline laboratory studies. Drug may cause mild lymphocyte suppression. Nadir: 7–10 days; recovery 14 days.
2. Obtain serum amylase levels and check periodically during therapy to detect for evidence of pancreatitis.
Interventions
1. Anticipate antiemetic administration prior to drug therapy.
2. If ordered, administer vincristine and prednisone before asparaginase to reduce the toxic effect.
3. Administration of asparaginase 9–10 days before or within 24 hr after methotrexate may be ordered to reduce the GI and hematologic effects of methotrexate.
4. Weigh weekly and monitor I&O; assess for any evidence of renal failure. Alkalinization of the urine and allopurinol therapy may help prevent urate stone formation.
5. Observe client for peripheral edema due to hypoalbuminemia triggered by asparaginase.
6. Monitor for hyperglycemia, glycosuria, and polyuria, all of which may be precipitated by asparaginase.
7. Have IV fluids and regular insulin available to treat hyperglycemia. Anticipate discontinuation of asparaginase.
8. Assess for shakiness or unusual body movements. A Parkinson-like condition may be precipitated by asparaginase.
Client/Family Teaching
1. Promptly report any stomach pain and N&V because these side effects may be symptoms of pancreatitis.
2. Report hyperthermia immediately.
3. Encourage client to consume 2–3 L/day of fluids.
4. Caution that the drug may cause drowsiness, even several weeks after administration; therefore, do not drive a car or operate hazardous machinery.
5. Avoid immunizations and contact with child who has recently taken polio vaccine.
6. Avoid crowds, especially during flu season.
7. Do not take any aspirin-containing compounds or drink alcoholic beverages.
Evaluate
- Improved hematologic parameters
- Inhibition of malignant cell proliferation

Etoposide (VP-16—213)

(eh-**TOH**-poh-syd)
Pregnancy Category: D
VePesid **(Rx)**

See also *Antineoplastic Agents,* Chapter 20.
How Supplied: *Capsule:* 50 mg; *Injection:* 20 mg/mL

Action/Kinetics: Etoposide is a semisynthetic derivative of podophyllotoxin. Etoposide acts as a mitotic inhibitor at the G_2 portion of the cell cycle to inhibit DNA synthesis. At high doses, cells entering mitosis are lysed, whereas at low doses, cells will not enter prophase. **t½:** biphasic; initial, 1.5 hr; final, 4–11 hr. **Effective plasma levels:** 0.3–10 mcg/mL. Poor penetration to the CNS. The drug is eliminated through both the urine and bile unchanged and as liver metabolites.

Uses: With combination therapy to treat refractory testicular tumors and small cell lung cancer. *Investigational:* Alone or in combination to treat acute monocytic leukemia, non-Hodgkin's lymphoma, Hodgkin's disease, AIDS-associated Kaposi's sarcoma, Ewing's sarcoma. Also, choriocarcinoma; hepatocellular carcinoma; nonsmall cell lung, breast, endometrial, and gastric cancers; acute lymphocytic leukemia; soft tissue carcinoma; rhabdomyosarcoma.

Dosage

• **IV**

Testicular carcinoma.

50–100 mg/m²/day on days 1–5 or 100 mg/m²/day on days 1, 3, and 5 q 3–4 weeks (i.e., after recovery from toxic effects). Used in combination with other agents.

Small cell lung carcinoma.

35 mg/m²/day for 4 days to 50 mg/m²/day for 5 days, repeated q 3–4 weeks.

• **Capsules**

Small cell lung carcinoma.

70 mg/m² (rounded to the nearest 50 mg) daily for 4 days to 100 mg/m² (rounded to the nearest 50 mg) daily for 5 days; repeat q 3–4 weeks.

Administration/Storage

1. For IV use, the drug should be diluted with either 5% dextrose or 0.9% sodium chloride injection for a final concentration of 0.2 or 0.4 mg/mL (5-mL vial in 250 or 500 mL of IV solution).
2. A slow IV infusion over 30–60 min will decrease the chance of hypotension. The drug should not be given by rapid IV push.
3. Medical personnel should wear gloves when preparing this medication; if the drug comes in contact with the skin or mucosa, the area should be washed immediately and thoroughly with soap and water.
4. Diluted solutions with a final concentration of 0.2 mg/mL are stable for 96 hr at room temperature; final concentrations of 0.4 mg/mL are stable for 48 hr at room temperature.
5. Capsules must be stored at 2°C–8°C (36°F–46°F) but should not be frozen.
6. Be prepared to treat anaphylactic reactions. Have available corticosteroids, pressor agents, antihistamines, and plasma expanders.

Contraindication: Lactation.

Special Concerns: Safety and efficacy in children have not been established. Severe myelosuppression may occur.

Additional Side Effects: ***Anaphylactic-type reactions,*** hypotension, peripheral neuropathy, somnolence.

NURSING CONSIDERATIONS

See also *Nursing Considerations* for *Antineoplastic Agents,* Chapter 20.

Assessment

1. Document onset of symptoms and any previous treatments.
2. Obtain baseline liver and renal function studies and CBC; drug may cause granulocyte and platelet suppression. Nadir: 14 days; recovery: 21 days.
3. Determine pregnancy if female and of childbearing years.
4. Drug may cause increased uric acid levels.
5. Assess nutritional status. Anticipate pretreatment with an antiemetic as drug may cause N&V.

Interventions

1. Monitor for signs of infection and bleeding, which are more likely to occur with this drug than with most antineoplastic agents.
2. When receiving infusions stress bed rest and supervise ambulation as orthostatic hypotension may oc-

cur. Record BP during infusions and at least twice a day with PO therapy; note any significant decreases.
3. Report any tingling sensations, numbness, and other signs of peripheral neuropathy.
4. Client may feel fatigued and be sleepy during and after drug administration. Schedule nursing activities to ensure adequate rest.

Client/Family Teaching

1. Report any flu-like symptoms because drug combination therapy may cause severe myelosuppression.
2. Provide a printed list of side effects that require immediate reporting.
3. Consume 2–3 L/day of fluids to prevent kidney damage.
4. Report if N&V impair intake.
5. Practice barrier contraception during treatment.

Evaluate

- Suppression of malignant cell proliferation
- Improved hematologic parameters with leukemia

Interferon alfa-2a recombinant (rI FN-A; IFLrA)

(in-ter-**FEER**-on **AL**-fah)
Pregnancy Category: C
Roferon-A **(Rx)**

How Supplied: *Injection:* 3 million U/mL, 6 million U/mL, 9 million U/0.9 mL, 36 million U/mL; *Powder for injection:* 18 million U

Action/Kinetics: Interferon alfa-2a is the product of recombinant DNA technology using strains of genetically engineered *Escherichia coli*. The activity of these drugs is expressed as International Units, which are determined by comparing the antiviral activity of recombinant interferons with the activity of the international reference standard of human leukocyte interferon. Interferons bind to specific receptors on the cell surface, resulting in inhibition of virus replication in virus-infected cells, suppression of cell proliferation, increase in the phagocytic activity of macrophages, and enhancement of the toxic effects of leukocytes for target cells. *Interferon A-2a.* **Peak serum levels:** 3.8–7.3 hr. **t½:** 3.7–8.5 hr. The drug is metabolized by the kidney.

Uses: Hairy cell leukemia in clients older than 18 years of age. Can be used in splenectomized and nonsplenectomized clients. AIDS-related Kaposi's sarcoma in clients older than 18 years of age. *Investigational:* The drug has been used for a large number of other conditions. Significant activity has been noted against the following neoplastic diseases: locally for superficial bladder tumors, carcinoid tumor, chronic myelogenous leukemia, cutaneous T-cell lymphoma, essential thrombocythemia, low-grade non-Hodgkin's lymphoma. Limited activity has been noted in acute leukemias, cervical carcinoma, chronic lymphocytic leukemia, Hodgkin's disease, malignant gliomas, melanoma, multiple myeloma, nasopharyngeal carcinoma, osteosarcoma, ovarian carcinoma, renal carcinoma. Interferon alfa-2a has also been used to treat the following viral infections: chronic non-A, non-B hepatitis, condylomata acuminata, cutaneous warts, cytomegaloviruses, herpes keratoconjunctivitis, herpes simplex, papillomaviruses, rhinoviruses, vaccinia virus, varicella zoster, and viral hepatitis B.

Dosage

- **IM, SC**

Hairy cell leukemia.

Induction: 3 million IU/day for 16–24 weeks; **maintenance,** 3 million IU 3 times/week. Doses higher than 3 million IU are not recommended.

AIDS-related Kaposi's sarcoma.

Induction: 36 million IU/day for 10–12 weeks; or, 3 million IU/day on days 1–3; 9 million IU/day on days 4–6; and 18 million IU/day on days 7–9 followed by 36 million IU/day for the remainder of the 10–12-week induction period. **Mainte-**

nance: 36 million IU 3 times/week. If severe side effects occur, the dose can be withheld or reduced by one-half.

Administration/Storage

1. Treatment should be discontinued if the hairy cell leukemia does not respond within 6 months.
2. If severe reactions occur, the dose of the drug can be reduced by one-half or individual doses may be withheld. Also, assess the effect on bone marrow of previous radiation or chemotherapy.
3. Although the optimal duration of treatment has not been established, clients have been treated for up to 20 consecutive months. Nadir: leukocytes, 20–40 days; platelets, 15–20 days.
4. The SC route of administration should be considered for clients who have a platelet count less than 50,000/mm^3.
5. Although not approved by the FDA, interferon alfa-2a has been given by continuous or intermittent IV infusion as well as ophthalmically and intravaginally.
6. The reconstituted solution is stable for 30 days when stored at 2°C–8°C and for 24 hr when stored at room temperature. The undiluted drug is not stable in syringes due to adhesion to syringe surfaces.

Contraindication: Lactation.

Special Concerns: Use with caution in clients with a history of unstable angina, uncontrolled CHF, COPD, diabetes mellitus prone to ketoacidosis, thrombophlebitis, pulmonary embolism, seizure disorders, severe renal and hepatic disease, compromised CNS function, and severe myelosuppression. Safety and efficacy in individuals less than 18 years of age have not been established.

Laboratory Test Interferences: ↑ AST, ALT, LDH, BUN, serum creatinine, alkaline phosphatase, bilirubin, uric acid, serum glucose, serum phosphorus. ↓ H&H. Hypocalcemia, proteinuria.

Side Effects: *Flu-like symptoms:* Fever, headache, fatigue, arthralgia, myalgias, chills. *CV:* Hypotension, ***arrhythmias,*** syncope, hypertension, edema, chest pain, palpitations, transient ischemic attacks, pulmonary edema, CHF, ***MI, stroke,*** hot flashes, Raynaud's phenomenon. *Respiratory:* Coughing, dyspnea, chest congestion, ***bronchospasm,*** tachypnea, rhinitis, rhinorrhea, sinusitis. *CNS:* Depression, confusion, dizziness, paresthesia, anxiety, nervousness, numbness, lethargy, sleep disturbances, visual disturbances, vertigo, decreased mental status, forgetfulness. *GI:* Anorexia, N&V, diarrhea, hypermotility, abdominal fullness, abdominal pain, flatulence, constipation, gastric distress. *Hematologic:* Thrombocytopenia, neutropenia, leukopenia, decreased hemoglobin. *Musculoskeletal:* Myalgia, arthralgia, muscle contractions. *Dermatologic:* Rash, inflammation or dryness of the oropharynx, pruritus, dry skin, skin flushing, alopecia, urticaria. *Other:* Taste alteration, hepatitis, weight loss, diaphoresis, transient impotence, conjunctivitis, night sweats, excessive salivation, reactivation of herpes labialis, muscle contractions, cyanosis, eye irritation, earache.

NURSING CONSIDERATIONS

Client/Family Teaching

1. Review the appropriate method for administration and have client or person designated to administer, return demonstrate. Explain the care and safe storage of drug and equipment and proper disposal of syringes.
2. The most common side effects are flu-like symptoms, such as fever, fatigue, headache, chills, nausea, and loss of appetite, and these symptoms may be minimized by taking the drug at bedtime. Report if pronounced.
3. Flu-like symptoms usually diminish in severity as treatment continues. Acetaminophen may be used to treat side effects of fever and headache.
4. Clients should be well hydrated, especially when therapy is initiated. Drink plenty of fluids (2–3 L/day) during therapy.

5. Stress that hypotension may occur up to 2 days following drug therapy so sit before standing and rise slowly.
6. Do not change brands of interferon without approval because changes in dosage may occur with a different brand.
7. Stress the importance of reporting for lab tests, including CBC, electrolyte levels, and liver function studies as scheduled.
8. Report any evidence of neurologic or psychologic disturbances.
9. Advise that hair loss may occur.
10. Practice safe sex and use contraception.
11. Avoid alcohol and any other unprescribed CNS depressants.

Evaluate

- ↓ Tumor size and spread
- Improved hematologic parameters
- ↓ Lesions with Kaposi's sarcoma

Interferon alfa-2b recombinant (rI FN-a2; a-2-interferon)

(in-ter-**FEER**-on **AL**-fah)
Pregnancy Category: C
Intron A, Wellferon ✱ **(Rx)**

How Supplied: *Injection:* 5 million IU/mL, 6 million IU/mL; *Powder for injection:* 3 million IU, 5 million IU, 10 million IU, 18 million IU, 25 million IU, 50 million IU

Action/Kinetics: Interferon alfa-2b is a product of recombinant DNA technology using strains of genetically engineered *Escherichia coli.* The activity is expressed as International Units, which are determined by comparing the antiviral activity of the recombinant interferon with the activity of the international reference standard of human leukocyte interferon. Interferons bind to specific receptors on the cell surface, resulting in inhibition of virus replication in virus-infected cells, suppression of cell proliferation, increase in the phagocytic activity of macrophages, and enhancement of the toxic effects of leukocytes for target cells. *Interferon alfa-2b.* **Peak serum levels after IM, SC:** up to 116 IU/mL after 3–12 hr. **t½, IM, SC:** 6–7 hr. **Peak serum levels after IV infusion:** up to 270 IU/mL at the end of the infusion. **t½, IV:** 2 hr. The main site of metabolism may be the kidney.

Uses: Hairy cell leukemia in clients older than 18 years of age (in both splenectomized and nonsplenectomized clients). Intralesional use for genital or venereal warts (*Condylomata acuminata.*) AIDS-related Kaposi's sarcoma in clients over 18 years of age. Chronic hepatitis non-A, non-B/C in clients at least 18 years of age with compensated liver disease and a history of blood or blood product exposure or who are HCV antibody positive. Chronic hepatitis B in clients over 18 years of age with compensated liver disease and HBV replication (clients must be serum HBsAg positive for at least 6 months and have HBV replication with elevated serum ALT). *Investigational:* The drug has been used for a large number of conditions. Significant activity has been noted against the following neoplastic diseases: locally for superficial bladder tumors, carcinoid tumor, chronic myelogenous leukemia, cutaneous T-cell lymphoma, essential thrombocythemia, and low-grade non-Hodgkin's lymphoma. Limited activity has been noted in acute leukemias, cervical carcinoma, chronic lymphocytic leukemia, Hodgkin's disease, malignant gliomas, melanoma, multiple myeloma, nasopharyngeal carcinoma, osteosarcoma, ovarian carcinoma, renal carcinoma. Interferon alfa-2b has also been used to treat the following viral infections: cutaneous warts, CMVs, herpes keratoconjunctivitis, herpes simplex, papillomaviruses, rhinoviruses, vaccinia virus, and varicella zoster. It has also been used to treat multiple sclerosis.

Dosage

- **IM, SC**

Hairy cell leukemia.

2 million IU/m^2 3 times/week. Higher doses are not recommended. May require 6 or more months of therapy for improvement.

AIDS-related Kaposi's sarcoma.

30 million IU/m^2 3 times/week using only the 50-million-IU vial. Using this dose, clients should tolerate an average dose of 110 million IU/week at the end of 12 weeks of therapy and 75 million IU/week at the end of 24 weeks of therapy.

Chronic hepatitis non-A, non-B/C.

3 million IU 3 times/week for up to 6 months. Therapy should be discontinued if there is no response after 16 weeks.

Chronic hepatitis B.

30–35 million IU/week given as either 5 million IU/day or 10 million IU 3 times/week for 16 weeks. If serious side effects occur, the dose may be decreased by 50%.

Intralesional

Genital or venereal warts.

1 million IU/lesion 3 times/week for 3 weeks. For this purpose, use only the vial containing 10 million units and reconstitute using no more than 1 mL diluent.

Administration/Storage

1. Prior to administration, the drug must be reconstituted with bacteriostatic water for injection, which is provided. After reconstitution, the solution is stable for 1 month at 2°C–8°C (36°F–46°F).
2. If severe side effects occur, the dose can be reduced as much as 50% or therapy can be discontinued until side effects improve. For example, if the granulocyte count is less than 750/mm^3 and the platelet count is less than 50,000/mm^3, the dose should be reduced by 50%; if the granulocyte count is less than 500/mm^3 and the platelet count is less than 30,000/mm^3, drug therapy should be interrupted until counts return to normal or baseline levels.
3. Treatment for hairy cell leukemia should be discontinued if the client does not respond within 6 months.
4. When used for venereal or genital warts, maximum response usually occurs 4–8 weeks after therapy is initiated. If results are not satisfactory after 12–16 weeks, a second course of therapy may be undertaken.
5. Although the optimal duration of treatment has not been established, clients have been treated for up to 20 consecutive months.
6. If the platelet count is less than 50,000/mm^3, the drug should be given SC rather than IM.
7. Although not approved by the FDA, interferon alfa-2a has been given by continuous or intermittent IV infusion as well as ophthalmically and intravaginally.
8. The reconstituted solution is stable for 30 days when stored from 2°C–8°C and for 48 hr when stored at 40°C or less. The undiluted drug is not stable in syringes due to adhesion to syringe surfaces.

Contraindications: Lactation. To treat rapidly progressive visceral disease in AIDS-related Kaposi's sarcoma.

Special Concerns: Use with caution in clients with a history of unstable angina, uncontrolled CHF, COPD, diabetes mellitus prone to ketoacidosis, thrombophlebitis, pulmonary embolism, seizure disorders, severe renal and hepatic disease, compromised CNS function, and severe myelosuppression. Safety and efficacy in individuals less than 18 years of age have not been established.

Laboratory Test Interferences: ↑ AST, ALT, LDH, BUN, serum creatinine, alkaline phosphatase. ↓ H&H.

Side Effects: *Flu-like symptoms:* Fever, headache, fatigue, myalgia, chills. *CV:* Hypotension, ***arrhythmias,*** tachycardia, syncope, hypertension, coagulation disorders, chest pain, palpitations, flushing, atrial fibrillation, bradycardia, ***cardiac failure, cardiomyopathy,*** extrasystoles, postural hypotension. *CNS:* Depression, confusion, somnolence, insomnia, migraine, dizziness, ataxia, irritability, paresthesia, anxiety, nervousness, emotional lability, amnesia, impaired concentration, weakness, tremor, syncope, abnormal coordination, hypesthesia, agitation, apathy, aphasia, dysphonia, extrapyramidal disorder, hot flashes, hyperesthesia, hyperkinesia, neurosis, paresis, paroniria, parosmia, personality disorder, ***seizures, coma,*** polyneuropathy, ***suicide attempt.*** *GI:* N&V, diarrhea, stomatitis, weight loss, anorexia, dyspepsia, flatulence, taste loss, thirst, dehydration, constipation, eructation, abdominal pain, loose stools, abdominal distention, dysphagia, esophagitis, gastric ulcer, ***GI hemorrhage,*** GI mucosal discoloration, gum hyperplasia, gingival bleeding, gingivitis, increased saliva, increased appetite, melena, oral leukoplakia, rectal bleeding after stool, ***rectal hemorrhage,*** ulcerative stomatitis. *Hematologic:* Thrombocytopenia, transient granulocytopenia, anemia, ***hemolytic anemia,*** leukopenia. *Musculoskeletal:* Arthralgia, leg cramps, asthenia, arthrosis, arthritis, muscle pain or weakness, back pain, bone pain, rigors. *Respiratory:* Pharyngitis, coughing, dyspnea, sinusitis, rhinitis, epistaxis, nasal congestion, dry mouth, ***bronchospasm,*** pleural pain, pneumonia, rhinorrhea, sneezing, wheezing. *EENT:* Alteration of taste, tinnitus, hearing disorders, conjunctivitis, photophobia, vision disorders, eye pain, diplopia, dry eyes, earache, lacrimal gland disorder, periorbital edema, vertigo. *Dermatologic:* Rash, pruritus, alopecia, urticaria, dry skin, dermatitis, purpura, photosensitivity, acne, nail disorder, facial edema, moniliasis, reaction at injection site, abnormal hair texture, cold/clammy skin, cyanosis of the hand, epidermal necrolysis, dermatitis lichenoides, furunculosis, increased hair growth, erythema, melanosis, nonherpetic cold sores, peripheral ischemia, skin depigmentation or discoloration, vitiligo. *GU:* Amenorrhea, hematuria, impotence, leukorrhea, menorrhagia, urinary frequency, nocturia, polyuria, uterine bleeding, increased BUN. *Other:* Pain, increased sweating, malaise, decreased libido, herpes simplex, lymphadenopathy, chest pain, abscess, cachexia, hypercalcemia, peripheral edema, stye, substernal chest pain, weakness, sepsis.

Drug Interactions

Aminophylline / ↓ Clearance of aminophylline due to ↓ breakdown by the liver

AZT / ↑ Risk of neutropenia

NURSING CONSIDERATIONS

See also *Nursing Considerations* for *Interferon alfa-2a recombinant* and *Interferon alfa-n3,* Chapter 25.

Client/Family Teaching

1. Flu-like symptoms may be minimized by administering the drug at bedtime.
2. Acetaminophen may be used to treat side effects of fever and headache.
3. Clients should be well hydrated, especially when therapy is initiated. Consume 2–3 L/day during therapy.
4. Report for scheduled lab studies. Prior to and periodically during therapy, the levels of hemoglobin, platelets, granulocytes and hairy cells, and bone marrow hairy cells should be determined. Nadir: 3–5 days.

Evaluate

- Improved hematologic response and disease regression (treatment should be continued until no further beneficial effects are observed and lab values have been stable for 3 months)
- ↓ Size and number of genital and/or venereal warts (reevaluate need for continued treatment if warts persist)

Interferon alfa-n3

(in-ter-**FEER**-on **AL**-fah)

Pregnancy Category: C

Alferon N **(Rx)**

How Supplied: *Injection:* 5 million IU/mL

Action/Kinetics: Interferon alfa-n3 is made from pooled human leukocytes induced by incomplete infection with Sendai (avian) virus. The product is a sterile, aqueous formulation of purified, natural, human interferon alpha proteins. The drug binds to receptors on cell surfaces leading to a sequence of events including inhibition of virus replication and suppression of cell proliferation. Also, interferon alfa-n3 causes immunomodulation characterized by enhanced phagocytosis by macrophages, augmentation of the cytotoxicity of lymphocytes, and enhancement of human leukocyte antigen expression. Intralesional use of interferon alfa-n3 does not result in detectable plasma levels of the drug.

Uses: Intralesional treatment of refractory or recurring external condylomata acuminata (genital or venereal warts) in clients 18 years of age or older. *Investigational:* Alpha interferons are being tested for use in a large number of neoplastic diseases and viral infections.

Dosage

- **Intralesional injection**

Condylomata acuminata.

0.05 mL (250,000 IU)/wart twice a week for up to 8 weeks. The maximum recommended dose per treatment session is 0.5 mL (2.5 million IU). The safety and effectiveness of a second course of treatment have not been determined.

Administration/Storage

1. The drug should be injected into the base of the wart using a 30-gauge needle.
2. For large warts, the drug can be injected at several points around the periphery of the wart using a total dose of 0.05 mL/wart.
3. The drug should be stored at 2°C–8°C (36°F–46°F). It should not be frozen or shaken.

Contraindications: Hypersensitivity to human interferon alpha; clients who are allergic to mouse immunoglobulin (IgG), egg protein, or neomycin (the production process involves a nutrient medium containing neomycin although it has not been detected in the final product). Lactation.

Special Concerns: Due to the manifestation of fever and flu-like symptoms with interferon alfa-n3 use, the drug should be used with caution in clients with debilitating diseases including unstable angina, uncontrolled CHF, COPD, diabetes mellitus with ketoacidosis, thrombophlebitis, pulmonary embolism, hemophilia, severe myelosuppression, or seizure disorders. Safety and effectiveness have not been determined in children less than 18 years of age.

Side Effects: *Flu-like symptoms:* Commonly, fever, headache, myalgias which decrease with repeated doses. Also, chills, fatigue, malaise. *CNS:* Dizziness, lightheadedness, insomnia, depression, nervousness, decreased ability to concentrate. *GI:* N&V, heartburn, diarrhea, tongue hyperesthesia, thirst, altered taste, increased salivation. *Musculoskeletal/Skin:* Arthralgia, back pain, hot sensation at bottom of feet, tingling of legs/feet, muscle cramps. *Respiratory:* Nose or sinus drainage, nose bleed, throat tightness, pharyngitis. *Miscellaneous:* Pruritus, swollen lymph nodes, heat intolerance, visual disturbances, sensitivity to allergens, papular rash on neck, hot flashes, herpes labialis, dysuria, photosensitivity, decreased WBC count.

NOTE: When used for treatment of cancer, the incidence of many of the above side effects was increased. Additional side effects were noted including: *GI:* Constipation, anorexia, stomatitis, dry mouth, mucositis, sore mouth. *Laboratory Test Values:* Abnormal hemoglobin, WBC count, alkaline phosphatase, total bilirubin, platelet count, AST, and GGT. *Miscellaneous:* Insomnia, blurred vision, ocular rotation pain, sore injection site, chest pains, low BP.

NURSING CONSIDERATIONS

See also *Nursing Considerations* for *Interferon alfa-2a* and *alfa-2b Recombinant,* Chapter 25.

Assessment

1. Document indications for therapy and type and onset of symptoms.
2. Review client history, especially noting any history of allergic reactions to egg protein or neomycin.

These could indicate an increased sensitivity to interferon alfa-n3.
3. Determine any client history of preexisting debilitating diseases and note functional level.
4. For condylomata therapy, measure and document the size of the wart(s) prior to initiating therapy.

Client/Family Teaching

1. Intralesional treatment should be continued for 8 weeks.
2. Genital warts may disappear both during treatment and after treatment has been discontinued. When this occurs, unless new warts appear or warts become enlarged, there should be a 3-month waiting period after the first 8-week course of therapy.
3. Do not change brands of interferon without approval because the manufacturing process, strength, and type of interferon may vary.
4. Women should use contraceptive practices if fertile.
5. Review the early signs of hypersensitivity reactions (e.g., hives, chest tightness, generalized urticaria, hypotension, wheezing, anaphylaxis) and instruct client to report immediately should these occur.

Evaluate

- ↓ Pain and regression of genital warts
- Suppression of malignant cell proliferation

Octreotide acetate

(ock-**TREE**-oh-tyd)
Pregnancy Category: B
Sandostatin **(Rx)**

How Supplied: *Injection:* 50 mcg/mL, 100 mcg/mL, 200 mcg/mL, 500 mcg/mL, 1000 mcg/mL

Action/Kinetics: Octreotide exerts effects similar to the natural hormone somatostatin. It suppresses secretions of serotonin and GI peptides including gastrin, insulin, glucagon, secretin, motilin, vasoactive intestinal peptide, and pancreatic polypeptide. The drug stimulates fluid and electrolyte absorption from the GI tract. It also inhibits growth hormone. The drug is rapidly absorbed from injection sites. **Peak levels:** Approximately 25 min. **$t^{1}/_{2}$:** 1.7 hr. **Duration:** Up to 12 hr. About one-third of a dose is excreted unchanged in the urine.

Uses: Metastatic carcinoid tumors; vasoactive intestinal tumors (VIPomas). The drug inhibits severe diarrhea in both situations and causes improvement in hypokalemia in VIPomas. Acromegaly. *Investigational:* Life-threatening hypotension. GI fistula, variceral bleeding, pancreatic fistula, irritable bowel syndrome, and dumping syndrome. Also, treatment of diarrhea due to AIDS, short bowel syndrome, diabetes, pancreatic cholera syndrome, chemotherapy or radiation therapy in cancer patients, and idiopathic secretory diarrhea.

Dosage

- **SC (Recommended), IV Bolus (Emergencies)**

Metastatic carcinoid tumors.

Initial, SC: 50 mcg 1–2 times/day. **Then,** 100–600 mcg/day in two to four divided doses for the first 2 weeks; **maintenance, usual:** 450 mcg/day (range: 50–1,500 mcg/day).

VIPomas.

Initial, SC: 50 mcg 1–2 times/day. **Then,** 200–300 mcg/day in two to four divided doses for the first 2 weeks; **maintenance:** 150–750 mcg/day. **Pediatric, SC:** 1–10 mcg/kg/day.

Acromegaly.

Initial: 50 mcg t.i.d.; **then,** 100–500 mcg t.i.d. The goal is to achieve growth hormone levels less than 5 ng/mL or IGF-1 levels less than 1.9 U/mL in males and less than 2.2 U/mL in females.

Administration/Storage

1. Experience is lacking for doses greater than 750 mcg/day.
2. Ampules should be inspected for particulate matter and discoloration; if present, the ampule must not be used.
3. Multiple injections at the same site should be avoided within a short period of time. Preferred sites for injection are the abdomen, hip, and thigh.

4. Reactions at the site of injection can be minimized by letting the solution warm to room temperature before administering the injection and by giving the injection slowly.
5. GI side effects can be minimized by giving the drug between meals and at bedtime.
6. Ampules should be stored for long periods at 2°C–8°C (36°F–46°F) although they may be stored at room temperature the day they will be used.
7. *Treatment of Overdose:* Withdraw drug temporarily and treat symptomatically.

Special Concerns: Use with caution in diabetics, in clients with gallbladder disease, in clients with severe renal failure requiring dialysis, and during lactation.

Side Effects: *GI:* Nausea, diarrhea or loose stools, abdominal pain or distention, malabsorption of fat, vomiting; less commonly, constipation, anorexia, dry mouth, flatulence, rectal spasm, swollen stomach, heartburn, cholelithiasis, GI bleeding, hemorrhoids. *CNS:* Headache, dizziness, lightheadedness, fatigue; less commonly, anxiety, seizures, depression, vertigo, hyperesthesia, drowsiness, pounding in head, irritability, decrease in libido, drowsiness, malaise, forgetfulness, nervousness, syncope, tremor, shakiness, Bell's palsy, paranoia, pituitary apoplexy. *CV:* Flushing, edema, sinus bradycardia; less commonly, hypertension, thrombophlebitis, SOB, CHF, ischemia, palpitations, orthostatic hypotension, chest pain. *Metabolic:* Hyperglycemia or hypoglycemia, hyperosmolarity of urine, increase in CPK. *Musculoskeletal:* Asthenia, weakness; less commonly, muscle pain or cramping, back pain; joint, shoulder, arm, and leg pain; leg cramps. *Dermatologic:* Less commonly, thinning or flaking of skin, bruising, bleeding from superficial wounds, hair loss, rash, pruritus. *GU:* Prostatitis, oliguria, pollakiuria. *Other:* Pain, wheal, or erythema at injection site; less commonly, rhinorrhea, galactorrhea, hypothyroidism, numbness, hyperhidrosis, hyperdipsia, warm feeling or burning sensation, visual disturbance, chills, fever, throat discomfort, eyes burning.

Symptoms of Overdose: Hyperglycemia and hypoglycemia manifested by dizziness, drowsiness, loss of sensory or motor function, incoordination, disturbed consciousness, and visual blurring.

Drug Interactions: Octreotide may interfere with drugs such as diazoxide, insulin, beta-adrenergic blocking agents, or sulfonylureas. Close monitoring is necessary.

NURSING CONSIDERATIONS

Interventions

1. Monitor serum electrolyte and glucose levels. The drug alters serum glucose levels and may require an adjustment of antidiabetic drug dosage in clients with diabetes.
2. Obtain baseline thyroid function studies and monitor throughout therapy. The drug may cause biochemical hypothyroidism, necessitating replacement therapy.
3. Because the drug may alter fat absorption and gallbladder function, assess client carefully and monitor the appropriate lab values (e.g., quantitative 72-hr fecal fat and serum carotene [fat malabsorption]) and ultrasonography studies during long-term therapy.
4. Monitor I&O. Perform abdominal assessments routinely, noting character and frequency of stools. Document and report any abnormal findings.

Client/Family Teaching

1. Demonstrate the appropriate technique for SC injection and have the client return demonstrate.
2. Explain that the drug is usually administered SC. There may be pain at the site of injection. Discuss the need to rotate administration sites and provide written guidelines for the administration, dose, and site rotation.
3. Explain that the dosage of drug is highly individualized. Therefore, it is important to take only as prescribed. Usually two injections a day are necessary when treating endocrine tumors.
4. Provide a printed list of side effects and advise of the more frequent side

effects, such as N&V, dizziness, headache, diarrhea, abdominal cramps, flatulence, steatorrhea with bulky bowel movements, and weakness. Advise client to report if any of these symptoms persist.
5. Keep the medication refrigerated.
6. Clients with diabetes should monitor blood sugars frequently and report significant variations.

Evaluate:

- Relief of severe diarrhea and control of secondary electrolyte imbalance in clients with metastatic disease (carcinoid, VIPomas).
- ↓ Tumor growth

Paclitaxel

(**PACK**-lih-**tax**-el)
Pregnancy Category: D
Taxol **(Rx)**

See also *Antineoplastic Agents,* Chapter 20.

How Supplied: *Injection:* 6 mg/mL

Action/Kinetics: Paclitaxel is a naturally occurring antineoplastic agent. It promotes the assembly of microtubules from tubulin dimers and stabilizes microtubules by preventing depolymerization. The stabilization results in the inhibition of the normal dynamic reorganization of the microtubule network that is required for vital interphase and mitotic cellular functions. Paclitaxel also induces abnormal "bundles" of microtubules throughout the cell cycle and multiple esters of microtubules during mitosis. Following IV administration, there is a biphasic decline in plasma levels. The initial rapid decline is due to distribution to the peripheral compartment and significant elimination, whereas the second phase is due, in part, to a slow efflux of the drug from the peripheral compartment. Paclitaxel is metabolized by the liver with small amounts of unchanged drug excreted in the urine.

Uses: Treatment of metastatic carcinoma of the ovary after failure of first-line or subsequent chemotherapy. Treatment of breast cancer after combination chemotherapy has failed or there has been relapse within 6 months of adjuvant chemotherapy (prior therapy must have included an anthracycline unless contraindicated). *Investigational:* Alone or in combination with other chemotherapeutic drugs for advanced head and neck cancer, previously untreated extensive-stage small-cell lung cancer, adenocarcinoma of the upper GI tract, hormone-refractory prostate cancer, advanced non-small-cell lung cancer, and leukemias.

Dosage

- **IV Infusion**

Metastatic carcinoma of the ovary.

Adults: 135 mg/m^2 given IV over 24 hr (some recommend over 72 hr) q 3 weeks.

Metastatic breast cancer.

Adults: 175 mg/m^2 given IV over 72 hr q 3 weeks.

Administration/Storage

1. The undiluted concentrate of paclitaxel should not come in contact with plasticized polyvinyl chloride equipment or devices used to prepare solutions for infusion.
2. All clients should be premedicated before use of paclitaxel to prevent severe hypersensitivity reactions. Premedication may consist of oral dexamethasone, 20 mg, given 12 and 6 hr before paclitaxel; diphenhydramine (or equivalent), 50 mg IV, 30–60 min before paclitaxel; and cimetidine, 300 mg IV, or ranitidine, 50 mg IV, 30–60 min before paclitaxel.
3. Paclitaxel concentrate must be diluted prior to infusion in 0.9% sodium chloride injection, 5% dextrose injection, 5% dextrose and 0.9% sodium chloride injection, or 5% dextrose in Ringer's injection to a final concentration of 0.3–1.2 mg/mL. Diluted solutions are stable for up to 24 hr at room temperature and lighting conditions.
4. The diluted solution should be administered through an in-line filter

with a microporous membrane not greater than 0.22 µm.
5. The dilutions may show haziness, which is due to the formulation vehicle. No significant loss of potency has been noted following simulated delivery of the solution through IV tubing containing an in-line (0.22-µm) filter.
6. To minimize client exposure to the plasticizer DHEP which may be leached from polyvinylchloride infusion bags or sets, diluted paclitaxel solutions should be stored in bottles (glass, polypropylene) or plastic bags (polypropylene, polyolefin) and administered through polyethylene-lined administration sets.
7. Unopened vials of the concentrate are stable when stored under refrigeration, protected from light, in the original package.
8. Repeat courses of paclitaxel should not be undertaken until the neutrophil count is at least 1,500 cells/mm^3 and the platelet count is at least 100,000 cells/mm^3. The dose should be reduced by 20% for subsequent courses in those who experience a neutrophil count below 500 cells/mm^3 for 1 week or more or if there is severe peripheral neuropathy during therapy.
9. The use of gloves is recommended in handling the drug. If the solution comes in contact with the skin, wash the skin immediately and thoroughly with soap and water. If the drug comes in contact with mucous membranes, thoroughly flush the membranes with water.
10. *Treatment of Overdose:* Treat symptomatically.
11. *Treatment of Hypersensitivity Reactions:* Stop the infusion and treat with bronchodilators (such as albuterol or theophylline), epinephrine, antihistamines, and corticosteroids.

Contraindications: Hypersensitivity to paclitaxel, in those with a hypersensitivity to products containing polyoxymethylated castor oil (Cremophor EL), and clients with a baseline neutropenia below 1,500 cells/mm^3. Lactation.

Special Concerns: Use with caution in clients with impaired hepatic function. Safety and efficacy have not been determined in children.

Laboratory Test Interferences: ↑ Bilirubin, alkaline phosphatase, ALT, AST.

Side Effects: *Hypersensitivity reactions:* Severe symptoms usually occur during the first hour of therapy and occur during both the first or second course of therapy despite premedication. Severe symptoms include ***dyspnea, angioedema,*** hypotension, or generalized urticaria all of which require immediate cessation of the drug and aggressive treatment therapy. Symptoms not requiring treatment include milder dyspnea, flushing, skin reactions, hypotension, or tachycardia. *Hematologic:* Neutropenia and leukopenia (common), thrombocytopenia, anemia, infections, bleeding, packed cell transfusions, platelet transfusions. *CV:* Bradycardia and hypotension (including during the infusion), ***severe CV events (including asymptomatic ventricular tachycardia, bigeminy, syncope, complete AV block),*** abnormal ECG (including nonspecific repolarization abnormalities, sinus tachycardia, premature beats). *Musculoskeletal:* Peripheral neuropathy (in- cluding mild paresthesia), myalgia, arthralgia. *GI:* N&V, diarrhea, mucositis. *Miscellaneous:* Alopecia, fever associated with severe neutropenia; infections of the urinary tract and upper respiratory tract as well as ***sepsis due to neutropenia.***

Symptoms of Overdose: ***Bone marrow suppression,*** peripheral neurotoxicity, mucositis.

Drug Interactions

Cisplatin / More profound myelosuppression when paclitaxel was given after cisplatin than when paclitaxel was given before cisplatin. Is due to a ⅓ decrease in paclitaxel clearance

Ketoconazole / Inhibition of metabolism of paclitaxel by ketoconazole

NURSING CONSIDERATIONS

See also *Nursing Considerations* for *Antineoplastic Agents,* Chapter 20.

Assessment

1. Document tumor location and all previous therapy (include agents, dosage, and duration), especially radiation because this may enhance myelosuppressive drug effects. Determine if client has received this drug and the response.
2. Obtain baseline CBC and liver and renal function studies and monitor during therapy.
3. Document CBC to ensure that neutrophil count is 1,500 cells/mm^3 before drug administration and that platelet count is at least 100,000 cells/mm^3. Neutrophil nadir: 11 days; platelet nadir 8–9 days.

Interventions

1. Administer paclitaxel in a carefully monitored environment.
2. Administer pretreatment medications, usually corticosteroids, diphenhydramine, and H_2 antagonists. After pretreatment medication, if symptoms of severe hypersensitivity reaction (dyspnea, hypotension, angioedema, or generalized urticaria) appear, interrupt infusion and report. Hypersensitivity reactions usually occur during the first hour and despite premedication.
3. Monitor VS and I&O frequently.
4. Assess CBC to evaluate response to drug therapy and to detect any bone marrow depression or neutropenia.
5. Document any severe hypersensitivity reaction so that client is *NOT* rechallenged with paclitaxel.

Client/Family Teaching

1. Anticipate and prepare client for loss of hair.
2. Advise that joint pain and discomfort may be experienced 2–3 days after therapy but should resolve in several days.
3. Report any CNS symptoms especially peripheral neuropathy, as drug dose should be reduced.

Evaluate: Evidence of ↓ tumor size and spread.

Pegaspargase (PEG-L-asparaginase)

(peg-**ASS**-pair-gays)
Pregnancy Category: C
Oncaspar **(Rx)**

See also *Antineoplastic Agents,* Chapter 20.

How Supplied: *Injection:* 750 IU/mL

Action/Kinetics: Pegaspargase is a modification of the enzyme L-asparaginase. L-asparaginase, derived from *Escherichia coli,* is modified by conjugating covalently units of monomethoxypolyethylene glycol (PEG), thus forming the active PEG-L-asparaginase. Leukemic cells are not able to synthesize asparagine due to a lack of the enzyme asparaginase synthetase and are thus dependent on exogenous asparaginase for survival. Rapid depletion of asparagine, due to administration of asparaginase, kills leukemic cells. Normal cells, which can synthesize their own asparagine, are less affected.

Uses: Clients with acute lymphoblastic leukemia who have developed hypersensitivity to the native forms of L-asparaginase. Pegaspargase is used in combination with other antineoplastic drugs including vincristine, methotrexate, cytarabine, daunorubicin, and doxorubicin. Use of pegaspargase as a single agent should only be undertaken when therapy with multiple drugs is determined to be inappropriate for the client.

Dosage

- **IM (preferred), IV**

  As a component of selected multidrug regimens.

Adults: 2,500 IU/m^2 q 14 days. This dose is also used if the drug is given as a sole agent. **Children with a BSA greater than 0.6 m^2:** 2,500 IU/m^2 q 14 days. **Children with a BSA less than 0.6 m^2:** 82.5 IU/kg q 14 days.

Administration/Storage

1. The preferred route of administration is IM because of a lower risk of hepatotoxicity, coagulopathy, and GI and renal disorders.
2. The product should not be given if there is any indication it has been frozen, as freezing destroys the activity of pegaspargase.
3. When given IM, the volume to a single injection site should not exceed 2 mL; if more than 2 mL is necessary, use multiple injection sites.
4. When used IV, administer over a 1–2-hr period in 100 mL of sodium chloride or D5W, through an infusion tube of a solution that is already running.
5. When remission is obtained, appropriate maintenance therapy may be instituted with pegaspargase as part of the maintenance regimen.
6. The drug should not be shaken and excessive agitation should be avoided. The product should not be used if it is cloudy, if a precipitate is present, or if it has been stored at room temperature for more than 48 hr.
7. The drug is kept refrigerated at 2°C–8°C (36°F– 46°F).
8. Use only one dose per vial; the vial should not be reentered. Any unused portions should be discarded.

Contraindications: Pancreatitis or history thereof. Clients who have had significant hemorrhagic events associated with prior L-asparaginase therapy. Previous allergic reactions, such as generalized urticaria, bronchospasm, laryngeal edema, hypotension, or other side effects to pegaspargase that are not acceptable. Lactation.

Special Concerns: Clients taking pegaspargase are at a higher risk for bleeding problems, especially with simultaneous use of other drugs that have anticoagulant properties (e.g., aspirin, NSAIDs). Safety and efficacy have not been determined in clients from 1 to 21 years of age with known previous hypersensitivity to L-asparaginase.

Laboratory Test Interferences: ↑ AST, amylase, lipase, gamma-glutamyltranspeptidase, BUN, creatinine. Bilirubinemia, hyperglycemia, hyperuricemia, hypoglycemia, hypoproteinemia, hyperammonemia, hyponatremia, hypoalbuminemia, proteinuria.

Side Effects: Most commonly hypersensitivity reactions, chemical hepatotoxicity, and coagulopathies. *Allergic reactions:* ***Hypersensitivity reactions*** (acute or delayed), including ***life-threatening anaphylaxis,*** may occur during therapy, especially in clients with known hypersensitivity to other forms of L-asparaginase. Also, skin rashes, erythema, edema, pain, fever, chills, urticaria, dyspnea, ***bronchospasm,*** increased ALT, N&V, malaise, arthralgia, induration, hives, tenderness, swelling, lip edema. *GI:* Pancreatitis (may be severe), abdominal pain, anorexia, diarrhea, constipation, flatulence, GI pain, indigestion, mucositis, mouth tenderness, severe colitis. *Coagulation disorders:* Decreased anticoagulant effect, ***disseminated intravascular coagulation,*** decreased fibrinogen, increased thromboplastin, increased coagulation time, prolonged PTs, prolonged PTTs, ***clinical hemorrhage (may be fatal),*** decreased antithrombin III, superficial and deep venous thrombosis, sagittal sinus thrombosis, venous catheter thrombosis, atrial thrombosis, decreased platelet count, purpura, ecchymosis, easy bruisability. *Hepatic:* Jaundice, abnormal liver function test, liver fatty deposits, hepatomegaly, ascites, ***liver failure.*** *CV:* Hypotension (may be severe), tachycardia, thrombosis, chest pain, hypertension, subacute bacterial endocarditis, edema. *Hematologic:* ***Hemolytic anemia,*** leukopenia, pancytopenia, thrombocytopenia, ***agranulocytosis,*** anemia. *CNS:* ***Convulsions, status epilepticus,*** temporal lobe seizures, headache, paresthesia, mild to severe confusion, disorientation, dizziness, emotional lability, somnolence, ***coma,*** mental status changes, Parkinson-like syndrome. *Respiratory:* Dyspnea, ***bronchospasm,*** increased cough, epistaxis, upper respiratory infection. *Dermatologic:* Injection site hypersensitivity, rash, petechial rash, erythema simplex, pruritus, itching, alopecia, fever blister, hand whiteness, fungal changes, nail whiteness and ridging. *GU:* Hematuria, increased urinary frequency, abnormal kidney function, severe hemorrhagic cystitis, ***renal failure,*** uric acid nephropathy. *Musculoskeletal:* Arthralgia, myalgia, bone pain, joint disorder, diffuse and local musculoskeletal pain, joint stiffness, cramps. *Miscellaneous:* Pain in the extremities, injection site reaction (including pain, swelling, or redness), night sweats, peripheral edema, increased or decreased appetite, excessive thirst, weight loss, face edema, lesional edema, ***septic shock, sepsis,*** infection, malaise, fatigue, metabolic acidosis.

Drug Interactions: Depletion of serum proteins by pegaspargase may ↑ the toxicity of other drugs which are protein bound. ↑ Predisposition to bleeding when used with warfarin, heparin, dipyridamole, aspirin, or NSAIDs. May ↓ the effect of methotrexate.

NURSING CONSIDERATIONS

See also *Nursing Considerations* for *Antineoplastic Agents,* Chapter 20.

Assessment

1. Note previous treatment modalities and any evidence of hypersensitivity to L-asparaginase.
2. Document any adverse effects noted with previous L-asparaginase therapy. Use the National Cancer Institute Common Toxic Criteria to grade the severity of any hypersensitivity reaction.
3. Anticipate concomitant administration with other antineoplastic agents.
4. Document baseline liver function studies, serum uric acid levels, and hematologic and coagulation profiles.

Interventions

1. Observe and monitor client continuously for anaphylaxis during the first hour of therapy.
2. Assess carefully for early S&S of infection due to the immunosuppressive effects of pegaspargase.
3. Anticipate that IM administration may decrease many of the drug-associated adverse systemic effects.

Client/Family Teaching

1. Any increased bruising or bleeding warrants immediate attention.
2. Any agents that may increase bleeding tendency (e.g., aspirin or NSAIDs) should not be taken without approval.
3. Review the drug side effects, stressing those that require immediate reporting.
4. Stress that any persistent N&V, yellow skin discoloration, or severe abdominal pain should be evaluated immediately.
5. Report any altered mental status or evidence of seizure activity.
6. Advise that drug lowers resistance to infections and to try to avoid situations that may put one at risk as well as to report any early S&S of infection.

Evaluate

- Improved hematologic parameters
- Remission of acute lymphoblastic leukemia (ALL)
- Evidence of a response in relapsed, hypersensitive clients with ALL

Procarbazine hydrochloride

(pro-**KAR**-bah-zeen)
Pregnancy Category: D
Matulane, MIH, N-Methylhydrazine, Natulan ✱ (Abbreviation: PCB) **(Rx)**

See also *Antineoplastic Agents,* Chapter 20.

How Supplied: *Capsule:* 50 mg

Action/Kinetics: Procarbazine is both an alkylating agent and an inhibitor of MAO. The drug is cell-cycle specific for the S phase of cell division. It inhibits synthesis of protein, RNA, and DNA, possibly because of autoxidation (production of hydrogen peroxide). Well absorbed from GI tract. Drug equilibrates between plasma and CSF (peak levels occur

within 30–90 min). **t½, after IV:** 10 min. About 70% eliminated in urine, mostly as metabolites, after 24 hr. Procarbazine is mostly used in combination with other drugs (MOPP therapy).
Uses: As an adjunct in the treatment of Hodgkin's disease (stage III and stage IV). *Investigational:* Non-Hodgkin's lymphomas, malignant melanoma, primary brain tumors, lung cancer, multiple myeloma, polycythemia vera.

Dosage

• Capsules

Adults: 2–4 mg/kg/day for first week; **then,** 4–6 mg/kg/day until leukocyte count falls below 4,000/mm³ or platelet count falls below 100,000/mm³. If toxic symptoms appear, discontinue drug and resume treatment at rate of 1–2 mg/kg/day; **maintenance:** 1–2 mg/kg/day. **Children, highly individualized:** 50 mg/m²/day for first week; then 100 mg/m² (to nearest 50 mg) until maximum response obtained.
Administration/Storage: *Treatment of Overdose:* Induce vomiting or undertake gastric lavage. IV fluids. Frequent blood counts and liver function tests should be performed.
Additional Contraindications: Hypersensitivity to drug. Depressed bone marrow. Low WBCs and RBCs or platelet counts. Lactation.
Special Concerns: Use with caution in impaired kidney or liver function.
Additional Side Effects: *GI:* Dysphagia, constipation or diarrhea. *CNS:* Psychosis, manic reactions, insomnia, nightmares, foot drop, decreased reflexes, tremors, delirium, ***coma, convulsions.*** *Dermatologic:* Hyperpigmentation, photosensitivity. *Miscellaneous:* Petechiae, purpura, arthralgia, hemolysis, ***acute myelocytic leukemia, malignant myelosclerosis,*** azoospermia. ***In geriatric clients, the MAO inhibitor effects may cause increased vascular accidents*** and increased sensitivity to hypotensive effects.

Symptoms of Overdose: N&V, diarrhea, enteritis, hypotension, tremors, seizures, coma, hematologic and hepatic toxicity.

Drug Interactions

Alcohol / Antabuse-like reaction
Antihistamines / Additive CNS depression
Antihypertensive drugs / Additive CNS depression
Barbiturates / Additive CNS depression
Digoxin / ↓ Digoxin plasma levels if combination therapy used
Guanethidine / Excitation and hypertension
Hypoglycemic agents, oral / ↑ Hypoglycemic effect
Insulin / ↑ Hypoglycemic effect
Levodopa / Flushing and hypertension
MAO inhibitors / Possibility of hypertensive crisis
Methyldopa / Excitation and hypertension
Narcotics / Additive CNS depression
Phenothiazines / Additive CNS depression; also, possibility of hypertensive crisis
Reserpine / Excitation and hypertension
Sympathomimetics / Possibility of hypertensive crisis
Tricyclic antidepressants / Possibility of hypertensive crisis
Tyramine-containing foods / Possibility of hypertensive crisis

NURSING CONSIDERATIONS

See also *Nursing Considerations* for *Antineoplastic Agents,* Chapter 20.

Assessment

1. Document indications for therapy and other agents prescribed.
2. Obtain baseline liver and renal function studies and hematologic profile and monitor throughout therapy. Drug may cause granulocyte and platelet suppression. Nadir: 14 days; recovery: 21–28 days.

Client/Family Teaching

1. Avoid any OTC preparations and other prescription drugs unless specifically approved. Consult provider before taking any other medication because procarbazine has MAO inhib-

itory activity. The use of sympathomimetic drugs and foods with a high tyramine content (yeasts, yogurt, caffeine, chocolate, aged cheese, liver, smoked or pickled fish, fermented sausage, etc.) is contraindicated during therapy and for 2 weeks after discontinuing therapy. Ingestion of these products may precipitate a hypertensive crisis.
2. Do not drive or perform tasks that require mental alertness until drug effects are realized.
3. Consume adequate fluids (2–3 L/day) to prevent dehydration.
4. Observe and report adverse CNS effects that may necessitate withdrawal of the drug, as noted under *Additional Side Effects.*
5. For clients with diabetes, procarbazine increases effect of insulin and oral hypoglycemic agents. Hypoglycemic symptoms should be reported because adjustment of antidiabetic medication may be necessary.
6. Avoid exposure to sun or to ultraviolet rays because a photosensitive skin reaction may occur. Wear sunscreen, sunglasses, and protective clothing if exposure is necessary.
7. Avoid alcohol because a disulfiram-type reaction may occur.
8. Contraception should be practiced by both men and women.
9. Report persistent constipation (especially if diet,increased fluids, and bulk are ineffective) as laxatives may be prescribed.

Evaluate: Suppression of malignant cell proliferation.

Strontium-89 Chloride

(STRON-shee-um)
Pregnancy Category: D
Metastron **(Rx)**

See also *Antineoplastic Agents,* Chapter 20.

How Supplied: *Injection:* 10.9-22.6 mg/mL

Action/Kinetics: Strontium-89 is taken up preferentially in sites of active osteogenesis leading to significant accumulation in primary bone tumors and areas of metastatic involvement. As a beta emitter, the drug selectively irradiates primary metastatic bone involvement with minimal irradiation of soft tissues distant from bone lesions. Strontium-89 is retained in metastatic areas significantly longer than in normal bone. **Physical t½:** 50.5 days. Two-thirds is excreted through the urine and one-third through the feces. Urinary excretion is greater in clients with no bone lesions.

Use: Relief of bone pain in clients with painful skeletal metastases.

Dosage

- **Slow IV injection**

  Pain from bone metastases.

148 MBq, 4 mCi, given by slow IV injection over 1–2 min. An alternative dose is 1.5–2.2 MBq/kg, 40–60 mcCi/kg.

Administration/Storage

1. Pain relief is usually noted within 7–10 days after a dose and should last for several months.
2. Repeat doses are usually not recommended at intervals of less than 90 days.
3. The vial is shipped in a transportation shield of about 3 mm lead wall thickness. The vial and its contents are stored inside the transportation container at room temperature (15°C–25°C; 59°F–77°F) until used.
4. The injection is preservative free.
5. Radiopharmaceuticals should be administered only by physicians who have been trained and have experience in the safe use and handling of such drugs.

Contraindications: Use in clients with seriously compromised bone marrow from previous therapy or disease without an assessment of benefit vs. risk. Use during lactation.

Special Concerns: The drug is a potential carcinogen. Use with caution in clients with platelet counts below 60,000 and WBC counts less than 2,400. Safety and efficacy in children less than 18 years of age have not been determined.

Side Effects: Calcium-like flushing following rapid (< 30 sec) administration. Increase in bone pain between 36 and 72 hr following injection. Bone marrow depression.

NURSING CONSIDERATIONS

See also *Nursing Considerations* for *Antineoplastic Agents,* Chapter 20.

Assessment

1. Confirm presence of bone metastases prior to therapy.
2. Note other procedures and agents utilized and the outcome.
3. Drug is bone marrow toxic. Obtain baseline hematologic profile and monitor. Platelet nadir: 12–16 weeks.
4. Strontium-89 delivers a high dose of radioactivity. Ensure client consent and carefully verify client and dose prior to administration.
5. Administration is not recommended in clients with a very short life expectancy as it takes from 7 to 20 days for relief of pain to be noted.

Client/Family Teaching

1. Explain that drug is an injectable radioisotope that accumulates in and irradiates metastatic bone lesions.
2. Stress that an increase in bone pain 36–72 hr after administration is usually mild and self-limiting and can be managed with analgesics.
3. Advise client to continue to take analgesics until the strontium-89 becomes effective and then to reduce the dose of the analgesic gradually.
4. Review the special precautions that must be taken in incontinent clients to minimize the risk of radioactive contamination of clothing, bed linen, and the client's environment. Strontium-89 will be present in urine and blood for the first week after an injection. Thus, proper precautions must be taken to avoid contamination. Provide written guidelines for the caregiver including:
   - Wear gloves if available.
   - Offer a toilet if client is able, and flush twice after use.
   - Thoroughly wash and rinse bed pan or urinal after each use.
   - If incontinence is a problem, a catheter may be considered to minimize the risk of radioactive contamination.
   - When urine is dripped or spilled, wipe up immediately with a tissue and flush it away.
   - Always wash hands thoroughly after toileting.
   - Any clothes or linens that become stained with urine or blood should be washed immediately. Wash separately from other clothes and rinse thoroughly.
   - Any cuts, scratches, or spilled blood should be washed and wiped with a tissue, which is then properly discarded.
5. Reinforce that the client can eat and drink normally and that there is no need to avoid alcohol or caffeine.
6. Stress the importance of practicing some form of reliable contraception as drug will cause fetal damage.
7. Advise that repeated administrations will be based on client response, current symptoms, and hematologic status. These are generally not repeated for approximately 90 days.

Evaluate: Relief of bone pain in clients with skeletal metastases.

Cardiovascular Drugs

CHAPTER TWENTY-SIX

Antiarrhythmic Agents

See also the following individual entries:

- Adenosine
- Amiodarone Hydrochloride
- Bretylium Tosylate
- Calcium Channel Blocking Agents - See Chapter 28 ✓
- Digitoxin - See Chapter 30
- Digoxin - See Chapter 30
- Diltiazem Hydrochloride - See Chapter 28
- Disopyramide Phosphate
- Flecainide Acetate
- Indecainide Hydrochloride
- Lidocaine Hydrochloride
- Mexiletine Hydrochloride
- Moricizine Hydrochloride
- Phenytoin - See Chapter 36
- Phenytoin Sodium - See Chapter 36
- Procainamide Hydrochloride
- Propafenone Hydrochloride
- Propranolol Hydrochloride - See Chapter 51
- Quinidine Bisulfate
- Quinidine Gluconate
- Quinidine Polygalacturonate
- Quinidine Sulfate
- Tocainide Hydrochloride
- Verapamil - See Chapter 28

General Statement: The orderly sequence of contraction of the heart chambers, at an efficient rate, is necessary so that the heart can pump enough blood to the body organs. Normally the atria contract first, then the ventricles. Altered patterns of contraction, or marked increases or decreases in the rate of the heart, reduce the ability of the heart to pump blood. Such altered patterns are called cardiac arrhythmias. Some examples of cardiac arrhythmias are:

1. *Premature ventricular beats* or beats that occasionally originate in the ventricles instead of in the sinus node region of the atrium. This causes the ventricles to contract before the atria and ultimately results in a decrease in the volume of blood pumped into the aorta.
2. *Ventricular tachycardia.* A rapid heartbeat with a succession of beats originating in the ventricles.
3. *Atrial flutter.* Rapid contraction of the atria at a rate too fast to enable it to force blood into the ventricles efficiently.
4. *Atrial fibrillation.* The rate of atrial contraction is even faster than that noted during atrial flutter and more disorganized.
5. *Ventricular fibrillation.* Rapid, irregular, and uncoordinated ventricular

contractions that are unable to pump any blood to the body. This condition will cause death if not corrected immediately.

6. *Atrioventricular heart block.* Slowing or failure of the transmission of the cardiac impulse from atria to ventricles, in the AV junction. This can result in atrial contraction *not* followed by ventricular contraction.

The effective treatment of arrhythmias depends on accurate diagnosis, changing the causative factors, and, if appropriate, selecting an antiarrhythmic drug. The various antiarrhythmic drugs are classified according to both their mechanism of action and their effects on the action potential of cardiac cells. Importantly, one drug in a particular class may be more effective and safer in an individual client. The antiarrhythmic drugs are classified as follows:

1. Group I. These drugs decrease the rate of entry of sodium during cardiac membrane depolarization, decrease the rate of rise of phase O of the cardiac membrane action potential, prolong the effective refractory period of fast-response fibers, and require that a more negative membrane potential be reached before the membrane becomes excitable (and thus can propagate to other membranes). Drugs classified as group I are further listed in subgroups (according to their effects on action potential duration) as follows:

• Group IA: Depress phase O and prolong the duration of the action potential. The drugs are disopyramide, procainamide, and quinidine.

• Group IB: Slightly depress phase O and are thought to shorten the action potential. The drugs include lidocaine, mexiletine, phenytoin, and tocainide.

• Group IC: Slight effect on repolarization but marked depression of phase O of the action potential. Significant slowing of conduction. The drugs in this group are flecainide, indecainide, and propafenone.

NOTE: Moricizine is classified as a group I agent but it has characteristics of agents in groups IA, B, and C.

2. Group II. The drugs of this group competitively block beta-adrenergic receptors and depress phase 4 depolarization. Acebutolol, esmolol, and propranolol are group II antiarrhythmics.

3. Group III. The drugs in this group prolong the duration of the membrane action potential (relative refractory period) without changing the phase of depolarization or the resting membrane potential. Drugs in this group include amiodarone and bretylium.

4. Group IV. The drug in this group (verapamil) is a calcium channel blocker, slows conduction velocity, and increases the refractoriness of the AV node.

Special Concerns: It is important to monitor serum levels of antiarrhythmic drugs since some drugs can cause toxic side effects which can be confused with the purpose for which the drug is used. For example, toxicity from quinidine can result in cardiac arrhythmias. Antiarrhythmic drugs may cause new or worsening of arrhythmias, ranging from an increase in frequency of PVCs to severe ventricular tachycardia, ventricular fibrillation, or tachycardia that is more sustained and rapid. Such situations (called proarrhythmic effect) may make it difficult to distinguish the proarrhythmic effect from the underlying rhythm disorder.

NURSING CONSIDERATIONS

Assessment

1. Obtain a thorough nursing history and note any reports of drug sensitivity and previous experiences with this class of drugs.

2. Assess the extent of the client's palpitations, fluttering sensations, or missed beats prior to initiating the therapy and obtain a pretreatment ECG with arrhythmia documentation.

3. Note client complaints of chest pains or fainting episodes.

4. Obtain BP, pulse, and apical HR; lis-

ten to heart sounds. Record findings as these should serve as baseline data against which to measure the outcome of the prescribed therapy.
5. Ensure that lab tests for liver and renal function and electrolytes and blood glucose levels have been completed.
6. Assess lab values to ensure that serum pH and electrolytes are within normal limits and that pO_2 and/or O_2 saturations are within desired range.
7. Determine if electrophysiologic studies will be conducted to assess the drug efficacy.
8. Review client life-style related to cigarettes and caffeine use, alcohol consumption, and a lack of regular exercise. Certain foods, emotional stress, and other environmental factors may trigger arrhythmias in certain individuals. These should be identified and if possible eliminated before instituting pharmacologic agents.

Interventions

1. Attach client to a cardiac monitor if administering antiarrhythmic drugs by IV route and use an electronic infusion device for safety.
2. Obtain specific written guidelines concerning what to do should the client develop unusual changes in HR or rhythm.
3. Monitor BP and pulse. A HR of less than 50 beats/min or greater than 120 should generally be avoided, depending on the client's baseline level. Request written parameters for BP and pulse.
4. Monitor for changes in cardiac rhythm. Document with rhythm strips and report as the drug therapy may need to be altered.
• Report any new onset of bradycardia, as this may be an early indicator of approaching cardiac collapse.
• Note any depression of cardiac activity, such as the prolongation of the PR interval, widening of the QRS complex, increased AV block, or aggravation of the arrhythmia.
• Have emergency drugs and equipment available in the event of an adverse reaction to therapy. Be prepared to help withdraw the medication, administer emergency drugs, and use resuscitative techniques.
5. Monitor serum concentrations of the antiarrhythmic agent to ensure therapeutic concentration ranges.
6. Monitor serum electrolyte levels, diet, and drug regimens to determine if the serum potassium levels are sufficient to enhance drug effectiveness.

Client/Family Teaching

1. Explain desired effects of the drug therapy (e.g., by controlling the irregular beats with the medication, the heart can pump more efficiently).
2. Provide a written list and review the S&S of adverse reactions that should be reported.
3. Stress the importance of taking the drugs as ordered. If a dose of medication is missed the client should not double up on the next dose unless this is specifically ordered by the provider.
4. Establish a time and a method of recording that would enable clients to remember to take the medications as prescribed.
5. Teach client/family how to take BP and pulse and instruct to maintain a record for review at each visit.
6. Stress the importance of eliminating caffeine, cigarettes, and alcohol, as these agents may alter drug absorption and may also precipitate arrhythmias.
7. Avoid any OTC products unless approved.
8. Stress the importance of returning for follow-up visits as scheduled so that drug therapy can be adjusted and evaluated.
9. Explore concerns and encourage client to verbalize any fears or concerns R/T sexual activity. Provide appropriate referrals and counselling as needed.
10. Remind clients to inform all health care providers that they are taking antiarrhythmic agents. A list of currently prescribed medications

and a Medic Alert bracelet may be helpful.

11. Encourage family/significant other to learn CPR and explain that survival rate is greatly increased when CPR is initiated immediately.

Evaluate

- Knowledge and understanding of cardiac arrhythmias and level of compliance with prescribed therapy
- ECG evidence of control of arrhythmias and restoration of stable cardiac rhythm
- Laboratory confirmation that serum drug concentrations are within therapeutic range
- Any adverse side effects that may be drug related

Adenosine

(ah-**DEN**-oh-seen)
Pregnancy Category: C
Adenocard **(Rx)**

How Supplied: *Injection:* 3 mg/mL

Action/Kinetics: Adenosine is found naturally in all cells of the body. The substance slows conduction time through the AV node, interrupts the reentry pathways through the AV node, and restores normal sinus rhythm in paroxysmal supraventricular tachycardia (including Wolff-Parkinson-White syndrome). **t½:** Less than 10 sec (taken up by erythrocytes and vascular endothelial cells). Exogenous adenosine becomes part of the body pool and is metabolized mainly to inosine and AMP.

Uses: Conversion of sinus rhythm of paroxysmal SVT (including that associated with accessory bypass tracts). Symptomatic relief of varicose vein complications with stasis dermatitis. *Investigational:* With ^{201}thallium tomography in noninvasive assessment of clients with suspected CAD.

Dosage

- **Rapid IV bolus only**

Initial: 6 mg over 1–2 sec. If the first dose does not reverse the SVT within 1–2 min, 12 mg should be given as a rapid IV bolus. The 12-mg dose may be repeated a second time, if necessary. Doses greater than 12 mg are not recommended.

Administration/Storage

1. Store at room temperature. Do not refrigerate as crystallization may occur.
2. The solution should be clear at the time of use.
3. Discard any unused portion because the product contains no preservatives.
4. The drug should be administered directly into a vein. If it is to be given into an IV line, introduce the drug in the most proximal line and follow with a rapid saline flush.

Contraindications: Second- or third-degree AV block or sick sinus syndrome (except in clients with a functioning artificial pacemaker). Also, atrial flutter, atrial fibrillation, ventricular tachycardia.

Special Concerns: At time of conversion to normal sinus rhythm, new rhythms (PVC, atrial premature contractions, sinus bradycardia, skipped beats, varying degrees of AV block, sinus tachycardia) lasting a few seconds may occur. Use with caution in clients with asthma.

Side Effects: *CV:* Short lasting first-, second-, or ***third-degree heart block***. Facial flushing (common), headache, chest pain, sweating, palpitations, hypotension. *CNS:* Lightheadedness, dizziness, numbness, tingling in arms, heaviness in arms, blurred vision, apprehension. *GI:* Nausea, metallic taste, tightness in throat. *Respiratory:* SOB or dyspnea (common), chest pressure, hyperventilation. *Miscellaneous:* Pressure in head, burning sensation, neck and back pain, pressure in groin.

Drug Interactions

Carbamazepine / ↑ Degree of heart block
Caffeine / Competitively antagonizes effect of adenosine
Dipyridamole / ↑ Effect of adenosine
Theophylline / Competitively antagonizes effect of adenosine

NURSING CONSIDERATIONS

See also *Nursing Considerations* for *Antiarrhythmic Agents,* Chapter 26.

Assessment

1. Document indications for therapy and onset of symptoms.
2. Client should be on a cardiac monitor during drug administration.
3. In stasis dermatitis assess extremities and note findings.

Interventions

1. Document client complaints of chest pressure, SOB, heaviness of the arms, palpitations, or dyspnea.
2. Report any facial flushing. Reassure client that this is a common side effect of therapy.
3. Monitor BP and pulse. If client complains of numbness, tingling in the arms, blurred vision, or appears apprehensive, report as this may be an indication to discontinue drug therapy.
4. Monitor ECG rhythm strips closely for evidence of varying degrees of AV block and increased arrhythmias during conversion to sinus rhythm. These are usually only transient.

Evaluate

- Conversion of paroxysmal SVT to NSR
- Symptomatic relief when used as therapy for stasis dermatitis

Amiodarone hydrochloride

(am-ee-**OH**-dah-rohn)
Pregnancy Category: D
Cordarone **(Rx)**

See also *Antiarrhythmic Agents,* Chapter 26.

How Supplied: *Tablet:* 200 mg

Action/Kinetics: The antiarrhythmic activity is due to an increase in the duration of the myocardial cell action potential as well as alpha- and beta-adrenergic blockade. The drug decreases sinus rate, increases PR and QT intervals, results in development of U waves, and changes T-wave contour. **Onset:** Several days up to 1–3 weeks. Drug may accumulate in the liver, lung, spleen, and adipose tissue. **Therapeutic serum levels:** 0.5–2.5 mcg/mL. **t½:** Biphasic: initial t½: 2.5–10 days; final t½: 40–55 days (usual). Effects may persist for several weeks or months after therapy is terminated. Effective plasma concentrations are difficult to predict although concentrations below 1 mg/L are usually ineffective, whereas those above 2.5 mg/L are not necessary. Neither amiodarone nor its metabolite, desethylamiodarone, is dialyzable.

Uses: This drug should be reserved for life-threatening ventricular arrhythmias unresponsive to other therapy, such as recurrent ventricular fibrillation and recurrent, hemodynamically unstable ventricular tachycardia. *Investigational:* Refractory sustained or paroxysmal atrial fibrillation, paroxysmal SVT, symptomatic atrial flutter. Also, in CHF with decreased LV ejection fraction, exercise tolerance and ventricular arrhythmias.

Dosage

Due to the drug's side effects, unusual pharmacokinetic properties, and difficult dosing schedule, amiodarone should be administered in a hospital only by physicians trained in treating life-threatening arrhythmias. Loading doses are required to ensure a reasonable onset of action.

- **Tablets**

Life-threatening arrhythmias.

Loading dose: 800–1,600 mg/day for 1–3 weeks (or until initial response occurs); **then,** reduce dose to 600–800 mg/day for 1 month. **Maintenance dose:** 400 mg/day (as low as 200 mg/day or as high as 600 mg/day may be needed in some clients).

Administration/Storage

1. Therapy should be initiated in a hospital by physicians who can treat or who have access to equipment for monitoring and treating recurrent life-threatening ventricular arrhythmias.
2. Daily doses of 1,000 mg or more should be administered in divided doses with meals.

3. To minimize side effects, the lowest effective dose should be determined. If side effects occur, the dose should be reduced.
4. If dosage adjustments are required, the client should be monitored for an extended period of time due to the long and variable half-life of the drug and the difficulty in predicting the time needed to achieve a new steady-state plasma drug level.
5. When initiating amiodarone therapy, other antiarrhythmic drugs should be gradually discontinued.
6. If additional antiarrhythmic therapy is required in clients on amiodarone, the initial dose of such drugs should be about one-half the usual recommended dose.
7. *Treatment of Overdose:* Use supportive treatment. A beta-adrenergic agonist or a pacemaker is used to treat bradycardia; hypotension due to insufficient tissue perfusion is treated with a vasopressor or positive inotropic agents. There is some evidence that cholestyramine hastens the reversal of side effects by increasing elimination. Drug is not dialyzable.

Contraindications: Marked sinus bradycardia due to severe sinus node dysfunction, second- or third-degree AV block, syncope caused by bradycardia (except when used with a pacemaker). Lactation.

Special Concerns: Safety and effectiveness in children have not been determined. The drug may be more sensitive in geriatric clients, especially on thyroid function.

Laboratory Test Interferences: ↑ AST, ALT. Alteration of thyroid function tests (↑ serum T_4, ↓ serum T_3).

Side Effects: Adverse reactions, some potentially fatal, are common with doses greater than 400 mg/day. *Pulmonary:* Interstitial pneumonitis, alveolitis, pulmonary infiltrates, pulmonary inflammation or fibrosis, ***ARDS,*** cough and progressive dyspnea. *CV:* ***Worsening of arrhythmias, paroxysmal ventricular tachycardia,*** symptomatic bradycardia, sinus arrest, SA node dysfunction, ***CHF,*** edema, hypotension, ***cardiac conduction abnormalities, coagulation abnormalities.*** *Hepatic:* Abnormal liver function tests, nonspecific hepatic disorders, cholestatic hepatitis, cirrhosis, hepatitis. *CNS:* Malaise, tremor, lack of coordination, fatigue, ataxia, paresthesias, peripheral neuropathy, abnormal involuntary movements, sleep disturbances, dizziness, insomnia, headache, decreased libido. *Ophthalmologic:* Corneal microdeposits (asymptomatic) in clients on therapy for 6 months or more, photophobia, dry eyes, visual disturbances, blurred vision, halos, optic neuritis. *GI:* N&V, constipation, anorexia, abdominal pain, abnormal smell and taste, abnormal salivation. *Dermatologic:* Photosensitivity, solar dermatitis, blue discoloration of skin, rash, alopecia, spontaneous ecchymosis, flushing. *Miscellaneous:* Hypothyroidism or hyperthyroidism, vasculitis, pseudotumor cerebri, epididymitis, thrombocytopenia.

Symptoms of Overdose: Bradycardia, hypotension, ***disorders of cardiac rhythm.***

Drug Interactions

Anticoagulants / ↑ Anticoagulant effect → bleeding disorders
Beta-adrenergic blocking agents / ↑ Chance of bradycardia, sinus arrest, or AV block
Digoxin / ↑ Serum digoxin levels → toxicity
Flecainide / ↑ Plasma levels of flecainide
Quinidine / ↑ Serum quinidine → toxicity, including fatal cardiac arrhythmias
Procainamide / ↑ Serum procainamide levels → toxicity
Phenytoin / ↑ Serum phenytoin levels → toxicity; also, ↑ levels of amiodarone
Theophylline / ↑ Serum theophylline levels → toxicity (effects may not be seen for 1 week and may last for a prolonged period after drug is discontinued)

NURSING CONSIDERATIONS

See also *Nursing Considerations* for *Antiarrhythmic Agents,* Chapter 26.

Assessment
1. Determine if client is taking any other antiarrhythmic medications.
2. Assess quality of respirations and breath sounds.
3. Note baseline VS and perfusion (skin temperature, color). Record pulse rate several times in similar circumstances, where possible, to establish a baseline against which to measure responses after initiating therapy.
4. Assess vision before starting therapy.
5. Determine that baseline CBC, electrolytes, CXR, and liver and renal function studies have been performed.
6. Obtain ECG and document rhythm strips.

Interventions
1. During administration, observe ECG for increased PR and QRS intervals, increased arrhythmias, and HR below 60 beats/min and report if evident.
2. Monitor BP and assess for evidence of hypotension.
3. Note client complaints of SOB, painful breathing, or cough. Assess pulmonary status for evidence of CHF.
4. Observe CNS symptoms such as tremor, lack of coordination, paresthesias, and dizziness.
5. Note client complaints of headaches, depression, or insomnia. Also observe for any change in client behavior such as decreased interest in personal appearance or apparent hallucinations. These findings may indicate a need for a change in drug therapy.
6. Anticipate reduced dosages of digoxin, warfarin, quinidine, procainamide, and phenytoin if administered concomitantly with amiodarone hydrochloride.
7. Monitor thyroid studies because drug inhibits conversion of T_4 to T_3.
8. Schedule periodic ophthalmic examinations because small yellow-brown granular corneal deposits may develop during prolonged therapy.

Client/Family Teaching
1. If client develops crystals on the skin, producing a bluish color, report so dosage of drug can be adjusted.
2. Avoid direct exposure to sunlight. Wear protective clothing, hat, sunglasses, and a sunscreen if exposure is necessary.
3. Report all side effects, especially any abnormal bleeding or bruising promptly.
4. Wheezing, fever, coughing, or dyspnea are all symptoms of pulmonary problems and require prompt attention.
5. Stress the importance of reporting for laboratory studies as scheduled.

Evaluate
- Termination and control of life-threatening ventricular arrhythmias
- Serum drug levels within therapeutic range (1.0–2.5 mcg/mL)

Bretylium tosylate

(breh-**TILL**-ee-um **TOZ**-ill-ayt)
Pregnancy Category: C
Bretylate Parenteral ✦, Bretylol **(Rx)**

How Supplied: *Injection:* 50 mg/mL

Action/Kinetics: Bretylium inhibits catecholamine release at nerve endings by decreasing excitability of the nerve terminal. Initially there is a release of norepinephrine, which may cause tachycardia and a rise in BP; this is followed by a blockade of release of catecholamines. The drug also increases the duration of the action potential and the effective refractory period, which may assist in reversing arrhythmias. **Peak plasma concentration and effect:** 1 hr after IM injection. Antifibrillatory effect within a few minutes after IV use. Suppression of ventricular tachycardia and ventricular arrhythmias takes 20–120 min, whereas suppression of PVCs does not occur for 6–9 hr. **Therapeutic serum levels:** 0.5–1.5 mcg/mL. **t½:** Approximately 7–8 hr. Up to

90% of drug is excreted unchanged in the urine after 24 hr.

Uses: Life-threatening ventricular arrhythmias that have failed to respond to other antiarrhythmics. Prophylaxis and treatment of ventricular fibrillation. For short-term use only. *Investigational:* Second-line drug (after lidocaine) for advanced cardiac life support during CPR.

Dosage

• **IV**

Ventricular fibrillation, hemodynamically unstable ventricular tachycardia.

Adults: 5 mg/kg of undiluted solution given rapidly. Can increase to 10 mg/kg if ventricular fibrillation persists; repeat as needed. **Maintenance, IV infusion:** 1–2 mg/min; or, 5–10 mg/kg q 6 hr of diluted drug infused over more than 8 min. **Children:** 5 mg/kg/dose IV followed by 10 mg/kg at 15–30-min intervals for a maximum total dose of 30 mg/kg; **maintenance:** 5–10 mg/kg q 6 hr.

Other ventricular arrhythmias.

• **IV infusion**

5–10 mg/kg of diluted solution over more than 8 min. **Maintenance:** 5–10 mg/kg q 6 hr over a period of 8 min or more or 1–2 mg/min by continuous IV infusion. **Children:** 5–10 mg/kg/dose q 6 hr.

• **IM**

Other ventricular arrhythmias.

Adults: 5–10 mg/kg of undiluted solution followed, if necessary, by the same dose at 1–2-hr intervals; **then,** give same dosage q 6–8 hr.

Administration/Storage

1. For IV infusion, bretylium is compatible with 5% dextrose injection, 0.9% sodium chloride, 5% dextrose and 0.45% sodium chloride, 5% dextrose in 0.9% sodium chloride, 5% dextrose in lactated Ringer's, 5% sodium bicarbonate, 20% mannitol, 1/6 molar sodium lactate, lactated Ringer's, calcium chloride (54.5 mEq/L) in 5% dextrose, and potassium chloride (40 mEq/L) in 5% dextrose.
2. For direct IV, administer undiluted over 15–30 sec; may repeat in 15–30 min if symptoms persist. May further dilute 500 mg in 50 cc and infuse over 10–30 min.
3. For IM injection, use the drug undiluted.
4. Rotate the injection sites so that no more than 5 mL of drug is given at any site. This avoids localized atrophy, necrosis, fibrosis, vascular degeneration, or inflammation.
5. The client should be kept supine during therapy or closely observed for postural hypotension.
6. The client should be placed on an oral antiarrhythmic medication as soon as possible.
7. *Treatment of Overdose:* Hypertension can be treated by nitroprusside or another short-acting IV antihypertensive. Hypotension can be treated with appropriate fluid therapy and pressor agents such as norepinephrine or dopamine.

Contraindications: Severe aortic stenosis, severe pulmonary hypertension.

Special Concerns: Safety and efficacy in children have not been established. Dosage adjustment is required in clients with impaired renal function.

Side Effects: *CV:* Hypotension (including postural hypotension), transient hypertension, increased frequency of PVCs, bradycardia, precipitation of anginal attacks, initial increase in arrhythmias, sensation of substernal pressure. *GI:* N&V (especially after rapid IV administration), diarrhea, abdominal pain, hiccoughs. *CNS:* Vertigo, dizziness, lightheadedness, syncope, anxiety, paranoid psychosis, confusion, mood swings. *Miscellaneous:* Renal dysfunction, flushing, hyperthermia, SOB, nasal stuffiness, diaphoresis, conjunctivitis, erythematous macular rash, lethargy, generalized tenderness.

Symptoms of Overdose: Marked hypertension followed by hypotension.

Drug Interactions

Digitoxin, Digoxin / Bretylium may aggravate digitalis toxicity due to initial release of norepinephrine

Procainamide, Quinidine / Concomitant use with bretylium ↓ inotropic effect of bretylium and ↑ hypotension

NURSING CONSIDERATIONS

See also *Nursing Considerations* for *Antiarrhythmic Agents,* Chapter 26.

Assessment

1. Document indications for therapy and pretreatment rhythm strips.
2. Note if client is taking digitalis. Bretylium tosylate may aggravate digitalis toxicity.

Interventions

1. Monitor VS and rhythm strips as the dose of bretylium to be administered is titrated based on the client's response to therapy.
2. To reduce N&V, administer the IV drug slowly over 10 min with the client supine.
3. Bretylium often causes a fall in supine BP within 1 hr of IV administration. If the SBP falls below 75 mm Hg, anticipate the need to use pressor agents.
4. Once the IV is finished, the client should continue to remain supine until the BP has stabilized.
5. Supervise clients once ambulation is permitted because they may develop lightheadedness and vertigo.
6. If clients develop side effects, stay with them, reassuring and reorienting as needed.

Evaluate

- Termination of life-threatening ventricular arrhythmia
- Restoration of stable cardiac rhythm
- Therapeutic serum drug levels (0.5–1.5 mcg/mL)

Disopyramide phosphate

(dye-so-**PEER**-ah-myd)
Pregnancy Category: C
Norpace, Norpace CR, Rythmodan ✱, Rythmodan-LA ✱ **(Rx)**

How Supplied: *Capsule:* 100 mg, 150 mg; *Capsule, Extended Release:* 100 mg, 150 mg

Action/Kinetics: Disopyramide decreases the rate of diastolic depolarization (phase 4), decreases the upstroke velocity (phase 0), increases the action potential duration (of normal cardiac cells), and prolongs the refractory period (phases 2 and 3). It manifests weak anticholinergic effects although it has fewer side effects than quinidine. The drug does not affect BP significantly, and it can be used in digitalized and nondigitalized clients. **Onset:** 30 min. **Peak plasma levels:** 2 hr. **Duration:** average of 6 hr (range 1.5–8 hr). **t½:** 4–10 hr. **Therapeutic serum levels:** 2–4 mcg/mL. Serum levels should not be used to adjust the dose because of variance in protein binding and potential toxicity of unbound drug. **Protein binding:** 40%–60%. The bioavailability of the controlled-release capsules appears to be similar to that of the immediate-release capsules. Both unchanged drug (50%) and metabolites (30%) are excreted through the urine. Approximately 15% is excreted through the bile.

Uses: Life-threatening ventricular arrhythmias (e.g., sustained ventricular tachycardia). *Investigational:* Paroxysmal SVT.

Dosage

- **Immediate-Release Capsules**

Antiarrhythmic.

Adults, initial loading dose: 300 mg of immediate-release capsule (200 mg if client weighs less than 50 kg); **maintenance:** 400–800 mg/day in four divided doses (usual: 150 mg q 6 hr). **For clients less than 50 kg, maintenance:** 100 mg q 6 hr. **Children, less than 1 year:** 10–30 mg/kg/day in divided doses q 6 hr; **1–4 years of age:** 10–20 mg/kg/day in divided doses q 6 hr; **4–12 years of age:** 10–15 mg/kg/day in divided doses q 6 hr; **12–18 years of age:** 6–15 mg/kg/day in divided doses q 6 hr.

Severe refractory tachycardia.

Up to 400 mg q 6 hr may be required.

Cardiomyopathy.

Do not administer a loading dose;

give 100 mg q 6 hr of immediate-release or 200 mg q 12 hr for controlled-release.

• **Extended-Release Capsules or Tablets**

Antiarrhythmic, maintenance only. **Adults:** 300 mg q 12 hr (200 mg q 12 hr for body weight less than 50 kg).

NOTE: For all uses, dosage must be decreased in clients with renal or hepatic insufficiency.

Moderate renal failure or hepatic failure.
100 mg q 6 hr (or 200 mg/12 hr of sustained-release form).

Severe renal failure.
100 mg q 8–24 hr depending on severity (with or without an initial loading dose of 150 mg).

Administration/Storage

1. Administer drug only after ECG assessment has been done.
2. Use with other antiarrhythmics (e.g., class IA or propranolol) should be reserved for life-threatening arrhythmias unresponsive to a single agent.
3. The controlled-release capsule should not be used for initial dosage. These are intended for maintenance therapy.
4. When the client is being transferred from the regular PO capsule, the first controlled-release capsule should be given 6 hr after the last regular dose.
5. For children, a 1–10-mg/mL suspension may be made by adding the contents of the immediate-release capsule (the controlled-release capsule should not be used) to cherry syrup. The syrup is stable for 1 month if refrigerated. The syrup should be shaken thoroughly before use and dispensed in an amber bottle.
6. *Treatment of Overdose:* Induction of vomiting, gastric lavage, or a cathartic followed by activated charcoal. Monitor ECG. IV isoproterenol, IV dopamine, cardiac glycosides, diuretics, intra-aortic balloon counterpulsation, artificial respiration, hemodialysis. Use endocardial pacing to treat AV block and neostigmine to treat anticholinergic symptoms.

Contraindications: Hypersensitivity to drug. Cardiogenic shock, heart failure, heart block (especially preexisting second- and third-degree AV block if no pacemaker is present), congenital QT prolongation, asymptomatic ventricular premature contractions, sick sinus syndrome, glaucoma, urinary retention, myasthenia gravis. Use of controlled-release capsules in clients with severe renal insufficiency. Lactation.

Special Concerns: Safe use during childhood, labor, and delivery has not been established. Use with caution in Wolff-Parkinson-White syndrome or bundle branch block. Dosage should be decreased in impaired hepatic function. Geriatric clients may be more sensitive to the anticholinergic effects of this drug. The drug may be ineffective in hypokalemia and toxic in hyperkalemia.

Laboratory Test Interferences: ↑ Creatinine, BUN, cholesterol, triglycerides, and liver enzymes.

Side Effects: *CV:* Hypotension, CHF, ***worsening of arrhythmias,*** edema, weight gain, cardiac conduction disturbances, SOB, syncope, chest pain, AV block, ***severe myocardial depression (with hypotension and increased venous pressure).*** *Anticholinergic:* Dry mouth, urinary retention, constipation, blurred vision, dry nose, eyes, and throat. *GU:* Urinary frequency and urgency, urinary retention, impotence, dysuria. *GI:* Nausea, pain, flatulence, anorexia, diarrhea, vomiting, severe epigastric pain. *CNS:* Headache, nervousness, dizziness, fatigue, depression, insomnia, psychoses. *Dermatologic:* Rash, dermatoses, itching. *Other:* Fever, respiratory problems, gynecomastia, ***anaphylaxis,*** malaise, muscle weakness, numbness, tingling, angle-closure glaucoma, hypoglycemia, reversible cholestatic jaundice, symptoms of lupus erythematosus (usually in clients switched to disopyramide from procainamide).

Symptoms of Overdose: Apnea, loss of consciousness, ***cardiac arrhythmias*** (widening of QRS complex and QT interval, conduction disturbances), hypotension, bradycardia, anticholinergic symptoms, ***loss of spontaneous respiration, death.***

Drug Interaction

Anticoagulants / ↓ PT after discontinuing disopyramide
Beta-adrenergic blockers / Possible ↓ clearance of disopyramide; sinus bradycardia, hypotension
Digoxin / ↑ Serum digoxin levels (may be beneficial)
Erythromycin / ↑ Disopyramide levels → arrhythmias and ↑ QTc intervals
Phenytoin / ↓ Effect due to ↑ breakdown by liver; ↑ anticholinergic effects
Quinidine / ↑ Disopyramide serum levels or ↓ quinidine levels
Rifampin / ↓ Effect due to ↑ breakdown by liver

NURSING CONSIDERATIONS

See also *Nursing Considerations* for *Antiarrhythmic Agents,* Chapter 26.

Assessment

1. Document indications for therapy and type and onset of symptoms.
2. If client has been taking other antiarrhythmic agents, identify and document response to that therapy.
3. Assess for any evidence of hypersensitivity to the drug.
4. Note any client complaint of dribbling urine, frequency of voiding, or sensation of bladder fullness. The condition may worsen once the client begins taking disopyramide.
5. Determine serum potassium levels and, if low, take corrective measures before initiating therapy.
6. Ensure that baseline ECG is available.

Interventions

1. Clients who have been receiving other antiarrhythmic agents and who are now being placed on disopyramide therapy need to be monitored closely for anticholinergic side effects.
2. Monitor BP frequently for hypotensive effect. Clients with poor LV function are more likely to develop hypotension and require close monitoring.
3. If the client is receiving the drug in the hospital, monitor ECG for QRS widening and QT prolongation. If this occurs, the drug should be discontinued.
4. Report symptoms of CHF, such as cough, dyspnea, moist rales, and cyanosis.
5. Monitor serum potassium levels to ensure effective response to disopyramide. Hyperkalemia increases drug toxicity.
6. Assess I&O and weights. Question clients about urinary hesitancy, difficulty voiding, or a sense of not completely emptying the bladder. This is particularly important in men with prostatic hypertrophy and in elderly clients who have had prior urinary tract problems; palpate bladder if hesitancy is severe.
7. If the ECG shows a new onset of first-degree heart block, do not administer the drug. Report and anticipate the dosage of drug will be reduced.

Client/Family Teaching

1. Take drug at the same time each day.
2. Instruct clients how to take their own BP and assist to develop a method to maintain a written record for evaluation and review by the provider.
3. Increase intake of fruit juices and other bulk foods to prevent constipation.
4. For complaints of dry mouth suggest using frequent mouth rinses, sugarless gum, or hard candy.
5. Avoid using alcohol in any form.
6. Review the symptoms of CHF (edema, cough, sudden weight gain, dyspnea) and stress the importance of reporting these findings immediately.
7. Change positions slowly and avoid hot showers, temperature extremes, exposure to the sun, or prolonged standing.
8. Report any evidence of mental confusion.

Evaluate

- Termination and control of ventricular arrhythmias
- Restoration of stable cardiac rhythm

Flecainide acetate

(fleh-**KAY**-nyd)
Pregnancy Category: C
Tambocor **(Rx)**

See also *Antiarrhythmic Agents,* Chapter 26.

How Supplied: *Tablet:* 50 mg, 100 mg, 150 mg

Action/Kinetics: Flecainide produces its antiarrhythmic effect by a local anesthetic action, especially on the His-Purkinje system in the ventricle. The drug decreases single and multiple PVCs and reduces the incidence of ventricular tachycardia. **Peak plasma levels:** 3 hr.; **steady state levels:** 3–5 days. **Effective plasma levels:** 0.2–1 mcg/mL (trough levels). **t½:** 20 hr (12–27 hr). Approximately 30% is excreted in urine unchanged. Impaired renal function decreases rate of elimination of unchanged drug. Food or antacids do not affect absorption.

Uses: Life-threatening arrhythmias manifested as sustained ventricular tachycardia. Prevention of paroxysmal supraventricular tachycardias (PSVT) and paroxysmal atrial fibrillation or flutter (PAF) associated with disabling symptoms but not structural heart disease.

Dosage

- **Tablets**

Sustained ventricular tachycardia.

Initial: 100 mg q 12 hr; **then,** increase by 50 mg b.i.d. q 4 days until effective dose reached. **Usual effective dose:** 150 mg q 12 hr; dose should not exceed 400 mg/day.

PSVT, PAF.

Initial: 50 mg q 12 hr; **then,** dose may be increased in increments of 50 mg b.i.d. q 4 days until effective dose reached. Maximum recommended dose: 300 mg/day. *NOTE:* For PAF clients, increasing the dose from 50 to 100 mg b.i.d. may increase efficacy without a significant increase in side effects.

NOTE: For clients with a creatinine clearance less than 35 mL/min/1.73 m^2, the starting dose is 100 mg once daily (or 50 mg b.i.d.). For less severe renal disease, the initial dose may be 100 mg q 12 hr.

Administration/Storage

1. For most situations, therapy should be started in a hospital setting (especially in clients with symptomatic CHF, sustained ventricular arrhythmias, compensated clients with significant myocardial dysfunction, or sinus node dysfunction).
2. For clients with renal impairment, the dosage should be increased at intervals greater than 4 days. The client should be monitored carefully for adverse toxic effects.
3. The chance of toxic effects increases if the trough plasma levels exceed 1 mcg/mL.
4. If client is being transferred to flecainide from another antiarrhythmic, at least two to four plasma half-lives should elapse for the drug being discontinued before initiating flecainide therapy.
5. An occasional client may benefit from dosing at 8-hr intervals.
6. To minimize toxicity, the dose may be reduced once the arrhythmia is controlled.
7. *Treatment of Overdose:* Charcoal will remove unabsorbed drug up to 90 min after drug ingestion. Administration of dopamine, dobutamine, or isoproterenol. Artificial respiration. Intra-aortic balloon pumping, transvenous pacing (to correct conduction block). Acidification of the urine may be beneficial, especially in those with an alkaline urine. Due to the long duration of action of the drug, treatment measures may have to be continued for a prolonged period of time.

Contraindications: Cardiogenic shock, preexisting second- or third-degree AV block, right bundle branch block when associated with bifascicular block (unless pacemaker is present to maintain cardiac rhythm). Recent MI. Cardiogenic shock.

Chronic atrial fibrillation. Frequent premature ventricular complexes and symptomatic nonsustained ventricular arrhythmias. Lactation.

Special Concerns: Use with caution in sick sinus syndrome, in clients with a history of CHF or MI, in disturbances of potassium levels, in clients with permanent pacemakers or temporary pacing electrodes, renal and liver impairment. Safety and efficacy in children less than 18 years of age are not established. The incidence of proarrhythmic effects may be increased in geriatric clients.

Side Effects: *CV:* ***New or worsened ventricular arrhythmias,*** new or worsened CHF, palpitations, chest pain, sinus bradycardia, sinus pause, sinus arrest, ***ventricular fibrillation, ventricular tachycardia that cannot be resuscitated,*** second- or third-degree AV block, tachycardia, hypertension, hypotension, bradycardia, angina pectoris. *CNS:* Dizziness, faintness, syncope, lightheadedness, neuropathy, unsteadiness, headache, fatigue, paresthesia, paresis, hypoesthesia, insomnia, anxiety, malaise, vertigo, depression, ***seizures,*** euphoria, confusion, depersonalization, apathy, morbid dreams, speech disorders, stupor, amnesia, weakness, somnolence. *GI:* Nausea, constipation, abdominal pain, vomiting, anorexia, dyspepsia, dry mouth, diarrhea, flatulence, change in taste. *Ophthalmic:* Blurred vision, difficulty in focusing, spots before eyes, diplopia, photophobia, eye pain, nystagmus, eye irritation, photophobia. *Hematologic:* Leukopenia, thrombocytopenia. *GU:* Decreased libido, impotence, urinary retention, polyuria. *Musculoskeletal:* Asthenia, tremor, ataxia, arthralgia, myalgia. *Dermatologic:* Skin rashes, urticaria, exfoliative dermatitis, pruritus, alopecia. *Other:* Edema, dyspnea, fever, ***bronchospasm,*** flushing, sweating, tinnitus, swollen mouth, lips, and tongue.

Symptoms of Overdose: Lengthening of PR interval; increase in QRS duration, QT interval, and amplitude of T wave; decrease in HR and contractility; conduction disturbances; hypotension; ***respiratory failure*** or asystole.

Drug Interactions

Acidifying agents / ↑ Renal excretion of flecainide
Alkalinizing agents / ↓ Renal excretion of flecainide
Amiodarone / ↑ Plasma levels of flecainide
Cimetidine / ↑ Bioavailability and renal excretion of flecainide
Digoxin / ↑ Digoxin plasma levels
Disopyramide / Additive negative inotropic effects
Propranolol / Additive negative inotropic effects; also, ↑ plasma levels of both drugs
Smoking (Tobacco) / ↑ Plasma clearance of flecainide
Verapamil / Additive negative inotropic effects

NURSING CONSIDERATIONS

See also *Nursing Considerations* for *Antiarrhythmic Agents,* Chapter 26.

Assessment

1. Obtain baseline ECG, CXR, electrolytes, and renal function studies prior to initiating therapy.
2. Review client history and ECGs for evidence of CHF, ventricular arrhythmias, sinus node dysfunction, or abnormal ejection fractions.

Interventions

1. Monitor ECG for increased arrhythmias or AV block and report if evident.
2. Check serum potassium levels. Preexisting hypokalemia or hyperkalemia may alter the effects of the drug and should be corrected before starting therapy with flecainide.
3. Monitor for labile BP.
4. Note adverse CNS effects, such as client complaints of dizziness, visual disturbances, headaches, nausea, or depression and report.
5. Obtain urinary pH to detect alkalinity or acidity. Alkalinity of the urine decreases renal excretion and acidity increases renal excretion, which in turn affects the rate of drug elimination.
6. Observe for any S&S of CHF.

7. Concomitant administration of flecainide with disopyramide, propranolol, or verapamil will promote additive negative inotropic effects.
8. Clients with pacemakers should have the pacing thresholds checked and adjusted before and 1 week following drug therapy.

Client/Family Teaching

1. Stress the importance of taking the medication in the dose and at the times prescribed.
2. Observe for and report changes in elimination patterns.
3. Report any bruising or increased bleeding tendencies.
4. Instruct to report for scheduled visits so that drug effectiveness can be monitored carefully.

Evaluate

- Termination of lethal ventricular arrhythmias
- Therapeutic serum (trough) drug levels (0.2–1.0 mcg/mL)

Indecainide hydrochloride

(in-deh-**KANE**-eyed)
Pregnancy Category: B
Decabid **(Rx)**

How Supplied: Information not available at time of printing.

Action/Kinetics: Although the mechanism of action is not known with certainty, indecainide is thought to block sodium movement into Purkinje and myocardial cells resulting in stabilization of the cell membrane and a slowing of conduction of cardiac impulses. Both AV and intraventricular conduction velocities are slowed with an increase in the AV nodal effective refractory period. At doses of 200 mg/day, the drug significantly reduces LV ejection fraction both at rest and during exercise. Food has no effect on absorption and there is no first-pass effect. **Peak serum levels:** 4 hr. **t½:** Approximately 8 hr in normal clients. Indecainide is metabolized in the liver to inactive and one active (desisopropylindecainide) metabolite. Approximately 80% excreted in the urine (65% unchanged) and 17% in the feces.

Uses: Treatment of life-threatening ventricular arrhythmias (such as sustained ventricular tachycardia). Use should be reserved for those clients in whom benefits outweigh the risks of using the drug.

Dosage

- **Extended-Release Tablets**

Adults, initial: 50 mg b.i.d. at 12-hr intervals. After a minimum of 4 days, dose can be increased to 75 mg b.i.d. if necessary. If the desired effect is not observed after 4 more days, the dosage may be increased to 100 mg b.i.d. Some clients may require as much as 300 mg/day and should be hospitalized for initial dosing at this level. In clients with a creatinine clearance of 30 mL/min or less, therapy should be initiated with a single daily dose of 50 mg; the dose may be increased to 75 mg/day after 7 days. Thereafter, increase dose slowly (no more frequently than q 7 days) up to a maximum of 150 mg/day if necessary.

Administration/Storage

1. Therapy should be initiated in a hospital with facilities for monitoring cardiac rhythm because many of the serious proarrhythmic effects are observed within the first 1–2 weeks of therapy.
2. Extended-release tablets should be swallowed whole and not crushed or chewed.
3. Increments in dosage should not be undertaken more often than q 4 days.
4. When transferring clients from other antiarrhythmic drugs, the drug should be withdrawn for 2–5 plasma half-lives before beginning indecainide therapy. If withdrawal is potentially life-threatening, the client should be hospitalized and closely monitored.

Contraindications: Use for less severe ventricular arrhythmias. Pre-existing second- or third-degree AV block or right bundle branch block associated with a left hemiblock (unless client has a pacemaker to sustain cardiac rhythm). Cardiogenic shock. Use during lactation.

Special Concerns: Safety and effectiveness have not been determined in children less than 18 years of age. Use with caution in clients with impaired renal function. Use with extreme caution in clients with sick sinus syndrome (drug may cause sinus bradycardia, sinus pause, or sinus arrest).

Laboratory Test Interferences: ↑ BUN, creatinine clearance, AST, ALT.

Side Effects: *CV: **Possibly increased mortality*** or nonfatal cardiac arrest in clients with asymptomatic non-life-threatening ventricular arrhythmias who experienced a MI between 6 days and 2 years before use of the drug (this effect noted with use of encainide or flecainide). ***Proarrhythmic effects including new or worsening of arrhythmias,*** causing or worsening CHF. Possibility of increased pacemaker thresholds. ***First- and third-degree AV block,*** syncope, sinus bradycardia, sinus pause, sinus arrest, angina pectoris, hypertension, hypotension, bundle branch block, palpitations. *GI:* Nausea, abdominal pain, constipation, diarrhea, dry mouth, dyspepsia, alteration in taste, vomiting. *CNS:* Dizziness, headache, circumoral paresthesia, insomnia, anxiety, emotional lability, vertigo, abnormal dreams, agitation, ataxia, confusion, nervousness, paresthesia, hypesthesia, ***seizures.*** *Respiratory:* Dyspnea, rhinitis, increased cough, chest pain. *Whole body:* Asthenia, back pain, general pain, fever, malaise. *Dermatologic:* Rash (including maculopapular or petechial), urticaria. *Hematologic:* Eosinophilia, anemia, leukopenia, thrombocytopenia. *Miscellaneous:* Hyperglycemia, tinnitus, diplopia, abnormal accommodation, arthralgia.

Drug Interactions

Antiarrhythmic drugs / Additive pharmacologic effects

Cimetidine / Significant ↑ in serum levels of indecainide

NURSING CONSIDERATIONS

See also *Nursing Considerations* for *Antiarrhythmic Agents,* Chapter 26.

Assessment

1. Document indications for therapy and other agents previously prescribed for this condition.
2. Obtain baseline ECG to determine if client has any evidence of advanced AV block because drug is contraindicated under these circumstances.
3. Note any client history of CHF.

Interventions

1. Indecainide is recommended only for the treatment of life-threatening ventricular arrhythmias. Client should be in a closely monitored environment and have rhythm strips to document these arrhythmias before, during, and throughout initial dosing adjustments.
2. Review serum electrolytes. Preexisting hypokalemia or hyperkalemia should be corrected before administration of indecainide.
3. Note renal function studies to determine if there is any evidence of impairment. Anticipate reduced dose and dosing intervals of 7 days when adjusting the dosage for clients with renal dysfunction.
4. Observe clients for complaints of dizziness, weakness, chest pain, or dyspnea because these are frequent side effects of drug therapy and should be documented and reported if evident.

Evaluate: Successful termination of lethal ventricular arrhythmias.

Lidocaine hydrochloride

(**LYE**-doh-kayn)

Pregnancy Category: B

IM: LidoPen Auto-Injector, **(Rx)**. **Direct IV or IV Admixtures:** Lidocaine HCl for Cardiac Arrhythmias, Xylocaine HCl IV for Cardiac Arrhythmias, Xylocard ✱ **(Rx)**. **IV Infusion:** Lidocaine HCl in 5% Dextrose **(Rx)**

See also *Antiarrhythmic Agents,* Chapter 26.

How Supplied: *Gel/jelly:* 2%; *Injection:* 0.5%, 1%, 1.5%, 2%, 4%, 10%, 20%; *Ointment:* 5%; *Set*; *Solution:* 2%, 4%, 5%

Action/Kinetics: Lidocaine shortens the refractory period and suppresses the automaticity of ectopic foci without affecting conduction of impulses through cardiac tissue. The drug increases the electrical stimulation threshold of the ventricle during diastole. It does not affect BP, CO, or myocardial contractility. **IV: Onset,** 45–90 sec; **duration:** 10–20 min. **IM, Onset,** 5–15 min; **duration,** 60–90 min. **t½:** 1–2 hr. **Therapeutic serum levels:** 1.5–6 mcg/mL. **Time to steady-state plasma levels:** 3–4 hr (8–10 hr in clients with AMI). **Protein-binding:** 40%–80%. Ninety percent of lidocaine is rapidly metabolized in the liver to active metabolites. Since lidocaine has little effect on conduction at normal antiarrhythmic doses, it should be used in acute situations (instead of procainamide) in instances in which heart block might occur.

Uses: IV: Treatment of acute ventricular arrhythmias such as those following MIs or occurring during surgery. The drug is ineffective against atrial arrhythmias. **IM:** Certain emergency situations (e.g., ECG equipment not available; mobile coronary care unit, under advice of a physician).

Investigational: IV in children who develop ventricular couplets or frequent premature ventricular beats.

Dosage

- **IV Bolus**

Antiarrhythmic.

Adults: 50–100 mg at rate of 25–50 mg/min. Bolus is used to establish rapid therapeutic plasma levels. Repeat if necessary after 5-min interval. Onset of action is 10 sec. **Maximum dose/hr:** 200–300 mg.

- **Infusion**

Antiarrhythmic.

20–50 mcg/kg at a rate of 1–4 mg/min. No more than 200–300 mg/hr should be given. **Pediatric, loading dose:** 1 mg/kg IV or intratracheally q 5–10 min until desired effect reached (maximum total dose: 5 mg/kg).

- **IV Continuous Infusion**

Maintain therapeutic plasma levels following loading doses.

Adults: Give at a rate of 1–4 mg/min (20–50 mcg/kg/min). Dose should be reduced in clients with heart failure, with liver disease, or who are taking drugs that interact with lidocaine. **Pediatric:** 20–50 mcg/kg/min (usual is 30 mcg/kg/min).

- **IM**

Antiarrhythmic.

Adults: 4.5 mg/kg (approximately 300 mg for a 70-kg adult). Switch to IV lidocaine or oral antiarrhythmics as soon as possible although an additional IM dose may be given after 60–90 min.

Administration/Storage

1. *Do not add lidocaine to blood transfusion assembly.*
2. Lidocaine solutions that contain epinephrine should not be used to treat arrhythmias. Make certain that vial states, "For Cardiac Arrhythmias." Check prefilled syringes closely to ensure the appropriate dose has been obtained. (Lidocaine prefilled syringes come in both milligrams and grams).
3. Use D5W to prepare solution; this is stable for 24 hr.
4. IV infusions should be administered with an electronic infusion device.
5. IV bolus dosage should be reduced in clients over 70 years of age, in those with CHF or liver disease, and in clients taking cimetidine or propranolol (i.e., where metabolism of lidocaine is reduced).
6. *Treatment of Overdose:* Discontinue the drug and begin emergency resuscitative procedures. Seizures can be treated with diazepam, thiopental, or thiamylal. Succinylcholine, IV, may be used if the client is anesthetized. IV fluids, vasopressors, and CPR are used to correct circulatory depression.

Contraindications: Hypersensitivity to amide-type local anesthetics,

Stokes-Adams syndrome, Wolff-Parkinson-White syndrome, severe SA, AV, or intraventricular block (when no pacemaker is present).

Special Concerns: Use with caution during labor and delivery, during lactation, and in the presence of liver or severe kidney disease, CHF, marked hypoxia, digitalis toxicity with AV block, severe respiratory depression, or shock. In geriatric clients, the rate and dose for IV infusion should be decreased by one-half and slowly adjusted. Safety and efficacy have not been determined in children; the IM autoinjector product should not be used for children.

Laboratory Test Interference: ↑ CPK following IM use.

Side Effects: *Body as a whole:* Malignant hyperthermia characterized by tachycardia, tachypnea, labile BP, metabolic acidosis, temperature elevation. *CV:* ***Precipitation or aggravation of arrhythmias (following IV use),*** hypotension, ***bradycardia (with possible cardiac arrest), CV collapse.*** *CNS:* Dizziness, apprehension, euphoria, lightheadedness, nervousness, drowsiness, confusion, changes in mood, hallucinations, twitching, "doom anxiety," ***convulsions,*** unconsciousness. *Respiratory:* Difficulties in breathing or swallowing, ***respiratory depression or arrest.*** *Allergic:* Rash, cutaneous lesions, urticaria, edema, ***anaphylaxis.*** *Other:* Tinnitus, blurred or double vision, vomiting, numbness, sensation of heat or cold, twitching, tremors, soreness at IM injection site, fever, ***venous thrombosis or phlebitis (extending from site of injection),*** extravasation. During anesthesia, CV depression may be the first sign of lidocaine toxicity. During other usage, convulsions are the first sign of lidocaine toxicity.

Symptoms of Overdose: Symptoms are dependent on plasma levels. If plasma levels range from 4 to 6 mcg/mL, mild CNS effects are observed. Levels of 6–8 mcg/mL may result in significant CNS and CV depression while levels greater than 8 mcg/mL cause hypotension, decreased CO, respiratory depression, obtundation, ***seizures, and coma.***

Drug Interactions

Aminoglycosides / ↑ Neuromuscular blockade

Beta-adrenergic blockers / ↑ Lidocaine levels with possible toxicity

Cimetidine / ↓ Clearance of lidocaine → possible toxicity

Phenytoin / IV phenytoin → excessive cardiac depression

Procainamide / Additive cardiodepressant effects

Succinylcholine / ↑ Action of succinylcholine by ↓ plasma protein binding

Tocainide / ↑ Risk of side effects

Tubocurarine / ↑ Neuromuscular blockade

NURSING CONSIDERATIONS

See also *Nursing Considerations* for *Antiarrhythmic Agents,* Chapter 26.

Assessment

1. Document indications for therapy and type and onset of symptoms.
2. Note any client history of hypersensitivity to amide-type local anesthetics.
3. Note client age. Elderly clients who have hepatic or renal disease or who weigh less than 45.5 kg will need to be watched especially closely for adverse side effects; adjust dosage as directed.

Interventions

1. Monitor VS frequently during IV therapy. Clients on antiarrhythmic drug therapy are particularly susceptible to hypotension and cardiac collapse.
2. Observe for myocardial depression, variations of rhythm, or aggravation of the arrhythmia and report as drug administration may need to be altered.
3. Note evidence of dizziness or visual disturbances, and report any CNS effects such as twitching and tremors. These symptoms may precede convulsions.
4. Assess for any respiratory depression, characterized by slow, shallow respirations.

5. Note any sudden changes in mental status and report immediately because the dose of drug may need to be decreased.
6. The administration of the drug should be titrated to the client's response and within established written guidelines.

Evaluate

- Control of ventricular arrhythmias
- Therapeutic serum drug levels (1.5–6 mcg/mL)

Mexiletine hydrochloride

(mex-**ILL**-eh-teen)
Pregnancy Category: C
Mexitil **(Rx)**

See also *Antiarrhythmic Drugs,* Chapter 26.

How Supplied: *Capsule:* 150 mg, 200 mg, 250 mg

Action/Kinetics: Mexiletine is similar to lidocaine but is effective PO. The drug inhibits the flow of sodium into the cell, thereby reducing the rate of rise of the action potential. The drug decreases the effective refractory period in Purkinje fibers. BP and pulse rate are not affected following use, but there may be a small decrease in CO and an increase in peripheral vascular resistance. The drug also has both local anesthetic and anticonvulsant effects. **Onset:** 30–120 min. **Peak blood levels:** 2–3 hr. **Therapeutic plasma levels:** 0.5–2 mcg/mL. **Plasma t½:** 10–12 hr. Approximately 10% excreted unchanged in the urine; acidification of the urine enhances excretion, whereas alkalinization decreases excretion.

Uses: Documented life-threatening ventricular arrhythmias (such as ventricular tachycardia). *Investigational:* Prophylactically to decrease the incidence of ventricular tachycardia and other ventricular arrhythmias in the acute phase of MI. To reduce pain, dysesthesia, and paresthesia associated with diabetic neuropathy.

Dosage

- **Capsules**

Antiarrhythmic.

Adults, individualized, initial: 200 mg q 8 hr if rapid control of arrhythmia not required; dosage adjustment may be made in 50- or 100-mg increments q 2–3 days, if required. **Maintenance:** 200-300 mg q 8 hr, depending on response and tolerance of client. If adequate response is not achieved with 300 mg or less q 8 hr, 400 mg q 8 hr may be tried although the incidence of CNS side effects increases. If the drug is effective at doses of 300 mg or less q 8 hr, the same total daily dose may be given in divided doses q 12 hr (e.g., 450 mg q 12 hr). Maximum total daily dose: 1,200 mg.

Rapid control of arrhythmias.

Initial loading dose: 400 mg followed by a 200-mg dose in 8 hr.

Diabetic neuropathy.

Initial: 150 mg/day for 3 days; **then,** 300 mg/day for 3 days. **Maintenance:** 10 mg/kg/day.

Administration/Storage

1. The dose should be reduced in clients with severe liver disease and marked right-sided CHF.
2. If transferring to mexiletine from other class I antiarrhythmics, mexiletine may be initiated at a dose of 200 mg and then titrated according to the response at the following times: 6–12 hr after the last dose of quinidine sulfate, 3–6 hr after the last dose of procainamide, 6–12 hr after the last dose of disopyramide, or 8–12 hr after the last dose of tocainide.
3. When transferring to mexiletine, the client should be hospitalized if there is a chance that withdrawal of the previous antiarrhythmic may produce life-threatening arrhythmias.
4. *Treatment of Overdose:* General supportive treatment. Give atropine to treat hypotension or bradycardia. Acidification of the urine may increase rate of excretion.

Contraindications: Cardiogenic shock, preexisting second- or third-degree AV block (if no pacemaker is present). Use with lesser arrhythmias. Lactation.

Special Concerns: Use with caution in hypotension, severe CHF, or known seizure disorders. Dosage has not been established in children.

Laboratory Test Interferences: ↑ AST. Positive ANA.

Side Effects: *CV:* ***Worsening of arrhythmias,*** palpitations, chest pain, increased ventricular arrhythmias (PVCs), CHF, angina or angina-like pain, hypotension, bradycardia, syncope, ***AV block or conduction disturbances,*** atrial arrhythmias, hypertension, ***cardiogenic shock,*** hot flashes, edema. *GI:* High incidence of N&V, heartburn. Also, diarrhea or constipation, changes in appetite, dry mouth, abdominal cramps or pain, abdominal discomfort, salivary changes, dysphagia, altered taste, pharyngitis, changes in oral mucous membranes, upper GI bleeding, peptic ulcer, esophageal ulceration. *CNS:* High incidence of lightheadedness, dizziness, tremor, coordination difficulties, and nervousness. Also, changes in sleep habits, headache, fatigue, weakness, tinnitus, paresthesias, numbness, depression, confusion, difficulty with speech, short-term memory loss, hallucinations, malaise, psychosis, ***seizures,*** loss of consciousness. *Hematologic:* Leukopenia, neutropenia, agranulocytosis, thrombocytopenia. *GU:* Decreased libido, impotence, urinary hesitancy or retention. *Dermatologic:* Rash, dry skin. Rarely, exfoliative dermatitis, and ***Stevens-Johnson syndrome.*** *Miscellaneous:* Blurred vision, visual disturbances, dyspnea, arthralgia, fever, diaphoresis, loss of hair, hiccoughs, laryngeal or pharyngeal changes, syndrome of SLE, myelofibrosis.

Symptoms of Overdose: CNS symptoms (dizziness, drowsiness, paresthesias, seizures) usually precede CV symptoms (hypotension, sinus bradycardia, intermittent left bundle branch block, ***temporary asystole). Massive overdoses cause coma and respiratory arrest.***

Drug Interactions

Aluminum hydroxide / ↓ Absorption of mexiletine
Atropine / ↓ Absorption of mexiletine
Cimetidine / ↑ or ↓ Plasma levels of mexiletine
Magnesium hydroxide / ↓ Absorption of mexiletine
Metoclopramide / ↑ Absorption of mexiletine
Narcotics / ↓ Absorption of mexiletine
Phenobarbital / ↓ Plasma levels of mexiletine
Phenytoin / ↑ Clearance → ↓ plasma levels of mexiletine
Rifampin / ↑ Clearance → ↓ plasma levels of mexiletine
Theophylline / ↑ Effect of theophylline due to ↑ serum levels
Urinary acidifiers / ↑ Rate of excretion of mexiletine
Urinary alkalinizers / ↓ Rate of excretion of mexiletine

NURSING CONSIDERATIONS

See also *Nursing Considerations* for *Antiarrhythmic Drugs,* Chapter 26.

Assessment

1. Document indications for therapy and type and onset of symptoms.
2. List any other agents used for this condition and the outcome.
3. Note any evidence of CHF and assess ECG for evidence of AV block.
4. Obtain baseline ECG, CXR, CBC, and liver and renal function studies and monitor throughout therapy.

Interventions

1. Review ECG for increased arrhythmias and report.
2. Observe for adverse CNS effects such as dizziness, tremor, impaired coordination, and N&V and supervise activity.
3. Obtain urinary pH to determine alkalinity or acidity. Alkalinity decreases renal excretion and acidity increases renal excretion of the drug.

Client/Family Teaching

1. Take medication with food or an antacid to ↓ GI upset.

2. Report any bruising, bleeding, fevers, or sore throat.
3. Note any increase in heart palpitations, irregularity, or rate less than 50 beats/min and report immediately.
4. Do not perform tasks that require mental alertness until drug effects are realized.
5. Carry identification that lists drugs currently prescribed.

Evaluate

- Control of ventricular arrhythmias
- Restoration of stable cardiac rhythm
- Therapeutic serum drug levels (0.5–2 mcg/mL)
- Control of symptoms of diabetic neuropathy

Moricizine hydrochloride

(mor-**IS**-ih-zeen)
Pregnancy Category: B
Ethmozine **(Rx)**

See also *Antiarrhythmic Agents,* Chapter 26.

How Supplied: *Tablet:* 200 mg, 250 mg, 300 mg

Action/Kinetics: Moricizine causes a stabilizing effect on the myocardial membranes as well as local anesthetic activity. The drug shortens phase II and III repolarization leading to a decreased duration of the action potential and an effective refractory period. Also, there is a decrease in the maximum rate of phase O depolarization and a prolongation of AV conduction in clients with ventricular tachycardia. Whether the client is at rest or is exercising, moricizine has minimal effects on cardiac index, stroke index volume, systemic or pulmonary vascular resistance or ejection fraction, and pulmonary capillary wedge pressure. There is a small increase in resting BP and HR. The time, course, and intensity of antiarrhythmic and electrophysiologic effects are not related to plasma levels of the drug. **Peak plasma levels:** 30–120 min. **t½:** 2–3 hr. Significant first-pass effect. Metabolized almost completely by the liver with metabolites excreted through both the urine and feces; the drug induces its own metabolism. Food delays the rate of absorption resulting in lower peak plasma levels; however, the total amount absorbed is not changed.

Uses: Documented life-threatening ventricular arrhythmias (e.g., sustained ventricular tachycardia) where benefits of the drug are determined to outweigh the risks. *Investigational:* Ventricular premature contractions, couplets, and nonsustained ventricular tachycardia.

Dosage

- **Tablets**

Antiarrhythmic.

Adults: 600–900 mg/day in equally divided doses q 8 hr. If needed, the dose can be increased in increments of 150 mg/day at 3-day intervals until the desired effect is obtained. In clients with hepatic or renal impairment, the initial dose should be 600 mg or less with close monitoring and dosage adjustment.

Administration/Storage

1. When transferring clients from other antiarrhythmics to moricizine, the previous drug should be withdrawn for one to two plasma half-lives before starting moricizine. For example, when transferring from quinidine or disopyramide, moricizine can be started 6–12 hr after the last dose; when transferring from procainamide, moricizine can be initiated 3–6 hr after the last dose; when transferring from mexiletine, propafenone, or tocainide, moricizine can be started 8–12 hr after the last dose; and, when transferring from flecainide, moricizine can be started 12–24 hr after the last dose.
2. If clients are well controlled on an 8-hr regimen, they might be given the same total daily dose q 12 hr to increase compliance.
3. *Treatment of Overdose:* In acute overdose, induce vomiting, taking care to prevent aspiration. Client should be hospitalized and closely monitored for cardiac, respiratory, and CNS changes. Provide life support, including an intracardiac pacing catheter, if necessary.

Contraindications: Preexisting second- or third-degree block, right bundle branch block when associated with bifascicular block (unless the client has a pacemaker), cardiogenic shock. Use during lactation.
Special Concerns: Safety and effectiveness in children less than 18 years of age have not been determined. Geriatric clients have a higher rate of side effects. Increased survival rates following use of antiarrhythmic drugs have not been proven in clients with ventricular arrhythmias. Use with caution in clients with sick sinus syndrome due to the possibility of sinus bradycardia, sinus pause, or sinus arrest. Use with caution in clients with CHF.
Laboratory Test Interferences: ↑ Bilirubin and liver transaminases.
Side Effects: *CV:* ***Proarrhythmias, including new rhythm disturbances or worsening of existing arrhythmias;*** ECG abnormalities, including conduction defects, sinus pause, function rhythm, AV block; palpitations, ***sustained ventricular tachycardia,*** cardiac chest pain, CHF, ***cardiac death,*** hypotension, hypertension, atrial fibrillation, atrial flutter, syncope, bradycardia, ***cardiac arrest, MI, pulmonary embolism,*** vasodilation, thrombophlebitis, ***cerebrovascular events.*** *CNS:* Dizziness (common), anxiety, headache, fatigue, nervousness, paresthesias, sleep disorders, tremor, anxiety, hypoesthesias, depression, euphoria, somnolence, agitation, confusion, ***seizures,*** hallucinations, loss of memory, vertigo, coma. *GI:* Nausea, dry mouth, abdominal pain, vomiting, diarrhea, dyspepsia, anorexia, ileus, flatulence, dysphagia, bitter taste. *Musculoskeletal:* Asthenia, abnormal gait, akathisia, ataxia, abnormal coordination, dyskinesia, pain. *GU:* Urinary retention, dysuria, urinary incontinence, urinary frequency, impotence, kidney pain, decreased libido. *Respiratory:* Dyspnea, apnea, asthma, hyperventilation, pharyngitis, cough, sinusitis. *Opthalmologic:* Nystagmus, diplopia, blurred vision, eye pain, periorbital edema. *Dermatologic:* Rash, pruritus, dry skin, urticaria. *Miscellaneous:* Sweating, drug fever, hypothermia, temperature intolerance, swelling of the lips and tongue, speech disorder, tinnitus, jaundice.

Symptoms of Overdose: Vomiting, hypotension, lethargy, worsening of CHF, ***MI, conduction disturbances, arrhythmias (e.g., junctional bradycardia, ventricular tachycardia, ventricular fibrillation, asystole), sinus arrest, respiratory failure.***

Drug Interactions
Cimetidine / ↑ Plasma levels of moricizine due to ↓ excretion
Digoxin / Additive prolongation of the PR interval (but no significant increase in the rate of second- or third-degree AV block)
Propranolol / Additive prolongation of the PR interval
Theophylline / ↓ Plasma levels of theophylline due to ↑ rate of clearance

NURSING CONSIDERATIONS

See also *Nursing Considerations* for *Antiarrhythmic Agents,* Chapter 26.

Assessment
1. Document cardiac history and note any preexisting conditions and ECG abnormalities.
2. Obtain baseline ECG, electrolytes, and liver and renal function studies.
3. List drugs client currently taking to determine any potential adverse interactions.

Interventions
1. Monitor cardiac rhythm closely to observe for drug-induced rhythm disturbances during therapy.
2. Anticipate lower initial doses in clients with impaired hepatic or renal function.
3. Clients should be hospitalized for initial dosing because they will be at high risk. Antiarrhythmic response may be determined by ECG, exercise testing, or programmed electrical stimulation testing.
4. Correct any electrolyte imbalance before initiating drug therapy.

5. Document and monitor pacing parameters in clients with pacemakers.
6. Monitor VS and report any persistent temperature elevations.

Client/Family Teaching

1. Take before meals because food delays the rate of absorption.
2. Provide a printed list of side effects that require immediate reporting.
3. Drug may cause dizziness. Use care when rising from a lying or sitting position.
4. Advise family member or significant other to learn CPR.

Evaluate: Termination of life-threatening ventricular arrhythmias.

Procainamide hydrochloride

(proh-**KAYN**-ah-myd)
Pregnancy Category: C
Procan SR, Pronestyl, Pronestyl-SR
(Rx)

See also *Antiarrhythmic Agents,* Chapter 26.

How Supplied: *Capsule:* 250 mg, 375 mg, 500 mg; *Injection:* 100 mg/mL, 500 mg/mL; *Tablet:* 250 mg, 375 mg, 500 mg; *Tablet, extended release:* 250 mg, 500 mg, 750 mg, 1000 mg

Action/Kinetics: Procainamide produces a direct cardiac effect to prolong the refractory period of the atria and to a lesser extent the bundle of His-Purkinje system and ventricles. Large doses may cause AV block. It has some anticholinergic and local anesthetic effects. Antiarrhythmic drugs have not been shown to increase the rate of survival in clients with ventricular arrhythmias. **Onset: PO,** 30 min; **IV,** 1–5 min. **Time to peak effect, PO:** 90–120 min; **IM,** 15–60 min; **IV,** immediate. **Duration:** 3 hr. **t½:** 3–4 hr. **Therapeutic serum level:** 4–8 mcg/mL. **Protein binding:** 15%. From 30% to 60% excreted unchanged. The drug may be metabolized in the liver (16%–21% by slow acetylators and 24%–33% by fast acetylators) to the active N-acetylprocainamide (NAPA).

Uses: Documented ventricular arrhythmias (e.g., sustained ventricular tachycardia) that may be life-threatening in clients where benefits of treatment clearly outweigh risks.

Dosage

• **Capsules, Tablets**

Adults, initial: 50 mg/kg/day in divided doses q 3 hr. **Usual, 40–50 kg:** 250 mg q 3 hr of standard formulation or 500 mg q 6 hr of sustained-release; **60–70 kg:** 375 mg q 3 hr of standard formulation or 750 mg q 6 hr of sustained-release; **80–90 kg:** 500 mg q 3 hr of standard formulation or 1 g q 6 hr of sustained-release; **over 100 kg:** 625 mg q 3 hr of standard formulation or 1.25 g q 6 hr of sustained-release. **Pediatric:** 15–50 mg/kg/day divided q 3–6 hr (up to a maximum of 4 g/day).

• **IM**

Ventricular arrhythmias.

Adults, initial: 50 mg/kg/day divided into fractional doses of 1/8–1/4 given q 3–6 hr until PO therapy is possible. **Pediatric:** 20–30 mg/kg/day divided q 4–6 hr (up to a maximum of 4 g/day).

Arrhythmias associated with surgery or anesthesia.

Adults: 100–500 mg.

• **IV**

Initial loading infusion: 20 mg/min (for up to 25–30 min). **Maintenance infusion:** 2–6 mg/min. **Pediatric, initial loading dose:** 3–5 mg/kg/dose over 5 min (maximum of 100 mg); **maintenance:** 20–80 mcg/kg/min continuous infusion (maximum of 2 g/day).

Administration/Storage

1. IV use should be reserved for emergency situations.
2. IM therapy may be used as an alternative to PO for clients with less threatening arrhythmias but who are nauseated or vomiting, who cannot take anything PO (e.g., preoperatively), or who have malabsorptive problems.
3. If more than three IM injections are required, the age and renal function of the client should be assessed as well as blood levels of procaina-

mide and NAPA; adjust dosage accordingly.
4. For IV initial therapy, the drug should be diluted with 5% dextrose solution and a maximum of 1 g administered slowly to minimize side effects by one of the following methods:
• Direct injection into a vein or into tubing of an established infusion line at a rate not to exceed 50 mg/min. Dilute either the 100- or 500-mg/mL vials prior to injection to facilitate control of the dosage rate. Doses of 100 mg may be given q 5 min until arrhythmia is suppressed or until 500 mg has been given (then wait 10 or more min before resuming administration).
• Loading infusion containing 20 mg/mL (1 g diluted with 50 mL of 5% dextrose injection) given at a constant rate of 1 mL/min for 25–30 min to deliver 500–600 mg.
5. For IV maintenance infusion, the dose is usually 2–6 mg/min. Drug solutions should be administered with an electronic infusion device for safety and accuracy.
6. Discard solutions of drug that are darker than light amber or otherwise colored. Solutions that have turned slightly yellow on standing may be used. Consult with pharmacist for clarification.
7. Extended-release tablets are not recommended for use in children or for initiating treatment.
8. Procainamide metabolite NAPA also has antiarrhythmic properties with a longer half-life than procainamide.
9. *Treatment of Overdose:*
• Induce emesis or perform gastric lavage followed by administration of activated charcoal.
• To treat hypotension, give IV fluids and/or a vasopressor (dopamine, phenylephrine, or norepinephrine).
• Infusion of 1/6 molar sodium lactate IV reduces the cardiotoxic effects.
• Hemodialysis (but not peritoneal dialysis) is effective in reducing serum levels.
• Renal clearance can be enhanced by acidification of the urine and with high flow rates.
• A ventricular pacing electrode can be inserted as a precaution in the event AV block develops.

Contraindications: Hypersensitivity to drug, complete AV heart block, lupus erythematosus, torsades de pointes, asymptomatic ventricular premature contractions. Lactation.

Special Concerns: Although used in children, safety and efficacy have not been established. Use with extreme caution in clients for whom a sudden drop in BP could be detrimental, in CHF, acute ischemic heart disease, or cardiomyopathy. Also, use with caution in clients with liver or kidney dysfunction, preexisting bone marrow failure or cytopenia of any type, development of first-degree heart block while on procainamide, myasthenia gravis, and those with bronchial asthma or other respiratory disorders. Procainamide may cause more hypotension in geriatric clients; also, in this population, the dose may have to be decreased due to age-related decreases in renal function.

Laboratory Test Interferences: May affect liver function tests. False + ↑ serum alkaline phosphatase. Positive ANA test. High levels of lidocaine and meprobamate may inhibit fluorescence of procainamide and NAPA.

Side Effects: *Body as a whole:* Lupus erythematosus–like syndrome especially in those on maintenance therapy and who are slow acetylators. Symptoms include arthralgia, pleural or abdominal pain, arthritis, pleural effusion, pericarditis, fever, chills, myalgia, skin lesions, hematologic changes. *CV:* Following IV use: Hypotension, ***ventricular asystole or fibrillation, partial or complete heart block.*** Rarely, second-degree heart block after PO use. *GI:* N&V, diarrhea, anorexia, bitter taste, abdominal pain. *Hematologic:* Thrombocytopenia,

agranulocytosis, neutropenia. ***Rarely, hemolytic anemia.*** *Dermatologic:* Urticaria, pruritus, angioneurotic edema, flushing, maculopapular rash. *CNS:* Depression, dizziness, weakness, giddiness, psychoses, hallucinations. *Other:* Granulomatous hepatitis, weakness, fever, chills.

Symptoms of Overdose: Plasma levels of 10–15 mcg/mL are associated with toxic symptoms. Progressive widening of the QRS complex, prolonged QT or PR intervals, lowering of R and T waves, increased AV block, increased ventricular extrasystoles, ***ventricular tachycardia or fibrillation. IV overdose may result in hypotension, CNS depression, tremor, respiratory depression.***

Drug Interactions

Acetazolamide / ↑ Effect of procainamide due to ↓ excretion by kidney

Anticholinergic agents, atropine / Additive anticholinergic effects

Antihypertensive agents / Additive hypotensive effect

Cholinergic agents / Anticholinergic activity of procainamide antagonizes effect of cholinergic drugs

Cimetidine / ↑ Effect of procainamide due to ↑ bioavailability

Disopyramide / ↑ Risk of enhanced prolongation of conduction or depression of contractility and hypotension

Ethanol / Effect of procainamide may be altered, but because the main metabolite is active as an antiarrhythmic, specific outcome not clear

Kanamycin / Procainamide ↑ muscle relaxation produced by kanamycin

Lidocaine / Additive cardiodepressant effects

Magnesium salts / Procainamide ↑ muscle relaxation produced by magnesium salts

Neomycin / Procainamide ↑ muscle relaxation produced by neomycin

Propranolol / ↑ Serum procainamide levels

Quinidine / ↑ Risk of enhanced prolongation of conduction or depression of contractility and hypotension

Ranitidine / ↑ Effect of procainamide due to ↑ bioavailability

Sodium bicarbonate / ↑ Effect of procainamide due to ↓ excretion by the kidney

Succinylcholine / Procainamide ↑ muscle relaxation produced by succinylcholine

Trimethoprim / ↑ Effect of procainamide due to ↑ serum levels

---

NURSING CONSIDERATIONS

See also *Nursing Considerations* for *Antiarrhythmic Agents,* Chapter 26.

Assessment

1. Document indications for therapy and type and onset of symptoms.
2. List other agents prescribed and the outcome.
3. Obtain baseline CBC, ANA titers, and liver and renal function studies and monitor throughout therapy.

Interventions

1. Place client in a supine position during IV infusion and monitor SBP frequently. Be prepared to discontinue infusion if SBP falls 15 mm Hg or more during administration or if increased SA or AV block is noted on ECG.
2. Assess clients on PO drug maintenance for symptoms of lupus erythematosus, as manifested by polyarthralgia, arthritis, pleuritic pain, fever, myalgia, and skin lesions.
3. Weigh clients and assess GI symptoms. If severe and persistent the provider may permit the client to take the medication with meals or with a snack to ensure compliance with drug therapy.

Client/Family Teaching

1. Take the medication with a full glass of water to lessen GI symptoms. The drug should be taken either 1 hr before or 2 hr after meals unless otherwise ordered.
2. Take medication only as directed. Set an alarm clock to awaken through the night to take the drug as ordered, if necessary.
3. Sustained-release preparations should be swallowed whole. They

should not be crushed, broken, or chewed. The wax matrix of sustained-release tablets may be evident in the stool and is considered normal.
4. Report any sore throat, fever, rash, chills, bruising, or diarrhea.
5. Do not take any OTC drugs without approval.
6. Stress the importance of reporting for scheduled lab studies and ECG evaluation.

Evaluate

- Termination of arrhythmias with restoration of stable cardiac rhythm
- Therapeutic serum drug levels (4–8 mcg/mL)

Propafenone hydrochloride

(proh-pah-**FEN**-ohn)
Pregnancy Category: C
Rythmol **(Rx)**

How Supplied: *Tablet:* 150 mg, 225 mg, 300 mg
Action/Kinetics: Propafenone manifests local anesthetic effects and a direct stabilizing action on the myocardium. The drug reduces upstroke velocity (Phase O) of the monophasic action potential, reduces the fast inward current carried by sodium ions in the Purkinje fibers, increases diastolic excitability threshold, and prolongs the effective refractory period. Also, spontaneous activity is decreased. The drug slows AV conduction and causes first-degree heart block. The drug has slight beta-adrenergic blocking activity. **Peak plasma levels:** 3.5 hr. **Therapeutic plasma levels:** 0.5–3 mcg/mL. Significant first-pass effect. Most clients metabolize propafenone rapidly (**t½:** 2–10 hr) to two active metabolites: 5-hydroxypropafenone and N-depropylpropafenone. However, approximately 10% of clients (as well as those taking quinidine) metabolize the drug more slowly (**t½:** 10–32 hr). However, because the 5-hydroxy metabolite is not formed in slow metabolizers and because steady-state levels are reached after 4–5 days in all clients, the recommended dosing regimen is the same for all clients.
Uses: Documented life-threatening ventricular arrhythmias such as sustained ventricular tachycardia where the benefits outweigh the risks. Should not be used in less severe ventricular arrhythmias even if the client is symptomatic. *Investigational:* SVTs including atrial fibrillation or flutter and arrhythmias associated with Wolff-Parkinson-White syndrome.

Dosage

- **Tablets**

Adults, initial: 150 mg q 8 hr; dose may be increased at a minimum of q 3–4 days to 225 mg q 8 hr and, if necessary, to 300 mg q 8 hr.

Administration/Storage

1. Initiation of propafenone therapy should always be undertaken in a hospital setting.
2. The effectiveness and safety of doses exceeding 900 mg/day have not been determined.
3. There is no evidence that the use of propafenone affects the survival or incidence of sudden death in clients with recent MI or SVT.
4. *Treatment of Overdose:* To control BP and cardiac rhythm, defibrillation and infusion of dopamine or isoproterenol. If seizures occur, diazepam, IV, can be given. External cardiac massage and mechanical respiratory assistance may be required.

Contraindications: Uncontrolled CHF, cardiogenic shock, sick sinus node syndrome or AV block in the absence of an artificial pacemaker, bradycardia, marked hypotension, bronchospastic disorders, electrolyte disorders, hypersensitivity to the drug. MI more than 6 days but less than 2 years previously. Lactation.
Special Concerns: Use with caution during labor and delivery. The safety and effectiveness have not been determined in children. Use with caution in clients with impaired

hepatic or renal function. Geriatric clients may require lower dosage.
Laboratory Test Interference: ↑ ANA titers.
Side Effects: *CV:* ***New or worsened arrhythmias.*** First-degree AV block, intraventricular conduction delay, palpitations, PVCs, proarrhythmia, bradycardia, atrial fibrillation, angina, syncope, CHF, ***ventricular tachycardia, second-degree AV block,*** increased QRS duration, chest pain, hypotension, bundle branch block. Less commonly, atrial flutter, AV dissociation, flushing, hot flashes, sick sinus syndrome, sinus pause or arrest, SVT, ***cardiac arrest.*** *CNS:* Dizziness, headache, anxiety, drowsiness, fatigue, loss of balance, ataxia, insomnia. Less commonly, abnormal speech, abnormal dreams, abnormal vision, confusion, depression, memory loss, ***apnea,*** psychosis/mania, vertigo, ***seizures, coma,*** numbness, paresthesias. *GI:* Unusual taste, constipation, nausea and/or vomiting, dry mouth, anorexia, flatulence, abdominal pain, cramps, diarrhea, dyspepsia. Less commonly, gastroenteritis and liver abnormalities (cholestasis, hepatitis, elevated enzymes, hepatitis). *Hematologic:* ***Agranulocytosis,*** increased bleeding time, anemia, granulocytopenia, bruising, leukopenia, purpura, anemia, thrombocytopenia. *Miscellaneous:* Blurred vision, dyspnea, weakness, rash, edema, tremors, diaphoresis, joint pain, possible decrease in spermatogenesis. Less commonly, tinnitus, unusual smell sensation, alopecia, eye irritation, hyponatremia, inappropriate ADH secretion, impotence, increased glucose, kidney failure, lupus erythematosus, muscle cramps or weakness, nephrotic syndrome, pain, pruritus.

Symptoms of Overdose: Bradycardia, hypotension, IA and intraventricular conduction disturbances, somnolence. ***Rarely, high-grade ventricular arrhythmias and seizures.***

Drug Interactions

Beta-adrenergic blockers / Propafenone ↑ plasma levels of beta blockers metabolized by the liver
Cimetidine / Cimetidine ↓ plasma levels of propafenone
Cyclosporine / ↑ Blood trough levels of cyclosporine; ↓ renal function
Digoxin / Propafenone ↑ plasma levels of digoxin necessitating a ↓ in the dose of digoxin
Local anesthetics / May ↑ risk of CNS side effects
Quinidine / ↑ Serum levels of propafenone in rapid metabolizers → possible ↑ effect
Rifampin / ↓ Effect of propafenone due to ↑ clearance
Warfarin / Propafenone may ↑ plasma levels of warfarin necessitating ↓ dose of warfarin

NURSING CONSIDERATIONS

See also *Nursing Considerations* for *Antiarrhythmic Agents,* Chapter 26.

Assessment

1. Assess ECG, document baseline arrhythmias, and note any client history of cardiac problems.
2. Determine if there is any history of renal or hepatic disease. Propafenone must be used with caution in these clients.

Interventions

1. Propafenone may induce new or more severe arrhythmias. Document ECG strips and monitor client response closely as the dose of propafenone should be titrated in each client on the basis of response and tolerance.
2. Report any significant widening of the QRS complex or second- or third-degree AV block immediately.
3. Anticipate that the dose of propafenone will be increased more gradually in elderly clients as well as in clients with previous myocardial damage.
4. Monitor VS. Weigh client and place on strict I&O.
5. Evaluate hematologic studies during drug therapy to determine the presence of anemia, agranulocytosis, leukopenia, thrombocytopenia, or altered prothrombin and coagulation times.
6. Client may complain of an unusual taste in the mouth. This may inter-

fere with eating and nutrition so observe closely.

Client/Family Teaching

1. Drink adequate quantities of fluid (2–3 L/day) and maintain adequate bulk in the diet to avoid constipation.
2. Report any incidence of increased or unusual bruising or bleeding.
3. Observe for indications of hepatic dysfunction such as yellow sclera, dark yellow urine, or yellow pigmentation of the skin.
4. Report any evidence of urinary tract problems such as decreased urinary output.
5. Instruct in how to take BP and pulse and advise what readings and symptoms to report.

Evaluate

- Termination of life-threatening ventricular tachycardia
- Therapeutic serum drug levels (0.5–3 mcg/mL)

Quinidine bisulfate

(**KWIN**-ih-deen)
Pregnancy Category: D
Biquin Durules ✱ **(Rx)**

Quinidine gluconate

(**KWIN**-ih-deen)
Pregnancy Category: C
Quinaglute Dura-Tabs, Quinalan, Quinate ✱ **(Rx)**

Quinidine polygalacturonate

(**KWIN**-ih-deen)
Pregnancy Category: C
Cardioquin **(Rx)**

Quinidine sulfate

(**KWIN**-ih-deen)
Pregnancy Category: C
Apo-Quinidine ✱, Novo-Quinidin ✱, Quinidex Extentabs, Quinora **(Rx)**

See also *Antiarrhythmic Agents*, Chapter 26.

How Supplied: Quinidine bisulfate: *Sustained-release tablet:* 250 mg.
Quinidine gluconate: *Injection:* 80 mg/mL; *Tablet, extended release:* 324 mg.
Quinidine polygalacturonate: *Tablet:* 275 mg.
Quinidine sulfate: *Tablet:* 200 mg, 300 mg; *Tablet, extended release:* 300 mg

Action/Kinetics: Quinidine reduces the excitability of the heart and depresses conduction velocity and contractility. The drug prolongs the refractory period and increases conduction time. It also decreases CO and possesses anticholinergic, antimalarial, antipyretic, and oxytocic properties. **PO: Onset:** 0.5–3 hr. **Maximum effects, after IM:** 30–90 min. **t½:** 6–7 hr. **Time to peak levels, PO:** 3–5 hr for gluconate salt, 1–1.5 hr for sulfate salt, and 6 hr for polygalacturonate salt; **IM:** 1 hr. **Therapeutic serum levels:** 2–6 mcg/mL. **Protein binding:** 60%–80%. **Duration:** 6–8 hr for tablets/capsules and 12 hr for extended-release tablets. Metabolized by liver. Rate of urinary excretion (10%–50% excreted unchanged) is affected by urinary pH.

Uses: Premature atrial, AV junctional, and ventricular contractions. Treatment and control of atrial flutter, established atrial fibrillation, paroxysmal atrial tachycardia, paroxysmal AV junctional rhythm, paroxysmal and chronic atrial fibrillation, paroxysmal ventricular tachycardia not associated with complete heart block, maintenance therapy after electrical conversion of atrial flutter or fibrillation. The parenteral route is indicated when PO therapy is not feasible or immediate effects are required. *Investigational:* Gluconate salt for life-threatening *Plasmodium falciparum* malaria.

Dosage

- **Quinidine Bisulfate Controlled-Release Tablets**

Antiarrhythmic.

Initial: Test dose of 200 mg in the morning (to ascertain hypersensitivity). In the evening, administer 500 mg. **Then,** beginning the next day, 500–750 mg/12 hr. **Maintenance:** 0.5–1.25 g morning and evening.

• Quinidine Polygalacturonate Tablets, Quinidine Sulfate Tablets

Premature atrial and ventricular contractions.

Adults: 200–300 mg t.i.d.–q.i.d.

Paroxysmal SVTs.

Adults: 400–600 mg/2–3 hr until the paroxysm is terminated.

Conversion of atrial flutter.

Adults: 200 mg/2–3 hr for five to eight doses; daily doses can be increased until rhythm is restored or toxic effects occur.

Conversion of atrial flutter, Maintenance therapy.

Adults: 200–300 mg t.i.d.–q.i.d. Large doses or more frequent administration may be required in some clients.

• Quinidine Gluconate Sustained-Release Tablets, Quinidine Sulfate Sustained-Release Tablets

All uses.

Adults: 300–600 mg/8–12 hr.

• Quinidine Gluconate Injection (IM or IV)

Acute tachycardia.

Adults, initial: 600 mg IM; **then,** 400 mg IM repeated as often as q 2 hr.

Arrhythmias.

Adults: 330 mg IM or less IV (as much as 500–750 mg may be required).

P. falciparum malaria.

Two regimens may be used. (1) *Loading dose:* 15 mg/kg in 250 mL NSS given over 4 hr; **then,** 24 hr after beginning the loading dose, institute 7.5 mg/kg infused over 4 hr and given q 8 hr for 7 days or until PO therapy can be started. (2) *Loading dose:* 10 mg/kg in 250 mL NSS infused over 1–2 hr followed immediately by 0.02 mg/kg/min for up to 72 hr or until parasitemia decreases to less than 1% or PO therapy can be started.

Administration/Storage

1. A preliminary test dose may be given before instituting quinidine therapy. **Adults:** 200 mg quinidine sulfate or quinidine gluconate administered PO or IM. **Children:** Test dose of 2 mg of quinidine sulfate per kilogram of body weight.
2. The sustained-release forms cannot be considered interchangeable.
3. IV solution can be prepared by diluting 10 mL of quinidine gluconate injection (800 mg) with 50 mL of 5% glucose solution; this should be given at a rate of 1 mL/min.
4. Use only colorless clear solution for injection because light may cause quinidine to crystallize, which turns solution brownish.
5. *Treatment of Overdose:*

• Perform gastric lavage, induce vomiting, and administer activated charcoal if ingestion is recent.
• Monitor ECG, blood gases, serum electrolytes, and BP.
• Institute cardiac pacing, if necessary.
• Acidify the urine.
• Use artificial respiration and other supportive measures.
• Infusions of 1/6 molar sodium lactate IV may decrease the cardiotoxic effects.
• Treat hypotension with metaraminol or norepinephrine after fluid volume replacement.
• Use phenytoin or lidocaine to treat tachydysrhythmias.
• Hemodialysis is effective but not often required.

Contraindications: Hypersensitivity to drug or other cinchona drugs. Myasthenia gravis, history of thrombocytopenic purpura associated with quinidine use, digitalis intoxication evidenced by arrhythmias or AV conduction disorders. Also, complete heart block, left bundle branch block, or other intraventricular conduction defects manifested by marked QRS widening or bizarre complexes. Complete AV block with an AV nodal or idioventricular pacemaker, aberrant ectopic impulses and abnormal rhythms due to escape mechanisms. History of drug-induced torsades de pointes or long QT syndrome.

Special Concerns: Safety in children and during lactation has not been established. Quinidine should be used with extreme caution in clients in whom a sudden change in BP might be detrimental or in those suffering from extensive myocardial damage, subacute endocarditis, bradycardia, coronary occlusion, disturbances in impulse conduction, chronic valvular disease, considerable cardiac enlargement, frank CHF, and renal or hepatic disease. Cautious use is also recommended in clients with acute infections, hyperthyroidism, muscular weakness, respiratory distress, and bronchial asthma. The dose in geriatric clients may have to be reduced due to age-related changes in renal function.

Laboratory Test Interferences: False + or ↑ PSP, 17-ketosteroids, PT.

Side Effects: *CV:* Widening of QRS complex, hypotension, cardiac asystole, ectopic ventricular beats, ***ventricular tachycardia or fibrillation, torsades de pointes,*** paradoxical tachycardia, ***arterial embolism,*** ventricular extrasystoles (one or more every 6 beats), prolonged QT interval, complete AV block, ventricular flutter. *GI:* N&V, abdominal pain, anorexia, diarrhea, urge to defecate as well as urinate, esophagitis (rare). *CNS:* Syncope, headache, confusion, excitement, vertigo, apprehension, delirium, dementia, ataxia, depression. *Dermatologic:* Rash, urticaria, exfoliative dermatitis, photosensitivity, flushing with intense pruritus, eczema, psoriasis, pigmentation abnormalities. *Allergic:* Acute asthma, angioneurotic edema, ***respiratory arrest,*** dyspnea, fever, ***vascular collapse,*** purpura, vasculitis, hepatic dysfunction (including granulomatous hepatitis), hepatic toxicity. *Hematologic:* Hypoprothrombinemia, acute hemolytic anemia, thrombocytopenic purpura, ***agranulocytosis,*** thrombocytopenia, leukocytosis, neutropenia, shift to left in WBC differential. *Ophthalmologic:* Blurred vision, mydriasis, alterations in color perception, decreased field of vision, double vision, photophobia, optic neuritis, night blindness, scotomata. *Other:* Liver toxicity including hepatitis, lupus nephritis, tinnitus, decreased hearing acuity, arthritis, myalgia, increase in serum skeletal muscle CPK, lupus erythematosus.

Symptoms of Overdose: CNS: Lethargy, confusion, ***coma, seizures, respiratory depression or arrest,*** headache, paresthesia, vertigo. CNS symptoms may be seen after onset of CV toxicity. *GI:* Vomiting, diarrhea, abdominal pain, hypokalemia, nausea. *CV:* Sinus tachycardia, ***ventricular tachycardia or fibrillation, torsades de pointes, depressed automaticity and conduction*** (including bundle branch block, sinus bradycardia, SA block, prolongation of QRS and QTc, sinus arrest, AV block, ST depression, T inversion), syncope, ***heart failure.*** Hypotension due to decreased conduction and CO and vasodilation. *Miscellaneous:* Cinchonism, visual and auditory disturbances, hypokalemia, tinnitus, acidosis.

Drug Interactions

Acetazolamide, Antacids / ↑ Effect of quinidine due to ↓ renal excretion

Amiodarone / ↑ Quinidine levels with possible fatal cardiac dysrhythmias

Anticholinergic agents, Atropine / Additive effect on blockade of vagus nerve action

Anticoagulants, oral / Additive hypoprothrombinemia with possible hemorrhage

Barbiturates / ↓ Effect of quinidine due to ↑ breakdown by liver

Cholinergic agents / Quinidine antagonizes effect of cholinergic drugs

Cimetidine / ↑ Effect of quinidine due to ↓ breakdown by liver

Digoxin, Digitoxin / ↑ Symptoms of digoxin or digitoxin toxicity

Disopyramide / Either ↑ disopyramide levels or ↓ quinidine levels

Guanethidine / Additive hypotensive effect

Methyldopa / Additive hypotensive effect

Metoprolol / ↑ Effect of propranolol in fast metabolizers

Neuromuscular blocking agents / ↑ Respiratory depression

Nifedipine / ↓ Effect of quinidine

Phenobarbital, Phenytoin / ↓ Effect of quinidine by ↑ rate of metabolism in liver
Potassium / ↑ Effect of quinidine
Procainamide / ↑ Effects of procainamide with possible toxicity
Propafenone / ↑ Serum propafenone levels in rapid metabolizers
Propranolol / ↑ Effect of propranolol in fast metabolizers
Reserpine / Additive cardiac depressant effects
Rifampin / ↓ Effect of quinidine due to ↑ breakdown by liver
Skeletal muscle relaxants / ↑ Skeletal muscle relaxation
Sodium bicarbonate / ↑ Effect of quinidine due to ↓ renal excretion
Sucralfate / ↓ Serum levels of quinidine → ↓ effect
Thiazide diuretics / ↑ Effect of quinidine due to ↓ renal excretion
Tricyclic antidepressants / ↑ Effect of antidepressant due to ↓ clearance
Verapamil / ↓ Clearance of verapamil ↑ hypotension, bradycardia, AV block, ventricular tachycardia, and pulmonary edema

---

NURSING CONSIDERATIONS

See also *Nursing Considerations* for *Antiarrhythmic Agents,* Chapter 26.

Assessment

1. Note any history of allergic reactions to antiarrhythmic drugs or tartrazine, which is found in some formulations. A test dose may be performed by administering one regular PO tablet before therapy is instituted. Observe client for hypersensitivity reactions to check for any intolerance.
2. Document indications for therapy, type, and onset of symptoms.
3. Determine that pretreatment lab tests including blood glucose, CBC, liver and renal function studies and CXR have been performed. Monitor serum electrolytes, CBC, and liver and renal function studies during prolonged therapy with quinidine.
4. Obtain VS and ECG and carefully assess heart and lung sounds.

Interventions

1. Evaluate ECG and report any evidence of increased AV block, cardiac irritability, or rhythm suppression during IV administration.
2. Monitor I&O and VS; observe closely for evidence of hypotension. The drug induces urinary alkalization.
3. Observe for neurologic deficits or sensory impairment and report if evident.
4. Report any persistent diarrhea.
5. Among the elderly, there is a higher risk of toxicity, reduced CO, and unpredictable effects from drug therapy.
6. Clients with long-standing atrial fibrillation or CHF with atrial fibrillation run a risk of embolization from mural thrombi when converting to sinus rhythm.

Client/Family Teaching

1. Administer with food to minimize GI effects.
2. Drug may cause dizziness or blurred vision. Activities that require mental alertness should be avoided until drug effects are realized.
3. Incorporate fruit and grain in the diet. A high intake of fruits and vegetables (alkaline-ash foods) may prolong the half-life of quinidine.
4. Palpitations or faintness may indicate quinidine-induced ventricular arrhythmias and should be reported immediately.
5. Advise client to report any of the following symptoms:
• Severe skin rash, hives or itching
• Severe headache
• Unexplained fever
• Ringing in the ears, buzzing, or hearing loss
• Unusual bruising or bleeding
• Blurred vision
• Irregular heart beat
• Continued diarrhea
6. Wear dark glasses if photophobia is experienced.
7. Stress the importance of reporting for lab studies and follow-up appointments as scheduled.

Evaluate

• Control of arrhythmia with restoration of stable cardiac rhythm
• Therapeutic serum drug levels (2–6 mcg/mL)

Tocainide hydrochloride

(toe-**KAY**-nyd)
Pregnancy Category: C
Tonocard **(Rx)**

See also *Antiarrhythmic Agents,* Chapter 26.
How Supplied: *Tablet:* 400 mg, 600 mg
Action/Kinetics: Tocainide, which is similar to lidocaine, decreases the excitability of cells in the myocardium by decreasing sodium and potassium conductance. Tocainide increases pulmonary and aortic arterial pressure and slightly increases peripheral resistance. Is effective in both digitalized and nondigitalized clients. **Peak plasma levels:** 0.5–2 hr. **t½:** 15 hr. **Therapeutic serum levels:** 4–10 mcg/mL. **Duration:** 8 hr. Approximately 10% is bound to plasma protein. Forty percent is excreted unchanged in the urine. Alkalinization decreases the excretion of the drug although acidification does not produce any changes in excretion.
Uses: Life-threatening ventricular arrhythmias, including ventricular tachycardia. *Investigational:* Myotonic dystrophy, trigeminal neuralgia.

Dosage

- **Tablets**

Antiarrhythmic.

Adults, individualized, initial: 400 mg q 8 hr, up to a maximum of 2,400 mg/day; **maintenance:** 1,200–1,800 mg/day in divided doses. Total daily dose of 1,200 mg may beadequate in clients with liver or kidney disease.

Myotonic dystrophy.

800–1,200 mg/day.

Trigeminal neuralgia.

20 mg/kg/day in three divided doses.
Administration/Storage: *Treatment of Overdose:* Gastric lavage and activated charcoal may be useful. In the event of respiratory depression or arrest or seizures, maintain airway and provide artificial ventilation. An IV anticonvulsant (e.g., diazepam, thiopental, thiamylal, pentobarbital, secobarbital) may be required if seizures are persistent.
Contraindications: Allergy to amide-type local anesthetics, second- or third-degree AV block in the absence of artificial ventricular pacemaker. Lactation.
Special Concern: Safety and efficacy have not been established in children. Use with caution in clients with impaired renal or hepatic function (dose may have to be decreased). Geriatric clients may have an increased risk of dizziness and hypotension; the dose may have to be reduced in these clients due to age-related impaired renal function.
Laboratory Test Interferences: Abnormal liver function tests (especially in early therapy). ↑ ANA.
Side Effects: *CV:* ***Increased arrhythmias,*** increased ventricular rate (when given for atrial flutter or fibrillation), CHF, tachycardia, hypotension, ***conduction disturbances,*** bradycardia, chest pain, LV failure, palpitations. *CNS:* Dizziness, vertigo, headache, tremors, confusion, disorientation, hallucinations, ataxia, paresthesias, numbness, nervousness, altered mood, anxiety, incoordination, walking disturbances. *GI:* N&V, anorexia, diarrhea. *Respiratory:* ***Pulmonary fibrosis, fibrosing alveolitis,*** interstitial pneumonitis, ***pulmonary edema,*** pneumonia. *Hematologic:* Leukopenia, ***agranulocytosis,*** hypoplastic anemia, ***aplastic anemia,*** bone marrow depression, neutropenia, ***thrombocytopenia and sequelae as septicemia and septic shock.*** *Musculoskeletal:* Arthritis, arthralgia, myalgia. *Dermatologic:* Rash, skin lesion, diaphoresis. *Other:* Blurred vision, visual disturbances, nystagmus, tinnitus, hearing loss, lupus-like syndrome.

Symptoms of Overdose: Initially are CNS symptoms including tremor (see above). GI symptoms may follow (see above).

Drug Interactions
Cimetidine / ↓ Bioavailability of tocainide
Metoprolol / Additive effects on wedge pressure and cardiac index
Rifampin / ↓ Bioavailability of tocainide

NURSING CONSIDERATIONS

See also *Nursing Considerations* for *Antiarrhythmic Agents*, Chapter 26.

Assessment

1. Document indications for therapy and type and onset of symptoms.
2. Obtain baseline CBC, electrolytes, and renal function studies. Potassium deficits should be corrected before initiating tocainide therapy.

Client/Family Teaching

1. Take with food to minimize GI upset.
2. Drug may cause drowsiness or dizziness. Do not drive or operate machinery until drug effects are realized.
3. Report any abnormal bruising, or bleeding, or signs of infection such as fever, sore throat, or chills. These symptoms may indicate a blood dyscrasia.
4. Pulmonary symptoms such as wheezing, coughing, or dyspnea should be reported immediately. These may indicate pulmonary fibrosis and in this case the drug must be discontinued.
5. Stress the importance of reporting for scheduled lab tests (CBC, hepatic and renal function) and follow-up visits.

Evaluate

- Control of lethal ventricular arrhythmias
- ↓ Muscle spasm and pain
- Therapeutic serum drug levels (4–10 mcg/mL)

CHAPTER TWENTY-SEVEN

Antianginal Drugs

See also the following individual entries:

- Amyl Nitrite
- Calcium Channel Blocking Agents —See Chapter 28
- Erythrityl Tetranitrate
- Isosorbide Dinitrate
- Isosorbide Mononitrate, Oral
- Nitroglycerin IV
- Nitroglycerin Sublingual
- Nitroglycerin Sustained Release
- Nitroglycerin Topical Ointment
- Nitroglycerin Transdermal System
- Nitroglycerin Translinqual Spray
- Nitroglycerin Transmucosal
- Pentaerythritol Tetranitrate

General Statement: Angina pectoris may occur as a result of coronary atherosclerotic disease where there is an imbalance between the demand for oxygen by the myocardium and the oxygen supply (called secondary angina). The oxygen supply is compromised due to the inability of coronary blood flow to increase proportionally to increases in myocardial oxygen requirements. Angina pectoris may also result from vasospasm of large, surface coronary vessels or one of their major branches (called primary angina). In some clients, angina is due to a combination of constriction of coronary vessels and an insufficient oxygen supply.

Three groups of drugs are currently used for the treatment of angina. These agents include the nitrates/nitrites, beta-adrenergic blocking agents, and calcium channel blocking drugs. These drugs reduce the frequency and/or severity of angina by either increasing myocardial oxygen supply and/or decreasing the oxygen demand of the myocardium.

Action/Kinetics: The main mechanism of action of nitrates is to relax vascular smooth muscle by stimulating production of intracellular cyclic guanosine monophosphate. Dilation of postcapillary vessels decreases venous return to the heart due to pooling of blood; thus, LV end-diastolic pressure (preload) is reduced. Relaxation of arterioles results in a decreased systemic vascular resistance and arterial pressure (afterload). The oxygen requirements of the myocardium are also reduced. There is also a more efficient redistribution of blood flow in myocardial tissue. Reflex tachycardia may occur due to the overall decrease in BP. For nitrates, several dosage forms are available, including sublingual, topical, transdermal, parenteral, oral, and buccal. The onset and duration depend on the product and route of administration.

Uses: Treatment and prophylaxis of acute angina pectoris (use sublingual, transmucosal, or translingual nitroglycerin; amyl nitrite). Nitrates are first-line therapy for unstable angina. Prophylaxis of chronic angina pectoris (topical, transdermal, translingual, transmucosal, or oral sustained-release nitroglycerin; isosorbide dinitrate and mononitrate; erythrityl tetranitrate; pentaerythritol tetranitrate). IV nitroglycerin is used to decrease BP in surgical procedures resulting in hypertension, as well as an adjunct in treating hypertension or CHF associated with MI. *Investigational:* Nitroglycerin ointment has

been used as an adjunct in treating Raynaud's disease. Also, isosorbide dinitrate with prostaglandin E_1 for peripheral vascular disease. Sublingual and topical nitroglycerin and oral nitrates have been used to decrease cardiac workload in clients with acute MI and in CHF.
Contraindications: Sensitivity to nitrites, which may result in severe hypotensive reactions, MI, or tolerance to nitrites. Severe anemia, cerebral hemorrhage, recent head trauma, postural hypotension, closed angle glaucoma, impaired hepatic function, hypertrophic cardiomyopathy, hypotension, recent MI. PO dosage forms should not be used in clients with GI hypermotility or with malabsorption syndrome. IV nitroglycerin should not be used in clients with hypotension, uncorrected hypovolemia, inadequate cerebral circulation, constrictive pericarditis, increased ICP, or pericardial tamponade.
Special Concerns: Use with caution during lactation and in glaucoma. Tolerance to the antianginal and vascular effects may occur. Safety and efficacy have not been determined during lactation and in children.
Side Effects: *CNS:* Headaches (most common) which may be severe and persistent, restlessness, dizziness, weakness, apprehension, vertigo, anxiety, insomnia, confusion, nightmares, hypoesthesia, hypokinesia, dyscoordination. *CV:* Postural hypotension (common) with or without paradoxical bradycardia and increased angina, tachycardia, palpitations, syncope, rebound hypertension, crescendo angina, retrosternal discomfort, ***CV collapse,*** atrial fibrillation, PVCs, ***arrhythmias.*** *GI:* N&V, dyspepsia, diarrhea, dry mouth, abdominal pain, involuntary passing of feces and urine, tenesmus, tooth disorder. *Dermatologic:* Crusty skin lesions, pruritus, rash, exfoliative dermatitis, cutaneous vasodilation with flushing. *GU:* Urinary frequency, impotence, dysuria. *Respiratory:* Upper respiratory tract infection, bronchitis, pneumonia. *Allergic:* Itching, wheezing, tracheobronchitis. *Miscellaneous:* Perspiration, muscle twitching, methemoglobinemia, cold sweating, blurred vision, diplopia, ***hemolytic anemia,*** arthralgia, edema, malaise, neck stiffness, increased appetite, rigors. **Topical use:** Peripheral edema, contact dermatitis.

Tolerance can occur following chronic use. Nitrites convert hemoglobin to methemoglobin, which impairs the oxygen-carrying capacity of the blood, resulting in ***anemic hypoxia.*** This interaction is dangerous in clients with preexisting anemia.

Symptoms of Overdose (Toxicity): Severe toxicity is rarely encountered with therapeutic use. Symptoms include hypotension, flushing, tachycardia, headache, palpitations, vertigo, perspiring skin followed by cold and cyanotic skin, visual disturbances, syncope, nausea, dizziness, diaphoresis, initial hyperpnea, dyspnea and slow breathing, slow pulse, ***heart block,*** vomiting with the possibility of bloody diarrhea and colic, anorexia, and increased ICP with symptoms of confusion, moderate fever, and paralysis. Tissue hypoxia (due to methemoglobinemia) may result in ***cyanosis, metabolic acidosis, coma, seizures, and death due to CV collapse.***

Drug Interactions

Acetylcholine / Effects ↓ when used with nitrates
Alcohol, ethyl / Hypotension and CV collapse due to vasodilator effect of both agents
Antihypertensive drugs / Additive hypotension
Aspirin / ↑ Serum levels and effects of nitrates
Beta-adrenergic blocking drugs / Additive hypotension
Calcium channel blocking drugs / Additive hypotension, including significant orthostatic hypotension
Dihydroergotamine / ↑ Effect of dihydroergotamine due to increased bioavailability or antagonism resulting in ↓ antianginal effects
Heparin / Possible ↓ effect of heparin
Narcotics / Additive hypotensive effect

Phenothiazines / Additive hypotension

Sympathomimetics / ↓ Effect of nitrates; also, nitrates may ↓ effect of sympathomimetics resulting in hypotension

Laboratory Test Interferences: ↑ Urinary catecholamines. False negative ↓ in serum cholesterol.

Dosage

See individual agents.

NURSING CONSIDERATIONS

Administration/Storage

1. Nitrites and nitrates are available in a variety of dosage forms including sublingual, chewable, topical, transdermal, PO, inhalation, and parenteral. It is important to understand the appropriate use of each of these dosage forms. Changing from one brand to another should not be undertaken without consulting the provider or pharmacist as products manufactured by different companies may not be equivalent.
2. Tablets and capsules should be stored tightly closed in their original container. Avoid exposure to air, heat, and moisture.
3. Oral nitrates should be taken on an empty stomach with a glass of water.
4. Inhalation products should be used with the client either lying or sitting down.
5. Inhalation products are flammable and should not be used under situations where they might ignite.
6. *Treatment of Overdose (Toxicity):*

- Induction of emesis or gastric lavage followed by activated charcoal (nitrates are usually rapidly absorbed from the stomach). Gastric lavage may be used if the drug has been recently ingested.
- Maintain client in a recumbent shock position and keep warm. Give oxygen and artificial respiration if required.
- Methemoglobin levels should be monitored.
- Elevate the legs and administer IV fluids to treat severe hypotension and reflex tachycardia. Phenylephrine or methoxamine may also be helpful.
- Epinephrine and similar drugs are ineffective in reversing severe hypotension and should not be used to treat overdosage.

Assessment

1. Note any history of sensitivity to nitrites.
2. Document indications for therapy, type and onset of symptoms, and other agents prescribed and the outcome.
3. Assess and document location, intensity, duration, extension, and any precipitating factors surrounding client's anginal pain. Use a pain-rating scale to enable the client to report pain levels more reliably and consistently.
4. If client has a history of anemia, document and administer this category of drugs with extreme caution. Nitrates are contraindicated with elevated intracranial pressure.
5. Determine client experience with self-administered medications and note if sublingual tablets were ordered for the bedside.

Interventions

1. If hospitalized clients are instructed to keep sublingual tablets at the bedside, instruct them so that accurate records of attacks, amounts and frequency of drug use, and the extent of medication relief are noted.
2. While caring for the client in the hospital, mutually record how much drug the client requires to keep angina under control. Record:

- How frequently the drug is given
- The intensity of pain (use a rating scale 1–10 to ensure consistent reporting; have client rate pain initially and 5 min after drug administration)
- The duration of the attacks
- Whether the relief is partial or complete
- How long it takes for relief to occur
- Whether or not there are any side effects

3. Remind client to notify someone when the medication is consumed so that effectiveness can be determined.
4. Monitor BP and pulse. Assess for symptoms of sensitivity to the hypotensive effects of nitrites. These may include the presence of N&V, pallor, restlessness, and CV collapse.
5. Monitor for the presence of hypotension when clients are receiving additional drugs that may cause hypotension. Adjustment of drug dosage may be necessary. Supervise activities and ambulation until drug effects are realized.
6. Be alert for signs of tolerance, which generally occur following chronic use but may begin several days after treatment is started. This is manifested by absence of response to the usual dose. (Nitrites may be discontinued temporarily until such tolerance is lost, and then reinstituted. During the interim, other vasodilators may be ordered.)
7. Observe clients for nausea, vomiting, complaints of drowsiness, headache, or visual disturbances during long-term prophylaxis. These are prolonged effects and may require a change in medication.
8. Note change in client activity and response to the drug therapy. Determine if client experiences less discomfort when performing regular activity.

Client/Family Teaching

1. PO medications should be taken on an empty stomach.
2. Explain the drug action— decreased myocardial oxygen demand and reduced workload of the heart.
3. To prevent the occurrence of postural hypotension, take sublingual tablet while sitting or lying down. Make position changes slowly and rise only after dangling feet for several minutes.
4. Elderly clients should be encouraged to sit or lie down when taking nitroglycerin. Elderly clients are more prone to hypotensive side effects and may become dizzy and fall.
5. Brand interchange is not recommended due to differences in effectiveness between products manufactured by different companies.
6. Always carry sublingual tablets for use in aborting an attack. Observe the expiration date on the bottle, and obtain a fresh bottle or prescription when needed or every 6 months.
7. The presence of a burning sensation under the tongue attests to the potency of the drug. If there is no burning sensation, the potency may have diminished and a fresh supply should be obtained.
8. Carry sublingual tablets in a *glass* bottle, tightly capped. Keep in original container as heat, moisture, and air cause deterioration of the drug. Do not use plastic containers because drug will deteriorate in plastic; also, do not use bottles with child-proof caps since client must get to the tablets quickly.
9. If anginal pain is not relieved in 5 min by first sublingual tablet, take up to 2 more tablets at 5-min intervals. If pain has not subsided 5 min after third tablet, client should be taken to emergency room by a family member or by ambulance. Client should **not** drive.
10. Take sublingual tablets 5–15 min prior to any situation likely to cause anginal pain (e.g., climbing stairs, sexual intercourse, exposure to cold weather).
11. Advise client to maintain a record of attacks and to report any increase in the frequency and intensity of attacks and/or loss of drug effectiveness.
12. Schedule frequent rest periods, pace activities, and avoid stressful situations.
13. Follow specific instructions on how to apply topical nitroglycerin. Some practitioners prescribe removing at bedtime and then replacing upon arising. Advise that some studies support that a nitrate-free period of at least 8 hr may reduce or prevent nitrate tolerance.

14. Do not drink alcohol. Nitrite syncope, a severe shock-like state, may occur.
15. Encourage family members or significant other to learn CPR. Explain that the survival rate is greatly increased when CPR is initiated immediately.
16. Clients should be advised to wear a Medic Alert bracelet and/or carry appropriate identification and a list of prescribed drugs at all times.

Evaluate
- Clinical evidence of ↓ myocardial oxygen requirements; ↑ activity tolerance
- Improved perfusion to ischemic myocardium
- Relief of coronary artery spasm

Amyl nitrite

(AM-ill)
Pregnancy Category: X
Amyl Nitrite Aspirols, Amyl Nitrite Vaporole **(Rx)**

See also *Antianginal Drugs* Chapter 27.
How Supplied: *Solution*
Action/Kinetics: Amyl nitrite is believed to act by reducing systemic and PA pressure (afterload) and by decreasing CO due to peripheral vasodilation as opposed to causing coronary artery dilation. Vascular relaxation occurs due to stimulation of intracellular cyclic guanosine monophosphate. As an antidote to cyanide poisoning, amyl nitrite promotes formation of methemoglobin which combines with cyanide to form the nontoxic cyanmethemoglobin. **Onset (inhalation):** 30 sec. **Duration:** 3–5 min. About 33% is excreted through the kidneys.
Uses: Prophylaxis or relief of acute attacks of angina pectoris; acute cyanide poisoning. *Investigational:* Diagnostic aid to assess reserve cardiac function.

Dosage
- **Inhalation**

Angina pectoris.
Usual: 0.3 mL (1 container crushed). Usually, 1–6 inhalations from one container produces relief. Dosage may be repeated after 3–5 min.
Antidote for cyanide poisoning. Administer for 30–60 sec q 5 min until client is conscious; is then repeated at longer intervals for up to 24 hr.

Administration/Storage
1. Administer only by inhalation.
2. Containers should be protected from light and stored at a temperature of 15°C–30°C (59°F–86°F).
3. ***Amyl nitrite vapors are highly flammable. Do not use near flame or intense heat.***

Contraindication: Lactation.
Special Concerns: Use of amyl nitrite in children has not been studied. Hypotensive effects are more likely to occur in geriatric clients.

NURSING CONSIDERATIONS

See also *Nursing Considerations* for *Antianginal Drugs* Chapter 27.

Assessment
1. Take a history of common precipitating incidents that immediately precede the onset of chest pain.
2. Determine and document the degree, location, type, and duration of chest pain, and the direction in which it radiates.
3. Note and identify the presence of any cardiac risk factors.
4. Determine and document source of cyanide poisoning and presenting symptoms.

Client/Family Teaching
1. Discuss with client and family and mutually set goals of therapy.
2. Assist client to identify changes in lifestyle that may reduce the need for amyl nitrite.
3. Advise to enclose fabric-covered ampule in a handkerchief or piece of cloth and crush by hand.
4. Sit down during inhalation to avoid hypotension.
5. Drug has a pungent odor, but several deep breaths must nevertheless be taken to attain drug effects.

6. Drug is inactivated when exposed to heat.
7. Always store medication out of reach of children.
8. The medication has the potential for abuse (sexual stimulant) and must be stored appropriately.

Evaluate

- Improved tissue perfusion with termination of angina attack
- Antidote for cyanide poisoning

Erythrityl tetranitrate

(er-**RIH**-thrih-till)
Pregnancy Category: C
Cardilate **(Rx)**

See also *Antianginal Drugs,* Chapter 27.

Action/Kinetics: Sublingual: Onset, 2–5 min; maximum effect: 30–45 min. **Duration:** 1–3 hr. **PO: Onset,** 20–40 min; maximum effect: 1–1.5 hr. **Duration:** 4–6 hr. **PO, Sustained-release, onset,** Up to 4 hr; **duration:** 6–8 hr. Tolerance may develop.

Uses: Prophylaxis and chronic treatment of angina. Diffuse esophageal spasm. May improve exercise tolerance. As a vasodilator in CHF.

Dosage

- **Sublingual Tablets**

5–10 mg prior to physical or emotional stress.

- **Oral Tablets**

10 mg before each meal as well as midmorning and midafternoon. An additional dose may be given at bedtime if nocturnal anginal attacks occur. Dose may be increased to 100 mg/day if necessary (chance of headache increases).

Additional Contraindication: To treat acute attacks of angina pectoris.

Special Concerns: Dosage has not been established for children.

NURSING CONSIDERATIONS

See also *Nursing Considerations* for *Antianginal Drugs,* p Chapter 27.

Client/Family Teaching

1. Explain that all restrictions on activity cannot be removed, even though drug may permit more normal activity.
2. Sublingual tingling sensations may be relieved by placing tablet in buccal pouch.
3. Report symptoms of headaches and/or GI upset. These symptoms call for a reduction in dosage early in therapy.
4. Analgesics will be ordered for headaches if needed.

Evaluate

- ↓ Frequency and severity of anginal episodes
- Improved exercise tolerance

Isosorbide dinitrate capsules

(eye-so-**SOR**-byd)
Pregnancy Category: C

Isosorbide dinitrate chewable tablets

(eye-so-**SOR**-byd)
Pregnancy Category: C

Isosorbide dinitrate extended-release capsules

(eye-so-**SOR**-byd)
Pregnancy Category: C
Dilatrate-SR, Iso-Bid, Isordil Tembids, Isotrate Timecelles, Sorbitrate **(Rx)**

Isosorbide dinitrate extended-release tablets

(eye-so-**SOR**-byd)
Pregnancy Category: C
Cedocard-SR ✱, Coradur ✱, Isordil Tembids, Sorbitrate SA **(Rx)**

Isosorbide dinitrate sublingual tablets

(eye-so-**SOR**-byd)
Pregnancy Category: C
Apo-ISDN ✱, Coronex ✱, Isordil, Sorbitrate **(Rx)**

Isosorbide dinitrate tablets

(eye-so-**SOR**-byd)
Pregnancy Category: C
Apo-ISDN ✱, Coronex ✱, Isordil Titradose, Sorbitrate **(Rx)**

See also *Antianginal Drugs,* Chapter 27.

How Supplied: *Chew Tablet:* 5 mg, 10 mg; *Capsule, Extended Release:* 40 mg; *Tablet, Extended Release:* 40 mg; *Sublingual tablet:* 2.5 mg, 5 mg, 10 mg; *Tablet:* 2.5 mg, 5 mg, 10 mg, 20 mg, 30 mg, 40 mg

Action/Kinetics: Sublingual, chewable. Onset: 2–5 min; **duration:** 1–3 hr. **Oral Capsules/Tablets. Onset:** 15–40 min; **duration:** 4–6 hr. **Extended-release. Onset:** up to 4 hr; **duration:** 6–8 hr.

Additional Uses: Diffuse esophageal spasm. Oral tablets are only for prophylaxis while sublingual and chewable forms may be used to terminate acute attacks of angina.

Dosage

- **Capsules, Tablets**

  Antianginal.

Initial: 5–20 mg q 6 hr; **maintenance:** 5–40 mg q 6 hr (usual: 20–40 mg q.i.d.

- **Chewable Tablets**

  Antianginal, acute attack.

Initial: 5 mg q 2–3 hr.

Prophylaxis.

5–10 mg q 2–3 hr.

- **Extended-Release Capsules**

  Antianginal.

40–80 mg q 8–12 hr.

- **Extended-Release Tablets**

  Antianginal.

Initial: 40 mg; **maintenance:** 20–80 mg q 8–12 hr.

- **Sublingual**

  Acute attack.

2.5–5 mg q 2–3 hr as required.

Prophylaxis.

5–10 mg q 2–3 hr.

Special Concerns: Use with caution during lactation. Safety and efficacy have not been established in children.

Additional Side Effect: Vascular headaches occur especially frequently.

Additional Drug Interactions

Acetylcholine / Isosorbide antagonizes the effect of acetylcholine

Norepinephrine / Isosorbide antagonizes the effect of norepinephrine

NURSING CONSIDERATIONS

See also *Nursing Considerations* for *Antianginal Drugs,* Chapter 27.

Client/Family Teaching

1. Administer with meals to eliminate or reduce headaches; otherwise, take on an empty stomach to facilitate absorption.
2. None of the products should be crushed or chewed, unless specifically ordered.
3. Review appropriate method for administration. Remind client not to chew sublingual tablets.
4. Stress that chewable tablets should be held in the mouth for 1–2 min to allow for absorption through the buccal membranes.
5. Avoid alcohol or alcohol-containing products.
6. Acetaminophen may assist to relieve drug-induced headaches.
7. Identify symptoms that require medical intervention.

Evaluate

- ↓ Frequency and severity of anginal attacks
- ↑ Exercise tolerance
- Resolution of esophageal spasm

Isosorbide mononitrate, oral

(eye-so-**SOR**-byd)

Pregnancy Category: C

Imdur, ISMO, Monoket **(Rx)**

See also *Antianginal Drugs* and *Isosorbide Dinitrate,* Chapter 27.

How Supplied: *Tablet:* 10 mg, 20 mg

Action/Kinetics: Isosorbide mononitrate is the major metabolite of isosorbide dinitrate. The mononitrate is not subject to first-pass metabolism. Bioavailability is nearly 100%. **Onset:** 30–60 min. **t½:** About 5 hr.

Uses: Prophylaxis of angina pectoris.

Dosage

IMDUR TABLETS

Prophylaxis of angina.
Initial: 30 mg (given as one-half of the 60-mg tablet) or 60 mg once daily; **then,** dosage may be increased to 120 mg given as 2–60-mg tablets once daily. Rarely, 240 mg daily may be needed.
ISMO, MONOKET TABLETS
Prevention and treatment of angina.
Adults: 20 mg b.i.d. with the doses 7 hr apart (it is preferable that first dose be given on awakening). An initial dose of 5 mg may be best for clients of small stature; the dose should then be increased to at least 10 mg by the second or third day of therapy.
Administration/Storage
1. The treatment regimen provided minimizes the development of refractory tolerance.
2. The extended release tablet should be given in the morning on arising. These tablets should not be crushed or chewed. They should be taken with a half glass of water.
3. *Treatment of Overdose:* Therapy should be directed toward an increase in central fluid volume. Vasoconstrictors should *not* be used.
Contraindication: To abort acute anginal attacks. Use in acute MI or CHF.
Special Concerns: Use with caution in clients who may be volume depleted or who are already hypotensive. Use with caution during lactation. Safety and effectiveness have not been determined in children. The benefits have not been established in acute MI or CHF.
Side Effects: *CV:* Hypotension (may be accompanied by paradoxical bradycardia and increased angina pectoris). *CNS:* Headache, lightheadedness, dizziness. *GI:* N&V. *Miscellaneous:* Possibility of methemoglobinemia.
Symptoms of Overdose: Increased intracranial pressure manifested by throbbing headache, confusion, moderate fever. Also, vertigo, palpitations, visual disturbances, N&V, syncope, air hunger, dyspnea (followed by reduced ventilatory effort), diaphoresis, skin either flushed or cold and clammy, heart block, bradycardia, paralysis, ***coma, seizures, death.***
Drug Interactions
Ethanol / Additive vasodilation
Calcium channel blockers / Severe orthostatic hypotension
Organic nitrates / Severe orthostatic hypotension

NURSING CONSIDERATIONS

See also *Nursing Considerations* for *Antianginal Drugs* and *Isosorbide Dinitrate,* Chapter 27.
Interventions
1. Determine that the client is adequately hydrated.
2. Ensure that SBP > 100 as drug may cause marked hypotension.
Evaluate: Desired prophylaxis of angina pectoris.

Nitroglycerin IV

(nye-troh-**GLIH**-sir-in)
Pregnancy Category: C
Nitro-Bid IV, Nitroglycerin in 5% Dextrose, Tridil **(Rx)**

See also *Antianginal Drugs,* Chapter 27.
How Supplied: *Injection:* 5 mg/mL
Action/Kinetics: Onset: 1–2 min; **duration:** 3–5 min (dose-dependent).
Uses: Hypertension associated with surgery (e.g., associated with ET intubation, skin incision, sternotomy, anesthesia, cardiac bypass, immediate postsurgical period). CHF associated with acute MI. Angina unresponsive to usual doses of organic nitrate or beta-adrenergic blocking agents. Cardiac-load reducing agent. Produce controlled hypotension during surgical procedures.

Dosage

- **IV infusion only**

Initial: 5 mcg/min delivered by precise infusion pump. May be increased by 5 mcg/min q 3–5 min until response is seen. If no response seen at 20 mcg/min, dose can be increased by 10–20 mcg/min until response noted. Monitor titration continuously until client reaches desired level of response.

Administration/Storage
1. Dilute with 5% dextrose USP, or 0.9% sodium chloride injection. Nitroglycerin injection is not for direct IV use; it must first be diluted.
2. Use only a glass IV bottle and administration set provided by the manufacturer because nitroglycerin is readily adsorbed onto many plastics. Avoid adding unnecessary plastic to IV system.
3. Aspirate medication into a syringe and then inject immediately into a glass bottle (or polyolefin bottle) to minimize contact with plastic.
4. Do not administer with any other medications in the IV system.
5. Do not interrupt IV nitroglycerin for administration of a bolus of any other medication.
6. To provide correct dosage, remove 15 mL of solution from the IV tubing if concentration of solution is changed.
7. Administer IV solution with an electronic infusion device (volumetric) and in a closely monitored environment.
8. Have emergency drugs readily available.

Special Concerns: Dosage has not been established in children.

NURSING CONSIDERATIONS

See also *Nursing Considerations* for *Antianginal Drugs,* Chapter 27.

Interventions
1. Obtain written parameters for BP and pulse and monitor closely throughout drug therapy.
2. Be prepared to monitor CVP and/or PA pressure as ordered.
3. Monitor VS. Note any evidence of hypotension, client complaint of nausea, sweating, and/or vomiting. Document presence of tachycardia or bradycardia. These symptoms may indicate that the dosage of drug is more than the client can tolerate.
• Elevate the legs to restore BP.
• Be prepared to reduce the rate of flow of the solution or to administer additional IV fluids.
4. Assess for thrombophlebitis at the IV site. Remove the IV from the reddened area.
5. Anticipate that after the initial positive response to therapy the dosage increments will be smaller. Adjustments in dosage will also be made at longer intervals.
6. Sinus tachycardia may occur in a client with angina pectoris who is receiving a maintenance dose of nitroglycerin (HR of 80 beats/min or less reduces myocardial demand).
7. Check that topical, PO, or sublingual doses are adjusted if client is on concomitant therapy with IV nitroglycerin.
8. Anticipate that client will be weaned from IV nitroglycerin by gradually decreasing doses to avoid posttherapy or CV distress. Tapering off is usually initiated when the client is receiving the peak effect from PO or topical vasodilators. The IV flow is usually reduced, and the client is monitored for hypertension and angina, which would require increased titration.
9. Obtain as needed order for a nonnarcotic analgesic (usually acetaminophen) because headache is a common side effect of drug therapy.

Evaluate
• Resolution or control of angina
• ↓ BP
• Improvement in S&S of CHF (↑ output, ↓ rales, ↓ CVP)
• ↑ Activity tolerance

Nitroglycerin sublingual

(nye-troh-**GLIH**-sir-in)
Pregnancy Category: C
Nitrostat **(Rx)**

See also *Antianginal Drugs,* Chapter 27.

How Supplied: *Tablet:* 0.3 mg, 0.4 mg, 0.6 mg

Action/Kinetics: Sublingual. Onset: 1–3 min; **duration:** 30–60 min.

Uses: Agents of choice for prophylaxis and treatment of angina pectoris.

Dosage

- **Sublingual Tablets**

150–600 mcg under the tongue or in the buccal pouch at first sign of attack; may be repeated in 5 min if necessary (no more than 3 tablets should be taken within 15 min). For prophylaxis, tablets may be taken 5–10 min prior to activities that may precipitate an attack.

Administration/Storage

1. Sublingual tablets should be placed under the tongue and allowed to dissolve; they should not be swallowed.
2. Sublingual tablets should be stored in the original container at room temperature protected from moisture. Unused tablets should be discarded if 6 months has elapsed since the original container was opened.

Special Concerns: Dosage has not been established in children.

NURSING CONSIDERATIONS

See also *Nursing Considerations* for *Antianginal Drugs,* Chapter 27.

Client/Family Teaching

1. Instruct to date sublingual container upon opening.
2. Advise to report immediately if pain is not controlled.

Evaluate

- Angina prophylaxis prior to strenuous activities
- Termination of anginal attack

Nitroglycerin sustained-release capsules

(nye-troh-**GLIH**-sir-in)
Pregnancy Category: C
Nitro-Bid Plateau Caps, Nitrocine Timecaps, Nitroglyn **(Rx)**

Nitroglycerin sustained-release tablets

(nye-troh-**GLIH**-sir-in)
Pregnancy Category: C
Nitrogard-SR ✱, Nitrong, Nitrong SR ✱ **(Rx)**

See also *Antianginal Drugs,* Chapter 27.

How Supplied: Nitroclycerin sustained-release capsules: *Capsule, Extended Release:* 2.5 mg, 6.5 mg, 9 mg.
Nitroglycerin sustained-release tablets: *Tablet, Extended Release:* 2.6 mg, 6.5 mg

Action/Kinetics: Sustained-release: Onset: 20–45 min; **duration:** 3–8 hr.

Uses: To prevent anginal attacks. "Possibly effective" for the prophylaxis or treatment of anginal attacks.

Dosage

- **Sustained-Release Capsules**

2.5, 6.5, or 9 mg q 8–12 hr.

- **Sustained-Release Tablets**

1.3, 2.6, or 6.5 mg q 8–12 hr.

Administration/Storage

1. Sustained-release tablets and capsules should not be chewed and are not intended for sublingual use.
2. The smallest effective dose should be given 2–4 times/day.
3. Tolerance may develop.

Special Concerns: Dosage has not been established in children.

NURSING CONSIDERATIONS

See also *Nursing Considerations* for *Antianginal Drugs,* Chapter 27.

Evaluate: Desired angina prophylaxis.

Nitroglycerin topical ointment

(nye-troh-**GLIH**-sir-in)
Pregnancy Category: C
Nitro-Bid, Nitrol, Nitrol TSAR Kit ✱, Nitrong ✱ **(Rx)**

See also *Antianginal Drugs,* Chapter 27.

How Supplied: *Ointment:* 2%

Action/Kinetics: Onset: 30–60 min; **duration:** 2–12 hr (depending on amount used per unit of surface area).

Uses: Prophylaxis and treatment of angina pectoris.

Dosage

- **Topical ointment (2%)**

1–2 in. (15–30 mg) q 8 hr [up to 5 in. (75 mg) q 4 hr may be necessary]. One inch equals approximately 15 mg nitroglycerin. Determine optimum dosage by starting with ½ in./8 hr and increasing by ½ in. with each successive dose until headache occurs; then, decrease to largest dose that does not cause headache. When ending treatment, reduce both the dose and frequency of administration over 4–6 weeks to prevent sudden withdrawal reactions.

Administration/Storage

1. Squeeze ointment carefully onto dose-measuring application papers, which are packaged with the medicine. Use applicator to spread ointment or fold paper in half and rub back and forth.
2. Use the paper to spread the ointment onto a nonhairy area of skin. Many clients find application to the chest psychologically helpful, but ointment may be applied to other nonhairy areas.
3. Rotate sites to prevent irritation. Keep a record of areas used to avoid unnecessary repetitive use of sites.
4. Apply ointment in a thin, even layer covering an area of skin 5–6 in. in diameter. Remember to remove last dose.
5. Tape the application paper over the area, or cover the area with a piece of plastic wrap-type material. A clear plastic cover causes less leakage of ointment, decreases skin irritation, increases the amount absorbed, and prevents clothing stains. Date, time, and initial tape at site.
6. Once the dose is established, use the same type of covering to ensure that the same amount of drug is absorbed during each application.
7. Clean around tube opening and tightly cap tube after use.
8. To prevent systemic absorption into nurse's system, the nurse should protect her own skin from contact with the ointment. Wash hands thoroughly after application to prevent headache.
9. Remove at bedtime or as directed to prevent tolerance or loss of drug effect. Remember to reapply upon awakening the next morning.

Special Concerns: Dosage has not been established in children.

NURSING CONSIDERATIONS

See also *Nursing Considerations* for *Antianginal Drugs,* Chapter 27.

Evaluate: Termination and prevention of acute anginal episodes.

Nitroglycerin transdermal system

(nye-troh-**GLIH**-sir-in)

Pregnancy Category: C

Deponit 0.2 mg/hr and 0.4 mg/hr; Minitran 0.1 mg/hr, 0.2 mg/hr, 0.4 mg/hr, and 0.6 mg/hr; Nitrocine 0.6 mg/hr; Nitrodisc 0.2 mg/hr, 0.3 mg/hr, and 0.4 mg/hr; Nitro-Dur 0.1 mg/hr, 0.2 mg/hr, 0.3 mg/hr, 0.4 mg/hr, 0.6 mg/hr, and 0.8 mg/hr; Transderm-Nitro 0.1 mg/hr, 0.2 mg/hr, 0.4 mg/hr, and 0.6 mg/hr **(Rx)**

See also *Antianginal Drugs,* Chapter 27.

How Supplied: *Film, Extended Release:* 0.1 mg/hr, 0.2 mg/hr, 0.3 mg/hr, 0.4 mg/hr, 0.6 mg/hr, 0.8 mg/hr

Action/Kinetics: **Onset:** 30–60 min; **duration:** 8–24 hr. The amount released each hour is indicated in the name.

Use: Prophylaxis of angina pectoris due to CAD. *NOTE:* There is some evidence that nitroglycerin patches stop preterm labor.

Dosage

• **Topical Patch**

Initial: 0.2–0.4 mg/hr (initially the smallest available dose in the dosage series) applied each day to skin site free of hair and free of excessive movement (e.g., chest, upper arm).

Maintenance: Additional systems or strengths may be added depending on the clinical response.

Administration/Storage

1. Follow instructions for specific products on package insert.

2. To avoid skin irritation, the application site should be slightly different each day.
3. Do not apply to distal areas of extremities.
4. If the pad loosens, apply a new pad.
5. It is important to note that there is a wide variety between clients in the actual amount of nitroglycerin absorbed each day. Physical exercise and increased ambient temperatures may increase the amount absorbed.
6. When terminating therapy, the dose and frequency of application should be gradually reduced over 4–6 weeks.
7. Tolerance is a significant factor affecting efficacy if the system is used continuously for more than 12 hr/day. Thus, a dosage regimen would include a daily period where the patch is on for 12–14 hr and a period of 10–12 hr when the patch is off.
8. Remove patch before defibrillating as patch may explode.

Special Concerns: Dosage has not been established in children.

NURSING CONSIDERATIONS

See also *Nursing Considerations* for *Antianginal Drugs,* Chapter 27.

Client/Family Teaching

1. Apply only as directed. Make sure skin is completely dry before applying.
2. Remember to remove old pad and rotate sites of application.
3. Date patch as a reminder that drug has been administered.
4. Once applied, do not disturb or open patch.
5. Remove at bedtime or as directed to prevent a diminished response (tolerance) to the drug. Remember to reapply a new system upon awakening the next morning.
6. Bathing or swimming should not interfere with therapy.
7. Do not stop therapy abruptly.

Evaluate: Control and prevention of anginal episodes.

Nitroglycerin translingual spray

(nye-troh-**GLIH**-sir-in)
Pregnancy Category: C
Nitrolingual **(Rx)**

See also *Antianginal Drugs,* Chapter 27.

How Supplied: *Spray:* 0.4 mg/Spray

Action/Kinetics: Onset: 2–4 min; **duration:** 30–60 min.

Uses: Coronary artery disease to relieve an acute attack or used prophylactically 10–15 min before beginning activities that can cause an acute anginal attack.

Dosage

- **Spray**

Termination of acute attack.

One to two metered doses (400–800 mcg) on or under the tongue q 5 min as needed; no more than three metered doses should be administered within a 15-min period.

Prophylaxis.

One to two metered doses 5–10 min before beginning activities that might precipitate an acute attack.

Administration/Storage

1. The spray should *not* be inhaled.
2. Immediate medical attention should be sought if chest pain persists.

Special Concerns: Dosage has not been established in children.

NURSING CONSIDERATIONS

See also *Nursing Considerations* for *Antianginal Drugs,* Chapter 27.

Evaluate: Control and prevention of acute anginal episodes.

Nitroglycerin transmucosal

(nye-troh-**GLIH**-sir-in)
Pregnancy Category: C
Nitrogard, Nitrogard-SR ✱ **(Rx)**

See also *Antianginal Drugs,* Chapter 27.

How Supplied: *Tablet:* 1 mg, 2 mg, 3 mg

Action/Kinetics: Onset: 3 min; **duration:** 3–5 hr.

Uses: Treatment and prophylaxis of angina.

Dosage

Initial: 1 mg q 3–5 hr during time client is awake. Dose may be increased if necessary.

Administration/Storage

1. Tablet should be placed either between the lip and gum above the upper incisors or between the gum and cheek in the buccal area.
2. Allow tablet to dissolve in the mouth. The client should be warned not to swallow the tablet.
3. From 3 to 5 hr is required for tablet dissolution.
4. Store properly to maintain potency.
• Do not expose to light, heat, or air.
• Keep in a tightly closed container below 30°C (86°F).
• *Do not* keep cotton in the container once the bottle has been opened.

Special Concerns: Dosage has not been established in children.

NURSING CONSIDERATIONS

See also *Nursing Considerations* for *Antianginal Drugs,* Chapter 27.

Client/Family Teaching

1. Demonstrate and review the appropriate method for buccal administration and proper storage of medication.
2. Stress that proper storage is imperative to maintain potency.
3. Instruct not to chew or swallow tablet and to expect 3–5 hr for complete dissolution.
4. Advise that drinking hot liquids or touching tablet with tongue will increase the rate of dissolution.

Evaluate: ↓ Frequency and ↓ intensity of anginal episodes.

Pentaerythritol tetranitrate sustained-release capsules

(pen-tah-er-**ITH**-rih-toll)
Pregnancy Category: C
Duotrate, Duotrate 45 **(Rx)**

Pentaerythritol tetranitrate sustained-release tablets

(pen-tah-er-**ITH**-rih-toll)
Pregnancy Category: C
Peritrate SA **(Rx)**

Pentaerythritol tetranitrate tablets

(pen-tah-er-**ITH**-rih-toll)
Pregnancy Category: C
Pentylan, Peritrate, Peritrate Forte ✱ **(Rx)**

See also *Antianginal Drugs,* Chapter 27.

How Supplied: *Capsule, Extended Release:* 45 mg

Action/Kinetics: Onset, Tablets: 20–60 min; **Sustained-release Capsules/Tablets:** 30 min. **Duration, Tablets:** 4–6 hr; **Sustained-release Capsules/Tablets:** 12 hr. Excreted in urine and feces.

Use: Prophylaxis of anginal attacks but is not to be used to terminate acute attacks.

Dosage

• **Tablets**

Initial: 10–20 mg t.i.d.–q.i.d.; **then,** up to 40 mg q.i.d.

• **Sustained-Release Capsules or Tablets**

1 capsule or tablet (30, 45, or 80 mg) q 12 hr.

Special Concerns: Dosage has not been established in children.

Additional Side Effects: Severe rash, exfoliative dermatitis.

Additional Drug Interactions

Acetylcholine / Pentaerythritol antagonizes the effect of acetylcholine
Norepinephrine / Pentaerythritol antagonizes the effect of norepinephrine

NURSING CONSIDERATIONS

See also *Nursing Considerations* for *Antianginal Drugs,* Chapter 27.

Client/Family Teaching

1. Drug is to be taken 30 min before or 1 hr after meals, as well as at bedtime. Sustained-release tablets are to be taken on an empty stomach and are not to be chewed or crushed.
2. Take only as directed and report any rash or bothersome side effects.
3. Remind client that this product is not for acute anginal attacks and advise to use other nitrates specifically prescribed in this event.

Evaluate: ↓ Frequency and severity of anginal attacks.

CHAPTER TWENTY-EIGHT

Antihypertensive Drugs

See also the following drug classes and individual drugs:

Agents Acting Directly on Vascular Smooth Muscle

Diazoxide IV
Hydralazine Hydrochloride
Nitroprusside Sodium

Alpha-1-Adrenergic Blocking Agents

Doxazosin Mesylate
Prazosin Hydrochloride
Terazosin

Angiotensin-Converting Enzyme Inhibitors

Benazepril Hydrochloride
Captopril
Enalapril Maleate
Fosinopril Sodium
Lisinopril
Quinapril Hydrochloride
Ramipril

Beta-Adrenergic Blocking Agents - See Chapter 51

Calcium Channel Blocking Agents

Amlodipine
Bepridil Hydrochloride
Diltiazem Hydrochloride
Felodipine
Isradipine
Nicardipine Hydrochloride
Nifedipine
Nimodipine
Verapamil

Centrally-Acting Agents

Clonidine Hydrochloride
Guanabenz Acetate
Guanfacine Hydrochloride
Methyldopa
Methyldopate Hydrochloride

Combination Drugs Used for Hypertension

Amiloride and Hydrochlorothiazide
Bisoprolol fumarate and Hydrochlorothiazide
Enalapril Maleate and Hydrochlorothiazide
Lisinopril and Hydrochlorothiazide
Methyldopa and Hydrochlorothiazide
Propranolol and Hydrochlorothiazide
Reserpine and Chlorothiazide
Reserpine, Hydralazine, and Hydrochlorothiazide
Spironolactone and Hydrochlorothiazide
Triamterene and Hydrochlorothiazide

Peripherally-Acting Agents

Guanadrel Sulfate
Guanethidine Sulfate
Phenoxybenzamine Hydrochloride—See Chapter 51
Phentolamine Mesylate—See Chapter 51

Miscellaneous Agents

Labetalol Hydrochloride
Mecamylamine Hydrochloride
Minoxidil, Oral

General Statement: Hypertension is a condition in which the mean arterial BP is elevated. It is one of the most widespread chronic conditions for which medication is prescribed and taken on a regular basis. Most cases of hypertension are of unknown etiology and result from a generalized increase in resistance to flow in the peripheral vessels (arterioles). Such cases are known as primary or essential hypertension. Treatment of essential hypertension is aimed at reducing BP to normal or near-normal levels, because this is believed to prevent or halt the slow, albeit permanent, damage caused by constant excess pressure.

Essential hypertension is commonly classified according to its severity as stage 1 (mild: systolic BP, 140–159 mm Hg; diastolic BP: 90–99 mm Hg), stage 2 (moderate: systolic BP, 160–179 mm Hg; diastolic BP: 100–109 mm Hg), stage 3 (severe: systolic BP, 180–209 mm Hg; diastolic BP: 110–119 mm Hg), or stage 4 (very severe: systolic BP, over 210 mm Hg; diastolic BP: over 120 mm Hg). Moderate or severe (malignant) hypertension can result in degenerative changes in the brain, heart, and kidneys and can be fatal.

Other types of hypertension (secondary hypertension) have a known etiology and can result from a complication of pregnancy (toxemic hypertension) or certain other diseases that cause impairment of kidney function. It can also be caused by a tumor of the adrenal gland (pheochromocytoma) or by blockage of certain arteries leading into the kidney (renal hypertension). The latter two cases can be corrected by surgery.

Most pharmacologic agents used to treat hypertension lower BP by relaxing the constricted arterioles leading to a decrease in the resistance to peripheral blood flow. These drugs exert this effect by decreasing the influence of the sympathetic nervous system on smooth muscle of arterioles, by directly relaxing arteriolar smooth muscle, or by acting on the centers in the brain that control BP.

Antihypertensive drug therapy is usually initiated when diastolic BP is greater than 90 mm Hg. Treatment of hypertension involves a stepped-care approach. The first step is life-style modifications that include weight reduction, reduction of sodium intake, regular exercise, cessation of smoking, and moderate alcohol intake. If these steps are not effective, step II approaches may be initiated that include continuation of life-style modifications and initiation of a diuretic or beta-adrenergic blocking agent (drugs from either group are preferred due to a decrease in morbidity and mortality). Other drugs that may be used include ACE inhibitors, calcium channel blockers, alpha-1 blockers, and an alpha-beta blocker. Step III therapy is initiated when there is inadequate response to step II approaches and includes increasing the drug dose, substituting another drug, or adding a second agent from a different drug class. Step IV therapy is initiated when step III therapy is inadequate; step IV therapy includes adding a second or third agent or diuretic (if not already prescribed). Supplemental antihypertensive drugs include clonidine, guanabenz, guanfacine, methyldopa, guanadrel, guanethidine, rauwolfia alkaloids, hydralazine, minoxidil.

Attempts should be made to decrease the dosage or number of antihypertensive drugs (step-down therapy) while maintaining life-style modifications. Step-down therapy may be tried if the client has been controlled effectively for 1 year or at least four visits to the physician. It should be noted that an antihypertensive drug withdrawal syndrome may occur after discontinuation of antihypertensives. The syndrome is due to catecholamine excess and may or may not include a rapid rise in BP; symptoms include nervousness, agitation, tremors, palpitations, insomnia, sweating, flushing, headache, N&V. Rarely, malignant hypertension, MI, angina, and cardiac arrhythmias may be seen. To prevent such problems, client compliance should be stressed and excessive doses and combining beta blockers with sympatholytics avoided. If the medication is to be discontinued, the dose should be tapered slowly, one drug at a time, with special caution taken in clients with coronary artery or cerebrovascular disease.

NURSING CONSIDERATIONS

Assessment

1. Obtain a complete nursing history and include any family history of hy-

pertension, stroke, CVD, CHD, dyslipidemia, and diabetes.
2. Determine baseline BP before starting any antihypertensive therapy. To ensure accuracy of baseline readings, take BP in both arms (lying, standing, and sitting) at least three times during one visit and on two subsequent visits.
3. Evaluate the extent of client's understanding of the disease of hypertension and the therapy as prescribed.
4. Ascertain life-style modifications (in the area of weight reduction, moderation of alcohol intake, obtaining regular physical activity, reduction of sodium intake, and smoking cessation) clients may have to make in order to achieve the goal of lowered BP.
5. Assess the probability of the client's willingness to adhere to prescribed therapy.
6. Determine client's ability to take own BP measurements.
7. Ensure that baseline electrolytes, fasting blood sugar, CBC, uric acid, urinalysis, and liver and renal function studies have been performed.
8. During complete PE include funduscopic and neurologic exam and note findings.
9. Assess for any thyroid enlargement.

Client/Family Teaching

1. Discuss goals of drug therapy in the management of hypertension and the goal of preventing CVD.
2. Instruct that medication controls but does not cure hypertension. Remind client to take medication despite feeling better and not to stop abruptly as rebound hypertension may occur.
3. Explain the importance of adhering to the treatment plan as prescribed. Review the importance of exercise, proper diet, and rest, and of complying with the prescribed drug therapy.
4. Teach clients and a family member how and when to take BP recordings. Explain the importance of keeping a written record to share with the health care provider so that prescribed therapy may be evaluated at each visit.
5. Adhere to a low-sodium, low-fat diet; obtain dietitian assistance in meal planning as needed.
6. Teach the client and family how to monitor fluid I&O and weights accurately. Advise to keep a record for review and to report any overt changes.
7. Discuss the expected drug responses and the toxic side effects of prescribed drugs. Report these symptoms immediately.
8. Explain that weakness, dizziness, and fainting may occur with rapid changes of position from supine to standing. Advise to rise slowly from a lying or sitting position and to dangle legs for several minutes before standing to minimize the occurrence of orthostatic hypotension.
9. If clients accidentally miss a dose of medication and if it is remembered at the time of the next dose of drug, they should not double up or take two doses close together.
10. Stress the importance of routine eye exams to detect early retinal changes.
11. Avoid the concomitant use of other medications that could lower BP (e.g., alcohol, barbiturates, CNS depressants) or that could elevate BP (e.g., OTC cold remedies, oral contraceptives, steroids, NSAIDs, appetite suppressants, tricyclic antidepressants, MAO inhibitors).
12. Avoid any OTC medications, especially cold remedies, without first consulting the physician or pharmacist. Sympathomimetic amines in products used to treat asthma, colds, and allergies are to be used with extreme caution.
13. Advise that exercising in hot weather may enhance the occurrence of hypotensive effects.
14. Avoid excessive amounts of caffeine (tea, coffee, chocolate, or colas).
15. Advise client if sexual dysfunction occurs to notify provider as medica-

tion can usually be changed to minimize symptoms.
16. Emphasize the importance and review additional holistic interventions and life-style modifications for BP control, some of which may include dietary restrictions of fat and sodium, weight reduction, decreased use of alcohol, discontinuation of tobacco products, increased physical activity, regular exercise programs (help identify ones with which the client may feel comfortable), and methods to reduce and deal with stress.

Evaluate

• Knowledge and understanding of illness and evidence of compliance with prescribed therapy
• Evidence of a consistent ↓ in BP to within desired range (SBP<140 and DBP<90)
• Evidence of ↓ weight, if on a reducing diet
• Freedom from complications/side effects of drug therapy

AGENTS ACTING DIRECTLY ON VASCULAR SMOOTH MUSCLE

See the following individual entries:

Diazoxide IV
Hydralazine Hydrochloride
Nitroprusside Sodium

Diazoxide IV

(dye-az-**OX**-eyed)
Pregnancy Category: C
Hyperstat IV **(Rx)**

How Supplied: *Injection:* 15 mg/mL

Action/Kinetics: Diazoxide is thought to exert a direct action on vascular smooth muscle to cause arteriolar vasodilation and decreased peripheral resistance. **Onset:** 1–5 min. **Time to peak effect:** 2–5 min. **Duration** (variable): usual, 3–12 hr. Excreted through the kidney (50% unchanged).

Uses: May be the drug of choice for hypertensive crisis (malignant and nonmalignant hypertension). Often given concomitantly with a diuretic. Especially suitable for clients with impaired renal function, hypertensive encephalopathy, hypertension complicated by LV failure, and eclampsia. Ineffective for hypertension due to pheochromocytoma.

Dosage

• **IV push (30 sec or less)**
Hypertensive crisis.

Adults: 1–3 mg/kg up to a maximum of 150 mg; may be repeated at 5–15-min intervals until adequate BP response obtained. Drug may then be repeated at 4–24-hr intervals for 4–5 days or until oral antihypertensive therapy can be initiated. **Pediatric:** 1–3 mg/kg (30–90 mg/m^2) using the same dosing intervals as adults.

Administration/Storage

1. Do not administer IM or SC. Medication is highly alkaline.
2. Ensure patency and inject rapidly (30 sec) undiluted into a peripheral vein to maximize response.
3. Assess site for signs of irritation or extravasation. If extravasation should occur, apply ice packs.
4. Protect from light, heat, and freezing.
5. Have a sympathomimetic drug, such as norepinephrine, available to treat severe hypotension should it occur.
6. *Treatment of Overdose:* Use the Trendelenburg maneuver to reverse hypotension.

Contraindications: Hypersensitivity to drug or thiazide diuretics.

Special Concerns: A decrease in dose may be necessary in geriatric clients due to age-related decreases in renal function.

Laboratory Test Interference: False + or ↑ uric acid.

Side Effects: *CV:* Hypotension (may be severe), sodium and water retention, ***arrhythmias, cerebral or myocardial ischemia,*** palpitations, bradycardia. *CNS:* Headache, dizziness, drowsiness, lightheadedness. Confusion, ***seizures,*** paralysis, unconsciousness, numbness (all due to cerebral ischemia). *Respiratory:* Tightness in chest, cough, dyspnea, sensation of choking. *GI:* N&V, diarrhea, anorexia, parotid swelling, change in sense of taste, salivation, dry mouth, ileus, constipation. *Other:* Hyperglycemia (may be serious enough to require treatment), sweating, flushing, sensation of warmth, tinnitus, hearing loss, retention of nitrogenous wastes, acute pancreatitis. Pain, cellulitis, phlebitis at injection site.

Symptoms of Overdose: Hypotension, excessive hyperglycemia.

Drug Interactions

Anticoagulants, oral / ↑ Effect of oral anticoagulants due to ↓ plasma protein binding
Nitrites / ↑ Hypotensive effect
Phenytoin / Diazoxide ↓ anticonvulsant effect of phenytoin
Reserpine / ↑ Hypotensive effect
Thiazide diuretics / ↑ Hyperglycemic, hyperuricemic, and antihypertensive effect of diazoxide
Vasodilators, peripheral / ↑ Hypotensive effect

NURSING CONSIDERATIONS

See also *Nursing Considerations* for *Antihypertensive Agents,* Chapter 28 and *Diazoxide oral,* Chapter 65.

Assessment

1. Note client history for hypersensitivity to thiazide diuretics, sulfa drugs, or diazoxide.
2. Particularly note if client has diabetes mellitus. Diazoxide can cause serious elevations in blood sugar levels.
3. Obtain uric acid level and assess for evidence of hyperuricemia.

Interventions

1. Monitor BP frequently until it has stabilized and then every hour thereafter until hypertensive crisis is resolved. Obtain final BP upon arising, prior to ambulation.
2. Explain to client the need to remain in a recumbent position during and for 30 min after injection to avoid orthostatic hypotension.
3. Maintain the client in a recumbent position for 8–10 hr if furosemide is administered as part of the therapy.
4. Note client complaints of sweating, flushing, or evidence of hyperglycemia and be prepared to treat.

Evaluate: Significant reduction in BP during hypertensive crisis.

Hydralazine hydrochloride

(hy-**DRAL**-ah-zeen)
Pregnancy Category: C
Apo-Hydralazine ✱, Apresoline, Novo-Hylazin ✱, Nu-Hydral ✱ **(Rx)**

How Supplied: *Injection:* 20 mg/mL; *Tablet:* 10 mg, 25 mg, 50 mg, 100 mg

Action/Kinetics: Exerts a direct vasodilating effect on vascular smooth muscle. The drug also alters cellular calcium metabolism that interferes with calcium movement within the vascular smooth muscle responsible for initiating or maintaining contraction. Hydralazine preferentially dilates arterioles compared with veins; this minimizes postural hypotension and increases CO. The drug increases renin activity in the kidney leading to an increase in angiotensin II, which then causes stimulation of aldosterone and thus sodium reabsorption. Because there is a reflex increase in cardiac function, hydralazine is commonly used with drugs that inhibit sympathetic activity (e.g., beta blockers, clonidine, methyldopa). The drug is rapdily absorbed after PO use. Food increases bioavailability of the drug. **PO: Onset,** 45 min; **peak plasma level:** 1–2 hr; **duration:** 3–8 hr. **$t^{1}/_{2}$:** 3–7 hr. **IM: Onset,** 10–30 min; **peak plasma level:** 1 hr; **duration:** 2–4 hr. **IV: Onset,** 10–20 min; **maximum effect:** 10–80 min; **duration:** 2–4 hr. Metabolized in the liver and excreted through the kidney (2%–5% unchanged after PO use and 11%–14% unchanged after IV administration).

Uses: *PO:* In combination with other drugs for essential hypertension. *Parenteral:* Severe essential hypertension when PO use is not possible or when there is an urgent need to lower BP. Hydralazine is the drug of choice for eclampsia. *Investigational:* To reduce afterload in CHF, severe aortic insufficiency, and after valve replacement.

Dosage

- **Tablets**

Hypertension.

Adult, initial: 10 mg q.i.d for 2–4 days; **then,** increase to 25 mg q.i.d. for rest of first week. For second and following weeks, increase to 50 mg q.i.d. **Maintenance:** individualized to lowest effective dose; maximum daily dose should not exceed 300 mg. **Pediatric, initial:** 0.75 mg/kg/day (25 mg/m^2/day) in two to four divided doses; dosage may be increased gradually up to 7.5 mg/kg/day (or 300 mg/day). Food increases the bioavailability of the drug.

- **IV, IM**

Hypertensive crisis.

Adults, usual: 20–40 mg, repeated as necessary. BP may fall within 5–10 min, with maximum response in 10–80 min. Usually switch to PO medication in 1–2 days. Dosage should be decreased in clients with renal damage. **Pediatric:** 0.1–0.2 mg/kg q 4–6 hr as needed.

Eclampsia.

5–10 mg q 20 min as an IV bolus. If no effect after 20 mg, another drug should be tried.

Administration/Storage

1. Parenteral injections should be made as quickly as possible after being drawn into the syringe. Administer undiluted at a rate of 10 mg over at least 1 min.
2. The presence of a metal filter will cause a change in color of hydralazine.
3. The liquid formulation for parenteral use has been withdrawn from the market, although limited supplies may be available for emergency situations. A lyophilized formulation of the drug is being developed.
4. To enhance bioavailability, the tablets should be taken with food.
5. *Treatment of Overdose:* If the CV status is stable, induce vomiting or perform gastric lavage followed by activated charcoal. Treat shock with volume expanders, without vasopressors; if a vasopressor is necessary, one should be used that is least likely to cause or aggravate tachycardia and cardiac arrhythmias. Renal function should be monitored.

Contraindications: Coronary artery disease, angina pectoris, advanced renal disease (as in chronic renal hypertension), rheumatic heart disease (e.g., mitral valvular) and chronic glomerulonephritis.

Special Concerns: Use with caution in stroke clients and in those with pulmonary hypertension. Use with caution during lactation, in clients with advanced renal disease, and in clients with tartrazine sensitivity. Safety and efficacy have not been established in children. Geriatric clients may be more sensitive to the hypotensive and hypothermic effects of hydralazine; also, a decrease in dose may be necessary in these clients due to age-related decreases in renal function.

Side Effects: *CV:* Orthostatic hypotension, hypotension, ***MI,*** angina pectoris, palpitations, paradoxical pressor reaction, tachycardia. *CNS:* Headache, dizziness, psychoses, tremors, depression, anxiety, disorientation. *GI:* N&V, diarrhea, anorexia, constipation, paralytic ileus. *Allergic:* Rash, urticaria, fever, chills, arthralgia, pruritus, eosinophilia. Rarely, hepatitis, obstructive jaundice. *Hematologic:* Decrease in hemoglobin and RBCs, purpura, agranulocytosis, leukopenia. *Other:* Peripheral neuritis (paresthesias, numbness, tingling), dyspnea, impotence, nasal congestion, edema, muscle cramps, lacrimation, flushing, conjunctivitis, difficulty in urination, lupus-like syndrome, lymphadenopathy, splenomegaly. Side effects are less severe when dosage is increased slowly. *NOTE:* Hydralazine may cause symptoms resembling system lupus erythematosus (e.g., arthralgia, dermatoses, fever, splenomegaly, glomerulonephritis). Residual effects may persist for several years and long-term treatment with steroids may be necessary.

Symptoms of Overdose: Hypotension, tachycardia, skin flushing, headache. Also, myocardial ischemia, ***cardiac arrhythmias, MI, and severe shock.***

Drug Interactions

Beta-adrenergic blocking agents / ↑ Effect of both drugs
Indomethacin / ↓ Effect of hydralazine
Methotrimeprazine / Additive hypotensive effect
Procainamide / Additive hypotensive effect
Quinidine / Additive hypotensive effect
Sympathomimetics / ↑ Risk of tachycardia and angina

NURSING CONSIDERATIONS

See also *Nursing Considerations* for *Antihypertensive Agents,* Chapter 28.

Assessment

1. Document indications for therapy, onset of symptoms, other agents trialed, and the outcome.
2. Assess VS, especially presenting BP (lying, sitting, and standing).
3. Note any client history of hypersensitivity to the drug.
4. List any other drugs prescribed that may interact unfavorably with hydralazine.
5. Note any history of coronary or renal disease.

Interventions

1. During parenteral administration, take the BP every 5 min until stable, then every 15 min during hypertensive crisis.
2. Monitor electrolytes and I&O; report any reduction in urine output or electrolyte abnormality.
3. The BP should be taken several times a day under standardized conditions, lying, sitting, and/or standing.
4. Clients with cardiac conditions may require closer monitoring during drug therapy.
5. Observe for the development of arthralgia, dermatoses, fever, anemia, or splenomegaly since these may require discontinuation of drug therapy.

Client/Family Teaching

1. Take tablets with meals to avoid gastric irritation.
2. Headaches, palpitations, and possibly mild postural hypotension may be experienced after the first dose and may persist for 7–10 days with continued treatment.
3. Record daily weights and report any evidence of rapid weight gain or edema.
4. Any evidence of a rheumatoid-like or influenza-like syndrome (fever, muscle, or joint aches) will necessitate discontinuing hydralazine therapy, so report promptly.
5. Tingling sensations or discomfort in the hands or feet generally are signs of peripheral neuropathies and should be reported since the problem may be reversed with the use of other drugs, usually pyridoxine.
6. Avoid the use of alcohol or other drugs that could also lower BP or interact unfavorably.
7. Reinforce the importance of lifestyle modifications in BP management with diet, exercise, quitting smoking, limiting alcohol use, and reducing stress.

Evaluate

- ↓ BP with control of hypertension
- Improvement in S&S of CHF (↓ afterload, ↑ CO)

Nitroprusside sodium

(nye-troh-**PRUS**-eyed)
Pregnancy Category: C
Nitropress **(Rx)**

How Supplied: *Powder for injection:* 50 mg

Action/Kinetics: Direct action on vascular smooth muscle, leading to peripheral vasodilation. The drug acts on excitation-contraction coupling of vascular smooth muscle by interfering with both influx and intracellular activation of calcium. Nitroprusside has no effect on smooth muscle of the duodenum or uterus and is more active on veins than on arteries. The drug may also improve CHF by decreasing systemic resistance, preload and afterload reduction, and improved CO. **Onset**

(drug must be given by IV infusion): 0.5–1 min; **peak effect:** 1–2 min; **t1/2:** 2 min; **duration:** Up to 10 min after infusion stopped. Nitroprusside reacts with hemoglobin to produce cyanmethemoglobin and cyanide ion. Caution must be exercised as nitroprusside injection can result in toxic levels of cyanide. However, when used briefly or at low infusion rates, the cyanide produced reacts with thiosulfate to produce thiocyanate, which is excreted in the urine.
Uses: Hypertensive crisis to reduce BP immediately. To produce controlled hypotension during anesthesia to reduce bleeding. *Investigational:* Severe refractory CHF (may be combined with dopamine); in combination with dopamine for AMI.

Dosage

- **IV infusion only**

Hypertensive crisis.

Adults: average, 3 mcg/kg/min. **Range:** 0.5–10 mcg/kg/min. Smaller dose is required for clients receiving other antihypertensives. **Pediatric:** 1.4 mcg/kg/min adjusted slowly depending on the response.

Monitor BP and use as guide to regulate rate of administration to maintain desired antihypertensive effect. Rate of administration should not exceed 10 mcg/kg/min.

Administration/Storage

1. Protect drug from heat, light, and moisture.
2. Protect dilute solutions during administration by wrapping flask with opaque material, such as aluminum foil.
3. The contents of the vial (50 mg) should be dissolved in 2–3 mL of D5W. This stock solution must be diluted further in 250–1,000 mL D5W.
4. If properly protected from light, the reconstituted solution is stable for 24 hr.
5. Discard solutions that are any color but light brown.
6. Do not add any other drug or preservative to solution.
7. Cover IV bag and tubing with aluminum foil or foil-lined bags and change setup every 24 hr, unless otherwise indicated. Explain that covering the IV bag protects the medication from light and maintains drug stability. Administer IV solution with an electronic infusion device in a monitored environment.
8. Cyanide toxicity is possible if more than 500 mcg/kg nitroprusside is given faster than 2 mcg/kg/min. To reduce this possibility, sodium thiosulfate can be co-infused with nitroprusside at rates of 5–10 times that of nitroprusside.
9. *Treatment of Overdose:*

• Measure cyanide levels and blood gases to determine venous hyperoxemia or acidosis.

• To treat cyanide toxicity, discontinue nitroprusside and give sodium nitrite, 4–6 mg/kg (about 0.2 mL/kg) over 2–4 min (to convert hemoglobin into methemoglobin); follow by sodium thiosulfate, 150–200 mg/kg (about 50 mL of the 25% solution). This regimen can be given again, at half the original doses, after 2 hr.

Contraindications: Compensatory hypertension. Use to produce controlled hypotension during surgery in clients with known inadequate cerebral circulation. Clients with congenital optic atrophy or tobacco amblyopia (both of which are rare).
Special Concerns: Use with caution in hypothyroidism, liver or kidney impairment, during lactation, and in the presence of increased ICP. Geriatric clients may be more sensitive to the hypotensive effects of nitroprusside; also, a decrease in dose may be necessary in these clients due to age-related decreases in renal function.
Side Effects: Excessive hypotension. ***Large doses may lead to cyanide toxicity.*** *Following rapid injection:* Dizziness, nausea, restlessness, headache, sweating, muscle twitching, palpitations, abdominal pain, apprehension, retching, retrosternal discomfort. *Other symptoms:* Bradycardia, tachycardia, increased ICP, ECG changes, venous streaking, rash, methemoglobinemia, decreased platelet aggregation, flushing, hypothyroidism, ileus. *Symptoms of thiocyanate toxicity:* Blurred vision, tinnitus, confusion, hyperreflexia, sei-

zures. *CNS symptoms (transitory):* Restlessness, agitation, and muscle twitching. Vomiting or skin rash.

Symptoms of Overdose: Excessive hypotension, cyanide toxicity, thiocyanate toxicity.

Drug Interactions: Concomitant use of other antihypertensives, volatile liquid anesthetics, or certain depressants ↑ response to nitroprusside.

NURSING CONSIDERATIONS

See also *Nursing Considerations* for *Antihypertensive Agents,* Chapter 28.

Assessment

1. Document indications for therapy, onset of symptoms, and other therapies used unsuccessfully.
2. Note any history of hypothyroidism or vitamin B_{12} deficiency.
3. Obtain baseline liver and renal function studies to assess function.

Interventions

1. Monitor VS, I&O, and ECG. Obtain written parameters for BP and monitor closely throughout drug therapy. Titrate infusion accordingly.
2. Observe for symptoms of thiocyanate toxicity listed under side effects. Evaluate lab values for thiocyanate levels q 24–48 hr or as directed. Levels should be less than 100 mcg thiocyanate/mL or 3 μmol cyanide/mL.
3. Metabolic acidosis may be an early indicator of cyanide toxicity. Interrupt infusion and report if evident.

Evaluate

- ↓ BP to within desired range
- Improvement in S&S of refractory CHF

ALPHA-1-ADRENERGIC BLOCKING AGENTS

See also the following individual entries:

Doxazosin Mesylate
Prazosin Hydrochloride
Terazosin

Action/Kinetics: The drugs in this group selectively block postsynaptic alpha-1-adrenergic receptors. This results in dilation of both arterioles and veins leading to a decrease in supine and standing BP. Diastolic BP is affected the most. Prazosin and terazosin do not produce reflex tachycardia. Terazosin also relaxes smooth muscle in the bladder neck and prostate, making it useful to treat benign prostatic hypertrophy.

Uses: Alone or in combination with diuretics or beta-adrenergic blocking agents to treat hypertension. Terazosin is used to treat benign prostatic hypertrophy. *Investigational:* Prazosin is used for refractory CHF, for management of Raynaud's vasospasm, and to treat prostatic outflow obstruction. Doxazosin, along with digoxin and diuretics, is used to treat CHF.

Contraindication: Hypersensitivity to these drugs (i.e., quinazolines).

Special Concerns: The first few doses may cause postural hypotension and syncope with sudden loss of consciousness. Use with caution in those with impaired hepatic function or in clients receiving drugs known to influence hepatic metabolism. Use with caution during lactation. Safety and efficacy have not been established in children.

Side Effects: The following side effects are common to alpha-1-adrenergic blockers. Please see individual drugs as well. *CV:* Palpitations, postural hypotension, hypotension, tachycardia, chest pain, arrhythmia. *GI:* N&V, dry mouth, diarrhea, constipation, abdominal discomfort or pain, flatulence. *CNS:* Dizziness, depression, decreased libido, sexual dysfunction, nervousness, paresthesia, somnolence, anxiety, insomnia, asthenia, drowsiness. *Musculoskeletal:* Pain in the shoulder, neck, or back; gout, arthritis, joint pain, arthralgia. *Respiratory:* Dyspnea, nasal congestion, sinusitis, bronchitis, ***bronchospasm,*** cold symptoms, epistaxis, increased cough, flu symptoms, pharyngitis, rhinitis. *Ophthalmic:*

Blurred vision, abnormal vision, reddened sclera, conjunctivitis. *GU:* Impotence, urinary frequency, incontinence. *Miscellaneous:* Tinnitus, vertigo, pruritus, sweating, alopecia, lichen planus, headache, edema, weight gain, facial edema, fever.

Symptoms of Overdose: Extension of the side effects, especially on BP.

Laboratory Test Interference: ↑ Urinary VMA.

Dosage

See individual agents.

NURSING CONSIDERATIONS

Administration/Storage

1. The first dose of prazosin and terazosin should be taken at bedtime.
2. *Treatment of Overdose:* Keep the client supine to restore BP and normalize heart rate. Shock may be treated with volume expanders or vasopressors; support renal function.

Interventions

1. Use cautiously in older clients due to possibility of orthostatic hypotension.
2. Initiate therapy with a low dose and at bedtime to prevent syncope and postural hypotensive effects.
3. Titration generally should be based on standing BP due to postural effects.
4. Drug does not affect glucose levels and may be useful in clients with diabetes.

Client/Family Teaching

1. Take first dose at bedtime to minimize first dose syncope and hypotensive effects. Use caution when performing activities that require mental alertness until drug effects are realized.
2. Do not drive or undertake hazardous tasks for 12–24 hr after the first dose and after increasing the dose or reinstituting therapy following an interruption of dosage.
3. Avoid symptoms of orthostatic hypotension associated with the medication by rising slowly from a sitting or lying position and waiting until symptoms subside.
4. Keep an accurate record of BP readings and record weight 2 times/week. Report any evidence of weight gain or ankle edema because without concomitant administration of a diuretic, one may experience retention of salt and water due to vasodilation.
5. Advise that dizziness, lassitude, headache, and palpitations may occur and should be reported if persistent or bothersome.
6. Report any other persistent side effects so dosage may be evaluated and adjusted accordingly.
7. Stress the importance of life-style modifications and review additional holistic interventions for BP control, some of which may include dietary restrictions of fat, sodium, and cholesterol; weight reduction; regular physical activity; decreased use of alcohol; stress reduction; and smoking cessation.
8. Avoid excessive amounts of caffeine and any OTC agents (especially cold remedies) unless approved by provider.
9. Do not interrupt therapy without approval.

Evaluate: Control of hypertension.

Doxazosin mesylate

(dox-**AYZ**-oh-sin)
Pregnancy Category: B
Cardura **(Rx)**

How Supplied: *Tablet:* 1 mg, 2 mg, 4 mg, 8 mg

Action/Kinetics: Doxazosin is a quinazoline compound that blocks the alpha-1 (postjunctional) adrenergic receptors resulting in a decrease in systemic vascular resistance and a corresponding decrease in BP. **Peak plasma levels:** 2–3 hr. **Peak effect:** 2–6 hr. Significantly bound (98%) to plasma proteins. Metabolized in the liver to active and inactive metabolites, which are excreted through the feces and urine. **$t^1/_2$:** 22 hr.

Uses: Alone or in combination with diuretics or beta-adrenergic blocking drugs for the treatment of hypertension.

Dosage

Tablets. Adults: initial, 1 mg once

daily at bedtime; **then,** depending on the response (client's standing BP both 2–6 hr and 24 hr after a dose), the dose may be increased to 2 mg/day. A maximum of 16 mg/day may be required to control BP.

Administration/Storage

1. To minimize the possibility of severe hypotension, initial dosage should be limited to 1 mg/day.
2. The drug should be given once daily at bedtime.
3. Increasing the dose higher than 4 mg/day increases the possibility of severe syncope, postural dizziness, vertigo, and postural hypotension.
4. *Treatment of Overdose:* IV fluids.

Contraindications: Use in clients allergic to prazosin or terazosin.

Special Concerns: Use with caution during lactation. Safety and effectiveness have not been demonstrated in children. Due to the possibility of severe hypotension, the 2-, 4-, and 8-mg tablets are not to be used for initial therapy. Use with caution in clients with impaired hepatic function or in those who are taking drugs known to influence hepatic metabolism.

Side Effects: *CV:* Dizziness (most frequent), syncope, vertigo, lightheadedness, edema, palpitation, arrhythmia, postural hypotension, tachycardia, peripheral ischemia. *CNS:* Fatigue, headache, paresthesia, kinetic disorders, ataxia, somnolence, nervousness, depression, insomnia. *Musculoskeletal:* Arthralgia, arthritis, muscle weakness, muscle cramps, myalgia, hypertonia. *GU:* Polyuria, sexual dysfunction, urinary incontinence, urinary frequency. *GI:* Nausea, diarrhea, dry mouth, constipation, dyspepsia, flatulence, abdominal pain, vomiting. *Respiratory:* Fatigue or malaise, rhinitis, epistaxis, dyspnea. *Miscellaneous:* Rash, pruritus, flushing, abnormal vision, conjunctivitis, eye pain, tinnitus, chest pain, asthenia, facial edema, generalized pain, slight weight gain.

Symptom of Overdose: Hypotension.

NURSING CONSIDERATIONS

Assessment

1. Document indications for therapy, other agents used, and the outcome.
2. Note any allergy to prazosin or terazosin as drug is a quinazoline derivative.
3. Determine hepatic function and note any history of liver failure.
4. List drugs client prescribed to ensure there will be no drug interactions.
5. Anticipate that it may take 4–5 days to achieve desired response.

Client/Family Teaching

1. Instruct client to take BP and to maintain a written record for review at each medical appointment.
2. Show client how to assess for edema and advise to initially record weight three times a week.
3. Provide a printed list of side effects and advise client to report any that are persistent or bothersome.
4. Review S&S of postural hypotension and advise client to rise slowly to a sitting position before attempting to stand.
5. Explain that postural effects are most likely to occur 2–6 hr after a dose.
6. Driving and hazardous tasks should be avoided for 24 hr after the first dose until effects are evident.
7. Provide recommendations concerning appropriate diet and activity schedules to follow and life style modifications necessary to control BP.

Evaluate

- Client knowledge and understanding of illness as well as desire to comply with mutually outlined goals of therapy
- Control of hypertension (e.g., maintaining SBP < 140 and DBP < 90 mm Hg)

Prazosin hydrochloride

(**PRAY**-zoh-sin)
Pregnancy Category: C
Apo-Prazo ✱, Minipress, Novo-Prazin ✱, Nu-Prazo ✱ **(Rx)**

How Supplied: *Capsule:* 1 mg, 2 mg, 5 mg

Action/Kinetics: Produces selective blockade of postsynaptic alpha-1-adrenergic receptors. Dilates arterioles and veins, thereby decreasing total peripheral resistance and decreasing DBP more than SBP. CO, HR, and renal blood flow are not affected. Can be used to initiate antihypertensive therapy and is most effective when used with other agents (e.g., diuretics, beta-adrenergic blocking agents). **Onset:** 2 hr. Absorption is not affected by food. **Maximum effect:** 2–3 hr; **duration:** 6–12 hr. **t½:** 2–3 hr. Full therapeutic effect: 4–6 weeks. Metabolized extensively; excreted primarily in feces.

Uses: Mild to moderate hypertension. *Investigational:* CHF refractory to other treatment. Raynaud's disease, ergot alkaloid toxicity, pheochromocytoma.

Dosage

- **Capsules**

  Hypertension.

Individualized: Initial, 1 mg b.i.d.–t.i.d.; **maintenance:** if necessary, increase gradually to 6–15 mg/day in two to three divided doses. Daily dose should not exceed 20 mg, although some clients have benefitted from doses of 40 mg daily. If used with diuretics or other antihypertensives, reduce dose to 1–2 mg t.i.d. **Pediatric, less than 7 years of age, initial:** 0.25 mg b.i.d.–t.i.d. adjusted according to response. **Pediatric, 7–12 years of age, initial:** 0.5 mg b.i.d.–t.i.d. adjusted according to response.

Administration/Storage

1. The first dose should be taken at bedtime. Also, the first dose of each increment should be given at bedtime to reduce the incidence of syncope.
2. Due to the first-dose effect, clients should not drive or operate machinery for 24 hr after the first dose.
3. *Treatment of Overdose:* Keep client supine to restore BP and HR. If shock is manifested, use volume expanders and vasopressors; maintain renal function.

Special Concerns: Safe use in children has not been established. Use with caution during lactation. Geriatric clients may be more sensitive to the hypotensive and hypothermic effects of prazosin; also, it may be necessary to decrease the dose in these clients due to age-related decreases in renal function.

Laboratory Test Interferences: ↑ Urinary metabolites of norepinephrine, VMA.

Side Effects: **First-dose effect:** ***Marked hypotension*** and syncope 30–90 min after administration of initial dose (usually 2 or more mg), increase of dosage, or addition of other antihypertensive agent. *CNS:* Dizziness, drowsiness, headache, fatigue, paresthesias, depression, vertigo, nervousness, hallucinations. *CV:* Palpitations, syncope, tachycardia, orthostatic hypotension, aggravation of angina. *GI:* N&V, diarrhea or constipation, dry mouth, abdominal pain, pancreatitis. *GU:* Urinary frequency or incontinence, impotence, priapism. *Respiratory:* Dyspnea, nasal congestion, epistaxis. *Dermatologic:* Pruritus, rash, sweating, alopecia, lichen planus. *Miscellaneous:* Asthenia, edema, symptoms of lupus erythematosus, blurred vision, tinnitus, arthralgia, reddening of sclera, conjunctivitis, edema, fever.

Symptoms of Overdose: Hypotension, ***shock.***

Drug Interactions

Antihypertensives (other) / ↑ Antihypertensive effect
Beta-adrenergic blocking agents / Enhanced acute postural hypotension following the first dose of prazosin
Clonidine / ↓Antihypertensive effect of clonidine
Diuretics / ↑ Antihypertensive effect
Indomethacin / ↓ Effect of prazosin
Nifedipine / ↑ Hypotensive effect
Propranolol / Especially pronounced additive hypotensive effect
Verapamil / ↑ Hypotensive effect; ↑ sensitivity to prazosin-induced postural hypotension

NURSING CONSIDERATIONS

See also *Nursing Considerations* for *Antihypertensive Agents,* Chapter 28.

Client/Family Teaching

1. Food may delay absorption and minimize side effects of the drug.
2. Do not engage in activities requiring alertness, such as operating machinery or driving a car, until drug effects are determined. The drug may cause dizziness and drowsiness.
3. Avoid rapid postural changes that may precipitate weakness, dizziness, and syncope.
4. Lie down or sit down and put head below knees to avoid fainting if a rapid heartbeat is felt.
5. Avoid dangerous situations that may lead to fainting.
6. Report any bothersome side effects because reduction in dosage may be indicated.
7. Do not discontinue medication unless directed by medical supervision.
8. Avoid cold, cough, and allergy medications, unless approved. The sympathomimetic component of such medications will interfere with the action of prazosin.
9. Comply with prescribed drug regimen because the full effect of drug may not be evident for 4–6 weeks.

Evaluate

- ↓ BP
- Improvement in symptoms of refractory CHF

Terazosin

(ter-**AY**-zoh-sin)
Pregnancy Category: C
Hytrin **(Rx)**

How Supplied: *Capsule:* 1 mg, 2 mg, 5 mg, 10 mg

Action/Kinetics: Terazosin blocks postsynaptic alpha-1-adrenergic receptors, leading to a dilation of both arterioles and veins, and ultimately, a reduction in BP. Both standing and supine BPs are lowered with no reflex tachycardia. The drug also relaxes smooth muscle of the prostate and bladder neck. Its usefulness in benign prostatic hypertrophy is due to alpha-1 receptor blockade, which relaxes the smooth muscle of the prostate and bladder neck and relieves pressure on the urethra. Bioavailability is not affected by food. **Onset:** 15 min. **Peak plasma levels:** 1–2 hr. **t½:** 9–12 hr. **Duration:** 24 hr. Terazosin is excreted as unchanged drug and inactive metabolites in both the urine and feces.

Uses: Alone or in combination with diuretics or beta-adrenergic blocking agents to treat hypertension. Treat symptoms of benign prostatic hyperplasia.

Dosage

- **Tablets**

Hypertension.

Individualized, initial: 1 mg at bedtime (this dose is not to be exceeded); **then,** increase dose slowly to obtain desired response. **Range:** 1–5 mg/day; doses as high as 20 mg may be required in some clients.

Benign prostatic hyperplasia.

Initial: 1 mg/day; dose should be increased to 2 mg, 5 mg, and then 10 mg once daily to improve symptoms and/or urinary flow rates.

Administration/Storage

1. The initial dosing regimen must be carefully observed to minimize severe hypotension.
2. Monitor BP 2–3 hr after dosing as well as at the end of the dosing interval to ensure BP control has been maintained.
3. An increase in dose or b.i.d. dosing should be considered if BP control is not maintained at 24-hr interval.
4. To prevent dizziness or fainting due to a drop in BP, the initial dose should be taken at bedtime; the daily dose can be given in the morning.
5. If terazosin must be discontinued for more than a few days, the initial dosing regimen should be used if therapy is reinstituted.
6. Due to additive effects, caution must be exercised when terazosin is combined with other antihypertensive agents.

7. When treating BPH, a minimum of 4– 6 weeks of 10 mg/day may be needed to determine if a beneficial effect has occurred.
8. *Treatment of Overdose:* Restore BP and HR. Client should be kept supine; vasopressors may be indicated. Volume expanders can be used to treat shock.

Special Concerns: Use with caution during lactation. Safety and efficacy have not been determined in children. Geriatric clients may be more sensitive to the hypotensive and hypothermic effects of terazosin.

Laboratory Test Interferences: ↓ H&H, WBCs, albumin.

Side Effects: *First-dose effect:* Marked postural hypotension and syncope. *CV:* Palpitations, tachycardia, postural hypotension, syncope, ***arrhythmias,*** vasodilation. *CNS:* Dizziness, headache, somnolence, nervousness, paresthesia, depression, anxiety, insomnia. *Respiratory:* Nasal congestion, dyspnea, sinusitis, epistaxis, bronchitis, cough, pharyngitis, rhinitis. *GI:* Nausea, constipation, diarrhea, dyspepsia, dry mouth, vomiting, flatulence. *Musculoskeletal:* Asthenia, arthritis, arthralgia, myalgia, joint disorders, back pain, pain in extremities, neck and shoulder pain. *Miscellaneous:* Peripheral edema, weight gain, blurred vision, impotence, chest pain, fever, gout, pruritus, rash, sweating, urinary frequency, tinnitus, conjunctivitis, abnormal vision.

Symptoms of Overdose: Hypotension, drowsiness, shock.

NURSING CONSIDERATIONS

See also *Nursing Considerations* for *Antihypertensive Agents,* Chapter 28.

Client/Family Teaching

1. Take initial dose of medication at bedtime to minimize side effects. Use caution when performing activities that require mental alertness until drug effects are realized.
2. Do not drive or undertake hazardous tasks for 12 hr after the first dose and after increasing the dose or reinstituting therapy following an interruption of dosage.
3. Avoid symptoms of orthostatic hypotension associated with the medication by rising slowly from a sitting or lying position and waiting until symptoms subside.
4. Record weight 2 times/week and report any evidence of weight gain or ankle edema.
5. Do not interrupt therapy without approval.
6. Report any persistent side effects so dosage may be evaluated and adjusted accordingly.

Evaluate

- Control of BP with hypertension
- Reports of improvement in symptoms R/T prostate enlargement

ANGIOTENSIN-CONVERTING ENZYME INHIBITORS

See also the following individual entries:

Benazepril Hydrochloride
Captopril
Enalapril Maleate
Fosinopril Sodium
Lisinopril
Quinapril Hydrochloride
Ramipril

Action/Kinetics: The ACE inhibitors are believed to act by suppressing the renin-angiotensin-aldosterone system. Renin, which is synthesized by the kidneys, is released into the general circulation where it produces angiotensin I, an inactive decapeptide derived from plasma globulin substrate. Angiotensin I is converted to angiotensin II by ACE. Angiotensin II is a potent vasoconstrictor that also stimulates secretion of aldosterone from the adrenal cortex, resulting in sodium and fluid retention. The ACE inhibitors prevent the conversion of angiotensin I to angiotensin II. This results in a decrease in plasma angiotensin II and subsequently a decrease in peripheral resistance and decreased aldosterone secretion (leading to sodium and fluid loss) and therefore a decrease in BP.

There may be either no change or an increase in CO. Several weeks of therapy may be required to achieve the maximum effect to reduce BP. Standing and supine BPs are lowered to about the same extent. The drugs are also antihypertensive in low renin hypertensive clients.

Uses: Alone or in combination with other antihypertensive agents (especially thiazide diuretics) for the treatment of hypertension. Captopril, enalapril, lisinopril, and quinapril are used for CHF. Captopril and enalapril are used for left ventricular dysfunction. See also individual drug entries.

Contraindication: History of angioedema due to previous treatment with an ACE inhibitor.

Special Concerns: Use of ACE inhibitors during the second and third trimesters of pregnancy can result in injury and even death to the developing fetus. ACE inhibitors may cause a profound drop in BP following the first dose; therapy should be initiated under close medical supervision. Use with caution in renal disease (especially renal artery stenosis) as increases in BUN and serum creatinine have occurred; thus, monitor carefully in clients with impaired renal function. Use with caution in clients with aortic stenosis due to possible decreased coronary perfusion following vasodilator use. With the exception of fosinopril (contraindicated), use with caution during lactation. Geriatric clients may show a greater sensitivity to the hypotensive effects of ACE inhibitors although these drugs may preserve or improve renal function and reverse LV hypertrophy. For most ACE inhibitors, safety and effectiveness have not been determined in children.

Side Effects: See individual entries. Side effects common to most ACE inhibitors include the following. *GI:* Abdominal pain, N&V, diarrhea, constipation. dry mouth. *CNS:* Sleep disturbances, insomnia, headache, dizziness, fatigue, nervousness, paresthesias. *CV:* Hypotension (especially following the first dose), palpitations, angina pectoris, ***MI,*** orthostatic hypotension, chest pain. *Hepatic:* Rarely, cholestatic jaundice progressing to ***hepatic necrosis and death.*** *Miscellaneous:* Chronic cough, dyspnea, increased sweating, diaphoresis, pruritus, rash, impotence, syncope, asthenia, arthralgia, myalgia. ***Angioedema*** of the face, lips, tongue, glottis, larynx, extremities, and mucous membranes. ***Anaphylaxis.***

Symptom of Overdose: Hypotension is the most common.

Drug Interactions

Allopurinol / ↑ Risk of hypersensitivity reactions
Anesthetics / ↑ Risk of hypotension if used with anesthetics that also cause hypotension
Antacids / Possible ↓ bioavailability of ACE inhibitors
Capsaicin / Capsaicin may cause or worsen cough associated with ACE inhibitor use
Digoxin / ↑ Plasma digoxin levels
Indomethacin / ↓ Hypotensive effects of ACE inhibitors, especially in low renin or volume-dependent hypertensive clients
Lithium / ↑ Serum lithium levels → ↑ risk of toxicity
Phenothiazines / ↑ Effect of ACE inhibitors
Potassium-sparing diuretics / ↑ Serum potassium levels
Potassium supplements / ↑ Serum potassium levels
Thiazide diuretics / Additive effect to ↓ BP

Laboratory Test Interferences: ↑ BUN and creatinine (both are transient and reversible). ↑ Liver enzymes, serum bilirubin, uric acid, blood glucose. Small ↑ in serum potassium.

Dosage

See individual drugs.

NURSING CONSIDERATIONS

Administration/Storage

1. ACE inhibitor therapy should not be interrupted or discontinued without consulting a physician.

2. *Treatment of Overdose:* Supportive measures. The treatment of choice to restore BP is volume expansion with an IV infusion of NSS. Certain of the ACE inhibitors (captopril, enalaprilat, lisinopril) may be removed by hemodialysis.

Assessment

1. Note any previous therapy with ACE inhibitors and antihypertensive agents and the results.
2. Obtain baseline VS (BP—both arms while lying, standing, and sitting). Assess electrolytes, CBC, and renal function studies, and check urine for proteins during therapy.
3. List other medications client currently prescribed noting any that may interact unfavorably.
4. Document any history of hereditary angioedema (especially if caused by a deficiency of C1 esterase inhibitor).
5. Assess mental status and evaluate extent of client's understanding of the disease of hypertension (or CHF) and the therapy as prescribed.
6. Determine client's ability to take own BP measurement and maintain a record as requested.
7. Ascertain life-style changes clients may need to make to achieve and maintain the goal of lowered BP; assess motivation.

Interventions

1. Monitor CBC and urine for protein every 2 weeks. Observe clients closely for evidence of neutropenia (especially in those receiving captopril), as this is an indication to discontinue drug therapy.
2. Monitor client for any evidence of angioedema (swelling of face, lips, extremities, tongue, mucous membranes, glottis, or larynx) especially after first dose of drug (but this may also be a delayed response). Symptoms may be relieved with antihistamines. If angioedema involves laryngeal edema, client warrants astute observation for airway obstruction. *Discontinue* drug therapy and have epinephrine (1:1000 SC) readily available.
3. Monitor VS, I&O, weight, and renal function studies, reporting any significant changes. Clients who are hypovolemic due to diuretics, GI fluid loss, or salt restriction may exhibit severe hypotension after initial doses of ACE inhibitors.
4. Monitor BP closely during initiation of therapy, assessing for the development of severe hypotension. Observe and supervise ambulation until drug response is evident.
5. For clients undergoing surgery or general anesthesia with drugs that cause hypotension, ACE inhibitors will block angiotensin II formation; thus, hypotension can be corrected by volume expansion.

Client/Family Teaching

1. Take 1 hr before meals and only as directed. Consult provider before interrupting or discontinuing drug therapy.
2. Review prescribed dietary guidelines and advise that salt substitutes containing potassium should *not* be used without approval.
3. Instruct that medication controls but does not cure hypertension. Remind client to take prescribed medication despite feeling better and not to stop abruptly.
4. Teach clients and a family member how to take BP recordings and to report any changes. Explain the importance of keeping a written record to share with the health care provider so that prescribed therapy may be evaluated at each visit.
5. Advise not to perform activities that require mental alertness until drug effects are realized as they may cause dizziness, fainting, or lightheadedness, especially during the first few days of therapy.
6. Instruct to rise slowly from a lying position and dangle feet before standing; avoid sudden changes in posture to minimize postural effects.
7. Practice birth control and report if pregnancy is suspected.
8. Discuss the expected drug responses and the adverse side effects. Advise client to report:

- The development of a nonproductive, persistent, chronic cough as this may be drug induced
- Symptoms of sore throat, fever, swelling of hands or feet, irregular

heartbeat, signs of angioedema, chest pains, difficulty breathing, or hoarseness immediately

- Excessive perspiration, dehydration, vomiting, and diarrhea as these will cause a reduction in BP
- Any itching, joint pain, fever, or skin rash

9. Explain the importance of and how to accurately assess fluid I&O and for edema and weight gain, advising to report any overt changes.
10. Advise clients with diabetes (with or without hypertension) that ACE inhibitors have been shown to reduce proteinuria and to slow the progression of renal disease.
11. Avoid any OTC medications, especially cold remedies, without first consulting the provider or pharmacist. Explain that NSAIDs include aspirin and may impair the hypotensive effects of ACE inhibitors while antacids may decrease bioavailability of these agents.
12. Avoid excessive amounts of caffeine (e.g., tea, coffee, cola).
13. Explain the importance of exercise, proper diet, weight loss, stress management, and adequate rest in conjunction with medications in the overall management of hypertension. Review additional interventions such as reducing the use of alcohol, discontinuing tobacco products, reducing salt intake, and methods to reduce stress that may assist client in the overall goal of BP control. Assist to identify ways in which these interventions may be easily incorporated into the clients' life-style.

Evaluate

- ↓ BP with evidence of control of hypertension
- Improvement in S&S of CHF

Benazepril hydrochloride

(beh-**NAYZ**-eh-prill)
Pregnancy Category: D
Lotensin **(Rx)**

See also *Angiotensin-Converting Enzyme Inhibitors,* Chapter 28.

How Supplied: *Tablet:* 5 mg, 10 mg, 20 mg, 40 mg

Action/Kinetics: Both supine and standing BPs are reduced in clients with mild-to-moderate hypertension with no compensatory tachycardia. Benazepril also has an antihypertensive effect in clients with low-renin hypertension. Food does not affect the extent of absorption. Benazepril is almost completely converted to the active benazeprilat, which has greater ACE inhibitor activity. **Onset:** 1 hr. **Duration:** 24 hr. **Peak plasma levels, benazepril:** 30–60 min. **Peak plasma levels, benazeprilat:** 1–2 hr if fasting and 2–4 hr if not fasting. **$t^{1/2}$, benazeprilat:** 10–11 hr. **Peak reduction in BP:** 2–4 hr after dosing. **Peak effect with chronic therapy:** 1–2 weeks. The drug is excreted through the urine with about 20% of a dose excreted as benazeprilat.

Uses: Used alone or in combination with thiazide diuretics to treat hypertension.

Dosage

- **Tablets**

Clients not receiving a diuretic.

Initial: 10 mg once daily; **maintenance:** 20–40 mg/day given as a single dose or in two equally divided doses. Total daily doses greater than 80 mg have not been evaluated.

Clients receiving a diuretic.

Initial: 5 mg/day.

Creatinine clearance <30 mL/min/1.73 m^2. The recommended starting dose is 5 mg/day; **maintenance:** titrate dose upward until BP is controlled or to a maximum total daily dose of 40 mg.

Administration/Storage

1. Dosage adjustment should be based on measuring peak (2–6 hr after dosing) and trough responses. If once daily dosing does not provide an adequate trough response, increasing the dose or giving divided doses should be considered.

2. If BP cannot be controlled by benazepril alone, a diuretic can be added.
3. If a client is receiving a diuretic, the diuretic, if possible, should be discontinued 2–3 days before beginning benazepril therapy.
4. The drug may be taken without regard to food.

Contraindications: Hypersensitivity to benazepril or any other ACE inhibitor.

Special Concerns: Use with caution during lactation. Safety and effectiveness have not been determined in children.

Laboratory Test Interferences: ↑ Serum creatinine, BUN, serum potassium. ↓ Hemoglobin. ECG changes.

Side Effects: *CNS:* Headache, dizziness, fatigue, anxiety, insomnia, nervousness. *GI:* N&V, constipation, abdominal pain, melena. *CV:* Symptomatic hypotension, postural hypotension, syncope, angina pectoris, palpitations, peripheral edema, ECG changes. *Dermatologic:* Dermatitis, pruritus, rash, flushing, diaphoresis. *GU:* Decreased libido, impotence, UTI. *Respiratory:* Cough, asthma, bronchitis, dyspnea, sinusitis, bronchospasm. *Neuromuscular:* Paresthesias, arthralgia, arthritis, asthenia, myalgia. *Hematologic:* Occasionally, eosinophilia, leukopenia, neutropenia, decreased hemoglobin. *Miscellaneous:* Angioedema, which may be associated with involvement of the tongue, glottis, or larynx; hypertonia; proteinuria; hyponatremia; infection.

Drug Interactions

Diuretics / Excessive ↓ in BP
Lithium / ↑ Serum lithium levels with ↑ risk of lithium toxicity
Potassium-sparing diuretics, potassium supplements / ↑ Risk of hyperkalemia

NURSING CONSIDERATIONS

See also *Nursing Considerations* for *Angiotensin-Converting Enzyme Inhibitors,* and *Antihypertensive Agents,* Chapter 28.

Assessment

1. Note any previous experience with this class of drugs.
2. Obtain baseline electrolytes and renal function studies and monitor throughout therapy.

Client/Family Teaching

1. Take only as directed.
2. Avoid concomitant administration of potassium supplements, potassium salt substitutes, or potassium-sparing diuretics as these can lead to increases of serum potassium.
3. Advise that the side effects of headache, fatigue, dizziness, and cough have been associated with this drug therapy and if persistent or bothersome should be reported.

Evaluate: Control of hypertension with a minimum of side effects.

Captopril

(**KAP**-toe-prill)
Pregnancy Category: C
Apo-Captopril ✱, Capoten, Novo-Capto ✱, Syn-Captopril ✱ **(Rx)**

See also *Angiotensin-Converting Enzyme Inhibitors,* Chapter 28.

How Supplied: *Tablet:* 12.5 mg, 25 mg, 50 mg, 100 mg

Action/Kinetics: Onset: 15 min. **Peak serum levels:** 30–90 min; presence of food decreases absorption by 30%–40%. **Plasma protein binding:** 25%–30%. **Time to peak effect:** 60–90 min. **Duration:** 6–12 hr. **t½, normal renal function:** 2 hr; **t½, impaired renal function:** 3.5–32 hr. More than 95% of absorbed dose excreted in urine (40%–50% unchanged). Food decreases bioavailability of captopril by 30%–40%.

Uses: Antihypertensive, step I therapy in clients with normal renal function. Concomitant use with diuretic therapy may, however, cause precipitous hypotension. In combination with diuretics and digitalis in treatment of CHF not responding to conventional therapy. To improve survival following MI in clinically stable clients with LV dysfunction manifested as an ejection fraction of 40% or less. Treatment of diabetic nephropathy (proteinuria > 500 mg/day) in those with type I insulin-dependent diabetes and retinopathy. *Investigational:* Rheumatoid arthritis, hypertensive crisis, neonatal and childhood hypertension, hypertension related to scleroderma renal crisis, diagnosis of anatomic renal artery stenosis, diagnosis of primary aldosteronism, Raynaud's syndrome, hypertension of Takayasu's disease, idiopathic edema, Bartter's syndrome, and glomerular hypertension).

Dosage

- **Tablets**

Hypertension.

Adults, initial: 25 mg b.i.d.–t.i.d. If unsatisfactory response after 1–2 weeks, increase to 50 mg b.i.d.–t.i.d.; if still unsatisfactory after another 1–2 weeks, thiazide diuretic should be added (e.g., hydrochlorothiazide, 25 mg/day). Dosage may be increased to 100–150 mg b.i.d.–t.i.d., not to exceed 450 mg/day.

Heart failure.

Initial: 25 mg t.i.d.; **then,** if necessary, increase dose to 50 mg t.i.d. and evaluate response; **maintenance:** 50–100 mg t.i.d., not to exceed 450 mg/day.

NOTE: For adults, an initial dose of 6.25–12.5 mg (0.15 mg/kg t.i.d. in children) should be given b.i.d.–t.i.d. to clients who are sodium- and water-depleted due to diuretics, who will continue to be on diuretic therapy, and who have renal impairment.

Hypertensive crisis.

Initial: 25 mg; **then,** 100 mg 90–120 min later, 200-300 mg/day for 2–5 days.

Rheumatoid arthritis.

75–150 mg/day in divided doses.

Prophylaxis of LV dysfunction following MI.

Initial: Give a test dose of 6.25 mg followed by 12.5 mg t.i.d.; **then,** increase the dose to 25 mg t.i.d. after several days. **Usual maintenance:** 50 mg t.i.d. (achieved after several weeks of therapy).

Diabetic nephropathy.

25 mg t.i.d. for chronic use. Other antihypertensive drugs (e.g., beta blockers, centrally-acting drugs, diuretics, vasodilators) may be used with captopril if additional drug therapy is needed to reduce BP.

NOTE: For all uses, doses should be reduced in clients with renal impairment.

Administration/Storage

1. Captopril should not be discontinued without the provider's consent.
2. The dose should be given 1 hr before meals.
3. If possible, previous antihypertensive medication should be discontinued 1 week before starting captopril.
4. In cases of overdosage, volume expansion with NSS (IV) is the treatment of choice to restore BP.

Special Concerns: Use with caution in cases of impaired renal function. Use in children only if other antihypertensive therapy has proven ineffective in controlling BP. Use with caution during lactation.

Laboratory Test Interference: False + test for urine acetone.

Side Effects: *Dermatologic:* Rash (usually maculopapular) with pruritus and occasionally fever, eosinophilia, and arthralgia. Alopecia, erythema multiforme, photosensitivity, exfoliative dermatitis, ***Stevens-Johnson syndrome,*** reversible pemphigoid-like lesions, bullous pemphigus, onycholysis, flushing, pallor, scalded mouth sensation. *GI:* N&V, anorexia, constipation or diarrhea, gastric irritation, abdominal pain, dysgeusia, peptic ulcers, aphthous ulcers, dyspepsia, dry mouth, glossitis, pancreatitis. *Hepatic:* Jaundice, cholestasis, hepatitis. *CNS:* Headache, dizziness, insomnia, malaise, fatigue, paresthesias, confusion, depression, nervousness, ataxia, somnolence. *CV:* Hypotension, angina, ***MI,*** Raynaud's phenomenon, chest pain, palpitations, tachycardia, ***CVA, CHF, cardiac arrest,*** orthostatic hypotension, rhythm disturbances. *Renal:* Renal insufficiency or failure, proteinuria, urinary frequency, oliguria, polyuria, nephrotic syndrome, interstitial nephritis. *Respiratory:* ***Bronchospasm,*** cough, dyspnea, asthma, ***pulmonary embolism, pulmonary infarction.*** *Hematologic:* Agranulocytosis, neutropenia, thrombocytopenia, pancytopenia, ***aplastic or hemolytic anemia.*** *Other:* Decrease or loss of taste perception with weight loss (reversible), angioedema, asthenia, syncope, fever, myalgia, arthralgia, vasculitis, blurred vision, impotence, hyperkalemia, hyponatremia, myasthenia, gynecomastia, rhinitis, eosinophilic pneumonitis.

Additional Drug Interaction: Probenecid increases blood levels of captopril due to decreased renal excretion.

NURSING CONSIDERATIONS

See also *Nursing Considerations* for *Angiotensin-Converting Enzyme Inhibitors,* and *Antihypertensive Agents,* Chapter 28.

Assessment

1. Obtain baseline hematologic studies and renal and liver function tests prior to beginning therapy.
2. Determine if the client is taking nitroglycerin or other antianginal nitrates. These may act in synergism with captopril and may cause a more pronounced response.
3. Determine the potential for the client to understand and comply with the prescribed therapy.
4. Document that ejection fraction is less than or equals 40% in stable, post-MI clients.

Interventions

1. Observe client closely for a precipitous drop in BP within 3 hr after initial dose of captopril if client has been on diuretic therapy and a sodium-restricted diet.
2. If BP falls rapidly, place the client in a supine position and be prepared to assist with an IV infusion of saline.
3. Check for proteinuria monthly after the onset of treatment and for at least 9 months during therapy.
4. Withhold potassium-sparing diuretics and report as hyperkalemia may result.
5. Be alert to hyperkalemia occurring several months after administration of spironolactone and captopril.

Client/Family Teaching

1. Take captopril 1 hr before meals, on an empty stomach. Food interferes with the absorption of the drug.
2. Report any fever, skin rash, sore throat, mouth sores, fast or irregular heartbeat, chest pain, or cough.
3. Some clients may develop dizziness, fainting, or lightheadedness. These symptoms usually disappear once the body adjusts to the medication. Avoid sudden changes in posture to prevent dizziness and fainting.
4. A loss of taste may be experienced for the first 2–3 months and then disappear. Report if this persists and interferes with nutrition.
5. Carry identification and a list of medications currently prescribed to share with all providers.
6. Call with any questions concerning symptoms or about the effects of drug therapy. Do not stop taking the medication without approval.
7. Insulin-dependent clients may experience hypoglycemia; monitor blood sugar levels closely.

Evaluate

- ↓ BP
- Improvement in symptoms of CHF
- Improved mortality post-MI

Enalapril maleate

(en-**AL**-ah-prill)
Pregnancy Category: D
Vasotec, Vasotec I.V. **(Rx)**

See also *Angiotensin-Converting Enzyme Inhibitors,* Chapter 28.

How Supplied: *Tablet:* 2.5 mg, 5 mg, 10 mg, 20 mg

Action/Kinetics: Enalapril is converted in the liver by hydrolysis to the active metabolite, enalaprilat. The parenteral product is enalaprilat injection. **Onset, PO:** 1 hr; **IV,** 15 min. **Time to peak action, PO:** 4–6 hr; **IV,** 1–4 hr. **Duration, PO:** 24 hr; **IV,** About 6 hr. Approximately 50%–60% is protein bound. **$t^1/_2$, PO:** 1.3 hr; **IV,** 15 min. Enalapril is excreted through the urine (half unchanged) and feces.

Uses: Alone or in combination with a thiazide diuretic for the treatment of hypertension (step I therapy). As adjunct with digitalis and diuretic in acute and chronic CHF. *Investigational:* Hypertension in children, hypertension related to scleroderma renal crisis, diabetic nephropathy, decrease in incidence of heart failure in clients with asymptomatic LV dysfunction following MI. Enalaprilat may be used for hypertensive emergencies (effect is variable).

Dosage

- **Tablets (Enalapril)**

Antihypertensive in clients not taking diuretics.

Initial: 5 mg/day; **then,** adjust dosage according to response (range: 10–40 mg/day in one to two doses).

Antihypertensive in clients taking diuretics.

Initial: 2.5 mg. Since hypotension may occur following the initiation of enalapril, the diuretic should be discontinued, if possible, for 2–3 days before initiating enalapril. If BP is not maintained with enalapril alone, diuretic therapy may be resumed.

Adjunct with diuretics and digitalis in heart failure.

Initial: 2.5 mg 1–2 times/day; **then,** depending on the response, 5–20 mg/day in two divided doses. Dose should not exceed 40 mg/day. Dosage must be adjusted in clients with renal impairment or hyponatremia.

Asymptomatic LV dysfunction following MI.

2.5–20 mg/day beginning 72 hr or longer after onset of MI. Therapy is continued for 1 yr or longer.

NOTE: Dosage should be decreased in clients with a creatinine clearance less than 30 mL/min and a serum creatinine level greater than 3 mg/dL.

- **IV (Enalaprilat)**

Hypertension.

1.25 mg over a 5-min period; repeat q 6 hr.

Antihypertensive in clients taking diuretics.

Initial: 0.625 mg over 5 min; if an adequate response is seen after 1 hr, administer another 0.625-mg dose. Thereafter, 1.25 mg q 6 hr.

Clients with impaired renal function.

Give enalaprit, 1.25 mg q 6 hr for clients with a creatinine clearance more than 30 mL/min and an initial dose of 0.625 mg for clients with a creatinine clearance less than 30 mL/min. If there is an adequate response, an additional 0.625 mg may be given after 1 hr; thereafter, additional 1.25-mg doses can be given q 6 hr. For dialysis clients, the initial dose is 0.625 mg q 6 hr.

Administration/Storage

1. Following IV administration, the peak effect after the first dose may not be observed for 4 hr (whether or not the client is on a diuretic). For subsequent doses, the peak effect is usually within 15 min.
2. Enalapril should be given as a slow IV infusion (over 5 min) either alone or diluted up to 50 mL with an appropriate diluent. Any of the following can be used: 5% dextrose injection, 5% dextrose in lactated Ringer's injection, Isolyte E, 0.9% sodium chloride injection, or 0.9% sodium chloride injection in 5% dextrose.
3. When used initially for heart failure, observe the client for at least 2 hr after the initial dose and until the BP has stabilized for an additional hour. If possible, the dose of diuretic should be reduced.
4. To convert from IV to PO therapy in clients on a diuretic, begin with 2.5 mg/day for clients responding to a 0.625-mg IV dose. Thereafter, 2.5 mg/day may be given.
5. To convert from PO to IV enalapril therapy in clients not on a diuretic, use the recommended IV dose (i.e., 1.25 mg/6 hr). To convert from IV to PO therapy, begin with 5 mg/day.
6. Anticipate lowered dosage for clients receiving diuretics and in those with impaired renal function.

Special Concerns: Use with caution during lactation. Safety and effectiveness have not been determined in children.

Side Effects: *CV:* Palpitations, hypotension, chest pain, syncope, angina, ***CVA, MI,*** orthostatic hypotension, disturbances in rhythm, tachycardia, ***cardiac arrest,*** orthostatic effects, atrial fibrillation, bradycardia. *GI:* N&V, diarrhea, abdominal pain, alterations in taste, anorexia, dry mouth, constipation, dyspepsia, glossitis, ileus, melena, stomatitis. *CNS:* Insomnia, headache, fatigue, dizziness, paresthesias, nervousness, sleepiness, ataxia, confusion, depression, vertigo. *Hepatic:* Hepatitis, hepatocellular or cholestatic jaundice, pancreatitis, elevated liver enzymes, hepatic failure. *Respiratory:* Bronchitis, cough, dyspnea, bronchospasm, upper respiratory infection, pneumonia, pulmonary infiltrates, asthma, ***pulmonary embolism and infarction, pulmonary edema.*** *Renal:* Renal dysfunction, oliguria, UTI, transient increases in creatinine and BUN. *Hematologic:* Rarely, neutropenia, thrombocytopenia, bone marrow depression, decreased H&H in hypertensive or CHF clients. *Dermatologic:* Rash, pruritus, alopecia, flushing, erythema multiform, exfoliative dermatitis, photosensitivity, urticaria, increased sweating, pemphigus, ***Stevens-Johnson syndrome,*** herpes zoster, toxic epidermal necrolysis. *Other:* Angioedema, asthenia, impotence, blurred vision, fever, arthralgia, arthritis, vasculitis, eosinophilia, tinnitus, myalgia, rhinorrhea, sore throat, hoarseness, conjunctivitis, tearing, dry eyes, loss of sense of smell, hearing loss, peripheral neuropathy, anosmia, myositis, flank pain, gynecomastia.

Additional Drug Interactions: Rifampin may ↓ the effects of enalapril. Explain that drug should not be discontinued without first reporting this side effect to the physician.

NURSING CONSIDERATIONS

See also *Nursing Considerations* for *Angiotensin-Converting Enzyme Inhibitors* and *Antihypertensive Agents,* Chapter 28.

Assessment

1. Document indications for therapy, presenting symptoms, and other agents previously used and the outcome.
2. List any prescribed drugs that may interact unfavorably with enalapril.
3. Record baseline VS and weight.
4. Obtain CBC, serum electrolytes, and liver and renal function studies as baseline data and monitor.

Client/Family Teaching

1. Use caution, may cause orthostatic effects and dizziness.
2. Emphasize the importance of maintaining a healthy diet, limiting the intake of caffeine, and avoiding alcohol.
3. Avoid salt substitutes or high-Na and high-K foods.
4. Report any weight loss that may result from the loss of taste or rapid weight gain that may result from fluid overload.
5. Any flu-like symptoms should be reported immediately.
6. Stress the importance of keeping scheduled lab and provider appointments. If there is a conflict, advise to reschedule as soon as possible.

Evaluate

- Resolution of S&S of CHF
- ↓ BP to within desired range

Fosinopril sodium

(foh-**SIN**-oh-prill)

Pregnancy Category: D

Monopril **(Rx)**

See also *Angiotensin-Converting Enzyme Inhibitors,* Chapter 28.

How Supplied: *Tablet:* 10 mg, 20 mg

Action/Kinetics: **Onset:** 1 hr. **Time to peak serum levels:** About 3 hr. Metabolized in the liver to the active fosinoprilat. Fosinoprilat is significantly bound to plasma proteins. **t½:** 12 hr (prolonged in impaired renal function) following IV administration. **Duration:** 24 hr. Approximately 50% excreted through the urine and 50% in the feces. Food decreases the rate, but not the extent, of absorption of fosinopril.

Use: Alone or in combination with other antihypertensive agents (especially thiazide diuretics) for the treatment of hypertension.

Dosage

- **Tablets**

Hypertension.

Initial: 10 mg/day **then,** adjust dose depending on BP response at peak (2–6 hr after dosing) and trough (24 hr after dosing) blood levels. **Maintenance:** Usually 20–40 mg/day, although some clients manifest beneficial effects at doses up to 80 mg.

In clients taking diuretics.

Discontinue diuretic 2–3 days before starting fosinopril. If diuretic cannot be discontinued, use an initial dose of 10 mg fosinopril.

Administration/Storage

1. If the antihypertensive effect decreases at the end of the dosing interval in clients taking the medication once daily, b.i.d. administration should be considered.
2. If the client is taking a diuretic, the diuretic should be discontinued 2–3 days prior to beginning fosinopril therapy. If the BP is not controlled, the diuretic should be reinstituted. If the diuretic cannot be discontinued, an initial dose of fosinopril should be 10 mg.
3. The dose of fosinopril does not have to be adjusted in clients with renal insufficiency.

Contraindication: Use during lactation.

Laboratory Test Interferences: Transient ↓ H&H. False low measurement of serum digoxin levels with DigiTab RIA Kit for Digoxin.

Side Effects: *CV:* Orthostatic hypotension, chest pain, hypotension, palpitations, angina pectoris, ***CVA, MI,*** rhythm disturbances, hypertensive crisis, claudication. *CNS:* Headache, dizziness, fatigue, confusion, memory disturbance, tremors, drowsiness, mood change, insomnia, vertigo, sleep disturbances. *GI:* N&V, diarrhea, abdominal pain, constipation, dry mouth, dysphagia, taste disturbance, abdominal distention, flatulence, heartburn, appetite changes, weight changes. *Respiratory:* Cough, sinusitis, ***bronchospasm,*** asthma, pharyngitis, laryngitis. *Hematologic:* Leukopenia, eosinophilia, decreases in hemoglobin (mean of 0.1 g/dL), neutropenia. *Dermatologic:* Diaphoresis, photosensitivity, flushing, pruritus, rash, urticaria. *Body as a whole:* Angioedema, muscle cramps, syncope, myalgia, arthralgia, edema, weakness, musculoskeletal pain. *GU:* Decreased libido, sexual dysfunction, renal insufficiency, urinary frequency. *Miscellaneous:* Paresthesias, hepatitis, pancreatitis, syncope, tinnitus, gout, lymphadenopathy, rhinitis, epistaxis, vision disturbances, eye irritation, laryngitis.

NURSING CONSIDERATIONS

See also *Nursing Considerations* for *Angiotensin-Converting Enzyme Inhibitors,* and *Antihypertensive Agents,* Chapter 28.

Evaluate: Control of hypertension.

Lisinopril

(lie-**SIN**-oh-prill)
Pregnancy Category: C
Prinivil, Zestril **(Rx)**

See also *Angiotensin-Converting Enzyme Inhibitors,* Chapter 28.

How Supplied: *Tablet:* 2.5 mg, 5 mg, 10 mg, 20 mg, 40 mg

Action/Kinetics: Both supine and standing BPs are reduced, although the drug is less effective in blacks than in Caucasians. Although food does not alter the bioavailability of lisinopril, only 25% of a PO dose is absorbed. **Onset:** 1 hr. **Peak serum levels:** 7 hr. **Duration:** 24 hr. **t½:** 12 hr. 100% of the drug is excreted unchanged in the urine.

Uses: Alone or in combination with a diuretic (usually a thiazide) to treat hypertension (step I therapy). In combination with digitalis and a diuretic for treating CHF not responding to other therapy.

Dosage

- **Tablets**

Essential hypertension, used alone.

10 mg/day. Adjust dosage depending on response (range: 20–40 mg/day given as a single dose). Doses greater than 80 mg/day do not give a greater effect.

Essential hypertension in combination with a diuretic.

Initial: 5 mg. The BP-lowering effects of the combination are additive. Dosage should be reduced in clients with renal impairment.

CHF.

Initial: 5 mg once daily (2.5 mg/day in clients with hyponatremia) in combination with diuretics and digitalis. **Dosage range:** 5–20 mg/day as a single dose.

Administration/Storage

1. When considering use of lisinopril in a client taking diuretics, discontinue the diuretic, if possible, 2–3 days before beginning lisinopril therapy. If the diuretic cannot be discontinued, the initial dose of lisinopril should be 5 mg and the client should be closely observed for at least 2 hr.
2. In some clients, maximum antihypertensive effects may not be observed for 2–4 weeks.
3. When starting treatment for CHF, give under medical supervision, especially in clients with a systolic blood pressure less than 100 mm Hg.
4. With clients whose BP is controlled with lisinopril, 20 mg plus hydrochlorothiazide, 25 mg given separately should be given a trial of Prinzide 12.5 mg or Zestoretic 20–12.5 mg before Prinzide 25 mg or Zestoretic 20–25 mg is used.
5. The maximum recommended daily dose of lisinopril is 80 mg in a single daily dose. However, clients usually do not require hydrochlorothiazide in doses exceeding 50 mg/day, especially if combined with other antihypertensives.
6. Use of potassium supplements, potassium-sparing diuretics, or potassium salt substitutes with Prinzide or Zestoretic may lead to increases in serum potassium.
7. Prinzide or Zestoretic is recommended for those clients with a creatinine clearance greater than 30 mL/min.
8. Anticipate reduced dosage if the client has renal insufficiency—initial dose of 10 mg/day if creatinine clearance is greater than 30 mL/min, 5 mg/day if creatinine clearance is between 10 and 30 mL/min, and 2.5 mg/day in dialysis clients (i.e., less than 10 mL/min).
9. *Treatment of Overdose:* Supportive. To correct hypotension, IV normal saline is treatment of choice. Lisinopril may be removed by hemodialysis.

Special Concerns: Use with caution during lactation. Safety and efficacy have not been established in children. Geriatric clients may manifest higher blood levels. Dosage should be reduced in clients with impaired renal function.

Laboratory Test Interferences: ↑ Serum potassium, BUN, serum creatinine. ↓ H&H.

Side Effects: *CNS:* Dizziness, headache, fatigue, vertigo, insomnia, depression, sleepiness, paresthesias, malaise, nervousness, confusion. *GI:* Diarrhea, N&V, dyspepsia, anorexia, constipation, dysgeusia, dry mouth, abdominal pain, flatulence. *Respiratory:* Cough, dyspnea, bronchitis, upper respiratory symptoms, nasal congestion, sinusitis, pharyngeal pain, ***bronchospasm, asthma.*** *CV:* Hypotension, orthostatic hypotension, angina, tachycardia, palpitations, rhythm disturbances, ***stroke,*** chest pain, orthostatic effects, peripheral edema, MI. *Musculoskeletal:* Asthenia, muscle cramps, joint pain, shoulder and back pain, myalgia, arthralgia, arthritis. *Hepatic:* Hepatitis, cholestatic jaundice, pancreatitis. *Dermatologic:* Rash, pruritus, flushing, increased sweating, urticaria. *GU:* Impotence, oliguria, progressive azotemia, acute renal failure, UTI. *Miscellaneous:* ***Angioedema (may be fatal if laryngeal edema occurs),*** hyperkalemia, neutropenia, anemia, ***bone marrow depression,*** decreased libido, chest pain, fever, blurred vision, syncope, vasculitis of the legs, gout.

Symptom of Overdose: Hypotension.

Drug Interactions

Diuretics / Excess ↓ BP
Indomethacin / Possible ↓ effect of lisinopril
Potassium-sparing diuretics / Significant ↑ serum potassium

NURSING CONSIDERATIONS

See also *Nursing Considerations* for *Angiotensin-Converting Enzyme Inhibitors,* and *Antihypertensive Agents,* Chapter 28.

Client/Family Teaching

1. Take medication at bedtime to minimize potential adverse side effects.
2. Explain how to avoid symptoms of orthostatic hypotension, (i.e., rise slowly from sitting or lying position and wait until symptoms subside).
3. Avoid all potassium supplements as well as foods high in potassium.
4. Review list of drug side effects stressing those that require immediate reporting.
5. Stress the importance of reporting for scheduled lab studies.

Evaluate

- ↓ BP to within desired range
- Resolution of S&S of CHF

Quinapril hydrochloride

(**KWIN**-ah-prill)
Pregnancy Category: D
Accupril **(Rx)**

See also *Angiotensin-Converting Enzyme Inhibitors,* Chapter 28.

How Supplied: *Tablet:* 5 mg, 10 mg, 20 mg, 40 mg

Action/Kinetics: **Onset:** 1 hr. **Time to peak serum levels:** 1 hr. The peak reduction of BP occurs within 2–4 hr after dosing. Quinapril is metabolized to quinaprilat, the active metabolite. **t½, quinaprilat:** 2 hr. **Duration:** 24 hr. The drug is metabolized with approximately 60% excreted through the urine and 37% excreted in the feces.

Uses: Alone or in combination with a thiazide diuretic for the treatment of hypertension. Adjunct with a diuretic or digitalis to treat CHF.

Dosage

- **Tablets**

Hypertension.

Initial: 10 mg/day; **then,** adjust dosage based on BP response at peak (2–6 hr) and trough (predose) blood levels. The dose should be adjusted at 2-week intervals. **Maintenance:** 20, 40, or 80 mg daily as a single dose or in two equally divided doses. In clients with impaired renal function, the initial dose should be 10 mg if the creatinine clearance is greater than 60 mL/min, 5 mg if the creatinine clearance is between 30 and 60 mL/min, and 2.5 mg if the creatinine clearance is between 10 and 30 mL/min. If the initial dose is well tolerated, the drug may be given the following day as a b.i.d. regimen.

CHF.

Initial: 5 mg b.i.d. If this dose is well tolerated, titrate clients at weekly intervals until an effective dose, usually 20–40 mg daily in two equally divided doses, is attained. Undesirable hypotension, orthostasis, or azotemia may prevent this dosage level from being reached.

Administration/Storage

1. If the client is taking a diuretic, the diuretic should be discontinued 2–3 days prior to beginning quinapril therapy. If the BP is not controlled, the diuretic should be reinstituted. If the diuretic cannot be discontinued, an initial dose of quinapril should be 1.25 mg.
2. If the antihypertensive effect decreases at the end of the dosing interval in clients taking the medication once daily, either twice daily administration should be considered or the dose should be increased.
3. The antihypertensive effect may not be observed for 1–2 weeks.

4. *Treatment of Overdose:* IV infusion of normal saline to restore blood pressure.

Special Concerns: Use with caution during lactation. Safety and effectiveness have not been determined in children. Geriatric clients may be more sensitive to the effects of quinapril and manifest higher peak quinaprilat blood levels.

Side Effects: *CV:* Vasodilation, tachycardia, ***heart failure,*** palpitations, ***MI, CVA, hypertensive crisis,*** angina pectoris, orthostatic hypotension, ***cardiac rhythm disturbances, cardiogenic shock***. *GI:* Dry mouth or throat, constipation, N&V, abdominal pain, ***GI hemorrhage.*** *CNS:* Somnolence, vertigo, nervousness, depression, headache, dizziness, fatigue. *Hematologic:* ***Agranulocytosis,*** bone marrow depression, thrombocytopenia. *Dermatologic:* ***Angioedema of the lips, tongue, glottis, and larynx;*** sweat ing, pruritus, exfoliative dermatitis, photosensitivity, dermatopolymyositis. *Body as a whole:* Malaise, back pain. *GU:* Oliguria and/or progressive azotemia and rarely ***acute renal failure and/or death in severe heart failure.*** Worsening renal failure. *Respiratory:* Pharyngitis, cough, asthma, bronchospasm. *Miscellaneous:* Oligohydramnios in fetuses exposed to the drug in utero. Abnormal liver function tests, pancreatitis, syncope, hyperkalemia, amblyopia, viral infections.

Symptoms of Overdose: Commonly, hypotension.

Drug Interactions

Potassium-containing salt substitutes / ↑ Risk of hyperkalemia
Potassium-sparing diuretics / ↑ Risk of hyperkalemia
Potassium supplements / ↑ Risk of hyperkalemia
Tetracyclines / ↓ Absorption of tetracycline due to high magnesium content of quinapril tablets

NURSING CONSIDERATIONS

See also *Angiotensin-Converting Enzyme Inhibitors,* and *Antihypertensive Agents,* Chapter 28.

Assessment

1. Obtain baseline electrolytes, CBC, and renal function studies and monitor throughout therapy. Agranulocytosis and bone marrow depression are seen more often in clients with renal impairment, especially if they also have a collagen vascular disease (e.g., SLE, scleroderma).
2. Clients with unilateral or bilateral renal artery stenosis may manifest increase BUN and serum creatinine if given quinapril. Thus, renal function should be monitored closely the first few weeks of therapy.

Interventions

1. Monitor VS, I&O, and weights.
2. If angioedema occurs, the drug should be discontinued immediately and the client observed until the swelling disappears. Antihistamines may be useful in relieving symptoms.
3. Infants exposed to quinapril *in utero* should be closely observed for the development of hypotension, oliguria, and hyperkalemia and managed symptomatically.

Client/Family Teaching

1. Review the appropriate time and frequency for administration.
2. Advise to report any evidence of unusual bruising or bleeding.
3. Any increased SOB, palpitations, or persistent nonproductive cough should be evaluated.

Evaluate: ↓ BP to within desired range.

Ramipril

(**RAM**-ih-prill)
Pregnancy Category: D
Altace **(Rx)**

See also *Angiotensin-Converting Enzyme Inhibitors,* Chapter 28.

How Supplied: *Capsule:* 1.25 mg, 2.5 mg, 5 mg, 10 mg

Action/Kinetics: Onset: 1–2 hr. **Time to peak serum levels:** 1 hr (1–2 hr for ramiprilat, the active metabolite). Ramiprilat has approximately six times the ACE inhibitory activity than ramipril. **t½:** 1–2 hr

(13–17 hr for ramiprilat); prolonged in impaired renal function. **Duration:** 24 hr. Metabolized in the liver with 60% excreted through the urine and 40% in the feces. Food decreases the rate, but not the extent, of absorption of ramipril.

Uses: Alone or in combination with other antihypertensive agents (especially thiazide diuretics) for the treatment of hypertension. *Investigational:* Used with digoxin and diuretics to treat CHF (increased survival has been documented).

Dosage

- **Capsules**

  Hypertension.

Initial: 2.5 mg once daily in clients not taking a diuretic; **maintenance:** 2.5–20 mg/day as a single dose or two equally divided doses. *Clients taking diuretics or who have a creatinine clearance less than 40 mL/min/1.73 m^2:* initially 1.25 mg/day; dose may then be increased to a maximum of 5 mg/day.

Administration/Storage

1. If the antihypertensive effect decreases at the end of the dosing interval in clients taking the medication once daily, either twice daily administration should be considered or the dose should be increased.
2. If the client is taking a diuretic, the diuretic should be discontinued 2–3 days prior to beginning ramipril therapy. If the BP is not controlled, the diuretic should be reinstituted. If the diuretic cannot be discontinued, an initial dose of ramipril should be 1.25 mg.

Contraindication: Use during lactation.

Special Concerns: Geriatric clients may manifest higher peak blood levels of ramiprilat.

Laboratory Test Interferences: ↓ H&H.

Side Effects: *CV:* Hypotension, chest pain, palpitations, angina pectoris, ***MI, arrhythmias.*** *GI:* N&V, abdominal pain, diarrhea, dysgeusia, anorexia, constipation, dry mouth, dyspepsia, enzyme changes suggesting pancreatitis, dysphagia, gastroenteritis, increased salivation. *CNS:* Headache, dizziness, fatigue, insomnia, sleep disturbances, somnolence, depression, nervousness, malaise, vertigo, anxiety, amnesia, ***convulsions,*** tremor. *Respiratory:* Cough, dyspnea, upper respiratory tract infection, asthma, ***bronchospasm***. *Hematologic:* Leukopenia, eosinophilia. Rarely, decreases in hemoglobin or hematocrit. *Dermatologic:* Diaphoresis, photosensitivity, pruritus, rash, dermatitis, purpura. *Body as a whole:* Paresthesias, angioedema, asthenia, syncope, fever, muscle cramps, myalgia, arthralgia, arthritis, neuralgia, neuropathy, influenza, edema. *Miscellaneous:* Impotence, tinnitus, hearing loss, vision disturbances, epistaxis, weight gain, proteinuria.

NURSING CONSIDERATIONS

See also *Nursing Considerations* for *Angiotensin-Converting Enzyme Inhibitors,* and *Antihypertensive Agents,* Chapter 28.

Client/Family Teaching

1. Use caution; drug may cause dizziness and postural effects with sudden changes in position.
2. Note any unusual bruising or bleeding.
3. Report any persistent dry nonproductive cough.
4. Anticipate periodic scheduled lab studies.

Evaluate

- ↓ BP to within desired range
- Resolution of S&S of CHF

BETA-ADRENERGIC BLOCKING AGENTS

See Chapter 51

CALCIUM CHANNEL BLOCKING AGENTS

See also the following individual entries:

Amlodipine
Bepridil Hydrochloride
Diltiazem Hydrochloride
Felodipine
Isradipine
Nicardipine Hydrochloride
Nifedipine
Nimodipine
Verapamil

Action/Kinetics: Calcium ions are important for generation of action potentials and for excitation/contraction of muscles. For contraction of cardiac and smooth muscle to occur, extracellular calcium must move into the cell through openings called *calcium channels*. The calcium channel blocking agents (also called *slow channel blockers* or *calcium antagonists*) inhibit the influx of calcium through the cell membrane, resulting in a depression of automaticity and conduction velocity in both smooth and cardiac muscle. This leads to a depression of contraction in these tissues. Although all drugs in this class act similarly, they have different degrees of selectivity on vascular smooth muscle, myocardium, and conduction and pacemaker tissues. In the myocardium, these drugs dilate coronary vessels and inhibit spasms of coronary arteries. They also decrease total peripheral resistance, thus reducing energy and oxygen requirements of the heart. These effects benefit various types of angina. These agents also are effective against certain cardiac arrhythmias by slowing AV conduction and prolonging repolarization. In addition, they depress the amplitude, rate of depolarization, and conduction in atria.

Uses: See individual drugs. Depending on the drug, calcium channel blockers are used for angina pectoris (chronic stable, unstable, or vasospastic) and essential hypertension. Selected drugs are used for arrhythmias (verapamil) or subarachnoid hemorrhage (nimodipine).

Contraindications: Sick sinus syndrome, second- or third-degree AV block (except with a functioning pacemaker). Use of bepridil, diltiazem, or verapamil for hypotension (<90 mm Hg systolic pressure). Lactation.

Special Concerns: Abrupt withdrawal of calcium channel blockers may result in increased frequency and duration of chest pain. Safety and effectiveness of bepridil, diltiazem, felodipine, and isradipine have not been established in children.

Side Effects: Side effects vary from one calcium channel blocker to another; refer to individual drugs.

Symptoms of Overdose: Nausea, weakness, drowsiness, dizziness, slurred speech, confusion, marked and prolonged hypotension, bradycardia, junctional rhythms, ***second- or third-degree block.***

Drug Interactions

Beta-adrenergic blocking agents / Beta blockers may cause depression of myocardial contractility and AV conduction

Cimetidine / ↑ Effect of calcium channel blockers due to ↓ first-pass metabolism

Fentanyl / Severe hypotension or increased fluid volume requirements

Ranitidine / ↑ Effect of calcium channel blockers due to ↓ first-pass metabolism

Dosage

See individual drugs.

NURSING CONSIDERATIONS

Administration/Storage: *Treatment of Overdosage:*

- Treatment is supportive. Monitor cardiac and respiratory function.
- If client is seen soon after ingestion, emetics or gastric lavage should be considered followed by cathartics.
- *Hypotension:* IV calcium, dopamine, isoproterenol, metaraminol, norepinephrine. Also, provide IV fluids. Place client in Trendelenburg position.
- *Ventricular tachycardia:* IV procainamide or lidocaine; also, cardioversion may be necessary. Also, provide slow-drip IV fluids.

• *Bradycardia, asystole, AV block:* IV atropine sulfate (0.6–1 mg), calcium gluconate (10% solution), isoproterenol, norepinephrine; also, cardiac pacing may be indicated. Provide slow-drip IV fluids.

Assessment

1. Document indications for therapy and type and onset of symptoms.
2. Note if the client has had any experience with calcium channel blocking drugs in the past and the response.
3. Assess and document mental status.
4. Determine that baseline weight and ECG have been performed.
5. Obtain baseline serum glucose, electrolytes, and liver and renal function studies.
6. Document pulse and BP in both arms with client lying, sitting, and standing.

Interventions

1. These drugs cause peripheral vasodilation. Therefore, clients should have their BP and pulse monitored during the initial administration of the drug. Any excessive hypotensive response and increased HR may precipitate angina. Request written parameters for safe drug administration.
2. Monitor I&O and daily weights. Assess for symptoms of CHF (weight gain, peripheral edema, dyspnea, rales, jugular vein distention).
3. During IV drug administration, monitor activities and hemodynamics closely until drug effects are realized.

Client/Family Teaching

1. Take calcium channel blocking agents with meals to reduce GI irritation.
2. Explain that these agents work by decreasing myocardial contractile force, which in turn decreases the myocardial oxygen requirements.
3. Discuss the goals of therapy (e.g., to decrease the DBP by 10 mm Hg, to decrease the heart rate by 20 beats/min).
4. Teach how to take pulse and BP at home and provide written instructions regarding when to withhold medication and when to contact the provider. Advise client that pulse and BP should be taken at the same time of day and at least twice a week as well as weights.
5. Develop a method to maintain a written record of BP and pulse and weights and to note any response after taking the drug. This record should be brought for review at each visit.
6. Evaluate client understanding and adherence to prescribed drug regimen. Correct any misunderstandings the client may have.
7. Review benefits of the drug and any possible side effects. Encourage the client to report any new S&S to the health care provider.
8. Advise not to perform activities that require mental alertness until drug effects are realized.
9. Report any side effects such as dizziness, vertigo, unusual flushing, facial warmth, edema, nausea, or persistent constipation, as they may be toxic drug effects and require discontinuation of therapy.
10. If postural hypotension occurs, advise the client to change positions slowly, especially when standing up from a reclining position. Sit down immediately if lightheadedness occurs. Move slowly from lying down to a sitting or standing position.
11. Explain that long periods of standing, excessive heat, hot showers or baths, and ingestion of alcohol may exacerbate postural hypotension and to take precautions to avoid these situations.
12. Avoid alcohol and any OTC preparations without approval.
13. Any swelling of the hands or feet, pronounced dizziness, or chest pain accompanied by diaphoresis, SOB, or severe headaches should be reported immediately.

Evaluate

- ↓ BP to within desired range
- ↓ HR

• Reports of ↓ frequency and intensity of anginal attacks
• ECG evidence of control of cardiac arrhythmias

Amlodipine

(am-**LOH**-dih-peen)
Pregnancy Category: C
Norvasc **(Rx)**

See also *Calcium Channel Blocking Agents,* Chapter 28.

How Supplied: *Tablet:* 2.5 mg, 5 mg, 10 mg

Action/Kinetics: Amlodipine increases myocardial contractility although this effect may be counteracted by reflex activity. Cardiac output is increased while there is a pronounced decrease in peripheral vascular resistance. **Peak plasma levels:** 6–12 hr. **t½, elimination:** 30–50 hr. 90% metabolized in the liver to inactive metabolites; 10% excreted unchanged in the urine.

Uses: Hypertension alone or in combination with other antihypertensives. Chronic stable angina alone or in combination with other antianginal drugs. Confirmed or suspected Prinzmetal's or variant angina alone or in combination with other antianginal drugs.

Dosage

• **Tablets**

Hypertension.

Adults, usual, individualized: 5 mg/day, up to a maximum of 10 mg/day. The dose should be titrated over 7–14 days.

Chronic stable or vasospastic angina.

Adults: 5–10 mg, using the lower dose for elderly clients and those with hepatic insufficiency. Most clients require 10 mg.

Administration/Storage

1. Food does not affect the bioavailability of amlodipine. Thus, the drug may be taken without regard to meals.
2. Elderly clients, small/fragile clients, or those with hepatic insufficiency may be started on 2.5 mg/day. This dose may also be used when adding amlodipine to other antihypertensive therapy.

Special Concerns: Use with caution in clients with CHF and in those with impaired hepatic function or reduced hepatic blood flow. Safety and efficacy have not been determined in children.

Side Effects: *CNS:* Headache, fatigue, lethargy, somnolence, dizziness, lightheadedness, sleep disturbances, depression, amnesia, psychosis, hallucinations, psychosis, paresthesia, asthenia, insomnia, abnormal dreams, malaise, anxiety, tremor, hand tremor, hypoesthesia, vertigo, depersonalization, migraine, apathy, agitation, amnesia. *GI:* Nausea, abdominal discomfort, cramps, dyspepsia, diarrhea, constipation, vomiting, dry mouth, thirst, flatulence, dysphagia, loose stools. *CV:* Peripheral edema, palpitations, hypotension, syncope, bradycardia, unspecified arrhythmias, tachycardia, ventricular extrasystoles, peripheral ischemia, ***cardiac failure,*** pulse irregularity. *Dermatologic:* Dermatitis, rash, pruritus, urticaria, photosensitivity, petechiae, ecchymosis, purpura, bruising, hematoma, cold/clammy skin, skin discoloration, dry skin. *Musculoskeletal:* Muscle cramps, pain, or inflammation; joint stiffness or pain, arthritis, twitching, ataxia, hypertonia. *GU:* Polyuria, dysuria, urinary frequency, nocturia, sexual difficulties. *Respiratory:* Nasal or chest congestion, sinusitis, rhinitis, SOB, dyspnea, wheezing, cough, chest pain. *Ophthalmologic:* Diplopia, abnormal vision, conjunctivitis, eye pain, abnormal visual accommodation, xerophthalmia. *Miscellaneous:* Tinnitus, flushing, sweating, weight gain, epistaxis, anorexia, increased appetite, taste perversion, parosmia.

NURSING CONSIDERATIONS

See also *Nursing Considerations* for *Calcium Channel Blocking Agents,* Chapter 28.

Assessment

1. Note any history of CAD or CHF.
2. Review list of drugs currently prescribed to prevent any unfavorable interactions.

3. Document baseline VS, ECG, and liver and renal function studies.

Interventions

1. Monitor and record VS and I&O.
2. Anticipate reduced dose in clients with cirrhosis.
3. Monitor BP and PR interval to assess drug response.

Client/Family Teaching

1. Take only as directed, once a day.
2. Report any symptoms of chest pain, SOB, dizziness, swelling of extremities, irregular pulse, or altered vision immediately.

Evaluate

- ↓ BP
- ↓ Frequency and intensity of anginal episodes

Bepridil hydrochloride

(BEH-prih-dill)
Pregnancy Category: C
Vascor **(Rx)**

See also *Calcium Channel Blocking Agents,* Chapter 28.

How Supplied: *Tablet:* 200 mg, 300 mg, 400 mg

Action/Kinetics: Bepridil inhibits the transmembrane influx of calcium ions into cardiac and vascular smooth muscle. The drug increases the effective refractory period of the atria, AV node, His-Purkinje fibers, and ventricles. The drug dilates peripheral arterioles and reduces total peripheral resistance; it reduces HR and arterial pressure at rest and at a given level of exercise. The drug is rapidly and completely absorbed following PO use. **Onset:** 60 min. **Time to peak plasma levels:** 2–3 hr. Greater than 99% bound to plasma protein. Food does not affect either the peak plasma levels or the extent of absorption. **Therapeutic serum levels:** 1–2 ng/mL. **t½, distribution:** 2 hr; **terminal elimination:** 24 hr.

Steady-state blood levels do not occur for 8 days. The drug is metabolized in the liver, and metabolites are excreted through both the kidney (70%) and the feces (22%).

Uses: Chronic stable angina (classic effort-associated angina) in clients who have failed to respond to other antianginal medications or who are intolerant to such medications. It may be used alone or with beta blockers or nitrates. An additive effect occurs if used with propranolol.

Dosage

- **Tablets**

Chronic stable angina.

Adults, initial: 200 mg once daily; after 10 days the dosage may be adjusted upward depending on the response of the client (e.g., ability to perform ADL, QT interval, HR, frequency and severity of angina). **Maintenance:** 300 mg/day, not to exceed 400 mg/day. The minimum effective dose is 200 mg.

Administration/Storage

1. Can be taken with meals or at bedtime if nausea occurs.
2. Bepridil should be taken at about the same time each day. If a dose is missed, the next dose should *not* be doubled.
3. Geriatric clients may require more frequent monitoring.

Contraindications: Clients with a history of serious ventricular arrhythmias, sick sinus syndrome, second- or third-degree heart block (except in the presence of a functioning ventricular pacemaker), hypotension (less than 90 mm Hg systolic), uncompensated cardiac insufficiency, congenital QT interval prolongation, and in those taking other drugs that prolong the QT interval (e.g., quinidine, procainamide, tricyclic antidepressants). Use in clients with MI during the previous 3 months. During lactation.

Special Concerns: Safety and effectiveness have not been determined in children. Use with caution in clients with CHF, left bundle block, sinus bradycardia (less than 50 beats/min), serious hepatic or renal disorders. New arrhythmias can be induced. Geriatric clients may require more frequent monitoring.

Side Effects: *CV:* ***Induction of new serious arrhythmias such as torsades de pointes type ventricular tachycardia, prolongation of QTc and QT interval, increased PVC rates, new sustained VT and VT/VF,*** sinus tachycardia, sinus bradycardia, hypertension vasodilation, palpitations. *GI:* Nausea (common), dyspepsia, GI distress, diarrhea, dry mouth, anorexia, abdominal pain, constipation, flatulence, gastritis, increased appetite. *CNS:* Nervousness, dizziness, drowsiness, insomnia, depression, vertigo, akathisia, anxiousness, tremor, hand tremor, syncope, paresthesia. *Respiratory:* Cough, pharyngitis, rhinitis, dyspnea, respiratory infection. *Body as a whole:* Asthenia, headache, flu syndrome, fever, pain, superinfection. *Dermatologic:* Rash, skin irritation, sweating. *Miscellaneous:* Tinnitus, arthritis, blurred vision, taste change, loss of libido, impotence, agranulocytosis.

Laboratory Test Interferences: ↑ ALT, transaminase. Abnormal liver function tests.

Drug Interactions

Cardiac glycosides / Exaggeration of the depression of AV nodal conduction

Digoxin / Possible ↑ serum digoxin levels

Potassium-wasting diuretics / Hypokalemia, which causes an ↑ risk of serious ventricular arrhythmias

Procainamide / ↑ Risk of serious side effects due to exaggerated prolongation of the QT interval

Quinidine / ↑ Risk of serious side effects due to exaggerated prolongation of the QT interval

Tricyclic antidepressants / ↑ Risk of serious side effects due to exaggerated prolongation of the QT interval

NURSING CONSIDERATIONS

See also *Nursing Considerations* for *Calcium Channel Blocking Agents,* Chapter 28.

Assessment

1. Determine which antianginal agents have been used in the past and their effects.
2. Perform baseline CBC, serum electrolytes (especially K) and ECG prior to initiating drug therapy.
3. List drugs currently prescribed to determine any potential drug interactions. Notify provider if the client is taking any medications that prolong the QT interval (e.g., procainamide, quinidine, tricyclic antidepressants).
4. QT intervals should be checked prior to initiating therapy with bepridil, 1–3 weeks after beginning therapy, and periodically thereafter, especially after any dosage adjustment. Clients with prolongation of QT intervals may be at greater risk for developing serious ventricular arrhythmias.
5. Document any evidence of AV block, arrhythmias, MI, and implanted ventricular pacemaker.

Interventions

1. Clients requiring diuretics should take a potassium-sparing agent.
2. Monitor VS. Observe closely for evidence of new arrhythmias, especially torsades de pointes tachycardia.
3. Clients should continue taking nitroglycerin if prescribed.

Evaluate

- Prophylaxis and control of angina
- Therapeutic serum drug levels (1–2 ng/mL)

Diltiazem hydrochloride

(dill-**TIE**-ah-zem)

Pregnancy Category: C

Apo-Diltiaz ✱, Cardizem, Cardizem CD, Cardizem Injectable, Cardizem-SR, Dilacor XR, Novo-Diltazem ✱, Nu-Diltiaz ✱, Syn-Diltiazem ✱ **(Rx)**

See also *Calcium Channel Blocking Agents,* Chapter 28.

How Supplied: *Capsule, Extended Release:* 60 mg, 90 mg, 120 mg, 180 mg, 240 mg, 300 mg; *Injection:* 5 mg/mL; *Tablet:* 30 mg, 60 mg, 90 mg, 120 mg

Action/Kinetics: Decreases SA and AV conduction and prolongs AV node effective and functional refractory periods. The drug also decreases myocardial contractility and peripheral vascular resistance. **Tablets: Onset,** 30–60 min; **time to peak plasma levels:** 2–3 hr; **t½, first phase:** 20–30 min; **second phase:** about 3–4.5 hr (5–8 hr with high and repetitive doses); **duration:** 4–8 hr. **Extended-Release Capsules: Onset,** 2–3 hr; **time to peak plasma levels:** 6–11 hr; **t½:** 5–7 hr; **duration:** 12 hr. **Therapeutic serum levels:** 0.05–0.2 mcg/mL. Metabolized to desacetyldiltiazem, which manifests 25%–50% of the activity of diltiazem. Excreted through both the bile and urine.

Uses: Tablets: Vasospastic angina (Prinzmetal's variant); chronic stable angina (especially in clients who cannot use beta-adrenergic blockers or nitrates or who remain symptomatic after clinical doses of these agents). **Sustained-Release Capsules:** Essential hypertension, angina. **Parenteral:** Atrial fibrillation or flutter. Paroxysmal SVT. *Investigational:* Prophylaxis of reinfarction of nonQ wave MI; tardive dyskinesia, Raynaud's syndrome.

Dosage

- **Tablets**

Angina.

Adults, initial: 30 mg q.i.d. before meals and at bedtime; **then,** increase gradually to total daily dose of 180–360 mg (given in three to four divided doses) q 1–2 days.

- **Capsules, Sustained-Release**

Angina.

Cardizem CD: Adults, initial: 120 or 180 mg once daily. Up to 480 mg/day may be required. Dosage adjustments should be carried out over a 7–14-day period.

Hypertension.

Cardizem CD: Adults, initial: 180–240 mg once daily. Maximum antihypertensive effect usually reached within 14 days. Usual range is 240–360 mg once daily.

Cardizem SR: Adults, initial: 60–120 mg b.i.d.; **then,** when maximum antihypertensive effect is reached (approximately 14 days), adjust dosage to a range of 240–360 mg/day.

Dilacor XR: Adults, initial: 180–240 mg once daily. Usual range is 180–480 mg once daily.

- **IV bolus**

Atrial fibrillation/flutter; paroxysmal SVT.

Adults, initial: 0.25 mg/kg (average 20 mg) given over 2 min; **then,** if response is inadequate, a second dose may be given after 15 min. The second bolus dose is 0.35 mg/kg (average 25 mg) given over 2 min. Subsequent doses should be individualized. Some clients may respond to an initial dose of 0.15 mg/kg (duration of action may be shorter).

- **IV infusion**

Atrial fibrillation/flutter.

Adults: 10 mg/hr following IV bolus dose(s) of 0.25 mg/kg or 0.35 mg/kg. Some clients may require 5 mg/hr while others may require 15 mg/hr. Infusion may be maintained for 24 hr.

Administration/Storage

1. Sublingual nitroglycerin may be taken concomitantly for acute angina.
2. Diltiazem may be taken together with long-acting nitrates.
3. The sustained-release capsules should be taken on an empty stomach.
4. Sustained-release capsules should not be opened, chewed, or crushed and should be swallowed whole.
5. Use with beta blockers or digitalis is usually well tolerated but the combined effects cannot be predicted, especially in clients with cardiac conduction abnormalities or LV dysfunction.
6. The infusion may be maintained for up to 24 hr. Use for more than 24 hr is not recommended.
7. May be administered by direct IV over 2 min or as an infusion (see *Dosage*). For IV infusion, the drug may be mixed with NSS, 5% dextrose, or 5% dextrose and 0.45% NaCl.
8. The injection should be refrigerated at 2°C–8°C (36°F–46°F). The solution may be stored at room temperature for

1 month, after which any remaining solution should be destroyed.

Contraindications: Hypotension. Second- or third-degree AV block and sick sinus syndrome except in presence of a functioning ventricular pacemaker. Acute MI, pulmonary congestion. Lactation.

Special Concerns: Safety and effectiveness in children have not been determined. The half-life may be increased in geriatric clients. Use with caution in hepatic disease and in CHF. Abrupt withdrawal may cause an increase in the frequency and duration of chest pain. Use with beta blockers or digitalis is usually well tolerated, although the effects of coadministration cannot be predicted (especially in clients with left ventricular dysfunction or cardiac conduction abnormalities).

Laboratory Test Interferences: ↑ Alkaline phosphatase, CPK, LDH, AST, ALT.

Side Effects: *CV:* AV block, bradycardia, CHF, hypotension, syncope, palpitations, peripheral edema, ***arrhythmias,*** angina, tachycardia, ***abnormal ECG, ventricular extrasystoles.*** *GI:* N&V, diarrhea, constipation, anorexia, abdominal discomfort, cramps, dry mouth, dysgeusia. *CNS:* Weakness, nervousness, dizziness, lightheadedness, headache, depression, psychoses, hallucinations, disturbances in sleep, somnolence, insomnia, amnesia, abnormal dreams. *Dermatologic:* Rashes, dermatitis, pruritus, urticaria, erythema multiforme, ***Stevens-Johnson syndrome.*** *Other:* Photosensitivity, joint pain or stiffness, flushing, nasal or chest congestion, dyspnea, SOB, nocturia/polyuria, sexual difficulties, weight gain, paresthesia, tinnitus, tremor, asthenia, gynecomastia, gingival hyperplasia, petechiae, ecchymosis, purpura, bruising, hematoma, leukopenia, double vision, epistaxis, eye irritation, thirst, alopecia, ***bundle branch block,*** abnormal gait, hyperglycemia.

Additional Drug Interactions

Anesthetics / ↑ Risk of depression of cardiac contractility, conductivity, and automaticity as well as vascular dilation

Carbamazepine / ↑ Effect of diltiazem due to ↓ breakdown by liver

Cimetidine / ↑ Bioavailability of diltiazem

Cyclosporine / ↑ Effect of cyclosporine possibly leading to renal toxicity

Digoxin / ↑ Serum digoxin levels are possible

Lithium / ↑ Risk of neurotoxicity

Ranitidine / ↑ Bioavailability of diltiazem

Theophyllines / ↑ Risk of pharmacologic and toxicologic effects of theophyllines

NURSING CONSIDERATIONS

See also *Nursing Considerations* for *Calcium Channel Blocking Agents,* Chapter 28.

Assessment

1. Document indications for therapy, onset of symptoms, and previous treatment modalities.
2. Note any evidence of peripheral edema or CHF.
3. Review ECG for any evidence of AV block.
4. Obtain baseline laboratory studies and note any evidence of hepatic and/or renal dysfunction.
5. Anticipate reduced dosage of diltiazem in clients with impaired renal or hepatic function.
6. The plasma half-life of the drug may be prolonged in elderly clients. Therefore, monitor these clients closely.

Client/Family Teaching

1. Drug may cause drowsiness or dizziness.
2. Review symptoms of postural hypotension and advise client to rise slowly from a lying to a sitting and to a standing position.
3. Report any persistent and bothersome side effects including constipation, unusual tiredness, or weakness.
4. Continue carrying short-acting nitrites (nitroglycerin) at all times and use as directed.

Evaluate

- ↓ Frequency and intensity of vasospastic anginal attacks
- ↓ BP
- Restoration of stable cardiac rhythm

Felodipine

(feh-**LOHD**-ih-peen)
Pregnancy Category: C
Plendil, Renedil ✱ **(Rx)**

See also *Calcium Channel Blocking Agents,* Chapter 28.

How Supplied: *Tablet, Extended Release:* 2.5 mg, 5 mg, 10 mg

Action/Kinetics: Onset after PO: 120–300 min. **Peak plasma levels:** 2.5–5 hr. Over 99% bound to plasma protein. **t½, elimination:** 11–16 hr. Metabolized in the liver.

Uses: Treatment of mild to moderate hypertension, alone or with other antihypertensives.

Dosage

- **Tablets**

Hypertension.

Initial: 5 mg once daily; **then:** adjust dose according to response, usually at 2-week intervals with the usual dosage range being 5–10 mg once daily, up to a maximum of 20 mg once daily.

Administration/Storage

1. Tablets should be swallowed whole and not chewed or crushed.
2. The bioavailability is not affected by food although it is increased more than twofold when taken with doubly concentrated grapefruit juice when compared with water or orange juice.

Contraindication: Use during lactation.

Special Concerns: Use with caution in clients with CHF or compromised ventricular function, especially in combination with a beta-adrenergic blocking agent. Use with caution in impaired hepatic function or reduced hepatic blood flow. Felodipine may cause a greater hypotensive effect in geriatric clients. Safety and effectiveness have not been determined in children.

Side Effects: *CV:* Significant hypotension, syncope, angina pectoris, peripheral edema, palpitations, AV block, ***MI, arrhythmias,*** tachycardia. *CNS:* Dizziness, lightheadedness, headache, nervousness, sleepiness, irritability, anxiety, insomnia, paresthesia, depression, amnesia, paranoia, psychosis, hallucinations. *Body as a whole:* Asthenia, flushing, muscle cramps, pain, inflammation, warm feeling, influenza. *GI:* Nausea, abdominal discomfort, cramps, dyspepsia, diarrhea, constipation, vomiting, dry mouth, flatulence. *Dermatologic:* Rash, dermatitis, urticaria, pruritus. *Respiratory:* Rhinitis, rhinorrhea, pharyngitis, sinusitis, nasal and chest congestion, SOB, wheezing, dyspnea, cough, bronchitis, sneezing, respiratory infection. *Miscellaneous:* Anemia, gingival hyperplasia, sexual difficulties, epistaxis, back pain, facial edema, erythema, urinary frequency or urgency, dysuria.

Additional Drug Interactions

Cimetidine / ↑ Bioavailability of felodipine
Digoxin / ↑ Peak plasma levels of digoxin
Fentanyl / Possible severe hypotension or ↑ fluid volume
Ranitidine / ↑ Bioavailability of felodipine

NURSING CONSIDERATIONS

See also *Nursing Considerations* for *Calcium Channel Blocking Agents,* Chapter 28.

Assessment

1. Document onset of symptoms and any other agents previously used and the outcome.
2. Note any history of heart failure or compromised ventricular function.
3. List drugs currently prescribed and note any potential interactions.
4. During any adjustment of dosage, BP should be closely monitored in clients over 65 years of age and in clients with impaired hepatic function.

Client/Family Teaching

1. Do not stop drug abruptly as abrupt withdrawal may cause an increased frequency and duration of chest pain.
2. Avoid activities that require mental alertness until drug effects are realized.
3. Rise slowly from a lying position and dangle feet before standing to minimize postural effects.
4. Practice frequent careful oral hygiene to minimize the incidence and severity of drug-induced gingival hyperplasia.

Evaluate: Control of hypertension.

Isradipine

(iss-**RAD**-ih-peen)
Pregnancy Category: C
DynaCirc **(Rx)**

See also *Calcium Channel Blocking Agents,* Chapter 28.

How Supplied: *Capsule:* 2.5 mg, 5 mg

Action/Kinetics: Isradipine binds to calcium channels resulting in the inhibition of calcium influx into cardiac and smooth muscle and subsequent arteriolar vasodilation. The reduced systemic resistance leads to a decrease in BP with a small increase in resting HR. In clients with normal ventricular function, the drug reduces afterload leading to some increase in CO. Isradipine is well absorbed from the GI tract although it undergoes significant first-pass metabolism. **Peak plasma levels:** 1 ng/mL after 1.5 hr. **Onset:** 2–3 hr. When taken with food, the time to peak effect is increased by approximately 1 hr, although the total bioavailability does not change. **t½, initial:** 1.5–2 hr; **terminal,** 8 hr. The drug is completely metabolized in the liver with 60%–65% excreted through the kidneys and 25%–30% through the feces. The maximum effect may not be observed for 2–4 wk.

Uses: Alone or with thiazide diuretics in the management of essential hypertension. *Investigational:* Chronic stable angina.

Dosage

• **Capsules**

Hypertension.

Adults, initial: 2.5 mg b.i.d. alone or in combination with a thiazide diuretic. If BP is not decreased satisfactorily after 2–4 weeks, the dose may be increased in increments of 5 mg/day at 2–4-week intervals up to a maximum of 20 mg/day. Adverse effects increase, however, at doses above 10 mg/day.

Administration/Storage: The drug should be stored in a tight container protected from light.

Contraindication: Lactation.

Special Concerns: Safety and effectiveness have not been determined in children. Use with caution in clients with CHF, especially those taking a beta-adrenergic blocking agent. The bioavailability of isradipine increases in geriatric clients over 65 years of age, clients with impaired hepatic function, and those with mild renal impairment.

Laboratory Test Interference: ↑ Liver function tests.

Side Effects: *CV:* Palpitations, edema, flushing, tachycardia, SOB, hypotension, transient ischemic attack, ***stroke,*** atrial fibrillation, ***ventricular fibrillation, MI,*** CHF, angina. *CNS:* Headache, dizziness, fatigue, drowsiness, insomnia, lethargy, nervousness, depression, syncope, amnesia, psychosis, hallucinations, weakness, jitteriness, paresthesia. *GI:* Nausea, abdominal discomfort, diarrhea, vomiting, constipation, dry mouth. *Respiratory:* Dyspnea, cough. *Dermatologic:* Pruritus, urticaria. *Miscellaneous:* Chest pain, rash, pollakiuria, cramps of the legs and feet, nocturia, polyuria, hyperhidrosis, visual disturbances, numbness, throat discomfort, leukopenia, sexual difficulties.

Drug Interaction: Severe hypotension has been observed during fentanyl anesthesia with concomitant use of a beta-blocker and a calcium channel blocking agent.

NURSING CONSIDERATIONS

See *Nursing Considerations* for *Cal-*

cium Channel Blocking Agents, Chapter 28.

Client/Family Teaching

1. Use caution, as drug may cause dizziness and confusion; assess drug effects.
2. Review drug side effects, stressing those that require immediate reporting.
3. Report for scheduled lab tests: liver and renal function studies.

Evaluate: ↓ BP with control of hypertension.

Nicardipine hydrochloride

(nye-**KAR**-dih-peen)
Pregnancy Category: C
Cardene, Cardene IV, Cardene SR
(Rx)

See also *Calcium Channel Blocking Agents,* Chapter 28.

How Supplied: *Capsule:* 20 mg, 30 mg; *Capsule, Extended Release:* 30 mg, 45 mg, 60 mg; *Injection:* 2.5 mg/mL

Action/Kinetics: The drug moderately increases CO and significantly decreases peripheral vascular resistance. **Onset of action:** 20 min. **Maximum plasma levels:** 30–120 min. Significant first-pass metabolism by the liver. Food (especially fats) will decrease the amount of drug absorbed from the GI tract. Steady-state plasma levels are reached after 2–3 days of therapy. **Therapeutic serum levels:** 0.028–0.050 mcg/mL. **t½, at steady state:** 8.6 hr. **Duration:** 8 hr. The drug is highly bound to plasma protein (>95%) and is metabolized by the liver with excretion through both the urine and feces.

Uses: *Immediate release:* Chronic stable angina (effort-associated angina) alone or in combination with beta-adrenergic blocking agents.

Immediate and sustained released: Hypertension alone or in combination with other antihypertensive drugs.

IV: Short-term treatment of hypertension when PO therapy is not desired or possible.

Investigational: CHF.

Dosage

- **Capsules, Immediate Release**

Angina, hypertension.

Initial, usual: 20 mg t.i.d. (range: 20–40 mg t.i.d.). Wait 3 days before increasing dose to ensure steady-state plasma levels.

- **Capsules, Sustained Release**

Hypertension.

Initial: 30 mg b.i.d. (range: 30–60 mg b.i.d.).

NOTE: In renal impairment, the initial dose should be 20 mg t.i.d. In hepatic impairment, the initial dose should be 20 mg b.i.d.

- **IV**

Hypertension.

Individualize dose. Initial: 5 mg/hr; the infusion rate may be increased to a maximum of 15 mg/hr (by 2.5-mg/hr increments q 15 min). For a more rapid reduction in BP, initiate at 5 mg/hr but increase the rate q 5 min in 2.5-mg/hr increments until a maximum of 15 mg/hr is reached. **Maintenance:** 3 mg/hr. The IV infusion rate to produce an average plasma level similar to a particular PO dose is as follows: 20 mg q 8 hr is equivalent to 0.5 mg/hr; 30 mg q 8 hr is equivalent to 1.2 mg/hr; and 40 mg q 8 hr is equivalent to 2.2 mg/hr.

Administration/Storage

1. The maximum BP-lowering effects for immediate release are seen 1–2 hr after dosing; the maximum BP-lowering effects for sustained release are seen in 2–6 hr.
2. When used for treating clients with angina, nicardipine may be administered safely along with sublingual nitroglycerin, prophylactic nitrates, or beta blockers.
3. When used to treat clients with hypertension, nicardipine may be administered safely along with diuretics or beta blockers.
4. During initial therapy and when dosage is increased, clients may expe-

rience an increase in the frequency, duration, or severity of angina.
5. If transfer to PO antihypertensives other than nicardipine is planned, therapy should be initiated after discontinuing the infusion. If PO nicardipine is to be used at a dosage regimen of three times daily, give the first dose 1 hr prior to discontinuing IV infusion.
6. Ampules must be diluted before infusion. Acceptable diluents are 5% dextrose, 5% dextrose and 0.45% sodium chloride, 5% dextrose with 40 mEq potassium, 0.45% sodium chloride, and 0.9% sodium chloride. Nicardipine is incompatible with 5% sodium bicarbonate and lactated Ringer's solution.
7. The infusion concentration should be 0.1 mg/mL. The diluted product is stable at room temperature for 24 hr.
8. Ampules should be stored at room temperature although freezing does not affect the product. Ampules should be protected from light and elevated temperatures.

Contraindications: Clients with advanced aortic stenosis due to the effect on reducing afterload. During lactation.

Special Concerns: Safety and efficacy in children less than 18 years of age have not been established. Use with caution in clients with CHF, especially in combination with a beta blocker due to the possibility of a negative inotropic effect. Use with caution in clients with impaired liver function, reduced hepatic blood flow, or impaired renal function. Initial increase in frequency, duration, or severity of angina.

Side Effects: *CV:* Pedal edema, flushing, increased angina, palpitations, tachycardia, other edema, abnormal ECG, hypotension, postural hypotension, syncope, ***MI, AV block,*** ventricular extrasystoles, peripheral vascular disease. *CNS:* Dizziness, headache, somnolence, malaise, nervousness, insomnia, abnormal dreams, vertigo, depression, confusion, amnesia, anxiety, weakness, psychoses, hallucinations, paranoia. *GI:* N&V, dyspepsia, dry mouth, constipation, sore throat. *Neuromuscular:* Asthenia, myalgia, paresthesia, hyperkinesia, arthralgia. *Miscellaneous:* Rash, dyspnea, SOB, nocturia, polyuria, allergic reactions, abnormal liver chemistries, hot flashes, impotence, rhinitis, sinusitis, nasal congestion, chest congestion, tinnitus, equilibrium disturbances, abnormal or blurred vision, infection, atypical chest pain.

Symptoms of Overdose: Marked hypotension, bradycardia, palpitations, flushing, drowsiness, confusion, and slurred speech following PO overdose. Lethal overdose may cause systemic hypotension, bradycardia (following initial tachycardia), and progressive AV block.

Drug Interactions
Cimetidine / ↑ Bioavailability of nicardipine → ↑ plasma levels
Cyclosporine / ↑ Plasma levels of cyclosporine possibly leading to renal toxicity
Ranitidine / ↑ Bioavailability of nicardipine

NURSING CONSIDERATIONS

See also *Nursing Considerations* for *Calcium Channel Blocking Agents,* Chapter 28.

Assessment
1. Document indications for therapy and type and onset of symptoms.
2. List other agents prescribed and the outcome.
3. Note any history of CHF and if beta blockers prescribed, as this warrants close monitoring.
4. Obtain baseline renal and liver function studies, noting any evidence of dysfunction.

Interventions
1. Monitor VS. When the immediate-release product is used for hypertension, the maximum lowering of BP occurs 1–2 hr after dosing. Thus, during initiation of therapy BP should be monitored at this interval. Also, BP should be evaluated at the trough (8 hr after dosing). When the sustained-release product is used, maximum lowering of BP occurs 2–6 hr after dosing.

2. Monitor BP frequently during and following IV infusion. Avoid too rapid or excessive decrease in BP and discontinue infusion if there is significant hypotension or tachycardia.

Client/Family Teaching

1. Take the medication at the same time each day.
2. Report any persistent and/or bothersome side effects such as dizziness, flushing, or increased incidents of angina or evidence of weight gain or edema.
3. Maintain a proper intake of fluids to avoid constipation.
4. Male clients may experience impotence; advise to report.
5. Explain that anginal attacks may persist up to 30 min following drug ingestion due to reflex tachycardia; advise to use nitrates as prescribed.
6. Report any evidence of change in psychologic state—depression, anxiety, or decreased mental acuity. This may be particularly important when working with elderly clients since there may be a tendency to misdiagnose the problem as senility.
7. Advise to report any altered sleep patterns as these could be drug related.

Evaluate

- Control of hypertension
- ↓ Frequency and intensity of anginal attacks
- Therapeutic serum drug levels (0.028–0.050 mcg/mL)

Nifedipine

(nye-**FED**-ih-peen)
Pregnancy Category: C
Adalat, Adalat CC, Adalat P.A. 10 and 20 ✹, Apo-Nifed ✹, Gen-Nifedipine ✹, Nu-Nifed ✹, Procardia, Procardia XL **(Rx)**

See also *Calcium Channel Blocking Agents,* Chapter 28.

How Supplied: *Capsule:* 10 mg, 20 mg; *Tablet, Extended Release:* 30 mg, 60 mg, 90 mg

Action/Kinetics: Variable effects on AV node effective and functional refractory periods. CO is moderately increased while peripheral vascular resistance is significantly decreased. **Onset:** 20 min. **Peak plasma levels:** 30 min (up to 4 hr for extended-release). **t½:** 2–5 hr. **Therapeutic serum levels:** 0.025–0.1 mcg/mL. **Duration:** 4–8 hr (12 hr for extended-release). Low-fat meals may slow the rate but not the extent of absorption. Metabolized in the liver to inactive metabolites.

Uses: Vasospastic (Prinzmetal's or variant) angina. Chronic stable angina without vasospasm, including angina due to increased effort (especially in clients who cannot take beta blockers or nitrates or who remain symptomatic following clinical doses of these drugs). Essential hypertension (sustained-release only). *Investigational:* PO, sublingually, or chewed in hypertensive emergencies. Also prophylaxis of migraine headaches, primary pulmonary hypertension, severe pregnancy-associated hypertension, esophageal diseases, Raynaud's phenomenon, CHF, asthma, premature labor, biliary and renal colic, and cardiomyopathy.

Dosage

- **Capsules**

Individualized. Initial: 10 mg t.i.d. (range: 10–20 mg t.i.d.); **maintenance:** 10–30 mg t.i.d.–q.i.d. Clients with coronary artery spasm may respond better to 20–30 mg t.i.d.–q.i.d. Doses greater than 120 mg/day are rarely needed while doses greater than 180 mg/day are not recommended.

- **Sustained-Release Tablets**

Initial: 30 or 60 mg once daily for Procardia XL and 30 mg once daily for Adalat CC. Titrate over a 7–14-day period. Dosage can be increased as required and as tolerated, to a maximum of 120 mg/day for Procardia XL and 90 mg/day for Adalat CC.

Investigational, hypertensive emergencies.

10–20 mg given PO, sublingually (by puncturing capsule and squeezing contents under the tongue), or chewed (capsule is punctured several times and then chewed).

Administration/Storage

1. A single dose (other than sustained-released) should not exceed 30 mg.
2. Before increasing the dose of drug, BP should be carefully monitored.
3. Only the sustained-release tablets should be used to treat hypertension.
4. Sublingual nitroglycerin and long-acting nitrates may be used concomitantly with nifedipine.
5. Concomitant therapy with beta-adrenergic blocking agents may be used. In these cases, note any potential drug interactions.
6. Clients withdrawn from beta blockers may manifest symptoms of increased angina which cannot be prevented by nifedipine; in fact, nifedipine may increase the severity of angina in this situation.
7. Clients with angina may be switched to the sustained-release product at the nearest equivalent total daily dose. However, doses greater than 90 mg/day should be used with caution.
8. Protect capsules from light and moisture and store at room temperature in the original container.
9. During initial therapy and when dosage is increased, clients may experience an increase in the frequency, duration, or severity of angina.
10. Food may decrease the rate but not the extent of absorption. Thus, the drug can be taken without regard to meals.

Contraindications: Hypersensitivity. Lactation.

Special Concerns: Use with caution in impaired hepatic or renal function and in elderly clients. Initial increase in frequency, duration, or severity of angina (may also be seen in clients being withdrawn from beta blockers and who begin taking nifedipine).

Laboratory Test Interferences: ↑ Alkaline phosphatase, CPK, LDH, AST, ALT. Positive Coombs' test.

Side Effects: *CV:* Peripheral and pulmonary edema, MI, hypotension, palpitations, syncope, CHF (especially if used with a beta blocker), decreased platelet aggregation, arrhythmias, tachycardia. Increased frequency, length, and duration of angina when beginning nifedipine therapy. *GI:* Nausea, diarrhea, constipation, flatulence, abdominal cramps, dysgeusia, vomiting, dry mouth, eructation, gastroesophageal reflux, melena. *CNS:* Dizziness, lightheadedness, giddiness, nervousness, sleep disturbances, headache, weakness, depression, migraine, psychoses, hallucinations, disturbances in equilibrium, somnolence, insomnia, abnormal dreams, malaise, anxiety. *Dermatologic:* Rash, dermatitis, urticaria, pruritus, photosensitivity, erythema multiforme, ***Stevens-Johnson syndrome.*** *Respiratory:* Dyspnea, cough, wheezing, SOB, respiratory infection, throat, nasal, or chest congestion. *Musculoskeletal:* Muscle cramps or inflammation, joint pain or stiffness, arthritis, ataxia, myoclonic dystonia, hypertonia, asthenia. *Hematologic:* Thrombocytopenia, leukopenia, purpura, anemia. *Other:* Fever, chills, sweating, blurred vision, sexual difficulties, flushing, transient blindness, hyperglycemia, hypokalemia, gingival hyperplasia, allergic hepatitis, hepatitis, tinnitus, gynecomastia, polyuria, nocturia, erythromelalgia, weight gain, epistaxis, facial and periorbital edema, hypoesthesia, gout, abnormal lacrimation, breast pain, dysuria, hematuria.

Additional Drug Interactions

Anticoagulants, oral / Possibility of ↑ PT

Cimetidine / ↑ Bioavailability of nifedipine

Digoxin / ↑ Effect of digoxin by ↓ excretion by kidney

Magnesium sulfate / ↑ Neuromuscular blockade and hypotension

Quinidine / Possible ↓ effect of quinidine due to ↓ plasma levels; ↑ risk of hypotension, bradycardia, AV block, pulmonary edema, and ventricular tachycardia

Ranitidine / ↑ Bioavailability of nifedipine
Theophylline / Possible ↑ effect of theophylline

NURSING CONSIDERATIONS

See also *Nursing Considerations* for *Calcium Channel Blocking Agents,* Chapter 28.

Assessment

1. Document any history of hypersensitivity to other calcium channel blocking agents.
2. Note any evidence of pulmonary edema, ECG abnormalities, or palpitations.
3. When working with women of childbearing age, determine if pregnant because drug is contraindicated.

Interventions

1. During the titration period, note evidence of hypotensive response and increased HR that result from peripheral vasodilation. These side effects may precipitate angina.
2. Although beta-blocking drugs may be used concomitantly in clients with chronic stable angina, the combined effects of the drugs cannot be predicted (especially in clients with compromised LV function or cardiac conduction abnormalities). Pronounced hypotension, heart block, and CHF may occur.
3. If therapy with a beta blocker is to be discontinued, gradually decrease dosage to prevent withdrawal syndrome.
4. Determine if client is able to swallow before administering sublingually.

Client/Family Teaching

1. Sustained-release tablets should not be chewed or divided.
2. There is no cause for concern if an empty tablet appears in the stool.
3. Maintain a fluid intake of 2–3 L/day to avoid constipation, unless contraindicated.
4. Do not use OTC agents unless approved.
5. Report any symptoms of persistent headache, flushing, nausea, palpitations, weight gain, dizziness, or lightheadedness.
6. Perform daily weights and note any extremity swelling. Advise that peripheral edema may result from arterial vasodilatation that is precipitated by nifedipine or that swelling may indicate increasing ventricular dysfunction and should be reported.
7. For clients also receiving beta-adrenergic blocking agents, review symptoms and advise to report any evidence of hypotension, exacerbation of angina, or evidence of heart failure.
8. Once beta-blocking agents have been discontinued, increased anginal pain may occur. This is a common withdrawal symptom and should be reported.

Evaluate

- ↓ Frequency and intensity of anginal episodes
- ↓ BP
- Improved peripheral circulation
- Therapeutic serum drug levels (0.025–0.1 mcg/mL)

Nimodipine

(nye-**MOH**-dih-peen)
Pregnancy Category: C
Nimotop, Nimotop I.V. ✱ **(Rx)**

See also *Calcium Channel Blocking Agents,* Chapter 28.

How Supplied: *Capsule:* 30 mg

Action/Kinetics: Nimodipine acts similarly to other calcium channel blocking agents although it has a greater effect on cerebral arteries than arteries elsewhere in the body (probably due to its highly lipophilic properties). Its mechanism, however, is not known when used to reduce neurologic deficits following subarachnoid hemorrhage. **Peak plasma levels:** 1 hr. **t½:** 1–2 hr. Significantly bound (over 95%) to plasma protein. Undergoes first-pass metabolism in the liver; metabolites are excreted through the urine.

Uses: Improvement of neurologic deficits due to spasm following subarachnoid hemorrhage from ruptured congenital intracranial aneurysms; clients should have Hunt and Hess grades of I–III. *Investigational:* Migraine headaches and cluster headaches.

Dosage

• **Capsules**

Adults: 60 mg q 4 hr beginning within 96 hr after subarachnoid hemorrhage and continuing for 21 consecutive days. The dosage should be reduced to 30 mg q 4 hr in clients with hepatic impairment.

Administration/Storage

1. If the client cannot swallow the capsule (e.g., unconscious or at time of surgery), a hole should be made in both ends of the capsule (soft gelatin) with an 18-gauge needle and the contents withdrawn into a syringe. The medication can then be administered into the NGT of the client and washed down the tube with 30 mL of NSS.
2. Adult clients should be given 60 mg q 4 hr for 21 consecutive days after subarachnoid hemorrhage. The drug dosage should be reduced to 30 mg q 4 hr if the client has hepatic failure.

Contraindication: Lactation.

Special Concerns: Safety and efficacy have not been established in children. Use with caution in clients with impaired hepatic function and reduced hepatic blood flow. The half-life may be increased in geriatric clients.

Laboratory Test Interferences: ↑ Nonfasting serum glucose, LDH, alkaline phosphatase, ALT. ↓ Platelet count.

Side Effects: *CV:* Hypotension, peripheral edema, CHF, ECG abnormalities, tachycardia, bradycardia, palpitations, rebound vasospasm, hypertension, hematoma, ***disseminated intravascular coagulation, deep vein thrombosis.*** *GI:* Nausea, dyspepsia, diarrhea, abdominal discomfort, cramps, ***GI hemorrhage,*** vomiting. *CNS:* Headache, depression, lightheadedness, dizziness. *Hepatic:* Abnormal liver function test, hepatitis, jaundice. *Hematologic:* Thrombocytopenia, anemia, purpura, ecchymosis. *Dermatologic:* Rash, dermatitis, pruritus, urticaria. *Miscellaneous:* Dyspnea, muscle pain or cramps, acne, itching, flushing, diaphoresis, wheezing, hyponatremia.

NURSING CONSIDERATIONS

See also *Nursing Considerations* for *Calcium Channel Blocking Agents,* Chapter 28.

Assessment

1. Obtain baseline lab studies and note any hepatic dysfunction, as dose should be reduced.
2. If the client is of childbearing age, ascertain if pregnant.
3. Perform baseline neurologic scores and thoroughly document deficits.

Interventions

1. Anticipate initiation of nimodipine therapy within 96 hr of subarachnoid hemorrhage.
2. Monitor VS and request written parameters for withholding drug.
3. Record I&O and weights throughout therapy.

Client/Family Teaching

1. Stress the importance of giving the drug on time. Sleep must be interrupted to give the medication q 4 hr RTC for 21 days.
2. Report any side effects of drug therapy, such as nausea, lightheadedness, dizziness, muscle cramps, or muscle pain.
3. Any SOB, the need to take deep breaths on occasion, wheezing, or other evidence of adverse effects should be reported.

Evaluate

• ↓ Neurologic deficits due to venospasm following subarachnoid hemorrhage

Verapamil

(ver-**AP**-ah-mil)

Pregnancy Category: C

Apo-Verap ✱, Calan, Calan SR, Isoptin, Isoptin I.V. ✱, Isoptin SR, Novo-Veramil ✱, Nu-Verap ✱, Verelan **(Rx)**

See also *Calcium Channel Blocking Agents,* Chapter 28.

How Supplied: *Capsule, extended release:* 120 mg, 180 mg, 240 mg; *Injection:* 2.5 mg/mL; *Tablet:* 40 mg,

80 mg, 120 mg; *Tablet, extended release:* 120 mg, 180 mg, 240 mg

Action/Kinetics: Slows AV conduction and prolongs effective refractory period. IV doses may slightly increase LV filling pressure. The drug moderately decreases myocardial contractility and peripheral vascular resistance. Worsening of heart failure may result if verapamil is given to clients with moderate to severe cardiac dysfunction. **Onset: PO,** 30 min; **IV,** 3–5 min. **Time to peak plasma levels (PO):** 1–2 hr (5–7 hr for extended-release). **t½, PO:** 4.5–12 hr with repetitive dosing; **IV, initial:** 4 min; **final:** 2–5 hr. **Therapeutic serum levels:** 0.08–0.3 mcg/mL. **Duration, PO:** 8–10 hr (24 hr for extended-release); **IV,** 10–20 min for hemodynamic effect and 2 hr for antiarrhythmic effect. Verapamil is metabolized to norverapamil, which possesses 20% of the activity of verapamil.

Uses: PO: Angina pectoris due to coronary artery spasm (Prinzmetal's variant), chronic stable angina including angina due to increased effort, unstable angina (preinfarction, crescendo). With digitalis to control rapid ventricular rate at rest and during stress in chronic atrial flutter or atrial fibrillation. Prophylaxis of repetitive paroxysmal supraventricular tachycardia. Essential hypertension. Sustained-release tablets are used to treat essential hypertension (Step I therapy). **IV:** Supraventricular tachyarrhythmias. Atrial flutter or fibrillation. *Investigational:* PO for prophylaxis of migraine, manic depression (alternate therapy), exercise-induced asthma, recumbent nocturnal leg cramps, hypertrophic cardiomyopathy, cluster headaches.

Dosage

• **Tablets**

Angina.

Individualized. Adults, initial: 80–120 mg t.i.d. (40 mg t.i.d. if client is sensitive to verapamil); **then,** increase dose to total of 240–480 mg/day.

Arrhythmias.

Dosage range in digitalized clients with chronic atrial fibrillation: 240–320 mg/day. For prophylaxis of nondigitalized clients: 240–480 mg/day in divided doses t.i.d.–q.i.d. Maximum effects are seen within 48 hr.

Essential hypertension.

Initial, when used alone: 80 mg t.i.d. Doses up to 360 mg daily may be used. Effects are seen in the first week of therapy. In the elderly or in people of small stature, initial dose should be 40 mg t.i.d.

• **Extended-Release Tablets**

Essential hypertension.

180–240 mg/day (120 mg/day in the elderly or people of small stature). If response is inadequate, 240 mg may be given b.i.d.

• **IV, Slow**

Supraventricular tachyarrhythmias.

Adults, initial: 5–10 mg (0.075–0.15 mg/kg) given over 2 min (over 3 min in older clients); **then,** 10 mg (0.15 mg/kg) 30 min later if response is not adequate. **Infants, up to 1 year:** 0.1–0.2 mg/kg over 2 min; **1–15 years:** 0.1–0.3 mg/kg (not to exceed 10 mg total dose) over 2 min. If response to initial dose is inadequate, it may be repeated after 30 min.

Administration/Storage

1. Before administration, ampules should be inspected for particulate matter or discoloration.
2. IV dosage should be administered under continuous ECG monitoring with resuscitation equipment readily available.
3. Give as a slow IV bolus (5–10 mg) over 2 min (3 min to elderly clients) to minimize toxic effects.
4. Ampules should be stored at 15°C–30°C (59°F–86°F) and protected from light.
5. Do not give verapamil in an infusion line containing 0.45% sodium chloride with sodium bicarbonate because a crystalline precipitate will form.

6. Do not give verapamil by IV push in the same line used for nafcillin infusion because a milky white precipitate will form.
7. Verapamil should not be mixed with albumin, amphotericin B, hydralazine, trimethoprim/sulfamethoxazole, or diluted with sodium lactate in polyvinyl chloride bags.
8. Verapamil will precipitate in any solution with a pH greater than 6.
9. Dosage of verapamil in the elderly should always be individualized because the pharmacologic effects are more pronounced and more prolonged.
10. The SR tablets (120 mg) may be useful for small stature and elderly clients who require less medication.
11. The sustained release tablets should be taken with food.
12. *Treatment of Overdose:* Beta-adrenergics, IV calcium, vasopressors, pacing, and resuscitation.

Contraindications: Severe hypotension, second- or third-degree AV block, cardiogenic shock, severe CHF, sick sinus syndrome (unless client has artificial pacemaker), severe LV dysfunction. Cardiogenic shock and severe CHF unless secondary to SVT that can be treated with verapamil. Lactation. Use of verapamil, IV, with beta-adrenergic blocking agents (as both depress myocardial contractility and AV conduction). Ventricular tachycardia.

Special Concerns: Infants less than 6 months of age may not respond to verapamil. Use with caution in hypertrophic cardiomyopathy, impaired hepatic and renal function, and in the elderly.

Laboratory Test Interferences: ↑ Alkaline phosphatase, transaminase.

Side Effects: *CV:* CHF, bradycardia, ***AV block, asystole,*** premature ventricular contractions and tachycardia (after IV use), peripheral and pulmonary edema, hypotension, syncope, palpitations, AV dissociation, ***MI, CVA.*** *GI:* Nausea, constipation, abdominal discomfort or cramps, dyspepsia, diarrhea, dry mouth. *CNS:* Dizziness, headache, sleep disturbances, depression, amnesia, paranoia, psychoses, hallucinations, jitteriness, confusion, drowsiness, vertigo. IV verapamil may increase intracranial pressure in clients with supratentorial tumors at the time of induction of anesthesia. *Dermatologic:* Rash, dermatitis, alopecia, urticaria, pruritus, erythema multiforme, ***Stevens-Johnson syndrome.*** *Respiratory:* Nasal or chest congestion, dyspnea, SOB, wheezing. *Musculoskeletal:* Paresthesia, asthenia, muscle cramps or inflammation, decreased neuromuscular transmission in Duchenne's muscular dystrophy. *Other:* Blurred vision, equilibrium disturbances, sexual difficulties, spotty menstruation, sweating, rotary nystagmus, flushing, gingival hyperplasia, polyuria, nocturia, gynecomastia, claudication, hyperkeratosis, purpura, petechiae, bruising, hematomas, tachyphylaxis.

Additional Drug Interactions

Antihypertensive agents / Additive hypotensive effects
Barbiturates / ↓ Bioavailability of verapamil
Calcium salts / ↓ Effect of verapamil
Carbamazepine / ↑ Effect of carbamazepine due to ↓ breakdown by liver
Cimetidine / ↑ Bioavailability of verapamil
Cyclosporine / ↑ Plasma levels of cyclosporine possibly leading to renal toxicity
Digoxin / ↑ Risk of digoxin toxicity due to ↑ plasma levels
Disopyramide / Additive depressant effects on myocardial contractility and AV conduction
Etomidate / Anesthetic effect of etomidate may be ↑ with prolonged respiratory depression and apnea
Lithium / ↓ Lithium plasma levels; lithium toxicity also observed
Muscle relaxants, nondepolarizing / ↑ Neuromuscular blockade due to effect of verapamil on calcium channels
Prazosin / Acute hypotensive effect
Quinidine / Possibility of bradycardia, hypotension, AV block, ventric-

ular tachycardia, and pulmonary edema
Ranitidine / ↑ Bioavailability of verapamil
Rifampin / ↓ Effect of verapamil
Sulfinpyrazone / ↑ Clearance of verapamil
Theophyllines / ↑ Effect of theophyllines
Vitamin D / ↓ Effect of verapamil
Warfarin / Possible ↑ effect of either drug due to ↓ plasma protein binding

NOTE: Since verapamil is significantly bound to plasma proteins, interaction with other drugs bound to plasma protein may occur.

NURSING CONSIDERATIONS

See also *Nursing Considerations* for *Calcium Channel Blocking Agents,* Chapter 28.

Assessment

1. Document indications for therapy and type and onset of symptoms.
2. List other agents prescribed and the outcome.
3. Review list of prescribed medications to ensure that none interact unfavorably.
4. Obtain baseline ECG and liver and renal function studies. Anticipate reduced dosage for clients with hepatic or renal impairment.

Interventions

1. Monitor VS and assess for bradycardia and hypotension, symptoms that may indicate overdosage. Verapamil may lower BP to dangerously low levels if the client already has a low BP.
2. *Do not* administer concurrently with IV beta-adrenergic blocking agents.
3. Unless treating verapamil overdosage, withhold any medication that elevates serum calcium levels and check with provider.
4. Clients receiving concurrent digoxin therapy should be assessed for symptoms of toxicity and have digoxin levels checked periodically.
5. If disopyramide is to be used, do not administer for at least 48 hr before verapamil to 24 hr after verapamil administration.
6. Administer extended-release tablets with food to minimize fluctuations in serum levels.

Client/Family Teaching

1. Review the appropriate method, frequency, and dose for administration.
2. Caution that drug may cause dizziness and orthostatic effects.
3. Instruct client in how to take BP and pulse and to maintain a record for provider review.
4. Avoid alcohol, CNS depressants, and any OTC preparations without provider approval.
5. Remind client to continue to follow lifestyle modifications (low-fat and low-salt diet, decreased alcohol consumption, no smoking, and regular exercise) in the overall goal of BP control.

Evaluate

- ↓ Frequency and severity of anginal attacks
- ↓ BP
- Restoration of normal sinus rhythm (usually 10 min after IV administration)
- Therapeutic serum drug levels (0.08–0.3 mcg/mL)

CENTRALLY-ACTING AGENTS

See the following individual entries:

Clonidine Hydrochloride
Guanabenz Acetate
Guanfacine Hydrochloride
Methyldopa
Methyldopate Hydrochloride

Clonidine hydrochloride

(**KLOH**-nih-deen)
Pregnancy Category: C
Apo-Clonidine ✱; Catapres; Catapres-TTS-1, -2, and -3; Dixarit ✱; Nu-Clonidine ✱ **(Rx)**

How Supplied: *Film, Extended Release:* 0.1 mg/24 hrs, 0.2 mg/24 hrs, 0.3 mg/24 hrs; *Tablet:* 0.1 mg, 0.2 mg, 0.3 mg

Action/Kinetics: Stimulates alpha-adrenergic receptors of the CNS, which results in inhibition of the sympathetic vasomotor centers and decreased nerve impulses. Thus, bradycardia and a fall in both SBP and DBP occur. Plasma renin levels are decreased, while peripheral venous pressure remains unchanged. The drug has few orthostatic effects. Although sodium chloride excretion is markedly decreased, potassium excretion remains unchanged. Tolerance to the drug may develop. **Onset, PO:** 30–60 min; **transdermal:** 2–3 days. **Peak plasma levels, PO:** 3–5 hr; **transdermal:** 2–3 days. **Maximum effect, PO:** 2–4 hr. **Duration, PO:** 12–24 hr; **transdermal:** 7 days (with system in place). **t½:** 12–16 hr. Approximately 50% excreted unchanged in the urine; 20% excreted through the feces.

The transdermal dosage form contains the following levels of drug: Catapres-TTS-1 contains 2.5 mg clonidine (surface area 3.5 cm^2), with 0.1 mg released daily; Catapres-TTS-2 contains 5 mg clonidine (surface area 7 cm^2), with 0.2 mg released daily; and Catapres-TTS-3 contains 7.5 mg clonidine (surface area 10.5 cm^2), with 0.3 mg released daily.

Uses: Mild to moderate hypertension. A diuretic or other antihypertensive drugs, or both, are often used concomitantly. *Investigational:* Diabetic diarrhea, alcohol withdrawal, treatment of Gilles de la Tourette syndrome, detoxification of opiate dependence, constitutional growth delay in children, hypertensive urgency (DBP greater than 120 mm Hg), menopausal flushing, diagnosis of pheochromocytoma, facilitate cessation of smoking, ulcerative colitis, postherpetic neuralgia, reduce allergen-induced inflammation in clients with extrinsic asthma.

Dosage

- **Tablets**

Hypertension.

Initial: 0.1 mg b.i.d.; **then,** increase by 0.1–0.2 mg/day until desired response is attained; **maintenance:** 0.2–0.6 mg/day in divided doses (maximum: 2.4 mg/day). Tolerance necessitates increased dosage or concomitant administration of a diuretic. Gradual increase of dosage after initiation minimizes side effects.

NOTE: In hypertensive clients unable to take PO medication, clonidine may be administered sublingually at doses of 0.2–0.4 mg/day. **Pediatric:** 0.005–0.025 mg/kg/day (5–25 mcg/kg/day) in divided doses q 6 hr; increase dose at 5–7-day intervals.

Gilles de la Tourette syndrome.

0.15–0.2 mg/day.

Withdrawal from opiate dependence.

0.015–0.016 mg/kg/day (15–16 mcg/kg/day).

Alcohol withdrawal.

0.3–0.6 mg q 6 hr.

Diabetic diarrhea.

0.15–1.2 mg/day.

Constitutional growth delay in children.

0.0375–0.15 mg/m^2/day.

Hypertensive urgency.

Initial: 0.1–0.2 mg; **then,** 0.05–0.1 mg q hr to a maximum of 0.8 mg.

Menopausal flushing.

0.1–0.4 mg.

Diagnosis of pheochromocytoma.

0.3 mg.

Postherpetic neuralgia.

0.2 mg/day.

Reduce allergen-induced inflammation in extrinsic asthma.

0.15 mg for 3 days.

Facilitate cessation of smoking.

0.15–0.4 mg/day or 0.2 mg/24 hr patch.

Ulcerative colitis.

0.3 mg t.i.d.

- **Transdermal**

Hypertension.

Initial: Use 0.1-mg system; **then,** if after 1–2 weeks adequate control has not been achieved, can use another 0.1-mg system or a larger system.

The antihypertensive effect may not be seen for 2–3 days. The system should be changed q 7 days.

Diabetic diarrhea.
0.3 mg/24 hr patch.

Menopausal flushing.
0.1 mg/24 hr patch.

Facilitate cessation of smoking.
0.2 mg/24 hr patch.

Administration/Storage

1. If the transdermal system is used, apply the medication to a hairless area of skin, such as upper arm or torso changing the system q 7 days.
2. Use a different site with each application.
3. It may take 2–3 days to achieve effective blood levels using the transdermal system. Therefore, any prior drug dosage should be reduced gradually.
4. If the drug is to be taken PO, administer the last dose of the day at bedtime to ensure overnight control of BP.
5. Clients with severe hypertension may require other antihypertensive drug therapy in addition to transdermal clonidine.
6. If the drug is to be discontinued, it should be done gradually over a period of 2–4 days.
7. *Treatment of Overdose:* Maintain respiration; perform gastric lavage followed by activated charcoal. Magnesium sulfate may be used to hasten the rate of transport through the GI tract. IV atropine sulfate (0.6 mg for adults; 0.01 mg/kg for children), epinephrine, tolazoline, or dopamine to treat persistent bradycardia. IV fluids and elevation of the legs are used to reverse hypotension; if unresponsive to these measures, dopamine (2–20 mcg/kg/min) or tolazoline (1 mg/kg IV, up to a maximum of 10 mg/dose) may be used. To treat hypertension, diazoxide, IV furosemide, or an alpha-adrenergic blocking drug may be used.

Special Concerns: Use with caution in presence of severe coronary insufficiency, recent MI, cerebrovascular disease, or chronic renal failure. Use with caution during lactation. Safe use in children not established. Geriatric clients may be more sensitive to the hypotensive effects; a decreased dosage may also be necessary in these clients due to age-related decreases in renal function.

Laboratory Test Interferences: Transient ↑ blood glucose and serum CPK. Weakly + Coombs' test. Alteration of electrolyte balance.

Side Effects: *CNS:* Drowsiness (common), sedation, dizziness, headache, fatigue, malaise, nightmares, nervousness, restlessness, anxiety, mental depression, increased dreaming, insomnia, hallucinations, delirium, agitation. *GI:* Dry mouth (common), constipation, anorexia, N&V, parotid pain, weight gain. *CV:* CHF, Raynaud's phenomenon, abnormalities in ECG, palpitations, tachycardia and bradycardia, orthostatic symptoms, conduction disturbances, sinus bradycardia. *Dermatologic:* Urticaria, skin rashes, ***angioneurotic edema,*** pruritus, thinning of hair, alopecia. *GU:* Impotence, urinary retention, decreased sexual activity, loss of libido, nocturia, difficulty in urination. *Musculoskeletal:* Muscle or joint pain, leg cramps, weakness. *Other:* Gynecomastia, increase in blood glucose (transient), increased sensitivity to alcohol, dryness of mucous membranes of nose; itching, burning, dryness of eyes; skin pallor, fever.

Transdermal products: Localized skin reactions, pruritus, erythema, allergic contact sensitization and contact dermatitis, localized vesiculation, hyperpigmentation, edema, excoriation, burning, papules, throbbing, blanching, generalized macular rash.

NOTE: Rebound hypertension may be manifested if clonidine is withdrawn abruptly.

Symptoms of Overdose: Hypotension, bradycardia, respiratory and CNS depression, hypoventilation, hypothermia, apnea, miosis, agitation, irritability, lethargy, ***seizures,***

cardiac conduction defects, arrhythmias, transient hypertension, diarrhea, vomiting.

Drug Interactions

Alcohol / ↑ Depressant effects
Beta-adrenergic blocking agents / Paradoxical hypertension; also, ↑ severity of rebound hypertension following clonidine withdrawal
CNS depressants / ↑ Depressant effect
Levodopa / ↓ Effect of levodopa
Tolazoline / Blocks antihypertensive effect
Tricyclic antidepressants / Blocks antihypertensive effect

NURSING CONSIDERATIONS

See also *Nursing Considerations* for *Antihypertensive Agents,* Chapter 28.

Assessment

1. Document indications for therapy, onset and type of symptoms, and previous treatments.
2. Note client's occupation as this drug may interfere with the ability to work and should be noted.
3. List drugs currently prescribed to prevent any unfavorable interactions.

Interventions

1. Monitor BP closely during the initial therapy. A decrease in BP occurs within 30–60 min after administration of clonidine and may persist for 8 hr.
2. Weigh the client daily, in the morning, in clothing of the same weight, to determine if there is edema caused by sodium retention. Any fluid retention should disappear after 3–4 days.
3. Note any fluctuations in BP to determine whether it is preferable to use clonidine alone or concomitantly with a diuretic. A stable BP reduces orthostatic effects of postural changes.
4. Observe for a paradoxical hypertensive response if client is also receiving propranolol.
5. Note any evidence of depression that may be precipitated by the drug, especially in those clients with a history of mental depression.
6. If the client is concomitantly receiving tolazoline or a tricyclic antidepressant, be aware that these drugs may block the antihypertensive action of clonidine. An increased dosage of clonidine may be indicated.

Client/Family Teaching

1. Do not engage in activities that require mental alertness, such as operating machinery or driving a car, because the drug may cause drowsiness.
2. Do not discontinue medication abruptly or without medical supervision. Also do not initiate any change in the medication regimen until cleared by the provider.
3. If the drug is to be withdrawn, explain the need for gradual withdrawal to prevent rebound hypertension.
4. If the client has Parkinson's disease and is controlled with levodopa, advise to report any increase in the S&S of the disease. Clonidine may reduce the effect of levodopa.

Evaluate

• Control of BP
• Control of withdrawal symptoms from opiates

Guanabenz acetate

(**GWON**-ah-benz)
Pregnancy Category: C
Wytensin **(Rx)**

See also *Antihypertensive Agents,* Chapter 28.

How Supplied: *Tablet:* 4 mg, 8 mg

Action/Kinetics: Guanabenz stimulates alpha-adrenergic receptors in the CNS, resulting in a decrease in sympathetic impulses and in sympathetic tone. It also decreases the pulse rate, but postural hypotension has not been manifested. **Onset:** 60 min. **Peak effect:** 2–4 hr. **Peak plasma levels:** 2–5 hr. **t½:** 6 hr. **Duration:** 8–12 hr.

Use: Hypertension, alone or as adjunct with thiazide diuretics.

Dosage

• **Tablets**

Hypertension.

Adults: initial, 4 mg b.i.d. alone or with a diuretic; **then,** increase by

4–8 mg q 1–2 weeks until control achieved. Maximum recommended dose: 32 mg b.i.d.

Administration/Storage

1. The drug should be kept tightly closed and protected from light.

2. *Treatment of Overdose:* Supportive treatment. VS and fluid balance should be monitored. Syrup of ipecac or gastric lavage followed by activated charcoal; administration of fluids, pressor agents, and atropine. Adequate airway should be maintained; artificial respiration may be required.

Contraindications: Lactation, children under 12 years of age.

Special Concerns: Use with caution in severe coronary insufficiency, cerebrovascular disease, recent MI, hepatic or renal disease. Geriatric clients may be more sensitive to the hypotensive and sedative effects of guanabenz; also, it may be necessary to decrease the dose in these clients due to age-related decreases in renal function.

Side Effects: *CNS:* Drowsiness and sedation (common), dizziness, weakness, headache, ataxia, depression, disturbances in sleep, excitement. *GI:* Dry mouth (common), N&V, diarrhea, constipation, abdominal pain or discomfort. *CV:* Palpitations, chest pain, arrhythmias. *Miscellaneous:* Edema, blurred vision, muscle aches, dyspnea, rash, pruritus, nasal congestion, urinary frequency, gynecomastia, alterations in taste, disturbances of sexual function, taste disorders, aches in extremities.

Symptoms of Overdose: Hypotension, sleepiness, irritability, miosis, lethargy, bradycardia.

Drug Interaction: Use with CNS depressants may result in significant sedation.

NURSING CONSIDERATIONS

See also *Nursing Considerations* for *Antihypertensive Agents,* Chapter 28.

Client/Family Teaching

1. Do not drive an automobile or operate machinery until the sedative effect of this drug has been assessed.

2. Be alert to disturbances in sleep that may indicate a depressive episode and report.

3. Avoid alcohol and any other CNS depressants.

Evaluate: ↓ BP with control of hypertension.

Guanfacine hydrochloride

(**GWON**-fah-seen)

Pregnancy Category: B

Tenex **(Rx)**

See also *Antihypertensive Agents,* Chapter 28.

How Supplied: *Tablet:* 1 mg, 2 mg

Action/Kinetics: Guanfacine is thought to act by central stimulation of alpha-2 receptors resulting in a decrease in peripheral sympathetic output and HR resulting in a decrease in BP. The drug may also manifest a direct peripheral alpha-2 receptor stimulant action. **Onset:** 2 hr. **Peak plasma levels:** 1–4 hr. **Peak effect:** 6–12 hr. **t½:** 12–23 hr. **Duration:** 24 hr. Approximately 50% is excreted through the kidneys unchanged.

Uses: Hypertension alone or with a thiazide diuretic. *Investigational:* Withdrawal from heroin use, to reduce the frequency of migraine headaches.

Dosage

- **Tablets**

Hypertension.

Initial: 1 mg/day alone or with other antihypertensives; if satisfactory results are not obtained in 3–4 weeks, dosage may be increased by 1 mg at 1–2-week intervals up to a maximum of 3 mg/day in one to two divided doses.

Heroin withdrawal.

0.03–1.5 mg/day.

Reduce frequency of migraine headaches.

1 mg/day for 12 weeks.

Administration/Storage

1. To minimize drowsiness, the daily dose should be given at bedtime.

2. If a decrease in BP is not maintained for over 24 hr, the daily dose may be more effective if divided, although the incidence of side effects increases.
3. Adverse effects increase significantly when the daily dose exceeds 3 mg.
4. Therapy for hypertension should be initiated in clients already taking a thiazide diuretic.
5. Abrupt cessation of therapy may result in increases in plasma and urinary catecholamines, symptoms of nervousness and anxiety, and increases in BP greater than those prior to therapy.
6. *Treatment of Overdose:* Gastric lavage. Supportive therapy, as needed. The drug is not dialyzable.

Contraindications: Hypersensitivity to guanfacine. Acute hypertension associated with toxemia. Children less than 12 years of age.

Special Concerns: Use with caution during lactation. Use with caution in clients with recent MI, cerebrovascular disease, chronic renal or hepatic failure, or severe coronary insufficiency. Geriatric clients may be more sensitive to the hypotensive and sedative effects. Safety and efficacy in children less than 12 years of age have not been determined.

Side Effects: *GI:* Dry mouth, constipation, nausea, abdominal pain, diarrhea, dyspepsia, dysphagia, taste perversion or alterations in taste. *CNS:* Sedation, weakness, dizziness, headache, fatigue, insomnia, amnesia, confusion, depression, vertigo, agitation, anxiety, malaise, nervousness, tremor. *CV:* Bradycardia, substernal pain, palpitations, syncope, chest pain, tachycarida, cardiac fibrillation, CHF, heart block, MI (rare), cardiovascular accident (rare). *Ophthalmic:* Visual disturbances, conjunctivitis, iritis, blurred vision. *Dermatologic:* Pruritus, dermatitis, purpura, sweating, skin rash with exfoliation, alopecia, rash. *GU:* Decreased libido, impotence, urinary incontinence or frequency, testicular disorder, nocturia, acute renal failure. *Musculoskeletal:* Leg cramps, hypokinesia, arthralgia, leg pain, myalgia. *Other:* Rhinitis, tinnitus, dyspnea, paresthesias, paresis, asthenia, edema, abnormal liver function tests.

Symptoms of Overdose: Drowsiness, bradycardia, lethargy, hypotension.

Drug Interactions: Additive sedative effects when used concomitantly with CNS depressants.

NURSING CONSIDERATIONS

See also *Nursing Considerations* for *Antihypertensive Agents,* Chapter 28.

Assessment

1. Document indications for therapy, onset of symptoms, and any previous agents used and the outcome.
2. Determine the extent of CAD, and note any evidence of renal or liver dysfunction.

Client/Family Teaching

1. Stress the importance of not discontinuing the drug abruptly.
2. Do not perform activities that require mental alertness until drug effects realized.

Evaluate

- ↓ BP to within desired range
- Control of S&S of heroin withdrawal
- ↓ Frequency of migraine headaches

Methyldopa

(meth-ill-**DOH**-pah)
Pregnancy Category: B
Aldomet, Apo-Methyldopa ✱, Novo-Medopa ✱, Nu-Medopa ✱
(Rx)

Methyldopate hydrochloride

(meth-ill-**DOH**-payt)
Pregnancy Category: B
Aldomet Hydrochloride **(Rx)**

How Supplied: Methyldopa: *Suspension:* 250 mg/5 mL; *Tablet:* 125 mg, 250 mg, 500 mg.
Methyldopate hydrochloride: *Injection:* 50 mg/mL

Action/Kinetics: Primary mechanism thought to be that the active metabolite, alpha-methyl-norepinephrine, lowers BP by stimulating central inhibitory alpha-adrenergic receptors, false neurotransmission, and/or reduction of plasma renin. It causes little change in CO. **PO: Onset:** 7–12 hr. **Duration:** 12–24 hr. All effects terminated within 48 hr. Absorption is variable. **IV: Onset:** 4–6 hr. **Duration:** 10–16 hr. Seventy percent of drug excreted in urine. **Full therapeutic effect:** 1–4 days. **t½:** 1.7 hr. *NOTE:* Methyldopa is a component of Aldoril.

Uses: Moderate to severe hypertension. Particularly useful for clients with impaired renal function, renal hypertension, resistant cases of hypertension complicated by stroke, CAD, or nitrogen retention, and for hypertensive crisis (parenterally).

Dosage

• **Methyldopa. Oral Suspension, Tablets.**

Hypertension.

Initial: 250 mg b.i.d.–t.i.d. for 2 days. Adjust dose q 2 days. If increased, start with evening dose. **Usual maintenance:** 0.5–3.0 g/day in two to four divided doses; **maximum:** 3 g/day. Transfer to and from other antihypertensive agents should occur gradually, with initial dose of methyldopa not exceeding 500 mg. *NOTE:* Do not use combination medication to initiate therapy. **Pediatric, initial:** 10 mg/kg/day in two to four divided doses, adjusting maintenance to a maximum of 65 mg/kg/day (or 3 g/day, whichever is less).

• **Methyldopate HCl. IV Infusion**

Hypertension.

Adults: 250–500 mg q 6 hr; **maximum:** 1 g q 6 hr for hypertensive crisis.

Switch to PO methyldopa, at same dosage level, when BP is brought under control. **Pediatric:** 20–40 mg/kg/day in divided doses q 6 hr; **maximum:** 65 mg/kg/day (or 3 g/day, whichever is less).

Administration/Storage

1. If the drug is to be administered by IV, methyldopate HCl should be mixed with 100 mL of 5% dextrose or administered in D5W at a concentration of 10 mg/mL.
2. The IV should be diluted in 100 mL of D5W and infused over a 30–60-min period.
3. Tolerance may occur following 2–3 months of therapy.
4. Increasing the dose or adding a diuretic often restores effect on BP.
5. *Treatment of Overdose:* Induction of vomiting or gastric lavage if detected early. General supportive treatment with special attention to HR, CO, blood volume, urinary function, electrolyte imbalance, paralytic ileus, and CNS activity. In severe cases, hemodialysis is effective.

Contraindications: Sensitivity to drug, labile and mild hypertension, pregnancy, active hepatic disease, or pheochromocytoma.

Special Concerns: Use with caution in clients with a history of liver or kidney disease. Geriatric clients may be more sensitive to the hypotensive and sedative effects of guanabenz; also, it may be necessary to decrease the dose in these clients due to age-related decreases in renal function.

Laboratory Test Interferences: False + or ↑ : Alkaline phosphatase, bilirubin, BUN, BSP, cephalin flocculation, creatinine, AST, ALT, uric acid, Coombs' test, PT. Positive lupus erythematosus cell preparation and antinuclear antibodies.

Side Effects: *CNS:* Sedation (disappears with use), weakness, headache, asthenia, dizziness, paresthesias, Parkinson-like symptoms, psychic disturbances, choreoathetotic movements, Bell's palsy, decreased mental acuity, verbal memory impairment. *CV:* Bradycardia, orthostatic hypotension, hypersensitivity of carotid sinus, worsening of angina, hypertensive response (paradoxical), myocarditis. *GI:* N&V, abdominal distention, diarrhea or constipation, flatus, colitis, dry mouth, "black tongue," pancreatitis, sialoadenitis. *Hematologic:* ***Hemolytic anemia,*** leukopenia, granulocytopenia, thrombocytopenia, ***bone marrow depression.*** *Endocrine:* Gynecomastia, amenorrhea, galactorrhea, lactation, hyperprolactinemia. *Miscellaneous:* Edema, jaundice, hepatitis, liver disorders, abnormal liver function tests, rash (eczema, lichenoid eruption), ***toxic epidermal necrolysis,*** fever, lupus-like symptoms, impotence, failure to ejaculate, decreased libido, nasal stuffiness, joint pain, myalgia, ***septic shock-like syndrome.***

Symptoms of Overdose: CNS, GI, and CV effects including sedation, weakness, lightheadedness, dizziness, coma, bradycardia, acute hypotension, impairment of AV conduction, constipation, diarrhea, distention, flatus, N&V.

Drug Interactions

Anesthetics, general / Additive hypotension
Antidepressants, tricyclic / Tricyclic antidepressants may block hypotensive effect of methyldopa
Ephedrine / ↓ Action of ephedrine in methyldopa-treated clients
Fenfluramine / ↑ Effect of methyldopa
Haloperidol / Methyldopa ↑ toxic effects of haloperidol
Levodopa / ↑ Effect of both drugs
Lithium / ↑ Possibility of lithium toxicity
MAO inhibitors / May reverse hypotensive effect of methyldopa and cause headache and hallucinations
Methotrimeprazine / Additive hypotensive effect
Norepinephrine / ↑ Pressor response to norepinephrine
Phenoxybenzamine / Urinary incontinence
Phenylpropanolamine / ↑ Pressor response to phenylpropanolamine
Propranolol / Paradoxical hypertension
Sympathomimetics / Potentiation of hypertensive effect of sympathomimetics
Thiazide diuretics / Additive hypotensive effect
Thioxanthenes / Additive hypotensive effect
Tolbutamide / ↑ Hypoglycemia due to ↓ breakdown by liver
Tricyclic antidepressants / ↓ Effect of methyldopa
Vasodilator drugs / Additive hypotensive effect
Verapamil / ↑ Effect of methyldopa

NURSING CONSIDERATIONS

See also *Nursing Considerations* for *Antihypertensive Agents,* Chapter 28.

Assessment

1. Document indications for therapy, onset of symptoms, and other agents prescribed and the outcome.
2. Ascertain that hematologic studies, liver function tests, and a Coombs' test are done before and during drug therapy.
3. If the client requires a blood transfusion, ascertain that both direct and indirect Coombs' tests are done. If the indirect and direct Coombs' tests are positive, anticipate consultation with a hematologist.
4. Assess for signs of drug tolerance. These may occur during the second or third month of drug therapy.
5. Note any evidence of jaundice. The drug is contraindicated when the client has active hepatic disease.

Client/Family Teaching

1. To prevent dizziness and fainting, rise from bed slowly to a sitting position and dangle legs over the edge of the bed.
2. Sedation may occur when therapy is first started, but should disappear once the maintenance dose is established.
3. In rare cases, methyldopa may darken urine or turn it blue, but this reaction is not harmful.
4. Withhold drug and report any of the following symptoms: tiredness, fever, or yellowing of skin and whites of eyes.
5. Remind client to continue to follow prescribed diet and exercise program in the overall goal of BP contol.
6. Do not take any other medications or remedies unless appoved by provider.
7. Always carry a card detailing current medication regimen.

Evaluate: ↓ BP with control of hypertension.

COMBINATION DRUGS USED FOR HYPERTENSION

See the following individual entries:

Amiloride and Hydrochlorothiazide
Bisoprolol Fumarate and Hydrochlorothiazide
Enalapril Maleate and Hydrochlorothiazide
Lisinopril and Hydrochlorothiazide
Methyldopa and Hydrochlorothiazide
Propranolol and Hydrochlorothiazide
Reserpine and Chlorothiazide
Reserpine, Hydralazine, and Hydrochlorothiazide
Spironolactone and Hydrochlorothiazide
Triamterene and Hydrochlorothiazide

—COMBINATION DRUG—

Amiloride and Hydrochlorothiazide

(ah-**MILL**-oh-ryd, hy-droh-klor-oh-**THIGH**-ah-zyd)
Pregnancy Category: C
Apo-Amilzide, Moduretic, Moduret ✱, Nu-Amilzide ✱ **(Rx)**

See also *Amiloride* and *Hydrochlorothiazide,* Chapter 75.

How Supplied: See Content

Content: *Diuretic, potassium-sparing:* Amiloride HCl, 5 mg. *Antihypertensive/diuretic:* Hydrochlorothiazide, 50 mg.

Uses: Hypertension or CHF, especially when hypokalemia occurs. May be used alone or with other antihypertensive drugs, such as beta-adrenergic blocking drugs and methyldopa.

Dosage

- **Tablets**

All uses.

Initial: 1 tablet/day; **then,** dosage may be increased to 2 tablets/day.

Administration/Storage

1. This drug should be taken with food.
2. The daily dose may be given as a single dose or in divided doses.
3. More than 2 tablets/day are not usually necessary.
4. Maintenance therapy may be intermittent.

Special Concerns: Use with caution during lactation. Geriatric clients may be more sensitive to the hypotensive and electrolyte effects of this combination; also, age-related decreases in renal function may require a decrease in dosage.

NURSING CONSIDERATIONS

See *Nursing Considerations* for *Antihypertensive Agents,* Chapter 28, and individual agents.

Assessment

1. Note indications for therapy and assess appropriate parameters.
2. Document age; obtain baseline electrolytes and renal function studies.

Evaluate

- Control of hypertension
- Desired diuresis

—COMBINATION DRUG—

Bisoprolol fumarate and Hydrochlorothiazide

(**BUY**-soh-**proh**-lol, **high**-droh-**klor**-oh-**THIGH**-ah-zyd)
Pregnancy Category: C
Ziac **(Rx)**

See also *Bisoprolol fumarate,* Chapter 51, and *Hydrochlorothiazide,* Chapter 75.

How Supplied: See Content

Content: *Beta-adrenergic blocking agent:* Bisoprolol fumarate: 2.5, 5, or 10 mg. *Diuretic/antihypertensive:* Hydrochlorothiazide: 6.25 mg in all tablets.

Uses: First-line therapy in mild to moderate hypertension.

Dosage

- **Tablets**

Antihypertensive.

Adults, initial: One 2.5/6.25-mg

tablet given once daily. If needed, the dose may be increased q 14 days to a maximum of two 10/6.25-mg tablets given once daily.

Administration/Storage

1. The combination of bisoprolol and hydrochlorothiazide may be substituted for the titrated individual components.
2. If withdrawal of this combination is necessary, it should be achieved gradually over a period of 2 weeks with clients being carefully monitored.
3. Clients whose BP is controlled adequately with 50 mg hydrochlorothiazide but who experience significant potassium loss may achieve similar control of BP without the electrolyte disturbances by using the combination of bisoprolol and hydrochlorothiazide.

Contraindications: Use in bronchospastic pulmonary disease, cardiogenic shock, overt CHF, second- or third-degree AV block, marked sinus bradycardia, anuria, hypersensitivity to either drug or to other sulfonamide-derived drugs. Use during lactation.

Special Concerns: Use with caution in clients with peripheral vascular disease, impaired renal or hepatic function, and progressive liver disease. Use with caution in clients also receiving myocardial depressants or inhibitors of AV conduction such as verapamil, diltiazem, and disopyramide. Elderly clients may be more sensitive to the effects of this drug product. Safety and effectiveness have not been determined in children.

Side Effects: See individual drugs. Most commonly, dizziness and fatigue. At higher doses, bisoprolol inhibits beta-2-adrenergic receptors located in bronchial and vascular muscle.

Drug Interactions

Antihypertensives / Additive effect to decrease BP
Cyclopropane / Additive depression of myocardium
Trichloroethylene / Additive depression of myocardium

NURSING CONSIDERATIONS

See also *Nursing Considerations* for *Beta-Adrenergic Blocking Agents,* Chapter 51, *Antihypertensive Agents,* Chapter 28, and *Diuretics, Thiazides,* Chapter 75.

Assessment

1. Document indications for therapy, other agents used, and the outcome.
2. Determine any sensitivity to drug components or sulfonamide-derived drugs.
3. List all drugs prescribed to ensure that none interacts unfavorably.
4. Obtain baseline electrolytes and liver and renal function studies.
5. Screen client carefully as drug is not for use with bronchospastic pulmonary disease, PVD, diabetes, thyrotoxicosis, compensated cardiac failure, and liver or renal disease.
6. Obtain baseline ECG to ensure that there are no cardiac rhythms (second- or third-degree AV block or bradycardia) that would preclude drug therapy.

Interventions

1. Monitor VS carefully; drug will cause a reduction in SBP and DBP and HR. Request parameters for administration (e.g., hold if SBP < 90; HR < 45) when necessary.
2. Monitor I&O and serum electrolytes; observe closely for any symptoms of fluid and electrolyte imbalance.
3. With cessation of therapy, anticipate tapering dosages over 2 weeks to prevent any adverse sequelae.
4. If therapy is to be discontinued in clients receiving both clonidine and Ziac, the Ziac should be withdrawn several days before withdrawal of clonidine.

Client/Family Teaching

1. Do not stop taking medication abruptly. In clients with CAD, a heart attack or ventricular arrhythmia may be precipitated.
2. Do not perform activities that require mental alertness until drug effects realized.
3. Review some of the S&S of heart failure (increased SOB, edema, fatigue) and advise to report should

they occur as alternative therapy may be indicated.
4. Advise client with diabetes to monitor blood sugars carefully as beta blockers may mask symptoms of hypoglycemia.
5. Review the list of drug side effects, stressing those that should be reported immediately and also advise to report those that are persistent or bothersome.
6. Ensure that someone can and will take client BP and pulse regularly and maintain a written record for review by the provider.
7. Address diet restrictions (e.g., low salt, low fat, and, when indicated, low calorie) as well as a regular exercise routine that client will tolerate and follow.

Evaluate: Control of BP in clients with hypertension.

—COMBINATION DRUG—

Enalapril maleate and Hydrochlorothiazide

(en-**AL**-ah-prill, **high**-droh-**KLO**-**R**oh-**THIGH**-ah-zyd)
Pregnancy Category: D
Vaseretic **(Rx)**

See also *Enalapril maleate,* Chapter 28, and *Hydrochlorothiazide,* Chapter 75.

How Supplied: See Content

Content: *ACE inhibitor:* Enalapril, 10 mg. *Diuretic:* Hydrochlorothiazide, 25 mg.

Use: Hypertension in clients in whom combination therapy is appropriate.

Dosage

- **Tablets**

Adults: 1–2 of the 10–25 tablets once daily.

Administration/Storage

1. The dose of Vaseretic must be individualized and is determined by the titration of the individual components. Once the client has been successfully titrated with the individual components, Vaseretic (1 or 2 of the 10–25 tablets) may be given once daily if the titrated doses are the same as those in the fixed combination.
2. The daily dose should not exceed 2 tablets.
3. In clients who are being treated with hydrochlorothiazide, hypotension may occur following the initial dose of enalapril. Thus, if possible, the diuretic should be discontinued for 2–3 days before beginning therapy with enalapril. If the diuretic cannot be discontinued, an initial dose of 2.5 mg enalapril should be used under close medical supervision for at least 2 hr and until BP has stabilized for at least 1 additional hr.
4. Administration of potassium supplements, potassium salt substitutes, or potassium-sparing drugs may increase serum potassium levels.
5. The usual dose of Vaseretic is recommended for clients with a creatinine clearance greater than 30 mL/min.

Contraindications: Use for initial therapy of hypertension. Anuria or severe renal dysfunction. History of angioedema related to use of ACE inhibitors. Lactation.

Special Concerns: Excessive hypotension may be observed in clients with severe salt or volume depletion such as those treated with diuretics or on dialysis. Significant hypotension may also be seen in clients with severe CHF, with or without associated renal insufficiency. A significant fall in BP may result in MI or CVA in clients with ischemic heart or cerebrovascular disease.

Safety and effectiveness have not been established in children.

NURSING CONSIDERATIONS

See also *Nursing Considerations* for *Antihypertensive Agents,* Chapter 28, and individual agents.

Assessment

1. Document baseline BP, CBC, electrolytes, and liver and renal function.
2. Note any evidence of heart failure, cerebrovascular disease, or angioedema.

3. Document any history of gout, elevated cholesterol levels, or diabetes.
Evaluate: Control of hypertension.

COMBINATION DRUG

Lisinopril and Hydrochlorothiazide

(lie-**SIN**-oh-pril, hy-droh-kloh-roh-**THIGH**-ah-zyd)
Pregnancy Category: C
Prinzide, Zestoretic **(Rx)**

See also *Lisinopril,* Chapter 28, and *Hydrochlorothiazide,* Chapter 75.
How Supplied: See Content
Content: Lisinopril is an ACE inhibitor and hydrochlorothiazide is a diuretic. Prinzide 12.5 and Zestoretic 20–12.5: Lisinopril, 20 mg, and hydrochlorothiazide, 12.5 mg. Prinzide 25 and Zestoretic 20–25: Lisinopril, 20 mg, and hydrochlorothiazide, 25 mg.
Uses: Hypertension in clients in whom combination therapy is appropriate. Not for initial therapy.

Dosage

- **Tablets**

Hypertension.

Individualized. Usual: 1 or 2 tablets once daily of Prinzide 12.5, Prinzide 25, Zestoretic 20–12.5, or Zestoretic 20–25.

Administration

1. With clients whose BP is controlled with lisinopril, 20 mg plus hydrochlorothiazide, 25 mg given separately should be given a trial of Prinzide 12.5 or Zestoretic 20–12.5 before Prinzide 25 or Zestoretic 20–25 mg is used.
2. The maximum recommended daily dose of lisinopril is 80 mg in a single daily dose. However, clients usually do not require hydrochlorothiazide in doses exceeding 50 mg/day, especially if combined with other antihypertensives.
3. Use of potassium supplements, potassium-sparing diuretics, or potassium salt substitutes with Prinzide or Zestoretic may lead to increases in serum potassium.
4. Prinzide or Zestoretic is recommended for those clients with a creatinine clearance greater than 30 mL/min.

NURSING CONSIDERATIONS

See also *Nursing Considerations* for *Antihypertensive Agents,* Chapter 28. and Individual Agents.

Client/Family Teaching

1. Instruct how to take BP and maintain written record for provider review.
2. Explain how to avoid symptoms of orthostatic hypotension (i.e., rise slowly from sitting or lying position and wait until symptoms subside).
3. Avoid all potassium supplements as well as foods high in potassium.
4. Stress the importance of reporting for scheduled lab studies.

Evaluate: Control of hypertension.

COMBINATION DRUG

Methyldopa and Hydrochlorothiazide

(meth-ill-**DOH**-pah, hy-droh-klor-oh-**THIGH**-ah-zyd)
Pregnancy Category: C
Aldoril 15, Aldoril 25, Aldoril D30, Aldoril D50, Apo-Methazide ✱ **(Rx)**

See also *Methyldopa,* Chapter 28, and *Hydrochlorothiazide,* Chapter 75.
How Supplied: See Content
Content: *Antihypertensive:* Methyldopa, 250–500 mg. *Diuretic/antihypertensive:* Hydrochlorothiazide, 15–50 mg.
Uses: Hypertension (not for initial treatment).

Dosage

- **Tablets**

Adults: 1 tablet b.i.d.–t.i.d. for first 48 hr; **then,** increase or decrease dose, depending on response, in intervals of not less than 2 days. Maximum daily dosage: methyldopa, 3.0 g; hydrochlorothiazide, 100–200 mg.

Administration/Storage

1. If Aldoril is given together with antihypertensives other than thiazides, the initial dose of methyldopa should not be more than 500 mg/day in divided doses.
2. Additional methyldopa may be

given separately if Aldoril alone does not control BP adequately.
3. If tolerance is observed after 2–3 months of therapy, the dose of either methyldopa and/or hydrochlorothiazide may be increased to restore control.
Contraindications: Active hepatic disease.
Special Concerns: Use in pregnancy only if benefits outweigh risks.

NURSING CONSIDERATIONS

See also *Nursing Considerations* for *Antihypertensive Agents,* Chapter 28, and individual agents.
Evaluate: ↓ BP with control of hypertension.

COMBINATION DRUG

Propranolol and Hydrochlorothiazide

(proh-**PRAN**-oh-lohl, hy-droh-**klor**-oh-**THIGH**-ah-zyd)
Pregnancy Category: C
Inderide 40/25, Inderide 80/25, Inderide LA 80/50, Inderide LA 120/50, Inderide LA 160/50 **(Rx)**

See also *Propranolol,* Chapter 51, and *Hydrochlorothiazide,* Chapter 75.
How Supplied: See Content
Content: *Antihypertensive/diuretic:* Hydrochlorothiazide, 25 mg (Inderide) or 50 mg (Inderide LA).
Beta-adrenergic blocking agent: Propranolol HCl, 40 or 80 mg (Inderide) or 80, 120, or 160 mg (Inderide LA).

Also see information on individual components.
Use: Hypertension (not indicated for initial therapy).

Dosage
- **Inderide Tablets**

Individualized: 1–2 tablets b.i.d., up to 320 mg propranolol HCl daily.
- **Inderide LA Capsules**

1 capsule once daily.
Administration/Storage
1. Because of side effects from hydrochlorothiazide, Inderide should not be used if propranolol must be given in excess of 320 mg/day.
2. If another antihypertensive agent is required, initial dosage should be one-half the usual recommended dose to prevent an excessive drop in BP.
3. Inderide LA should not be considered a milligram-to-milligram substitute for Inderide because the LA produces lower blood levels.
Special Concerns: Use with caution during lactation. Safety and effectiveness have not been established in children. The risk of hypothermia is increased in geriatric clients.

NURSING CONSIDERATIONS

See also *Nursing Considerations* for *Antihypertensive Agents,* Chapter 28, and Individual Agents.
Evaluate: ↓ BP with control of hypertension.

COMBINATION DRUG

Reserpine and Chlorothiazide

(reh-**SIR**-peen, klor-oh-**THIGH**-ah-zyd)
Pregnancy Category: C
Diupres, Diurigen with Reserpine **(Rx)**

See also *Chlorothiazide,* Chapter 75.
How Supplied: See Content
Content: *Antihypertensive:* Reserpine, 0.125 mg. *Antihypertensive/diuretic:* Chlorothiazide, 250 or 500 mg.
Uses: Hypertension—not to be used for initial treatment.

Dosage
- **Tablets**

1–2 tablets 1–2 times/day.
Contraindications: Pregnancy, lactation, anuria. Reserpine is contraindicated in active peptic ulcer, ulcerative colitis, active mental depression, and clients with suicidal tendencies.
Special Concerns: Safety and effectiveness have not been determined in children. Use with caution in severe renal disease, in impaired hepatic function, and progressive liver dis-

ease. Geriatric clients may be more sensitive to the usual adult dose.

NURSING CONSIDERATIONS

See also *Nursing Considerations* for *Antihypertensive Agents,* Chapter 28, and Individual Agents.

Client/Family Teaching

1. Administer with or after meals.
2. Drug may cause dizziness and drowsiness.
3. Maintain a record of BP and bring to each visit, especially when used with other antihypertensive agents.
4. Report any nightmares or depression.
5. Advise women of childbearing age to use birth control.

Evaluate: Control of BP with hypertension.

—COMBINATION DRUG—

Reserpine, Hydralazine, and Hydrochlorothiazide

(reh-**SIR**-peen, hy-**DRAL**-ah-zeen, **hy**-droh-**klor**-oh-**THIGH**-ah-zyd)

Pregnancy Category: C

Cam-Ap-Es, Cherapas, Ser-A-Gen, Seralazide, Ser-Ap-Es, Serpazide, Tri-Hydroserpine, Unipres **(Rx)**

See also *Hydralazine,* Chapter 28, and *Hydrochlorothiazide,* Chapter 75.

How Supplied: See Content

Content: *Antihypertensive:* Hydralazine, 25 mg. *Antihypertensive:* Reserpine, 0.1 mg. *Antihypertensive/diuretic:* Hydrochlorothiazide, 15 mg.

Uses: Treatment of hypertension (not to be used for initial therapy).

Dosage

- **Tablets**

Individualized. Usual: 1–2 tablets t.i.d.

Administration/Storage

1. It may take up to 2 weeks to manifest the maximum effect on BP reduction.
2. Clients should be maintained on the lowest dose possible (requires titration).
3. If additional antihypertensive medication is necessary, initial doses should be 50% of the usual recommended dose.

Contraindications: Pregnancy, lactation, anuria. Reserpine is contraindicated in active peptic ulcer, ulcerative colitis, active mental depression, in clients with suicidal tendencies or in those receiving electroconvulsive shock therapy, CAD, mitral valvular rheumatic heart disease.

Special Concerns: Safety and effectiveness have not been determined in children. Geriatric clients may be more sensitive to the adult dose.

NURSING CONSIDERATIONS

See also *Nursing Considerations* for *Antihypertensive Agents,* Chapter 28, and Individual Agents.

Assessment

1. Note any history of mental depression or electroshock therapy.
2. Determine presence of ulcerative colitis or PUD.

Evaluate: Control of BP with hypertension.

—COMBINATION DRUG—

Spironolactone and Hydrochlorothiazide

(speer-oh-no-**LAK**-tohn, hy-droh-**klor**-oh-**THIGH**-ah-zyd)

Aldactazide, Novo-Spirozine ✱ **(Rx)**

How Supplied: See Content

Content: This drug is a combination of a thiazide and potassium-sparing diuretic. *Diuretic:* Spironolactone, 25 or 50 mg. *Diuretic/antihypertensive:* Hydrochlorothiazide, 25 or 50 mg. Also see information on individual components.

Uses: Congestive heart failure, essential hypertension, nephrotic syndrome. Edema and/or ascites in cirrhosis of the liver.

Dosage

- **Tablets**

Edema.

Adults, usual: 100 mg of each drug daily (range: 25–200 mg), given as single or divided doses. **Pediatric, usual:** equivalent to 1.65–3.3 mg/kg spironolactone.

Essential hypertension.
Adults, usual: 50–100 mg of each drug daily in single or divided doses.
Contraindication: Use in pregnancy only if benefits outweigh risks.

NURSING CONSIDERATIONS

See *Nursing Considerations* for *Diuretics, Antihypertensive Agents,* Chapter 28, and individual components.

Evaluate

- Enhanced diuresis with ↓ edema
- ↓ BP

COMBINATION DRUG

Triamterene and Hydrochlorothiazide Capsules

(try-**AM**-ter-een, hy-droh-**klor**-oh-**THIGH**-ah-zyd)
Pregnancy Category: C
Dyazide **(Rx)**

Triamterene and Hydrochlorothiazide Tablets

(try-**AM**-teh-reen, hy-droh-**kloh**-roh-**THIGH**-ah-zyd)
Pregnancy Category: C
Apo-Triazide ✱, Dyazide, Maxzide, Maxide-25MG, Novo-Triamzide ✱, Nu-Triazide ✱ **(Rx)**

See also *Hydrochlorothiazide* and *Triamterene,* Chapter 75.
How Supplied: See Content
Content: Capsules. *Diuretic:* Hydrochlorothiazide, 25 or 50 mg. *Diuretic:* Triamterene, 50 or 100 mg. **Tablets.** *Diuretic:* Hydrochlorothiazide, 25 or 50 mg. *Diuretic:* Triamterene, 37.5 or 75 mg. (In Canada the tablets contain 25 mg of hydrochlorothiazide and 50 mg triamterene.)
Uses: To treat hypertension or edema in clients who manifest hypokalemia on hydrochlorothiazide alone. In clients requiring a diuretic and in whom hypokalemia cannot be risked (i.e., clients with cardiac arrhythmias or those taking digitalis). Usually not the first line of therapy, except for clients in whom hypokalemia should be avoided.

Dosage

- **Capsules**

Hypertension or Edema.
Adults: Triamterene/hydrochlorothiazide: 37.5/25 mg—1–2 capsules given once daily with monitoring of serum potassium and clinical effect. Triamterene/hydrochlorothiazide: 50 mg/25 mg—1–2 capsules b.i.d. after meals. Some clients may be controlled using 1 capsule every day or every other day. No more than 4 capsules should be taken daily.

- **Tablets**

Hypertension or Edema.
Adults: Triamterene/hydrochlorothiazide: 37.5/25 mg—1–2 tablets/day (determined by individual titration with the components). Or, triamterene/hydrochlorothiazide: 75 mg/50 mg—1 tablet daily.
Administration: Clients who are transferred from less bioavailable formulations of triamterene and hydrochlorothiazide should be monitored for serum potassium levels following the transfer.
Contraindications: Clients receiving other potassium-sparing drugs such as amiloride and spironolactone. Use in anuria, acute or chronic renal insufficiency, significant renal impairment, preexisting elevated serum potassium.
Special Concerns: Use with caution during lactation. Geriatric clients may be more sensitive to the hypotensive and electrolyte effects of this combination; also, age-related decreases in renal function may require a decrease in dosage.

NURSING CONSIDERATIONS

See also *Nursing Considerations* for *Antihypertensive Agents,* Chapter 28. and Individual Agents.

Evaluate

- Control of hypertension
- Resolution of edema with serum potassium levels within desired range

PERIPHERALLY-ACTING AGENTS

See the following individual entries:

Guanadrel Sulfate
Guanethidine Sulfate
Phenoxybenzamine Hydrochloride - see Chapter 51
Phentolamine Mesylate - see Chapter 51

Guanadrel sulfate

(**GWON**-ah-drell)
Pregnancy Category: B
Hylorel **(Rx)**

See also *Antihypertensive Agents,* Chapter 28.

How Supplied: *Tablet:* 10 mg, 25 mg

Action/Kinetics: Similar to that of guanethidine. Inhibits vasoconstriction by blocking efferent, peripheral sympathetic pathways by depleting norepinephrine reserves and inhibiting norepinephrine release. Causes increased sensitivity to norepinephrine. **Onset:** 2 hr. **Peak plasma levels:** 1.5–2 hr. **Peak effect:** 4–6 hr. $t^{1}/_{2}$**:** Approximately 10 hr. **Duration:** 4–14 hr. Excreted through the urine as unchanged drug (40%) and metabolites.

Use: Hypertension (usually step 2 therapy) in those not responding to a thiazide diuretic.

Dosage

- **Tablets**

Hypertension.

Individualized. Initial: 5 mg b.i.d.; **then,** increase dosage to maintenance level of 20–75 mg/day in two to four divided doses. For clients with a creatinine clearance of 30–60 mL/min, the initial dose should be 5 mg q 24 hr. If the creatinine clearance is less than 30 mL/min, the dosing interval should be increased to q 48 hr. Dose changes should be made carefully q 7 or more days for moderate renal insufficiency and q 14 or more days for severe insufficiency.

Administration/Storage

1. Tolerance may occur with long-term therapy, necessitating a dosage increase.
2. While adjusting dosage, both supine and standing BP should be monitored.
3. *Treatment of Overdose:* Administration of a vasoconstrictor (e.g., phenylephrine) if hypotension persists. If used, monitor carefully as client may be hypersensitive.

Contraindications: Pheochromocytoma, CHF, within 1 week of MAO drug use, within 2–3 days of elective surgery, lactation.

Special Concerns: Use with caution in bronchial asthma and peptic ulcer. Safety and efficacy not established in children. Geriatric clients may be more sensitive to the hypotensive effects.

Side Effects: *CNS:* Fainting, fatigue, headache, drowsiness, paresthesias, confusion, psychological problems, depression, syncope, sleep disorders, visual disturbances. *CV:* Chest pain, orthostatic hypotension, palpitations, peripheral edema. *Respiratory:* Exertional or resting SOB, coughing. *GI:* Increase in number of bowel movements, constipation, anorexia, indigestion, flatus, glossitis, N&V, dry mouth and throat, abdominal distress or pain. *GU:* Difficulty in ejaculation, impotence, nocturia, hematuria, urinary urgency or frequency. *Miscellaneous:* Leg cramps during both the day and night, excessive weight gain or loss, backache, neckache, joint pain or inflammation, aching limbs.

Symptoms of Overdose: Postural hypotension, syncope, dizziness, blurred vision.

Drug Interactions

Beta-adrenergic blocking agents / Excessive hypotension, bradycardia
Phenothiazines / Reverses effect of guanadrel
Phenylpropanolamine / ↓ Effect of guanadrel
Reserpine / Excessive hypotension, bradycardia
Sympathomimetics / Hypotensive effect of guanadrel may be reversed; also, guanadrel may ↑ the

effects of directly acting sympathomimetics
Tricyclic antidepressants / Reverses effect of guanadrel
Vasodilators / ↑ Risk of orthostatic hypotension

NURSING CONSIDERATIONS

See also *Nursing Considerations* for *Antihypertensive Agents,* Chapter 28.

Client/Family Teaching

1. Warn clients that they may develop a dry mouth and become drowsy. Care should be taken not to perform any tasks that require mental alertness, such as driving a car, until drug effects realized.
2. Clients may develop diarrhea. If this is persistent, the condition should be reported as a severe electrolyte imbalance may occur. This is particularly true with elderly clients.

Evaluate: Control of hypertension.

Guanethidine sulfate

(gwon-**ETH**-ih-deen)
Pregnancy Category: C
Apo-Guanethidine ✦, Ismelin Sulfate
(Rx)

See also *Antihypertensive Agents,* Chapter 28.
How Supplied: *Tablet:* 10 mg, 25 mg
Action/Kinetics: Guanethidine produces selective adrenergic blockade of efferent, peripheral sympathetic pathways by depleting norepinephrine reserve and inhibiting norepinephrine release. It induces a gradual, prolonged drop in both SBP and DBP, usually associated with bradycardia, decreased pulse pressure, a decrease in peripheral resistance, and small changes in CO. The drug is not a ganglionic blocking agent and does not produce central or parasympathetic blockade. In clients with depleted catecholamines, guanethidine can directly depress the myocardium and can cause an increase in the sensitivity of tissues to catecholamines. Incompletely and variably absorbed from the GI tract (3%–30%) but is relatively constant for any given client. **Peak effect:** 6–8 hr. **Duration:** 24–48 hr. **Maximum effect:** 1–3 weeks. **Duration:** 7–10 days after discontinuation. **t½:** 4–8 days. From 25% to 50% excreted through the kidneys unchanged. The drug is slowly excreted due to extensive tissue binding.
Uses: Moderate to severe hypertension—used alone or in combination. *NOTE:* The use of a thiazide diuretic may increase the effectiveness of guanethidine and reduce the incidence of edema. Also used for renal hypertension, including that secondary to pyelonephritis, renal artery stenosis, and renal amyloidosis.

Dosage

- **Tablets**

Ambulatory clients.
Initial: 10–12.5 mg/day; increase in 10–12.5-mg increments q 5–7 days; **maintenance:** 25–50 mg/day.

Hospitalized clients.
Initial: 25–50 mg; increase by 25 or 50 mg/day or every other day; **maintenance:** estimated to be approximately one-seventh of loading dose. **Pediatric, initial:** 0.2 mg/kg/day (6 mg/m^2) given in one dose; **then,** dose may be increased by 0.2 mg/kg/day q 7–10 days to maximum of 3 mg/kg/day.

Administration/Storage

1. The loading dose for severe hypertension is given t.i.d. at 6-hr intervals with no nighttime dose.
2. The effects of guanethidine are cumulative; thus, initial doses should be small and increased gradually in small increments.
3. Often used concomitantly with thiazide diuretics to reduce severity of sodium and water retention caused by guanethidine. When used together, the dose of guanethidine should be reduced.
4. When control is achieved, dosage should be reduced to the minimal dose required to maintain lowest possible BP.
5. Guanethidine sulfate should be

discontinued or dosage decreased at least 2 weeks before surgery and MAO inhibitors should be discontinued at least 1 week before starting guanethidine.

6. *Treatment of Overdose:* If the client was previously normotensive, keep in a supine position (symptoms usually subside within 72 hr). If the client was previously hypertensive (especially with impaired cardiac reserve or other CV problems or renal disease), intensive treatment may be needed. Vasopressors may be required. Severe diarrhea should be treated.

Contraindications: Mild, labile hypertension; pheochromocytoma, CHF not due to hypertension, use of MAO inhibitors, lactation.

Special Concerns: Administer with caution and at a reduced rate to clients with impaired renal function, coronary disease, CV disease especially when associated with encephalopathy, or severe cardiac failure or to those who have suffered a recent MI. Use with caution in hypertensive clients with renal disease and nitrogen retention or increasing BUN levels. Fever decreases dosage requirements. During prolonged therapy, cardiac, renal, and blood tests should be performed. Used with caution in peptic ulcer. Geriatric clients may be more sensitive to the hypotensive effects of guanethidine; also, it may be necessary to decrease the dose in these clients due to age-related decreases in renal function. Safety and efficacy have not been determined in children.

Laboratory Test Interferences: ↑ BUN, AST, and ALT. ↓ PT, serum glucose, and urine catecholamines. Alteration of electrolyte balance.

Side Effects: *CNS:* Dizziness, weakness, lassitude. Rarely, fatigue, psychic depression. *CV:* Syncope due to exertional or postural hypotension, bradycardia, fluid retention and edema with possible CHF. Less commonly, angina. *Respiratory:* Dyspnea, nasal congestion, asthma in susceptible individuals. *GI:* Persistent diarrhea (may be severe enough to cause discontinuation of use), increased frequency of bowel movements. N&V, dry mouth, and parotid tenderness are less common. *GU:* Inhibition of ejaculation, nocturia, urinary incontinence, priapism, impotence. *Hematologic:* Anemia, thrombocytopenia, leukopenia (rare). *Miscellaneous:* Dermatitis, scalp hair loss, blurred vision, myalgia, muscle tremors, chest paresthesia, weight gain, ptosis of the lids.

Symptoms of Overdose: Bradycardia, postural hypotension, diarrhea (may be severe).

Drug Interactions

Alcohol, ethyl / Additive orthostatic hypotension
Amphetamines / ↓ Effect of guanethidine by ↓ uptake of the drug to its site of action
Anesthetics, general / Additive hypotension
Antidepressants, tricyclic / ↓ Effect of guanethidine by ↓ uptake of the drug to its site of action
Antidiabetic drugs / Additive effect ↓ in blood glucose
Cocaine / ↓ Effect of guanethidine by ↓ uptake of the drug at its site of action
Digitalis / Additive slowing of HR
Ephedrine / ↓ Effect of guanethidine by ↓ uptake of the drug at its site of action
Epinephrine / Guanethidine ↑ effect of epinephrine
Haloperidol / ↓ Effect of guanethidine by ↓ uptake of the drug at its site of action
Levarterenol / See *Norepinephrine*
MAO inhibitors / Reverse effect of guanethidine
Metaraminol / Guanethidine ↑ effect of metaraminol
Methotrimeprazine / Additive hypotensive effect
Methoxamine / Guanethidine ↑ effect of methoxamine
Methylphenidate / ↓ Effect of guanethidine
Minoxidil / Profound drop in BP
Norepinephrine / ↑ Effect of norepinephrine probably due to ↑ sensitivity of norepinephrine receptor and ↓ uptake of norepinephrine by the neuron

Oral contraceptives / ↓ Effect of guanethidine by ↓ uptake of the drug to its site of action
Phenothiazines / ↓ Effect of guanethidine by ↓ uptake of the drug to its site of action
Phenylephrine / ↑ Response to phenylephrine in guanethidine-treated clients
Phenylpropanolamine / ↓ Effect of guanethidine by ↓ uptake of the drug to its site of action
Procainamide / Additive hypotensive effect
Procarbazine / Additive hypotensive effect
Propranolol / Additive hypotensive effect
Pseudoephedrine / ↓ Effect of guanethidine by ↓ uptake of the drug at its site of action
Quinidine / Additive hypotensive effect
Reserpine / Excessive bradycardia, postural hypotension, and mental depression
Sympathomimetics / ↓ Effect of guanethidine; also, guanethidine potentiates the effects of directly acting sympathomimetics
Thiazide diuretics / Additive hypotensive effect
Thioxanthenes / ↓ Effect of guanethidine by ↓ uptake of the drug at its site of action
Tricyclic antidepressants / Inhibition of the effects of guanethidine
Vasodilator drugs, peripheral / Additive hypotensive effect
Vasopressor drugs / ↑ Effect of vasopressor agents probably due to ↑ sensitivity of norepinephrine receptor and ↓ uptake of vasopressor agent by the neuron

NURSING CONSIDERATIONS

See also *Nursing Considerations* for *Antihypertensive Agents,* Chapter 28.

Assessment

1. Ascertain that baseline hepatic and renal function studies are completed.
2. List drugs currently prescribed to ensure none interact unfavorably.
3. Perform baseline VS and report the presence of bradycardia. An anticholinergic drug, such as atropine, may be indicated for severe bradycardia.
4. Assess client for any undue stress, which could precipitate CV collapse. Assist to identify and reduce such stress whenever possible.

Client/Family Teaching

1. Limit alcohol intake; otherwise, orthostatic hypotension may be further precipitated. Postural hypotension is more prevalent in the morning and may be worsened by hot weather, alcohol, or exercise.
2. Avoid any sudden or prolonged standing or exercise.
3. Report any persistent nausea, vomiting, or diarrhea because severe electrolyte imbalances may occur.
4. Perform daily weights. Report any sudden increases in weight or any reduction in urine volume because this could indicate the presence of edema.

Evaluate: ↓ BP with control of hypertension.

MISCELLANEOUS AGENTS

See the following individual entries:

Labetalol Hydrochloride
Mecamylamine Hydrochloride
Minoxidil, Oral

Labetalol hydrochloride

(lah-**BET**-ah-lohl)
Pregnancy Category: C
Normodyne, Trandate **(Rx)**

How Supplied: *Injection:* 5 mg/mL; *Tablet:* 100 mg, 200 mg, 300 mg
Action/Kinetics: Labetalol decreases BP by blocking both alpha- and beta-adrenergic receptors. Significant reflex tachycardia and bradycardia do not occur although AV conduction may be prolonged. **Onset: PO,** 2–4 hr; **IV,** 5 min. **Peak plasma**

levels, PO: 1–2 hr. **Duration: PO,** 8–12 hr. **t½: PO,** 6–8 hr; **IV,** 5.5 hr. Significant first-pass effect; metabolized in liver. Food increases bioavailability of the drug.

Uses: PO: Alone or in combination with other drugs for hypertension. **IV:** Hypertensive emergencies. *Investigational:* Pheochromocytoma, clonidine withdrawal hypertension.

Dosage

- **Tablets**

Hypertension.

Initial: 100 mg b.i.d. alone or with a diuretic; **maintenance:** 200–400 mg b.i.d. up to 1,200–2,400 mg/day for severe cases.

- **IV**

Hypertension.

Individualize. Initial: 20 mg slowly over 2 min; **then,** 40–80 mg q 10 min until desired effect occurs or a total of 300 mg has been given.

- **IV infusion**

Hypertension.

Initial: 2 mg/min; **then,** adjust rate according to response. **Usual dose range:** 50–300 mg.

Transfer from IV to PO therapy.

Initial: 200 mg; **then,** 200–400 mg 6–12 hr later, depending on response. Thereafter, dosage based on response.

Administration/Storage

1. When transferring to oral labetalol from other antihypertensive therapy, slowly reduce dosage of current therapy.
2. To transfer from IV to PO therapy in hospitalized clients, begin when supine BP begins to increase.
3. Labetalol is not compatible with 5% sodium bicarbonate injection.
4. The full antihypertensive effect of labetalol is usually seen within the first 1–3 hr after the initial dose or dose increment.
5. May give IV undiluted (20 mg over 2 min) or reconstituted with dextrose or saline solutions (infuse at a rate of 2 mg/min). When given by IV infusion, labetalol should be administered using an infusion pump, a micro-drip regulator, or similar type device that allows precise control of flow rate.
6. *Treatment of Overdose:* Induce vomiting or perform gastric lavage. Clients should be placed in a supine position with legs elevated. If required, the following treatment can be used:

- Epinephrine or a beta-2 agonist (aerosol) to treat bronchospasm.
- Atropine or epinephrine to treat bradycardia.
- Digitalis glycoside and a diuretic for cardiac failure; dopamine or dobutamine may also be used.
- Diazepam to treat seizures.
- Norepinephrine (or another vasopressor) to treat hypotension.
- Administration of glucagon (5–10 mg rapidly over 30 sec), followed by continuous infusion of 5 mg/hr, may be effective in treating severe hypotension and bradycardia.

Contraindications: Cardiogenic shock, cardiac failure, bronchial asthma, bradycardia, greater than first-degree heart block.

Special Concerns: Use with caution during lactation, in impaired renal and hepatic function, and diabetes (may prevent premonitory signs of acute hypoglycemia). Safety and efficacy in children have not been established.

Laboratory Test Interference: False + increase in urinary catecholamines.

Side Effects: *CV:* Postural hypotension, edema, flushing, ***ventricular arrhythmias, intensification of AV block.*** *GI:* N&V, diarrhea, altered taste, dyspepsia. *CNS:* Headache, drowsiness, fatigue, sleepiness, dizziness, vertigo, paresthesias, numbness. *GU:* Impotence, urinary bladder retention, difficulty in urination, failure to ejaculate, priapism, Peyronie's disease. *Dermatologic:* Rashes, facial erythema, alopecia, urticaria, pruritus, psoriasis-like syndrome, bullous lichen planus. *Respiratory:* ***Bronchospasm,*** dyspnea, wheezing. *Musculoskeletal:* Muscle cramps, asthenia, toxic myopathy. *Other:* SLE, jaundice, cholestasis, difficulties with vision, dry eyes, nasal stuffiness, tingling of skin or scalp, sweating, fever. Possible changes in laboratory values include increased serum transaminase, positive antinuclear factor, antimitochondrial antibodies, and increases in blood urea and creatine.

Symptoms of Overdose: Excessive hypotension and bradycardia.

Drug Interactions

Beta-adrenergic bronchodilators / Labetalol ↓ bronchodilator effect of these drugs
Cimetidine / ↑ Bioavailability of oral labetalol
Glutethimide / ↓ Effects of labetalol due to ↑ breakdown by liver
Halothane / ↑ Risk of severe myocardial depression → hypotension
Nitroglycerin / Additive hypotension
Tricyclic antidepressants / ↑ Risk of tremors

NURSING CONSIDERATIONS

See also *Nursing Considerations* for *Beta-Adrenergic Blocking Agents,* Chapter 51, and *Antihypertensive Agents,* Chapter 28.

Interventions

1. The effect of labetalol tablets on standing BP should be assessed before the client is discharged from the hospital. Perform measurements with the client standing at several different times during the day to determine full effects of the drug.
2. To reduce the chance of orthostatic hypotension, clients should remain supine for 3 hr after receiving parenteral labetalol.

Client/Family Teaching

1. Use caution as drug may precipitate orthostatic hypotension.
2. May cause increased sensitivity to cold; dress appropriately.

Evaluate: ↓ BP and control of hypertension.

Mecamylamine hydrochloride

(mek-ah-**MILL**-ah-meen)
Pregnancy Category: C
Inversine **(Rx)**

How Supplied: *Tablet:* 2.5 mg

Action/Kinetics: The drug is less apt than other ganglionic blocking agents to induce tolerance. Withdraw or substitute mecamylamine slowly because sudden withdrawal or switching to other antihypertensive agents may result in severe hypertensive rebound. Since mecamylamine reduces peristalsis, it is a useful addition to a thiazide-guanethidine regimen in clients who experience persistent diarrhea with guanethidine. **Onset (gradual):** ½–2 hr. **Duration:** 6–12 hr. May take 2–3 days to achieve full therapeutic potential. Mecamylamine is excreted unchanged by the kidneys. The rate of excretion is influenced by urinary pH in that alkalinization of the urine decreases, and acidification increases, renal excretion.

Use: Moderate to severe hypertension including uncomplicated malignant hypertension.

Dosage

- **Tablets**

  Hypertension.

Adults, initial: 2.5 mg b.i.d. Increase by increments of 2.5 mg q 2 or more days; **maintenance:** 25 mg/day in three divided doses.

Administration/Storage

1. For better control of hypertension, administer after meals.
2. The morning dose may be small or omitted; larger doses are given at noon and in the evening.
3. *Treatment of Overdose:* Vasopressors to treat hypotension.

Contraindications: Mild, moderate, labile hypertension; coronary insufficiency, clients with recent MI, uremia, clients being treated with antibiotics and sulfonamides, glaucoma, pyloric stenosis, uncooperative clients.

Special Concerns: Safe use during lactation has not been established. Dosage has not been established in children. Geriatric clients may be more sensitive to the hypotensive effects of mecamylamine; also, a de-

crease in dose may be required in these clients due to age-related decreases in renal function. Use with caution in marked cerebral and coronary arteriosclerosis, after recent CVA, prostatic hypertrophy, urethral stricture, bladder neck obstruction. Abdominal distention, decreased bowel signs, and other symptoms of adynamic ileus are reasons for discontinuing the drug.
Side Effects: *GI:* N&V, constipation (may be preceded by small, frequent, liquid stools), dry mouth, glossitis, anorexia, ileus. *CNS:* Sedation, weakness, fatigue. Rarely, choreiform movements, mental aberrations, tremors, ***seizures.*** *Respiratory:* Fibrosis, interstitial pulmonary edema. *CV:* Postural hypotension, orthostatic dizziness, syncope. *GU:* Urinary retention, decreased libido, impotence. *Miscellaneous:* Paresthesia, blurred vision, dilated pupils.

Symptoms of Overdose: Hypotension, ***peripheral vascular collapse,*** N&V, diarrhea, constipation, paralytic ileus, dizziness, anxiety, dry mouth, mydriasis, blurred vision, palpitations, increased intraocular pressure, urinary retention.

NURSING CONSIDERATIONS

See also *Nursing Considerations* for *Antihypertensive Agents,* Chapter 28.
Client/Family Teaching
1. Allow more time to prepare for the day's activities than usual to permit the body time to adjust to postural effects of drug therapy.
2. If weak, dizzy, or faint after standing or exercising for a long time, lie down if possible or otherwise sit down and lower head between knees.
3. Eat a diet high in fiber and provide a list of food and fluids that will help to avoid constipation.
Evaluate: ↓ BP with control of hypertension.

Minoxidil, oral

(mih-**NOX**-ih-dil)
Pregnancy Category: C
Loniten **(Rx)**

See also *Antihypertensive Agents,* Chapter 28.
How Supplied: *Tablet:* 2.5 mg, 10 mg
Action/Kinetics: Decreases elevated BP by decreasing peripheral resistance by a direct effect. Drug causes increase in renin secretion, increase in cardiac rate and output, and salt/water retention. It does not cause orthostatic hypotension. **Onset:** 30 min. **Peak plasma levels:** reached within 60 min; **plasma t½:** 4.2 hr. **Duration:** 24–48 hr. Ninety percent absorbed from GI tract; excretion: renal (90% metabolites). The time needed to reach the maximum effect is inversely related to the dose.
Uses: Severe hypertension not controllable by the use of a diuretic plus two other antihypertensive drugs. Usually taken with at least two other antihypertensive drugs (a diuretic and a drug to minimize tachycardia such as a beta-adrenergic blocking agent). Minoxidil can produce severe side effects; it should be reserved for resistant cases of hypertension. Close medical supervision required, including possible hospitalization during initial administration. Topically to promote hair growth in balding men (see *Minoxidil, topical solution,* Chapter 83).

Dosage

- **Tablets**

Hypertension.
Adults and children over 12 years, Initial: 5 mg/day. For optimum control, dose can be increased to 10, 20, and then 40 mg in single or divided doses/day. Daily dosage should not exceed 100 mg. **Children under 12 years: Initial,** 0.2 mg/kg/day. Effective dose range: 0.25–1.0 mg/kg/day. Dosage must be titrated to individual response. Daily dosage should not exceed 50 mg.
Administration/Storage
1. Can be taken with fluids and without regard to meals.
2. The drug should be given once daily if the supine diastolic pressure has been reduced less than 30 mm Hg and twice daily (in two equal doses)

if it has been reduced more than 30 mm Hg.
3. The interval between dosage adjustments should be at least 3 days as the full response is not obtained until then. However, if more rapid control is required, adjustments can be made q 6 hr but with careful monitoring.
4. *Treatment of Overdose:* Give NSS IV (to maintain BP and urine output). Vasopressors, such as phenylephrine and dopamine, can be used but only in underperfusion of a vital organ.
Contraindications: Pheochromocytoma. Within 1 month after a MI. Dissecting aortic aneurysm.
Special Concerns: Safe use during lactation not established. Use with caution and at reduced dosage in impaired renal function. Geriatric clients may be more sensitive to the hypotensive and hypothermic effects of minoxidil; also, it may be necessary to decrease the dose in these clients due to age-related decreases in renal function. BP controlled too rapidly may cause syncope, stroke, MI, and ischemia of affected organs. Experience with use in children is limited.
Laboratory Test Interferences: Nonspecific changes in ECG. ↑ Alkaline phosphatase, serum creatinine, and BUN.
Side Effects: *CV:* Edema, ***pericardial effusion that may progress to tamponade*** (acute compression of heart caused by fluid or blood in pericardium), CHF, angina pectoris, changes in direction of T waves, increased HR. In children, rebound hypertension following slow withdrawal. *GI:* N&V. *CNS:* Headache, fatigue. *Hypersensitivity:* Rashes, including bullous eruptions and ***Stevens-Johnson syndrome.*** *Hematologic:* Initially, decrease in hematocrit, hemoglobin, and erythrocyte count but all return to normal. Rarely, thrombocytopenia and leukopenia. *Other:* Hypertrichosis (enhanced hair growth, pigmentation and thickening of fine body hair 3–6 weeks after initiation of therapy), breast tenderness, darkening of skin.

Symptom of Overdose: Excessive hypotension.
Drug Interaction: Concomitant use with guanethidine may result in severe hypotension.

NURSING CONSIDERATIONS

See also *Nursing Considerations* for *Antihypertensive Agents,* Chapter 28.
Assessment
1. Anticipate that minoxidil therapy will be initiated in the hospital. After medication administration, BP decreases within 30 min and the client reaches minimum BP within 2–3 hr.
2. List all agents prescribed for this condition, length of use, and the outcome.
3. Determine if concomitant diruetic is prescribed.
4. Clients receiving guanethidine concomitantly may experience severe hypotensive effects that may be precipitated by a drug interaction.
Client/Family Teaching
1. Use only in the dose and form prescribed.
2. Record weight daily and report any S&S of fluid overload (gain of over 2.3 kg within 3 days as well as any edema of extremities, face, and abdomen, or dyspnea).
3. Symptoms of angina, dizziness, or fainting and any dyspnea that occurs, especially when lying down, should be reported.
4. Drug may cause elongation, thickening, and increased pigmentation of body hair, but a return to pretreatment norm should occur when the drug is discontinued.
Evaluate: ↓ BP with control of refractory hypertension.

CHAPTER TWENTY-NINE

Antihyperlipidemic/ Hypocholesterolemic Agents

See also the following drug classes and individual drugs:

HMG-CoA Reductase Inhibitors

Fluvastatin Sodium
Lovastatin
Pravastatin sodium
Simvastatin

Miscellaneous Agents

Cholestyramine Resin
Clofibrate
Colestipol Hydrochloride
Dextrothyroxine Sodium
Probucol

HMG-CoA REDUCTASE INHIBITORS

See the following individual entries:

Fluvastatin sodium
Lovastatin
Pravastatin sodium
Simvastatin

Action/Kinetics: These drugs competitively inhibit 3-hydroxy-3-methylglutaryl-coenzyme A (HMG-CoA) reductase; this enzyme catalyzes the early rate-limiting step in the synthesis of cholesterol. HMG-CoA reductase inhibitors increase HDL cholesterol and decrease LDL cholesterol, VLDL cholesterol, and plasma triglycerides. The mechanism to lower LDL cholesterol may be due to both a decrease in VLDL cholesterol levels and induction of the LDL receptor, leading to reduced production or increased catabolism of LDL cholesterol. The maximum therapeutic response is seen in 4–6 weeks.

Use: Adjunct to diet to decrease elevated and total LDL cholesterol in clients with primary hypercholesterolemia (types IIa and IIb) when the response to diet and other nondrug approaches have not been adequate.

Contraindications: Active liver disease or unexplained persistent elevated liver function tests. Pregnancy, lactation. Use in children.

Special Concerns: Use with caution in those who ingest large quantities of alcohol or who have a history of liver disease. Safety and efficacy have not been established in children less than 18 years of age.

Side Effects: The following side effects are common to most HMG-CoA reductase inhibitors. Also see individual drugs. *GI:* N&V, diarrhea, constipation, abdominal cramps or pain, flatulence, dyspepsia, heartburn. *CNS:* Headache, dizziness, dysfunction of certain cranial nerves (e.g., alteration of taste, facial paresis, impairment of extraocular movement), tremor, vertigo, memory loss, paresthesia, anxiety, insomnia, depression. *Musculoskeletal:* Localized pain, myalgia, muscle cramps or pain, myopathy, rhabdomyolysis, arthralgia. *Respiratory:* Upper respiratory infection, rhinitis, cough. *Ophthalmic:* Progression of cataracts (lens opacities), ophthalmoplegia. *Hypersensitivity:* ***Anaphylaxis, angioedema,*** vasculitis, purpura, thrombocytopenia, leukopenia, ***hemolytic anemia,*** lupus erythematosus-like syndrome, polymyalgia rheumatica, positive ANA, ESR increase, arthritis, arthralgia, eosinophilia, urticaria, photosensitivity, fever, chills, flushing, malaise, dyspnea, ***toxic dermal necrolysis, Stevens-Johnson syndrome.*** *Miscellaneous:* Rash, pruritus, cardiac chest pain, fatigue, influenza, alopecia, edema, dryness of skin and mucous membranes, changes to hair and nails, skin discoloration.

Drug Interactions

Gemfibrozil / Severe myopathy or rhabdomyolysis

Warfarin / ↑ Anticoagulant effect of warfarin.

Laboratory Test Interferences: ↑ AST, ALT, CPK, alkaline phosphatase, bilirubin. Abnormal thyroid function tests.

Dosage

See individual drugs.

NURSING CONSIDERATIONS

Administration/Storage: Lovastatin should be taken with meals; fluvastatin, pravastatin, and simavastatin may be taken without regard to meals.

Assessment

1. Review client life-style, duration of illness, and all attempts made to control hypercholesterolemia with diet, exercise, and weight reduction.
2. Note any history of alcohol abuse or liver disease.
3. Perform a complete history, review of systems, and physical examination; ensure that any underlying medical conditions have been addressed and treated.
4. Obtain baseline serum CK and liver function studies and monitor q 4–6 weeks during the first 3 months of therapy, q 6–12 weeks during the next 12 months or after any increase in dose, and then at 6-month intervals.
5. If transaminase levels exceed 3 times the normal limit, drug must be discontinued because it may precipitate severe hepatic toxicity.
6. If CK is elevated, assess renal function and discontinue drug, as rhabdomyolsis may lead to myoglobinuria, which could cause renal shutdown.

Client/Family Teaching

1. Take only as directed and with meals if prescribed.
2. Drugs may cause photosensitivity. Prolonged exposure to the sun or ultraviolet light should be avoided. Use sunscreens, sunglasses, and protective clothing when exposure is necessary.
3. Report any significant generalized pain in skeletal muscles or unexplained muscle pain, tenderness, or weakness promptly, especially if accompanied by fever or malaise, as drug should be discontinued.
4. Stress the importance of continuing life-style modifications that include low-fat, low-cholesterol, and low-sodium diets, weight reduction with obese clients, and regular exercise in the overall goal of cholesterol reduction.
5. Do not take niacin while on drug therapy as this may increase the risk of hepatic failure.
6. Avoid any unprescribed or OTC agents without provider approval.
7. Advise that with any major trauma, surgery, or serious illness, drug should be discontinued.
8. Remind client of the importance of reporting for scheduled lab studies to prevent toxic drug effects and to assess drug effectiveness.

Evaluate

- ↓Levels of LDL
- ↓Total serum cholesterol levels

Fluvastatin sodium

(flu-vah-**STAH**-tin)
Pregnancy Category: X
Lescol **(Rx)**

See also *Antihyperlipidemic Agents —HMG-CoA Reductase Inhibitors,* Chapter 29.

How Supplied: *Capsule:* 20 mg, 40 mg

Action/Kinetics: **t½:** 1.2 hr. The drug undergoes extensive first-pass metabolism. The drug is metabolized in the liver with 90% excretion through the feces and 5% through the urine.

Special Concern: Use with caution in clients with severe renal impairment.

Use: Adjunct to diet for the reduction of elevated total and LDL cholesterol levels in clients with primary hypercholesterolemia. The lipid-lowering effects of fluvastatin are enhanced when it is combined with a bile-acid binding resin or with niacin.

Dosage

- **Capsules**

Antihyperlipidemic.

Adults: 20 mg once daily at bedtime. **Dose range:** 20–40 mg/day as a single dose in the evening. Splitting the 40-mg dose into a twice-daily regimen results in a modest improvement in LDL cholesterol.

Administration/Storage

1. The client should be placed on a standard cholesterol-lowering diet before receiving fluvastatin. The diet should be continued during treatment.
2. The drug may be taken without regard to meals, although it is usually taken with the evening meal.
3. Maximum reductions of LDL cholesterol are usually seen within 4 weeks; periodic lipid determinations should be made during this time, with dosage adjusted accordingly.
4. When a bile-acid binding resin is given with fluvastatin, in order to avoid the fluvastatin binding to the resin, the fluvastatin should be given at bedtime and the resin given at least 2 hr before.

Side Effects: Side effects listed are those most common with fluvastatin. A complete list of possible side effects is provided under *Antihyperlipidemic Agents—HMG-CoA Reductase Inhibitors. GI:* N&V, diarrhea, abdominal pain or cramps, constipation, flatulence, dyspepsia, tooth disorder. *Musculoskeletal:* Muscle cramps or pain, back pain, arthropathy. *CNS:* Headache, dizziness, insomnia. *Respiratory:* Upper respiratory infection, rhinitis, cough, pharyngitis, sinusitis, bronchitis. *Miscellaneous:* Rash, pruritus, fatigue, influenza, allergy, accidental trauma.

NURSING CONSIDERATIONS

See also *Nursing Considerations* for *Antihyperlipidemic Agents—HMG-CoA Reductase Inhibitors,* Chapter 29.

Assessment: Obtain baseline CPK, LDL, HDL, and total serum cholesterol and triglyceride levels and monitor periodically.

Client/Family Teaching

1. May be taken with or without food but is usually consumed with the evening meal.
2. Explain that these drugs are used to help lower blood cholesterol and fat levels, which have been proven to promote CAD.
3. Stress the importance of continuing dietary restrictions of saturated fat and cholesterol and regular exercise programs in addition to this therapy in the overall goal of lowering serum cholesterol levels.

Evaluate: ↓Levels of triglycerides, LDL, and total serum cholesterol levels.

Lovastatin (Mevinolin)

(**LOW**-vah-**STAT**-in, me-**VIN**-oh-lin)
Pregnancy Category: X
Mevacor **(Rx)**

How Supplied: *Tablet:* 10 mg, 20 mg, 40 mg

Action/Kinetics: Lovastatin is a drug isolated from a strain of *Aspergillus terreus.* It specifically inhibits HMG–coenzyme A reductase, an enzyme that is necessary to convert HMG–coenzyme A to mevalonate (an early step in the biosynthesis of cholesterol). The levels of VLDL, LDL, cholesterol, and plasma triglycerides are reduced, while the plasma concentration of HDL cholesterol is increased. Since the enzyme is not completely inhibited, mevalonate is available in amounts necessary to maintain homeostasis. Approximately 35% of a dose is absorbed; there is an extensive first-pass effect so that less than 5% of an oral dose actually reaches the general circulation. Absorption is decreased by about one-third if the drug is given on an empty stomach rather than with food.

Onset: within 2 weeks using multiple doses. **Time to peak plasma levels:** 2–4 hr. **Time to peak effect:** 4–6 weeks using multiple doses. **Duration:** 4–6 weeks after termination of therapy. Over 95% is bound to plasma proteins. The drug is metabolized in the liver (its main site of action) to active metabolites. Over 80% of a PO dose is excreted in the feces, via the bile, and approximately 10% is excreted through the urine.

Uses: As an adjunct to diet in primary hypercholesterolemia (types IIa and IIb) in clients with a significant risk of CAD and who have not responded to diet or other measures. May also be useful in clients with combined hypercholesterolemia and hypertriglyceridemia. *Investigational:* Diabetic dyslipidemia, nephrotic hyperlipidemia, familial dysbetalipoproteinemia, and familial combined hyperlipidemia.

Dosage

• **Tablets**

Adults/adolescents, initial: 20 mg once daily with the evening meal. If serum cholesterol levels are greater than 300 mg/dL, initial dose should be 40 mg/day. **Maintenance:** 20–80 mg/day, individualized and adjusted at intervals of every 4 weeks, if necessary.

Administration/Storage

1. Dosage modification is not necessary in clients with renal insufficiency.
2. The maximum dose for clients on immunosuppressive therapy is 20 mg/day.

Contraindications: During pregnancy and lactation, active liver disease, persistent unexplained elevations of serum transaminases. Use in children less than 18 years of age.

Special Concerns: Safety and efficacy have not been determined in children less than 18 years of age. Use with caution in clients who have a history of liver disease or who are known heavy consumers of alcohol. Carefully monitor clients with impaired renal function.

Laboratory Test Interferences: ↑ AST, ALT, CPK, alkaline phosphatase, bilirubin. Thyroid function test abnormalities.

Side Effects: *GI:* Flatus (most common), abdominal pain, cramps, diarrhea, constipation, dyspepsia, N&V, heartburn, anorexia, stomatitis, acid regurgitation, dry mouth. *CNS:* Headache, dizziness, tremor, vertigo, memory loss, paresthesia, anxiety, depression, insomnia. *Musculoskeletal:* Myalgia, muscle cramps, localized pain, arthralgia, myopathy, rhabdomyolysis with renal dysfunction secondary to myoglobinuria. *Hypersensitivity reaction:* Vasculitis, purpura, polymyalgia rheumatica, angioedema, lupus erythematosus-like syndrome, thrombocytopenia, ***hemolytic anemia,*** leukopenia, eosinophilia, positive ANA, arthritis, arthralgia, urticaria, asthenia, ESR increase, fever, chills, flushing, photosensitivity, malaise, dyspnea, ***toxic epidermal necrolysis, anaphylaxis, erythema multiforme including Stevens-Johnson syndrome.*** *Dermatologic:* Alopecia, pruritus, rash, skin changes, including nodules, discoloration, dryness, changes to hair and nails. *Hepatic:* Hepatitis (including chronic active hepatitis), cholestatic jaundice, fatty change in liver, cirrhosis, ***fulminant hepatic necrosis,*** hepatoma, pancreatitis. *GU:* Gynecomastia, loss of libido, erectile dysfunction. *Ophthalmic:* Blurred vision, progression of cataracts, lens opacities, ophthalmoplegia. *Hematologic:* Anemia, leukopenia, transient asymptomatic eosinophilia, thrombocytopenia. *Miscellaneous:* Cardiac chest pain, dysgeusia, edema, alteration of taste, impairment of extraocular movement, facial paresis, peripheral neuropathy, peripheral nerve palsy.

Drug Interactions

Cyclosporine / ↑ Risk of rhabdomyolysis or severe myopathy
Erythromycin / ↑ Risk of rhabdomyolysis or severe myopathy
Gemfibrozil / ↑ Risk of rhabdomyolysis or severe myopathy

Niacin / ↑ Risk of rhabdomyolysis or severe myopathy
Warfarin / ↑ PT

NURSING CONSIDERATIONS

Assessment

1. Document indications for therapy and baseline serum cholesterol levels. Note any other agents used for this condition and the outcome.
2. Note hepatic disease and any heavy consumption of alcohol.
3. Determine if pregnant.
4. Note if the client has had recent eye examinations. If not, request a baseline report since slight changes have been noted in the lenses of some clients.
5. Assess liver function tests every 4–6 weeks for the first 15 months of therapy. A threefold increase in serum transaminase or new-onset abnormal liver function is an indication to discontinue therapy.

Client/Family Teaching

1. Take with meals. Continue cholesterol-lowering diet as prescribed.
2. Adhering to dietary restrictions, daily exercise, and weight loss in the overall management and control of hypercholesterolemia and hyperlipidemia should be stressed.
3. If of childbearing age, practice some form of birth control; drug is pregnancy category X.
4. Report the development of malaise, muscle spasms, or fever. These may be mistaken for the flu, but the symptoms could be serious side effects of drug therapy and should not be ignored.
5. Any right upper quadrant abdominal pain or change in color and consistency of the stool should be reported.
6. Stress the importance of periodic eye exams and to report any early visual disturbances.

Evaluate: ↓ Serum cholesterol and triglyceride levels.

Pravastatin sodium

(prah-vah-**STAH**-tin)
Pregnancy Category: X
Pravachol **(Rx)**

How Supplied: *Tablet:* 10 mg, 20 mg, 40 mg

Action/Kinetics: Pravastatin competitively inhibits HMG-CoA reductase, the enzyme catalyzing the conversion of HMG-CoA to mevalonate in the biosynthesis of cholesterol. This results in an increased number of LDL receptors on cell surfaces and enhanced receptor-mediated catabolism and clearance of circulating LDL. The drug also inhibits LDL production by inhibiting hepatic synthesis of VLDL, the precursor of LDL. Elevated levels of total cholesterol, dLDL cholesterol, and apolipoprotein B (a membrane transport complex for LDL) promote development of atherosclerosis and are lowered by pravastatin. Pravastatin is rapidly absorbed from the GI tract. **Peak plasma levels:** 1–1.5 hr. The drug undergoes significant first-pass extraction and metabolism in the liver, which is the site of action of the drug; thus, plasma levels may not correlate well with lipid-lowering effectiveness. **t½, elimination:** 77 hr. The drug is metabolized in the liver and approximately 20% of a PO dose is excreted through the urine and 70% in the feces.

Uses: Adjunct to diet for reducing elevated total and LDL cholesterol levels in clients with primary hypercholesterolemia (type IIa and IIb) when the response to a diet with restricted saturated fat and cholesterol has not been effective.

Dosage

• Tablets

Initial: 10–20 mg once daily at bedtime (geriatric clients should take 10 mg once daily at bedtime). **Maintenance dose:** 10–40 mg once daily at bedtime (maximum dose for geriatric clients is 20 mg/day).

Administration/Storage

1. Client should be placed on a standard cholesterol-lowering diet for 3–6 months before beginning pravastatin therapy. The diet should be continued during therapy.
2. Drug may be taken without regard to meals.
3. The maximum effect is seen with-

in 4 weeks during which time periodic lipid determinations should be undertaken.

Contraindications: Use to treat hypercholesterolemia due to hyperalphaproteinemia. Active liver disease; unexplained, persistent elevations in liver function tests. Use during pregnancy and lactation and in children less than 18 years of age.

Special Concerns: Use with caution in clients with a history of liver disease, renal insufficiency, or heavy alcohol use.

Laboratory Test Interferences: ↑ CPK, AST, ALT, alkaline phosphatase, bilirubin. Abnormalities in thyroid function tests.

Side Effects: *Musculoskeletal:* Rhabdomyolysis with renal dysfunction secondary to myoglobinuria, myalgia, myopathy, arthralgias, localized pain. *CNS:*CNS vascular lesions characterized by ***perivascular hemorrhage,*** edema, and mononuclear cell infiltration of perivascular spaces; headache, dizziness, psychic disturbances. Dizziness, vertigo, memory loss, anxiety, insomnia, depression. *GI:* N&V, diarrhea, abdominal pain, cramps, constipation, flatulence, heartburn, anorexia. *Hepatic:* Hepatitis (including chronic active hepatitis), fatty change in liver, cirrhosis, ***fulminant hepatic necrosis, hepatoma,*** pancreatitis, cholestatic jaundice. *GU:* Gynecomastia, erectile dysfunction, loss of libido. *Ophthalmic:* Progression of cataracts, lens opacities, ophthalmoplegia. *Hypersensitivity reaction:* Vasculitis, purpura, polymyalgia rheumatica, ***angioedema,*** lupus erythematosus–like syndrome, thrombocytopenia, ***hemolytic anemia,*** leukopenia, positive ANA, arthritis, arthralgia, urticaria, asthenia, ESR increase, fever, chills, photosensitivity, malaise, dyspnea, ***toxic epidermal necrolysis, Stevens-Johnson syndrome.*** *Dermatologic:* Alopecia, pruritus, skin nodules, discoloration of skin, dryness of skin and mucous membranes, changes in hair and nails. *Neurologic:*Dysfunction of certain cranial nerves resulting in alteration of taste, impairment of extraocular movement, and facial paresis; paresthesia, peripheral neuropathy, tremor, vertigo, memory loss peripheral nerve palsy. *Respiratory:* Common cold, rhinitis, cough. *Hematologic:* Anemia, transient asymptomatic eosinophilia, thrombocytopenia, leukopenia. *Miscellaneous:* Rash, pruritus, cardiac chest pain, fatigue, influenza.

Drug Interactions

Bile acid sequestrants / ↓ Bioavailability of pravastatin

Clofibrate / ↑ Risk of myopathy

Cyclosporine / ↑ Risk of myopathy or rhabdomyolysis

Erythromycin / ↑ Risk of myopathy or rhabdomyolysis

Gemfibrozil / ↑ Risk of myopathy or rhabdomyolysis

Niacin / ↑ Risk of myopathy or rhabdomyolysis

Warfarin / ↑ Anticoagulant effect of warfarin

NURSING CONSIDERATIONS

See also *Nursing Considerations* for *Antihyperlipidemic Agents—HMG-CoA Reductase Inhibitors,* Chapter 29.

Assessment

1. Determine that secondary causes for hypercholesterolemia are ruled out. Secondary causes include hypothyroidism, poorly controlled diabetes mellitus, dysproteinemias, obstructive liver disease, nephrotic syndrome, alcoholism, and other drug therapy.
2. If female of childbearing age and sexually active, determine if pregnant.
3. Assess for any evidence of liver disease or alcohol abuse.
4. Obtain baseline lab values including a lipid profile, serum cholesterol level, CBC, and liver and renal function studies.

Interventions

1. Liver function tests should be performed prior to pravastatin therapy q 6 weeks during the first 3 months of therapy, q 8 weeks during the re-

mainder of the first year, and at about 6-month intervals thereafter.
2. Pravastatin should be discontinued if markedly elevated CPK levels occur or myopathy is diagnosed or suspected.
3. Pravastatin should be discontinued temporarily in clients experiencing an acute or serious condition (e.g., sepsis, hypotension, major surgery, trauma, uncontrolled epilepsy, or severe metabolic, endocrine, or electrolyte disorders) predisposing to the development of renal failure secondary to rhabdomyolysis.

Client/Family Teaching
1. Review the prescribed dietary recommendations (restricted cholesterol and saturated fats), assess client understanding of dietary guidelines, and refer to a dietitian as needed.
2. Instruct to report any unexplained muscle pain, tenderness, or weakness, especially if accompanied by malaise or fever.
3. Advise to practice birth control and to report if pregnancy is suspected. Review potential hazards of drug therapy to a developing fetus.

Evaluate: ↓ Serum cholesterol levels.

Simvastatin

(**sim**-vah-**STAH**-tin)
Pregnancy Category: X
Zocor **(Rx)**

How Supplied: *Tablet:* 5 mg, 10 mg, 20 mg, 40 mg

Action/Kinetics: Simvastatin inhibits HMG-CoA reductase, an enzyme that is necessary to convert HMG-CoA to mevalonate (an early step in the biosynthesis of cholesterol). The levels of VLDL and LDL cholesterol and plasma triglycerides are reduced while the plasma concentration of HDL cholesterol is increased. Simvastatin does not reduce basal plasma cortisol or testosterone levels or impair renal reserve. **Peak therapeutic response:** 4–6 weeks. Approximately 85% is absorbed although there is a significant first-pass effect with less than 5% of a PO dose reaching the general circulation. Liver metabolites are excreted in the feces (60%) and urine (13%).

Uses: Adjunct to diet for the reduction of elevated total and LDL cholesterol levels in types IIa and IIb hypercholesterolemia when the response to diet and other approaches have been inadequate. *Investigational:* Heterozygous familial hypercholesterolemia, familial combined hyperlipidemia, diabetic dyslipidemia in non-insulin-dependent diabetes, hyperlipidemia secondary to the nephrotic syndrome, and homozygous familial hypercholesterolemia in clients with defective LDL receptors.

Dosage

• Tablets

Adults, initially: 5–10 mg once daily in the evening; **maintenance:** 5–40 mg/day as a single dose in the evening. A starting dose of 5 mg/day should be considered for clients with LDL less than 190 mg/dL and 10 mg/day for clients with LDL greater than 190 mg/dL. For geriatric clients, the starting dose should be 5 mg/day with maximum LDL reductions seen with 20 mg or less daily.

Administration/Storage
1. The client should be placed on a standard cholesterol-lowering diet for 3–6 months before starting simvastatin. The diet should be continued during drug therapy.
2. May be given without regard to meals.
3. Dosage may be adjusted at intervals of at least 4 weeks.

Contraindications: Active liver disease or unexplained persistent increases in liver function tests. Use in pregnancy, during lactation, or in children.

Special Concerns: Use with caution in clients who have a history of liver disease or who consume large quantities of alcohol. Use with caution with drugs that affect steroid levels or activity. Higher plasma levels may be observed in clients with severe renal insufficiency. Safety and efficacy have not been determined in children less than 18 years of age.

Laboratory Test Interferences: ↑ CPK, AST, ALT.

Side Effects: *Musculoskeletal:* Rhabdomyolysis with renal dysfunction secondary to myoglobinuria, myopathy, arthralgias. *GI:* N&V, diarrhea, abdominal pain, constipation, flatulence, dyspepsia, pancreatitis, anorexia, stomatitis. *Hepatic:* Hepatitis (including chronic active hepatitis), cholestatic jaundice, cirrhosis, fatty change in liver, ***fulminant hepatic necrosis, hepatoma.*** *Neurologic:* Dysfunction of certain cranial nerves resulting in alteration of taste, impairment of extraocular movement, and facial paresis. Paresthesia, peripheral neuropathy, peripheral nerve palsy. *CNS:* Headache, tremor, vertigo, memory loss, anxiety, insomnia, depression. *Hypersensitivity Reactions:* Although rare, the following symptoms have been noted. ***Angioedema, anaphylaxis,*** lupus erythematous–like syndrome, vasculitis, purpura, thrombocytopenia, leukopenia, ***hemolytic anemia,*** polymyalgia rheumatica, positive ANA, ESR increase, arthritis, arthralgia, asthenia, urticaria, photosensitivity, chills, fever, flushing, malaise, dyspnea, ***toxic epidermal necrolysis, erythema multiforme (including Stevens-Johnson syndrome).*** *GU:* Gynecomastia, loss of libido, erectile dysfunction. *Ophthalmologic:* Lens opacities, ophthalmoplegia. *Hematologic:* Transient asymptomatic eosinophilia, anemia, thrombocytopenia, leukopenia. *Miscellaneous:* Upper respiratory infection, asthenia, alopecia, edema.

Drug Interactions

Gemfibrozil / Possible severe myopathy or rhabdomyolysis

Warfarin / ↑ Anticoagulant effect of warfarin

NURSING CONSIDERATIONS

Assessment

1. Document baseline CBC and liver and renal function studies. Schedule liver function studies q 4–6 weeks during the first 3 months of therapy, q 6–8 weeks during the next 12 months, and at approximately 6-month intervals thereafter. Special attention should be paid to elevated serum transaminase levels.
2. List all medications currently prescribed to prevent any unfavorable interactions.
3. Determine that weight reduction, exercise, and cholesterol-lowering diet were all used in an attempt to lower total serum cholesterol and LDL levels; assess level of client compliance.
4. Note any history or evidence of alcohol abuse.

Client/Family Teaching

1. Advise that a low-cholesterol diet must continue to be followed during drug therapy. Refer to a dietitian for assistance in meal planning and food preparation.
2. Remind clients that liver function tests will be performed often during drug therapy and to report as scheduled (every 4–6 weeks during the first 3 months of therapy, every 6–8 weeks during the next 12 months, and then every 6 months).
3. Provide a printed list of drug side effects. Advise to report any S&S of infections, unexplained muscle pain, tenderness or weakness (especially if accompanied by fever or malaise), surgery, trauma, or metabolic disorders.

Evaluate: Desired ↓ serum cholesterol levels.

MISCELLANEOUS AGENTS

See the following individual entries:

Cholestyramine Resin
Clofibrate
Colestipol Hydrochloride
Dextrothyroxine Sodium
Probucol

Cholestyramine resin

(koh-less-**TEER**-ah-meen)
Cholybar, Questran, Questran Light
(Rx)

How Supplied: *Powder for Reconstitution:* 4 g/5 g, 4 g/9 g

Action/Kinetics: Cholestyramine binds sodium cholate (bile salts) in the intestine; thus, the principal precursor of cholesterol is not absorbed due to formation of an insoluble complex, which is excreted in the feces. The drug decreases cholesterol and LDL and has either no effect or increases triglycerides, VLDL, and HDL. Also, itching is relieved as a result of removing irritating bile salts. The antidiarrheal effect results from the binding and removal of bile acids. **Onset, to reduce plasma cholesterol:** Within 24–48 hr but levels may continue to fall for 1 yr; **to relieve pruritus:** 1–3 weeks; **relief of diarrhea associated with bile acids:** 24 hr. Cholesterol levels return to pretreatment levels 2–4 wks after discontinuance. Fat-soluble vitamins (A, D, K) and possibly folic acid may have to be administered IM during long-term therapy because cholestyramine binds these vitamins in the intestine.

Uses: Pruritus associated with partial biliary obstruction. As adjunctive therapy in hyperlipoproteinemia (types IIA and IIB) to reduce serum cholesterol in clients who do not respond adequately to diet. Diarrhea due to bile acids. *Investigational:* Treatment of poisoning by chlordecone (Kepone), antibiotic-induced pseudomembranous colitis (i.e., due to toxin produced by *Clostridium difficile*), digitalis toxicity, postvagotomy diarrhea, and hyperoxaluria.

Dosage

• Powder

Adults: 4 g 1–6 times/day. After relief of pruritus, dosage may be reduced. Doses greater than 24 g/day result in an increased incidence of side effects. **Pediatric, 6–12 years:** 80 mg (anhydrous cholestyramine)/kg (2.35 g/m^2) t.i.d. The adult dose should be used in children older than 12 years. Not recommended for children less than 6 years of age.

• Tablets

Initial: 4 g 1–2 times/day; **maintenance:** 8–16 g/day divided into two doses. Dose may be increased gradually (based on lipid/lipoprotein levels) at intervals of 4 or more weeks. Maximum recommended dose: 24 g/day.

Administration/Storage

1. Always mix powder with 60–180 mL water or noncarbonated beverage before administering because resin may cause esophageal irritation or blockage. Highly liquid soups or pulpy fruits such as applesauce or crushed pineapple may also be used.
2. After placing contents of 1 packet of resin on the surface of 4–6 oz of fluid, allow it to stand without stirring for 2 min, occasionally twirling the glass, and then stir slowly (to prevent foaming) to form a suspension.
3. Avoid inhaling the powder while mixing as it may be irritating to mucous membranes.
4. The bar should be chewed thoroughly and taken with plenty of fluids.
5. Cholestyramine may interfere with the absorption of other drugs taken orally; thus, take other drug(s) 1 hr before or 4–6 hr after cholestyramine.

Contraindications: Complete obstruction or atresia of bile duct.

Special Concerns: Use during pregnancy only if benefits outweigh risks. Use with caution during lactation and in children. Geriatric clients may be more likely to manifest GI side effects as well as adverse nutritional effects.

Side Effects: *GI:* Constipation (may be severe), N&V, diarrhea, heartburn, GI bleeding, anorexia, flatulence, belching, abdominal distention, abdominal pain or cramping, loose stools, indigestion, aggravation of hemorrhoids, rectal bleeding or pain, black stools, bleeding duodenal ulcer, peptic ulceration, GI irritation, dysphagia, dental bleeding, hiccoughs, sour taste, pancreatitis, diverticulitis, cholescystitis, cholelithiasis. Fecal impaction in elderly clients. Large doses may cause steatorrhea. *CNS:* Migraine or sinus headaches, dizziness, anxiety, vertigo, insomnia, fatigue, lightheadedness, syncope, drowsiness, femoral nerve pain, paresthesia. *Hypersensitivity:* Urticaria, dermatitis, asthma, wheezing, rash. *Hematologic:* Increased PT, ecchymosis, anemia. *Musculoskeletal:* Muscle or joint pain, backache, arthritis, osteoporosis. *GU:* Hematuria, dysuria, burnt odor to urine, diuresis. *Other:* Bleeding tendencies (due to hypoprothrombinemia). Deficiencies of vitamins A and D. Uveitis, weight loss or gain, osteoporosis, swollen glands, increased libido, weakness, SOB, edema, swelling of hands/feet; hyperchloremic acidosis in children, rash and irritation of the skin, tongue, and perianal area.

Symptoms of Overdose: GI tract obstruction.

Drug Interactions

Acetaminophen / ↓ Effect of acetaminophen due to ↓ absorption from GI tract
Amiodarone / ↓ Effect of amiodarone due to ↓ absorption from GI tract
Anticoagulants, oral / ↓ Anticoagulant effect due to ↓ absorption from GI tract
Cephalexin / ↓ Absorption of cephalexin from GI tract
Chenodiol / ↓ Effect of chenodiol due to ↓ absorption from GI tract
Chlorothiazide / ↓ Effect of chlorothiazide due to ↓ absorption from GI tract
Clindamycin / ↓ Absorption of clindamycin from GI tract
Corticosteroids / ↓ Effect of corticosteroids due to ↓ absorption from GI tract
Digitalis glycosides / Cholestyramine binds digitoxin in the intestine and ↓ its half-life
Gemfibrozil / ↓ Bioavailability of gemfibrozil
Glipizide / ↓ Serum glipizide levels
Iopanoic acid / Results in abnormal cholecystography
Iron preparations / ↓ Effect of iron preparations due to ↓ absorption from GI tract
Lovastatin / Effects may be additive
Naproxen / ↓ Effect of naproxen due to ↓ absorption from GI tract
Penicillin G / ↓ Effect of penicillin G due to ↓ absorption from GI tract
Phenobarbital / ↓ Absorption of phenobarbital from GI tract
Phenylbutazone / Absorption of phenylbutazone delayed by cholestyramine—may ↓ effect
Piroxicam / ↓ Effect of piroxicam due to ↓ absorption from GI tract
Propranolol / ↓ Effect of propranolol due to ↓ absorption from GI tract
Tetracyclines / ↓ Effect of tetracyclines due to ↓ absorption from GI tract
Thiazide diuretics / ↓ Effect of thiazides due to ↓ absorption from GI tract
Thyroid hormones / ↓ Effect of thyroid hormones due to ↓ absorption from GI tract
Trimethoprim / ↓ Effect of trimethoprim due to ↓ absorption from GI tract
Ursodiol / ↓ Effect of ursodiol due to ↓ absorption from GI tract
Vitamins A, D, E, K / Malabsorption of fat-soluble vitamins
Warfarin / ↓ Effect of warfarin due to ↓ absorption from GI tract
NOTE: These drug interactions may also be observed with colestipol.

NURSING CONSIDERATIONS

Assessment

1. Document indications for therapy and note type and onset of symptoms.
2. Determine onset of pruritus and obtain bile acid level.
3. Perform baseline CBC and liver and renal function studies.
4. Note color of client's skin and eyes for evidence of jaundice.

Interventions

1. Anticipate that vitamins A, D, K, and folic acid will be administered in a water-miscible form during long-term therapy.
2. Note client complaints of constipation, abdominal pain, or abdominal bloating. Encourage daily exercise and a fluid intake of 2.5–3 L/day. An increased intake of citrus fruits, fruit juices, and high fiber foods may serve as preventive measures. Also, a stool softener may be indicated.

3. If symptoms are severe or if they persist, discuss a change in the dosage or form of drug, or a change of medication with the provider.
4. If the client complains of diarrhea, monitor I&O, electrolytes, and weight. Note any evidence of dehydration and/or electrolyte imbalance.
5. Monitor serum cholesterol and triglyceride levels. Serum transaminase and other liver function tests should be conducted routinely.
6. To ensure that the clients are not developing anemia, leukopenia, eosinophilia, potential anticoagulant effects, or renal dysfunction, blood counts and renal function tests should be done routinely.
7. If clients develop bleeding from any orifice or develop purpura, they should receive parenteral vitamin K.

Client/Family Teaching

1. Other prescribed medications should be taken at least 1 hr before or 4 hr after taking antihyperlipidemic medication. These drugs interfere with the absorption and desired effects of other medications.
2. Discuss the constipating effects the drug may have and ways to control this problem. Exercise daily, drink extra fluids, and include extra roughage in the diet.
3. If the client has problems with persistent constipation despite efforts to avoid the problem, a stool softener may be required.
4. Report tarry stools or abnormal bleeding as supplemental vitamin K (10 mg/week) may be necessary.
5. Pruritus may subside 1–3 weeks after taking the drug but may return after the medication is discontinued. Corn starch or oatmeal baths may assist to alleviate this discomfort.

Evaluate

- Control of pruritus
- ↓ Serum cholesterol levels
- ↓ Diarrheal stools

Clofibrate

(kloh-**FYE**-brayt)
Pregnancy Category: C
Atromid-S, Novo-Fibrate ✱ **(Rx)**

How Supplied: *Capsule:* 500 mg

Action/Kinetics: Clofibrate decreases triglycerides, VLDL, and, cholesterol and either does not change or increases HDL and does not change or decreases LDL. The mechanism is not known with certainty but may be due to increased catabolism of VLDL to LDL and decreased synthesis of VLDL by the liver. The higher the cholesterol level, the more effective the drug. The drug may also increase the release of ADH from the posterior pituitary. **Peak plasma levels:** 2–6 hr. **t½:** 6–25 hr. **Therapeutic effect: Onset,** 2–5 days; **maximum effect:** 3 weeks. Triglycerides return to pretreatment levels 2–3 weeks after therapy is terminated. Clofibrate is hydrolyzed to the active *p*-chlorophenoxyisobutyric acid which is further metabolized and excreted in the urine. The drug may concentrate in fetal blood. Liver function tests should be performed during therapy.

Uses: As adjunct treatment for type III hyperlipidemia in clients with a significant risk of coronary heart disease who have not responded to diet or other measures. Limited use in type II hyperlipidemia. *Investigational:* Partial central diabetes insipidus in clients with some residual posterior pituitary function.

Dosage

- **Capsules**

Antihyperlipidemic.

Adults: 500 mg q.i.d. Therapeutic response may take several weeks to become apparent. Drug must be administered on a continuous basis because lowered levels of cholesterol and other lipids will return to elevated state within several weeks after administration is stopped. Discontinue after 3 months if response is poor.

Contraindications: Impaired hepatic or renal function, primary biliary cirrhosis, lactation, children.

Special Concerns: Use with caution in clients with gout and peptic ulcer. Reduced dosage may be required in geriatric clients due to age-related decreases in renal function.

Dosage has not been established in children.

Side Effects: *GI:* Nausea, dyspepsia, weight gain, gastritis, vomiting,bloating, flatulence, abdominal distress, stomatitis, loose stools, hepatomegaly. *CNS:* Headaches, dizziness, fatigue, weakness, drowsiness. *CV:* Changes in blood-clotting time, arrhythmias, increased or decreased angina, thrombophlebitis, swelling and phlebitis at xanthoma site, pulmonary embolism. *Skeletal muscle:* Myositis, asthenia, myalgia, weakness, muscle aches, cramps. *GU:* Impotence, dysuria, hematuria, decreased urine output, decreased libido, proteinuria. *Hematologic:* Anemia, leukopenia, eosinophilia. *Dermatologic:* Urticaria, skin rash, dry skin, pruritus, dry brittle hair, alopecia. *Enzyme changes:* ↑ CPK, increased serum transaminase (if levels continue to increase after maximum therapeutic response has been achieved, therapy should be discontinued). *Other:* Increased incidence of gallstones, dyspnea, polyphagia.

Drug Interactions

Anticoagulants / Clofibrate ↑ anticoagulant effect by ↓ plasma protein binding

Antidiabetics (sulfonylureas) / Clofibrate ↑ effect of antidiabetics

Furosemide / Concurrent use may ↑ effects of both drugs

Insulin / Clofibrate ↑ effect of insulin

Probenecid / ↑ Effect of clofibrate due to ↓ breakdown by liver and ↓ kidney excretion

Rifampin / ↓ Effect of clofibrate due to ↑ breakdown by liver

---

NURSING CONSIDERATIONS

Assessment

1. If client is of childbearing age, determine if pregnant.
2. Obtain baseline CBC and liver and renal function studies; document triglycerides, VLDL, and cholesterol levels.

Client/Family Teaching

1. Drug may be taken with food if GI upset occurs. Nausea usually decreases with continued therapy or reduced dosage.
2. A reduction in anticoagulant drug dosage is customary if clofibrate therapy is instituted. Advise client to report any abnormal bleeding.
3. Report symptoms of hypoglycemia because of possible drug interactions with oral antidiabetic agents.
4. Use contraception if appropriate because clofibrate may be teratogenic. Do not discontinue contraception for several months after discontinuing drug therapy if pregnancy is planned.
5. Review the potential risks of drug therapy (e.g., gallstones, tumors) and advise to report any side effects so that drug therapy can be evaluated.
6. Stress the importance of adhering to dietary restrictions, daily exercise, and weight loss in the overall management and control of hypercholesterolemia and hyperlipidemia.

Evaluate: Significant ↓ in serum cholesterol and lipid levels.

Colestipol hydrochloride

(koh-**LESS**-tih-poll)

Colestid **(Rx)**

How Supplied: *Granule for Reconstitution:* 5 g/7.5 g, 5 g/packet, 5 g/scoopful; *Tablet:* 1 g

Action/Kinetics: Colestipol, an anion exchange resin, binds bile acids in the intestine, forming an insoluble complex excreted in the feces. The loss of bile acids results in increased oxidation of cholesterol to bile acids and a decrease in LDL and serum cholesterol. Colestipol does not affect (or may increase) triglycerides or HDL and may increase VLDL. The drug is not absorbed from the GI tract. **Onset:** 1–2 days; **maximum effect:** 1 month. Return to pretreatment cholesterol levels after discontinuance of therapy: 1 month.

Uses: As adjunctive therapy in hyperlipoproteinemia (types IIA and IIB) to reduce serum cholesterol in clients who do not respond adequately to diet. *Investigational:* Digitalis toxicity, pruritus associated with partial biliary obstruction, diarrhea due to bile acids, hyperoxaluria.

Dosage

- **Oral Granules**

Antihyperlipidemic.

Adults, initial: 5 g 1–2 times/day; **then,** can increase 5 g/day at 1–2-month intervals. **Total dose:** 5–30 g/day given once or in two to three divided doses.

- **Tablets**

Adults, initial: 2 g 1–2 times/day. Dose can be increased by 2 g, once or twice daily, at 1–2-month intervals. **Total dose:** 2–16 g/day given once or in divided doses.

Digitalis toxicity.

10 g followed by 5 g q 6–8 hr.

Administration/Storage

1. Always mix the granules with 90 mL or more of fluid before administering because resin may cause esophageal irritation or blockage.
2. Disguise unpalatable taste of drug by mixing it with fruit juice, soup, cereal, milk, water, applesauce, pureed fruit, or carbonated beverages. Granules are available in an orange-flavored product.
3. The glass should be rinsed with a small amount of additional beverage to ensure the total amount of the drug is taken.
4. If compliance is good and side effects acceptable but the desired effect is not obtained with 2–16 g/day using the tablets, combined therapy or alternative treatment should be considered.
5. Tablets should be swallowed whole (i.e., they should not be cut, crushed, or chewed). Tablets may be taken with water or other fluids.
6. Take other drugs 1 hr before or 4 hr after colestipol to reduce interference with their absorption.

Contraindication: Complete obstruction or atresia of bile duct.

Special Concerns: Use during pregnancy only if benefits outweigh risks. Use with caution during lactation and in children. Children may be more likely to develop hyperchloremic acidosis although dosage has not been established. Clients over 60 years of age may be at greater risk of GI side effects and adverse nutritional effects.

Side Effects: *GI:* Constipation (may be severe), N&V, diarrhea, heartburn, GI bleeding, anorexia, flatulence, belching, abdominal distention, aggravation of hemorrhoids. Fecal impaction in elderly clients. Large doses may cause steatorrhea. *Other:* Bleeding tendencies (due to hypoprothrombinemia). Osteoporosis, electrolyte imbalance, and CNS and musculoskeletal manifestations. Prolonged administration may interfere with absorption of fat-soluble vitamins. Irritation and rash of skin, tongue, and perianal area.

Drug Interactions

See *Cholestyramine,* Chapter 29.

NURSING CONSIDERATIONS

See also *Nursing Considerations* for *Cholestyramine,* Chapter 29.

Client/Family Teaching

1. Take 30 min before meals. Do not take at the same time as other medications as drug may alter their absorption.
2. Never take dose in dry form. Review mixing and proper method of administration.
3. Consume adequate amounts of fluids, fruits, and fiber to diminish constipating effects of drug.
4. Explain that serum cholesterol level will return to pretreatment levels within 1 month if drug is discontinued.

Evaluate: Desired ↓ in serum cholesterol and LDL levels.

Dextrothyroxine sodium

(dek-stroh-thigh-**ROX**-een)

Choloxin **(Rx)**

How Supplied: *Tablet:* 1 mg, 2 mg, 4 mg

Action/Kinetics: Dextrothyroxine (the dextro isomer of thyroid hormone) increases the rate at which cholesterol is metabolized in the liver; excretion of cholesterol and metabolites is increased, leading to decreased serum levels of cholesterol and LDL; there is no change in levels of triglycerides or HDL. Dextrothyroxine has little effect on the BMR but is otherwise similar physiologically to levothyroxine. The effectiveness increases as cholesterol levels increase. Approximately 25% is absorbed from the GI tract; almost completely bound to plasma proteins. **t½:** 18 hr. **Duration:** Serum lipid levels return to pretreatment levels from 6 to 12 weeks after termination of drug therapy. Eliminated through both the kidneys and feces.

Uses: Only for clients with primary hypercholesterolemia (type IIa hyperlipidemia) who are at a significant risk for CAD and who have not responded to diet or other measures.

Dosage

- **Tablets**

Primary hypercholesterolemia.

Adults, initial: 1–2 mg/day. Daily dosage can be increased q 4 weeks by 1–2 mg; **maintenance:** 4–8 mg/day. **Maximum daily dosage:** 8 mg. It may take 2–4 weeks for the therapeutic response to become manifested. **Pediatric, initial:** 0.05 mg/kg (1.5 mg/m^2) daily. Increase by 0.05 mg/kg q month, up to maximum of 4 mg/day, until satisfactory control is established. **Maintenance:** 0.1 mg/kg (3 mg/m^2) daily. Withdraw drug 2 weeks before surgery.

Contraindications: Euthyroid clients with hypertensive organic heart disease, including angina pectoris, history of MI, cardiac arrhythmias or tachycardia, rheumatic disease, CHF, decompensated or borderline compensated cardiac status, hypertension (other than mild, labile, systolic). Pregnancy, lactation, advanced liver or kidney disease, or a history of hypersensitivity to iodine.

Special Concerns: Use with caution in impaired liver and kidney function. Clients intolerant to lactose, milk, or milk products may be intolerant to the tablet since it also contains lactose. Geriatric clients may be more sensitive to the effects of dextrothyroxine.

Side Effects: *CNS:* Insomnia, nervousness, fever, headache, decreased sensorium, paresthesia, dizziness, malaise, tiredness, psychic changes, tremors. *CV:* Angina pectoris, increase in heart size, ischemic myocardial changes (ECG changes), ***arrhythmias*** including ectopic beats, SVT, extrasystoles, worsening of peripheral vascular disease, possibility of ***fatal*** or nonfatal ***MI*** (relationship to drug uncertain). *GI:* N&V, diarrhea, constipation, anorexia, dyspepsia, weight loss, bitter taste, GI hemorrhages. *Other:* Drooping eyelids, changes in libido, sweating, hair loss, diuresis, menstrual irregularities, hoarseness, tinnitus, peripheral edema, visual disturbances, muscle pain, gallstones, increases in blood sugar of diabetic clients, skin rashes, itching, flushing.

Aggravation of existing cardiac disease is cause for discontinuation.

Symptoms of Overdose: Hyperthyroidism, diarrhea, cramps, vomiting, nervousness, twitching, tachycardia, and weight loss.

Drug Interactions

Anticoagulants, oral / ↑ Effect of anticoagulants by ↑ hypoprothrombinemia

Antidiabetics, oral / ↓ Diabetic control as dextrothyroxine ↑ blood glucose

Beta-adrenergic blocking agents / Dextrothyroxine ↓ effect of beta blockers

Cholestyramine / ↓ Effect of dextrothyroxine due to ↓ absorption from GI tract

Colestipol / ↓ Effect of dextrothyroxine due to ↓ absorption from GI tract

Digitalis / Additive stimulation of myocardium

Epinephrine / In CAD, concomitant use → coronary insufficiency
Insulin / ↓ Diabetic control as dextrothyroxine ↑ blood glucose
Thyroid drugs / ↑ Sensitivity of hypothyroid clients to thyroid drugs
Tricyclic antidepressants / Use with dextrothyroxine → CNS stimulation, ↑ HR, cardiac arrhythmias, nervousness

NURSING CONSIDERATIONS

Assessment

1. Note any history of hypersensitivity to tartrazine, history of CAD or thyroid disorder. Use should be discontinued if symptoms of cardiac disease develop.
2. Obtain baseline ECG prior to starting the client on therapy.
3. Determine if taking cardiac glycosides or oral anticoagulants as dextrothyroxine may enhance the action of these agents.
4. Document serum cholesterol, LDL, and HDL levels.
5. Note other therapies and medications utilized for this problem and the outcome.

Interventions

1. Assess for and note client complaints of chest pain or any attacks of angina.
2. Monitor pulse and if it remains 120 beats/min, withhold the dosage (unless otherwise indicated) and report.
3. Dextrothyroxine may increase blood glucose levels. An adjustment in oral hypoglycemic agents or insulin dosage may be necessary in clients with diabetes.
4. Check eyes routinely for exophthalmos.

Client/Family Teaching

1. If nausea or a decrease in appetite is evident, taking the drug with meals may reduce the gastric irritation and ensure better compliance with therapy.
2. Provide a printed list of drug side effects. Advise to report any new S&S to prevent the development of serious side effects.
3. Stress the importance of adhering to dietary restrictions, daily exercise, and weight loss in the overall management and control of hypercholesterolemia and hyperlipidemia.
4. Report for all scheduled laboratory studies so the drug effectiveness can be evaluated.

Evaluate: ↓ Serum cholesterol levels.

Probucol

(**PROH**-byou-kohl)
Pregnancy Category: B
Lorelco **(Rx)**

How Supplied: *Tablet:* 250 mg, 500 mg

Action/Kinetics: Mechanism for alteration of cholesterol metabolism unknown, although the drug increases excretion of fecal bile acids, inhibits early stages of cholesterol synthesis, and slightly inhibits absorption of cholesterol from the diet. Decreases LDL cholesterol and HDL; produces no change in triglycerides and either does not change or increases VLDL levels. After prolonged administration, the drug becomes deposited in the adipose tissues and, after discontinuation, persists in the body for up to 6 months. Absorption from the GI tract is variable (usually less than 10%). Food increases peak blood levels. **t½ (biphasic): initial** 24 hr; **final:** 20 days. **Therapeutic onset:** 2–4 weeks; maximum: 20–50 days. Excreted through the feces and the urine (mainly unchanged).

Uses: Primary hypercholesterolemia, especially of type IIa, not responding to diet or weight control and clients who have a significant risk of CAD.

Dosage

• **Tablets**

Adults only: 500 mg b.i.d. with morning and evening meals. In some clients, 500 mg/day may be as effective as giving the drug b.i.d.

Administration/Storage

1. To be taken with morning and evening meals because food seems to increase absorption from the GI tract.
2. Clofibrate and probucol should not be given together because the

combination may cause a significant decrease of HDL.
3. Store in a dry place, in light-resistant containers away from excessive heat.

Contraindications: Hypersensitivity. Serious ventricular arrhythmias, unexplained syncope or syncope of CV origin, recent or progressive myocardial damage. In situations where the QT interval at an observed HR is more than 15% above the upper limit of normal (see package insert). Should not be used in treatment of elevated blood lipids to prevent coronary heart disease.

Special Concerns: Safe use during pregnancy and lactation and in childhood has not been established.

Laboratory Test Interferences: Transient ↑ AST, ALT, alkaline phosphatase, uric acid, bilirubin, creatine phosphatase, alkaline phosphatase, blood glucose, BUN.

Side Effects: *CV:* Prolongation of the QT interval on the ECG, syncope, ***ventricular arrhythmias; sudden death may occur.*** *GI:* Most common: diarrhea, anorexia, indigestion, flatulence, GI bleeding, abdominal pain, N&V. *Ophthalmic:* Blurred vision, tearing, conjunctivitis. *CNS:* Headache, dizziness, insomnia, paresthesia. *Hematologic:* Thrombocytopenia, eosinophilia, low H&H. *Dermatologic:* Rash, pruritus, hyperhidrosis, fetid sweat, petechiae, ecchymosis. *Miscellaneous:* Angioneurotic edema, decreased taste and smell sensations, enlargement of multinodular goiter, tinnitus, peripheral neuritis.

During the beginning of therapy certain clients have manifested anidiosyncratic reaction including dizziness, syncope, N&V, palpitations, and chest pain.

NURSING CONSIDERATIONS

Client/Family Teaching

1. Take with food, as directed, to enhance absorption. Continue to follow the prescribed dietary restrictions.
2. If diarrhea occurs, it is usually transient. Roughage should be eliminated until diarrhea stops. Report any bothersome or persistent GI symptoms.
3. Stress the importance of reporting any unexplained bruising or bleeding.
4. Clients may develop insomnia, dizziness, and/or headaches. These should be reported and a record kept of the frequency of occurrences.
5. If blurred vision occurs or if dizziness develops, client should avoid driving or using heavy equipment.
6. Nocturia and impotence may occur. Discuss this when therapy is initiated. Report these developments at once because another medication may be necessary.

Evaluate: ↓ Serum cholesterol levels.

CHAPTER THIRTY

Drugs Used for Congestive Heart Failure/Inotropic Agents

See the following individual entries:

Amiloride and
Hydrochlorothiazide - See Chapter 28
Amrinone Lactate
Cardiac Glycosides
Digitoxin
Digoxin
Milrinone Lactate

Amrinone lactate

(**AM**-rih-nohn)
Pregnancy Category: C
Inocor **(Rx)**

How Supplied: *Injection:* 5 mg/mL
Action/Kinetics: Amrinone causes an increase in CO by increasing the force of contraction of the heart, probably by inhibiting phosphodiesterase. It reduces afterload and preload by directly relaxing vascular smooth muscle. **Time to peak effect:** 10 min. **t½, after rapid IV:** 3.6 hr; **after IV infusion:** 5.8 hr. **Plasma levels:** 3.0 mcg/mL. **Duration:** 30 min–2 hr, depending on the dose. The drug is excreted primarily in the urine both unchanged and as metabolites.
Uses: Congestive heart failure (short-term therapy in clients unresponsive to digitalis, diuretics, and/or vasodilators). Can be used in digitalized clients.

Dosage

• **IV**

Initial: 0.75 mg/kg as a bolus given slowly over 2–3 min; may be repeated after 30 min if necessary. **Maintenance, IV infusion:** 5–10 mcg/kg/min. Daily dose should not exceed 10 mg/kg although up to 18 mg/kg/day has been used in some clients for short periods.

Administration/Storage

1. Amrinone may be administered undiluted or diluted in 0.9% or 0.45% saline to a concentration of 1–3 mg/mL. Diluted solutions should be used within 24 hr.
2. Amrinone should not be diluted with solutions containing dextrose (glucose) prior to injection. However, the drug may be injected into running dextrose (glucose) infusions through a Y connector or directly into the tubing.
3. Administer loading dose over 2–3 min; may be repeated in 30 min.
4. Solutions should appear clear yellow.
5. Administer solution with an electronic infusion device.
6. Amrinone should not be administered in an IV line containing furosemide because a precipitate will form.
7. Protect from light and store at room temperature.
8. *Treatment of Overdose:* Reduce or discontinue drug administration and begin general supportive measures.

Contraindications: Hypersensitivity to bisulfites. Severe aortic or pulmonary valvular disease in lieu of surgery. Acute MI.
Special Concerns: Safety and effica-

cy not established during lactation and in children.

Side Effects: *GI:* N&V, abdominal pain, anorexia. *CV:* Hypotension, ***arrhythmias.*** *Allergic:* Pericarditis, pleuritis, ascites. *Other:* Thrombocytopenia, ***hepatotoxicity,*** fever, chest pain, burning at site of injection.

Symptom of Overdose: Hypotension.

Drug Interaction: Excessive hypotension when used with disopyramide.

NURSING CONSIDERATIONS

Assessment

1. Determine that baseline VS, CXR, and ECG have been performed.
2. Obtain baseline electrolytes, CBC, and platelet count.
3. Identify previous pharmacologic agents used for these symptoms and the results.

Interventions

1. Clients should be monitored while receiving amrinone.
2. Monitor serum potassium levels, CBC, and platelets; report any bruises or bleeding.
3. Monitor VS, I&O, weights, and urine output. Document CVP, CO, and PA pressures if Swan Ganz catheter in place.
4. Observe for any hypersensitivity reactions, including pericarditis, pleuritis, or ascites.

Evaluate

- ↓ Preload and afterload; ↑ CO
- Improvement in S&S of CHF

CARDIAC GLYCOSIDES

See also the following individual entries:

Digitoxin
Digoxin

General Statement: Cardiac glycosides, such as digitoxin, are plant alkaloids. They are probably the oldest, yet still the most effective, drugs for treating CHF. By improving myocardial contraction, they improve blood supply to all organs, including the kidney, thereby improving function. This action results in diuresis, thereby correcting the edema often associated with cardiac insufficiency. Digitalis glycosides are also used for the treatment of cardiac arrhythmias, since they decrease pulse rate as well. The cardiac glycosides are cumulative in action. This effect is partially responsible for the difficulties associated with their use.

Action/Kinetics: Cardiac glycosides increase the force of myocardial contraction (positive inotropic effect). This effect is due to inhibition of movement of sodium and potassium ions across myocardial cell membranes due to complexing with adenosine triphosphatase. This results in an increase of calcium influx and an increased release of free calcium ions within the myocardial cells, which then potentiate the contractility of cardiac muscle fibers. The digitalis glycosides also decrease the rate of conduction and increase the refractory period of the AV node. This effect is due to an increase in parasympathetic tone and a decrease in sympathetic tone. The cardiac glycosides are absorbed from the GI tract. Absorption varies from 40% to 90%, depending on the preparation and *brand.* With most preparations, peak plasma concentrations are reached within 2–3 hr. Half-life ranges from 1.7 days for digoxin to 7 days for digitoxin. The drugs are primarily excreted through the kidneys, either unchanged (digoxin) or metabolized (digitoxin). The initial dose of digitalis glycosides is larger (loading dose) and is traditionally referred to as the *digitalizing dose;* subsequent doses are referred to as *maintenance doses.*

Uses: Congestive heart failure, especially secondary to hypertension, coronary artery or atherosclerotic heart disease, or valvular heart disease. Control of rapid ventricular contraction rate in clients with atrial fibrillation or flutter. Slow HR in sinus tachycardia due to CHF. Supraventricular tachycardia. Prophylaxis and treatment of recurrent paroxysmal atrial tachycardia with paroxysmal AV junctional rhythm. In conjunction with propranolol for angina. Cardiogenic shock (value not established).

Contraindications: Coronary occlusion or angina pectoris in the absence of CHF or hypersensitivity to cardiogenic glycosides.

Special Concerns: Use with caution in clients with ischemic heart disease, acute myocarditis, ventricular tachycardia, hypertrophic subaortic stenosis, hypoxic or myxedemic states, Adams-Stokes or carotid sinus syndromes, cardiac amyloidosis, or cyanotic heart and lung disease, including emphysema and partial heart block. Electric pacemakers may sensitize the myocardium to cardiac glycosides. The cardiac glycosides should also be given cautiously and at reduced dosage to elderly, debilitated clients, pregnant women and nursing mothers, and newborn, term, or premature infants who have immature renal and hepatic function. Similar precautions also should be observed for clients with reduced renal and/or hepatic function, since such impairment retards excretion of cardiac glycosides.

Side Effects: Cardiac glycosides are extremely toxic and have caused death even in clients who have received the drugs for long periods of time. There is a narrow margin of safety between an effective therapeutic dose and a toxic dose. Overdosage caused by the cumulative effects of the drug is a constant danger in therapy with cardiac glycosides. Digitalis toxicity is characterized by a wide variety of symptoms, which are hard to differentiate from those of the cardiac disease itself.

CV: Changes in the rate, rhythm, and irritability of the heart and the mechanism of the heartbeat. Extrasystoles, bigeminal pulse, coupled rhythm, ectopic beat, and other forms of arrhythmias have been noted. ***Death most often results from ventricular fibrillation.*** Cardiac glycosides should be discontinued in adults when pulse rate falls below 60 beats/min. All cardiac changes are best detected by the ECG, which is also most useful in clients suffering from intoxication. ***Acute hemorrhage.*** *GI:* Anorexia, N&V, excessive salivation, epigastric distress, abdominal pain, diarrhea, bowel necrosis. Clients on digitalis therapy may experience two vomiting stages. The first is an early sign of toxicity and is a direct effect of digitalis on the GI tract. Late vomiting indicates stimulation of the vomiting center of the brain, which occurs after the heart muscle has been saturated with digitalis. *CNS:* Headaches, fatigue, lassitude, irritability, malaise, muscle weakness, insomnia, stupor. Psychotomimetic effects (especially in elderly or arteriosclerotic clients or neonates) including disorientation, confusion, depression, aphasia, delirium, hallucinations, and, rarely, ***convulsions.*** *Neuromuscular:* Neurologic pain involving the lower third of the face and lumbar areas, paresthesia. *Visual disturbances:* Blurred vision, flickering dots, white halos, borders around dark objects, diplopia, amblyopia, color perception changes. *Hypersensitivity (5–7 days after starting therapy):* Skin reactions (urticaria, fever, pruritus, facial and ***angioneurotic edema***). *Other:* Chest pain, coldness of extremities.

Symptoms of Overdose (Toxicity): GI symptoms include anorexia, N&V, diarrhea, abdominal discomfort. CNS symptoms include blurred, yellow, or green vision and halo effect; headache, weakness, drowsiness, mental depression, apathy, restlessness, disorientation, confusion, ***seizures,*** EEG abnormalities, delirium, hallucinations, psychosis. Cardiac effects include ventricular tachycardia, unifocal or multiform PVCs, paroxysmal and nonparoxysmal nodal rhythms, AV dissociation, accelerated junctional rhythm, excessive slowing of the pulse, ***AV block (may proceed to complete block),*** atrial fibrillation, ***ventricular fibrillation (most common cause of death).*** *Children:* Atrial arrhythmias and atrial tachycardia with ***AV block*** are the most common signs of toxicity; in neonates excessive slowing of sinus rate, SA arrest, and prolongation of PR interval occur.

Drug Interactions: One of the most serious side effects of digitalis-type drugs is hypokalemia (lowering of serum potassium levels). This may lead to cardiac arrhythmias, muscle weakness, hypotension, and respiratory distress. Other agents causing hypokalemia reinforce this effect and increase the chance of digitalis toxicity. Such reactions may occur in clients who have been on digitalis maintenance for a long time.

Aminoglycosides / ↓ Effect of digitalis glycosides due to ↓ absorption from GI tract
PAS / ↓ Effect of digitalis glycosides due to ↓ absorption from GI tract
Amphotericin B / ↑ K depletion caused by digitalis; ↑ incidence of digitalis toxicity
Antacids / ↓ Effect of digitalis glycosides due to ↓ absorption from GI tract
Calcium preparations / Cardiac arrhythmias if parenteral calcium given with digitalis
Chlorthalidone / ↑ K and Mg loss with ↑ chance of digitalis toxicity
Cholestyramine / Binds digitoxin in the intestine and ↓ its absorption
Colestipol / Binds digitoxin in the intestine and ↓ its absorption
Ephedrine / ↑ Chance of cardiac arrhythmias
Epinephrine / ↑ Chance of cardiac arrhythmias
Ethacrynic acid / ↑ K and Mg loss with ↑ chance of digitalis toxicity
Furosemide / ↑ K and Mg loss with ↑ chance of digitalis toxicity
Glucose infusions / Large infusions of glucose may cause ↓ in serum potassium and ↑ chance of digitalis toxicity
Hypoglycemic drugs / ↓ Effect of digitalis glycosides due to ↑ breakdown by liver
Methimazole / ↑ Chance of toxic effects of digitalis
Metoclopramide / ↓ Effect of digitalis glycosides by ↓ absorption from GI tract
Muscle relaxants, nondepolarizing / ↑ Risk of cardiac arrhythmias
Propranolol / Potentiates digitalis-induced bradycardia
Reserpine / ↑ Chance of cardiac arrhythmias
Spironolactone / Either ↑ or ↓ toxic effects of digitalis glycosides
Succinylcholine / ↑ Chance of cardiac arrhythmias
Sulfasalazine / ↓ Effect of digitalis glycosides by ↓ absorption from GI tract
Sympathomimetics / ↑ Chance of cardiac arrhythmias
Thiazides / ↑ K and Mg loss with ↑ chance of digitalis toxicity
Thyroid hormones / ↑ Effectiveness of digitalis glycosides

Laboratory Test Interferences: May ↓ PT. Alters tests for 17-ketosteroids and 17-hydroxycorticosteroids.

Dosage

PO, IM, or IV. *Highly individualized.* See individual drugs: digitoxin, digoxin. Initially, the drugs are usually given at higher ("digitalizing" or loading) doses. These are reduced as soon as the desired therapeutic effect is achieved or undesirable toxic reactions develop. The client's response to cardiac glycosides is gauged by clinical and ECG observations. The rates at which clients become digitalized vary considerably. Clients with mild signs of congestion can often be digitalized gradually over a period of several days. Clients suffering from more serious congestion, for example, those showing signs of acute LV failure, dyspnea, or lung edema, can be digitalized more rapidly by parenteral administration of a fast-acting cardiac glycoside. Once digitalization has been attained (pulse 68–80 beats/min) and symptoms of CHF have subsided, the client is put on maintenance dosage. Depending on the drug and the age of the client, the daily maintenance dose is often approximately 10% of the digitalizing dose.

NURSING CONSIDERATIONS

Administration/Storage

1. Many cardiac glycosides have similar names. However, their dosage and duration of their effect differ markedly. Therefore, check the order, the medication administration record/card, and the bottle label of the medication to be administered. If a client questions the drug (size, color, etc.) recheck the drug order, bottle label, and the name of the client to whom the drug is to be given.
2. Measure all oral liquid cardiac medications precisely, using a calibrated dropper or a syringe.
3. The half-life of cardiac glycosides is prolonged in the elderly. When working with elderly clients, anticipate the doses of drug will be smaller than for those in other age groups.
4. Obtain written parameters indicating the pulse rates, both high and low, at which cardiac glycosides are to be withheld. Any change in rate or rhythm may indicate digitalis toxicity.
5. *Treatment of Overdose in Adults:*
• Discontinue drug and admit to the intensive care area for continuous monitoring of ECG.
• If serum potassium is below normal, potassium chloride should be administered in divided PO doses totaling 3–6 g (40–80 mEq). Potassium should not be used when severe or complete heart block is due to digitalis and not related to tachycardia.
• *Atropine:* A dose of 0.01 mg/kg IV to treat severe sinus bradycardia or slow ventricular rate due to secondary AV block.
• *Cholestyramine, colestipol, activated charcoal:* To bind digitalis in the intestine thus preventing enterohepatic recirculation.
• *Digoxin immune FAB:* See drug entry. Given in approximate equimolar quantities as digoxin, it reverses S&S of toxicity.
• *Lidocaine:* A dose of 1 mg/kg given over 5 min followed by an infusion of 15–50 mcg/kg/min to maintain normal cardiac rhythm.
• *Phenytoin:* For cases unresponsive to potassium, can give a dose of 0.5 mg/kg at a rate not exceeding 50 mg/min (given at 1–2 hr intervals). The maximum dose should not exceed 10 mg/kg/day.
• *Countershock:* A direct-current countershock can be used **only as a last resort.**
6. *Treatment of Overdose in Children:* Give potassium in divided doses totaling 1–1.5 mEq/kg (if correction of arrhythmia is urgent, a dose of 0.5 mEq/kg/hr can be used) with careful monitoring of the ECG. The potassium IV solution should be dilute to avoid local irritation although IV fluid overload must be avoided. Digoxin immune FAB may also be used.

FOR CLIENTS STARTING ON A DIGITALIZING DOSE

Assessment

1. Document indications for therapy, type and onset of symptoms, and other agents prescribed.
2. Note any drugs the client may be taking that would adversely interact with digitalis glycosides.
3. Obtain and review the following lab tests before administering the medication: CBC, serum electrolytes, calcium, magnesium, and liver and renal function tests.
4. Ascertain that an ECG has been completed and reviewed before administration.

FOR CLIENTS BEING DIGITALIZED AND FOR CLIENTS ON A MAINTENANCE DOSE OF A CARDIAC GLYCOSIDE

Interventions

1. Observe cardiac monitor for evidence of bradycardia and/or arrhythmias, or count the apical pulse rate for at least 1 min before administering the drug. Obtain written parameters (e.g., HR > 50) for drug administration.
• Document if the adult pulse rate is below 50 beats/min or if an arrhyth-

mia (irregular heart beat/pulse) not previously noted occurs, withhold the drug, and report.

• If a child's pulse rate is 90–110 beats/min or if an arrhythmia is present, withhold the drug and report.

2. With another nurse simultaneously take the client's apical/radial pulse for 1 min, report if there is a pulse deficit (e.g., the wrist rate is less than the apical rate). A pulse deficit may indicate that the client is having an adverse reaction to the drug.

3. Monitor weights and place the client on I&O. Determine that the client is adequately hydrated and that elimination is in line with the intake. Weight gain may indicate edema. Adequate intake will help prevent cumulative toxic effects of the drug.

4. Anticipate that clients taking non-potassium-sparing diuretics as well as a cardiac glycoside will require potassium supplements.

5. When a potassium supplement is needed, ask the pharmacist to provide the client with the most palatable preparation available. (Liquid potassium preparations are usually bitter.)

6. If the client complains of gastric distress, an antacid preparation may be ordered.

• Antacids containing aluminum or magnesium and kaolin/pectin mixtures should be given 6 hr before or 6 hr after dose of cardiac glycoside to prevent decreased therapeutic effect of glycoside.

7. When the drug is given to newborns, use a cardiac monitor to identify early evidence of toxicity. Any excessive slowing of sinus rate, sinoatrial arrest, or prolonged PR interval should be reported immediately and the drug withheld.

8. Monitor serum digoxin levels (therapeutic range 0.5–2.0 ng/mL) and become familiar with medications that enhance the effects of digoxin.

9. During digitalization the client should be in a closely monitored environment where emergency equipment is readily available.

10. Anticipate more than once daily dosing in most children (up to age 10) due to higher metabolic activity.

11. Have digoxin antidote available (digoxin immune FAB) for management of clients with severe toxicity.

Client/Family Teaching

1. Take medication after meals to lessen gastric irritation.

2. Stress the need for close medical and nursing supervision and the importance of reporting any changes, however minor they may seem.

3. Provide written guidelines for withholding medication and reporting abnormal pulse rates.

4. Review how to count the pulse accurately before taking the medication and observe client technique. Review all written instructions several times in the days prior to discharge.

5. Initially, instruct client to maintain a written record of pulse rates, weights, and medication administration for review by health care provider.

6. Develop a checklist to be marked after taking medications. This is particularly important when working with elderly clients who may be more forgetful.

7. Weigh in every morning at the same time before breakfast, and in similar clothing.

8. Due to its narrow safety margin, use the same brand of cardiac glycoside administered in the hospital. Different preparations have variations in bioavailability and could cause toxicity or loss of effect.

9. Follow directions carefully for taking the medication. If one dose of drug is accidentally missed, do not double up on the next dose. Provider should address this event as well as sick days individually with written guidelines to follow.

10. Discard any previously prescribed cardiac glycoside to avoid taking medications by mistake.

11. Review the toxic symptoms of prescribed drugs. Provide a printed list of the toxic symptoms, stressing early recognition and prompt reporting. Anorexia, N&V, and diarrhea are often early symptoms and are due to the toxic effects on the GI tract and CTZ stimulation. Also, disorientation, agitation, visual disturbances, changes in color perception, and hallucinations may be evident.
12. Review and explain any dietary and activity restrictions.
13. Maintain a sodium-restricted diet. Provide a printed list of foods low in sodium and refer to dietician for assistance in shopping, meal planning, and preparation.
14. Follow a potassium-rich diet (unless already prescribed potassium supplementation) and provide a list of potassium-rich foods. This is particularly important when working with clients on a limited income because it enables them to make choices they can afford. Consult dietitian as needed to assist with shopping and meal planning.
15. Consult with the provider before taking any other medications, whether prescribed or OTC, because drug interactions occur frequently with cardiac glycosides.
16. Report any persistent cough, difficulty breathing, or edema, as these are all signs of CHF, and demand immediate medical attention.
17. Help clients contact community health agencies designed to assist them in maintaining health.
18. Stress the importance of returning for scheduled follow-up visits and lab tests.

Evaluate

• A positive response to digitalization, as evidenced by a stable cardiac rate and rhythm, improved breathing patterns, ↓ severity of S&S of CHF, improved CO, ↓ weight, and improved diuresis

• Laboratory confirmation that serum levels of drug are within therapeutic range (e.g., digoxin 0.5–2.0 ng/mL)

Special Concerns

1. Elderly clients must be observed for early S&S of toxicity, because their rate of drug elimination is slower than with other clients. N&V, anorexia, confusion, and visual disturbances may be signs of toxicity and should be reported immediately.
2. The half-life of cardiac glycosides is prolonged in the elderly. When working with elderly clients, anticipate the doses of drug will be smaller than for those in other age groups.
3. Be especially alert to cardiac arrhythmias in children. This sign of toxicity occurs more frequently in children than in adults.

Digitoxin

(dih-jih-**TOX**-in)
Pregnancy Category: C
Digitaline ✱ **(Rx)**

See also *Cardiac Glycosides,* Chapter 30.

How Supplied: *Tablet:* 0.1 mg

Action/Kinetics: Most potent of the digitalis glycosides. Its slow onset of action makes it unsuitable for emergency use. Almost completely absorbed from GI tract. **Onset: PO,** 1–4 hr; maximum effect: 8–12 hr. **t½:** 5–9 days; **Duration:** 2 weeks. Significant protein binding (over 90%). Metabolized by the liver and excreted as inactive metabolites through the urine. **Therapeutic serum levels:** 14–26 ng/mL. Withhold drug and check with physician if serum level exceeds 35 ng/mL, indicating toxicity.

Use: Drug of choice for maintenance in CHF.

Dosage

• **Tablets**

Digitalizing dose: Rapid.

Adults: 0.6 mg followed by 0.4 mg in 4–6 hr; **then,** 0.2 mg q 4–6 hr until therapeutic effect achieved.

Digitalizing dose: Slow.

Adults: 0.2 mg b.i.d. for 4 days.

Maintenance dose: PO.

Adults: 0.05–0.3 mg/day (**usual:** 0.15 mg/day).

Administration/Storage
1. Incompatible with acids and alkali.
2. Protect from light.

Special Concerns: Digitalis tablets may not be suitable for small children; thus, other digitalis products should be considered.

Additional Drug Interactions
Aminoglutethimide / ↓ Effect of digitoxin due to ↑ breakdown by liver
Barbiturates / ↓ Effect of digitoxin due to ↑ breakdown by liver
Diltiazem / May ↑ serum levels of digitoxin
Phenylbutazone / ↓ Effect of digitoxin due to ↑ breakdown by liver
Phenytoin / ↓ Effect of digitoxin due to ↑ breakdown by liver
Quinidine / May ↑ serum levels of digitoxin
Rifampin / ↓ Effect of digitoxin due to ↑ breakdown by liver
Verapamil / May ↑ serum levels of digitoxin

NURSING CONSIDERATIONS

See also *Nursing Considerations* for *Cardiac Glycosides,* Chapter 30.

Evaluate
- Control of S&S of CHF
- Serum digitoxin level within desired range (14–26 ng/mL)

Digoxin

(dih-**JOX**-in)
Pregnancy Category: A
Lanoxicaps, Lanoxin, Novo-Digoxin ✱ **(Rx)**

See also *Cardiac Glycosides,* Chapter 30.

How Supplied: *Capsule:* 0.05 mg, 0.1 mg, 0.2 mg; *Elixir:* 0.05 mg/mL; *Injection:* 0.1 mg/mL, 0.25 mg/mL; *Tablet:* 0.125 mg, 0.25 mg, 0.5 mg

Action/Kinetics: Action prompter and shorter than that of digitoxin. **Onset: PO,** 0.5–2 hr; **time to peak effect:** 2–6 hr. **Duration:** 6 days. **Onset, IV:** 5–30 min; **time to peak effect:** 1–4 hr. **Duration:** 6 days. **t½:** 35 hr. **Therapeutic serum level:** 0.5–2.0 ng/mL. Serum levels above 2.5 ng/mL indicate toxicity. Fifty percent to 70% is excreted unchanged by the kidneys. Bioavailability depends on the dosage form: tablets (60%–80%), capsules (90%–100%), and elixir (70%–85%). Thus, changing dosage forms may require dosage adjustments.

Uses: May be drug of choice for CHF because of rapid onset, relatively short duration, and ability to be administered PO or IV.

Dosage

- **Capsules**

Digitalization: Rapid.

Adults: 0.4–0.6 mg initially followed by 0.1–0.3 mg q 6–8 hr until desired effect achieved.

Digitalization: Slow.

Adults: A total of 0.05–0.35 mg/day divided in two doses for a period of 7–22 days to reach steady-state serum levels. **Pediatric.** Digitalizing dosage is divided into three or more doses with the initial dose being about one-half the total dose; doses are given q 4–8 hr. **Children, 10 years and older:** 0.008–0.012 mg/kg. **5–10 years:** 0.015–0.03 mg/kg. **2–5 years:** 0.025–0.035 mg/kg. **1 month–2 years:** 0.03–0.05 mg/kg. **Neonates, full-term:** 0.02–0.03 mg/kg. **Neonates, premature:** 0.015–0.025 mg/kg.

Maintenance.

Adults: 0.05–0.35 mg once or twice daily. **Premature neonates:** 20%–30% of total digitalizing dose divided and given in two to three daily doses. **Neonates to 10 years:** 25%–35% of the total digitalizing dose divided and given in two to three daily doses.

- **Elixir, Tablets**

Digitalization: Rapid.

Adults: A total of 0.75–1.25 mg divided into two or more doses each given at 6–8-hr intervals.

Digitalization: Slow.

Adults: 0.125–0.5 mg/day for 7 days. **Pediatric.** (Digitalizing dose is divided into two or more doses and given at 6–8-hr intervals.) **Children,**

10 years and older, rapid or slow: Same as adult dose. **5–10 years:** 0.02–0.035 mg/kg. **2–5 years:** 0.03–0.05 mg/kg. **1 month–2 years:** 0.035–0.06 mg/kg. **Premature and newborn infants to 1 month:** 0.02–0.035 mg/kg.

Maintenance.

Adults: 0.125–0.5 mg/day. **Pediatric:** One-fifth to one-third the total digitalizing dose daily. *NOTE:* An alternate regimen (referred to as the "small-dose" method) is 0.017 mg/kg/day. This dose causes less toxicity.

• **IV**

Digitalization.

Adults: Same as tablets. **Maintenance:** 0.125–0.5 mg/day in divided doses or as a single dose. **Pediatric:** Same as tablets.

Administration/Storage

1. IV injections should be given over 5 min (or longer) either undiluted or diluted fourfold or greater with sterile water for injection, 0.9% sodium chloride injection, lactated Ringer's injection, or 5% dextrose injection.
2. Lanoxicaps gelatin capsules are more bioavailable than tablets. Thus, the 0.05-mg capsule is equivalent to the 0.0625-mg tablet; the 0.1-mg capsule is equivalent to the 0.125-mg tablet, and the 0.2-mg capsule is equivalent to the 0.25-mg tablet.
3. Differences in bioavailability have been noted between products; thus, clients should be monitored when changing from one product to another.
4. Protect from light.
5. *Treatment of Overdose:* Use digoxin immune Fab (see Chapter 84).

Additional Drug Interactions

1. The following drugs increase serum digoxin levels, leading to possible toxicity: Aminoglycosides, amiodarone, anticholinergics, benzodiazepines, captopril, diltiazem, erythromycin, esmolol, flecainide, hydroxychloroquine, ibuprofen, indomethacin, nifedipine, quinidine, quinine, tetracyclines, tolbutamide, verapamil.
2. Disopyramide may alter the pharmacologic effect of digoxin.
3. Penicillamine decreases serum digoxin levels.

NURSING CONSIDERATIONS

See also *Nursing Considerations* for *Cardiac Glycosides,* Chapter 30.

Client/Family Teaching

1. Take pulse before taking medication. Provide written parameters for holding digoxin and notifying provider, i.e., HR below 45 or above 150.
2. Review S&S of digoxin toxicity: abdominal pain, N&V, visual disturbances, arrhythmias, etc., and instruct to report when evident.
3. Return as scheduled for lab and ECG studies.

Evaluate

• Control of S&S of CHF (↑ CO, ↓ HR, ↑ urine output, ↓ rales)

• Therapeutic serum digoxin level (0.5–2.0 ng/mL)

Milrinone lactate

(**MILL**-rih-nohn)

Pregnancy Category: C

Primacor **(Rx)**

How Supplied: *Injection:* 1 mg/mL

Action/Kinetics: Milrinone is a selective inhibitor of peak III cyclic AMP phosphodiesterase isozyme in cardiac and vascular muscle. This results in a direct inotropic effect and a direct arterial vasodilator activity. In addition to improving myocardial contractility, milrinone improves diastolic function as manifested by improvements in LV diastolic relaxation. In clients with depressed myocardial function, the drug produces a prompt increase in CO and a decrease in pulmonary wedge pressure and vascular resistance, without a significant increase in HR or myocardial oxygen consumption. Milrinone has an inotropic effect in clients who are fully digitalized without causing signs of glycoside toxicity. Also, LV function has improved in clients with ischemic heart disease. **Therapeutic plasma levels:** 150–250 ng/mL. **t½:** 2.3 hr following doses of 12.5–125 mcg/kg to clients with

CHF. The drug is metabolized in the liver and excreted primarily through the urine.

Use: Short-term treatment of CHF, usually in clients receiving digoxin and diuretics.

Dosage

- **IV Infusion**

Adults, loading dose: 50 mcg/kg administered slowly over 10 min. **Maintenance, minimum:** 0.59 mg/kg/24 hr (infused at a rate of 0.375 mcg/kg/min); **maintenance, standard:** 0.77 mg/kg/24 hr (infused at a rate of 0.5 mcg/kg/min; **maintenance, maximum:** 1.13 mg/kg/24 hr (infused at a rate of 0.75 mcg/kg/min).

Administration/Storage

1. IV infusions should be administered at rates described in the package insert.
2. The infusion rate should be adjusted depending on the hemodynamic and clinical response.
3. Dilutions of milrinone may be prepared using 0.45% or 0.9% sodium chloride injection or 5% dextrose injection.
4. Clients with renal impairment require a reduced infusion rate (see package insert for chart).
5. Furosemide should not be given in IV lines containing milrinone as a precipitate will form.
6. *Treatment of Overdose:* If hypotension occurs, reduce or temporarily discontinue administration of milrinone until the condition of the client stabilizes. General measures should be used for supporting circulation.

Contraindications: Hypersensitivity to the drug. Use in severe obstructive aortic or pulmonic valvular disease in lieu of surgical relief of the obstruction.

Special Concerns: Use with caution during lactation. Safety and efficacy have not been determined in children.

Side Effects: *CV:* ***Ventricular and supraventricular arrhythmias, including ventricular ectopic activity, nonsustained ventricular tachycardia, sustained ventricular tachycardia, and ventricular fibrillation. Infrequently, life-threatening arrhythmias associated with preexisting arrhythmias,*** metabolic abnormalities, abnormal digoxin levels, and catheter insertion. Also, hypotension, angina, chest pain. *Miscellaneous:* Mild to moderately severe headaches, hypokalemia, tremor, thrombocytopenia.

Symptom of Overdose: Hypotension.

NURSING CONSIDERATIONS

Assessment

1. Document indications for therapy and type and onset of symptoms.
2. Identify other medications used to manage the condition and the outcome.
3. Obtain baseline CBC, electrolytes, and liver and renal function studies.
4. Document baseline ECG, CO, and PCWP and ensure that AMI has been ruled out.

Interventions

1. Monitor and record I&O, electrolyte levels, and renal function. If diuresis is excessive, assess for hypokalemia.
2. Potassium loss due to excessive diuresis may result in arrhythmias in digitalized clients. Thus, hypokalemia must be corrected before or during milrinone use.
3. Monitor VS closely during milrinone infusion. Obtain written parameters for interruption of infusion (e.g., SBP < 80; HR < 50).
4. Observe cardiac rhythm for evidence of increased supraventricular and ventricular arrhythmias.

Evaluate

- ↑ CO and ↓ PCWP
- Resolution of S&S of CHF
- Therapeutic serum drug levels (150–250 ng/mL)

CHAPTER THIRTY-ONE

Drugs Used For Peripheral Vascular Disease

See the following individual drugs:

Isoxsuprine
Papaverine
Pentoxifylline

Isoxsuprine

(eye-**SOX**-you-preen)
Vasodilan, Vasoprine **(Rx)**

How Supplied: *Tablet:* 10 mg, 20 mg

Action/Kinetics: Direct relaxation of vascular smooth muscle in skeletal muscle, increasing peripheral blood flow. The drug has alpha-adrenergic receptor blocking activity and beta-adrenergic receptor stimulant properties. Isoxsuprine also causes cardiac stimulation and uterine relaxation. Peripheral resistance decreases while both HR and CO increase. Drug crosses placenta. In high doses it lowers blood viscosity and inhibits platelet aggregation. **Onset, PO:** 1 hr; **IV,** 10 min. **Peak serum levels:** 1 hr, persisting for approximately 3 hr. **t½:** 75 min. Mostly excreted in urine.

Uses: Symptomatic treatment of cerebrovascular insufficiency. Improves peripheral blood circulation in arteriosclerosis obliterans, Buerger's disease, and Raynaud's disease. *Investigational:* Dysmenorrhea, threatened premature labor.

Dosage

- **Tablets**

  All uses.

10–20 mg t.i.d.–q.i.d.

- **IM**

  Premature labor.

5–10 mg b.i.d.–t.i.d. (Injection not available in the U.S.).

Contraindications: Postpartum period, arterial bleeding.

Special Concerns: Use with caution parenterally in clients with hypotension and tachycardia. Safety for use during pregnancy has not been determined. Risk of drug-induced hypothermia may be increased in geriatric clients.

Side Effects: *CV:* Tachycardia, hypotension, chest pain. *GI:* Abdominal distress, N&V. *CNS:* Lightheadedness, dizziness, nervousness, weakness. *Miscellaneous:* Severe rash.

NURSING CONSIDERATIONS

Assessment

1. Document indications for therapy and type and onset of symptoms.
2. Note if client is taking a beta-blocking agent because this may diminish response to isoxsuprine.
3. List any other drugs such as diuretics or hypotensive agents that are prescribed.
4. Document circulation noting extremity color, warmth, and quality of pulses.
5. Assess mental status.

Interventions

1. When used to control premature labor, monitor the intensity, frequency, and duration of uterine contractions.
2. If used to counteract a threatened spontaneous abortion, monitor the fetal HR at regular intervals.

Client/Family Teaching

1. Review the goals of drug therapy.
2. Discuss the potential of the drug to cause hypotension, lightheadedness,

and dizziness and advise appropriate safely precautions.

3. Emphasize that drug-induced hypothermia is an added risk for geriatric clients and to dress appropriately.

4. Avoid alcohol in any form.

Evaluate

- Improvement in extremity color, warmth, and quality of pulses
- Termination of premature labor

Papaverine

(pah-**PAV**-er-een)

Pregnancy Category: C

Cerespan, Genabid, Pavabid HP Capsulet, Pavabid Plateau Caps, Pavacap, Pavacen, Pavagen, Pavarine Spancaps, Pavased, Pavatine, Paverolan Lanacaps **(Rx)**

How Supplied: *Capsule, Extended Release:* 150 mg; *Injection:* 30 mg/mL

Action/Kinetics: Direct spasmolytic effect on smooth muscle, possibly by inhibiting cyclic nucleotide phosphodiesterase, thus increasing levels of cyclic AMP. This effect is seen in the vascular system, bronchial muscle, and in the GI, biliary, and urinary tracts. Large doses produce CNS sedation and sleepiness as well as depressing AV nodal and intraventricular conduction. The drug may also directly relax cerebral vessels as it increases cerebral blood flow and decreases cerebral vascular resistance. Absorbed fairly rapidly. Localized in fat tissues and liver. Steady plasma concentration maintained when drug is given q 6 hr. **Peak plasma levels:** 1–2 hr. **t½:** 30–120 min. Sustained-release products may be poorly and erratically absorbed. Metabolized in the liver and inactive metabolites excreted in the urine.

Uses: PO. Cerebral and peripheral ischemia due to arterial spasm and myocardial ischemia complicated by arrhythmias. Smooth muscle relaxant. **Parenteral.** Various conditions in which muscle spasm is observed including AMI, angina pectoris, peripheral vascular disease (with a vasospastic element), peripheral and pulmonary embolism, certain cerebral angiospastic states; ureteral, biliary, and GI colic. *Investigational:* Alone or with phentolamine as an intracavernous injection for impotence.

NOTE: The FDA has determined that papaverine is not effective for its claimed indications.

Dosage

- **Capsules, Extended-Release**

  Vasospastic therapy.

150 mg/ q 12 hr up to 150 mg/ q 8 hr or 300 mg/ q 12 hr for severe cases.

- **Tablets**

  Vasospastic therapy.

100–300 mg 3–5 times/day.

- **IM, IV**

  Vasospastic therapy.

30–120 mg given slowly (over 1–2 min, if IV) q 3 hr.

Cardiac extrasystoles.

30–120 mg. Two doses 10 min apart either IM or IV (given slowly over 2 min). **Pediatric:** 6 mg/kg.

- **Intra-arterial**

  Vasospastic therapy.

40 mg given slowly over 1–2 min.

- **Intracavernosal**

  Impotence therapy.

30 mg (of the injectable) mixed with 0.5–1 mg phentolamine mesylate for injection.

Administration/Storage

1. IV injections must be given by the physician or under physician's immediate supervision.

2. Do not mix with Ringer's lactate solution because a precipitate will form.

3. *Treatment of Acute Poisoning:* Delay absorption by giving tap water, milk, or activated charcoal followed by gastric lavage or induction of vomiting and then a cathartic. BP should be maintained and measures taken to treat respiratory depression and coma. Hemodialysis is effective.

4. *Treatment of Chronic Poisoning:* Discontinue medication. Monitor and treat blood dyscrasias. Provide symptomatic treatment. Treat hypotension by IV fluids, elevation of

legs, and a vasopressor with inotropic effects.

Contraindications: Complete AV block; administer with extreme caution in presence of coronary insufficiency and glaucoma.

Special Concerns: Safe use during lactation or for children not established.

Laboratory Test Interferences: ↑ AST, ALT, and bilirubin.

Side Effects: *CV:* Flushing of face, hypertension, increase in HR. *GI:* Nausea, anorexia, abdominal distress, constipation or diarrhea, dry mouth and throat. *CNS:* Headache, drowsiness, sedation, vertigo. *Miscellaneous:* Sweating, malaise, pruritus, skin rashes, increase in depth of respiration, hepatitis, jaundice, eosinophilia, altered liver function tests.

NOTE: Both acute and chronic poisoning may result from use of papaverine. Symptoms are extensions of side effects.

Symptoms of Acute Poisoning: Nystagmus, diplopia, drowsiness, weakness, lassitude, incoordination, coma, cyanosis, ***respiratory depression.***

Symptoms of Chronic Poisoning: Ataxia, blurred vision, drowsiness, anxiety, headache, GI upset, depression, urticaria, erythematous macular eruptions, blood dyscrasias, hypotension.

Drug Interactions

Diazoxide IV / Additive hypotensive effect

Levodopa / Papaverine ↓ effect of levodopa by blocking dopamine receptors

NURSING CONSIDERATIONS

Assessment

1. Document indications for therapy and type and onset of symptoms.
2. Note any drugs prescribed that would interact unfavorably with papaverine.
3. Determine any evidence of cardiac dysfunction and obtain baseline ECG.
4. Document baseline mental status and assess all extremities for color, warmth, and pulses.

Interventions

1. Monitor VS closely for at least 30 min after IV injection.
2. Report any symptoms of autonomic nervous system distress such as nystagmus, diplopia, or blurred vision.
3. Assess for GI reactions such as nausea or anorexia as these may be symptoms of acute poisoning and require the immediate withdrawal of the drug and institution of emergency measures.

Client/Family Teaching

1. Take with meals or milk to minimize GI upset.
2. Do not perform activities that require mental alertness until drug effects are realized as drug may cause dizziness or drowsiness.
3. Avoid tobacco products as nicotine may cause vasospasm.

Evaluate

- ↓ Pain symptoms
- Improvement in extremity color, warmth, and pulse quality
- ↑ Levels of mental alertness

Pentoxifylline

(pen-tox-**EYE**-fih-leen)
Pregnancy Category: C
Trental **(Rx)**

How Supplied: *Tablet, Extended Release:* 400 mg

Action/Kinetics: Pentoxifylline and its active metabolites decrease the viscosity of blood. This results in increased blood flow to the microcirculation and an increase in tissue oxygen levels. Although not known with certainty, the mechanism may include (1) decreased synthesis of thromboxane A_2, thus decreasing platelet aggregation, (2) increased blood fibrinolytic activity (decreasing fibrinogen levels), and (3) decreased RBC aggregation and local hyperviscosity by increasing cellular ATP. **Peak plasma levels:** 1 hr. Significant first-pass effect. **t½:** pentoxifylline, 0.4–0.8 hr; metabolites, 1–1.6

hr. **Time to peak levels;** 2–4 hr. Excretion is via the urine.

Uses: Peripheral vascular disease including intermittent claudication. The drug is not intended to replace surgery. *Investigational:* To improve circulation in clients with cerebrovascular insufficiency, transient ischemic attacks, sickle cell thalassemia, diabetic angiopathies and neuropathies, high-altitude sickness, strokes, hearing disorders, circulation disorders of the eye, and Raynaud's phenomenon.

Dosage

- **Extended-Release Tablets**

Peripheral vascular disease.

Adults: 400 mg t.i.d. with meals. Treatment should be continued for at least 8 weeks. If side effects occur, dosage can be reduced to 400 mg b.i.d.

Administration/Storage: *Treatment of Overdose:* Gastric lavage followed by activated charcoal. Monitor BP and ECG. Support respiration, control seizures, and treat arrhythmias.

Contraindications: Intolerance to pentoxifylline, caffeine, theophylline, or theobromine.

Special Concerns: Use with caution in impaired renal function and during lactation. Safety and efficacy in children less than 18 years of age not established. Geriatric clients may be at greater risk for manifesting side effects.

Side Effects: *CV:* Angina, chest pain, hypotension, edema. *GI:* Abdominal pain, flatus/bloating, dyspepsia, salivation, bad taste in mouth, N&V, anorexia, constipation, dry mouth and thirst. *CNS:* Dizziness, headache, tremor, malaise, anxiety, confusion. *Ophthalmologic:* Blurred vision, conjunctivitis, scotomata. *Dermatologic:* Pruritus, rash, urticaria, brittle fingernails. *Respiratory:* Dyspnea, laryngitis, nasal congestion, epistaxis. *Miscellaneous:* Flu-like symptoms, leukopenia, sore throat, swollen neck glands, change in weight.

Symptoms of Overdose: Agitation, fever, flushing, hypotension, nervousness, ***seizures,*** somnolence, tremors, loss of consciousness.

Drug Interaction: Prothrombin times should be monitored carefully if the client is on warfarin therapy.

NURSING CONSIDERATIONS

Assessment

1. Note any client history of sensitivity to caffeine, theophylline, or theobromine.
2. If client is female, sexually active, and of childbearing age, determine if pregnant.
3. Obtain baseline CBC and renal function studies and monitor during therapy.

Client/Family Teaching

1. Take the medication with meals to minimize GI upset.
2. Provide written instructions concerning adverse side effects, such as angina and palpitations, that should be reported if evident.
3. Discuss the need to continue the treatment for at least 8 weeks, even though effectiveness may not yet be apparent.
4. Do not perform activities that require mental alertness until drug effects are realized as dizziness and blurred vision may occur.
5. Avoid nicotine-containing products as nicotine constricts blood vessels.
6. Explain the importance of follow-up visits and reporting for lab studies to evaluate the effectiveness of the drug.

Evaluate: Reports of ↓ pain and cramping in lower extremities during activity.

Hematologic Drugs

CHAPTER THIRTY-TWO

Antianemic Drugs

See also the following individual entries:

Ferrous Fumarate
Ferrous Gluconate
Ferrous Sulfate
Ferrous Sulfate, Dried

General Statement: Anemia refers to the many clinical conditions in which there is a deficiency in the number of RBCs or in the hemoglobin level within those cells. Hemoglobin is a complex substance consisting of a large protein (globin) and an iron-containing chemical referred to as heme. The hemoglobin is contained inside the RBCs. Its function is to combine with oxygen in the lungs and transport it to all tissues of the body, where it is exchanged for carbon dioxide (which is transported back to the lungs where it can be excreted). A lack of either RBCs or hemoglobin may result in an inadequate supply of oxygen to various tissues.

The average life span of a RBC is 120 days; thus, new ones have to be constantly formed. They are produced in the bone marrow, with both vitamin B_{12} and folic acid playing an important role in their formation. In addition, a sufficient amount of iron is necessary for the formation and maturation of RBCs. This iron is supplied in a normal diet and is also salvaged from old RBCs. There are many types of anemia. However, the two main categories are (1) iron-deficiency anemias, resulting from greater than normal loss or destruction of blood cells, and (2) megaloblastic anemias, resulting from deficient production of blood cells. Iron-deficiency anemia can result from hemorrhage or blood loss; the bone marrow is unable to replace the quantity of RBCs lost even when working at maximum capacity (due to iron-deficient diet or failure to absorb iron from the GI tract). The RBCs in iron-deficiency anemias (also called *microcytic* or *hypochromic anemias*) contain too little hemoglobin. When examined under the microscope, they are paler and sometimes smaller than normal. The cause of the iron deficiency must be determined before therapy is started.

Therapy consists of administering compounds containing iron so as to increase the body's supplies.

Megaloblastic anemias may result from insufficient supplies of the necessary vitamins and minerals needed by the bone marrow to manufacture blood cells. Pernicious anemia, for example, results from inadequate vitamin B_{12}. The RBCs characteristic of the megaloblastic anemias are enlarged and particularly rich in hemoglobin. However, the blood contains fewer mature RBCs than normal and usually contains a relatively higher number of immature RBCs (megaloblasts), which have been prematurely released from the bone marrow.

Iron Preparations: These agents are usually a complex of iron and another substance and are normally taken by mouth. The amount absorbed from the GI tract depends on the dose administered; therefore the largest dose that can be tolerated without causing side effects is given. Under certain conditions, iron compounds must be given parenterally, particularly (1) when there is some disorder limiting the amount of drug absorbed from the intestine or (2) when the client is unable to tolerate oral iron.

Iron preparations are effective only in the treatment of anemias specifically resulting from iron deficiency. Blood loss is almost always the only cause of iron deficiency in adult males and postmenopausal females. The daily iron requirement is increased by growth and pregnancy, and iron deficiency is, therefore, particularly common in infants and young children on diets low in iron. Pregnant women and women with heavy menstrual blood loss may also be deficient in iron.

Iron is available for therapy in two forms: bivalent and trivalent. Bivalent (ferrous) iron salts are administered more often than trivalent (ferric) salts because they are less astringent and less irritating than ferric salts and are better absorbed.

Iron preparations are particularly suitable for the treatment of anemias in infants and children, in blood donors, during pregnancy, and in clients with chronic blood loss. Optimum therapeutic responses are usually noted within 2–4 weeks of treatment.

The RDA for iron is 90–300 mg/day.

Action/Kinetics: Iron is an essential mineral normally supplied in the diet. Iron salts and other preparations supply additional iron to meet the needs of the client. Iron is absorbed from the GI tract through the mucosal cells where it combines with the protein transferrin. This complex is transported in the body to bone marrow where iron is incorporated into hemoglobin. Absorption kinetics depend on the iron salt ingested and on the degree of deficiency. Under normal circumstances, iron is well conserved by the body although small amounts are lost through shedding of skin, hair, and nails and in feces, perspiration, urine, breast milk, and during menstruation. Iron is highly bound to protein.

Uses: Prophylaxis and treatment of iron-deficiency anemia. *Investigational:* Clients receiving epoetin therapy (failure to give iron supplements either IV or PO can impair the hematologic response to epoetin).

Contraindications: Clients with hemosiderosis, hemochromatosis, peptic ulcer, regional enteritis, and ulcerative colitis. Hemolytic anemia, pyridoxine-responsive anemia, and cirrhosis of the liver.

Special Concerns: Allergic reactions may result due to certain products containing tartrazine and some products containing sulfites.

Side Effects: *GI:* Constipation, gastric irritation, nausea, abdominal cramps, anorexia, vomiting, and diarrhea. These effects may be minimized by administering preparations as a coated tablet. Soluble iron preparations may stain the teeth.

Symptoms of Overdose: Symptoms occur in four stages—(1) Lethargy, N&V, abdominal pain, weak and rapid pulse, tarry stools, dehydration, acidosis, hypotension, and ***coma*** within 1–6 hr. (2) If client survives, symptoms subside for about 24 hr. (3) Within 24–48 hr symptoms return with ***diffuse vascular congestion, shock, pulmonary edema, acido-***

sis, seizures, anuria, hyperthermia, and death. (4) If client survives, pyloric or antral stenosis, hepatic cirrhosis, and CNS damage are seen within 2–6 weeks. Toxic reactions are more likely to occur after parenteral administration.

Drug Interactions

Allopurinol / May ↑ hepatic iron levels
Antacids, oral / ↓ Effect of iron preparations due to ↓ absorption from GI tract
Chloramphenicol / Chloramphenicol ↑ serum iron levels
Cholestyramine / ↓ Effect of iron preparations due to ↓ absorption from GI tract
Cimetidine / ↓ Effect of iron preparations due to ↓ absorption from GI tract
Pancreatic extracts / ↓ Effect of iron preparations due to ↓ absorption from GI tract
Penicillamine / ↓ Effect of penicillamine due to ↓ absorption from GI tract
Fluoroquinolones / ↓ Effect of fluoroquinolones due to ↓ absorption from GI tract due to formation of a ferric ion-quinolone complex
Levodopa / ↓ GI absorption and ↓ effect of levodopa due to formation of chelates with iron salts
Methyldopa / ↓ Effect of methyldopa due to ↓ absorption from GI tract
Tetracyclines / ↓ Effect of tetracyclines due to ↓ absorption from GI tract; also, ↓ absorption of iron salts
Vitamin E / Vitamin E ↓ response to iron therapy

Laboratory Test Interference: Iron-containing drugs may affect electrolyte balance determinations.

Dosage

See individual drugs. Most replacement iron is given PO in daily doses of 90–300 mg elemental iron. Duration of therapy: 2–4 months longer than the time needed to reverse anemia, usually 6 or more months.

NURSING CONSIDERATIONS

Administration/Storage

1. For infants and young children, administer liquid preparation with a dropper. Deposit liquid well back against the cheek.
2. Eggs and milk inhibit absorption of iron. Also, coffee and tea consumed with a meal or 1 hr after may significantly inhibit absorption of dietary iron.
3. Ingestion of calcium and iron supplements with food can decrease iron absorption by one-third; iron absorption is not decreased if calcium carbonate is used and it is taken between meals.
4. Sustained-release products should not be crushed or chewed.
5. *Treatment of Iron Toxicity:*
• General supportive measures.
• Maintain a patent airway, respiration, and circulation.
• Induce vomiting with syrup of ipecac followed by gastric lavage using tepid water or 1%–5% sodium bicarbonate (to convert from ferrous sulfate to ferrous carbonate, which is poorly absorbed and less irritating). Saline cathartics can also be used.
• Deferoxamine is indicated for clients with serum iron levels greater than 300 mg/dL. Deferoxamine is usually given IM, but in severe cases of poisoning it may be given IV. Hydration should be maintained.
• It may be necessary to treat for shock, acidosis, renal failure, and seizures.

Assessment

1. Prior to administering medication, assess client and take a complete drug history, including:
• Client use of antacids and any other drugs that may interact with these preparations
• Any OTC drugs, such as iron compounds or vitamin E, which are being used
• Allergy to sulfites or tartrazines, as these may be present in some products.
2. Ask client about any evidence of GI

bleeding such as tarry stools or bright red blood in stool or vomitus.
3. Note any complaints of fatigue, pallor, poor skin turgor, or change in mental status, especially among the elderly.
4. Assess nutritional status and diet history through questioning as well as observation of intake if possible.
5. Pregnancy has generally been considered an indication for prescribing iron prophylactically.
6. Review pregnancies and menstruation history and note frequency of, amounts of, and any heavy or abnormal bleeding.
7. Obtain baseline CBC, stool for occult blood, iron, and total iron binding capacity results. Note if iron-deficient or megaloblastic anemia.

Interventions

1. Establish goals of therapy with client and other members of the health care team.
2. Check for occult blood if GI bleeding is suspected, as drugs may alter stool color.
3. Encourage persons with symptoms of anemia to seek medical assistance; discourage self-medication with iron based on symptoms only.
4. Coated tablets may be prescribed to diminish effects on the GI tract such as nausea, constipation or diarrhea, gastric irritation, and abdominal cramps.
5. Be prepared to assist with treatment of clients who may develop symptoms of iron intoxication (most likely to occur after parenteral administration; see symptoms of iron toxicity). If a client has symptoms of iron poisoning:
• Stop parenteral iron administration.
• Notify physician.
• Monitor VS for 48 hr since a second crisis is likely to occur within 12–48 hr of the first one.
• Follow guidelines for *Treatment of Iron Toxicity*.
6. Anticipate that the medication will be discontinued if 500 mg of iron daily does not cause a rise of at least 2 mg/100 mL of hemoglobin in 3 weeks.
7. Iron will reduce the absorption of tetracycline. If a client is to receive tetracyclines as well as iron products, establish a schedule that allows at least 2 hr to elapse between administering the iron product and the tetracycline.

Client/Family Teaching

1. Many clients will be taking their medications at home and without constant supervision. Therefore, it is important to teach them to adhere to the prescribed regimen and to report any problems with medication therapy immediately.
2. Review the form of iron prescribed (bi- or trivalent) and carefully explain the frequency of administration.
3. Take iron preparations with meals to reduce gastric irritation. Identify foods (milk, eggs) that inhibit the absorption of iron and unless taking ferrous lactate, advise the client *NOT* to take iron compounds with milk products or antacids. Also, coffee and tea consumed within 1 hr of meals may inhibit the absorption of dietary iron.
4. Taking iron preparations with citrus juices enhances the absorption of iron.
5. Discuss the possibility of indigestion, change in stool color (black and tarry or dark green), and constipation.
6. Advise to increase the intake of fruit, fiber, and fluids to minimize drug's constipating effects.
7. Explain the possible side effects that may occur (gastric irritation, constipation or diarrhea, abdominal cramps) and encourage reporting because they may be relieved by changing the medication, dosage, or time of administration.
8. Encourage clients to eat a well-balanced diet, stressing the intake of foods high in iron (i.e., meat proteins). When working with poor families, explore the kinds of foods they can afford to ensure that the

diet prescribed is one they have access to (e.g., raisins, green vegetables, and liver may be more affordable than apricots or prunes).

9. Iron preparations are extremely dangerous for children. An overdosage can be fatal so keep iron preparations out of the reach of children.

10. When administering liquid iron medications to young children, dilute well with water or fruit juice and use a straw to minimize the possibility of staining the teeth.

11. When working with pregnant women, review their need for an iron-rich diet. Also, The American Academy of Pediatrics recommends an iron supplement for infants during their first year of life.

12. Follow administration guidelines for each product to minimize side effects. Advise against self-medicating with vitamins and mineral supplements and review the potential risks associated with chronic iron ingestion.

Evaluate

- Laboratory confirmation of resolution of anemia (hemoglobin within desired range). Generally, if hemoglobin has not increased 1 g/100 mL in 2 weeks then the diagnosis of iron deficiency anemia should be reconfirmed.
- Reports of improvement in exercise tolerance and level of fatigue
- Resolution of S&S of anemia (skin pallor, color of nail beds, hemoglobin and iron levels, changes in stool color, etc.)
- Successful treatment and prevention of iron deficiency anemia

Ferrous fumarate

(**FAIR**-us **FYOU**-mar-ayt)

Femiron, Feostat, Feostat Drops and Suspension, Fumasorb, Fumerin, Hemocyte, Ircon, Nephro-Fer, Palafer ✦, Palafer Pediatric Drops ✦, Span-FF **(OTC)**

See also *Antianemic Drugs,* Chapter 32.

How Supplied: *Chew Tablet:* 100 mg; *Liquid:* 45 mg/0.6 mL; *Suspension:* 100 mg/5 mL; *Tablet:* 63 mg, 200 mg, 325 mg, 350 mg

Action/Kinetics: Better tolerated than ferrous gluconate or ferrous sulfate. Contains 33% elemental iron.

Dosage

- **Extended-Release Capsules**

Prophylaxis.

Adults: 325 mg/day.

Anemia.

Adults: 325 mg b.i.d. Capsules are not recommended for use in children.

- **Oral Solution, Oral Suspension, Tablets, Chewable Tablets**

Prophylaxis.

Adults: 200 mg/day. **Pediatric:** 3 mg/kg/day.

Anemia.

Adults: 200 mg t.i.d.–q.i.d. **Pediatric:** 3 mg/kg t.i.d., up to 6 mg/kg/day, if needed.

NURSING CONSIDERATIONS

See *Nursing Considerations* for *Antianemic Drugs,* Chapter 32.

Evaluate: Restoration of serum iron stores.

Ferrous gluconate

(**FAIR**-us **GLUE**-kon-ayt)

Apo-Ferrous Gluconate ✦, Fergon, Ferralet, Ferralet Slow Release, Simron **(OTC)**

See also *Antianemic Drugs,* Chapter 32.

How Supplied: *Capsule, Extended Release:* 320 mg; *Elixir:* 300 mg/5 mL; *Enteric Coated Tablet:* 325 mg; *Tablet:* 300 mg, 320 mg, 324 mg, 325 mg; *Tablet, Extended Release:* 320 mg

Use: Particularly indicated for clients who cannot tolerate ferrous sulfate because of gastric irritation. Preparation contains 11.6% elemental iron.

Dosage

- **Capsules, Tablets**

Prophylaxis.

Adults: 325 mg/day. **Pediatric, 2 years and older:** 8 mg/kg/day.

Anemia.

Adults: 325 mg q.i.d. Can be increased to 650 mg q.i.d. if needed and tolerated. **Pediatric, 2 years and older:** 16 mg/kg t.i.d.

• **Elixir, Syrup**

Prophylaxis.

Adults: 300 mg/day. **Pediatric, 2 years and older:** 8 mg/kg/day.

Anemia.

Adults: 300 mg q.i.d. Can be increased to 600 mg q.i.d. as needed and tolerated. **Pediatric, 2 years and older:** 16 mg/kg t.i.d. The physician must determine dosage for children less than 2 years of age.

NURSING CONSIDERATIONS

See *Nursing Considerations* for *Antianemic Drugs,* Chapter 32.

Evaluate

- Restoration of serum iron stores
- H&H within desired range

Ferrous sulfate

(**FAIR**-us **SUL**-fayt)

Apo-Ferrous Sulfate ✱, Feosol, Fer-In-Sol, Fer-Iron, Fero-Gradumet, Ferospace, Feratab, Mol-Iron, PMS Ferrous Sulfate ✱ **(OTC)**

Ferrous sulfate, dried

(**FAIR**-us **SUL**-fayt)

Feosol, Fer-in-Sol, Ferralyn Lanacaps, Ferra-TD, Slow-Fe **(OTC)**

See also *Antianemic Drugs,* Chapter 32.

How Supplied: Ferrous sulfate: *Capsule:* 250 mg, 324 mg; *Capsule, Extended Release:* 250 mg; *Elixir:* 220 mg/5 mL; *Enteric Coated Tablet:* 325 mg; *Liquid:* 25 mg/mL, 75 mg/0.6 mL, 300 mg/5 mL; *Solution:* 300 mg/5 mL; *Syrup:* 90 mg/5 mL; *Tablet:* 195 mg, 300 mg, 324 mg, 325 mg; *Tablet, Extended Release:* 250 mg, 525 mg

Ferrous sulfate, dried: *Capsule:* 159 mg; *Capsule, Extended Release:* 150 mg, 159 mg, 190 mg; *Enteric Coated Tablet:* 200 mg; *Tablet:* 200 mg; *Tablet, Extended Release:* 152 mg, 159 mg, 160 mg

Action/Kinetics: Least expensive, most effective iron salt for PO therapy. Ferrous sulfate products contain 20% elemental iron, whereas ferrous sulfate dried products contain 30% elemental iron. The exsiccated form is more stable in air.

Dosage

Ferrous Sulfate.

• **Extended-Release Capsules**

Adults: 150–250 mg 1–2 times/day. This dosage form is not recommended for children.

• **Elixir, Oral Solution, Tablets, Enteric-coated Tablets**

Prophylaxis.

Adults: 300 mg/day. **Pediatric:** 5 mg/kg/day.

Anemia.

Adults: 300 mg b.i.d. increased to 300 mg q.i.d. as needed and tolerated. **Pediatric:** 10 mg/kg t.i.d. The enteric-coated tablets are not recommended for use in children.

• **Extended-Release Tablets**

Adults: 525 mg 1–2 times/day. This dosage form is not recommended for use in children.

Ferrous Sulfate, Dried.

• **Capsules**

Prophylaxis.

Adults: 300 mg/day. **Pediatric:** 5 mg/kg/day.

Anemia.

Adults: 300 mg b.i.d. up to 300 mg q.i.d. as needed and tolerated. **Pediatric:** 10 mg/kg t.i.d.

• **Tablets**

Prophylaxis.

Adults: 200 mg/day. **Pediatric:** 5 mg/kg/day.

Anemia.

Adults: 200 mg t.i.d. up to 200 mg q.i.d. as needed and tolerated. **Pediatric:** 10 mg/kg t.i.d.

• **Extended-Release Tablets**

Adults: 160 mg 1–2 times/day. This dosage form is not recommended for use in children.

NURSING CONSIDERATIONS

See *Nursing Considerations* for *Antianemic Drugs,* Chapter 32.

Evaluate

- Restoration of serum iron levels
- Resolution of S&S of anemia

CHAPTER THIRTY-THREE

Anticoagulants

See also the following individual entries:

Antithrombin III (Human)
Enoxaparin Injection
Heparin Sodium Injection
Heparin Sodium and Sodium Chloride
Heparin Sodium Lock Flush Solution
Warfarin Sodium

General Statement: Blood coagulation is a precise mechanism that results in the formation of a stable fibrin clot. The process is dependent upon a number of reactions involving interaction of clotting factors, platelets, and tissue materials. Both intrinsic and extrinsic pathways lead to formation of a fibrin clot and both pathways are necessary for hemostasis. For the intrinsic pathway, all protein factors required for coagulation are present in circulating blood; the process is initiated by activation of factor XII and clot formation may take several minutes. Coagulation is activated for the extrinsic pathway by release of tissue thromboplastin; clotting occurs rapidly (seconds) because factor III (thromboplastin, tissue factor) bypasses early reactions in the coagulation pathway. The coagulation pathway may be summarized as follows:

1. Thromboplastin and other blood clotting factors help convert the protein prothrombin to thrombin.
2. Thrombin mediates the formation of soluble fibrinogen to soluble fibrin.
3. Soluble fibrin is converted to insoluble fibrin by activated fibrin-stabilizing factor. The insoluble fibrin forms a clot, trapping blood cells and platelets.

Once formed, the blood clot is dissolved by another enzymatic chain reaction involving a substance called fibrinolysin. Blood coagulation can be affected by a number of diseases. An excessive tendency to form blood clots is one of the main factors involved in CV disorders, and a defect in the clotting mechanism is the cause of hemophilia and related diseases. Since several of the factors that participate in blood clotting are manufactured by the liver, severe liver disease can also affect blood clotting, as does vitamin K deficiency. Drugs that influence blood coagulation can be divided into three classes: (1) *anticoagulants,* or drugs that prevent or slow blood coagulation; (2) *thrombolytic agents,* which increase the rate at which an existing blood clot dissolves; and (3) *hemostatics,* which prevent or stop internal bleeding. The dosage of all agents discussed must be carefully adjusted since overdosage can have serious consequences. The three major types of anticoagulants are: (1) warfarin, (2) anisindione (indanedione-type), and (3) heparin. The following considerations are pertinent to each type. Anticoagulant drugs are used mainly in the management of clients with thromboembolic disease; they do not dissolve previously formed clots, but they do forestall their enlargement and prevent new clots from forming.

Uses: Venous thrombosis, pulmonary embolism, acute coronary occlusions with MIs, and strokes caused by emboli or cerebral thrombi. Prophylactically for rheumatic heart disease, atrial fibrillation, traumatic injuries of blood vessels, vascular surgery, major abdominal, thoracic, and pelvic surgery, prevention of strokes in clients with transient attacks of cerebral ischemia, or other signs of impending stroke.

Heparin is often used concurrently during the therapeutic initiation period. *Investigational (Coumarin anticoagulants):* Reduce risk of postconversion emboli; prophylaxis of recurrent, cerebral thromboembolism; prophylaxis of myocardial reinfarction; treatment of transient ischemic attacks; reduce the risk of thromboembolic complications in clients with certain types of prosthetic heart valves; reduced risk of thrombosis and/or occlusion following coronary bypass surgery.

Contraindications: Hemorrhagic tendencies (including hemophilia), clients with frail or weakened blood vessels, blood dyscrasias, ulcerative lesions of the GI tract (including peptic ulcer), diverticulitis, colitis, SBE, threatened abortion, recent operations on the eye, brain, or spinal cord, regional anesthesia and lumbar block, vitamin K deficiency, leukemia with bleeding tendencies, thrombocytopenic purpura, open wounds or ulcerations, acute nephritis, impaired hepatic or renal function, or severe hypertension. Hepatic and renal dysfunction. In the presence of drainage tubes in any orifice. Alcoholism.

Special Concerns: The drugs should be used with caution in menstruating women, in pregnant women (because they may cause hypoprothrombinemia in the infant), during lactation, during the postpartum period, and following cerebrovascular accidents. Geriatric clients may be more susceptible to the effects of anticoagulants.

Side Effects: See individual drugs.

Dosage

See individual drugs.

NURSING CONSIDERATIONS

See also *Nursing Considerations* for individual agents.

Assessment

1. Obtain a thorough nursing history and complete drug profile prior to initiating therapy. Assess drugs currently prescribed to ensure none interact unfavorably.
2. Through the health history profile identify client complaints that may indicate defects in the clotting mechanism.
3. Observe for any evidence of weakened blood vessel walls (capillary fragility).
4. Review past health problems (peptic ulcer, evidence of chronic ulcerations of the GI tract, renal or liver dysfunction, infections of the endocardium, hypertension) as evidence for contraindications to this therapy.
5. Note any evidence of alcoholism as anticoagulants are contraindicated. This is particularly important when working with clients who are homeless. Also, such evidence suggests the client may have problems with drug compliance.
6. Determine that appropriate lab studies [especially PT, International Normalized Ratio (INR), PTT] have been conducted to serve as a baseline against which to measure response to treatment.
7. Note if the client is a woman in the childbearing years and sexually active. Include in the history if the woman is postpartum or if nursing a baby. In these instances, anticoagulant therapy must be used with caution.

Interventions

1. Post and advise all personnel caring for the client that client is receiving anticoagulant therapy.
2. Assist the health team in evaluating the client's ability to take medication without supervision.
3. Monitor PT or INR and PTT levels closely; anticipate dose adjustment of the anticoagulant if the client is also receiving one of the many drugs known to interact or compete with anticoagulants.
4. Question client for any evidence of bleeding (bleeding gums, hematuria, tarry stools, hematemesis, ecchymosis,

and/or petechiae) during initial therapy and also during therapy with any medication that increases the anticoagulant effect. If clients have discolored urine, determine cause, i.e., if discoloration is from drug therapy or if it is hematuria.

5. Report the sudden appearance of lumbar pain in clients receiving anticoagulant therapy, since this symptom may indicate retroperitoneal hemorrhage.

6. Report symptoms of GI dysfunction in clients on anticoagulant therapy since these symptoms may indicate intestinal hemorrhage. Anticipate that a client who has a history of ulcers or who has recently undergone surgery should have frequent tests for blood in the urine and feces, as well as measurements of hemoglobin and hematocrit to assess for abnormal bleeding.

7. Have large doses of phytonadione (vitamin K_1, fresh frozen plasma, or Factor IX concentrate for warfarin overdoses and protamine sulfate for heparin overdose (generally for every 100 U of heparin remaining in client administer 1 mg IV) available for parenteral emergency use.

8. Apply pressure to all venipuncture and injection sites to prevent bleeding and hematoma formation.

9. Request written parameters and report any abnormal lab findings especially before administering the next prescribed dose of anticoagulant.

Client/Family Teaching

1. Establish a routine that allows the medication to be taken at the same time every day or as otherwise prescribed and advise client to maintain a written record to discourage any confusion as to whether the medication had in fact been taken.

2. Discuss the possibility of bleeding and symptoms of impending hemorrhage. Report immediately if dizziness, headaches, bleeding gums or wounds, or vomiting of coffee ground material are evident. This is particularly important with elderly clients.

3. Bleeding or the presence of black and blue areas on the skin, heavy menstrual flow, or blood in the urine, is an indication that the medication should be held and the provider notified.

4. Indanedione-type anticoagulants turn alkaline urine a red-orange color. Discoloration that results from the drug can be differentiated from hematuria by acidifying urine and reevaluating its color or testing it for occult blood.

5. Other medications and changes in diet or physical state may affect the action of anticoagulants. Illness should be reported promptly.

6. Avoid contact sports and any unsafe situations or activities that may result in injury, falls, bumps, or cuts.

7. To prevent cuts, clients should use an electric razor for shaving instead of a razor blade.

8. To reduce the potential of bleeding gums, use a soft bristle toothbrush and brush gently. Remind dentist of drug therapy prior to any procedures.

9. When the client has severe problems with sight, teach family members that it is important that furniture not be moved from usual places. This creates confusion for someone without full vision and can cause accidents resulting in bleeding and/or bruising. Advise client to wear shoes and to use a night light to prevent falls and bumps in the dark.

10. Review the dietary sources of vitamin K (asparagus, spinach, broccoli, brussels sprouts, cabbage, collards, turnips, mustard greens, milk, yogurt, and cheese) that should be consumed in limited quantities because these foods will alter PT.

11. Check with provider and pharmacist prior to taking any nonprescription drugs that have anticoagulant-type effects such as aspirin, ibuprofen compounds, vitamin preparations with high levels of vitamin K, mineral preparations from health food stores, or alcohol.

12. The client should be instructed to always wear a Medic Alert bracelet and carry identification noting pre-

scribed drug therapy, and the name and number of the person providing care so that appropriate persons may be contacted if excessive bleeding occurs or if emergency surgery is required.
13. Determine social and economic situations that may alter compliance with prescribed drug therapy and assist to identify resources to help the client and family.
14. Clients and families need to be aware of the necessity of remaining under medical supervision for periodic blood tests and adjustment of drug dosages. If necessary, ask a reliable relative or friend to report any adverse effects and to make sure that the client takes the medication and comes in for scheduled lab tests.
15. Stress the importance of follow-up visits and lab studies to evaluate the effectiveness of drug therapy and to ensure proper dosage.

Evaluate

- With warfarin therapy, PT ratios of usually 1.5–2 times the control, or an INR range of 2.0–3.0 (for standard anticoagulant therapy)
- With heparin therapy, PTT within desired range, usually 2–2.5 times the control/normal
- Prevention of thrombus formation
- Freedom from complications of drug therapy and abnormal bleeding

Special Concerns

1. Elderly people are more prone to developing bleeding complications than are other groups. Therefore, special attention must be given to this problem.
2. Unusual hair loss and itching are common problems with the elderly during drug therapy and should be reported immediately.
3. Since many elderly people use many different pharmacies to fill prescriptions, make sure that they have a printed form with the name and dosage of all drugs they are currently taking.

Antithrombin III (Human)

(an-tee-**THROM**-bin)
Pregnancy Category: C
ATnativ **(Rx)**

How Supplied: *Powder for injection*

Action/Kinetics: Antithrombin III (human) is derived from pooled human plasma obtained from healthy donors. It is identical with heparin cofactor I, which is a component of plasma necessary for heparin to exert its anticoagulant effect. Plasma used for antithrombin III (human) has been found to be nonreactive for hepatitis B surface antigen and negative for antibody to HIV. The drug also undergoes heat treatment for 10 hr to prevent transmittal of viral infections. One unit is the amount of antithrombin III (AT-III) in 1 mL of normal pooled human plasma. Antithrombin III inactivates all coagulation enzymes except factor VIIa and factor XIII.

Uses: Hereditary AT-III deficiency in pregnant clients, in clients requiring surgery, and in individuals with thromboembolism.

Dosage

- **IV**

The dose must be individualized depending on the status of the client. Assuming a plasma volume of 40 mL/kg, an initial loading dose may be calculated as follows:

Dosage units = [desired AT-III level (%) – baseline AT-III level (%)] × body weight (kg)/1% (IU/kg)

Administration of 1 IU/kg raises the level of AT-III by 1%–2.1%. The drug may be infused slowly over 5–10 min at a rate of 50 IU (1 mL)/min, not to exceed 100 IU (2 mL)/min.

Administration/Storage

1. To reconstitute, the powder should be dissolved by gently swirling in 10 mL sterile water for injection, 0.9% sodium chloride injection, or 5% dextrose injection. The product should not be shaken.

2. After reconstitution, the drug should be brought to room temperature and administered within 3 hr.
3. After the initial dose (which may increase AT-III levels to 120% of normal), the dose should be adjusted to maintain AT-III levels greater than 80% of normal.
4. AT-III levels should be measured at least b.i.d. initially and until the client is stabilized and then once daily, immediately before the next infusion.
5. Anticipate a loading dose followed by once daily dosing, based on frequent plasma AT-III levels. Dosing recommendations are only guidelines; the exact loading and maintenance doses must be individualized depending on the status of the client, response to therapy, and actual plasma AT-III levels achieved.

Special Concerns: Safety and effectiveness have not been determined in children. Even though special precautions are taken, individuals may develop S&S of viral infections, including non-A, non-B hepatitis.

Side Effects: No side effects have been reported to date.

Drug Interactions: The anticoagulant effect of heparin is increased when used concomitantly with AT-III; the dose of heparin should be decreased during AT-III therapy.

NURSING CONSIDERATIONS

Assessment

1. Perform a complete nursing history on clients with hereditary AT-III deficiency, noting any positive family history of venous thrombosis.
2. Determine that AT-III levels have been obtained prior to drug therapy and before each subsequent infusion.
3. Document pretreatment weight.

Interventions

1. Observe for elevated BP and dyspnea during IV administration; slow infusion rate and report if evident.
2. Monitor VS closely (q 5–15 min) during infusion.
3. Note early S&S of acute thrombosis. Perform routine vascular checks and monitor AT-III levels.
4. Observe for any evidence of bleeding. Anticipate a reduced dose of heparin when administered concomitantly with AT-III.
5. Anticipate that when AT-III is given for clients with heredity deficiency to control an acute thrombosis or to prevent thrombosis due to surgery or in obstetrics, that levels should be maintained for 2–8 days, depending on the status of the client.

Client/Family Teaching

1. Explain the high risk of thrombosis during pregnancy and surgery in clients with hereditary deficiencies because their AT-III levels are generally 50% of the level of normal.
2. Stress that the disease is inherited and refer for appropriate medical follow-up, counseling, and family planning.
3. Discuss the associated risks of drug therapy because product is derived from pooled human plasma.

Evaluate

- Serum AT-III levels > 80% of normal during therapy for high-risk procedures
- Prevention of thrombus formation

Enoxaparin injection

(ee-**nox**-ah-**PAIR**-in)
Pregnancy Category: B
Lovenox **(Rx)**

How Supplied: *Injection:* 30 mg/0.3 mL

Action/Kinetics: Enoxaparin is a low molecular weight heparin with antithrombotic properties. The drug is characterized by a higher ratio of anti–Factor Xa to anti–Factor IIa activity than unfractionated heparin. **t½, elimination:** 4.5 hr after SC use. **Duration:** 12 hr following a 40-mg dose. The drug is excreted mainly through the urine.

Use: Prophylaxis of deep vein thrombosis, which may lead to pulmonary embolism, after hip replacement surgery.

Dosage

- **SC**

Clients undergoing hip replacement.

Adults: 30 mg b.i.d. with the initial dose given not more than 24 hr after surgery for 7–10 days (usually).

Administration/Storage
1. Treatment should be continued throughout the postsurgical period until the risk of deep vein thrombosis has decreased.
2. Enoxaparin injection should not be mixed with other injections or infusions.
3. Discard any unused solution.
4. Do *not* interchange (unit for unit) with unfractionated heparin or other low molecular weight heparins.
5. *Treatment of Overdose:* Slow IV injection of protamine sulfate (1% solution). One mg protamine sulfate should be given to neutralize 1 mg enoxaparin injection. A second infusion of 0.5 mg protamine sulfate may be given if the APTT measured 2–4 hr after the first infusion remains prolonged. However, even with higher doses of protamine sulfate, the APTT may remain more prolonged than under normal conditions. Care should be taken to avoid overdosage with protamine sulfate.

Contraindications: In clients with active major bleeding; clients with thrombocytopenia associated with a positive in vitro test for antiplatelet antibody in the presence of enoxaparin; or in those with hypersensitivity to enoxaparin, heparin, or pork products. IM use. Interchangeable (unit for unit) use with unfractionated heparin or other low molecular weight heparins.

Special Concerns: Use with caution during lactation. Use with extreme caution in clients with a history of heparin-induced thrombocytopenia and in conditions with increased risk of hemorrhage (e.g., bacterial endocarditis, congenital or acquired bleeding disorders, active ulcer and angiodysplastic GI disease, hemorrhagic stroke, or shortly after brain, spinal, or ophthalmic surgery). Use with caution in clients with a bleeding diathesis, uncontrolled arterial hypertension, or a history of recent GI ulceration and hemorrhage. Elderly clients and those with renal insufficiency may have delayed elimination of the drug. Safety and efficacy have not been determined in children.

Laboratory Test Interferences: ↑ AST, ALT.

Side Effects: *Hematologic:* Thrombocytopenia, ***hemorrhage,*** hypochromic anemia, ecchymosis. *At site of injection:* Mild local irritation, pain, hematoma, erythema. *GI:* Nausea. *CNS:* Confusion. *Miscellaneous:* Fever, pain, edema, peripheral edema.

Symptoms of Overdose: ***Hemorrhagic complications.***

Drug Interactions: Enoxaparin should be used with caution in clients receiving oral anticoagulants and/or platelet inhibitors.

NURSING CONSIDERATIONS

See also *Nursing Considerations* for *Anticoagulants,* Chapter 33.

Assessment
1. Obtain a thorough nursing history, noting any disorders that may preclude therapy with enoxaparin.
2. Note any history of heparin or pork product sensitivity as drug is contraindicated.
3. Determine that pretreatment screening has been performed to rule out any bleeding disorders.
4. Document baseline hematologic parameters, liver function, and coagulation studies; monitor throughout therapy.
5. Review drug profile to determine any concurrently prescribed anticoagulants and/or platelet inhibitors.

Interventions
1. Monitor VS closely and report any sudden drop in BP.
2. Observe carefully for early S&S of abnormal bleeding; test stools regularly for occult blood; monitor CBC and platelets. An unexplained fall in hematocrit or BP should lead to a search for a bleeding site.
3. Anticipate that enoxaparin may cause significant, nonsymptomatic increases in SGOT and SGPT.
4. Report and discontinue enoxaparin therapy with any clinical evidence of a thromboembolic event.
5. Monitor clients with renal dys-

function and the elderly closely during therapy.

Client/Family Teaching

1. Instruct client in the proper technique for self- administration if prescribed:
• Use prefilled syringes.
• Alternate sites between the left and right anterolateral and left and right posterolateral abdominal wall; provide picture/guidelines for client to follow.
• Lie down during self-administration.
• Pull up a skin fold between the thumb and forefinger.
• Hold the skin fold throughout the injection and insert the whole needle directly into the skin fold to deliver the medication.
2. Observe client technique to ensure proper administration.
3. Advise that client may experience mild discomfort, irritation, and hematoma at injection site.
4. Explain that anticipated duration of therapy is 7–10 days and to report as scheduled for follow-up.

Evaluate: Deep vein thrombosis prophylaxis following hip replacement surgery.

Heparin sodium injection

(**HEP**-ah-rin)
Pregnancy Category: C
Hepalean ✱, Heparin Leo ✱, Liquaemin Sodium, Liquaemin Sodium Preservative Free **(Rx)**

Heparin sodium and sodium chloride

(**HEP**-ah-rin)
Pregnancy Category: C
Heparin Sodium and 0.45% Sodium Chloride, Heparin Sodium and 0.9% Sodium Chloride **(Rx)**

Heparin sodium lock flush solution

(**HEP**-ah-rin)
Pregnancy Category: C
Hepalean-Lok ✱, Heparin lock flush, Hep-Lock, Hep-Lock U/P **(Rx)**

See also *Anticoagulants,* Chapter 33.

How Supplied: Heparin sodium injection: *Injection:* 1000 U/mL, 2500 U/mL, 5000 U/mL, 7500 U/mL, 10,000 U/mL, 12,500 U/mL, 20,000 U/mL, 25,000 U/mL, 40,000 U/mL
Heparin sodium and sodium chloride: *Injection:* 200 U/100 mL-0.9%, 5000 U/100 mL-0.45%, 10,000 U/100 mL-0.45%
Heparin sodium lock flush solution: *Injection:* 10 U/mL, 100 U/mL; *Kit:* 10 U/mL, 100 U/mL

General Statement: Heparin is a naturally occurring substance isolated from porcine intestinal mucosa or bovine lung, although there is no difference in the pharmacologic effects between the two. Must be given parenterally. Heparin does not interfere with wound healing. Leukocyte counts should be performed in heparinized blood within 2 hr after adding heparin. Heparinized blood should not be used for complement, isoagglutinin, erythrocyte fragility test, or platelet counts.

Action/Kinetics: Heparin potentiates the inhibitory action of antithrombin III on various coagulation factors including factors IIa, IXa, Xa, XIa, and XIIa. This occurs due to the formation of a complex with and causing a conformational change in the antithrombin III molecule. Inhibition of factor Xa results in interference with thrombin generation; thus, the action of thrombin in coagulation is inhibited. Heparin also increases the rate of formation of antithrombin III–thrombin complex causing inactivation of thrombin and preventing the conversion of fibrinogen to fibrin. By inhibiting the activation of fibrin-stabilizing factor by thrombin, heparin also prevents formation of a stable fibrin clot. Therapeutic doses of heparin prolong thrombin time, whole blood clotting time, activated clotting time, and PTT. Heparin also decreases the levels of triglycerides by releasing lipoprotein lipase from tissues; the resultant hydrolysis of triglycerides causes increased blood levels of free fatty acids. **Onset: IV**; immediate; **deep SC:** 20–60 min. **t½:** 30–180 min in healthy persons. **t½** increases with dose, severe renal disease, and cirrhosis and in anephric clients and decreases with pulmonary embolism and liver impairment other than cirrhosis. *Metabolism:* Probably by reticuloendothelial system although up to 50% is excreted unchanged in the urine. Clotting time returns to normal within 2–6 hr.

Uses: Pulmonary embolism, peripheral arterial embolism, prophylaxis, and treatment of venous thrombosis and its extension. Atrial fibrillation with embolization. Diagnosis and treatment of disseminated intravascular coagulation. Low doses to prevent deep venous thrombosis and pulmonary embolism in pregnant clients with a history of thromboembolism, urology clients over 40 years of age, clients with stroke or heart failure, AMI or pulmonary infection, high-risk surgery clients, moderate and high-risk gynecologic clients with no malignancy, neurology clients with extracranial problems, and clients with severe musculoskeletal trauma. Prophylaxis of clotting in blood transfusions, extracorporeal circulation, dialysis procedures, blood samples for lab tests, and arterial and heart surgery. *Investigational:* Prophylaxis of post-MI, CVAs, and LV thrombi. By continuous infusion to treat myocardial ischemia in unstable angina refractory to usual treatment. Adjunct to treat coronary occlusion with AMI. Prophylaxis of cerebral thrombosis in evolving stroke.

Heparin lock flush solution: Dilute solutions are used to maintain patency of indwelling catheters used for IV therapy or blood sampling. Not to be used therapeutically.

Dosage

NOTE: Adjusted for each client on the basis of laboratory tests.

• **Deep SC**

General heparin dosage.

Initial loading dose: 10,000–20,000 units; **maintenance:** 8,000–10,000 units q 8 hr or 15,000–20,000 units q 12 hr. *Use concentrated solution.*

Prophylaxis of postoperative thromboembolism.

5,000 units of concentrated solution 2 hr before surgery and 5,000 units q 8–12 hr thereafter for 7 days or until client is ambulatory.

• **Intermittent IV**

General heparin dosage.

Initial loading dose: 10,000 units undiluted or in 50–100 mL saline; **then,** 5,000–10,000 units q 4–6 hr undiluted or in 50–100 mL saline.

• **Continuous IV infusion**

General heparin dosage.

Initial loading dose: 20,000–40,000 units/day in 1,000 mL saline (preceded initially by 5,000 units IV).

• **Special Uses**

Surgery of heart and blood vessels.

Initial, 150–400 units/kg to clients undergoing total body perfusion for open heart surgery. *NOTE:* 300 units/kg may be used for procedures less than 60 min while 400 units/kg is used for procedures lasting more than 60 min. To prevent clotting in the tube system, add heparin to fluids in pump oxygenator.

Extracorporeal renal dialysis.

See instructions on equipment.

Blood transfusion.

400–600 units/100 mL whole blood. 7500 units should be added to 100 mL 0.9% sodium chloride injection; from this dilution, add 6–8 mL/100 mL whole blood.

Laboratory samples.

70–150 units/10- to 20-mL sample to prevent coagulation.

Heparin lock sets.

To prevent clot formation in a heparin lock set, inject 10–100 units/mL heparin solution through the injection hub in a sufficient quantity to fill the entire set to the needle tip.

Administration/Storage

1. Client should be hospitalized for IV heparin therapy.
2. Drug may be diluted in dextrose,

NSS, or Ringer's solution and administered over 4–24 hr with an infusion pump.
3. Protect solutions from freezing.
4. Heparin should **not** be administered IM.
5. Administer by deep SC injection to minimize local irritation, hematoma, and tissue sloughing and to prolong action of drug.
• Z-track method: Use any fat roll, but abdominal fat rolls are preferred. Use a ½-in. or ⅝-in., 25- or 27-gauge needle. Grasp the skin layer of the fat roll and lift it up. Insert the needle at about a 45° angle to the skin's fat layer and then administer the medication. With this medication, it is not necessary to aspirate to check whether or not the needle is in a blood vessel. Rapidly withdraw the needle while releasing the skin.
• "Bunch technique" method: Grasp the tissue around the injection site, creating a tissue roll of about ½ in. in diameter. Insert the needle into the tissue roll at a 90° angle to the skin surface and inject the medication. Again, it is not necessary to aspirate to check whether or not the needle is in a blood vessel. Withdraw the needle rapidly when the skin is released.
• Do not administer within 2 in. of the umbilicus because of increased vascularity of area.
6. Do not massage before or after injection.
7. Change sites of administration.
8. Caution should be used to prevent negative pressure (with a roller pump), which would increase the rate at which heparin is injected into the system. Administer with a constant rate infusion pump.
9. Dose is individualized and will depend on client age, indications, and response.
10. Slight discoloration does not affect potency.
11. Have protamine sulfate, a heparin antagonist, available should the client develop excessive bleeding and anticoagulant effects.
12. *Treatment of Overdose:* Drug withdrawal is usually sufficient to correct heparin overdosage. In some cases, blood transfusion or the administration of protamine sulfate may be necessary.

Contraindications: Active bleeding, blood dyscrasias (or other disorders characterized by bleeding tendencies such as hemophilia), purpura, thrombocytopenia, liver disease with hypoprothrombinemia, suspected intracranial hemorrhage, suppurative thrombophlebitis, inaccessible ulcerative lesions (especially of the GI tract), open wounds, extensive denudation of the skin, and increased capillary permeability (as in ascorbic acid deficiency). IM use.

The drug should not be administered during surgery of the eye, brain, or spinal cord or during continuous tube drainage of the stomach or small intestine. Use is also contraindicated in subacute endocarditis, shock, advanced kidney disease, threatened abortion, severe hypertension, or hypersensitivity to drug. Premature neonates due to the possibility of a fatal "gasping syndrome."

Special Concerns: Women over age 60 may be more susceptible to hemorrhage during heparin therapy. Increased resistance to heparin is observed in thrombosis, thrombophlebitis, fever, cancer, MI, postoperatively, and infections with thrombosing tendencies. Use with caution in clients with allergies, diabetes, and renal insufficiency and during menses and in the postpartum period. Use heparin lock flush solution with caution in infants with diseases prone to hemorrhage.

Laboratory Test Interferences: ↑ AST and ALT.

Side Effects: *CV:* ***Hemorrhage ranging from minor local ecchymoses to major hemorrhagic complications from any organ or tissue.*** Higher incidence is seen in women over 60 years of age. Hemorrhagic reactions are more likely to occur in prophylactic administration during surgery than in the treatment of thromboembolic disease. White clot syndrome. *Hematologic:* Thrombocytopenia (both early and late). *Hypersensitivity:* Chills, fever, urticaria are the most common. Rarely, asthma, lacrimation, headache, N&V, rhinitis, ***shock, anaphylaxis.*** Allergic vasospastic reaction within 6–10 days after initiation of therapy (lasts 4–6 hr) including painful, ischemic, cyanotic limbs. Use a test dose of 1,000 units in clients with a history of asthma or allergic disease. *Miscellaneous:* Hyperkalemia, cutaneous necrosis, osteoporosis (after long-term use), delayed transient alopecia, priapism, suppressed aldosterone synthesis. Discontinuance of heparin has resulted in rebound hyperlipemia. *Following IM injection:* Local irritation, erythema, mild pain, ulceration, hematoma, and tissue sloughing.

Symptoms of Overdose: Nosebleeds, hematuria, tarry stools, petechiae, and easy bruising may be the first signs.

Drug Interactions

ACTH / Heparin antagonizes effect of ACTH
Alteplase, recombinant / ↑ Risk of bleeding, especially at arterial puncture sites
Anticoagulants, oral / Additive ↑ PT
Antihistamines / ↓ Effect of heparin
Aspirin / Additive ↑ PT
Cephalosporins / ↑ Risk of bleeding due to additive effect
Corticosteroids / Heparin antagonizes effect of corticosteroids
Dextran / Additive ↑ PT
Diazepam / Heparin ↑ plasma levels of diazepam
Digitalis / ↓ Effect of heparin
Dipyridamole / Additive ↑ PT
Hydroxychloroquine / Additive ↑ PT
Ibuprofen / Additive ↑ PT
Indomethacin / Additive ↑ PT
Insulin / Heparin antagonizes effect of insulin
Nitroglycerin / ↓ Effect of heparin
Penicillins / ↑ Risk of bleeding due to possible additive effects
Phenylbutazone / Additive ↑ PT
Quinine / Additive ↑ PT
Salicylates / ↑ Risk of bleeding
Tetracyclines / ↓ Effect of heparin

NURSING CONSIDERATIONS

See also *Nursing Considerations* for *Anticoagulants,* Chapter 33.

Assessment

1. Inquire about any bleeding incidents a client may have had, i.e., bleeding tendencies, family history, or any other incidents of unexplained or active bleeding.
2. Determine history of PUD. This may be an indication for a potential site of bleeding.
3. Determine that a test dose (1,000 units SC) has been administered to clients with multiple allergies or asthma history.
4. Note any evidence of possible intracranial hemorrhage.
5. If the client is receiving one of the many drugs that interact with anticoagulants, document and anticipate an adjustment in the dosage of heparin.
6. Obtain baseline hematologic (CBC, PT, PTT) parameters and liver and renal function studies.

Interventions

1. If given by continuous IV infusion, coagulation tests should be performed q 4 hr during early therapy and then daily when PTT is stabilized to within desired range. When given by intermittent IV infusion, coagulation tests should be drawn 30 min before the next scheduled dose and from the site/extremity opposite the infusion. Coagulation tests should be performed 4–6 hr after SC injections as needed.
2. Apply pressure to all venipuncture sites to minimize hematoma formation; avoid IM injections. Post at bedside that client is receiving anticoagulation therapy.

Client/Family Teaching

1. Review the appropriate technique for administration.
2. Stress the importance of reporting any signs of active bleeding.
3. Women of childbearing age should report any excessive menstrual flow as a reduction in dosage may be necessary.

4. Alopecia, if evident, is generally only temporary.
5. Alterations in GU function, urine color, or any injury should be immediately reported.
6. Use an electric razor for shaving and a soft-bristle toothbrush to decrease gum irritation.
7. Arrange furniture to allow open space for unimpeded ambulation and to diminish chances of bumping into objects that may cause bruising and bleeding.
8. Use a night light to provide illumination during trips to the bathroom at night.
9. Avoid any activity where excessive bumping or bruising or injury may be experienced.
10. Eat potassium-rich foods (e.g., baked potato, orange juice, bananas, beef, flounder, haddock, sweet potato, turkey, raw tomato).
11. Advise against eating large amounts of vitamin K foods. These are mostly yellow and dark green vegetables.
12. Report any evidence of increased bruising, bleeding of nose, mouth, gums, tarry stools, or GI upset.
13. Avoid using alcohol, aspirin, and NSAIDs as these create an increased anticoagulant response.
14. Warn other providers of prescribed anticoagulant therapy.
15. Wear or carry appropriate identification.

Evaluate
- Prevention of thrombus formation
- PTT within desired range (1.5–2.5 times control)

Interventions: for *Heparin Lock Flush Solution*.
1. Aspirate lock to determine patency. Maintain patency by injecting 1 mL of heparin lock flush solution into the diaphragm of the device after each use. This dose should maintain patency for up to 24 hr for a converted (capped) catheter.
2. When a drug incompatible with heparin is to be administered, flush the device with 0.9% sodium chloride injection or sterile water for injection before and immediately after the incompatible drug is administered. After the final flush, inject another dose of heparin lock flush solution.
3. Clients with underlying coagulation disorders may be at a risk for bleeding; observe coagulation times carefully.
4. When repeated blood samples are drawn from the venipuncture device, the presence of heparin or NSS may cause interference with lab tests.
- Clear the heparin lock flush solution by aspirating and discarding 1 mL of fluid from the device before withdrawing the blood sample.
- Inject another 1 mL of heparin lock flush solution into the device after blood samples are drawn.
- Because this is not the most reliable method of acquiring serum levels, if there are any excessively abnormal results, obtain a repeat sample from another site before initiating treatment.

5. Monitor for any allergic reactions to heparin due to various biologic sources of the product.

Special Concerns: Studies have shown that 0.9% NaCl is effective in maintaining patency of peripheral (noncentral) intermittent infusion devices and in reducing added medical costs. The following procedure has been recommended:
- Determine patency by aspirating lock.
- Flush with 2 mL NSS.
- Administer medication therapy. (Flush between drugs.)
- Flush with 2 mL NSS.
- Frequency of flushing to maintain patency when not actively in use varies from every 8 hr to every 24–48 hr.
- This does *NOT* apply to any central venous access devices.

Evaluate
- IV access for desired route of therapy
- Patency of indwelling catheter

Warfarin sodium

(**WAR**-far-in)
Pregnancy Category: X
Coumadin, Sofarin, Warfilone ✱ **(Rx)**

See also *Anticoagulants,* Chapter 33.
How Supplied: *Powder for injection:* 5 mg; *Tablet:* 1 mg, 2 mg, 2.5 mg, 4 mg, 5 mg, 7.5 mg, 10 mg
Action/Kinetics: Interferes with synthesis of vitamin K–dependent clotting factors resulting in depletion of clotting factors VII, IX, X, and II. Has no direct effect on an established thrombus although therapy may prevent further extension of a formed clot as well as secondary thromboembolic problems. Well absorbed from the GI tract although food affects the rate (but not the extent) of absorption. Suitable for parenteral administration. **Peak activity:** 1.5–3 days; **duration:** 2–5 days. **t½:** 1–2.5 days. Highly bound to plasma proteins. Metabolized in the liver and inactive metabolites are excreted through the urine and feces.
Uses: Prophylaxis and treatment of venous thrombosis and pulmonary embolism. Prophylaxis and treatment of atrial fibrillation with embolization. Adjunct in the prophylaxis of systemic embolism after MI. To prevent blood clots associated with prosthetic heart valve replacement. *Investigational:* Adjunct to treat small cell carcinoma of the lung with chemotherapy and radiation. Prophylaxis of recurrent transient ischemic attacks, reduce risk of recurrent MI.

Dosage

- **Tablets**

Induction.
Adults, initial: 10 mg/day for 2–4 days; **then,** adjust dose based on prothrombin or INR determinations. A lower dose should be used in geriatric or debilitated clients or clients with increased sensitivity. Dosage has not been established for children.

Maintenance.
Adults: 2–10 mg, based on prothrombin or INR.

Prevent blood clots with prosthetic heart valve replacement.
2–5 mg daily.

Administration/Storage
1. Daily monitoring of PT is recommended during the first week of therapy, or during adjustment periods, and weekly thereafter.
2. Client should not change brands of warfarin sodium. There may be differences in bioavailability.
3. If receiving anticoagulants, intramuscular injections should be avoided.
4. To transfer from heparin therapy, heparin and warfarin should be given together from the first day (as there is a delayed onset of oral anticoagulant effects). Alternatively, warfarin may be started on the third to sixth day of heparin therapy.
5. Levels of anticoagulation that are recommended for specific indications by the American College of Chest Physicians and the National Heart, Lung, and Blood Institute should be followed.
6. *Treatment of Overdose:* Discontinue therapy. Administer oral or parenteral phytonadione (e.g., 2.5–10 mg PO or 5–25 mg parenterally). In emergency situations, 200–250 mL fresh frozen plasma or commercial factor IX complex. Fresh whole blood may be needed in clients unresponsive to phytonadione.
Additional Contraindications: Lactation. Use of a large loading dose (30 mg) is not recommended due to increased risk of hemorrhage and lack of more rapid protection.
Special Concerns: Geriatric clients may be more sensitive. Anticoagulant use in the following clients leads to increased risk: trauma, infection, renal insufficiency, sprue, vitamin K deficiency, severe to moderate hypertension, polycythemia vera, severe allergic disorders, vasculitis, indwelling catheters, severe diabetes, anaphylactic disorders,

surgery or trauma resulting in large exposed raw surfaces. Use with caution in impaired hepatic and renal function. Safety and efficacy have not been determined in children less than 18 years of age. Careful monitoring and dosage regulation are required during dentistry and surgery.

Laboratory Test Interferences: False ↓ levels of serum theophylline determined by Schack and Waxler UV method (warfarin and dicumarol). Metabolites of indanedione derivatives may color alkaline urine red; color disappears upon acidification.

Side Effects: *CV: **Hemorrhage*** is the main side effect and may occur from any tissue or organ. Symptoms of hemorrhage include headache, paralysis; pain in the joints, abdomen, or chest; difficulty in breathing or swallowing; SOB, unexplained swelling or shock. *GI:* N&V, diarrhea, sore mouth, mouth ulcers, anorexia, abdominal cramping, paralytic ileus, intestinal obstruction (due to intramural or submucosal hemorrhage). *Hepatic:* Hepatotoxicity, cholestatic jaundice. *Dermatologic:* Dermatitis, exfoliative dermatitis, urticaria, alopecia, necrosis or gangrene of the skin and other tissues (due to protein C deficiency). *Miscellaneous:* Pyrexia, red-orange urine, priapism, leukopenia, systemic cholesterol microembolization ("purple toes" syndrome), hypersensitivity reactions, compressive neuropathy secondary to hemorrhage adjacent to a nerve (rare).

Symptoms of Overdose: Early symptoms include melena, petechiae, microscopic hematuria, oozing from superficial injuries (e.g., nicks from shaving, excessive bruising, bleeding from gums after teeth brushing), excessive menstrual bleeding.

Drug Interactions: Warfarin and anisindione are responsible for more adverse drug interactions than any other group. Clients on anticoagulant therapy must be monitored carefully each time a drug is added or withdrawn. Monitoring usually involves determination of PT. In general, a lengthened PT means potentiation of the anticoagulant. Since potentiation may mean hemorrhages, a lengthened PT warrants **reduction of the dosage of the anticoagulant.** However, the anticoagulant dosage must again be increased when the second drug is discontinued. A shortened PT means inhibition of the anticoagulant and may require an increase in dosage.

Acetaminophen / ↑ Anticoagulant effect

Alcohol, ethyl / Chronic alcohol use ↓ effect of oral anticoagulants

Aminoglutethimide / ↓ Effect of anticoagulants due to ↑ breakdown by liver

Aminoglycoside antibiotics / Potentiate pharmacologic effect of anticoagulants due to interference with vitamin K

Amiodarone / ↑ Effect of anticoagulants due to ↓ breakdown by liver

Androgens / ↑ Effect of anticoagulants

Ascorbic acid / ↓ Effect of anticoagulants by unknown mechanism

Barbiturates / ↓ Effect of anticoagulants due to ↑ breakdown by liver

Beta-adrenergic blockers / ↑ Effect of anticoagulants

Carbamazepine / ↓ Effect of anticoagulants due to ↑ breakdown by liver

Cephalosporins / ↑ Effect of anticoagulants due to effects on platelet function

Chloral hydrate / ↑ Effect of anticoagulant due to ↓ binding to plasma proteins

Chloramphenicol / ↑ Effect of anticoagulant due to ↓ breakdown by liver

Cholestyramine / ↓ Anticoagulant effect due to binding in and ↓ absorption from GI tract

Cimetidine / ↑ Anticoagulant effect due to ↓ breakdown by liver

Clofibrate / ↑ Anticoagulant effect

Contraceptives, oral / ↓ Anticoagulant effect by ↑ activity of certain clotting factors (VII and X); rarely, the opposite effect of ↑ risk of thromboembolism

Contrast media containing iodine / ↑ Effect of anticoagulants by ↑ PT
Corticosteroids / ↑ Effect of anticoagulants; also ↑ risk of GI bleeding due to ulcerogenic effect of steroids
Cyclophosphamide / ↑ Anticoagulant effect
Dextrothyroxine / ↑ Effect of anticoagulants
Dicloxacillin / ↓ Effect of anticoagulants
Diflunisal / ↑ Anticoagulant effect and ↑ risk of bleeding due to effect on platelet function and GI irritation
Disulfiram / ↑ Effect of anticoagulants
Erythromycin / ↓ Effect of anticoagulants
Estrogens / ↓ Anticoagulant response by ↑ activity of certain clotting factors; rarely, the opposite effect of ↑ risk of thromboembolism
Ethchlorvynol / ↓ Effect of anticoagulants
Etretinate / ↓ Effect of anticoagulants due to ↑ breakdown by liver
Fluconazole / ↑ Effect of anticoagulants
Gemfibrozil / ↑ Effect of anticoagulants
Glucagon / ↑ Effect of anticoagulants
Glutethimide / ↓ Effect of anticoagulants due to ↑ breakdown by liver
Griseofulvin / ↓ Effect of anticoagulants
Hydantoins / ↑ Effect of anticoagulants; also, ↑ hydantoin serum levels
Hypoglycemics, oral / ↑ Effect of anticoagulants due to ↓ plasma protein binding; also, ↑ effect of sulfonylureas
Ifosfamide / ↑ Effect of anticoagulants due to ↓ breakdown by liver and displacement from protein binding sites
Indomethacin / ↑ Effect of anticoagulants by an effect on platelet function; also, indomethacin is ulcerogenic cause GI hemorrhage
Isoniazid / ↑ Effect of anticoagulants
Ketoconazole / ↑ Effect of anticoagulants
Loop diuretics / ↑ Effect of anticoagulants by displacement from protein binding sites
Lovastatin / ↑ Effect of anticoagulants due to ↓ breakdown by liver
Metronidazole / ↑ Effect of anticoagulants due to ↓ breakdown by liver
Miconazole / ↑ Effect of anticoagulants
Mineral oil / ↑ Hypoprothrombinemia by ↓ absorption of vitamin K from GI tract; also mineral oil may ↓ absorption of anticoagulants from GI tract
Moricizine / ↑ Effect of anticoagulants
Nafcillin / ↓ Effect of anticoagulants
Nalidixic acid / ↑ Effect of anticoagulants due to displacement from protein binding sites
Nonsteroidal anti-inflammatory agents / ↑ Effect of anticoagulants and ↑ risk of bleeding due to effects on platelet function and GI irritation
Omeprazole / ↑ Effect of anticoagulant due to ↓ breakdown by liver
Penicillin / ↑ Effect of anticoagulants and ↑ risk of bleeding due to effects on platelet function
Phenylbutazone / ↑ Effect of anticoagulants due to ↓ breakdown by liver and ↑ displacement from protein binding sites
Propafenone / ↑ Effect of anticoagulant due to ↓ breakdown by liver
Propoxyphene / ↑ Effect of anticoagulants
Quinidine, quinine / ↑ Effect of anticoagulants due to ↓ breakdown by liver
Quinolones / ↑ Effect of anticoagulants
Rifampin / ↓ Anticoagulant effect due to ↑ breakdown by liver
Salicylates / ↑ Effect of anticoagulants and ↑ risk of bleeding due to effect on platelet function and GI irritation
Spironolactone / ↓ Effect of antico-

agulants due to hemoconcentration of clotting factors due to diuresis
Sucralfate / ↓ Effect of anticoagulants
Sulfamethoxazole and Trimethoprim / ↑ Effect of anticoagulants due to ↓ breakdown by liver
Sulfinpyrazone / ↑ Anticoagulant effect due to ↓ breakdown by liver and inhibition of platelet aggregation
Sulfonamides / ↑ Effect of sulfonamides
Sulindac / ↑ Effect of anticoagulants
Tamoxifen / ↑ Effect of anticoagulants
Tetracyclines / ↑ Effect of anticoagulants due to interference with vitamin K
Thioamines / ↑ Effect of anticoagulants
Thiopurines / ↓ Effect of anticoagulants due to ↑ synthesis or activation of prothrombin
Thyroid hormones / ↑ Anticoagulant effect
Trazodone / ↓ Effect of anticoagulants
Thiazide diuretics / ↓ Effect of anticoagulants due to hemoconcentration of clotting factors due to diuresis
Vitamin E / ↑ Effect of anticoagulants due to interference with vitamin K
Vitamin K / ↓ Effect of anticoagulants

NURSING CONSIDERATIONS

See also *Nursing Considerations* for *Anticoagulants,* Chapter 33.

Assessment

1. Document indications for therapy and type and onset of symptoms.
2. List drugs currently prescribed to ensure that none interacts unfavorably by increasing or decreasing PT as a result of competition for protein binding at receptor sites.
3. Note any history of bleeding tendencies.
4. When working with sexually active females check for pregnancy. Fetal malformations have been documented; additionally, there is danger of neonatal hemorrhage.
5. Obtain baseline CBC, PT, PTT, and liver and renal function studies.
6. Monitor PT [or International Normalized Ratio (INR)] and check the most recent lab findings prior to administering warfarin.

Interventions

1. Request written parameters noting the desired range for client PT or INR, once client is stably anticoagulated (orally). It usually takes 36–48 hr for drug to reach steady state; therefore allow time to equilibrate. The INR is the PT ratio (test/control) obtained from human brain thromboplastin and is universally considered most accurate for monitoring to calculate dosage.
2. Drug inhibits production of factors II, VII, IX, and X; onset in response is delayed because of degradation of clotting factors that have already been synthesized.
3. Test all nasogastric drainage, stool, and urine for occult blood.
4. Observe for "purple toe syndrome" related to inhibition of protein C and S.

Client/Family Teaching

1. Take oral warfarin as prescribed and at the same time each day.
2. Explain that this medicine does not dissolve clots but decreases the clotting ability of the blood and helps to prevent the formation of harmful blood clots in the blood vessels and heart valves.
3. Avoid activities and contact sports that may cause injury or cuts and bruises. Use a soft toothbrush, use an electric razor to shave, wear shoes and use a night light to avoid falls at night.
4. Review side effects that require immediate reporting, such as any unusual bruising or bleeding, dark brown or blood tinged body secretions, dizziness, abdominal pain or swelling, back pain, severe headaches, and joint swelling and pain.
5. Carry vitamin K for emergency use. The usual dosage is 5–20 mg, to

be used in the event of excessive bleeding.

6. Provide a list of foods high in vitamin K (asparagus, broccoli, cabbage, brussels sprouts, spinach, turnips, milk, cheese, etc.) that should be avoided during drug therapy.

7. Advise sexually active women to use reliable birth control measures because there are added risks in pregnancy.

8. Menstruation may be prolonged and flow slightly increased. Report if excessive and unusual.

9. Skin eruptions may develop as an allergic reaction and should be reported.

10. Do not change brands of drug unless approved because response may be altered.

11. Wear identification and alert all providers that you are on anticoagulant therapy.

12. Stress the importance of reporting as scheduled for lab studies to evaluate the effectiveness of therapy, as dosage may need to be adjusted.

Evaluate

- Prevention of thrombus formation
- PT within desired range (usually 1.5–2 times the control)
- INR within desired therapeutic range (2.0–3.0 with standard therapy; 2.5–3.5 with high-dose therapy)

CHAPTER THIRTY-FOUR

Thrombolytic Drugs/Platelet Aggregation Inhibitors

See the following individual entries:

Alteplase, Recombinant
Anistreplase
Streptokinase
Ticlopidine Hydrochloride
Urokinase

Alteplase, recombinant

(**AL**-teh-playz)
Pregnancy Category: C
Activase, Activase rt-PA ✱ **(Rx)**

How Supplied: *Powder for injection:* 20 mg, 50 mg, 100 mg
Action/Kinetics: Alteplase, a tissue plasminogen activator, is synthesized by a human melanoma cell line using recombinant DNA technology. This enzyme binds to fibrin in a thrombus, causing a conversion of plasminogen to plasmin. This conversion results in local fibrinolysis and a decrease in circulating fibrinogen. Within 10 min following termination of an infusion, 80% of the alteplase has been cleared from the plasma by the liver. The enzyme activity of alteplase is 580,000 IU/mg. **t½, initial:** 4 min; **final:** 35 min (elimination phase).
Uses: Lysis of coronary thrombi following AMI. The drug thus reduces the incidence of CHF and improves ventricular function. Acute pulmonary thromboembolism. *Investigational:* Unstable angina pectoris.

Dosage

- **IV infusion only.**

AMI.

100 mg total dose subdivided as follows: 60 mg (34.8 million IU) the first hour with 6–10 mg given in a bolus over the first 1–2 min and the remaining 50–54 mg given over the hour; 20 mg (11.6 million IU) over the second hour and 20 mg (11.6 million IU) given over the third hour. **Clients less than 65 kg:** 1.25 mg/kg given over 3 hr, with 60% given the first hour with 6%–10% given by direct IV injection within the first 1–2 min; 20% is given the second hour and 20% during the third hour. Doses of 150 mg have caused an increase in intracranial bleeding.

Pulmonary embolism.

100 mg over 2 hr; heparin therapy should be instituted near the end of or right after the alteplase infusion when the partial thromboplastin or thrombin time returns to twice that of normal or less.

Administration/Storage

1. Alteplase therapy should be initiated as soon as possible after onset of symptoms.
2. Nearly 90% of clients also receive heparin concomitantly with alteplase and either aspirin or dipyridamole during or after heparin therapy.
3. The product must be reconstituted with only sterile water for injection without preservatives immediately prior to use. The reconstituted preparation contains 1 mg/mL and is a colorless to pale yellow transparent solution.
4. Using an 18-gauge needle, the stream of sterile water for injection

should be directed into the lyophilized cake. The product should be left undisturbed for several minutes to allow dissipation of any large bubbles.
5. If necessary, the reconstituted solution may be further diluted immediately prior to use in an equal volume of 0.9% sodium chloride injection or 5% dextrose injection to yield a concentration of 0.5 mg/mL. Dilution should be accomplished by gentle swirling or slow inversion.
6. Either glass bottles or polyvinyl chloride bags may be used for administration.
7. The usual dose is given over 3 hr with 60% of the dose administered in the first hour, 20% of the dose over the second hour, and 20% over the third hour.
8. Alteplase is stable for up to 8 hr following reconstitution or dilution. Stability will not be affected by light.
9. Use an electronic infusion device for medication administration. Do not add any other medications to the line. Anticipate 3 lines for access (1–alteplase; 1–heparin and other drugs such as lidocaine; 1–blood drawing and transfusions).
10. Lyophilized alteplase should be stored at room temperatures not to exceed 30°C or under refrigeration between 2°C–8°C.
11. Have available emergency drugs (especially aminocaproic acid) and resuscitative equipment.
12. *Treatment of Overdose:* Discontinue therapy immediately as well as any concomitant heparin therapy.

Contraindications: Severe (uncontrolled) hypertension. Clients with a risk of internal bleeding and history of CVA, intracranial or intraspinal surgery or trauma (within 2 months), aneurysm, bleeding diathesis, intracranial neoplasm, arteriovenous malformation or aneurysm, severe uncontrolled hypertension, and active internal bleeding.

Special Concerns: Use with caution in the presence of recent GI or GU bleeding (within 10 days), subacute bacterial endocarditis, acute pericarditis, significant liver dysfunction, concomitant use of oral anticoagulants, diabetic hemorrhagic retinopathy, septic thrombophlebitis or occluded arteriovenous cannula (at infected site), lactation, mitral stenosis with atrial fibrillation. Since fibrin will be lysed during therapy, careful attention should be given to potential bleeding sites such as sites of catheter insertion and needle puncture sites. Use with caution within 10 days of major surgery (e.g., obstetrics, coronary artery bypass) and in clients over 75 years of age. Safety and efficacy have not been established in children. *NOTE:* Doses greater than 150 mg have been associated with an increase in intracranial bleeding.

Side Effects: *Bleeding tendencies:* ***Internal bleeding*** (including the GI and GU tracts and intracranial or retroperitoneal site). Superficial bleeding (e.g., gums, sites of recent surgery, venous cutdowns, arterial punctures). Ecchymosis, epistaxis. *GI:* N&V. *Miscellaneous:* Fever, urticaria, hypotension.

Drug Interactions
Acetylsalicylic acid / ↑ Risk of bleeding
Dipyridamole / ↑ Risk of bleeding
Heparin / ↑ Risk of bleeding, especially at arterial puncture sites

NURSING CONSIDERATIONS

Assessment

1. Note any history of hypertension, internal bleeding, or PUD.
2. Record client age and determine whether or not client has had recent surgery.
3. Document characteristics of chest pain, especially onset, and assess throughout therapy.
4. Assess and document client's overall physical condition; obtain weight.
5. Obtain a drug history and determine what client is currently taking; especially note any oral anticoagulant drugs.
6. Obtain baseline hematologic pa-

rameters, type and cross, coagulation times, cardiac isoenzymes, and renal function studies.

Interventions

1. Carefully review and follow instructions for drug reconstitution and review the contraindications before initiating therapy.
2. Record VS q 15 min during infusion and for 2 hr following.
3. Clients receiving therapy should be observed in a closely monitored environment. Review and document monitor strips.
4. Anticipate and assess for reperfusion reactions such as:
• Reperfusion arrhythmias usually of short duration. These may include accelerated idioventricular rhythm and sinus bradycardia.
• A reduction of chest pain
• A return of the elevated ST segment to near baseline levels
• Smaller Q waves
5. Check all access sites for any evidence of bleeding.
6. During IV therapy, arterial sticks require 30 min of manual pressure followed by application of a pressure dressing.
7. In the event of any uncontrolled bleeding, terminate the alteplase and heparin infusions and report immediately.
8. Monitor neurologic status and record findings q 15–30 min during infusion.
9. During treatment for pulmonary embolism, ensure that the PTT or PT is no more than twice that of normal before heparin therapy is added.
10. Keep on bed rest and observe for S&S of abnormal bleeding (hematuria, hematemesis, melena, CVA, cardiac tamponade).
11. Obtain appropriate postinfusion laboratory studies (isoenzymes, platelets, H&H, PTT) as directed.

Client/Family Teaching

1. Review the inherent risks of drug therapy during acute coronary artery occlusion.
2. Stress that to be effective, the therapy should be instituted within 4–6 hr of onset of symptoms of AMI.

Evaluate

• Lysis of thrombi with reperfusion of ischemic tissue
• ↓ Infarct size with restoration of coronary perfusion and improved ventricular function (↑ CO, ↓ HR)

Anistreplase

(an-ih-**STREP**-layz)
Pregnancy Category: C
Eminase **(Rx)**

How Supplied: *Powder for injection:* 30 U

Action/Kinetics: Anistreplase is prepared by acylating human plasma derived from lys-plasminogen and purified streptokinase derived from group C beta-hemolytic streptococci. When prepared, anistreplase is an inactive derivative of a fibrinolytic enzyme although the compound can still bind to fibrin. Anistreplase is activated by deacylation and subsequent release of the anisoyl group in the blood stream. The production of plasmin from plasminogen occurs in both the blood stream and the thrombus leading to thrombolysis. The drug will lyse thrombi obstructing coronary arteries and reduce the size of infarcts. **t½:** 70–120 min.

Uses: Management of AMI in adults, resulting in improvement of ventricular function and reduction of mortality. Treatment should be initiated as soon as possible after the onset of symptoms of AMI.

Dosage

IV only: 30 units over 2–5 min into an IV line or vein as soon as possible after onset of symptoms.

Administration/Storage

1. The drug is reconstituted by slowly adding 5 mL of sterile water for injection. To minimize foaming, gently roll the vial after directing the stream of sterile water against the side of the vial. The vial should not be shaken.
2. The reconstituted solution should be colorless to pale yellow without any particulate matter or discoloration.
3. The reconstituted solution should

not be further diluted before administration.
4. The reconstituted solution should not be added to any infusion fluids and no other medications should be added to the vial or syringe containing anistreplase.
5. The solution should be discarded if not administered within 30 min of reconstitution.
Contraindications: Use in active internal bleeding; within 2 months of intracranial or intraspinal surgery or trauma; history of CVA; intracranial neoplasm, arteriovenous malformation, or aneurysm; known bleeding diathesis; severe, uncontrolled hypertension; severe allergic reactions to streptokinase.
Special Concerns: Use with caution in nursing mothers. Safety and effectiveness have not been determined in children.

NOTE: The risks of anistreplase therapy may be increased in the following conditions; thus, benefit versus risk must be assessed prior to use. Within 10 days of major surgery (e.g., CABG, obstetric delivery, organ biopsy, previous puncture of noncompressible vessels); cerebrovascular disease; within 10 days of GI or GU bleeding; within 10 days of trauma including cardiopulmonary resuscitation; SBP > 180 mm Hg or DBP > 110 mm Hg; likelihood of left heart thrombus (e.g., mitral stenosis with atrial fibrillation); SBE; acute pericarditis; hemostatic defects including those secondary to severe hepatic or renal disease; pregnancy; clients older than 75 years of age; diabetic hemorrhagic retinopathy or other hemorrhagic ophthalmic conditions; septic thrombophlebitis or occluded arteriovenous cannula at seriously infected site; clients on oral anticoagulant therapy; any condition in which bleeding constitutes a significant hazard or would be difficult to manage due to its location.
Laboratory Test Interferences: ↑ Transaminase levels, thrombin time, activated PTT, and PT. ↓ Plasminogen and fibrinogen.
Side Effects: *Bleeding:* Including at the puncture site (most common), nonpuncture site hematoma, hematuria, hemoptysis, ***GI hemorrhage, intracranial bleeding,*** gum/mouth hemorrhage, epistaxis, anemia, eye hemorrhage. *CV:* ***Arrhythmias,*** conduction disorders, hypotension; ***cardiac rupture,*** chest pain, emboli (causal relationship to use of anistreplase unknown). *Allergic:* ***Anaphylaxis, bronchospasm,*** angioedema, urticaria, itching, flushing, rashes, eosinophilia, delayed purpuric rash which may be associated with arthralgia, ankle edema, mild hematuria, GI symptoms, and proteinuria. *GI:* N&V. *Hematologic:* Thrombocytopenia. *CNS:* Agitation, dizziness, paresthesia, tremor, vertigo. *Respiratory:* Dyspnea, lung edema. *Miscellaneous:* Chills, fever, headache, shock.
Drug Interactions: Increased risk of bleeding or hemorrhage if used with heparin, oral anticoagulants, vitamin K antagonists, aspirin, or dipyridamole.

NURSING CONSIDERATIONS

See also *Nursing Considerations* for *Alteplase, Recombinant,* Chapter 34.
Assessment
1. Note any history and any evidence of bleeding.
2. Take a full drug history. Note especially if client has been taking aspirin, anticoagulants, or vitamin K antagonists.
3. Note resistance to the effects of anistreplase, which may be observed if the drug is given more than 5 days after a previous dose, after streptokinase therapy, or after a streptococcal infection.
4. Increased antistreptokinase antibody levels between 5 days and 6 months after anistreplase or streptokinase administration may increase the risk of allergic reactions.
5. Determine that appropriate laboratory studies have been completed prior to starting drug therapy.

Interventions

1. Invasive procedures should be avoided to minimize bleeding tendencies. Incorporate bleeding precautions.
2. If an arterial puncture is necessary following use of anistreplase, an upper extremity vessel accessible to manual compression should be used. Apply 30 min of manual pressure followed by application of a pressure dressing. Puncture site should be checked frequently for any evidence of bleeding.
3. Monitor ECG closely and document any reperfusion arrhythmias.

Evaluate

- Restoration of blood flow to ischemic cardiac tissue
- ↓ Infarct size and improved ventricular function

Streptokinase

(strep-toe-**KYE**-nayz)
Pregnancy Category: C
Kabikinase, Streptase **(Rx)**

How Supplied: *Powder for injection:* 250,000 IU, 750,000 IU, 1.5 million IU

Action/Kinetics: Most clients have a natural resistance to streptokinase that must be overcome with the loading dose before the drug becomes effective. Thrombin time and streptokinase resistance should be determined before initiation of the therapy. Streptokinase acts with plasminogen to produce an "activator complex," which enhances the conversion of plasminogen to plasmin. Plasmin then breaks down fibrinogen, fibrin clots, and other plasma proteins. Thus, the drug promotes the dissolution (lysis) of the insoluble fibrin trapped in intravascular emboli and thrombi. Also, inhibitors of streptokinase, such as alpha-2-macroglobulin, are rapidly inactivated by streptokinase. **Onset:** rapid; **duration:** 12 hr. **t½, activator complex:** 23 min.

Uses: Deep vein thrombosis; arterial thrombosis and embolism; acute evolving transmural MI. Also, clearing of occluded arteriovenous and IV cannulae.

Dosage

- **IV infusion**

Venous or arterial thrombosis, arterial or pulmonary embolism.
Initial: 250,000 IU over 30 min (use the 1,500,000 IU vial diluted to 90 mL); **maintenance:** 100,000 IU/hr for 24–72 hr for arterial thrombosis or embolism, 72 hr for deep vein thrombosis, and 24 hr for pulmonary embolism.

Acute evolving transmural MI.
1,500,000 IU within 60 min (use the 1,500,000 IU vial diluted to a total of 45 mL).

Arteriovenous cannula occlusion.
250,000 IU in 2-mL IV solution into each occluded limb of cannula; **then,** after 2 hr aspirate cannula limbs, flush with saline, and reconnect cannula.

- **Intracoronary infusion**

Venous or arterial thrombosis, arterial or pulmonary embolism.
Same dose as IV infusion; however, the 1,500,000 IU vial should be diluted to 45 mL with a rate of infusion of 15 mL/hr for the loading dose and 3 mL/hr for maintenance doses. May be followed by continuous IV heparin infusion to prevent recurrent thrombosis (start only after thrombin time has decreased to less than twice the normal control value, usually 3–4 hr).

Acute evolving transmural MI.
20,000 IU by bolus; **then,** 2,000 IU/min for 60 min (total dose of 140,000 IU). Use the 250,000 IU vial diluted to 125 mL.

Administration/Storage

1. Sodium chloride injection USP or 5% dextrose injection is the preferred diluent for IV use.
2. For AV cannulae, dilute 250,000 units with 2 mL of sodium chloride injection or 5% dextrose injection.
3. Reconstitute gently, as directed by manufacturer, without shaking vial.
4. Use within 24 hr after reconstitution.
5. Use an electronic infusion device to administer streptokinase and do not

add any other medications to the line. Note any redness and/or pain at the site of infusion. It may be necessary to further dilute the solution to prevent phlebitis.
6. Have emergency drugs and equipment available. Have corticosteroids and aminocaproic acid available in the event bleeding is excessive.

Contraindications: Any condition presenting a risk of hemorrhage, such as recent surgery or biopsies, delivery within 10 days, ulcerative disease. Arterial emboli originating from the left side of the heart. Also, hepatic or renal insufficiency, tuberculosis, recent cerebral embolism, thrombosis, hemorrhage, SBE, rheumatic valvular disease, thrombocytopenia. Streptokinase resistance in excess of 1 million IU.

Special Concerns: The use of streptokinase in septic thrombophlebitis may be hazardous. History of significant allergic response. Safety in children has not been established.

Laboratory Test Interferences: ↓ Fibrinogen, plasminogen. ↑ Thrombin time, PT, and activated PTT.

Side Effects: *CV:* Superficial bleeding, ***severe internal bleeding.*** *Allergic:* Nausea, headache, breathing difficulties, ***bronchospasm, angioneurotic edema,*** urticaria, flushing, musculoskeletal pain, vasculitis, interstitial nephritis, periorbital swelling. *Other:* Fever, possible development of Guillain-Barre syndrome, development of antistreptokinase antibody (i.e., streptokinase may be ineffective if administered between 5 days and 6 months following prior use of streptokinase or following streptococcal infections).

Drug Interactions: The following drugs increase the chance of bleeding when given concomitantly with streptokinase: anticoagulants, aspirin, heparin, indomethacin, and phenylbutazone.

NURSING CONSIDERATIONS

See also *Nursing Considerations* for *Alteplase, Recombinant,* Chapter 34.

Assessment

1. Document indications for therapy and type and onset of symptoms.
2. During the nursing history, note any history of prior conditions that might contraindicate the use of streptokinase. (e.g., tuberculosis, SBE, ulcerative disease, recent surgery or streptococcal infection).
3. Determine any history or evidence of bleeding tendencies, heart disease, and/or allergic reaction to any drugs.
4. Identify other drugs the client may be taking such as aspirin or similar products that could increase bleeding times.
5. Clients with high allergy potential or high streptokinase antibody titer may benefit by skin testing prior to administering therapy. Drug may not be effective if administered within 5 days to 6 months of a strep infection.
6. Ensure that baseline bleeding studies, type, and crossmatch have been completed prior to initiation of therapy.

Interventions

1. Ensure that the client understands the purpose of the therapy and possible side effects.
2. Review all contraindications before initiating therapy.
3. Clients receiving therapy should be observed in a closely monitored environment; document rhythm strips and VS q 15–30 min initially.
4. Check access sites for evidence of bleeding. Check stools, urine, and emesis for evidence of occult blood.
5. During IV therapy, arterial sticks require 30 min of manual pressure followed by application of a pressure dressing.
6. To prevent bruising, avoid unnecessary handling of client.
7. If an IM injection is necessary, apply pressure after withdrawing the needle to prevent a hematoma and bleeding from the puncture site.
8. If excessive bleeding develops from an invasive procedure, discontinue therapy and call for packed

RBCs and plasma expanders *other than dextran*.

9. To prevent new thrombus formation, or rethrombosis, anticipate the use of IV heparin and oral anticoagulants when the thrombolytic therapy is concluded.

10. Geriatric clients have an increased risk of bleeding during therapy.

11. Observe injection sites and postoperative wounds for bleeding during thrombolytic therapy. Document and report.

12. Note evidence of allergic reactions, ranging from anaphylaxis to moderate and mild reactions. These usually can be controlled with antihistamines and corticosteroids.

13. Provide symptomatic treatment for fever reaction; may be treated with acetaminophen.

14. Following recanalization of an occluded coronary artery, clients may develop reperfusion reactions; these may include:

- Reperfusion arrhythmias, usually of short duration. These may include accelerated idioventricular rhythm and sinus bradycardia.
- A reduction of chest pain
- A return of the elevated ST segment to near baseline levels

Client/Family Teaching

1. Review the inherent benefits and risks of drug therapy.
2. Answer all questions and assist to decrease anxiety levels.
3. Stress that to be effective, the therapy should be instituted within 4–6 hr of onset of symptoms of acute MI.
4. Explain the importance of reporting any symptoms or side effects immediately.
5. With CAD, encourage family members or significant other to learn CPR.

Evaluate

- Lysis of emboli and thrombi with restoration of normal blood flow
- ↓ Myocardial infarct size and improved ventricular function
- Evidence of catheter patency in previously occluded AV or IV cannulae

Ticlopidine hydrochloride

(tie-**KLOH**-pih-deen)
Pregnancy Category: B
Ticlid **(Rx)**

How Supplied: *Tablet:* 250 mg

Action/Kinetics: Ticlopidine irreversibly inhibits ADP-induced platelet-fibrinogen binding and subsequent platelet-platelet interactions. This results in inhibition of both platelet aggregation and release of platelet granule constituents as well as prolongation of bleeding time. **Peak plasma levels:** 2 hr. **Maximum platelet inhibition:** 8–11 days after 250 mg b.i.d. **Steady-state plasma levels:** 14–21 days. **t½, elimination:** 4–5 days. After discontinuing therapy, bleeding time and other platelet function tests return to normal within 14 days. The drug is rapidly absorbed; bioavailability is increased by food. Highly bound (98%) to plasma proteins. Extensively metabolized by the liver with approximately 60% excreted through the kidneys; 23% is excreted in the feces (with one-third excreted unchanged). Clearance of the drug decreases with age.

Uses: To reduce the risk of fatal or nonfatal thrombotic stroke in clients who have manifested precursors of stroke or who have had a completed thrombotic stroke. Due to the risk of neutropenia or agranulocytosis, use should be reserved for clients who are intolerant to aspirin therapy. *Investigational:* Chronic arterial occlusion, coronary artery bypass grafts, intermittent claudication, open heart surgery, primary glomerulonephritis, subarachnoid hemorrhage, sickle cell disease, uremic clients with AV shunts or fistulas.

Dosage

- **Tablets**

Reduce risk of thrombotic stroke.
250 mg b.i.d.

Administration/Storage

1. To increase bioavailability and decrease GI discomfort, ticlopidine

should be taken with food or just after eating.
2. If a client is switched from an anticoagulant or fibrinolytic drug to ticlopidine, the former drug should be discontinued before initiation of ticlopidine therapy.
3. IV methylprednisolone (20 mg) may normalize prolonged bleeding times, usually within 2 hr.

Contraindications: In the presence of neutropenia and thrombocytopenia, hemostatic disorder, or active pathologic bleeding such as bleeding peptic ulcer or intracranial bleeding. Severe liver impairment. Lactation.

Special Concerns: Use with caution in clients with ulcers (i.e., where there is a propensity for bleeding). Reduced dosage should be considered in impaired renal function. Geriatric clients may be more sensitive to the effects of the drug. Safety and effectiveness have not been established in children less than 18 years of age.

Laboratory Test Interferences: ↑ Alkaline phosphatase, ALT, AST, serum cholesterol, and triglycerides.

Side Effects: *Hematologic:* Neutropenia, ***agranulocytosis,*** thrombocytopenia, pancytopenia, thrombotic thrombocytopenia purpura, immune thrombocytopenia, ***hemolytic anemia with reticulocytosis.*** *GI:* Diarrhea, N&V, GI pain, dyspepsia, flatulence, anorexia, GI fullness. *Bleeding complications:* Ecchymosis, hematuria, epistaxis, conjunctival hemorrhage, ***GI bleeding,*** perioperative bleeding, ***intracerebral bleeding (rare).*** *Dermatologic:* Maculopapular or urticarial rash, pruritus, urticaria. *CNS:* Dizziness, headache. *Neuromuscular:* Asthenia, SLE, peripheral neuropathy, arthropathy, myositis. *Miscellaneous:* Tinnitus, pain, allergic pneumonitis, vasculitis, hepatitis, cholestatic jaundice, nephrotic syndrome, hyponatremia, serum sickness.

Drug Interactions
Antacids / ↓ Plasma levels of ticlopidine
Aspirin / Ticlopidine ↑ effect of aspirin on collagen-induced platelet aggregation
Cimetidine / ↓ Clearance of ticlopidine probably due to ↓ breakdown by liver
Digoxin / Slight ↓ in digoxin plasma levels
Theophylline / ↑ Plasma levels of theophylline due to ↓ clearance

---

NURSING CONSIDERATIONS

Assessment
1. Note any history of liver disease, bleeding disorders, or ulcer disease.
2. Ascertain aspirin intolerance.
3. Determine baseline hematologic profile (e.g., CBC, PT, PTT, platelets).

Client/Family Teaching
1. Take with food or after meals to minimize GI upset.
2. It may take longer than usual to stop bleeding; unusual bleeding should be reported. Inform all providers that ticlopidine is prescribed.
3. Brush teeth with a soft-bristle tooth brush, use an electric razor for shaving, wear shoes when ambulating, use caution and avoid injury as bleeding times may be prolonged.
4. During the first 3 months of therapy, neutropenia can occur, resulting in an increased risk of infection. Come for scheduled blood tests and report any symptoms of infection (e.g., fever, chills, sore throat).
5. Any severe or persistent diarrhea, SC bleeding, skin rashes, or any evidence of cholestasis (e.g., yellow skin or sclera, dark urine, light-colored stools) should be reported.

Evaluate: Successful pharmacologic prevention of a complete or recurrent cerebral thrombotic event.

Urokinase

(your-oh-**KYE**-nayz)
Pregnancy Category: B
Abbokinase, Abbokinase Open-Cath
(Rx)

How Supplied: *Powder for injection:* 5000 IU, 9000 IU, 250,000 IU

Action/Kinetics: Urokinase converts plasminogen to plasmin; plasmin then breaks down fibrin clots and fibrinogen. **Onset:** rapid; **duration:** 12 hr. **t½:** <20 min, although effect on coagulation disappears after a few hours.

Uses: Acute pulmonary thromboembolism. To clear IV catheters that are blocked by fibrin or clotted blood. *Investigational:* Acute arterial thromboembolism, acute arterial thrombosis, acute arterial coronary thrombosis, to clear arteriovenous cannula.

Dosage

- **IV infusion only**

Acute pulmonary embolism.

Loading dose: 4,400 IU/kg administered over 10 min at a rate of 90 mL/hr; **maintenance:** 4,400 IU/kg administered continuously at a rate of 15 mL/hr for 12 hr. May be followed by continuous IV heparin infusion to prevent recurrent thrombosis (start only after thrombin time has decreased to less than twice the normal control value).

Coronary artery thrombi.

Initial: Heparin, as a bolus of 2,500–10,000 units **IV; then,** begin infusion of urokinase at a rate of 6,000 IU/min (4 mL/min) for up to 2 hr (average total dose of urokinase may be 500,000 IU). Urokinase should be administered until the artery is opened maximally (15–30 min after initial opening although it has been given for up to 2 hr).

Clear IV catheter.

Instill into the catheter 1–1.8 mL of a solution containing 5,000 IU/mL.

Administration/Storage

1. Reconstitute only with sterile water for injection without preservatives. Do not use bacteriostatic water.
2. The vial should be rolled and tilted, but not shaken, during reconstitution.
3. Reconstitute immediately before using.
4. Discard any unused portion.
5. Dilute reconstituted urokinase before IV administration in 0.9% NSS or 5% dextrose injection.
6. Type and cross and have blood for transfusion available. Aminocaproic acid may be employed with severe bleeding or hemorrhage.

Contraindications: Any condition presenting a risk of hemorrhage, such as recent surgery or biopsies, delivery within 10 days, pregnancy, ulcerative disease. Also hepatic or renal insufficiency, tuberculosis, recent cerebral embolism, thrombosis, hemorrhage, SBE, rheumatic valvular disease, thrombocytopenia.

Special Concerns: The use of the drugs in septic thrombophlebitis may be hazardous. Use with caution during lactation. Safe use in children has not been established.

Side Effects: *CV:* Superficial bleeding, ***severe internal bleeding.*** *Allergic:* Rarely, skin rashes, ***bronchospasm.*** *Other:* Fever.

Drug Interactions: The following drugs increase the chance of bleeding when given concomitantly with urokinase: Anticoagulants, aspirin, heparin, indomethacin, and phenylbutazone.

NURSING CONSIDERATIONS

See also *Nursing Considerations* for *Streptokinase* and *Alteplase, Recombinant,* Chapter 34.

Evaluate

- Evidence of successful lysis of thrombi with restoration of blood flow and prevention of tissue infarction
- Evidence of the restoration of catheter or cannula patency in previously occluded AV or IV cannulae

CHAPTER THIRTY-FIVE

Hemostatics—Systemic/Topical

See the following individual entries:

Aminocaproic Acid
Antihemophilic Factor (AHF, Factor VIII)
Factor IX Complex (Human)
Microfibrillar Collagen Hemostat

Aminocaproic acid

(ah-**ME**-noh-kah-**PROH**-ick **AH**-sid)

Amicar, Epsikapron **(Rx)**

How Supplied: *Injection:* 250 mg/mL; *Syrup:* 1.25 g/5 mL; *Tablet:* 500 mg

Action/Kinetics: Inhibits action of plasminogen (clotting factor), thereby preventing fibrinolysis (clot dissolution). Rapidly absorbed from the GI tract. **Peak plasma levels:** 2 hr. **Effective plasma levels:** 0.13 mg/mL. **Duration (after IV):** 3 hr or less. Rapidly excreted through the kidney, mostly unchanged.

Uses: Excessive bleeding associated with systemic hyperfibrinolysis and urinary fibrinolysis. Surgical complications following heart surgery and portacaval shunt in cancer of the lung, prostate, cervix, stomach, and other types of surgery associated with heavy postoperative bleeding. Aplastic anemia. *Investigational:* Prevention of recurrence of subarachnoid hemorrhage, megakaryocytic thrombocytopenia, prophylaxis and treatment of hereditary angioneurotic edema, acute promyelocytic leukemia with accompanying coagulopathy.

Dosage

- **Syrup, Tablets**

Acute bleeding.

Initial priming dose: 5 g during first hour; **then,** 1–1.25 g q hr for 8 hr or until bleeding is controlled. **Maximum daily dose:** 30 g.

After prostatic surgery.

6 g over the first 24 hr may be sufficient.

Prevention of hemorrhage after dental surgery.

6 g immediately after surgery followed by 6 g q 6 hr for 9–19 days.

- **IV infusion**

Acute bleeding.

Initial priming dose: 4–5 g during first hour; **then,** 1 g q hr for 8 hr (or until desired response is obtained).

Subarachnoid hemorrhage, recurrent.

36 g/day (18 g in 400 mL 5 % dextrose solution infused over 12 hr) for 10 days. Switch to PO therapy after this time.

Administration/Storage

1. For IV use, may be mixed with saline, 5% dextrose, sterile water, or Ringer's solution. It should *never* be injected undiluted.
2. For IV, priming dose (4–5 g) is dissolved in 250 mL of solution; continuous infusion is at the rate of 1–1.25 g/hr for 8 hr in 50–100 mL of diluent.
3. Infusions should be administered utilizing an electronic infusion device.
4. Keep tablets and raspberry-flavored syrup out of the reach of children.
5. Have available vitamin K or protamine sulfate for emergency use.

Contraindication: Clients with active, intravascular clotting possibly associated with fibrinolysis and bleeding.

Special Concerns: Use with caution, or not at all, in clients with uremia or cardiac, renal, or hepatic disease. Use during pregnancy only if benefits clearly outweigh risks.

Laboratory Test Interferences: ↑ Serum aldolase, AST, CPK, and potassium.

Side Effects: *GI:* Nausea, cramping, diarrhea. *CNS:* Dizziness, malaise, headache, delirium; auditory, visual, and kinesthetic hallucinations. *CV:* Hypotension, thrombophlebitis. *Other:* Tinnitus, conjunctival suffusion, myopathies, nasal stuffiness, skin rash, prolongation of menses, reversible acute renal failure.

Drug Interactions

Anticoagulants, oral / ↓ Anticoagulant effects

Contraceptives, oral (Estrogen) / Combination with aminocaproic acid may lead to hypercoagulable condition

---

NURSING CONSIDERATIONS

Assessment

1. Note any history of prior incidence of cardiac, renal, or hepatic disease.
2. Determine if client is taking any oral contraceptives (estrogen). Interaction with aminocaproic acid can lead to hypercoagulable condition. Note presence of menses.
3. Obtain baseline CBC, platelet count, bleeding parameters, and liver and renal function studies.

Interventions

1. Monitor VS q 15 min during infusion. Observe for hypotension, bradycardia, and arrhythmias; symptoms indicating that the rate is too fast. Slow rate of IV infusion and report.
2. Monitor color, temperature, and pulses in all extremities. Observe carefully for S&S of thrombosis, such as leg pain, chest pain, positive Homan's sign or respiratory distress.
3. Note presence of adverse side effects such as nausea, cramping, or diarrhea and report.
4. If client is experiencing menses, observe for excessive bleeding.

Evaluate

- Control of bleeding
- Prevention of rebleeding in subarachnoid hemorrhage
- Hematologic parameters and coagulation factors within desired range

---

Antihemophilic factor (AHF, Factor VIII)

(an-tie-hee-moh-**FILL**-ick)

Pregnancy Category: C

Hemofil M, Koate-HP ✱, Koate-HS, Koate-HT, Monoclate **(Rx)**

How Supplied: *Powder for injection*

Action/Kinetics: Antihemophilic factor is either isolated from pooled normal human blood or is derived from monoclonal antibodies. AHF is essential for blood coagulation. The potency and purity of preparation vary but each lot is standardized. Details on the package should be noted. Plasma protein (factor VIII) accelerates abnormally slow transformation of prothrombin to thrombin. **t½:** 9–15 hr. One AHF unit is the activity found in 1 mL of normal pooled human plasma.

Use: Control of bleeding in clients suffering from hemophilia A (factor VIII deficiency and acquired factor VIII inhibitors).

Dosage

- **IV only**

Individualized, depending on severity of bleeding, degree of deficiency, body weight, and presence of inhibitors of factor VIII. *NOTE:* AHF levels may rise 2% for every unit of AHF per kilogram administered. Dosages given are only guidelines.

Mild hemorrhage.

Single infusion to achieve AHF levels of at least 30%. Dosage should not be repeated.

Minor surgery, moderate hemorrhage.

AHF levels should be raised to 30%–50% of normal. **Initial:** 15–25

IU/kg; **maintenance:** 10–15 IU/kg q 8–12 hr.

Severe hemorrhage.
Increase AHF levels to 80%–100% of normal. **Initial:** 40–50 IU/kg; **maintenance:** 20–25 IU/kg q 8–12 hr.

Major surgery.
Raise AHF levels to 80%–100% of normal. Administer 1 hr before surgery; one-half the priming dose may be given 5 hr after the first dose. AHF levels should be maintained at 30% of normal for at least 10–14 days.

Administration/Storage
1. AHF is labile and is inactivated rapidly: within 10 min at 56°C and within 3 hr at 49°C. Store vials at 2°C–8°C. Check expiration date. **Do not freeze.**
2. Warm the concentrate and diluent to room temperature before reconstitution.
3. Place one needle in the concentrate to act as an airway and then aseptically with a syringe and needle add the diluent to the concentrate.
4. Gently agitate or roll the vial containing diluent and concentrate to dissolve the drug. **Do not shake vigorously.**
5. Administer drug within 3 hr of reconstitution, to avoid incubation if contamination occurred during mixing.
6. Do not refrigerate drug after reconstitution, because the active ingredient may precipitate out.
7. Keep reconstituted drug at room temperature during infusion because, at a lower temperature, precipitation of active ingredients may occur.
8. Administer IV only using a plastic syringe (solutions stick to glass syringes). Medication should be administered at a rate of 2 mL/min although rates up to 10 mL/min can be used if necessary.

Contraindication: Use of monoclonal antibody-derived AHF in clients hypersensitive to mouse protein.

Side Effects: *Allergic:* Nausea, fever, hives, chills, urticaria, wheezing, hypotension, chest tightness, stinging at infusion site, ***anaphylaxis.*** Antibodies may form to the mouse protein found in AHF derived from monoclonal antibodies.

Antihemophilic factor contains traces of blood group A and B isohemagglutins. These may cause ***intravascular hemolysis*** in clients with types A, B, or AB blood.

Both hepatitis and AIDS may be transmitted from AHF prepared from human plasma.

NURSING CONSIDERATIONS

Assessment
1. Note blood type. Clients with A, B, and AB are more prone to hemolytic reactions.
2. Determine any recent trauma or injury.

Interventions
1. Document baseline VS and monitor q 5–15 min during infusion. If tachycardia and hypotension occur, slow IV and report.
2. Monitor H&H and factor levels and perform Coombs' test during therapy.
3. Document I&O. Assess urine for color and occult blood.
4. If the client complains of headaches, flushing, numbness, back pain, visual disturbances, or chest constriction or if you notice the client flushing, slow the IV, document, and report.
5. Premedicate with diphenhydramine to reduce allergic reactions.

Client/Family Teaching
1. Review the appropriate method for storing and administering AHF at home.
2. Explain that the product is prepared from human plasma and identify the associated potential risks, such as hepatitis and HIV.
3. Determine client knowledge concerning disease process and hereditary transmission. Identify and reinforce any areas in need of clarification or emphasis to ensure compliance with therapy.
4. Local support groups may assist client to understand and cope with this illness; provide appropriate referrals.

Evaluate

- Prevention and control of bleeding with hemophilia A
- Promotion of normal clotting mechanisms
- Coagulation times and factor VIII levels within desired range

Factor IX Complex (Human)

(**FAK**-tor 9)
Pregnancy Category: C
Konyne-HT, Profilnine Heat-Treated, Proplex SX-T, Proplex T **(Rx)**

How Supplied: *Powder for injection*

Action/Kinetics: This product provides factors II, VII, IX, and X; thus, homeostasis can be restored. **t½:** 24 hr. A unit is the activity present (as factor IX) in 1 mL of normal plasma less than 1 hr old.

Uses: For clients with factor IX deficiency, especially hemophilia B and Christmas disease. Clients with inhibitors to factor VIII. To reverse hemorrhage induced by coumarin. To control or prevent bleeding in clients with factor VII deficiency (Proplex T only).

Dosage

• IV

Individualized, depending on severity of bleeding, degree of deficiency, body weight, and level of factor required. Minimum factor IX level required in surgery or following trauma is 25% of normal, which is maintained for 1 week after surgery. As a guide in determining the units required to raise blood level percentages of factor IX, use the following formula:

1 unit/kg × body weight (kg) × desired increase (% of normal).

For factor VII deficiency, use 0.5 unit/kg × body weight (kg) × desired increase (% of normal). The dose may be repeated q 4–6 hr. The package insert should be checked carefully as a guideline for doses for various factor deficiencies.

Bleeding in hemophilia A clients with factor VIII inhibitors.

75 IU/kg followed in 12 hr by a second dose.

Prophylaxis of bleeding in hemophilia B clients.

10–20 IU/kg once or twice a week.

Administration/Storage

1. The rate of administration varies with the product. As a general guideline, infuse about 100 IU/min at a rate of 2–3 mL/min, not to exceed 3 mL/min.
2. Store at 2°C–8°C.
3. Avoid freezing the diluent provided with drug.
4. Discard 2 years after date of manufacture.
5. Before reconstitution, warm diluent to room temperature but not above 40°C.
6. Agitate the solution gently until the powder is dissolved.
7. Administer drug within 3 hr of reconstitution to avoid incubation in case contamination occurred during preparation.
8. Do not refrigerate after reconstitution, because the active ingredient may precipitate out.

Contraindications: Factor VII deficiency, except for Proplex T. Liver disease with suspected intravascular coagulation or fibrinolysis.

Special Concerns: Assess benefit versus risk prior to use in liver disease or elective surgery.

Side Effects: *CV:* ***Disseminated intravascular coagulation, thrombosis. High doses may cause MI, venous or pulmonary thrombosis.*** *Miscellaneous:* Chills, fever. *Symptoms due to rapid infusion:* N&V, headache, fever, chills, tingling, flushing, urticaria, and changes in BP.

Most of these side effects disappear when rate of administration is slowed.

The preparation also contains trace amounts of blood groups A and B and isohemagglutinins, which may cause intravascular hemolysis when administered in large amounts to clients with blood groups A, B, and AB.

Both hepatitis and AIDS may be transmitted using factor IX Complex since it is derived from pooled human plasma.

Drug Interaction: ↑ Risk of thrombosis if administered with aminocaproic acid.

NURSING CONSIDERATIONS

Assessment

1. Document previous experience and treatment with factor replacement and outcome.
2. Obtain client's weight, height, and blood type.
3. Note any complaints suggestive of liver disease (urticaria, fever, pruritus, anorexia, N&V) and monitor LFTs.
4. Determine that baseline CBC, coagulation, and factor levels are available and monitor throughout therapy.

Interventions

1. Obtain baseline BP and pulse and monitor q 30 min during infusion.
2. Observe for increased bleeding and joint swelling. Use rest, ice, and elevation with affected joints.
3. If a tingling sensation, headache, chills, or a fever occur, reduce the rate of flow and report.
4. Avoid aminocaproic acid administration. It may precipitate the development of thrombosis.
5. Monitor closely for disseminated intravascular coagulation if factor IX level is increased above 50% of normal. At 50% or greater, there is an increased risk for the development of a thromboembolic event and/or disseminated intravascular coagulation.
6. Make sure client has received hepatitis B vaccine.
7. Monitor I&O and test urine for occult blood. Hemolytic reactions are more pronounced in clients with A, B, and AB type blood.

Client/Family Teaching

1. Explain that product is prepared from human plasma and outline the associated potential risks.
2. Avoid contact sports and any activities that may lead to injury or excessive jostling.
3. Ensure that family members are screened as disease is hereditary.
4. Avoid aspirin-containing products.
5. Local support groups may assist client to understand and cope with this disease; provide appropriate referrals.

Evaluate

- Control of bleeding episodes with stable H&H and coagulation studies
- Factor levels within desired range

Microfibrillar Collagen Hemostat

(my-kroh-**FIB**-rih-lar **KOLL**-ah-jen **HEE**-moh-stat)
Avitene **(Rx)**

How Supplied: *Pad*; *Powder*; *Sponge*

Action/Kinetics: This product is purified bovine corium collagen prepared as the partial hydrochloric acid salt. Attracts platelets, which then release clotting factors that initiate formation of a fibrinous mass. Absorbable, water insoluble.

Uses: During surgery to control capillary bleeding and as an adjunct to hemostasis when conventional procedures are ineffectual or insufficient. It is ineffective in controlling systemic coagulation disorders.

Dosage

- **Topical**

Individualized depending on severity of bleeding.

Usual dose for capillary bleeding.

1 g for 50 cm^2. More for heavier flow.

Administration/Storage

1. Before applying dry product, compress surface to be treated with dry sponge. Use dry smooth forceps to handle.
2. Apply collagen hemostat directly to source of bleeding.
3. Once in place, apply pressure with a dry sponge (not a gloved hand) for up to 5 min, depending on severity of bleeding.
4. When controlling oozing from porous (cancellous) bone, pack collagen hemostat tightly into affected area. Tease off excess material after

5–10 min. Apply more in case of breakthrough bleeding.
5. Avoid spillage on nonbleeding surfaces, especially in the abdomen or thorax.
6. Remove excess material after a few minutes.
7. Do not reautoclave. Discard any unused portion.
8. Avoid contacting nonbleeding surfaces with microfibrillar collagen hemostat.
9. Dry forceps should be used to handle collagen hemostat as it will adhere to wet gloves or instruments.

Contraindications: Closure of skin incisions, because preparation may interfere with healing. On bone surfaces to which prosthetic materials will be attached. Intraocular use or for injection.

Special Concerns: Use during pregnancy only when benefits clearly outweigh risks.

Side Effects: Potentiation of infections, abscess formation, hematomas, wound dehiscence, mediastinitis. Formation of adhesions, foreign body or allergic reactions. *Following dental use:* Alveolalgia. *Following tonsillectomy:* ***Laryngospasm*** due to inhalation of dry material.

NURSING CONSIDERATIONS

Assessment

1. Document indications for therapy and type and onset of symptoms.
2. Obtain BP and pulse and assess for shock because collagen hemostat may mask a deeper hemorrhage by sealing off its exit site.

Evaluate: Promotion of clot formation with control of bleeding.

Central Nervous System Drugs

CHAPTER THIRTY-SIX

Anticonvulsants

See also the following individual entries:

- Acetazolamide
- Acetazolamide Sodium
- Carbamazepine
- Clonazepam
- Clorazepate Dipotassium—See Chapter 40
- Diazepam—See Chapter 40
- Felbamate
- Gabapentin
- Magnesium Sulfate—See Chapter 60
- Phenobarbital
- Phenobarbital Sodium
- Phenytoin (Diphenylhydantoin)
- Phenytoin Sodium, Extended
- Phenytoin Sodium, Parenteral
- Phenytoin Sodium Prompt
- Primidone
- *Succinimides*
  - Ethosuximide
  - Methsuximide
  - Phensuximide
- Valproic Acid

General Statement: Anticonvulsant agents are used for the control of the chronic seizures and involuntary muscle spasms or movements characteristic of certain neurologic diseases. They are most frequently used in the therapy of epilepsy, which results from disorders of nerve impulse transmission in the brain. Therapeutic agents cannot cure these convulsive disorders, but do control seizures without impairing the normal functions of the CNS. This is often accomplished by selective depression of hyperactive areas of the brain responsible for the convulsions. Therefore, these drugs are taken at all times (prophylactically) to prevent the occurrence of the seizures. There are several different types of epileptic disorders; the International Classification of Epileptic Seizures is as follows: I. Partial seizures which usually involve one brain hemisphere at onset. Seizures are either simple (where consciousness is not impaired) or complex (where consciousness is impaired). Simple seizures may be accompanied by motor symptoms (Jacksonian, adversive), somatosensory (or other sensory) symptoms, autonomic symptoms, or psychic symptoms. Complex seizures may be manifested by simple partial seizures at onset (followed by impaired consciousness) or impaired consciousness at onset. Either simple or complex seizures may evolve to generalized tonic-clonic seizures. II. Generalized seizures which involve both hemispheres of the brain at onset and where consciousness is usually impaired. Generalized seizures are further categorized as (a) absence (typical or atypical), (b) myoclonic, (c) clonic, (d) tonic, (e) tonic-clonic, or (f) atonic. III. Localization-related (focal) which are categorized as either idiopathic (benign focal epilepsy of childhood) or symptomatic (chronic progressive epilepsia partialis continua, temporal-lobe, or extratemporal). IV. Generalized epilepsy which is further categorized as (a) idiopathic (benign neonatal, childhood absence, or juvenile myoclonic convulsions) or (b) cryptogenic or symptomatic (infantile spasms–West syndrome, early myoclonic encephalopathy, Lennox–Gestaut syndrome, progressive myoclonic epilepsy). V. Special syndromes which includes febrile seizures. No single drug can control all types of epilepsy; thus, accurate diagnosis is important. Drugs effective against one type of epilepsy may not be effective against another. Anticonvulsant therapy must be individualized. Therapy begins with a small dose of the drug, which is continuously increased until either the seizures disappear or drug toxicity occurs. If a certain drug decreases the frequency of seizures but does not completely prevent them, another drug can be added to the dosage regimen and administered concomitantly with the first. Often a drug is ineffective and then another agent must be given. Failure of therapy most often results from the administration of doses too small to have a therapeutic effect or from failure to use two or more drugs together. If for any reason drug therapy is discontinued, the anticonvulsant drugs must be withdrawn gradually over a period of days or weeks to avoid severe, prolonged convulsions. This guideline also applies when one anticonvulsant is substituted for another; the dosage of the second drug is slowly increased at the same time that the dosage of the first drug is being reduced. With appropriate diagnosis and selection of drugs, four out of five cases of epilepsy can be controlled adequately, but it may take the physician some time to find the best drug or combination of drugs with which to treat the client.

Dosage

Dosage is highly individualized. However, trauma or emotional stress may necessitate an increase in drug dosage requirements (e.g., if the client requires surgery and starts having seizures). For details, see individual agents.

NURSING CONSIDERATIONS

Administration/Storage

1. Oral suspensions of drugs should be shaken thoroughly before pouring to ensure uniform mixing.
2. Drug therapy must be individualized according to the needs of the client.
3. Medication should not be discontinued abruptly unless the physician advises it. Withdrawal should occur over a period of days or weeks to avoid severe, prolonged convulsions.
4. If there is reason to substitute one anticonvulsant drug for another, the first drug should be withdrawn slowly at the same time the dosage of the second drug is being increased.
5. Be prepared, in case of acute oral toxicity, to assist with inducing emesis (provided the client is not comatose) and with gastric lavage, along with other supportive measures such as administration of fluids and oxygen.
6. *Treatment of Overdose:* Anticipate that peritoneal dialysis or hemodialysis may be instituted in the treatment of acute toxicity for barbiturates, hydantoins, and succinimides (hemodialysis only).

Assessment

1. Check the client's medical history for hypersensitivity to particular types of anticonvulsant drugs. Note the derivatives of that particular type as they should also be avoided.
2. Note the client's orientation as to

time and place, affect, reflexes, and VS and record as baseline data.
3. Document seizure classification because the medication is prescribed based on the type of seizure group (partial or generalized). Determine the frequency and severity of client's seizures, noting location, duration, consciousness, type, frequency and any precipitating factors, the presence of an aura, and any other reportable characteristics.
4. Assess the condition of the client's skin and mucous membranes.
5. If female and of childbearing age, determine the likelihood of pregnancy. Some of these drugs have been linked to fetal abnormalities.
6. Obtain CBC, blood glucose level, liver and renal function studies, and urinalysis prior to initiating therapy.
7. Determine why client is receiving therapy and when it was instituted. Seizure-free clients (i.e., those clients who have not experienced a seizure for over 1 year) receiving prophylactic therapy may generally have drugs gradually discontinued.

Interventions

1. During initial therapy, monitor BP, pulse, and respirations. Observe for S&S of impending seizures.
2. For clients who require IV administration of anticonvulsant drugs, monitor closely for respiratory depression and CV collapse.
3. Note any evidence of CNS side effects, such as complaints of blurred vision, dimmed vision, slurred speech, nystagmus, or confusion. Supervise ambulation until drug effects resolved.
4. Observe for muscle twitching, loss of muscle tone, episodes of bizarre behavior, and/or subsequent amnesia.
5. Frequently check for decreased levels of serum calcium since phenytoin can contribute to demineralization of bone. This can result in osteomalacia in adults and rickets in children. The risk is particularly great in clients who are inactive.
6. Check if client is to receive vitamin D supplementation to prevent hypocalcemia. The usual dose is 4,000 units of vitamin D weekly.
7. Clients who are to be on prolonged therapy need to have a diet rich in vitamin D.
8. Determine if the client is to receive folic acid supplements to prevent megaloblastic anemia.
9. Anticipate that vitamin K will be prescribed for pregnant women 1 month before delivery. This is to prevent postpartum hemorrhage and bleeding in the newborn and the mother.

Client/Family Teaching

1. Take the prescribed amount of drug ordered. The doses of anticonvulsant drugs are not to be increased, decreased, or discontinued without the provider's approval. There is a danger that convulsions may result.
2. During the initiation of therapy the anticonvulsant drugs may cause a decrease in mental alertness, drowsiness, headache, vertigo, and ataxia. CNS symptoms are often dose-related and may disappear with a change of dosage or continued therapy. Therefore, the client should be warned to avoid hazardous tasks until the drug therapy has been regulated and the symptoms disappear.
3. GI distress may be lessened by taking the drugs with large amounts of fluid or with food.
4. Provide a list of drug and food interactions as well as side effects associated with drug therapy. Explain what to do and when to report should these occur.
5. Instruct clients to report any unusual incidents in their life. The dosage of drug may require adjusting, especially if the client is undergoing physical trauma or emotional distress.
6. Avoid the use of alcohol and any other CNS depressants because they may interfere with the action of anticonvulsants.
7. For complaints of altered sleep patterns, explore the nature of the

disturbance and suggest ways to counteract the problem.
8. For alteration in bowel habits, suggest increased fluid intake and include fruit and other foods with roughage and bulk in the diet.
9. For clients who develop gingival hyperplasia, advocate the use of intensified oral hygiene, the use of a soft tooth brush, massage of the gums, and daily use of dental floss. It is also important to have routine dental visits.
10. If slurred speech develops, advocate slowing speech patterns to avoid the problem.
11. Review the importance of avoiding situations that result in fever, low glucose and low sodium levels as these conditions lower the seizure threshold.
12. If rash, fever, severe headaches, stomatitis, rhinitis, urethritis, or balanitis (inflammation of the glans penis) occur, instruct clients to report immediately. These are early symptoms of hypersensitivity and may require a change in medication.
13. Report sore throat, easy bruising, petechiae, or nosebleeds, all of which are signs of hematologic toxicity.
14. Instruct client to report jaundice, dark urine, anorexia, and abdominal pain. These may be signs of hepatotoxicity.
15. If the client is female and likely to become pregnant, discuss the possible effects of the medication on pregnancy.
16. If the client is a lactating mother, observe and report signs of toxicity in the nursing infant.
17. Stress the importance of regular liver function studies so as to detect early signs of hepatitis, hepatocellular degeneration, and fatal hepatocellular necrosis. Remind the client of the importance of reporting for all scheduled lab studies including CBC, renal and liver function studies as well as drug levels on a regular basis.
18. Individuals on anticonvulsant therapy should carry identification indicating the form of epilepsy and the prescribed drug therapy.
19. Encourage family/significant other to learn CPR. Explain how to protect client during a seizure.
20. Identify support groups (Epilepsy Foundation; National Head Injury Group) that may assist client and family to understand and cope with disorder.

Evaluate

- Evidence of compliance with the prescribed medication regimen
- ↓ Frequency of seizures with an improved level of seizure control
- Evidence of freedom from complications of drug therapy
- Laboratory confirmation that serum drug levels are within desired therapeutic range

Acetazolamide

(ah-set-ah-**ZOE**-la-myd)
Pregnancy Category: C
AK-Zol, Apo-Acetazolamide ✱, Dazamide, Diamox, Diamox Sequels
(Rx)

Acetazolamide sodium

(ah-set-ah-**ZOE**-la-myd)
Diamox **(Rx)**

See also *Anticonvulsants,* Chapter 36.

How Supplied: Acetazolamide: *Capsule, Extended Release:* 500 mg; *Tablet:* 125 mg, 250 mg
Acetazolamide sodium: *Powder for injection:* 500 mg

Action/Kinetics: Acetazolamide is a sulfonamide derivative possessing carbonic anhydrase inhibitor activity. As an anticonvulsant, beneficial effects may be due to inhibition of carbonic anhydrase in the CNS, which increases carbon dioxide tension resulting in a decrease in neuronal conduction. Systemic acidosis may also be involved. As a diuretic, the drug inhibits carbonic anhydrase in the kidney, which decreases formation of bicarbonate and hydrogen ions from carbon dioxide, thus reducing the availability of these ions for active transport. Use as a diuretic is limited because the drug promotes metabolic acidosis, which inhibits diuretic activity. This may be partially circumvented by giving acetazolamide on alternate days. Acetazolamide also reduces intraocular pressure.

Absorbed from the GI tract and widely distributed throughout the body, including the CNS. Excreted unchanged in the urine. **Tablets: Onset,** 60–90 min; **peak:** 1–4 hr; **duration:** 8–12 hr. **Sustained-release capsules: Onset,** 2 hr; **peak:** 3–6 hr; **duration:** 18–24 hr. **Injection (IV): Onset,** 2 min; **peak:** 15 min; **duration:** 4–5 hr. The drug is eliminated mainly unchanged through the kidneys.

Uses: Adjunct in the treatment of edema due to congestive heart failure, drug-induced edema. Absence (petit mal) and unlocalized seizures. Open-angle, secondary, or acute-angle closure glaucoma when delay of surgery is desired to lower intraocular pressure. Prophylaxis or treatment of acute mountain sickness in climbers attempting a rapid ascent or in those who are susceptible to mountain sickness even with gradual ascent.

Dosage

• **Extended-Release Capsules, Tablets, IV**

Epilepsy.

Adults/children: 8–30 mg/kg/day in divided doses. Optimum daily dosage: 375–1,000 mg (doses higher than 1,000 mg do not increase therapeutic effect).

If used as adjunct to other anticonvulsants.

Initial: 250 mg/day; dose can be increased up to 1,000 mg/day in divided doses if necessary.

Glaucoma, simple open-angle.

Adults: 250–1,000 mg/day in divided doses. Doses greater than 1 g/day do not increase the effect.

Glaucoma, closed-angle prior to surgery or secondary.

Adults, short-term therapy: 250 mg q 4 hr or 250 mg b.i.d. **Adults, acute therapy:** 500 mg followed by 125–250 mg q 4 hr using tablets. For extended-release capsules, give 500 mg b.i.d. in the morning and evening. IV therapy may be used for rapid decrease in intraocular pressure. **Pediatric:** 5–10 mg/kg/dose IM or IV q 6 hr or 10–15 mg/kg/day in divided doses q 6–8 hr using tablets.

Acute mountain sickness.

Adults: 250 mg b.i.d.–q.i.d. (500 mg 1–2 times/day of extended-release capsules). During rapid ascent, 1 g/day is recommended.

Diuresis in CHF.

Adults, initial: 250–375 mg (5 mg/kg) once daily in the morning. If the client stops losing edema fluid after an initial response, the dose should not be increased; rather, medication should be skipped for a day to allow the kidney to recover. The best diuretic effect occurs when the drug is given on alternate days or for 2 days alternative with a day of rest.

Drug-induced edema.

Adults: 250–375 mg once daily for 1 or 2 days. The drug is most effective if given every other day or for 2 days followed by a day of rest. **Children:** 5 mg/kg/dose orally or IV once daily in the morning.

Administration/Storage

1. Change over from other anticonvulsant therapy to acetazolamide should be gradual.
2. Acetazolamide tablets may be crushed and suspended in a cherry, chocolate, raspberry, or other sweet syrup. Vehicles containing glycerin or alcohol should not be used. As an alternative, 1 tablet may be submerged in 10 mL of hot water and added to 10 mL of honey or syrup.
3. For parenteral use, reconstitute each 500-mg vial with at least 5 mL of sterile water for injection. Use parenteral solutions within 24 hr after reconstitution, although reconstituted solutions retain potency for 1 week if refrigerated.
4. IV administration is preferred; IM administration is painful due to alkalinity of solution.

5. Reconstitute each 500-mg vial with at least 5 mL of sterile water for injection. For direct IV use, administer over at least 1 min. For intermittent IV use, further dilute in dextrose or saline solution and infuse over 4–8 hr.
6. Tolerance after prolonged use may necessitate dosage increase.
7. Do not administer the sustained-release dosage form as an anticonvulsant; it should be used only for glaucoma and acute mountain sickness.
8. When used for prophylaxis of mountain sickness, dosage should be initiated 1–2 days before ascent and should be continued for at least 2 days while at high altitudes.
9. Due to possible differences in bioavailability, brands should not be interchanged.
10. *Treatment of Overdose:* Emesis or gastric lavage. Hyperchloremic acidosis may respond to bicarbonate. Administration of potassium may also be necessary. Client should be observed carefully with supportive treatment given.

Contraindications: Low serum sodium and potassium levels. Renal and hepatic dysfunction. Hyperchloremic acidosis, adrenal insufficiency, suprarenal gland failure, hypersensitivity to thiazide diuretics, cirrhosis. Not to be used chronically in presence of noncongestive angle-closure glaucoma.

Special Concerns: Use with caution in the presence of mild acidosis and advanced pulmonary disease and during lactation. Increasing the dose of acetazolamide does not increase effectiveness and may increase the risk of drowsiness or paresthesia. Safety and efficacy have not been established in children.

Side Effects: *GI:* Anorexia, N&V, melena, constipation, alteration in taste, diarrhea. *GU:* Hematuria, glycosuria, urinary frequency, renal colic, renal calculi, crystalluria, polyuria, phosphaturia, decreased or absent libido, impotence. *CNS:* ***Seizures,*** weakness, malaise, fatigue, nervousness, drowsiness, depression, dizziness, disorientation, confusion, ataxia, tremor, headache, tinnitus, flaccid paralysis, lassitude, paresthesia of the extremities. *Hematologic:* ***Bone marrow depression,*** thrombocytopenic purpura, thrombocytopenia, ***hemolytic anemia,*** leukopenia, pancytopenia, agranulocytosis. *Dermatologic:* Pruritus, urticaria, skin rashes, erythema multiforme, ***Stevens-Johnson syndrome, toxic epidermal necrolysis,***photosensitivity. *Other:* Weight loss, fever, acidosis, electrolyte imbalance, transient myopia, hepatic insufficiency. *NOTE:* Side effects similar to those produced by sulfonamides may also occur.

Symptoms of Overdose: Drowsiness, anorexia, N&V, dizziness, ataxia, tremor, paresthesias, tinnitus.

Drug Interactions

Also see *Diuretics,* Chapter 75.
Amphetamine / ↑ Effect of amphetamine by ↑ renal tubular reabsorption
Cyclosporine / ↑ Levels of cyclosporine → possible nephrotoxicity and neurotoxicity
Diflunisal / Significant ↓ in intraocular pressure with ↑ side effects
Ephedrine / ↑ Effect of ephedrine by ↑ renal tubular reabsorption
Lithium carbonate / ↓ Effect of lithium by ↑ renal excretion
Methotrexate / ↓ Effect of methotrexate due to ↑ renal excretion
Primidone / ↓ Effect of primidone due to ↓ GI absorption
Pseudoephedrine / ↑ Effect of pseudoephedrine by ↑ renal tubular reabsorption
Quinidine / ↑ Effect of quinidine by ↑ renal tubular reabsorption
Salicylates / Accumulation and toxicity of acetazolamide (including CNS depression and metabolic acidosis). Also, acidosis due to acetazolamide may ↑ CNS penetration of salicylates

NURSING CONSIDERATIONS

See also *Nursing Considerations* for *Anticonvulsants,* Chapter 36.

Assessment

1. Obtain a complete nursing history, noting indications for drug use and type and onset of symptoms.

2. Review laboratory findings for levels of electrolytes, uric acid, and glucose. Document any evidence of liver and renal dysfunction prior to administering the medication.
3. Obtain a thorough drug history to ensure that the client is not receiving any drug therapy that interacts unfavorably with acetazolamide.
4. When administered for glaucoma, obtain baseline intraocular pressure recordings and assess for visual effects.
5. Perform a thorough pulmonary assessment in clients with CHF.

Client/Family Teaching

1. Taking the drug with food may decrease gastric irritation and GI upset.
2. The drug increases the frequency of voiding. Therefore, take the medication early in the day to avoid interrupting sleep.
3. Increase fluid intake (2–3 L/day) to prevent crystalluria and stone formation.
4. Take only as directed. If prescribed every other day or with rest days in between (as with CHF), utilize a log for documenting administration to enhance compliance.
5. Clients with diabetes should be warned that the drug may increase blood glucose levels. Therefore, they should monitor serum glucose levels carefully and report increases because the dose of hypoglycemic agent may require adjustment.
6. If nausea, dizziness, muscle weakness, or cramps occur, notify provider.
7. Report any changes in the color and consistency of stools.
8. Emphasize importance of reporting for scheduled laboratory studies.
9. Determine drug effects before undertaking tasks that require mental alertness.

Evaluate

- ↓ Seizure activity
- ↓ Intraocular pressure
- ↓ CHF-associated edema
- Prevention of mountain sickness

Carbamazepine

(kar-bah-**MAYZ**-eh-peen)
Pregnancy Category: C
Apo-Carbamazepine ✱, Epitol, Novo-Carbamaz ✱, Tegretol, Tegretol Chewtabs ✱, Tegretol CR ✱ **(Rx)**

See also *Anticonvulsants,* Chapter 36.

How Supplied: *Chew Tablet:* 100 mg; *Suspension:* 100 mg/5 mL; *Tablet:* 200 mg

Action/Kinetics: Carbamazepine is chemically similar to the cyclic antidepressants. It also manifests antimanic, antineuralgic, antidiuretic, anticholinergic, antiarrhythmic, and antipsychotic effects. The anticonvulsant action is not known but may involve depressing activity in the nucleus ventralis anterior of the thalamus. Due to the potentially serious blood dyscrasias, a benefit-to-risk evaluation should be undertaken before the drug is instituted. **Peak serum levels:** 4–5 hr. **t½** (serum): 12–17 hr with repeated doses. **Therapeutic serum levels:** 4–12 mcg/mL. Carbamazepine is metabolized in the liver to an active metabolite (epoxide derivative) with a half-life of 5–8 hr. Metabolites are excreted through the feces and urine.

Uses: Epilepsy, especially partial seizures with simple or complex symptomatology. Clonic-tonic seizures, psychomotor epilepsy, and diseases with mixed seizure patterns. Carbamazepine is often a drug of choice due to its low incidence of side effects. To treat pain associated with tic douloureux (trigeminal neuralgia) and glossopharyngeal neuralgia. *Investigational:* Neurogenic diabetes insipidus, alcohol and benzodiazepine withdrawal, cocaine withdrawal, herpes zoster, selected psychiatric disorders such as resistant schizophrenia, dyscontrol syndrome with limbic system dysfunction, bipolar disorders, explosive disorder, borderline personality disorder, poststroke pain, restless leg syndrome.

Dosage

• **Oral Suspension, Tablets, Chewable Tablets, Extended-Release Tablets**

Anticonvulsant.

Adults and children over 12 years, initial: 200 mg b.i.d. on day 1. Increase by 200 mg/day at weekly intervals until best response is attained. Divide total dose and administer q 6–8 hr. **Maximum dose, children 12–15 years:** 1,000 mg/day; **adults and children over 15 years:** 1,200 mg/day. **Maintenance:** decrease dose gradually to 800–1,200 mg/day. **Children, 6–12 years: initial,** 100 mg b.i.d. on day 1; **then,** increase slowly, at weekly intervals, by 100 mg/day; dose is divided and given q 6–8 hr. Daily dose should not exceed 1,000 mg. **Maintenance:** 400–800 mg/day. **Children, less than 6 years:** 10–20 mg/kg/day in two to three divided doses; dose can be increased slowly in weekly increments to maintenance levels of 250–300 mg/day (not to exceed 400 mg/day).

Trigeminal neuralgia.

Initial: 100 mg b.i.d. on day 1; increase by no more than 200 mg/day, using increments of 100 mg q 12 hr as needed, up to maximum of 1,200 mg/day. **Maintenance: Usual:** 400–800 mg/day (range: 200–1,200 mg/day). Attempt discontinuation of drug at least 1 time q 3 months.

Administration/Storage

1. Do not administer for a minimum of 2 weeks after client has received MAO inhibitor drugs.
2. Protect tablets from moisture.
3. The therapy should be started gradually with the lowest doses of drug to minimize adverse reactions.
4. Carbamazepine should be added gradually to other anticonvulsant therapy. The other anticonvulsant dosage may be maintained or decreased except for phenytoin, which may need to be increased.
5. *Treatment of Overdose:* Stomach should be irrigated completely even if more than 4 hr has elapsed following drug ingestion. Activated charcoal, 50–100 g initially, using a NGT (dose of 12.5 or more g/hr until client is symptom free). Diazepam or phenobarbital may be used to treat seizures (although they may aggravate respiratory depression, hypotension, and coma). Respirations should be monitored.

Contraindications: History of bone marrow depression. Hypersensitivity to drug or tricyclic antidepressants. Lactation. In clients taking MAO inhibitors. Should not be used to relieve general aches and pains.

Special Concerns: Safety and effectiveness have not been established in children less than 6 years of age. Use with caution in glaucoma and in hepatic, renal, and CV disease. Use with caution in clients with mixed seizure disorder that includes atypical absence seizures (carbamazepine not effective). Use in geriatric clients may cause an increased incidence of confusion, agitation, AV heart block, syndrome of inappropriate antidiuretic hormone, and bradycardia.

Side Effects: *GI:* N&V (common), diarrhea, constipation, abdominal pain or upset, anorexia, glossitis, stomatitis, dryness of mouth and pharynx. *Hematologic:* ***Aplastic anemia,*** leukopenia, eosinophilia, thrombocytopenia, purpura, ***agranulocytosis,*** leukocytosis, pancytopenia, ***bone marrow depression.*** *CNS:* Dizziness, drowsiness and unsteadiness (common); headache, fatigue, confusion, speech disturbances, visual hallucinations, depression with agitation, talkativeness, hyperacusis, abnormal involuntary movements, behavioral changes in children. *CV:* CHF, hypertension, hypotension, syncope, thrombophlebitis, worsening of angina, ***arrhythmias (including AV block).*** *GU:* Urinary frequency or retention, oliguria, impotence, renal failure, azotemia, albuminuria, glycosuria, increased BUN. *Dermatologic:* Pruritus, urticaria, photosensitivity, exfoliative dermatitis, erythematous rashes, alterations in pigmentation, alopecia, sweating, purpura, aggravation of toxic epidermal necrolysis (Lyell's syndrome), ***Stevens-Johnson syn-***

drome, aggravation of SLE, alopecia, erythema nodosum or multiforme. *Ophthalmologic:* Nystagmus, double vision, blurred vision, oculomotor disturbances, conjunctivitis; scattered, punctate lens opacities. *Other:* Peripheral neuritis, paresthesias, tinnitus, fever, chills, joint and muscle aches and cramps, adenopathy or lymphadenopathy, dyspnea, pneumonitis, pneumonia, inappropriate ADH secretion syndrome.

Symptoms of Overdose: Neuromuscular disturbances, irregular breathing, ***respiratory depression,*** tachycardia, hypo- or hypertension, conduction disorders, ***shock, seizures, impaired consciousness (deep coma possible),*** motor restlessness, muscle twitching or tremors, athetoid movements, ataxia, drowsiness, dizziness, nystagmus, mydriasis, psychomotor disturbances, hyperreflexia followed by hyporeflexia, opisthotonos, dysmetria, urinary retention, N&V, anuria or oliguria.

Drug Interactions

Acetaminophen / ↑ Breakdown of acetaminophen → ↓ effect and ↑ risk of hepatotoxicity
Charcoal / ↓ Effect of carbamazepine due to ↓ absorption from GI tract
Cimetidine / ↑ Effect of carbamazepine due to ↓ breakdown by liver
Contraceptives, oral / ↓ Effect of contraceptives due to ↑ breakdown by liver
Danazol / ↑ Effect of carbamazepine due to ↓ breakdown by liver
Desmopressin / ↑ Effect of desmopressin
Diltiazem / ↑ Effect of carbamazepine due to ↓ breakdown by liver
Doxycycline / ↓ Effect of doxycycline due to ↑ breakdown by liver
Erythromycin / ↑ Effect of carbamazepine due to ↓ breakdown by liver
Ethosuximide / ↓ Effect of ethosuximide due to ↑ breakdown by liver
Haloperidol / ↓ Effect of haloperidol due to ↑ breakdown by liver
Isoniazid / ↑ Effect of carbamazepine due to ↓ breakdown by liver; also, carbamazepine may ↑ risk of isoniazid-induced hepatotoxicity
Lithium / ↑ CNS toxicity
Lypressin / ↑ Effect of lypressin
MAO inhibitors / Exaggerated side effects of carbamazepine
Muscle relaxants, nondepolarizing / ↓ Effect of muscle relaxants
Nicotinamide / ↑ Effect of carbamazepine due to ↓ breakdown by liver
Phenobarbital / ↓ Effect of carbamazepine due to ↑ breakdown by liver
Phenytoin / ↓ Effect of carbamazepine due to ↑ breakdown by liver; also, phenytoin levels may ↑ or ↓
Primidone / ↓ Effect of carbamazepine due to ↑ breakdown by liver
Propoxyphene / ↑ Effect of carbamazepine due to ↓ breakdown by liver
Theophyllines / ↓ Effect of theophylline
Tricyclic antidepressants / ↓ Effect of tricyclic antidepressants due to ↑ breakdown by liver
Troleandomycin / ↑ Effect of carbamazepine due to ↓ breakdown by liver
Valproic acid / ↓ Effect of valproic acid due to ↑ breakdown by liver; half-life of carbamazepine may be ↑
Vasopressin / ↑ Effect of vasopressin
Verapamil / ↑ Effect of carbamazepine due to ↓ breakdown by liver
Warfarin sodium / ↓ Effect of anticoagulant due to ↑ breakdown by liver

NURSING CONSIDERATIONS

See also *Nursing Considerations* for *Anticonvulsants,* Chapter 36.

Assessment

1. Obtain baseline hematologic, liver, and renal function tests. Do not initiate therapy until significant abnormalities have been ruled out.
2. Note eye examinations for evidence of opacities and baseline intraocular pressure measurement.

3. Assess for a history of psychosis because drug may activate symptoms.
4. Document indications for therapy and include pretreatment findings.

Interventions

1. CNS depression may impair client functions. If the client becomes agitated, side rails should be used.
2. CBC evaluation should be done on a weekly basis for the first 3 months of therapy, and monthly thereafter. The following guide should be used to determine the extent of bone marrow depression:
• Erythrocyte count less than 4 million/mm^3
• Hematocrit less than 32%
• Hemoglobin less than 11 g%
• Leukocytes less than 4,000/mm^3
• Reticulocytes less than 0.3% of erythrocytes (20,000/mm^3)
• Serum iron greater than 150 mcg%
3. Carbamazepine should be discontinued slowly at the first sign of a blood cell disorder.
4. Monitor I&O ratios and VS for evidence of fluid retention, renal failure, or CV complications during the period of dosage adjustment.
5. An EEG should be obtained periodically throughout the therapy.
6. If the drug has been withdrawn quickly, use seizure precautions. Quick withdrawal may precipitate status epilepticus.

Client/Family Teaching

1. Take drug with meals to minimize GI upset.
2. Withhold drug and report if any of the following symptoms occur:
• Fever, sore throat, mouth ulcers, easy bruising, petechial and purpuric hemorrhages. These are early signs of bone marrow depression.
• Urinary frequency, acute urinary retention, oliguria, and sexual impotence. These are early signs of GU dysfunction.
• Symptoms of CHF, syncope, collapse, edema, thrombophlebitis, or cyanosis. These are CV side effects that require immediate attention.
3. Use caution in operating an automobile or other dangerous machinery because the drug may interfere with vision and coordination.
4. Report any skin eruptions or changes in skin pigmentation. These may require withdrawal of the drug.
5. Avoid excessive sunlight and wear protective clothing and sunscreen because of the risk of photosensitivity.
6. Stress the importance of reporting for scheduled laboratory studies to assess for early organ dysfunction.

Evaluate

• Control of refractory seizures
• ↓ Manic and psychotic manifestations
• ↓ Pain associated with trigeminal neuralgia

Clonazepam

(kloh-**NAY**-zeh-pam)
Klonopin, Rivotril ✦ **(C-IV) (Rx)**

See also *Anticonvulsants,* Chapter 36. and *Anti-Anxiety/Antimanic Drugs,* Chapter 40.

How Supplied: *Tablet:* 0.5 mg, 1 mg, 2 mg

Action/Kinetics: Benzodiazepine derivative. Clonazepam increases presynaptic inhibition and suppresses the spread of seizure activity. **Peak plasma levels:** 1–2 hr. **t½:** 18–50 hr. **Peak serum levels:** 20–80 ng/mL. The drug is more than 80% bound to plasma protein; it is metabolized almost completely in the liver to inactive metabolites, which are excreted in the urine.

Even though a benzodiazepine, clonazepam, is used only as an anticonvulsant. However, contraindications, side effects, and so forth are similar to those for diazepam.

Uses: Absence seizures (petit mal) including Lennox-Gastaut syndrome, akinetic and myoclonic seizures. Some effectiveness in clients resistant to succinimide therapy. *Investigational:* Parkinsonian dysarthria, acute manic episodes of bipolar affective disorder, leg movements (periodic) during sleep, adjunct in treating schizophrenia, neuralgias, multifocal tic disorders.

Dosage

• **Tablets**

Seizure disorders.
Adults, initial: 0.5 mg t.i.d. Increase by 0.5–1 mg/day q 3 days until seizures are under control or side effects become excessive; **maximum:** 20 mg/day. **Pediatric up to 10 years or 30 kg:** 0.01–0.03 mg/kg/day in two to three divided doses up to a maximum of 0.05 mg/kg/day. Increase by increments of 0.25–0.5 mg q 3 days until seizures are under control or maintenance of 0.1–0.2 mg/kg is attained.

Parkinsonian dysarthria.
Adults: 0.25–0.5 mg/day.

Acute manic episodes of bipolar affective disorder.
Adults: 0.75–16 mg/day.

Periodic leg movements during sleep.
Adults: 0.5–2 mg nightly.

Adjunct to treat schizophrenia.
Adults: 0.5–2 mg/day.

Neuralgias.
Adults: 2–4 mg/day.

Multifocal tic disorders.
Adults: 1.5–12 mg/day.

Administration/Storage
1. Approximately one-third of clients show some loss of anticonvulsant activity within 3 months; adjustment of dose may reestablish effectiveness.
2. Adding clonazepam to existing anticonvulsant therapy may increase the depressant effects.
3. The daily dose should be divided into three equal doses; if doses cannot be divided equally, the largest dose should be given at bedtime.

Contraindications: Sensitivity to benzodiazepines. Severe liver disease, acute narrow-angle glaucoma. Pregnancy.

Special Concern: Effects during pregnancy and lactation are not known.

Additional Side Effects: In clients in whom different types of seizure disorders exist, clonazepam may elicit or precipitate ***grand mal seizures.***

Drug Interactions
CNS depressants / Potentiation of CNS depressant effect of clonazepam
Phenobarbital / ↓ Effect of clonazepam due to ↑ breakdown by liver
Phenytoin / ↓ Effect of clonazepam due to ↑ breakdown by liver
Valproic acid / ↑ Chance of absence seizures

NURSING CONSIDERATIONS

See also *Nursing Considerations* for *Anti-Anxiety/Antimanic Drugs,* Chapter 40. and *Anticonvulsants,* Chapter 36.

Assessment: Document indications for therapy and onset/cause of symptoms; list other agents prescribed and the outcome.

Evaluate: ↓ Number and frequency of seizures.

Felbamate

(**FELL**-bah-mayt)
Pregnancy Category: C
Felbatol **(Rx)**

See also *Anticonvulsants* Chapter 36.

NOTE: In August 1994 it was recommended that felbamate treatment be discontinued for epilepsy clients due to several cases of aplastic anemia. Revised labeling states, "...Felbatol should only be used in patients whose epilepsy is so severe that the risk of aplastic anemia is deemed acceptable in light of the benefits conferred by its use..."

How Supplied: *Suspension:* 600 mg/5 mL; *Tablet:* 400 mg, 600 mg

Action/Kinetics: The precise mechanism of action is not known, but felbamate may reduce seizure spread and increase seizure threshold. The drug has weak inhibitory effects on GABA receptor binding and benzodiazepine receptor binding. Felbamate is well absorbed after PO use. **Terminal $t^1/_2$:** 20–23 hr. Trough blood levels are dose dependent. From 40% to 50% of an absorbed dose is excreted unchanged in the urine.

Uses: Alone or as part of adjunctive therapy for the treatment of partial seizures with and without generalization in adults with epilepsy. As an adjunct in the treatment of partial and generalized seizures associated with Lennox-Gastaut syndrome in children.

Dosage

• **Suspenion, Tablets**

Monotherapy, initial therapy.

Adults over 14 years of age, initial: 1,200 mg/day in divided doses t.i.d.–q.i.d. The dose may be increased in 600-mg increments q 2 weeks to 2,400 mg/day based on clinical response and thereafter to 3,600 mg/day, if needed.

Conversion to monotherapy.

Adults: Initiate at 1,200 mg/day in divided doses t.i.d.–q.i.d. Reduce the dose of concomitant antiepileptic drugs by ⅓ at initiation of felbamate therapy. At week 2, the felbamate dose should be increased to 2,400 mg/day while reducing the dose of other antiepileptic drugs up to another ⅓ of the original dose. At week 3, increase the felbamate dose to 3,600 mg/day and continue to decrease the dose of other antiepileptic drugs as indicated by response.

Adjunctive therapy.

Adults: Add felbamate at a dose of 1,200 mg/day in divided doses t.i.d.–q.i.d. while reducing current antiepileptic drugs by 20%. Further decreases of concomitant antiepileptic drugs may be needed to minimize side effects due to drug interactions. The dose of felbamate can be increased by 1,200-mg/day increments at weekly intervals to 3,600 mg/day.

Lennox-Gastaut syndrome in children, aged 2–14 years.

As an adjunct, add felbamate at a dose of 15 mg/kg/day in divided doses t.i.d.–q.i.d. while decreasing present antiepileptic drugs by 20%. Further decreases in antiepileptic drug dosage may be needed to minimize side effects due to drug interactions. The dose of felbamate may be increased by 15-mg/kg/day increments at weekly intervals to 45 mg/kg/day.

Administration/Storage

1. The suspension should be shaken well before using.
2. The medication should be stored in a tightly closed container at room temperature away from heat, direct sunlight, or moisture and away from children.
3. Most side effects seen during adjunctive therapy are resolved as the dose of concomitant antiepileptic drugs is decreased.

Special Concerns: Use with caution in clients who are hypersensitive to carbamates. Use with caution during lactation. Safety and efficacy have not been established in children other than those with Lennox-Gastaut syndrome.

Laboratory Test Interferences: ↑ ALT, AST, gamma-glutamyl transpeptidase, LDH, alkaline phosphatase, CPK. Hypophosphatemia, hypokalemia, hyponatremia.

Side Effects: May differ depending on whether the drug is used as monotherapy or adjunctive therapy in adults or for Lennox-Gastaut syndrome in children. *CNS:* Insomnia, headache, anxiety, somnolence, dizziness, nervousness, tremor, abnormal gait, depression, paresthesia, ataxia, stupor, abnormal thinking, emotional lability, agitation, psychologic disturbance, aggressive reaction, hallucinations, euphoria, ***suicide attempt,*** migraine. *GI:* Dyspepsia, vomiting, constipation, diarrhea, dry mouth, nausea, anorexia, abdominal pain, hiccoughs, esophagitis, increased appetite. *Respiratory:* Upper respiratory tract infection, rhinitis, sinusitis, pharyngitis, coughing. *CV:* Palpitation, tachycardia, SVT. *Body as a whole:* Fatigue, weight decrease or increase, facial edema, fever, chest pain, pain, asthenia, malaise, flu-like symptoms, ***anaphylaxis.*** *Ophthalmologic:* Miosis, diplopia, abnormal vision. *GU:* Urinary incontinence, intramenstrual bleeding, UTI. *Hematologic:* ***Aplastic anemia,*** purpura, leukopenia, lymphadenopathy, leukopenia, leukocytosis, thrombocytopenia, granulocytopenia, positive antinuclear factor test, ***agranulocytosis,*** qualitative platelet disorder. *Dermatologic:* Pruritus, urticaria, bullous eruption, buccal mucous membrane swelling, ***Stevens-***

Johnson syndrome. *Miscellaneous:* Otitis media, ***acute liver failure,*** taste perversion, hypophosphatemia, myalgia, photosensitivity, substernal chest pain, dystonia, allergic reaction.

Drug Interactions

Carbamazepine / Felbamate ↓ steady-state carbamazepine levels and ↑ steady-state carbamazepine epoxide (metabolite) levels. Also, carbamazepine → 50% ↑ in felbamate clearance

Phenytoin / Felbamate ↑ steady-state phenytoin levels necessitating a 40% decrease in phenytoin dose. Also, phenytoin ↑ felbamate clearance

Valproic acid / Felbamate ↑ steady-state valproic acid levels

NURSING CONSIDERATIONS

Assessment

1. Document indications for therapy and type and onset of seizures.
2. List all other medications prescribed for this condition and the outcome.
3. Note any hypersensitivity reactions to other carbamates.
4. Review other drugs prescribed to ensure none interact unfavorably and to determine the need for dosage adjustments.
5. Determine if monotherapy or adjunctive therapy is needed.

Client/Family Teaching

1. Take only as prescribed and store appropriately to prevent loss of felbamate effectiveness.
2. Explain side effects that are drug associated (e.g., anorexia, vomiting, insomnia, nausea, and headaches); instruct to report if persistent or bothersome.
3. Report any changes in mental status or loss of seizure control. Explain that dosage is determined by clinical response.
4. Do not stop taking medication suddenly without provider approval due to the possibility of increasing seizure frequency.
5. Explain the potentially lethal side effects of this drug therapy. Stress that the seizure control benefit should far outweigh the potential for development of aplastic anemia.

Evaluate: Control of seizures.

Gabapentin

(**gab**-ah-**PEN**-tin)

Pregnancy Category: C

Neurontin **(Rx)**

See also *Anticonvulsants,* Chapter 36.

How Supplied: *Capsule:* 100 mg, 300 mg, 400 mg

Action/Kinetics: The mechanism of action of gabapentin against seizures is not known. Food has no effect on the rate and extent of absorption; however, as the dose increases, the bioavailability decreases. **t½:** 5–7 hr. The drug is excreted unchanged through the urine.

Uses: In adults as an adjunct in the treatment of partial seizures with and without secondary generalization.

Dosage

- **Capsules**

  Anticonvulsant.

Adults: Dose range of 900–1,800 mg/day in three divided doses. Titration to an effective dose can begin on day 1 with 300 mg followed by 300 mg b.i.d. on day 2 and 300 mg t.i.d. on day 3. If necessary, the dose may be increased to 300–400 mg t.i.d., up to 1,800 mg/day. In clients with a creatinine clearance of 30–60 mL/min, the dose is 300 mg b.i.d.; if the creatinine clearance is 15–30 mL/min, the dose is 300 mg/day; if the creatinine clearance is less than 15 mL/min, the dose is 300 mg every other day.

Administration/Storage

1. Gabapentin should be taken at least 2 hr following antacid administration.
2. May be taken with or without food.
3. The first dose on day 1 may be taken at bedtime to minimize somnolence, dizziness, fatigue, and ataxia.
4. The maximum time between dos-

es in the t.i.d. daily schedule should not exceed 12 hr.
5. If gabapentin is discontinued or an alternate anticonvulsant is added to the regimen, this should be done gradually over a 1-week period.
6. *Treatment of Overdose:* Hemodialysis.

Special Concerns: Use during lactation only if benefits outweigh risks. Plasma clearance is reduced in geriatric clients and in those with impaired renal function. Safety and efficacy have not been determined in children less than 12 years of age.

Laboratory Test Interference: False + reading with Ames N-Multistix SG dipstick test for urinary protein.

Side Effects: Side effects listed are those with an incidence of 0.1% or greater.

CNS: Most commonly: somnolence, ataxia, dizziness, and fatigue. Also, nystagmus, tremor, nervousness, dysarthria, amnesia, depression, abnormal thinking, twitching, abnormal coordination, headache, ***convulsions (including the possibility of precipitation of status epilepticus),*** confusion, insomnia, emotional lability, vertigo, hyperkinesia, paresthesia, decreased/increased/absent reflexes, anxiety, hostility, CNS tumors, syncope, abnormal dreaming, aphasia, hypesthesia, ***intracranial hemorrhage,*** hypotonia, dysesthesia, paresis, dystonia, hemiplegia, facial paralysis, stupor, cerebellar dysfunction, positive Babinski sign, decreased position sense, subdural hematoma, apathy, hallucinations, decreased or loss of libido, agitation depersonalization, euphoria, "doped-up" sensation, ***suicidal tendencies,*** psychoses. *GI:* Most commonly: N&V. Also, dyspepsia, dry mouth and throat, constipation, dental abnormalities, increased appetite, abdominal pain, diarrhea, anorexia, flatulence, gingivitis, glossitis, gum hemorrhage, thirst, stomatitis, taste loss, unusual taste, increased salivation, gastroenteritis, hemorrhoids, bloody stools, fecal incontinence, hepatomegaly. *CV:* Hypertension, vasodilation, hypotension, angina pectoris, peripheral vascular disorder, palpitation, tachycardia, migraine, murmur. *Musculoskeletal:* Myalgia, fracture, tendinitis, arthritis, joint stiffness or swelling, positive Romberg test. *Respiratory:* Rhinitis, pharyngitis, coughing, pneumonia, epistaxis, dyspnea, apnea. *Dermatologic:* Pruritus, abrasion, rash, acne, alopecia, eczema, dry skin, increased sweating, urticaria, hirsutism, seborrhea, cyst, herpes simplex. *Body as a whole:* Weight increase, back pain, peripheral edema, asthenia, facial edema, allergy, weight decrease, chills. *GU:* Hematuria, dysuria, frequent urination, cystitis, urinary retention, urinary incontinence, vaginal hemorrhage, amenorrhea, dysmenorrhea, menorrhagia, breast cancer, inability to climax, abnormal ejaculation, impotence. *Hematologic:* Leukopenia, decreased WBCs, purpura, anemia, thrombocytopenia, lymphadenopathy. *Ophthalmologic:* Diplopia, amblyopia, abnormal vision, cataract, conjunctivitis, dry eyes, eye pain, visual field defect, photophobia, bilateral or unilateral ptosis, eye hemorrhage, hordeolum, eye twitching. *Otic:* Hearing loss, earache, tinnitus, inner ear infection, otitis, ear fullness.

Symptoms of Overdose: Double vision, slurred speech, drowsiness, lethargy, diarrhea.

Drug Interactions

Antacids / Antacids ↓ bioavailability of gabapentin
Cimetidine / Cimetidine ↓ renal excretion of gabapentin

NURSING CONSIDERATIONS

See also *Nursing Considerations* for *Anticonvulsants,* Chapter 36.

Assessment

1. Document indications for therapy and type and onset of symptoms, any other agents prescribed, and the outcome.
2. List other drugs prescribed to ensure that none interact unfavorably.
3. Obtain baseline renal function studies and anticipate reduced dose with impaired creatine clearance.

Interventions

1. When drug therapy is discontinued

or supplemental therapy is added, do so gradually over at least 1 week.
2. Anticipate reduced dosing in the elderly and those with impaired renal function.

Client/Family Teaching

1. Do not stop taking the drug abruptly.
2. Avoid antacids for 1 hr before or 2 hr after taking drug.
3. Drug may cause dizziness, fatigue, drowsiness, ataxia, and nystagmus. Do not perform any activities that require mental alertness until full drug effects are realized.
4. Report any unusual side effects or those that are not tolerable.

Evaluate: Control of seizure activity.

Phenobarbital

(fee-no-**BAR**-bih-tal)
Pregnancy Category: D
Solfoton **(C-IV) (Rx)**

Phenobarbital sodium

(fee-no-**BAR**-bih-tal)
Pregnancy Category: D
Luminal Sodium **(C-IV) (Rx)**

See also *Hypnotics,* Chapter 39.

How Supplied: Phenobarbital: *Capsule:* 16 mg; *Elixir:* 15 mg/5 mL, 20 mg/5 mL, 30 mg/5 mL; *Tablet:* 15 mg, 16 mg, 16.2 mg, 30 mg, 60 mg, 100 mg.
Phenobarbital sodium: *Injection:* 30 mg/mL, 60 mg/mL, 65 mg/mL, 130 mg/mL

Action/Kinetics: Long-acting. **t½:** 53–118 hr. **Onset:** 30 to more than 60 min. **Duration:** 10–16 hr. **Anticonvulsant therapeutic serum levels:** 10–40 mcg/mL. **Time for peak effect, after IV:** up to 15 min. Distributed more slowly than other barbiturates due to lower lipid solubility. Is 50%–60% protein bound.

Uses: PO: Sedative, hypnotic (short-term), anticonvulsant (partial and generalized tonic-clonic or cortical focal seizures); emergency control of acute seizure disorders such as status epilepticus, meningitis, tetanus, eclampsia, toxicity of local anesthetics. **Parenteral:** Sedative, hypnotic (short- term), preanesthetic, anticonvulsant, emergency control of acute seizure disorders.

Dosage

Phenobarbital, Phenobarbital Sodium.

• **Capsules, Elixir, Tablets**

Sedation.

Adults: 30–120 mg/day in two to three divided doses. **Pediatric:** 2 mg/kg (60 mg/m^2) t.i.d.

Hypnotic.

Adults: 100–200 mg at bedtime. **Pediatric:** Dose should be determined by physician, based on age and weight.

Anticonvulsant.

Adults: 60–100 mg/day in single or divided doses. **Pediatric:** 3–6 mg/kg/day in single or divided doses.

• **IM, IV**

Sedation.

Adults: 30–120 mg/day in two to three divided doses.

Preoperative sedation.

Adults: 100–200 mg IM only, 60–90 min before surgery. **Pediatric:** 1–3 mg/kg IM or IV 60–90 min prior to surgery.

Hypnotic.

Adults: 100–320 mg IM or IV.

Acute convulsions.

Adults: 200–320 mg IM or IV; may be repeated in 6 hr if needed. **Pediatric:** 4–6 mg/kg/day for 7–10 days to achieve a blood level of 10–15 mcg/mL (or 15 mg/kg/day, IV or IM).

Status epilepticus.

Adults: 15–20 mg/kg IV (given over 10–15 min); may be repeated if needed. **Pediatric:** 15–20 mg/kg given over a 10–15-min period.

Administration/Storage

1. When used for seizures, give the major fraction of the dose according to when seizures are likely to occur (i.e., on arising for daytime seizures and at bedtime when seizures occur at night).
2. When used as an anticonvulsant in infants and children, a loading dose of 15–20 mg/kg achieves blood levels of about 20 mcg/mL shortly after administration. In order to achieve therapeutic blood levels of 10–20 mcg/mL,

higher doses per kilogram may be necessary compared with adults.
3. When used IM, inject into a large muscle (e.g., gluteus maximus, vastus lateralis). Injection into or near peripheral nerves may cause permanent neurological deficit.
4. IV use should be reserved for conditions when other routes are not feasible. There is the possibility of overdose, including respiratory depression, even with slow injection of fractional doses.
5. In most cases, when used for epilepsy, drug must be taken regularly to avoid seizures, even when no seizures are imminent.
6. When used for seizures, the dose should be as low as possible in order to avoid adding to the depression that may follow seizures.
7. The aqueous solution for injection must be freshly prepared.
8. Some ready-dissolved solutions for injection are available; the vehicle is propylene glycol, water, and alcohol.
9. For IV administration, inject slowly at a rate of 50 mg/min.
10. Avoid extravasation as tissue damage and necrosis may result.

Special Concerns: The dose should be reduced in geriatric and debilitated clients as well as those with impaired hepatic or renal function.

Additional Side Effects: Chronic use may result in headache, fever, and megaloblastic anemia.

NURSING CONSIDERATIONS

See also *Nursing Considerations* for *Hypnotics,* Chapter 39.

Assessment

1. Document indications for therapy and type and onset of symptoms.
2. List other agents prescribed and the outcome.
3. Obtain baseline liver and renal function studies. Anticipate reduced dose with impairment in debilitated and elderly clients.

Client/Family Teaching

1. Take only as directed and do not stop abruptly.
2. Caution that drug may initially cause drowsiness and to assess drug effects before performing tasks that require mental alertness.
3. Phenobarbital may require an increase in vitamin D consumption. Review and encourage intake of foods that are high in vitamin D.
4. Drug decreases the effect of oral contraceptives. Other nonhormonal forms of birth control should be practiced during drug therapy.
5. Provide a printed list of side effects. Report any that are unusual, bothersome, or persistent.
6. Avoid alcohol and any OTC agents without approval.

Evaluate

- Desired level of sedation
- Control of seizures
- ↓ Serum bilirubin in the newborn
- Therapeutic anticonvulsant serum drug levels (10–40 mcg/mL)

Phenytoin (Diphenylhydantoin)

(**FEN**-ih-toyn, dye-**fen**-ill-hy-**DAN**-toyn)

Dilantin Infatab, Dilantin-30 Pediatric, Dilantin-125 **(Rx)**

Phenytoin sodium, extended

(**FEN**-ih-toyn)

Dilantin Kapseals **(Rx)**

Phenytoin sodium, parenteral

(**FEN**-ih-toyn)

Dilantin Sodium **(Rx)**

Phenytoin sodium prompt

(**FEN**-ih-toyn)

Diphenylan Sodium **(Rx)**

See also *Anticonvulsants* Chapter 36, and *Antiarrhythmic Agents,* Chapter 26.

How Supplied: Phenytoin: *Chew Tablet:* 50 mg; *Suspension:* 100 mg/4 mL, 125 mg/5 mL
Phenytoin sodium, extended: *Capsule, Extended Release:* 30 mg, 100 mg
Phenytoin sodium, parenteral: *Injection:* 50 mg/mL

Phenytoin sodium prompt: *Capsule:* 100 mg

Action/Kinetics: Phenytoin acts in the motor cortex of the brain to reduce the spread of electrical discharges from the rapidly firing epileptic foci in this area. This is accomplished by stabilizing hyperexcitable cells possibly by affecting sodium efflux. Also, phenytoin decreases activity of centers in the brain stem responsible for the tonic phase of grand mal seizures. This drug has few sedative effects.

Serum levels must be monitored because the serum concentrations of phenytoin increase disproportionately as the dosage is increased. Phenytoin extended is designed for once-a-day dosage. It has a slow dissolution rate—no more than 35% in 30 min, 30%–70% in 60 min, and less than 85% in 120 min. Absorption is variable following PO dosage. **Peak serum levels: PO,** 4–8 hr. Since the rate and extent of absorption depend on the particular preparation, the same product should be used for a particular client. **Peak serum levels (following IM):** 24 hr (wide variation). **Therapeutic serum levels:** 10–20 mcg/mL. **t½:** 8–60 hr (average: 20–30 hr). Steady state attained 7–10 days after initiation. Phenytoin is biotransformed in the liver. Both inactive metabolites and unchanged drug are excreted in the urine.

As an antiarrhythmic, phenytoin increases the electrical stimulation threshold of heart muscle, although it is less effective than quinidine, procainamide, or lidocaine. **Onset:** 30–60 min. **Duration:** 24 hr or more. **t½:** 22–36 hr. **Therapeutic serum level:** 10–20 mcg/mL.

Uses: Chronic epilepsy, especially of the tonic-clonic, psychomotor type. Not effective against absence seizures and may even increase the frequency of seizures in this disorder. Parenteral phenytoin is sometimes used to treat status epilepticus and to control seizures during neurosurgery. PO for certain PVCs and IV for PVCs and tachycardia. The drug is particularly useful for arrhythmias produced by digitalis overdosage.

Investigational: Paroxysmal choreoathetosis; to treat blistering and erosions in clients with recessive dystrophic epidermolysis bullosa; episodic dyscontrol; trigeminal neuralgia; as a muscle relaxant in neuromyotonia, myotonia congenita, or myotonic muscular dystrophy; to treat cardiac symptoms in overdosage of tricyclic antidepressants. Severe preeclampsia.

Dosage

• Oral Suspension, Chewable Tablets

Seizures.

Adults: 125 mg t.i.d. initially; adjust dosage at 7–10-day intervals until seizures are controlled; **usual, maintenance:** 300–400 mg/day, although 600 mg/day may be required in some. **Pediatric, initial:** 5 mg/kg/day in two to three divided doses; **maintenance,** 4–8 mg/kg (up to maximum of 300 mg/day). Children over 6 years may require up to 300 mg/day. **Geriatric:** 3 mg/kg initially in divided doses; **then,** adjust dosage according to serum levels and response. Once dosage level has been established, the extended capsules may be used for once-a-day dosage.

• Capsules, Extended-Release Capsules

Seizures.

Adults, initial: 100 mg t.i.d.; adjust dose at 7–10-day intervals until control is achieved. An initial loading dose of 12–15 mg/kg divided into two to three doses over 6 hr followed by 100 mg t.i.d. on subsequent days may be preferred if seizures are frequent. **Pediatric:** See dose for Oral Suspension and Chewable Tablets.

Arrhythmias.

Adults: 200–400 mg/day.

• IV

Status epilepticus.
Adults, loading dose: 10–15 mg/kg at a rate not to exceed 50 mg/min; **then,** 100 mg/ q 6–8 hr at a rate not exceeding 50 mg/min. PO administration at a dose of 5 mg/kg/day divided into two to four doses should begin 12–24 hr after a loading dose is given. **Pediatric, loading dose:** 15–20 mg/kg given at a rate of 1 mg/kg, not to exceed 50 mg/min.

Arrhythmias.
Adults: 100 mg/ q 5 min up to maximum of 1 g.

• **IM**
Dose should be 50% greater than the PO dose.

Neurosurgery.
100–200 mg/ q 4 hr during and after surgery (during first 24 hr, no more than 1,000 mg should be administered; after first day, give maintenance dosage).

Administration/Storage
1. Full effectiveness of PO administered hydantoins is delayed and may take 6–9 days to be fully established. A similar period of time will elapse before effects disappear completely.
2. When hydantoins are substituted for or added to another anticonvulsant medication, their dosage is gradually increased, while dosage of the other drug is decreased proportionally.
3. For parenteral preparations:
• Only a clear solution of the drug may be used.
• Dilute with special diluent supplied by manufacturer.
• Shake the vials until the solution is clear. It may take about 10 min for the drug to dissolve.
• To hasten the process, warm the vial in warm water after adding the diluent.
• The drug is incompatible with acid solutions.
4. IV phenytoin may form a precipitate. Therefore, flush tubing thoroughly with 0.9% NaCl before and after IV administration. *Do not* use dextrose solutions. Use an in-line filter to collect microscopic particulate matter.
5. *Do not* add phenytoin to an already running IV solution.
6. Following the IV administration of the drug, administer sodium chloride injection through the same needle or IV catheter to avoid local irritation of the vein. This is caused by alkalinity of the solution.
7. Avoid subcutaneous or perivascular injections. Pain, inflammation, and necrosis may be caused by the highly alkaline solutions.
8. For treatment of status epilepticus, inject the IV slowly at a rate not to exceed 50 mg/min. If necessary, the dose may be repeated 30 min after the initial administration.
9. If the client is receiving tube feedings of Isocal or Osmolite, there may be interference with the absorption of PO phenytoin. Therefore, do not administer them together.
10. *Treatment of Overdose:* Treat symptoms. Hemodialysis may be effective. In children, total exchange transfusion has been used.

Contraindications: Hypersensitivity to hydantoins, exfoliative dermatitis, sinus bradycardia, second- and third-degree AV block, clients with Adams-Stokes syndrome, SA block. Lactation.

Special Concerns: Use with caution in acute, intermittent porphyria. Administer with extreme caution to clients with a history of asthma or other allergies, impaired renal or hepatic function, and heart disease (hypotension, severe myocardial insufficiency). Abrupt withdrawal may cause status epilepticus. Combined drug therapy is required if petit mal seizures are also present.

Laboratory Test Interferences: Alters liver function tests, ↑ blood glucose values, and ↓ PBI values. ↑ Gamma globulins. Phenytoin ↓ immunoglobulins A and G. False + Coombs' test.

Side Effects: *CNS:* Most commonly, drowsiness, ataxia, dysarthria, confusion, insomnia, nervousness, irritability, depression, tremor, numbness, headache, psychoses, ***increased seizures.*** Choreoathetosis following IV use. *GI:* Gingival hyperplasia, N&V, either diarrhea or constipation. *Dermatologic:* Various dermatoses including a measles-like rash (common), scarlatiniform, maculopapular, and urticarial rashes. Rarely, drug-induced lupus erythematosus, ***Stevens-Johnson syndrome,*** exfoliative or purpuric dermatitis, and ***toxic epidermal necrolysis.*** Alopecia, hirsutism. Skin reactions may necessitate withdrawal of therapy. *Hematopoietic:* Leukopenia, granulocytopenia, thrombocytopenia, pancytopenia, ***agranulocytosis,*** macrocytosis, megaloblastic anemia, leukocytosis, monocytosis, eosinophilia, simple anemia, ***aplastic anemia, hemolytic anemia.*** *Hepatic:* Liver damage, toxic hepatitis, hypersensitivity reactions involving the liver including hepatocellular degeneration and ***fatal hepatocellular necrosis.*** *Ophthalmic:* Diplopia, nystagmus, conjunctivitis. *Miscellaneous:* Hyperglycemia, chest pain, edema, fever, photophobia, weight gain, ***pulmonary fibrosis,*** lymph node hyperplasia, gynecomastia, periarteritis nodosa, depression of IgA, soft tissue injury at injection site, coarsening of facial features, Peyronie's disease, enlarged lips.

Rapid parenteral administration may cause serious CV effects, including hypotension, arrhythmias, CV collapse, and heart block, as well as CNS depression.

Many clients have a partial deficiency in the ability of the liver to degrade phenytoin, and as a result, toxicity may develop after a small PO dose. Liver and kidney function tests and hematopoietic studies are indicated prior to and periodically during drug therapy.

Symptoms of Overdose: Initially, ataxia, dysarthria, and nystagmus followed by unresponsive pupils, hypotension, and ***coma.*** Plasma levels greater than 40 mcg/mL result in significant decreases in mental capacity.

Drug Interactions

Acetaminophen / ↓ Effect of acetaminophen due to ↑ breakdown by liver; however, hepatotoxicity may be ↑

Alcohol, ethyl / In alcoholics, ↓ effect of phenytoin due to ↑ breakdown by liver

Allopurinol / ↑ Effect of phenytoin due to ↓ breakdown in liver

Amiodarone / ↑ Effect of phenytoin or amiodarone due to ↓ breakdown by liver

Antacids / ↓ Effect of phenytoin due to ↓ GI absorption

Anticoagulants, oral / ↑ Effect of phenytoin due to ↓ breakdown by liver. Also, possible ↑ anticoagulant effect due to ↓ plasma protein binding

Antidepressants, tricyclic / May ↑ incidence of epileptic seizures or ↑ effect of phenytoin by ↓ plasma protein binding

Barbiturates / Effect of phenytoin may be ↑, ↓, or not changed; possible ↑ effect of barbiturates

Benzodiazepines / ↑ Effect of phenytoin due to ↓ breakdown by liver

Carbamazepine / ↓ Effect of phenytoin or carbamazepine due to ↑ breakdown by liver

Charcoal / ↓ Effect of phenytoin due to ↓ absorption from GI tract

Chloramphenicol / ↑ Effect of phenytoin due to ↓ breakdown by liver

Chlorpheniramine / ↑ Effect of phenytoin

Cimetidine / ↑ Effect of phenytoin due to ↓ breakdown by liver

Clonazepam / ↓ Plasma levels of clonazepam or phenytoin; or, ↑ risk of phenytoin toxicity

Contraceptives, oral / Estrogen-induced fluid retention may precipitate seizures; also, ↓ effect of contraceptives due to ↑ breakdown by liver

Corticosteroids / Effect of corticosteroids ↓ due to ↑ breakdown by liver; also, corticosteroids may mask hypersensitivity reactions due to phenytoin

Cyclosporine / ↓ Effect of cyclosporine due to ↑ breakdown by liver

Diazoxide / ↓ Effect of phenytoin due to ↑ breakdown by liver
Dicumarol / Phenytoin ↓ effect of dicumarol due to ↑ breakdown by liver
Digitalis glycosides / ↓ Effect of digitalis glycosides due to ↑ breakdown by liver
Disopyrimide / ↓ Effect of disopyramide due to ↑ breakdown by liver
Disulfiram / ↑ Effect of phenytoin due to ↓ breakdown by liver
Dopamine / IV phenytoin results in hypotension and bradycardia; also, ↓ effect of dopamine
Doxycycline / ↓ Effect of doxycycline due to ↑ breakdown by liver
Estrogens / See *Contraceptives, Oral*
Fluconazole / ↑ Effect of phenytoin due to ↓ breakdown by liver
Folic acid / ↓ Effect of phenytoin
Furosemide / ↓ Effect of furosemide due to ↓ absorption
Haloperidol / ↓ Effect of haloperidol due to ↑ breakdown by liver
Ibuprofen / ↑ Effect of phenytoin
Isoniazid / ↑ Effect of phenytoin due to ↓ breakdown by liver
Levodopa / Phenytoin ↓ effect of levodopa
Levonorgestrel / ↓ Effect of norgestrel
Lithium / ↑ Risk of lithium toxicity
Loxapine / ↓ Effect of phenytoin
Mebendazole / ↓ Effect of mebendazole
Meperidine / ↓ Effect of meperidine due to ↑ breakdown by liver; toxic effects of meperidine may ↑ due to accumulation of active metabolite (normeperidine)
Methadone / ↓ Effect of methadone due to ↑ breakdown by liver
Metronidazole / ↑ Effect of phenytoin due to ↓ breakdown by liver
Metyrapone / ↓ Effect of metyrapone due to ↑ breakdown by liver
Mexiletine / ↓ Effect of mexiletine due to ↑ breakdown by liver
Miconazole / ↑ Effect of phenytoin due to ↓ breakdown by liver
Nitrofurantoin / ↓ Effect of phenytoin
Omeprazole / ↑ Effect of phenytoin due to ↓ breakdown by liver
Phenacemide / ↑ Effect of phenytoin due to ↓ breakdown by liver
Phenothiazines / ↑ Effect of phenytoin due to ↓ breakdown by liver
Phenylbutazone / ↑ Effect of phenytoin due to ↓ breakdown by liver and ↓ plasma protein binding
Primidone / Possible ↑ effect of primidone
Pyridoxine / ↓ Effect of phenytoin
Quinidine / ↓ Effect of quinidine due to ↑ breakdown by liver
Rifampin / ↓ Effect of phenytoin due to ↑ breakdown by liver
Salicylates / ↑ Effect of phenytoin by ↓ plasma protein binding
Sucralfate / ↓ Effect of phenytoin due to ↓ absorption from GI tract
Sulfonamides / ↑ Effect of phenytoin due to ↓ breakdown in liver
Sulfonylureas / ↓ Effect of sulfonylureas
Theophylline / ↓ Effect of both drugs due to ↑ breakdown by liver
Trimethoprim / ↑ Effect of phenytoin due to ↓ breakdown by liver
Valproic acid / ↑ Effect of phenytoin due to ↓ breakdown by liver and ↓ plasma protein binding; phenytoin may also ↓ effect of valproic acid due to ↑ breakdown by liver

NURSING CONSIDERATIONS

See also *Nursing Considerations* for *Anticonvulsants,* Chapter 36, and *Antiarrhythmic Agents,* Chapter 26.

Assessment

1. Document indications for therapy and type and onset of symptoms.
2. Note the history and nature of the client's seizures, addressing location, frequency, duration, causes, and characteristics.
3. Determine if the client is hypersensitive to hydantoins or has exfoliative dermatitis.
4. If the client is female and pregnant, note that she should not breast-feed the baby following delivery.
5. Obtain baseline ECG hematologic, liver, and renal function studies and monitor throughout therapy.

Interventions

1. During IV administration, monitor BP closely for hypotension.

2. Monitor serum drug levels on a routine basis:

• Seven to 10 days may be required to achieve recommended serum levels. Drug is highly protein bound; may consider requesting free and bound drug levels to better assess response. The drug is metabolized much more slowly by elderly clients; thus most may be managed with once a day dosing.

• If the client is receiving drugs that interact with hydantoins or has impaired liver function, the level should be done more frequently. Dilantin induces hepatic microsomal enzymes for drug metabolism.

3. Oral form has variable absorption; do not administer with tube feedings. Administer separately, flush, and clamp tube for 20 min to ensure absorption.

Client/Family Teaching

1. May take with food to minimize GI upset. Do not take within 2–3 hr of antacid ingestion.

2. Refer to a dietitian as needed to review food intake and diet.

3. Review symptoms of overdose and instruct client to report if evident.

4. Use care when performing tasks that require mental alertness. Drug may cause drowsiness, dizziness, and blurred vision.

5. Do not substitute phenytoin products or exchange brands because bioavailability of phenytoin may vary. Seizure control may be lost or toxic blood levels may develop if a substitution is made.

6. Prompt-release forms of the medication cannot be substituted for another unless the dosage is also adjusted.

• If taking phenytoin extended, do not substitute chewable tablets for capsules. The strengths of the medications are not equal.

• Clients taking phenytoin extended should check the labels of the bottle carefully. Chewable tablets are never in the extended form.

• Clients taking phenytoin extended should take only a single dose of medication a day. It should be taken only as directed and only in the brand prescribed.

7. If the client misses a dose of medication, take the dose as soon as it is remembered. Then resume the usual schedule. Do not, however, double up to make up for the missed dose of drug. If the doses of drug are scheduled throughout the day, and one of the doses is missed, take the drug as soon as it is realized that the dose has been missed unless it is within 4 hr of the next dose of drug. In that case, omit the missed dose unless otherwise instructed.

8. Do not take any other medication without medical supervision. Hydantoins interact with many other medications, and the addition of other drugs may require adjustment of the anticonvulsant dose.

9. Avoid ingestion of alcohol in any form.

10. If the client has diabetes mellitus, blood glucose levels should be monitored frequently when initiating therapy or when the dosage of phenytoin is being adjusted. Report any changes in glucose determinations as it may be necessary to adjust insulin dosage and/or diet.

11. Warn that hydantoin may cause the urine to appear pink, red, or brown and not to be alarmed.

12. To minimize bleeding from the gums, practice good oral hygiene. Brush teeth with a soft toothbrush, massage the gums, and floss every day. Advise dentist of prescribed drug.

13. Hydantoin has an androgenic effect on the hair follicle. Clients may develop acne and should be encouraged to practice good skin care.

14. Report any excessive growth of hair on the face and trunk and any discolorations or skin rash as a dermatologist referral may be necessary.

15. Complaints of weakness, ease of fatigue, headaches, or feeling faint may be signs of folic acid deficiency or megaloblastic anemia. Dietitian evalu-

ation of food intake may be indicated as well as hematologic evaluations.
16. Stress the importance of reporting for lab studies as ordered, including a CBC, drug levels, and renal and liver function studies on a regular basis.
17. Explain that the drug may alter thyroid function results. If thyroid studies are conducted, for ensured accuracy, they should be repeated 10 days after therapy has been discontinued.
18. Do not abruptly stop medications. Report all bothersome side effects because these effects may be dose-related.
19. Provide sexually active women of childbearing age with birth control information as drug may interfere with oral contraceptives.

Evaluate

- Control of seizures
- Termination of ventricular arrhythmias
- Restoration of stable cardiac rhythm
- Therapeutic serum drug levels (10–20 mcg/mL)

Primidone

(PRIH-mih-dohn)
Apo-Primidone ✱, Mysoline **(Rx)**

How Supplied: *Suspension:* 250 mg/5 mL; *Tablet:* 50 mg, 250 mg
Action/Kinetics: Primidone is closely related to the barbiturates; however, the mechanism for its anticonvulsant effects is unknown. Primidone produces a greater sedative effect than barbiturates when used for seizure treatment. Side effects usually subside with use. **Peak plasma levels:** 3 hr. Primidone is converted in the liver to two active metabolites, phenobarbital and phenylethylmalonamide (PEMA). **Peak plasma levels (PEMA):** 7–8 hr. **t½ (primidone):** 3–24 hr; **t½ (PEMA):** 24–48 hr; **t½ (phenobarbital):** 72–144 hr. The appearance of phenobarbital in the plasma may be delayed several days after initiation of therapy. **Therapeutic plasma levels, primadone:** 5–12 mcg/mL; **phenobarbital,** 10–30 mcg/mL. Primidone and metabolites are excreted through the kidneys.
Uses: Psychomotor seizures, focal seizures, or refractory tonic-clonic seizures. May be used alone or with other drugs. Often reserved for client refractory to barbiturate-hydantoin regimen. *Investigational:* Benign familial tremor.

Dosage

- **Oral Suspension, Tablets**

Seizures, in clients on no other anticonvulsant medication.

Adults and children over 8 years, initial: Days 1–3, 100–125 mg at bedtime; days 4–6, 100–125 mg b.i.d.; days 7–9, 100–125 mg t.i.d.; **maintenance:** 250 mg t.i.d. (may be increased to 250 mg 5–6 times/day; daily dosage should not exceed 500 mg q.i.d.). **Children under 8 years, initial:** days 1–3, 50 mg at bedtime; days 4–6, 50 mg b.i.d.; days 7–9, 100 mg b.i.d.; **maintenance:** 125 mg b.i.d.–250 mg t.i.d. (10–25 mg/kg in divided doses).

Seizures, in clients receiving other anticonvulsants.

Initial: 100–125 mg at bedtime; **then,** increase to maintenance levels as other drug is slowly withdrawn (transition should take at least 2 weeks).
Contraindications: Porphyria. Hypersensitivity to phenobarbital. Lactation.
Special Concerns: Safe use during pregnancy has not been determined. Use during lactation may result in drowsiness in the neonate. Children and geriatric clients may react to primidone with restlessness and excitement. Due to differences in bioavailability, brand interchange is not recommended.
Side Effects: *CNS:* Drowsiness, ataxia, vertigo, irritability, general malaise, headache, fatigue, emotional disturbances, including mood changes and paranoia. *GI:* N&V, anorexia, painful gums. *Hematologic:* Megaloblastic anemia, leukopenia, thrombocytopenia. *Ophthalmologic:* Diplopia, nystagmus. *Miscellaneous:* Skin rash, edema of eyelids and legs, alopecia, impotence, morbilliform and maculopapular skin rashes. Occa-

sionally has caused hyperexcitability, especially in children. ***Postpartum hemorrhage and hemorrhagic disease of the newborn.*** Symptoms of SLE.

Drug Interactions

See also *Hypnotics,* Chapter 39.

Acetazolamide / ↓ Effect of primidone

Carbamazepine / ↑ Plasma levels of primidone and phenobarbital and ↑ plasma levels of carbamazepine

Hydantoins / ↑ Plasma levels of primidone, phenobarbital, and PEMA

Isoniazid / ↑ Effect of primidone due to ↓ breakdown by liver

Nicotinamide / ↑ Effect of primidone due to ↓ rate of clearance from body

Succinimides / ↓ Plasma levels of primidone and phenobarbital

NURSING CONSIDERATIONS

See also *Nursing Considerations* for *Anticonvulsants,* Chapter 36.

Assessment

1. Document age at onset of seizures and cause if known.
2. List any other agents prescribed and the outcome.

Client/Family Teaching

1. May be taken with food if GI upset occurs.
2. Review the goals of therapy and associated side effects of drug therapy. Instruct that the following conditions should be reported:
• Hyperexcitability in children
• Excessive loss of hair
• Edema of eyelids and legs
• Impotence
• Loss of seizure control
3. Remind the pregnant client that vitamin K may be prescribed during the last month of pregnancy. This is to prevent postpartum hemorrhage in the mother and hemorrhagic disease of the newborn.

Evaluate

• Control of refractory seizures
• Therapeutic serum drug levels (5–12 mcg/mL)

SUCCINIMIDES

See also the following individual entries:

Ethosuximide
Methsuximide
Phensuximide

General Statement: Three succinimide derivatives are currently used primarily for the treatment of absence seizures (petit mal): ethosuximide, methsuximide, and phensuximide. Ethosuximide is currently the drug of choice. Methsuximide should be used only when the client is refractory to other drugs. These drugs may be given concomitantly with other anticonvulsants if other types of epilepsy are manifested with absence seizures.

Action/Kinetics: The succinimide derivatives suppress the paroxysmal 3-cycle/sec spike and wave activity that is associated with lapses of consciousness seen in absence seizures. They apparently do so by depressing the motor cortex and by raising the threshold of the CNS to convulsive stimuli. The drugs are rapidly absorbed from the GI tract.

Use: Primarily absence seizures (petit mal).

Contraindications: Hypersensitivity to succinimides.

Special Concerns: Safe use during pregnancy has not been established. Must be used with caution in clients with abnormal liver and kidney function.

Side Effects: *CNS:* Drowsiness, ataxia, dizziness, headaches, euphoria, lethargy, fatigue, insomnia, irritability, nervousness, dream-like state, hyperactivity. Psychiatric or psychologic aberrations such as mental slowing, hypochondriasis, sleep disturbances, inability to concentrate, depression, night terrors, instability, confusion, aggressiveness. Rarely, auditory hallucinations, paranoid psychosis, increased libido, suicidal behavior. *GI:* N&V, hiccoughs, anorexia, diarrhea, gastric distress, weight loss, abdominal and epigastric pain, cramps, constipation. *Hematologic:* Leukopenia, granulocytopenia, eosinophilia, ***agranulocytosis,*** pancytopenia with or without bone marrow suppression, monocytosis. *Dermatologic:* Pruritus, urticaria, erythema multiforme, lupus erythematosus, ***Stevens-Johnson syndrome,*** pruritic erythematous rashes, skin eruptions, alopecia, hirsutism, photophobia. *GU:* Urinary frequency, vaginal bleeding, renal damage, microscopic hematuria. *Miscellaneous:* Blurred vision, muscle weakness, hyperemia, hypertrophy of gums, swollen tongue, myopia, periorbital edema.

Symptoms of Acute Overdose: Confusion, sleepiness, slow shallow respiration, N&V, ***CNS depression with coma and respiratory depression,*** hypotension, cyanosis, hyper- or hypothermia, absence of reflexes, unsteadiness, flaccid muscles.

Symptoms of Chronic Overdose: Ataxia, dizziness, drowsiness, confusion, depression, proteinuria, skin rashes, hangover, irritability, poor judgment, N&V, muscle weakness, periorbital edema, hepatic dysfunction, ***fatal bone marrow aplasia, delayed onset of coma,*** nephrosis, hematuria, casts.

Drug Interactions: Succinimides may increase the effects of hydantoins by decreasing breakdown by the liver.

Dosage

Individualized. See individual agents. Succinimides may be given in combination with other anticonvulsants if two or more types of seizures are present.

NURSING CONSIDERATIONS

See also *Nursing Considerations* for *Anticonvulsants,* Chapter 36.

Administration/Storage: *Treatment of Overdose:* General supportive measures. Charcoal hemoperfusion may be helpful.

Client/Family Teaching

1. Take as directed and do not stop abruptly as this may cause an increase in the severity and frequency of seizures.
2. Report any increase in frequency of tonic-clonic (grand mal) seizures immediately.
3. Alert the family to the possibility of transient personality changes, hypochondriacal behavior, and aggressiveness. Stress the need to report these changes immediately to the provider.
4. Any persistent fever, swollen glands, and bleeding gums should be reported. These may be symptoms of a blood dyscrasia and warrant medical evaluation.
5. Advise that drugs may discolor urine pinkish brown.
6. Caution should be exercised while driving or performing other tasks requiring alertness and coordination as the drugs may cause, dizziness, blurred vision, headaches, N&V, and drowsiness. These should subside after several weeks of therapy.
7. Report for CBC and liver and renal function studies on a routinely scheduled basis.

Evaluate

- Evidence of ↓ frequency of petit mal seizures
- Freedom from side effects of drug therapy

Ethosuximide

(eth-oh-**SUCKS**-ih-myd)
Zarontin **(Rx)**

See also *Anticonvulsants* and *Succinimides,* Chapter 36.

How Supplied: *Capsule:* 250 mg; *Syrup:* 250 mg/5 mL

Action/Kinetics: Peak serum levels: 3–7 hr. **t½: adults,** 60 hr; **t½: children,** 30 hr. Steady serum levels reached in 7–10 days. **Therapeutic serum levels:** 40–100 mcg/mL. The drug is metabolized in the liver. Both inactive metabolites and unchanged drug are excreted in the urine.

Use: To control absence (petit mal) seizures.

Dosage

- **Capsules, Syrup**

Absence seizures.

Adults and children over 6 years, initial: 250 mg b.i.d.; the dose may be increased by 250 mg/day at 4–7-day intervals until seizures are controlled or until total daily dose reaches 1.5 g.

Children under 6 years, initial: 250 mg/day; dosage may be increased by 250 mg/day every 4–7 days until control is established or total daily dose reaches 1 g.

Administration/Storage: The drug may be given with other anticonvulsants when other forms of epilepsy are present.

Additional Drug Interaction: Both isoniazid and valproic acid may ↑ the effects of ethosuximide.

NURSING CONSIDERATIONS

See also *Nursing Considerations* for *Anticonvulsants* and *Succinimides,* Chapter 36.

Client/Family Teaching

1. Take medication with meals to minimize GI upset.
2. Do not engage in hazardous activities while on drug therapy.
3. Do not stop drug abruptly because this may precipitate withdrawal seizures.
4. Report any loss of evidence of seizure control.
5. Stress the importance of reporting for lab studies every 3 months to assess hematologic, liver, and renal function.

Evaluate

- Control of petit mal seizures
- Therapeutic serum drug levels (40–100 mcg/mL)

Methsuximide

(meth-**SUCKS**-ih-myd)
Celontin **(Rx)**

See also *Anticonvulsants* and *Succinimides,* Chapter 36.

How Supplied: *Capsule:* 300 mg

Action/Kinetics: Peak levels: 1–4 hr. **t½:** 1–3 hr for methsuximide and 36–45 hr for the active metabolite. **Therapeutic serum levels:** 10–40 mcg/mL.

Uses: Methsuximide is used for absence seizures refractory to other drugs. May be given with other anticonvulsants when absence seizures coexist with other types of epilepsy.

Dosage

- **Capsules**

Absence seizures.

Adults and children, initial: 300 mg/day for first week; **then,** if necessary, increase dosage by 300 mg/day at weekly intervals until control established. **Maximum daily dose:** 1.2 g in divided doses.

Administration/Storage: The 150-mg dosage form can be used for children.

Additional Side Effects: Most common are ataxia, dizziness, and drowsiness.

Additional Drug Interaction: Methsuximide may ↑ the effect of primidone.

NURSING CONSIDERATIONS

See also *Nursing Considerations* for *Anticonvulsants* and *Succinimides,* Chapter 36.

Assessment

1. Document indications for therapy, type of seizures experienced, and other drugs prescribed and the outcome.
2. Determine baseline level of consciousness and balance, as drug may impair.

Evaluate

- Control of refractory petit mal seizures
- Therapeutic serum drug levels (10–40 mcg/mL)

Phensuximide

(fen-**SUCKS**-ih-myd)
Milontin **(Rx)**

See also *Anticonvulsants* and *Succinimides,* Chapter 36.

How Supplied: *Capsule:* 0.5 g

Action/Kinetics: Phensuximide is said to be less effective as well as less toxic than other succinimides. May color the urine pink, red, or red-brown. **t½:** 5–12 hr. **Peak effect:** 1–4 hr.

Dosage

- **Capsules**

Absence seizures.

Adults and children, initial: 0.5 g b.i.d.; **then,** dose can be increased by 0.5 g/day at 1-week intervals until seizures are controlled or the daily dosage reaches 3 g. May be used with other anticonvulsants in the presence of multiple types of epilepsy.

Special Concern: Use with caution in clients with intermittent porphyria.

Additional Side Effects: Kidney damage, hematuria, urinary frequency.

NURSING CONSIDERATIONS

See also *Nursing Considerations* for *Anticonvulsants* and *Succinimides,* Chapter 36.

Client/Family Teaching

1. Drug may discolor urine a pink-brown.
2. Report changes in urinary elimination such as pain, frequency, or blood.
3. Any loss of seizure control should be reported.

Evaluate: Control of seizures.

Valproic acid

(val-**PROH**-ick)

Pregnancy Category: D

Depakene **(Rx)**

How Supplied: *Capsule:* 250 mg; *Syrup:* 250 mg/5 mL

Action/Kinetics: The following information also applies to divalproex sodium. The precise anticonvulsant action is unknown, but activity is believed to be caused by increased brain levels of the neurotransmitter GABA. Other possibilities include acting on postsynaptic receptor sites to mimic or enhance the inhibitory effect of GABA, inhibiting an enzyme that catabolizes GABA, affecting the potassium channel, or directly affecting membrane stability. Absorption from the GI tract is more rapid following administration of the syrup (sodium salt) than capsules. **Peak serum levels, capsules and syrup:** 1–4 hr (delayed if the drug is taken with food); **peak serum levels, enteric-coated tablet (divalproex sodium):** 3–4 hr. **t½:** 6–16 hr. **Therapeutic serum levels:** 50–100 mcg/mL. The drug is approximately 90% bound to plasma protein. It is metabolized in the liver and inactive metabolites are excreted in the urine; small amounts of valproic acid are excreted in the feces.

Uses: Alone (preferred) or in combination with other anticonvulsants for treatment of epilepsy characterized by simple and complex absence seizures (petit mal). As an adjunct in mixed seizure patterns. *Investigational:* Alone or in combination to treat atypical absence, myoclonic, and grand mal seizures; also, atonic, complex partial, elementary partial, and infantile spasm seizures. Prophylaxis of febrile seizures in children, manic-depressive illness, and subchronically to treat minor incontinence after ileoanal anastomosis. Treatment of migraine headaches.

Dosage

- **Capsules, Syrup, Enteric-Coated Tablets (Divalproex)**

Seizures using monotherapy.

Adults and adolescents, initial: 15 mg/kg/day. Increase at 1-week intervals by 5–10 mg/kg/day; **maximum:** 60 mg/kg/day. If the total daily dose exceeds 250 mg, the dosage should be divided. **Pediatric, 1–12 years of age, initial:** 15–45 mg/kg/day; dose can be increased by 5–10 mg/kg/day at 1-week intervals.

Seizures, using polytherapy.

Adults and adolescents, initial: 10–30 mg/kg/day; dose can be increased by 5–10 mg/kg/day at 1-week intervals. **Pediatric, 1–12 years of age, initial:** 30–100 mg/kg/day; dose can be increased by 5–10 mg/kg/day at 1-week intervals.

Administration/Storage

1. Divide daily dosage if it exceeds 250 mg/day.
2. Initiate at lower dosage level or give with food to clients who suffer from GI irritation.
3. Valproic acid capsules should be swallowed whole to avoid local irritation. However, divalproex sodium capsules can either be swallowed whole or the contents sprinkled on a teaspoonful of a soft food (e.g., applesauce, pudding) and swallowed immediately without chewing.
4. Depakote is enteric coated and may decrease GI upset.
5. Do not administer valproic acid syrup to clients whose *sodium* intake must be restricted. Consult provider if a sodium-restricted client is unable to swallow capsules.
6. In clients taking valproic acid, conversion to divalproex sodium can be undertaken at the same total daily dose and dosing schedule.
7. *Treatment of Overdose:* Perform gastric lavage if client is seen early enough (valproic acid is absorbed rapidly). Undertake general supportive measures making sure urinary output is maintained. Naloxone has been used to reverse the CNS depression (however, it could also reverse the anticonvulsant effect). Hemodialysis and hemoperfusion have been used with success.

Contraindications: Liver disease or dysfunction.

Special Concerns: Safe use during lactation has not been established. Use with caution in children 2 years of age or less as they are at greater risk for developing fatal hepatotoxicity. Geriatric clients should receive a lower daily dose because they may have increased free, unbound valproic acid levels in the serum.

Laboratory Test Interferences: False + for ketonuria. Altered thyroid function tests.

Side Effects: *GI:* (most frequent): N&V, indigestion. Also, abdominal cramps, diarrhea, constipation, anorexia with weight loss or increased appetite with weight gain. *CNS:* Sedation, psychosis, depression, emotional upset, aggression, hyperactivity, deterioration of behavior, tremor, headache, dizziness, dysarthria, incoordination, coma (rare). *Ophthalmologic:* Nystagmus, diplopia, "spots before eyes." *Hematologic:* Thrombocytopenia, leukopenia, eosinophilia, anemia, bone marrow suppression, relative lymphocytosis, hypofibrinogenemia myelodysplastic-type syndrome. *Dermatologic:* Transient alopecia, petechiae, erythema multiforme, skin rashes. photosensitivity, pruritus. *Hepatic:* **Hepatotoxicity.** Also, minor increases in AST, ALT, LDH, serum bilirubin, and serum alkaline phosphatase values. *Endocrine:* Menstrual irregularities, breast enlargement, galactorrhea, swelling of parotid gland, abnormal thyroid function tests. *Miscellaneous:* Also asterixis, weakness, bruising, hematoma formation, frank hemorrhage, acute pancreatitis, hyperammonemia, hyperglycinemia, hypocarnitinemia, edema of arms and legs, weakness.

Symptoms of Overdose: Motor restlessness, asterixis, visual hallucinations, ***deep coma.***

Drug Interactions

Alcohol / ↑ Incidence of CNS depression
Aspirin / ↑ Effect of valproic acid due to ↓ plasma protein binding. Also, additive anticoagulant effect
Benzodiazepines / ↑ Effect of benzodiazepines due to ↓ breakdown by liver
Carbamazepine / Variable changes in levels of carbamazepine with possible loss of seizure control
Charcoal / ↓ Absorption of valproic acid from the GI tract
Chlorpromazine / ↓ Clearance and ↑ t½ of valproic acid → ↑ pharmacologic effects
Cimetidine / ↓ Clearance and ↑ t½ of valproic acid → ↑ pharmacologic effects
Clonazepam / ↑ Chance of absence

seizures (petit mal) and ↑ toxicity due to clonazepam
CNS depressants / ↑ Incidence of CNS depression
Ethosuximide / ↑ or ↓ Effect of ethosuximide
Phenobarbital / ↑ Effect of phenobarbital due to ↓ breakdown by liver
Phenytoin / ↑ Effect of phenytoin due to ↓ breakdown by liver or ↓ effect of phenytoin due to ↓ total serum phenytoin
Primidone / ↑ Effect of primidone due to ↓ breakdown by liver
Warfarin sodium / ↑ Effect of valproic acid due to ↓ plasma protein binding. Also, additive anticoagulant effect

NURSING CONSIDERATIONS

See also *Nursing Considerations* for *Anticonvulsants,* Chapter 36.

Assessment

1. Document characteristics of seizure activity, prodrome, onset, and any other agents prescribed.
2. Obtain baseline liver function tests and monitor due to increased potential for hepatoxicity.

Client/Family Teaching

1. Take with or after meals to minimize GI upset and at bedtime to minimize sedative effects.
2. Take only as directed and do not stop suddenly because seizures may occur.
3. Do not drive or perform activities that require mental alertness until drug effects realized and seizure control verified by the provider.
4. Any unexplained fever, sore throat, skin rash, yellow skin discoloration, or unusual bruising or bleeding should be reported immediately.
5. Advise clients with diabetes that the drug may cause a false positive urine test for ketones. Review some of the symptoms of ketoacidosis (dry mouth, thirst, and dry flushed skin) so that clients can determine if they are acidotic. Instruct to report the development of any of these symptoms.
6. Report any loss of seizure control.
7. Avoid alcohol and any other CNS depressants or OTC products without provider approval.
8. Stress the importance of reporting as scheduled for periodic CBC, serum glucose and acetone, and liver function studies throughout drug therapy.

Evaluate

- Control of seizures
- Relief of migraine headache
- Therapeutic serum drug levels (50–100 mcg/mL)

CHAPTER THIRTY-SEVEN

Antidepressants

See also the following drug classes and individual drugs:

Tricyclic Antidepressants

Amitriptyline Hydrochloride
Amitriptyline and Perphenazine
Amoxapine
Clomipramine Hydrochloride
Desipramine Hydrochloride
Doxepin Hydrochloride
Imipramine Hydrochloride
Imipramine Pamoate
Maprotiline Hydrochloride
Nortriptyline Hydrochloride
Protriptyline Hydrochloride
Trimipramine Maleate

Miscellaneous Antidepressants

Bupropion Hydrochloride
Fluoxetine Hydrochloride
Paroxetine Hydrochloride
Sertraline Hydrochloride
Trazodone Hydrochloride
Venlafaxine Hydrochloride

TRICYCLIC ANTIDEPRESSANTS

See the following individual entries:

Amitriptyline Hydrochloride
Amitriptyline and Perphenazine
Amoxapine
Clomipramine Hydrochloride
Desipramine Hydrochloride
Doxepin Hydrochloride
Imipramine Pamoate
Maprotiline Hydrochloride
Nortriptyline Hydrochloride
Protriptyline Hydrochloride
Trimipramine Maleate

General Statement: The tricyclic antidepressants are chemically related to the phenothiazines and, as such, they exhibit many of the same pharmacologic effects (e.g., anticholinergic, antiserotonin, sedative, antihistaminic, and hypotensive). The tricyclic antidepressants are less effective for depressed clients in the presence of organic brain damage or schizophrenia. Also, they can induce mania; this possibility should be kept in mind when given to clients with manic-depressive psychoses.

Action/Kinetics: Tricyclic antidepressants prevent the reuptake of norepinephrine or serotonin, or both, into the storage granules of the presynaptic nerves. This results in increased concentrations of these neurotransmitters in the synapses, which alleviates depression. (*NOTE:* Endogenous depression is thought to be caused by low concentrations of norepinephrine and/or serotonin.) The tricyclic antidepressants are well absorbed from the GI tract. All these drugs have a long serum half-life. Up to 4–6 days may be required to reach steady plasma levels, and maximum therapeutic effects may not be noted for 2–4 weeks. Because of the long half-life, single daily dosage may suffice. The tricyclic antidepressants are more than 90% bound to plasma protein. They are partially metabolized in the liver and excreted primarily in the urine.

Uses: Endogenous and reactive depressions. Preferred over MAO inhibitors because they are less toxic. See individual drugs for special uses, such as use in depression associated with anxiety and disturbances in sleep.

Contraindications: Severely impaired liver function. Use during acute recovery phase from MI. Concomitant use with MAO inhibitors.

Special Concerns: Use with caution in clients with epilepsy, CV diseases, glaucoma, BPH, suicidal tendencies, a history of urinary retention, and the elderly. Concomitant use with MAO inhibitors should be undertaken with caution. Use during pregnancy only when benefits clearly outweigh risks. Use with caution during lactation. Generally not recommended for children less than 12 years of age. Geriatric clients may be more sensitive to the anticholinergic and sedative side effects.

Side Effects: Most frequent side effects are sedation and atropine-like reactions. *CNS:* Confusion, anxiety, restlessness, insomnia, nightmares, hallucinations, delusions, mania or hypomania, headache, dizziness, inability to concentrate, panic reaction, worsening of psychoses, fatigue, weakness. *Anticholinergic:* Dry mouth, blurred vision, mydriasis, constipation, paralytic ileus, urinary retention or difficulty in urination. *GI:* N&V, anorexia, gastric distress, unpleasant taste, stomatitis, glossitis, cramps, increased salivation, black tongue. *CV:* Fainting, tachycardia, hypo- or hypertension, arrhythmias, ***heart block,*** possibility of palpitations, ***MI, stroke.*** *Neurologic:* Paresthesias, numbness, incoordination, neuropathies, extrapyramidal symptoms including tardive dyskinesia, dysarthria, seizures. *Dermatologic:* Skin rashes, urticaria, flushing, pruritus, petechiae, photosensitivity, edema. *Endocrine:* Testicular swelling and gynecomastia in males, increase or decrease in libido, impotence, menstrual irregularities and galactorrhea in females, hypo- or hyperglycemia, changes in secretion of ADH. *Miscellaneous:* Sweating, alopecia, nasal congestion, lacrimation, increase in body temperature, chills, urinary frequency including nocturia. Bone marrow depression including thrombocytopenia, leukopenia, ***agranulocytosis,*** eosinophilia.

High dosage increases the frequency of seizures in epileptic clients and may cause epileptiform attacks in normal subjects.

Symptoms of Overdose: CNS symptoms include agitation, confusion, hallucinations, hyperactive reflexes, choreoathetosis, ***seizures, coma.*** Anticholinergic symptoms include dilated pupils, dry mouth, flushing, and ***hyperpyrexia.*** CV toxicity includes depressed myocardial contractility, decreased HR, decreased coronary blood flow, tachycardia, intraventricular block, ***complete AV block, re-entry ventricular arrhythmias, PVCs, ventricular tachycardia or fibrillation, sudden cardiac arrest, hypotension, pulmonary edema.***

Drug Interactions

Acetazolamide / ↑ Effect of tricyclics by ↑ renal tubular reabsorption of the drug

Alcohol, ethyl / Concomitant use may lead to ↑ GI complications and ↓ performance on motor skill tests—death has been reported

Ammonium chloride / ↓ Effect of tricyclics by ↓ renal tubular reabsorption of the drug

Anticholinergic drugs / Additive anticholinergic side effects

Anticoagulants, oral / ↑ Hypoprothrombinemia due to ↓ breakdown by liver

Anticonvulsants / Tricyclics may ↑ incidence of epileptic seizures

Antihistamines / Additive anticholinergic side effects

Ascorbic acid / ↓ Effect of tricyclics by ↓ renal tubular reabsorption of the drug

Barbiturates / Additive depressant effects; also, barbiturates may ↑ breakdown of antidepressants by liver

Benzodiazepines / Tricyclic antidepressants ↑ effect of benzodiazepines

Beta-adrenergic blocking agents / Tricyclic antidepressants ↓ effect of the blocking agents

Charcoal / ↓ Absorption of tricyclic antidepressants → ↓ effectiveness (or toxicity)

Chlordiazepoxide / Concomitant use may cause additive sedative ef-

fects and/or additive atropine-like side effects
Cimetidine / ↑ Effect of tricyclics (especially serious anticholinergic symptoms) due to ↓ breakdown by liver
Clonidine / Dangerous ↑ BP and hypertensive crisis
Diazepam / Concomitant use may cause additive sedative effects and/or additive atropine-like side effects
Dicumarol / Tricyclic antidepressants may ↑ the t½ of dicumarol → ↑ anticoagulation effects
Disulfiram / ↑ Levels of tricyclic antidepressant; also, possibility of acute organic brain syndrome
Ephedrine / Tricyclics ↓ effects of ephedrine by preventing uptake at its site of action
Estrogens / Depending on the dose, estrogens may ↑ or ↓ the effects of tricyclics
Ethchlorvynol / Combination may result in transient delirium
Fluoxetine / Fluoxetine ↑ pharmacologic and toxic effects of tricyclic antidepressants (effect may persist for several weeks after fluoxetine is discontinued)
Furazolidone / Toxic psychoses possible
Glutethimide / Additive anticholinergic side effects
Guanethidine / Tricyclics ↓ antihypertensive effect of guanethidine by preventing uptake at its site of action
Haloperidol / ↑ Effect of tricyclics due to ↓ breakdown by liver
Levodopa / ↓ Effect of levodopa due to ↓ absorption
MAO inhibitors / Concomitant use may result in excitation, increase in body temperature, delirium, tremors, and convulsions although combinations have been used successfully
Meperidine / Tricyclics enhance narcotic-induced respiratory depression; also, additive anticholinergic side effects
Methyldopa / Tricyclics may block hypotensive effects of methyldopa
Methylphenidate / ↑ Effect of tricyclics due to ↓ breakdown by liver
Narcotic analgesics / Tricyclics enhance narcotic-induced respiratory depression; also, additive anticholinergic effects
Oral contraceptives / ↑ Plasma levels of tricyclic antidepressants due to ↓ breakdown by liver
Oxazepam / Concomitant use may cause additive sedative effects and/or atropine-like side effects
Phenothiazines / Additive anticholinergic side effects; also, phenothiazines ↑ effects of tricyclics due to ↓ breakdown by liver
Procainamide / Additive cardiac effects
Quinidine / Additive cardiac effects
Reserpine / Tricyclics ↓ hypotensive effect of reserpine
Sodium bicarbonate / ↑ Effect of tricyclics by ↑ renal tubular reabsorption of the drug
Sympathomimetics / Potentiation of sympathomimetic effects → hypertension or cardiac arrhythmias
Tobacco (smoking) / ↓ Serum levels of tricyclic antidepressants due to ↑ breakdown by liver
Thyroid preparations / Mutually potentiating effects observed
Vasodilators / Additive hypotensive effect

Laboratory Test Interferences: ↑ Alkaline phosphatase, bilirubin; ↑ or ↓ blood glucose. False + or ↑ urinary catecholamines.

Dosage

See individual drugs.

Dosage levels vary greatly in effectiveness from one client to another; therefore, dosage regimens must be carefully individualized.

NURSING CONSIDERATIONS

Administration/Storage

1. In adolescents and elderly clients, initial dosage should be lower than in adults; the dose may then be gradually increased as required.

2. The dosage of drug should be highly individualized according to the client's age, weight, physical and mental condition, and response to the therapy.
3. For maintenance therapy, a single daily dose may suffice.
4. The dose is usually administered at bedtime, so any anticholinergic and/or sedative effects will not be bothersome.
5. To reduce incidence of sedation and anticholinergic effects, small dosages of the drug should be used first and then gradually increased to the desired dosage levels.
6. *Treatment of Overdose:*
• Admit client to hospital and monitor ECG closely for 3–5 days.
• Empty stomach in alert clients by inducing vomiting followed by gastric lavage and charcoal administration **after insertion of cuffed ET tube.** Maintain respiration and avoid the use of respiratory stimulants.
• Normal or half-normal saline is used to prevent water intoxication.
• To reverse the CV effects (e.g., hypotension and cardiac dysrhythmias), hypertonic sodium bicarbonate, IM, is given by IV infusion. The usual dose is 0.5–2 mEq/kg by IV bolus followed by IV infusion to maintain the blood at pH 7.5. If hypotension is not reversed by bicarbonate, vasopressors (e.g., dopamine) and fluid expansion may be needed. If the cardiac dysrhythmias do not respond to bicarbonate, lidocaine or phenytoin may be used.
• Isoproterenol may be effective in controlling bradyarrhythmias and torsades de pointes ventricular tachycardia. Propranolol, 0.1 mg/kg IV (up to 0.25 mg by IV bolus) is used to treat life-threatening ventricular arrhythmias in children.
• Shock and metabolic acidosis are treated with IV fluids, oxygen, bicarbonate, and corticosteroids.
• Control hyperpyrexia by external means (ice pack, cool baths, spongings).
• To reduce possibility of convulsions, minimize external stimulation. If necessary, use diazepam or phenytoin to control convulsions. Avoid barbiturates if MAO inhibitors have been used recently.

Assessment

1. Document indications for therapy, behavioral manifestations, onset of symptoms, and any potential causative factors.
2. Assess for evidence of suicide ideations, extent of dysphoric mood, appetite, and any reports of excessive weight changes.
3. Note client reports of sleep disturbances, lethargy, apathy, impaired thought processes, or lack of responses.
4. Note client past history of the drugs experienced and the response.
5. Obtain baseline CBC and liver function studies before initiating therapy.
6. Record baseline ECG, assess heart sounds, and evaluate neurologic functioning.
7. Obtain baseline ophthalmic exam and note any reports of visual disturbances and note the presence of glaucoma.
8. Determine any evidence of urinary retention, especially among the elderly.
9. Attempt to differentiate type of depression based on diagnostic features related to reactive, major depressive, or bipolar affective disorders.

Interventions

1. Monitor clients for any changes in vision, such as client complaint of headaches, halos, or eye pain.
2. Assess clients closely if they also develop dilated pupils or complain of nausea. These symptoms may be serious, especially if the client has angle-closure glaucoma and may require a change in medication.
3. Provide a diet high in fiber, an increased fluid intake, and a stool softener to prevent constipation.
4. Assess GI complaints of anorexia, N&V, epigastric distress, diarrhea, a blackened tongue, and a peculiar taste in the mouth. Document and report because these symptoms require an adjustment of dosage. Ad-

ministering the medication with or immediately following meals may reduce gastric irritation.
5. Monitor I&O. Check for abdominal distention, urinary retention, and the absence of bowel sounds (as in paralytic ileus) because these conditions may require immediate attention and a reduction in drug dose.
6. Note any signs of an allergic response to the drug, such as skin rash, alopecia, and eosinophilia.
7. Note complaints of sore throat, fever, easy bruising, unusual bleeding, presence of petechiae or purpura. Withhold drug and report as these are symptoms of blood dyscrasias. Place client in protective isolation and practice universal precautions until the CBC with leukocyte counts has been evaluated.
8. Routinely check client's CBC for eosinophil count, thrombocytes, and leukocytes. Check for evidence of agranulocytosis, especially common among elderly women and during the second month of drug therapy. Report abnormal findings as the drug may need to be withheld.
9. Obtain ECGs periodically throughout drug therapy and compare to the baseline ECG. If the client has a history of CV disorders, assess for tachycardia and any increase in attacks of angina because these may lead to a MI or stroke.
10. In clients with a history of hyperthyroidism, be alert for cardiac arrhythmias that may be precipitated by tricyclic drugs.
11. Assess clients for changes in baseline behavior, indicating further psychologic disturbances such as mood swings, increases in agitation, and anxiety. Document and report because a change in medication may be indicated.
12. Query client concerning adverse endocrine disturbances such as increased or decreased libido, gynecomastia, testicular swelling, and impotence. Discuss and mutually devise a plan to assist client to deal with the problem.
13. Note symptoms of cholestatic jaundice and biliary tract obstruction such as high fever, yellowing of the skin, mucous membranes and sclera, pruritus, and upper abdominal pain. Document and report because a change in therapy may be indicated.
14. Monitor clients with diabetes mellitus, especially when tricyclic therapy is initiated or discontinued. These drugs may alter blood sugar levels in either direction and require an adjustment in the dose of hypoglycemic agent.
15. If the client has been receiving electroshock therapy, check with the physician before administering tricyclic drugs. The combination may be hazardous.
16. Ascertain if the drug is to be discontinued several days prior to surgery. The tricyclic compounds may adversely affect BP during surgery.
17. If withdrawal of the drug is required for any reason, expect the procedure to occur slowly to avoid any withdrawal symptoms.
18. MAO inhibitors are usually contraindicated with tricyclic antidepressants. If used in conjunction with tricyclic drugs, the dosages should be small and the client should be under close medical supervision.
19. Note if any epileptiform seizures are precipitated by the drug. Incorporate seizure precautions when evident.

Client/Family Teaching

1. Explain the drug action; it reduces the depression that inhibits one's ability to make decisions and to cope effectively.
2. Advise to take medications that may cause sedation at bedtime to minimize excess daytime sedation and to take medications that cause insomnia in the morning or upon arising.
3. Stress the importance of maintaining an environment conducive to regular sleep patterns during the initiation of tricyclic therapy.

4. Do not ingest any other drugs or alcohol while taking tricyclic antidepressants without the express consent of the physician. This rule should also be followed for 2 weeks after completing tricyclic drug therapy.
5. Use caution when performing hazardous tasks requiring mental alertness or physical coordination because the drug may cause drowsiness or ataxia.
6. Rise gradually from a supine position and do not remain standing in one place for any length of time. If feeling faint, lie down to minimize orthostatic hypotension. Review appropriate safety measures.
7. Provide nutritional guidance to avoid or counteract problems associated with drug therapy such as anorexia, nausea, or nervous eating. Take medication with meals to decrease GI upset.
8. Increase oral hygiene and take frequent sips of water, suck on hard candy, or chew sugarless gum to maintain a moist mouth.
9. Advise clients with diabetes to monitor blood glucose levels carefully because drug may affect carbohydrate metabolism, and adjustment of hypoglycemic drugs and diet may be indicated.
10. If the client becomes photosensitive, stay out of the sun. Wear protective clothing, sunglasses, and a sunscreen if exposure is necessary.
11. Discuss changes in libido or reproductive function. Encourage involvement in marital and family therapy.
12. Advise women of childbearing age to practice birth control and to report immediately if pregnancy is suspected.
13. Report any alterations in perceptions, such as the development of hallucinations, blurred vision, or excessive stimulations. Especially evaluate clients recovering from depression for suicidal tendencies.
14. It may require 2–4 weeks for the client to realize a maximum clinical response. Apprise clients of the delay in response and encourage them to stay on the treatment regimen.
15. Explain that the prescriptions will be for only small amounts of drug to ensure return visits for close follow-up and to prevent quantities that may be used for an overdose, as excess consumption of some of these agents can be lethal.
16. Instruct the family on methods to help clients alter their behavior. Encourage participation in prescribed psychotherapy programs.

Evaluate

- Resolution or ↓ symptoms of depression as evidenced by any of the following: improved appetite, a renewed interest in outside activities, ↑ socialization, reports of improved sleeping patterns, ↑ energy, and a general sense of well being
- Knowledge and understanding of illness; prescribed dosing parameters and the need for continued drug therapy
- Reports of improved coping skills and less experienced fear
- Evidence of ↓ anxiety levels

Amitriptyline hydrochloride

(ah-me-**TRIP**-tih-leen)
Pregnancy Category: C
Amitril, Apo-Amitriptyline ✱, Elavil, Endep, Enovil, Levate ✱ **(Rx)**

See also *Antidepressants, Tricyclic,* Chapter 37.

How Supplied: *Injection:* 10 mg/mL; *Tablet:* 10 mg, 25 mg, 50 mg, 75 mg, 100 mg, 150 mg

Action/Kinetics: Amitriptyline is metabolized to an active metabolite, nortriptyline. Has significant anticholinergic and sedative effects with moderate activity to cause orthostatic hypotension. **Effective plasma levels of amitriptyline and nortriptyline:** Approximately 110–250 ng/mL. **t½:** 31–46 hr. Up to 1 month may be required for beneficial effects to be manifested.

Amitriptyline is also found in Limbritrol and Triavil.

Uses: Relief of symptoms of depression including depression accompanied by anxiety and insomnia. Chronic pain due to cancer or other pain syndromes. Prophylaxis of cluster and migraine headaches. *Investigational:* Pathologic laughing and crying secondary to forebrain disease, bulimia nervosa, antiulcer agent, enuresis.

Dosage

- **Syrup, Tablets**

Antidepressant.

Adults (outpatients): 75 mg/day in divided doses; may be increased to 150 mg/day. *Alternate dosage:* **Initial,** 50–100 mg at bedtime; **then,** increase by 25–50 mg, if necessary, up to 150 mg/day. **Hospitalized clients: initial,** 100 mg/day; may be increased to 200–300 mg/day. **Maintenance: usual,** 40–100 mg/day (may be given as a single dose at bedtime). **Adolescent and geriatric:** 10 mg t.i.d. and 20 mg at bedtime up to a maximum of 100 mg/day. **Pediatric, 6–12 years:** 10–30 mg (1–5 mg/kg) daily in two divided doses.

Chronic pain.

50–100 mg/day.

Enuresis.

Pediatric, over 6 years: 10 mg/day as a single dose at bedtime; dose may be increased up to a maximum of 25 mg. **Less than 6 years:** 10 mg/day as a single dose at bedtime.

- **IM Only**

Antidepressant.

Adults: 20–30 mg q.i.d.; switch to **PO** therapy as soon as possible.

Administration/Storage

1. Increases in dosage should be made in late afternoon or at bedtime.
2. Beneficial antidepressant effects may not be noted for 30 days.
3. Sedative effects may be manifested prior to antidepressant effects.

NURSING CONSIDERATIONS

See also *Nursing Considerations* for *Antidepressants, Tricyclic,* Chapter 37.

Client/Family Teaching

1. Take with food to minimize gastric upset.
2. Warn clients not to drive a car or operate hazardous machinery until drug effects are realized because drug causes a high degree of sedation.
3. Client may take entire dose at bedtime if sedation is manifested during waking hours.
4. Rise slowly from a lying to a sitting position to reduce orthostatic drug effects.
5. Urine may appear blue-green in color; this is harmless.

Evaluate

- ↓ Symptoms of depression with improved sleeping and eating patterns, ↓ fatigue, and ↑ interest in self and others
- Control of incontinence
- Enhanced pain control with chronic pain management

COMBINATION DRUG

Amitriptyline and Perphenazine

(ah-me-**TRIP**-tih-leen, per-**FEN**-ah-zeen)

Elavil Plus ✱, Etrafon 2-10 ✱, Etrafon-A ✱, Etrafon-D ✱, Etrafon-F ✱, PMS-Levazine 2/25 ✱, PMS-Levazine 4/25 ✱, Triavil 2-10, 2-25, 4-10, 4-25, and 4-50 **(Rx)**

How Supplied: See Content

Content: See also information on individual components.

Antidepressant: Amitriptyline HCl, 10, 25, or 50 mg. *Antipsychotic:* Perphenazine, 2 or 4 mg.

There are five different strengths of Triavil: Triavil 2–10, Triavil 2–25, Triavil 4–10, Triavil 4–25, and Triavil 4–50. *NOTE:* The first number refers to the number of milligrams of perphenazine and the second number refers to the number of milligrams of amitriptyline.

Uses: Depression with moderate to severe anxiety and/or agitation. Depression and anxiety in clients with chronic physical disease. Also schizophrenic clients with symptoms of depression.

Dosage

- **Tablets**

Antidepressant.

Adults, initial: One tablet of Triavil 2–25 or 4–25 t.i.d.–q.i.d. or 1 tablet of Triavil 4–50 b.i.d. Schizophrenic clients should receive an initial dose of 2 tablets of Triavil 4–50 t.i.d., with a fourth dose at bedtime, if necessary. Initial dosage for geriatric or adolescent clients in whom anxiety dominates is Triavil 4–10 t.i.d.–q.i.d., with dosage adjusted as required. **Maintenance:** One tablet Triavil 2–25 or 4–25 b.i.d.–q.i.d. or 1 tablet Triavil 4–50 b.i.d.

Administration/Storage

1. Triavil is not recommended for children.
2. Total daily dosage of Triavil should not exceed 4 of the 4–50 tablets or 8 tablets of all other dosage strengths.
3. The therapeutic effect may take up to several weeks to be manifested.
4. Once a satisfactory response has been observed, the dose should be reduced to the smallest amount required for relief of symptoms.

Contraindications: Use during pregnancy is not recommended. CNS depression due to drugs. In presence of bone marrow depression. Concomitant use with MAO inhibitors. During acute recovery phase from MI. Use in children.

NURSING CONSIDERATIONS

See also *Nursing Considerations* for *Antidepressants, Tricyclic* and *Amitriptyline,* Chapter 37.

Evaluate: Relief of symptoms of depression and associated anxiety.

Amoxapine

(ah-**MOX**-ah-peen)
Pregnancy Category: C
Asendin **(Rx)**

See also *Antidepressants, Tricyclic,* Chapter 37.

How Supplied: *Tablet:* 25 mg, 50 mg, 100 mg, 150 mg

Action/Kinetics: In addition to its effect on monoamines, this drug also blocks dopamine receptors. Is metabolized to the active metabolites 7-hydroxy- and 8-hydroxyamoxapine. **Peak blood levels:** 90 min. **Effective plasma levels:** 200–500 ng/mL. **t½:** 8 hr; t½ of major metabolite: 30 hr. Excreted in urine.

Uses: Endogenous and reactive depression. Antianxiety agent.

Dosage

• **Tablets**

Antidepressant.

Adults, individualized, initial: 50 mg t.i.d. Can be increased to 100 mg t.i.d. during first week. Doses greater than 300 mg/day should not be used unless this dose has been ineffective for at least 14 days. **Maintenance:** 300 mg as a single dose at bedtime. **Hospitalized clients:** Up to 150 mg q.i.d. **Geriatric, initial:** 25 mg b.i.d.–t.i.d. If necessary, increase to 50 mg b.i.d.–t.i.d. after first week. **Maintenance:** Up to 300 mg/day at bedtime.

Contraindications: Avoid high dose levels in clients with a history of convulsive seizures. Not to be used during acute recovery period after MI.

Special Concerns: Safe use in children under 16 years of age and during lactation not established.

Additional Side Effects: Tardive dyskinesia. ***Overdosage may cause seizures (common), neuroleptic malignant syndrome,*** testicular swelling, impairment of sexual function, and breast enlargement in males and females. Also, renal failure may be seen 2–5 days after overdosage.

NURSING CONSIDERATIONS

See also *Nursing Considerations* for *Antidepressants, Tricyclic* Chapter 37.

Client/Family Teaching

1. Take with food to minimize gastric upset.
2. Administer entire dose at bedtime if daytime sedation persists.
3. Review and advise to report early CNS manifestations of tardive dyskinesia.
4. Review list of toxic side effects R/T overdosage that require immediate medical intervention.

Evaluate

• Improved coping mechanisms
• Control of depression with ↓ anxiety levels

Clomipramine hydrochloride

(kloh-**MIP**-rah-meen)
Pregnancy Category: C
Anafranil **(Rx)**

See also *Antidepressants, Tricyclic,* Chapter 37.
How Supplied: *Capsule:* 25 mg, 50 mg, 75 mg
Action/Kinetics: Clomipramine possesses a high degree of anticholinergic and sedative effects as well as moderate orthostatic hypotension. **t½:** 19–37 hr. **Effective plasma levels:** 80–100 ng/mL. The drug is metabolized to the active desmethylclomipramine.
Uses: Treatment of obsessive-compulsive disorder in which the obsessions or compulsions cause marked distress, significantly interfere with social or occupational activities, or are time-consuming. Also, to treat panic attacks and cataplexy associated with narcolepsy.

Dosage

- **Capsules**

Adult, initial: 25 mg/day; **then,** increase gradually to approximately 100 mg during the first 2 weeks (depending on client tolerance). The dose may then be increased slowly to a maximum of 250 mg/day over the next several weeks. **Adolescents, children, initial:** 25 mg/day; **then,** increase gradually during the first 2 weeks to a maximum of 100 mg or 3 mg/kg, whichever is less. The dose may then be increased to a maximum daily dose of 3 mg/kg or 200 mg, whichever is less.
Administration/Storage
1. Initially, the daily dosage should be divided and given with meals to reduce GI side effects.
2. After the optimum dose is determined, the total daily dose can be given at bedtime to minimize daytime sedation.
3. The dose for all ages should be adjusted to the lowest effective dose and be evaluated periodically to determine the continued need for treatment.
4. Although the efficacy of clomipramine has not been determined after 10 weeks of therapy, clients have successfully used the drug for up to 1 year without loss of beneficial effects.
Contraindication: To relieve symptoms of depression.
Special Concerns: Safety has not been established for use during lactation. Safety has not been established in children less than 10 years of age.
Additional Side Effects: Hyperthermia, especially when used with other drugs. Increased risk of ***seizures.*** Aggressive reactions, asthenia, anemia, eructation, failure to ejaculate, laryngitis, vestibular disorders, muscle weakness.

NURSING CONSIDERATIONS

See also *Nursing Considerations* for *Antidepressants, Tricyclic,* Chapter 37.
Assessment
1. Document indications for therapy and baseline behavorial findings.
2. List drugs currently prescribed, those used previously for this disorder, and the outcome.
Client/Family Teaching
1. Take only as directed.
2. Review anticipated results of therapy and the time frame for follow-up.
3. Rise slowly to prevent orthostatic drug effects.
4. Advise that symptoms of depression should be reported.
5. Suggest that fluids and lozenges may relieve symptoms of dry mouth.
Evaluate: Control of obsessive-compulsive behaviors that interfere with normal social or occupational functioning.

Desipramine hydrochloride

(dess-**IP**-rah-meen)
Norpramin, Pertofrane **(Rx)**

See also *Antidepressants, Tricyclic,* Chapter 37.

How Supplied: *Tablet:* 10 mg, 25 mg, 50 mg, 75 mg, 100 mg, 150 mg
Action/Kinetics: Has minimal anticholinergic and sedative effects and slight ability to cause orthostatic hypotension. **Effective plasma levels:** 125–300 ng/mL. **t½:** 12–24 hr. Clients who will respond to drug usually do so within the first week.
Uses: Symptoms of depression. Bulimia nervosa. To decrease craving and depression during cocaine withdrawal. To treat severe neurogenic pain. Cataplexy associated with narcolepsy. Attention deficit disorders with or without hyperactivity in children over 6 years of age.

Dosage

- **Capsules, Tablets**

Antidepressant.

Initial: 100–200 mg in single or divided doses. **Maximum daily dose:** 300 mg. **Maintenance:** 50–100 mg/day. **Geriatric clients:** 25–50 mg/day in divided doses up to a maximum of 150 mg/day. **Children, 6–12 years:** 10–30 mg/day (1–5 mg/kg) in divided doses. **Adolescents:** 25–50 mg/day in divided doses up to a maximum of 100 mg.

Cocaine withdrawal.

50–200 mg/day.

Administration/Storage

1. Clients requiring 300 mg/day should have treatment initiated in a hospital setting.
2. Maintenance doses should be given for at least 2 months following a satisfactory response.
3. Administration of a single daily dose or any increases in the dosage should be administered at bedtime in order to reduce daytime sedation.

Special Concerns: Safe use during pregnancy has not been established. Safety and efficacy have not been established in children.
Additional Side Effects: Bad taste in mouth, hypertension during surgery.

NURSING CONSIDERATIONS

See also *Nursing Considerations* for *Antidepressants, Tricyclic,* Chapter 37.

Evaluate

- Reports of less perceived depression with an improved sense of self
- Relief of neurogenic pain
- Therapeutic serum drug levels (125–300 ng/mL)

Doxepin hydrochloride

(**DOX**-eh-pin)
Adapin, Sinequan, Triadapin ✱ **(Rx)**

See also *Antidepressants, Tricyclic,* Chapter 37.
How Supplied: *Capsule:* 10 mg, 25 mg, 50 mg, 75 mg, 100 mg, 150 mg; *Concentrate:* 10 mg/mL; *Cream:* 5%
Action/Kinetics: Doxepin is metabolized to the active metabolite, desmethyldoxepin. It has moderate anticholinergic effects and ability to cause orthostatic hypotension and high sedative effects. **Minimum effective plasma level of both doxepin and desmethyldoxepin:** 100–200 ng/mL. **t½:** 8–24 hr.
Uses: Symptoms of depression. Antianxiety agent, depression accompanied by anxiety and insomnia, depression in clients with manic-depressive illness. Depression or anxiety due to organic disease or alcoholism. Chronic, severe neurogenic pain. Peptic ulcer disease. Dermatologic disorders including chronic urticaria, angioedema, and nocturnal pruritus due to atopic eczema.

Dosage

- **Capsules, Oral Solution**

Antidepressant, mild to moderate anxiety or depression.

Adults: 25 mg t.i.d. (or up to 150 mg can be given at bedtime); **then,** adjust dosage to individual response (usual optimum dosage: 75–150 mg/day). **Geriatric clients, initially:** 25–50 mg/day; dose can be increased as needed and tolerated.

Severe symptoms.

Initial: 50 mg t.i.d.; **then,** gradually increase to 300 mg/day.

Emotional symptoms with organic disease.

25–50 mg/day.

Antipruritic.
10–30 mg at bedtime.
Administration/Storage: Oral concentrate is to be diluted with 4 oz water, fruit juice, or milk just before ingestion. The concentrate should not be mixed with carbonated beverages or grape juice.
Additional Contraindications: Glaucoma or a tendency for urinary retention.
Special Concerns: Safety has not been determined in pregnancy. Not recommended for use in children less than 12 years of age.
Additional Side Effects: Doxepin has a high incidence of side effects, including a high degree of sedation, decreased libido, extrapyramidal symptoms, dermatitis, pruritus, fatigue, weight gain, edema, paresthesia, breast engorgement, insomnia, tremor, chills, tinnitus, and photophobia.

NURSING CONSIDERATIONS

See also *Nursing Considerations* for *Antidepressants, Tricyclic,* Chapter 37.
Assessment
1. Document indications for therapy and type and onset of symptoms.
2. List any other prescribed therapy for this problem and the outcome.
3. Document clinical presentation and attempt to identify any factors that may be contributing to this disorder.
Evaluate
- ↓ Symptoms of anxiety and depression
- Improved sleeping patterns
- Control of chronic neurogenic pain
- Relief of nocturnal pruritus

Imipramine hydrochloride

(im-**IHP**-rah-meen)
Pregnancy Category: B
Apo-Imipramine ✦, Janimine, Tofranil **(Rx)**

Imipramine pamoate

(im-**IHP**-rah-meen)
Pregnancy Category: B
Tofranil-PM **(Rx)**

See also *Antidepressants, Tricyclic,* Chapter 37.
How Supplied: Imipramine hydrochloride: *Injection:* 12.5 mg/mL; *Tablet:* 10 mg, 25 mg, 50 mg.
Imipramine pamoate: *Capsule:* 75 mg, 100 mg, 125 mg, 150 mg
Action/Kinetics: Imipramine is biotransformed into its active metabolite, desmethylimipramine (desipramine). **Effective plasma level of imipramine and desmethylimipramine:** 200–350 ng/mL. **t½:** 11–25 hr.
Uses: Symptoms of depression. Enuresis in children. Chronic, severe neurogenic pain. Bulimia nervosa.

Dosage

- **Tablets, Capsules**

Depression.
Hospitalized clients: 50 mg b.i.d.–t.i.d. Can be increased by 25 mg every few days up to 200 mg/day. After 2 weeks, dosage may be increased gradually to maximum of 250–300 mg/day at bedtime. **Outpatients:** 75–150 mg/day. Maximum dose for outpatients is 200 mg. Decrease when feasible to maintenance dosage: 50–150 mg/day at bedtime. **Adolescent and geriatric clients:** 30–40 mg/day up to maximum of 100 mg/day. **Pediatric:** 1.5 mg/kg/day in three divided doses; can be increased 1–1.5 mg/kg/day q 3–5 days to a maximum of 5 mg/kg/day.
Childhood enuresis.
Age 6 years and over: 25 mg/day 1 hr before bedtime. Dose can be increased to 50 mg/day up to 12 years of age and to 75 mg/day in children over 12 years of age.

- **IM**

Antidepressant.
Adults: Up to 100 mg/day in divided doses. IM route not recommended for use in children less than 12 years of age.

Administration/Storage

1. Crystals, which may be present in the injectable form, can be dissolved by immersing closed ampules into hot water for 1 min.
2. Total daily dose can be given once daily at bedtime.
3. Protect from direct sunlight and strong artificial light.
4. Parenteral therapy should be used only in clients unwilling or unable to take PO medication. Switch to PO medication as soon as possible.
5. Imipramine injection should not be given IV.
6. When used for the treatment of enuresis, the drug can be given in doses of 25 mg in midafternoon and 25 mg at bedtime (this regimen may increase effectiveness).
7. When used as an enuretic in children, the dose should not exceed 2.5 mg/kg/day.

Laboratory Test Interferences: ↑ Metanephrine (Pisano test); ↓ Urinary 5-HIAA.

Additional Side Effects: ***High therapeutic dosage may increase frequency of seizures in epileptic clients and cause seizures in nonepileptic clients.*** Elderly and adolescent clients may have low tolerance to the drug.

NURSING CONSIDERATIONS

See also *Nursing Considerations* for *Antidepressants, Tricyclic,* Chapter 37.

Client/Family Teaching

1. Review appropriate times and methods for administration.
2. Report any increase in frequency of seizures in epileptics and any occurrence of seizures in nonepileptics.
3. Advise parents that children may experience mild N&V, unusual tiredness, nervousness, or insomnia. If pronounced, these symptoms should be reported.
4. Drug may cause sedation. Do not perform activities that require mental alertness until drug effects realized.
5. With enuresis, refer parents to regional centers with incontinence programs if bed-wetting persists.

Evaluate

- Improvement in symptoms of depression (improved appetite, ↑ sense of well being, and ↑ socialization)
- Prevention of bed-wetting
- Control of severe neurogenic pain
- Therapeutic serum drug levels (200–350 ng/mL)

Maprotiline hydrochloride

(mah-**PROH**-tih-leen)
Pregnancy Category: B
Ludiomil **(Rx)**

See also *Antidepressants, Tricyclic,* Chapter 37.

How Supplied: *Tablet:* 25 mg, 50 mg, 75 mg

Action/Kinetics: Maprotiline is actually a tetracyclic compound but has many similarities to the tricyclic drugs. It causes moderate anticholinergic, sedative, and orthostatic hypotensive effects. **Effective plasma levels:** 200–300 ng/mL. **t½:** Approximately 21–25 hr. **Peak effect:** 12 hr. Beneficial effects may not be observed for 2–3 weeks.

Uses: Treat symptoms of depression. Depressive neuroses, depression in clients with manic-depressive illness, depression with anxiety.

Dosage

- **Tablets**

Mild to moderate depression.

Adult outpatients, initial: 75 mg/day; can be increased to 150–225 mg/day if necessary.

Severe depression.

Adults, hospitalized, initial: 100–150 mg/day; can be increased to 225 mg if necessary. Dosage should not exceed 225 mg/day. **Maintenance:** For all uses, 75–150 mg/day, adjusted depending on therapeutic response. **Geriatric clients:** 50–75 mg/day.

Administration/Storage

1. May be given in single or divided doses.
2. If daytime sedation is a problem, may take at bedtime.
3. Should be discontinued as long as possible before elective surgery.

Assessment

1. Document indications for therapy and onset of symptoms.

2. List any agents previously used for this condition and the outcome.
3. Document any evidence of seizure disorder.
4. Attempt to identify and address underlying reasons for depression.

Additional Contraindications: Known or suspected seizure disorders.
Special Concerns: Not recommended for clients under 18 years of age.
Additional Side Effect: Overdosage may cause ***increased incidence of seizures.***

NURSING CONSIDERATIONS

See also *Nursing Considerations* for *Antidepressants, Tricyclic,* Chapter 37.

Evaluate

- Reports of less depression and anxiety
- ↓ Fatigue, improved sleeping and eating patterns, ↑ sense of self-worth
- Therapeutic serum drug levels (200–300 ng/mL)

Nortriptyline hydrochloride

(nor-**TRIP**-tih-leen)
Pregnancy Category: C
Aventyl, Pamelor **(Rx)**

See also *Antidepressants, Tricyclic,* Chapter 37.
How Supplied: *Capsule:* 10 mg, 25 mg, 50 mg, 75 mg; *Solution:* 10 mg/5 mL
Action/Kinetics: Nortriptyline manifests moderate anticholinergic and sedative effects but slight orthostatic hypotensive effects. **Effective plasma levels:** 50–150 ng/mL. **t½:** 18–44 hr.
Uses: Treatment of symptoms of depression. Chronic, severe neurogenic pain. Dermatologic disorders including chronic urticaria, angioedema, and nocturnal pruritus in atopic eczema.

Dosage

- **Capsules, Oral Solution**

Depression.
Adults: 25 mg t.i.d.–q.i.d. Dose individualized. **Doses above 150 mg/day are not recommended. Elderly clients:** 30–50 mg/day in divided doses. **Not recommended for children.**

Dermatologic disorders.
75 mg/day.
Administration/Storage: Give after meals and at bedtime to minimize GI upset.
Special Concerns: Safety and efficacy have not been determined in children.
Laboratory Test Interference: ↓ Urinary 5-HIAA.

NURSING CONSIDERATIONS

See also *Nursing Considerations* for *Antidepressants, Tricyclic,* Chapter 37.

Assessment

1. Document indications for therapy and type and onset of symptoms.
2. Assist client to identify any causative factors.

Evaluate

- Control of symptoms of depression (↓ fatigue, improved sleeping and eating patterns, effective coping)
- ↓ Nocturnal pruritus
- Relief of chronic neurogenic pain

Protriptyline hydrochloride

(proh-**TRIP**-tih-leen)
Triptil ✱, Vivactil **(Rx)**

See also *Antidepressants, Tricyclic,* Chapter 37.
How Supplied: *Tablet:* 5 mg, 10 mg
Action/Kinetics: Significant anticholinergic effects but low sedative and orthostatic hypotensive effects. **Effective plasma levels:** 100–200 ng/mL. **t½:** Approximately 67–89 hr.
Uses: Symptoms of depression. Withdrawn and anergic clients. Obstructive sleep apnea. Has also been used with amphetamines to treat cataplexy associated with narcolepsy and to relieve symptoms of attention deficit disorders in some children over 6 years of age with or without hyperactivity.

Dosage

- **Tablets**

Antidepressant.

Adults, individualized: 15–40 mg/day in three to four divided doses. Up to 60 mg/day (maximum) may be given. **Elderly clients, adolescents, initial:** 5 mg t.i.d.; increase dose slowly. Monitor CV system closely if dose exceeds 20 mg/day in the elderly. **Not recommended for children.**

Anticataleptic.

15–20 mg/day at bedtime.

Administration/Storage: If drug causes insomnia, give last dose no less than 8 hr before bedtime.

Special Concerns: Use with caution during pregnancy. Administer with caution to clients with myocardial insufficiency and those in whom tachycardia or a drop in BP might lead to serious complications. Safety and efficacy for treating depression have not been determined in children.

NURSING CONSIDERATIONS

See also *Nursing Considerations* for *Antidepressants, Tricyclic,* Chapter 37.

Assessment

1. Document indications for therapy, onset of symptoms, and presenting behaviors.
2. Closely assess VS and mental status until response established.

Evaluate

- ↓ Depressive and withdrawn behaviors
- Reports of improved attention span (in attention deficit disorder [ADD])

Trimipramine maleate

(try-**MIP**-rah-meen)
Pregnancy Category: C
Apo-Trimip ✱, Novo-Tripramine ✱, Rhotrimine ✱, Surmontil **(Rx)**

See also *Antidepressants, Tricyclic,* Chapter 37.

How Supplied: *Capsule:* 25 mg, 50 mg, 100 mg

Action/Kinetics: Trimipramine causes moderate anticholinergic and orthostatic hypotensive effects and significant sedative effects. **Effective plasma levels:** 180 ng/mL. **t½:** 7–30 hr. Seems more effective in endogenous depression than in other types of depression.

Uses: Treatment of symptoms of depression. PUD.

Dosage

- **Capsules**

Antidepressant.

Adults, outpatients, initial: 75 mg/day in divided doses up to 150 mg/day. Daily dosage should not exceed 200 mg; **maintenance:** 50–150 mg/day. Total dose can be given at bedtime. **Adults, hospitalized, initial:** 100 mg/day in divided doses up to 200 mg/day. If no improvement in 2–3 weeks, increase to 250–300 mg/day. **Adolescent/geriatric clients, initial:** 50 mg/day up to 100 mg/day. Not recommended for children.

Special Concerns: Not recommended for use in children less than 12 years of age.

NURSING CONSIDERATIONS

See also *Nursing Considerations* for *Antidepressants, Tricyclic,* Chapter 37.

Assessment: Document indications for therapy and type and onset of symptoms.

Evaluate

- Evidence of behaviors that reflect ↓ levels of depression (such as improved eating and sleeping patterns, ↓ fatigue, ↑ social interactions)
- Control of symptoms of PUD

MISCELLANEOUS ANTIDEPRESSANTS

See the following individual entries:

Bupropion Hydrochloride
Fluoxetine Hydrochloride
Paroxetine Hydrochloride
Sertraline Hydrochloride
Trazodone Hydrochloride
Venlafaxine Hydrochloride

Bupropion hydrochloride

(byou-**PROH**-pee-on)
Pregnancy Category: B
Wellbutrin

How Supplied: *Tablet:* 75 mg, 100 mg
Action/Kinetics: Bupropion is an antidepressant whose mechanism of action is not known; the drug does not inhibit MAO and it only weakly blocks neuronal uptake of epinephrine, serotonin, and dopamine. **Peak plasma levels:** 2 hr. **t½:** 8–24 hr. Metabolized to both active and inactive metabolites. During chronic use the plasma levels of two active metabolites may be higher than bupropion. Excreted through both the urine (87%) and the feces (10%).
Uses: Short-term (6 weeks or less) treatment of depression.

Dosage

- **Tablets**

Antidepressant.

Adults, initial: 100 mg in the morning and evening for the first 3 days; **then,** 100 mg t.i.d., given in the morning, midday, and in the evening (6 hr should elapse between doses). If no response is observed after 4 weeks or longer, the dose may be increased to 450 mg/day with individual doses not to exceed 150 mg. Doses higher than 450 mg should not be administered. **Maintenance:** Lowest dose to control depression.
Administration/Storage
1. To reduce the risk of seizures, the total daily dose should not exceed 450 mg, each single dose should not exceed 150 mg, and doses of drug should be increased gradually.
2. Several months of treatment may be necessary to control acute depression.
3. Review list of drugs with which this medication interacts.
4. *Treatment of Overdose:* Client should be hospitalized. If conscious, syrup of ipecac is given to induce vomiting followed by activated charcoal q 6 hr during the first 12 hr after ingestion. Both ECG and EEG should be monitored for 48 hr and fluid intake must be adequate. If the client is in a stupor, is comatose, or is convulsing, gastric lavage may be undertaken provided intubation of the airway has been performed. Seizures may be treated with IV benzodiazepines and other supportive procedures.
Contraindications: Seizure disorders; presence or history of bulimia or anorexia nervosa due to the higher incidence of seizures in such clients. Concomitant use of an MAO inhibitor.
Special Concerns: Use with caution in clients with a history of seizures, cranial trauma, with drugs that lower the seizure threshold, and other situations that might cause seizures (e.g., abrupt cessation of a benzodiazepine). Use with caution and in lower doses in clients with liver or kidney disease and in those with a recent history of MI or unstable heart disease. Assess benefits versus risks during lactation. Safety and efficacy have not been established in clients less than 18 years of age.
Side Effects: *CNS:* ***Dose-dependent risk of seizures,*** restlessness, agitation, hostility, sedation, headache or migraine, insomnia, decreased libido, decreased concentration, euphoria, ataxia, incoordination, delusions, hallucinations, impaired sleep quality, psychotic epidsodes, confusion, paranoia, anxiety, manic episodes in bipolar manic depression, ***suicide.*** *GI:* N&V, constipation, anorexia, weight loss (up to 2.3 kg), diarrhea, dyspepsia, increased appetite, weight gain, dry mouth, increased salivation, stomatitis. *Neurologic:* Akinesia, bradykinesia, tremor, sensory disturbances, pseudoparkinsonism, akathisia, dyskinesia, dystonia, muscle spasms. *CV:* Dizziness, tachycardia, hypertension, hypotension, palpitations, ***cardiac arrhythmias,*** edema, syncope. *GU:* Impotence, menstrual irregularities, urinary fre-

quency or retention, nocturia. *Miscellaneous:* Excessive sweating, blurred vision, auditory disturbances, alteration in taste, rash, pruritus, fever, chills, arthritis, fatigue, flu-like symptoms, upper respiratory problems, temperature disturbances of the skin.

Symptoms of Overdose: Seizures, hallucinations, loss of consciousness, tachycardia, multiple uncontrolled seizures, bradycardia, cardiac failure and cardiac arrest prior to death.

Drug Interactions

Alcohol / Alcohol ↓ seizure threshold; use with bupropion may precipitate seizures
Carbamazepine / Possible additive effect to ↑ drug metabolizing enzymes in the liver
Cimetidine / See *Carbamazepine* Chapter 36
Levodopa / ↑ Risk of side effects
MAO inhibitors / Acute toxicity to bupropion may ↑, especially if used with phenelzine
Phenobarbital / See *Carbamazepine* Chapter 36
Phenytoin / See *Carbamazepine* Chapter 36

NURSING CONSIDERATIONS

Assessment

1. Document indications for therapy, presenting behaviors, and length of time this has been evident.
2. Determine if client has a history of seizures and/or recent MI. Dose of bupropion may need to be reduced.
3. Note any client history of bulimia or anorexia nervosa.
4. Determine if the woman client is of childbearing age and lactating.
5. Obtain baseline weight, ECG, and liver and renal function studies. Anticipate reduced dose with renal and/or liver dysfunction.
6. Assess client mental stability and potential for compliance. There are fewer side effects (no CV effects, drug interactions, sedation, and weight gain) with bupropion than with other agents used for this disorder.

Client/Family Teaching

1. Discuss the side effects associated with drug therapy and advise to report any that are bothersome or persistent, especially marked weight loss or diarrhea.
2. Explain the potential for a change in taste perceptions. The result could be loss of appetite and weight loss. Record weights and report any significant changes.
3. Inform client of possible menstrual irregularities.
4. Men should be warned about the possibility of impotence.
5. The beneficial effects of the drug may not be noticed for 5–21 days. Continue taking the medication and do not be discouraged by the delayed response.
6. Any changes in urinary output should be reported.
7. Dizziness may occur. Therefore, clients should not arise from a supine position suddenly. If dizziness occurs during the day, the client should sit down until the sensation subsides and report if it persists.
8. Stress the importance of reporting for follow-up laboratory studies and medical visits so that drug therapy and dosage may be evaluated and adjusted as needed.
9. Report any mood swings or suicidal ideations immediately.

Evaluate: Improvement in symptoms of depression such as ↓ fatigue, improved eating and sleeping patterns, and ↑ socialization.

Fluoxetine hydrochloride

(flew-**OX**-eh-teen)
Pregnancy Category: B
Prozac **(Rx)**

How Supplied: *Capsule:* 10 mg, 20 mg; *Solution:* 20 mg/5 mL
Action/Kinetics: Fluoxetine is not related chemically to tricyclic, tetracyclic, or other antidepressants. The antidepressant effect is thought to be due to inhibition of uptake of serotonin into CNS neurons. The drug also binds to muscarinic, histaminer-

gic, and alpha-1-adrenergic receptors, accounting for many of the side effects. Fluoxetine is metabolized in the liver to norfluoxetine, a metabolite with equal potency to fluoxetine. Norfluoxetine is further metabolized by the liver to inactive metabolites that are excreted by the kidneys. **t½, fluoxetine:** 2–7 days; **t½, norfluoxetine:** 7–9 days. Steady-state plasma levels are achieved after 4–5 weeks. Active drug will be maintained in the body for weeks after withdrawal.

Uses: Depression manifested by outpatients. Use in hospitalized clients or for longer than 5–6 weeks has not been studied adequately. Obsessive-compulsive disorders. *Investigational:* Treatment of obesity and bulimia nervosa.

Dosage

- **Capsules, Liquid**

Antidepressant.

Adults, initial: 20 mg/day in the morning. If clinical improvement is not observed after several weeks, the dose may be increased to a maximum of 80 mg/day in two equally divided doses.

Obsessive-compulsive disorder.

Initial:20 mg/day in the morning. If improvement is not significant after several weeks, the dose may be increased. **Usual dosage range:** 20–60 mg/day; total daily dosage should not exceed 80 mg.

Treatment of obesity.

20–60 mg/day.

Treatment of bulimia nervosa.

60–80 mg/day.

Administration/Storage

1. Doses greater than 20 mg/day should be divided and given in the morning and at noon.
2. If doses lower than 20 mg are necessary, the drug may be emptied from the capsule into cranberry, orange, or apple juice; this should not be refrigerated (is stable for 2 weeks). *NOTE:* A liquid preparation (20 mg/5 mL) is also available.
3. The maximum therapeutic effect may not be observed until 4 weeks after beginning therapy.
4. Elderly clients or clients taking multiple medications should take lower or less frequent doses.
5. Lower doses should be used in clients with liver or kidney dysfunction.
6. When used for obsessive-compulsive disorders, therapy has been continued for over 6 months. However, the client should be reassessed periodically to determine if continued drug therapy is needed.

Special Concerns: Use with caution during lactation and in clients with impaired liver or kidney function. Safety and efficacy have not been determined in children. A lower initial dose may be necessary in geriatric clients.

Side Effects: A large number of side effects have been reported for this drug. Listed are those with a reported frequency of greater than 1%. *CNS:* Headache (most common), activation of mania or hypomania, insomnia, anxiety, nervousness, dizziness, fatigue, sedation, decreased libido, drowsiness, lightheadedness, decreased ability to concentrate, tremor, disturbances in sensation, agitation, abnormal dreams. Although less frequent than 1%, ***some clients may experience seizures or attempt suicide.*** *GI:* Nausea (most common), diarrhea, vomiting, constipation, dry mouth, dyspepsia, anorexia, abdominal pain, flatulence, alteration in taste, gastroenteritis, increased appetite. *CV:* Hot flashes, palpitations. *GU:* Sexual dysfunction, frequent urination, infection of the urinary tract, dysmenorrhea. *Respiratory:* Upper respiratory tract infections, pharyngitis, cough, dyspnea, rhinitis, bronchitis, nasal congestion. *Skin:* Rash, pruritus, sweating. *Musculoskeletal:* Muscle, joint, or back pain. *Miscellaneous:* Flu-like symptoms, asthenia, fever, chest pain, allergy, visual disturbances, weight loss.

Drug Interactions

Diazepam / Fluoxetine ↑ half-life of diazepam → excessive sedation or impaired psychomotor skills

Digoxin / ↑ Effect of fluoxetine due to ↓ plasma protein binding
Lithium / ↑ Serum levels of lithium → possible neurotoxicity
MAO inhibitors / MAO inhibitors should be discontinued 14 days before initiation of fluoxetine therapy
Tricyclic antidepressants / ↑ Pharmacologic and toxicologic effects of tricyclics due to ↓ breakdown by liver
Tryptophan / Symptoms of agitation, GI distress, restlessness
Warfarin / ↑ Effect of fluoxetine due to ↓ plasma protein binding

NURSING CONSIDERATIONS

Assessment

1. Document indications for therapy and type and onset of symptoms.
2. Review drugs currently prescribed to detect any that may interact unfavorably.
3. In women of childbearing age, determine if pregnant or lactating.
4. Obtain baseline liver and renal function studies before initiating therapy. Anticipate reduced dose in clients with hepatic and/or renal insufficiency.
5. Periodically reassess client to determine need for continued therapy.

Client/Family Teaching

1. Use caution when driving or performing tasks that require mental alertness because drug may cause drowsiness and/or dizziness.
2. Report any side effects, especially rashes, hives, increased anxiety, and loss of appetite.
3. Stress the importance of taking the medication at the specific times designated as nervousness and insomnia may occur.
4. Remind client that it usually takes 1 month to note any significant benefits from therapy and not to become discouraged and discontinue the medication before benefits are attained and evaluated.
5. Avoid ingestion of alcohol and do not take any OTC medications without approval.
6. Stress the importance of reporting for all scheduled lab and medical visits.
7. Any thoughts of suicide or evidence of increased suicide ideations should be reported immediately.
8. Use birth control during therapy.

Evaluate

- ↓ Symptoms of depression, as evidenced by improved sleeping and eating patterns, ↓ fatigue, and ↑ social involvement and activity.
- Control of repetitive behavioral manifestations

Paroxetine hydrochloride

(pah-**ROX**-eh-teen)
Pregnancy Category: B
Paxil **(Rx)**

How Supplied: *Tablet:* 20 mg, 30 mg

Action/Kinetics: Paroxetine acts by inhibiting neuronal reuptake of serotonin in the CNS resulting in potentiation of serotonergic activity in the CNS. It appears to have weak effects on neuronal uptake of norepinephrine and dopamine. The drug is completely absorbed from the GI tract. **Time to peak plasma levels:** 5.2 hr. **Peak plasma levels:** 61.7 ng/mL. Approximately 10 days is required to reach steady-state levels. **t½:** 21 hr. Plasma levels are increased in clients with impaired renal and hepatic function as well as in geriatric clients. The drug is extensively metabolized in the liver to inactive metabolites. Approximately two-thirds of the drug is excreted through the urine and one-third is excreted in the feces.

Uses: Treatment of major depressive episodes. To treat premature ejaculation in men.

Dosage

- **Tablets**

Treatment of Depression.

Adults: 20 mg/day, usually given as a single dose in the morning. Some clients not responding to the 20-mg dose may benefit from increasing the dose in 10-mg/day increments, up to a maximum of 50 mg/day. Dose changes should be made at intervals of at least 1 week. **Geriatric or debilitated clients, those with se-**

vere hepatic or renal impairment, initial: 10 mg/day, up to a maximum of 40 mg/day.

Premature ejaculation in men. 20 mg/day.

Administration/Storage

1. Even though beneficial effects may be seen in 1–4 weeks, therapy should be continued as directed by the physician.

2. Studies have shown that effectiveness is maintained for up to 1 year with daily doses averaging 30 mg.

3. *Treatment of Overdose:*

- Establish and maintain an airway
- Ensure adequate oxygenation and ventilation
- Induction of emesis, lavage, or both; following evacuation, 20–30 g activated charcoal may be given q 4–6 hr during the first 24–48 hr after ingestion
- An ECG should be taken and cardiac function monitored if there is any evidence of abnormality
- Provide supportive care with monitoring of VS

Contraindications: Use in clients taking MAO inhibitors. Use of alcohol.

Special Concerns: Use with caution and initially at reduced dosage in elderly clients as well as in those with impaired hepatic or renal function, with a history of mania, with a history of seizures, in clients with diseases or conditions that could affect metabolism or hemodynamic responses, and during lactation. Concurrent administration of paroxetine with lithium or digoxin should be undertaken with caution. Safety and efficacy have not been determined in children.

Side Effects: The side effects listed were observed with a frequency up to 1 in 1,000 clients.

CNS: Headache, somnolence, insomnia, agitation, ***seizures,*** tremor, anxiety, activation of mania or hypomania, dizziness, nervousness, paresthesia, agitation, drugged feeling, myoclonus, CNS stimulation, confusion, amnesia, impaired concentration, depression, emotional lability, vertigo, abnormal thinking, akinesia, alcohol abuse, ataxia, ***convulsions,*** depersonalization, hallucinations, hyperkinesia, hypertonia, incoordination, lack of emotion, manic reaction, paranoid reaction. *GI:* Nausea, abdominal pain, diarrhea, dry mouth, vomiting, constipation, decreased appetite, flatulence, oropharynx disorder ("lump" in throat, tightness in throat), dyspepsia, increased appetite, bruxism, dysphagia, eructation, gastritis, glossitis, increased salivation, mouth ulceration, ***rectal hemorrhage,*** abnormal liver function tests. *Hematologic:* Anemia, leukopenia, lymphadenopathy, purpura. *CV:* Palpitation, vasodilation, postural hypotension, hypertension, syncope, tachycardia, bradycardia, conduction abnormalities, abnormal ECG, hypotension, migraine, peripheral vascular disorder. *Dermatologic:* Sweating, rash, pruritus, acne, alopecia, dry skin, ecchymosis, eczema, furunculosis, urticaria. *Metabolic/ Nutritional:* Edema, weight gain, weight loss, hyperglycemia, peripheral edema, thirst. *Respiratory:* Respiratory disorder (cold symptoms or upper respiratory infection), increased cough, rhinitis, asthma, bronchitis, dyspnea, epistaxis, hyperventilation, pneumonia, respiratory flu, sinusitis. *GU:* Abnormal ejaculation (usually delay), erectile difficulties, sexual dysfunction, impotence, urinary frequency, urinary difficulty or hesitancy, decreased libido, anorgasmia in women, difficulty in reaching climax/orgasm in women, abortion, amenorrhea, breast pain, cystitis, dysmenorrhea, dysuria, menorrhagia, nocturia, polyuria, urethritis, urinary incontinence, urinary retention, vaginitis. *Musculoskeletal:* Asthenia, back pain, myopathy, myalgia, myasthenia, neck pain, arthralgia, arthritis. *Ophthalmologic:* Blurred vision, abnormality of accommodation, eye pain, mydriasis. *Otic:* Ear pain, otitis media, tinnitus. *Miscellaneous:* Fever, chest pain, trauma, taste perversion, chills, malaise, allergic reaction, ***carcinoma,*** face edema, moniliasis.

NOTE: Over 4–6-week period, there was evidence of adaptation to side effects such as nausea and dizziness but less adaptation to dry mouth, somnolence, and asthenia.

Symptoms of Overdose: N&V, drowsiness, sinus tachycardia, dilated pupils.

Drug Interactions

Antiarrhythmics, Type IC / Possible ↑ effect due to ↓ breakdown by the liver
Cimetidine / ↑ Effect of paroxetine due to ↓ breakdown by the liver
Digoxin / Possible ↓plasma levels
Monoamine oxidase inhibitors / Possibility of serious, and sometimes fatal, reactions including hyperthermia, rigidity, myoclonus, autonomic instability with possible rapid fluctuations in VS, and mental status changes including extreme agitation progressing to delirium and coma
Phenobarbital / Possible ↓ effect of paroxetine due to ↑ breakdown by the liver
Phenytoin / Possible ↓ effect of paroxetine due to ↑ breakdown by the liver; also, paroxetine ↓levels of phenytoin
Procyclidine / ↓ Dose of procyclidine as significant anticholinergic effects are seen
Tryptophan / Possibility of headache, nausea, sweating, and dizziness when taken together
Warfarin / Possibility of ↑ bleeding tendencies

NURSING CONSIDERATIONS

Assessment

1. Obtain a thorough nursing history, noting onset and type of symptoms, any previous treatment, and the outcome.
2. Document any history of mania, altered metabolic or hemodynamic states, or seizures.
3. List drugs currently prescribed to ensure no unfavorable interactions.
4. Determine that client is not taking a MAO inhibitor. Paroxetine should not be used in combination with a MAO or within 14 days of discontinuing treatment with a MAO.
5. Concomitant use with tryptophan may cause headaches, nausea, dizziness, and sweating.
6. During management of overdose, always entertain the possibility of multiple drug involvement.
7. Obtain baseline electrolytes, CBC, and liver and renal function studies and note any evidence of dysfunction.

Client/Family Teaching

1. Take only as directed. Prescriptions will be for a small quantity of medication to ensure compliance and discourage overdose.
2. Do not engage in tasks that require mental alertness until drug effects are realized.
3. Avoid alcohol. Do not take any OTC products without provider approval.
4. Provide a printed list of drug side effects advising client to report those that are persistent or not tolerable.
5. Report excessive weight gain or loss.
6. Notify provider if pregnancy is suspected or planned.
7. Advise family not to leave severely depressed individuals alone. The possibility of a suicide attempt is inherent in depression and may persist until significant remission is observed. Report any thoughts of suicide or increased suicide ideations.
8. Encourage participation in therapy sessions designed to assist with underlying client problem.

Evaluate

- ↓ Level of experienced depression
- Improved eating and sleeping patterns
- Evidence of ↑ social involvement and activity

Sertraline hydrochloride

(**SIR**-trah-leen)
Pregnancy Category: B
Zoloft **(Rx)**

How Supplied: *Tablet:* 50 mg, 100 mg

Action/Kinetics: Sertraline is believed to act by inhibiting CNS neuronal uptake of serotonin. The drug is not believed to have any significant affinity for adrenergic, cholinergic, dopaminergic, histaminergic, serotonergic, GABA, or benzodiazepine receptors. Steady-state plasma levels are usually reached after 1 week of once daily dosing but is increased to 2–3 weeks in older clients. **Time to peak plasma levels:** 4.5–8.4 hr. **Peak plasma levels:** 20–55 ng/mL. **Terminal elimination t½:** 26 hr. Washout period is 7 days. Food will decrease the time to reach peak plasma levels. The drug undergoes significant first-pass metabolism; there is significant (98%) binding to serum proteins. The routes of elimination are renal (40%–45%) and hepatic (40%–45%). Drug is metabolized to n-desmethyl-sertraline, which has minimal antidepressant activity.

Uses: Treatment of depression with reduced psychomotor agitation, anxiety, and insomnia. *Investigational:* Obsessive-compulsive disorders.

Dosage

• **Tablets**

Adults, initial: 50 mg/day once daily either in the morning or evening. Clients not responding to a 50-mg dose may benefit from doses up to a maximum of 200 mg/day.

Administration/Storage

1. Clients responding during an initial 8-week treatment period will likely benefit during an additional 8-week treatment period. The effectiveness of sertraline has not been evaluated for more than 16 weeks, although it is generally recognized that acute periods of depression require several months or longer of sustained drug therapy.
2. Dosage increases should not occur at intervals of less than 1 week.
3. Beneficial effects may not be observed for 2–4 weeks after treatment is started.
4. *Treatment of Overdose:*

• Establish and maintain an airway, ensuring adequate oxygenation and ventilation.
• Activated charcoal, with or without sorbitol, may be as or more effective than emesis or lavage.
• Cardiac and VS should be monitored.
• Provide general supportive measures and symptomatic treatment.
• Since sertraline has a large volume of distribution, it is unlikely that dialysis, forced diuresis, hemoperfusion, or exchange transfusion will be beneficial.

Contraindications: Use in combination with a MAO inhibitor or within 14 days of discontinuing treatment with a MAO inhibitor.

Special Concerns: Use with caution in clients with impaired hepatic or renal function, in clients with seizure disorders, and during lactation. Safety and efficacy have not been determined in children. The plasma clearance may be lower in elderly clients. The possibility of a suicide attempt is possible in depression and may persist until significant remission occurs. Use with caution in clients with diseases or conditions that may affect hemodynamic responses or metabolism.

Laboratory Test Interferences: ↑ AST or ALT, total cholesterol, triglycerides. ↓ Serum uric acid.

Side Effects: A large number of side effects is possible; listed are those side effects with a frequency of 0.1% or greater. *GI:* Nausea and diarrhea (common), dry mouth, constipation, dyspepsia, vomiting, flatulence, anorexia, abdominal pain, thirst, increased salivation, increased appetite, teeth-grinding, dysphagia, eructation. *CV:* Palpitations, hot flushes, chest pain, edema, hypertension, hypotension, peripheral ischemia, postural hypotension or dizziness, syncope, tachycardia. *CNS:* Headache (common), insomnia (common), somnolence, agitation, nervousness, anxiety, dizziness, tremor, fatigue, impaired concentration, yawning, paresthesia, hypoesthesia, twitching, hypertonia, confusion, ataxia or abnormal coordination, abnormal gait, hyperesthesia, hyperkinesia, abnormal dreams, aggressive reaction, amnesia, apathy, delusion, depersonalization, depression, aggravated depression, emotional lability, euphoria, activation of mania or hypomania, hallucinations, neurosis, paranoid reaction, ***suicide ideation or attempt,*** abnormal thinking, hypokinesia, migraine, nystagmus, vertigo. *Dermatologic:* Rash, acne, excessive sweating, alopecia, pruritus, cold and clammy skin, facial edema, erythematous rash, maculopapular rash, dry skin. *Musculoskeletal:* Myalgia, arthralgia, arthrosis, dystonia, muscle cramps or weakness. *GU:* Urinary frequency, micturition disorders, menstrual disorders, dysmenorrhea, dysuria, painful menstruation, intermenstrual bleeding, sexual dysfunction and decreased libido, nocturia, polyuria, urinary incontinence. *Respiratory:* Rhinitis, pharyngitis, bronchospasm, coughing, dyspnea, epistaxis. *Ophthalmologic:* Blurred vision, abnormal vision, abnormal accommodation, conjunctivitis, diplopia, eye pain, xerophthalmia. *Otic:* Tinnitus, earache. *Body as a whole:* Asthenia, fever, chest pain, chills, back pain, weight loss or weight gain, malaise, flushing, hot flashes, rigors, lymphadenopathy, purpura.

Symptoms of Overdose: Intensification of side effects.

Drug Interactions: Because sertraline is highly bound to plasma proteins, its use with other drugs that are also highly protein bound may lead to displacement, resulting in higher plasma levels of the drug and possibly increased side effects.

Alcohol / Concurrent use is not recommended in depressed clients

Diazepam / ↑ Plasma levels of desmethyldiazepam (significance not known)

MAO inhibitors / Serious and possibly fatal reactions including hyperthermia, rigidity, autonomic instability with possible rapid fluctuation of VS, myoclonus, changes in mental status (e.g., extreme agitation, delirium, coma)

Tolbutamide / ↓ Clearance of tolbutamide (significance unknown)

Warfarin / ↑ PT and delayed normalization of PT

NURSING CONSIDERATIONS

Assessment

1. Obtain a thorough nursing history. Document indications for therapy and type and onset of symptoms.
2. List other medications used to treat symptoms and the outcome.
3. Note any history of seizure disorder.
4. Review list of drugs currently prescribed to prevent any unfavorable interactions.
5. Obtain baseline liver and renal function studies.

Client/Family Teaching

1. Take only as directed and remain under close medical supervision.
2. Do not perform activities that require mental and physical alertness until drug effects are realized.
3. Provide a printed list of side effects stressing those that require immediate medical attention.
4. Loss of appetite, persistent nausea, and diarrhea with excessive weight loss should be reported.
5. Advise family to maintain contact with severely depressed client and to observe medication utilization as the risk of suicide is tantamount in a depressive phase. Report any evidence of suicidal thoughts or aggression.
6. Avoid alcohol and any other CNS depressants.
7. Request provider approval before ingesting any OTC products.
8. Practice contraception and notify provider if pregnancy is suspected.

Evaluate

- Improved eating and sleeping patterns
- Evidence of ↑ social involvement and activity
- ↓ Levels of agitation and anxiety
- Relief of symptoms of depression

Trazodone hydrochloride

(**TRAYZ**-oh-dohn)
Pregnancy Category: C
Desyrel, Desyrel Dividose, PMS-Trazodone ✱, Trazon, Trialodine **(Rx)**

How Supplied: *Tablet:* 50 mg, 100 mg, 150 mg, 300 mg

Action/Kinetics: Trazodone is a novel antidepressant that does not inhibit MAO and is also devoid of amphetamine-like effects. Response usually occurs after 2 weeks (75% of clients), with the remainder responding after 2–4 weeks. The drug may inhibit serotonin uptake by brain cells, therefore increasing serotonin concentrations in the synapse. It may also cause changes in binding of serotonin to receptors. The drug causes moderate sedative and orthostatic hypotensive effects and slight anticholinergic effects. **Peak plasma levels:** 1 hr (empty stomach). **t½:** initial, 3–6 hr; final, 5–9 hr. **Effective plasma levels:** 800–1,600 ng/mL. Metabolized in liver and excreted through both the urine and feces.

Uses: Depression with or without accompanying anxiety. *Investigational:* In combination with tryptophan for treating aggressive behavior. Treatment of cocaine withdrawal. Chronic pain including diabetic neuropathy.

Dosage

- **Tablets**

Antidepressant.

Adults and adolescents, initial: 150 mg/day; **then,** increase by 50 mg/day every 3–4 days to maximum of 400 mg/day in divided doses (outpatients). Inpatients may require up to, but not exceeding, 600 mg/day in divided doses. **Maintenance:** Use lowest effective dose. **Geriatric clients:** 75 mg/day in divided doses; dose can then be increased, as needed and tolerated, at 3–4-day intervals.

Administration/Storage

1. Dose should be initiated at the lowest possible level and increased gradually.
2. Beneficial effects may be observed within 1 week with optimal effects in most clients seen within 2 weeks.
3. *Treatment of Overdose:* Treat symptoms (especially hypotension and sedation). Gastric lavage and forced diuresis to remove the drug from the body.

Contraindications: During the initial recovery period following MI. Concurrently with electroshock therapy.

Special Concerns: Use with caution during lactation. Safety and efficacy in children less than 18 years of age have not been established. Geriatric clients are more prone to the sedative and hypotensive effects.

Side Effects: *General:* Dermatitis, edema, blurred vision, constipation, dry mouth, nasal congestion, skeletal muscle aches and pains. *CV:* Hypertension or hypotension, syncope, palpitations, tachycardia, SOB, chest pain. *GI:* Diarrhea, N&V, bad taste in mouth, flatulence. *GU:* Delayed urine flow, priapism, hematuria, increased urinary frequency. *CNS:* Nightmares, confusion, anger, excitement, decreased ability to concentrate, dizziness, disorientation, drowsiness, lightheadedness, fatigue, insomnia, nervousness, impaired memory. Rarely, hallucinations, impaired speech, hypomania. *Other:* Incoordination, tremors, paresthesias, decreased libido, appetite disturbances, red eyes, sweating or clamminess, tinnitus, weight gain or loss, anemia, hypersalivation. Rarely, akathisia, muscle twitching, increased libido, impotence, retrograde ejaculation, early menses, missed periods.

Symptoms of Overdose: ***Respiratory arrest, seizures,*** ECG changes, hypotension, priapism as well as an increase in the incidence and severity of side effects noted above (vomiting and drowsiness are the most common).

Drug Interactions
Alcohol / ↑ Depressant effects of alcohol
Antihypertensives / Additive hypotension
Barbiturates / ↑ Depressant effects of barbiturates
Clonidine / Trazodone ↓ effect of clonidine
CNS depressants / ↑ CNS depression
Digoxin / Trazodone may ↑ serum digoxin levels
MAO inhibitors / Initiate therapy cautiously if trazodone is to be used together with MAO inhibitors
Phenytoin / Trazodone may ↑ serum phenytoin levels

NURSING CONSIDERATIONS

Assessment

1. Document indications for therapy, onset of symptoms, and any associated causative factors.
2. Take a complete medication history noting any that may interact unfavorably (e.g., MAO inhibitors, antihypertensives).
3. Note any history of recent MI.
4. Obtain baseline CBC and renal and liver function studies; obtain ECG with history of CV diseases.

Client/Family Teaching

1. Take with food to enhance absorption and minimize dizziness and/or lightheadedness.
2. To reduce side effects during the day, take major portion of dose at bedtime.
3. Use caution when driving or when performing other hazardous tasks because trazodone may cause drowsiness or dizziness.
4. Avoid alcohol and do not take any other depressant drugs during therapy with trazodone.
5. Provide a printed list of drug side effects and advise client to report any that are persistent or bothersome.
6. Use sugarless gum or candies and frequent mouth rinses to diminish the dry mouth drug effects.
7. Inform surgeon if elective surgery is planned to minimize interaction of trazodone with anesthetic agent.
8. Encourage family to observe client closely for any suicidal cues. Clients taking antidepressants and emerging from the deepest phases of depression are more prone to suicide.
9. Encourage family to share responsibility for drug therapy to optimize treatment and to prevent overdosage.
10. Advise that it may take 2–4 weeks for full drug effects to be realized.

Evaluate: ↓ Symptoms of depression (e.g., improved sleeping and eating patterns, ↓ fatigue, and ↑ social interactions).

Venlafaxine hydrochloride

(ven-lah-**FAX**-een)
Pregnancy Category: C
Effexor **(Rx)**

How Supplied: *Tablet:* 25 mg, 37.5 mg, 50 mg, 75 mg, 100 mg
Action/Kinetics: Venlafaxine is not related chemically to any of the currently available antidepressants. The drug is a potent inhibitor of the uptake of neuronal serotonin and norepinephrine in the CNS and a weak inhibitor of the uptake of dopamine. The major metabolite—O-desmethylvenlafaxine (ODV)—is active. The drug and metabolite are eliminated through the kidneys. **t½, venlafaxine:** 5 hr; **t½, ODV:** 11 hr. The half-life of the drug and metabolite are increased in clients with impaired liver or renal function. Food has no effect on the absorption of venlafaxine.
Use: Treatment of depression.

Dosage

- **Tablets**

Depression.

Adults, initial: 75 mg/day given in two or three divided doses. Depending on the response, the dose can be increased to 150–225 mg/day in divided doses. Dosage increments should be made up to 75 mg/day at intervals of 4 or more days. Severely depressed clients may require 375 mg/day in divided doses. **Maintenance:** Sufficient studies have not been undertaken to determine how long a client should continue to take venlafaxine.

Administration/Storage

1. The drug should be taken with food.
2. The dose should be reduced by 50% in clients with moderate hepatic impairment and by 25% in clients with mild to moderate renal impairment.
3. When discontinuing venlafaxine after more than 1 week of therapy, the dose should be tapered to minimize the risk of symptoms of discontinuation. Clients receiving venlafaxine for 6 or more weeks should have their doses tapered over a 2-week period.
4. At least 14 days should elapse between discontinuation of a MAO inhibitor and initiation of venlafaxine therapy; at least 7 days should elapse after stopping venlafaxine before starting a MAO inhibitor.
5. *Treatment of Overdose:* General supportive measures; treat symptoms. Ensure an adequate airway, oxygenation, and ventilation. Monitor cardiac rhythm and VS. Activated charcoal, induction of emesis, or gastric lavage may be helpful.

Contraindications: Use with a MAO inhibitor or within 14 days of discontinuation of a MAO inhibitor. Use of alcohol.

Special Concerns: Use with caution in clients with impaired hepatic or renal function. Use with caution during lactation, in clients with a history of mania, and in those with diseases or conditions that could affect the hemodynamic responses or metabolism. Although it is possible for a geriatric client to be more sensitive, dosage adjustment is not necessary. The use of venlafaxine for more than 4–6 weeks has not been evaluated.

Laboratory Test Interferences: ↑ Alkaline phosphatase, creatinine, AST, ALT. Glycosuria, hyperglycemia, hyperlipemia, bilirubinemia, hyperuricemia, hypercholesterolemia, hypoglycemia, hypokalemia, hyperkalemia, hyperphosphatemia, hyponatremia, hypophosphatemia, hypoproteinemia, uremia, albuminuria.

Side Effects: Side effects with an incidence of 0.1% or greater are listed.

CNS: Anxiety, nervousness, insomnia, mania, hypomania, ***seizures, suicide attempts,*** dizziness, somnolence, tremors, abnormal dreams, hypertonia, paresthesia, decreased libido, agitation, confusion, abnormal thinking, depersonalization, depression, twitching, migraine, emotional lability, trismus, vertigo, apathy, ataxia, circumoral paresthesia, CNS stimulation, euphoria, hallucinations, hostility, hyperesthesia, hyperkinesia, hypertonia, hypotonia, incoordination, increased libido, myoclonus, neuralgia, neuropathy, paranoid reaction, psychosis, psychotic depression, sleep disturbance, abnormal speech, stupor, torticollis. *CV:* Sustained increase in BP (hypertension), vasodilation, tachycardia, postural hypotension, angina pectoris, extrasystoles, hypotension, peripheral vascular disorder, syncope, thrombophlebitis, peripheral edema. *GI:* Anorexia, N&V, dry mouth, constipation, diarrhea, dyspepsia, flatulence, dysphagia, eructation, colitis, edema of tongue, esophagitis, gastroenteritis, gastritis, glossitis, gingivitis, hemorrhoids, ***rectal hemorrhage,*** melena, stomatitis, stomach ulcer, mouth ulceration. *Body as a whole:* Headache, asthenia, infection, chills, chest pain, trauma, yawn, weight loss, accidental injury, malaise, neck pain, enlarged abdomen, allergic reaction, cyst, facial edema, generalized edema, hangover effect, hernia, intentional injury, neck rigidity, moniliasis, substernal chest pain, pelvic pain, photosensitivity reaction. *Respiratory:* Bronchitis, dyspnea, asthma, chest congestion, epistaxis, hyperventilation, laryngismus, laryngitis, pneumonia, voice alteration. *Dermatologic:* Acne, alopecia, brittle nails, contact dermatitis, dry skin, herpes simplex, herpes zoster, maculopapular rash, urticaria. *Hematologic:* Ecchymosis, anemia, leukocytosis, leukopenia, lymphadenopathy, lymphocytosis, thrombocytopenia, thrombocythemia, abnormal WBCs. *Endocrine:* Hypothyroidism, hyperthyroidism, goiter. *Musculoskeletal:* Arthritis, arthrosis, bone pain, bone spurs, bursitis, joint disorder, myasthenia, tenosynovitis. *Ophthalmic:* Blurred vision, mydriasis, abnormal accommodation, abnormal vision, cataract, conjunctivitis, corneal lesion, diplopia, dry eyes, exophthalmos, eye pain, photophobia, subconjunctival hemorrhage, visual field defect. *GU:* Urinary retention, abnormal ejaculation, impotence, urinary frequency, impaired urination, disturbed orgasm, menstrual disorder, anorgasmia, dysuria, hematuria, metrorrhagia, vaginitis, amenorrhea, kidney calculus, cystitis, leukorrhea, menorrhagia, nocturia, bladder pain, breast pain, kidney pain, polyuria, prostatitis, pyelonephritis, pyuria, urinary incontinence, urinary urgency, enlarged uterine fibroids, ***uterine hemorrhage, vaginal hemorrhage,*** vaginal moniliasis. *Miscellaneous:* Sweating, tinnitus, taste perversion, thirst, diabetes mellitus, alcohol intolerance, gout, hypoglycemic reaction, hemochromatosis, ear pain, otitis media.

Symptoms of Overdose: Extensions of side effects, especially somnolence. Other symptoms include prolongation of QTc, mild sinus tachycardia, and ***seizures.***

Drug Interactions

Cimetidine / ↓ First-pass metabolism of venlafaxine

MAO inhibitors / Serious and possibly fatal reaction, including hyperthermia, rigidity, myoclonus, autonomic instability with rapid changes in VS, extreme agitation, coma

NURSING CONSIDERATIONS

Assessment

1. Document indications for therapy and type and onset of symptoms.
2. List other agents prescribed to ensure none interact unfavorably.
3. Obtain baseline serum lipid levels and hepatic and renal function studies. Anticipate reduced dosage with hepatic or renal impairment.

Intervention: Due to possible sustained hypertension, HR and BP of clients should be monitored regularly.

Client/Family Teaching

1. Take only as directed; *do not* stop abruptly.
2. Drug may cause dizziness or drowsiness. Do not perform activities that require mental alertness until drug effects realized.
3. Any rash, hives, or other allergic manifestations should be reported immediately.
4. Drug may impair appetite and induce weight loss; report if excessive.
5. May experience anxiety, palpitations, headaches, and constipation; report if persistent or intolerable.
6. Avoid alcohol. Do not take any unprescribed or OTC preparations without provider approval.
7. Advise to use birth control. Notify provider if client is pregnant or intends to become pregnant while taking venlafaxine.
8. Any suicide ideations or abnormal behaviors should be reported. Explain that due to the possibility of suicide, high-risk clients should be observed closely during initial therapy. Prescriptions should be written for the smallest quantity to reduce the risk of overdose. Advise family to supervise medication administration with severely depressed clients.

Evaluate

- Reports of symptomatic improvement
- Evidence of improvement in symptoms of depression by changes in attention, concentration, memory, fine motor ability, reaction time, performance, drive, and wakefulness

CHAPTER THIRTY-EIGHT

Antipsychotic Agents

See also the following drug classes and individual drugs:

Phenothiazines

Acetophenazine Maleate
Chlorpromazine
Chlorpromazine Hydrochloride
Fluphenazine Decanoate
Fluphenazine Enanthate
Fluphenazine Hydrochloride
Mesoridazine Besylate
Perphenazine
Prochlorperazine
Prochlorperazine Edisylate
Prochlorperazine Maleate
Promazine Hydrochloride
Thioridazine Hydrochloride
Trifluoperazine
Triflupromazine Hydrochloride

Miscellaneous Antipsychotic Agents

Clozapine
Droperidol
Haloperidol
Haloperidol Decanoate
Haloperidol Lactate
Loxapine Hydrochloride
Risperidone
Thiothixene

PHENOTHIAZINES

See the following individual entries:

Acetophenazine Maleate
Chlorpromazine
Chlorpromazine Hydrochloride
Fluphenazine Decanoate
Fluphenazine Enanthate
Fluphenazine Hydrochloride
Mesoridazine Besylate
Perphenazine
Prochlorperazlne
Prochlorperazine Edisylate
Prochlorperazine Maleate
Promazine Hydrochloride
Thioridazine Hydrochloride
Trifluoperazine
Triflupromazine Hydrochloride

General Statement: The advent of antipsychotic drugs was responsible for a major change in the treatment of the mentally ill. Reserpine, an alkaloid derived from *Rauwolfia serpentina,* and chlorpromazine, both of which appeared during the early 1950s, almost singlehandedly revolutionized the care of the mentally ill both inside and outside the hospital. Clients who had not been helped for decades with electroshock, insulin therapy, and/or other forms of treatment could now often be discharged from the hospital. Antipsychotic drugs do not cure mental illness, but they calm the intractable client, relieve the despondency of the severely depressed, activate the immobile and withdrawn, and make some clients more accessible to psychotherapy.

Most phenothiazines induce some sedation, especially during the initial phase of the treatment. Medicated clients can, however, be easily roused. In this manner, the phenothiazines differ markedly from the narcotic analgesics and sedative hypnotics. However, phenothiazines potentiate the analgesic properties of opiates and prolong the action of CNS depressant drugs.

The drugs also decrease spontaneous motor activity, as in parkinsonism, and many lower BP.

According to their detailed chemical structure, the phenothiazines belong to three subgroups:

1. Dimethylaminopropyl compounds

2. Piperazine compounds
3. Piperidine compounds

Drugs belonging to the *dimethylaminopropyl subgroup,* which includes chlorpromazine, are often the first choice for clients in acute excitatory states. Drugs belonging to this subgroup cause more sedation than other phenothiazines and are especially indicated for clients exhausted by lack of sleep.

Members of the *piperazine subgroup* act most selectively on the subcortical sites. This accounts for the fact that they can be administered in relatively small doses. This, in turn, results in minimal drowsiness and undesirable motor effects. The piperazines also have the greatest antiemetic effects because they specifically depress the CTZ of the vomiting center. Members of the *piperidyl subgroup* are less toxic in terms of extrapyramidal effects. Mellaril, a member of this group, has little effectiveness as an antiemetic drug.

Action/Kinetics: It has been postulated that excess amounts of dopamine in certain areas of the CNS cause psychoses. Phenothiazines are thought to act by blocking postsynaptic mesolimbic dopamine receptors, leading to a reduction in psychotic symptoms. Phenothiazines block both D_1 and D_2 dopamine receptors. The antiemetic effects are thought to be due to inhibition or blockade of dopamine (D_2) receptors in the chemoreceptor trigger zone in the medulla as well as by peripheral blockade of the vagus nerve in the GI tract. Relief of anxiety is manifested as a result of an indirect decrease in arousal and increased filtering of internal stimuli to the brain stem reticular system. Alpha blockade produces sedation. Phenothiazines also raise pain threshold and produce amnesia due to suppression of sensory impulses. In addition, these drugs produce anticholinergic and antihistaminic effects and depress the release of hypothalamic and hypophyseal hormones. Peripheral effects include anticholinergic and alpha-adrenergic blocking properties. Kinetic information on the phenothiazines is scarce and often unreliable.

Generally, peak plasma levels occur 2–4 hr after PO administration. Phenothiazines are widely distributed throughout the body. They have an average half-life of 10–20 hr. Most are metabolized in the liver and excreted by the kidney. Studies have shown that both PO dosage forms and suppositories from different manufacturers differ in their bioavailability. It is recommended that brands not be interchanged unless data indicating bioequivalance are available.

Uses: Psychoses, especially if excessive psychomotor activity manifested. Involutional, toxic, or senile psychoses. Used in combination with MAO inhibitors in depressed clients manifesting anxiety, agitation, or panic (use with caution). With lithium in acute manic phase of manic-depressive illness. As an adjunct in alcohol withdrawal to reduce anxiety, tension, depression, nausea, and/or vomiting. For severe behavioral problems in children, manifested by hyperexcitable and/or combative behavior; also, for short-term use in hyperactive children who exhibit excess motor activity and conduct disorders.

Prophylaxis and control of severe N&V due to cancer chemotherapy, radiation therapy, postoperatively. Intractable hiccoughs, intermittent porphyria, tetanus (as adjunct). As preoperative and/or postoperative medications. Some phenothiazines are antipruritics. See also individual drugs.

Contraindications: Severe CNS depression, coma, clients with subcortical brain damage, bone marrow depression, lactation. In clients with a history of seizures and in those on anticonvulsant drugs. Geriatric or debilitated clients, hepatic or renal disease, CV disorders, glaucoma, prostatic hypertrophy. Contraindicated in children with chickenpox, CNS infections, measles, gastroenteritis, dehydration due to increased risk of extrapyramidal symptoms.

Special Concerns: Phenothiazines should be used with caution in clients exposed to extreme heat or cold and in those with asthma, emphysema, or acute respiratory tract infections. Safe use during pregnancy not established; thus use only when benefits outweigh risks. Children may be more sensitive to the neuromuscular or extrapyramidal effects (especially dystonias); those especially at risk include children with chickenpox, CNS infections, measles, dehydration, or gastroenteritis. Thus, generally, phenothiazines are not recommended for use in children less than 12 years of age. Geriatric clients often manifest higher plasma levels due to decreases in lean body mass, total body water, and albumin and an increase in total body fat. Also, geriatric clients may be more likely to manifest orthostatic hypotension, anticholinergic effects, sedative effects, and extrapyramidal side effects.

Side Effects: *CNS:* Depression, drowsiness, dizziness, lethargy, fatigue. Extrapyramidal effects, Parkinson-like symptoms including shuffling gait or tic-like movements of head and face, tardive dyskinesia (see below), akathisia, dystonia. ***Seizures,*** especially in clients with a history thereof. ***Neuroleptic malignant syndrome (rare).*** *CV:* Orthostatic hypotension, increase or decrease in BP, tachycardia, fainting. *GI:* Dry mouth, anorexia, constipation, paralytic ileus, diarrhea. *Endocrine:* Breast engorgement, galactorrhea, gynecomastia, increased appetite, weight gain, hyper- or hypoglycemia, glycosuria. Delayed ejaculation, increased or decreased libido. *GU:* Menstrual irregularities, loss of bladder control, urinary difficulty. *Dermatologic:* Photosensitivity, pruritus, erythema, eczema, exfoliative dermatitis, pigment changes in skin (long-term use of high doses). *Hematologic:* ***Aplastic anemia,*** leukopenia, ***agranulocytosis,*** eosinophilia, thrombocytopenia. *Ophthalmologic:* Deposition of fine particulate matter in lens and cornea leading to blurred vision, changes in vision. *Respiratory:* ***Laryngospasm, bronchospasm, laryngeal edema,*** breathing difficulties. *Miscellaneous:* Fever, muscle stiffness, decreased sweating, muscle spasm of face, neck, or back, obstructive jaundice, nasal congestion, pale skin, mydriasis, systemic lupus-like syndrome.

Tardive dyskinesia has been observed with all classes of antipsychotic drugs, although the precise cause is not known. The syndrome is most commonly seen in older clients, especially women, and in individuals with organic brain syndrome. It is often aggravated or precipitated by the sudden discontinuance of antipsychotic drugs and may persist indefinitely after the drug is discontinued. Early signs of tardive dyskinesia include fine vermicular movements of the tongue and grimacing or tic-like movements of the head and neck. Although there is no known cure for the syndrome, it may not progress if the dosage of the drug is slowly reduced. Also, a few drug-free days may unmask the symptoms of tardive dyskinesia and help in early diagnosis.

Symptoms of Overdose: CNS depression including deep sleep and ***coma,*** hypotension, extrapyramidal symptoms, agitation, restlessness, seizures, hypothermia, ***hyperthermia,*** autonomic symptoms, ***cardiac arrhythmias,*** ECG changes.

Drug Interactions

Alcohol, ethyl / Potentiation or addition of CNS depressant effects. Concomitant use may lead to drowsiness, lethargy, stupor, respiratory collapse, coma, or death

Aluminum salts (antacids) / ↓ Absorption from GI tract

Amphetamine / ↓ Effect of amphetamine by ↓ uptake of drug to the site of action

Anesthetics, general / See *Alcohol*

Antacids, oral / ↓ Effect of phenothiazines due to ↓ absorption from GI tract
Antianxiety drugs / See *Alcohol*
Anticholinergic drugs / Additive anticholinergic side effects and/or ↓ antipsychotic effect
Antidepressants, tricyclic / Additive anticholinergic side effects
Antidiabetic agents / ↓ Effect of antidiabetic agents, since phenothiazines ↑ blood sugar
Bacitracin / Additive respiratory depression
Barbiturate anesthetics / ↑ Chance of tremor, involuntary muscle activity, and hypotension
Barbiturates / See *Alcohol;* also, barbiturates may ↓ effect due to ↑ breakdown by liver
Bromocriptine / Phenothiazines ↓ effect
Capreomycin / Additive respiratory depression
Charcoal / ↓ Effect of phenothiazines due to ↓ absorption from GI tract
CNS depressants / See *Alcohol;* also, ↓ effect of phenothiazines due to ↑ breakdown by liver
Colistimethate / Additive respiratory depression
Diazoxide / Additive hyperglycemic effect
Guanethidine / ↓ Effect of guanethidine by ↓ uptake of drug at the site of action
Hydantoins / ↑ Risk of hydantoin toxicity
Lithium carbonate / ↑ Risk of extrapyramidal symptoms, disorientation, or unconsciousness
MAO inhibitors / ↑ Effect of phenothiazines due to ↓ breakdown by liver
Meperidine / ↑ Risk of hypotension and sedation
Metoprolol / Additive hypotensive effects
Narcotics / See *Alcohol*
Phenytoin / ↑ Effect of phenytoin due to ↓ breakdown by liver
Polymyxin B / Additive respiratory depression
Propranolol / Additive hypotensive effects
Quinidine / Additive cardiac depressant effect
Sedative-hypnotics, nonbarbiturate / See *Alcohol*
Succinylcholine / ↑ Muscle relaxation
Tricyclic antidepressants / ↑ Serum levels of tricyclic antidepressant

Laboratory Test Interferences: False +: Bile (urine dipstick), ferric chloride, pregnancy tests, urinary porphobilinogen, urinary steroids, urobilinogen (urine dipstick). False –: Inorganic phosphorus, urinary steroids. *Caused by pharmacologic effects:* ↑ Alkaline phosphatase, bilirubin, serum transaminases, serum cholesterol, urinary catecholamines. ↓ Glucose tolerance, serum uric acid, 5-HIAA, FSH, growth hormone, LH, vanillylmandelic acid.

Dosage

See individual drugs.

The phenothiazines are effective over a wide dosage range. Dosage is usually increased gradually to minimize side effects over 7 days until the minimal effective dose is attained. Dosage is increased more gradually in elderly or debilitated clients because they are more susceptible to the effects and side effects of drugs. After symptoms are controlled, dosage is gradually reduced to maintenance levels. It is usually desirable to keep chronically ill clients on maintenance levels indefinitely.

Medication, especially in clients on high dosages, should not be discontinued abruptly.

NURSING CONSIDERATIONS

Administration/Storage

1. Do not interchange brands of PO form of drug or suppositories. They may differ in bioavailability.
2. Do not use pink or markedly discolored solutions.
3. When preparing or administering parenteral solutions, both nurse and client should avoid contact of drug with skin, eyes, and clothing to prevent contact dermatitis.

4. Do not mix antipsychotic drugs with other drugs in the same syringe.
5. A specific rate of flow of drug should be ordered when administering parenteral solutions.
6. To lessen the pain of the injection, dilute commercially available injectable solutions in saline or local anesthetic.
7. When administering the drug IM, inject the drug deeply into the muscle.
8. Massage the area of the injection site after IM administration to reduce the pain.
9. Prevent extravasation of the IV solution.
10. Store solutions in a cool dry place in amber-colored containers.
11. *Treatment of Overdose:* Emetics are not to be used as they are of little value and may cause a dystonic reaction of the head or neck that may result in aspiration of vomitus.

- Hypotension: Volume replacement; norepinephrine or phenylephrine may be used (do not use epinephrine).
- Ventricular arrhythmias: phenytoin, 1 mg/kg IV, not to exceed 50 mg/min; may be repeated q 5 min up to 10 mg/kg.
- Seizures or hyperactivity: Diazepam or pentobarbital.
- Extrapyramidal symptoms: Antiparkinson drugs, diphenhydramine, barbiturates.

NOTE: These *Nursing Considerations* apply to all antipsychotic agents except lithium.

Assessment

1. Take a complete family and drug history noting any past incidence of drug hypersensitivity or genetic predisposition. (These agents are referred to as neuroleptics in Europe.)
2. Determine if there is any history of seizures as drugs in this class may lower the seizure threshold.
3. Document indications for therapy. Assess baseline mental status, noting mood, behavior, and any evidence of depression.
4. When working with elderly clients, carefully assess their baseline level of mental acuity.
5. If administering the drug to children, note the extent of the client's hyperexcitability.
6. If the client is a child, assess the possibility of the child having chickenpox or measles.
7. Note any history of asthma or emphysema.
8. Obtain baseline readings of BP and pulse before administering any antipsychotic drug. Assess the BP in both arms when the client is in a reclining position, standing position, and sitting position.
9. Ensure that the client has baseline hematologic profile, liver and renal function studies, urinalysis, an EEG, and ocular examination prior to initiating therapy.
10. Note all medications the client may be taking to determine if any may interact unfavorably with the antipsychotic agent being considered.

Interventions

1. If the medication is to be administered IV, the rate of flow should be monitored carefully and the BP taken at frequent intervals. Keep the client recumbent for at least 1 hr after the IV is completed, then slowly elevate the head of the bed, and observe for tachycardia, faintness, or complaint of dizziness.
2. If clients are in a hospital setting, remain with them to ensure that the medication has been swallowed. It may be advisable to give a liquid preparation of the drug to permit better control over drug taking and improve compliance.
3. Note client complaints of undue distress when in a hot or cold room. The client's heat regulating mechanism may be affected by the drug.

- If the client complains of feeling cold, provide extra blankets.
- If the client complains of feeling too warm, suggest bathing in tepid water.

• Clients should *NOT* use heating pads or hot water bottles if they feel cold.

4. If the client becomes excessively active or depressed, document and report as the medication may need to be changed.

5. Note the presence of spasms of the client's face, neck, back, or tongue. The physician may determine that the condition can be treated with antihistamines, or the decision may be to discontinue the drug.

6. If the client develops a sore throat, persistent fever, malaise, and weakness, document and report. These may be signs associated with agranulocytosis. The drug should be withheld until the appropriate blood work has been performed and the tests evaluated.

7. Measure I&O and observe for abdominal distention. Report any urinary retention. The dosage of medication may need to be reduced, antispasmodics may be indicated, or the drug may need to be changed.

8. Question clients concerning constipation. Encourage them to maintain an adequate fluid intake (2 L/day) and to eat a diet high in roughage. Laxatives may be required.

9. Conduct periodic ocular examinations to detect any early visual disturbances.

10. Note any changes in carbohydrate metabolism (e.g., glycosuria, weight loss, polyphagia, increased appetite, or excessive weight gain). These signs may require a change in diet or medication therapy. These symptoms can be particularly significant if the client has diabetes.

11. Premenopausal women need to know that the menstrual cycle may become irregular. They may develop engorged breasts and begin lactating. The client needs to be reassured that this condition may be altered by a change in the medication therapy.

12. Some clients may develop a hypersensitivity reaction such as fever, asthma, laryngeal edema, angioneurotic edema, and anaphylactic reaction. **Stop** medication, notify physician, and treat symptomatically.

13. Be aware that clients on long-term therapy may develop a yellow-brown skin reaction that may turn grayish purple.

14. Note evidence of early cholestatic jaundice, such as high fever, client complaint of upper abdominal pain, nausea, diarrhea, itching, and rash. Obtain liver function studies and compare with the baseline measurements.

15. If the client develops yellowing of the sclera, skin, or mucous membranes, withhold the drug. Record these observations and report because these signs may indicate that the client has a biliary obstruction.

16. The antiemetic effects of phenothiazines may mask other pathology such as toxicity to other drugs, intestinal obstruction, or brain lesions. Careful observations of the client are therefore essential.

17. If the client is receiving barbiturates to relieve anxiety during phenothiazine therapy, anticipate the dose of the barbiturate will be reduced.

18. If barbiturates are being administered as an anticonvulsant, the dosage of barbiturates will not be reduced.

19. If the drug is to be discontinued, it should be done gradually to minimize the possible onset of severe GI disturbances or symptoms of tardive dyskinesia.

20. If clients develop respiratory symptoms, instruct them to take slow, deep breaths. The drug may depress the cough reflex.

21. When clients are being seen on an outpatient basis, check on the number of times they request prescription refills. They may be hoarding medication, especially if they are depressed.

Client/Family Teaching

1. May take with food or milk to minimize GI upset.

2. Stress the importance of taking the drug(s) exactly as prescribed.

3. Review the goals of therapy with client and family and assess degree to which they have been attained. Remind the client and family that it may be weeks or months before the

full effects of the medication will be noticed.

4. Take as prescribed, even if feeling well. Do not stop taking the drug abruptly. An abrupt cessation of high doses of phenothiazines can cause N&V, tremors, sensations of warmth and cold, sweating, tachycardia, headache, and insomnia.

5. Advise young women that the drug may cause menstrual irregularity and can cause false positive pregnancy tests. Encourage them to keep an accurate record of their menstrual periods and to report if pregnancy is suspected.

6. Male clients should be told they may experience decreased libido and develop breast enlargement. Reassure client and instruct him to report the development of these symptoms so that the medication can be adjusted.

7. Many clients develop photosensitivity reactions. Advise them to wear protective clothing and sunglasses when in the sun and to avoid sunbathing. They should also use large quantities of sun screens for added protection.

8. Drug may discolor the urine pink or reddish brown.

9. Avoid driving a car or operating heavy machinery or engaging in any activities that require mental alertness for at least 2 weeks after the therapy has started. Consult with provider for evaluation of client's response to treatment before resuming any of these activities.

10. If the client develops blurred vision, avoid driving and report.

11. Remind clients that long-term therapy may affect their vision. Therefore, they should schedule regular ophthalmic examinations.

12. To prevent a dry mouth, rinse the mouth frequently, increase fluid intake, chew sugarless gum, and/or suck on sour hard candies.

13. Increase fluids and bulk in the diet to minimize the constipating effects of these drugs. Report any evidence of urinary retention or persistent constipation.

14. Rise slowly from a lying or sitting position and dangle legs before standing to avoid orthostatic symptoms.

15. Report any elevation of body temperature, feeling of weakness, or sore throat. These may be indications of blood dyscrasias and require immediate attention.

16. Stress the importance of taking the drug as prescribed after discharge and remind client to advise all health care providers of the medications they are currently taking.

17. Avoid alcohol, OTC drugs, and any other CNS depressants without approval.

18. Stress the importance of reporting for periodic lab studies and follow-up care for evaluation and adjustment of drug dosage.

Evaluate

- Evidence of ↓ excitable, withdrawn, agitated, or paranoid behaviors (comparing baseline evaluations of behavior with current presentation)
- Orientation to time and place, and an understanding of illness
- Evidence of adherence to the prescribed drug regimen
- Evidence of any extrapyramidal effects of drug therapy
- Reports of relief of N&V

Special Concerns

1. When working with elderly clients be particularly observant for symptoms of tardive dyskinesia. Clients may exhibit puffing of the cheeks or tongue, develop chewing movements, and involuntary movements of the extremities and trunk. Such symptoms should be reported immediately and the drug discontinued.

2. If administering phenothiazines to a child, note neuromuscular reactions, especially if the child is dehydrated or has an acute infection. These children are more susceptible to side effects.

Acetophenazine maleate

(ah-**SEAT**-oh-**FEN**-ah-zeen)
Tindal **(Rx)**

See also *Phenothiazines,* Chapter 38.
How Supplied: *Tablet:* 20 mg
Action/Kinetics: Acetophenazine manifests a low incidence of orthostatic hypotension, moderate sedation and anticholinergic effects but a high incidence of extrapyramidal effects.
Use: Psychoses.

Dosage

- **Tablets**

Psychoses.

Adults and children over 12 years, usual: 20 mg t.i.d. (range: 40–80 mg/day in divided doses); 80–120 mg/day in divided doses for hospitalized schizophrenic clients (doses as high as 400–600 mg/day may be needed in severe schizophrenia). Emaciated, geriatric, and debilitated clients require a lower initial dose.
Special Concerns: Dosage has not been established in children less than 12 years of age.

NURSING CONSIDERATIONS

See also *Nursing Considerations* for *Antipsychotic Agents, Phenothiazines,* Chapter 38.
Assessment
1. Note the age of the client since elderly clients usually require lower drug dosage.
2. Identify if the client is taking lithium. Acetophenazine potentiates CNS toxicity.

Client/Family Teaching
1. Administer 1 hr before bedtime if client has difficulty sleeping.
2. Provide clients with a list of potential drug reactions that should be reported.
3. Do *not* stop taking the medication abruptly.
4. Drug may cause a photosensitivity reaction; use appropriate precautions.
5. Avoid activities that require mental alertness until drug effects realized.

Evaluate: Control of hyperactive and agitated behaviors with evidence of reality orientation.

Chlorpromazine

(klor-**PROH**-mah-zeen)
Largactil ✱, Thorazine **(Rx)**

Chlorpromazine hydrochloride

(klor-**PROH**-mah-zeen)
Largactil ✱, Ormazine, Thorazine, Thor-Prom **(Rx)**

See also *Antipsychotic Agents, Phenothiazines,* Chapter 38.
How Supplied: Chlorpromazine: *Suppository:* 25 mg, 100 mg.
Chlorpromazine hydrochloride: *Capsule, Extended Release:* 30 mg, 75 mg, 150 mg; *Concentrate:* 30 mg/mL, 100 mg/mL; *Injection:* 25 mg/mL; *Syrup:* 10 mg/5 mL; *Tablet:* 10 mg, 25 mg, 50 mg, 100 mg, 200 mg
Action/Kinetics: Chlorpromazine has significant antiemetic, hypotensive, and sedative effects; moderate to strong anticholinergic effects and weak to moderate extrapyramidal effects. **Peak plasma levels:** 2–3 hr after both PO and IM administration. **t½** (after IV, IM): **Initial,** 4–5 hr; **final,** 3–40 hr. Chlorpromazine is extensively metabolized in the intestinal wall and liver; certain of the metabolites are active. **Steady-state plasma levels** (in psychotics): 10–1,300 ng /mL. After 2–3 weeks of therapy, plasma levels decline, possibly because of reduction in drug absorption and/or increase in drug metabolism.
Uses: Acute and chronic psychoses, including schizophrenia; manic phase of manic-depressive illness. Acute intermittent porphyria. Preanesthetic, adjunct to treat tetanus, intractable hiccoughs, severe behavioral problems in children, neuroses, and N&V. Treatment of choreiform movements in Huntington's disease.

Dosage

- **Tablets, Extended-Release Capsules, Oral Concentrate, Syrup**

Psychotic disorders.

Adults and adolescents: 10–25 mg (of the base) b.i.d.–q.i.d.; dosage may be increased by 20–50 mg/day q 3–4 days as needed. Or, 30–300 mg (of the base) using the extended-release capsules 1–3 times/day (the 300-mg extended-release capsules are used only in severe neuropsychiatric situations). **Pediatric:** 0.55 mg/kg (15 mg/m²) q 4–6 hr.

N&V.

Adults and adolescents: 10–25 mg (of the base) q 4 hr; dosage may be increased as needed. **Pediatric:** 0.55 mg/kg (15 mg/m²) q 4–6 hr.

Preoperative sedation.

Adults and adolescents: 25–50 mg (of the base) 2–3 hr before surgery. **Pediatric:** 0.55 mg/kg (15 mg/m²) 2–3 hr before surgery.

Hiccoughs or porphyria.

Adults and adolescents: 25–50 mg (of the base) t.i.d.–q.i.d.

• **IM**

Severe psychoses.

Adults: 25–50 mg (of the base) repeated in 1 hr if needed; **then,** repeat the dose q 3–4 hr as needed and tolerated (the dose may be increased gradually over several days). **Pediatric, over 6 months:** 0.55 mg/kg (15 mg/m²) q 6–8 hr as needed.

N&V.

Adults: 25 mg (base) as a single dose; **then,** increase to 25–50 mg q 3–4 hr as needed until vomiting ceases. **Pediatric:** 0.55 mg/kg q 6–8 hr as needed.

N&V during surgery.

Adults: 12.5 mg (base) as a single dose; repeat in 30 min if needed. **Pediatric,** 0.275 mg/kg; repeat in 30 min if needed.

Preoperative sedative.

Adults: 12.5–25 mg (base) 1–2 hr before surgery. **Pediatric:** 0.55 mg/kg 1–2 hr before surgery.

Hiccoughs.

Adults: 25–50 mg (base) t.i.d.–q.i.d.

Porphyria.

Adults: 25 mg (base) q 6–8 hr until client can take PO therapy.

Tetanus.

Adults: 25–50 mg (base) t.i.d.–q.i.d. (dose can be increased as needed and tolerated).

• **IV**

N&V during surgery.

Adults: 25 mg (base) diluted to 1 mg/mL with 0.9% sodium chloride injection given at a rate of no more than 2 mg/2 min. **Pediatric:** 0.275 mg/kg diluted to 1 mg/mL with 0.9% sodium chloride injection given at a rate of no more than 1 mg q 2 min.

Tetanus.

Adults: 25–50 mg (base) diluted to 1 mg/mL with 0.9% sodium chloride injection and given at a rate of 1 mg/min. **Pediatric:** 0.55 mg/kg diluted to 1 mg/mL with 0.9% sodium chloride injection and given at a rate of 1 mg/2 min.

• **Suppositories**

N&V.

Adults and adolescents: 50–100 mg q 6–8 hr as needed up to a maximum of 400 mg/day. **Pediatric:** 1 mg/kg q 6–8 hr as needed (the 100-mg suppository should not be used in children).

Administration/Storage

1. Chlorpromazine should not be used to treat N&V in children less than 6 months of age.
2. The maximum daily PO and parenteral dose for adults and adolescents should be 1 g of the base.
3. The maximum IM dose should be 40 mg/day for children up to 5 years of age and 75 mg/day for children 5–12 years of age.
4. Sustained-release capsules should be swallowed whole.
5. Solutions of chlorpromazine may cause contact dermatitis; thus, medical personnel should avoid getting solution on hands or clothing.
6. When used IV in children for tetanus, the preparation should be diluted to 1 mg/mL and given at a rate of 1 mg/2 min.
7. The concentrate (to be used in hospitals only) can be mixed with 60 mL or more of fruit or tomato juice, orange or simple syrup, milk, carbonated drinks, coffee, tea, water, or semisolid foods (e.g., soup, pudding).

8. Slight discoloration of injection or PO solutions will not affect the action of the drug.
9. Solutions with marked discoloration should be discarded. Consult with pharmacist if unsure of drug potency.
10. When administering the drug IM, select a large, well-developed muscle mass. Use the dorsogluteal site or rectus femoris in adults and the vastus lateralis in children.
11. Document and rotate injection sites.

Special Concerns: Use during pregnancy only if benefits outweigh risks. PO dosage for psychoses and N&V has not been established in children less than 6 months of age.

Additional Drug Interactions
Epinephrine / Chlorpromazine ↓ peripheral vasoconstriction and may reverse action of epinephrine
Norepinephrine / Chlorpromazine ↓ pressor effect and eliminates bradycardia due to norepinephrine
Valproic acid / ↑ Effect of valproic acid due to ↓ clearance

NURSING CONSIDERATIONS

See also *Nursing Considerations* for *Antipsychotic Agents, Phenothiazines,* Chapter 38.

Assessment
1. Note any history of seizure disorders as the drug is contraindicated in these instances.
2. Conduct baseline studies of liver and kidney function.
3. Determine age of male clients and assess for prostatic hypertrophy.

Client/Family Teaching
1. Provide a printed list of side effects and advise client to immediately report any extrapyramidal symptoms, especially tardive dyskinesia.
2. Advise that urine may become discolored pinkish to brown.
3. Protect self during sun exposure as exposed skin surfaces may develop pigmentation changes.
4. Use caution when performing activities that require mental alertness.
5. Avoid alcohol and any other CNS depressants. May potentiate orthostatic hypotension.
6. Perform frequent toothbrushing and flossing to discourage oral infections.
7. Report any unusual bruising or bleeding.
8. Advise to avoid temperature extremes because drug may impair the body's ability to regulate temperature.
9. Explain that therapeutic psychologic effects may require 7–8 weeks of therapy.

Evaluate
- ↓ Psychotic and manic manifestations
- Control of N&V
- Cessation of hiccoughs
- Desired level of sedation
- Control of muscular twitching

Fluphenazine decanoate

(flew-**FEN**-ah-zeen)
Modecate Decanoate ✱, Modecate Concentrate ✱, Prolixin Decanoate **(Rx)**

Fluphenazine enanthate

(flew-**FEN**-ah-zeen)
Moditen Enanthate ✱, Prolixin Enanthate **(Rx)**

Fluphenazine hydrochloride

(flew-**FEN**-ah-zeen)
Apo-Fluphenazine ✱, Permitil, Prolixin, Moditen HCl ✱, Moditen HCl-H.P. ✱, PMS-Fluphenazine ✱ **(Rx)**

See also *Antipsychotic Agents, Phenothiazines,* Chapter 38.

How Supplied: Fluphenazine decanoate: *Injection:* 25 mg/mL
Fluphenazine enanthate: *Injection:* 25 mg/mL
Fluphenazine hydrochloride: *Concentrate:* 5 mg/mL; *Elixir:* 2.5 mg/5 mL; *Injection:* 2.5 mg/mL; *Tablet:* 1 mg, 2.5 mg, 5 mg

Action/Kinetics: Fluphenazine is accompanied by a high incidence of extrapyramidal symptoms and a low incidence of sedation, anticholinergic effects, antiemetic effects, and orthostatic hypotension. The enanthate and decanoate esters dramatically increase the duration of action. *Decanoate:* **Onset,** 24–72 hr; **peak plasma levels,** 24–48 hr; **t¹/₂** (approximate), 14 days; **duration:** up to 4 weeks. *Enanthate:* **Onset,** 24–72 hr; **peak plasma levels,** 48–72 hr; **t¹/₂** (approximate): 3.6 days; **duration:** 1–3 weeks.

Fluphenazine hydrochloride can be cautiously administered to clients with known hypersensitivity to other phenothiazines.

Fluphenazine enanthate may replace fluphenazine hydrochloride if desired response occurs with hypersensitivity reaction to fluphenazine.

Uses: Psychotic disorders. Adjunct to tricyclic antidepressants for chronic pain states (e.g., diabetic neuropathy, and clients trying to withdraw from narcotics).

Dosage

Fluphenazine hydrochloride is administered **PO and IM.** Fluphenazine enanthate or decanoate is administered **SC and IM.**

Hydrochloride.

- **Elixir, Oral Solution, Tablets**

Psychotic disorders.

Adults and adolescents, initial: 2.5–10 mg/day in divided doses q 6–8 hr; **then,** reduce gradually to maintenance dose of 1–5 mg/day (usually given as a single dose, not to exceed 20 mg/day).

Psychotic disorders.

Geriatric, emaciated, debilitated clients, initial: 1–2.5 mg/day; **then,** dosage determined by response. **Pediatric:** 0.25–0.75 mg 1–4 times/day.

Hydrochloride.

- **IM**

Psychotic disorders.

Adults and adolescents: 1.25–2.5 mg q 6–8 hr as needed. Maximum daily dose: 10 mg. Elderly, debilitated, or emaciated clients should start with 1–2.5 mg/day.

Decanoate.

- **IM, SC**

Psychotic disorders.

Adults, initial: 12.5–25 mg; **then,** the dose may be repeated or increased q 1–3 weeks. The usual maintenance dose is 50 mg/1–4 weeks. Maximum adult dose: 100 mg/dose. **Pediatric, 12 years and older:** 6.25–18.75 mg/week; the dose can be increased to 12.5–25 mg given q 1–3 weeks. **Pediatric, 5–12 years:** 3.125–12.5 mg with this dose being repeated q 1–3 weeks.

Enanthate.

- **IM, SC**

Psychotic disorders.

Adults and adolescents: 25 mg; dose can be repeated or increased q 1–3 weeks. For doses greater than 50 mg, increases should be made in increments of 12.5 mg. Maximum adult dose: 100 mg.

Administration/Storage

1. Protect all forms of medication from light.
2. Store at room temperature and avoid freezing.
3. Color of parenteral solution may vary from colorless to light amber. Do not use solutions that are darker than light amber.
4. The hydrochloride concentrate should not be mixed with any beverage containing caffeine, tannates (e.g., tea), or pectins (e.g., apple juice) due to a physical incompatibility.
5. Clients beginning therapy with phenothiazines should first receive a short-acting form of the drug; the decanoate and enanthate can be considered after the response to the drug has been evaluated and for those that demonstrate compliance problems.

NURSING CONSIDERATIONS

See also *Nursing Considerations* for *Antipsychotic Agents, Phenothiazines,* Chapter 38.

Assessment

1. Document indications for therapy, presenting symptoms, and any other previous treatments utilized.
2. Note the age and condition of the client. Elderly and debilitated clients are particularly at risk for acute extrapyramidal symptoms.
3. Plasma protein binding is reduced

resulting in increased circulating free drug.

Client/Family Teaching

1. Review administration techniques and determine if client is able to assume the responsibility for self-medication.
2. Provide written guidelines concerning side effects that should be reported and when client should return for the next follow-up appointment.

Evaluate

- Improved behavior patterns with ↓ agitation
- Control of tics
- ↓ Paranoid and withdrawal behaviors

Mesoridazine besylate

(mez-oh-**RID**-ah-zeen)
Serentil **(Rx)**

See also *Antipsychotic Agents, Phenothiazines,* Chapter 38.

How Supplied: *Concentrate:* 25 mg/mL; *Injection:* 25 mg/mL; *Tablet:* 10 mg, 25 mg, 50 mg, 100 mg

Action/Kinetics: Mesoridazine has pronounced sedative and hypotensive effects, moderate anticholinergic effects, and a low incidence of extrapyramidal symptoms and antiemetic effects.

Uses: Schizophrenia, acute and chronic alcoholism, behavior problems in clients with mental deficiency and chronic brain syndrome, psychoneurosis.

Dosage

- **Oral Solution, Tablets**

Psychotic disorders.

Adults and adolescents: 30–150 mg/day in two to three divided doses.

Alcoholism.

Adults, initial: 25 mg b.i.d.; **optimum total dose:** 50–200 mg/day.

- **IM**

Psychotic disorders.

Adults and adolescents: 25 mg (base); **then,** repeat the dose in 30–60 min as needed.

Administration/Storage

1. Maintain client supine for minimum of 30 min after parenteral administration to minimize orthostatic effect.
2. Acidified tap or distilled water, orange juice, or grape juice may be used to dilute the concentrate prior to use.
3. Bulk dilutions should not be prepared or stored.
4. For IM administration, give 25 mg initially, repeated at 30–60-min intervals as needed.

Special Concerns: Use during pregnancy only if benefits clearly outweigh risks. Dosage has not been established in children less than 12 years of age. Geriatric, debilitated, and emaciated clients require a lower initial dose.

NURSING CONSIDERATIONS

See also *Nursing Considerations* for *Antipsychotic Agents, Phenothiazines,* Chapter 38.

Assessment

1. Document onset of symptoms and describe behaviors necessitating treatment.
2. List any other agents prescribed and the outcome.
3. Observe for increased sedation and orthostatic and cholinergic effects.

Evaluate: Improved patterns of behavior with ↓ agitation, ↓ hyperactivity, and reality orientation.

Perphenazine

(per-**FEN**-ah-zeen)
Apo-Perphenazine ✱, Trilafon **(Rx)**

See also *Antipsychotic Agents, Phenothiazines,* Chapter 38.

How Supplied: *Concentrate:* 16 mg/5 mL; *Injection:* 5 mg/mL; *Tablet:* 2 mg, 4 mg, 8 mg, 16 mg

Action/Kinetics: Resembles chlorpromazine. Use accompanied by a high incidence of extrapyramidal effects; strong antiemetic effects; moderate anticholinergic effects; and a low incidence of orthostatic hypotension and sedation. Perphenazine is also found in Triavil. **Onset, IM:** 10

min. **Maximum effect, IM:** 1–2 hr. **Duration, IM:** 6 hr (up to 24 hr).
Uses: Psychotic disorders. To treat severe N&V.

Dosage

• **Oral Solution, Syrup, Tablets, Repeat-Action Tablets**

Psychoses.

Nonhospitalized clients: 4–8 mg t.i.d. or 8–16 mg repeat-action tablets b.i.d. **Hospitalized clients:** 8–16 mg b.i.d.–q.i.d. or 8–32 mg repeat-action tablets b.i.d. Total daily dosage should not exceed 64 mg.

Severe N&V.

Adults: 8–16 mg/day in divided doses (24 mg/day may be required in some clients).

• **IM**

Psychotic disorders.

Adults and adolescents, nonhospitalized: 5 mg/ q 6 hr, not to exceed 15 mg/day. **Hospitalized clients: initial,** 5–10 mg; total daily dose should not exceed 30 mg.

Severe N&V.

Adults and adolescents: 5 mg (initially, 10 mg in severe cases) q 6 hr, not to exceed 15 mg in ambulatory clients or 30 mg in hospitalized clients.

• **IV**

Severe N&V.

Adults: Up to 5 mg diluted to 0.5 mg/mL with 0.9% sodium chloride injection. Should be given in divided doses of not more than 1 mg/ q 1–3 hr. Can also be given as an infusion at a rate not to exceed 1 mg/min. Use should be restricted to hospitalized recumbent adults. Maximum single dose should not exceed 5 mg.

Administration/Storage

1. Each 5.0 mL of oral concentrate should be diluted with 60 mL of diluent, such as water, milk, carbonated beverage, or orange juice.
2. Do not mix with tea, coffee, cola, grape juice, or apple juice as it will precipitate.
3. When rapid action is required, administer IM using 5 mg. Inject deep into the muscle, and repeat at 6-hr intervals as needed. The client should be in a recumbent position and remain in that position for at least 1 hr after IM administration.
4. For IV use dilute with NSS to a concentration of 0.5 mg/mL and administer 1 mg over at least 1 min.
5. Protect from light.
6. Store solutions in an amber-colored container.

Special Concerns: Use during pregnancy only if benefits clearly outweigh risks. Dosage has not been established in children less than 12 years of age. Geriatric, emaciated, or debilitated clients usually require a lower initial dose.

NURSING CONSIDERATIONS

See also *Nursing Considerations* for *Antipsychotic Agents, Phenothiazines,* Chapter 38.

Assessment

1. Document indications for therapy and type and onset of symptoms.
2. List other agents prescribed, duration of therapy, and the outcome.

Interventions

1. Monitor VS closely since the drug may cause hypotension, tachycardia, and/or bradycardia.
2. Supervise client activity until drug effects realized.
3. Observe for tardive dyskinesia and other extrapyramidal symptoms as this would require a reduction in dose or discontinuation of therapy.

Client/Family Teaching

1. Caution that drug may cause drowsiness and dizziness.
2. Report any rash, fever, or urinary retention.
3. Drug may discolor urine pinkish brown.
4. Review symptoms of tardive dyskinesia and extrapyramidal symptoms and advise to report.
5. Wear protective clothes and sunscreen when sun exposure necessary; may discolor skin a bluish color.
6. Dress appropriately, as drug impairs body temperature regulation; avoid temperature extremes.

7. Avoid alcohol and any other CNS depressants unless approved by provider.

Evaluate

- ↓ Agitation, excitability, or withdrawn behaviors
- Control of severe N&V

Prochlorperazine

(proh-klor-**PAIR**-ah-zeen)
Compazine, Nu-Prochlor ✱, Stemetil ✱ **(Rx)**

Prochlorperazine edisylate

(proh-klor-**PAIR**-ah-zeen)
Compazine Edisylate **(Rx)**

Prochlorperazine maleate

(proh-klor-**PAIR**-ah-zeen)
Compazine Maleate, PMS Prochlorperazine ✱, Stemetil ✱ **(Rx)**

See also *Antipsychotic Agents, Phenothiazines,* Chapter 38.

How Supplied: Prochlorperazine: *Suppository:* 2.5 mg, 5 mg, 25 mg Prochlorperazine Edisylate: *Injection:* 5 mg/mL; *Syrup:* 5 mg/5 mL Prochlorperazine maleate: *Capsule, extended release:* 10 mg, 15 mg; *Tablet:* 5 mg, 10 mg, 25 mg

Action/Kinetics: Prochlorperazine causes a high incidence of extrapyramidal and antiemetic effects, moderate sedative effects, and a low incidence of anticholinergic effects and orthostatic hypotension. It also possesses significant antiemetic effects.

Uses: Psychoneuroses. Postoperative N&V, radiation sickness, vomiting due to toxins. Generally not used for clients who weigh less than 44 kg or who are under 2 years of age. Severe N&V.

Dosage

- **Edisylate Syrup, Maleate Extended-Release Capsules, Tablets**

Psychotic disorders.

Adults and adolescents: 5–10 mg (base) t.i.d.–q.i.d. (dose can be increased gradually q 2–3 days as needed and tolerated). For extended-release capsules, up to 100–150 mg/day can be given. **Pediatric, 2–12 years:** 2.5 mg (base) b.i.d.–t.i.d.

N&V.

Adults and adolescents: 5–10 mg (base) t.i.d.–q.i.d. (up to 40 mg/day). For extended-release capsules, the dose is 15–30 mg once daily in the morning (or 10 mg q 12 hr, up to 40 mg/day). **Pediatric, 18–39 kg:** 2.5 mg (base) t.i.d. (or 5 mg b.i.d.), not to exceed 15 mg/day; **14–17 kg:** 2.5 mg (base) b.i.d.–t.i.d., not to exceed 10 mg/day; **9–13 kg:** 2.5 mg (base) 1–2 times/day, not to exceed 7.5 mg/day. The total daily dose for children should not exceed 10 mg the first day; on subsequent days, the total daily dose should not exceed 20 mg for children 2–5 years of age or 25 mg for children 6–12 years of age.

Anxiety.

Adults and adolescents: 5 mg (base) t.i.d.–q.i.d. up to 20 mg/day for no longer than 12 weeks.

- **IM, Edisylate Injection**

Psychotic disorders, for immediate control of severely disturbed clients.

Adults and adolescents: 10–20 mg (base); dose can be repeated q 2–4 hr as needed (usually up to three or four doses). **Maintenance:** 10–20 mg (base) q 4–6 hr. **Pediatric:** 0.132 mg/kg.

Anxiety.

Adults and adolescents: 5–10 mg (base); dose can be repeated q 2–4 hr as needed.

N&V.

Adults and adolescents: 5–10 mg with the dose repeated q 3–4 hr as needed. **Pediatric, 2–12 years:** 0.132 mg/kg.

N&V during surgery.

Adults and adolescents: 5–10 mg (base) 1–2 hr before induction of anesthesia; to control symptoms during or after surgery, the dose can be repeated once after 30 min.

- **IV, Edisylate Injection**

N&V.

Adults and adolescents: 2.5–10 mg as a slow injection or infusion (rate should not exceed 5 mg/min up to 40 mg/day).

N&V during surgery.
Adults and adolescents: 5–10 mg (base) given as a slow injection or infusion 15–30 min before induction of anesthesia; to control symptoms during or after surgery the dose can be repeated once. The rate of infusion should not exceed 5 mg/mL/min.

• **Rectal Suppositories**
Pediatric, 2–12 years: 2.5 mg b.i.d.–t.i.d. with no more than 10 mg given on the first day. No more than 20 mg/day for children 2–5 years and 25 mg/day for children 6–12 years of age.

Administration/Storage
1. Store all forms of the drug in tight-closing amber-colored bottles; store the suppositories below 37°C (98.6°F).
2. Add the desired dosage of concentrate to 60 mL of beverage (e.g., tomato or fruit juice, milk, soup) or semisolid food just before administration to disguise the taste.
3. Drug should not be administered SC due to local irritation.
4. Prochlorperazine should not be mixed with other agents in a syringe.
5. Prochlorperazine should not be diluted with any material containing the preservative parabens.
6. When given IM to children for N&V, the duration of action may be 12 hr.
7. Parenteral prescribing limits are 20 mg/day for children 2–5 years of age and 25 mg/day for children 6–12 years of age.

Special Concerns: Safe use during pregnancy has not been established. Dosage has not been established in children less than 2 years of age or 9.1 kg body weight. Geriatric, emaciated, and debilitated clients usually require a lower initial dose.

NURSING CONSIDERATIONS

See also *Nursing Considerations* for *Antipsychotic Agents, Phenothiazines,* Chapter 38.

Assessment
1. Document indications for therapy, onset of symptoms, and presenting behaviors.
2. List other agents prescribed and the outcome.

Interventions
1. Monitor I&O and prevent dehydration.
2. Auscultate bowel sounds and assess function.
3. Have emergency equipment and drugs available when treating an overdose.
4. Monitor VS and incorporate safety precautions during the treatment of an overdose.
5. If the client was taking spansules, continue the treatment until all signs of overdosage are no longer evident.
6. In treating clients for an overdosage, anticipate that saline laxatives may be used to hasten the evacuation of pellets that have not yet released their medication.

Client/Family Teaching
1. Advise parents not to exceed the prescribed dose of drug.
2. If the child shows signs of restlessness and excitement, withhold the medication and report.
3. Do not drive or operate machinery until drug effects are realized because drowsiness or dizziness may occur.
4. Review symptoms of extrapyramidal effects and tardive dyskinesia and advise to report immediately if evident.

Evaluate
• Control of N&V
• Evidence of a reduction in agitation, excitability, or withdrawn behaviors

Promazine hydrochloride

(**PROH**-mah-zeen)
Prozine-50, Sparine **(Rx)**

See also *Antipsychotic Agents, Phenothiazines,* Chapter 38.

How Supplied: *Injection:* 25 mg/mL, 50 mg/mL; *Tablet:* 25 mg, 50 mg

Action/Kinetics: The use of promazine is accompanied by significant anticholinergic, sedative, and hypotensive effects; moderate antiemetic effect; and weak extrapyramidal effects. This drug is ineffective in reducing destructive behavior in acutely agitated psychotic clients.
Uses: Psychotic disorders.

Dosage

- **Tablets**

Psychotic disorders.
Adults: 10–200 mg q 4–6 hr; adjust dose as needed and tolerated. Total daily dose should not exceed 1,000 mg. **Pediatric, 12 years and older:** 10–25 mg q 4–6 hr; adjust dose as needed and tolerated.

- **IM**

Psychotic disorders, severe and moderate agitation.
Adults, initial: 50–150 mg; adjust dose if necessary after 30 min. **Maintenance:** 10–200 mg q 4–6 hr as needed and tolerated. Switch to PO therapy as soon as possible. **Pediatric over 12 years:** 10–25 mg q 4–6 hr for chronic psychotic disorders (maximum dose: 1 g/day).

IM doses may be given IV continuously.

Administration/Storage
1. Dilute concentrate as directed on bottle. Taste can be disguised when given with citrus fruit juice, milk, or flavored drinks.
2. IM injections should be given in the gluteal region.
3. IV doses should be diluted to 25 mg/mL with 0.9% sodium chloride injection and given slowly.

Special Concerns: Safe use during pregnancy has not been established. Dosage has not been established in children less than 12 years of age. Geriatric, emaciated, and debilitated clients may require a lower initial dosage.

NURSING CONSIDERATIONS

See also *Nursing Considerations* for *Antipsychotic Agents, Phenothiazines,* Chapter 38.

Assessment: Document indications for therapy, onset of symptoms, and presenting behaviors.
Evaluate: Improved behavior patterns with a reduction in agitation, excitability, or withdrawn behaviors.

Thioridazine hydrochloride

(thigh-oh-**RID**-ah-zeen)
Apo-Thioridazine ✱, Mellaril, Mellaril-S, Thioridazine HCl Intensol Oral **(Rx)**

See also *Antipsychotic Agents, Phenothiazines,* Chapter 38.
How Supplied: *Concentrate:* 30 mg/mL, 100 mg/mL; *Tablet:* 10 mg, 15 mg, 25 mg, 50 mg, 100 mg, 150 mg, 200 mg
Action/Kinetics: The use of thioridazine is accompanied by a high incidence of hypotensive effects; a moderate incidence of sedative and anticholinergic effects and weak antiemetic and extrapyramidal effects. Thioridazine can often be used in clients intolerant of other phenothiazines. It has little or no antiemetic effects. **Peak plasma levels** (after PO administration): 1–4 hr. Thioridazine may impair its own absorption at higher doses due to the strong anticholinergic effects. **t½:** 10 hr. Metabolized in the liver to both active and inactive metabolites.
Uses: Acute and chronic schizophrenia; moderate to marked depression with anxiety; sleep disturbances. *In children:* Treatment of hyperactivity in clients and those with retarded and behavior problems. Geriatric clients with organic brain syndrome. Alcohol withdrawal. Intractable pain.

Dosage

- **Oral Suspension, Oral Solution, Tablets**

Highly individualized.

Neurosis, anxiety states, sleep disturbances, tension, alcohol withdrawal, senility.
Adults, range: 20–200 mg/day; **initial:** 25 mg t.i.d. **Maintenance,** mild cases: 10 mg b.i.d.–q.i.d.; severe cases: 50 mg t.i.d.–q.i.d.

Psychotic, severely disturbed hospitalized clients.
Adults, initial, 50–100 mg t.i.d. If necessary, increase to maximum of 200 mg q.i.d. When control is achieved, reduce gradually to minimum effective dosage. **Pediatric above 2 years:** 0.25–3.0 mg/kg/day.
Hospitalized psychotic children.
Initial: 25 mg b.i.d.–t.i.d. *Moderate problems:* **initial,** 10 mg b.i.d.–t.i.d. Increase gradually if necessary. **Not recommended for children under 2 years of age.**
Administration/Storage: Dilute each dose just before administration with distilled water, acidified tap water, or suitable juices. Preparation and storage of bulk dilutions are not recommended.
Special Concerns: Safe use during pregnancy has not been established. Dosage has not been established in children less than 2 years of age. Geriatric, emaciated, or debilitated clients usually require a lower initial dose.
Additional Side Effect: More likely to cause pigmentary retinopathy than other phenothiazines.

NURSING CONSIDERATIONS

See also *Nursing Considerations* for *Antipsychotic Agents, Phenothiazines,* Chapter 38.
Client/Family Teaching
1. Take only as directed and do not stop abruptly as withdrawal may activate N&V, gastritis, dizziness, tachycardia, headache, and insomnia.
2. Use caution as drug may cause drowsiness.
3. Wear protective clothing and sunscreens to prevent a photosensitivity reaction.
4. May cause retinal deposits viewed as a "browning of vision."
5. Drug may impair temperature regulation so avoid temperature extremes and dress appropriately.
6. Doses exceeding 300 mg/day may cause reversible T-wave abnormalities on ECG. Doses in excess of 800 mg/day have been associated with retinal deposits and cardiac toxicity.

Evaluate
- Improved behavioral patterns with ↓ agitation and improved coping mechanisms
- ↓ Anxiety levels with ↓ depression
- ↓ Sleep disturbances

Trifluoperazine

(try-**flew**-oh-**PER**-ah-zeen)
Apo-Trifluoperazine ✦, Stelazine **(Rx)**

See also *Antipsychotic Agents, Phenothiazines,* Chapter 38.
How Supplied: *Concentrate:* 10 mg/mL; *Injection:* 2 mg/mL; *Tablet:* 1 mg, 2 mg, 5 mg, 10 mg
Action/Kinetics: Trifluoperazine is accompanied by a high incidence of extrapyramidal symptoms and antiemetic effects and a low incidence of sedation, orthostatic hypotension, and anticholinergic side effects. Recommended only for hospitalized or well-supervised clients. **Maximum therapeutic effect:** Usually 2–3 weeks after initiation of therapy.
Uses: Schizophrenia. Suitable for clients with apathy or withdrawal. Anxiety, tension, agitation in neuroses.

Dosage
- **Oral Solution, Tablets**

Psychoses.
Adults and adolescents, initial: 2–5 mg (base) b.i.d.; **maintenance:** 15–20 mg/day in two or three divided doses. **Pediatric, 6–12 years:** 1 mg (base) 1–2 times/day; adjust dose as required and tolerated.
Anxiety/tension.
Adults and adolescents: 1–2 mg/day up to 6 mg/day. Not to be given for this purpose longer than 12 weeks.
- **IM**

Pyschoses.
Adults: 1–2 mg q 4–6 hr, not to exceed 10 mg/day. Switch to PO therapy as soon as possible. **Pediatric:** *Severe symptoms only:* 1 mg 1–2 times/day.

Administration/Storage
1. Dilute concentrate with 60 mL of juice (tomato or fruit), carbonated drinks, water, milk, orange or simple syrup, coffee, tea, or semisolid foods (e.g., applesauce, pudding, soup).
2. Dilute just before administration.
3. Protect liquid forms from light.
4. Discard strongly colored solutions.
5. Avoid skin contact with liquid form to prevent contact dermatitis.
6. To prevent cumulative effects, at least 4 hr should elapse between IM injections.

Special Concerns: Use during pregnancy only when benefits clearly outweigh risks. Dosage has not been established in children less than 6 years of age. Geriatric, emaciated, or debilitated clients usually require a lower initial dose.

NURSING CONSIDERATIONS

See also *Nursing Considerations* for *Antipsychotic Agents, Phenothiazines,* Chapter 38.

Assessment
1. Document indications for therapy, onset of symptoms, and behavioral presentations.
2. Note other agents prescribed and the outcome.

Evaluate
• Reduction in paranoid, excitable, or withdrawn behaviors
• ↓ Levels of anxiety, agitation, and tension in those with neuroses

Triflupromazine hydrochloride

(try-flew-**PROH**-mah-zeen)
Vesprin **(Rx)**

See also *Antipsychotic Agents, Phenothiazines,* Chapter 38.

How Supplied: *Injection:* 10 mg/mL, 20 mg/mL

Action/Kinetics: This drug produces significant anticholinergic and antiemetic effects; moderate to strong extrapyramidal and sedative effects; and moderate hypotensive effects.

Uses: Severe N&V. Psychotic disorders (should not be used for psychotic disorders with depression).

Dosage

• **IM**

Psychoses.

Adults and adolescents: 60 mg up to maximum of 150 mg/day. **Pediatric,** 0.2–0.25 mg/kg to maximum of 10 mg/day.

N&V.

Adults and adolescents: 5–15 mg as single dose repeated q 4 hr up to maximum of 60 mg/day (for elderly or debilitated clients: 2.5 mg up to maximum of 15 mg/day). **Pediatric, over 2½ years:** 0.2–0.25 mg/kg up to maximum of 10 mg/day.

• **IV**

Psychoses.

Adults and adolescents: 1 mg as required, up to a maximum of 3 mg/day.

Administration/Storage
1. Avoid excessive heat and freezing.
2. Store in amber-colored containers.
3. Do not use discolored (darker than light amber) solutions.
4. Avoid skin contact with liquid form to prevent contact dermatitis.
5. When used in children for N&V, the duration may be 12 hr.
6. May discolor urine reddish brown.

Special Concerns: Use during pregnancy only if benefits clearly outweigh risks. Dosage has not been established for children less than 30 months of age. IV use not recommended for children because of hypotension and rapid onset of extrapyramidal side effects. Geriatric, emaciated, or debilitated clients may require a lower initial dose.

NURSING CONSIDERATIONS

See also *Nursing Considerations* for *Antipsychotic Agents, Phenothiazines,* Chapter 38.

Assessment
1. Document indications for therapy and source and duration of symptoms.

2. Note other agents prescribed and the outcome.

Evaluate

- Control of N&V
- ↓ Agitated and hyperactive behaviors

MISCELLANEOUS ANTIPSYCHOTIC AGENTS

See the following individual entries:

Clozapine
Droperidol
Haloperidol
Haloperidol Decanoate
Haloperidol Lactate
Loxapine Hydrochloride
Risperidone
Thiothixene

Clozapine

(**KLOH**-zah-peen)
Pregnancy Category: B
Clozaril **(Rx)**

How Supplied: *Tablet:* 25 mg, 100 mg

Action/Kinetics: Clozapine interferes with the binding of dopamine to both D-1 and D-2 receptors; it is more active at limbic than at striatal dopamine receptors. Thus, it is relatively free from extrapyramidal side effects and it does not induce catalepsy. The drug also acts as an antagonist at adrenergic, cholinergic, histaminergic, and serotonergic receptors. Clozapine increases the amount of time spent in REM sleep. Food does not affect the bioavailability of clozapine. **Peak plasma levels:** 2.5 hr. **Average maximum concentration at steady state:** 122 ng/mL plasma after 100 mg b.i.d. Highly bound to plasma proteins. **t½:** 12 hr. Metabolized in the liver to inactive compounds and excreted through the urine (50%) and feces (30%).

Uses: Severely ill schizophrenic clients who do not respond adequately to conventional antipsychotic therapy, either because of ineffectiveness or intolerable side effects from other drugs. Due to the possibility of development of agranulocytosis and seizures, continued use should be avoided in clients failing to respond.

Dosage

- **Tablets**

Schizophrenia.

Adults, initial: 25 mg 1–2 times/day; **then,** if drug is tolerated, the dose can be increased by 25–50 mg/day to a dose of 300–450 mg/day at the end of 2 weeks. Subsequent dosage increments should occur no more often than once or twice a week in increments not to exceed 100 mg. **Usual maintenance dose:** 300–600 mg/day (although doses up to 900 mg/day may be required in some clients). Total daily dose should not exceed 900 mg.

Administration

1. Clozapine is available through independent "Clozaril treatment systems" based on a plan developed by physicians and pharmacists to ensure safe use of the drug with respect to weekly blood monitoring, data reporting, and drug dispensing. Prescriptions are limited to 1-week supplies, and the drug may only be dispensed following receipt, by the pharmacist, of weekly WBC test results that fall within the established limits. All weekly blood test results must be reported by participating pharmacists to the Clozaril National Registry.
2. If the drug is effective, the lowest maintenance doses possible should be sought to maintain remission.
3. If termination of therapy is planned, the dose should be gradually reduced over a 1–2-week period. If cessation of therapy is abrupt due to toxicity, the client should be observed carefully for recurrence of psychotic symptoms.
4. Clozapine therapy may be initiated immediately upon discontinuation of other antipsychotic medication;

however, a 24-hr "washout period" is desirable.

5. *Treatment of Overdose:* An airway should be established and maintained with adequate oxygenation and ventilation. Give activated charcoal and sorbitol. Cardiac status and VS should be monitored. General supportive measures.

Contraindications: Myeloproliferative disorders. Use in conjunction with other agents known to suppress bone marrow function. Severe CNS depression or coma due to any cause. Lactation.

Special Concerns: Use with caution in clients with known CV disease, prostatic hypertrophy, narrow angle glaucoma, hepatic or renal disease.

Side Effects: *Hematologic:* ***Agranulocytosis,*** leukopenia, neutropenia, eosinophilia. *CNS:* ***Seizures*** (appear to be dose dependent), drowsiness or sedation, dizziness, vertigo, headache, tremor, restlessness, nightmares, hypokinesia, akinesia, agitation, akathisia, confusion, rigidity, fatigue, insomnia, hyperkinesia, weakness, lethargy, slurred speech, ataxia, depression, anxiety, epileptiform movements. *CV:* Orthostatic hypotension (especially initially), tachycardia, syncope, hypertension, angina, chest pain, ***cardiac abnormalities,*** changes in ECG. *Neuroleptic malignant syndrome:* ***Hyperpyrexia,*** muscle rigidity, altered mental status, irregular pulse or BP, tachycardia, diaphoresis, cardiac dysrhythmias. *GI:* Constipation, nausea, heartburn, abdominal discomfort, vomiting, diarrhea, anorexia. *GU:* Urinary abnormalities, incontinence, abnormal ejaculation, urinary frequency or urgency, urinary retention. *Musculoskeletal:* Muscle weakness, pain (back, legs, neck), muscle spasm, muscle ache. *Respiratory:* Dyspnea, SOB, throat discomfort, nasal congestion. *Miscellaneous:* Salivation, sweating, visual disturbances, fever (transient), dry mouth, rash, weight gain, numb or sore tongue.

Symptoms of Overdose: Drowsiness, delirium, tachycardia, ***respiratory depression,*** hypotension, hypersalivation, ***seizures, coma.***

Drug Interactions

Anticholinergic drugs / Additive anticholinergic effects

Antihypertensive drugs / Additive hypotensive effects

Benzodiazepines / Possible respiratory depression and collapse

Digoxin / ↑ Effect of digoxin due to ↓ binding to plasma protein

Epinephrine / Clozapine may reverse effects if epinephrine is given for hypotension

Warfarin / ↑ Effect of warfarin due to ↓ binding to plasma protein

NURSING CONSIDERATIONS

Assessment

1. Document indications for therapy and assess client's behavior to gain baseline information.
2. List previous therapies tried and the outcome.
3. Note any history of seizure disorder.
4. Document baseline VS and ECG.
5. Obtain laboratory studies, including CBC, prior to initiating therapy.

Interventions

1. Monitor VS; report any irregular pulse, tachycardia, hyperpyrexia, or hypotension.
2. If WBCs fall below 2,000/mm^3 or granulocyte counts fall below 1,000/mm^3, the drug should be discontinued. Such clients should *not* be restarted on clozapine therapy.
3. Periodically reassess client to determine continued need for drug therapy.

Client/Family Teaching

1. Take only as directed; use supervision as needed.
2. Report immediately symptoms of lethargy, weakness, fever, sore throat, malaise, mucous membrane ulceration, or other signs of infection.
3. Avoid driving or other potentially hazardous activity while taking clozapine due to the possibility of seizures.
4. Because of a risk of orthostatic hypotension, especially during initial

dosing, use care when rising from a supine or sitting position.
5. Women of childbearing age should report if they become pregnant or intend to become pregnant during therapy.
6. Do not breast-feed when taking clozaril.
7. Do not take any prescription drugs, OTC drugs, or alcohol without approval.
8. Stress the importance of periodic laboratory studies to monitor for the occurrence of agranulocytosis.

Evaluate: Improved behavior patterns with ↓ agitation, ↓ hyperactivity, and improved coping behaviors.

Droperidol

(droh-**PER**-ih-dol)
Pregnancy Category: C
Inapsine **(Rx)**

How Supplied: *Injection:* 2.5 mg/mL

Action/Kinetics: Droperidol causes sedation, alpha-adrenergic blockade, peripheral vascular dilation, and has antiemetic properties. For other details, see *Haloperidol,* p. 693, and *Phenothiazines,* p. 97. **Onset** (after IM, IV): 3–10 min. **Peak effect:** 30 min. **Duration:** 2–4 hr, although alteration of consciousness may last up to 12 hr. **t½:** 2.2 hr. Metabolized in the liver and excreted in both the feces and urine.

Uses: Preoperatively; induction and maintenance of anesthesia. To relieve N&V and reduce anxiety in diagnostic procedures or surgery. Neuroleptanalgesia. Antiemetic in cancer chemotherapy (used IV).

Dosage

- **IM**

Preoperatively.

Adults: 2.5–10 mg 30–60 min before surgery (modify dosage in elderly, debilitated); **pediatric, 2–12 years,** 88–165 mcg/kg.

Diagnostic procedures.

Adults: 2.5–10 mg 30–60 min before procedure; **then,** if necessary, **IV,** 1.25–2.5 mg.

- **IV**

Adjunct to general anesthesia.

Adults: 0.28 mg/kg with analgesic or anesthetic; **maintenance:** 1.25–2.5 mg (total dose).

- **IV (Slow) or IM**

Adjunct to regional anesthesia.

Adults: 2.5–5 mg.

Administration/Storage

1. May be administered by direct IV slowly over 1 min; may also be reconstituted in 250 mL of D5%/W or NSS and administered slowly via infusion control device as prescribed.
2. At a concentration of 1 mg/50 mL, droperidol is stable for 7–10 days in glass bottles with 5% dextrose injection, lactated Ringer's injection, and 0.9% sodium chloride injection. Droperidol is stable for 7 days in polyvinyl chloride bags containing 5% dextrose injection or 0.9% sodium chloride injection.
3. If droperidol is used with Innovar injection (fentanyl plus droperidol), the dose of droperidol in the injection must be taken into consideration.
4. Droperidol is compatible at a concentration of 2.5 mg/mL for 15 min when combined in a syringe with the following: atropine sulfate, butorphanol tartrate, chlorpromazine hydrochloride, diphenhydramine hydrochloride, fentanyl citrate, glycopyrrolate, hydroxyzine hydrochloride, meperidine hydrochloride, morphine sulfate, perphenazine, promazine hydrochloride, promethazine hydrochloride, and scopolamine hydrobromide.
5. A precipitate will form if droperidol is mixed with barbiturates.

Special Concerns: Use with caution during lactation; in the elderly, debilitated, or poor risk client; and in renal or hepatic impairment. Safety for use during labor has not been established. Safety and efficacy have not been established in children less than 2 years of age.

Side Effects: *CNS:* Postoperative drowsiness (common), restlessness, hyperactivity, anxiety, dizziness, postoperative hallucinations; extrapyramidal symptoms (e.g., akathisia, dystonia, oculogyric crisis). *CV:* Hypotension and tachycardia (common), increase in BP (when combined with fentanyl or other parenteral analgesics). *Respiratory:* ***Respiratory depression (when combined with fentanyl), laryngospasm, bronchospasm.*** *Miscellaneous:* Chills, shivering.

Drug Interactions

Anesthetics, conduction (e.g., spinal) / Peripheral vasodilation and hypotension
CNS depressants / Additive or potentiating effects
Narcotic analgesics / ↑ Respiratory depressant effects

NURSING CONSIDERATIONS

See also *Nursing Considerations* for *Antipsychotic Agents and Phenothiazines,* Chapter 38.

Interventions

1. Monitor VS during the immediate postoperative period until stabilized.
2. Observe for extrapyramidal symptoms up to 48 hr after therapy.
3. Keep on bed rest and supervise activities until VS stable. Drug causes orthostatic hypotension and drowsiness.

Evaluate

- ↓ Procedure anxiety
- Control of N&V
- Desired sedative effect

Haloperidol

(hah-low-**PAIR**-ih-dohl)
Apo-Haloperidol ✤, Haldol, Novo-Peridol ✤, Peridol ✤, PMS Haloperidol ✤ **(Rx)**

Haloperidol decanoate

(hah-low-**PAIR**-ih-dohl)
Pregnancy Category: C (decanoate form)
Haldol Decanoate 50 and 100, Haldol LA ✤ **(Rx)**

Haloperidol lactate

(hah-low-**PAIR**-ih-dohl)
Haldol Lactate **(Rx)**

How Supplied: Haloperidol: *Tablet:* 0.5 mg, 1 mg, 2 mg, 5 mg, 10 mg, 20 mg.
Haloperidol decanoate: *Injection:* 50 mg/mL, 100 mg/mL.
Haloperidol lactate: *Concentrate:* 2 mg/mL; *Injection:* 5 mg/mL

Action/Kinetics: Although the precise mechanism is not known, haloperidol does competitively block dopamine receptors in the tuberoinfundibular system to cause sedation. The drug also causes alpha-adrenergic blockade, decreases release of growth hormone, and increases prolactin release by the pituitary. Haloperidol causes significant extrapyramidal effects, as well as a low incidence of sedation, anticholinergic effects, and orthostatic hypotension. The margin between the therapeutically effective dose and that causing extrapyramidal symptoms is narrow. The drug also has antiemetic effects. **Peak plasma levels: PO,** 3–5 hr; **IM,** 20 min; **IM, decanoate:** approximately 6 days. **Therapeutic serum levels:** 3–10 ng/mL. **t½, PO:** 12–38 hr; **IM:** 13–36 hr; **IM, decanoate:** 3 weeks; **IV:** approximately 14 hr. **Plasma protein binding:** 90%. Metabolized in liver, slowly excreted in urine and bile.

Uses: Psychotic disorders including manic states, drug-induced psychoses, and schizophrenia. Aggressive and agitated clients, including chronic brain syndrome or mental retardation. Severe behavior problems in children (those with combative, explosive hyperexcitability not accounted for by immediate provocation). Short-term treatment of hyperactive children. Control of tics and vocal utterances associated with Gilles de la Tourette's syndrome in adults and children. The decanoate is used for prolonged therapy in chronic schizophrenia.

Investigational: Antiemetic for cancer chemotherapy, phencyclidine (PCP) psychosis, infantile autism. IV for acute psychiatric conditions.

Dosage

- **Oral Solution, Tablets**

Psychoses.

Adults: 0.5–2 mg b.i.d.–t.i.d. up to 3–5 mg b.i.d.–t.i.d. for severe symptoms; **maintenance:** reduce dosage to lowest effective level. Up to 100 mg/day may be required in some. **Geriatric or debilitated clients:** 0.5–2 mg b.i.d.–t.i.d. **Pediatric, 3–12 years or 15–40 kg:** 0.5 mg/day in two to three divided doses; if necessary the daily dose may be increased by 0.5-mg increments q 5–7 days for a total of 0.15 mg/kg/day for psychotic disorders and 0.075 mg/kg for nonpsychotic behavior disorders and Tourette's syndrome. Doses for children 3–6 years of age are 0.01–0.03 mg/kg/day PO for agitation and hyperkinesia and 0.5–4 mg/day for infantile autism.

- **IM**

  Acute psychoses.

Adults and adolescents, initial: 2–5 mg; may be repeated if necessary q 4–8 hr to a total of 100 mg/day. Switch to **PO** therapy as soon as possible.

- **IM, Decanoate**

  Chronic therapy.

Adults, initial dose: 10–15 times the daily PO dose, not to exceed 100 mg initially, regardless of the previous oral antipsychotic dose; **then,** repeat q 4 weeks (decanoate is not to be given IV).

Administration/Storage

1. The decanoate should be given by deep IM injection using a 21-gauge needle. The maximum volume per site should not exceed 3 mL.
2. The decanoate product should not be given IV.
3. *Treatment of Overdose:* Treat symptomatically. Antiparkinson drugs, diphenhydramine, or barbiturates can be used to treat extrapyramidal symptoms. Fluid replacement and vasoconstrictors (either norepinephrine or phenylephrine) can be used to treat hypotension. Ventricular arrhythmias can be treated with phenytoin. To treat seizures, use pentobarbital or diazepam. A saline cathartic can be used to hasten the excretion of sustained-release products.

Contraindications: Use with extreme caution, or not at all, in clients with parkinsonism. Lactation.

Special Concerns: PO dosage has not been determined in children less than 3 years of age; IM dosage is not recommended in children. Geriatric clients are more likely to exhibit orthostatic hypotension, anticholinergic effects, sedation, and extrapyramidal side effects (such as parkinsonism and tardive dyskinesia).

Laboratory Test Interferences: ↑ Alkaline phosphatase, bilirubin, serum transaminase; ↓ PT (clients on coumarin), serum cholesterol.

Side Effects: Extrapyramidal symptoms, especially akathisia and dystonias, occur more frequently than with the phenothiazines. Overdosage is characterized by severe extrapyramidal reactions, hypotension, or sedation. The drug does not elicit photosensitivity reactions like those of the phenothiazines.

Symptoms of Overdose: CNS depression, hypertension or hypotension, extrapyramidal symptoms, agitation, restlessness, fever, hypothermia, hyperthermia, ***seizures, cardiac arrhythmias,*** changes in the ECG, autonomic reactions, ***coma.***

Drug Interactions

Amphetamine / ↓ Effect of amphetamine by ↓ uptake of drug at its site of action
Anticholinergics / ↓ Effect of haloperidol
Antidepressants, tricyclic / ↑ Effect of antidepressants due to ↓ breakdown by liver
Barbiturates / ↓ Effect of haloperidol due to ↑ breakdown by liver
Guanethidine / ↓ Effect of guanethidine by ↓ uptake of drug at site of action
Lithium / ↑ Toxicity of haloperidol
Methyldopa / ↑ Toxicity of haloperidol
Phenytoin / ↓ Effect of haloperidol due to ↑ breakdown by liver

NURSING CONSIDERATIONS

See also *Nursing Considerations* for *Antipsychotic Agents, Phenothiazines,* Chapter 38.

Assessment

1. Document indications for therapy, describing type and onset of symptoms.
2. Note age and use with caution in the elderly as they tend to exhibit toxicity more frequently and may benefit from a periodic "drug holiday."
3. Document any evidence of new onset of extra pyramidal symptoms because drug may induce these.

Evaluate

- Improved patterns of behavior with ↓ agitation, ↓ hostility, and ↓ delusions
- Control of tics and vocal utterances in Tourette's syndrome
- ↓ Hyperactive behaviors and motor activity

Loxapine hydrochloride

(**LOX**-ah-peen)
Pregnancy Category: C
Loxapac ✱, Loxitane C, Loxitane IM **(Rx)**

Loxapine succinate

(**LOX**-ah-peen)
Pregnancy Category: C
Loxapac ✱, Loxitane **(Rx)**

See also *Antipsychotic Agents, Phenothiazines,* Chapter 38.

How Supplied: Loxapine hydrochloride: *Concentrate:* 25 mg/mL; *Injection:* 50 mg/mL
Loxapine succinate: *Capsule:* 5 mg, 10 mg, 25 mg, 50 mg

Action/Kinetics: Loxapine belongs to a new subclass of tricyclic antipsychotic agents. The drug is thought to act by blocking dopamine at postsynaptic brain receptors. It causes significant extrapyramidal symptoms, moderate sedative effects, and a low incidence of anticholinergic effects, as well as orthostatic hypotension. **Onset:** 20–30 min. **Peak effects:** 1.5–3 hr. **Duration:** about 12 hr. **t½:** 3–4 hr. Partially metabolized in the liver; excreted in urine, and unchanged in feces.

Uses: Psychoses. *Investigational:* Anxiety neurosis with depression.

Dosage

- **Capsules, Oral Solution**

Psychoses.

Adults, initial: 10 mg (of the base) b.i.d. For severe cases, up to 50 mg/day may be required. Increase dosage rapidly over 7–10 days until symptoms are controlled. **Range:** 60–100 mg up to 250 mg/day. **Maintenance:** If possible reduce dosage to 15–25 mg b.i.d.–q.i.d.

- **IM**

Psychoses.

Adults: 12.5–50 mg (of the base) q 4–6 hr; once adequate control has been established, switch to PO medication after control achieved (usually within 5 days).

Administration/Storage

1. Measure the dosage of the concentrate *only* with the enclosed calibrated dropper.
2. Mix oral concentrate with orange or grapefruit juice immediately before administration to disguise unpleasant taste.

Additional Contraindication: History of convulsive disorders.

Special Concerns: Use with caution in clients with CV disease. Use during lactation only if benefits outweigh risks. Dosage has not been established in children less than 16 years of age. Geriatric clients may be more prone to developing orthostatic hypotension, anticholinergic, sedative, and extrapyramidal side effects.

Additional Side Effects: Tachycardia, hypertension, hypotension, lightheadedness, and syncope.

NURSING CONSIDERATIONS

See also *Nursing Considerations* for *Antipsychotic Agents, Phenothiazines,* Chapter 38.

Assessment

1. Document indications for therapy and type and onset of symptoms.

2. List any agents used previously for these symptoms and the outcome.

Client/Family Teaching: Caution client about orthostatic drug effects.

Evaluate: ↓ Agitated and hyperactive behaviors.

Risperidone

(ris-**PAIR**-ih-dohn)
Pregnancy Category: C
Risperdal **(Rx)**

How Supplied: *Tablet:* 1 mg, 2 mg, 3 mg, 4 mg

Action/Kinetics: Although the mechanism of action is not known, it may be due to a combination of antagonism of dopamine (D_2) and serotonin (5-HT_2) receptors. The drug also has high affinity for the alpha-1, alpha-2, and histamine-1 receptors. Risperidone is metabolized significantly in the liver to the active metabolite 9-hydroxyrisperidone, which is equally effective as risperidone to receptor binding activity. Thus, the effect of the drug is likely due to both the parent compound and the metabolite. Food does not affect either the rate or extent of absorption. The ability to convert risperidone to 9-hydroxyrisperidone is subject to genetic variation. A low percentage of Asians have the ability to metabolize the drug. **Peak plasma levels, risperidone:** 1 hr; **peak plasma levels, 9-hydroxyrisperidone:** 3 hr for extensive metabolizers and 17 hr for poor metabolizers. **t½, risperidone and 9-methylrisperidone:** 3 and 21 hr, respectively, for extensive metabolizers and 20 and 30 hr, respectively, for poor metabolizers. The clearance of the drug is decreased in geriatric clients and in clients with hepatic and renal impairment.

Use: Treatment of psychotic disorders.

Dosage

• **Tablets**

Antipsychotic.

Adults, initial: 1 mg b.i.d. Can be increased by 1 mg b.i.d. on the second and third day as tolerated to reach a dose of 3 mg b.i.d. by the third day. Further increases in dose should occur at intervals of about 1 week. **Maximal effect:** 4–6 mg/day. Doses greater than 6 mg/day were not shown to be more effective and were associated with greater incidence of side effects. Safety of doses greater than 16 mg/day have not been studied. The initial dose is 0.5 mg b.i.d. for clients who are elderly or debilitated, those with severe renal or hepatic impairment, and those predisposed to hypotension or in whom hypotension would pose a risk. Dosage increases in these clients should be in increments of 0.5 mg b.i.d. Dosage increases above 1.5 mg b.i.d. should occur at intervals of about 1 week.

Administration/Storage

1. A lower starting dose should be used in geriatric clients and in clients with impaired renal or hepatic function.
2. When restarting clients who have had an interval of risperidone, the initial 3-day dose titration schedule should be followed.
3. If switching from other antipsychotic drugs to risperidone, immediate discontinuation of the previous antipsychotic drug is recommended when starting risperidone therapy. When switching clients from a depot antipsychotic injection, risperidone should be initiated in place of the next scheduled injection.
4. *Treatment of Overdose:* Establish and secure airway, and ensure adequate oxygenation and ventilation. Gastric lavage should be followed by activated charcoal and a laxative. Monitor CV system, including continuous ECG readings. Provide general supportive measures. Hypotension and circulatory collapse can be treated with IV fluids or sympathomimetic drugs; however, epinephrine and dopamine should not be used, as beta stimulation may worsen hypotension due to risperidone-induced alpha blockade. Anticholinergic drugs can

be given for severe extrapyramidal symptoms.

Contraindication: Use during lactation.

Special Concerns: Use with caution in clients with known CV disease (including history of MI or ischemia, heart failure, conduction abnormalities), cerebrovascular disease, and conditions that predispose the client to hypotension (e.g., dehydration, hypovolemia, use of antihypertensive drugs). Use with caution in clients who will be exposed to extreme heat. The effectiveness of risperidone for more than 6–8 weeks has not been studied. Safety and effectiveness have not been established for children.

Laboratory Test Interferences: ↑ CPK, serum prolactin, AST, ALT. Hyponatremia.

Side Effects: ***Neuroleptic malignant syndrome:*** Hyperpyrexia, muscle rigidity, altered mental status, autonomic instability (i.e., irregular pulse or BP, tachycardia, diaphoresis, cardiac dysrhythmia), elevated CPK, rhabdomyolysis, ***acute renal failure, death.*** *CNS:* Tardive dyskinesia (especially in geriatric clients), somnolence, insomnia, agitation, anxiety, aggressive reaction, extrapyramidal symptoms, headache, dizziness, increased dream activity, decreased sexual desire, nervousness, impaired concentration, depression, apathy, catatonia, euphoria, increased libido, amnesia, increased duration of sleep, dysarthria, vertigo, stupor, paresthesia, confusion. *GI:* Constipation, nausea, dyspepsia, vomiting, abdominal pain, increased or decreased salivation, toothache, anorexia, flatulence, diarrhea, increased appetite, stomatitis, melena, dysphagia, hemorrhoids, gastritis. *CV:* Prolongation of the QT interval that might lead to ***torsades de pointes***. Orthostatic hypotension, tachycardia, palpitation, hypertension or hypotension, ***AV block, MI.*** *Respiratory:* Rhinitis, coughing, upper respiratory infection, sinusitis, pharyngitis, dyspnea. *Body as a whole:* Arthralgia, back pain, chest pain, fever, fatigue, rigors, malaise, edema, flu-like symptoms, increase or decrease in weight. *Hematologic:* Purpura, anemia, hypochromic anemia. *GU:* Polyuria, polydipsia, urinary incontinence, hematuria, dysuria, menorrhagia, orgastic dysfunction, dry vagina, erectile dysfunction, nonpuerperal lactation, amenorrhea, female breast pain, leukorrhea, mastitis, dysmenorrhea, female perineal pain, intermenstrual bleeding, ***vaginal hemorrhage,*** failure to ejaculate. *Dermatologic:* Rash, dry skin, seborrhea, increased pigmentation, increased or decreased sweating, acne, alopecia, hyperkeratosis, pruritus, skin exfoliation. *Ophthalmic:* Abnormal vision, abnormal accommodation, xerophthalmia. *Miscellaneous:* Increased prolactin, photosensitivity, diabetes mellitus, thirst, myalgia, epistaxis.

Symptoms of Overdose: Exaggeration of known effects, especially drowsiness, sedation, tachycardia, hypotension, and extrapyramidal symptoms.

Drug Interactions

Carbamazepine / ↑ Clearance of risperidone following chronic use of carbamazepine

Clozapine / ↓ Clearance of risperidone following chronic use of clozapine

Levodopa / Risperidone antagonizes the effects of levodopa and dopamine antagonists

NURSING CONSIDERATIONS

See also *Nursing Considerations* for *Antipsychotic Drugs,* Chapter 38.

Assessment

1. Document indications for therapy and describe presenting behavioral manifestations.
2. List other drugs prescribed to ensure none interact unfavorably.
3. Perform appropriate baseline assessments. Electrolyte imbalance, bradycardia, and concomitant administration with drugs that prolong the QT interval may increase the risk of torsades de pointes.
4. Anticipate reduced dosage in clients with severe liver, cardiac, or renal dysfunction.

5. Note any history of drug dependency.

Interventions

1. Observe for any evidence of altered mental status, muscle rigidity, dyskinetic movements, or overt changes in VS.
2. Assess client carefully because the antiemetic effect of risperidone may mask the S&S of overdose with certain drugs or of conditions such as intestinal obstruction, Reye's syndrome, and brain tumor.

Client/Family Teaching

1. Take only as directed and do not share medications.
2. Drug may impair judgment, motor skills, and thinking and cause blurred vision, so determine drug effects before engaging in activities that require mental alertness.
3. Rise slowly from a lying to a sitting position and dangle legs before standing, as drug may cause orthostatic hypotension.
4. Drug may alter temperature regulation. Avoid situations where exposure to extreme heat may occur.
5. Wear protective clothing, sunscreen, a hat, and sunglasses when sun exposure is necessary, as drug may cause a photosensitivity reaction.
6. Report any abnormal bruising or bleeding or yellow discoloration of the skin.
7. Practice birth control during drug therapy. Notify provider if pregnancy is suspected or desired.
8. Avoid alcohol and any other OTC agents during drug therapy.
9. Review the list of drug side effects, stressing those that require immediate attention, and advise to report any that are persistent or bothersome.
10. Warn that risperidone elevates serum prolactin levels. Explain the potential relationship of prolactin and human breast cancer development, and screen carefully for any evidence or history of breast cancer.
11. Any suicide ideations or bizarre behavior should be reported immediately. Due to the possibility of suicide attempts in clients with schizophrenia, advise family that close supervision of high-risk clients is necessary and that prescriptions will be written for the smallest quantity of tablets. Stress the importance of close follow-up.

Evaluate: Improved patterns of behavior with ↓ agitation, ↓ hyperactivity, and evidence of reality orientation.

Thiothixene

(thigh-oh-**THICKS**-een)
Navane **(Rx)**

See also *Antipsychotic Agents, Phenothiazines,* Chapter 38.

How Supplied: *Capsule:* 1 mg, 2 mg, 5 mg, 10 mg, 20 mg

Action/Kinetics: The antipsychotic action is due to blockade of postsynaptic dopamine receptors in the brain. Thiothixene causes significant extrapyramidal symptoms and antiemetic effects; minimal sedation, orthostatic hypotension, and anticholinergic effects. Its actions closely resemble those of chlorprothixene with respect to postural reflexes and motor coordination. The margin between a therapeutically effective dose and one that causes extrapyramidal symptoms is narrow. **Peak plasma levels, PO:** 1–3 hr. **t½:** 34 hr. **Therapeutic plasma levels** (during chronic treatment): 10–150 ng/mL.

Use: Symptomatic treatment of acute and chronic schizophrenia, especially when condition is accompanied by florid symptoms.

Dosage

- **Capsules, Oral Solution**
  Antipsychotic.

Adults and adolescents, initial: 2 mg t.i.d. for mild conditions and 5 mg b.i.d. for severe conditions; can be increased gradually to usual maintenance dose of 20–30 mg/day, although some clients require 60 mg/day.

- **IM**

Antipsychotic.

Adults and adolescents: 4 mg b.i.d.–q.i.d.; **usual maintenance:** 16–20 mg/day, although up to 30 mg/day may be required in some cases. Switch to **PO** form as soon as possible. **Not recommended for children under 12 years of age.**

Administration/Storage

1. The powder for injection can be reconstituted by adding 2.2 mL of sterile water for injection.
2. Thiothixene is well absorbed.
3. Assess behavior for a therapeutic response in 1–6 hr after an IM injection, whereas PO medications will require several days to observe therapeutic effects.

Special Concerns: Safe use during pregnancy has not been established. Dosage has not been established for children under 12 years of age. Children are more prone to develop neuromuscular and extrapyramidal side effects (especially dystonias). Adolescents may experience a higher incidence of hypotensive and extrapyramidal reactions than adults. Geriatric clients may be more prone to orthostatic hypotension and manifest an increased sensitivity to tardive dyskinesia and Parkinson-like symptoms. Geriatric or debilitated clients usually require a lower starting dose.

Laboratory Test Interference: ↓ Serum uric acid.

Side Effects: Drowsiness, lethargy, orthostatic hypotension, tachycardia, dizziness, and dry mouth occur especially frequently.

Drug Interactions: May cause additive hyypotensive effects with methyldopa or reserpine.

NURSING CONSIDERATIONS

See also *Nursing Considerations* for *Antipsychotic Agents, Phenothiazines,* Chapter 38.

Assessment

1. Document indications for therapy, onset of symptoms, and behavioral presentation.
2. Describe location and character of any associated dermatologic discoloration.
3. Note any history of seizure disorder as drug may lower seizure threshold.

Client/Family Teaching

1. Take with milk or food to diminish GI upset.
2. Caution that drug may cause drowsiness or dizziness.
3. Dress appropriately as drug may alter temperature regulation and may also cause a photosensitivity reaction in the sun.

Evaluate: Evidence of ↓ agitated, hyperactive behaviors.

CHAPTER THIRTY-NINE

Hypnotics

See the following individual entries:

Chloral Hydrate
Estazolam
Ethchlorvynol
Flurazepam Hydrochloride
Paraldehyde
Barbiturates
Pentobarbital
Pentobarbital Sodium
Secobarbital Sodium
Triazolam
Zolpidem Tartrate

Chloral hydrate

(**KLOH**-ral **HY**-drayt)
Pregnancy Category: C
Aquachloral Supprettes, Noctec
(C-IV) (Rx)

How Supplied: *Capsule:* 500 mg; *Suppository:* 325 mg, 500 mg, 650 mg; *Syrup:* 250 mg/5 mL, 500 mg/5 mL

Action/Kinetics: Chloral hydrate is metabolized to trichloroethanol, which is the active metabolite causing CNS depression. Chloral hydrate produces only slight hangover effects and is said not to affect REM sleep. High doses lead to severe CNS depression, as well as depression of respiratory and vasomotor centers (hypotension). Both psychologic and physical dependence develop. **Onset:** Within 30 min. **Duration:** 4–8 hr. **t½, trichloroethanol:** 7–10 hr. The drug is readily absorbed from the GI tract and is distributed to all tissues; it passes the placental barrier and appears in breast milk as well. Metabolites excreted by kidney.

Uses: Short-term hypnotic. Daytime sedative and sedation prior to EEG procedures. Preoperative sedative and postoperative as adjunct to analgesics. Prevent or reduce symptoms of alcohol withdrawal.

Dosage

- **Capsules, Syrup**

Daytime sedative.

Adults: 250 mg t.i.d. after meals.

Preoperative sedative.

Adults: 0.5–1.0 g 30 min before surgery.

Hypnotic.

Adults: 0.5–1 g 15–30 min before bedtime. **Pediatric:** 50 mg/kg (1.5 g/m^2) at bedtime (up to 1 g may be given as a single dose).

Daytime sedative.

Pediatric: 8.3 mg/kg (250 mg/m^2) up to a maximum of 500 mg t.i.d. after meals.

Premedication prior to EEG procedures.

Pediatric: 20–25 mg/kg.

- **Suppositories, rectal**

Daytime sedative.

Adults: 325 mg t.i.d. **Pediatric:** 8.3 mg/kg (250 mg/m^2) t.i.d.

Hypnotic.

Adults: 0.5–1 g at bedtime. **Pediatric:** 50 mg/kg (1.5 g/m^2) at bedtime (up to 1 g as a single dose).

Administration/Storage

1. PO: give capsules after meals with a full glass of water. Give the syrup with half a glass of juice, water, or ginger ale.
2. PO syrups have an unpleasant taste, which can be reduced by chilling the syrup before administration.
3. Have emergency drugs and equipment available should the client require supportive, physiologic treatment of acute poisoning.

Contraindications: Marked hepatic or renal impairment, severe cardiac disease, lactation. Drugs should not be given PO to clients with esophagitis, gastritis, or gastric or duodenal ulcer.

Special Concerns: Use by nursing mothers may cause sedation in the infant. A decrease in dose may be necessary in geriatric clients due to age-related decrease in both hepatic and renal function.

Laboratory Test Interferences: ↑ 17-Hydroxycorticosteroids. Interference with fluorescence tests for catecholamines and copper sulfate test for glucose.

Side Effects: *CNS:* Paradoxical paranoid reactions. Sudden withdrawal in dependent clients may result in "chloral delirium." ***Sudden intolerance to the drug following prolonged use may result in respiratory depression, hypotension, cardiac effects, and possibly death.*** *GI:* N&V, diarrhea, bad taste in mouth, gastritis, increased peristalsis. *GU:* Renal damage, decreased urine flow and uric acid excretion. *Miscellaneous:* Skin reactions, hepatic damage, allergic reactions, leukopenia, eosinophilia.

Chronic toxicity is treated by gradual withdrawal and rehabilitative measures such as those used in treatment of the chronic alcoholic. Poisoning by chloral hydrate resembles acute barbiturate intoxication; the same supportive treatment is indicated (see *Hypnotics,* Chapter 39).

Drug Interactions

Anticoagulants, oral / ↑ Effect of anticoagulants by ↓ plasma protein binding

CNS depressants / Additive CNS depression; concomitant use may lead to drowsiness, lethargy, stupor, respiratory collapse, coma, or death

Furosemide (IV) / Concomitant use results in diaphoresis, tachycardia, hypertension, flushing

NURSING CONSIDERATIONS

See also *Nursing Considerations* for *Hypnotics,* Chapter 39.

Assessment

1. Document indications for therapy and evaluate sleep habits and patterns.
2. Assess mental status and response to stimuli.
3. Note any history of cardiac disease, liver or renal dysfunction. Drug is metabolized to an alcohol component.

Interventions

1. Monitor level and pattern of alertness and compare with the premedication history.
2. Observe respiratory and cardiac responses. Document any evidence of vasomotor depression and dilatation of cutaneous blood vessels.
3. Periodically perform liver and renal function studies to determine any evidence of impairment.
4. Observe for psychologic and physical dependence and report if evident. Symptoms of dependence resemble those of acute alcoholism, but with more severe gastritis.
5. Offer measures to promote comfort and relaxation.
6. Protect from injury. Assist with ambulation, side rails up, call bell within reach, and night light.
7. Administer analgesics as needed for pain relief.

Client/Family Teaching

1. Take only as directed.
2. Store away from the bedside.
3. Stress that drug is for short-term use only as drug may cause psychologic and physical dependence.
4. Review list of drug side effects, noting those that require immediate attention.

Evaluate

- Desired level of sedation
- Control of symptoms of alcohol withdrawal
- Improved sleep patterns

Estazolam

(es-**TAYZ**-oh-lam)
Pregnancy Category: X
ProSom **(C-IV) (Rx)**

See also *Anti-Anxiety/Antimanic Drugs,* Chapter 40.

How Supplied: *Tablet:* 1 mg, 2 mg

Action/Kinetics: Peak plasma levels: 2 hr. **t1/2:** 10–24 hr. The clearance is increased in smokers compared with nonsmokers. Metabolized in the liver and excreted mainly in the urine. Two metabolites—4'-hydroxy estazolam and 1-oxo-estazolam—have minimal pharmacologic activity although at the levels present they do not contribute significantly to the hypnotic effect of estazolam.

Uses: Short-term use for insomnia characterized by difficulty in falling asleep, frequent awakenings, and/or early morning awakenings.

Dosage

• Tablets

Adults: 1 mg at bedtime (although some clients may require 2 mg). The initial dose in small or debilitated geriatric clients is 0.5 mg. Prolonged use is not recommended or necessary.

Contraindications: Pregnancy. Use during labor and delivery and during lactation.

Special Concerns: Use with caution in geriatric or debilitated clients, in those with impaired renal or hepatic function, in those with compromised respiratory function, and in those with depression or who show suicidal tendencies. Safety and efficacy have not been determined in children less than 18 years of age.

NURSING CONSIDERATIONS

See also *Nursing Considerations* for *Anti-Anxiety/Antimanic Drugs,* Chapter 40.

Assessment

1. Determine any history of depression or suicidal tendencies.
2. Obtain baseline liver and renal function studies and monitor if impairment evident.
3. Note any history or evidence of compromised respiratory status.
4. Attempt to determine the underlying cause(s) for insomnia because alternative nonpharmacologic methods for sleep inducement may be useful.

Interventions

1. Observe closely and anticipate reduced dosage in geriatric and debilitated clients and those with impaired renal and hepatic function.
2. Identify if client is a smoker because this may alter drug absorption.
3. Estazolam may enhance the duration and quality of sleep for up to 12 weeks. Carefully assess the need for continued therapy for insomnia after this period of time.

Client/Family Teaching

1. Provide a printed list of adverse drug effects and stress those symptoms that require immediate reporting.
2. Instruct females of childbearing age to practice contraception. Advise client to discontinue the use of estazolam before becoming pregnant.
3. Do not perform tasks that require mental alertness until drug effects are realized. The ability to drive or operate dangerous machinery may be impaired.
4. Avoid alcohol during drug therapy and do not take any OTC medications without consent.
5. Take only as directed because estazolam may produce psychologic and physical dependence.
6. Do not stop taking the drug abruptly. After prolonged treatment, gradual withdrawal is recommended.

Evaluate: Enhanced duration and quality of sleep with less frequent awakenings.

Ethchlorvynol

(eth-klor-**VYE**-nohl)

Pregnancy Category: C

Placidyl **(C-IV) (Rx)**

How Supplied: *Capsule:* 200 mg, 500 mg, 750 mg

Action/Kinetics: Manifests anticonvulsant and muscle relaxant properties, as well as sedative and hypnotic effects. Said to depress REM sleep. Chronic use produces psychologic and physical dependence. Produces less respiratory depression than occurs with barbiturates. **Onset:** 15–60 min. **Peak blood levels:** 1–1.5 hr. **Duration:** 5 hr. **t1/2:** initial, 1–3 hr; final, 10–25 hr. Approximately 90% metabolized in liver and excreted in urine.

Uses: Short-term treatment of insomnia (treatment not to exceed 1 week). Has generally been replaced by other sedative-hypnotic drugs. *Investigational:* Sedation.

Dosage

- **Capsules**

Hypnotic.

Adult, usual: 500 mg at bedtime; up to 1,000 mg may be required if insomnia is severe. If client awakens, a 100–200-mg supplemental dose can be given. Adjust dose carefully in geriatric or debilitated clients.

Sedation.

Adults: 100–200 mg b.i.d.–t.i.d.

Contraindications: Porphyria, hypersensitivity.

Special Concerns: Use during the third trimester may result in CNS depression and withdrawal symptoms in the neonate. Geriatric clients may be more sensitive to the effects of this drug; also, a decrease in dose may be necessary in these clients due to age-related decreases in both hepatic and renal function.

Laboratory Test Interference: ↓ PT (clients on Coumadin).

Side Effects: *CNS:* Initial excitement, giddiness, vertigo, mental confusion, headache, blurred vision, hangover, fatigue, ataxia. *GI:* Bad aftertaste, N&V, gastric upset. *CV:* Hypotension, fainting. *Miscellaneous:* Skin rash, thrombocytopenia, jaundice, pulmonary edema (following IV abuse). Overdose produces symptoms similar to those of barbiturate intoxication.

Drug Interactions

Anticoagulants, oral / ↓ Effect of anticoagulants due to ↑ breakdown by liver

Antidepressants, tricyclic / Combination may result in transient delirium

NURSING CONSIDERATIONS

See also *Nursing Considerations* for *Hypnotics,* Chapter 39.

Interventions

1. Monitor liver and renal function studies and anticipate a decreased dose in clients with altered function.
2. Advise client to use caution in driving or operating machinery until daytime sedative effects are evaluated. Milk or food taken with the medication may reduce these symptoms.
3. Explore alternative methods for inducing sleep.
4. Assess closely for tolerance and for psychologic and physical dependence.

Evaluate

- Enhanced duration and quality of sleep with less frequent awakenings
- Desired level of sedation

Flurazepam hydrochloride

(flur-**AYZ**-eh-pam)

Apo-Flurazepam ✱, Dalmane, Durapam, Somnol ✱ **(C-IV) (Rx)**

See also *Anti-Anxiety/Antimanic Drugs,* Chapter 40.

How Supplied: *Capsule:* 15 mg, 30 mg

Action/Kinetics: Flurazepam acts at benzodiazepine receptors, which are part of the benzodiazepine-GABA receptor-chloride ionophore complex. Interaction with the complex enhances the inhibitory action of GABA leading to interference of transmission of nerve impulses in the reticular activating system. **Onset:** 17 min. The major active metabolite, *N*-desalkyl-flurazepam, is active and has a **t½** of 47–100 hr. **Time to peak plasma levels, flurazepam:** 0.5–1 hr; **active metabolite:** 1–3 hr. **Duration:** 7–8 hr. **Maximum effectiveness:** 2–3 days (due to slow accumulation of active metabolite). Significantly bound to plasma protein. Elimination is slow because metabolites remain in the blood for several days. Exceeding the recommended dose may result in development of tolerance and dependence.

Use: Insomnia (all types). Flurazepam is increasingly effective on the second or third night of consecutive use and for one or two nights after the drug is discontinued.

Dosage

- **Capsules**

Adults: 15–30 mg at bedtime; 15 mg for geriatric and/or debilitated clients.

Contraindications: Hypersensitivity. Pregnancy or in women wishing to become pregnant. Depression, renal or hepatic disease, chronic pulmonary insufficiency, children under 15 years.

Special Concerns: Use during the last few weeks of pregnancy may result in CNS depression of the neonate. Use during lactation may cause sedation and feeding problems in the infant. Geriatric clients may be more sensitive to the effects of flurazepam.

Laboratory Test Interferences: ↑ Alkaline phosphatase, bilirubin, serum transaminases.

Side Effects: *CNS:* Ataxia, dizziness, drowsiness/sedation, headache, disorientation. Symptoms of stimulation including nervousness, apprehension, irritability, and talkativeness. *GI:* N&V, diarrhea, gastric upset or pain, heartburn, constipation. *Miscellaneous:* Arthralgia, chest pains, or palpitations. Rarely, symptoms of allergy, SOB, jaundice, anorexia, blurred vision.

Drug Interactions

Cimetidine / ↑ Effect of flurazepam due to ↓ breakdown by liver
CNS depressants / Addition or potentiation of CNS depressant effects—drowsiness, lethargy, stupor, respiratory depression or collapse, coma, and possible death
Disulfiram / ↑ Effect of flurazepam due to ↓ breakdown by liver
Ethanol / Additive depressant effects up to the day following flurazepam administration
Isoniazid / ↑ Effect of flurazepam due to ↓ breakdown by liver
Oral contraceptives / Either ↑ or ↓ effect of benzodiazepines due to effect on breakdown by liver
Rifampin / ↓ Effect of benzodiazepines due to ↑ breakdown by liver

NURSING CONSIDERATIONS

See also *Nursing Considerations* for *Anti-Anxiety/Antimanic Drugs,* Chapter 40.

Assessment

1. Document indications for therapy, onset of symptoms, and any other agents prescribed for this condition and the results.
2. Anticipate short-term therapy. Attempt to identify and address causative factors.

Client/Family Teaching

1. Use caution in driving or operating machinery until daytime sedative effects are evaluated. Report persistent morning "hangover."
2. Clients suffering from simple insomnia should be instructed to try warm baths, warm drinks, soft music, white noise simulator, and other relaxation methods to induce sleep.
3. Avoid ingestion of alcohol.
4. Report tolerance and any symptoms of psychologic and/or physical dependence. Advise client that drug is for short-term therapy and that continued use causes a tolerance and a decrease in drug responsiveness.

Evaluate: Improved sleeping patterns and less frequent awakenings.

Paraldehyde

(par-**AL**-deh-hyd)
Pregnancy Category: C
Paral **(C-IV) (Rx)**

How Supplied: *Liquid:* 1 g/mL

Action/Kinetics: Paraldehyde is bitter tasting (liquid) and has a strong, unpleasant odor. In usual doses, it has little effect on either respiration or BP. In the presence of pain, paraldehyde may induce excitement or delirium; it is not analgesic. **Onset:** 10–15 min. **Duration:** 8–12 hr. **Peak serum levels:** After oral, 30–60 min; after rectal administration, 2.5 hr. Approximately 70%–90% is detoxified in the liver, with the remainder excreted unchanged by the lungs. **t½:** 3.4–9.8 hr.

Uses: Sedative and hypnotic, although such use has generally been replaced by other sedative-hypnotics. Delirium tremens and other excited states. Prior to EEG to induce artificial sleep. Emergency treatment of seizures, eclampsia, tetanus, status epilepticus, and overdose of stimulant or convulsant drugs.

Dosage

- **Liquid, Oral or Rectal**

Hypnotic.

Adults, PO: 10–30 mL; **Rectal:** 10–20 mL with 1–2 parts olive oil or isotonic sodium chloride. **Pediatric, PO, rectal:** 0.3 mL/kg.

Sedation.

Adults, PO, rectal: 5–10 mL. **Pediatric, PO, rectal:** 0.15 mL/kg.

Delirium tremens.

Adults, PO: 10–35 mL.

Anticonvulsant.

Adults, PO: Up to 12 mL via gastric tube q 4 hr, if needed; **Rectal:** 10–20 mL. **Pediatric, PO, rectal:** 0.3 mL/kg.

- **IM, IV**

Anticonvulsant.

Adults, IM: 5–10 mL; **IV infusion:** 5 mL diluted with at least 100 mL 0.9% sodium chloride given at a rate not to exceed 1 mL/min. **Pediatric, IM, IV,** 0.1–0.15 mL/kg.

Administration/Storage

1. *PO:* Drug should be cold to minimize odor and taste as well as gastric irritation. Mask the taste and odor by mixing drug with syrup, milk, or fruit juice.
2. *Rectal:* Mix with olive oil, cottonseed oil, or isotonic sodium chloride solution to minimize irritation—1 part medication to 2 parts diluent.
3. *IM:* A pure sterile preparation should be used. Inject deeply into gluteus maximus and avoid extravasation into SC tissue because drug is irritating and may cause sterile abscesses and nerve injury and paralysis.
4. *IV:* Only in an emergency, dilute with 20 volumes of 0.9% sodium chloride injection and inject at a rate not to exceed 1 mL/min because circulatory collapse or pulmonary edema may occur. Use glass syringe and metal needles because the drug may react with the plastic used in disposable syringes and needles.
5. Store in a tight, light-resistant container, at temperatures not to exceed 25°C (77°F).
6. Should not be used if paraldehyde has a strong vinegar odor or is brownish in color.
7. Paraldehyde should not be used if the container has been opened for more than 24 hr.
8. *Treatment of Overdose:* See *Hypnotics,* Chapter 39.

Contraindications: Gastroenteritis, bronchopulmonary disease, hepatic insufficiency. Use with caution during labor and during lactation.

Special Concerns: Use during labor may lead to respiratory depression in the neonate.

Laboratory Test Interferences: 17-Hydroxycorticosteroids; 17-ketogenic steroids.

Side Effects: *Dermatologic:* Skin rash, redness, swelling or pain at injection site; nerve damage (may be severe and permanent), especially of the sciatic nerve if drug injected too close to nerve. *Respiratory:* Rarely, difficulty in breathing, SOB. *Miscellaneous:* Bradycardia, strong odor to breath up to 24 hr following use. *Following IV use:* Coughing; ***right heart edema, dilation and failure; massive pulmonary hemorrhage.*** *Following prolonged use:* Dependence, similar to alcoholism leading to withdrawal syndrome including hallucinations and delirium tremens. Also, prolonged use may result in hepatitis.

Symptoms of Overdose: See *Hypnotics,* Chapter 39.

Drug Interactions

Disulfiram / Combination may produce an Antabuse-like reaction
Sulfonamides / ↑ Chance of sulfonamide crystalluria

NURSING CONSIDERATIONS

See also *Nursing Considerations* for *Chloral Hydrate,* Chapter 39.

Assessment

1. Determine indications for therapy and list other agents prescribed and the outcome.
2. Document baseline neurological assessment and mental status.
3. Obtain baseline CXR and liver and renal function studies and monitor periodically.

Interventions

1. Ensure that the room is well ventilated so as to remove exhaled paraldehyde.
2. Offer reassurance if the client is disturbed by the odor of the drug.
3. Assess for evidence of dependency and toxicity. Do not withdraw the drug abruptly.
4. Report any evidence of coughing during IV administration. This symptom can indicate deleterious effects on pulmonary capillaries.
5. Note any evidence of pulmonary edema or respiratory depression, document, and report immediately.
6. Report any excessive sedation, respiratory depression, decrease in BP, or odor of paraldehyde on the breath.
7. Keep on bed rest and supervise ambulation as drug causes drowsiness.

Evaluate

- Desired level of sedation
- Control of symptoms of alcohol withdrawal
- Termination of seizures

BARBITURATES

See also the following individual entries:

Pentobarbital
Pentobarbital Sodium
Phenobarbital - see Chapter 36
Phenobarbital Sodium - see Chapter 36
Secobarbital Sodium

Action/Kinetics: Barbiturates produce all levels of CNS depression, ranging from mild depression (sedation) following low doses to hypnotic (sleep-inducing) effects, and even coma and death, as dosage is increased. Certain barbiturates are also effective anticonvulsants. The depressant and anticonvulsant effects may be related to their ability to increase and/or mimic the inhibitory activity of the neurotransmitter GABA on nerve synapses. For example, the sedative-hypnotic effects of barbiturates may be due to an effect in the thalamus to inhibit ascending conduction in the reticular activating system, thus interfering with the transmission of impulses to the cerebral cortex. Barbiturates decrease the amount of time spent in REM sleep (dreaming stage). The anticonvulsant effects are believed to result from depression of monosynaptic and polysynaptic impulses in the CNS; barbiturates may also increase the threshold for electrical stimulation in the motor cortex. Toxic doses depress the activity of tissues in addition to the CNS, including the CV system. In some clients, barbiturates manifest an unusual action, including an excitatory response. Importantly, barbiturates are not analgesics and therefore should not be given to clients for the purpose of ameliorating pain.

The barbiturates, especially their sodium salts, are readily absorbed after PO, rectal, or parenteral administration. They are distributed throughout all tissues, cross the placental barrier, and appear in breast milk. The main difference between the various barbiturates is in the onset of action. *Ultrashort-acting:* **Onset: IV,** immediate; **duration:** up to 30 min. *Short-acting:* **Onset: PO,** 10–15 min; **peak effect:** 3–4 hr. *Intermediate-acting:* **Onset: PO,** 45–60 min; **peak effect:** 6–8 hr. *Long-acting:* **Onset: PO,** 60 or more min; **peak effect:** 10–12 hr. **Rectal administration:** Onset times are similar to PO. **IV administration:** From immediate for short-acting drugs up to 5 min for long-acting drugs. **Duration of sedation:** 3–6 hr after **IV;** 6–8 hr, for all other routes. *NOTE:* It is currently believed that there is little difference in the duration of hypnosis after the use of any barbiturate; however, there is a difference in the time of onset. Thus, although widely used, the classification by duration of action may be outdated. Barbiturates are bound to both plasma and tissue proteins; the higher the lipid solubility, the greater the extent of protein binding. Barbiturates are metabolized almost completely in the liver (except for barbital and phenobarbital) and are excreted in the urine.

Uses: Preanesthetic medication. Thiobarbiturates are used for induction of anesthesia, to supplement other anesthetics, and as IV anesthetics for short surgical procedures with minimal painful stimuli. Sedation, hypnotic, anticonvulsant (phenobarbital, mephobarbital) and for the control of acute convulsive conditions (only phenobarbital, mephobarbital), as in epilepsy, tetanus, meningitis, eclampsia, and toxic reactions to local anesthetics or strychnine. The benzodiazepines have replaced barbiturates for the treatment of many conditions, especially daytime sedation. See also information on individual drugs.

Contraindications: Hypersensitivity to barbiturates, severe trauma, pulmonary disease when dyspnea or obstruction is present, edema, uncontrolled diabetes, history of porphyria, and impaired liver function and for clients in whom they produce an excitatory response. Also, clients who have been addicted previously to sedative-hypnotics. Thiobarbiturates should not be used in severe CV disease, hypotension or shock, increased intracranial pressure, asthma, myasthenia gravis, and conditions in which hypnotic effects may be prolonged or potentiated (e.g., Addison's disease, liver or kidney dysfunction, myxedema, excessive premedication, increased blood urea, and severe anemia).

Special Concerns: Use with caution during lactation and in clients with CNS depression, hypotension, marked asthenia (characteristic of Addison's disease, hypoadrenalism, and severe myxedema), porphyria, fever, anemia, hemorrhagic shock, cardiac, hepatic or renal damage, and a history of alcoholism in suicidal clients. Geriatric clients usually manifest increased sensitivity to barbiturates, as evidenced by confusion, excitement, mental depression, and hypothermia. When given in the presence of pain, restlessness, excitement, and delirium may result. Intra-arterial use may cause symptoms from transient pain to gangrene; SC use produces tissue irritation, including tenderness and redness to necrosis.

Side Effects: *CNS:* Sleepiness, drowsiness, agitation, confusion, hyperkinesia, ataxia, CNS depression, nightmares, nervousness, psychiatric disturbances, hallucinations, insomnia, anxiety, dizziness, headache, abnormal thinking, vertigo, lethargy, hangover, excitement, appearance of being inebriated. Irritability and hyperactivity in children. *Musculoskeletal:* Localized or diffuse myalgic, neuralgic, or arthritic pain, especially in psychoneurotic clients. Pain is often most intense in the morning and is frequently located in the neck, shoulder girdle, and arms. *Respiratory:* Hypoventilation, ***apnea, respiratory depression.*** *CV:* Bradycardia, hypotension, syncope, ***circulatory collapse.*** *GI:* N&V, constipation, liver damage (especially with chronic use of phenobarbital). *Allergic:* Skin rashes, ***angioedema,*** exfoliative dermatitis (including ***Stevens-Johnson syndrome and toxic epidermal necrolysis***). Allergic reactions are most common in clients who have asthma, urticaria, angioedema, and similar conditions. Symptoms include localized swelling (especially of the lips, cheeks, or eyelids) and erythematous dermatitis).

After SC use: Tissue necrosis, pain, tenderness, redness, permanent neurologic damage if injected near peripheral nerves.

After IV use. CV: Circulatory depression, thrombophlebitis, ***peripher-***

al vascular collapse, seizures with cardiorespiratory arrest, myocardial depression, cardiac arrhythymias. *Respiratory:* ***Apnea, laryngospasm, bronchospasm,*** dyspnea, rhinitis, sneezing, coughing. *CNS:* Emergence delirium, headache, anxiety, prolonged somnolence and recovery, restlessness, ***seizures.*** *GI:* N&V, abdominal pain, diarrhea, cramping. *Hypersensitivity:* ***Acute allergic reactions, including erythema, pruritus, anaphylaxis.*** *Miscellaneous:* Pain or nerve injury at injection site, salivation, hiccups, skin rashes, shivering, skeletal muscle hyperactivity, ***immune hemolytic anemia with renal failure***, and radial nerve palsy.

After IM use: Pain at injection site.

Barbiturates can induce physical and psychologic dependence if high doses are used regularly for long periods of time. Withdrawal symptoms usually begin after 12–16 hr of abstinence. Manifestations of withdrawal include anxiety, weakness, N&V, muscle cramps, delirium, and even ***tonic-clonic seizures.***

Symptoms of Acute Toxicity: Characterized by cortical and ***respiratory depression; anoxia; peripheral vascular collapse;*** feeble, rapid pulse; pulmonary edema; decreased body temperature; clammy, cyanotic skin; depressed reflexes; stupor; and ***coma.*** After initial constriction the pupils become dilated. ***Death results from respiratory failure or arrest followed by cardiac arrest.***

Symptoms of Chronic Toxicity: Prolonged use of barbiturates at high doses may lead to physical and psychologic dependence, as well as tolerance. Doses of 600–800 mg daily for 8 weeks may lead to physical dependence. The addict usually ingests 1.5 g/day. Addicts prefer short-acting barbiturates. Symptoms of dependence are similar to those associated with chronic alcoholism, and withdrawal symptoms are equally severe. Withdrawal symptoms usually last for 5–10 days and are terminated by a long sleep.

Drug Interactions

GENERAL CONSIDERATIONS

1. Barbiturates stimulate the activity of enzymes responsible for the metabolism of a large number of other drugs by a process known as *enzyme induction*. As a result, when barbiturates are given to clients receiving such drugs, their therapeutic effectiveness is markedly reduced or even abolished.
2. The CNS depressant effect of the barbiturates is potentiated by many drugs. Concomitant administration may result in coma or fatal CNS depression. Barbiturate dosage should either be reduced or eliminated when other CNS drugs are given.
3. Barbiturates also potentiate the toxic effects of many other agents.

Acetaminophen / ↑ Risk of hepatotoxicity when used with large or chronic doses of barbiturates
Alcohol / Potentiation or addition of CNS depressant effects. Concomitant use may lead to drowsiness, lethargy, stupor, respiratory collapse, coma, or death
Anesthetics, general / See *Alcohol*
Anorexiants / ↓ Effect of anorexiants due to opposite activities
Antianxiety drugs / See *Alcohol*
Anticoagulants, oral / ↓ Effect of anticoagulants due to ↓ absorption from GI tract and ↑ breakdown by liver
Antidepressants, tricyclic / ↓ Effect of antidepressants due to ↑ breakdown by liver
Antidiabetic agents / Prolong the effects of barbiturates
Antihistamines / See *Alcohol*
Beta-adrenergic agents / ↓ Beta blockade due to ↑ breakdown by the liver
Carbamazepine / ↓ Serum carbazepine levels may occur
Charcoal / ↓ Absorption of barbiturates from the GI tract
Chloramphenicol / ↑ Effect of barbiturates by ↓ breakdown by the liver and ↓ effect of chloramphenicol by ↑ breakdown by liver

Clonazepam / Barbiturates may ↑ excretion of clonazepam → loss of efficacy
CNS depressants / See *Alcohol*
Corticosteroids / ↓ Effect of corticosteroids due to ↑ breakdown by liver
Digitoxin / ↓ Effect of digitoxin due to ↑ breakdown by liver
Doxorubicin / ↓ Effect of doxorubicin due to ↑ excretion
Doxycycline / ↓ Effect of doxycycline due to ↑ breakdown by liver (effect may last up to 2 weeks after barbiturates are discontinued)
Estrogens / ↓ Effect of estrogen due to ↑ breakdown by liver
Felodipine / ↓ Plasma levels of felodipine → ↓ effect
Fenoprofen / ↓ Bioavailability of fenoprofen
Furosemide / ↑ Risk or intensity of orthostatic hypotension
Griseofulvin / ↓ Effect of griseofulvin due to ↓ absorption from GI tract
Haloperidol / ↓ Effect of haloperidol due to ↑ breakdown by liver
MAO inhibitors / ↑ Effect of barbiturates due to ↓ breakdown by liver
Meperidine / CNS depressant effects may be prolonged
Methadone / ↓ Effect of methadone
Methoxyflurane / ↑ Kidney toxicity due to ↑ breakdown of methoxyflurane by liver to toxic metabolites
Metronidazole / ↓ Effect of metronidazole
Narcotic analgesics / See *Alcohol*
Oral contraceptives / ↓ Effect of contraceptives due to ↑ breakdown by liver
Phenothiazines / ↓ Effect of phenothiazines due to ↑ breakdown by liver; also see *Alcohol*
Phenylbutazone / ↓ Elimination t½ of phenylbutazone
Phenytoin / Effect variable and unpredictable; monitor carefully
Probenecid / Anesthesia with thiobarbiturates may be ↑ or achieved at lower doses
Procarbazine / ↑ Effect of barbiturates
Quinidine / ↓ Effect of quinidine due to ↑ breakdown by liver
Rifampin / ↓ Effect of barbiturates due to ↑ breakdown by liver
Sedative-hypnotics, nonbarbiturate / See *Alcohol*
Sulfisoxazole / Sulfisoxazole may ↑the anesthetic effects of thiobarbiturates
Theophyllines / ↓ Effect of theophyllines due to ↑ breakdown by liver
Valproic acid / ↑ Effect of barbiturates due to ↓ breakdown by liver
Verapamil / ↑ Excretion of verapamil → ↓ effect
Vitamin D / Barbiturates may ↑ requirements for vitamin D due to ↑ breakdown by the liver

Laboratory Test Interferences

1. **Interference with test method:** ↑ 17-Hydroxycorticosteroids.
2. **Caused by pharmacologic effects:** ↑ Creatinine phosphokinase, alkaline phosphatase, serum transaminase, serum testosterone (in certain women), urinary estriol, porphobilinogen, coproporphyrin, uroporphyrin. ↓ PT in clients on coumarin. ↑ or ↓ Bilirubin. False + lupus erythematosus test.

Dosage

See individual drugs. Aim for minimum effective dosage. As hypnotics, barbiturates should be administered intermittently because tolerance develops. Elderly clients should receive one-half of the adult dose, and children should receive one-quarter to one-half the adult dose.

NURSING CONSIDERATIONS

Administration/Storage

1. When used as hypnotics, barbiturates should not be given for more than 14–28 days.
2. Aqueous solutions of sodium salts are unstable and must be used within 30 min after preparation.
3. Discard parenteral solutions that contain precipitate.
4. During IV administration:

• Closely monitor the IV administration for the correct rate of flow. A too rapid injection may produce respiratory depression, dyspnea, and shock.

• Monitor the site of the IV injection closely for extravasation, which may cause pain, nerve damage, and necrosis.

• Note any redness or swelling along the site of the vein. This is evidence of thrombophlebitis.

5. Maintain an accurate record of the barbiturates on hand and the amounts dispensed following appropriate institutional and Drug Enforcement Agency guidelines.

6. *Treatment of Acute Toxicity:*

• Maintenance of an adequate airway, oxygen intake, and carbon dioxide removal are essential.

• After PO ingestion, gastric lavage or gastric aspiration may delay absorption. Emesis should not be induced once the symptoms of overdosage are manifested, as the client may aspirate the vomitus into the lungs. Also, if the dose of barbiturate is high enough, the vomiting center in the brain may be depressed.

• Absorption following SC or IM administration of the drug may be delayed by the use of ice packs or tourniquets.

• Maintain renal function.

• Removal of the drug by peritoneal dialysis or an artificial kidney should be carried out.

• Supportive physiologic methods have proven superior to use of analeptics.

7. *Treatment of Chronic Toxicity:* Cautious withdrawal of the hospitalized addict over a 2–4-week period. A stabilizing dose of 200–300 mg of a short-acting barbiturate is administered q 6 hr. The dose is then reduced by 100 mg/day until the stabilizing dose is reduced by one-half. The client is then maintained on this dose for 2–3 days before further reduction. The same procedure is repeated when the initial stabilizing dose has been reduced by three-quarters. If a mixed spike and slow activity appear on the EEG, or if insomnia, anxiety, tremor, or weakness is observed, the dosage is maintained at a constant level or increased slightly until symptoms disappear.

Assessment

1. Note any history of adverse side effects to any of the barbiturate family of drugs.

2. Identify indications for therapy, associated symptoms, and anticipated time frame for administration.

3. When used for sleep disorders, discuss sleeping patterns with the client and family. This information is important in the decision concerning the type of barbiturate to prescribe.

• Determine the client's usual bedtime and the usual wakening hours

• Determine the cause of the client's inability to sleep. A person in pain who gains relief of the pain may not need sleeping medication. Note evidence of fear and anxiety that may interfere with sleep.

• Assess the client's environmental preferences for sleep, such as room temperature, lights, and sounds.

• Note presence of sensory alterations that could cause sleeplessness or disruptions in sleep time.

4. If the client is of childbearing age determine if pregnancy is likely. Other measures should be found to encourage sleep if pregnancy is a probability.

5. Document any evidence or history of previous dependence on any sedative-hypnotics.

6. Assess for any physical conditions that may preclude drug therapy.

Interventions

1. Prior to administering the drug, discuss the goals of the medication therapy with the client.

2. Review the treatment for chronic and acute toxicity associated with barbiturates.

3. Do not awaken a client to administer a sleeping medication.

4. Assist the client during ambulation and use side rails once the client is in bed. Clients who receive hypnotic medications may become confused and unsteady. This is a particular problem among the elderly and

"at risk for fall" should be prominently posted.

5. Use supportive measures such as a back rub, warm drinks, a quiet atmosphere and a calm attitude to encourage relaxation.

6. When the drug is administered PO, remain with the client to determine that the drug has been swallowed. If the client is disoriented and/or wearing dentures, check the buccal cavity, under the tongue, and under denture plates. Routinely check the bedside area to ensure that the client is not hoarding medication.

7. Anticipate that some clients may experience a period of transitory elation, confusion, or euphoria before sedation, and provide appropriate nursing measures to calm the client and prevent injury.

8. If clients become confused after taking the barbiturate, do not apply cuffs or other restraints. Remain with them and try to soothe and orient them by turning on a light and talking quietly and calmly until they are relaxed.

9. If the client asks for a second sleeping medication during the night, try to determine the cause of the sleeplessness. Institute comfort measures. If the client has pain, relieve the pain first. Wait approximately 20–30 min and then give the second dose of sleeping medication if the client has not yet fallen asleep.

10. Keep a careful check of the length of time the client has been receiving barbiturates. Therapy that requires sedative doses of medication over an 8-week period of time will cause physical dependence. Remind the medical staff of the amount of time the client has been taking the medication. If the client is not responding as anticipated, review the need to alter the dose and explore other related factors, such as the environment, the existence of psychologic stress, or possibly drug dependence.

11. Assess the client for evidence of physical and/or psychologic dependence and tolerance. Document any changes in the VS and condition of the client's skin and report.

12. Be alert to S&S of porphyria, a metabolic disorder characterized by N&V, abdominal pain, and muscle spasms. Document and report, anticipating that the drug will be discontinued.

13. If the client receiving barbiturates is a child, supervise the child's play activity, especially if child is riding a bicycle or engaging in other potentially dangerous forms of play.

14. At each visit, review the goals of therapy with the client and the effectiveness of the medication regimen. Investigate any problems noted by the client. When clients are receiving barbiturates on an outpatient basis, be alert to the number of times they return for prescription refills. Frequency of refills may indicate the client has developed a dependency or that the client may be selling the drug for profit.

15. Monitor the client's CBC, differential, and platelet count. Some clients may develop hematologic disorders such as agranulocytosis, megaloblastic anemia, and/or thrombocytopenia.

16. If the barbiturate is administered IV to counteract acute convulsions or for anesthesia anticipate that the therapy will be of limited duration.

Client/Family Teaching

1. Avoid the use of alcoholic beverages. These potentiate the effects of barbiturates.

2. Do not drive a car or operate other hazardous machinery after taking the medication.

3. Take the medication only as prescribed.

4. Avoid the use of all OTC drugs or any other medications unless prescribed.

5. If the client is taking barbiturates for insomnia, suggest that the drug be taken a half hour before bedtime.

6. To avoid an accidental overdose, keep the medication in a medicine closet or in a drawer *away from* the bedside.

7. Keep all medications out of the reach of children. Large doses may be fatal and the potential for abuse exists.
8. If taking a barbiturate for 8 or more weeks, client should not discontinue the drug suddenly without supervision. To do so may result in withdrawal symptoms such as weakness, anxiety, delirium, and tonic-clonic seizures.
9. Dosages of drug should not be reduced without first checking with the provider.
10. Report immediately any signs of hematologic toxicity such as signs of infection (sore throat or fever) or increased bleeding tendencies (nosebleeds or easy bruising).
11. Assist client to identify factors contributing to insomnia. Identify alternative methods to promote relaxation and sleep (such as progressive muscle relaxation, guided imagery, white noise simulator, or soft music); support the client in exploring these methods.
12. Explain the importance of daily exercise in promoting rest and assist the client to identify a program and establish a daily routine such as with daily walks in the development or mall.
13. Advise that intake of caffeine should be very minimal, if at all, and avoided after midafternoon.
14. Establish a regular routine for bedtime and discourage any dozing during the afternoon or early evening hours.
15. Advise client to take any prescribed analgesics for adequate relief of pain and to provide sufficient time to unwind from a busy or overstimulating day, before attempting to sleep.
16. Explain that with continous use of these drugs a decrease in responsiveness to the drug (tolerance) may develop. Abuse and physical dependence with these drugs limit their usefulness in long-term therapy.

Evaluate

- Reports of ↓ muscle spasms, ↓ tremulousness, and ↓ level of anxiety in preparation for anesthesia
- Evidence of effective sedation
- Reports of improved sleeping patterns with less frequent awakenings
- Evidence of effective control of seizures

Pentobarbital

(pen-toe-**BAR**-bih-tal)
Pregnancy Category: D
Nembutal **(C-II) (Rx)**

Pentobarbital sodium

(pen-toe-**BAR**-bih-tal)
Pregnancy Category: D
Nembutal Sodium, Nova-Rectal ✱
(C-II) (Rx)

See also *Hypnotics*, Chapter 39.

How Supplied: Pentobarbital: *Elixir:* 18.2 mg/5 mL.
Pentobarbital sodium: *Capsule:* 50 mg, 100 mg; *Injection:* 50 mg/mL; *Suppository:* 30 mg, 60 mg, 120 mg, 200 mg

Action/Kinetics: Short-acting. t½: 19–34 hr. Is 60%–70% protein bound.

Uses: PO: Sedative. Short-term treatment of insomnia (no more than 2 weeks). Preanesthetic. **Rectal:** Sedation, short-term treatment of insomnia (no more than 2 weeks). **Parenteral:** Short-term treatment of insomnia (no more than 2 weeks). Preanesthetic. Anticonvulsant in anesthetic doses for emergency treatment of acute convulsive states (e.g., status epilepticus, eclampsia, meningitis, tetanus, and toxic reactions to strychnine or local anesthetics). *Investigational:* Parenterally to induce coma to protect the brain from ischemia and increased ICP following stroke and head trauma.

Dosage

- **Capsules**

Sedation.

Adults: 20 mg t.i.d.–q.i.d. **Pediatric:** 2–6 mg/kg/day, depending on age, weight, and degree of sedation desired.

Preoperative sedation.
Adults: 100 mg. **Pediatric:** 2–6 mg/kg/day (maximum of 100 mg), depending on age, weight, and degree of sedation desired.
Hypnotic.
Adults: 100 mg at bedtime.
• **Suppositories, Rectal**
Hypnotic.
Adults: 120–200 mg at bedtime; **infants, 2–12 months (4.5–9 kg):** 30 mg; **1–4 years (9–18.2 kg):** 30 or 60 mg; **5–12 years (18.2–36.4 kg):** 60 mg; **12–14 years (36.4–50 kg):** 60 or 120 mg.
• **IM**
Hypnotic/preoperative sedation.
Adults: 150–200 mg; **pediatric:** 2–6 mg/kg (not to exceed 100 mg).
Anticonvulsant.
Pediatric, initially: 50 mg; **then,** after 1 min, additional small doses may be given, if needed, until the desired effect is achieved.
• **IV**
Sedative/hypnotic.
Adults: 100 mg followed in 1 min by additional small doses, if required, up to a total of 500 mg.
Anticonvulsant.
Adults, initial: 100 mg; **then,** after 1 min, additional small doses may be given, if needed, up to a total of 500 mg. **Pediatric, initially:** 50 mg; **then,** after 1 min, additional small doses may be given, if needed, until the desired effect is achieved.

Administration/Storage

1. The IV dose is given in fractions because pentobarbital is a potent CNS depressant that may cause adverse respiratory and circulatory responses. Adults generally receive 100 mg initially; children and debilitated clients, 50 mg. Subsequent fractions are administered after 1-min observation periods. Overdose or too rapid administration may cause spasms of the larynx or pharynx, or both.
2. The rate of IV injection should not exceed 50 mg/min.
3. Pentobarbital solutions are highly alkaline.
4. If the medication is administered IV, assess site for patency. Note client complaint of pain at the site of injection or in the limb and interrupt the injection, and report.
5. The parenteral product is not for SC use.
6. Parental pentobarbital is incompatible with most other drugs; therefore, do not mix other drugs in the same syringe.
7. Administer no more than 5 mL at one site **IM** because of possible tissue irritation (pain, necrosis, gangrene).
8. Suppositories are not to be divided.
9. The parenteral solution should not be used if it is discolored or contains a precipitate.

Special Concerns: Dosage should be reduced in geriatric and debilitated clients and in those with impaired hepatic or renal function.

NURSING CONSIDERATIONS

See also *Nursing Considerations* for *Hypnotics,* Chapter 39.

Assessment

1. Document indications for therapy, onset and type of symptoms, source (if known), and any other agents prescribed.
2. Assist client to identify type and any causative factors R/T insomnia. Review sleep patterns.
3. Obtain baseline liver and renal function studies and anticipate reduced dosage with impairment as well as with the debilitated and elderly.

Interventions

1. Observe for signs of respiratory depression. This is usually the first sign of drug overdose.
2. During treatment of cerebral edema (barbiturate coma), monitor and document ICP readings, and neurologic status.
3. Initiate appropriate safety measures once the medication has been administered. This is particularly important when working with confused or elderly clients.
4. Administer analgesics as needed since sedatives and hypnotics do not control pain.

Client/Family Teaching
1. Caution that drug may cause drowsiness and morning-after "hangover."
2. Avoid alcohol or any other CNS depressants.
3. Emphasize with insomnia that drug is for short-term use only; with long-term use one can experience rebound insomnia.

Evaluate
- Improved sleeping patterns with less frequent awakenings
- Desired level of sedation
- Control of seizures and acute convulsive states

Secobarbital sodium

(see-koh-**BAR**-bih-tal)
Pregnancy Category: D
Seconal Sodium **(C-II) (Rx)**

See also *Hypnotics,* Chapter 39.
How Supplied: *Capsule:* 100 mg; *Injection:* 50 mg/mL
Action/Kinetics: Short-acting. Distributed quickly as it has the highest lipid solubility of the barbiturates. **Onset:** 10–15 min. **t½:** 15–40 hr. **Duration:** 3–4 hr. Is 46%–70% protein bound.
Uses: Parenteral: Intermittent use as a sedative, hypnotic, or preanesthetic.

Dosage
- **IM, IV**

Hypnotic.
Adults: 100–200 mg IM or 50–250 mg IV.

Preoperative sedative.
Adults: 1 mg/kg IM 10–15 min before procedure. **Children:** 4–5 mg/kg IM.

Dentistry in clients who will receive nerve block.
100–150 mg IV.

Status epilepticus.
Children: 15–20 mg/kg IV over 10–15 min.

Administration/Storage
1. For adults, the aqueous parenteral solution is preferred to polyethylene glycol, which may be irritating to the kidneys, especially in clients with signs of renal insufficiency.
2. Aqueous solutions for injection should be freshly prepared from dry-packed ampules.
3. Rapid IV administration may precipitate hypotension, respiratory depression, laryngospasm or apnea; do not exceed recommended rate (50 mg/15 sec).
4. Parenteral form may damage or necrose tissue if infiltrated due to high solution alkalinity.
5. Following prolonged use, taper dosage and withdraw drug slowly to prevent precipitating withdrawal symptoms.
6. Refrigerate the parenteral solution and protect from light. The solution should not be used if it contains a precipitate.
7. Dosage should be reduced in clients with impaired hepatic or renal function.

Special Concerns: Elderly or debilitated clients may be more sensitive to the drug and require reduced dosage.

NURSING CONSIDERATIONS

See also *Nursing Considerations* for *Hypnotics,* Chapter 39.

Client/Family Teaching
1. Do not perform activities that require mental alertness until drug effects realized.
2. Avoid alcohol and any other CNS depressants without approval.
3. Take analgesics as prescribed as drug does not control pain.
4. Drug may cause dependency. Review alternative methods that assist with sleeping, such as relaxation techniques, daily exercise, stress reduction, no caffeine, and/or white noise simulator.

Evaluate
- Improved sleeping patterns with less frequent awakenings
- Effective sedation

Triazolam

(try-**AYZ**-oh-lam)

Pregnancy Category: X
Apo-Triazo ✱, Gen-Triazolam ✱, Halcion, Novo-Triolam ✱, Nu-Triazo ✱
(C-IV) (Rx)

See also *Anti-Anxiety/Antimanic Drugs,* Chapter 40.
How Supplied: *Tablet:* 0.125 mg, 0.25 mg
Action/Kinetics: Triazolam decreases sleep latency, increases the duration of sleep, and decreases the number of awakenings. **Time to peak plasma levels:** 0.5–2 hr. **t½:** 1.5–5.5 hr. Metabolized in liver and inactive metabolites excreted in the urine.
Uses: Insomnia (short-term management, not to exceed 1 month). May be beneficial in preventing or treating transient insomnia from a sudden change in sleep schedule.

Dosage

- **Tablets**

Adults, initial: 0.25–0.5 mg before bedtime. **Geriatric or debilitated clients, initial:** 0.125 mg; **then,** depending on response, 0.125–0.25 mg before bedtime.
Special Concerns: Safety and efficacy in children under 18 years of age not established. Use during lactation may cause sedation and feeding problems in the infant. Geriatric clients may be more sensitive to the effects of triazolam.
Side Effects: *CNS:* Rebound insomnia, anterograde amnesia, headache, ataxia, decreased coordination. Psychologic and physical dependence. *GI:* N&V.

NURSING CONSIDERATIONS

See also *Nursing Considerations* for *Anti-Anxiety/Antimanic Drugs,* Chapter 40.

Interventions

1. Assess client for tolerance and for psychologic and physical dependence.
2. When client suffers from simple insomnia, try warm baths, warm milk, and other interventions to induce sleep, such as soft music, guided imagery, or progressive muscle relaxation.
3. Evaluate and document sleep patterns. Attempt to determine underlying cause of insomnia so that source may be removed.
4. Initiate safety precautions (i.e., side rails up, supervised ambulation, frequent observations) at bedtime, especially with elderly clients and confused clients.
5. Monitor closely for CNS toxic effects especially during prolonged therapy (longer than 2 weeks).

Client/Family Teaching

1. Avoid the use of alcoholic beverages and other CNS depressants.
2. Use caution when driving or operating machinery until daytime sedative effects have been evaluated.
3. Advise that drug is for short-term use only, as it may cause physical and psychologic dependence. Try warm baths, warm milk, and other methods to induce sleep, such as white noise simulator, guided imagery, or progressive muscle relaxation rather than become dependent on drugs for insomnia.
4. Report immediately any unusual side effects including hallucinations, nightmares, depression, or periods of confusion.

Evaluate: Improved sleeping patterns with relief from insomnia.

Zolpidem tartrate

(**ZOL**-pih-dem)
Pregnancy Category: B
Ambien **(C-IV) (Rx)**

How Supplied: *Tablet:* 5 mg, 10 mg
Action/Kinetics: The drug is believed to act by subunit modulation of the GABA receptor chloride channel macromolecular complex resulting in sedative, anticonvulsant, anxiolytic, and myorelaxant properties. Although zolpidem's chemical structure is unrelated to the benzodiazepines or barbiturates, it interacts with a GABA-benzodiazepine receptor complex and shares some of the pharmacologic effects of the benzodiazepines. Specifically, zolpidem binds the omega-1 receptor prefe-

rentially. There is no evidence of residual next-day effects or rebound insomnia at recommended doses; there is little evidence for memory impairment. Sleep time spent in stage 3 to 4 (deep sleep) was comparable to placebo with only inconsistent, minor changes in REM sleep at recommended doses. The drug is rapidly absorbed from the GI tract. **t½:** About 2.5 hr (increased in geriatric clients and those with impaired hepatic function). The drug is bound significantly (92.5%) to plasma proteins. Food decreases the bioavailability of zolpidem. The drug is metabolized in the liver and inactive metabolites are excreted primarily through the urine.

Use: Short-term treatment of insomnia.

Dosage

- **Tablets**

Hypnotic.

Adults, individualized, usual: 10 mg just before bedtime. An initial dose of 5 mg is recommended in clients with hepatic insufficiency.

Administration/Storage

1. Therapy should be limited to 7–10 days. Clients should be reevaluated if the drug is required for more than 2–3 weeks.
2. The drug should not be prescribed in quantities exceeding a 1-month supply.
3. The total daily dose should not exceed 10 mg.
4. *Treatment of Overdose:* Gastric lavage if appropriate. General symptomatic and supportive measures. IV fluids as needed. Flumazenil may be effective in reversing CNS depression. Monitor hypotension and CNS depression and treat appropriately. Sedative drugs should not be used, even if excitation occurs. Zolpidem is not dialyzable.

Contraindication: Lactation.

Special Concerns: Use with caution and at reduced dosage in clients with impaired hepatic function. Impaired motor or cognitive performance after repeated use or unusual sensitivity to hypnotic drugs may be noted in geriatric or debilitated clients. Use with caution in clients with compromised respiratory function, in those with impaired renal function, and in clients with S&S of depression. Closely observe individuals with a history of dependence on or abuse of drugs or alcohol. Safety and efficacy have not been determined in children less than 18 years of age.

Laboratory Test Interferences: ↑ ALT, AST, BUN. Hyperglycemia, hypercholesterolemia, hyperlipidemia, abnormal hepatic function.

Side Effects: *Symptoms of withdrawal:* Although there is no clear evidence of a withdrawal syndrome, the following symptoms were noted with zolpidem following placebo substitution. Fatigue, nausea, flushing, lightheadedness, uncontrolled crying, emesis, stomach cramps, panic attack, nervousness, abdominal discomfort.

The most common side effects following use for up to 10 nights included drowsiness, dizziness, and diarrhea. The side effects listed below are for an incidence of 1% or greater. *CNS:* Headache, drowsiness, dizziness, lethargy, drugged feeling, lightheadedness, depression, abnormal dreams, amnesia, anxiety, nervousness, sleep disorder, ataxia, confusion, euphoria, insomnia, vertigo. *GI:* Nausea, diarrhea, dyspepsia, abdominal pain, constipation, anorexia, vomiting. *Musculoskeletal:* Myalgia, arthralgia. *Respiratory:* Upper respiratory infection, sinusitis, pharyngitis, rhinitis. *Body as a whole:* Allergy, back pain, flu-like symptoms, chest pain, fatigue. *Ophthalmologic:* Diplopia, abnormal vision. *Miscellaneous:* Rash, UTI, palpitations, dry mouth, infection.

Symptoms of Overdose: Symptoms ranging from somnolence to light coma. Rarely, CV and respiratory compromise.

Drug Interaction: Additive CNS depressant effects are possible when combined with alcohol and other drugs with CNS depressant effects.

NURSING CONSIDERATIONS

Assessment

1. Document indications for therapy and onset of symptoms; assist client to identify any causative factors.
2. Note any history or evidence of respiratory dysfunction.
3. Determine any drug or alcohol dependence and assess for symptoms of depression.
4. Obtain baseline liver function studies.
5. Review sleep patterns and life style. Assist client to identify underlying cause(s) of insomnia.

Client/Family Teaching

1. Take only as directed, on an empty stomach at bedtime.
2. Do not perform any activities that require mental or physical alertness after ingesting medication. Evaluate response the following day to ensure that no residual depressant effects are evident.
3. Avoid alcohol and any unprescribed or OTC drugs.
4. Explain that the drug is only for short-term use and assist the client in identifying factors that may be contributing to the insomnia.
5. Review alternative methods for inducing sleep such as relaxation techniques, daily exercise, soft music, no daytime napping, white noise or special effects simulator, etc.
6. Clients with symptoms of depression are at a higher risk for suicide or intentional overdose. Advise family that these clients warrant closer observation and limited prescriptions. Report any evidence of suicidal thoughts or aggressive behavior.
7. Keep out of reach of children and store in a safe place as drug has a high potential for abuse.

Evaluate: Improved sleeping patterns with less frequent awakenings.

CHAPTER FORTY

Anti-Anxiety/ Antimanic Drugs

See also the following individual entries:

Alprazolam
Buspirone Hydrochloride
Chlordiazepoxide
Clorazepate Dipotassium
Diazepam
Halazepam
Hydroxyzine Hydrochloride
Hydroxyzine Pamoate
Lithium Carbonate
Lithium Citrate
Lorazepam
Meprobamate
Midazolam Hydrochloride
Oxazepam
Quazepam
Temazepam
Triazolam

General Statement: The tranquilizers exhibit a wide margin of safety between therapeutic and toxic doses. For example, ataxia and sedation are observed at doses higher than those required to achieve antianxiety effects. The major difference among benzodiazepines and other tranquilizers appears to be a function of duration of action and other pharmacokinetic properties. All antianxiety agents have the ability to cause psychologic and physical dependence. Withdrawal symptoms usually start within 12–48 hr after stopping the drug and last for 12–48 hr. When the client has received large doses of these drugs for weeks or months, dosage should be reduced gradually over a period of 1–2 weeks. Alternatively, a short-acting barbiturate may be substituted and then withdrawn gradually. Abrupt withdrawal of high dosage of the drug may be accompanied by coma, convulsions, and even death.

Action/Kinetics: The major antianxiety agents include the benzodiazepines and meprobamate. The benzodiazepines are thought to affect the limbic system and reticular formation to reduce anxiety. This effect is believed to be mediated through the action of the benzodiazepines to increase or facilitate the inhibitory neurotransmitter activity of GABA, which is one of the inhibitory CNS neurotransmitters. Two benzodiazepine receptor subtypes have been identified in the brain–BZ_1 and BZ_2. Receptor subtype BZ_1 is believed to be associated with sleep mechanisms, whereas receptor subtype BZ_2 is associated with memory, motor, sensory, and cognitive function. When used for 3–4 weeks for sleep, certain benzodiazepines may cause REM rebound when discontinued. Meprobamate and the benzodiazepines also possess varying degrees of anticonvulsant activity, skeletal muscle relaxation, and the ability to alleviate tension. The rate of absorption from the GI tract will determine the onset and intensity of action of the various benzodiazepines. The benzodiazepines generally have long half-lives (1–8 days); thus cumulative effects can occur. Also, several of the benzodiazepines are metabolized to active metabolites in the liver, which prolongs their duration of action. Benzodiazepines are widely distributed throughout the body. Approximately 70%–99% of an administered dose is bound to plasma protein. Metabolites of benzodiazepines are excreted through the kidneys.

Uses: Management of anxiety and tension occurring alone or as a side effect of other conditions, including menopausal syndrome, premenstrual tension, asthma, and angina pectoris. Neurologic conditions involving muscle spasm and tetanus. Insomnia (recurring or due to poor sleeping habits) characterized by difficulty in falling asleep, frequent awakenings during the night, or early morning awakening. Adjunct in treatment of rheumatoid arthritis, osteoarthritis, trauma, low back pain, torticollis, and selected convulsive disorders including status epilepticus. Premedication for surgery or electric cardioversion. Rehabilitation of chronic alcoholics, delirium tremens, nocturnal enuresis in childhood. *Investigational:* Irritable bowel syndrome.

Contraindications: Hypersensitivity, acute narrow-angle glaucoma, psychoses. Use of flurazepam for insomnia in children less than 15 years of age and use of estazolam, quazepam, temazepam, or triazolam for insomnia in children less than 18 years of age.

Special Concerns: Use with caution in impaired hepatic or renal function and in the geriatric or debilitated client. Use during lactation may cause sedation, weight loss, and possibly feeding difficulties in the infant. Geriatric clients may be more sensitive to the effects of benzodiazepines; symptoms may include oversedation, dizziness, confusion, or ataxia. When used for insomnia, rebound sleep disorders may occur following abrupt withdrawal of certain benzodiazepines.

Side Effects: *CNS:* Drowsiness, fatigue, confusion, ataxia, sedation, dizziness, vertigo, depression, apathy, lightheadedness, delirium, headache, lethargy, disorientation, hypoactivity, crying, anterograde amnesia, slurred speech, stupor, ***coma,*** fainting, difficulty in concentration, euphoria, nervousness, irritability, akathisia, hypotonia, vivid dreams, "glassy-eyed," hysteria, ***suicide attempt,*** psychosis. Paradoxical excitement manifested by anxiety, acute hyperexcitability, increased muscle spasticity, insomnia, hallucinations, sleep disturbances, rage, and stimulation. *GI:* Increased appetite, constipation, diarrhea, anorexia, N&V, weight gain or loss, dry mouth, bitter or metallic taste, increased salivation, coated tongue, sore gums, difficulty in swallowing, gastritis, fecal incontinence. *Respiratory:* ***Respiratory depression and sleep apnea,*** especially in clients with compromised respiratory function. *Dermatologic:* Urticaria, rash, pruritus, alopecia, hirsutism, dermatitis, edema of ankles and face. *Endocrine:* Increased or decreased libido, gynecomastia, menstrual irregularities. *GU:* Difficulty in urination, urinary retention, incontinence, dysuria, enuresis. *CV:* Hypertension, hypotension, bradycardia, tachycardia, palpitations, edema, ***CV collapse.*** *Hematologic:* Anemia, ***agranulocytosis,*** leukopenia, eosinophilia, thrombocytopenia. *Ophthalmologic:* Diplopia, conjunctivitis, nystagmus, blurred vision. *Miscellaneous:* Joint pain, lymphadenopathy, muscle cramps, paresthesia, dehydration, lupus-like symptoms, sweating, SOB, flushing, hiccoughs, fever, hepatic dysfunction. *Following IM use:* Redness, pain, burning. *Following IV use:* Thrombosis and phlebitis at site.

Symptoms of Overdose: Severe drowsiness, confusion with reduced or absent reflexes, tremors, slurred speech, staggering, hypotension, SOB, labored breathing, ***respiratory depression,*** impaired coordination, ***seizures,*** weakness, slow HR, ***coma.*** *NOTE:* Geriatric clients, debilitated clients, young children, and clients with liver disease are more sensitive to the CNS effects of benzodiazepines.

Drug Interactions
Alcohol / Potentiation or addition of CNS depressant effects. Concomitant use may lead to drowsiness, lethargy, stupor, respiratory collapse, coma, or death
Anesthetics, general / See *Alcohol*
Antacids / ↓ Rate of absorption of benzodiazepines
Antidepressants, tricyclic / Concomitant use with benzodiazepines may cause additive sedative effect and/or atropine-like side effects
Antihistamines / See *Alcohol*
Barbiturates / See *Alcohol*
Cimetidine / ↑ Effect of benzodiazepines by ↓ breakdown in liver
CNS depressants / See *Alcohol*
Digoxin / Benzodiazepines ↑ effect of digoxin by ↑ serum levels
Disulfiram / ↑ Effect of benzodiazepines by ↓ breakdown in liver
Erythromycin / ↑ Effect of benzodiazepines by ↓ breakdown in liver
Fluoxetine / ↑ Effect of benzodiazepines due to ↓ breakdown in liver
Isoniazid / ↑ Effect of benzodiazepines due to ↓ breakdown in liver
Ketoconazole / ↑ Effect of benzodiazepines due to ↓ breakdown in liver
Levodopa / Effect may be ↓ by benzodiazepines
Metoprolol / ↑ Effect of benzodiazepines due to ↓ breakdown in liver
Narcotics / See *Alcohol*
Neuromuscular blocking agents / Benzodiazepines may ↑, ↓, or have no effect on the action of neuromuscular blocking agents
Oral contraceptives / ↑ Effect of benzodiazepines due to ↓ breakdown in liver; or, ↑ rate of clearance of benzodiazepines that undergo glucuronidation (e.g., lorazepam, oxazepam)
Phenothiazines / See *Alcohol*
Phenytoin / Concomitant use with benzodiazepines may cause ↑ effect of phenytoin due to ↓ breakdown by liver
Probenecid / ↑ Effect of selected benzodiazepines due to ↓ breakdown by liver
Propoxyphene / ↑ Effect of benzodiazepines due to ↓ breakdown by liver
Propranolol / ↑ Effect of benzodiazepines due to ↓ breakdown by liver
Ranitidine / May ↓ absorption of benzodiazepines from the GI tract
Rifampin / ↓ Effect of benzodiazepines due to ↑ breakdown by liver
Sedative-hypnotics, nonbarbiturate / See *Alcohol*
Theophyllines / ↓ Sedative effect of benzodiazepines
Valproic acid / ↑ Effect of benzodiazepines due to ↓ breakdown by liver

Laboratory Test Interferences: ↑ AST, ALT, LDH, alkaline phosphatase.

Dosage

See individual drugs.

NURSING CONSIDERATIONS

Administration/Storage

1. Persistent drowsiness, ataxia, or visual disturbances may require dosage adjustment.
2. Lower dosage is usually indicated for older clients.
3. GI effects are decreased when drugs are given with meals or shortly afterward.
4. Withdraw drugs gradually.
5. Review the list of drug interactions prior to taking the client's history and beginning drug therapy.
6. In case of overdose, a benzodiazepine antagonist (flumazenil) should be readily available.
7. *Treatment of Overdose:* Supportive therapy. Gastric lavage, provided that an ET tube with an inflated cuff is used to prevent aspiration of vomitus. Emesis only if drug ingestion was recent and client is fully conscious. Activated charcoal and saline cathartic may be given after emesis or lavage. Adequate respiratory function must be maintained. Hypotension may be reversed by IV fluids, norepinephrine, or metaraminol. Excitation should **not** be treated with barbiturates.

Assessment

1. Note any history of adverse reactions to this class of drugs.
2. Document indications for therapy, onset of symptoms, and behavioral manifestations.
3. Determine if the client has had any prior treatment for the same problems, what was used, and the outcome.
4. Assess the client's life-style and general level of health noting any situations that may be contributing to this presentation.
5. Note the manner in which the client responds to questions and discusses the problem.
6. Obtain baseline CBC and liver and renal function studies to determine potential problems or impaired function.
7. Review the client's physical history for any contraindications to drug therapy.
8. List drugs currently prescribed to ensure none interact unfavorably.

Interventions

1. Document any symptoms consistent with overdosage.
2. Determine the presence of any blood dyscrasias that could preclude administering the drug.
3. Report any complaints of sore throat (other than those caused by NG or ET tubes), fever, or weakness and assess for blood dyscrasias. Obtain a CBC and anticipate that the drug may be withheld until appropriate data can be evaluated.
4. Monitor the BP before and after the client receives an IV dose of antianxiety medication. Keep the client in a recumbent position for 2–3 hr after IV administration. Determine the presence and degree of hypotension and document.
5. Anticipate that the dosage of drug will be the lowest possible effective one, especially if client is elderly or debilitated.
6. When the drug is administered PO to a hospitalized client, remain with client until the drug is swallowed.
7. If the client exhibits ataxia, or complains of weakness or lack of coordination when ambulating, provide supervision and assistance. Use side rails once the client is back in bed and identify if at risk for fall.
8. Note any early symptoms of cholestatic jaundice, such as client complaints of nausea, diarrhea, upper abdominal pain, or the presence of high fever or rash. Check liver functions studies and report.
9. If there is any yellowing of the client's sclera, skin, or mucous membranes, the client is exhibiting a late sign of cholestatic jaundice and biliary tract obstruction. Withhold the medication, and report.
10. If the client appears overly sleepy or confused or becomes comatose, withhold the drug and report.
11. If the client has suicidal tendencies, anticipate that the drug will be prescribed in small doses. Be alert to signs of increased depression and report immediately.
12. If the prescription is for a client who has a history of alcoholism or of taking excessive quantities of drug, carefully supervise the amount of drug prescribed and dispensed.
13. Note any other evidences of client physical or psychologic dependence.
14. Assess for manifestations of ataxia, slurred speech, and vertigo. Such symptoms are characteristic of chronic intoxication and are usually indications that the client is taking more than the recommended dose of drug.
15. For clients receiving the medication on an outpatient basis, determine the frequency of the requests for medication. If the renewal frequency seems unusual, count the number of pills or capsules left at the time of the request for refills or renewal of the prescription, as the client may be taking larger doses than are recommended.

Client/Family Teaching

1. Stress that these drugs may reduce the ability to handle potentially dangerous equipment, such as automobiles and other machinery.
2. Advise client to take most of the daily dose at bedtime with smaller

doses during the waking hours to minimize mental and motor impairment if situation permits.
3. Avoid alcohol while taking anti-anxiety agents. Alcohol potentiates the depressant effects of both the alcohol and the medication.
4. Do not take any unprescribed or OTC medications without approval.
5. Arise slowly from a supine position and dangle the legs over the side of the bed for a few minutes before standing up.
6. If feeling faint client should sit or lie down immediately and lower the head.
7. Encourage working clients to allow extra time to prepare for their daily activities to enable them to take the necessary precautions before arising, thereby reducing one source of anxiety and stress.
8. Do not stop taking the drug suddenly. Any sudden withdrawal of the drug after a prolonged period of therapy or after excessive use may cause a recurrence of the preexisting symptoms of anxiety. It may also cause a withdrawal syndrome, manifested by increased anxiety, anorexia, insomnia, vomiting, ataxia, muscle twitching, confusion, and hallucinations. Some clients may develop seizures and convulsions.
9. Instruct the client and family in several relaxation techniques that may assist in lowering their anxiety levels.
10. Advise that these drugs are generally for short-term therapy and that follow-up is imperative to evaluate response and the need for continued therapy.
11. Refer for appropriate counselling as condition and length of therapy determine.

Evaluate

- Symptomatic improvement with ↓ frequency in the occurrence of anxiety and tension episodes
- Reports of effective coping with evidence of new coping strategies
- ↓ Frequency and intensity of muscle spasms and tremor
- Reports of improved sleeping patterns with less frequent awakenings, especially early morning
- Effective control of seizures
- Control of symptoms of alcohol withdrawal

Alprazolam

(al-**PRAYZ**-oh-lam)
Pregnancy Category: D
Apo-Alpraz ✱, Novo-Alprazol ✱, Nu-Alpraz ✱, Xanax **(C-IV) (Rx)**

See also *Anti-Anxiety/Antimanic Drugs,* Chapter 40.

How Supplied: *Concentrate:* 1 mg/mL; *Solution:* 0.5 mg/5 mL; *Tablet:* 0.25 mg, 0.5 mg, 1 mg, 2 mg

Action/Kinetics: Peak plasma levels: PO, 8–37 ng/mL after 1–2 hr. **t½:** 12–15 hr. 80% plasma protein bound. Metabolized to alpha-hydroxyalprazolam, an active metabolite. **t½:** 12–15 hr. Excreted in urine.

Uses: Anxiety. Anxiety associated with depression with or without agoraphobia. *Investigational:* Agoraphobia with social phobia, depression, PMS.

Dosage

- **Tablets**

Anxiety disorder.

Adults, initial: 0.25–0.5 mg t.i.d.; **then,** titrate to needs of client, with total daily dosage not to exceed 4 mg. **In elderly or debilitated: initial;** 0.25 mg b.i.d.–t.i.d.; **then,** adjust dosage to needs of client.

Antipanic agent.

Adults: 0.5 mg t.i.d.; increase dose as needed up to a maximum of 10 mg/day.

Agoraphobia with social phobia.

Adults: 2–8 mg/day.

PMS.

0.25 mg t.i.d.

Administration/Storage

1. The daily dose should not be decreased more than 0.5 mg over 3 days if therapy is terminated or the dose decreased.
2. May be given with milk or food to decrease GI upset.

NURSING CONSIDERATIONS

See also *Nursing Considerations* for *Anti-Anxiety/Antimanic Drugs,* Chapter 40.

Interventions

1. Anticipate reduced dosage in elderly and debilitated clients.
2. Use side rails and support devices as needed, especially at night, because elderly clients tend to become confused.
3. Provide extra fluids and bulk in the diet to minimize constipation.

Evaluate

- Positive behaviors in clients being treated for phobias
- ↓ Anxiety and evidence of new coping strategies
- Control of panic disorder
- Improvement in symptoms of PMS

Buspirone hydrochloride

(byou-**SPYE**-rohn)
Pregnancy Category: B
BuSpar **(Rx)**

How Supplied: *Tablet:* 5 mg, 10 mg

Action/Kinetics: The mechanism of action is unknown. Buspirone is not chemically related to the benzodiazepines; it does not manifest anticonvulsant or muscle relaxant properties. Significant sedation has not been observed. The drug binds to serotonin ($5\text{-}HT_{1A}$) and dopamine (D_2) receptors in the CNS; it is thus possible that dopamine-mediated neurologic disorders may occur. These include dystonia, Parkinson-like symptoms, akathisia, and tardive dyskinesia. **Peak plasma levels:** 1–6 ng/mL 40–90 min after a single PO dose of 20 mg. **t½:** 2–3 hr. The drug undergoes extensive first-pass metabolism, and active and inactive metabolites are excreted in the urine and through the feces.

Uses: Anxiety disorders, short-term use to relieve symptoms of anxiety due to motor tension, apprehension, autonomic hyperactivity, or hyperattentiveness. Not usually indicated for treatment of anxiety and tension due to stress of everyday living.

Dosage

- **Tablets**

Adults: 5 mg t.i.d. Dosage may be increased in increments of 5 mg/day q 2–3 days to achieve optimum effects; the total daily dose should not exceed 60 mg.

Administration/Storage

1. Buspirone does not manifest cross-tolerance with other sedative-hypnotic drugs, including benzodiazepines.
2. Buspirone will not block the withdrawal syndrome, which may occur following cessation of sedative-hypnotics. Thus, clients on chronic sedative-hypnotic therapy should be withdrawn gradually prior to beginning buspirone therapy.
3. To date, buspirone has not manifested potential for abuse, tolerance, or either physical or psychologic dependence.
4. Up to 2 weeks may be required before beneficial antianxiety effects are manifested.
5. *Treatment of Overdose:* Immediate gastric lavage; general symptomatic and supportive measures.

Contraindications: Psychoses, severe liver or kidney impairment, lactation.

Special Concerns: Safety and efficacy in children less than 18 years of age not established. A decrease in dose may be necessary in geriatric clients due to age-related impairment of renal function.

Side Effects: *CNS:* Dizziness, drowsiness, insomnia, fatigue, nervousness, excitement, dream disturbances, dysphoria, noise intolerance, euphoria, depersonalization, akathisia, hallucinations, suicidal ideation, seizures, decreased concentration, confusion, anger or hostility, depression. *CV:* Nonspecific chest pain, hypotension, palpitations, tachycardia, syncope, hypertension. *GI:* N&V, diarrhea, constipation, abdominal distress, dry mouth, altered taste, increased appetite, irritable colon. *Ophthalmologic:* Redness and itching of eyes, conjunctivitis, photophobia, eye pain. *Dermatologic:* Skin rash, pruritus, dry skin, edema of face, acne, easy bruising, flushing. *Neurologic:* Paresthesia, tremor, numbness, incoordination. *GU:* Urinary hesitancy or frequency, enuresis, amenorrhea, pelvic inflammatory disease. *Miscellaneous:* Tinnitus, sore throat, nasal congestion, altered smell, muscle aches or pains, skin rash, headache, sweating, hyperventilation, SOB, hair loss, galactorrhea, decreased or increased libido, delayed ejaculation.

Symptoms of Overdose: Dizziness, drowsiness, N&V, gastric distress, miosis.

Drug Interactions: Use with MAO inhibitors may cause an increase in BP.

NURSING CONSIDERATIONS

Assessment

1. Document indications for therapy and pretreatment assessments.
2. Determine support systems and encourage active family involvement in treatment plan.
3. Assess for any history of recent benzodiazepine therapy as buspar may be less effective in these clients.
4. Note age; good agent to use in elderly because of less CNS suppression.
5. Attempt to determine causative factor or event that precipitated problems.

Client/Family Teaching

1. Take with food or snack to decrease nausea, which is a common side effect. Report if the nausea persists or is severe.
2. Review the goals of therapy and possible side effects. Advise to report any persistent, bothersome side effects.
3. The drug may cause drowsiness or dizziness. Use with caution when operating a motor vehicle or performing tasks that require mental alertness.
4. Report any involuntary, repetitive movements of the face or neck muscles immediately.
5. Avoid the use of alcohol.
6. Do not stop taking the drug as withdrawal symptoms such as nausea, vomiting, dry mouth, nasal congestion, or sore throat may occur.
7. Report any complaints of weakness, restlessness, nervousness, headaches, or feelings of depression.
8. The development of Parkinson-like symptoms or suicide ideations should be reported immediately and anticipate withdrawal of the drug.
9. Avoid any OTC preparations without approval.

Evaluate: Relief of symptoms of agitated depression and anxiety states with depression.

Chlordiazepoxide

(klor-dye-**AYZ**-eh-**POX**-eyed)

Pregnancy Category: D

Apo-Chlordiazepoxide ✱, Libritabs, Librium, Lipoxide, Mitran, Reposans-10, Solium ✱ **(C-IV) (Rx)**

See also *Anti-Anxiety/Antimanic Drugs,* Chapter 40.

How Supplied: *Capsule:* 5 mg, 10 mg, 25 mg; *Powder for injection:* 100 mg; *Tablet:* 5 mg, 25 mg

Action/Kinetics: Onset: PO, 30–60 min; **IM,** 15–30 min (absorption may be slow and erratic); **IV,** 3–30 min. **Peak plasma levels (PO):** 0.5–4 hr. **Duration: t½:** 5–30 hr. Is metabolized to four active metabolites: desmethylchlordiazepoxide, desmethyldiazepam, oxazepam, and demoxepam. Chlordiazepoxide has less anticonvulsant activity and is less potent than diazepam.

Uses: Anxiety, acute withdrawal symptoms in chronic alcoholics. Sedative-hypnotic. Preoperatively to reduce anxiety and tension. Tension headache. Antitremor agent (PO). Antipanic (parenteral).

Dosage

- **Capsules, Tablets**

Anxiety and tension.

Adults: 5–10 mg t.i.d.–q.i.d. (up to 20–25 mg t.i.d.–q.i.d. in severe cases). Reduce dose to 5 mg b.i.d.–q.i.d. in geriatric or debilitated clients. **Pediatric, over 6 years, initial,** 5 mg b.i.d.–q.i.d. May be increased to 10 mg b.i.d.–q.i.d.

Preoperatively.

Adults: 5–10 mg t.i.d.–q.i.d. on day before surgery.

Alcohol withdrawal/Sedative-hypnotic.

Adults: 50–100 mg; may be increased to 300 mg/day; **then,** reduce to maintenance levels.

• **IM, IV (not recommended for children under 12 years)**

Acute/severe agitation, anxiety.

Initial: 50–100 mg; **then,** 25–50 mg t.i.d.–q.i.d.

Preoperatively.

Adults: 50–100 mg IM 1 hr before surgery.

Alcohol withdrawal.

Adults: 50–100 mg IM or IV; repeat in 2–4 hr if necessary. Dosage should not exceed 300 mg/day.

Antipanic.

Adults, initial: 50–100 mg; dose may be repeated in 4–6 hr if needed

Administration/Storage

1. **IM:** Prepare solution immediately before administration by adding diluent, which is provided, to ampule. Shake until dissolved. Discard any unused solution. Inject slowly into upper, outer quadrant of gluteal muscle.
2. **IV:** Prepare immediately before administration by diluting with 5 mL of sterile water for injection or sterile 0.9% sodium chloride solution. Inject directly into vein over 1-min period. Do not add to IV infusion because of instability of drug. Do not use IV solution for IM.

Laboratory Test Interferences

1. *Interference with test methods:* ↑ 17-Hydroxycorticosteroids, 17-ketosteroids.
2. *Caused by pharmacologic effects:* ↑ Alkaline phosphatase, bilirubin, serum transaminase, porphobilinogen. ↓ PT (clients on Coumarin).

Additional Side Effects: Jaundice, acute hepatic necrosis, hepatic dysfunction.

NURSING CONSIDERATIONS

See also *Nursing Considerations* for *Anti-Anxiety/Antimanic Drugs,* Chapter 40.

Assessment

1. Document indications for therapy and pretreatment findings.
2. Obtain liver function studies if impairment is suspected.

Interventions

1. Maintain a quiet, supervised environment. Observe and have client remain recumbent for 3 hr following parenteral administration.
2. Provide extra fluids and bulk to minimize constipating effects.

Client/Family Teaching

1. Drug may cause dizziness and drowsiness; use caution.
2. Avoid alcohol and any other CNS depressants.

Evaluate

- ↓ Tremors
- ↓ Symptoms of anxiety
- Desired level of sedation
- Control of panic episodes
- Control of symptoms of alcohol withdrawal

Clorazepate dipotassium

(klor-**AYZ**-eh-payt)
Pregnancy Category: D
Apo-Clorazepate ✱, Gen-Xene, Novo-Clopate ✱, Nu-Clopate ✱, Tranxene, Tranxene-SD, Tranxene-SD Half **(C-IV) (Rx)**

See also *Anti-Anxiety/Antimanic Drugs,* Chapter 40.

How Supplied: *Tablet:* 3.75 mg, 7.5 mg, 11.25 mg, 15 mg, 22.5 mg

Action/Kinetics: Peak plasma levels: 1–2 hr. **t½:** 30–100 hr. Clorazepate is hydrolyzed in the stomach to desmethyldiazepam, the active metabolite. Oxazepam is also an active metabolite. **t½, desmethyldiazepam:** 30–100 hr; **t½, oxazepam:** 5–15 hr. **Time to peak plasma levels:** 0.5–2 hr. The drug is slowly excreted by the kidneys.

Uses: Anxiety, tension. Acute alcohol withdrawal, as adjunct in treatment of seizures. Adjunct for treating partial seizures.

Dosage

• **Capsules, Tablets**

Anxiety.

Initial: 7.5–15 mg b.i.d.–q.i.d.; **maintenance:** 15–60 mg/day in divided doses. **Elderly or debilitated clients, initial:** 7.5–15 mg/day. **Alternative.** Single daily dosage: **Adult, initial,** 15 mg; **then,** 11.25–22.5 mg once daily.

Acute alcohol withdrawal.

Day 1, initial: 30 mg; **then,** 15 mg b.i.d.–q.i.d. the first day; **day 2:** 45–90 mg/day; **day 3:** 22.5–45 mg/day; **day 4:** 15–30 mg/day. Thereafter, reduce to 7.5–15 mg/day and discontinue as soon as possible.

Anticonvulsant, adjunct.

Adults and children over 12 years, initial: 7.5 mg t.i.d.; increase no more than 7.5 mg/week to maximum of 90 mg/day. **Children (9–12 years), initial:** 7.5 mg b.i.d.; increase by no more than 7.5 mg/week to maximum of 60 mg/day. Not recommended for children under 9 years of age.

Additional Contraindications: Depressed clients, nursing mothers. Give cautiously to clients with impaired renal or hepatic function.

NURSING CONSIDERATIONS

See also *Nursing Considerations* for *Anti-Anxiety/Antimanic Drugs,* Chapter 40.

Assessment

1. Note any evidence of depression because drug is contraindicated.
2. In clients with excessive alcohol intake, determine when they had their last drink.

Evaluate

- ↓ Anxiety and tension
- Control of symptoms of alcohol withdrawal
- Control of seizures

Diazepam

(dye-**AYZ**-eh-pam)
Pregnancy Category: D
Apo-Diazepam ♣, Diazemuls ♣, Diazepam Intensol, Rival ♣, Valium, Valrelease, Vivol ♣, Zetran **(C-IV) (Rx)**

See also *Anti-Anxiety/Antimanic Drugs,* Chapter 40.

How Supplied: *Capsule, Extended Release:* 15 mg; *Concentrate:* 5 mg/mL; *Injection:* 5 mg/mL; *Solution:* 5 mg/5 mL; *Tablet:* 2 mg, 5 mg, 10 mg

Action/Kinetics: The skeletal muscle relaxant effect of diazepam may be due to enhancement of GABA-mediated presynaptic inhibition at the spinal level as well as in the brain stem reticular formation. **Onset: PO,** 30–60 min; **IM,** 15–30 min; **IV,** more rapid. **Peak plasma levels: PO,** 0.5–2 hr; **IM,** 0.5–1.5; **IV,** 0.25 hr. **Duration:** 3 hr. **t½:** 20–70 hr. Diazepam is broken down in the liver to the active metabolites desmethyldiazepam, oxazepam, and temazepam. Diazepam and metabolites are excreted through the urine.

Uses: Anxiety, tension (more effective than chlordiazepoxide), alcohol withdrawal, muscle relaxant, adjunct to treat seizure disorders, antipanic drug. Used prior to gastroscopy and esophagoscopy, preoperatively and prior to cardioversion. In dentistry to induce sedation. Treatment of status epilepticus. Relief of skeletal muscle spasm due to inflammation of muscles or joints or trauma; spasticity caused by upper motor neuron disorders such as cerebral palsy and paraplegia; athetotis; and stiff-man syndrome. Relieve spasms of facial muscles in occlusion and temporomandibular joint disorders. IV to treat status epilepticus, severe recurrent seizures, and tetanus.

Dosage

- **Tablets, Oral Solution**

Antianxiety, anticonvulsant, adjunct to skeletal muscle relaxants.

Adults: 2–10 mg b.i.d.–q.i.d. **Elderly, debilitated clients:** 2–2.5 mg 1–2 times/day. May be gradually increased to adult level. **Pediatric, over 6 months, initial:** 1–2.5 mg (0.04–0.2 mg/kg or 1.17–6 mg/m^2) t.i.d.–b.i.d.

Alcohol withdrawal.

Adults: 10 mg t.i.d.–q.i.d. during the first 24 hr; **then,** decrease to 5 mg t.i.d.–q.i.d. as required.

• **Extended-Release Capsules**

Antianxiety, skeletal muscle relaxant.

Adults: 15–30 mg once daily. To be used in children over 6 months of age only if the dose has been determined to be 5 mg t.i.d. (use one 15-mg capsule/day).

• **IM, IV**

Preoperative or diagnostic use.

Adults: 10 mg IM 5–30 min before procedure.

Adjunct to treat skeletal muscle spasm.

Adults, initial: 5–10 mg IM; **then,** repeat in 3–4 hr if needed (larger doses may be required for tetanus).

Moderate anxiety.

Adults: 2–5 mg IM q 3–4 hr if necessary.

Severe anxiety, muscle spasm.

Adults: 5–10 mg IM q 3–4 hr, if necessary.

Acute alcohol withdrawal.

Initial: 10 mg IM; **then,** 5–10 mg q 3–4 hr.

Preoperatively.

Adults: 10 mg IM prior to surgery.

Endoscopy.

IV: 10 mg or less although doses up to 20 mg can be used; **IM:** 5–10 mg 30 min prior to procedure.

Cardioversion.

IV: 5–15 mg 5–10 min prior to procedure.

Tetanus in children.

IM, IV, over 1 month: 1–2 mg, repeated q 3–4 hr as necessary; **5 years and over:** 5–10 mg q 3–4 hr.

• **IV**

Status epilepticus.

Adults, initial: 5–10 mg; **then,** dose may be repeated at 10–15-min intervals up to a maximum dose of 30 mg. Dosage may be repeated after 2–4 hr. **Children, 1 month–5 years:** 0.2–0.5 mg q 2–5 min, up to maximum of 5 mg. Can be repeated in 2–4 hr. **5 years and older:** 1 mg q 2–5 min up to a maximum of 10 mg; dose can be repeated in 2–4 hr, if needed.

NOTE: Elderly or debilitated clients should not receive more than 5 mg parenterally at any one time.

Administration/Storage

1. One 15-mg sustained-release diazepam capsule may be used if the daily dosage is 5 mg t.i.d.
2. The Intensol solution should be mixed with beverages such as water, soda, and juices or soft foods such as applesauce or puddings. Only the calibrated dropper provided with the product should be used to withdraw the medication. Once the medication is withdrawn and mixed, it should be used immediately.
3. To reduce reactions at the site of IV administration, diazepam should be given slowly (5 mg/min). Also, small veins or intra-arterial administration should be avoided.
4. Due to the possibility of precipitation and instability, diazepam should not be infused. Also, the drug should not be mixed or diluted with other solutions or drugs in the syringe or infusion container.
5. When administering the drug IV, have emergency equipment and drugs available.
6. Diazepam interacts with plastic; therefore, introducing diazepam into plastic containers or administration sets will decrease availability of the drug.
7. Except for the deltoid muscle, absorption from IM sites is slow and erratic.
8. Review the drug interaction chart before administering the drug.
9. The IV route is preferred in the convulsing client.

Additional Contraindications: Narrow-angle glaucoma, children under 6 months, and parenterally in children under 12 years. During lactation.

Additional Drug Interactions

1. Diazepam potentiates antihypertensive effects of thiazides and other diuretics.
2. Diazepam potentiates muscle relaxant effects of *d*-tubocurarine and gallamine.
3. Ranitidine ↓ GI absorption of diazepam.
4. Isoniazid ↑ half-life of diazepam.
5. Fluoxetine ↑ half-life of diazepam.

NURSING CONSIDERATIONS

See also *Nursing Considerations* for *Anti-Anxiety/Antimanic Drugs,* Chapter 40.

Assessment

1. Obtain baseline CBC, platelet count, and liver and renal function studies.
2. Note if the client has diabetes and the type of agent used for testing the urine as diazepam interferes with many of these agents. Have client convert to finger sticks for a more accurate blood glucose determination.
3. Determine any history of depression or drug abuse.
4. Document indications for therapy and time frame for anticipated results.

Interventions

1. Parenteral administration may cause bradycardia, respiratory or cardiac arrest. Monitor client and VS closely.
2. Elderly clients may experience adverse reactions more quickly than younger clients. Therefore, anticipate a lower dose of drug in this group.
3. Simultaneous use of CNS depressants should be avoided.
4. Anticipate a gradual reduction of drug to avoid withdrawal symptoms such as anxiety, tremors, anorexia, insomnia, weakness, headache, and N&V.

Client/Family Teaching

1. Drug may cause dizziness and drowsiness.
2. Avoid activities that require mental alertness until drug effects are realized.
3. Avoid alcohol and any other CNS depressants.
4. Notify provider if pregnancy is suspected.

Evaluate

- ↓ Frequency of anxiety and tension episodes
- Control of symptoms of alcohol withdrawal
- Interruption and control of seizures
- Relief of muscle spasms
- Effective sedation

Halazepam

(hal-**AYZ**-eh-pam)
Pregnancy Category: D
Paxipam **(C-IV) (Rx)**

See also *Anti-Anxiety/Antimanic Drugs,* Chapter 40.

How Supplied: *Tablet:* 20 mg, 40 mg

Action/Kinetics: t½: 14 hr. Metabolized in liver to *N*-desmethyldiazepam (active with a **t½:** of 30–100 hr) and to inactive conjugates. **Maximum plasma levels of active metabolite:** 3–6 hr. Excreted through the kidneys.

Use: Short-term relief of anxiety.

Dosage

- **Tablets**

Adults: 20–40 mg t.i.d.–q.i.d. In elderly or debilitated clients: **initial,** 20 mg 1–2 times/day.

Additional Contraindication: Acute narrow-angle glaucoma.

Special Concerns: Dose has not been established in children less than 18 years of age.

NURSING CONSIDERATIONS

See also *Nursing Considerations* for *Anti-Anxiety/Antimanic Drugs,* Chapter 40.

Evaluate: ↓ Anxiety levels and improved coping ability.

Hydroxyzine hydrochloride

(hy-**DROX**-ih-zeen)
Anxanil, Apo-Hydroxyzine ✱, Atarax, Atozine, E-Vista, Hyzine-50, Multipax ✱, Novo-Hydroxyzin ✱, PMS Hydroxyzine ✱, Quiess, Vistaject-25 and -50, Vistaquel 50, Vistaril, Vistazine 50 **(Rx)**

Hydroxyzine pamoate

(hy-**DROX**-ih-zeen)
Vamate, Vistaril **(Rx)**

How Supplied: Hydroxyzine hydrochloride: *Injection:* 25 mg/mL, 50 mg/mL; *Syrup:* 10 mg/5 mL; *Tablet:* 10 mg, 20 mg, 25 mg, 50 mg, 100 mg. Hydroxyzine pamoate: *Capsule:* 25 mg, 50 mg, 100 mg; *Suspension:* 25 mg/5 mL

Action/Kinetics: The action of hydroxyzine may be due to a depression of activity in selected important regions of the subcortical areas of the CNS. Hydroxyzine manifests anticholinergic, antiemetic, antispasmodic, local anesthetic, antihistaminic, and skeletal relaxant effects. The drug also has mild antiarrhythmic activity and mild analgesic effects. **Onset:** 15–30 min. **$t^{1}/_{2}$:** 3 hr. **Duration:** 4–6 hr. Metabolized by the liver and excreted through the urine. The pamoate salt is believed to be converted to the hydrochloride in the stomach.

Uses: PO use: Psychoneurosis and tension states, anxiety, and agitation. Anxiety observed in organic disease. Adjunct in the treatment of chronic urticaria. Control of N&V accompanying various diseases. Preanesthetic medication. **IM use:** Acute hysteria or agitation, withdrawal symptoms (including delirium tremens) in the acute or chronic alcoholic, asthma, N&V (except that due to pregnancy), pre- or postoperative and pre- or postpartum to allow decrease in dosage of narcotics.

Dosage

• **Capsules, Oral Suspension, Syrup. Hydroxyzine hydrochloride and hydroxyzine pamoate**

Antianxiety.

Adults: 50–100 mg q.i.d.; **pediatric under 6 years:** 50 mg/day; **over 6 years:** 50–100 mg/day in divided doses.

Pruritus.

Adults: 25 mg t.i.d.–q.i.d.; **children under 6 years:** 50 mg/day in divided doses; **children over 6 years:** 50–100 mg/day in divided doses.

Preoperatively.

Adults: 50–100 mg; **children:** 0.6 mg/kg.

• **IM. Hydroxyzine hydrochloride**

Acute anxiety, including alcohol withdrawal.

Adults, initial: 50–100 mg repeated q 4–6 hr as needed.

N&V, pre- and postoperative, pre- and postpartum.

Adults: 25–100 mg; **pediatric,** 1.1 mg/kg. Switch to **PO** as soon as possible.

Administration/Storage

1. Inject IM only. Injection should be made into the upper, outer quadrant of the buttocks or the midlateral muscles of the thigh. In children the drug should be injected into the midlateral muscles of the thigh.

2. *Treatment of Overdose:* Immediate induction of vomiting or performance of gastric lavage. General supportive care with monitoring of VS. Control hypotension with IV fluids and either norepinephrine or metaraminol (epinephrine should not be used).

Contraindications: Pregnancy (especially early) or lactation; not recommended for the treatment of morning sickness during pregnancy or as sole agent for treatment of psychoses or depression. Hypersensitivity to drug. Not to be used IV, SC, or intra-arterially.

Special Concerns: Geriatric clients may manifest increased anticholinergic and sedative effects.

Laboratory Test Interference: Hydroxycorticosteroids.

Side Effects: Low incidence at recommended dosages. Drowsiness, dryness of mouth, involuntary motor activity, dizziness, urticaria, or skin reactions. Marked discomfort, induration, and even gangrene have been reported at site of IM injection.

Symptom of Overdose: Oversedation.

Drug Interactions: Additive effects when used with other CNS depressants. See *Drug Interactions* for *Anti-Anxiety/Antimanic Drugs,* Chapter 40.

NURSING CONSIDERATIONS

See also *Nursing Considerations* for *Anti-Anxiety/Antimanic Drugs,* Chapter 40.

Client/Family Teaching

1. Frequent rinsing of the mouth and increased fluid intake may relieve dryness of the mouth.

2. Wait and evaluate the sedative effects of hydroxyzine before perform-

ing any tasks that require mental alertness.
3. Avoid ingestion of alcohol or any other CNS depressants.
4. Report as scheduled for follow-up and evaluation. Drug is only for short-term management of anxiety.

Evaluate

- ↓ Symptoms of anxiety and agitation
- Relief of itching and allergic symptoms
- Control of N&V

Lithium carbonate

(**LITH**-ee-um)
Pregnancy Category: D
Carbolith ✱, Duralith ✱, Eskalith, Eskalith CR, Lithane, Lithizine ✱, Lithobid, Lithonate, Lithotabs **(Rx)**

Lithium citrate

(**LITH**-ee-um)
Pregnancy Category: D

How Supplied: Lithium carbonate: *Capsule:* 150 mg, 300 mg, 600 mg; *Tablet:* 300 mg; *Tablet, Extended Release:* 300 mg, 450 mg.
Lithium citrate: *Syrup:* 300 mg/5 mL

Action/Kinetics: Although the precise mechanism for the antimanic effect of lithium is not known, various hypotheses have been put forth. These include: (a) a decrease in catecholamine neurotransmitter levels caused by lithium's effect on Na^+–K^+ ATPase to improve transneuronal membrane transport of sodium ion; (b) a decrease in cyclic AMP levels caused by lithium which decreases sensitivity of hormonal-sensitive adenyl cyclase receptors; or (c) interference by lithium with lipid inositol metabolism ultimately leading to insensitivity of cells in the CNS to stimulation by inositol.

Lithium also affects the distribution of calcium, magnesium, and sodium ions and affects glucose metabolism. **Peak serum levels** (regular release): 1–4 hr; (slow-release): 4–6 hr. **Onset:** 5–14 days. **Therapeutic serum levels:** 0.4–1.0 mEq/L (must be carefully monitored because toxic effects may occur at these levels and significant toxic reactions occur at serum lithium levels of 2 mEq/L). **t½** (plasma): 24 hr (longer in presence of renal impairment and in the elderly). Lithium and sodium are excreted by the same mechanism in the proximal tubule. Thus, to reduce the danger of lithium intoxication, sodium intake must remain at normal levels.

Uses: Control of manic and hypomanic episodes in manic-depressive clients. Prophylaxis of bipolar depression. *Investigational:* To reverse neutropenia induced by cancer chemotherapy and in children with chronic neutropenia. Prophylaxis of cluster headaches and cyclic migraine headaches. Treatment of certain types of mental depression (e.g., schizoaffective disorder, augment the antidepressant effect of tricyclic or MAO drugs in treating unipolar depression). Also for premenstrual tension, alcoholism accompanied by depression, tardive dyskinesia, bulimia, hyperthyroidism, excess ADH secretion. Lithium succinate, in a topical form, has been used for the treatment of genital herpes and seborrheic dermatitis.

Dosage

- **Capsules, Slow-Release Capsules, Tablets, Extended-Release Tablets, Syrup**

Acute mania.

Adults: Individualized and according to lithium serum level (not to exceed 1.4 mEq/L) and clinical response. **Usual initial:** 300–600 mg t.i.d. or 600–900 mg b.i.d. of slow-release form; **elderly and debilitated clients:** 0.6–1.2 g/day in three doses. **Maintenance:** 300 mg t.i.d.–q.i.d.

Administration of drug is discontinued when lithium serum level exceeds 1.2 mEq/L and resumed 24 hr after it has fallen below that level.

To reverse neutropenia.

300–1,000 mg/day (to achieve serum levels of 0.5–1.0 mEq/L) for 7–10 days.

Prophylaxis of cluster headaches. 600–900 mg/day.

Administration/Storage

1. To prevent toxic serum levels from occurring, blood levels should be determined 1–2 times/week during initiation of therapy, and monthly thereafter, on blood samples taken 8–12 hr after dosage.
2. Full beneficial effects of lithium therapy may not be noted for 6–10 days after initiation.
3. *Treatment of Overdose:* Early symptoms are treated by decreasing the dose or stopping treatment for 24–48 hr.

- Use gastric lavage.
- Restore fluid and electrolyte balance (can use saline) and maintain kidney function.
- Increase lithium excretion by giving aminophylline, mannitol, or urea.
- Prevent infection. Maintain adequate respiration.
- Monitor thyroid function.
- Institute hemodialysis.

Contraindications: Cardiovascular or renal disease. Brain damage. Dehydration, sodium depletion, clients receiving diuretics. Lactation.

Special Concerns: Safety and efficacy have not been established for children less than 12 years of age. Use with caution in geriatric clients because lithium is more toxic to the CNS in these clients; also, geriatric clients are more likely to develop lithium-induced goiter and clinical hypothyroidism and are more likely to manifest excessive thirst and larger volumes of urine.

Laboratory Test Interferences: False + urinary glucose test (Benedict's), ↑ serum glucose, creatinine kinase. False – or ↓ serum PBI, uric acid; ↑ TSH; ↓ T_4.

Side Effects: These are related to the blood lithium level. *CNS:* Fainting, drowsiness, slurred speech, confusion, dizziness, tiredness, lethargy, ataxia, dysarthria, aphasia, vertigo, stupor, restlessness, ***coma, seizures.*** Pseudotumor cerebri leading to papilledema and increased ICP. *GI:* Anorexia, N&V, diarrhea, thirst, dry mouth, bloated stomach. *Muscular:* Tremors (especially of hand), muscle weakness, fasciculations and/or twitching, clonic movements of limbs, increased deep tendon reflexes, choreoathetoid movements, cogwheel rigidity. *Renal:* Nephrogenic diabetes insipidus (polyuria, polydypsia), oliguria, albuminuria. *Endocrine:* Hypothyroidism, goiter, hyperparathyroidism. *CV:* Changes in ECG, edema, hypotension, ***CV collapse,*** irregular pulse, tachycardia. *Ophthalmologic:* Blurred vision, downbeat nystagmus. *Dermatologic:* Acneform eruptions, pruritic-maculopapular rashes, drying and thinning of hair, alopecia, paresthesia, cutaneous ulcers, lupus-like symptoms. *Miscellaneous:* Hoarseness; swelling of feet, lower legs, or neck; cold sensitivity; leukemia; leukocytosis; dyspnea on exertion.

Symptoms of Overdose: Symptoms dependent on serum lithium levels. Levels less than 2 mEq/L: N&V, diarrhea, muscle weakness, drowsiness, loss of coordination.

Levels of 2–3 mEq/L: agitation, ataxia, blackouts, blurred vision, choreoathetoid movements, confusion, dysarthria, fasciculations, giddiness, hyperreflexia, hypertonia, manic-like behavior, myoclonic twitching or movement of entire limbs, slurred speech, tinnitus, urinary or fecal incontinence, vertigo.

Levels over 3 mEq/L: ***arrhythmias, coma,*** hypotension, ***peripheral vascular collapse, seizures (focal and generalized),*** spasticity, stupor, twitching of muscle groups.

Drug Interactions

Acetazolamide / ↓ Lithium effect by ↑ renal excretion
Aminophylline / ↓ Lithium effect by ↑ renal excretion
Bumetanide / ↑ Lithium toxicity due to ↓ renal clearance
Carbamazepine / ↑ Risk of lithium toxicity
Diazepam / ↑ Risk of hypothermia
Ethacrynic acid / ↑ Lithium toxicity due to ↓ renal clearance
Fluoxetine / ↑ Serum levels of lithium

Furosemide / ↑ Lithium toxicity due to ↓ renal clearance
Haloperidol / ↑ Risk of neurologic toxicity
Ibuprofen / ↑ Chance of lithium toxicity due to ↓ renal clearance
Indomethacin / ↑ Chance of lithium toxicity due to ↓ renal clearance
Iodide salts / Additive effect to cause hypothyroidism
Mannitol / ↓ Lithium effect by ↑ renal excretion
Mazindol / ↑ Chance of lithium toxicity due to ↑ serum levels
Methyldopa / ↑ Chance of lithium toxicity due to ↑ serum levels
Naproxen / ↑ Chance of lithium toxicity due to ↑ serum levels
Neuromuscular blocking agents / Lithium ↑ effect of these agents → respiratory depression and apnea
Phenothiazines / ↓ Levels of phenothiazines and ↑ neurotoxicity
Phenylbutazone / ↑ Chance of lithium toxicity due to ↓ renal clearance
Phenytoin / ↑ Chance of lithium toxicity
Piroxicam / ↑ Chance of lithium toxicity due to ↓ renal clearance
Probenecid / ↑ Chance of lithium toxicity due to ↑ serum levels
Sodium bicarbonate / ↓ Lithium effect by ↑ renal excretion
Sodium chloride / Excretion of lithium is proportional to amount of sodium chloride ingested; if client is on salt-free diet, may develop lithium toxicity since less lithium excreted
Spironolactone / ↑ Chance of lithium toxicity due to ↑ serum levels
Succinylcholine / ↑ Muscle relaxation
Sympathomimetics / ↓ Pressor effect of sympathomimetics
Tetracyclines / ↑ Chance of lithium toxicity due to ↑ serum levels
Theophyllines / ↓ Effect of lithium due to ↑ renal excretion
Thiazide diuretics, triamterene / ↑ Chance of lithium toxicity due to ↓ renal clearance
Tricyclic antidepressants / ↑ Effect of tricyclic antidepressants
Urea / ↓ Lithium effect by ↑ renal excretion

NURSING CONSIDERATIONS

Assessment

1. Document indications for therapy and type and onset of symptoms.
2. Conduct a drug history and determine if the client is taking other medications that are likely to interact with lithium.
3. If clients have arthritic conditions, determine if they are taking any anti-inflammatory agents and document.
4. Obtain pretreatment thyroid function studies and assess for decreased function.
5. Document baseline ECG and monitor CV function periodically during drug therapy.

Client/Family Teaching

1. Take drug with food or immediately after meals. Report any episodes of persistent diarrhea because these symptoms may indicate a need for supplemental fluids or salt.
2. Avoid any caffeinated beverages/foods because these may aggravate mania.
3. Explain the relationship between lithium activity and dietary sodium. Instruct clients to maintain a constant level of salt intake to avoid fluctuations in lithium activity. Weight gain and edema may be related to sodium retention; report if excessive.
4. Advise client to drink 10–12 glasses of water each day and to avoid dehydration (e.g., vigorous exercise, sunbathing, sauna) to prevent increased concentrations of lithium in urine.
5. Review the goals of therapy. Provide printed instructions regarding medication administration and side effects that require immediate reporting.
6. If diarrhea, vomiting, drowsiness, muscular weakness, and lack of coordination occur, lithium therapy must be discontinued immediately, and

client must report for medical supervision.
7. Do not engage in physical activities that require alertness or physical coordination until drug effects are realized. Lithium therapy causes drowsiness and may impair these abilities.
8. Reassure the client and family that it will take several weeks to realize a behavioral benefit from lithium therapy.
9. Do not change brands of medication.
10. Explain that lithium usually works well in the manic phase and concomitant use of an antidepressant may be necessary during depressive phases.
11. Advise that transient acneiform eruptions, folliculitis, and altered sexual function in men has been noted with this drug.
12. Provide the name and telephone number of persons to contact if the client has problems or if family members note behavioral changes or physical changes contrary to expectations.
13. Advise to report for serum drug levels on day 5 and day 10 and if levels are adequate the frequency can be diminished. Establish a schedule of follow-up lab and medical appointments and stress the importance of adhering to this schedule.
14. Instruct clients to carry identification indicating the diagnosis and prescribed medication regimen.

Evaluate

- Stabilization of mood swings and affect
- ↓ Symptoms of mania (↓ hyperactivity, ↓ sleeplessness, and improved judgment)
- Therapeutic serum drug levels (0.4–1.0 mEq/L)

Lorazepam

(lor-**AYZ**-eh-pam)
Pregnancy Category: D
Apo-Lorazepam ✦, Ativan, Lorazepam Intensol, Novo-Lorazem ✦, Nu-Loraz ✦ **(C-IV) (Rx)**

See also *Anti-Anxiety/Antimanic Drugs,* Chapter 40.

How Supplied: *Concentrate:* 2 mg/mL; *Injection:* 2 mg/mL, 4 mg/mL; *Tablet:* 0.5 mg, 1 mg, 2 mg

Action/Kinetics: Absorbed and eliminated faster than other benzodiazepines. **Peak plasma levels: PO,** 1–6 hr; **IM,** 1–1.5 hr. **t½:** 10–20 hr. Is metabolized to inactive compounds, which are excreted through the kidneys.

Uses: PO: Anxiety, tension, anxiety with depression, insomnia, acute alcohol withdrawal symptoms. **Parenteral:** Amnesic agent, anticonvulsant, antitremor drug, adjunct to skeletal muscle relaxants, preanesthetic medication, adjunct prior to endoscopic procedures, treatment of status epilepticus, relief of acute alcohol withdrawal symptoms. *Investigational:* Antiemetic in cancer chemotherapy.

Dosage

- **Tablets**

Anxiety.

Adults: 1–3 mg b.i.d.–t.i.d.

Hypnotic.

Adults: 2–4 mg at bedtime. **Geriatric/debilitated clients, initial:** 0.5–2 mg/day in divided doses. Dose can be adjusted as required.

- **IM**

Preoperatively.

Adults: 0.05 mg/kg up to maximum of 4 mg 2 hr before surgery for maximum amnesic effect.

- **IV**

Preoperatively.

Adults, initial: 0.044 mg/kg or a total dose of 2 mg, whichever is less.

Amnesic effect.

Adults: 0.05 mg/kg up to a maximum of 4 mg administered 15–20 min prior to surgery.

Antiemetic in cancer chemotherapy.

Initial: 2 mg 30 min before beginning chemotherapy; **then,** 2 mg q 4 hr as needed.

Administration/Storage

1. For IV use, dilute just before use with equal amounts of either sterile

water for injection, sodium chloride injection, or 5% dextrose injection.
2. The IV rate of administration should not exceed 2 mg/min.
3. The solution should not be used if it is discolored or contains a precipitate.
4. If higher doses are required, the evening dose should be increased before the daytime doses.
Additional Contraindications: Narrow-angle glaucoma. Use cautiously in presence of renal and hepatic disease. Parenterally in children less than 18 years.
Special Concerns: PO dosage has not been established in children less than 12 years of age and IV dosage has not been established in children less than 18 years of age.
Additional Drug Interactions: With parenteral lorazepam, scopolamine → sedation, hallucinations, and behavioral abnormalities.

NURSING CONSIDERATIONS

See also *Nursing Considerations* for *Anti-Anxiety/Antimanic Drugs,* Chapter 40.
Assessment
1. Document indications for therapy and type and onset of symptoms.
2. List any other agents used to treat this condition and the outcome.
Client/Family Teaching
1. Take only as directed and report any loss of effectiveness.
2. Drug may cause dizziness and drowsiness; use with caution until drug effects realized.
3. Report immediately any increased depression or suicidal ideations.
4. Avoid alcohol and any other CNS depressants.
Evaluate
- Improvement in levels of anxiety, tension, and depression
- Control of alcohol withdrawal symptoms
- Desired level of muscle relaxation and amnesia

Meprobamate

(meh-proh-**BAM**-ayt)

Apo-Meprobamate ✱; Equanil; Equanil Wyseals; Meprospan 200 and 400; Miltown 200, 400, and 600; Neuramate **(C-IV) (Rx)**

How Supplied: *Capsule, Extended Release:* 200 mg, 400 mg; *Tablet:* 200 mg, 400 mg, 600 mg
Action/Kinetics: Meprobamate is a carbamate derivative that also possesses muscle relaxant and anticonvulsant effects. It acts on the limbic system and the thalamus, as well as to inhibit polysynaptic spinal reflexes. **Onset:** 1 hr. **Blood levels, chronic therapy:** 5–20 mcg/mL. **t½:** 6–24 hr. Extensively metabolized in liver and inactive metabolites and some unchanged drug (8%–19%) are excreted in the urine. Meprobamate is also found in *Equagesic.*
Use: Short-term treatment (no more than 4 months) of anxiety.

Dosage

- **Tablets**

Anxiety.

Adults, initial: 400 mg t.i.d.–q.i.d. (or 600 mg b.i.d.). May be increased, if necessary, up to maximum of 2.4 g/day. **Pediatric, 6–12 years of age:** 100–200 mg b.i.d.–t.i.d. (the 600-mg tablet is not recommended for use in children).

- **Extended-Release Capsules**

Anxiety.

Adults: 400–800 mg in the morning and at bedtime. **Pediatric 6–12 years:** 200 mg in the morning and at bedtime.
Administration/Storage
1. Tablets and sustained-release capsules should not be crushed or chewed.
2. *Treatment of Overdose:* Induction of vomiting or gastric lavage if detected shortly after ingestion. It is imperative that gastric lavage be continued or gastroscopy be performed as incomplete gastric emptying can cause relapse and death.
- Give fluids to treat hypotension. Avoid fluid overload.
- Institute artificial respiration.

• Use care in treating seizures due to combined CNS depressant effects.
• Use forced diuresis and vasopressors followed by hemodialysis or hemoperfusion if condition deteriorates.

Contraindications: Hypersensitivity to meprobamate or carisoprodol. Porphyria. Children less than 6 years of age.

Special Concerns: Use with caution in pregnancy, lactation, epilepsy, liver and kidney disease. Geriatric clients may be more sensitive to the depressant effects of meprobamate; also, due to age-related impaired renal function, the dose of meprobamate may have to be reduced.

Laboratory Test Interferences: *With test methods:* ↑ 17-Hydroxycorticosteroids, 17-ketogenic steroids, and 17-ketosteroids. *Pharmacologic effects:* ↑ Alkaline phosphatase, bilirubin, serum transaminase, urinary estriol (calorimetric tests), porphobilinogen. ↓ PT in clients on Coumarin.

Side Effects: *CNS:* Ataxia, drowsiness, dizziness, weakness headache, paradoxical excitement, euphoria, slurred speech, vertigo. *GI:* N&V, diarrhea. *Miscellaneous:* Visual disturbances, allergic reactions including hematologic and dermatologic symptoms, paresthesias.

Symptoms of Overdose: Drowsiness, stupor, lethargy, ataxia, ***shock, coma, respiratory collapse, death.*** Also, arrhythmias, tachycardia or bradycardia, reduced venous return, ***profound hypotension, CV collapse.*** Excessive oronasal secretions, ***relaxation of pharyngeal wall leading to obstruction of airway.***

Drug Interactions: Additive depressant effects when used with CNS depressants, MAO inhibitors, and tricyclic antidepressants.

NURSING CONSIDERATIONS

See also *Nursing Considerations* for *Anti-Anxiety/Antimanic Drugs,* Chapter 40.

Assessment

1. Document indications for therapy and onset of symptoms.
2. Assist client to identify any causative factors.

Evaluate: Control of anxiety symptoms.

Midazolam hydrochloride

(my-**DAYZ**-oh-lam)
Pregnancy Category: D
Versed **(C-IV) (Rx)**

See also *Anti-Anxiety/Antimanic Drugs,* Chapter 40.

How Supplied: *Injection:* 1 mg/mL, 5 mg/mL

Action/Kinetics: Midazolam is a short-acting benzodiazepine with sedative–general anesthetic properties. The drug depresses the response of the respiratory system to carbon dioxide stimulation; this effect is more pronounced in clients with COPD. There may be mild to moderate decreases in CO, mean arterial BP, SV, and systemic vascular resistance. The effect on HR may rise somewhat in clients with slow HRs (<65/min) and decrease in others (especially those with HRs more than 85/min). **Onset, IM:** 15 min; **IV:** 2–2.5 min for induction (if combined with a preanesthetic narcotic, induction is about 1.5 min). If preanesthetic medication (morphine) is given, the **Peak plasma levels, IM:** 45 min. **Maximum effect:** 30–60 min. **Time to recovery:** Usually within 2 hr, although up to 6 hr may be required. About 97% bound to plasma protein. **t½, elimination:** 1.2–12.3 hr. The drug is rapidly metabolized in the liver to inactive compounds which are excreted through the urine.

Uses: IV: Induction of general anesthesia; before administration of other anesthetics; supplement to balanced anesthesia for surgical procedures of short duration. Midazolam should be used for conscious sedation (e.g., prior to short diagnostic or endoscopic procdures) only by personnel skilled in early detection of underventilation, maintaining a patent airway, and supporting ventilation. **IM:**

Preoperative sedation; to impair memory of events surrounding surgery. *Investigational:* IV for conscious sedation prior to certain dental or minor surgical procedures (may be preferable to diazepam due to faster onset, more consistent anterograde amnesia, and lack of venous complications). IV as an adjunct to local or regional anesthesia for some diagnostic and therapeutic procedures (e.g., sedation in clients receiving subarachnoid or epidural anesthesia).

Dosage

- **IM, IV**

Preoperative sedation, memory impairment for events surrounding surgery.

Adults: 0.07–0.08 mg/kg IM (average: 5 mg) 1 hr before surgery. **Children:** 0.08–0.2 mg/kg.

Conscious sedation for endoscopic or CV procedures in healthy adults, less than 60 years of age.

Using the 1 mg/mL (can be diluted with 0.9% sodium chloride or D5W) product, titrate slowly to the desired effect (usually slurred speech); initial dose should be no higher than 2.5 mg IV (may as low as 1 mg IV) within a 2-min period, after which an additional 2 min should be waited to evaluate the sedative effect. If additional sedation is necessary, small increments should be given waiting an additional 2 min or more after each increment to evaluate the effect. Total doses greater than 5 mg are usually not required. **Children:** Dosage must be individualized by the physician.

Conscious sedation for endoscopic or CV procedures in debilitated or chronically ill clients or clients aged 60 or over.

Slowly titrate to the desired effect using no more than 1.5 mg initially IV (may be as little as 1 mg IV) given over a 2-min period after which an additional 2 min or more should be waited to evaluate the effect. If additional sedation is needed, no more than 1 mg should be given over 2 min; wait an additional 2 min or more after each increment in dose. Total doses greater than 3.5 mg are usually not needed.

Induction of general anesthesia, before use of other general anesthetics, in unmedicated clients.

Adults, unmedicated clients up to 55 years of age, IV, initial: 0.2–0.35 mg/kg given over 5–30 sec, waiting 2 min for effects to occur. If needed, increments of about 25% of the initial dose can be used to complete induction; or, induction can be completed using a volatile liquid anesthetic. Up to 0.6 mg/kg may be used but recovery will be prolonged. **Adults, unmedicated clients over 55 years of age who are good risk surgical clients, initial IV:** 0.15–0.3 mg/kg given over 20–30 sec. **Adults, unmedicated clients over 55 years of age with severe systemic disease or debilitation, initial IV:** 0.15–0.25 mg/kg given over 20–30 sec. **Pediatric:** 0.05–0.2 mg/kg IV.

Induction of general anesthesia, before use of other general anesthetics, in medicated clients.

Adults, premedicated clients up to 55 years of age, IV, initial: 0.15–0.35 mg/kg. If less than 55 years of age, 0.25 mg/kg may be given over 20–30 sec allowing 2 min for effect. **Adults, premedicated over 55 years of age who are good risk surgical clients, initial, IV:** 0.2 mg/kg. **Adults, premedicated over 55 years of age with severe systemic disease or debilitation, initial, IV:** 0.15 mg/kg may be sufficient.

Maintenance of balanced anesthesia for short surgical procedures.

IV: Incremental injections about 25% of the dose used for induction when signs indicate anesthesia is lightening.

NOTE: Narcotic preanesthetic medication may include fentanyl, 1.5–2 mcg/kg IV 5 min before induction; morphine, up to 0.15 mg/kg IM; meperidine, up to 1 mg/kg IM; or, Innovar, 0.02 mL/kg IM. Sedative preanesthetic medication may include secobarbital sodium, 200 mg

PO or hydroxyzine pamoate, 100 mg PO. Except for fentanyl, all preanesthetic medications should be given 1 hr prior to midazolam. Doses should always be individualized.

Administration/Storage

1. When used for conscious sedation, the drug should not be given by rapid or single bolus IV administration.
2. When used for induction of general anesthesia, the initial dose of midazolam should be given over 20–30 sec.
3. If preanesthetic medications with a depressant component are given (e.g., narcotic analgesics or CNS depressants), the midazolam dosage should be reduced by 50% compared with healthy, young unmedicated clients.
4. Maintenance doses to all clients should be given in increments of 25% of the dose first required to achieve the sedative endpoint.
5. When used for procedures via the mouth, a topical anesthetic should also be used.
6. A narcotic preanesthetic should be given for bronchoscopic procedures.
7. All IV doses should be carefully monitored with the immediate availability of oxygen, resuscitative equipment, and personnel who are skilled in maintaining a patent airway and for support of ventilation.
8. IM doses should be given in a large muscle mass.

Contraindications: Hypersensitivity to benzodiazepines. Acute narrow-angle glaucoma. Use in obstetrics. Not to be given to clients in coma, shock, or in acute alcohol intoxication where VS are depressed. IA injection.

Special Concerns: Use with caution during lactation. Safety and effectiveness have not been determined in children less than 18 years of age. Hypotension may be more common in conscious sedation clients who have received a preanesthetic narcotic. Geriatric and debilitated clients require lower doses to induce anesthesia and they are more prone to side effects. IV midazolam should be used with extreme caution in clients with severe fluid or electrolyte disturbances.

Side Effects: Fluctuations in VS (including decreased respiratory rate and tidal volume) are common. The following are general side effects regardless of the route of administration. *Respiratory:* ***IV use has resulted in respiratory depression and respiratory arrest when used for conscious sedation.*** *CV:* Hypotension, cardiac arrest. *CNS:* Confusion, retrograde amnesia, euphoria, nervousness, agitation, anxiety, argumentativeness, restlessness, emergence delirium, increased time for emergence, dreaming during emergence, nightmares, insomnia, ***tonic-clonic seizures,*** ataxia, muscle tremor, involuntary or athetoid movements, dizziness, dysphoria, dysphonia, slurred speech, paresthesia. *GI:* Acid taste, retching, excessive salivation. *Ophthalmologic:* Double vision, blurred vision, nystagmus, pinpoint pupils, visual disturbances, cyclic eyelid movements, difficulty in focusing. *Dermatologic:* Hives, swelling or feeling of burning, warmth or cold feeling at injection site, hive-like wheal at injection site, pruritus, rash. *Miscellaneous:* Blocked ears, loss of balance, chills, weakness, faint feeling, lethargy, yawning, toothache, hematoma.

More common following IM use: Pain at injection site, headache, induration and redness, muscle stiffness.

More common following IV use: *Respiratory:* ***Bronchospasm,*** dyspnea, laryngospasm, hyperventilation, shallow respirations, tachypnea, airway obstruction, wheezing. *CV:* PVCs, bigeminy, tachycardia, vasovagal episode, nodal rhythm. *GI:* Hiccoughs, N&V. *At injection site:* Tenderness, pain, redness, induration, phlebitis. *Miscellaneous:* Drowsiness, oversedation, coughing, headache.

Drug Interactions

Alcohol / ↑ Risk of apnea or underventilation

Anesthetics, inhalation / Dose should be reduced if midazolam used as an induction agent

CNS Depressants / ↑ Risk of apnea or underventilation
Droperidol / ↑ Hypnotic effect of midazolam when used as a premedication
Fentanyl / ↑ Hypnotic effect of midazolam when used as a premedication
Meperidine / See *Narcotics;* also, ↑ Risk of hypotension
Narcotics / ↑ Hypnotic effect of midazolam when used as premedications

NURSING CONSIDERATIONS

See also *Nursing Considerations* for *Anti-Anxiety/Antimanic Drugs,* Chapter 40.

Interventions

1. Ensure that client understands reasons for medication and reassure that memory of procedure may be minimal.
2. The client should be monitored constantly for early signs of respiratory distress or apnea, which can lead to cardiac arrest or hypoxia. Monitoring should continue during the recovery period.

Client/Family Teaching

1. Drug may cause dizziness and drowsiness. Avoid activities that require mental alertness for 24 hr following drug administration.
2. Avoid alcohol and any other CNS depressants for 24 hr following drug administration unless specifically prescribed.

Evaluate: Desired level of sedation and amnesia.

Oxazepam

(ox-**AY**-zeh-pam)
Pregnancy Category: D
Apo-Oxazepam ✱, Serax **(C-IV) (Rx)**

See also *Anti-Anxiety/Antimanic Drugs,* Chapter 40.

How Supplied: *Capsule:* 10 mg, 15 mg, 30 mg; *Tablet:* 15 mg

Action/Kinetics: Absorbed more slowly than most benzodiazepines. **Peak plasma levels:** 2–4 hr. **$t^{1}/_{2}$:** 5–20 hr. Broken down in the liver to inactive metabolites, which are excreted through both the urine and feces. Drug is reputed to cause less drowsiness than chlordiazepoxide.

Uses: Anxiety, tension, anxiety with depression. Adjunct in acute alcohol withdrawal.

Dosage

- **Capsules, Tablets**

Anxiety, mild to moderate.

Adults: 10–30 mg t.i.d.–q.i.d.

Anxiety, tension, irritability, agitation.

Geriatric and debilitated clients: 10 mg t.i.d.; can be increased to 15 mg t.i.d.–q.i.d.

Alcohol withdrawal.

Adults: 15–30 mg t.i.d.–q.i.d.

Special Concerns: Dosage has not been established in children less than 12 years of age; use is not recommended in children less than 6 years of age.

Additional Side Effects: Paradoxical reactions characterized by sleep disorders and hyperexcitability during first weeks of therapy. Hypotension has occurred with parenteral administration.

NURSING CONSIDERATIONS

See also *Nursing Considerations* for *Anti-Anxiety/Antimanic Drugs,* Chapter 40.

Client/Family Teaching

1. Caution that drug may cause dizziness and drowsiness and to use caution until drug effects realized.
2. Report any persistant insomnia or hyperactivity.

Evaluate

- Reports of ↓ symptoms of anxiety and tension
- Control of alcohol withdrawal symptoms

Quazepam

(**KWAY**-zeh-pam)
Pregnancy Category: X
Doral **(Rx) (C-IV)**

See also *Anti-Anxiety/Antimanic Drugs,* Chapter 40.

How Supplied: *Tablet:* 7.5 mg, 15 mg

Action/Kinetics: The drug will improve sleep induction time, duration of sleep, number of nocturnal awakenings, occurrence of early morning awakening, and sleep quality without producing an effect on REM sleep. Hangover effects are minimal. **Peak plasma levels:** 2 hr. Quazepam and two of its metabolites (2-oxoquazepam and N-desalkyl-2-oxoquazepam) are active on the CNS. **t½, quazepam and 2-oxoquazepam:** 39 hr; **t½, N-desalkyl-2-oxoquazepam:** 73 hr. Significantly (95%) bound to plasma protein.

Use: Insomnia characterized by difficulty in falling asleep, frequent nocturnal awakenings, and/or early morning awakenings.

Dosage

• **Tablets**

Adults, initial: 15 mg until individual response has been determined. The dose may be reduced to 7.5 mg in some clients (especially in geriatric or debilitated clients).

Contraindications: Clients with established sleep apnea. Lactation.

Special Concerns: Use with caution in clients with impaired renal or hepatic function, in chronic pulmonary insufficiency, and in depression. Safety and effectiveness have not been established in children less than 18 years of age. Use during lactation may cause sedation and feeding problems in the infant. Geriatric and debilitated clients may be more sensitive to the effects of quazepam.

NURSING CONSIDERATIONS

See also *Nursing Considerations* for *Anti-Anxiety/Antimanic Drugs,* Chapter 40.

Client/Family Teaching

1. Take only as directed. Do not increase the dose of quazepam without approval.
2. Do not drive a car or operate potentially dangerous machinery until sedative effects are realized.
3. The drug may produce daytime sedation even for several days after it has been discontinued.
4. Do not use alcohol or any other drugs having CNS depressant effects.
5. Drug is generally for short-term use. Stress not to stop taking the drug abruptly following prolonged and regular use.
6. Explore sleeping habits and offer alternative methods to induce sleep and ensure adequate rest such as relaxation techniques or white noise simulators.

Evaluate: Improved sleeping patterns with less frequent night time awakenings.

Temazepam

(teh-**MAZ**-eh-pam)

Pregnancy Category: X

Restoril **(C-IV) (Rx)**

See also *Anti-Anxiety/Antimanic Drugs,* Chapter 40.

How Supplied: *Capsule:* 7.5 mg, 15 mg, 30 mg

Action/Kinetics: Temazepam is a benzodiazepine derivative. Disturbed nocturnal sleep may occur the first one or two nights following discontinuance of the drug. Prolonged administration is not recommended because physical dependence and tolerance may develop. See also *Flurazepam,* p. 650. **Peak blood levels:** 2–4 hr. **t½, initial:** 0.4–0.6 hr; **final:** 10 hr. **Steady-state plasma levels:** 382 ng/mL (2.5 hr after 30-mg dose). Accumulation of the drug is minimal following multiple dosage. Significantly bound (98%) to plasma protein. The drug is metabolized in the liver to inactive metabolites.

Uses: Insomnia in clients unable to fall asleep, with frequent awakenings during the night and/or early morning awakenings.

Dosage

• **Capsules**

Adults, usual: 15–30 mg at bedtime. **In elderly or debilitated clients, initial:** 15 mg; **then,** adjust dosage to response.

Contraindications: Pregnancy (category: X).
Special Concerns: Use with caution in severely depressed clients. Use during lactation may cause sedation and feeding problems in the infant. Geriatric clients may be more sensitive to the effects of temazepam.
Side Effects: *CNS:* Drowsiness (after daytime use) and dizziness are common. Lethargy, confusion, euphoria, weakness, ataxia, lack of concentration, hallucinations. In some clients, paradoxical excitement (less than 0.5%), including stimulation and hyperactivity, occurs. *GI:* Anorexia, diarrhea. *Other:* Tremors, horizontal nystagmus, falling, palpitations. Rarely, blood dyscrasias.

NURSING CONSIDERATIONS

See also *Nursing Considerations* for *Anti-Anxiety/Antimanic Drugs,* Chapter 40.
Assessment
1. Document indications for therapy and onset of symptoms.
2. Assess sleep patterns, and assist client to identify factors that may cause insomnia and frequent awakenings.
Client/Family Teaching
1. Take only as directed. Do not increase dose as improvement may not be evident for several days.
2. May cause daytime drowsiness. Avoid activities that require mental alertness until drug effects are realized.
3. Avoid alcohol and CNS depressants because they tend to increase feelings of depression.
4. Avoid cigarette smoking because this decreases drug's effect.
5. For short-term use only. Long-term use can cause dependence and withdrawal symptoms. After more than 3 weeks of continuous use client may experience rebound insomnia.
Evaluate: Improved sleeping patterns with less frequent awakenings.

Triazolam

(try-**AYZ**-oh-lam)
Pregnancy Category: X
Apo-Triazo ✱, Gen-Triazolam ✱, Halcion, Novo-Triolam ✱, Nu-Triazo ✱
(C-IV) (Rx)

See also *Anti-Anxiety/Antimanic Drugs,* Chapter 40.
How Supplied: *Tablet:* 0.125 mg, 0.25 mg
Action/Kinetics: Triazolam decreases sleep latency, increases the duration of sleep, and decreases the number of awakenings. **Time to peak plasma levels:** 0.5–2 hr. **t½:** 1.5–5.5 hr. Metabolized in liver and inactive metabolites excreted in the urine.
Uses: Insomnia (short-term management, not to exceed 1 month). May be beneficial in preventing or treating transient insomnia from a sudden change in sleep schedule.

Dosage
- **Tablets**

Adults, initial: 0.25–0.5 mg before bedtime. **Geriatric or debilitated clients, initial:** 0.125 mg; **then,** depending on response, 0.125–0.25 mg before bedtime.
Special Concerns: Safety and efficacy in children under 18 years of age not established. Use during lactation may cause sedation and feeding problems in the infant. Geriatric clients may be more sensitive to the effects of triazolam.
Side Effects: *CNS:* Rebound insomnia, anterograde amnesia, headache, ataxia, decreased coordination. Psychologic and physical dependence. *GI:* N&V.

NURSING CONSIDERATIONS

See also *Nursing Considerations* for *Anti-Anxiety/Antimanic Drugs,* Chapter 40.
Interventions
1. Assess client for tolerance and for psychologic and physical dependence.

2. When client suffers from simple insomnia, try warm baths, warm milk, and other interventions to induce sleep, such as soft music, guided imagery, or progressive muscle relaxation.
3. Evaluate and document sleep patterns. Attempt to determine underlying cause of insomnia so that source may be removed.
4. Initiate safety precautions (i.e., side rails up, supervised ambulation, frequent observations) at bedtime, especially with elderly clients and confused clients.
5. Monitor closely for CNS toxic effects especially during prolonged therapy (longer than 2 weeks).

Client/Family Teaching

1. Avoid the use of alcoholic beverages and other CNS depressants.
2. Use caution when driving or operating machinery until daytime sedative effects have been evaluated.
3. Advise that drug is for short-term use only, as it may cause physical and psychologic dependence. Try warm baths, warm milk, and other methods to induce sleep, such as white noise simulator, guided imagery, or progressive muscle relaxation rather than become dependent on drugs for insomnia.
4. Report immediately any unusual side effects including hallucinations, nightmares, depression, or periods of confusion.

Evaluate: Improved sleeping patterns with relief from insomnia.

CHAPTER FORTY-ONE

Non-Narcotic Analgesics/ Antipyretics

See the following individual entries:

Acetaminophen
Acetaminophen Buffered
Acetylsalicylic Acid
Acetylsalicylic Acid Buffered
Aspirin Free Excedrin
Darvocet-N 50 and 100
Darvon Compound 65
Equagesic
Excedrin Extra Strength
Excedrin P.M.
Mesalamine
Olsalazine Sodium
Sinus Excedrin

Acetaminophen (Apap, Paracetamol)

(ah-**SEAT**-ah-**MIN**-oh-fen)

Capsules: Anacin-3 ♣, Anacin-3 Extra Strength ♣, Panadol, Apacet Extra Strength, Meda Cap, Ty-Tab. **Granules:** Snaplets-FR Granules. **Oral Solution/Elixir:** Aceta, Actamin, Actamin Extra, Alba-Temp 300, Apacet Oral Solution, Atasol ♣, Children's Anacin-3 Elixir, Children's Genapap Elixir, Children's Panadol, Children's Tylenol Elixir, Children's Tylenol Suspension Liquid, Dolanex, Dorcal Children's Fever and Pain Reducer, Genapap, Halenol Elixir, Infants' Anacin-3, Infants' Genapap, Infants' Tylenol, Infants' Tylenol Suspension Drops, Liquiprin Children's Elixir, Myapap, Myapap Elixir, Oraphen-PD, Panadol, Pedric, PMS Acetaminophen ♣, Robigesic ♣, St. Joseph Aspirin-Free Fever Reducer for Children, Tempra, Tenol, Tylenol, Tylenol Extra Strength, Valdol Liquid. **Oral Suspension:** Liquiprin Infants' Drops. **Tablets:** 222 AF ♣, Aceta, Actamin, Actamin Extra, Aminofen, Aminofen Max, Anacin-3, Anacin-3 Extra Strength, Anacin-3 Maximum Strength Caplets, Apacet, Apacet Extra Strength, Apacet Extra Strength Caplets, Apo-Acetaminophen ♣, Atasol ♣, Atasol Caplets ♣, Atasol Forte ♣, Atasol Forte Caplets ♣, Banesin, Conacetol, Dapa, Datril Extra-Strength, Datril Extra-Strength Caplets, Genapap, Genapap Extra Strength, Genapap Extra Strength Caplets, Genebs, Genebs Extra Strength, Genebs Extra Strength Caplets, Halenol, Halenol Extra Strength, Halenol Extra Strength Caplets, Meda Tab, Neo-Dol ♣, Panadol, Panadol Caplets, Panadol Junior Strength Caplets, Panex, Panex-500, Phenaphen Caplets, PMS-Acetaminophen ♣, Robigesic ♣, Rounox ♣, Tapanol, Tapanol Extra Strength, Tapanol Extra Strength Caplets, Tapar, Tenol, Tylenol, Tylenol Caplets, Tylenol Extended Relief Caplets, Tylenol Extra Strength, Tylenol Extra Strength Caplets, Tylenol Extra Strength Gelcaps, Tylenol Junior Strength Caplets, Ty-Tab, Ty-Tab Caplets, Ty-Tab Extra Strength, Valadol, Valorin, Valorin Extra. **Tablets, Chewable:** Children's Anacin-3, Children's Genapap, Children's Panadol, Children's Tylenol, Children's Ty-Tab, Panadol ♣, St. Joseph Aspirin-Free Fever Reducer for Children, Tempra, Tempra Double Strength. **Suppositories:** Abenol ♣, Acephen, Children's Feverall, Feverall, Infant's Feverall, Junior Strength Feverall, Neopap, Suppap-120, Suppap-325, Suppap-650. **Wafers:** Pedric. **(OTC)**

Acetaminophen, buffered

(ah-**SEAT**-ah-**MIN**-oh-fen)
Bromo Seltzer **(OTC)**

How Supplied: *Capsule:* 80 mg, 160 mg, 325 mg, 500 mg, 650 mg; *Chew tablet:* 80 mg, 160 mg; *Elixir:* 120 mg/5 mL, 160 mg/5 mL; *Liquid:* 80 mg/2.5 mL, 120 mg/3.75 mL, 160 mg/5 mL, 325 mg/5 mL, 500 mg/15 mL; *Powder for reconstitution:* 950 mg; *Solution:* 80 mg/0.8 mL, 120 mg/2.5 mL, 160 mg/mL; *Suppository:* 80 mg, 120 mg, 325 mg, 650 mg; *Suspension:* 160 mg/5 mL; *Tablet:* 65 mg, 80 mg, 160 mg, 325 mg, 500 mg, 648 mg, 650 mg; *Tablet, Extended Release:* 650 mg

Acetaminophen, buffered: *Granule, effervescent*

Action/Kinetics: The only para-aminophenol derivative currently used is acetaminophen. It decreases fever by an effect on the hypothalamus leading to sweating and vasodilation. Acetaminophen also inhibits the effect of pyrogens on the hypothalamic heat-regulating centers. It may cause analgesia by inhibiting CNS prostaglandin synthesis; however, due to minimal effects on peripheral prostaglandin synthesis, acetaminophen has no anti-inflammatory or uricosuric effects. It does not manifest any anticoagulant effect and does not produce ulceration of the GI tract. The magnitude of its antipyretic and analgesic effects is comparable to that of aspirin.

Peak plasma levels: 30–120 min. **t½:** 45 min–3 hr. **Therapeutic serum levels** (analgesia): 5–20 mcg/mL. **Plasma protein binding:** Approximately 25%. Acetaminophen is metabolized in the liver and is excreted in the urine as glucuronide and sulfate conjugates. However, an intermediate hydroxylated metabolite is hepatotoxic following large doses of acetaminophen.

Acetaminophen is often combined with other drugs, as in Darvocet-N, Parafon Forte, Phenaphen with Codeine, and Tylenol with Codeine.

The buffered product is a mixture of acetaminophen, sodium bicarbonate, and citric acid that effervesces when placed in water. This product has a high sodium content (0.76 g/¾ capful).

Uses: Control of pain due to headache, dysmenorrhea, arthralgia, myalgia, musculoskeletal pain, immunizations, teething, tonsillectomy. To reduce fever in bacterial or viral infections. As a substitute for aspirin in upper GI disease, aspirin allergy, bleeding disorders, clients on anticoagulant therapy, and gouty arthritis. *Investigational:* In children receiving diptheria-pertussis-tetany vaccination to decrease incidence of fever and pain at injection site.

Dosage

- **Capsules, Granules, Elixir, Oral Solution, Oral Suspension, Tablets, Wafers**

Analgesic, antipyretic.

Adults: 325–650 mg q 4 hr; doses up to 1 g q.i.d. may be used. Daily dosage should not exceed 4 g. **Pediatric:** Doses given 4–5 times/day. **Up to 3 months:** 40 mg/dose; **4–12 months:** 80 mg/dose; **1–2 years:** 120 mg/dose; **2–3 years:** 160 mg/dose; **4–5 years:** 240 mg/dose; **6–8 years:** 320 mg/dose; **9–10 years:** 400 mg/dose; **11–12 years:** 480 mg/dose. *Alternative pediatric dose:* 10 mg/kg q 4 hr.

- **Extended Relief Caplets**

Analgesic, antipyretic.

Adults: 2 caplets (1,300 mg) q 8 hr.

- **Suppositories**

Analgesic, antipyretic.

Adults: 325–650 mg q 4 hr or 650–1,000 mg q 6 hr, not to exceed 4 g/day for up to 10 days. Clients on long-term therapy should not exceed 2.6 g/day. **Pediatric, up to 2 years:** Physician should be consulted; **2–4 years:** 160 mg q 4 hr; **4–6 years:** 240 mg q 4 hr; **6–9 years:** 320 mg q 4 hr; **9–11 years:** 320–400 mg q 4 hr; **11–12 years:** 320– 480 mg q 4 hr. Dosage should be given as needed while symptoms persist. Children up to 12 years of age should receive no more than five doses in a 24-hr period unless prescribed by a physician.

BUFFERED

Analgesic, antipyretic.

Adult, usual: 1 or 2 three-quarter capfuls are placed into an empty glass; add half a glass of cool water. May be taken while fizzing or after settling. Can be repeated q 4 hr as required or directed by physician.

Administration/Storage

1. Suppositories should be stored below 80°F (27°C).

2. *Treatment of Overdose:* Initially, induction of emesis, gastric lavage, activated charcoal. Oral *N*-acetylcysteine (see p. 238) is said to reduce or prevent hepatic damage by inactivating acetaminophen metabolites, which cause liver toxicity. CNS stimulation, excitement, and delirium are symptoms of toxicity.

Contraindications: Renal insufficiency, anemia. Clients with cardiac or pulmonary disease are more susceptible to toxic effects of acetaminophen.

Special Concern: Evidence indicates that acetaminophen may have to be used with caution in pregnancy.

Side Effects: Few when taken in usual therapeutic doses. Chronic and even acute toxicity can develop after long symptom-free usage. *Hematologic:* Methemoglobinemia, ***hemolytic anemia***, neutropenia, thrombocytopenia, pancytopenia, leukopenia. *Allergic:* Skin rashes, fever. *Miscellaneous:* CNS stimulation, hypoglycemia, jaundice, drowsiness, glossitis.

Symptoms of Overdose: There may be few initial symptoms. ***Hepatic toxicity.*** *CNS:* CNS stimulation, general malaise, delirium followed by depression, ***seizures, coma, death.*** *GI:* N&V, diarrhea, gastric upset. *Miscellaneous:* Sweating, chills, fever, vascular collapse.

Drug Interactions

Alcohol, ethyl / Chronic use of alcohol ↑ toxicity of larger therapeutic doses of acetaminophen

Anticoagulants, oral / Acetaminophen may ↑ hypoprothrombinemic effect

Barbiturates / ↑ Potential of hepatotoxicity due to ↑ breakdown of acetaminophen by liver

Carbamazepine / ↓ Potential of hepatotoxicity due to ↑ breakdown of acetaminophen by liver

Diflunisal / ↑ Plasma levels of acetaminophen

Caffeine / ↑ Analgesic effect of acetaminophen

Chloramphenicol / Acetaminophen ↑ serum chloramphenicol levels

Hydantoins / ↑ Potential of hepatotoxicity due to ↑ breakdown of acetaminophen by liver

Oral contraceptives / ↑ Breakdown of acetaminophen by liver

Phenobarbital / ↑ Potential of hepatotoxicity due to ↑ breakdown of acetaminophen by liver

Phenytoin / ↑ Potential of hepatotoxicity due to ↑ breakdown of acetaminophen by liver

Sulfinpyrazone / ↑ Potential of hepatotoxicity due to ↑ breakdown of acetaminophen by liver

NURSING CONSIDERATIONS

Assessment

1. If the client is to receive long-term therapy, liver function studies should be conducted prior to initiating drug therapy.

2. Document presence of fever. Question client concerning pain, noting type, location, duration, and intensity.

Interventions

1. Note any bluish coloration of the mucosa and nailbeds or client complaints of dyspnea, weakness, headache, or vertigo. These symptoms of methemoglobinemia are caused by anoxia and require immediate attention.

2. Observe for pallor, weakness, and complaints of heart palpitations. Document and report as these symptoms may signal the presence of hemolytic anemia.

3. To assess for evidence of nephritis, check urine for occult blood and the presence of albumin, especially when client is receiving long-term drug therapy.

4. Clients complaining of dyspnea; rapid, weak pulse; cold extremities; or feeling clammy or sweaty; or with subnormal temperatures may be displaying symptoms of chronic poisoning. Any unusual complaints and symptoms observed during drug therapy should be reported immediately.

Client/Family Teaching

1. Provide printed information and teach symptoms of acute toxicity that require immediate reporting such as N&V and abdominal pain.
2. Review signs that may indicate possible chronic overdose of medication, such as unexplained bleeding, bruising, sore throat, malaise, and fever.
3. Phenacetin, the major active metabolite of acetaminophen, may cause the urine to become dark brown or wine-colored.
4. Teach clients to read the labels on all OTC preparations they consume. Many contain acetaminophen and, as a result, can produce toxic reactions if taken over time with the prescribed drug.
5. Explain that so-called headache and minor pain relievers containing combinations of salicylates, acetaminophen, and caffeine may be no more beneficial than aspirin alone and that such combinations may be more dangerous. When in doubt consult provider.
6. Any pain or fever that persists for longer than 3–5 days requires medical evaluation.

Evaluate

- ↓ Fever
- Relief of pain

Acetylsalicylic acid (ASA, Aspirin)

(ah-**SEE**-till-sal-ih-**SILL**-ick **AH**-sid)

Pregnancy Category: C

Apo-Asa 🍁, Artria SR 🍁, Aspergum, Aspirin, Bayer Children's Aspirin, Easprin, Ecotrin Caplets and Tablets, Ecotrin Maximum Strength Caplets and Tablets, Empirin, Entrophen 🍁, Genprin, Genuine Bayer Aspirin Caplets and Tablets, Halfprin, 8-Hour Bayer Timed-Release Caplets, Maximum Bayer Aspirin Caplets and Tablets, Norwich Aspirin, Norwich Extra Strength, Novasen 🍁, PMS-ASA 🍁, St. Joseph Adult Chewable Aspirin, Supasa 🍁, Therapy Bayer Caplets, ZOR-prin **(OTC)** (Easprin and ZOR-prin are Rx)

Acetylsalicylic acid, buffered

(ah-**SEE**-till-sal-ih-**SILL**-ick **AH**-sid)

Pregnancy Category: C

Alka-Seltzer with Aspirin, Alka-Seltzer with Aspirin (flavored), Alka-Seltzer Extra Strength with Aspirin, Arthritis Pain Formula, Arthritis Strength Bufferin, Ascriptin Regular Strength, Ascriptin A/D, Bayer Buffered, Buffered Aspirin, Bufferin, Bufferin Extra Strength, Buffex, Cama Arthritis Pain Reliever, Magnaprin, Magnaprin Arthritis Strength Captabs, Tri-Buffered Bufferin Caplets and Tablets, Wesprin Buffered **(OTC)**

How Supplied: *Capsule:* 325 mg; *Chew tablet:* 80 mg, 81 mg; *Enteric coated tablet:* 81 mg, 162 mg, 324 mg, 325 mg, 500 mg, 650 mg, 975 mg; *Gum:* 227 mg; *Suppository:* 60 mg, 120 mg, 125 mg, 200 mg, 300 mg, 325 mg, 600 mg, 650 mg; *Tablet:* 81 mg, 324 mg, 325 mg, 486 mg, 500 mg, 650 mg; *Tablet, Extended Release:* 650 mg, 800 mg, 975 mg

Action/Kinetics: Aspirin manifests antipyretic, anti-inflammatory, and analgesic effects. The antipyretic effect is due to an action on the hypothalamus, resulting in heat loss by vasodilation of peripheral blood vessels and promoting sweating. The anti-inflammatory effects are probably mediated through inhibition of cyclo-oxygenase, which results in a decrease in prostaglandin synthesis and other mediators of the pain response. Prostaglandins have been implicated in the inflammatory process, as well as in mediation of pain. Thus, if levels are decreased, the inflammatory reaction may subside. The mechanism of action for the analgesic effects of aspirin is not known fully but is partly attributable to improvement of the inflammatory condition. Aspirin also produces inhibition of platelet aggregation by decreasing the synthesis of endoperoxides and thromboxanes—substances that mediate platelet aggregation.

Large doses of aspirin (5 g/day or more) increase uric acid secretion, while low doses (2 g/day or less) decrease uric acid secretion. However, aspirin antagonizes drugs used to treat gout.

Aspirin is rapidly absorbed after PO administration. Aspirin is hydrolyzed to the active salicylic acid, which is 70%–90% protein bound. For arthritis and rheumatic disease, blood levels of 150–300 mcg/mL should be maintained. For analgesic and antipyretic, blood levels of 25– 50 mcg/mL should be achieved. For acute rheumatic fever, blood levels of 150–300 mcg/mL should be achieved. **Therapeutic salicylic acid serum levels:** 150–300 mcg/mL, although tinnitus occurs at serum levels above 200 mcg/mL and serious toxicity above 400 mcg/mL. **t½:** aspirin, 15–20 min; salicylic acid, 2–20 hr, depending on the dose. Salicylic acid and metabolites are excreted by the kidney. The bioavailability of enteric-coated salicylate products may be poor. The addition of antacids (buffered aspirin) may decrease GI irritation and increase the dissolution and absorption of such products.

Aspirin is found in many combination products including Darvon Compound, Empirin Compound Plain and with Codeine, Equagesic, Fiorinal Plain and with Codeine, Norgesic and Norgesic Forte, and Synalgos DC.

Uses: Pain arising from integumental structures, myalgias, neuralgias, arthralgias, headache, dysmenorrhea, and similar types of pain. Antipyretic. Anti-inflammatory agent in conditions such as arthritis, osteoarthritis, SLE, acute rheumatic fever, gout, and many other conditions. Mucocutaneous lymph node syndrome (Kawasaki disease). Aspirin is also used to reduce the risk of recurrent transient ischemic attacks and strokes in men. Decrease risk of death from nonfatal MI in clients who have a history of infarction or who manifest unstable angina; aortocoronary bypass surgery. Gout. May be effective in less severe postoperative and postpartum pain; pain secondary to trauma and cancer. *Investigational:* Chronic use to prevent cataract formation; low doses to prevent toxemia of pregnancy; in pregnant women with inadequate uteroplacental blood flow. Reduce colon cancer mortality (low doses).

Dosage

• Gum, Chewable Tablets, Coated Tablets, Effervescent Tablets, Enteric-Coated Tablets, Suppositories, Tablets, Timed (Controlled) Release Tablets

Analgesic, antipyretic.

Adults: 325–500 mg q 3 hr, 325–600 mg q 4 hr, or 650–1,000 mg q 6 hr. As an alternative, the adult chewable tablet (81 mg each) may be used in doses of 4–8 tablets q 4 hr as needed. **Pediatric:** 65 mg/kg/day (alternate dose: 1.5 g/m²/day) in divided doses q 4–6 hr, not to exceed 3.6 g/day. Alternatively, the following dosage regimen can be used: **Pediatric, 2–3 years:** 162 mg q 4 hr as needed; **4–5 years:** 243 mg q 4 hr as needed; **6–8 years:** 320–325 mg q 4 hr as needed; **9–10 years:** 405 mg q 4 hr as needed; **11 years:** 486 mg q 4 hr as needed; **12–14 years:** 648 mg q 4 hr.

Arthritis, rheumatic diseases.

Adults: 3.2–6 g/day in divided doses.

Juvenile rheumatoid arthritis.

60–110 mg/kg/day (alternate dose: 3 g/m²) in divided doses q 6–8 hr. When initiating therapy at 60 mg/kg/day, dose may be increased by 20 mg/kg/day after 5–7 days and by 10 mg/kg/day after another 5–7 days.

Acute rheumatic fever.

Adults, initial: 5–8 g/day. **Pediatric, initial,** 100 mg/kg/day (3 g/m²/day) for 2 weeks; **then,** decrease to 75 mg/kg/day for 4–6 weeks.

Transient ischemic attacks in men.

Adults: 650 mg b.i.d. or 325 mg q.i.d. A dose of 300 mg/day may be as effective and with fewer side effects.

Prophylaxis of MI.

Adults: 300 or 325 mg/day (both solid PO dosage forms–regular and buffered as well as buffered aspirin in solution). The adult chewable tablets be also be used.

Kawasaki disease.

Adults: 80–180 mg/kg/day during the febrile period. After the fever resolves, the dose may be adjusted to 10 mg/kg/day.

NOTE: Doses as low as 80–100 mg/day are being studied for use in unstable angina, MI, and aortocoronary bypass surgery.

Administration/Storage

1. Enteric-coated tablets or buffered tablets are better tolerated by some clients.
2. Aspirin should be taken with a full glass of water to prevent lodging of the drug in the esophagus.
3. Have epinephrine available to counteract hypersensitivity reactions should they occur. Asthma caused by hypersensitive reaction to salicylates may be refractory to epinephrine, so antihistamines should also be available for parenteral and PO use.
4. *Treatment of Overdose:* Initially induce vomiting or perform gastric lavage followed by activated charcoal (most effective if given within 2 hr of ingestion). Monitor salicylate levels, acid-base and fluid and electrolyte balance. For seizures, give diazepam. Treat hyperthermia if present. Alkaline diuresis will enhance renal excretion. Hemodialysis is effective but should be reserved for severe poisonings.

Contraindications: Hypersensitivity to salicylates. Clients with asthma, hay fever, or nasal polyps have a higher incidence of hypersensitivity reactions. Severe anemia, history of blood coagulation defects, in conjunction with anticoagulant therapy. Salicylates can cause congestive failure when taken in the large doses used for rheumatic diseases. Vitamin K deficiency; 1 week before and after surgery. In pregnancy, especially the last trimester as the drug may cause problems in the newborn child or complications during delivery. In children or teenagers with chickenpox or flu due to possibility of development of Reye's syndrome.

Controlled-release aspirin is not recommended for use as an antipyretic or short-term analgesic because adequate blood levels may not be reached. Also, controlled-release products are not recommended for children less than 12 years of age and in children with fever accompanied by dehydration.

Special Concerns: Use with caution during lactation. Salicylates are to be used with caution in the presence of gastric or peptic ulcers, in mild diabetes, erosive gastritis or bleeding tendencies, and in clients with cardiac disease. Use with caution in liver or kidney disease. Aspirin products now carry the following labeling: "It is especially important not to use aspirin during the last three months of pregnancy unless specifically directed to do so by a doctor because it may cause problems in the newborn child or complications during delivery."

Laboratory Test Interferences: False + or ↑ : Amylase, AST, ALT, uric acid, PBI, urinary VMA (most tests), catecholamines, urinary glucose (Benedict's, Clinitest), and urinary uric acid (at high doses) values. False – or ↓ : CO_2 content, glucose (fasting), potassium, urinary VMA (Pisano method), and thrombocyte values.

Side Effects: The toxic effects of the salicylates are dose-related. *GI:* Dyspepsia, heartburn, anorexia, nausea, occult blood loss, epigastric discomfort, ***massive GI bleeding, potentiation of peptic ulcer***. *Allergic:* ***Bronchospasm, asthma-like symptoms, anaphylaxis,*** skin rashes, angioedema, urticaria, rhinitis, nasal polyps. *Hematologic:* Prolongation of bleeding time, thrombocytopenia, leukopenia, purpura, shortened erythrocyte survival time, decreased plasma iron levels. *Miscel-*

laneous: Thirst, fever, dimness of vision.

NOTE: Use of aspirin in children and teenagers with flu or chickenpox may result in the development of ***Reye's syndrome***. Also, dehydrated, febrile children are more prone to salicylate intoxication.

Salicylism—mild toxicity. Seen at serum levels between 150 and 200 mcg/mL. *GI:* N&V, diarrhea, thirst. *CNS:* Tinnitus (most common), dizziness, difficulty in hearing, mental confusion, lassitude. *Miscellaneous:* Flushing, sweating, tachycardia. Symptoms of salicylism may be observed with doses used for inflammatory disease or rheumatic fever.

Severe salicylate poisoning. Seen at serum levels over 400 mcg/mL. *CNS:* Excitement, confusion, disorientation, irritability, hallucinations, lethargy, stupor, ***coma, respiratory failure, seizures.*** *Metabolic:* Respiratory alkalosis (initially), respiratory acidosis and metabolic acidosis, dehydration. *GI:* N&V. *Hematologic:* Platelet dysfunction, hypoprothrombinemia, increased capillary fragility. *Miscellaneous:* ***Hyperthermia, hemorrhage, CV collapse, renal failure,*** hyperventilation, pulmonary edema, tetany, hypoglycemia (late).

For treatment, see *Nursing Considerations, Interventions for Salicylate Toxicity.*

Drug Interactions

Acetazolamide / ↑ CNS toxicity of salicylates; also, ↑ excretion of salicylic acid if urine kept alkaline
Alcohol, ethyl / ↑ Chance of GI bleeding caused by salicylates
Alteplase, recombinant / ↑ Risk of bleeding
PAS / Possible ↑ effect of PAS due to ↓ excretion by kidney or ↓ plasma protein binding
Ammonium chloride / ↑ Effect of salicylates by ↑ renal tubular reabsorption
ACE inhibitors / ↓ Effect of ACE inhibitors possibly due to prostaglandin inhibition
Antacids / ↓ Salicylate levels in plasma due to ↑ rate of renal excretion
Anticoagulants, oral / ↑ Effect of anticoagulant by ↓ plasma protein binding and plasma prothrombin
Antirheumatics / Both are ulcerogenic and may cause ↑ GI bleeding
Ascorbic acid / ↑ Effect of salicylates by ↑ renal tubular reabsorption
Beta-adrenergic blocking agents / Salicylates ↓ action of beta-blockers, possibly due to prostaglandin inhibition
Charcoal, activated / ↓ Absorption of salicylates from GI tract
Corticosteroids / Both are ulcerogenic; also, corticosteroids may ↓ blood salicylate levels by ↑ breakdown by liver and ↑ excretion
Dipyridamole / Additive anticoagulant effects
Furosemide / ↑ Chance of salicylate toxicity due to ↓ renal excretion; also, salicylates may ↓ effect of furosemide in clients with impaired renal function or cirrhosis with ascites
Heparin / Inhibition of platelet adhesiveness by aspirin may result in bleeding tendencies
Hypoglycemics, oral / ↑ Hypoglycemia due to ↓ plasma protein binding and ↓ excretion
Indomethacin / Both are ulcerogenic and may cause ↑ GI bleeding
Insulin / Salicylates ↑ hypoglycemic effect of insulin
Methionine / ↑ Effect of salicylates by ↑ renal tubular reabsorption
Methotrexate / ↑ Effect of methotrexate by ↓ plasma protein binding; also, salicylates block renal excretion of methotrexate
Nitroglycerin / Combination may result in unexpected hypotension
Nizatidine / ↑ Serum levels of salicylates
NSAIDs / Additive ulcerogenic effects; also, aspirin may ↓ serum levels of NSAIDs
Phenylbutazone / Combination may produce hyperuricemia

Phenytoin / ↑ Effect of phenytoin by ↓ plasma protein binding
Probenecid / Salicylates inhibit uricosuric activity of probenecid
Sodium bicarbonate / ↓ Effect of salicylates by ↑ rate of excretion
Spironolactone / Aspirin ↓ diuretic effect of spironolactone
Sulfinpyrazone / Salicylates inhibit uricosuric activity of sulfinpyrazone
Sulfonamides / ↑ Effect of sulfonamides by ↑ blood levels of salicylates
Valproic acid / ↑ Effect of valproic acid due to ↓ plasma protein binding

---

NURSING CONSIDERATIONS

Interventions for Salicylate Toxicity

1. If the client has had repeated administration of large doses of salicylates, document and report evidence of hyperventilation or complaints of auditory or visual disturbances (symptoms of salicylism).
2. Severe salicylate poisoning, whether due to overdose or accumulation, will have an exaggerated effect on the CNS and the metabolic system.
• Clients may develop a salicylate jag characterized by garrulous behavior. They may act as if they were inebriated.
• Convulsions and coma may follow.
3. When working with febrile children or the elderly who have been treated with aspirin, maintain adequate fluid intake. These clients are more susceptible to salicylate intoxication if they are dehydrated.
4. Have the following emergency supplies available for treatment of *acute salicylate toxicity:*
• Apomorphine
• Emetics and equipment for gastric lavage
• IV equipment and solutions of dextrose, saline, potassium, and sodium bicarbonate; vitamin K
• Short-acting barbiturates such as pentobarbital or secobarbital to treat convulsions
• Oxygen and a ventilator

Assessment

1. Take a complete drug history and note any evidence of hypersensitivity. Individuals allergic to tartrazine should not take aspirin. Clients who have tolerated salicylates well in the past may suddenly have an allergic or anaphylactoid reaction.
2. If aspirin is being administered for pain, determine the type and pattern of pain, if the pain is unusual, or if it is recurring. Use a rating scale to assess the level of pain. Note the effectiveness of aspirin if used in the past for pain control.
3. Note if client has asthma, hay fever, ulcer disease or nasal polyps.
4. Document age; drug is discouraged in those under 12. Assess the child for chickenpox or the flu.
5. Note any history of peptic ulcers or other conditions that could suggest potential problems with the use of salicylates.
6. Determine if client is to have diagnostic tests. Drug causes irreversible platelet effects. Anticipate 4–7 days for the body to replace these once drug discontinued; hence no salicylates one week prior to procedure.
7. Determine any history of bleeding tendencies. Obtain baseline bleeding parameters if prolonged use is anticipated.
8. Review drugs currently prescribed to determine the potential for drug interactions.
9. The therapeutic serum level of salicylate is 150–300 mcg/mL for adult and juvenile rheumatoid arthritis and acute rheumatic fever.Reassure that the higher dosage is necessary for anti-inflammatory effects.

Interventions

1. Administer salicylates only as specified.
2. Minimize distress by assisting the client to preserve energy and provide a comforting, relaxing environment.
3. When administering for antipyretic effect, obtain written parameters for temperature at which the drug should be administered.
• Obtain temperature 1 hr after ad-

ministering the medication to assess outcome.

• Check for marked diaphoresis, and if present, dry client, change linens, provide fluids, and prevent chilling.

4. Test for blood in the stool and urine and monitor CBC routinely during high-dose and chronic therapy.

5. Observe client receiving anticoagulant therapy for bruises or bleeding of the mucous membranes. Large doses of salicylates may increase the PT and should be avoided.

6. Assess for gastric irritation and related pain.

Client/Family Teaching

1. To reduce gastric irritation, administer with meals, milk, or crackers.

2. Explain that if sodium bicarbonate is to be taken concurrently to lessen gastric irritation it must be prescribed. Sodium bicarbonate may decrease the serum level of aspirin more rapidly than normal, thus reducing the effectiveness of the aspirin.

3. Do not take salicylates if product is off-color or has a strange odor. Note expiration date.

4. Discuss the toxic symptoms to be reported: ringing in the ears, difficulty hearing, dizziness or fainting spells, unusual increase in sweating, severe abdominal pain, or mental confusion.

5. Salicylates potentiate the effects of antidiabetic drugs. Clients with pharmacologically controlled diabetes should monitor their blood glucose levels carefully and report if hypoglycemia occurs.

6. Cardiac clients on large doses of drug should be alert to symptoms of CHF and should report if evident.

7. Remind clients to tell their dentist and other health providers that they are taking salicylates and the reasons for this therapy.

8. Before purchasing other OTC preparations, notify the provider and note the quantity used per day.

9. Salicylates should be administered to children only upon specific medical recommendation.

10. If a child refuses to take the medication or vomits it, discuss the possibility of using aspirin suppositories or acetaminophen.

11. Children who are dehydrated and who have a fever are especially susceptible to aspirin intoxication from even small amounts of aspirin.

12. Report any gastric irritation and pain experienced by the child. These may be symptoms of hypersensitivity or toxicity.

13. Aspirin and aspirin NSAIDs that may interfere with blood-clotting mechanisms (antiplatelet effects) are usually discontinued 1 week before surgery to prevent the risk of postoperative bleeding.

14. Warn clients to avoid indiscriminate use of salicylate drugs.

Evaluate

• Relief of pain and discomfort
• ↓ Fever
• Improved joint mobility and level of functioning

COMBINATION DRUG

Aspirin Free Excedrin
(OTC)

Excedrin Extra Strength
(OTC)

Excedrin P.M.
(OTC)

Sinus Excedrin
(OTC)

See also information on individual components.

How Supplied: See Content

Content: Each Aspirin Free Excedrin caplet contains: *Analgesic/antipyretic:* Acetaminophen, 500 mg. *CNS stimulant:* Caffeine, 65 mg.

Each Excedrin Extra Strength caplet contains: *Analgesic/antipyretic:* Acetaminophen, 250 mg, and Aspirin, 250 mg. *CNS stimulant:* Caffeine, 65 mg.

Each Excedrin P.M. caplet or tablet

contains: *Analgesic/antipyretic:* Acetaminophen, 500 mg. *Antihistamine:* Diphenhydramine citrate, 38 mg.

Each 30 mL Excedrin P.M. liquid contains: *Analgesic/antipyretic:* Acetaminophen, 1000 mg. *Antihistamine:* Diphenhydramine HCl, 50 mg.

Each Sinus Excedrin caplet or tablet contains: *Analgesic/antipyretic:* Acetaminophen, 500 mg. *Decongestant:* Pseudoephedrine HCl, 30 mg.

Uses: *Aspirin Free Excedrin and Excedrin Extra Strength:* Relief of the pain due to headache, sinusitis, colds, muscular aches, menstrual discomfort, toothaches, and minor arthritis pain. *Excedrin P.M.:* Relief of headaches and minor aches and pains with accompanying sleeplessness. *Sinus Excedrin:* Relief of headache, sinus pain and sinus pressure, and congestion due to sinusitis or the common cold.

Dosage

• **Caplets, Tablets**

Aspirin Free Excedrin

Adults and children over 12 years of age: 2 caplets q 6 hr, not to exceed 8 caplets in a 24-hr period.

Excedrin Extra Strength

Adults and children over 12 years of age: 2 caplets or tablets with water q 6 hr, not to exceed 8 caplets or tablets in a 24-hr period.

Excedrin P.M.

Adults: 2 caplets or tablets or 30 mL (2 tablespoons) at bedtime.

Sinus Excedrin

Adults and children over 12 years of age: 2 caplets or tablets q 6 hr, not to exceed 8 caplets or tablets in a 24-hr period.

Administration/Storage

1. These products should not be taken for more than 10 days (for more than 3 days if fever is present).
2. These products should only be taken while symptoms persist.
3. For children under 12 years of age, a physician should be consulted before use.

Contraindications: Aspirin-containing products should not be used in children and teenagers with chickenpox or flu symptoms or in women during the last 3 months of pregnancy. Pseudoephedrine-containing products should not be taken by clients with heart disease, hypertension, thyroid disease, diabetes, or difficulty in urination due to an enlarged prostate. Also, pseudoephedrine-containing products should not be taken by clients on medication for hypertension or depression.

Special Concerns: A physician should be consulted before using these products during pregnancy or lactation.

Side Effects: Higher doses of pseudophedrine-containing products may cause dizziness, nervousness, and sleeplessness.

NURSING CONSIDERATIONS

See also *Nursing Considerations* for individual components.

Assessment

1. Document indications for therapy and type and onset of symptoms.
2. Determine any conditions that may preclude drug therapy.

Evaluate: Relief of pain and discomfort.

COMBINATION DRUG

Darvocet-N 50 and Darvocet-N 100

(**DAR**-voh-set)

(Rx)

How Supplied: See Content

Content: *Nonnarcotic analgesic:* Acetaminophen, 325 (Darvocet-N 50) or 650 mg (Darvocet-N 100). *Analgesic:* Propoxyphene napsylate, 50 or 100 mg.

Uses: Mild to moderate pain (may be used if fever is present).

Dosage

• **Tablets**

Analgesia.

Two Darvocet-N 50 tablets or 1 Darvocet-N 100 tablet q 4 hr. Maximum daily dose of propoxyphene napsylate should not exceed 600 mg. Total daily dose should be reduced in clients with impaired hepatic or renal function.

Special Concern: Use during pregnancy only if benefits outweigh risks. Safety and a suitable dosage regimen have not been established in children. Increased dosing intervals should be considered in geriatric clients.

NURSING CONSIDERATIONS

See *Nursing Considerations* for *Acetaminophen,* Chapter 41, and *Propoxyphene napsylate,* Chapter 43.

Assessment

1. Document indications for therapy and type and onset of symptoms.
2. Anticipate reduced dose with renal and hepatic dysfunction.

Evaluate: Relief of pain and discomfort.

—COMBINATION DRUG—

Darvon Compound 65

(**DAR**-von)

(Rx)

See also *Acetylsalicylic Acid,* Chapter 41, and *Propoxyphene,* Chapter 43.

How Supplied: See Content

Content: *Analgesic:* Propoxyphene HCl, 65 mg. *Nonnarcotic analgesic:* Aspirin, 389 mg. *CNS stimulant:* Caffeine, 32.4 mg.

Uses: Mild to moderate pain, with or without accompanying fever.

Dosage

• **Capsules**

Analgesia.

One capsule q 4 hr. Total daily dose of propoxyphene HCl should not exceed 390 mg. Total daily dosage should be decreased in clients with hepatic or renal impairment.

Special Concern: Use during pregnancy only if benefits outweigh risks.

NURSING CONSIDERATIONS

See also *Nursing Considerations* for *Acetylsalicylic Acid,* Chapter 41, and *Propoxyphene Napsylate,* Chapter 43.

Assessment

1. Document indications for therapy and onset of symptoms.
2. Anticipate reduced dose in clients with renal or liver dysfunction.

Client/Family Teaching

1. Use with caution when performing tasks that require mental alertness because drug may cause dizziness and sedation.
2. Do *NOT* ingest alcohol.
3. Keep out of the reach of children.
4. Use cautiously as psychologic and physical dependence may occur.

Evaluate: Relief of pain and discomfort.

—COMBINATION DRUG—

Equagesic

(eh-kwah-**JEE**-sik)

(Rx)

How Supplied: See Content

Content: *Nonnarcotic Analgesic:* Aspirin, 325 mg. *Antianxiety agent:* Meprobamate, 200 mg. See also information on individual components.

Uses: Treatment (short-term only) of pain due to musculoskeletal disease accompanied by anxiety and tension.

Dosage

• **Tablets**

Pain due to musculoskeletal disease.

Adults: 1–2 tablets t.i.d.–q.i.d.

Additional Contraindications: Pregnancy. Children under 12 years of age. Use for longer than 4 months.

NURSING CONSIDERATIONS

See also *Nursing Considerations* for *Acetylsalicylic Acid,* Chapter 41, and *Tranquilizers,* Chapter 40.

Assessment: Document indications for therapy, noting type and onset of symptoms.

Evaluate: Relief of musculoskeletal pain and associated anxiety and tension.

Mesalamine (5-aminosalicylic acid)

(mes-**AL**-ah-meen)
Pregnancy Category: B
Asacol, Mesasal, Pentasa, Rowasa, Salofalk ✱ **(Rx)**

How Supplied: *Capsule, Extended Release:* 250 mg; *Enema:* 4 g/60 mL; *Enteric Coated Tablet:* 400 mg; *Suppository:* 500 mg

Action/Kinetics: Chemically, mesalamine is related to acetylsalicylic acid. Mesalamine is believed to act locally in the colon to inhibit cyclooxygenase and therefore prostaglandin synthesis resulting in a reduction of inflammation of colitis. Mesalamine is administered PO and rectal. Following rectal administration, between 10% and 30% is absorbed and is excreted through the urine as the N-acetyl-5-aminosalicylic acid metabolite; the remainder is excreted in the feces. The PO tablets are coated with an acrylic-based resin that prevents release of mesalamine until it reaches the terminal ileum and beyond. Approximately 28% of the drug found in tablets is absorbed with the remaining drug available for action in the colon. Capsules are ethylcellulose coated, controlled release designed to release the drug throughout the GI tract; from 20% to 30% is absorbed. **t¹/₂, mesalamine:** 0.5–1.5 hr; **t¹/₂, n-acetyl mesalamine:** 5–10 hr. **Time to reach maximum plasma levels:** 4–12 hr for both mesalamine and metabolite. The drug is excreted mainly through the kidneys.

Uses: PO: Remission and treatment of mild to moderate active ulcerative colitis. **Rectal:**Treatment of active mild to moderate distal ulcerative colitis, proctosigmoiditis, or proctitis.

Dosage

- **Suppository**

One suppository (500 mg) b.i.d.

- **Rectal Suspension Enema**

4 g in 60 mL once daily for 3–6 weeks, usually given at bedtime. For maintenance, the drug can be given every other day or every third day at doses of 1–2 g.

- **Capsules, Controlled-Release**

1 g (4 capsules) q.i.d. for a total daily dose of 4 g for up to 8 weeks.

- **Tablets, Delayed-Release**

800 mg t.i.d. for a total dose of 2.4 g/day for 6 weeks.

Administration/Storage

1. Shake the bottle well to ensure that the suspension is homogeneous.
2. Have the client lie on the left side with the lower leg extended and the upper right leg flexed forward. The knee-chest position may also be used.
3. Insert the applicator tip and squeeze the bottle steadily to allow the bottle to empty.
4. The client should retain the enema for approximately 8 hr.
5. The suppository should remain in the rectum for 1–3 hr or more for maximal effect.
6. Beneficial effects using the suppository or enema may be seen within 3–21 days with a full course of therapy lasting up to 6 weeks.
7. Tablets should be taken whole, being careful not to break the outer coating.
8. *Treatment of Overdose:* Therapy to treat salicylate toxicity, including emesis, gastric lavage, fluid and electrolyte replacement (if necessary), maintenance of adequate renal function.

Contraindications: Hypersensitivity to salicylates.

Special Concerns: Use with caution in clients with sulfasalazine sensitivity, in those with impaired renal function, and during lactation. Safety and efficacy have not been established in children. Pyloric stenosis may delay the drug in reaching the colon.

Laboratory Test Interferences: ↑ AST, ALT, BUN, LDH, alkaline phosphatase, serum creatinine, amylase, lipase, GTTP.

Side Effects: *Sulfite sensitivity:* Hives, wheezing, itching, ***anaphylaxis.*** *Intolerance syndrome:* Acute abdominal pain, cramping, bloody diarrhea, rash, fever, headache. *GI:* Abdominal pain or discomfort, flatulence, cramps, dyspepsia, nausea, diarrhea, hemorrhoids, rectal pain or burning, rectal urgency, constipation, bloating, worsening of colitis, eructation, pain following insertion of enema, vomiting (after PO use). *CNS:* Headache, dizziness, insomnia, fatigue, malaise, chills, fever, asthenia. *Respiratory:* Cold, sore throat; increased cough, pharyngitis, rhinitis following PO use. *Dermatologic:* Acne, pruritus, itching, rash. *Musculoskeletal:* Back pain, hypertonia, arthralgia, myalgia, leg and joint pain, arthritis. *Miscellaneous:* Flu-like symptoms, hair loss, anorexia, peripheral edema, urinary burning, sweating, pain, chest pain, conjunctivitis, dysmenorrhea, pancreatitis.

In addition to the above, PO use may result in the following side effects. *GI:* Anorexia, gastritis, gastroenteritis, cholecystitis, dry mouth, increased appetite, oral ulcers, tenesmus, perforated peptic ulcer, bloody diarrhea, tenesmus, duodenal ulcer, dysphagia, esophageal ulcer, fecal incontinence, GI bleeding, oral moniliasis, rectal bleeding, abnormal stool color and texture. *CNS:* Anxiety, depression, hyperesthesia, nervousness, confusion, peripheral neuropathy, somnolence, emotional lability, vertigo, paresthesia, migraine, tremor, transverse myelitis, Guillain-Barre syndrome. *Dermatologic:* Dry skin, psoriasis, pyoderma gangrenosum, urticaria, erythema nodosum, eczema, photosensitivity, lichen planus, nail disorder. *CV:* Pericarditis, myocarditis, vasodilation, palpitations, ***fatal myocarditis***, chest pain, T-wave abnormalities. *GU:* Nephropathy, interstitial nephritis, urinary urgency, dysuria, hematuria, menorrhagia, epididymitis, amenorrhea, hypomenorrhea, metrorrhagia, nephrotic syndrome, urinary frequency, albuminuria, nephrotoxicity. *Hematologic:* ***Agranulocytosis,*** anemia, eosinophilia, leukopenia, thrombocytopenia, lymphadenopathy, thrombocythemia, ecchymosis. *Respiratory:* Worsening of asthma, sinusitis, interstitial pneumonitis, pulmonary infiltrates, fibrosing alveolitis. *Ophthalmologic:* Eye pain, blurred vision. *Miscellaneous:* Ear pain, tinnitus, taste perversion, neck pain, enlargement of abdomen, facial edema, gout, hypersensitivity pneumonitis, breast pain, Kawasaki-like syndrome.

Symptoms of Overdose: Salicylate toxicity manifested by tinnitus, vertigo, headache, confusion, drowsiness, sweating, hyperventilation, vomiting, and diarrhea. Severe toxicity results in disruption of electrolyte balance and blood pH, ***hyperthermia, and dehydration.***

NURSING CONSIDERATIONS

Assessment

1. Determine any sulfite sensitivity.
2. Document character and frequency of stools. Assess abdomen and describe bowel sounds.
3. Obtain baseline electrolytes and renal function studies.

Client/Family Teaching

1. Demonstrate the proper technique for administering the suspension enema. Have the client/family do a return demonstration to ensure that they understand the procedure.
   • Explain that prior to use, the bottle should be shaken until all contents are thoroughly mixed. Remove cap from applicator tip, insert tip into rectum, and squeeze steadily to discharge contents.
   • Review the appropriate positions that facilitate enema administration (lying on left side).
   • Describe how to protect the bed linens.
2. To ensure the proper absorption of the drug in enema form, it must be retained for 8 hr. This may best be accomplished by administering at bedtime, after bowel movement, and retaining it throughout the sleep cycle.
3. If any severe abdominal pain, cramping, bloody diarrhea, rash, fever, or headache occurs, discontinue the drug, and report.
4. Review the potential drug-related side effects that require immediate medical intervention.

5. Avoid smoking and cold foods as these tend to increase bowel motility.
6. The therapy may last 3–6 weeks. Therefore, it is important to continue taking as prescribed.

Evaluate

- Relief of pain and diarrhea R/T colitis
- Restoration of normal bowel patterns

Olsalazine sodium

(ohl-**SAL**-ah-zeen)
Pregnancy Category: C
Dipentum **(Rx)**

How Supplied: *Capsule:* 250 mg
Action/Kinetics: Olsalazine is a salicylate that is converted by bacteria in the colon to 5-PAS, which exerts an anti-inflammatory effect for the treatment of ulcerative colitis. The 5-PAS is slowly absorbed resulting in a high concentration of drug in the colon. The anti-inflammatory activity is likely due to inhibition of synthesis of prostaglandins in the colon. After PO use the drug is only slightly absorbed (2.4%) into systemic circulation where it has a short half-life (<1 hr) and is more than 99% bound to plasma proteins.
Use: To maintain remission of ulcerative colitis in clients who cannot take sulfasalazine.

Dosage

- **Capsules**

Adults: Total of 1 g/day in two divided doses.
Contraindication: Hypersensitivity to salicylates.
Special Concerns: Use with caution during lactation. Safety and efficacy have not been established in children. May cause worsening of symptoms of colitis.
Side Effects: *GI:* Diarrhea (common), pain or cramps, nausea, dyspepsia, bloating, anorexia, vomiting, stomatitis. *CNS:* Headache, drowsiness, lethargy, fatigue, dizziness, vertigo. *Miscellaneous:* Arthralgia, rash, itching, upper respiratory tract infection. *NOTE:* The following symptoms have been reported on withdrawal of therapy: diarrhea, nausea, abdominal pain, rash, itching, headache, heartburn, insomnia, anorexia, dizziness, lightheadedness, rectal bleeding, depression.

Symptoms of Overdose: Diarrhea, decreased motor activity.

NURSING CONSIDERATIONS

Assessment

1. Note any history of sensitivity to salicylates and/or an intolerance to sulfasalazine.
2. Document indications for therapy and type and onset of symptoms.
3. In clients with renal disease, obtain pretreatment urinalysis, BUN, and creatinine and monitor throughout drug therapy. With chronic therapy obtain a CBC and renal function studies and monitor periodically.

Client/Family Teaching

1. Drug should be taken with food and in evenly divided doses.
2. Provide a printed list of drug side effects and stress those, such as persistent diarrhea, that should be immediately reported.

Evaluate

- Remission of symptoms in ulcerative colitis
- Freedom from adverse side effects of drug therapy

CHAPTER FORTY-TWO

Nonsteroidal Anti-Inflammatory Drugs

See also the following individual entries:

Auranofin
Aurothioglucose Suspension
Carprofen
Diclofenac Potassium
Diclofenac Sodium
Diflunisal
Etodolac
Fenoprofen Calcium
Flurbiprofen
Flurbiprofen Sodium
Golden Sodium Thiomalate
Ibuprofen
Indomethacin
Indomethacin Sodium Trihydrate
Ketoprofen
Ketorolac Tromethamine
Meclofenamate Sodium
Mefenamic Acid
Nabumetone
Naproxen
Naproxen Sodium
Oxaprozin
Piroxicam
Sulindac
Suprofen
Tolmetin Sodium

General Statement: Arthritis, which means inflammation of the joints, refers to approximately 80 different conditions also called rheumatic, collagen, or connective tissue diseases. The most prominent symptoms of these conditions are painful, inflamed joints, but the cause for this joint inflammation varies from disease to disease. The joint pain of gout, for example, results from sodium urate crystals formed as a consequence of the overproduction or underelimination of uric acid. Osteoarthritis is caused by the degeneration of the joint; rheumatoid arthritis and SLE are autoimmune diseases. Immune factors trigger the release of corrosive enzymes in the joints in a complex manner. Infectious arthritis is the result of rapid joint destruction by microorganisms like gonococci that invade the joint cavity. Treatment must be aimed at the cause of the particular form of arthritis, and a thorough diagnostic evaluation must therefore precede the initiation of therapy. Gout is treated with uricosuric agents, which alter uric acid metabolism; infectious arthritis responds to antibiotics; osteoarthritis, rheumatoid arthritis, ankylosing spondylitis, and SLE respond to anti-inflammatory drugs. Rheumatoid arthritis may also be treated with two remitting agents (gold and penicillamine) or to hydroxychloroquine sulfate. Aspirin is an important agent in the treatment of all rheumatic diseases. Corticosteroids are used, preferably for short-term therapy only, for some of the more resistant cases of rheumatoid arthritis and SLE or for situations of exacerbation of these diseases. Corticosteroids also are used for intra-articular injection. Drug therapy of the arthritides must be supplemented by a physical therapy program, as well as proper rest and diet. Total joint replacement is also an important mode of therapy to correct the ravages of arthritis.

Action/Kinetics: Over the past decade, a growing number of NSAIDs have been developed, with anti-inflammatory, analgesic, and antipyretic effects. Chemically, these drugs are related to indene, indole, or propionic acid. As in the case of aspirin, the therapeutic actions of these agents are believed to result from the inhibition of the enzyme cyclooxygenase, resulting in decreased prostaglandin synthesis. The agents are effective in reducing joint swelling, pain, and morning stiffness, as well as in increasing mobility in individuals with arthritis. They do not alter the course of the disease, however. Their anti-inflammatory activity is comparable to that of aspirin.

The analgesic activity is due, in part, to relief of inflammation. Also, the drugs may inhibit lipoxygenase, inhibit synthesis of leukotrienes, inhibit release of lysosomal enzymes, and inhibit neutrophil aggregation. Rheumatoid factor production may also be inhibited. The antipyretic action is believed to occur by decreasing prostaglandin synthesis in the hypothalamus, resulting in an increase in peripheral blood flow and heat loss as well as promoting sweating.

The NSAIDs have an irritating effect on the GI tract. They differ from one another slightly with respect to their rate of absorption, length of action, anti-inflammatory activity, and effect on the GI mucosa. Most are rapidly and completely absorbed from the GI tract; food delays the rate, but not the total amount, of drug absorbed. These drugs are metabolized in the kidney and are excreted through the urine, mainly as metabolites.

Uses: Rheumatoid arthritis (acute flares and long-term management in adults and children), osteoarthritis, ankylosing spondylitis, gout, and other musculoskeletal diseases. Treatment of nonrheumatic inflammatory conditions including bursitis, acute painful shoulder, synovitis, tendinitis, or tenosynovitis. Mild to moderate pain including primary dysmenorrhea, episiotomy pain, strains and sprains, postextraction dental pain. Primary dysmenorrhea. *Investigational:* Depending on the drug, can be used for juvenile rheumatoid arthritis, for sunburn, to abort an acute migraine attack, for prophylaxis of migraine, and for PMS.

Contraindications: Most for children under 14 years of age. Lactation. Hypersensitivity to any of these agents or to aspirin. Individuals in whom aspirin, NSAIDs, or iodides have caused acute asthma, rhinitis, urticaria, nasal polyps, bronchospasm, angioedema or other symptoms of allergy or anaphylaxis. Use during lactation.

Special Concerns: Clients intolerant to one of the NSAIDs may be intolerant to others in this group. Use with caution in clients with a history of GI disease, reduced renal function, in geriatric clients, in clients with intrinsic coagulation defects or those on anticoagulant therapy, in compromised cardiac function, in hypertension, in conditions predisposing to fluid retention, and in the presence of existing controlled infection. The safety and efficacy of most NSAIDs have not been determined in children. Safety and efficacy have not been determined in functional class IV rheumatoid arthritis (i.e., clients incapacitated, bedridden, or confined to a wheelchair).

Side Effects: *GI (most common):* Peptic or duodenal ulceration and GI bleeding, intestinal ulceration with obstruction and stenosis, reactivation of preexisting ulcers. Heartburn, dyspepsia, N&V, anorexia, diarrhea, constipation, increased or decreased appetite, indigestion, stomatitis, epigastric pain, abdominal cramps or pain, gastroenteritis, paralytic ileus, salivation, dry mouth, glossitis, pyrosis, icterus, rectal irritation, gingival ulcer, occult blood in stool, hematemesis, gastritis, proctitis, eructation, sore or dry mucous membranes, ulcerative colitis, rectal bleeding, melena, ***perforation and hemorrhage of esophagus, stomach, duodenum, small or large intestine.*** *CNS:* Dizziness, drowsiness, vertigo, headaches, nervousness, migraine, anxiety, mental confusion, aggravation of parkinsonism and epilepsy, lightheadedness, paresthesia, peripheral neuropathy, akathisia, excitation, tremor, ***seizures,*** myalgia, asthenia, malaise, insomnia, fatigue, drowsiness, confusion, emotional lability, depression, inability to concentrate, psychoses, hallucinations, depersonalization, amnesia, ***coma,*** syncope. *CV:* CHF, hypotension, hypertension, arrhythmias, peripheral edema and fluid retention, vasodilation, exacerbation of angiitis, palpitations, tachycardia, chest pain, sinus bradycardia, peripheral vascular disease, peripheral edema. *Respiratory:* ***Bronchospasm, laryngeal edema,*** rhinitis, dyspnea, pharyngitis, hemoptysis, SOB, eosinophilic pneumonitis. *Hematologic:* Bone marrow depression, neutropenia, leukopenia, pancytopenia, eosinophila, thrombocytopenia, granulocytopenia, ***agranulocytosis, aplastic anemia, hemolytic anemia,*** decreased H&H, hypocoagulability, epistaxis. *Ophthalmologic:* Amblyopia, visual disturbances, corneal deposits, retinal hemorrhage, scotomata, retinal pigmentation changes or degeneration, blurred vision, photophobia, diplopia, iritis, loss of color vision (reversible), optic neuritis, cataracts, swollen, dry, or irritated eyes. *Dermatologic:* Pruritus, skin eruptions, sweating, erythema, eczema, hyperpigmentation, ecchymoses, petechiae, rashes, urticaria, purpura, onycholysis, vesiculobullous eruptions, cutaneous vasculitis, ***toxic epidermal necrolysis, angioneurotic edema,*** erythema nodosum, ***Stevens-Johnson syndrome,*** exfoliative dermatitis, photosensitivity, alopecia, skin irritation, peeling, erythema multiforme, desquamation, skin discoloration. *GU:* Menometrorrhagia, menorrhagia, impotence, menstrual disorders, hematuria, cystitis, azotemia, nocturia, proteinuria, UTIs, polyuria, dysuria, urinary frequency, oliguria, pyuria, anuria, renal insufficiency, nephrosis, nephrotic syndrome, glomerular and interstitial nephritis, urinary casts, acute renal failure in clients with impaired renal function, renal papillary necrosis *Metabolic:* Hyperglycemia, hypoglycemia, glycosuria, hyperkalemia, hyponatremia, diabetes mellitus. *Other:* Tinnitus, hearing loss or disturbances, ear pain, deafness, metallic or bitter taste in mouth, thirst, chills, fever, flushing, jaundice, sweating, breast changes, gynecomastia, muscle cramps, dyspnea, involuntary muscle movements, muscle weakness, facial edema, pain, serum sickness, aseptic meningitis, hypersensitivity reactions including asthma, acute respiratory distress, ***shock-like syndrome, angioedema,*** angiitis, dyspnea, ***anaphylaxis.***

Symptoms of Overdose: CNS symptoms include dizziness, drowsiness, mental confusion, lethargy, disorientation, intense headache, paresthesia, and ***seizures.*** GI symptoms include N&V, gastric irritation, and abdominal pain. Miscellaneous symptoms include tinnitus, sweating, blurred vision, increased serum creatinine and BUN, and acute renal failure.

Drug Interactions

Anticoagulants / Concomitant use results in ↑ PT

Aspirin / ↓ Effect of NSAIDs due to ↓ blood levels; also, ↑ risk of adverse GI effects

Beta-adrenergic blocking agents / ↓ Antihypertensive effect of blocking agents

Cimetidine / ↑ or ↓ Plasma levels of NSAIDs

Cyclosporine / ↑ Risk of nephrotoxicity

Lithium / ↑ Serum lithium levels

Loop diuretics / ↓ Effect of loop diuretics

Methotrexate / ↑ Risk of methotrexate toxicity (i.e., bone marrow suppression, nephrotoxicity, stomatitis)

Phenobarbital / ↓ Effect of NSAIDs due to ↑ breakdown by liver

Phenytoin / ↑ Effect of phenytoin due to ↓ plasma protein binding

Probenecid / ↑ Effect of NSAIDs due to ↑ plasma levels
Salicylates / Plasma levels of NSAIDs may be ↓ ; also, ↑ risk of GI side effects
Sulfonamides / ↑ Effect of sulfonamides due to ↓ plasma protein binding
Sulfonylureas / ↑ Effect of sulfonylureas due to ↓ plasma protein binding

Dosage

See individual drugs.

NURSING CONSIDERATIONS

Administration/Storage

1. Alcohol and aspirin should not be taken together with NSAIDs.
2. Can be taken with food, milk, or antacids should GI upset occur.
3. NSAIDs may have an additive analgesic effect when administered with narcotic analgesics, thus permitting lower narcotic dosages.
4. Clients who do not respond clinically to one NSAID may respond to another.
5. *Treatment of Overdose:* There are no antidotes; treatment includes general supportive measures. Since the drugs are acidic, it may be beneficial to alkalinize the urine and induce diuresis to hasten excretion.

Assessment

1. Note any history of allergic responses to aspirin or other anti-inflammatory agents. These drugs are contraindicated in this event.
2. Document indications for therapy, and type and onset of symptoms. Note other agents prescribed and the outcome.
3. Document location, intensity, and type of pain experienced. Assess joint mobility and ROM.
4. Review indications and dosage prescribed. For anti-inflammatory effects, high doses are required whereas analgesia and pain relief may be achieved with much lower dosages.
5. Determine if the client has asthma or nasal polyps. This condition may be exacerbated by the use of NSAIDs.
6. Note the age of the client. Children under 14 years of age generally should not receive drugs in this category.
7. Document if the client is taking oral hypoglycemic agents or insulin.
8. Interview clients concerning other medications they are currently taking. Determine if any of these drugs may interact unfavorably.
9. Determine that baseline hematologic studies have been performed and stool tested for occult blood; monitor periodically with long-term therapy. These agents cause platelet inhibition which is reversible in 24–48 hr, whereas aspirin requires 4–5 days to reverse its antiplatelet effects.

Client/Family Teaching

1. Take NSAIDs with a full glass of water or milk, with meals, or with a prescribed antacid and remain upright 30 min following administration to reduce gastric irritation.
2. Consume large quantities of water (2–3 L/day).
3. Report any changes in stool consistency or symptoms of GI irritation not relieved by adhering to the prescribed protocol. Sustained GI effects may need to be managed with misoprostol.
4. Stress compliance since regular intake of drug is necessary to sustain anti-inflammatory effects. Advise clients that if they do not obtain the desired response from this drug, another drug in this class may provide the desired response.
5. Discuss the need for regular medical supervision so that dosages of drug can be adjusted based on the client's condition, age, changes in disease activity, and overall drug response.
6. Report any episodes of bleeding, blurred vision or other eye symptoms, tinnitus, skin rashes, purpura, weight gain or edema.
7. Use caution in operating machinery or in driving a car because medication may cause dizziness or drowsiness.
8. Avoid alcohol, aspirin, acetaminophen, and any other OTC preparations without first consulting the

provider or pharmacist because of the increased risk for GI bleeding.
9. If the client has diabetes mellitus, explain the possible increase in hypoglycemic effect of NSAIDs on hypoglycemic agents. Advise clients to pay particular attention to urine and blood testing and to report any symptoms of hypoglycemic effects, as the dosage of agent and NSAID may need to be adjusted.
10. Advise to perform periodic weight measurements and to report any significant changes. Explain that NSAIDs cause Na and water retention.
11. Remind clients to tell other physicians and health care providers of the medication being taken to avoid having prescriptions written for drugs that would interact unfavorably with NSAIDs.

Evaluate

- Evidence of ↑ joint mobility and ROM
- Reports of ↓ levels of experienced discomfort and pain
- Clinical evidence of improvement in pretreatment symptoms

Auranofin

(or-**AN**-oh-fin)
Pregnancy Category: C
Ridaura **(Rx)**

How Supplied: *Capsule:* 3 mg
Action/Kinetics: Auranofin is a gold-containing (29%) compound that was developed for PO administration. The oral drug has fewer side effects than injectable gold products. Although the mechanism is not known, auranofin will improve symptoms of rheumatoid arthritis; it is most effective in the early stages of active synovitis and may act by inhibiting sulfhydryl systems. Other possible mechanisms include inhibition of phagocytic activity of macrophages and polymorphonuclear leukocytes, alteration of biosynthesis of collagen, and alteration of the immune response. Gold will not reverse damage to joints caused by disease. Approximately 25% of an oral dose is absorbed. **Plasma t½ of auranofin gold:** 26 days. **Onset:** 3–4 months (up to 6 months in certain clients). Approximately 3 months are required for steady-state blood levels to be achieved. The drug is metabolized and excreted in both the urine and feces.
Uses: Adults and children with rheumatoid arthritis that has not responded to other drugs. Up to 6 months may be required for beneficial effects to occur. Auranofin should be part of a total treatment regimen for rheumatoid arthritis, including nondrug treatments.

Dosage

- **Capsules**

Rhematoid arthritis.
Adults, initial: Either 6 mg/day or 3 mg b.i.d. If response is unsatisfactory after 6 months, increase to 3 mg t.i.d. If response is still inadequate after 3 additional months, the drug should be discontinued. Dosages greater than 9 mg/day are not recommended.

Transfer from injectable gold.
Discontinue injectable gold and begin auranofin at a dose of 6 mg/day.

Administration/Storage

1. This is the only gold compound administered PO.
2. A positive response should be noted after 6 months of therapy.
3. *Treatment of Overdose:* Discontinue and give dimercaprol. Supportive therapy should be provided for renal and hematologic symptoms. In acute overdosage, induction of emesis or gastric lavage should be performed immediately.

Contraindications: History of gold-induced disorders including necrotizing enterocolitis, pulmonary fibrosis, exfoliative dermatitis, bone marrow aplasia, or other hematologic disorders. Use during lactation.
Special Concerns: Use with caution in renal or hepatic disease, skin rashes, or history of bone marrow depression. Although used in chil-

dren, a recommended dosage has not been established.

Laboratory Test Interference: ↑ Liver enzymes.

Side Effects: *GI:* N&V, diarrhea (common), abdominal pain, metallic taste, stomatitis, glossitis, gingivitis, anorexia, constipation, flatulence, dyspepsia, dysgeusia. Rarely, melena, dysphagia, ***GI bleeding, ulcerative enterocolitis.*** *Dermatologic:* Skin rashes, pruritus, alopecia, urticaria, angioedema. *Hematologic:* Leukopenia, anemia, thrombocytopenia, hematuria, neutropenia, agranulocytosis. *Renal:* Proteinuria, hematuria. *Other:* Conjunctivitis, cholestatic jaundice, fever, interstitial pneumonia and fibrosis, peripheral neuropathy.

Symptoms of Overdose: Rapid appearance of hematuria, proteinuria, thrombocytopenia, granulocytopenia. Also, N&V, diarrhea, fever, urticaria, papulovesicular lesions, exfoliative dermatitis, pruritus.

NURSING CONSIDERATIONS

Assessment

1. Review client history and note any other severe systemic diseases such as renal, hepatic, or cardiac dysfunction.
2. Document the extent of the client's debilitation (functional class), ROM, and active synovitis.
3. Note onset of disease, course, other agents including disease-modifying agents used, and the outcome.
4. Inspect skin prior to initiating therapy to determine if there are any skin eruptions.
5. Assess gums and oral mucosa noting any lesions or need for treatment of oral problems.
6. Obtain baseline CBC, ESR, X rays, and liver and renal function studies.

Interventions

1. Determine if a dermal test dose has ever been performed with a gold salt.
2. Monitor and record I&O and weight.
3. If client complains of diarrhea, monitor electrolytes and report any evidence of abnormality.
4. Monitor liver and renal function studies and send urine to test for evidence of protein and blood.
5. Observe for the presence of peripheral neuropathy.
6. Encourage to return for appropriate follow-up evaluation and provide with only a 2-week supply of medication.

Client/Family Teaching

1. Avoid sunlight. If exposure is necessary, wear long sleeves, a hat, keep legs covered, and apply a sunscreen.
2. Inspect mouth regularly. Advise on a regular program of oral hygiene including regular brushing of the teeth, daily flossing, and mouth washes, avoiding those with alcohol or other drying ingredients.
3. Provide a printed list of the signs of toxicity that require immediate attention and reporting (skin rash, pruritus, metallic taste, stomatitis, diarrhea, leukopenia, and thrombocytopenia). Remind clients that side effects can occur at any time and must not be ignored.
4. Advise that it may take weeks to several months of therapy before improvement will be noticed.
5. Women of childbearing age who are sexually active should use some form of contraception.
6. Skin irritation (puritic dermatitis) and mouth ulcers may persist for months after discontinuing medication.
7. Expect to continue anti-inflammatory doses of NSAIDs for several weeks to months until auranofin takes effect.

Evaluate

- Improved mobility and ROM
- ↓ Pain, swelling, and stiffness in joints
- Slowing of the progression and degenerative effects of rheumatoid arthritis

Aurothioglucose suspension

(or-oh-thigh-oh-**GLOO**-kohz)

Pregnancy Category: C
Solganol **(Rx)**

For additional information regarding aurothioglucose, see *Gold Sodium Thiomalate,* Chapter 42.
How Supplied: *Injection:* 50 mg/mL

Dosage
- **IM Only**

Rheumatoid arthritis.
Adults: *Week 1:* 10 mg; *weeks 2 and 3:* 25 mg; **then,** 25–50 (maximum) mg/week until a total of 0.8–1 g has been administered. If client tolerates the dose and has improved, 50 mg may be given q 3–4 weeks for several months. **Pediatric, 6–12 years:** *Week 1:* 2.5 mg; *weeks 2 and 3:* 6.25 mg; **then,** 12.5 mg/week until a total dose of 200–250 mg has been administered. **Maintenance:** 6.25–12.5 mg q 3–4 weeks.
Administration/Storage
1. The client should remain lying down for 10 min after the injection and should be observed for 15 min following drug administration for evidence of flushing, dizziness, sweating, and hypotension (nitritoid reaction).
2. IM injections should be made only in the upper outer quadrant of the gluteal region; an 18-gauge, 1½-in. needle (or 2 in. for obese clients) should be used.
3. To obtain a uniform suspension, the vial should be shaken carefully before the dose is withdrawn.
4. Both the syringe and needle used to withdraw the dose should be dry.
5. The vial can be immersed in warm water to assist with withdrawing the appropriate dose of the suspension.
6. *Treatment of Overdose:* Discontinue and give dimercaprol. Supportive therapy should be provided for renal and hematologic symptoms. In acute overdose, induction of emesis or gastric lavage should be performed immediately.

NURSING CONSIDERATIONS

See also *Nursing Considerations* for *Gold Sodium Thiomalate,* Chapter 42.
Assessment
1. Document any sensitivity to sesame oil.
2. Determine if a dermal test dose has been performed.
3. Obtain baseline CBC and liver and renal function studies and monitor throughout therapy. Assess for blood dyscrasias, photosensitivity reactions, hepatic dysfunction, nephrotoxicity and fibrosis of the lungs (pneumonitis).
4. Carefully determine dosage and track until maximum total level administered.
5. Assess client mobility and stress the need to continue anti-inflammatory doses of NSAIDs for several more months.
Evaluate
- ↓ Joint pain, swelling, and stiffness with improved ROM
- Slowing of the progression and degenerative effects of rheumatoid arthritis

Carprofen
(kar-**PROH**-fen)
Pregnancy Category: C
Rimadyl **(Rx)**

See also *Nonsteroidal Anti-Inflammatory Drugs,* Chapter 42.
Action/Kinetics: t½: 6–17 hr. **Time to peak levels:** 1 hr.
Uses: Acute and chronic rheumatoid arthritis and osteoarthritis; acute gouty arthritis.

Dosage
- **Tablets**

Chronic rheumatoid arthritis and osteoarthritis.
Not to exceed 150 mg b.i.d. or 100 mg t.i.d.
Acute gouty arthritis.
600 mg/day in divided doses for 3–10 days. If ineffective after 2 days,

the drug should be discontinued and other treatment started.

Administration/Storage

1. When the client is to use the drug to treat chronic conditions, attempts should be made to reduce the dosage of drug after taking it for several weeks.
2. Lower doses of medication should be used for elderly clients and those with renal disease.
3. The maximum recommended dose is 300 mg/day.

Additional Side Effects: Compared with other NSAIDs, carprofen causes increased incidence of rashes, lower urinary tract symptoms, and leukopenia. Also, there is a greater incidence of abnormalities in levels of transaminase and alkaline phosphatase.

NURSING CONSIDERATIONS

See also *Nursing Considerations* for *Nonsteroidal Anti-Inflammatory Drugs,* Chapter 42.

Assessment

1. Determine that baseline transaminase, alkaline phosphatase, CBC, and renal function studies have been completed.
2. Document indications for therapy noting pretreatment findings.

Client/Family Teaching

1. Take with a full glass of water and remain upright.
2. Report if no improvements are noted after 2 days of therapy.
3. Provide a printed list of side effects, including GU reactions (such as cystitis, nocturia, oliguria, anuria, or urinary frequency) and skin rashes, which should be reported immediately should they occur.
4. Provide the names and addresses or phone numbers of local support groups that may assist clients in understanding and coping with chronic arthritic disorders.

Evaluate: Relief of joint pain and discomfort with ↑ ROM and improved mobility.

Diclofenac potassium

(dye-**KLOH**-fen-ack)
Pregnancy Category: B
Cataflam **(Rx)**

Diclofenac sodium

(dye-**KLOH**-fen-ack)
Pregnancy Category: B
Apo-Diclo ✦, Novo-Difenac ✦, Nu-Diclo ✦, Voltaren, Voltaren Ophtha ✦ **(Rx)**

See also *Nonsteroidal Anti-Inflammatory Drugs,* Chapter 42.

How Supplied: Diclofenac potassium: *Tablet:* 50 mg
Diclofenac sodium: *Enteric Coated Tablet:* 25 mg, 50 mg, 75 mg; *Ophthalmic solution:* 0.1%

Action/Kinetics: Diclofenac is a phenylacetic acid derivative; it is available as both the potassium (immediate-release) and sodium (delayed-release) salts. *Immediate-release product.* **Onset:** 30 min. **Peak plasma levels:** 1 hr. **Duration:** 8 hr. *Delayed-release product.* **Peak plasma levels:** 2–3 hr. **t½:** 1–2 hr. For all dosage forms, food will affect the rate, but not the amount, of drug absorbed from the GI tract. The drug is metabolized in the liver and excreted by the kidneys.

Uses: *PO, Immediate-release:* Analgesic, primary dysmenorrhea. *PO, Immediate- or delayed-release:* Rheumatoid arthritis, osteoarthritis, ankylosing spondylitis. *Investigational:* Mild to moderate pain, juvenile rheumatoid arthritis, acute painful shoulder, sunburn. *Ophthalmic:* Postoperative inflammation following cataract extraction.

Dosage

- **Immediate Release Tablets**

Analgesia, primary dysmenorrhea.

Adults: 50 mg t.i.d. In some clients, an initial dose of 100 mg followed by 50-mg doses may achieve better results. After the first day, the total daily dose should not exceed 150 mg.

- **Enteric-Coated (Delayed-Release) Tablets**

Rheumatoid arthritis.

Adults: 150–200 mg/day in two to four divided doses.

Osteoarthritis.

Adults: 100–150 mg/day in two to three divided doses.

Ankylosing spondylitis.

Adults: 25 mg q.i.d. with an extra 25-mg dose at bedtime, if necessary.

• **Ophthalmic Solution**

1 gtt of the 0.1% solution in the affected eye q.i.d. beginning 24 hr after cataract surgery and for 2 weeks thereafter.

Administration/Storage

1. Up to 3 weeks may be required for beneficial effects to be realized when used for rheumatoid arthritis or osteoarthritis.
2. The delayed-release tablets should not be crushed or chewed.

Contraindications: Ophthalmically in clients who wear soft contact lenses.

Special Concerns: Use with caution during lactation. Safety and effectiveness has not been determined in children. When used ophthalmically, may cause increased bleeding of ocular tissues in conjunction with ocular surgery. Healing may be slowed or delayed.

Side Effects: *Following ophthalmic use:* Keratitis, increased intraocular pressure, ocular allergy, N&V, anterior chamber reaction, viral infections, transient burning and stinging on administration.

NURSING CONSIDERATIONS

See also *Nursing Considerations* for *Nonsteroidal Anti-Inflammatory Drugs,* Chapter 42.

Assessment

1. Document indications for therapy and onset of symptoms.
2. Perform baseline liver and renal function studies and monitor during long-term therapy.
3. Ensure that drug is administered in high enough doses for anti-inflammatory effect when needed and in the lower doses for an analgesic effect.
4. With long-term therapy, test stool for occult blood and obtain periodic CBC.

Client/Family Teaching

1. May be taken with meals, a full glass of water or milk if GI upset occurs.
2. Limit intake of sodium, monitor weights, and report any evidence of edema or unusual weight gain.
3. Clients with diabetes should monitor blood sugar levels closely as drug may alter response to antidiabetic agents.
4. Avoid all OTC products unless approved.
5. Maintain fluid intake of 2 L/day.
6. Report any change in stool color and/or composition.

Evaluate

• Relief of joint pain with improved mobility

• Control of eye inflammation following cataract surgery

Diflunisal

(dye-**FLEW**-nih-sal)
Pregnancy Category: C
Dolobid (Rx)

How Supplied: *Tablet:* 250 mg, 500 mg

Action/Kinetics: Diflunisal is a salicylic acid derivative although it is not metabolized to salicylic acid. Its mechanism is not known although it is thought to be an inhibitor of prostaglandin synthetase. **Onset:** 1 hr. **Peak plasma levels:** 2–3 hr. **Peak effect:** 2–3 hr. **t½:** 8–12 hr. Ninety-nine percent protein bound. Metabolites excreted in urine.

Uses: Analgesic, rheumatoid arthritis, osteoarthritis, ankylosing spondylitis, psoriatic arthritis, musculoskeletal pain. Prophylaxis and treatment of vascular headaches.

Dosage

• **Tablets**

Mild to moderate pain.

Adults, initial: 1,000 mg; **then,** 250–500 mg q 8–12 hr.

Rheumatoid arthritis, osteoarthritis.

Adults: 250–500 mg b.i.d. Doses in excess of 1,500 mg/day are not recommended. For some clients, an initial dose of 500 mg followed by 250 mg q 8–12 hr may be effective. Dosage should be reduced in clients with impaired renal function.

Administration/Storage

1. When given for analgesic or antipyretic effect, expect the onset of action to occur within 20 min and to last for 4–6 hr.
2. If administering the drug to counteract the pain and swelling of arthritis, expect maximum relief to occur in 2–3 weeks.
3. Diflunisal may be given with water, milk, or meals to reduce gastric irritation.
4. Do not give acetaminophen or aspirin with diflunisal.
5. Tablets should not be crushed or chewed.
6. Serum salicylate levels are not used as a guide to dosage or toxicity because the drug is not hydrolyzed to salicylic acid.
7. *Treatment of Overdose:* Supportive measures. To empty the stomach, induce vomiting, or perform gastric lavage. Hemodialysis may not be effective since the drug is significantly bound to plasma protein.

Contraindications: Hypersensitivity to diflunisal, aspirin, or other anti-inflammatory drugs. Acute asthmatic attacks, urticaria, or rhinitis precipitated by aspirin. During lactation and in children less than 12 years of age.

Special Concerns: Use with caution in presence of ulcers or in clients with a history thereof, in clients with hypertension, compromised cardiac function, or in conditions leading to fluid retention. Use with caution in only first two trimesters of pregnancy. Geriatric clients may be at greater risk of GI toxicity.

Side Effects: *GI:* Nausea, dyspepsia, GI pain and bleeding, diarrhea, vomiting, constipation, flatulence, peptic ulcer, eructation, anorexia. *CNS:* Headache, fatigue, fever, malaise, dizziness, somnolence, insomnia, nervousness, vertigo, depression, paresthesias. *Dermatologic:* Rashes, pruritus, sweating, ***Stevens-Johnson syndrome,*** dry mucous membranes, erythema multiforme. *CV:* Palpitations, syncope, edema. *Other:* Tinnitus, asthenia, chest pain, hypersensitivity reactions, ***anaphylaxis,*** dyspnea, dysuria, muscle cramps, thrombocytopenia.

Symptoms of Overdose: Drowsiness, N&V, diarrhea, tachycardia, hyperventilation, stupor, disorientation, diminished urine output, ***coma, cardiorespiratory arrest.***

Drug Interactions

Acetaminophen / ↑ Plasma levels of acetaminophen
Antacids / ↓ Plasma levels of diflunisal
Anticoagulants / ↑ PT
Furosemide / ↓ Hyperuricemic effect of furosemide
Hydrochlorothiazide / ↑ Plasma levels and ↓ hyperuricemic effect of hydrochlorothiazide
Indomethacin / ↓ Renal clearance of indomethacin → ↑ plasma levels
Naproxen / ↓ Urinary excretion of naproxen and metabolite

NURSING CONSIDERATIONS

Assessment

1. Note any hypersensitivity to salicylates or other anti-inflammatory drugs.
2. Document indications for therapy, presenting symptoms, other agents prescribed, and the outcome.
3. Determine any history of peptic ulcers, hypertension, or compromised cardiac function.
4. Females of childbearing age should be questioned concerning the possibility of pregnancy. The drug should be avoided or used with extreme caution during the first two trimesters of pregnancy.
5. If receiving anticoagulant therapy, have prothrombin and coagulation times checked prior to administering drug.
6. Ensure that drug is administered in high enough doses for anti-inflammatory effects when needed and that the lower dose is prescribed for analgesic effects.
7. Obtain baseline CBC and liver

and renal function studies with long-term therapy.

Interventions

1. Assess clients for increased tendencies of bleeding when receiving high doses of diflunisal. This drug may inhibit platelet aggregation which is reversible with drug discontinuation.
2. Report complaints of diarrhea, especially in the elderly. This can cause an electrolyte imbalance and should be corrected. Test stool for occult blood periodically.

Client/Family Teaching

1. To minimize gastric irritation, take the medication with meals, milk, or a snack. If these measures do not work, consult provider concerning the use of an antacid. Antacids may lower plasma levels of diflunisal, reducing the effectiveness of the drug.
2. Taking the medication on a regular basis is necessary to sustain the anti-inflammatory effect of the drug. Therefore, compliance with the prescribed regimen is of utmost importance.
3. Urge client to report for medical follow-up and supervision on a regular basis. The medication needs to be adjusted according to the client's age, condition, and changes in disease activity.
4. The medication may cause dizziness or drowsiness; use care when operating machinery or driving an automobile.
5. Report any change in stool color or composition.
6. Advise parents to avoid aspirin or salicylates when treating children with a fever, children infected with varicella, or children who have influenza-like symptoms. Stress the importance of consulting with the child's provider before administering any OTC or unprescribed drugs.

Evaluate

- ↓ Pain and inflammation with ↑ joint mobility
- Prevention of vascular headaches

Etodolac

(ee-toh-**DOH**-lack)
Pregnancy Category: C
Lodine **(Rx)**

See also *Nonsteroidal Anti-Inflammatory Drugs,* Chapter 42.

How Supplied: *Capsule:* 200 mg, 300 mg; *Tablet:* 400 mg

Action/Kinetics: Etodolac is a NSAID in a class called the pyranocarboxylic acids. **Time to peak levels:** 1–2 hr. **Onset of analgesic action:** 30 min; **duration:** 4–12 hr. **t½:** 7.3 hr. The drug is metabolized by the liver and metabolites are excreted through the kidneys.

Uses: Acute and chronic treatment of osteoarthritis, mild to moderate pain.

Dosage

- **Capsules**

Osteoarthritis.

Adults, initial: 800–1,200 mg/day in divided doses; **then,** adjust dose within the range of 600–1,200 mg/day in divided doses (400 mg b.i.d.–t.i.d.; 300 mg b.i.d., t.i.d., or q.i.d.; 200 mg t.i.d. or q.i.d.). Total daily dose should not exceed 1,200 mg.

Acute pain.

Adults: 200–400 mg q 6–8 hr as needed, not to exceed 1,200 mg/day. For clients weighing less than 60 kg, the dose should not exceed 20 mg/kg.

Administration/Storage

1. The capsules should be protected from moisture.
2. *Treatment of Overdose:* Since there are no antidotes, treatment is supportive and symptomatic. If discovered within 4 hr, emesis followed by activated charcoal and an osmotic cathartic may be tried.

Contraindications: Clients in whom etodolac, aspirin, or other NSAIDs have caused asthma, rhinitis, urticaria, or other allergic reactions. Use during lactation, during labor and delivery, and in children.

Special Concerns: Use with caution in impaired renal or hepatic function, heart failure, those on diu-

retics, and in geriatric clients. Safety and effectiveness have not been determined in children.
Laboratory Test Interferences: False + reaction for urinary bilirubin and for urinary ketones (using the dip-stick method). ↑ Liver enzymes, serum creatinine. ↑ Bleeding time.
Additional Side Effects: *GI:* Diarrhea, gastritis, thirst, ulcerative stomatitis, anorexia. *CNS:* Nervousness, depression. *CV:* Syncope. *Respiratory:* Asthma. *Dermatologic:* Angioedema, vesiculobullous rash, cutaneous vasculitis with purpura, hyperpigmentation. *Miscellaneous:* Jaundice, hepatitis.

Symptoms of Overdose: N&V, drowsiness, lethargy, epigastric pain, ***anaphylaxis.*** Rarely, hypertension, acute renal failure, respiratory depression.
Additional Drug Interactions
Cyclosporine / ↑ Serum levels of cyclosporine due to ↓ renal excretion; ↑ risk of cyclosporine-induced nephrotoxicity
Digoxin / ↑ Serum levels of digoxin due to ↓ renal excretion
Lithium / ↑ Serum levels of lithium due to ↓ renal excretion
Methotrexate / ↑ Serum levels of methotrexate due to ↓ renal excretion

NURSING CONSIDERATIONS

See also *Nursing Considerations* for *Nonsteroidal Anti-Inflammatory Drugs,* Chapter 42.
Assessment
1. Note any previous experience with NSAIDs or acetylsalicylic acid and the results.
2. Document indications for therapy (i.e., analgesic or anti-inflammatory),include onset of symptoms and status of ROM.
3. With long-term therapy, obtain baseline bleeding parameters, platelets, and liver and renal function studies.
4. Determine any history of heart disease or cardiac failure.
5. Note age and weight of client and if currently prescribed diuretics.

Evaluate: Control of pain and inflammation with improved joint mobility.

Fenoprofen calcium

(fen-oh-**PROH**-fen)
Pregnancy Category: B
Fenopron, Nalfon **(Rx)**

See also *Nonsteroidal Anti-Inflammatory Drugs,* Chapter 42.
How Supplied: *Capsule:* 200 mg, 300 mg; *Tablet:* 600 mg
Action/Kinetics: Peak serum levels: 1–2 hr; **t½:** 2–3 hr. Ninety-nine percent protein bound. Food (but not antacids) delays absorption and decreases the total amount absorbed. When used for arthritis, onset of action is within 2 days but 2–3 weeks may be necessary to assess full therapeutic effects. Safety and efficacy in children have not been established.
Uses: Rheumatoid arthritis, osteoarthritis, mild to moderate pain. *Investigational:* Juvenile rheumatoid arthritis, prophylaxis of migraine, migraine due to menses, sunburn.

Dosage

- **Capsules, Tablets**

Rheumatoid and osteoarthritis.
Adults: 300–600 mg t.i.d.–q.i.d. Adjust dose according to response of client.

Mild to moderate pain.
Adults: 200 mg q 4–6 hr. Maximum daily dose for all uses: 3,200 mg.
Administration/Storage
1. Expect the peak effect to be realized in 2–3 hr and to last for 4–6 hr.
2. Two to 3 weeks of therapy may be required before a beneficial effect is noted.
3. Elderly clients over 70 years of age generally require half the usual adult dose of fenoprofen.
4. The drug is not recommended for children under 12 years of age or for pregnant women.
5. For clients who have difficulty swallowing, the tablets can be crushed and the contents mixed with applesauce or other similar foods.
6. If fenoprofen is given chronically, periodic auditory tests should be performed.

Additional Contraindication: Renal dysfunction.
Special Concerns: Dosage has not been determined in children.
Additional Side Effects: *GU:* Dysuria, hematuria, cystitis, interstitial nephritis, nephrotic syndrome. Overdosage has caused tachycardia and hypotension.

NURSING CONSIDERATIONS

See also *Nursing Considerations* for *Nonsteroidal Anti-Inflammatory Drugs,* Chapter 42.

Assessment

1. Document indications for therapy and type and onset of symptoms.
2. Note drugs currently prescribed to ensure that there are no potential drug interactions.
3. Obtain baseline ophthalmic and auditory examinations against which to measure any auditory or visual changes with long-term therapy.
4. Document baseline values and monitor CBC with differential, platelet counts, PT/PTT, and liver and renal function during therapy.

Client/Family Teaching

1. Take 30 min before or 2 hr after meals. Food decreases the rate and extent of absorption of fenoprofen.
2. Do not take aspirin or any other OTC agents without approval.
3. If vomiting or diarrhea occurs, monitor appetite, intake, and weights and report if persistent.
4. Note and report any evidence of easy bruising or bleeding as well as petechiae, oozing of blood from the gums, nosebleeds, sore throat, or fever.
5. Report any complaints of headache, sleepiness, dizziness, nervousness, weakness, or fatigue as these may be adverse drug effects.
6. Report any evidence of liver toxicity, such as jaundice, right upper quadrant abdominal pain, or a change in the color and consistency of stools.

Evaluate: ↓ Joint pain and inflammation with ↑ mobility.

Flurbiprofen

(flur-**BIH**-proh-fen)
Pregnancy Category: B
Ansaid, Apo-Flurbiprofen ✱, Froben ✱, Froben SR ✱ **(Rx)**

Flurbiprofen sodium

(flur-**BIH**-proh-fen)
Pregnancy Category: C
Ocufen **(Rx)**

See also *Nonsteroidal Anti-Inflammatory Drugs* Chapter 42.
How Supplied: Flurbiprofen: *Tablet:* 50 mg, 100 mg
Flurbiprofen sodium: *Ophthalmic solution:* 0.03%
Action/Kinetics: By inhibiting prostaglandin synthesis, flurbiprofen reverses prostaglandin-induced vasodilation, leukocytosis, increased vascular permeability, and increased intraocular pressure. The drug also inhibits miosis, which occurs during cataract surgery. **PO form, time to peak levels:** 1.5 hr; **t½:** 5.7 hr.
Uses: *Ophthalmic:* Prevention of intraoperative miosis. *PO:* Rheumatoid arthritis, osteoarthritis. *Investigational:* Inflammation following cataract surgery, uveitis syndromes. Topically to treat cystoid macular edema. Primary dysmenorrhea, sunburn, mild to moderate pain.

Dosage

• **Ophthalmic Drops**

Beginning 2 hr before surgery, instill 1 gtt q 30 min (i.e., total of 4 gtt of 0.03% solution).

• **Tablets**

Rheumatoid arthritis, osteoarthritis.

Adults, initial: 200–300 mg/day in divided doses b.i.d.–q.i.d.; **then,** adjust dose to client response. Doses greater than 300 mg/day are not recommended.

Dysmenorrhea.

50 mg q.i.d.

Administration/Storage: The maximum dose of 300 mg should be used only for initiating therapy or for treating acute exacerbations of the disease.
Contraindication: Dendritic keratitis.
Special Concerns: Use with caution in clients hypersensitive to aspi-

rin or other NSAIDs. Use with caution during lactation. Safety and efficacy in children have not been established.
Additional Side Effects: *Ophthalmic:* Ocular irritation, transient stinging or burning following use, delay in wound healing.

NURSING CONSIDERATIONS

See also *Nursing Considerations* for *Nonsteroidal Anti-Inflammatory Drugs,* Chapter 42.

Assessment

1. Document indications for therapy and type and onset of symptoms.
2. Prior to eye surgery, carefully follow the prescribed dosing intervals.

Client/Family Teaching

1. May take tablets with food to decrease GI upset.
2. Instruct client and family in the appropriate method of administering the eye medication.
3. Avoid rubbing the eyes after the medication has been administered and report any stinging, burning, or irritation immediately.
4. Report any delays in wound healing.

Evaluate

- ↓ Pain and inflammation with ↑ joint mobility
- Relief of pain and discomfort
- ↓ Optic inflammation
- Prevention of abnormal pupillary contractions

Gold sodium thiomalate

(gold **SO**-dee-um thigh-oh-**MAH**-layt)
Pregnancy Category: C
Myochrysine **(Rx)**

How Supplied: *Injection:* 50 mg/mL
Action/Kinetics: Although the exact mechanism is not known, gold salts may inhibit lysosomal enzyme activity in macrophages and decrease macrophage phagocytic activity. Other mechanisms may include alteration of the immune response and alteration of biosynthesis of collagen. Gold salts suppress, but do not cure, arthritis and synovitis. The beneficial effects may not be seen for 3–12 months. Most clients experience transient side effects, although serious effects may be manifested in some. **Peak blood levels (IM):** 4–6 hr. **t½:** increases with continued therapy. Gold may accumulate in tissues and persist for years. Significantly bound to plasma proteins. The drug is eliminated slowly through both the urine (60%–90%) and feces (10%–40%). This preparation contains 50% gold.
Uses: Adjunct to the treatment of rheumatoid arthritis (active and progressive stages) in children and adults. It is most effective in the early stages of the disease.

Dosage

- **IM**

Rheumatoid arthritis.

Adults: *week 1:* 10 mg as a single injection; *week 2:* 25 mg as a single dose. Then, 25–50 mg/week until 0.8–1 g total has been given. Thereafter according to individual response. *Usual maintenance:* 25–50 mg every other week for up to 20 weeks. If condition remains stable, the dose can be given every third or fourth week indefinitely. **Pediatric, initial:** *week 1,* 10 mg; **then,** usual dose is 1 mg/kg, not to exceed 50 mg/injection using the same spacing of doses as for adults.

Administration/Storage

1. Shake vial well to ensure uniformity of suspension before withdrawing medication.
2. Inject into gluteus maximus.
3. Gold therapy may be reinstituted following mild toxic symptoms but not after severe symptoms.
4. Geriatric clients manifest a lower tolerance to gold.
5. *Treatment of Overdose:* Discontinue use of the drug immediately. Give dimercaprol. Provide supportive treatment for hematologic or renal complications.

Contraindications: Hepatic disease, CV problems such as hypertension or CHF, severe diabetes, debilitated clients, renal disease, blood dyscrasias, agranulocytosis, hemorrhagic diathesis, clients receiving radiation treatments, colitis, lupus erythematosus, pregnancy, lactation, children under 6 years of age. Clients with eczema or urticaria.

Laboratory Test Interferences: Alters liver function tests. Urinary protein and RBCs, altered blood counts (indicative of toxic effect of drug).

Side Effects: *Skin:* Dermatitis (most common), pruritus, erythema, dermatoses, gray to blue pigmentation of tissues, alopecia, loss of nails. *GI:* Stomatitis (second most common), metallic taste, gastritis, colitis, gingivitis, glossitis, N&V, diarrhea (may be persistent), colic, anorexia, cramps, enterocolitis. *Hematologic:* Anemia, thrombocytopenia, granulocytopenia, leukopenia, eosinophilia, hemorrhagic diathesis. *Allergic:* Flushing, fainting, sweating, dizziness, ***anaphylaxis,*** syncope, bradycardia, angioneurotic edema, respiratory difficulties. *Other:* Interstitial pneumonitis, pulmonary fibrosis, nephrotic syndrome, glomerulitis (with hematuria), proteinuria, hepatitis, fever, headache, arthralgia, ophthalmologic problems including corneal ulcers, iritis, gold deposits, EEG abnormalities, peripheral neuritis. Corticosteroids may be used to treat symptoms such as stomatitis, dermatitis, GI, renal, hematologic, or pulmonary problems. Also, if symptoms are severe and do not respond to corticosteroids, a chelating agent such as dimercaprol may be used. Clients should be monitored carefully.

Symptoms of Overdose: Hematuria, proteinuria, thrombocytopenia, granulocytopenia, N&V, diarrhea, fever, papulovesicular lesions, urticaria, exfoliative dermatitis, severe pruritus.

Drug Interactions: Concomitant use contraindicated with drugs known to cause blood dyscrasias (e.g., antimalarials, cytotoxic drugs, pyrazolone derivatives, immunosuppressive drugs).

NURSING CONSIDERATIONS

Assessment

1. Document indications for therapy, previous treatments utilized for this condition, and the outcome.
2. Determine ROM and describe all areas of limitation and pain as well as active synovitis.
3. Obtain baseline urinalysis, CBC, platelets, and liver function tests; monitor every 2 weeks.

Interventions

1. Have the client remain in a recumbent position for at least 20 min after the injection to prevent falls resulting from transient vertigo or giddiness. Observe for flushing, dizziness, sweating, and hypotension (nitritoid reaction).
2. Monitor I&O and electrolytes if diarrhea occurs and is prolonged.

Client/Family Teaching

1. Close medical supervision is required during gold therapy.
2. Do not become discouraged. Stress that beneficial effects are slow to appear but that therapy may be continued for up to 12 months in anticipation of relief.
3. Provide a printed list of adverse drug effects. Identify those that require immediate reporting.
4. Practice contraception during therapy.
5. Avoid direct sun exposure as a photosensitivity reaction may occur. Wear sunscreen, protective clothing, and a hat if exposure is necessary.
6. Report any evidence of abnormal bruising or bleeding as well as any skin or mucous membrane lesions.
7. Advise to continue anti-inflammatory doses of NSAIDs for several weeks into therapy.

Evaluate: ↓ Joint pain, swelling, and stiffness with ↑ ROM and mobility.

Ibuprofen

(eye-byou-**PROH**-fen)

Rx: Actiprofen ✱, Apo-Ibuprofen ✱, Children's Advil, Children's Motrin, Ibuprohm, Ibu-Tab, Motrin, Novo-Profen ✱, Rufen, Saleto-400, -600, and -800. **OTC:** Aches-N-Pain, Advil Caplets and Tablets, Excedrin IB Caplets and Tablets, Genpril Caplets and Tablets, Haltran, Ibuprin,

Ibuprohm Caplets and Tablets, Ibu-Tab, Medipren Caplets and Tablets, Midol 200, Motrin-IB Caplets and Tablets, Nuprin Caplets and Tablets, Saleto-200, Trendar

---

See also *Nonsteroidal Anti-Inflammatory Drugs,* Chapter 42.

How Supplied: *Chew Tablet:* 50 mg, 100 mg; *Suspension:* 100 mg/5 mL; *Tablet:* 100 mg, 200 mg, 300 mg, 400 mg, 600 mg, 800 mg

Action/Kinetics: Time to peak levels: 1–2 hr. **Onset:** 30 min for analgesia and approximately 1 week for anti-inflammatory effect. **Peak serum levels:** 1–2 hr. **t½:** 2 hr. **Duration:** 4–6 hr for analgesia and 1–2 weeks for anti-inflammatory effect. Food delays absorption rate but not total amount of drug absorbed.

The OTC products each contain 200 mg of ibuprofen; tablets containing 300 mg, 400 mg, 600 mg, 800 mg or the oral suspension containing 100 mg/5 mL are all available by prescription only.

Uses: Analgesic for mild to moderate pain. Primary dysmenorrhea, rheumatoid arthritis, osteoarthritis, antipyretic. *Investigational:* Resistant acne vulgaris (with tetracyclines); inflammation due to ultraviolet-B exposure (sunburn), juvenile rheumatoid arthritis.

Dosage

- **Suspension, Tablets**

Rheumatoid arthritis, osteoarthritis.

Either 300 mg q.i.d. or 400, 600, or 800 mg t.i.d.–q.i.d.; adjust dosage according to client response. Full therapeutic response may not be noted for 2 or more weeks.

Juvenile arthritis.

30–40 mg/kg/day in three to four divided doses (20 mg/kg/day may be adequate for mild cases).

Mild to moderate pain.

Adults: 400 mg q 4–6 hr, as needed.

Antipyretic.

Pediatric, 2–12 years of age: 5 mg /kg if baseline temperature is 102.5°F (39.1°C) or below or 10 mg/kg if baseline temperature is greater than 102.5°F (39.1°C). Maximum daily dose: 40 mg/kg.

Dysmenorrhea.

Adults: 400 mg q 4 hr, as needed.

- **Tablets for OTC Use**

Mild to moderate pain, antipyretic, dysmenorrhea.

200 mg q 4–6 hr; dose may be increased to 400 mg if pain or fever persist. Dose should not exceed 1,200 mg/day.

Administration/Storage

1. Ibuprofen purchased OTC should not be used as an antipyretic for more than 3 days.
2. This drug should not be used as an analgesic for more than 10 days unless medically cleared.
3. Anticipate an onset of action in 30 min and that the effect will last 2–4 hr.
4. No more than 3.2 g/day should be taken of prescription products and no more than 1.2 g/day should be taken of OTC products.

Contraindications: Use of ibuprofen is not recommended during pregnancy, especially during the last trimester.

Special Concerns: The dosage must be individually determined for children less than 12 years of age as safety and effectiveness have not been established.

Additional Side Effects: Dermatitis (maculopapular type), rash. Hypersensitivity reaction consisting of abdominal pain, fever, headache, ***meningitis,*** nausea, signs of liver damage, and vomiting; especially seen in clients with SLE.

Additional Drug Interactions

Furosemide / Ibuprofen ↓ diuretic effect of furosemide due to ↓ renal prostaglandin synthesis

Lithium / Ibuprofen ↑ plasma levels of lithium

Thiazide diuretics / Ibuprofen ↓ diuretic effect of furosemide due to ↓ renal prostaglandin synthesis

---

NURSING CONSIDERATIONS

See also *Nursing Considerations* for *Nonsteroidal Anti-Inflammatory Drugs,* Chapter 42.

Assessment
1. Document indications for therapy, onset and type of symptoms, and any previous treatments used.
2. Take a complete drug history, noting if the client is taking any drugs with which ibuprofen interacts unfavorably.
3. Determine any evidence of lupus.
4. Obtain baseline CBC, liver and renal function studies, X rays if applicable, and eye examination prior to initiating long-term drug therapy.

Client/Family Teaching
1. Take with a snack, milk, antacid, or meals to decrease GI upset. Report if N&V, diarrhea, or constipation persists, because the drug may need to be discontinued.
2. Stress the importance of taking the dosage prescribed to ensure best results.
3. Clients with a history of CHF or compromised cardiac function should keep careful records of weight and report any evidence of edema as drug causes Na retention. (Records of BP and I&O may additionally be requested with some individuals.)
4. Report any evidence of blurred vision. Periodic eye examinations should be performed on clients undergoing long-term therapy.
5. Report as scheduled for follow-up evaluations: ROM, CBC, renal function, X rays, and stool for occult blood.

Evaluate
- Relief of pain
- ↓ Joint pain and ↑ mobility
- ↓ Fever
- ↓ Uterine cramping

Indomethacin

(in-doh-**METH**-ah-sin)
Apo-Indomethacin ✦, Indochron E-R, Indocid ✦, Indocid Ophthalmic Suspension ✦, Indocid PDA ✦, Indocin, Indocin SR, Novo-Methacin ✦, Nu-Indo ✦ **(Rx)**

Indomethacin sodium trihydrate

(in-doh-**METH**-ah-sin)
Indocin I.V. **(Rx)**

See also *Nonsteroidal Anti-Inflammatory Drugs,* Chapter 42.

How Supplied: Indomethacin: *Capsule:* 25 mg, 50 mg; *Capsule, Extended Release:* 75 mg; *Suppository:* 50 mg; *Suspension:* 25 mg/5 mL
Indomethacin sodium trihydrate: *Powder for injection:* 1 mg

Action/Kinetics: Indomethacin is not considered to be a simple analgesic and should only be used for the conditions listed. **PO. Onset:** 30 min for analgesia and up to 1 week for anti-inflammatory effect. **Peak plasma levels:** 1–2 hr (2–4 hr for sustained-release). **Duration:** 4–6 hr for analgesia and 1–2 weeks for anti-inflammatory effect. **Therapeutic plasma levels:** 10–18 mcg/mL. **t½:** Approximately 5 hr (up to 6 hr for sustained-release). **Plasma t½ following IV in infants:** 12–20 hr, depending on age and dose. Approximately 90% plasma protein bound. The drug is metabolized in the liver and excreted in both the urine and feces.

Uses: Moderate to severe rheumatoid arthritis, osteoarthritis, and ankylosing spondylitis (drug of choice). Acute gouty arthritis and acute painful shoulder (tendinitis, bursitis). *IV:* Pharmacologic closure of persistent patent ductus arteriosus in premature infants. *Investigational:* Topically to treat cystoid macular edema (0.5% and 1% drops), sunburn, primary dysmenorrhea, prophylaxis of migraine, cluster headache, polyhydramnios.

Dosage

- **Capsules, Oral Suspension**

Moderate to severe arthritis, osteoarthritis, ankylosing spondylitis.

Adults, initial: 25 mg b.i.d.–t.i.d.; may be increased by 25–50 mg at weekly intervals, according to condition and, if tolerated, until satisfactory response is obtained. In those with persistent night pain or morning stiffness, a maximum of 100 mg of the total daily dose can be given at bedtime. **Maximum daily dosage:** 150–200 mg. In acute flares of chronic rheumatoid arthritis, the dose may need to be increased by 25–50 mg/day until the acute phase is under control.

Acute gouty arthritis.

Adults, initial: 50 mg t.i.d. until pain is tolerable; **then,** reduce dosage rapidly until drug is withdrawn. Pain relief usually occurs within 2–4 hr, tenderness and heat subside in 24–36hr, and swelling disappears in 3–4 days.

Acute painful shoulder (bursitis/tendinitis).

75–150 mg/day in three to four divided doses for 1–2 weeks.

• **Sustained-release Capsules**

Antirheumatic, anti-inflammatory.

Adults: 75 mg, of which 25 mg is released immediately, 1–2 times/day.

• **Suppositories**

Anti-inflammatory, antirheumatic, antigout.

Adults: 50 mg up to q.i.d. **Pediatric:** 1.5–2.5 mg/kg/day in three to four divided doses (up to a maximum of 4 mg/kg or 250–300 mg/day, whichever is less).

• **IV Only**

Patent ductus arteriosus.

3 IV doses, depending on age of the infant, are given at 12–24-hr intervals. **Infants less than 2 days:** first dose, 0.2 mg/kg, followed by two doses of 0.1 mg/kg each; **infants 2–7 days:** three doses of 0.2 mg/kg each; **infants more than 7 days:** first dose, 0.2 mg/kg, followed by two doses of 0.25 mg/kg each. If patent ductus arteriosus reopens, a second course of one to three doses may be given. Surgery may be required if there is no response after two courses of therapy.

Administration/Storage

1. Store in amber-colored containers.
2. The IV solution should be prepared with 1–2 mL of preservative-free sodium chloride injection or sterile water for injection.
3. IV solutions should be freshly prepared prior to use.
4. Reconstitute to 0.1 mg/mL or 0.05 mg/mL immediately before use and infuse over 5–10 sec.
5. Up to 100 mg of the total daily dose can be given at bedtime for clients with night pain or morning stiffness.
6. The sustained-release form should not be crushed and should not be used in clients with acute gouty arthritis.
7. If the client has difficulty swallowing capsules, the contents may be emptied into applesauce, food, or liquid to ensure that the client receives the prescribed dose.
8. Suppositories (50 mg) may be used in clients unable to take PO medication. They should be stored below 30°C (86°F).
9. Anticipate a peak action of drug to occur in 24–36 hr in clients taking the medication for gout. Swelling gradually disappears in 3–5 days. The sustained-release form should not be used to treat gout.
10. Peak drug activity in clients taking the medication for antirheumatic effect will occur in about 4 weeks.
11. The smallest effective dose of the drug should be administered, based on individual need. Adverse reactions are dose related.

Additional Contraindications: Pregnancy and lactation. PO indomethacin in children under 14 years of age. GI lesions or history of recurrent GI lesions. *IV use:* GI or intracranial bleeding, thrombocytopenia, renal disease, defects of coagulation, necrotizing enterocolitis. *Suppositories:* Recent rectal bleeding, history of proctitis.

Special Concerns: Use in children should be restricted to those unresponsive to or intolerant of other anti-inflammatory agents; efficacy has not been determined in children less than 14 years of age. Geriatric clients are at greater risk of developing CNS side effects, especially confusion. To be used with caution in clients with history of epilepsy, psychiatric illness, or parkinsonism and in the elderly. Indomethacin should be used with extreme caution in the presence of existing, controlled infections.

Additional Side Effects: Reactivation of latent infections may mask signs of infection. More marked CNS manifestations than for other drugs of this group. Aggravation of depression or other psychiatric problems, epilepsy, and parkinsonism.

Additional Drug Interactions

Captopril / Indomethacin ↓ effect of captopril, probably due to inhibition of prostaglandin synthesis

Diflunisal / ↑ Plasma levels of indomethacin; also, possible fatal GI hemorrhage

Diuretics (loop, potassium-sparing, thiazide) / Indomethacin may reduce the antihypertensive and natriuretic action of diuretics

Lisinopril / Possible ↓ effect of lisinopril

Prazosin / Indomethacin ↓ antihypertensive effects of prazosin

NURSING CONSIDERATIONS

See also *Nursing Considerations* for *Nonsteroidal Anti-Inflammatory Drugs,* Chapter 42.

Assessment

1. Document indications for therapy and type and onset of symptoms.
2. Determine any agents used for this condition and the outcome.
3. List other drugs prescribed to ensure none interact unfavorably.

Client/Family Teaching

1. Take with food or milk to decrease GI upset.
2. Use caution when operating potentially hazardous equipment because of possible lightheadedness and decreased alertness.
3. Stress the importance of reporting any adverse drug effects immediately. If any adverse side effects occur, withhold the drug and report since many may be serious enough to discontinue the medication.
4. Advise to record weights, especially if nausea or vomiting occurs and to report any abdominal pain or diarrhea.
5. Explain that urine and stool will be tested for occult blood periodically and advise to report any S&S of anemia.
6. Explain that indomethacin masks infections so they should report any incidence of fever.
7. Report for scheduled ophthalmologic examinations and lab studies, especially if receiving long-term therapy.
8. Remind clients that it will take from 2–4 weeks of therapy before they will see significant improvement in arthritic conditions. Therefore, they should follow the prescribed dosing regimen carefully and refrain from becoming discouraged.

Evaluate

- Control of pain and inflammation with improved joint mobility
- Successful closure of patent ductus arteriosus with IV therapy
- Therapeutic serum drug levels (10–18 mg/mL)

Ketoprofen

(kee-toe-**PROH**-fen)

Pregnancy Category: B

Apo-Keto ✱, Apo-Keto-E ✱, Novo-Keto-EC ✱, Orudis, Orudis-E ✱, Orudis-SR ✱, Oruvail, PMS-Ketoprofen ✱, Rhodis ✱, Rhodis EC ✱ **(Rx)**

See also *Nonsteroidal Anti-Inflammatory Drugs,* Chapter 42.

How Supplied: *Capsule:* 25 mg, 50 mg, 75 mg; *Capsule, Extended Release:* 100 mg, 150 mg, 200 mg

Action/Kinetics: The drug possesses anti-inflammatory, antipyretic, and analgesic properties. It is known to inhibit both prostaglandin and leukotriene synthesis, to have antibradykinin activity, and to stabilize lysosomal membranes. **Onset:** 15–30 min. **Peak plasma levels:** 0.5–2 hr. **Duration:** 4–6 hr. **t½:** 2–4 hr. The **t½** is increased to approximately 5 hr in geriatric clients. Ketoprofen is 99% bound to plasma proteins. Food does not alter the bioavailability; however, the rate of absorption is reduced.

Uses: Acute or chronic rheumatoid arthritis and osteoarthritis (both capsules and sustained-release capsules). Primary dysmenorrhea. Analgesic for mild to moderate pain. *Investigational:* Juvenile rheumatoid arthritis, sunburn, prophylaxis of migraine, migraine due to menses.

Dosage

- **Capsules**

Rheumatoid arthritis, osteoarthritis.

Adults, initial: 75 mg t.i.d. or 50 mg q.i.d.; **maintenance:** 150–300 mg in three to four divided doses daily. Doses above 300 mg/day are not recommended. Alternatively, 200 mg once daily using the sustained-release formulation (Oruvail). Dosage should be decreased by one-half to one-third in clients with impaired renal function or in geriatric clients.

Mild to moderate pain, dysmenorrhea.

Adults: 25–50 mg q 6–8 hr as required, not to exceed 300 mg/day. Dosage should be reduced in smaller or geriatric clients and in those with liver or renal dysfunction.

Administration/Storage: The sustained-release form should not be used for initial therapy in clients who are small, are elderly, or who have renal or hepatic impairment. Also, the sustained-release form should not be used to treat pain in any client.

Contraindications: Should not be used during late pregnancy. Use should be avoided during lactation and in children. Use of the extended-release product for acute pain.

Special Concerns: Safety and effectiveness have not been established in children. Geriatric clients may manifest increased and prolonged serum levels due to decreased protein binding and clearance. Use with caution in clients with a history of GI tract disorders, in fluid retention, hypertension, and heart failure.

Additional Side Effects: *GI:* Peptic ulcer, ***GI bleeding,*** dyspepsia, nausea, diarrhea, constipation, abdominal pain, flatulence, anorexia, vomiting, stomatitis. *CNS:* Headache. *CV:* Peripheral edema, fluid retention.

Additional Drug Interactions

Acetylsalicylic acid / ↑ Plasma ketoprofen levels due to ↓ plasma protein binding

Hydrochlorothiazide / ↓ Chloride and potassium excretion

Methotrexate / Concomitant use → toxic plasma levels of methotrexate

Probenecid / ↓ Plasma clearance of ketoprofen and ↓ plasma protein binding

Warfarin / Additive effect to cause bleeding

NURSING CONSIDERATIONS

See also *Nursing Considerations* for *Nonsteroidal Anti-Inflammatory Drugs,* Chapter 42.

Assessment

1. Document indications for therapy and type and onset of symptoms.
2. Note any history of GI disorders, cardiac failure, hypertension, or fluid retention.
3. Determine if pregnant and document age. The drug is not recommended for children under 12 years of age.
4. Obtain baseline bleeding profiles and liver and renal function studies. Monitor hematologic profile and test urine and stools for occult blood. The drug may prolong bleeding times by decreasing platelet aggregation.
5. Anticipate a reduced dosage of drug in elderly clients and those with impaired renal function.

Client/Family Teaching

1. GI side effects may be minimized by taking ketoprofen with antacids, milk, or food.
2. Avoid alcohol.
3. Do not take any aspirin products unless specifically prescribed.
4. Report any new symptoms such as rash, headaches, black stools, disturbances in vision, petechiae, unexplained bruising, bleeding from the gums, or nose bleeds.
5. Advise to report any evidence of liver dysfunction such as jaundice, upper right quadrant pain, clay-colored

stools, or yellowing of the skin and sclera.
6. Stress the importance of reporting for scheduled lab studies and eye exams throughout therapy.

Evaluate

- Improvement in joint pain, inflammation, and mobility
- Control of pain and discomfort
- ↓ Uterine cramping

Ketorolac tromethamine

(kee-toh-**ROH**-lack)
Pregnancy Category: C
Acular, Toradol, Toradol IM **(Rx)**

See also *Nonsteroidal Anti-Inflammatory Drugs,* Chapter 42.

How Supplied: *Injection:* 15 mg/mL, 30 mg/mL; *Ophthalmic solution:* 0.5%; *Tablet:* 10 mg

Action/Kinetics: Ketorolac tromethamine is a NSAID that possesses anti-inflammatory, analgesic, and antipyretic effects. It is completely absorbed following an IM dose. **Onset:** Within 10 min. **Peak plasma levels:** 2.2–3.0 mcg/mL 50 min after a dose of 30 mg. **t½, terminal:** 3.8–6.3 hr in young adults and 4.7–8.6 hr in geriatric clients. Over 99% is bound to plasma proteins. The drug is metabolized in the liver with over 90% excreted in the urine and the remainder excreted in the feces.

Uses: Intramuscular for short-term management of pain. Ophthalmically to relieve itching caused by seasonal allergic conjunctivitis.

Dosage

- **IM**

Analgesic.

Adults, initial loading dose: 30 or 60 mg; **then,** 15 or 30 mg q 6 hr as needed to control pain. **Maximum daily dose:** 150 mg for the first day and 120 mg thereafter.

- **Ophthalmic Solution**

Seasonal allergic conjunctivitis.

1 gtt (0.25 mg) q.i.d.

Administration/Storage

1. Ketorolac should be used as part of a regular analgesic schedule rather than on an as needed basis.
2. To minimize a time delay in reaching adequate analgesic effects, an initial loading dose is recommended equal to twice the maintenance dose.
3. If the drug is given on an as needed basis, the size of a repeat dose should be based on the duration of pain relief from the previous dose. If the pain returns within 3–5 hr, the next dose could be increased by up to 50% (as long as the total daily dose is not exceeded). If the pain does not return for 8–12 hr, the next dose could be decreased by as much as 50% or the dosing interval could be increased to q 8–12 hr.
4. Lower doses should be considered for clients under 50 kg, over 65 years of age, and with reduced renal function.

Contraindications: Hypersensitivity to the drug, incomplete or partial syndrome of nasal polyps, angioedema, and bronchospasm due to aspirin or other NSAIDs. Use as an obstetric preoperative medication or for obstetric analgesia. Routine use with other NSAIDs. The ophthalmic solution should not be used in clients wearing soft contact lenses.

Special Concerns: Use with caution in impaired hepatic or renal function, during lactation, in geriatric clients, and in clients on high-dose salicylate regimens. The age, dosage, and duration of therapy should receive special consideration when using this drug. Safety and effectiveness have not been determined in children.

Additional Side Effects: *CV:* Vasodilation, pallor. *GI:* GI pain, nausea, dyspepsia, flatulence, GI fullness, stomatitis, excessive thirst, GI bleeding (higher in geriatric clients). *CNS:* Headache, nervousness, abnormal thinking, depression, euphoria. *Miscellaneous:* Purpura, asthma, abnormal vision, abnormal liver function.

Use of the ophthalmic solution: Transient stinging and burning following instillation, ocular irritation, allergic reactions, superficial ocular infections, superficial keratitis.
Drug Interaction: Ketorolac may ↑ plasma levels of salicylates due to ↓ plasma protein binding.

NURSING CONSIDERATIONS

See also *Nursing Considerations* for *Nonsteroidal Anti-Inflammatory Drugs,* Chapter 42.
Assessment
1. Document indications for therapy and type and onset of symptoms.
2. Note any previous experience with NSAIDs and the results.
3. Determine any evidence of liver or renal dysfunction.
Evaluate
- Effective pain control
- Relief of ocular allergic manifestations

Meclofenamate sodium

(me-kloh-fen-**AM**-ayt)
Meclofen, Meclomen **(Rx)**

See also *Nonsteroidal Anti-Inflammatory Drugs,* Chapter 42.
How Supplied: *Capsule:* 50 mg, 100 mg
Action/Kinetics: Peak plasma levels: 30–60 min. **t$^{1/2}$:** 2–3.3 hr. Peak anti-inflammatory activity may not be observed for 2–3 weeks. Excreted through urine and feces.
Uses: Acute and chronic rheumatoid arthritis and osteoarthritis. Not indicated as the initial drug for rheumatoid arthritis due to GI side effects. Has been used in combination with gold salts or corticosteroids. Mild to moderate pain. Primary dysmenorrhea, excessive menstrual blood loss. *Investigational:* Sunburn, prophylaxis of migraine, migraine due to menses.

Dosage

- **Capsules**

Rheumatoid arthritis, osteoarthritis.
Adults, usual: 200–400 mg/day in three to four equal doses. Initiate at lower dose and increase to maximum of 400 mg/day if necessary. After initial satisfactory response, lower dosage to decrease severity of side effects.

Mild to moderate pain.
Adults: 50 mg q 4–6 hr (100 mg may be required in some clients), not to exceed 400 mg/day.

Excessive menstrual blood loss and primary dysmenorrhea.
Adults: 100 mg t.i.d. for up to 6 days, starting at the onset of menses.
Administration/Storage
1. Lower doses may be effective for chronic use.
2. Reduce dose or discontinue temporarily if diarrhea occurs.
Additional Contraindications: Not recommended for use during pregnancy or lactation. Use in children less than 14 years of age.
Special Concerns: Safe use during lactation not established. Safety and efficacy not established in functional class IV rheumatoid arthritis.
Laboratory Test Interferences: ↑ Serum transaminase, alkaline phosphatase; rarely, ↑ serum creatinine or BUN.
Additional Side Effects: Severe diarrhea, nausea, headache, rash, dermatitis, abdominal pain, pyrosis, flatulence, malaise, fatigue, paresthesia, insomnia, depression, taste disturbances, nocturia, blood loss (through feces: 2 mL/day).
Drug Interactions
Aspirin / ↓ Plasma levels of meclofenamate
Warfarin / ↑ Effect of warfarin

NURSING CONSIDERATIONS

See also *Nursing Considerations* for *Nonsteroidal Anti-Inflammatory Drugs,* Chapter 42.
Client/Family Teaching
1. May take with food or milk to diminish GI effects.
2. Report any changes in stool color. Anticipate periodic CBC, renal function studies, and stool specimens for occult blood.
3. Continue to take the drug as ordered and do not become discouraged because beneficial effects are not readily evident and it may take

2–3 weeks to see improvement in arthritic conditions.

Evaluate

- Improvement in joint pain and mobility
- Relief of pain and dysmenorrhea

Mefenamic acid

(meh-fen-**NAM**-ick **AH**-sid)

Pregnancy Category: C

Ponstan ✱, Ponstel **(Rx)**

See also *Nonsteroidal Anti-Inflammatory Drugs,* Chapter 42.

How Supplied: *Capsule:* 250 mg

Action/Kinetics: Mefenamic acid inhibits prostaglandin synthesis. It possesses anti-inflammatory, antipyretic, and analgesic effects. **Peak plasma levels:** 2–4 hr; **t½:** 2–4 hr; **duration:** 4–6 hr. The drug is slowly absorbed from the GI tract, metabolized by the liver, and excreted in the urine and feces.

Uses: Short-term relief (<1 week) of mild to moderate pain (e.g., pain associated with tooth extraction and musculoskeletal disorders). Primary dysmenorrhea. *Investigational:* PMS, sunburn.

Dosage

- **Capsules**

Analgesia, primary dysmenorrhea.

Adults and children over 14 years of age, initial: 500 mg; **then,** 250 mg q 6 hr.

Administration/Storage

1. Give with food.
2. The drug should not be used for more than a week at a time.

Contraindications: Ulceration or chronic inflammation of the GI tract, pregnancy or possibility thereof, children under 14, and hypersensitivity to the drug.

Special Concerns: Dosage has not been established in children less than 14 years of age. Use with caution in clients with impaired renal or hepatic function, asthma, or clients on anticoagulant therapy.

Laboratory Test Interference: False + test for urinary bile using diazo tablets.

Additional Side Effects: ***Autoimmune hemolytic anemia if used more than 12 months.*** Diarrhea may be significant. Rash (maculopapular type).

Drug Interactions

Anticoagulants / ↑ Hypoprothrombinemia due to ↓ plasma protein binding

Insulin / ↑ Insulin requirement

Lithium / ↑ Plasma levels of lithium

NURSING CONSIDERATIONS

See also *Nursing Considerations* for *Nonsteroidal Anti-inflammatory Drugs,* Chapter 42.

Client/Family Teaching

1. Take with meals to minimize GI upset.
2. Use caution when operating potentially hazardous machinery, as in driving, because drug may cause dizziness, lightheadedness, or confusion.
3. Review anticipated benefits and possible side effects that may be associated with drug therapy.
4. Report any signs of bleeding or any evidence of rashes, diarrhea, urticaria, or increased sweating as therapy may need to be adjusted.
5. Anticipate periodic CBC, renal function studies, and stool for occult blood.

Evaluate

- Relief of pain
- Control of uterine cramping

Nabumetone

(nah-**BYOU**-meh-tohn)

Pregnancy Category: B

Relafen **(Rx)**

See also *Nonsteroidal Anti-Inflammatory Drugs,* Chapter 42.

How Supplied: *Tablet:* 500 mg, 750 mg

Action/Kinetics: Time to peak plasma levels: 2.5–4 hr. **t½ of active metabolite:** 22.5–30 hr.

Uses: Acute and chronic treatment of osteoarthritis and rheumatoid arthritis. Has also been used to treat mild to moderate pain including postextraction dental pain, postsurgical episiotomy pain, and soft-tissue athletic injuries.

Dosage

- **Tablets**

Osteoarthritis, rheumatoid arthritis.

Adults, initial: 1,000 mg as a single dose; **maintenance:** 1,500–2,000 mg/day. Doses greater than 2,000 mg/day have not been studied.

Administration/Storage

1. May be taken with or without food.
2. The total daily dose may be given either once or in two divided doses.
3. The lowest effective dose should be used for chronic treatment.

Contraindication: Lactation.

Special Concerns: Safety and efficacy have not been determined in children.

NURSING CONSIDERATIONS

See also *Nursing Considerations* for *Nonsteroidal Anti-Inflammatory Drugs,* Chapter 42.

Assessment

1. Document indications for therapy and type and onset of symptoms.
2. List any other drugs used and the outcome.
3. Obtain baseline CBC and liver and renal function studies and monitor values with chronic therapy.

Client/Family Teaching

1. Take only as directed. May take with food to decrease GI upset.
2. Review drug side effects that require immediate reporting: persistent headaches, altered vision, rash, swelling of extremities, blood in stools.
3. Do not perform tasks that require mental alertness until drug effects are realized.
4. Avoid alcohol and alcohol-containing products.
5. Do not use aspirin or aspirin-containing products.

Evaluate

- Symptomatic relief of pain
- Improved joint mobility and ↑ ROM

Naproxen

(nah-**PROX**-en)
Pregnancy Category: B
Apo-Naproxen ✱, Naprosyn, Naxen ✱, Novo-Naprox ✱, Nu-Naprox ✱, PMS-Naproxen ✱ **(Rx)**

Naproxen sodium

(nah-**PROX**-en)
Pregnancy Category: B
Anaprox, Anaprox DS, Apo-Napro-Na ✱, Novo-Naprox Sodium ✱, Synflex ✱, Synflex DS ✱ **(Rx)**, Aleve **(OTC)**

See also *Nonsteroidal Anti-Inflammatory Drugs,* Chapter 42.

How Supplied: Naproxen: *Enteric Coated Tablet:* 375 mg, 500 mg; *Suspension:* 25 mg/mL; *Tablet:* 250 mg, 375 mg, 500 mg
Naproxen sodium: *Tablet:* 220 mg, 275 mg, 550 mg

Action/Kinetics: Peak serum levels of naproxen: 2–4 hr; **for sodium salt:** 1–2 hr. **$t^1/_2$ for naproxen:** 12–15 hr; **for sodium salt:** 12–13 hr. **Onset, analgesia:** 1 hr. **Duration, analgesia:** Approximately 7 hr. The onset of anti-inflammatory effects may take up to 2 weeks and may last 2–4 weeks. Naproxen is more than 90% bound to plasma protein. Food delays the rate but not the amount of drug absorbed. Clinical improvement for inflammatory disease may not be observed for 2 weeks.

Uses: Rx. Mild to moderate pain. Musculoskeletal and soft tissue inflammation including rheumatoid arthritis, osteoarthritis, bursitis, tendinitis, ankylosing spondylitis. Primary dysmenorrhea, acute gout. Juvenile rheumatoid arthritis (naproxen only). *Investigational:* Antipyretic in cancer clients, sunburn, acute migraine (sodium salt only), prophylaxis of migraine, migraine due to menses, PMS (sodium salt only). **OTC.** Relief of minor aches and pains due to the common cold, headache, toothache, muscular aches, backache, minor arthritis pain, pain due to menstrual cramps. Decrease fever.

Dosage

NAPROXEN

• **Oral Suspension, Tablets**

Antirheumatic (rheumatoid arthritis, osteoarthritis, ankylosing spondylitis).

Adults, individualized, usual: 250, 375, or 500 mg b.i.d. in the morning and evening. Improvement should be observed within 2 weeks; if no improvement is seen, an additional 2-week course of therapy should be considered. May increase to 1.5 g for short periods of time.

Acute gout.

Adults, initial: 750 mg; **then,** 250 mg naproxen q 8 hr until symptoms subside.

Mild to moderate pain, primary dysmenorrhea, acute bursitis and tendinitis.

Adults, initial: 500 mg; **then,** 250 mg/6–8 hr. Total daily dosage should not exceed 1,250 mg.

Juvenile rheumatoid arthritis.

Naproxen only, 10 mg/kg/day in two divided doses. If the suspension is used, the following dosage can be used: **13 kg:** 2.5 mL b.i.d.; **25 kg:** 5 mL b.i.d.; **38 kg:** 7.5 mL b.i.d.

NAPROXEN SODIUM

• **Tablets (Rx)**

Anti-rheumatic.

Adults: 275 mg b.i.d. in the morning and evening (alternate dosage: 275 mg in the morning and 550 mg at night).

Acute gout.

Adults, initial: 825 mg; **then,** 275 mg q 8 hr until symptoms subside.

Mild to moderate pain, primary dysmenorrhea, acute bursitis and tendinitis.

Adults, initial: 550 mg; **then,** 275 mg q 6–8 hr as needed. Total daily dose should not exceed 1,375 mg.

• **Tablets (OTC)**

Adults: 200 mg q 8–12 hr with a full glass of liquid. For some clients, 400 mg initially followed by 200 mg 12 hr later will provide better relief. Dose should not exceed 600 mg in a 24-hr period. Geriatric clients should not take more than 200 mg q 12 hr. Not for use in children less than 12 years of age unless directed by a physician.

Administration/Storage

1. The onset of action is 1–2 hr. The duration of action is 7 hr.
2. It is recommended that the medication be taken in the morning and in the evening. The doses do not have to be equal.
3. Naproxen sodium should not be administered to children.
4. Naproxen suspension can be used to treat children with rheumatoid arthritis.

Contraindications: Use of naproxen and naproxen sodium simultaneously. Lactation.

Special Concerns: Safety and effectiveness of naproxen have not been determined in children less than 2 years of age; the safety and effectiveness of naproxen sodium have not been established in children. Geriatric clients may manifest increased total plasma levels of naproxen.

Laboratory Test Interferences: Naproxen may increase urinary 17-ketosteroid values. Both forms may interfere with urinary assays for 5-HIAA.

Drug Interactions

Methotrexate / Possibility of a fatal interaction

Probenecid / ↓ Plasma clearance of naproxen

NURSING CONSIDERATIONS

See also *Nursing Considerations* for *Nonsteroidal Anti-Inflammatory Drugs,* Chapter 42.

Assessment

1. Note any history of hypersensitivity to naproxen or other NSAIDs.
2. Document indications for therapy and type and onset of symptoms.
3. List other drugs prescribed and the outcome.
4. Determine any evidence of GI bleeding or ulcers.
5. Obtain baseline CBC and liver and renal function studies and monitor with chronic therapy.

Client/Family Teaching

1. May take with food to minimize GI upset.

2. Take as directed in the morning and evening for optimal effects.
3. Report any persistent abdominal pain or dark-colored stools immediately.

Evaluate

- Improvement in joint pain and mobility
- Relief of headaches
- ↓ Uterine cramping

Oxaprozin

(**ox**-ah-**PROH**-zin)
Pregnancy Category: C
Daypro **(Rx)**

See also *Nonsteroidal Anti-Inflammatory Drugs,* Chapter 42.
How Supplied: *Tablet:* 600 mg
Uses: Acute and chronic use to manage rheumatoid arthritis and osteoarthritis.

Dosage

- **Tablets**

Rheumatoid arthritis.
Adults: 1,200 mg/day. Lower and higher doses may be required in certain clients.

Osteoarthritis.
Adults: 1,200 mg/day. For clients with a lower body weight or with a milder disease, 600 mg/day may be appropriate.

The maximum daily use for either rheumatoid arthritis or osteoarthritis is 1,800 mg (or 26 mg/kg, whichever is lower) given in divided doses.
Administration/Storage: Regardless of the use, the dose must be individualized so the lowest effective dose is given to minimize side effects.

NURSING CONSIDERATIONS

See also *Nursing Considerations* for *Nonsteroidal Anti-Inflammatory Drugs,* Chapter 42.

Assessment

1. Document indications for therapy and type and onset of symptoms.
2. Assess involved joint(s) and determine baseline ROM and the extent of any inflammation.
3. Obtain baseline CBC and liver and renal function studies with chronic therapy and monitor (q 6–12 months).

Evaluate: Relief of joint pain with improved mobility.

Piroxicam

(peer-**OX**-ih-kam)
Apo-Piroxicam ✱, Feldene, Novo-Pirocam ✱, Nu-Pirox ✱ **(Rx)**

See also *Nonsteroidal Anti-Inflammatory Drugs,* Chapter 42.
How Supplied: *Capsule:* 10 mg, 20 mg
Action/Kinetics: Piroxicam may inhibit prostaglandin synthesis. **Peak plasma levels:** 1.5–2 mcg/mL after 3–5 hr (single dose). **Steady-state plasma levels** (after 7–12 days):3–8 mcg/mL. **t½:** 50 hr. **Analgesia, onset:** 1 hr; **duration:** 2–3 days. **Anti-inflammatory activity, onset:** 7–12 days; **duration:** 2–3 weeks. Metabolites and unchanged drug excreted in urine and feces.

The effect of piroxicam is comparable to that of aspirin, but with fewer GI side effects and less tinnitus. May be used with gold, corticosteroids, and antacids.
Uses: Acute and chronic treatment of rheumatoid arthritis and osteoarthritis. *Investigational:* Juvenile rheumatoid arthritis, primary dysmenorrhea, sunburn.

Dosage

- **Capsules**

Anti-inflammatory, antirheumatic.
Adults: 20 mg/day in one or more divided doses. Effect of therapy should not be assessed for 2 weeks.

Administration/Storage

1. Steady-state plasma levels may not be reached for 2 weeks.
2. Clients over 70 years of age generally require one-half the usual adult dose of medication.
3. The drug is not recommended for children under 14 years of age.

Contraindications: Safe use during pregnancy has not been determined. Lactation.
Special Concerns: Safety and efficacy have not been established in chil-

dren. Increased plasma levels and elimination half-life may be observed in geriatric clients (especially women).
Laboratory Test Interference: Reversible ↑ BUN.

NURSING CONSIDERATIONS

See also *Nursing Considerations* for *Nonsteroidal Anti-Inflammatory Drugs,* Chapter 42.

Assessment

1. Document indications for therapy, type of symptoms, other agents prescribed, and the outcome.
2. Assess involved joints and note ROM and the presence of any inflammation.

Client/Family Teaching

1. May take with food to decrease GI upset.
2. Stress the importance of taking at anti-inflammatory dose to prevent further joint destruction during acute exacerbations.
3. Therapeutic effects of the medication cannot be evaluated fully for at least 2 weeks after beginning treatment.
4. Aspirin decreases the effectiveness of piroxicam and may increase the occurrence of side effects. Avoid aspirin and any other OTC products unless directed.
5. Report any increased abdominal pain or changes in the color of the stool immediately.
6. Drug side effects may not be evident for 7–10 days.
7. Report as scheduled for lab studies including CBC and liver and renal function studies and stool and urine for occult blood during long-term therapy.

Evaluate: Control of joint pain and inflammation with improved mobility.

Sulindac

(sul-**IN**-dak)
Apo-Sulin ✱, Clinoril, Novo-Sudac ✱
(Rx)

See also *Nonsteroidal Anti-Inflammatory Drugs,* Chapter 42.

How Supplied: *Tablet:* 150 mg, 200 mg
Action/Kinetics: Sulindac is biotransformed in the liver to a sulfide, the active metabolite. **Peak plasma levels of sulfide:** after fasting, 2 hr; after food, 3–4 hr. **Onset, anti-inflammatory effect:** within 1 week; **duration, anti-inflammatory effect:** 1–2 weeks. **t½,** of sulindac: 7.8 hr; of metabolite: 16.4 hr. Excreted in both urine and feces.
Uses: Acute and chronic treatment of rheumatoid arthritis, osteoarthritis, ankylosing spondylitis, acute gouty arthritis; acute, painful shoulder; tendinitis, bursitis. *Investigational:* Juvenile rheumatoid arthritis, sunburn.

Dosage

- **Tablets**

Osteoarthritis, rheumatoid arthritis, ankylosing spondylitis.
Adults: 150 mg b.i.d.
Acute painful shoulder, acute gouty arthritis.
Adults: 200 mg b.i.d. for 7–14 days.
Antigout.
Adults: 200 mg b.i.d. for 7 days.

Administration/Storage

1. When used for arthritis, a favorable response usually occurs within 1 week.
2. For acute conditions, reduce dosage when satisfactory response is attained.

Contraindication: Use with active GI lesions or a history of recurrent GI lesions.
Special Concerns: Safety and efficacy have not been established for children. Safe use during pregnancy has not been established. Use with caution during lactation.
Additional Side Effects: Hypersensitivity, pancreatitis, GI pain (common), maculopapular rash. Stupor, ***coma,*** hypotension, and diminished urine output.
Additional Drug Interaction: Sulindac ↑ effect of warfarin due to ↓ plasma protein binding.

NURSING CONSIDERATIONS

See also *Nursing Considerations* for *Nonsteroidal Anti-Inflammatory Drugs,* Chapter 42.

Assessment

1. Document indications for therapy and type and onset of symptoms.
2. Determine baseline ROM, include a description and the location of clients' pain and discomfort; include functional class of arthritis.
3. If I&O or lab studies indicate renal dysfunction, anticipate a reduction in dosage of drug.
4. Obtain baseline CBC and liver and renal function studies with long-term therapy and monitor periodically; assess stools for occult blood.

Client/Family Teaching

1. Take with food to decrease GI upset and consume plenty of water.
2. Do not take aspirin because plasma levels of sulindac will be reduced.
3. Report any incidence of unexplained bleeding such as oozing of blood from the gums, nosebleeds, or excessive bruising.
4. Drug may cause dizziness; assess response prior to any activity requiring mental alertness.

Evaluate: Reports of ↓ joint pain and inflammation with ↑ mobility.

Suprofen

(sue-**PROH**-fen)
Pregnancy Category: C
Profenal **(Rx)**

See also *Nonsteroidal Anti-Inflammatory Drugs,* Chapter 42.

How Supplied: *Solution:* 1%

Action/Kinetics: By inhibiting prostaglandin synthesis, suprofen reverses prostaglandin-induced vasodilation, leukocytosis, increased vascular permeability, and increased intraocular pressure. The drug also inhibits miosis, which occurs during cataract surgery.

Use: Inhibition of intraoperative miosis.

Dosage

- **Ophthalmic**

Day before surgery.

2 gtt into the conjunctival sac q 4 hr during waking hours.

Day of surgery.

2 gtt into the conjunctival sac 3, 2, and 1 hr prior to surgery.

Administration: For best results, follow administration guidelines carefully.

Contraindication: Dendritic keratitis.

Special Concerns: Use with caution in clients sensitive to aspirin and other NSAIDs. Use with caution in surgical clients with a history of bleeding tendencies or who are on drugs that prolong bleeding time. Use with caution during lactation. Safety and efficacy have not been established in children.

Side Effects: *Ophthalmic:* Ocular irritation, transient burning, and stinging on installation. Redness, itching, discomfort, pain, iritis, allergy, chemosis, photophobia, punctate epithelial staining.

Drug Interactions: Acetylcholine and carbachol may be ineffective if used in combination with suprofen.

NURSING CONSIDERATIONS

See also *Nursing Considerations* for *Nonsteroidal Anti-Inflammatory Drugs,* Chapter 42.

Evaluate: Control of inflammation and inhibition of abnormal pupillary contractions.

Tolmetin sodium

(**TOLL**-met-in)
Pregnancy Category: C
Tolectin ✱, Tolectin 200, Tolectin 600, Tolectin DS **(Rx)**

See also *Nonsteroidal Anti-Inflammatory Drugs,* Chapter 42.

How Supplied: *Capsule:* 400 mg; *Tablet:* 200 mg, 600 mg

Action/Kinetics: Peak plasma levels: 30–60 min. **t½:** 1 hr. **Therapeutic plasma levels:** 40 mcg/mL. **Onset, anti-inflammatory effect:** within 1 week; **duration, anti-inflammatory effect:** 1–2 weeks. Inactivated in liver and excreted in urine.

Uses: Acute and chronic treatment of rheumatoid arthritis and osteoarthritis. Juvenile rheumatoid arthritis. *Investigational:* Sunburn.

Dosage

- **Capsules, Tablets**

Rheumatoid arthritis, osteoarthritis.

Adults: 400 mg t.i.d. (one dose on arising and one at bedtime); adjust dosage according to client response. **Maintenance:** *rheumatoid arthritis,* 600–1,800 mg/day in three to four divided doses; *osteoarthritis,* 600–1,600 mg/day in three to four divided doses. Doses larger than 1,800 mg/day for rheumatoid arthritis and osteoarthritis are not recommended.

Juvenile rheumatoid arthritis.

2 years and older, initial: 20 mg/kg/day in three to four divided doses to start; **then,** 15–30 mg/kg/day. Doses higher than 30 mg/kg/day are not recommended. Beneficial effects may not be observed for several days to a week.

Special Concerns: Use with caution during lactation. Dosage has not been determined in children less than 2 years of age.

Laboratory Test Interference: Tolmetin metabolites give a false + test for proteinuria using sulfosalicylic acid.

NURSING CONSIDERATIONS

See also *Nursing Considerations* for *Nonsteroidal Anti-Inflammatory Drugs,* Chapter 42.

Client/Family Teaching

1. Doses of medication should be spaced so that one dose is taken in the morning on arising, one during the day, and one at bedtime.
2. Caution that drug may cause drowsiness or dizziness.
3. Administer the drug with meals, milk, a full glass of water, or antacids (other than sodium bicarbonate) if the client develops symptoms of gastric irritation. Never administer the medication with sodium bicarbonate.
4. Elderly clients are particularly susceptible to gastric irritation. Therefore, they should receive their medication with milk, meals, or an antacid.
5. Report any unusual bruising or bleeding or evidence of edema.
6. Advise that it may take several weeks before effects are evident.
7. Avoid alcohol and any OTC medications without provider approval.

Evaluate: Reports of ↓ joint pain and inflammation with ↑ mobility.

CHAPTER FORTY-THREE

Narcotic Analgesics

See also the following individual entries:

Alfentanil Hydrochloride
Buprenorphine Hydrochloride
Butorphanol Tartrate
Codeine Phosphate
Codeine Sulfate
Dezocine
Empirin with Codeine
Fentanyl Citrate
Fentanyl Transdermal System
Fiorinal
Fiorinal with Codeine
Hydrocodone Bitartrate and Acetaminophen
Hydromorphone Hydrochloride
Levomethadyl Acetate Hydrochloride
Meperidine Hydrochloride (Pethidine Hydrochloride)
Methadone Hydrochloride
Morphine Hydrochloride
Morphine Sulfate
Nalbuphine Hydrochloride
Oxycodone Hydrochloride
Oxycodone Terephthalate
Oxymorphone Hydrochloride
Paregoric (Camphorated Opium Tincture)
Pentazocine Hydrochloride with Naloxone Hydrochloride
Pentazocine Lactate
Percocet
Percodan and Percodan-Demi
Phenaphen with Codeine No. 2, No. 3, and No. 4
Phenaphen-650 with Codeine Tablets
Propoxyphene Hydrochloride
Propoxyphene Napsylate
Sufentanil
Synalgos-DC
Tylenol with Codeine Elixir or Tablets
Tylox
Vicodin

General Statement: The narcotic analgesics include opium, morphine, codeine, various opium derivatives, and totally synthetic substances with similar pharmacologic properties. Of these, meperidine (Demerol) is the best known. The relative activity of all narcotic analgesics is measured against morphine.

Opium itself is a mixture of alkaloids obtained since ancient times from the poppy plant. Morphine and codeine are two of the pure chemical substances isolated from opium. Certain drugs (pentazocine, butorphanol, nalbuphine) have both narcotic agonist and antagonist properties. Such drugs may precipitate a withdrawal syndrome if given to clients dependent on narcotics.

Action/Kinetics: The most important effect of the narcotic analgesics is on the CNS. In addition to an alteration of pain perception (analgesia), the drugs, especially at higher doses, induce euphoria, drowsiness, changes in mood, mental clouding, and deep sleep.

The narcotic analgesics also depress respiration. The effect is noticeable with small doses. Death by overdosage is almost always the result of respiratory arrest.

The narcotic analgesics have a nauseant and emetic effect (direct stimulation of the CTZ). They depress the cough reflex, and small doses of narcotic analgesics (codeine) are part of several antitussive preparations.

The narcotic analgesics have little effect on BP when the client is in a supine position. However, most narcotics decrease the capacity of the client to respond to stress. Morphine and other narcotic analgesics induce peripheral vasodilation, which may result in hypotension.

Many narcotic analgesics constrict the pupil. With such drugs, pupillary constriction is the most obvious sign of dependence.

The narcotic analgesics also decrease peristaltic motility. The constipating effects of these agents (Paregoric) are sometimes used therapeutically in severe diarrhea. The narcotic analgesics also increase the pressure within the biliary tract.

The narcotic analgesics attach to specific receptors located in the CNS (cortex, brain stem, and spinal cord), resulting in analgesia. Although the details are unknown, the mechanism is believed to involve decreased permeability of the cell membrane to sodium, which results in diminished transmission of pain impulses. Five categories of opioid receptors have been identified: mu, kappa, sigma, delta, and epsilon. Narcotic analgesics are believed to exert their activity at mu, kappa, and sigma receptors. Mu receptors are thought to mediate supraspinal analgesia, euphoria, and respiratory depression. Pentazocine-like spinal analgesia, miosis, and sedation are mediated by kappa receptors while sigma receptors mediate dysphoria, hallucinations, as well as respiratory and vasomotor stimulation (caused by drugs with antagonist activity). For kinetics, see individual agents.

Uses: Severe pain, especially of coronary, pulmonary, or peripheral origin. Hepatic and renal colic. Preanesthetic medication and adjuncts to anesthesia. Postsurgical pain. Acute vascular occlusion, especially of coronary, pulmonary, and peripheral origin. Diarrhea and dysentery. Pain from MI, carcinoma, burns. Postpartum pain. Some members of this group are primarily used as antitussives. Methadone is used for heroin withdrawal and maintenance.

Contraindications: Asthmatic conditions, emphysema, kyphoscoliosis, severe obesity, convulsive states as in epilepsy, delirium tremens, tetanus and strychnine poisoning, diabetic acidosis, myxedema, Addison's disease, hepatic cirrhosis, and children under 6 months.

Special Concerns: Use cautiously in clients with head injury or after head surgery because of morphine's capacity to elevate ICP and mask the pupillary response.

Use with caution in the elderly, in the debilitated, in young children, in individuals with increased ICP, in obstetrics, and with clients in shock or during acute alcoholic intoxication.

Morphine should be used with extreme caution in clients with pulmonary heart disease (cor pulmonale). Deaths following ordinary therapeutic doses have been reported. Use cautiously in clients with prostatic hypertrophy, because it may precipitate acute urinary retention.

Use cautiously in clients with reduced blood volume, such as in hemorrhaging clients who are more susceptible to the hypotensive effects of morphine.

Since the drugs depress the respiratory center, they should be given early in labor, at least 2 hr before delivery, to reduce the danger of respiratory depression in the newborn. When given before surgery, the narcotic analgesics should be given at least 1–2 hr preoperatively so that the danger of maximum depression of respiratory function will have passed before anesthesia is initiated.

These drugs should sometimes be withheld prior to diagnostic procedures so that the physician can use pain to locate dysfunction.

Side Effects: *Respiratory:* ***Respiratory depression, apnea.*** *CNS:* Dizziness, lightheadedness, sedation, lethargy, headache, euphoria, mental clouding, fainting. Idiosyncratic effects including excitement, restlessness, tremors, delirium, insomnia. *GI:* N&V, vomiting, constipation, increased pressure in biliary tract, dry mouth, anorexia. *CV:* Flushing, changes in HR and BP, circulatory collapse. *Allergic:* Skin rashes including pruritus and urticaria. Sweating, ***laryngospasm,*** edema. *Miscellaneous:* Urinary retention, oliguria, reduced libido, changes in body temperature. Narcotics cross the placental barrier and depress respiration of the fetus or newborn.

DEPENDENCE AND TOLERANCE: It is important to remember that all drugs of this group are addictive. Psychologic and physical dependence and tolerance develop even when clients use clinical doses. Tolerance is characterized by the fact that the client requires shorter periods of time between doses or larger doses for relief of pain. Tolerance usually develops faster when the narcotic analgesic is administered regularly and when the dose is large.

Symptoms of Acute Toxicity: Severe toxicity is characterized by ***profound respiratory depression, apnea, deep sleep, stupor or coma, circulatory collapse, seizures, cardiopulmonary arrest, and death.*** Less severe toxicity results in symptoms including CNS depression, miosis, respiratory depression, deep sleep, flaccidity of skeletal muscles, hypotension, bradycardia, hypothermia, pulmonary edema, pneumonia, shock. The respiratory rate may be as low as 2–4 breaths/min. The client may be cyanotic. Urine output is decreased, the skin feels clammy, and body temperature decreases. If death occurs, it almost always results from ***respiratory depression.***

Symptoms of Chronic Toxicity: The problem of chronic dependence on narcotics occurs not only as a result of "street" use but is also found often among those who have easy access to narcotics (physicians, nurses, pharmacists). All the principal narcotic analgesics (morphine, opium, heroin, codeine, meperidine, and others) have, at times, been used for nontherapeutic purposes.

The nurse must be aware of the problem and be able to recognize signs of chronic dependence. These are constricted pupils, GI effects (constipation), skin infections, needle scars, abscesses, and itching, especially on the anterior surfaces of the body, where the client may inject the drug.

Withdrawal signs appear after drug is withheld for 4–12 hr. They are characterized by intense craving for the drug, insomnia, yawning, sneezing, vomiting, diarrhea, tremors, sweating, mental depression, muscular aches and pains, chills, and anxiety. Although the symptoms of narcotic withdrawal are uncomfortable, they are rarely life-threatening. This is in contrast to the withdrawal syndrome from depressants, where the life of the individual may be endangered because of the possibility of tonic-clonic seizures.

Drug Interactions

Alcohol, ethyl / Potentiation or addition of CNS depressant effects; concomitant use may lead to drowsiness, lethargy, stupor, respiratory collapse, coma, or death
Anesthetics, general / See *Alcohol*
Antianxiety drugs / See *Alcohol*
Antidepressants, tricyclic / ↑ Narcotic-induced respiratory depression
Antihistamines / See *Alcohol*
Barbiturates / See *Alcohol*
Cimetidine / ↑ CNS toxicity (e.g., disorientation, confusion, respiratory depression, apnea, seizures) with narcotics
CNS depressants / See *Alcohol*
MAO inhibitors / Possible potentiation of either MAO inhibitor (excitation, hypertension) or narcotic (hypotension, coma) effects; death has resulted
Methotrimeprazine / Potentiation of CNS depression
Phenothiazines / See *Alcohol*
Sedative-hypnotics, nonbarbiturate / See *Alcohol*
Skeletal muscle relaxants (surgical) / ↑ Respiratory depression and ↑ muscle relaxation

Laboratory Test Interferences: Altered liver function tests. False + or ↑ urinary glucose test (Benedict's). ↑ Plasma amylase or lipase.

Dosage

See individual drugs.

The dosage of narcotics and the reaction of a client to the dosage depend on the amount of pain. Two to four times the usual dose may be tolerated for relief of excruciating pain. However, the nurse should be aware that if, for some reason, the pain disappears, severe respiratory depression may result. This respiratory depression is not apparent while the pain is still present.

NURSING CONSIDERATIONS

Administration/Storage

1. Review the list of drugs with which narcotics interact and their associated effects.
2. Request that the orders be rewritten at timed intervals as required for continued administration.
3. Record the amount of narcotic used on the narcotic inventory sheet, indicating what was administered, the date, the time, the dose, and to whom, or if the drug was wasted and include an appropriate witness as necessary, addressing all requirements for documentation.
4. *Treatment of Acute Overdose:* Initial treatment is aimed at combating progressive respiratory depression by maintaining a patent airway and by artificial respiration. Gastric lavage and induced emesis are indicated in case of oral poisoning. The narcotic antagonist naloxone (Narcan), 0.4 mg IV, is effective in the treatment of acute overdosage. Respiratory stimulants (e.g., caffeine) should not be used to treat depression from the narcotic overdosage.

Assessment

1. Document indications for therapy and type and onset of symptoms. Differentiate acute vs chronic syndromes.
2. Note if the client has had any prior experience with narcotic analgesics such as an adverse reaction with the drug or category of drugs prescribed.
3. Identify clinical conditions that would precipitate pain syndromes, i.e., cancer, neuropathic as in diabetic neuropathy, postherpetic neuralgia, or musculoskeletal injury.
4. Determine the cause and document the amount of pain or discomfort, its location, intensity, and duration, frequency of occurrence, and what drug has been effective in the past. The amount and type of narcotic ordered should be individualized according to the client's response.
5. Use a pain rating scale (e.g., 1–10) so that clients can accurately and consistently calculate or describe their level of pain and measure the effectiveness of drug therapy.
6. Obtain baseline VS prior to administering the drug. Generally, if the respiratory rate is less than 12 breaths/min or the SBP is less than 90 mm Hg, a narcotic should not be administered unless there is ventilatory support or specific written guidelines, with parameters for administration.
7. Note the client's weight, age, and general body size. Too large a dosage of medication for the client's weight and age can result in serious side effects.
8. Document the amount of time that has elapsed between the doses for the client to have relief from recurring pain.
9. Note precipitating factors as well as the impact of the pain on the client's ability to function.
10. Document any history of asthma or other conditions that tend to compromise respirations.
11. If the client is of childbearing age, discuss the possibility of pregnancy. Narcotics cross the placental barrier and depress the respirations of the fetus. The drugs may be contraindicated under certain circumstances.
12. Baseline CBC, liver and renal functions studies, as well as electrolytes should be considered, especially when long-term therapy is anticipated.

Interventions

1. Determine when to use supportive nursing measures, such as relaxation techniques, repositioning the client, and reassurance to assist in relieving pain. Listen to the client and/or family and attempt to answer their questions honestly.
2. Explore the problem and source of the client's pain. Use nonnarcotic analgesic medications when possible. Coadministration (such as with NSAIDs) may increase analgesic effects and permit lower doses of the narcotic analgesic.
3. Administer the medication when it is needed. *Prolonging the medication until the client experiences the maximum amount of pain reduces the effectiveness of the medication.*
4. Monitor VS and mental status. During parenteral therapy:
   - Monitor the respiratory rate for signs of respiratory depression. Obtain written parameters for administration of narcotic analgesics, as necessary.
   - Narcotic analgesics depress the cough reflex. Therefore, turn clients q 2 hr, have them cough and take deep breaths to prevent atelectasis. Splinting incisions and painful areas may assist in client compliance. Ensure that narcotic is administered at least 30–60 min prior to activities or painful procedures.
   - Monitor BP. Hypotension is more apt to occur in the elderly and in those who are receiving other medications with hypotension as a side effect.
   - Monitor the HR. If the pulse drops below 60 beats/min in the adult or 110 beats/min in an infant, withhold the drug and report.
   - Observe the client for any decrease in BP, deep sleep, or constricted pupils. Withhold the drug if any of these symptoms occur, document and report.
   - Assess closely during meals to ensure that client does not choke and aspirate.
   - Note the effects of the drug on the client's mental status. A client who has experienced pain, fear, or anxiety may become euphoric and excited. Record this and report.
5. Report if the client develops N&V. If this occurs, the provider may order an antiemetic or change the medication therapy.
6. If the client is taking a narcotic medication by mouth, a snack or milk may decrease gastric irritation and lessen nausea.
7. Monitor bowel function. Narcotics, especially morphine, can have a depressant effect on the GI tract. Clients may become constipated as a consequence. If their condition permits, increase the fluid intake to 2,500–3,000 mL/day and increase their intake of fruit juices, fruits, and fiber as well as level and frequency of exercise as tolerated.
8. Narcotic drugs may cause urinary retention. Monitor the client's intake and urinary output and palpate the abdomen to detect for evidence of bladder distention. Encourage the client to attempt to empty the bladder q 3–4 hr. Question clients about difficulty voiding, pain in the bladder area, sensation of not emptying the bladder, or any unusual odors.
9. Note client complaint of difficulty with vision. Examine the client's pupillary response to light. If the client's pupils remain constricted, document and report.
10. Monitor mental status. If the client is bedridden, put up side rails and provide other protective safety measures. Assist with ambulation, BR, and transfers.
11. When administering medication, reassure client that flushing and a feeling of warmth sometimes may occur with therapeutic doses of drug.
12. Because clients may perspire profusely when receiving a narcotic, be prepared to bathe them and change their clothes and linens frequently.
13. If a client is to be receiving a narcotic preparation over a period of time, monitor renal and liver function studies.

14. Assess hospitalized clients receiving ATC therapy for evidence of tolerance and addiction.
15. In clients with terminal disease states, dependence on drug therapy is not a consideration, whereas *adequate pain control is of the utmost concern.*

Client/Family Teaching

1. Inform the client and family that the drug may become habit forming and include them in exploring alternative methods for pain control (with conditions that are not considered terminal).
2. Review the side effects of the drug and discuss the goals of therapy. Advise client to take the medication as prescribed before the pain becomes too severe.
3. Provide a printed list of the possible side effects of drug therapy. Review these with the client on discharge and again when the client returns for follow-up care.
4. Avoid consuming alcohol in any form.
5. Do not take OTC drugs without approval, as many contain small amounts of alcohol. Also, they may interact unfavorably with the prescribed medication.
6. For fecal impaction, describe preventive actions, such as increased fluid intake, increased use of fruit and fruit juices, and the possible need for a stool softener.
7. If the client is to go home on a narcotic medication, explain that the drug can cause drowsiness and dizziness. Therefore, client should use caution when operating a motor vehicle or performing other tasks that require mental alertness.
8. Advise to rise slowly from a lying to sitting position and to dangle legs before standing, to minimize orthostatic effects.
9. If the client is to be treated by someone other than the one prescribing the medication, tell that person about the drug being used and the reason for the prescribed therapy.
10. Stress the importance of storing all drugs in a safe place, out of the reach of children. Always store away from the bedside to prevent accidental overdosage.
11. During prolonged usage, advise client not to stop medications abruptly as withdrawal symptoms may occur.
12. Stress the importance of follow-up care and review the anticipated goals of the therapy with the client and family and determine whether or not these have been achieved.
13. Determine the extent of the pain relief achieved with each dosage of medication (e.g., pain level decreased from a level 5 to a level 2, 20 min after administration of medication).
14. If the goals have not been achieved, determine the source of the problem and modify the next plan of action.
15. Review techniques to enhance pain relief such as relaxation techniques, splinting incision, supporting painful areas, and taking medication before strenuous activities and before pain becomes severe.
16. Refer to appropriate support groups for assistance with the understanding, acceptance, and management of chronic pain. Determine locale of regional pain management center and refer as necessary.
17. For those with terminal diseases, refer client and family to the appropriate local support group for assistance with understanding and acceptance and to provide contact with those experiencing similar symptoms and treatments.

Special Concerns: For the elderly client, the blood levels of narcotic may be higher, resulting in longer periods of pain relief. Assess physical parameters and client complaints carefully before readministering narcotic for short-term pain control on the prescribed as-needed frequency.

Evaluate

• Reports of effective control of severe pain without altered hemodynamics or impaired level of consciousness

• The absence of symptoms of acute toxicity, tolerance, or addiction, during short-term therapy

Alfentanil hydrochloride

(al-**FEN**-tah-nil)

Pregnancy Category: C

Alfenta **(C-II) (Rx)**

See also *Narcotic Analgesics,* Chapter 43.

How Supplied: *Injection:* 0.5 mg/mL

Action/Kinetics: Onset: Immediate. **t½:** 1–2 hr (after IV use).

Uses: *Continuous infusion:* With nitrous oxide/oxygen to maintain general anesthesia. *Incremental doses:* Adjunct with barbiturate/nitrous oxide/oxygen to maintain general anesthesia. *Anesthetic induction:* As primary agent when ET intubation and mechanical ventilation are necessary.

Dosage

• **IV**

Continuous infusion, duration 45 min or more.

Initial for induction: 50–75 mcg/kg; **maintenance, with nitrous oxide/oxygen:** 0.5–3 mcg/kg/min. Following the induction dose, the infusion rate requirement should be reduced by 30%–50% for the first hour of maintenance.

Induction of anesthesia, duration 45 min or more.

Initial for induction: 130–245 mcg/kg; **maintenance:** 0.5–1.5 mcg/kg/min. If a general anesthetic is used for maintenance, the concentration of inhalation agents should be reduced by 30%–50% for the first hour.

Anesthetic adjunct, 30–60 min duration.

Initial for induction: 20–50 mcg/kg; **maintenance:** 5–15 mcg/kg, up to a total dose of 75 mcg/kg.

Anesthetic adjunct, less than 30 min duration.

Initial for induction: 8–20 mcg/kg; **maintenance:** 3–5 mcg/kg (or 0.5–1 mcg/kg/min, up to a total dose of 8–40 mcg/kg). If there is a lightening of general anesthesia or the client manifests signs of surgical stress, the rate of administration of alfentanil may be increased to 4 mcg/kg/min or a bolus dose of 7 mcg/kg may be used. If the situation is not controlled following three bolus doses over 5 min, an inhalation anesthetic, a barbiturate, or a vasodilator should be used. If signs of lightening anesthesia are noted within the last 15 min of surgery, a bolus dose of 7 mcg/kg should be given rather than increasing the infusion rate. A potent inhalation anesthetic may be used as an alternative.

Administration/Storage

1. The dosage of drug must be individualized for each client and for each use.

• For elderly or debilitated clients the dosage of drug should be reduced.

• For obese clients who are more than 20% above their ideal body weight, the dosage should be based on lean body weight.

2. The injectable form may be reconstituted with either normal saline, 5% dextrose in normal saline, lactated Ringer's solution, or 5% dextrose in water. Direct IV administration over 1½–3 min. For continous IV administration dilute 20 cc of Alfentanil in 230 mL diluent to provide a solution of 40 mcg/mL.

3. The infusion should be discontinued 10–15 min prior to the end of surgery.

Contraindication: Use during labor.

Special Concerns: Use in children less than 12 years of age is not recommended. Use with caution during lactation.

Additional Side Effects: Bradycardia, postoperative confusion, blurred vision, hypercapnia, shivering, and ***asystole***. Neonates with respiratory distress syndrome have manifested hypotension with doses of 20 mcg/ kg.

VISUAL IDENTIFICATION GUIDE

Use this section to quickly verify the identity of a capsule, tablet, or other solid oral medication. More than 200 leading products are shown in actual size and color, organized alphabetically by generic name. Each product is labeled with its brand name, if applicable, as well as its strength and the name of its supplier.

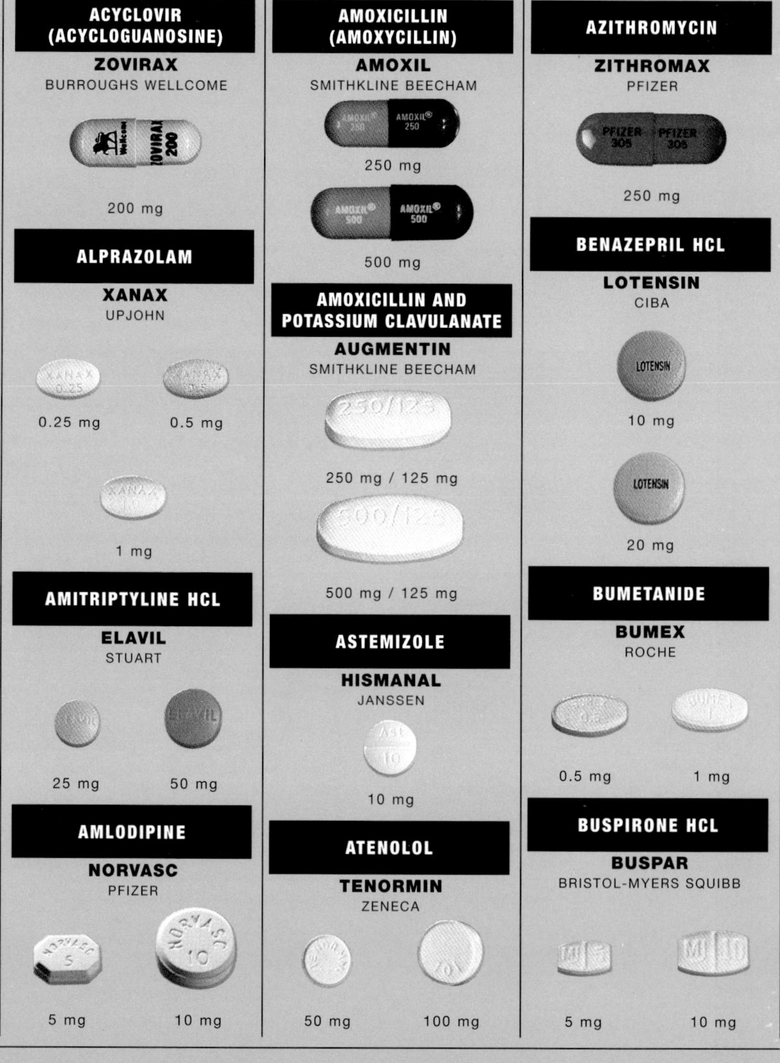

CAPTOPRIL

CAPOTEN
BRISTOL-MYERS SQUIBB

12.5 mg

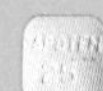

25 mg

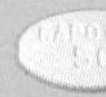

50 mg

CARBAMAZEPINE

TEGRETOL
BASEL

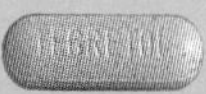

200 mg

CEFACLOR

CECLOR
ELI LILLY

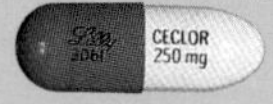

250 mg

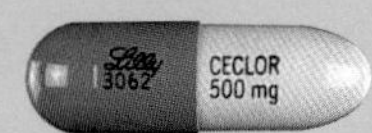

500 mg

CEFADROXIL MONOHYDRATE

DURICEF
BRISTOL-MYERS SQUIBB

500 mg

CEFIXIME

SUPRAX
LEDERLE

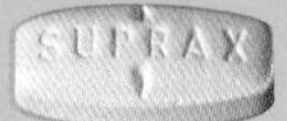

400 mg

CEFPROZIL

CEFZIL
BRISTOL-MYERS SQUIBB

250 mg

CEFUROXIME AXETIL

CEFTIN
GLAXO

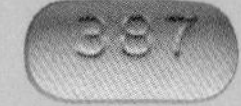

250 mg

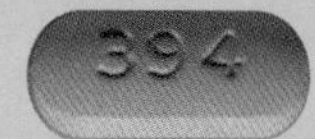

500 mg

CEPHALEXIN MONOHYDRATE

KEFLEX
DISTA

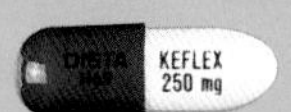

250 mg

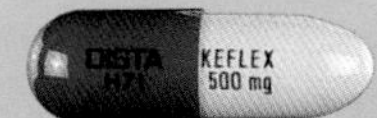

500 mg

CIMETIDINE

TAGAMET
SMITHKLINE BEECHAM

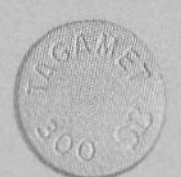

300 mg

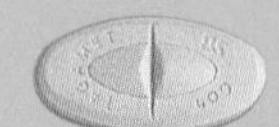

400 mg

CIPROFLOXACIN HCL

CIPRO
MILES

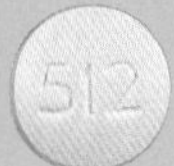

250 mg

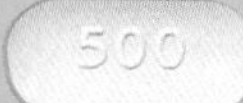

500 mg

CLARITHROMYCIN

BIAXIN
ABBOTT

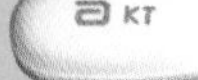

250 mg

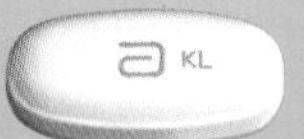

500 mg

CLONAZEPAM

KLONOPIN
ROCHE

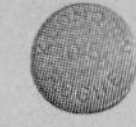

0.5 mg

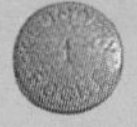

1 mg

CYCLOBENZAPRINE HCL

FLEXERIL
MERCK

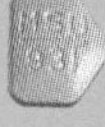

10 mg

DARVOCET-N 100

ACETAMINOPHEN AND PROPOXYPHENE NAPSYLATE
ELI LILLY

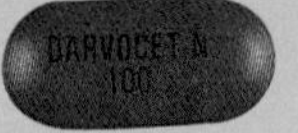

650 mg / 100 mg

DIAZEPAM

VALIUM
ROCHE

2 mg

5 mg

10 mg

DICLOFENAC SODIUM

VOLTAREN
GEIGY

50 mg

75 mg

DICYCLOMINE HCL

BENTYL
MARION MERRELL DOW

10 mg

20 mg

DIGOXIN

LANOXIN
BURROUGHS WELLCOME

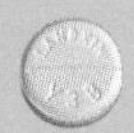

0.125 mg

0.25 mg

DILTIAZEM HCL

CARDIZEM CD
MARION MERRELL DOW

120 mg

180 mg

240 mg

DIVALPROEX SODIUM

DEPAKOTE
ABBOTT

250 mg

500 mg

DOXAZOSIN MESYLATE

CARDURA
ROERIG

1 mg

2 mg

ENALAPRIL MALEATE

VASOTEC
MERCK

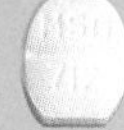

5 mg

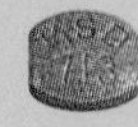

10 mg

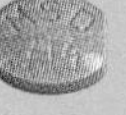

20 mg

ERYTHROMYCIN BASE

ERY-TAB
ABBOTT

250 mg

333 mg

ERYTHROMYCIN
ABBOTT

250 mg

PCE
ABBOTT

333 mg

500 mg

ERYTHROMYCIN STEARATE

ERYTHROCIN STEARATE FILMTAB
ABBOTT

250 mg

500 mg

ESTROGENS CONJUGATED

PREMARIN
WYETH-AYERST

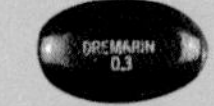

0.3 mg

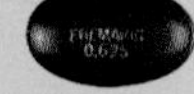

0.625 mg

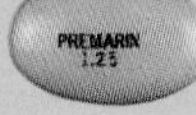

1.25 mg

ESTROPIPATE (PIPERAZINE ESTRONE SULFATE)

OGEN
UPJOHN

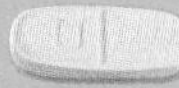

0.625 mg

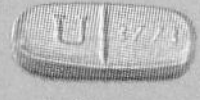

1.25 mg

ETODOLAC

LODINE
WYETH-AYERST

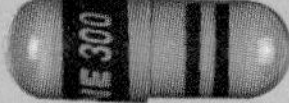

300 mg

400 mg

FAMOTIDINE

PEPCID
MERCK

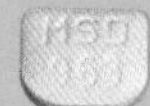

20 mg

40 mg

FINASTERIDE

PROSCAR
MERCK

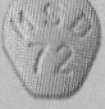

5 mg

FIORINAL

BUTALBITAL AND ASPIRIN AND CAFFEINE
SANDOZ

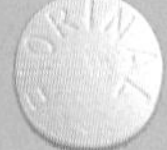

50 mg / 325 mg / 40 mg

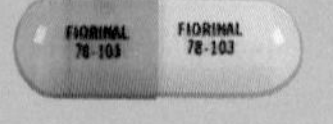

50 mg / 325 mg / 40 mg

FLUOXETINE HCL

PROZAC
DISTA

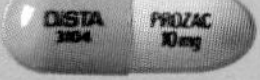

10 mg

20 mg

FLURBIPROFEN

ANSAID
UPJOHN

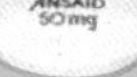

50 mg

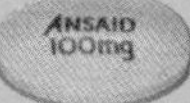

100 mg

FOSINOPRIL SODIUM

MONOPRIL
BRISTOL-MYERS SQUIBB

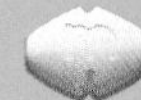

10 mg

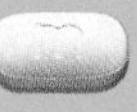

20 mg

FUROSEMIDE

LASIX
HOECHST-ROUSSEL

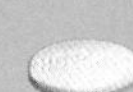

20 mg

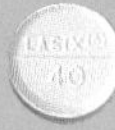

40 mg

GEMFIBROZIL

LOPID
PARKE-DAVIS

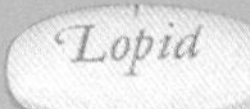

600 mg

GLIPIZIDE

GLUCOTROL
PRATT

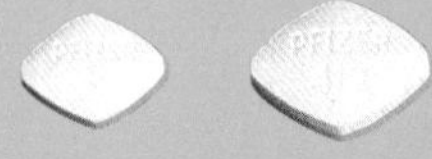

5 mg

10 mg

GLYBURIDE

DIABETA
HOECHST-ROUSSEL

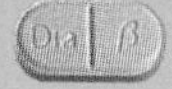

2.5 mg

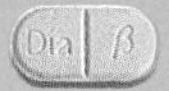

5 mg

GLYNASE PRESTAB
UPJOHN

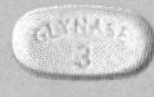

3 mg

MICRONASE
UPJOHN

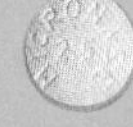

2.5 mg

5 mg

GUANFACINE HCL

TENEX
A. H. ROBINS

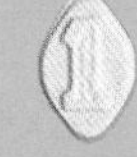

1 mg

HYDROCODONE BITARTRATE AND ACETAMINOPHEN

VICODIN
KNOLL

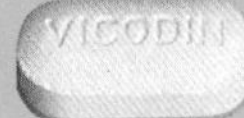

5 mg / 500 mg

IBUPROFEN

MOTRIN
UPJOHN

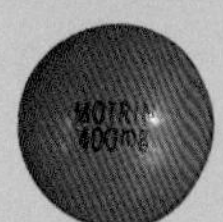

400 mg

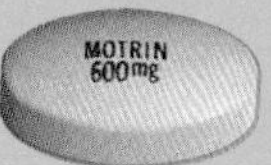

600 mg

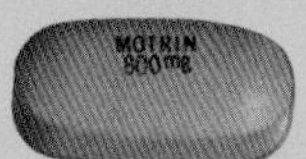

800 mg

INDAPAMIDE

LOZOL
RHONE-POULENC RORER

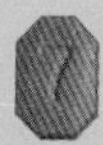

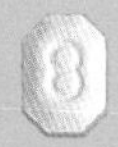

1.25 mg 2.5 mg

ISOSORBIDE DINITRATE TABLETS

ISORDIL TITRADOSE
WYETH-AYERST

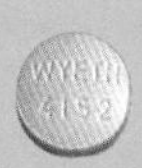

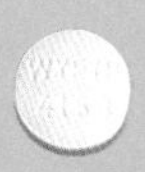

5 mg 10 mg

ISRADIPINE

DYNACIRC
SANDOZ

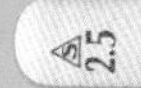

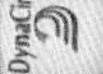

2.5 mg

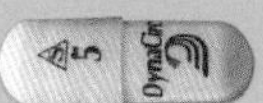

5 mg

KETOCONAZOLE

NIZORAL
JANSSEN

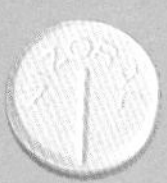

200 mg

KETOROLAC TROMETHAMINE

TORADOL
SYNTEX

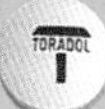

10 mg

LABETALOL HCL

NORMODYNE
SCHERING

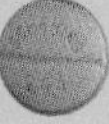

100 mg

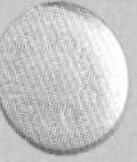

200 mg

LEVOTHYROXINE SODIUM

SYNTHROID
BOOTS

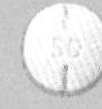

0.05 mg 0.1 mg

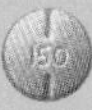

0.15 mg

LISINOPRIL

PRINIVIL
MERCK

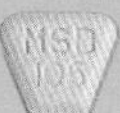

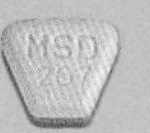

10 mg 20 mg

LISINOPRIL

ZESTRIL
STUART

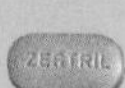

5 mg

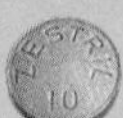

10 mg

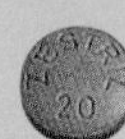

20 mg

LORACARBEF

LORABID
ELI LILLY

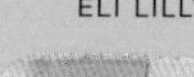

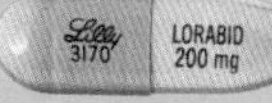

200 mg

LORATADINE

CLARITIN
SCHERING

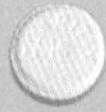

10 mg

LORAZEPAM

ATIVAN
WYETH-AYERST

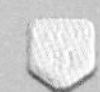

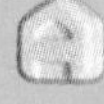

0.5 mg 1 mg

LOVASTATIN (MEVINOLIN)

MEVACOR
MERCK

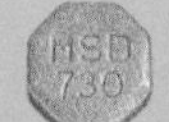

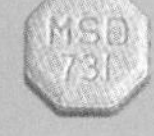

10 mg 20 mg

MEDROXYPROGESTERONE ACETATE

PROVERA
UPJOHN

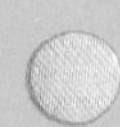
2.5 mg

10 mg

METHYLPHENIDATE HCL

RITALIN
CIBA

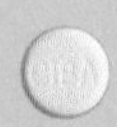
5 mg

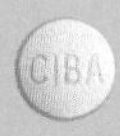

10 mg

METHYLPREDNISOLONE

MEDROL
UPJOHN

4 mg

METOPROLOL TARTRATE

LOPRESSOR
GEIGY

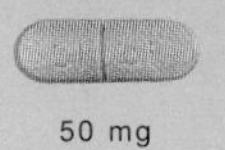
50 mg

100 mg

MISOPROSTOL

CYTOTEC
G. D. SEARLE

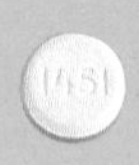

100 mcg

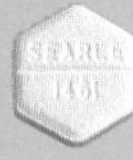
200 mcg

NABUMETONE

RELAFEN
SMITHKLINE BEECHAM

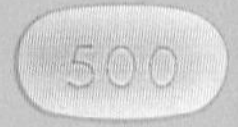

500 mg

NADOLOL

CORGARD
BRISTOL-MYERS SQUIBB

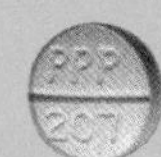

40 mg

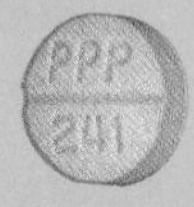

80 mg

NAPROXEN

NAPROSYN
SYNTEX

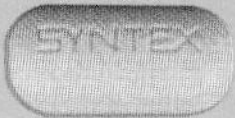

375 mg

500 mg

NAPROXEN SODIUM

ANAPROX
SYNTEX

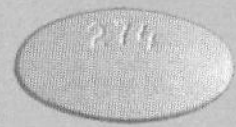

275 mg

ANAPROX DS
SYNTEX

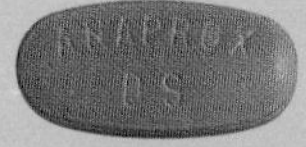

550 mg

NIFEDIPINE

PROCARDIA XL
PRATT

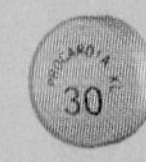

30 mg

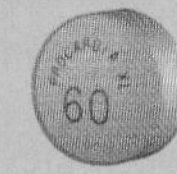

60 mg

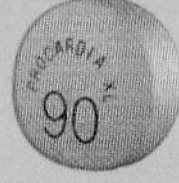

90 mg

NITROFURANTOIN MACROCRYSTALS

MACROBID
PROCTER & GAMBLE

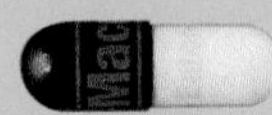
75 mg / 25 mg

NIZATIDINE

AXID
ELI LILLY

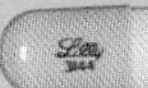
150 mg

NORTRIPTYLINE HCL

PAMELOR
SANDOZ

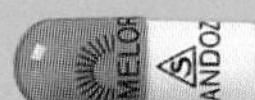

25 mg

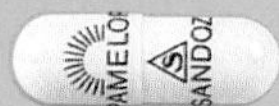

50 mg

OFLOXACIN

FLOXIN
MCNEIL

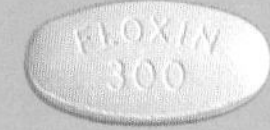

300 mg

OMEPRAZOLE

PRILOSEC
ASTRA MERCK

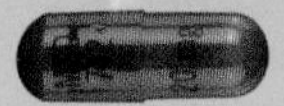
20 mg

OXAPROZIN

DAYPRO
G. D. SEARLE

600 mg

OXYCODONE AND ACETAMINOPHEN

PERCOCET
DUPONT

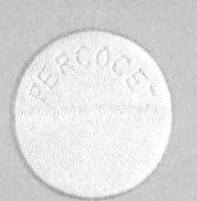

5 mg / 325 mg

PAROXETINE HCL

PAXIL
SMITHKLINE BEECHAM

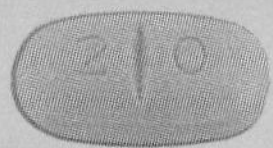

20 mg

PENICILLIN V POTASSIUM (PHENOXYMETHYL PENICILLIN POTASSIUM)

PEN-VEE K
WYETH-AYERST

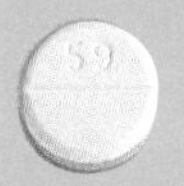

250 mg 500 mg

PENTOXIFYLLINE

TRENTAL
HOECHST-ROUSSEL

400 mg

PHENYTOIN SODIUM, EXTENDED

DILANTIN KAPSEALS
PARKE-DAVIS

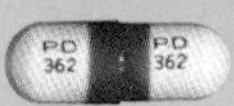

100 mg

PIROXICAM

FELDENE
PRATT

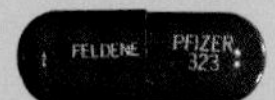

20 mg

POTASSIUM CHLORIDE

K-DUR
KEY

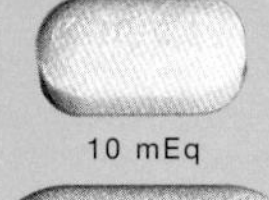

10 mEq

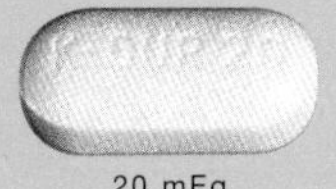

20 mEq

KLOR-CON 10
UPSHER-SMITH

10 mEq

MICRO-K 10 EXTENCAPS
A. H. ROBINS

10 mEq

PRAVASTATIN SODIUM

PRAVACHOL
BRISTOL-MYERS SQUIBB

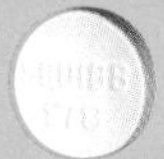

20 mg

PREDNISONE

DELTASONE
UPJOHN

5 mg

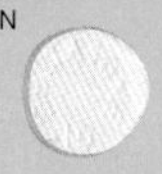

10 mg

20 mg

PROPRANOLOL HCL

INDERAL
WYETH-AYERST

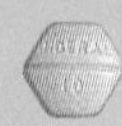

10 mg

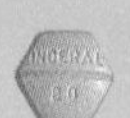

20 mg

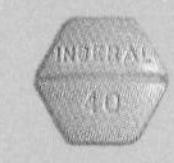

40 mg

INDERAL LA
WYETH-AYERST

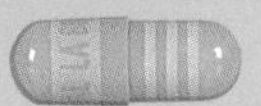

80 mg

QUINAPRIL HCL

ACCUPRIL
PARKE-DAVIS

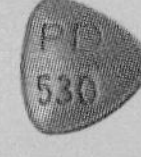

10 mg 20 mg

RAMIPRIL

ALTACE
HOECHST-ROUSSEL

2.5 mg

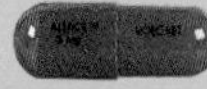

5 mg

RANITIDINE HCL

ZANTAC
GLAXO

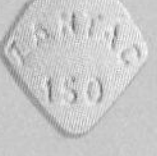

150 mg

300 mg

SERTRALINE HCL

ZOLOFT
ROERIG

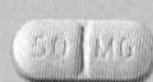

50 mg

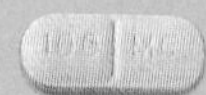

100 mg

SIMVASTATIN

ZOCOR
MERCK

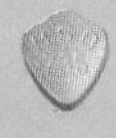

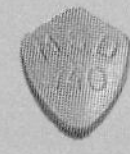

10 mg 20 mg

SUCRALFATE

CARAFATE
MARION MERRELL DOW

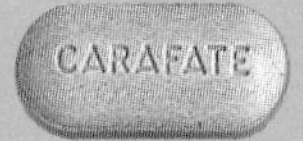

1 gm

TAMOXIFEN

NOLVADEX
ZENECA

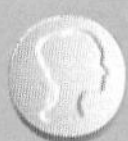

10 mg

TEMAZEPAM

RESTORIL
SANDOZ

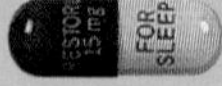

15 mg

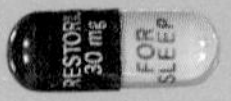

30 mg

TERAZOSIN

HYTRIN
ABBOTT

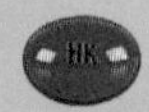

2 mg 5 mg

TERFENADINE

SELDANE
MARION MERRELL DOW

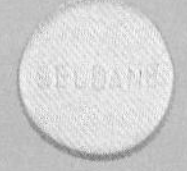

60 mg

TERFENADINE AND PSEUDOEPHEDRINE HCL

SELDANE-D
MARION MERRELL DOW

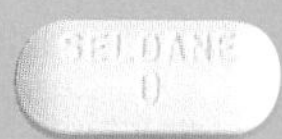

60 mg / 120 mg

THEOPHYLLINE

THEO-DUR
KEY

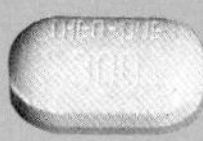

200 mg 300 mg

TRIAMTERENE AND HYDROCHLOROTHIAZIDE TABLETS

MAXZIDE
LEDERLE

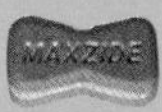

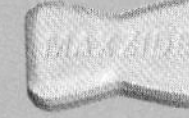

37.5 mg/ 25 mg 75 mg/ 50 mg

TRIAMTERENE AND HYDROCHLOROTHIAZIDE CAPSULES

DYAZIDE
SMITHKLINE BEECHAM

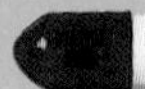

37.5 mg / 25 mg

TRIAZOLAM

HALCION
UPJOHN

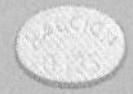

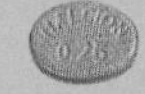

0.125 mg 0.25 mg

TRIMETHOPRIM AND SULFAMETHOXAZOLE

BACTRIM DS
ROCHE

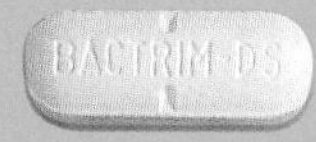

160 mg / 800 mg

TYLENOL WITH CODEINE TABLETS

ACETAMINOPHEN AND CODEINE PHOSPHATE
MCNEIL

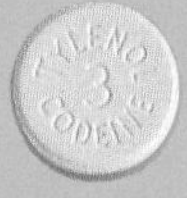

300 mg / 30 mg

VERAPAMIL

CALAN SR
G. D. SEARLE

CALAN

240 mg

WARFARIN SODIUM

COUMADIN
DUPONT PHARMA

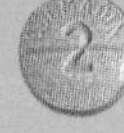

2 mg

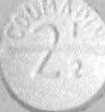

2.5 mg

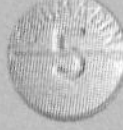

5 mg

NURSING CONSIDERATIONS

See also *Nursing Considerations* for *Narcotic Analgesics,* Chapter 43.

Assessment

1. Note any history of drug hypersensitivity.
2. Obtain baseline weight and VS prior to administering the medication. (Assisted or controlled ventilation may be required.)
3. Note any evidence of muscular rigidity and report before proceeding with the next dose of medication.

Client/Family Teaching

1. Perform preoperative teaching and determine level of understanding.
2. Stress that client may experience dizziness, drowsiness, and orthostatic hypotension.
3. Avoid alcohol or any CNS depressants for at least 24 hr following drug administration.

Evaluate

- Induction and maintenance of anesthesia
- ↓ Motor activity

Buprenorphine hydrochloride

(byou-pren-**OR**-feen)
Pregnancy Category: C
Buprenex **(C-V) (Rx)**

See also *Narcotic Analgesics,* Chapter 43.

How Supplied: *Injection:* 0.3 mg/mL

Action/Kinetics: Semisynthetic opiate possessing both narcotic agonist and antagonist activity. It has limited activity at the mu receptor. **IM, onset:** 15 min; **Peak effect:** 1 hr; **Duration:** 6 hr. **t½:** 2–3 hr. May also be given IV with shorter onset and peak effect. Buprenorphine is about equipotent with naloxone as a narcotic antagonist.

Uses: Moderate to severe pain.

Dosage

- **IM, Slow IV**

Analgesia.

Over 13 years of age: 0.3 mg q 6 hr. Up to 0.6 mg may be given; doses greater than 0.6 mg not recommended. **Children, 2–12 years of age:** 2–6 mcg/kg q 4–6 hr. Single doses greater than 6 mcg/kg should not be given.

Administration/Storage

1. Buprenorphine may be mixed with isotonic saline, lactated Ringer's solution, and 5% dextrose and 0.9% saline.
2. May be administered undiluted IV, slowly.
3. Buprenorphine may be mixed with solutions containing haloperidol, glycopyrrolate, scopolamine hydrobromide, hydroxyzine chloride, or droperidol.
4. Buprenorphine should not be mixed with solutions containing diazepam or lorazepam.
5. Storage in excessive heat and light should be avoided.
6. Not all children may clear buprenorphine faster than adults. Thus, fixed interval or "round the clock" dosing should not be undertaken until the proper interdose interval has been established.
7. Some pediatric clients may not need to be remedicated for 6–8 hr.
8. Have naloxone available to reverse drug-induced respiratory depression.

Special Concerns: Use during lactation only if benefits outweigh risks. Use in children less than 2 years of age has not been established. Use with caution in clients with compromised respiratory function, in head injuries, in impairment of liver or renal function, Addison's disease, prostatic hypertrophy, biliary tract dysfunction, urethral stricture, myxedema, and hypothyroidism. Administration to individuals physically dependent on narcotics may result in precipitation of a withdrawal syndrome.

Side Effects: *CNS:* Sedation, dizziness, confusion, headache, euphoria, slurred speech, depression, paresthesia, psychosis, malaise, hallucinations, coma, dysphoria, agitation, seizures. *GI:* N&V, constipation, dyspepsia, loss of appetite, dry mouth. *Ophthalmologic:* Miosis, blurred vision, double vision, conjunctivitis. *CV:* Hypotension, bradycardia, tachycardia, Wenckebach block. *Respiratory:* Decreased respiratory rate, cyanosis, dyspepsia. *Dermatologic:* Sweating, rash, pruritus, flushing. *Other:* Urinary retention, chills, tinnitus.

Drug Interactions: Additive CNS depression with alcohol, general anesthetics, antianxiety agents, sedative-hypnotics, phenothiazines, and other narcotic analgesics.

NURSING CONSIDERATIONS

See also *Nursing Considerations* for *Narcotic Analgesics,* Chapter 43.

Assessment

1. Determine if the client has evidence of respiratory depression and report because drug is contraindicated.
2. Report any evidence of head injuries immediately.
3. If the client has been receiving narcotics, observe for withdrawal symptoms and document.
4. Note any evidence of liver or renal dysfunction, diseases of the biliary tract, or prostatic hypertrophy.

Client/Family Teaching

1. Caution that drug may cause drowsiness, dizziness, and orthostatic effects.
2. Encourage to cough and deep breathe every 2 hr to prevent atelectasis.
3. Avoid alcohol.

Evaluate: Relief of pain.

Butorphanol tartrate

(byou-**TOR**-fah-nohl)
Pregnancy Category: C
Stadol, Stadol NS **(Rx)**

See also *Narcotic Analgesics,* Chapter 43.

How Supplied: *Injection:* 1 mg/mL, 2 mg/mL; *Nasal spray:* 10 mg/mL

Action/Kinetics: Butorphanol has both narcotic agonist and antagonist properties. Its analgesic potency is said to be up to 7 times that of morphine and 30–40 times that of meperidine. Overdosage responds to naloxone. After IV use, CV effects include increased PA pressure, pulmonary wedge pressure, LV end-diastolic pressure, system arterial pressure, pulmonary vascular resistance, and increased cardiac work load. **Onset, IM:** 10–15 min; **IV:** rapid; **nasal:** within 15 min. **Duration, IM, IV:** 3–4 hr; **nasal:** 4–5 hr. **Peak analgesia, IM, IV:** 30–60 min; **nasal:** 1–2 hr. **t½, IM:** 2.1–8.8 hr; **nasal:** 2.9–9.2 hr. The t½ is increased up to 25% in clients over 65 years of age. Butorphanol is metabolized in the liver and excreted by the kidney. The drug has about 1/40 the narcotic antagonist activity as naloxone. A metered-dose nasal spray is now available for this drug.

Uses: Parenteral and nasal: Moderate to severe pain, especially after surgery. **Parenteral:** Preoperative medication (as part of balanced anesthesia). Pain during labor. **Nasal:** Treatment of migraine headaches.

Dosage

• **IM**

Analgesia.

Adults, usual: 2 mg q 3–4 hr, as necessary; **range:** 1–4 mg q 3–4 hr. Single doses should not exceed 4 mg.

Preoperative/preanesthetic.

Adults: 2 mg 60–90 min before surgery. Individualize dosage.

Labor.

Adults: 1–2 mg if at full term and during early labor. May be repeated after 4 hr.

• **IV**

Analgesia.

Adults, usual: 1 mg q 3–4 hr; **range:** 0.5–2 mg q 3–4 hr. **Not recommended for use in children.**

Balanced anesthesia.

Adults: 2 mg just before induction or 0.5–1 mg in increments during anesthesia. The increment may be up to 0.06 mg/kg, depending on drugs previously given. Total dose range: less than 4 mg to less than 12.5 mg.

Labor.

Adults: 1–2 mg if at full term and during early labor. May be repeated after 4 hr.

- **Nasal Spray**

Analgesia.

Adults: 1 spray (1 mg) in one nostril. If pain relief is not reached within 60–90 min, an additional 1 mg may be given. The two-dose sequence may be repeated in 3–4 hr if necessary. In severe pain, 2 mg (1 spray in each nostril) may be given initially followed in 3–4 hr by additional 2-mg doses if needed. **Geriatric clients, initial:** 1 mg; wait 90–120 min before determining if a second 1-mg dose is required.

Administration/Storage

1. Geriatric clients should receive one-half the usual dose at twice the usual interval.
2. For clients with renal/hepatic impairment, increase the initial dosage interval to 6–8 hr with subsequent intervals determined by client response.
3. If the drug is to be administered by direct IV infusion, it may be given undiluted. Administer it at a rate of 2 mg or less over a 3–5-min period of time.
4. Have naloxone available for treatment of overdose.
5. The nasal product should be stored below 86°F (30°C).

Contraindication: The nasal form should not be used during labor or delivery.

Special Concerns: Safe use during pregnancy, during labor for premature infants, or in children under 18 years not established. Use with extreme caution in clients with AMI, ventricular dysfunction, and coronary insufficiency (morphine or meperidine are preferred). Use in clients physically dependent on narcotics will result in precipitation of a withdrawal syndrome. Geriatric clients may be more sensitive to side effects, especially dizziness.

Additional Side Effects: The most common side effects are somnolence, dizziness, N&V. The nasal product commonly causes nasal congestion and insomnia.

Additional Drug Interactions: Barbiturate anesthetics may increase respiratory and CNS depression of butorphanol.

NURSING CONSIDERATIONS

See also *Nursing Considerations* for *Narcotic Analgesics,* Chapter 43.

Assessment

1. Determine if the client is likely to be dependent on narcotics. Antagonist property of drug may precipitate withdrawal symptoms.
2. Document any history of CV problems as morphine may be a preferred drug to use.

Evaluate

- Relief of pain
- Treatment of migraine headache

Codeine phosphate

(**KOH**-deen)

Pregnancy Category: C

Paveral ✦ **(C-II) (Rx)**

Codeine sulfate

(**KOH**-deen)

Pregnancy Category: C

(C-II) (Rx)

See also *Narcotic Analgesics,* Chapter 43.

How Supplied: Codeine Phosphate: *Injection:* 30 mg/mL, 60 mg/mL; *Solution:* 15 mg/5 mL; *Tablet:* 30 mg, 60 mg

Codeine Sulfate: *Tablet:* 15 mg, 30 mg, 60 mg

Action/Kinetics: Codeine resembles morphine pharmacologically but produces less respiratory depression and N&V. It is moderately habit-forming and constipating. Dosages over 60 mg often cause restlessness and excitement and irritate the cough center. However, in lower doses, it is a potent antitussive and is an ingredient in many cough syrups. **Onset:** 10–30 min. **Peak effect:**

30–60 min. **Duration:** 4–6 hr. **t½:** 3–4 hr. Codeine is two-thirds as effective PO as parenterally.

It is often used to supplement the effect of nonnarcotic analgesics such as aspirin and acetaminophen. Codeine is also found in many combination cough/cold products.

Uses: Relief of mild to moderate pain. Antitussive to relieve chemical or mechanical respiratory tract irritation.

Dosage

- **Tablets, IM, IV, SC**

Analgesia.

Adults: 15–60 mg q 4–6 hr, not to exceed 360 mg/day. **Pediatric, over 1 year:** 0.5 mg/kg q 4–6 hr. IV should not be used in children.

Antitussive.

Adults: 10–20 mg q 4–6 hr, up to maximum of 120 mg/day. **Pediatric, 2–6 years:** 2.5–5 mg PO q 4–6 hr, not to exceed 30 mg/day; **6–12 years:** 5–10 mg q 4–6 hr, not to exceed 60 mg/day.

Contraindications: Premature infants or during labor when delivery of a premature infant is expected.

Special Concerns: May increase the duration of labor. Use with caution and reduce the initial dose in clients with seizure disorders, acute abdominal conditions, renal or hepatic disease, fever, Addison's disease, hypothyroidism, prostatic hypertrophy, ulcerative colitis, urethral stricture, following recent GI or GU tract surgery, and in the young, geriatric, or debilitated clients.

Additional Drug Interaction: Combination with chlordiazepoxide may induce coma.

NURSING CONSIDERATIONS

See also *Nursing Considerations* for *Narcotic Analgesics,* Chapter 43.

Client/Family Teaching

1. Take only as directed. Explain that acetaminophen and aspirin act synergistically with codeine and are therefore usually given together.
2. Increase intake of fluids, fruits, and fiber to diminish drug's constipating effects.
3. Clients taking codeine syrups to suppress coughs should be discouraged from overuse. Productive coughing is suppressed and may result in additional congestion.

Evaluate

- Relief of pain
- Control of coughing with improved sleeping patterns

Dezocine

(**DEZ**-oh-seen)
Pregnancy Category: C
Dalgan **(Rx)**

See also *Narcotic Analgesics,* Chapter 43.

How Supplied: *Injection:* 5 mg/mL, 10 mg/mL, 15 mg/mL

Action/Kinetics: Dezocine is a parenteral narcotic analgesic possessing both agonist and antagonist activity. It is similar to morphine with respect to analgesic potency and onset and duration of action. However, there is less risk of abuse due to the mixed agonist-antagonist properties of the drug. The narcotic antagonist activity is greater than that of pentazocine. **Onset:** Approximately 30 min after IM and approximately 15 min after IV. **Peak effect:** 30–150 min. **Peak plasma levels:** 10–38 ng/mL after a 10-mg dose. **Duration:** 2–4 hr. **t½, after IV:** 2.4 hr. Approximately two-thirds of a dose is excreted in the urine mostly as the glucuronide conjugate.

Use: Analgesic when use of a narcotic is desirable.

Dosage

- **IM**

Analgesia.

Adults: 5–20 mg (usual is 10 mg) as a single dose; dose may be repeated q 3–6 hr with dosage adjusted, if necessary, depending on the status of the client.

- **IV**

Analgesia.

Adults: 2.5–10 mg (usual initial dose is 5 mg) repeated q 2–4 hr.

Administration/Storage

1. The maximum single dose should not exceed 20 mg and the maximum

daily dose should not exceed 120 mg.
2. Dezocine can be stored at room temperature protected from light.
3. The solution should not be used if it contains a precipitate.
4. *Treatment of Overdose:* Naloxone IV with appropriate supportive measures including oxygen, IV fluids, vasopressors, and artificial respiration.

Contraindications: Lactation. Individuals dependent on narcotics. SC administration.

Special Concerns: Use in labor and delivery only if benefits outweigh risks. Safety and effectiveness have not been determined in children less than 18 years of age. Use with caution in clients with impaired renal or hepatic function. Use with caution in clients with head injury or increased intracranial pressure, in COPD, and in biliary surgery. Geriatric clients are at an increased risk for depressed respiration, reduced ventilatory drive, alteration of mental status, and delirium. Dezocine should not be used in clients who are tolerant to opiate drugs since there is a risk of precipitating an acute withdrawal syndrome.

Side Effects: *CNS:* Sedation (common), dizziness, vertigo, confusion, anxiety, crying, sleep disturbances, delusions, headache, depression, delirium. *Respiratory:* Respiratory depression, atelectasis. *CV:* Hypotension, irregular heart or pulse, hypertension, chest pain, pallor, thrombophlebitis. *GI:* N&V, dry mouth, constipation, abdominal pain, diarrhea. *Dermatologic:* Reactions at the injection site, pruritus, rash, erythema. *EENT:* Diplopia, blurred vision, congestion in ears, tinnitus. *GU:* Urinary frequency, retention, or hesitancy. *Miscellaneous:* Sweating, chills, edema, flushing, low hemoglobin, muscle cramps or aches, muscle pain, slurred speech.

Drug Interactions: Additive depressant effect when used with general anesthetics, sedatives, antianxiety drugs, hypnotics, alcohol, and other opiate analgesics.

NURSING CONSIDERATIONS

See also *Nursing Considerations* for *Narcotic Analgesics,* Chapter 43.

Assessment

1. Note any client sulfite sensitivity because drug contains sodium metabisulfite.
2. Determine any history or current use of opiate drugs because dezocine may precipitate an acute withdrawal syndrome.
3. Note any evidence of impaired renal or liver function; obtain pretreatment laboratory values.
4. Assess for any evidence of head injury or increased ICP.

Interventions

1. Monitor for evidence of allergic reaction.
2. Record VS and assess mental status and respiratory patterns.
3. Anticipate reduced dosage in clients with renal or hepatic dysfunction.
4. Geriatric clients should receive reduced doses and be individually evaluated for subsequent dose levels.
5. If dezocine is administered with CNS depressants, anticipate the dose of one or both agents should be reduced.

Client/Family Teaching

1. Provide a printed list of drug side effects instructing client to report those that are bothersome or persistent.
2. Do not drive or operate dangerous machinery until the drug effects have worn off.
3. Avoid alcohol and the use of any unprescribed sedatives, hypnotics, or antianxiety agents.

Special Concerns: Elderly clients are at an increased risk for altered respiratory patterns and mental changes.

Evaluate: Satisfactory pain management as evidenced by ↑ activity, improved appetite, and reports of effective pain control.

—COMBINATION DRUG—

Empirin with Codeine

(**EM**-pih-rin, **KOH**-deen)
Pregnancy Category: C
(C-III) (Rx)

See also *Narcotic Analgesics,* Chapter 43, and *Acetylsalicylic Acid,* Chapter 41.

How Supplied: See Content

Content: *Nonnarcotic analgesic:* Aspirin, 325 mg (in all tablets). *Narcotic analgesic:* Codeine, 15 mg (No. 2), 30 mg (No. 3), 60 mg (No. 4).

Uses: Relief of mild, moderate, or moderate-severe pain.

Dosage

- **Tablets**

Analgesia.

Adults, usual: 1–2 tablets of No. 2 or No. 3 q 4 hr as needed; 1 tablet of No. 4 q 4 hr as needed.

NURSING CONSIDERATIONS

See also *Nursing Considerations* for *Narcotic Analgesics,* Chapter 43, and *Acetylsalicylic Acid,* Chapter 41.

Client/Family Teaching

1. Take with food, milk, or water to decrease gastric irritation.
2. May be habit-forming; take only as directed.
3. The dose is adjusted according to the severity of the pain and the response of the client. Explain that the dose may exceed the recommended dosage if pain is severe or tolerance to the analgesic effect has developed.

Evaluate: Relief of pain and discomfort.

Fentanyl citrate

(**FEN**-tah-nil)
Pregnancy Category: C
Fentanyl Oralet, Sublimaze **(C-II) (Rx)**

See also *Narcotic Analgesics,* Chapter 43.

How Supplied: *Injection:* 0.05 mg/mL, 1.5 mg/mL, 2.5 mg/mL; *Lozenge/Troche:* 200 mcg, 300 mcg, 400 mcg

Action/Kinetics: Similar to those of morphine and meperidine. **IV. Onset:** 7–8 min. **Peak effect:** Approximately 30 min. **Duration:** 1–2 hr. **$t^{1/2}$:** 1.5–6 hr. When the oral form (lozenge) is sucked, fentanyl citrate is absorbed through the mucosal tissues of the mouth and GI tract. **Peak effect, transmucosal:** 20–30 min. The drug is faster-acting and of shorter duration than morphine or meperidine.

Uses: Parenteral. Preanesthetic medication, induction, and maintenance of anesthesia of short duration and immediate postoperative period. Supplement in general or regional anesthesia. Combined with droperidol for preanesthetic medication, induction of anesthesia, or as adjunct in maintenance of general or regional anesthesia. Combined with oxygen for anesthesia in high-risk clients undergoing open heart surgery, orthopedic procedures, or complicated neurologic procedures.

Oral (transmucosal). Anesthetic premedication in children and adults in an operating room setting. Prevent anxiety or fearlessness before diagnostic or medical procedures (use only in closely monitored situations due to the risk of hypoventilation).

Dosage

- **IM, IV**

Preoperatively.

Adults: 0.05–0.1 mg IM 30–60 min before surgery.

Adjunct to anesthesia, induction.

Adults: 0.002–0.05 mg/kg IV, depending on length and depth of anesthesia desired; **maintenance:** 0.025–0.1 mg/kg when indicated.

Adjunct to regional anesthesia.

Adults: 0.05–0.1 mg IM or IV over 1–2 min when indicated.

Postoperatively.

Adults: 0.05–0.1 mg IM q 1–2 hr for control of pain.

As general anesthetic with oxygen and a muscle relaxant.

0.05–0.1 mg/kg (up to 0.15 mg/kg may be required).

Induction and maintenance of anesthesia.
Pediatric, 2–12 years: 1.7–3.3 mcg/kg.
• **Transmucosal (Oral Lozenge)**
Individualize according to weight, age, physical status, general condition and medical status, underlying pathology, use of other drugs, type of anesthetic to be used, and the type and length of the surgical procedure. Doses of 5 mcg/kg are equivalent to IM fentanyl, 0.75–1.25 mcg/kg. Clients receiving more than 5 mcg/kg should be under the direct observation of medical personnel. Children may require up to 15 mcg/kg. Clients over 65 years of age should receive a dose from 2.5 to 5 mcg/kg. The maximum dose for adults and children, regardless of weight, is 400 mcg.
Administration/Storage
1. Direct IV infusions may be given, undiluted, over a period of 2–3 min.
2. After an IV injection, onset of action should occur within a few minutes and should last for 30–60 min.
3. Clients receiving an IM injection of drug can expect to have relief within 15 min and expect a duration of 1–2 hr.
4. Protect drug from light. The transmucosal product should be protected from freezing and moisture; it should be stored below 30°C (86°F).
5. Oral form is supplied as a raspberry-flavored lozenge mounted on a handle and comes in strengths of 200, 300, and 400 mcg.
6. The foil overwrap of the oral form is to be removed just prior to administration. After removing the plastic overcap, the client should be instructed to place the transmucosal unit in the mouth and to suck (not chew) it. After the drug is consumed or the client shows signs of respiratory depression, the unit is removed from the mouth by the handle. If any of the medication remains, it should be placed in the plastic overcap and disposed of properly for Schedule II drugs.
7. The transmucosal product should be given 20–40 min prior to time for the desired effect.
8. Lower doses of the transmucosal form should be considered in clients with head injury, cardiovascular or pulmonary disease, liver dysfunction, or hepatic disease.
9. When using the transmucosal form, the client must be attended to at all times by an individual skilled in airway management and resuscitative techniques.
10. Have naloxone available in the event of an overdose.
Additional Contraindications: Myasthenia gravis and other conditions in which muscle relaxants should not be used. Clients particularly sensitive to respiratory depression. Use during labor.

The transmucosal form is contraindicated in children who weigh less than 15 kg, for the treatment of acute or chronic pain (safety for this use not established), and for doses in excess of 15 mcg/kg in children and in excess of 5 mcg/kg in adults. Use outside the hospital setting is contraindicated.
Special Concerns: Safety and effectiveness have not been determined in children less than 2 years of age. Use with caution and at reduced dosage in poor-risk clients, children, the elderly, and when other CNS depressants are used. Use of the transmucosal form carries a risk of hypoventilation that may result in death.
Additional Side Effects: Skeletal and thoracic muscle rigidity, especially after rapid IV administration. Bradycardia, ***seizures,*** diaphoresis.
Additional Drug Interaction: ↑ Risk of CV depression when high doses of fentanyl are combined with nitrous oxide or diazepam.

NURSING CONSIDERATIONS

See also *Nursing Considerations* for *Narcotic Analgesics,* Chapter 43.
Assessment
1. Note any history of neurovascular disease.
2. Document any evidence of pulmonary disease.
Client/Family Teaching
1. May experience orthostatic hypotension.
2. Drug causes dizziness and drowsiness.

3. Avoid alcohol and any other CNS depressant for at least 24 hr.

Evaluate: Desired level of analgesia and relaxation.

Fentanyl Transdermal System

(**FEN**-tah-nil)

Pregnancy Category: C

Duragesic-25, -50, -75, and -100 **(C-II)** **(Rx)**

See also *Narcotic Analgesics* and *Fentanyl citrate,* Chapter 43.

How Supplied: *Film, Extended Release:* 25 mcg/hr, 50 mcg/hr, 75 mcg/hr, 100 mcg/hr

Action/Kinetics: The system provides continuous delivery of fentanyl for up to 72 hr. The amount of fentanyl released from each system each hour depends on the surface area (25 mcg/hr is released from each 10 cm^2). Each system also contains 0.1 mL of alcohol/10 cm^2; the alcohol enhances the rate of drug flux through the copolymer membrane and also increases the permeability of the skin to fentanyl. Following application of the system, the skin under the system absorbs fentanyl, resulting in a depot of the drug in the upper skin layers, which is then available to the general circulation. After the system is removed, the residual drug in the skin continues to be absorbed so that serum levels fall 50% in about 17 hr. The drug is metabolized in the liver and excreted mainly in the urine.

Use: Use should be restricted for the management of severe chronic pain that cannot be managed with less powerful drugs. The patch should only be used on clients who are already on and tolerant to narcotic analgesics and who require continuous narcotic administration.

Dosage

- **Transdermal System**

  Analgesia.

Adults, usual initial: 25 mcg/hr unless the client is tolerant to opioids (Duragesic-50, -75, and -100 are intended for use only in clients tolerant to opioids). Initial dose should be based on (1) the daily dose, potency, and characteristics (i.e., pure agonist, mixed agonist/antagonist) of the drug the client has been taking; (2) the reliability of the relative potency estimates used to calculate the dose as estimates vary depending on the route of administration; (3) the degree, if any, of tolerance to narcotics; and (4) the general condition and status of the client.

To convert clients from PO or parenteral opioids to the transdermal system, the following method should be used: (1) the previous 24-hr analgesic requirement should be calculated; (2) convert this amount to the equianalgesic PO morphine dose; (3) find the calculated 24-hr morphine dose and the corresponding transdermal fentanyl dose using the table provided with the product; and (4) initiate treatment using the recommended fentanyl dose. The dose may be increased no more frequently than 3 days after the initial dose or q 6 days thereafter. The ratio of 90 mg/24 hr of PO morphine to 25 mcg/hr increase in transdermal fentanyl dose should be used to base appropriate dosage increments on the daily dose of supplementary opioids.

If the dose of the fentanyl transdermal system exceeds 300 mcg/hr, it may be necessary to change clients to another narcotic analgesic. In such cases, the transdermal system should be removed and treatment initiated with one-half the equianalgesic dose of the new opioid 12–18 hr later. The dose of the new analgesic should be titrated based on the level of pain reported by the client.

Administration/Storage

1. The system should be applied to a nonirritated and nonirradiated fatty, flat surface of the skin, preferably on the upper torso. If needed, hair should be clipped (not shaved) from the site prior to application.

2. Only clear water, if needed, should be used to cleanse the site prior to application. Soaps, oils, lotions, alcohol, or other agents that

might irritate the skin should not be used. The skin should be allowed to dry completely prior to applying the system. If liquid comes in contact with the skin, use clear water only to remove.

3. The system should be removed from the sealed package and applied immediately by pressing firmly in place (for 10–20 sec) with the palm of the hand. **Never cut the system.** Ensure that contact of the system is complete, especially around the edges. Tape the patch to prevent dislodgement.

4. Each system should remain in place for 72 hr; if additional analgesia is required, a new system can be applied to a different skin site after removal of the previous system.

5. Systems removed from a skin site should be folded so that the adhesive side adheres to itself; it should then be flushed down the toilet immediately after removal.

6. Any unused systems should be disposed of as soon as they are no longer needed by removing them from their package and flushing down the toilet. During hospitalization, appropriate institutional guidelines for disposing of controlled substances should be addressed.

7. Multiple systems may be used if the delivery rate needs to exceed 100 mcg/hr.

8. The initial evaluation of the maximum analgesic effect should not be undertaken until 24 hr after the system is applied.

9. If required, clients can use a short-acting analgesic for the first 24 hr (i.e., until analgesic efficacy is reached with the transdermal system).

10. Clients may continue to require periodic supplemental doses of a short-acting analgesic to treat breakthrough pain.

11. If opioid therapy is to be discontinued, a gradual decrease in dose is recommended to minimize S&S of abrupt narcotic withdrawal.

Contraindications: Use for acute or postoperative pain (including out-patient surgeries). To manage mild or intermittent pain that can be managed by acetaminophen-opioid combinations, NSAIDs, or short-acting opioids. Hypersensitivity to fentanyl or adhesives. ICP, impaired consciousness, coma, medical conditions causing hypoventilation. Use during labor and delivery. Use of initial doses exceeding 25 mcg/hr, use in children less than 12 years of age and clients under 18 years of age who weigh less than 50 kg. Lactation.

Special Concerns: Use with caution in clients with brain tumors and bradyarrhythmias, as well as in elderly, cachectic, or debilitated individuals. Safety and efficacy have not been determined in children. The systems should be kept out of the reach of children; used systems should be disposed of properly.

Additional Side Effect: Sustained hypoventilation.

NURSING CONSIDERATIONS

See also *Nursing Considerations* for *Narcotic Analgesics* and *Fentanyl citrate,* Chapter 43.

Assessment

1. Document indications for therapy, noting onset of symptoms and previous agents used and the outcome.

2. Rate pain level at various times throughout the day to ensure adequate dosing. Determine that dose required is based on conversion guidelines provided by manufacturer.

3. Note any history or evidence of increased ICP or brain tumors.

Client/Family Teaching

1. Review and demonstrate the appropriate method for fentanyl transdermal patch application.

2. Assist client to develop a written record of drug administration for the transdermal system and for short-acting analgesics. Advise to date and time the patches and tape securely on when they are applied to avoid any confusion or dislodgement.

3. **Never** cut or open the system.
4. Provide a printed list of adverse drug effects that require immediate reporting.
5. Advise client not to stop drug system suddenly.
6. Stress the importance of administering *only* as prescribed.
7. Review the safe, appropriate method for drug storage and disposal.
8. Note time and frequency of use for a prescribed short-acting analgesic for breakthrough pain. Report if use exceeds expected needs because transdermal dosage may require adjustment.

Evaluate

- Reports of symptomatic improvement R/T pain management
- Relief of pain as evidenced by improved appetite, ↑ activity, and ↑ socialization

—COMBINATION DRUG—

Fiorinal

(fee-**OR**-in-al)
(Rx)

Fiorinal with Codeine

(fee-**OR**-in-al, **KOH**-deen)
Pregnancy Category: C
(C-III) (Rx)

See also *Narcotic Analgesics,* Chapter 43, *Acetylsalicylic Acid,* Chapter 41, and *Barbiturates,* Chapter 39.

How Supplied: Fiorinal: See Content.
Fiorinal with Codeine: See Content

Content: Each Fiorinal capsule or tablet contains:

Nonnarcotic analgesic: Aspirin, 325 mg.

Sedative barbiturate: Butalbital, 50 mg.

CNS stimulant: Caffeine, 40 mg.

In addition to the above, Fiorinal with Codeine capsules contain codeine phosphate, 7.5 mg (No. 1), 15 mg (No. 2), or 30 mg (No. 3).

Uses: Fiorinal is indicated for tension headaches. Fiorinal with Codeine is indicated as an analgesic for all types of pain.

Dosage

- **Capsules, Tablets**

FIORINAL

1–2 tablets or capsules q 4 hr, not to exceed 6 tablets or capsules/day.

FIORINAL WITH CODEINE

Initial: 1–2 capsules; **then,** dose may be repeated, if necessary, up to maximum of 6 capsules/day.

NURSING CONSIDERATIONS

See *Nursing Considerations* for *Acetylsalicylic Acid,* Chapter 41, and *Narcotic Analgesics,* Chapter 43.

Assessment

1. Document indications for therapy and onset and type of symptoms.
2. List any agents previously used for this condition and the outcome.

Evaluate

- Control of pain
- Relief of tension headaches

—COMBINATION DRUG—

Hydrocodone bitartrate and Acetaminophen

(**high**-droh-**KOH**-dohn, ah-**seat**-ah-**MIN**-oh-fen)
Pregnancy Category: C
Anexia 5/500, Anexia 7.5/650, Lorcet 10/650, Lorcet Plus **(Rx) (C-III)**

See also *Narcotic Analgesics,* Chapter 43, and *Acetaminophen,* Chapter 41.

How Supplied: See Content

Content: Anexia 5/500: *Narcotic analgesic:* Hydrocodone bitartrate, 5 mg, and *Nonnarcotic analgesic:* Acetaminophen, 500 mg.

Lorcet 10/650: *Narcotic analgesic:* Hydrocodone bitartrate, 10 mg, and *Nonnarcotic analgesic:* Acetaminophen, 650 mg. Anexia 7.5/650 and Lorcet Plus: *Narcotic analgesic:* Hydrocodone bitartrate, 7.5 mg, and *Nonnarcotic analgesic:* Acetaminophen, 650 mg.

Action/Kinetics: Hydrocodone produces its analgesic activity by an action on the CNS via opiate receptors. The analgesic action of acetaminophen is produced by both peripheral and central mechanisms.

Use: Relief of moderate to moderately severe pain.

Dosage

- **Tablets**

Analgesia.

1 tablet of Anexia 7.5/650, Lorcet 10/650, or Lorcet Plus q 4–6 hr as needed for pain. The total 24-hr dose should not exceed 6 tablets. 1–2 tablets of Anexia 5/500 q 4–6 hr as needed for pain. The total 24-hr dose should not exceed 8 tablets.

Administration/Storage

1. *Treatment of overdose of acetaminophen:*

- Empty stomach promptly by lavage or induction of emesis with syrup of ipecac.
- Serum acetaminophen levels should be determined as early as possible but no sooner than 4 hr after ingestion.
- Determine liver function initially and at 24-hr intervals.
- The antidote, *N*-acetylcysteine, should be given within 16 hr of overdose for optimal results.

2. *Treatment of overdose of hydrocodone:*

- Reestablish adequate respiratory exchange with a patent airway and assisted or controlled ventilation.
- Respiratory depression can be reversed by giving naloxone IV.
- Oxygen, IV fluids, vasopressors, and other supportive measures may be instituted as required.

Contraindications: Hypersensitivity to acetaminophen or hydrocodone. Lactation.

Special Concerns: Use with caution, if at all, in clients with head injuries as the CSF pressure may be increased further. Use with caution in geriatric or debilitated clients; in those with impaired hepatic or renal function; in hypothyroidism, Addison's disease, prostatic hypertrophy, or urethral stricture; and in clients with pulmonary disease. Use shortly before delivery may cause respiratory depression in the newborn. Safety and efficacy have not been determined in children.

Side Effects: *CNS:* Lightheadedness, dizziness, sedation, drowsiness, mental clouding, lethargy, impaired mental and physical performance, anxiety, fear, dysphoria, psychologic dependence, mood changes. *GI:* N&V. *Respiratory:* Respiratory depression (dose-related), irregular and periodic breathing. *GU:* Ureteral spasm, spasm of vesical sphincters, urinary retention.

Symptoms of Overdose: ***Acetaminophen overdose may result in potentially fatal hepatic necrosis.*** Also, renal tubular necrosis, hypoglycemic coma, and thrombocytopenia. Symptoms of hepatotoxic overdose include N&V, diaphoresis, and malaise. Symptoms of hydrocodone overdose include respiratory depression, somnolence progressing to stupor or ***coma,*** skeletal muscle flaccidity, cold and clammy skin, bradycardia, and hypotension. ***Severe overdose may cause apnea, circulatory collapse, cardiac arrest, and death.***

Drug Interactions

Anticholinergics / ↑ Risk of paralytic ileus

CNS depressants, including other narcotic analgesics, antianxiety agents, antipsychotics, alcohol / Additive CNS depression

MAO inhibitors / ↑ Effect of either the narcotic or the antidepressant

Tricyclic antidepressants / ↑ Effect of either the narcotic or the antidepressant

NURSING CONSIDERATIONS

See also *Nursing Considerations* for *Narcotic Analgesics,* Chapter 43, and *Acetaminophen,* Chapter 41.

Assessment

1. Document indications for therapy, onset of symptoms, any other agents prescribed, and the outcome. Determine if pain is acute or chronic in nature.
2. Note any history of hypothyroidism, prostatic hypertrophy or urethral stricture, Addison's disease, or pulmonary disease.
3. Obtain baseline liver and renal function studies.
4. Coadministration of an NSAID may reduce the dosage required for pain relief.

Client/Family Teaching
1. Take only as prescribed.
2. Do not perform activities that require mental alertness as drug causes dizziness, lethargy, and impaired physical and mental performance.
3. Report any evidence of abnormal bleeding or bruising, respiratory difficulties, N&V, urinary difficulty, or excessive sedation.
4. Avoid alcohol and any other medications without provider approval.
5. Store drug appropriately, away from the bedside and safely out of the reach of children.

Evaluate: Desired level of pain control.

Hydromorphone hydrochloride

(hy-droh-**MOR**-fohn)
Pregnancy Category: C
Dilaudid, Dilaudid-HP, PMS-Hydromorphone ✱ **(C-II) (Rx)**

See also *Narcotic Analgesics,* Chapter 43.

How Supplied: *Injection:* 1 mg/mL, 2 mg/mL, 3 mg/mL, 4 mg/mL, 10 mg/mL; *Liquid:* 1 mg/mL; *Suppository:* 3 mg; *Tablet:* 2 mg, 4 mg, 8 mg

Action/Kinetics: Hydromorphone is 7–10 times more analgesic than morphine, with a shorter duration of action. It manifests less sedation, less vomiting, and less nausea than morphine, although it induces pronounced respiratory depression. **Onset:** 15–30 min. **Peak effect:** 30–60 min. **Duration:** 4–5 hr. **t½:** 2–3 hr. The drug can be given rectally for prolonged activity.

Uses: Analgesia for moderate to severe pain (e.g., surgery, cancer, biliary colic, burns, renal colic, MI, bone trauma). Dilaudid-HP is a concentrated solution intended for clients who are tolerant to narcotics.

Dosage

- **Tablets**

  Analgesia.

Adults: 2 mg q 4–6 hr as necessary. For severe pain, 4 or more mg q 4–6 hr.

- **Suppositories**

  Analgesia.

Adults: 3 mg q 6–8 hr.

- **SC, IM, IV**

  Analgesia.

Adults: 1–2 mg q 4–6 hr. For severe pain, 3–4 mg q 4–6 hr.

Administration/Storage
1. May be administered by slow IV injection. When using this route, administer the drug slowly to minimize hypotensive effects and respiratory depression. Dilute with 5 mL of sterile water or NSS and administer at a rate of 2 mg over 5 min.
2. Suppositories should be refrigerated.
3. Drug may be administered as Dilaudid brand cough syrup. Be alert to the possibility of an allergic response in people sensitive to yellow dye number 5.
4. Have naloxone available in the event of overdosage.

Additional Contraindications: Migraine headaches. Use in children. Status asthmaticus, obstetrics, respiratory depression in absence of resuscitative equipment. Lactation.

Special Concerns: Do not confuse Dilaudid-HP with standard parenteral solutions of Dilaudid or with other narcotics as overdose and death can result. Use Dilaudid-HP with caution in clients with circulatory shock.

Additional Side Effect: Nystagmus.

NURSING CONSIDERATIONS

See also *Nursing Considerations* for *Narcotic Analgesics,* Chapter 43.

Interventions
1. Observe closely for respiratory depression, as it is more profound with hydromorphone than with other narcotic analgesics. Encourage client to turn, cough, and deep breathe or use incentive spirometry every 2 hr to prevent atelectasis.
2. Assess abdomen carefully as drug may mask symptoms of acute pathology.

Evaluate: Relief of pain.

Levomethadyl acetate hydrochloride

(lee-voh-**METH**-ah-dill)
ORLAAM **(Rx)**

See also *Narcotic Analgesics,* Chapter 43.

How Supplied: *Concentrate:* 10 mg/mL

Uses: Treatment of opiate dependence. *NOTE:* This drug can be dispensed only by treatment programs approved by the FDA, DEA, and the designated state authority. The drug can be dispensed only in the oral form and according to treatment requirements stated in federal regulations. The drug has no approved uses outside of the treatment of opiate dependence.

Dosage

- **Oral solution**

Induction.

Initial: 20–40 mg administered at 48–72-hr intervals; **then,** dose may be increased in increments of 5–10 mg until steady state is reached (usually within 1–2 weeks). Clients dependent on methadone may require higher initial doses of levomethadyl; the suggested initial 3-times/week dose for such clients is 1.2–1.3 times the daily methadone maintenance dose being replaced. This initial dose should not exceed 120 mg with subsequent doses given at 48- or 72-hr intervals, depending on the response. If additional opioids are required, supplemental amounts of methadone should be given rather than giving levomethadyl on 2 consecutive days.

Maintenance.

Most clients are stabilized on doses of 60–90 mg 3 times/week although the dose may range from 10 to 140 mg 3 times/week. The maximum *total* amount of levomethadyl recommended for any client is either 140, 140, 140 mg or 130, 130, 180 mg on a thrice-weekly schedule.

Reinduction after an unplanned lapse in dosing: following a lapse of one levomethadyl dose.

If the client comes to the clinic the day following a missed scheduled dose (e.g., misses Monday and arrives at clinic on Tuesday), the regular Monday dose is given, with the scheduled Wednesday dose given on Thursday and the Friday dose given on Saturday. The client's regular schedule can be resumed the following Monday. If the client misses one dose and comes to the clinic the day of the next scheduled dose (i.e., misses Monday, comes to clinic on Wednesday), the usual dose will be well tolerated in most cases although some clients will need a reduced dose.

Reintroduction after a lapse of more than one levomethadyl dose.

Restart the client at an initial dose of 50%–75% of the previous dose, followed by increases of 5–10 mg every dosing day (i.e., intervals of 48–72 hr) until the previous maintenance dose is reached.

Transfer from levomethadyl to methadone.

Transfer can be done directly, although the dose of methadone should be 80% of the levomethadyl dose being replaced. The first methadone dose should not be given sooner than 48 hr after the last levomethadyl dose. Increases or decreases of 5–10 mg may be made in the daily methadone dose to control symptoms of withdrawal or symptoms of excessive sedation.

Detoxification from levomethadyl.

Both gradual reduction (i.e., 5%–10% a week) and abrupt withdrawal have been used successfully.

Administration/Storage

1. The drug is usually given 3 times/week—either on Monday, Wednesday, and Friday or on Tuesday, Thursday, and Saturday. If withdrawal is a problem with this interval, the preceding dose may be increased.
2. If the degree of tolerance is not

known, clients can be started on methadone to facilitate more rapid titration to an effective dose. They can then be converted to levomethadyl after a few weeks. The crossover from methadone to levomethadyl should be accomplished in a single dose.
3. If clients on maintenance therapy complain of withdrawal symptoms (e.g., those on a Monday, Wednesday, and Friday schedule) on Sunday, the Friday dose may be increased in 5–10-mg increments up to 40% over the Monday/Wednesday dose up to a maximum of 140 mg.
4. Levomethadyl take-home doses are not permitted. If a situation arises where the client cannot come to the clinic for a regular dose of levomethadyl, that client may be switched to receive one or more doses of methadone. Methadone doses should be 80% of the client's Monday/Wednesday levomethadyl dose; the first dose of methadone should be taken no sooner than 48 hr after the last dose of levomethadyl. The number of take-home doses of methadone should be two less than the number of days expected absence and should not exceed the number of take-home doses allowed in the methadone regulations. Upon return to the clinic, the client should resume levomethadyl maintenance following the same dosage schedule prior to the temporary interruption. If more than 48 hr has elapsed since the last methadone dose, the client should be reintroduced on levomethadyl at a dose determined by the clinical evaluation.

Special Concerns: Usual dose must not be given on consecutive days due to the risk of fatal overdosage.

Side Effects: See *Narcotic Analgesics,* Chapter 43. Induction with levomethadyl that is too rapid for the level of tolerance of the client may result in overdosage, including symptoms of both ***respiratory and CV depression.***

NURSING CONSIDERATIONS

Assessment

1. Document that client is opiate dependent, length of dependence, and specific drugs used.
2. Determine methadone usage as drug requirements may be higher.
3. Identify that client has been accepted/approved for drug through a federally approved treatment protocol.
4. In clients who have missed scheduled doses, follow administration guidelines carefully.

Client/Family Teaching

1. Stress the importance of complying with regularly scheduled doses of levomethadyl.
2. Although the program does not require daily dosing, it does require that the client physically come to clinic for scheduled medication administration (usually every other day).
3. Identify additional support groups/persons who may assist clients in their goal of freedom from addiction.
4. Determine other resources (child care, job retraining, food stamps, etc.) that clients may qualify for and that would support them in their goal to live drug free.

Evaluate: Freedom from drug (opiate) dependence.

Meperidine hydrochloride (Pethidine hydrochloride)

(meh-**PER**-ih-deen)
Pregnancy Category: C
Demerol Hydrochloride **(C-II) (Rx)**

See also *Narcotic Analgesics,* Chapter 43.

How Supplied: *Injection:* 10 mg/mL, 25 mg/mL, 50 mg/mL, 75 mg/mL, 100 mg/mL; *Syrup:* 50 mg/5 mL; *Tablet:* 50 mg, 100 mg

Action/Kinetics: The pharmacologic activity of meperidine is similar to that of the opiates; however, meperidine is only one-tenth as potent an analgesic as morphine. Its analgesic effect is only one-half when given PO rather than parenterally. Meperidine has no antitussive effects and does not produce miosis. The drug does produce moderate spasmogenic effects on smooth muscle. The duration of action of meperidine is less than that of most opiates, and this must be kept in mind when a dosing schedule is being established. Meperidine will produce both psychological and physical dependence; overdosage is manifested by severe respiratory depression (see *Narcotic Overdose,* Chapter 43). **Onset:** 10–45 min. **Peak effect:** 30–60 min. **Duration:** 2–4 hr. **t½:** 3–4 hr.

Uses: Any situation that requires a narcotic analgesic: severe pain, hepatic and renal colic, obstetrics, preanesthetic medication, adjunct to anesthesia. These drugs are particularly useful for minor surgery, as in orthopedics, ophthalmology, rhinology, laryngology, and dentistry, and for diagnostic procedures such as cystoscopy, retrograde pyelography, and gastroscopy. Spasms of GI tract, uterus, urinary bladder. Anginal syndrome and distress of CHF.

Dosage

- **Tablets, Syrup, IM, SC**

Analgesic.

Adults: 50–100 mg q 3–4 hr as needed; **pediatric:** 1.1–1.8 mg/kg, up to adult dosage, q 3–4 hr as needed.

Preoperatively.

Adults, IM, SC: 50–100 mg 30–90 min before anesthesia; **pediatric, IM, SC:** 1–2 mg/kg 30–90 min before anesthesia.

Obstetrics.

Adults, IM, SC: 50–100 mg q 1–3 hr.

- **IV**

Support of anesthesia.

IV infusion: 1 mg/mL or **slow IV injection:** 10 mg/mL until client needs met.

Administration/Storage

1. For repeated doses, IM administration is preferred over SC use.
2. Meperidine is more effective when given parenterally than when given PO.
3. The syrup should be taken with ½ glass of water to minimize anesthetic effect on mucous membranes.
4. If used concomitantly with phenothiazines or antianxiety agents, the dose of meperidine should be reduced by 25%–50%.
5. Meperidine for IV use is incompatible with the following drugs: aminophylline, barbiturates, heparin, iodide, methicillin, morphine sulfate, phenytoin, sodium bicarbonate, sulfadiazine, and sulfisoxazole.
6. *Treatment of Overdose:* Naloxone 0.4 mg IV is effective in the treatment of acute overdosage. In PO overdose, gastric lavage and induced emesis are indicated. Treatment, however, is aimed at combating the progressive respiratory depression usually through artificial ventilation.

Additional Contraindications: Hypersensitivity to drug, convulsive states as in epilepsy, tetanus and strychnine poisoning, children under 6 months, diabetic acidosis, head injuries, shock, liver disease, respiratory depression, increased cranial pressure, and before labor during pregnancy.

Special Concerns: To be used with caution in lactating mothers and in older or debilitated clients. Use with extreme caution in clients with asthma. Meperidine has atropine-like effects that may aggravate glaucoma, especially when given with other drugs, which should be used with caution in glaucoma.

Additional Side Effects: Transient hallucinations, transient hypotension (high doses), visual disturbances. Meperidine may accumulate in clients with renal dysfunction, leading to an increased risk of CNS toxicity.

Additional Drug Interactions

Antidepressants, tricyclic / Additive anticholinergic side effects
Hydantoins / ↓ Effect of meperidine due to ↑ breakdown by liver
MAO inhibitors / ↑ Risk of severe symptoms including hyperpyrexia,

restlessness, hyper- or hypotension, convulsions, or coma

NURSING CONSIDERATIONS

See also *Nursing Considerations* for *Narcotic Analgesics,* Chapter 43.

Assessment

1. Note any evidence of head injury or history of seizure disorder.
2. Record any history of asthma or other conditions that tend to compromise respirations.
3. Obtain baseline renal function studies and note any history of glaucoma.
4. Determine if client is a candidate for PCA via pump.

Evaluate: Desired level of analgesia without compromise in level of consciousness or respirations.

Methadone hydrochloride

(**METH**-ah-dohn)
Pregnancy Category: C
Dolophine, Methadose **(C-II) (Rx)**

See also *Narcotic Analgesics,* Chapter 43.

How Supplied: *Concentrate:* 10 mg/mL; *Injection:* 10 mg/mL; *Solution:* 5 mg/5 mL, 10 mg/5 mL; *Tablet:* 5 mg, 10 mg, 40 mg

Action/Kinetics: Methadone produces only mild euphoria, which is the reason it is used as a heroin withdrawal substitute and for maintenance programs. Methadone produces physical dependence, but the abstinence syndrome develops more slowly upon termination of therapy; also, withdrawal symptoms are less intense but more prolonged than those associated with morphine. Methadone does not produce sedation or narcosis. Methadone is not effective for preoperative or obstetric anesthesia. When administered PO, it is only one-half as potent as when given parenterally. **Onset:** 30–60 min. **Peak effects:** 30–60 min. **Duration:** 4–6 hr. **t½:** 15–30 hr. Both the duration and half-life increase with repeated use due to cumulative effects.

Uses: Severe pain. Drug withdrawal and maintenance of narcotic dependence.

Dosage

• Tablets, Oral Solution, Oral Concentrate, IM, SC

Analgesia.

Adults, individualized: 2.5–10 mg q 3–4 hr, although higher doses may be necessary for severe pain or due to development of tolerance.

Narcotic withdrawal.

Initial: 15–20 mg/day PO (some may require 40 mg/day); **then,** depending on need of the client, slowly decrease dosage.

Maintenance following narcotic withdrawal.

Adults, individualized, initial: 20–40 mg PO 4–8 hr after heroin is stopped; **then,** adjust dosage as required up to 120 mg/day.

Administration/Storage

1. PO concentrations of solution should be diluted in at least 90 mL of water prior to administration.
2. If the client is taking dispersible tablets, the tablets should be diluted in 120 mL of water, orange juice, citrus flavored drink, or other acidic fruit drink. Allow at least 1 min for complete dispersion of the drug.
3. For repeated analgesic doses, IM administration is preferred over SC administration. Inspect injection sites for signs of irritation.
4. Clients receiving methadone for detoxification purposes should be on the drug no longer than 21 days. The treatment should not be repeated until 4 weeks have elapsed.

Additional Contraindications: Intravenous use, liver disease; give rarely, if at all, during pregnancy. Use in children. Use in obstetrics (due to long duration of action and chance of respiratory depression in the neonate).

Special Concerns: Use with caution during lactation.

Laboratory Test Interference: ↑ Immunoglobulin G.

Additional Side Effects: Marked constipation, excessive sweating, pulmonary edema, choreic movements.

Drug Interactions: Rifampin and phenytoin ↓ plasma methadone levels by ↑ breakdown by liver; thus, possible symptoms of narcotic withdrawal may develop.

NURSING CONSIDERATIONS

See also *Nursing Considerations* for *Narcotic Analgesics,* Chapter 43.

Client/Family Teaching

1. Review potential side effects with the client and family. Note that if the client is ambulatory and not suffering acute pain, side effects may be more pronounced.
2. Report if N&V develop because a lower dose of drug may relieve these symptoms.
3. To minimize drug's constipating effects, advise to exercise regularly and increase intake of fluids, fruit, and bulk in the diet.
4. For clients on narcotic withdrawal therapy, specifically advise storing drug out of the reach of children.
5. Evaluate needs and refer methadone-addicted parents to social services for assistance in child care.

Evaluate

- Control of severe pain
- Successful detoxification and maintenance of narcotic dependence

Morphine hydrochloride

(**MOR**-feen)

Pregnancy Category: C

Morphitec ✤, M.O.S. ✤, M.O.S.-S.R. ✤ **(Rx)**

Morphine sulfate

(**MOR**-feen **SUL**-fayt)

Pregnancy Category: C

Astramorph PF, Duramorph, Epimorph ✤, Infumorph, M-Eslon ✤, Morphine HP ✤, MS Contin, MS-IR, MSIR Capsules, Oramorph SR, RMS, RMS Rectal Suppositories, Roxanol, Roxanol 100, Roxanol Rescudose, Roxanol UD, Statex ✤ **(C-II) (Rx)**

See also *Narcotic Analgesics,* Chapter 43.

How Supplied: Morphine hydrochloride: *Syrup:* 1 mg/mL, 5 mg/mL, 10 mg/mL, 20 mg/mL; *Concentrate:* 20 mg/mL, 50 mg/mL; *Suppository:* 10 mg, 20 mg, 30 mg; *Tablets:* 10 mg, 20 mg, 40 mg, 60 mg; *Slow-release tablets:* 30 mg, 60 mg.

Morphine sulfate: *Capsule:* 15 mg, 30 mg; *Concentrate:* 20 mg/mL; *Injection:* 0.5 mg/mL, 1 mg/mL, 2 mg/mL, 4 mg/mL, 5 mg/mL, 8 mg/mL, 10 mg/mL, 15 mg/mL, 25 mg/mL, 50 mg/mL; *Solution:* 10 mg/5 mL, 20 mg/5 mL; *Suppository:* 5 mg, 10 mg, 20 mg, 30 mg; *Tablet:* 10 mg, 15 mg, 30 mg; *Tablet, Extended Release:* 15 mg, 30 mg, 60 mg, 100 mg, 200 mg

Action/Kinetics: Morphine is the prototype for opiate analgesics. **Onset:** approximately 15–60 min. **Peak effect:** 30–60 min. **Duration:** 3–7 hr. **t½:** 1.5–2 hr. Oral morphine is only one-third to one-sixth as effective as parenteral products.

Uses: Intrathecally, epidurally, PO, or by continuous IV infusion for acute or chronic pain. In low doses, morphine is more effective against dull, continuous pain than against intermittent, sharp pain. Large doses, however, will dull almost any kind of pain. Preoperative medication. To facilitate induction of anesthesia and reduce dose of anesthetic. *Investigational:* Acute LV failure (for dyspneic seizures) and pulmonary edema. Morphine should not be used with papaverine for analgesia in biliary spasms but may be used with papaverine in acute vascular occlusions.

Dosage

- **Tablets, Oral Solution, Soluble Tablets**

Analgesia.

10–30 mg q 4 hr.

- **Sustained-Release Tablets**

Analgesia.

30 mg q 8–12 hr, depending on client needs and response.

- **IM, SC**

Analgesia.

Adults: 5–20 mg/70 kg q 4 hr as needed; **pediatric:** 100–200 mcg/kg up to a maximum of 15 mg.

- **IV Infusion**

Analgesia.

Adults: 2.5–15 mg/70 kg in 4–5 mL of water for injection (should be administered slowly over 4–5 min).

- **IV Infusion, Continuous**

Analgesia.

Adults: 0.1–1 mg/mL in D5W by a controlled-infusion pump.

- **Rectal Suppositories**

Adults: 10–20 mg q 4 hr.

- **Intrathecal**

Adults: 0.2–1 mg as a single daily injection.

- **Epidural**

Initial: 5 mg/day in the lumbar region; if analgesia is not manifested in 1 hr, increasing doses of 1–2 mg can be given, not to exceed 10 mg/day. For continuous infusion, 2–4 mg/day with additional doses of 1–2 mg if analgesia is not satisfactory.

Additional Contraindications: Epidural or intrathecal morphine if infection is present at injection site, in clients on anticoagulant therapy, bleeding diathesis, if client has received parenteral corticosteroids within the past 2 weeks.

Special Concerns: Morphine may increase the length of labor. Clients with known seizure disorders may be at greater risk for morphine-induced seizure activity.

Administration/Storage

1. May be administered with food to diminish GI upset. Controlled-release tablets should not be crushed or chewed.
2. Immediate-release capsules may be swallowed intact or the contents of the capsule may be sprinkled on food or stirred in juice to avoid the bitter taste. The contents of the capsule may also be delivered through a nasogastric or a gastric tube.
3. For IV use, dilute 2–10 mg with at least 5 mL sterile water or NSS and administer over 4–5 min. For continous infusions, reconstitute to a concentration of 0.1–1 mg/mL and administer as prescribed to control symptoms.
4. Rapid IV administration increases the risk of adverse effects; a narcotic antagonist (e.g., naloxone) should be available at all times if morphine is given IV.
5. For intrathecal use, no more than 2 mL of the 5-mg/10 mL preparation or 1 mL of the 10-mg/10 mL product should be given.
6. Intrathecal administration should be only in the lumbar region; repeated injections are not recommended.
7. To reduce the chance of side effects with intrathecal administration, a constant IV infusion of naloxone (0.6 mg/hr for 24 hr after intrathecal injection) is recommended.
8. In certain circumstances (e.g., tolerance, severe pain), the physician may prescribe doses higher than those listed under *Dosage*.
9. Use an electronic infusion device for IV solutions. May also be administered by PCA pump.
10. Obtain written parameters for BP and respirations during IV infusions.
11. Dose may be lower in geriatric clients or those with respiratory disease.
12. Have respiratory support and naloxone available in the event of overdose.

NURSING CONSIDERATIONS

See also *Nursing Considerations* for *Narcotic Analgesics,* Chapter 43.

Assessment

1. Document indications for therapy and type and onset of symptoms.
2. List other agents prescribed and the outcome.
3. Note any history of seizure disorder.

Client/Family Teaching

1. Drug may cause dizziness and drowsiness. Avoid activities that require mental alertness during drug therapy.
2. Stress the importance of cough and deep breathing or incentive spirometry to minimize the development of atelectasis.

3. Avoid alcohol and any other CNS depressants unless specifically prescribed.

Evaluate

- Relief of pain
- Control of respirations during mechanical ventilation

Nalbuphine hydrochloride

(**NAL**-byou-feen)
Nubain **(Rx)**

See also *Narcotic Analgesics,* Chapter 43.

How Supplied: *Injection:* 10 mg/mL, 20 mg/mL

Action/Kinetics: Nalbuphine, a synthetic compound resembling oxymorphone and naloxone, is a potent analgesic with both narcotic agonist and antagonist actions. Its analgesic potency is approximately equal to that of morphine, while its antagonistic potency is approximately one-fourth that of nalorphine. **Onset: IV,** 2–3 min; **SC or IM,** <15 min. **Peak effect:** 30–60 min. **Duration:** 3–6 hr; **t½:** 5 hr.

Uses: Moderate to severe pain. Preoperative analgesia, anesthesia adjunct, obstetric analgesia.

Dosage

- **SC, IM, IV**

Analgesia.

Adults: 10 mg/70 kg q 3–6 hr as needed (single dose should not exceed 20 mg q 3–6 hr; total daily dose should not exceed 160 mg).

Administration/Storage: Nalbuphine hydrochloride may be administered IV, undiluted. Administer each 10 mg or less over a 3–5-min period.

Contraindications: Hypersensitivity to drug. Children under 18 years.

Special Concerns: Safe use during pregnancy (except for delivery) and lactation not established. Use with caution in presence of head injuries and asthma, MI (if client is nauseous or vomiting), biliary tract surgery (may induce spasms of sphincter of Oddi), renal insufficiency. Clients dependent on narcotics may experience withdrawal symptoms following use of nalbuphine.

Additional Side Effects: Even though nalbuphine is an agonist-antagonist, it may cause dependence and may precipitate withdrawal symptoms in an individual physically dependent on narcotics. *CNS:* Sedation is common. Crying, feelings of unreality, and other psychologic reactions. *GI:* Cramps, dry mouth, bitter taste, dyspepsia. *Skin:* Itching, burning, urticaria, sweaty, clammy skin. *Other:* Blurred vision, difficulty with speech, urinary frequency.

Drug Interactions: Concomitant use with CNS depressants, other narcotics, phenothiazines, may result in additive depressant effects.

NURSING CONSIDERATIONS

See also *Nursing Considerations* for *Narcotic Analgesics,* Chapter 43.

Assessment

1. Take a complete nursing history, noting any evidence of dependence on narcotics. Nalbuphine may precipitate withdrawal symptoms in clients with narcotic addiction.
2. Note any history of head injuries, asthma, or cardiac dysfunction because the drug may be contraindicated.
3. Document any sulfite sensitivity.

Evaluate: Relief of pain.

Oxycodone hydrochloride

(ox-ee-**KOH**-dohn)
Pregnancy Category: C
Roxicodone, Roxicodone Intensol, Supeudol ✱ **(C-II) (Rx)**

Oxycodone terephthalate

(ox-ee-**KOH**-dohn teh-ref-**THAL**-ayt)
Pregnancy Category: C
(C-II) (Rx)

See also *Narcotic Analgesics,* Chapter 43.

How Supplied: Oxycodone hydrochloride: *Concentrate:* 20 mg/mL; *Solution:* 5 mg/5 mL; *Tablet:* 5 mg.

Action/Kinetics: A semisynthetic opiate, oxycodone produces mild sedation with little or no antitussive effect. It is most effective in relieving acute pain. **Onset:** 15–30 min. **Peak effect:** 60 min. **Duration:** 4–6 hr. Dependence liability is moderate. Oxycodone terephthalate is only available in combination with aspirin (e.g., Percodan) or acetaminophen.

Use: Moderate to severe pain.

Dosage

- **Oral Solution, Concentrated Solution, Tablets**

Analgesia.

Adults: 5 mg q 6 hr.

Additional Contraindication: Use in children.

Additional Drug Interactions: Clients with gastric distress, such as colitis or gastric or duodenal ulcer, and clients who have glaucoma should not receive Percodan, which also contains aspirin.

NURSING CONSIDERATIONS

See also *Nursing Considerations* for *Narcotic Analgesics,* Chapter 43.

Client/Family Teaching

1. Take medication with food to minimize GI upset.
2. Use caution and do not perform activities that require mental alertness.
3. Avoid alcohol in any form.

Evaluate: Reports of relief of pain.

Oxymorphone hydrochloride

(ox-ee-**MOR**-fohn)

Pregnancy Category: C

Numorphan **(C-I) (Rx)**

See also *Narcotic Analgesics,* Chapter 43.

How Supplied: *Injection:* 1 mg/mL, 1.5 mg/mL; *Suppository:* 5 mg

Action/Kinetics: Oxymorphone, on a weight basis, is said to be 2–10 times more potent as an analgesic than morphine although potency depends on the route of administration. It produces mild sedation and moderate depression of the cough reflex. **Onset:** 5–10 min. **Peak effect:** 30–60 min. **Duration:** 3–6 hr.

Uses: Moderate to severe pain. Parenteral: Preoperative analgesia, to support anesthesia, obstetrics, relief of anxiety in clients with dyspnea associated with acute LV failure and pulmonary edema.

Dosage

- **SC, IM**

Analgesia.

Adults, initial: 1–1.5 mg q 4–6 hr; dose can be increased carefully until analgesic response obtained.

Analgesia during labor.

Adults: 0.5–1.0 mg IM.

- **IV**

Analgesia.

Adults, initial: 0.5 mg.

- **Suppositories**

Analgesia.

Adults: 5 mg q 4–6 hr. **Not recommended for children under 12 years of age.**

Administration/Storage

1. If the drug is to be administered IV, dilute the dosage in 5 mL of sterile water or NSS and administer over 2–3 min.
2. Suppositories should be stored in the refrigerator.

NURSING CONSIDERATIONS

See also *Nursing Considerations* for *Narcotic Analgesics,* Chapter 43.

Interventions

1. Encourage to C&DB several times each hour while awake to prevent atelectasis; incentive spirometry may be useful.
2. This particular drug may aggravate gallbladder conditions so carefully assess any client complaint that resembles gallbladder pain.
3. Use safety precautions and assist client with activities as drug causes drowsiness and dizziness.

Evaluate: Relief of pain and control of anxiety.

Paregoric (Camphorated opium tincture)

(pair-eh-**GOR**-ick)
Pregnancy Category: C
(C-III) (Rx)

See also *Narcotic Analgesics,* Chapter 43.
How Supplied: *Liquid*
Action/Kinetics: The active principle of the mixture is opium (0.04% morphine). The preparation also contains benzoic acid, camphor, and anise oil. Morphine increases the muscular tone of the intestinal tract, decreases digestive secretions, and inhibits normal peristalsis. The slowed passage of the feces through the intestines promotes desiccation, which is a function of the time the feces spend in the intestine. **t½:** 2–3 hr. **Duration:** 4–5 hr.
Use: Acute diarrhea.

Dosage

- **Liquid**

Adult: 5–10 mL 1–4 times/day (5 mL contains 2 mg of morphine). **Pediatric:** 0.25–0.5 mL/kg 1–4 times/day.
Administration/Storage
1. Administer paregoric with water to ensure that it will reach the stomach. The mixture will have a milky appearance.
2. Store the medication in a light-resistant container.
3. Carefully distinguish between paregoric and tincture of opium. Tincture of opium contains 25 times more morphine than paregoric.
4. Paregoric preparations are subject to the Controlled Substances Act and must be charted accordingly.
5. Have naloxone available to treat any overdosage.
Contraindications: See *Morphine Sulfate,* Chapter 43. Do not use in clients with diarrhea caused by poisoning until toxic substance has been eliminated. Treatment of pseudomembranous colitis due to lincomycin, penicillins, and cephalosporins. Rubbing paregoric on the gums of a teething child is no longer recommended.
Special Concerns: Many physicians do not recommend use of paregoric in treating neonatal opioid dependence.
Side Effects: See *Narcotic Analgesics,* Chapter 43.
Drug Interactions: See *Narcotic Analgesics,* Chapter 43.

NURSING CONSIDERATIONS

See also *Nursing Considerations* for *Narcotic Analgesics,* Chapter 43.
Assessment
1. Document type of condition and length of time the client has been taking paregoric, its level of effectiveness, and any other agents prescribed and the outcome.
2. Note any history of hepatic dysfunction or drug dependence.
Client/Family Teaching
1. Advise client to adhere to the prescribed regimen.
2. Report if the diarrhea persists.
3. Stop medication once diarrhea has abated. Continued use of paregoric may result in constipation.
Evaluate: Relief of diarrhea.

COMBINATION DRUG

Pentazocine hydrochloride with Naloxone hydrochloride

(pen-**TAZ**-oh-seen, nah-**LOX**-ohn)
Pregnancy Category: C
Talwin NX **(C-IV) (Rx)**

Pentazocine lactate

(pen-**TAZ**-oh-seen)
Pregnancy Category: C
Talwin **(C-IV) (Rx)**

See also *Narcotic Analgesics,* Chapter 43.
How Supplied: Pentazocine hydrochloride with Naloxone hydrochloride: See Content.
Pentazocine lactate: *Injection:* 30 mg/mL

Content: Pentazocine hydrochloride with Naloxone hydrochloride: Each tablet contains: 50 mg pentazocine hydrochloride, 0.5 mg naloxone hydrochloride.

General Statement: When administered preoperatively for pain, pentazocine is approximately one-third as potent as morphine. It is a weak antagonist of the analgesic effects of meperidine, morphine, and other narcotic analgesics. It also manifests sedative effects.

Pentazocine has been abused by combining it with the antihistamine tripelennamine (a combination known as *T's and Blues*). This combination has been injected IV as a substitute for heroin. To reduce this possibility, the PO dosage form of pentazocine has been combined with naloxone (Talwin NX), which will prevent the effects of IV administered pentazocine but will not affect the efficacy of pentazocine when taken PO. If pentazocine with naloxone is used IV, fatal reactions may occur, which include vascular occlusion, pulmonary emboli, ulceration, and abscesses, and withdrawal in narcotic-dependent individuals.

Action/Kinetics: Pentazocine manifests both narcotic agonist and antagonist properties. It exerts its agonist effects by an action on kappa and sigma opioid receptors and its antagonistic effect by an action on mu opioid receptors. The drug also elevates systemic and pulmonary arterial pressure, systemic vascular resistance, and LV end-diastolic pressure, which results in an increased cardiac workload. **Onset: IM,** 15–20 min; **PO,** 15–30 min; **IV,** 2–3 min. **Peak effect: IM,** 15–60 min; **PO:** 60–180 min. **Duration, all routes:** 3 hr. However, onset, duration, and degree of relief depend on both dose and severity of pain. **t½:** 2–3 hr. Extensive first-pass metabolism in the liver.

Uses: PO: Moderate to severe pain. **Parenteral:** Preoperative or preanesthetic medication, obstetrics, supplement to surgical anesthesia. Moderate to severe pain.

Dosage

PENTAZOCINE HYDROCHLORIDE WITH NALOXONE HYDROCHLORIDE

• **Tablets**

Analgesia.

Adults: 50 mg/q 3–4 hr, up to 100 mg. Daily dose should not exceed 600 mg.

PENTAZOCINE LACTATE

• **IM, IV, SC**

Analgesia.

Adults: 30 mg/ q 3–4 hr; doses exceeding 30 mg IV or 60 mg IM not recommended. Total daily dosage should not exceed 360 mg.

Obstetric analgesia.

Adults: 30 mg IM given once; or, 20 mg IV q 2–3 hr for two or three doses.

Administration/Storage

1. Do not mix soluble barbiturates in the same syringe with pentazocine. It will form a precipitate.
2. IV pentazocine may be administered undiluted. However, if the drug is to be diluted, place 5 mg of drug into 5 mL of sterile water for injection. Administer each 5 mg or less over a 1-min period.
3. Review the list of drugs with which the medication interacts.

Additional Contraindications: Increased ICP or head injury. Not recommended for use in children under 12 years of age. Avoid using methadone or other narcotics for pentazocine withdrawal.

Special Concerns: Use with caution in impaired renal or hepatic function, as well as after MI, when N&V are present. Use with caution in women delivering premature infants and in clients with respiratory depression. Safety and efficacy in children less than 12 years of age have not been determined.

Additional Side Effects: *CNS:* Syncope, dysphoria, nightmares, hallucinations, disorientation, paresthesias, confusion, ***seizures.*** *Miscellaneous;* Decreased WBCs, edema of the face, chills. Both psychologic and physical dependence are possible, although the addiction liability is thought to be no greater than for codeine. Multiple parenteral doses may cause severe sclerosis of the skin, SC tissues, and underlying muscle.

NURSING CONSIDERATIONS

See also *Nursing Considerations* for *Narcotic Analgesics,* Chapter 43.

Assessment

1. Document indications for therapy, any other agents used, and the outcome.
2. Note any evidence of head injury or increased ICP.
3. Determine any history of hepatic, renal, or cardiac dysfunction.

Client/Family Teaching

1. Caution that drug may cause dizziness and drowsiness.
2. Avoid alcohol and any other CNS depressants.

Evaluate: Relief of pain.

—COMBINATION DRUG—

Percocet

(**PER**-koh-set)
Pregnancy Category: C
(C-II) (Rx)

See also *Acetaminophen,* Chapter 41, and *Narcotic Analgesics,* Chapter 43.

How Supplied: See Content

Content: Each tablet contains: *Nonnarcotic analgesic:* Acetaminophen, 325 mg. *Narcotic analgesic:* Oxycodone HCl, 5 mg. Also see information on individual components.

Use: Moderate to moderately severe pain.

Dosage

- **Tablets**

Adults, usual: 1 tablet q 6 hr as required for pain.

Administration/Storage

1. It may be necessary to increase the dose if tolerance occurs or if the pain is severe.
2. Dosage should be adjusted depending on the response of the client and the severity of the pain.

Special Concerns: Use with caution during lactation. Safety and effectiveness have not been determined in children. Dependence to oxycodone can occur.

NURSING CONSIDERATIONS

See also *Nursing Considerations* for *Narcotic Analgesics,* Chapter 43, and *Acetaminophen,* Chapter 41.

Client/Family Teaching

1. Caution that drug may cause dizziness and drowsiness.
2. Advise that drug is for short-term use; chronic pain conditions require alternative pharmacologic agents.
3. Avoid alcohol and any other CNS depressants.

Evaluate: Relief of pain.

—COMBINATION DRUG—

Percodan and Percodan-Demi

(**PER**-koh-dan, **PER**-koh-dan **DEH**-mee)
(C-II) (Rx)

See also *Acetylsalicylic Acid,* Chapter 41, and *Narcotic Analgesics,* Chapter 43.

How Supplied: See Content

Content: Each tablet of Percodan contains: *Nonnarcotic Analgesic:* Aspirin, 325 mg. *Narcotic Analgesics:* Oxycodone HCl, 4.5 mg; Oxycodone Terephthalate, 0.38 mg. Percodan-Demi contains the same amount of aspirin as Percodan but one-half the amount of oxycodone HCl and oxycodone terephthalate.

Use: Treatment of moderate to moderately severe pain.

Dosage

- **Percodan Tablets**
  Analgesia.

Adults, usual: 1 tablet q 6 hr as required for pain.

- **Percodan-Demi Tablets**
  Analgesia.

Adults, usual: 1–2 tablets/ q 6 hr; **pediatric, over 12 years:** ½ tablet/ q 6 hr; **pediatric, 6–12 years:** ¼ tablet/ q 6 hr.

Administration/Storage

1. It may be necessary to increase the dose if tolerance occurs or if the pain is severe.

2. Dosage should be adjusted depending on the response of the client and the severity of the pain.
Contraindication: Percodan should not be used in children although Percodan-Demi may be considered for use in children 6–12 years of age.
Special Concern: Use during pregnancy only if benefits outweigh risks. Dependence on oxycodone can occur.

NURSING CONSIDERATIONS

See also *Nursing Considerations* for *Narcotic Analgesics,* Chapter 43, and *Acetylsalicylic Acid,* Chapter 41.
Client/Family Teaching
1. Caution that drug causes dizziness and drowsiness.
2. Stress that drug does contain aspirin.
Evaluate: Relief of pain.

COMBINATION DRUG

Phenaphen with Codeine No. 2, No. 3, and No. 4

(**FEN**-ah-fen, **KOH**-deen)
Pregnancy Category: C
(C-III) (Rx)

Phenaphen-650 with Codeine Tablets

(**FEN**-ah-fen, **KOH**-deen)
Pregnancy Category: C
(C-III) (Rx)

See also *Acetaminophen,* Chapter 41, and *Narcotic Analgesics,* Chapter 43.
How Supplied: Phenaphen with Codeine No. 2, No. 3, and No. 4: See Content
Phenaphen-650 with Codeine Tablets: See Content
Content: *Nonnarcotic analgesic:* Acetaminophen, 325 mg (in each strength). *Narcotic analgesic:* Codeine phosphate, 15 mg (No. 2), 30 mg (No. 3), and 60 mg (No. 4). Each Phenaphen-650 with Codeine tablet contains: Acetaminophen, 650 mg, and codeine phosphate, 30 mg. Also see information on individual components.
Use: Mild to moderately severe pain.

Dosage

- **Phenapen with Codeine Capsules**

Analgesia.
Adults, usual: 1–2 capsules of Phenaphen with Codeine No. 2 or No. 3 q 4 hr as required for pain. Or, 1 capsule of Phenaphen No. 4 q 4 hr as required for pain. Maximum 24-hr adult dose is 360 mg codeine and 4,000 mg acetaminophen. **Pediatric:** Dose of codeine equivalent to 0.5 mg/kg/ q 4 hr as required for pain.

- **Phenaphen-650 with Codeine Tablets**

Analgesia.
Adults, usual: 1–2 tablets/ q 4 hr as needed for pain up to a maximum of 360 mg codeine and 4,000 mg acetaminophen in a 24-hr period.
Administration/Storage
1. Dosage should be based on the response of the client and the severity of the pain.
2. Doses of codeine greater than 60 mg do not increase the analgesic effect but may increase the incidence of unpleasant side effects.
Special Concerns: Use with caution during lactation.

NURSING CONSIDERATIONS

See also *Nursing Considerations* for *Narcotic Analgesics,* Chapter 43, and *Acetaminophen,* Chapter 41.
Client/Family Teaching
1. Caution that drug may cause dizziness and drowsiness.
2. Avoid alcohol and any other CNS depressants.
Evaluate: Relief of pain.

Propoxyphene hydrochloride

(proh-**POX**-ih-feen)
Pregnancy Category: C
642 Tablets ✱, Darvon, Dolene, Doloxene, Doraphen, Doxaphene, Profene, Progesic, Pro Pox, Propoxycon
(C-IV) (Rx)

Propoxyphene napsylate

(proh-**POX**-ih-feen)
Pregnancy Category: C
Darvon-N **(C-IV) (Rx)**

How Supplied: Propoxyphene hydrochloride: *Capsule:* 65 mg. Propoxyphene napsylate: *Tablet:* 100 mg

Action/Kinetics: Propoxyphene resembles the narcotics with respect to its mechanism and analgesic effect; it is one-half to one-third as potent as codeine. It is devoid of antitussive, anti-inflammatory, or antipyretic activity. When taken in excessive doses for long periods, psychologic dependence and occasionally physical dependence and tolerance will be manifested. **Peak plasma levels:** *hydrochloride:* 2–2.5 hr; *napsylate:* 3–4 hr. **Analgesic onset:** up to 1 hr. **Peak analgesic effect:** 2 hr. **Duration:** 4–6 hr. **Therapeutic serum levels:** 0.05–0.12 mcg/mL. **t½, propoxyphene:** 6–12 hr; **norpropoxyphene:** 30–36 hr. Extensive first-pass effect; metabolites are excreted in the urine.

Propoxyphene is often prescribed in combination with salicylates. In such instances, the information on salicylates should also be consulted. Propoxyphene hydrochloride is found in Darvon Compound and Wygesic, while propoxyphene napsylate is found in Darvocet-N.

Uses: To relieve mild to moderate pain. Propoxyphene napsylate has been used experimentally to suppress the withdrawal syndrome from narcotics.

Dosage

- **Capsules (Hydrochloride)**

  Analgesia.

Adults: 65 mg q 4 hr, not to exceed 390 mg/day.

- **Tablets (Napsylate)**

  Analgesia.

Adults: 100 mg q 4 hr, not to exceed 600 mg/day. Dose of propoxyphene should be reduced in clients with renal or hepatic impairment.

Administration/Storage: *Treatment of Overdose:* Maintain an adequate airway, artificial respiration, and naloxone, 0.4–2 mg IV (repeat at 2–3-min intervals) to combat respiratory depression. Gastric lavage or administration of activated charcoal may be helpful. Correct acidosis and electrolyte imbalance. Acidosis due to lactic acid may require IV sodium bicarbonate.

Contraindications: Hypersensitivity to drug. Not recommended for use in children.

Special Concerns: Safe use during pregnancy has not been established. Use with caution during lactation. Safety and efficacy have not been established in children.

Side Effects: *GI:* N&V, constipation, abdominal pain. *CNS:* Sedation, dizziness, lightheadedness, headache, weakness, euphoria, dysphoria. *Other:* Skin rashes, visual disturbances. Propoxyphene can produce psychologic dependence, as well as physical dependence and tolerance.

Symptoms of Overdose: Stupor, respiratory depression, apnea, hypotension, pulmonary edema, ***circulatory collapse, cardiac arrhythmias,*** conduction abnormalities, ***coma, seizures,*** respiratory-metabolic acidosis.

Drug Interactions

Alcohol, antianxiety drugs, antipsychotic agents, narcotics, sedative-hypnotics / Concomitant use may lead to drowsiness, lethargy, stupor, respiratory, depression, and coma

Carbamazepine / ↑ Effect of carbamazepine due to ↓ breakdown by liver

CNS depressants / Additive CNS depression

Orphenadrine / Concomitant use may lead to confusion, anxiety, and tremors

Phenobarbital / ↑ Effect of phenobarbital due to ↓ breakdown by liver

Skeletal muscle relaxants / Additive respiratory depression

Warfarin / ↑ Hypoprothrombinemic effects of warfarin

NURSING CONSIDERATIONS

See also *Nursing Considerations* for *Narcotic Analgesics,* Chapter 43.

Assessment

1. Note any history of opiate or alcohol dependency.
2. Obtain baseline liver and renal function studies. Anticipate reduced dose with renal and liver dysfunction.
3. Determine if client smokes. Smoking reduces drug effect by increasing metabolism.
4. Document indications for therapy, other agents prescribed, and the outcome.
5. Use with caution in the elderly and review drug profile to ensure other prescribed agents do not cause additive CNS effects.

Evaluate: Relief of pain.

Sufentanil

(soo-**FEN**-tah-nil)
Pregnancy Category: C
Sufenta **(Rx)**

See also *Narcotic Analgesics,* Chapter 43.

How Supplied: *Injection:* 50 mcg/mL

Action/Kinetics: Onset, IV: 1.3–8 min. **Anesthetic blood concentration:** 8–30 mcg/kg. **t½:** 2.5 hr. Allows appropriate oxygenation of the heart and brain during prolonged surgical procedures. May be used in children.

Uses: Narcotic analgesic used as an adjunct to maintain balanced general anesthesia. To induce and maintain general anesthesia (with 100% oxygen), especially in neurosurgery or CV surgery.

Dosage

- **IV**

Analgesia.

Adults, individualized, usual initial: 1–2 mcg/kg with oxygen and nitrous oxide; **maintenance:** 10–25 mcg as required.

For complicated surgery.

Adults: 2–8 mcg/kg with oxygen and nitrous oxide; **maintenance:** 10–50 mcg.

To induce and maintain general anesthesia.

Adults: 8–30 mcg/kg with 100% oxygen and a muscle relaxant; **maintenance:** 25–50 mcg. **Pediatric, less than 12 years:** 10–25 mcg/kg with 100% oxygen; **maintenance:** 25–50 mcg.

Induction and maintenance of general anesthesia in children less than 12 years of age undergoing CV surgery.

Initial: 10–25 mcg/kg with 100% oxygen; **maintenance:** 25–50 mcg.

Administration/Storage

1. Dose should be reduced in the debilitated or elderly client.
2. The dose should be calculated based on lean body weight.

Additional Contraindication: Use during labor.

Special Concerns: Dosage must be decreased in the obese, elderly, or debilitated client.

Additional Side Effects: Erythema, chills, intraoperative muscle movement. ***Extended postoperative respiratory depression.***

NURSING CONSIDERATIONS

See also *Nursing Considerations* for *Narcotic Analgesics,* Chapter 43.

Client/Family Teaching

1. Avoid activities that require mental alertness for at least 24 hr following surgery.
2. Call for assistance with ambulation and transfers.
3. Avoid alcohol and any other CNS depressants for 24 hr following surgery.

Evaluate: Desired level of analgesia.

—COMBINATION DRUG—

Synalgos-DC

(sigh-**NAL**-gohs)
(C-III) (Rx)

See also *Acetylsalicylic Acid,* Chapter 41, *Narcotic Analgesics,* Chapter 43.

How Supplied: See Content

Content: *Nonnarcotic analgesic:* Aspirin, 356.4 mg. *Narcotic analgesic:* Dihydrocodeine bitartrate, 16 mg.

CNS stimulant: Caffeine, 30 mg. See also information on individual components.
Use: Relief of moderate to moderately severe pain.

Dosage
- **Capsules**
  Analgesia.

Adults, individualized, usual: 2 capsules q 4 hr as required for pain.
Administration/Storage: The dosage can be adjusted depending on the response of the client.
Contraindication: Use in children less than 12 years of age.
Special Concerns: Safe use during pregnancy has not been established. Use with caution in presence of peptic ulcer or coagulation abnormalities and in geriatric and debilitated clients.

NURSING CONSIDERATIONS

See also *Nursing Considerations* for *Narcotic Analgesics,* Chapter 43, and *Acetylsalicylic Acid,* Chapter 41.
Assessment
1. Document indications for therapy, onset of symptoms, other agents prescribed, and the outcome.
2. Note any conditions that may preclude therapy with this drug.

Evaluate: Reports of desired pain relief.

—COMBINATION DRUG—

Tylenol with Codeine Elixir or Tablets

(**TIE**-leh-noll, **KOH**-deen)
Pregnancy Category: C
(Tablets are C-III and Elixir is C-V) **(Rx)**

See also *Acetaminophen,* Chapter 41, and *Narcotic Analgesics,* Chapter 43.
How Supplied: See Content
Content: *Nonnarcotic analgesic:* Acetaminophen, 300 mg in each tablet, and 120 mg/5 mL elixir. *Narcotic analgesic:* Codeine phosphate, 7.5 mg (No. 1 Tablets), 15 mg (No. 2 Tablets), 30 mg (No. 3 Tablets), 60 mg (No. 4 Tablets), and 12 mg/5 mL (Elixir).
Uses: The tablets are used for mild to moderately severe pain while the elixir is used for mild to moderate pain.

Dosage
- **Tablets, Capsules**
  Analgesia.

Adults, individualized, usual: 1–2 No. 1, No. 2, or No. 3 Tablets or No. 3 Capsules q 2–4 hr as needed for pain. Or, 1 No. 4 Tablet or Capsule q 4 hr as required. Maximum 24-hr dose is 360 mg codeine phosphate and 4,000 mg acetaminophen. **Pediatric:** Dosage equivalent to 0.5 mg/kg codeine.
- **Elixir**
  Analgesia.

Adults, individualized, usual: 15 mL q 4 hr as needed; **pediatric, 7–12 years:** 10 mL t.i.d.–q.i.d.; **3–6 years:** 5 mL t.i.d.–q.i.d.
Administration/Storage
1. Dosage should be adjusted depending on the response of the client and the severity of the pain.
2. Doses of codeine greater than 60 mg do not provide additional analgesia but may lead to an increased incidence of side effects.

Special Concerns: Use with caution during lactation. Safety has not been determined in children less than 3 years of age. This product may be habit-forming due to the codeine component.

NURSING CONSIDERATIONS

See also *Nursing Considerations* for *Narcotic Analgesics,* Chapter 43, and *Acetaminophen,* Chapter 41.
Client/Family Teaching
1. Take only as directed.
2. Report any loss of pain control because drug and/or dosage may require adjustment.

Evaluate: Reports of relief of pain.

COMBINATION DRUG

Tylox

(**TIE**-lox)
Pregnancy Category: C
(C-II) (Rx)

See also *Acetaminophen,* Chapter 41, and *Narcotic Analgesics,* Chapter 43.
How Supplied: See Content
Content: Each capsule contains: *Nonnarcotic analgesic:* Acetaminophen, 500 mg. *Narcotic analgesic:* Oxycodone HCl, 5 mg.
Uses: Relief of moderate to moderately severe pain.

Dosage

- **Capsules**

  Analgesia.

Adults, individualized, usual: 1 capsule q 6 hr as required for pain.
Administration/Storage
1. The dose should be adjusted depending on the response of the client and the severity of the pain.
2. As the dose of oxycodone is increased, the incidence of side effects increases. The drug should not be used in high doses for severe or intractable pain.
Special Concerns: Use with caution during lactation. Safety and effectiveness have not been determined in children. Drug dependence can develop due to the oxycodone component.

NURSING CONSIDERATIONS

See also *Nursing Considerations* for *Narcotic Analgesics,* Chapter 43, and *Acetaminophen,* Chapter 41.
Evaluate: Reports of effective control of pain.

COMBINATION DRUG

Vicodin

(**VYE**-koh-din)
Pregnancy Category: C
(C-III) (Rx)

See also *Acetaminophen,* Chapter 41, and *Narcotic Analgesics,* Chapter 43.
How Supplied: See Content
Content: Each tablet contains: *Nonnarcotic analgesic:* Acetaminophen, 500 mg. *Narcotic analgesic:* Hydrocodone bitartrate, 5 mg.
Uses: Moderate to moderately severe pain.

Dosage

- **Tablets**

  Analgesia.

Adults, individualized, usual: 1–2 tablets q 4–6 hr as needed for pain, up to maximum of 8 tablets in 24 hr.
Administration/Storage: The dose should be adjusted depending on the response of the client and the severity of the pain.
Contraindication: Lactation.
Special Concerns: May cause dependence due to hydrocodone. Safety and effectiveness have not been determined in children.

NURSING CONSIDERATIONS

See also *Nursing Considerations* for *Acetaminophen,* Chapter 41, and *Narcotic Analgesics,* Chapter 43.
Evaluate: Reports of relief of pain.

CHAPTER FORTY-FOUR

Narcotic Antagonists

See also the following individual entries:

Naloxone Hydrochloride
Naltrexone

General Statement: The narcotic antagonists are able to prevent or reverse many of the pharmacologic actions of morphine-type analgesics and meperidine. For example, respiratory depression induced by these drugs is reversed within minutes. Naloxone is considered a pure antagonist in that it does not produce morphine-like effects.

The narcotic antagonists are not effective in reversing the respiratory depression induced by barbiturates, anesthetics, or other nonnarcotic agents. Narcotic antagonists almost immediately induce withdrawal symptoms in narcotic addicts and are sometimes used to unmask dependence.

Action/Kinetics: Narcotic antagonists block the action of narcotic analgesics by displacing previously given narcotics from their receptor sites or by preventing narcotics from attaching to the opiate receptors, thereby preventing access by the analgesic. This type of antagonism is competitive.

NURSING CONSIDERATIONS

Assessment

1. Determine the etiology of respiratory depression. Narcotic antagonists do not relieve the toxicity of nonnarcotic CNS depressants.
2. Assess and obtain baseline VS before administering any narcotic antagonist.

Interventions

1. Monitor respirations closely after the duration of action of the narcotic antagonist. Additional doses of drug may be necessary.
2. Observe for the appearance of withdrawal symptoms after administration of the narcotic antagonist. Withdrawal symptoms are characterized by restlessness, crying out due to sudden loss of pain control, lacrimation, rhinorrhea, yawning, perspiration, vomiting, diarrhea, sweating, writhing, anxiety, pain, chills, and an intense craving for the drug.
3. Have emergency drugs and equipment readily available and observe for symptoms of airway obstruction.
4. If the client is comatose, turn frequently and position on the side to prevent aspiration.
5. Maintain a safe, protective environment. Use side rails, supervise ambulation, and use soft supports as needed.
6. Assess VS after drug administration to determine the effectiveness of the drug.
7. Note the appearance of narcotic withdrawal symptoms after the antagonist has been administered.
8. If the narcotic antagonist is being used to diagnose narcotic use or dependence, observe the initial dilation of the client's pupils, followed by constriction.
9. Note agent being reversed. If narcotic is sustained release, anticipate that repeated doses will be required in order to continue to counteract drug effects.
10. Anticipate readministration of smaller doses of narcotic (once depressant symptoms reversed) in clients with terminal pain and conditions that warrant narcotic pain management.

Evaluate

- Effective reversal of toxic effects of narcotic analgesic as evidenced by ↑ level of consciousness and improved respiratory rate and pattern
- Confirmation of narcotic dependence as evidenced by withdrawal symptoms

Naloxone hydrochloride

(nal-**OX**-ohn)
Pregnancy Category: B
Narcan **(Rx)**

See also *Narcotic Antagonists,* Chapter 44.

How Supplied: *Injection:* 0.02 mg/mL, 0.4 mg/mL, 1 mg/mL

Action/Kinetics: Naloxone, administered by itself, does not produce significant pharmacologic activity. Since the duration of action of naloxone is shorter than that of the narcotic analgesics, the respiratory depression may return when the narcotic antagonist has worn off. **Onset: IV,** 2 min; **SC, IM:** <5 min. **Time to peak effect:** 5–15 min. **Duration:** Dependent on dose and route of administration but may be as short as 45 min. **t½:** 60–100 min. Metabolized in the liver to inactive products that are eliminated through the kidneys.

Uses: Respiratory depression induced by natural and synthetic narcotics, including butorphanol, methadone, nalbuphine, pentazocine, and propoxyphene. Drug of choice when nature of depressant drug is not known. Diagnosis of acute opiate overdosage. Not effective when respiratory depression is induced by hypnotics, sedatives, or anesthetics and other nonnarcotic CNS depressants. Adjunct to increase BP in septic shock. *Investigational:* Treatment of Alzheimer's dementia, alcoholic coma, and schizophrenia.

Dosage

- **IV, IM, SC**

Narcotic overdose.

Initial: 0.4–2 mg; if necessary, additional IV doses may be repeated at 2–3-min intervals. If no response after 10 mg, reevaluate diagnosis. **Pediatric, initial:** 0.01 mg/kg; **then,** 0.1 mg/kg, if needed.

To reverse postoperative narcotic depression.

IV, initial, 0.1–0.2-mg increments at 2–3-min intervals; **then,** repeat at 1–2-hr intervals if necessary. Supplemental IM dosage increases the duration of reversal.

To reverse postoperative narcotic depression.

Initial: Increments of 0.005–0.01 mg **IV** q 2–3 min to desired effect.

To reverse narcotic depression.

Initial: 0.01 mg/kg IV, IM, or SC; may be repeated if necessary.

Administration/Storage

1. May administer undiluted at a rate of 0.4 mg over 15 sec with narcotic overdosage. The drug may be reconstituted, 2 mg in 500 mL of NSS or 5% dextrose to provide a concentration of 4 mcg/mL or 0.004 mg/mL. The rate of administration varies with the response of the client.
2. Do not mix naloxone with preparations containing bisulfite, metabisulfite, long-chain or high molecular weight anions, or solutions with an alkaline pH.
3. When naloxone is mixed with other solutions, they should be used within 24 hr.
4. Naloxone is effective within 2 min after IV administration.

Contraindications: Sensitivity to drug. Narcotic addicts (drug may cause severe withdrawal symptoms). Not recommended for use in neonates.

Special Concerns: Safe use during lactation and in children is not established.

Side Effects: N&V, sweating, hypertension, tremors, sweating due to reversal of narcotic depression. If used postoperatively, excessive doses may cause tachycardia, fibrillation, hypo- or hypertension, pulmonary edema.

NURSING CONSIDERATIONS

See also *Nursing Considerations* for *Narcotic Antagonists,* Chapter 44.

Assessment
1. Document indications for therapy and type and onset of symptoms.
2. Identify any evidence of narcotic addiction.

Interventions
1. The duration of the effects of the narcotic may exceed the effects of naloxone (the antagonist). Therefore, more than one dose may be necessary to counteract the effects of the narcotic. Observe client closely and determine narcotic half-life.
2. Monitor VS at 5-min intervals, then every 30 min once stabilized.
3. For acutely ill clients or those who are in a coma, attach to a cardiac monitor and have a suction machine immediately available.
4. Titrate drug to avoid interfering with pain control or readminister narcotic at a lower dosage to maintain desired level of pain control.

Evaluate: Reversal of narcotic-induced respiratory depression.

Naltrexone

(nal-**TREX**-ohn)
Pregnancy Category: C
ReVia **(Rx)**

See also *Narcotic Antagonists,* Chapter 44.

How Supplied: *Tablet:* 50 mg

Action/Kinetics: Naltrexone binds to opiate receptors, thereby reversing or preventing the effects of narcotics. This is an example of competitive inhibition. **Peak plasma levels:** 1 hr. **Duration:** 24–72 hr. Metabolized in the liver; a major metabolite—6-beta-naltrexol—is active. **Peak serum levels, after 50 mg: naltrexone,** 8.6 ng/mL; **6-beta-naltrexol,** 99.3 ng/mL. **$t^1/_2$: naltrexone,** approximately 4 hr; **6-beta-naltrexol,** 13 hr. Naltrexone and its metabolites are excreted in the urine.

Uses: To prevent narcotic use in former narcotic addicts. Alcoholism. *Investigational:* To treat eating disorders and postconcussional syndrome not responding to other approaches.

Dosage

- **Tablets**

To produce blockade of opiate actions.

Initial: 25 mg followed by an additional 25 mg in 1 hr if no withdrawal symptoms occur. **Maintenance:** 50 mg/day.

Alternate dosing schedule.

The weekly dose of 350 mg may be given as: (a) 50 mg/day on weekdays and 100 mg on Saturday; (b) 100 mg/48 hr; (c) 100 mg every Monday and Wednesday and 150 mg on Friday; or, (d) 150 mg q 72 hr.

Administration/Storage
1. Naltrexone therapy should **never** be initiated until it has been determined that the individual is not dependent on narcotics (i.e., a naloxone challenge test should be completed).
2. The client should be opiate free for at least 7–10 days before beginning naltrexone therapy.
3. When initiating naltrexone therapy, begin with 25 mg and observe for 1 hr for any signs of narcotic withdrawal.
4. The blockade produced by naltrexone may be overcome by taking large doses of narcotics. Such doses may be fatal.
5. Clients taking naltrexone may not respond to preparations containing narcotics for use in coughs, diarrhea, or pain.

Contraindications: Clients taking narcotic analgesics, those dependent on narcotics, those in acute withdrawal from narcotics. Liver disease, acute hepatitis.

Special Concerns: Safety during lactation and in children under 18 years of age has not been established.

Side Effects: *CNS:* Headache, anxiety, nervousness, sleep disorders, dizziness, change in energy level, depression, confusion, restlessness, disorientation, hallucinations, nightmares, paranoia, fatigue, drowsiness. *GI:* N&V, diarrhea, constipation, anorexia, abdominal pain or cramps, flatulence, ulcers, increased appetite, weight gain or loss, increased thirst, xerostomia. *CV:* Phlebitis, edema, increased BP, changes in ECG, palpitations, epistaxis, tachycardia. *GU:*

Delayed ejaculation, increased urinary frequency or urinary discomfort, changes in interest in sex. *Respiratory:* Cough, sore throat, nasal congestion, rhinorrhea, sneezing, excess secretions, hoarseness, SOB, heaving breathing, sinus trouble. *Dermatologic:* Rash, oily skin, itching, pruritus, acne, cold sores, alopecia, athlete's foot. *Musculoskeletal:* Joint/muscle pain, muscle twitches, tremors, pain in legs, knees, or shoulders. *Other:* Hepatotoxicity, blurred vision, tinnitus, painful ears, aching or strained eyes, chills, swollen glands, inguinal pain, cold feet, "hot" spells, "pounding" head, fever.

A severe narcotic withdrawal syndrome may be precipitated if naltrexone is administered to a dependent individual. The syndrome may begin within 5 min and may last for up to 2 days.

NURSING CONSIDERATIONS

See also *Nursing Considerations* for *Narcotic Antagonists,* Chapter 44.

Assessment

1. Determine if addicted to opiates and when the last dose was ingested as client must be opiate free for 7–10 days before initiating therapy.
2. Obtain VS and monitor daily. Report if the respirations are severely lowered or if the client complains of difficulty breathing.
3. Obtain baseline ECG prior to initiating therapy.
4. Perform baseline liver function studies and monitor monthly during the first 6 months of therapy.
5. Ensure that urinalysis confirms absence of opiates and that naloxone challenge test has been performed before initiating drug therapy.

Client/Family Teaching

1. May take with food or milk to diminish GI upset.
2. Review the goals of therapy. Advise that headaches, restlessness, and irritability may be due to the effects of naltrexone.
3. Identify adverse side effects to be reported if they occur, such as loss of appetite, unusual fatigue, yellowing of skin or sclera, or itching.
4. Complaints of abdominal pain or difficulty with bowel function may warrant a reduction in the dosage of naltrexone; advise reporting.
5. Encourage to remain drug free. Provide clients with the names of health care agencies and support groups that may assist them in remaining drug free.
6. Stress the importance of active participation in support groups and behavioral therapy.
7. Inform health care providers and wear or carry appropriate identification indicating that client is taking naltrexone.

Evaluate: Maintenance of narcotic-free state in detoxified addicts.

CHAPTER FORTY-FIVE

Drugs Used for Vascular and Migraine Headaches

See the following individual entries:

Methysergide Maleate
Sumatriptan Succinate

Methysergide maleate

(meth-ih-**SIR**-jyd)
Sansert **(Rx)**

How Supplied: *Tablet:* 2 mg
Action/Kinetics: Methysergide is an ergot alkaloid derivative structurally related to LSD. It is thought to act by directly stimulating smooth muscle leading to vasoconstriction. The drug blocks the effects of serotonin, a powerful vasodilator believed to play a role in vascular headaches; it also inhibits the release of histamine from mast cells and prevents the release of serotonin from platelets. It has weak emetic and oxytocic activity. **Onset:** 1–2 days. **Peak plasma levels:** 60 ng/mL. **Duration:** 1–2 days. Excreted through the urine as unchanged drugs and metabolites.
Uses: Prophylaxis of vascular headache (in clients having one or more per week or in cases where headaches are so severe preventive therapy is indicated). Clients should remain under supervision.

Dosage

- **Tablets**

Adults: Administer 4–8 mg/day in divided doses. Continuous administration should not exceed 6 months. Drug may be readministered after a 3–4-week rest period.

Administration/Storage

1. Administer the drug with meals or milk to minimize GI irritation due to increased hydrochloric acid production.
2. The drug must be discontinued gradually to avoid migraine headache rebound.
3. If the drug is not effective after 3 weeks, it is not likely to be beneficial and should be discontinued.

Contraindications: Severe renal or hepatic disease, severe hypertension, CAD, peripheral vascular disease, or tendency toward thromboembolic disease, cachexia (profound ill health or malnutrition), severe arteriosclerosis, phlebitis or cellulitis of lower limbs, collagen diseases, valvular heart disease, infectious disease, or peptic ulcer. Pregnancy, lactation, use in children.
Special Concerns: Geriatric clients may be more affected by peripheral vasoconstriction leading to the possibility of hypothermia.
Side Effects: The drug is associated with a high incidence of side effects. *Fibrosis:* ***Retroperitoneal fibrosis, cardiac fibrosis, pleuropulmonary fibrosis,*** Peyronie's-like disease. The fibrotic condition may result in vascular insufficiency in the lower legs. *CV:* Vasoconstriction of arteries leading to paresthesia, chest pain, abdominal pain, or extremities that are cold, numb, or painful. Tachycardia, postural hypotension. *CNS:* Dizzi-

ness, ataxia, drowsiness, vertigo, insomnia, euphoria, lightheadedness, and psychic reactions such as depersonalization, depression, and hallucinations. *GI:* N&V, diarrhea, heartburn, abdominal pain, increased gastric acid, constipation. *Hematologic:* Eosinophilia, neutropenia. *Other:* Peripheral edema, flushing of face, skin rashes, transient alopecia, myalgia, arthralgia, weakness, weight gain, telangiectasia.

Drug Interaction: Narcotic analgesics are inhibited by methysergide.

NURSING CONSIDERATIONS

Assessment

1. Note the frequency and severity of the client's headaches and efforts made in the past to control or prevent them.
2. Note any history of renal or hepatic disease. Obtain baseline liver and renal function studies.
3. Assess behavior prior to initiating therapy. Review diet, activity, and stress levels. Determine any recent ingestion of agents that may have precipitated event.
4. Obtain baseline eosinophil and neutrophil counts.

Client/Family Teaching

1. Take with meals or milk to minimize GI upset.
2. Report symptoms of nervousness, weakness, insomnia, rashes, alopecia, or peripheral edema.
3. Record weights daily and report any unusual weight gain. Check the extremities for edema and report if evident.
4. If the weight gain becomes excessive, instruct the client on how to adjust the caloric intake. Maintain a low-salt diet and refer to a dietitian for assistance.
5. Advise to keep a diary noting any events, foods, or activities that may relate to the onset of these headaches.
6. Administration of methysergide should not be continued on a regular basis for longer than 6 months.
7. Remind the client to remain under medical supervision. Stress that blood tests must be done at periodic intervals to detect complications of drug therapy.
8. General malaise, fatigue, weight loss, low-grade fever, or urinary tract problems may be symptoms of fibrosis (cardiac or pleuropulmonary), and the drug should be discontinued. Report any of these symptoms immediately.
9. Do not drive a car or engage in other hazardous tasks until drug effects are realized because drug may cause drowsiness.
10. If dizziness or lightheadedness occurs upon arising, rise slowly from a supine position and dangle the legs for a few minutes before standing erect.
11. If feeling faint, lie down with the legs elevated.
12. Avoid alcohol, caffeine, and cannabalis, as these may precipitate vascular headaches.
13. Discuss with the family unusual psychologic changes that may occur, especially hallucinations that require reporting if evident.
14. Do not discontinue medication abruptly. Rebound migraine headaches may occur. Medication must be discontinued gradually.

Evaluate: ↓ Occurrence of severe vascular headaches.

Sumatriptan succinate

(**soo**-mah-**TRIP**-tan)
Pregnancy Category: C
Imitrex Injection

How Supplied: *Injection:* 6 mg/0.5 mL; *Kit:* 6 mg/0.5 mL

Action/Kinetics: Sumatriptan is a selective agonist for a vascular 5-HT_1 receptor subtype (probably 5-HT_{1D}. These receptors are located on cranial arteries, on the basilar artery, and the vasculature of the dura mater. In these tissues, sumatriptan activates the 5-HT_1 receptor, causing vasoconstriction and therefore relief of migraine. Transient increases in BP may be observed. It has no significant activity at 5-HT_2 or 5-HT_3 receptor subtypes; alpha-1-, alpha-2-, or beta-adrenergic receptors; dopamine-1 or dopamine-2 receptors; muscarinic receptors; or benzodiazepine receptors. **Distribution t½:** 15 min; **terminal t½:** 115 min. Approximately 22% is excreted in the urine as unchanged drug and 38% as metabolites. **Time to peak effect:** 12 min after a 6-mg SC dose.

Uses: Treatment of acute migraine attacks with or without aura. Photophobia, phonophobia, nausea, and vomiting associated with migraine attacks are also relieved.

Dosage

- **SC**

Migraine headaches.

Adults: 6 mg. **Maximum recommended dose:** Two 6-mg injections/24 hr.

Administration/Storage

1. No increased beneficial effect has been found with the administration of a second 6-mg dose in clients not responding to the first injection.
2. If side effects are dose limiting, a dose lower than 6 mg may be given; in such cases, only the single-dose vial dosage form should be used as the autoinjection form delivers 6 mg.
3. Consideration should be given to administering the first dose of sumatriptan in a physician's office due to the possibility (although rare) of coronary events.
4. Sumatriptan should be stored away from heat (no higher than 30°C; 86°F) and light.

Contraindications: Hypersensitivity to sumatriptan. IV use due to the possibility of coronary vasospasm. SC use in clients with ischemic heart disease, history of MI, documented silent ischemia, Prinzmetal's angina, or uncontrolled hypertension. Concomitant use with ergotamine-containing products. Use in clients with hemiplegic or basilar migraine.

Special Concerns: Use with caution during lactation, in clients with impaired hepatic or renal function, and in clients with heart conditions. Clients with risk factors for CAD (e.g., men over 40, smokers, postmenopausal women, hypertension, obesity, diabetes, hypercholesterolemia, family history of heart disease) should be screened before initiating treatment. Safety and efficacy have not been determined for use for cluster headache or in children.

Laboratory Test Interference: Disturbance of liver function tests.

Side Effects: *CV:* Coronary vasospasm in clients with a history of CAD. ***Serious and/or life-threatening arrhythmias, including atrial fibrillation, ventricular fibrillation, ventricular tachycardia, MI, marked ischemic ST elevations,*** chest and arm discomfort representing angina pectoris. Flushing, hypertension, hypotension, bradycardia, tachycardia, palpitations, pulsating sensations, EEG changes, sinus arrhythmia, nonsustained ventricular premature beats, isolated junctional ectopic beats, atrial ectopic beats, syncope, pallor, abnormal pulse, vasodilatation, Raynaud's syndrome. *At injection site:* Pain, redness. *Atypical sensations:* Sensation of warmth, cold, tingling, or paresthesia. Localized or generalized feeling of pressure, burning, numbness, and tightness. Feeling of heaviness, feeling strange, tight feeling in head. *CNS:* Fatigue, dizziness, drowsiness, vertigo, sedation, headache, anxiety, malaise, confusion, euphoria, agitation, relaxation, chills, tremor, shivering, prickling or stinging sensations. *EENT:* Throat discomfort, discomfort in nasal cavity or sinuses. Vision alterations, eye irritation, photophobia, lacrimation. *GI:* Abdominal discomfort, dysphagia, discomfort of mouth and tongue, gastroesophageal reflux, diarrhea, peptic ulcer, retching, flatulence, eructation, gallstones, taste disturbances. *Respiratory:* Dyspnea, diseases of the lower respiratory tract, hiccoughs, influenza. *Dermatologic:* Erythema, pruritus, skin rashes, skin eruptions, skin tenderness. *GU:* Dysuria, dysmenorrhea, urinary frequency, renal calculus. *Musculoskeletal:* Weakness, neck pain or stiffness, myalgia, muscle cramps, joint disturbances, muscle stiffness, need to flex calf muscles, backache, muscle tiredness, swelling of the extremities. *Miscellaneous:* Chest, jaw, or neck tightness. Sweating, thirst, polydipsia, chills.

Drug Interactions

Ergot drugs / Prolonged vasospastic reactions

Monoamine oxidase A inhibitors / MAO-A inhibitors → ↑ t½ of sumatriptan

---

NURSING CONSIDERATIONS

Assessment

1. Document onset and type of symptoms and list other agents used and the outcome.
2. Determine any history of cardiac problems or evidence of ischemic CV disease, as drug is contraindicated.
3. Ensure that neurologic exam has been performed to identify migraine category.
4. Obtain baseline ECG, liver, and renal function studies.
5. Prior to prescribing sumatriptan, a clear diagnosis of migraine should be made; the drug should not be given for headache due to other neurologic events.

Interventions

1. Administer (or have client self-administer) first dose in a monitored environment in order to carefully assess client response.
2. Monitor VS and anticipate transient increases in BP.
3. Drug is for SC use only. IV use may cause coronary vasospasm.

Client/Family Teaching

1. Review the appropriate method for administration and observe client in self-administration to ensure familiarity and comfort with the autoinjector.
2. Printed instructions concerning how to load the autoinjector, administer the medication, and remove the syringe, are enclosed and provided by the manufacturer. Advise client to keep these handy for reference.
3. Advise client that the injection is given just below the skin as soon as the symptoms of migraine appear or any time during the attack. A second injection may be administered 1 hr later if migraine symptoms return but do *not* exceed 2 injections in 24 hr.
4. Review safe handling and proper disposal of syringes; provide proper receptacle as needed.
5. Advise that pain and tenderness may be evident at injection site for up to an hour after administration.
6. Check expiration date before use and discard all outdated drugs.
7. Advise that chest, jaw, throat, and neck pain may occur after injection and that this should be shared with the provider and medically evaluated before using any more Imitrex Injection.
8. Provide a printed list of side effects that require immediate reporting such as severe chest pain or tightness, wheezing, palpitations, facial swelling, or rashes/hives.
9. Symptoms of flushing, tingling, heat and heaviness, as well as dizziness or drowsiness may occur and should be shared with provider before taking any more sumatriptan injections.
10. Practice barrier contraception and do not use Imitrex Injection if pregnancy is suspected.

Evaluate: Reversal of acute migraine attack and relief of associated symptoms.

CHAPTER FORTY-SIX

Antiparkinson Drugs

See also the following individual entries:

Amantadine Hydrochloride - See Chapter 19
Benztropine Mesylate - See Chapter 49
Biperiden Hydrochloride - See Chapter 49
Biperiden Lactate - See Chapter 49
Bromocriptine Mesylate
Carbidopa
Carbidopa/Levodopa
Diphenhydramine Hydrochloride - See Chapter 55
Levodopa
Pergolide Mesylate
Procyclidine Hydrochloride - See Chapter 49
Selegiline Hydrochloride (Deprenyl)
Trihexyphenidyl Hydrochloride - See Chapter 49

General Statement: Parkinson's disease is a progressive disorder of the nervous system, affecting mostly people over the age of 50. The symptoms include slowness of motor movements (bradykinesia and akinesia), stiffness or resistance to passive movements (rigidity), muscle weakness, tremors, speech impairment, sialorrhea (salivation), and postural instability. Parkinsonism is a frequent side effect of certain antipsychotic drugs, including prochlorperazine, chlorpromazine, and reserpine. Drug-induced symptoms usually disappear when the responsible agent is discontinued. Extrapyramidal Parkinson-like symptoms can accompany brain injuries (strokes, tumors) or other diseases of the nervous system. The cause of Parkinson's disease is unknown; however, it is associated with a depletion of the neurotransmitter dopamine in the nervous system. Administration of levodopa—the precursor of dopamine—relieves symptoms in 75%–80% of the clients. Anticholinergic agents also have a beneficial effect by reducing tremors and rigidity and improving mobility, muscular coordination, and motor performance. They are often administered together with levodopa. Certain antihistamines, notably diphenhydramine (Benadryl), are also useful in the treatment of parkinsonism. Clients suffering from Parkinson's disease need emotional support and encouragement because the debilitating nature of the disorder often causes depression. Comprehensive treatment also includes physical therapy.

NURSING CONSIDERATIONS

See *Nursing Considerations* for individual drugs.

Assessment

1. Document PMH, onset of symptoms, and their progression.
2. Determine if symptoms are drug induced with agents such as haldol or phenothiazines.

Client/Family Teaching

1. Explain that this is a movement disorder of unknown origin but is usually progressive and leads to disability if untreated.
2. Advise that drug therapy is aimed at restoring normal balances of cholinergic and dopaminergic influences in the brain (basal ganglia).
3. Caution to administer only as prescribed as some of the drugs have many adverse side effects.

4. Stress that close medical follow-up is imperative, as some of these drugs may lose their effectiveness.

Evaluate

- Improved motor function
- Evidence of a reduction in pretreatment symptoms such as ↓ drooling, ↓ rigidity, ↓ tremors
- Reports of improvement in gait, posture, and muscle spasms

Bromocriptine mesylate

(broh-moh-**KRIP**-teen)
Parlodel **(Rx)**

How Supplied: *Capsule:* 5 mg; *Tablet:* 2.5 mg

Action/Kinetics: Bromocriptine is a nonhormonal agent that inhibits the release of the hormone prolactin by the pituitary. The drug should be used only when prolactin production by pituitary tumors has been ruled out. Its effect in parkinsonism is due to a direct stimulating effect on dopamine type 2 receptors in the corpus striatum. Use for parkinsonism may allow the dose of levodopa to be decreased, thus decreasing the incidence of severe side effects following long-term levodopa therapy. Less than 30% of the drug is absorbed from the GI tract. **Onset, lower prolactin:** 2 hr; **antiparkinson:** 30–90 min; **decrease growth hormone:** 1–2 hr. **Peak plasma concentration:** 1–3 hr. **t½, plasma:** 3 hr; **terminal:** 15 hr. **Duration, lower prolactin:** 24 hr (after a single dose; **decrease growth hormone:** 4–8 hr. Significant first-pass effect. Metabolized in liver, excreted mainly through bile and thus the feces.

Uses: Short-term treatment of amenorrhea/galactorrhea associated with hyperprolactinemia. Acromegaly. As adjunctive therapy with levodopa in the treatment of idiopathic or postencephalitic Parkinson's disease. Bromocriptine may provide additional benefit in clients who are taking optimal doses of levodopa, in those who are developing tolerance to levodopa therapy, or in those who are manifesting levodopa "end of dose failure." Clients unresponsive to levodopa are not good candidates for bromocriptine therapy. Female infertility associated with hyperprolactinemia. The drug is no longer recommended to suppress postpartum lactation. *Investigational:* Hyperprolactinemia due to pituitary adenoma; male infertility.

Dosage

- **Capsules, Tablets**

Amenorrhea/galactorrhea/female or male infertility due to hyperprolactinemia.

Adults, initial: 1.25–2.5 mg/day with meals; **then,** increase dose by 2.5 mg q 3–7 days until optimum response observed (usual: 5–7.5 mg/day; range: 2.5–15 mg/day). For amenorrhea/galactorrhea, do not use for more than 6 months.

Parkinsonism.

Initial: 1.25 mg (½ tablet) b.i.d. with meals while maintaining dose of levodopa, if possible. Dosage may be increased q 14–28 days by 2.5 mg/day with meals. The usual dosage range is 10–40 mg/day. Any decrease in dosage should be done gradually in 2.5-mg decrements.

Acromegaly.

Initial: 1.25–2.5 mg for 3 days with food and on retiring; **then,** increased by 1.25–2.5 mg q 3–7 days until optimum response observed. Usual optimum therapeutic range: 20–30 mg/day, not to exceed 100 mg/day. Clients should be reevaluated monthly and dosage adjusted accordingly.

Administration/Storage

1. Before administering the first dose of drug, have the client lie down because of the possibility of fainting or dizziness.
2. For doses less than 5 mg, tablets should be used.

Contraindications: Sensitivity to ergot alkaloids. Pregnancy, lactation, children under 15 years of age. Peripheral vascular disease, ischemic heart disease.

Special Concerns: Geriatric clients may manifest more CNS effects. Use with caution in liver or kidney disease. The use of bromocriptine for the prevention of physiologic lactation is being questioned due to the potential for side effects.

Laboratory Test Interferences: ↑ BUN, AST, ALT, GGPT, CPT, alkaline phosphatase, uric acid.

Side Effects: The type and incidence of side effects depend on the use of the drug. *When used for hyperprolactinemia. GI:* N&V, abdominal cramps, diarrhea, constipation. *CNS:* Headache, dizziness, fatigue, drowsiness, lightheadedness, psychoses. *Other:* Nasal congestion, mild hypotension.

When used for acromegaly. GI: N&V, anorexia, dry mouth, dyspepsia, indigestion, GI bleeding. *CNS:* Dizziness, syncope, drowsiness, tiredness, headache; rarely, lightheadedness, lassitude, vertigo, sluggishness, paranoia, insomnia, decreased sleep requirement, delusional psychosis, visual hallucinations. *CV:* Orthostatic hypotension, digital vasospasm, worsening of Raynaud's syndrome; rarely, arrhythmias, ventricular tachycardia, bradycardia, vasovagal attack. *Other:* Rarely, potentiation of effects of alcohol, hair loss, SOB, paresthesia, tingling of ears, muscle cramps, facial pallor, reduced tolerance to cold.

When used for parkinsonism. GI: N&V, abdominal discomfort, constipation, anorexia, dry mouth, dysphagia. *CNS:* Confusion, hallucinations, fainting, drowsiness, dizziness, insomnia, depression, vertigo, anxiety, fatigue, headache, lethargy, nightmares. *GU:* Urinary incontinence, urinary retention, urinary frequency. *Other:* Abnormal involuntary movements, asthenia, visual disturbances, ataxia, hypotension, SOB, edema of feet and ankles, blepharospasm, erythromelalgia, skin mottling, nasal stuffiness, paresthesia, skin rash, S&S.

Drug Interactions

Alcohol / ↑ Chance of GI toxicity; alcohol intolerance
Antihypertensives / Additive ↓ BP
Butyrophenones / ↓ Effect of bromocriptine because butyrophenones are dopamine antagonists
Diuretics / Should be avoided during bromocriptine therapy
Phenothiazines / ↓ Effect of bromocriptine because phenothiazines are dopamine antagonists

NURSING CONSIDERATIONS

Assessment

1. In taking a drug history, inquire about any sensitivity to ergot alkaloids.
2. Document indications for therapy, onset and type of symptoms, any other agents used, and the outcome.
3. Note the age of the client, if she is female and sexually active and likely to become pregnant.
4. If the client has any history of liver or kidney dysfunction, obtain baseline liver and renal function studies.
5. List other drugs the client is taking to determine the potential for drug interactions.
6. With Parkinson's disease, assess and document baseline physical ability and areas of disability. This permits distinction between desired response and drug-induced side effects, which may be severe initially before subsiding with therapy. Also document pharmacologic agents currently in use and their dosage.

Client/Family Teaching

1. Take the drug with food to minimize GI upset.
2. Caution that drug may cause dizziness, drowsiness, or syncope and to lie down if evident. Avoid activities that require mental alertness.
3. Report any complaints of fatigue, headache, nausea, drowsiness, cramps, or diarrhea.
4. If using oral contraceptives, advise client to use other contraceptive measures while taking bromocriptine.
5. When a menstrual period is missed, schedule the sexually active client for pregnancy tests every 4

weeks during the period of amenorrhea and after resumption of menses.
6. Discuss the S&S of pregnancy. If pregnancy is likely, advise withholding the drug and reporting. Explain that pregnancy tests may fail to diagnose early pregnancy and the medication may harm the fetus.
7. Review side effects, stressing those that require immediate medical intervention.

Evaluate

- Resumption of normal menstrual cycle
- Reduction of growth hormone in acromegaly
- ↓ Muscle rigidity and tremor in Parkinson's disease

Carbidopa

(**KAR**-bih-doh-pah)
Lodosyn **(Rx)**

—COMBINATION DRUG—

Carbidopa/Levodopa

(**KAR**-bih-doh-pah/**LEE**-voh-doh-pah)
Sinemet-10/100, -25/100, or -25/250, Sinemet CR **(Rx)**

How Supplied: Carbodopa: *Tablet:* 25 mg.
Carbidopa/Levodopa: See Content
Content: Each 10/100 tablet contains: 10 mg carbidopa, 100 mg levodopa. Each 25/100 tablet contains: 25 mg carbidopa, 100 mg levodopa. Each 25/250 tablet contains: 25 mg carbidopa, 250 mg levodopa.
Each sustained-release tablet contains: 50 mg carbidopa, 200 mg levodopa.
Action/Kinetics: Carbidopa inhibits peripheral decarboxylation of levodopa but not central decarboxylation because it does not cross the blood-brain barrier. Since peripheral decarboxylation is inhibited, this allows more levodopa to be available for transport to the brain, where it will be converted to dopamine, thus relieving the symptoms of parkinsonism. It is recommended that both carbidopa and levodopa be given together (e.g., Sinemet). However, *the dosage of levodopa must be reduced by up to 80% when combined with carbidopa*. This decreases the incidence of levodopa-induced side effects. *NOTE:* Pyridoxine will not reverse the action of carbidopa/levodopa. **t½, carbidopa:** 1–2 hr; when given with levodopa, the t½ of levodopa increases from 1 hr to 2 hr (may be as high as 15 hr in some clients). About 30% carbidopa is excreted unchanged in the urine.
Uses: All types of parkinsonism (idiopathic, postencephalitic, following injury to the nervous system due to carbon monoxide and manganese intoxication). Carbidopa alone is used in clients who require individual titration of carbidopa and levodopa. *Investigational:* Postanoxic intention myoclonus. See *Levodopa,* Chapter 46. **Warning:** Levodopa must be discontinued at least 8 hr before carbidopa/levodopa therapy is initiated. Also, clients taking carbidopa/levodopa must not take levodopa concomitantly, because the former is a combination of carbidopa and levodopa.

Dosage

- **Tablets**

Parkinsonism, clients not receiving levodopa.

Initial: 1 tablet of 10 mg carbidopa/100 mg levodopa t.i.d.–q.i.d. or 25 mg carbidopa/100 mg levodopa t.i.d.; **then,** increase by 1 tablet q 1–2 days until a total of 8 tablets/day is taken. If additional levodopa is required, substitute 1 tablet of 25 mg carbidopa/250 mg levodopa t.i.d.–q.i.d.

Parkinsonism, clients receiving levodopa.

Initial: Carbidopa/levodopa dosage should be about 25% of prior levodopa dosage (levodopa dosage is discontinued 8 hr before carbidopa/levodopa is initiated); **then,** adjust dosage as required. Suggested starting dose is 1 tablet of 25 mg carbidopa/250 mg levodopa t.i.d.–q.i.d. for clients taking more than 1500 mg levodopa or 25 mg carbidopa/100 mg levodopa for clients taking less than 1500 mg levodopa.

• **Sustained-Release Tablets**

Parkinsonism, clients not receiving levodopa.

1 tablet b.i.d. at intervals of not less than 6 hr. Depending on the response, dosage may be increased or decreased. Usual dose is 2–8 tablets/day in divided doses at intervals of 4–8 hr during waking hours (if divided doses are not equal, the smaller dose should be given at the end of the day).

Parkinsonism, clients receiving levodopa.

1 tablet b.i.d. Carbidopa is available alone for clients requiring additional carbidopa (i.e., inadequate reduction in N&V); in such clients, carbidopa may be given at a dose of 25 mg with the first daily dose of carbidopa/levodopa. If necessary, additional carbidopa, at doses of 12.5 or 25 mg, may be given with each dose of carbidopa/levodopa.

Clients receiving carbidopa/levodopa who require additional carbidopa

In clients taking 10 mg carbidopa/100 mg levodopa, 25 mg carbidopa may be given with the first dose each day. Additional doses of 12.5 or 25 mg may be given during the day with each dose. If the client is taking 25 mg carbidopa/250 mg levodopa, a dose of 25 mg carbidopa may be given with any dose, as needed. The maximum daily dose of carbidopa is 200 mg.

Administration

1. The dosage of these drugs must be individualized.
2. Note any potential drug interactions prior to starting drug therapy.
3. Do not administer carbidopa/levodopa with levodopa.
4. Administration of the sustained-release form of carbidopa/levodopa with food results in increased availability of levodopa by 50% and increased peak levodopa levels by 25%.
5. The sustained-release form of Sinemet should not be crushed or chewed but can be administered as whole or half tablets.
6. A minimum of 3 days should elapse between dosage adjustments of the sustained-release product.
7. When carbidopa is used as a supplement to carbidopa/levodopa, 1 tablet of carbidopa may be added or omitted per day.
8. If general anesthesia is necessary, therapy should be continued as long as PO fluids and other medication are allowed. Therapy should be resumed as soon as the client can take PO medication.

Contraindications: See *Levodopa,* Chapter 46. History of melanoma. MAO inhibitors should be stopped 2 weeks before therapy. Lactation.

Special Concerns: Use during pregnancy only if benefits outweigh risks. Safety and efficacy in children less than 18 years of age have not been determined. Lower doses may be necessary in geriatric clients due to aged-related decreases in peripheral dopa decarboxylase.

Laboratory Test Interferences: ↓ Creatinine, BUN, and uric acid.

Side Effects: See *Levodopa*

Also, because more levodopa reaches the brain, dyskinesias may occur at lower doses with carbidopa/levodopa than with levodopa alone. Clients abruptly withdrawn from levodopa may experience neuroleptic malignant-like syndrome including symptoms of muscular rigidity, hyperthermia, increased serum phosphokinase, and changes in mental status.

Drug Interaction: Use with tricyclic antidepressants may cause hypertension and dyskinesia.

NURSING CONSIDERATIONS

Assessment

1. Assess and document motor function, reflexes, gait, strength of grip, and amount of tremor.
2. Observe the extent of the tremors, noting muscle weakness, muscle rigidity, difficulty walking, or changing directions.

3. Determine the client's usual sleep patterns.
4. Note any history of CV disease, cardiac arrhythmias, or COPD.
5. Document age as elderly clients may require a reduced dosage.
6. Obtain baseline ECG, VS, and respiratory assessment and determine level of bladder function.

Interventions

1. Monitor BP with the client supine and standing to facilitate the detection of postural hypotension.
2. Observe closely during the dosage adjustment period. Note any involuntary movement that may require dosage reduction.
3. Assess for blepharospasm as this may be an early sign of excessive dosage.
4. To facilitate adjustment to changes in medication, administer the last dose of levodopa at bedtime and start carbidopa/levodopa on arising in the morning.

Client/Family Teaching

1. Review the side effects that may occur and advise the client to report as the dose of drug may need to be reduced or temporarily discontinued. The client may be asked to tolerate certain side effects because of the overall benefits gained with therapy.
2. As clients improve with drug therapy, they may resume normal activity gradually. Also, remind clients that with increased activity, they must take other medical conditions into consideration.
3. Antiparkinson drugs should not be withdrawn abruptly. When changing medication, one drug should be withdrawn slowly and the other started in small doses under medical supervision.
4. Drug may discolor or darken urine and/or sweat.
5. Muscle and eyelid twitching may indicate toxicity and should be reported immediately.

Evaluate

- Control of parkinsonian symptoms (e.g., improvement in motor function, reflexes, gait, strength of grip, and amount of tremor)
- The need for a drug "holiday" based on ↓ drug response

Levodopa

(lee-voh-**DOH**-pah)
Dopar, Larodopa, L-Dopa **(Rx)**

How Supplied: *Capsule:* 100 mg, 250 mg, 500 mg; *Tablet:* 100 mg, 250 mg, 500 mg

Action/Kinetics: Depletion of dopamine in the striatum of the brain is thought to cause the symptoms of Parkinson's disease. Levodopa, a dopamine precursor, is able to cross the blood-brain barrier to enter the CNS. It is decarboxylated to dopamine in the basal ganglia, thus replenishing depleted dopamine stores. **Peak plasma levels:** 0.5–2 hr (may be delayed if ingested with food). **t½, plasma:** 1–3 hr. Onset occurs in 2–3 weeks although some clients may require up to 6 months. Levodopa is extensively metabolized both in the GI tract, and the liver and metabolites are excreted in the urine.

Uses: Idiopathic, arteriosclerotic, or postencephalitic parkinsonism. Parkinsonism due to carbon monoxide or manganese intoxication. Levodopa only provides symptomatic relief and does not alter the course of the disease. When effective, it relieves rigidity, bradykinesia, tremors, dysphagia, seborrhea, sialorrhea, and postural instability. Used in combination with carbidopa. *Investigational:* Pain from herpes zoster; restless legs syndrome.

Dosage

- **Capsules, Tablets**

  Parkinsonism.

Adults, initial: 250 mg b.i.d.–q.i.d. taken with food; **then,** increase total daily dose by 100–750 mg/3–7 days until optimum dosage reached (should not exceed 8 g/day). Up to 6 months may be required to achieve a significant therapeutic effect.

Administration/Storage

1. Administer to clients unable to swallow tablets or capsules by crushing tablets or emptying the

capsule into a small amount of fruit juice at the time of administration.
2. Levodopa is often administered together with an anticholinergic agent.
3. *Treatment of Overdose:* Immediate gastric lavage for acute overdose. Maintain airway and give IV fluids carefully. General supportive measures.

Contraindications: Concomitant use with MAO inhibitors. History of melanoma or in clients with undiagnosed skin lesions. Lactation. Hypersensitivity to drug, narrow-angle glaucoma, blood dyscrasias, hypertension, coronary sclerosis.

Special Concerns: Use with extreme caution in clients with history of MIs, convulsions, arrhythmias, bronchial asthma, emphysema, active peptic ulcer, psychosis or neurosis, wide-angle glaucoma, and renal, hepatic, or endocrine diseases. Use during pregnancy only if benefits clearly outweigh risks. Safety has not been established in children less than 12 years of age. Geriatric clients may require a lower dose as they have a reduced tolerance for the drug and its side effects (including cardiac effects). Clients may experience an "on-off" phenomenon in which they experience an improved clinical status followed by loss of therapeutic effect.

Laboratory Test Interferences: ↑ BUN, AST, LDH, ALT, bilirubin, alkaline phosphatase, protein-bound iodine. ↓ H&H, WBCs. False + Coombs' test. Interference with tests for urinary glucose and ketones.

Side Effects: The side effects of levodopa are numerous and usually dose related. Some may abate with usage. *CNS:* Choreiform and/or dystonic movements, paranoid ideation, psychotic episodes, ***depression (with possibility of suicidal tendencies),*** dementia, ***seizures (rare),*** dizziness, headache, faintness, confusion, insomnia, nightmares, hallucinations, delusions, agitation, anxiety, malaise, fatigue, euphoria. *GI:* N&V, anorexia, abdominal pain, dry mouth, sialorrhea, dysphagia, dysgeusia, hiccups, diarrhea, constipation, burning sensation of tongue, bitter taste, flatulence, weight gain or loss, GI bleeding (rare), duodenal ulcer (rare). *CV:* Cardiac irregularities, palpitations, orthostatic hypotension, hypertension, phlebitis, hot flashes. *Ophthalmologic:* Diplopia, dilated pupils, blurred vision, development of Horner's syndrome, oculogyric crisis. *Hematologic:* ***Hemolytic anemia, agranulocytosis,*** leukopenia. *Musculoskeletal:* Muscle twitching (early sign of overdose), tonic contraction of the muscles of mastication, increased hand tremor, ataxia. *Miscellaneous:* Blepharospasm (early sign of overdose), urinary retention, urinary incontinence, increased sweating, unusual breathing patterns, weakness, numbness, bruxism, alopecia, priapism, hoarseness, edema, dark sweat and/or urine, flushing, skin rash, sense of stimulation. Levodopa interacts with many other drugs (see below) and must be administered cautiously.

Symptoms of Overdose: Muscle twitching, blepharospasm. Also see *Side Effects,* above.

Drug Interactions

Amphetamines / Levodopa potentiates the effect of indirectly acting sympathomimetics
Antacids / ↑ Effect of levodopa due to ↑ absorption from GI tract
Anticholinergic drugs / Possible ↓ effect of levodopa due to ↑ breakdown of levodopa in stomach (due to delayed gastric emptying time)
Antidepressants, tricyclic / ↓ Effect of levodopa due to ↓ absorption from GI tract; also, ↑ risk of hypertension
Benzodiazepines / ↓ Effect of levodopa
Clonidine / ↓ Effect of levodopa
Digoxin / ↓ Effect of digoxin
Ephedrine / Levodopa potentiates the effect of indirectly acting sympathomimetics

Furazolidone / ↑ Effect of levodopa due to ↓ breakdown by liver
Guanethidine / ↑ Hypotensive effect of guanethidine
Hypoglycemic drugs / Levodopa upsets diabetic control with hypoglycemic agents
MAO inhibitors / Concomitant administration may result in hypertension, lightheadedness, and flushing due to ↓ breakdown of dopamine and norepinephrine formed from levodopa
Methionine / ↓ Effect of levodopa
Methyldopa / Additive effects including hypotension
Metoclopramide / ↑ Bioavailability of levodopa; ↓ effect of metoclopramide
Papaverine / ↓ Effect of levodopa
Phenothiazines / ↓ Effect of levodopa due to ↓ uptake of dopamine into neurons
Phenytoin / Antagonizes the effect of levodopa
Propranolol / May antagonize the hypotensive and positive inotropic effect of levodopa
Pyridoxine / Reverses levodopa-induced improvement in Parkinson's disease
Reserpine / Inhibits response to levodopa by ↓ dopamine in the brain
Thioxanthines / ↓ Effect of levodopa in Parkinson clients
Tricyclic antidepressants / ↓ Absorption of levodopa → ↓ effect

NURSING CONSIDERATIONS

See also *Nursing Considerations* for *Cholinergic Blocking Agents,* Chapter 49.

Assessment

1. Obtain baseline ECG, CBC, liver and renal function studies, and protein bound iodine tests prior to beginning therapy.
2. Review the client's medical history for contraindications to the drug therapy.
3. Assess and document baseline rigidity and tremors.

Interventions

1. Monitor VS, CBC, and liver and renal function studies during long-term therapy.
2. If the client is to have surgery, check to determine if the drug is to be stopped 24 hr before surgery. Also, note when the drug is to be restarted.
3. Observe and document any evidence of the client becoming depressed, psychotic, or exhibiting any other unusual behavioral changes.
4. Offer client and family emotional support and encouragement.
5. Monitor motor function and tremor, noting response to drug therapy as well as any sudden change in symptoms.

Client/Family Teaching

1. Take levodopa with food.
2. Report the occurrence of headaches because these may indicate drug-induced glaucoma.
3. Stress that dosage of drug is not to exceed 8 g/day.
4. Avoid taking multivitamin preparations containing 10–25 mg of vitamin B_6. This vitamin rapidly reverses the antiparkinson effect of levodopa.
5. Significant results may take up to 6 months to be realized. Therefore, continue taking the drug even though immediate results are not evident.
6. Instruct in how to take BP and pulse readings and to monitor these during drug therapy. Provide parameters for reporting.
7. Drug may cause dizziness or drowsiness. Do not perform tasks that require mental alertness until drug effects realized.
8. Sweat and urine may appear dark; this is not harmful.
9. Warn male clients that priapism may occur and should be reported immediately.
10. Stress the importance of reporting for all scheduled lab and medical visits so that the effectiveness of drug therapy can be evaluated and dosage adjusted as needed.

Evaluate

- Improvement in motor function, reflexes, gait, strength of grip, and amount of tremor

• Adverse side effects that may require ↓ drug dose or "drug holiday"

Pergolide mesylate

(**PER**-go-lyd)
Pregnancy Category: B
Permax **(Rx)**

How Supplied: *Tablet:* 0.05 mg, 0.25 mg, 1 mg
Action/Kinetics: Pergolide is a potent dopamine receptor (both D_1 and D_2) agonist. The drug is believed to act by directly stimulating postsynaptic dopamine receptors in the nigrostriatal system, thus relieving symptoms of parkinsonism. The drug also inhibits prolactin secretion, causes a transient rise in serum levels of growth hormone, and a decrease in serum levels of luteinizing hormone. About 90% of the drug is bound to plasma proteins. The drug is metabolized in the liver and excreted through the urine.
Uses: Adjunctive treatment to levodopa/carbidopa in Parkinson's disease.

Dosage

• **Tablets**

Parkinsonism.

Adults, initial: 0.05 mg/day for the first 2 days; **then,** increase dose gradually by 0.1 or 0.15 mg/day every third day over the next 12 days. The dosage may then be increased by 0.25 mg/day every third day until the therapeutic dosage level is reached. The mean therapeutic daily dosage is 3 mg used concurrently with levodopa/carbidopa (expressed as levodopa) at a dose of 650 mg/day. The effectiveness of doses of pergolide greater than 5 mg/day has not been evaluated.

Administration/Storage

1. Pergolide is usually given in divided doses 3 times/day.
2. When determining the therapeutic dose for pergolide, the dosage of concurrent levodopa/carbidopa may be decreased cautiously.
3. *Treatment of Overdose:* Activated charcoal (usually recommended instead of or in addition to gastric lavage or induction of vomiting). Maintain BP. An antiarrhythmic drug may be helpful. A phenothiazine or butyrophenone may help any CNS stimulation. Support ventilation.

Special Concerns: Benefit versus risk should be assessed when considered for use during lactation. Use with caution in clients prone to cardiac dysrhythmias, preexisting dyskinesia, and preexisting states of confusion or hallucinations. Safety and efficacy have not been determined in children.
Side Effects: The most common side effects are listed. *CV:* Postural hypotension, palpitation, vasodilation, syncope, hypotension, hypertension, ***arrhythmias, MI.*** *GI:* Nausea (common), vomiting, diarrhea, constipation, dyspepsia, anorexia, dry mouth. *CNS:* Dyskinesia (common), dizziness, dystonia, hallucinations, confusion, insomnia, somnolence, anxiety, tremor, depression, abnormal dreams, psychosis, personality disorder, extrapyramidal syndrome, akathisia, paresthesia, incoordination, akinesia, neuralgia, hypertonia, speech disorders. *Musculoskeletal:* Arthralgia, bursitis, twitching, myalgia. *Respiratory:* Rhinitis, dyspnea, hiccup, epistaxis. *Dermatologic:* Sweating, rash. *Ophthalmologic:* Abnormal vision, double vision, eye disorders. *GU:* UTI, urinary frequency, hematuria. *Whole body:* Pain in chest, abdomen, neck, or back; headache, asthenia, flu syndrome, chills, facial edema, infection. *Miscellaneous:* Taste alteration, peripheral edema, anemia, weight gain.

Symptoms of Overdose: Might include agitation, hypotension, vomiting, hallucinations, involuntary movements, palpitations, tingling of arms and legs.

Drug Interactions

Butyrophenones / ↓ Effect of pergolide due to dopamine antagonist effect
Metoclopramide / ↓ Effect of pergolide due to dopamine antagonist effect
Phenothiazines / ↓ Effect of pergo-

lide due to dopamine antagonist effect

Thioxanthines / ↓ Effect of pergolide due to dopamine antagonist effect

NURSING CONSIDERATIONS

See also *Nursing Considerations* for *Antiparkinson Agents,* Chapter 46.

Assessment

1. Note any sensitivity to ergot derivatives.
2. Document any evidence of cardiac arrhythmias.

Client/Family Teaching

1. Pergolide is to be taken concurrently with a prescribed dose of levodopa/carbidopa.
2. Do not exceed prescribed daily dose.
3. Review the list of side effects associated with pergolide therapy and instruct to report any persistent and/or bothersome symptoms. Activities may need to be curtailed until side effects subside.
4. Do not perform tasks that require mental alertness until drug effects realized. Drug may cause drowsiness or dizziness.
5. Rise slowly from a sitting or lying position to minimize hypotensive effects of pergolide.
6. Stress the importance of reporting for all scheduled lab and medical appointments so that drug therapy may be evaluated and adjusted as needed.

Evaluate: Improved response to levodopa/carbidopa as evidenced by ↓ muscle weakness, ↓ rigidity, ↓ salivation, and improved mobility.

Selegiline hydrochloride (Deprenyl)

(seh-**LEH**-jih-leen)
Pregnancy Category: C
Eldepryl **(Rx)**

How Supplied: *Tablet:* 5 mg

Action/Kinetics: Although the precise mechanism of action is not known, selegiline is known to inhibit MAO, type B. Also, selegiline may act through other mechanisms to increase dopaminergic activity, including interference with dopamine uptake at the synapse. Selegiline metabolites include amphetamine and methamphetamine, which may contribute to the effects of the drug. Rapidly absorbed and metabolized. Maximum plasma levels: 0.5–2 hr.

Uses: Adjunct in the treatment of Parkinson's disease in clients being treated with levodopa/carbidopa who have manifested a decreased response to this therapy. *NOTE:* There is no evidence that selegiline is effective in clients not taking levodopa.

Dosage

- **Tablets**

Parkinsonism in those receiving levodopa/carbidopa.

Adults: 5 mg taken at breakfast and lunch, not to exceed 10 mg/day.

Administration/Storage

1. No evidence exists that doses higher than 10 mg/day will result in additional beneficial effects.
2. Following 2 or 3 days of selegiline therapy, attempts may be made to decrease the dose of levodopa/carbidopa (10%–30%).
3. *Treatment of Overdose:* IV fluids and a dilute pressor agent to treat hypotension and vascular collapse. Treat symptoms.

Contraindications: Hypersensitivity to the drug. Doses greater than 10 mg/day. Use with meperidine (and usually other opiates).

Special Concerns: Use with caution during lactation. Safety and efficacy in children have not been established.

Side Effects: *CNS:* Dizziness, lightheadedness, fainting, confusion, hallucinations, vivid dreams/nightmares, headache, anxiety, drowsiness, depression, mood changes, delusions, fatigue, disorientation, apathy, malaise, vertigo, overstimulation, sleep disturbance, transient irritability, weakness, lethary, personality change. *Skeletal Muscle:* Tremor, chorea, loss of balance, blepharospasm, restlessness, increased bradykinesia, facial grimace, dystonic symptoms, tardive dyskinesia, dyskinesia, involuntary movements, muscle cramps, heavy leg, falling down, stiff neck, freezing, festination, increased apraxia. *Altered Sensations/pain:* Headache, tinnitus, migraine, back or leg pain, supraorbital pain, burning throat, chills, numbness of fingers/toes, taste disturbance, generalized aches. *CV:* Orthostatic hypotension, hypertension, arrhythmia, angina pectoris, palpitations, hypotension, tachycardia, syncope, peripheral edema, sinus bradycardia. *GI:* N&V, constipation, anorexia, weight loss, dry mouth, poor appetite, dysphagia, diarrhea, rectal bleeding, ***GI bleeding (worsening of pre-existing ulcer disease),*** heartburn. *GU:* Nocturia, slow urination, urinary hesitancy or retention, prostatic hypertrophy, urinary frequency, sexual dysfunction. *Miscellaneous:* Blurred vision, increased sweating, diaphoresis, facial hair, hair loss, rash, photosensitivity, hematoma, asthma, diplopia, SOB, speech affected.

Symptoms of Overdose: Hypotension, psychomotor agitation. Also, symptoms from overdose of nonselective MAO inhibitors (e.g., isocarboxazid, phenelzine, tranylcypromine).

Drug Interactions

Fluoxetine (Prozac) / Possibility of death—five weeks should elapse between discontinuing fluoxetine and beginning selegiline and 14 days between discontinuing selegiline and initiation of fluoxetine

Meperidine / Symptoms include stupor, muscle rigidity, severe agitation, hyperthermia, hallucinations, death.

NURSING CONSIDERATIONS

Assessment: List agents currently prescribed or used within the last 2 weeks to ensure that none interact unfavorably.

Client/Family Teaching

1. Do not exceed prescribed daily dose. Take with breakfast and lunch.
2. Selegiline is to be taken concurrently with prescribed dose of levodopa/carbidopa. Explain that drug enhances and prolongs the antiparkinsonism effects of levodopa, which thereby permits a reduction in dosage.
3. Review list of side effects associated with drug therapy and instruct to report any bothersome and/or persistent symptoms.
4. Rise slowly from a sitting or lying position to minimize the hypotensive effects of drug therapy.
5. Do not drive or operate hazardous machinery until drug effects are realized.
6. Avoid tyramine-containing foods as they may precipitate a hypertensive crisis.

Evaluate: Improved response to levodopa/carbidopa as evidenced by ↓ muscle weakness, ↓ rigidity, ↓ salivation, and improved mobility.

CHAPTER FORTY-SEVEN

Stimulants

See also the following individual entries:

Amphetamine Sulfate
Benzphetamine Hydrochloride
Dextroamphetamine Sulfate
Diethylpropion Hydrochloride
Doxapram Hydrochloride
Fenfluramine
Mazindol
Methamphetamine Hydrochloride
Methylphenidate Hydrochloride
Pemoline
Phendimetrazine Tartrate
Phentermine
Phentermine Resin
Phenylpropanolamine Hydrochloride - See Chapter 50

Action/Kinetics: Response to amphetamines is individualized. Psychic stimulation is often followed by a rebound effect manifested as fatigue. Tolerance will develop to all drugs of this class. The slight differences in the pharmacologic reactions and side effects of the different anorexiants (appetite suppression, respiratory stimulation, length of action) dictate their principal use.

These drugs are thought to act on the cerebral cortex and reticular activating system (including the medullary, respiratory, and vasomotor centers) by releasing norepinephrine from central adrenergic neurons. High doses cause release of dopamine from the mesolimbic system. The stimulatory effect on the CNS causes an increase in motor activity and mental alertness, a mood-elevating effect, a slight euphoric effect, and an anorexigenic effect. The anorexigenic effect is thought to be produced by direct stimulation of the satiety center in the lateral hypothalamic feeding center of the brain. Peripheral effects are mediated by alpha- and beta-adrenergic receptors and include increases in both systolic and diastolic BP and respiratory stimulation. Amphetamines are readily absorbed from the GI tract and are distributed throughout most tissues, with the highest concentrations in the brain and CSF. Duration of anorexia (PO): 3–6 hr. Metabolized in liver and excreted by kidneys.

There is a relatively wide margin of safety between the therapeutic and toxic doses of amphetamines. However, amphetamines can cause both acute and chronic toxicity. Amphetamines are excreted slowly (5–7 days), and cumulative effects may occur with continued administration.

Uses: See individual drugs.

Contraindications: Hyperthyroidism, advanced arteriosclerosis, nephritis, diabetes mellitus, hypertension, narrow-angle glaucoma, angina pectoris, CV disease, and individuals with hypersensitivity to these drugs. Use in emotionally unstable persons susceptible to drug abuse and in agitated states. Psychotic children. Lactation. Appetite suppressants in children less than 12 years of age. Within 14 days of MAO inhibitors.

Special Concerns: To be used with caution in clients suffering from hyperexcitability states; in elderly, debilitated, or asthenic clients; and in clients with psychopathic personality traits or a history of homicidal or suicidal tendencies.

Side Effects: *CNS:* Nervousness, dizziness, depression, headache, insomnia, euphoria, symptoms of excitation. Rarely, psychoses. In children, manifestation of vocal and motor tics and Tourette's syndrome. *GI:* N&V, cramps, diarrhea, dry mouth, constipation, metallic taste, anorexia. *CV:* Arrhythmias, palpitations, dyspnea, pulmonary hypertension, peripheral hyper- or hypotension, precordial pain, fainting. *Dermatologic:* Symptoms of allergy including rash, urticaria, erythema, burning. Pallor. *GU:* Urinary frequency, dysuria. *Ophthalmologic:* Blurred vision, mydriasis. *Hematologic:* ***Agranulocytosis,*** leukopenia. *Endocrine:* Menstrual irregularities, gynecomastia, impotence, and changes in libido. *Miscellaneous:* Alopecia, increased motor activity, fever, sweating, chills, muscle pain, chest pain.

Long-term use results in psychic dependence, as well as a high degree of tolerance.

Symptoms of Acute Overdose (Toxicity): Restlessness, irritability, insomnia, tremor, hyperreflexia, rhabdomyolysis, rapid respiration, ***hyperpyrexia,*** assaultiveness, hallucinations, panic states, sweating, mydriasis, flushing, hyperactivity, confusion, hypertension or hypotension, extrasystoles, tachypnea, fever, delirium, self-injury, arrhythmias, ***seizures, coma, circulatory collapse, death. Death usually results from CV collapse or convulsions.***

Symptoms of Chronic Toxicity: Chronic use/abuse is characterized by emotional lability, loss of appetite, severe dermatoses, hyperactivity, insomnia, irritability, somnolence, mental impairment, occupational deterioration, a tendency to withdraw from social contact, teeth grinding, continuous chewing, and ulcers of the tongue and lips. Prolonged use of high doses can elicit symptoms of paranoid schizophrenia, including auditory and visual hallucinations and paranoid ideation.

Drug Interactions

Acetazolamide / ↑ Effect of amphetamine by ↑ renal tubular reabsorption

Ammonium chloride / ↓ Effect of amphetamine by ↓ renal tubular reabsorption

Anesthetics, general / ↑ Risk of cardiac arrhythmias

Antihypertensives / Amphetamines ↓ effect of antihypertensives

Ascorbic acid / ↓ Effect of amphetamine by ↓ renal tubular reabsorption

Furazolidone / ↑ Toxicity of anorexiants due to MAO activity of furazolidone

Guanethidine / ↓ Effect of guanethidine by displacement from its site of action

Haloperidol / ↓ Effect of amphetamine by ↓ uptake of drug at its site of action

Insulin / Amphetamines alter insulin requirements

MAO inhibitors / All peripheral, metabolic, cardiac, and central effects of amphetamine are potentiated for up to 2 weeks after termination of MAO inhibitor therapy (symptoms include hypertensive crisis with possible intracranial hemorrhage, hyperthermia, convulsions, coma); death may occur. ↓ Effect of amphetamine by ↓ uptake of drug into its site of action

Methyldopa / ↓ Hypotensive effect of methyldopa by ↑ sympathomimetic activity

Phenothiazines / ↓ Effect of amphetamine by ↓ uptake of drug at its site of action

Sodium bicarbonate / ↑ Effect of amphetamine by ↑ renal tubular reabsorption

Thiazide diuretics / ↑ Effect of amphetamine by ↑ renal tubular reabsorption

Tricyclic antidepressants / ↓ Effect of amphetamines

Laboratory Test Interferences: ↑ Urinary catecholamines, ↑ plasma corticosteroid levels.

Dosage

See individual drugs. Many compounds are timed-release preparations.

NURSING CONSIDERATIONS

Administration/Storage

1. If the drug is prescribed to suppress the appetite, administer 30 min before meals.
2. The initial dose should be small, then increased gradually as necessary, for the individual.
3. Unless otherwise ordered, the last dose of drug for the day should be administered at least 6 hr before the client retires.
4. *Treatment of Acute Toxicity (Overdosage):*
• Symptomatic treatment. After oral ingestion, induce emesis or perform gastric lavage, followed by use of activated charcoal. Acidification of the urine increases the rate of excretion. Fluids should be given until urine flow is 3–6 mL/kg/hr; furosemide or mannitol may be beneficial.
• Adequate circulation and respiration should be maintained.
• CNS stimulation can be treated with chlorpromazine and psychotic symptoms with haloperidol. Hyperactivity can be treated with diazepam or a barbiturate. Stimuli should be reduced and the client maintained in a quiet, dim environment. Clients who have ingested an overdose of long-acting products should be treated for toxicity until all symptoms of overdosage have disappeared.
• IV phentolamine may be used for hypertension, whereas hypotension may be reversed by IV fluids and possibly vasopressors (used with caution).

Assessment

1. Obtain a complete drug history. Identify the medications the client is currently taking, the reasons, and the effectiveness of these medications in treating the problem.
2. Note any physical conditions that would contraindicate the client receiving drugs in this category.
3. Note the client's age and whether debilitated.
4. Drugs in this category are under the Controlled Substances Act. Therefore, follow appropriate policy for handling amphetamines to restrict availability and discourage abuse.

Interventions

1. Note if the client appears agitated or complains of sleeplessness. Notify the provider and anticipate a reduction in the dosage of drug.
2. Clients who have been receiving MAO inhibitors or who have received them 7–14 days before starting amphetamine therapy are susceptible to hypertensive crisis. Monitor for the development of fever, marked sweating, excitation, delirium, tremors, or twitching; document and report immediately. If hospitalized, observe client closely, pad the side rails, and have a suction machine available at the bedside.
3. Monitor VS and BP. Assess for evidence of arrhythmias, tachycardia, or hypertension. CV changes accompanied by psychotic syndrome usually indicate acute toxicity.
4. If the client complains of loss of appetite, somnolence, appears mentally impaired, and experiences occupational impairment, the drug should be discontinued.
5. Observe for signs of psychologic dependence and drug tolerance as the drug should be discontinued.
6. Initially, record food intake and weight daily and then at least once a week, to assess weight loss. Clients receiving amphetamines may become anorexic so any persistent, severe weight loss should be reported as the dosage or drug therapy may need to be adjusted.
7. Perform periodic determinations of height to assess for growth inhibition in children.
8. Report any changes in attention span and ability to concentrate.
9. Observe for any evidence of sleep disturbance and schedule last dose at least 6 hr before bedtime.

Client/Family Teaching

1. When anorexiants are used for weight reduction, their effect lasts only 4–6 weeks. Stress that use is short term. Follow an established dietary and exercise regimen to maintain weight loss and encourage participation in a behavioral modification weight control program.

2. Advise to take 1 hr before meals. Have a dietitian discuss a weight control and/or reducing diet with clients and assist them with meal planning when weight loss is the goal.
3. Explain that diets high in fiber, fruit, and fluids may assist to reduce the constipating effects of drug therapy.
4. Advise to take only as directed and never to share medications. Provide a printed list of symptoms of drug tolerance and explain that these may develop rapidly. If tolerance does develop, notify the provider who may begin decreasing the dose of medication.
5. Warn that amphetamines may cause a false sense of euphoria and well being and mask extreme fatigue. These may impair judgment and ability to perform potentially hazardous tasks, such as operating a machine or an automobile. Using amphetamines to treat fatigue is inappropriate because rebound effects may be severe.
6. Advise clients that they should seek medical assistance if they experience extreme fatigue and depression once the drug is discontinued. Periodic "drug holidays" may be ordered to assess progress and prevent dependence.
7. Avoid OTC medications and ingesting large amounts of caffeine in any form. Teach client how to scan and read labels for the detection of caffeine since this contributes to cardiovascular side effects.
8. Advise that symptoms of drug-induced dry mouth may be decreased by frequently rinsing the mouth, chewing sugarless gum, or sucking sugarless hard candies.
9. Amphetamines may alter insulin and dietary requirements. Therefore, clients with diabetes mellitus need to be warned to monitor their blood sugar closely as they may require a change in the dose of insulin, oral hypoglycemic agent, and/or dietary requirements.
10. Advise clients to take medication only as prescribed and remind them of the importance of keeping all appointments for regular medical follow-up.
11. Instruct not to stop medication abruptly as this may precipitate withdrawal symptoms.
12. Store all medications safely out of the reach of children.

Evaluate

- Improved attention span and ability to concentrate
- ↓ Weight
- ↓ Episodes of narcolepsy

Amphetamine sulfate

(am-**FET**-ah-meen)
Pregnancy Category: C
(C-II) (Rx)

See also *Stimulants,* Chapter 47.

How Supplied: *Tablet:* 5 mg, 10 mg

Action/Kinetics: After PO administration, completely absorbed in 3 hr. **Duration: PO,** 4–24 hr; **t½:** 10–30 hr, depending on urinary pH. Excreted in urine. Acidification will increase excretion, whereas alkalinization will decrease it. For every one unit increase in pH, the plasma half-life will increase by 7 hr.

Uses: Attention deficit disorders in children, narcolepsy.

Dosage

- **Tablets**

Narcolepsy.

Adults: 5–20 mg 1–3 times/day. **Children over 12 years, initial:** 5 mg b.i.d.; increase in increments of 10 mg/day at weekly intervals until optimum dose is reached. **Children, 6–12 years, initial:** 2.5 mg b.i.d.; increase in increments of 5 mg at weekly intervals until optimum dose is reached (maximum is 60 mg/day).

Attention deficit disorders in children.

3–6 years, initial: 2.5 mg/day; increase by 2.5 mg/day at weekly intervals until optimum dose is achieved (usual range 0.1–0.5 mg/kg/dose each morning). **6 years**

and older, initial: 5 mg 1–2 times/day; increase in increments of 5 mg/week until optimum dose is achieved (rarely over 40 mg/day).

Administration/Storage

1. When used as an anorexiant, the drug should be used only for short-term therapy.
2. When used for attention deficit disorders or narcolepsy, the first dose should be given on awakening with an additional one or two doses given at intervals of 4–6 hr.
3. The last dose of medication should be given 6 hr before bedtime.
4. The peak effects of the drug are observed 2–3 hr after administration. The effects last from 4 to 24 hr.

Special Concerns: Use is not recommended in children less than 3 years of age for attention deficit disorders and in children less than 6 years of age for narcolepsy. Use is no longer recommended as an appetite suppressant.

NURSING CONSIDERATIONS

See also *Nursing Considerations* for *Stimulants,* Chapter 47.

Assessment

1. Obtain baseline CNS/neurologic status prior to initiating therapy.
2. If female and of childbearing age, determine the possibility of pregnancy because amphetamines are contraindicated.
3. Obtain a baseline ECG before starting therapy.

Interventions

1. Document any symptoms of impaired mental processes or emotional lability.
2. Children receiving amphetamines may have their growth retarded. Drug should periodically be discontinued to allow growth to proceed normally and to evaluate the need for continued drug therapy.

Client/Family Teaching

1. Report any changes in mood or affect.
2. Do not use caffeine or caffeine-containing products.
3. Avoid any OTC preparations that contain caffeine, phenylpropanolamine, and other drugs that can affect the CV system.
4. Avoid using heavy machinery or driving a car until the effects of the medication can be evaluated.
5. Monitor weight and maintain a written record to share with the health care provider at each visit.
6. To prevent constipation, drink at least 2.5 L/day of fluids and increase intake of high-fiber foods, including fruits, in the diet.
7. Chew sugarless gum or candies and rinse the mouth frequently with nonalcoholic mouth rinses to offset dry mouth.

Evaluate

- Improved attention span
- ↓ Episodes of narcolepsy

Benzphetamine hydrochloride

(bens-**FET**-ah-meen)
Pregnancy Category: X
Didrex **(C-III) (Rx)**

See also *Stimulants,* Chapter 47.

How Supplied: *Tablet:* 50 mg

Action/Kinetics: $t^{1/2}$**:** 6–12 hr.

Use: Short-term (8–12 weeks) treatment of exogenous obesity in conjunction with a weight reduction regimen such as exercise, restriction of calories, and behavior modification.

Dosage

- **Tablets**

  Obesity.

Adults, initial: 25–50 mg once daily; **then,** increase dose according to response (dose ranges from 25–50 mg 1–3 times/day 1 hr before meals).

Administration/Storage

1. It is preferable to administer a single dose in midmorning or midafternoon, depending on the eating habits of the client.
2. Anorexiant effects occur within 1–2 hr and last approximately 4 hr.

NURSING CONSIDERATIONS

See also *Nursing Considerations* for *Stimulants,* Chapter 47.

Assessment
1. Note any history of glaucoma, advanced arteriosclerosis, cardiac disease, or mental instability.
2. Determine if pregnant. Benzphetamine is toxic to the fetus and should not be administered to pregnant women or nursing mothers.
3. Assess client's willingness to comply with behavioral modification approaches to weight loss, which include regular exercise and reduced caloric intake.
4. Determine support systems and encourage family participation in the overall goal of weight loss.
Evaluate: Control of appetite with resultant weight loss.

Dextroamphetamine sulfate

(dex-troh-am-**FET**-ah-meen)
Pregnancy Category: C
Dexedrine, Ferndex, Oxydess II, Spancap No. 1 **(C-II) (Rx)**

See also *Stimulants,* Chapter 47.
How Supplied: *Capsule, Extended Release:* 5 mg, 10 mg, 15 mg; *Tablet:* 5 mg, 10 mg
Action/Kinetics: Dextroamphetamine has stronger CNS effects and weaker peripheral action than does amphetamine; thus, dextroamphetamine manifests fewer undesirable CV effects. After PO administration, completely absorbed in 3 hr. **Duration: PO,** 4–24 hr; **t½, adults:** 10–12 hr; **children:** 6–8 hr. Excreted in urine. Acidification will increase excretion, while alkalinization will decrease it.
Uses: Attention deficit disorders in children, narcolepsy.

Dosage
• **Elixir, Tablets**
Attention deficit disorders in children.
3–5 years, initial: 2.5 mg/day; increase by 2.5 mg/day at weekly intervals until optimum dose is achieved (usual range 0.1–0.5 mg/kg/dose each morning). **6 years and older, initial:** 5 mg 1–2 times/day; increase in increments of 5 mg/week until optimum dose is achieved (rarely over 40 mg/day).
Narcolepsy.
Adults: 5–60 mg in divided doses daily. **Children over 12 years, initial:** 10 mg/day; increase in increments of 10 mg/day at weekly intervals until optimum dose is reached. **Children, 6–12 years, initial:** 5 mg/day; increase in increments of 5 mg/week until optimum dose is reached (maximum is 60 mg/day).
• **Extended-Release Capsule**
Attention deficit disorders.
Children, 6 years and older: 5–15 mg/day.
Narcolepsy.
Adults: 5–30 mg/day. **Children, 6–12 years:** 5–15 mg/day; **12 years and older:** 10–15 mg/day.
Administration/Storage
1. Long-acting products may be used for once-a-day dosing in attention deficit disorders and narcolepsy.
2. When tablets or the elixir are used for attention deficit disorders or narcolepsy, the first dose should be given on awakening with additional one or two doses given at intervals of 4–6 hr. If possible, the last dose should be given 6 hr before bedtime.
3. If the client is already receiving an MAO inhibitor, a period of at least 14 days should elapse before dextroamphetamine is initiated.
Additional Contraindications: Lactation. Use for obesity.
Special Concerns: Use of extended-release capsules for attention deficit disorders in children less than 6 years of age and the elixir or tablets for attention deficit disorders in children less than 3 years of age is not recommended. Dosage for narcolepsy has not been determined in children less than 6 years of age.

NURSING CONSIDERATIONS

See also *Nursing Considerations* for *Stimulants,* Chapter 47.

Evaluate

- Improved attention span and concentration levels
- ↓ Episodes of narcolepsy

Diethylpropion hydrochloride

(dye-eth-ill-**PROH**-pee-on)
Pregnancy Category: B
M-Orexic, Tenuate, Tenuate Dospan, Tepanil, Tepanil Ten-Tab **(C-IV) (Rx)**

See also *Stimulants,* Chapter 47.
How Supplied: *Tablet:* 25 mg; *Tablet, Extended Release:* 75 mg
Action/Kinetics: Duration, tablets: 4 hr; **extended-release tablets:** 12 hr.
Use: Short-term (8–12 weeks) treatment of exogenous obesity in conjunction with a weight reduction regimen including exercise, reduced caloric intake, and behavior modification.

Dosage

- **Tablets**

Adults: 25 mg t.i.d. 1 hr before meals.

- **Extended-Release Tablets**

Adults: 75 mg at midmorning.

Administration/Storage

1. Give extended-release tablets in the midmorning.
2. The drug may be taken in the midevening to reduce night hunger.

Special Concerns: Use with caution during lactation.
Additional Side Effect: May cause increased risk of seizures in epileptics.

NURSING CONSIDERATIONS

See also *Nursing Considerations* for *Stimulants,* Chapter 47.

Assessment

1. Document indications for therapy, any previous therapies, and the outcome.
2. Note any history of seizure disorder.
3. Assess client lifestyle and willingness to change negative eating behaviors.
4. Identify support persons. Determine client motivation and ability to exercise and comply with a behavior modification program.

Evaluate: ↓ Weight and compliance with overall weight loss program.

Doxapram hydrochloride

(**DOX**-ah-pram)
Pregnancy Category: B
Dopram **(Rx)**

How Supplied: *Injection:* 20 mg/mL
Action/Kinetics: Doxapram increases the rate and depth of respiration by stimulating carotid chemoreceptors. Higher doses also stimulate respiratory centers in the medulla with progressive stimulation of other CNS centers as well (toxic doses may induce tonic-clonic convulsions). An increase in BP may also occur due to increased CO. The drug will antagonize respiratory depression, but not analgesia, induced by narcotics. An increased salivation and release of both gastric acid and catecholamines may be seen. **Onset** (after IV): 20–40 sec. **Peak effect:** 1–2 min. **Duration:** 5–12 min. **t½:** Approximately 2.5–4 hr. Doxapram is metabolized in the liver and is excreted in the urine.
Uses: Respiratory stimulant in mild to moderate drug overdose, drug-induced postanesthetic respiratory depression, apnea not associated with muscle relaxants, acute respiratory insufficiency in COPD (used for 2 hr). The analeptic agents are no longer considered drugs of choice in the treatment of CNS depression caused by a severe overdose of sedatives and hypnotics. Current therapy for overdose of sedative-hypnotics relies largely on supportive therapy, such as establishing a patent airway, administering oxygen, assisting or controlling respiration when necessary, and maintaining BP and blood volume.

Dosage

- **IV**

After anesthesia.
Single IV injection: 0.5–1.0 mg/kg, not to exceed 1.5–2.0 mg/kg; may be given in several injections at 5-min intervals. **IV infusion:** 1 mg/mL of dextrose or saline solution, initially at a rate of 5 mg/min; **then,** 1–3 mg/min. Total recommended dose: 4 mg/kg (approximately 300 mg).

Chronic obstructive lung disease with acute hypercapnia.
IV infusion: 1–2 mg/min up to maximum of 3 mg/min for no longer than 2 hr.

Drug-induced CNS depression.
IV injection, initial: 1–2 mg/kg as a single dose; repeat in 5 min and q 1–2 hr to a maximum of 3 g/day. **Intermittent IV infusion, initial:** 2 mg/kg; **then,** if client not responsive, continue supportive treatment for 1–2 hr and repeat doxapram dose to a maximum of 3 g/day. If response occurs, infuse 1 mg/mL at a rate of 1–3 mg/min. The infusion should be discontinued at the end of 2 hr or if the client awakens.

Administration/Storage
1. For direct IV administration give over 5 min. For intermittent administration, dilute 250 mg in 250 mL of D5%/W or NSS and administer via infusion control device as prescribed.
2. Allow a minimum of 10 min between the discontinuation of anesthetic and the administration of doxapram.
3. Drug contains benzyl alcohol.
4. Children under 12 years of age should not receive doxapram.
5. *Treatment of Overdose:* Have short-acting barbiturates, oxygen, and resuscitative equipment available.

Contraindications: Epilepsy, convulsive states, respiratory incompetence due to muscle paresis, flail chest, pneumothorax, pulmonary fibrosis, acute bronchial asthma, extreme dyspnea, severe hypertension, and CVAs. Hypersensitivity. Use in newborns or immature infants (the benzoyl alcohol present may cause a fatal toxic reaction).

Special Concerns: Use with caution during lactation. Safety and efficacy have not been established in children less than 12 years of age. Use with caution in clients with cerebral edema, asthma, severe CV disease, hyperthyroidism, and pheochromocytoma (cancer of adrenals), peptic ulcer, or gastric surgery.

Laboratory Test Interferences: ↓ H&H, RBCs. ↑ BUN, proteinuria.

Side Effects: *CNS:* Excess stimulation including hyperactivity, clonus, ***convulsions.*** Headache, apprehension, dizziness, disorientation. *Autonomic:* Flushing, sweating, paresthesia, feeling of warmth, burning, or hot sensation in area of perineum and genitalia, mydriasis. *GI:* N&V, diarrhea, urge to defecate. *Respiratory:* ***Bronchospasm,*** dyspnea, cough, hiccoughs, rebound hypoventilation, ***laryngospasm,*** tachypnea. *CV:* ***Arrhythmias,*** abnormal ECG, tightness in chest or chest pain, phlebitis, change in HR, increase in BP. *GU:* Spontaneous micturition, urinary retention, proteinuria. *Miscellaneous:* Muscle spasms, involuntary movements, pruritus, increased deep tendon reflexes, pyrexia.

Symptoms of Overdose: Respiratory alkalosis and hypocapnia (too little CO_2 in blood) with tetany and apnea. Also excessive stimulation of CNS, which may result in ***convulsions.*** Hypertension, tachycardia, hyperactivity of skeletal muscle, enhanced deep tendon reflexes.

Drug Interactions
Anesthetics, general / Since doxapram ↑ epinephrine release, do not give until 10 min after anesthetic discontinued if halothane, cyclopropane, or enflurane used to minimize cardiac arrhythmias
MAO inhibitors / Additive pressor effects
Muscle relaxants / Doxapram may mask effects of muscle relaxants
Sympathomimetic amines / Additive pressor effects

NURSING CONSIDERATIONS

Assessment

1. Note any history of epilepsy or other convulsive disorders.
2. Obtain a complete baseline CNS/neurological assessment (noting deep tendon reflexes) prior to the client receiving therapy.
3. Note age of clients. Elderly people and debilitated clients may be unable to tolerate the increase in respirations caused by doxapram.
4. Document baseline ABGs, ECG, and VS.
5. Identify any drugs the client is taking that may interact unfavorably with doxapram.

Interventions

1. Drug should only be administered in a closely monitored environment.
2. For at least ½–1 hr after the client is alert, assess for possible poststimulation respiratory depression or increased SOB.
3. Ensure a patent airway. Administer oxygen along with the drug to clients suffering from chronic pulmonary insufficiency.
4. Follow seizure precautions after administration of drug. Have available IV diazepam.
5. Position on side to prevent aspiration. Report any persistent diarrhea or vomiting.
6. Monitor I&O. If the client has not voided in 2–4 hr, palpate the bladder to detect urinary retention and catheterize as needed.

Evaluate

- Reversal of drug-induced respiratory and CNS depression
- Prevention of hypercapnea in COPD

Fenfluramine

(fen-**FLUR**-ah-meen)
Pregnancy Category: C
Ponderal ✱, Pondimin **(C-IV) (Rx)**

See also *Stimulants,* Chapter 47.

How Supplied: *Tablet:* 20 mg

Action/Kinetics: This drug produces more CNS depression and less stimulation than does amphetamine. It may exert its activity by affecting turnover of serotonin in the brain or increasing the use of glucose. The abuse potential of fenfluramine appears to be different from other anorexiants in that it produces euphoria, derealization, and perceptual changes with doses of 80–400 mg. **Onset:** 1–2 hr. **Maximum effect:** 2–4 hr. **Duration:** 4–6 hr. **t½:** 11–30 hr. Excretion is pH dependent and is through the urine (alkaline urine decreases excretion).

Uses: Short-term treatment (8–12 weeks) of exogenous obesity in conjunction with a weight reduction program including reduced caloric intake, exercise, and behavior modification. To treat autistic children with high serotonin levels.

Dosage

- **Tablets**

Adults: 20 mg t.i.d. 30–60 min before meals. May be increased weekly to a maximum of 40 mg t.i.d. If initial dose is not well tolerated, reduce to 40 mg/day and increase gradually. Total daily dose should not exceed 120 mg.

- **Extended-Release Capsules**

Adults: 60 mg/day; the dose may be increased to a maximum of 120 mg/day, if needed.

Administration/Storage

1. Anticipate the drug will produce anorexiant effects within 1–2 hr after ingestion.
2. The effects of the drug should last approximately 4–6 hr.
3. The drug should not be abruptly withdrawn because depression may occur.

Additional Contraindication: Alcoholism.

Additional Side Effects: Hypoglycemia, CNS depression, impotence, drowsiness. Following long-term use (1 month), withdrawal symptoms have been observed, including tremor, ataxia, loss of sense of reality, visual hallucinations, depression, disturbed concentration and memory, suicidal feelings.

Symptoms of Overdose: CNS: Agitation, drowsiness, confusion, ***convulsions, coma.*** *Musculoskeletal:* Tremor, shivering, increased or decreased reflexes. *CV:* Tachycardia, ***ventricular extra systoles, culminating in ventricular fibril-***

lation and cardiac arrest (at high doses). *Miscellaneous:* Flushing, fever, sweating, abdominal pain, hyperventilation, rotary nystagmus, dilated nonreactive pupils. Treatment should be symptomatic and supportive; however, emesis should not be induced due to the depressant effects of the drug.
Additional Drug Interactions: Fenfluramine may ↑ effect of alcohol, CNS depressants, guanethidine, methyldopa, reserpine, thiazide diuretics, and tricyclic antidepressants.

NURSING CONSIDERATIONS

See also *Nursing Considerations* for *Stimulants,* Chapter 47.
Client/Family Teaching
1. Review the importance of diet and exercise in the overall management of obesity.
2. Avoid alcohol and any other CNS depressants.
Evaluate
- ↓ Weight and compliance with weight reduction program
- ↓ Serotonin levels (in autistic children)

Mazindol

(**MAYZ**-in-dohl)
Pregnancy Category: C
Mazanor, Sanorex **(C-IV) (Rx)**

See also *Stimulants,* Chapter 47.
How Supplied: *Tablet:* 1 mg, 2 mg
Action/Kinetics: Onset: 30–60 min; **duration:** 8–15 hr. **t½:** Less than 24 hr. **Therapeutic blood levels:** 0.003–0.012 mcg/mL. Excreted in urine partially unchanged.
Use: Short-term (8–12 weeks) treatment of exogenous obesity in conjunction with a weight reduction program including exercise, reduced caloric intake, and behavior modification.

Dosage
- **Tablets**

Adults, initial: 1 mg once daily 1 hr before the first meal of the day; **then,** dose can be increased to 1 mg t.i.d. or 2 mg once daily 1 hr before lunch.
Administration/Storage: Clients may take medication with meals if they experience GI distress.
Additional Side Effect: Testicular pain.

NURSING CONSIDERATIONS

See also *Nursing Considerations* for *Stimulants,* Chapter 47.
Client/Family Teaching
1. Review mutual goals of therapy and the anticipated time frame for achieving.
2. Stress the importance of diet, regular exercise, and reduced caloric intake in the overall management of obesity.
3. Refer for diet counseling and appropriate support groups.
Evaluate: ↓ Body weight.

Methamphetamine hydrochloride

(meth-am-**FET**-ah-meen)
Pregnancy Category: C
Desoxyn **(C-II) (Rx)**

See also *Stimulants,* Chapter 47.
How Supplied: *Tablet:* 5 mg, 10 mg; *Tablet, Extended Release:* 5 mg, 10 mg, 15 mg
Action/Kinetics: t½: 4–5 hr, depending on urinary pH.
Uses: Attention deficit disorders in children over 6 years of age.

Dosage
- **Tablets**

Attention deficit disorders in children, 6 years and older.
Initial: 5 mg 1–2 times/day; increase in increments of 5 mg/day at weekly intervals until optimum dose is reached (usually 20–25 mg/day).
- **Extended-Release Tablets**

Attention deficit disorders in children, 6 years and older.
20–25 mg once daily.
Administration/Storage
1. When used to facilitate verbalization during psychotherapeutic interview, give second dose only if the first dose has proven effective.
2. When used for attention deficit disorders, the total daily dose can be

given in two divided doses or once a day using the long-acting product. The long-acting product should not be used to initiate therapy. Evaluate client progress periodically to determine the need for continued treatment.
Contraindications: Use for obesity. Attention deficit disorders in children less than 6 years of age.

NURSING CONSIDERATIONS

See also *Nursing Considerations* for *Stimulants,* Chapter 47.
Assessment
1. Document indications for therapy and type and onset of symptoms.
2. List other agents prescribed and the outcome.
Evaluate: ↑ Attention span and the ability to sit quietly and concentrate.

Methylphenidate hydrochloride

(meth-ill-**FEN**-ih-dayt)
PMS-Methylphenidate ✦, Ritalin, Ritalin-SR **(C-II) (Rx)**

How Supplied: *Tablet:* 5 mg, 10 mg, 20 mg; *Tablet, Extended Release:* 20 mg
Action/Kinetics: The mechanism of action of methylphenidate is not known with certainty although it may act by blocking the reuptake mechanism of dopaminergic neurons. In children with attention deficit disorders, methylphenidate causes decreases in motor restlessness with an increased attention span. In narcolepsy the drug acts on the cerebral cortex and subcortical structures (e.g., thalamus) to increase motor activity and mental alertness and decrease fatigue. **Peak blood levels, children:** 1.9 hr for tablets and 4.7 hr for extended-release tablets. **Duration:** 4–6 hr. **t½:** 1–3 hr. The drug is metabolized by the liver and excreted by the kidney.
Uses: Attention deficit disorders in children as part of overall treatment regimen. Narcolepsy.

Dosage
- **Tablets**

Narcolepsy.
Adults: 5–20 mg b.i.d.–t.i.d. preferably 30–45 min before meals.
Attention deficit disorders.
Pediatric, 6 years and older, initial: 5 mg b.i.d. before breakfast and lunch; **then,** increase by 5–10 mg/week to a maximum of 60 mg/day.
- **Extended-Release Tablets**

Narcolepsy.
Adults: 20 mg 1–3 times/day q 8 hr, preferably on an empty stomach.
Attention deficit disorders.
Pediatric, 6 years and older: 20 mg 1–3 times/day.

Administration/Storage
1. Administer the drug before breakfast and lunch to avoid interference with sleep.
2. If the client is receiving the medication for attention deficit disorders and no improvement is noticed in 1 month, or if stimulation occurs, discontinue the medication.
3. The drug should be discontinued periodically to assess the condition of the client because drug therapy is not considered to be indefinite. Drug therapy should be terminated at the time of puberty.
4. Sustained-release tablets are effective for 8 hr and may be substituted for regular-release tablets if the 8-hr dosage of the sustained-release tablets is the same as the titrated 8-hr dosage of regular tablets.
5. *Treatment of Overdose:* Symptomatic. Excess CNS stimulation may be treated by keeping the client in quiet, dim surroundings to reduce external stimuli. Protect the client from self-injury. A short-acting barbiturate may be used. Emesis or gastric lavage should be undertaken if the client is conscious. Adequate circulatory and respiratory function must be maintained. Hyperpyrexia may be treated by cooling the client (e.g., cool bath, hypothermia blanket).
Contraindications: Marked anxiety, tension and agitation, glaucoma. Severe depression, use for preventing normal fatigue. Tourette's syndrome, motor tics. Should not be used in children who manifest symptoms of

primary psychiatric disorders (psychoses) or acute stress.

Special Concerns: Use during pregnancy only if benefits clearly outweigh risks. Use with caution during lactation. Safety and efficacy in children less than 6 years of age have not been established. Use with great caution in clients with history of hypertension or convulsive disease.

Laboratory Test Interference: ↑ Urinary excretion of epinephrine.

Side Effects: *CNS:* Nervousness, insomnia, headaches, dizziness, drowsiness, chorea. Toxic psychoses, dyskinesia, Tourette's syndrome. Psychologic dependence. *CV:* Palpitations, tachycardia, angina, arrhythmias, hyper- or hypotension. *GI:* Nausea, anorexia, abdominal pain, weight loss (chronic use). *Allergic:* Skin rashes, fever, urticaria, arthralgia, dermatoses, erythema. *Hematologic:* Thrombocytopenic purpura, leukopenia, anemia. *Miscellaneous:* Hair loss.

In children, the following side effects are more common: anorexia, abdominal pain, weight loss (chronic use), tachycardia, insomnia.

Symptoms of Overdose: Characterized by CV symptoms (hypertension, cardiac arrhythmias, tachycardia), mental disturbances, agitation, headaches, vomiting, hyperreflexia, ***hyperpyrexia, convulsions, and coma.***

Drug Interactions

Anticoagulants, oral / ↑ Effect of anticoagulants due to ↓ breakdown by liver

Anticonvulsants (phenobarbital, phenytoin, primidone) / ↑ Effect of anticonvulsants due to ↓ breakdown by liver

Guanethidine / ↓ Effect of guanethidine by displacement from its site of action

MAO inhibitors / Possibility of hypertensive crisis, hyperthermia, convulsions, coma

Phenylbutazone / ↑ Effect of phenylbutazone due to ↓ breakdown by liver

Tricyclic antidepressants / ↑ Effect of antidepressants due to ↓ breakdown by liver

NURSING CONSIDERATIONS

See also *Nursing Considerations* for *Pemoline,* Chapter 47.

Assessment

1. Document indications for therapy and type and onset of symptoms.
2. Note other drugs the client is prescribed that may interact unfavorably with methylphenidate.
3. Ensure that psychologic evaluations show no evidence of a psychotic disorder or severe stress.
4. Obtain baseline CNS evaluation and ECG prior to starting therapy.

Client/Family Teaching

1. Use caution when driving or operating hazardous machinery as drug may mask fatigue and/or cause physical incoordination, dizziness, or drowsiness.
2. Record weight 2 times/week and report any significant loss. Clients tend to lose weight while they are taking the medication.
3. Monitor attention span and report any overt changes in client mood.
4. Skin rashes, fever, or pain in the joints should be reported immediately.
5. Advise that children who do respond to the therapy may have the therapy interrupted every few months ("drug holiday") to determine if the drug therapy is still necessary.
6. Avoid caffeine in any form.

Evaluate

- ↑ Ability to sit quietly and concentrate
- ↓ Episodes of narcolepsy

Pemoline

(**PEM**-oh-leen)
Pregnancy Category: B
Cylert, Cylert Chewable **(C-IV) (Rx)**

How Supplied: *Chew Tablet:* 37.5 mg; *Tablet:* 18.75 mg, 37.5 mg, 75 mg

Action/Kinetics: Although pemoline resembles amphetamine and methylphenidate pharmacologically, its mechanism of action is not fully known. Pemoline is believed to act by dopaminergic mechanisms. The drug will result in a decrease in hyper

activity and a prolonged attention span in children. **Peak serum levels:** 2–4 hr. **t½:** 12 hr. Steady state reached in 2–3 days, and beneficial effects may not be noted for 3–4 weeks. Approximately 50% is bound to plasma protein. Pemoline is metabolized by the liver, and approximately 50% is excreted unchanged by the kidneys.
Uses: Attention deficit disorders. *Investigational:* Narcolepsy.

Dosage

- **Tablets, Chewable Tablets**

Attention deficit disorders.

Children, 6 years and older, initial: 37.5 mg/day as a single dose in the morning; increase at 1-week intervals by 18.75 mg until desired response is attained up to maximum of 112.5 mg/day. **Usual maintenance:** 56.25–75 mg/day.

Narcolepsy.

Adults: 50–200 mg/day in two divided doses.

Administration/Storage

1. Administer as a single dose in the morning.
2. Interrupt treatment once or twice annually to determine whether behavioral symptoms still necessitate drug therapy.
3. Anticipate the drug will reach peak activity in 2–4 hr and last up to 8 hr.
4. *Treatment of Overdose:* Reduce external stimuli. If symptoms are not severe, induce vomiting or undertake gastric lavage. Chlorpromazine can be used to decrease the CNS stimulation and sympathomimetic effects.

Contraindications: Hypersensitivity to drug. Tourette's syndrome. Children under 6 years of age.
Special Concerns: Safe use during lactation has not been established. Use with caution in impaired renal or kidney function. Chronic use in children may cause growth suppression.
Laboratory Test Interferences: ↑ AST, ALT, serum LDH.
Side Effects: *CNS:* Insomnia (most common). Dyskinesia of the face, tongue, lips, and extremities; precipitation of Tourette's syndrome. Mild depression, headache, nystagmus, dizziness, hallucinations, irritability, ***seizures.*** Exacerbation of behavior disturbances and thought disorders in psychotic children. *GI:* Transient weight loss, gastric upset, nausea. *Miscellaneous:* Skin rash.

Symptoms of Overdose: Symptoms of CNS stimulation and sympathomimetic effects including agitation, confusion, delirium, euphoria, headache, muscle twitching, mydriasis, vomiting, hallucinations, flushing, sweating, tachycardia, hyperreflexia, tremors, ***hyperpyrexia,*** hypertension, ***seizures (may be followed by coma).***

NURSING CONSIDERATIONS

Assessment

1. Document indications for therapy and type and onset of symptoms.
2. List other agents prescribed and the outcome.

Client/Family Teaching

1. Administer early in the morning to minimize insomnia.
2. Report any noted weight loss or failure to grow as soon as evident.
3. Advise child's school health department of medication regimen.
4. Measure height every month, and weigh child twice a week. Record all measurements on a graph, and bring to each follow-up medical visit.
5. Advise family to continue with therapy, because behavioral changes take 3–4 weeks to occur.
6. Instruct the family when to interrupt drug administration, as recommended by the physician. Then, observe and record behavior without the medication, to determine whether therapy should be resumed.
7. Stress the importance of bringing the child in periodically for liver function tests to detect adverse effects that would necessitate withdrawal of pemoline.
8. Provide a printed list of drug side effects. Instruct family to identify signs of overdosage, such as agitation, restlessness, hallucinations, and tachycardia. Instruct parents to withhold the drug, to protect child, and to report immediately.

9. Do not perform activities that require mental alertness until drug effects are realized.
10. Avoid excessive consumption of caffeine-containing products.
Evaluate
- Improved attention span
- ↓ Hyperactivity with ability to sit quietly and concentrate

Phendimetrazine tartrate

(fen-dye-**ME**-trah-zeen)
Pregnancy Category: C
Anorex, Bontrol PDM and Slow-Release, Dital, Dyrexan-OD, Marlibar A, Melfiat-105 Unicelles, Neocurab, Obalan, Obe-Del, Obezine, Panrexin M, Panrexin MTP, Parzine, Phendiet, Phendiet-105, Phendimet, Phentra, Prelu-2, PT 105, Rexigen, Rexigen Forte, Tega-Nil, Trimstat, Trimtabs, Uni Trim, Wehless Timecelles, Weightrol, Wescoid, X-Trozine, X-Trozine LA **(C-III) (Rx)**

See also *Stimulants,* Chapter 47.
How Supplied: *Capsule:* 35 mg; *Capsule, Extended Release:* 105 mg; *Tablet:* 35 mg
Action/Kinetics: Duration, tablets: 4 hr. **t½:** 5.5 hr (average).
Use: Short-term (8–12 weeks) treatment of exogenous obesity in conjunction with a weight reduction program including exercise, reduced caloric intake, and behavior modification.

Dosage
- **Capsules, Tablets**

Adults: 17.5–35 mg 2–3 times/day 1 hr before meals. **Maximum daily dose:** 70 mg t.i.d.
- **Extended-Release Capsules, Extended-Release Tablets**

Adults: 105 mg/day 30–60 min before the morning meal.

NURSING CONSIDERATIONS

See *Nursing Considerations* for *Stimulants,* Chapter 47.
Client/Family Teaching
1. Stress importance of combining therapy with exercise and reduced caloric intake in the overall management of obesity.
2. Advise that this agent is for short-term therapy only. Encourage attendance at formal behavioral modification programs.
Evaluate: Control of appetite with desired weight loss.

Phentermine

(**FEN**-ter-meen)
Pregnancy Category: C
Adipex-P, Anoxine-AM, Dapex-37.5, Fastin, Obe-Mar, Obe-Nix 30, Obephen, Oby-Trim, Panshape, Phentercot, Phenterxene, Phentride, Phentrol, Phentrol 2, 4, and 5, Span-RD, T-Diet, Teramin, Wilpowr, Zatryl **(C-IV) (Rx)**

Phentermine resin

(**FEN**-ter-meen)
Pregnancy Category: C
Ionamin **(C-IV) (Rx)**

See also *Stimulants,* Chapter 47.
How Supplied: Phentermine *Capsule:* 15 mg, 18.75 mg, 30 mg, 37.5 mg; *Capsule, Extended Release:* 30 mg; *Tablet:* 8 mg, 37.5 mg.
Phentermine resin: *Capsule, Extended Release:* 15 mg, 30 mg
Action/Kinetics: Duration, 8-mg tablets: 4 hr; **duration, 30-mg capsules, 37.5-mg tablets, resin:** 12–14 hr.
Use: Short-term (8–12 weeks) treatment of exogenous obesity in conjunction with a weight reduction program including exercise, reduced caloric intake, and behavior modification.

Dosage
- **Capsules, Tablets**

Adults: 15–37.5 mg/day either before breakfast, 1–2 hr after breakfast, or in divided doses 30 min before meals.
- **Resin Capsules**

Adults: 15–30 mg once daily before breakfast.

NURSING CONSIDERATIONS

See *Nursing Considerations* for *Stimulants,* Chapter 47.

Client/Family Teaching

1. Stress the importance of a regular exercise program, lowered caloric intake, and behavorial modification therapy counseling programs in the overall goal of weight loss.

2. Advise client that therapy of this nature is for short-term use only and that life style changes should be the focus for continued progress toward this goal.

Evaluate: ↓ Appetite and evidence of desired weight loss.

Autonomic Nervous System Drugs

CHAPTER FORTY-EIGHT

Cholinergic Drugs/Cholinesterase Inhibitors

See the following individual entries:

Bethanechol Chloride
Edrophonium Chloride
Edrophonium Chloride and Atropine Sulfate
Guanidine Hydrochloride
Neostigmine Bromide
Neostigmine Methylsulfate
Ophthalmic Cholinergic Agents
Physostigmine Salicylate
Physostigmine Sulfate
Pilocarpine Hydrochloride
Pilocarpine Nitrate
Pilocarpine Ocular Therapeutic System
Pilocarpine and Epinephrine
Pyridostigmine Bromide

Bethanechol chloride

(beh-**THAN**-eh-kohl)
Pregnancy Category: C
Duvoid, Myotonachol, PMS-Bethanechol Chloride ♣, Urecholine **(Rx)**

How Supplied: *Injection:* 5 mg/mL; *Tablet:* 5 mg, 10 mg, 25 mg, 50 mg

Action/Kinetics: Directly stimulates cholinergic receptors, primarily muscarinic type. This results in stimulation of gastric motility, increases gastric tone, and stimulates the detrusor muscle of the urinary bladder. Bethanechol produces a slight transient fall of DBP, accompanied by minor reflex tachycardia. The drug is resistant to hydrolysis by acetylcholinesterase, which increases its duration of action. **PO: Onset,** 30–90 min; **maximum:** 60–90 min; **duration:** up to 6 hr. **SC: Onset,** 5–15 min; **maximum:** 15–30 min; **duration:** 2 hr.

Uses: Postpartum or postoperative urinary retention, atony of the bladder with urinary retention. *Investigational:* Reflux esophagitis.

Dosage

• **Tablets**

Adults, usual: 10–50 mg t.i.d.–q.i.d. The minimum effective dose can be determined by giving 5–10 mg initially and repeating this dose q 1–2 hr until a satisfactory response is observed or a maximum of 50 mg has been given. **Pediatric:** 0.2 mg/kg (6.7 mg/m2) 4–5 times/day.

• **SC**

Adults, usual: 5 mg t.i.d.–q.i.d. The minimum effective dose is determined by giving 2.5 mg initially and repeating this dose at 15–30-min intervals to a maximum of four doses or until a satisfactory response is obtained. **Pediatric:** 0.15–0.2 mg/kg (5–6.7 mg/m2) t.i.d.

Administration/Storage

1. To avoid N&V, bethanechol tablets should be taken on an empty stomach. Usually, 1 hr before or 2 hr after meals.
2. Administer PO or SC only.
3. The client should be observed closely for 30–60 min after drug administration for possible severe side effects. Have atropine available during SC therapy to counteract manifestations of acute toxicity.
4. *Treatment of Overdose:* Atropine, 0.6 mg SC for adults; a dose of 0.01 mg/kg atropine SC (up to a maximum of 0.4 mg) is recommended for infants and children up to 12 years of age. IV atropine may be used in emergency situations.

Contraindications: Hypotension, hypertension, CAD, coronary occlusion, AV conduction defects, vasomotor instability, bradycardia. Also, peptic ulcer, asthma (latent or active), hyperthyroidism, parkinsonism, epilepsy, obstruction of the bladder, if the strength or integrity of the GI or bladder wall is questionable, peritonitis, GI spastic disease, inflammatory lesions of the GI tract, vagotonia. Not to be used IM or IV.

Special Concerns: Use with caution during lactation. Safety and effectiveness have not been determined in children.

Side Effects: Serious side effects are uncommon with PO dosage but more common following SC use. *GI:* Nausea, diarrhea, salivation, GI upset, involuntary defecation, cramps, colic, belching, rumbling/gurgling of stomach. *CV:* Hypotension with reflex tachycardia, vasomotor response. *CNS:* Headache, malaise. *Other:* Flushing, sensation of heat about the face, sweating, urinary urgency, attacks of asthma, bronchial constriction, miosis, lacrimation.

Symptoms of Overdose: Early signs include N&V, abdominal discomfort, salivation, sweating, flushing.

Drug Interactions

Cholinergic inhibitors / Additive cholinergic effects
Ganglionic blocking agents / Critical hypotensive response preceded by severe abdominal symptoms
Procainamide / Antagonism of cholinergic effects
Quinidine / Antagonism of cholinergic effects

NURSING CONSIDERATIONS

Assessment

1. Take a complete nursing history.
2. Note drugs currently prescribed to determine if any are likely to interact with bethanecol.
3. Obtain baseline data concerning I&O when the drug is used to treat urinary tract problems.
4. When used to treat GI atony, obtain baseline data concerning bowel sounds and habits.
5. If taking antacids, investigate the reasons to determine if the client has a history of peptic ulcers.

Interventions

1. Monitor VS and I&O until it can be determined what the effects of the drug will be.
2. Report if the urinary output is inadequate because the drug should be discontinued.
3. If the drug is to be administered SC, administer 2 hr before eating to reduce the potential for nausea.
4. Monitor for bowel sounds when the drug is being administered for GI atony.
5. Complaints of gnawing, aching, burning, or epigastric pain in the left epigastric area should be reported and further investigated.

Evaluate

• Improved bladder tone and function
• ↑ GI tract motility

Edrophonium chloride

(ed-roh-**FOH**-nee-um)
Pregnancy Category: C
Enlon, Reversol, Tensilon **(Rx)**

Edrophonium chloride and Atropine sulfate

(ed-roh-**FOH**-nee-um)
Pregnancy Category: C
Enlon-Plus **(Rx)**

For additional information, see *Neostigmine,* Chapter 48.

How Supplied: Edrophonium chloride: *Injection:* 10 mg/mL.
Edrophonium chloride and Atropine sulfate: *Injection:* 10 mg-0.14 mg/mL

Action/Kinetics: Edrophonium is a short-acting agent mostly used for diagnosis and not for maintenance therapy. By increasing the duration of action at the motor end plate, edrophonium causes a transient increase in muscle strength in myasthenia gravis clients and either no change or a slight weakness in muscle strength in clients with other disorders. Atropine has been added to edrophonium to counteract the muscarinic side effects that will occur due to edrophonium (e.g., increased secretions, bradycardia, bronchoconstriction). **Onset: IM,** 2–10 min; **IV,** <1 min. **Duration: IM,** 5–30 min; **IV,** 10 min. Eliminated through the kidneys.

Uses: *Edrophonium.* Differential diagnosis of myasthenia gravis. Adjunct to evaluate requirements for treating myasthenia gravis. Adjunct to treat respiratory depression due to curare and similar nondepolarizing agents such as gallamine, pancuronium, and tubocurarine.

Edrophonium and Atropine. To antagonize or reverse nondepolarizing neuromuscular blocking agents. Adjunct to treat respiratory depression caused by overdosage of curare.

Dosage

- **Edrophonium. IV**

Differential diagnosis of myasthenia gravis.

IV, Adults: 2 mg initially over 15–30 sec; with needle in place, wait 45 sec; if no response occurs after 45 sec inject an additional 8 mg. If a cholinergic reaction is obtained following 2 mg (muscarinic side effects, skeletal muscle fasciculations, increased muscle weakness), test is discontinued and atropine, 0.4–0.5 mg, is given IV. The test may be repeated in 30 min. **Pediatric, up to 34 kg, IV:** 1 mg; if no response after 45 sec, can give up to 5 mg. **Pediatric, over 34 kg, IV:** 2 mg; if no response after 45 sec, can give up to 10 mg in 1-mg increments q 30–45 sec. **Infants:** 0.5 mg. If IV injection is not feasible, IM can be used.

To evaluate treatment needs in myasthenic clients.

1 hr after PO administration of drug used to treat myasthenia, give edrophonium IV, 1–2 mg. (*NOTE:* Response will be myasthenic in undertreated clients, adequate in controlled clients, and cholinergic in overtreated clients.)

Curare antagonist.

Slow IV: 10 mg over 30–45 sec to detect onset of cholinergic reaction; repeat if necessary to maximum of 40 mg. Should not be given before use of curare, gallamine, or tubocurarine.

- **Edrophonium. IM**

Differential diagnosis of myasthenia gravis.

Adults: 10 mg; if hyperreactivity occurs, retest after 30 min with 2 mg IM to rule out false negative. **Pediatric, up to 34 kg:** 2 mg; **more than 34 kg:** 5 mg. (There is a 2–10-min delay in reaction with IM route.)

- **Edrophonium and Atropine. IV**

Adults: 0.5–1 mg/kg edrophonium and 0.007–0.014 mg/kg atropine.

Administration/Storage

1. Edrophonium should not be given before curare or curare-like drugs.
2. Have IV atropine sulfate available to use as an antagonist.
3. When atropine is combined with edrophonium, the response should be monitored carefully and assisted or

controlled ventilation should be undertaken.
4. Recurarization has not been noted following satisfactory reversal with edrophonium and atropine.
Contraindications: Edrophonium combined with atropine is not recommended for use in the differential diagnosis of myasthenia gravis.
Special Concerns: Edrophonium combined with atropine is not effective against depolarizing neuromuscular blocking agents.

NURSING CONSIDERATIONS

See also *Nursing Considerations* for *Neostigmine,* Chapter 48.
Assessment
1. Document indications for therapy.
2. List drugs client currently prescribed.
3. Note any history of asthma, seizures, CAD, or hyperthyroidism.
Interventions
1. Observe closely in a monitored environment during drug administration; drug effects last up to 30 min.
2. Monitor VS and I&O at least q 4 hr.
3. Document and report side effects such as increased salivation, bronchial spasm, bradycardia, and cardiac arrhythmia. This is particularly important when working with elderly clients.
4. When the drug is being administered as an antidote for curare, assess client for the effects of each dose of drug. Do not administer the next dose of drug unless the prior effects have been observed and recorded. Larger doses of medication may potentiate effects.
5. Evaluate respiratory effort and provide assisted ventilation as needed.
6. During cholinergic crisis, monitor state of consciousness closely.
Evaluate
• Diagnosis of myasthenia gravis (transient ↑ muscle strength)
• Reversal of respiratory depression R/T nondepolarizing neuromuscular blocking agents

Guanidine hydrochloride
(**GWON**-ih-deen)
(Rx)

How Supplied: *Tablet:* 125 mg
Action/Kinetics: Guanidine hydrochloride increases the release of acetylcholine at the synapses following nerve impulse transmission; it slows the rate of depolarization and repolarization of the muscle cell membrane, therefore acting as a cholinergic muscle stimulant.
Uses: Reduction of muscle weakness and relief of fatigue associated with Eaton-Lambert syndrome. It is ineffective in the treatment of myasthenia gravis.

Dosage
• **Tablets**
Adults, individualized, initial: 10–15 mg/kg/day in three to four divided doses; **then,** increase dose gradually to 35 mg/kg/day or up to the development of side effects.
Administration/Storage
1. Removal of the primary neoplastic lesion may improve the condition sufficiently to allow drug discontinuation.
2. *Treatment of Overdose:* Calcium gluconate given IV to control neuromuscular and convulsive symptoms. Atropine will help the GI symptoms, hypoglycemia, and circulatory disturbances.
Contraindications: Hypersensitivity to and intolerance of drug. Lactation. Use in myasthenia gravis.
Special Concerns: Use during pregnancy only if benefits clearly outweigh risks. Safety for use in children not established. Renal function may be affected in some clients.
Laboratory Test Interferences: Increase in blood creatinine, abnormal liver function tests.
Side Effects: *CNS:* Nervousness, tremors, irritability, lightheadedness, ataxia, jitteriness, psychoses, confusion, changes in mood and emo-

tions, hallucinations. *Neurologic:* Paresthesia of face, feet, hands, and lips; hands and feet feel cold; trembling sensation. *GI:* Nausea, cramps, diarrhea, anorexia, dry mouth, gastric irritation. *Dermatologic:* Rashes, petechiae, ecchymoses, sweating, dry skin, scaling of skin, folliculitis, purpura, flushing. *CV:* Hypotension, atrial fibrillation, tachycardia, palpitations. *Hematologic:* Bone marrow suppression with anemia, leukopenia, thrombocytopenia. *Renal:* Uremia, renal tubular necrosis, chronic interstitial nephritis. *Other:* Sore throat, fever.

Symptoms of Overdose: Anorexia, diarrhea, increased peristalsis. If intoxication is severe, symptoms include salivation, vomiting, diarrhea, hypoglycemia, nervous hyperirritability, fibrillary tremors and convulsive contractions of muscle, circulatory disturbances.

NURSING CONSIDERATIONS

Assessment

1. Take a complete nursing history.
2. Note any history of myasthenia gravis as the drug is contraindicated.
3. Obtain baseline CBC and liver and renal function studies and monitor periodically while client is receiving the drug because damage may be dose-related.

Client/Family Teaching

1. Report if anorexia or increased peristalsis is experienced. These are early warnings that suggest the drug should be discontinued.
2. Advise that symptoms of hyperirritability, tremors, convulsive contractions of muscles, increased salivation, vomiting, diarrhea, and hypoglycemia are usually toxic manifestations of drug therapy. The drug is highly toxic and treatment should continue only as long as necessary.

Evaluate: Reports of ↓ muscle weakness and relief of fatigue in clients with Eaton-Lambert syndrome.

Neostigmine bromide

(nee-oh-**STIG**-meen)
Pregnancy Category: C
Prostigmin Bromide **(Rx)**

Neostigmine methylsulfate

(nee-oh-**STIG**-meen)
Pregnancy Category: C
Prostigmin Injection **(Rx)**

How Supplied: Neostigmine bromide: *Tablet:* 15 mg.
Neostigmine methylsulfate: *Injection:* 0.25 mg/mL; 0.5 mg/mL, 1 mg/mL

Action/Kinetics: By inhibiting the enzyme acetylcholinesterase, these drugs cause an increase in the concentration of acetylcholine at the myoneural junction, thus facilitating transmission of impulses across the myoneural junction. In myasthenia gravis, muscle strength is increased. The drug may also act on the autonomic ganglia of the CNS. Neostigmine also prevents or relieves postoperative distention by increasing gastric motility and tone and prevents or relieves urinary retention by increasing the tone of the detrusor muscle of the bladder. Shorter acting than ambenonium chloride and pyridostigmine. Atropine is often given concomitantly to control side effects. **Onset: PO,** 45–75 min; **IM,** 20–30 min; **IV,** 4–8 min. **Time to peak effect, parenteral:** 20–30 min. **Duration:** All routes, 2–4 hr. **t½, PO:** 42–60 min; **IM:** 51–90 min; **IV:** 47–60 min. Eliminated through the urine (about 40% unchanged).

Uses: Diagnosis and treatment of myasthenia gravis. Prophylaxis and treatment of postoperative GI ileus or urinary retention. Antidote for tubocurarine and other nondepolarizing drugs.

Dosage

NEOSTIGMINE BROMIDE

• **Tablets**

Treat myasthenia gravis.
Adults: 15 mg q 3–4 hr; adjust dose and frequency as needed. **Usual maintenance:** 150 mg/day with dosing intervals determined by client response. **Pediatric,** 2 mg/kg (60 mg/m^2) daily in six to eight divided doses.

NEOSTIGMINE METHYLSULFATE

• **IM, IV, SC**

Diagnosis of myasthenia gravis.
Adults, IM, SC: 1.5 mg given with 0.6 mg atropine; **pediatric, IM:** 0.04 mg/kg (1 mg/m^2); or, **IV:** 0.02 mg/kg (0.5 mg/m^2).

Treat myasthenia gravis.
Adults, IM, SC: 0.5 mg. **Pediatric, IM, SC:** 0.01–0.04 mg/kg q 2–3 hr.

Antidote for tubocurarine.
Adults, IV: 0.5–2 mg slowly with 0.6–1.2 mg atropine sulfate. Can repeat if necessary up to total dose of 5 mg. **Pediatric, IV:** 0.04 mg/kg with 0.02 mg/kg atropine sulfate.

Prevention of postoperative GI distention or urinary retention.
Adults, IM, SC: 0.25 mg (1 mL of the 1:4,000 solution) immediately after surgery repeated q 4–6 hr for 2–3 days.

Treatment of postoperative GI distention.
Adults, IM, SC: 0.5 mg (1 mL of the 1:2,000 solution) as required.

Treatment of urinary retention.
Adults, IM, SC: 0.5 mg (1 mL of the 1:2,000 solution). If urination does not occur within 1 hr after 0.5 mg, the client should be catheterized. After the bladder is emptied, 0.5 mg is given q 3 hr for at least five injections.

Administration/Storage

1. The interval between doses must be individually determined to achieve optimum effects.
2. If greater fatigue occurs at certain times of the day, a larger part of the daily dose can be administered at these times.
3. Neostigmine should not be given if high concentrations of halothane or cyclopropane are present.
4. May administer IV form undiluted at a rate of 0.5 mg/min.
5. *Treatment of Overdose:* Discontinue medication temporarily. Give atropine, 0.5–1 mg IV (up to 5–10 or more mg may be needed to get the HR to 80 beats/min). Supportive treatment including artificial respiration and oxygen.

Contraindications: Hypersensitivity, mechanical obstruction of GI or urinary tract, peritonitis, history of bromide sensitivity. Vesical neck obstruction of urinary bladder.

Special Concerns: Safe use during lactation not established. Safety and effectiveness in children have not been established. Use with caution in clients with bronchial asthma, bradycardia, vagotonia, epilepsy, hyperthyroidism, peptic ulcer, cardiac arrhythmias, or recent coronary occlusion. May cause uterine irritability and premature labor if given IV to pregnant women near term. In geriatric clients, the duration of action may be increased.

Side Effects: *GI:* N&V, diarrhea, abdominal cramps, involuntary defecation, salivation, dysphagia, flatulence, increased gastric and intestinal secretions. *CV:* Bradycardia, tachycardia, hypotension, ECG changes, nodal rhythm, ***cardiac arrest,*** syncope, ***AV block,*** substernal pain, thrombophlebitis after IV use. *CNS:* Headache, ***seizures,*** malaise, weakness, dysarthria, dizziness, drowsiness, loss of consciousness. *Respiratory:* Increased oral, pharyngeal, and bronchial secretions; ***bronchospasms, skeletal muscle paralysis, laryngospasm, central respiratory paralysis, respiratory depression or arrest,*** dyspnea. *Ophthalmologic:* Miosis, double vision, lacrimation, accommodation difficulties, hyperemia of conjunctiva, visual changes. *Musculoskeletal:* Muscle fasciculations or weakness, muscle cramps or spasms, arthralgia. *Other:* Skin rashes, urinary frequency and incontinence, sweating, flushing, allergic reactions, anaphylaxis, urticaria. These effects can usually be reversed by parenteral administration of 0.6 mg of atropine sulfate, which should be readily available.

Cholinergic crisis, due to overdosage, must be distinguished from myasthenic crisis (worsening of the disease), since cholinergic crisis involves removal of drug therapy, while myasthenic crisis involves an increase in anticholinesterase therapy.

Symptoms of Overdose: Abdominal cramps, vomiting, diarrhea, epigastric distress, excessive salivation, cold sweating, pallor, blurred vision, urinary urgency, fasciculation and ***paralysis of voluntary muscles (including the tongue),*** miosis, increased BP (may be accompanied by bradycardia), sensation of internal trembling, panic, severe anxiety.

Drug Interactions

Aminoglycosides / ↑ Neuromuscular blockade

Atropine / Atropine suppresses symptoms of excess GI stimulation caused by cholinergic drugs

Corticosteroids / ↓ Effect of neostigmine

Magnesium salts / Antagonize the effects of anticholinesterases

Mecamylamine / Intense hypotensive response

Organophosphate-type insecticides/pesticides / Added systemic effects with cholinesterase inhibitors

Succinylcholine / ↑ Neuromuscular blocking effects

NURSING CONSIDERATIONS

Assessment

1. Note any history of hypersensitivity to drugs in this category.
2. Identify any drugs the client is taking to determine if they may interact unfavorably with neostigmine.
3. Note any history of bromide sensitivity. The drug is contraindicated in these instances.

Interventions

1. Observe and report symptoms of generalized cholinergic stimulation as this is evidence of a toxic reaction.
2. Assess for stability and vision. If the client has difficulty with coordination or vision caution him to avoid use of heavy machinery until the effects of the medication wear off.
3. Monitor the pulse and BP for the first hour after drug administration. Report if the pulse is less than 80 as the drug should be withheld. If hypotension occurs, have the client remain recumbent until the BP stabilizes.
4. When the medication is used as an antidote for nondepolarizing drugs, assist in the ventilation of the client and maintain a patent airway.
5. If the client is taking the medication for treatment of myasthenia gravis, any onset of weakness 1 hr after administration usually indicates overdosage of drug. The onset of weakness 3 hr or more after administration usually indicates underdosage and/or resistance and should also be documented as well as any associated difficulty with respirations or increase in muscle weakness.

Client/Family Teaching

1. Provide a printed list of adverse drug effects, stressing those that require immediate reporting.
2. Advise clients with myasthenia to maintain a written record of periods of muscle strength or weakness so that dosage can be evaluated and adjusted accordingly. Encourage client to space activities to avoid excessive fatigue.
3. Take the dose exactly as prescribed. Explain that taking the dose late may result in myasthenic crisis whereas taking it early may result in cholinergic crisis.
4. Stress that any increasing weakness should be reported immediately because drug tolerance can develop.
5. Wear a Medic Alert bracelet and/or carry identification indicating that client is receiving neostigmine and for what reasons.

Evaluate

- ↑ Muscle strength and function
- Relief of postoperative ileus or urinary retention
- Reversal of respiratory depression R/T nondepolarizing drugs

OPHTHALMIC CHOLINERGIC (MIOTIC) AGENTS

See also the following individual entries:

Physostigmine Salicylate
Physostigmine Sulfate
Pilocarpine Hydrochloride
Pilocarpine Nitrate
Pilocarpine Ocular Therapeutic System
Pilocarpine and Epinephrine

General Statement: Cholinergic agents are commonly used for the treatment of glaucoma and less frequently for the correction of accommodative esotropia.

Action/Kinetics: The ophthalmic cholinergic drugs fall into two classes: direct-acting (carbachol, pilocarpine) and indirect-acting (demecarium, echothiophate, isoflurophate, neostigmine, physostigmine), which inhibit the enzyme acetylcholinesterase. In the treatment of glaucoma, the drugs lead to an accumulation of acetylcholine, which stimulates the ciliary muscles and increases contraction of the iris sphincter muscle. This opens the angle of the eye and results in increased outflow of aqueous humor and consequently in a decrease of intraocular pressure. This effect is of particular importance in narrow-angle glaucoma. Hourly tonometric measurements are recommended during initiation of therapy. The drugs also cause spasms of accommodation.

Uses: *Glaucoma:* Primary acute narrow-angle glaucoma (acute therapy) and primary chronic wide-angle glaucoma (chronic therapy). Selected cases of secondary glaucoma. Diagnosis and treatment of accommodative esotropia. Antidote against harmful effects of atropine-like drugs in clients with glaucoma. Alternately with a mydriatic drug to break adhesions between lens and iris. See also individual drugs.

Contraindications: *Direct-acting drugs:* Inflammatory eye disease (iritis), asthma, hypertension. *Indirect-acting drugs:* Same as for *direct-acting drugs,* as well as acute-angle glaucoma, history of retinal detachment, ocular hypotension accompanied by intraocular inflammatory processes, intestinal or urinary obstruction, peptic ulcer, epilepsy, parkinsonism, spastic GI conditions, vasomotor instability, severe bradycardia or hypotension, and recent MIs. During lactation.

Special Concerns: Geriatric clients must be carefully monitored.

Side Effects: *Local:* Painful contraction of ciliary muscle, pain in eye, blurred vision, spasms of accommodation, darkened vision, failure to accommodate to darkness, twitching, headaches, painful brow. Most of these symptoms lessen with prolonged usage. Iris cysts and retinal detachment (indirect-acting drugs only).

Systemic: Systemic absorption of drug may cause nausea, GI discomfort, diarrhea, hypotension, bronchial constriction, and increased salivation.

Dosage

See individual drugs.

NURSING CONSIDERATIONS

Administration

1. To prevent the overflow of solution into the nasopharynx after topical instillation of drops, exert pressure on the nasolacrimal duct for 1–2 min before the client closes the eyelids.
2. Have epinephrine and atropine available for emergency treatment of increased intraocular pressure.

Assessment

1. Document indications for therapy and type and onset of symptoms. List other agents prescribed and the outcome.
2. Ensure that complete ophthalmologic exam and findings are available.
3. Review list of drugs and existing medical conditions that may preclude drug therapy to ensure that none are present.

Interventions

1. Report redness around the cornea. Epinephrine or phenylephrine hydrochloride (10%) may be ordered with demecarium bromide, echothiophate iodide, or isoflurophate to minimize this kind of reaction.
2. Instruct client to report any changes in vision, eye irritation, or evidence of severe headaches.

Client/Family Teaching

1. Explain why the medications have been prescribed and stress the importance of compliance in order to maintain vision by reducing intraocular pressures.
2. Review and demonstrate the appropriate method for instilling eye drops or ointment. Observe client self-administering prescribed medications to ensure appropriate, safe technique.
3. Stress the importance of taking the eye drops exactly as prescribed. Advise that side effects can be minimized by taking at least one dose of medication at bedtime.
4. Advise the client not to drive for 1–2 hr after instilling cholinergic agents. Caution that night vision may be impaired.
5. Pain and blurred vision may occur. This problem usually diminishes with continued use of the drug but should be reported if these symptoms persist, as the dosage of medication may need to be changed.
6. Explain that painful eye spasms may be relieved by applying cold compresses.
7. Provide the client with a schedule for eye examinations. Stress the importance of adhering to the schedule and refilling the prescriptions as needed.

Evaluate

- A positive clinical response based on ophthalmic examinations that show improved visual fields and tonometric measurements that show evidence of ↓ intraocular pressures
- Evidence of compliance with prescribed therapy
- Reports of side effects that may require a change in the dosage or agent

---

Physostigmine salicylate

(fye-zoh-**STIG**-meen)
Pregnancy Category: C
Antilirium, Eserine Salicylate **(Rx)**

Physostigmine sulfate

(fye-zoh-**STIG**-meen)
Pregnancy Category: C
Eserine Sulfate **(Rx)**

See also *Neostigmine,* and *Ophthalmic Cholinergic Agents,* Chapter 48.

How Supplied: Physostigmine salicylate: *Injection:* 1 mg/mL. Physostigmine sulfate: *Ophthalmic Ointment:* 0.25%

Action/Kinetics: Physostigmine is a reversible acetylcholinesterase inhibitor, resulting in an increased concentration of acetylcholine at nerve endings, which can antagonize anticholinergic drugs. It produces miosis, increased accommodation, and a decrease in intraocular pressure with decreased resistance to outflow of aqueous humor. When used for chronic open-angle glaucoma, ciliary muscle contraction may open the intertrabecular spaces, facilitating aqueous humor outflow. **Onset, IV:** 3–5 min. **Duration, IV:** 1–2 hr. **t½:** 1–2 hr. No dosage alteration is necessary in clients with renal impairment. **Onset, miosis:** 20–30 min; **duration, miosis:** 12–36 hr. **Reduction of intraocular pressure, peak:** 2–6 hr; **duration:** 12–36 hr.

Uses: Overdosage due to cholinergic blocking drugs (e.g., atropine) and tricyclic antidepressant overdosage. Reduce intraocular pressure in primary glaucoma. Friedreich's and other inherited ataxias (FDA has granted orphan status for this use). *Investigational:* Angle-closure glaucoma during or after iridectomy, secondary glaucoma if no inflammation present.

Dosage

- **IM, IV**

Anticholinergic drug overdose.

Adults, IM, IV: 0.5–2 mg at a rate of 1 mg/min; may be repeated if necessary. **Pediatric, IV:** 0.5 mg given over a period of at least 1 min. Dose may be repeated at 5–10 min if needed to a maximum of 2 mg if no toxic effects are manifested.

- **Ophthalmic Solution**

Glaucoma.

Adults and children: 2 gtt of the 0.25% or 0.5% salicylate solution in the eye up to q.i.d.

- **Ophthalmic Ointment**

Glaucoma.

Adults and children: 1 cm of the 0.25% sulfate ointment applied to the lower fornix up to t.i.d.

Administration/Storage

1. Following use of the ophthalmic solution, the lacrimal sac should be pressed for 1–2 min to avoid excessive systemic absorption.
2. The ophthalmic ointment may be used at night for prolonged effect of the medication.
3. The ophthalmic solution should be stored at 8°C–27°C (46°F–80°F) and kept tightly closed. The solution should not be used if it is cloudy or dark brown.
4. The ophthalmic ointment should be stored tightly closed and protected from heat.
5. May administer IV undiluted: 1 mg/min (0.5 mg/min for children).
6. *Treatment of Overdose:* IV atropine sulfate: **Adults:** 0.4–0.6 mg; **infants and children up to 12 years of age:** 0.01 mg/kg q 2 hr as needed (maximum single dose should not exceed 0.4 mg). A short-acting barbiturate may be used for seizures not relieved by atropine.

Special Concerns: Use with caution during lactation, in clients with chronic angle-closure glaucoma, or in clients with narrow angles. Safety and efficacy have not been established for ophthalmic use in children.

Additional Side Effects: If IV administration is too rapid, bradycardia, hypersalivation, breathing difficulties, and ***seizures*** may occur. Conjunctivitis when used for glaucoma.

Symptoms of Overdose: Cholinergic crisis.

NURSING CONSIDERATIONS

See also *Nursing Considerations* for *Neostigmine,* Chapter 48, *Cholinergic Blocking Agents,* Chapter 49, and *Ophthalmic Cholinergic Agents,* Chapter 48.

Assessment

1. Document indications for therapy and type and onset of symptoms.
2. Determine cause of overdosage (drug or plant ingestion), amount, and time ingested.

Interventions

1. During IV administration, monitor ECG and record VS; report any evidence of bradycardia, hypersalivation, respiratory difficulty, or seizure activity.
2. Have the client void prior to administering the medication. If the client develops incontinence, it may be caused by too high a dose.

Client/Family Teaching

1. During ophthalmic instillation, wipe away any excess solution from around the eyes.
2. Wash hands after administration to prevent systemic absorption.
3. Some stinging and burning of the eyes may occur. These symptoms should disappear as the use of the drug continues. If painful spasms occur, apply cold compresses. If itching, pain, or tearing persists, do not continue using the medication until medically cleared.
4. Do not use the ophthalmic solution if it is discolored.
5. Advise that night vision may be impaired.
6. N&V may occur; report if the symptoms persist or are severe.

Evaluate

- Reversal of toxic CNS symptoms R/T overdosage with cholinergic blocking agents or tricyclic antidepressants or from ingestion of poisonous plants
- ↓ Intraocular pressures

Pilocarpine hydrochloride

(pie-low-**CAR**-peen)
Pregnancy Category: C
Adsorbocarpine, Akarpine, Diocarpine M, Isopto Carpine, Minims Pilocarpine M, Miocarpine M, Ocu-Carpine, Pilocar, Pilopine HS, Piloptic-½, -1, -2, -3, -4, and -6, Pilopto-Carpine, Pilostat, R.O.–Carpine ✦, Salagen, Spersacarpine ✦ (Rx)

Pilocarpine nitrate

(pie-low-**CAR**-peen)
Pregnancy Category: C
Minims Pilocarpine ✦, Pilagan, P.V. Carpine Liquifilm ✦ **(Rx)**

Pilocarpine ocular therapeutic system

(pie-low-**CAR**-peen)
Pregnancy Category: C
Ocusert Pilo-20 and -40 **(Rx)**

See also *Ophthalmic Cholinergic Agents,* Chapter 48.

How Supplied: Pilocarpine hydrochloride: *Device:* 20 mcg/hr, 40 mcg/hr; *Ophthalmic gel:* 4%; *Ophthalmic Solution:* 0.25%, 0.5%, 1%, 2%, 3%, 4%, 5%, 6%, 8%; *Tablet:* 5 mg. Pilocarpine nitrate: *Ophthalmic Solution:* 1%, 2%, 4%
Pilocarpine ocular therapeutic system: *Device:* 20 mcg/hr, 40 mcg/hr

Action/Kinetics: *Hydrochloride or Nitrate Solution:* **Onset:** 45–60 min; **peak effect:** 75 min; **duration:** 4–14 hr. *Hydrochloride Gel:* **Onset:** 60 min; **peak effect:** 3–12 hr; **duration:** 18–24 hr. *Nitrate:* The ocular therapeutic system is a unit designed to be placed in the cul-de-sac of the eye for release of pilocarpine. The drug is released from the ocular therapeutic system three times faster during the first few hours and then decreases (within 6 hr) to a rate of 20 or 40 mcg/hr for 1 week. *Ocular system:* **onset:** 60 min. **peak effect:** 1.5–2 hr; **duration:** 7 days. When used to treat dry mouth due to radiotherapy in head and neck cancer clients, pilocarpine stimulates residual functioning salivary gland tissue to increase saliva production.

Uses: HCl, Nitrate: Chronic simple glaucoma (especially open-angle). Chronic angle-closure glaucoma, including after iridectomy. Acute angle-closure glaucoma (alone or with other miotics, epinephrine, beta-adrenergic blocking agents, carbonic anhydrase inhibitors, or hyperosmotic agents). To reverse mydriasis (i.e., after cycloplegic and mydriatic drugs). Pre- and postoperative intraocular tension. The nitrate product is also used for emergency miosis. Salagen (Pilocarpine HCl) has been approved for treatment of radiation-induced dry mouth in head and neck cancer clients. **Ocular Therapeutic System:** Glaucoma alone or with other ophthalmic medications. *Investigational:* Hydrochloride used to treat xerostomia in clients with malfunctioning salivary glands.

Dosage

- **Ophthalmic Gel.**

PILOCARPINE HYDROCHLORIDE

Glaucoma.

Adults and adolescents: ½-in. strip of 4% gel once daily at bedtime.

- **Ophthalmic Solution.**

PILOCARPINE HYDROCHLORIDE

Doses listed are all for adults and adolescents.

Chronic glaucoma.

1 gtt of a 0.5%–4% solution q.i.d.

Acute angle-closure glaucoma.

1 gtt of a 1% or 2% solution q 5–10 min for three to six doses; **then,** 1 gtt q 1–3 hr until pressure is decreased.

Miotic, to counteract sympathomimetics.

1 gtt of a 1% solution.

Miosis, prior to surgery.

1 gtt of a 2% solution q 4–6 hr for one or two doses before surgery.

Miosis before iridectomy.

1 gtt of a 2% solution for four doses immediately before surgery.

PILOCARPINE NITRATE

Doses listed are all for adults and adolescents.

Chronic glaucoma.

1–2 gtt of a 1%–4% solution b.i.d.–q.i.d.

Acute angle-closure glaucoma.

1 gtt of a 1% or 2% solution q 5–10 min for three to six doses; **then,** 1 gtt q 1–3 hr until pressure is decreased.

Miosis, to counteract sympathomimetics.

1 gtt of a 1% solution.

Miosis, before surgery for glaucoma.

1 gtt of a 2% solution q 4–6 hr (usually for one or two doses) before surgery.

Miosis, before surgery for iridectomy.

1 gtt of a 2% solution for four doses immediately before surgery.

• **Ocular System**

Insert and remove as directed by physician or package insert. Ocusert Pilo-20 is approximately equal to the 0.5% or 1% drops, while Ocusert Pilo-40 is approximately equal to the 2% or 3% solution.

• **Tablets (Salagen)**

Treat radiation-induced dry mouth in head and neck cancer clients.

Initial: 5 mg t.i.d.; **then,** up to 10 mg t.i.d., if needed.

Administration/Storage

1. The hydrochloride is available as 0.25%, 0.5%, 1%, 2%, 3%, 4%, 6%, 8%, and 10% solutions and as a 4% gel.
2. Concentrations greater than 4% of pilocarpine HCl may be more effective in clients with dark pigmented eyes; however, the incidence of side effects increases.
3. The nitrate is available as 1%, 2%, and 4% solutions.
4. If other glaucoma medication (i.e., drops) is used with the gel at bedtime, the drops should be instilled at least 5 min before the gel.
5. Myopia may be observed during the first several hours of therapy with the ocular therapeutic system.
6. Client should check for presence of the ocular therapeutic system before bed and upon arising.
7. For acute, narrow-angle glaucoma, pilocarpine should also be administered in the unaffected eye to prevent angle-closure glaucoma.
8. The solution should be stored, protected from light, at 8°C–30°C (46°F–86°F) while the gel should be refrigerated at 2°C–8°C (36°F–46°F) until dispensed to the client. The gel should not be frozen and any unused portion should be discarded after 8 weeks. The ocular therapeutic system should be refrigerated at 2°C–8°C (36°F–46° F).
9. *Treatment of Overdose:* Titrate with atropine (0.5–1 mg SC or IM) and supportive measures to maintain circulation and respiration. If there is severe cardiovascular depression or bronchoconstriction, epinephrine (0.3–1 mg SC or IV) may be used.

Contraindications: Lactation.

Special Concerns: Use with caution during lacation. Use with caution in clients with narrow angles (angle closure may result) or in those with known or suspected cholelithiasis or biliary tract disease. Use with caution in clients with controlled asthma, chronic bronchitis, or COPD. Safety and efficacy have not been established in children.

Additional Side Effects: The following side effects have been attributed to the pilocarpine ocular system. *Opthalmic:* Conjunctival irritation, including mild erythema with or without a slight increase in mucous secretion upon initial use.

Oral use (tablets). *Dermatologic:* Sweating, flushing, rash, pruritus. *GI:* N&V, dyspepsia, diarrhea, abdominal pain, taste perversion, anorexia, increased appetite, esophagitis, tongue disorder. *CV:* Hypertension, tachycardia, bradycardia, ECG abnormality, palpitations, syncope. *CNS:* Dizziness, asthenia, headache, tremor, anxiety, confusion, depression, abnormal dreams, hyperkinesia, hypesthesia, nervousness, paresthesias, speech disorder, twitching. *Respiratory:* Sinusitis, rhinitis, pharyngitis, epistaxis, increased sputum, stridor, yawning. *Ophthalmic:* Lacrimation, amblyopia, conjunctivitis, abnormal vision, eye pain, glaucoma. *GU:* Urinary frequency, dysuria, metrorrhagia, urinary impairment. *Body as a whole:* Chills, edema, body odor, hypothermia, mucous membrane abnormality. *Miscellaneous:* Dysphagia, voice alteration, myalgias, seborrhea.

NURSING CONSIDERATIONS

See also *Nursing Considerations* for *Ophthalmic Cholinergic Agents,* Chapter 48.

Assessment

1. Document indications for therapy, onset of symptoms, and baseline ophthalmic assessment when indicated.
2. List other agents prescribed, the duration of therapy, and the outcome.
3. Clients with acute infectious conjunctivitis or keratitis should be carefully evaluated before use of the pilocarpine ocular system.

Client/Family Teaching

1. Review how to insert drug and how to check the conjunctival sac for presence of the ocular system.
2. Advise client to follow these general guidelines for insertion:
- Wash hands.
- Do not permit drug to touch any surface.
- Rinse with cool water.
- Pull down lower eyelid.
- Place according to manufacturer's directions.
- System may be moved under closed eyelids to upper eyelid for sleep. Use caution and report any pain as corneal abrasion or irritation may be present.

3. Instruct to insert drug at bedtime to diminish side effects. Advise to check for the presence of ocular system at bedtime and also upon awakening each day.
4. Instruct client to report if eye irritation, redness, or mucus production persist with the ocular system.
5. Explain the importance of periodic tonometric readings to evaluate effectiveness of the drug.
6. Review the dose and frequency when prescribed orally for radiation-induced dry mouth.
7. Review the side effects of drug therapy, stressing those that require medical intervention.

Evaluate

- Tonometric evidence of ↓ intraocular pressures
- Desired pupillary constriction
- ↑Saliva production with relief of radiation-induced dry mouth symptoms
- Evidence of successful reversal of sympathomimetic drug effects

—COMBINATION DRUG—

Pilocarpine and Epinephrine

(pie-low-**CAR**-peen, ep-ih-**NEF**-rin)

E-Pilo-1, E-Pilo-2, E-Pilo-3, E-Pilo-4, E-Pilo-6, P1E1, P2E1, P3E1, P4E1, P6E1 **(Rx)**

See also *Ophthalmic Cholinergic Agents,* and *Pilocarpine Hydrochloride,* Chapter 48.

How Supplied: See Content

Content: E-Pilo-1 and P1E1 solutions contain: 1% pilocarpine hydrochloride, 1% epinephrine bitartrate. E-Pilo-2 and P2E1 solutions contain: 2% pilocarpine hydrochloride, 1% epinephrine bitartrate. P3E1 solution contains: 3% pilocarpine hydrochloride, 1% epinephrine bitartrate. E-Pilo-4 and P4E1 solutions contain: 4% pilocarpine hydrochloride, 1% epinephrine bitartrate. E-Pilo-6 and P6E1 solutions contain: 6% pilocarpine hydrochloride and 1% epinephrine bitartrate.

Action/Kinetics: Pilocarpine improves outflow of intraocular fluid by a direct cholinergic action whereas epinephrine increases outflow facility. Pilocarpine and epinephrine exert an additive effect to reduce intraocular pressure; the combination exerts opposite effects on the pupil which prevents significant mydriasis or miosis. The solutions all contain ep-

inephrine, 1%, with varying concentrations of pilocarpine, indicated by the number in the name (e.g., E-Pilo-1 contains 1% pilocarpine and P2E1 contains 2% pilocarpine).
Use: Glaucoma.

Dosage

- **Solution**

Glaucoma.
1–2 gtt into the eye(s) 1–4 times/day.

Administration/Storage
1. The concentration and frequency of use are determined by the severity of the glaucoma and client response.
2. Clients with heavily pigmented irides may require larger doses.
3. Solutions should not be used if they are brown or contain a precipitate.
4. Solutions should be stored, protected from heat and light, at 8°C–30°C (46°F–86°F).

NURSING CONSIDERATIONS

See also *Nursing Considerations* for *Ophthalmic Cholinergic Agents,* and *Pilocarpine,* Chapter 48.

Client/Family Teaching
1. Review appropriate method for instillation.
2. Advise that blurred vision will occur for a short time after drug administration and not to drive or attempt to operate machinery until vision clears.
Evaluate: ↓ Intraocular pressures.

Pyridostigmine bromide

(peer-id-oh-**STIG**-meen)
Mestinon, Regonol **(Rx)**

For all information, see also *Neostigmine,* Chapter 48.
How Supplied: *Injection:* 5 mg/mL; *Syrup:* 60 mg/5 mL; *Tablet:* 60 mg; *Tablet, extended release:* 180 mg
Action/Kinetics: Has a slower onset, longer duration of action, and fewer side effects than neostigmine. **Onset, PO:** 30–45 min for syrup and tablets and 30–60 min for extended-release tablets; **IM:** 15 min; **IV:** 2–5 min. **Duration, PO:** 3–6 hr for syrup and tablets and 6–12 hr for extended-release tablets; **IM, IV:** 2–4 hr. Poorly absorbed from the GI tract; excreted in urine up to 72 hr after administration.
Uses: Myasthenia gravis. Antidote for nondepolarizing muscle relaxants (e.g., tubocurarine).

Dosage

- **Syrup, Tablets**

Myasthenia gravis.
Adults: 60–120 mg q 3–4 hr with dosage adjusted to client response. **Maintenance:** 600 mg/day (range: 60 mg–1.5 g). **Pediatric:** 7 mg/kg (200 mg/m^2) daily in five to six divided doses.

- **Sustained-Release Tablets**

Myasthenia gravis.
Adults: 180–540 mg 1–2 times/day with at least 6 hr between doses. Sustained-release tablets not recommended for use in children.

- **IM, IV**

Myasthenia gravis.
Adults, IM, IV: 2 mg (about 1/30 the adult dose) q 2–3 hr.
Neonates of myasthenic mothers.
IM: 0.05–0.15 mg/kg q 4–6 hr.
Antidote for nondepolarizing drugs.
Adults, IV: 10–20 mg with 0.6–1.2 mg atropine sulfate given IV.

Administration/Storage
1. During dosage adjustment, administer the drug to the client in a closely monitored environment.
2. Parenteral medication dosage is 1/30 of the PO dose. May give undiluted at a rate of 0.5 mg IV over 1 min for myasthenia and at a rate of 5 mg IV over 1 min (with atropine) for reversal of nondepolarizing drug effects.
3. After PO administration, onset of action occurs in 30–45 min and lasts for 3–6 hr. When administered IM, the onset of action occurs within 15 min. When administered IV, the onset of action occurs within 2–5 min.
4. *Treatment of Overdose:* Discontinue medication temporarily. Give atropine, 0.5–1 mg IV (up to 5–10 mg or more may be needed to get HR to 80

beats/min). Supportive treatment including artificial respiration and oxygen.

Additional Contraindication: Sensitivity to bromides.

Special Concerns: Safe use during pregnancy and during lactation has not been established. May cause uterine irritability and premature labor if given IV to pregnant women near term. In geriatric clients, the duration of action may be increased.

Additional Side Effects: Skin rash. Thrombophlebitis after IV use.

Symptoms of Overdose: Abdominal cramps, vomiting, diarrhea, epigastric distress, excessive salivation, cold sweating, pallor, blurred vision, urinary urgency, fasciculation and ***paralysis of voluntary muscles*** (including the tongue), miosis, increased BP (may be accompanied by bradycardia), sensation of internal trembling, panic, severe anxiety.

NURSING CONSIDERATIONS

See also *Nursing Considerations* for *Neostigmine,* Chapter 48.

Interventions

1. Monitor VS and observe client for toxic reactions demonstrated by generalized cholinergic stimulation.
2. Assess for muscular weakness. This may be a sign of impending myasthenic crisis and cholinergic overdose.
3. Work with the client to determine the best individualized medication administration schedule according to their routines and lifestyle.

Client/Family Teaching

1. Explain how extended-release tablets work. Caution not to crush them and not to take these tablets more often than q 6 hr.
2. Extended-release tablets may be taken with conventional tablets, if prescribed.
3. Explain how to recognize symptoms of toxic reaction and myasthenic crisis.
4. Stress the importance of taking medication as prescribed since too early administration may result in cholinergic crisis, whereas too late administration may result in myasthenic crisis.
5. Provide with printed instructions and a list of toxic side effects that should be reported if evident.
6. Clients may develop resistance to the drug. Explain the importance of close medical supervision as well as the prompt reporting of all side effects so that drug therapy can be evaluated.
7. Identify local support groups that may assist the client and family to understand and cope with this disorder.

Evaluate

- Improvement in muscle strength and function
- Reversal of nondepolarizing muscle relaxants

CHAPTER FORTY-NINE

Cholinergic Blocking Agents

See also the following individual entries:

Atropine Sulfate
Benztropine Mesylate
Biperiden Hydrochloride
Biperiden Lactate
Dicyclomine Hydrochloride
Glycopyrrolate
Methantheline Bromide
Procyclidine Hydrochloride
Propantheline Bromide
Scopolamine Hydrobromide
Scopolamine Transdermal Therapeutic System
Trihexyphenidyl Hydrochloride

Action/Kinetics: The cholinergic blocking agents prevent the neurotransmitter acetylcholine from combining with receptors on the postganglionic parasympathetic nerve terminal (muscarinic site). In therapeutic doses, these drugs have little effect on transmission of nerve impulses across ganglia (nicotinic sites) or at the neuromuscular junction.

The main effects of cholinergic blocking agents are:

1. To reduce spasms of smooth muscles like those controlling the urinary bladder or spasms of bronchial and intestinal smooth muscle.
2. To block vagal impulses to the heart, resulting in an increase in the rate and speed of impulse conduction through the AV conducting system.
3. To suppress or decrease gastric secretions, perspiration, salivation, and secretion of bronchial mucus.
4. To relax the sphincter muscles of the iris and cause pupillary dilation (mydriasis) and loss of accommodation for near vision (cycloplegia).
5. To act in diverse ways on the CNS, producing such reactions as depression (scopolamine) or stimulation (toxic doses of atropine). Many of the anticholinergic drugs also have antiparkinsonism effects. They abolish or reduce the S&S of Parkinson's disease, such as tremors and rigidity, and result in some improvement in mobility, muscular coordination, and motor performance. These effects may be due to blockade of the effects of acetylcholine in the CNS. This section also discusses miscellaneous synthetic antispasmodics related to anticholinergic drugs.

The anticholinergics that are related to atropine are quickly absorbed following PO ingestion. These agents cross the blood-brain barrier and may exert significant CNS effects. Examples of these drugs are scopolamine, l-hyoscyamine, and belladonna alkaloids. The drugs classified as quaternary ammonium anticholinergic drugs are erratically absorbed from the GI tract and exert minimal CNS effects, since they do not cross the blood-brain barrier. Examples of these drugs are glycopyrrolate, methantheline, propantheline, tridihexethyl chloride, clidinium bromide, isopropamide, and others.

Uses: See individual drugs.

Contraindications: Glaucoma, adhesions between iris and lens of the eye, tachycardia, myocardial ischemia, unstable CV state in acute hemorrhage, partial obstruction of the GI and biliary tracts, prostatic hypertrophy, renal disease, myasthenia gravis, hepatic disease, paralytic ileus, pyloroduodenal stenosis, pyloric obstruction, intestinal atony, ulcerative colitis, obstructive uropathy. Cardiac clients, especially when there is danger of tachycardia; older persons suffering from atherosclerosis or mental impairment. Lactation.

Special Concerns: Use with caution in pregnancy. Infants and young children are more susceptible to the toxic side effects of anticholinergic drugs. Of particular importance is use of such drugs in children when the ambient temperature is high; due to suppression of sweat glands, the body temperature may increase rapidly. Geriatric clients are particularly likely to manifest anticholinergic side effects such as dry mouth, constipation, and urinary retention (especially in males). Geriatric clients are also more likely to experience agitation, confusion, drowsiness, excitement, glaucoma, and impaired memory. Use with caution in hyperthyroidism, CHF, cardiac arrhythmias, hypertension, Down syndrome, asthma, spastic paralysis, blonde individuals, allergies, and chronic lung disease.

Side Effects: These are desirable in some conditions and undesirable in others. Thus, the anticholinergics have an antisalivary effect that is useful in parkinsonism. This same effect is unpleasant when the drug is used for spastic conditions of the GI tract.

Most side effects are dose-related and decrease when dosage decreases. Sometimes it helps to discontinue the medication for several days. With this in mind, anticholinergic drugs have the following side effects. *GI:* N&V, dry mouth, dysphagia, constipation, heartburn, change in taste perception, bloated feeling, paralytic ileus. *CNS:* Dizziness, drowsiness, nervousness, disorientation, headache, weakness, insomnia, fever (especially in children). Large doses may produce CNS stimulation including tremor and restlessness. Anticholinergic psychoses: ataxia, euphoria, confusion, disorientation, loss of short-term memory, decreased anxiety, fatigue, insomnia, hallucinations, dysarthria, agitation. *CV:* Palpitations. *GU:* Urinary retention or hesitancy, impotence. *Ophthalmologic:* Blurred vision, dilated pupils, photophobia, cycloplegia, precipitation of acute glaucoma. *Allergic:* Urticaria, skin rashes, ***anaphylaxis.*** *Other:* Flushing, decreased sweating, nasal congestion, suppression of glandular secretions including lactation. Heat prostration (fever and heat stroke) in presence of high environmental temperatures due to decreased sweating.

Symptoms of Overdose (Belladonna poisoning): Infants and children are especially susceptible to the toxic effects of atropine and scopolamine. Poisoning (dose-dependent) is characterized by the following symptoms: dry mouth, burning sensation of the mouth, difficulty in swallowing and speaking, blurred vision, photophobia, rash, tachycardia, increased respiration, ***increased body temperature*** (up to 109°F, 42.7°C), restlessness, irritability, confusion, muscle incoordination, dilated pupils, hot dry skin, ***respiratory depression and paralysis,*** tremors, ***seizures,*** hallucinations, and ***death.***

Drug Interactions

Amantadine / Additive anticholinergic side effects
Antacids / ↓ Absorption of anticholinergics from GI tract
Antidepressants, tricyclic / Additive anticholinergic side effects
Antihistamines / Additive anticholinergic side effects
Atenolol / Anticholinergics ↑ effects of atenolol
Benzodiazepines / Additive anticholinergic side effects
Corticosteroids / Additive ↑ intraocular pressure
Cyclopropane / ↑ Chance of ventricular arrhythmias
Digoxin / ↑ Effect of digoxin due to ↑ absorption from GI tract
Disopyramide / Potentiation of anticholinergic side effects
Guanethidine / Reversal of inhibition of gastric acid secretion caused by anticholinergics

Haloperidol / Additive ↑ intraocular pressure
Histamine / Reversal of inhibition of gastric acid secretion caused by anticholinergics
Levodopa / Possible ↓ effect of levodopa due to ↑ breakdown of levodopa in stomach (due to delayed gastric emptying time)
MAO inhibitors / ↑ Effect of anticholinergics due to ↓ breakdown by liver
Meperidine / Additive anticholinergic side effects
Methylphenidate / Potentiation of anticholinergic side effects
Metoclopramide / Anticholinergics block action of metoclopramide
Nitrates, nitrites / Potentiation of anticholinergic side effects
Nitrofurantoin / ↑ Bioavailability of nitrofurantoin
Orphenadrine / Additive anticholinergic side effects
Phenothiazines / Additive anticholinergic side effects; also, effects of phenothiazines may ↓
Primidone / Potentiation of anticholinergic side effects
Procainamide / Additive anticholinergic side effects
Quinidine / Additive anticholinergic side effects
Reserpine / Reversal of inhibition of gastric acid secretion caused by anticholinergics
Sympathomimetics / ↑ Bronchial relaxation
Thiazide diuretics / ↑ Bioavailability of thiazide diuretics
Thioxanthines / Potentiation of anticholinergic side effects

Dosage

See individual drugs.

NURSING CONSIDERATIONS

Administration/Storage

1. Check dosage and measure the drug exactly. Some drugs in this category are given in small amounts. As a consequence, overdosage is quickly achieved and can lead to toxicity.
2. Review the list of drugs with which drugs in this category interact.
3. *Treatment of Overdose (Belladonna poisoning):*
   - Gastric lavage or induction of vomiting followed by activated charcoal. General supportive measures.
   - Anticholinergic effects can be reversed by physostigmine (Eserine), 1–3 mg IV (effectiveness uncertain; thus use other agents if possible). Neostigmine methylsulfate, 0.5–2 mg IV, repeated as necessary.
   - If there is excitation, diazepam, a short-acting barbiturate, IV sodium thiopental (2% solution), or chloral hydrate (100–200 mL of a 2% solution by rectal infusion) may be given.
   - For fever, cool baths may be used. Keep client in a darkened room if photophobia is manifested.
   - Artificial respiration should be instituted if there is paralysis of respiratory muscles.

Assessment

1. Document indications for therapy and assess client for a history of asthma, glaucoma, or duodenal ulcer, all of which contraindicate the use of these drugs.
2. Note client history of renal disease, cardiac problems, or hepatic disease.
3. Determine the age of the client. Elderly clients, especially those with mental impairment or atherosclerosis, should not receive these drugs.

Interventions

1. If the client complains of a dry mouth, provide frequent mouth care and cold drinks, especially postoperatively. Sugarless hard candies and chewing gum may also be of some benefit.
2. Observe the client for evidence of drug interactions that may occur. A reduction in dosage of one of the medications may be necessary.
3. Drugs such as atropine may suppress thermoregulatory sweating; counsel client concerning activity (especially in hot weather) and appropriate clothing. Also, children and infants may exhibit "atropine fever."

Client/Family Teaching

1. Explain that certain side effects are to be expected and describe. These should be reported to the

provider who may alleviate symptoms by reducing the dose of drug or by temporarily stopping the drug. Sometimes the client may be expected to tolerate certain side effects such as dry mouth or blurred vision because of the overall beneficial effects of drug therapy.
2. Remind the client that antiparkinsonism drugs are not to be withdrawn abruptly. If the medication is changed, one drug should be withdrawn slowly and the other started in small doses.

ADDITIONAL NURSING CONSIDERATIONS RELATED TO PATHOLOGIC CONDITIONS FOR WHICH THE DRUG IS ADMINISTERED

CARDIOVASCULAR

Interventions

1. Monitor VS and ECG. Assess for any hemodynamic changes and intraventricular conduction blocks.
2. Note any client complaints of palpitations.

OCULAR

Assessment

1. Determine any previous experience with this class of drugs and the results.
2. Document intraocular pressures and assess accommodation and pupillary response.

Interventions

1. Note any client complaint of dizziness or blurred vision. Provide assistance with ambulation and institute safety measures.
2. Hold medication and report any complaints of eye pain after drug administration.

Client/Family Teaching

1. Review the appropriate methods for instillation of drops or ointment and observe client administration technique.
2. Explain how long vision will be affected by the medication and assist the client in planning activities for safety.
3. Advise that temporary stinging and blurred vision will occur.
4. Caution that night vision may be impaired.
5. Explain that photophobia, which may occur, can be relieved by wearing dark glasses.
6. Report any marked changes in vision, eye irritation, or persistent headaches immediately.
7. With large doses, lacrimal secretion may be diminished and client may experience dry or "sandy" eyes.

GASTROINTESTINAL

Client/Family Teaching

1. Advise clients receiving medication for treatment of GI pathology to take the medication early enough before a meal (at least 20 min) so that the medication will be effective when needed.
2. Clients with GI pathology should be instructed on how to maintain the prescribed diet. Provide printed information related to the diet and refer to the dietitian for assistance in meal planning and preparation as needed.
3. Instruct the client to continue taking the medication as ordered and to notify the provider of any adverse effects.
4. Advise that gastric emptying times may be prolonged and intestinal transit time lengthened. Drug-induced intestinal paralysis is temporary and should resolve after 1–3 days of therapy.

GENITOURINARY

Interventions

1. Assess middle-aged male clients in particular for infrequent voiding. This is evidence of urinary retention and should be addressed. It may be more pronounced in elderly men with prostatic hypertrophy.
2. Monitor I&O. Palpate abdomen for evidence of bladder distention and determine the need for catheterization.
3. If impotence occurs, it may be drug-related. The client should be encouraged to consult with the provider for medication adjustment.

Evaluate

- Successful dilation of pupils

• Reports of ↓ bowel motility with improved elimination patterns
• ↑ HR
• Evidence of ↓ production of secretions
• Reports of ↓ muscle tremors, rigidity, and spasticity with parkinsonism

Atropine sulfate

(**AH**-troh-peen)
Pregnancy Category: C
Atropair, Atropine-1 Ophthalmic, Atropine A.K. ✱, Atropine Minims ✱, Atropine Sulfate Ophthalmic, Atropine Sulfate S.O.P., Atropine-Care Ophthalmic, Atropisol Ophthalmic, Isopto Atropine Ophthalmic, I-Tropine, Ocu-Tropine **(Rx)**

See also *Cholinergic Blocking Agents,* Chapter 49.

How Supplied: *Injection:* 0.05 mg/mL, 0.1 mg/mL, 0.4 mg/mL, 0.5 mg/mL, 0.8 mg/mL, 1 mg/mL; *Ophthalmic Ointment:* 1%; *Ophthalmic Solution:* 0.5%, 1%; Tablet: 0.4 *mg*

Action/Kinetics: Atropine blocks the action of acetylcholine on postganglionic cholinergic receptors in smooth muscle, cardiac muscle, exocrine glands, urinary bladder, and the AV and SA nodes in the heart. Ophthalmologically, atropine blocks the effect of acetylcholine on the sphincter muscle of the iris and the accommodative muscle of the ciliary body. This results in dilation of the pupil (mydriasis) and paralysis of the muscles required to accommodate for close vision (cycloplegia). This enables the physician to examine the inner structure of the eye, including the retina. It also permits examination of refractive errors of the lens without the client automatically accommodating. **Peak effect:** *Mydriasis,* 30–40 min; *cycloplegia,* 1–3 hr. **Recovery:** Up to 12 days. **Duration, PO:** 4–6 hr. **t½:** 2.5 hr. Metabolized by the liver although 30%–50% is excreted through the kidneys unchanged.

Uses: PO: Adjunct in peptic ulcer treatment. Irritable bowel syndrome. Adjunct in treatment of spastic disorders of the biliary tract. Urologic disorders, urinary incontinence. During anesthesia to control salivation and bronchial secretions. Has been used for parkinsonism but more effective drugs are available.

Parenteral: Antiarrhythmic, adjunct in GI radiography. Prophylaxis of arrhythmias induced by succinylcholine or surgical procedures. Reduce sinus bradycardia (severe) and syncope in hyperactive carotid sinus reflex. Prophylaxis and treatment of toxicity due to cholinesterase inhibitors, including organophosphate pesticides. Treatment of curariform block. As a preanesthetic or in dentistry to decrease secretions.

Ophthalmologic: Cycloplegic refraction or pupillary dilation in acute inflammatory conditions of the iris and uveal tract. *Investigational:* Treatment and prophylaxis of posterior synechiae; pre- and postoperative mydriasis; treatment of malignant glaucoma.

Dosage

• **Tablets, Soluble Tablets**

Anticholinergic or antispasmodic.

Adults: 0.3–1.2 mg q 4–6 hr. **Pediatric, over 41 kg:** same as adult; **29.5–41 kg:** 0.4 mg q 4–6 hr; **18.2–29.5 kg:** 0.3 mg q 4–6 hr; **10.9–18.2 kg:** 0.2 mg q 4–6 hr; **7.3–10.9 kg:** 0.15 mg q 4–6 hr; **3.2–7.3 kg:** 0.1 mg q 4–6 hr.

Prophylaxis of respiratory tract secretions and excess salivation during anesthesia.

Adults: 2 mg.

Parkinsonism.

Adults: 0.1–0.25 mg q.i.d.

• **IM, IV, SC**

Anticholinergic.

Adults, IM, IV, SC: 0.4–0.6 mg q 4–6 hr. **Pediatric, SC:** 0.01 mg/kg, not to exceed 0.4 mg (or 0.3 mg/m²).

To reverse curariform blockade.

Adults, IV: 0.6–1.2 mg given at the same time or a few minutes before 0.5–2 mg neostigmine methylsulfate (use separate syringes).

Treatment of toxicity from cholinesterase inhibitors.

Adults, IV, initial: 2–4 mg; **then,** 2 mg repeated q 5–10 min until muscarinic symptoms disappear and signs of atropine toxicity begin to appear. **Pediatric, IM, IV, initial:** 1 mg; **then,** 0.5–1 mg q 5–10 min until muscarinic symptoms disappear and signs of atropine toxicity appear.

Treatment of mushroom poisoning due to muscarine.

Adults, IM, IV: 1–2 mg q hr until respiratory effects decrease.

Treatment of organophosphate poisoning.

Adults, IM, IV, initial: 1–2 mg; **then,** repeat in 20–30 min (as soon as cyanosis has disappeared). Dosage may be continued for up to 2 days until symptoms improve.

Arrhythmias.

Pediatric, IV: 0.01–0.03 mg/kg.

Prophylaxis of respiratory tract secretions, excessive salivation, succinylcholine- or surgical procedure-induced arrhythmias.

Pediatric, up to 3 kg, SC: 0.1 mg; **7–9 kg:** 0.2 mg; **12–16 kg:** 0.3 mg; **20–27 kg:** 0.4 mg; **32 kg:** 0.5 mg; **41 kg:** 0.6 mg.

- **Ophthalmic Solution**

Uveitis.

Adults: 1–2 gtt instilled into the eye(s) up to q.i.d. **Children:** 1–2 gtt of the 0.05% solution into the eye(s) up to t.i.d.

Refraction.

Adults: 1–2 gtt of the 1% solution into the eye(s) 1 hr before refracting. **Children:** 1–2 gtt of the 0.5% solution into the eye(s) b.i.d. for 1–3 days before refraction.

- **Ophthalmic Ointment**

Instill a small amount into the conjunctival sac up to t.i.d.

Administration/Storage

1. For ophthalmic use, atropine sulfate is available in 0.5%, 1%, or 2% solutions or 0.5% and 1% ointment.
2. After instillation of the ophthalmic ointment, compress the lacrimal sac by digital pressure for 1–3 min.
3. Have physostigmine available in the event of overdose.
4. *Treatment of Ocular Overdose:* Eyes should be flushed with water or normal saline. A topical miotic may be necessary.

Additional Contraindications: Ophthalmic use: Infants less than 3 months of age, primary glaucoma or a tendency toward glaucoma, adhesions between the iris and the lens, geriatric clients and others where undiagnosed glaucoma or excessive pressure in the eye may be present, in children who have had a previous severe systemic reaction to atropine.

Special Concerns: Use with caution in infants, small children, geriatric clients, diabetes, hypo- or hyperthyroidism, narrow anterior chamber angle, individuals with Down syndrome.

Additional Side Effects: *Ophthalmologic:* Blurred vision, stinging, increased intraocular pressure, contact dermatitis. Long-term use may cause irritation, photophobia, eczematoid dermatitis, conjunctivitis, hyperemia, or edema.

NURSING CONSIDERATIONS

See also *Nursing Considerations* for *Cholinergic Blocking Agents,* Chapter 49.

Assessment

1. Document presenting symptoms and indications for therapy.
2. Check for a history of angle-closure glaucoma before administering the drug in the eye because atropine may precipitate an acute crisis.
3. Obtain VS and monitor ECG during IV therapy.

Client/Family Teaching

1. When atropine is used in the eye, vision will be temporarily impaired. Therefore, close work, operating machinery, or driving a car should be avoided until the effects of the medication have worn off.
2. Drug impairs heat regulation; avoid strenuous activity in hot environments.
3. Males with prostatic hypertrophy may experience urinary retention and hesitancy.
4. Increase fluids and add bulk to diet to diminish constipating drug effects.

5. Use sugarless candies and gums to decrease dry mouth symptoms.

Evaluate

- ↑ HR
- Desired pupillary dilatation
- ↓ GI activity
- Reversal of muscarinic effects of anticholinesterase agents
- ↓ Salivation

Benztropine mesylate

(BENS-troh-peen)

Pregnancy Category: C

Apo-Benztropine ✦, Cogentin, PMS-Benztropine ✦ **(Rx)**

See also *Cholinergic Blocking Agents,* Chapter 49.

How Supplied: *Injection:* 1 mg/mL; *Tablet:* 0.5 mg, 1 mg, 2 mg

Action/Kinetics: Benztropine is a synthetic anticholinergic possessing antihistamine and local anesthetic properties. **Onset, PO:** 1–2 hr; **IM, IV:** Within a few minutes. Its effects are cumulative, and it is long-acting (24 hr). Full effects are manifested in 2–3 days. The drug produces a low incidence of side effects.

Uses: As adjunct in the treatment of parkinsonism (all types). Used to reduce severity of extrapyramidal effects in phenothiazine or other antipsychotic drug therapy (not effective in tardive dyskinesia).

Dosage

- **Tablets**

Parkinsonism.

Adults: 1–2 mg/day (range: 0.5–6 mg/day).

Idiopathic parkinsonism.

Adults, initial: 0.5–1 mg/day, increased gradually to 4–6 mg/day, if necessary.

Postencephalitic parkinsonism.

Adults: 2 mg/day in one or more doses.

Drug-induced extrapyramidal effects.

Adults: 1–4 mg 1–2 times/day.

- **IM, IV (rarely)**

Acute dystonic reactions.

Adults, initial: 1–2 mg; **then,** 1–2 mg PO b.i.d. usually prevents recurrence. Clients can rarely tolerate full dosage.

Administration/Storage

1. When used as replacement for or supplement to other antiparkinsonism drugs, substitute or add gradually.
2. For clients who have difficulty swallowing tablets, the tablets may be crushed and mixed with a small amount of food or liquid.
3. Some clients may benefit by taking the entire dose at bedtime while others are best treated by taking divided doses, b.i.d.–q.i.d.
4. Therapy should be initiated with a low dose (e.g., 0.5 mg) and then increased in increments of 0.5 mg at 5–6-day intervals. The maximum daily dose should not exceed 6 mg.
5. If the drug is to be administered IV, it may be given undiluted at a rate of 1 mg over 1 min.

Special Concerns: Not recommended for children under 3 years of age. Geriatric and emaciated clients cannot tolerate large doses. Certain drug-induced extrapyramidal symptoms may not respond to benztropine.

NURSING CONSIDERATIONS

See also *Nursing Considerations* for *Cholinergic Blocking Agents,* Chapter 49.

Assessment

1. When taking the client's drug history, note if phenothiazines or tricyclic antidepressants are being used. When taken with benztropine mesylate, these drugs may cause a paralytic ileus.
2. Assess for any evidence of medical conditions that would preclude beginning the drug therapy.
3. Note the age of the client. Anticipate that elderly clients will require a lower dosage.

Interventions

1. If the client develops excitation or vomiting, the drug may need to be withdrawn temporarily. When treatment is resumed the dosage should be lowered.
2. Monitor I&O. Auscultate for bowel sounds. This is especially important if the client has limited mobility.
3. Inspect the client's skin at regular intervals for any evidence of skin changes.

Client/Family Teaching
1. Review the goals of therapy and the possible side effects.
2. Use caution when performing tasks that require mental alertness because drug has a sedative effect and may also cause postural hypotension.
3. Remind clients that it usually takes 2–3 days for the drug to exert a desired effect. The drug should be taken as ordered unless side effects occur; these should be reported. Reassure that side effects usually subside with continued use of the drug.
4. Avoid strenuous activity and increased heat exposure. Plan rest periods during the day as ability to tolerate heat will be reduced and heat stroke may occur.
5. Report any difficulty in voiding or inadequate emptying of the bladder.
6. Avoid alcohol and any other CNS depressants.

Evaluate
- ↓ Abnormal muscle movement and rigidity with improved gait and balance
- Control of extrapyramidal side effects of antipsychotic agents (esp. ↓ drooling)

Biperiden hydrochloride
(bye-**PER**-ih-den)
Pregnancy Category: C
Akineton Hydrochloride **(Rx)**

Biperiden lactate
(bye-**PER**-ih-den)
Akineton Lactate **(Rx)**(PC: C)

See also *Antiparkinson Agents,* Chapter 46, and *Cholinergic Blocking Agents,* Chapter 49.

How Supplied: Biperiden hydrochloride: *Tablet:* 2 mg.
Biperiden lactate: *Injection:* 5 mg/mL

Action/Kinetics: Tolerance may develop to this synthetic anticholinergic. Tremor may increase as spasticity is relieved. The drug has slight respiratory and CV effects. **Time to peak levels:** 60–90 min. **Peak levels:** 4–5 mcg/L. **t½:** About 18–24 hr.

Uses: Parkinsonism, especially of the postencephalitic, arteriosclerotic, and idiopathic types. Drug-induced (e.g., phenothiazines) extrapyramidal manifestations.

Dosage
- **Tablets (Hydrochloride)**

Parkinsonism.

Adults: 2 mg t.i.d.–q.i.d., to a maximum of 16 mg/day.

Drug-induced extrapyramidal effects.

Adults: 2 mg 1–3 times/day. Maximum daily dose: 16 mg.
- **IM, Slow IV (Lactate)**

Drug-induced extrapyramidal effects.

Adults: 2 mg; repeat q 30 min until symptoms improve, but not more than four doses daily. **Pediatric:** 0.04 mg/kg (1.2 mg/m^2); repeat q 30 min until symptoms improve, but not more than four doses daily.

Administration/Storage
1. If the drug is administered IM, supervise and assist the client in walking because of the possibility of transient incoordination.
2. If the drug is administered IV, have the client remain recumbent during the procedure and for 15 min after it is completed. Once the IV is finished, assist clients to get up by having them dangle their legs at the bedside prior to standing and walking, to lower the potential for hypotension, syncope, and falling.

Additional Contraindications: Children under the age of 3 years.

Special Concerns: Use with caution in older children.

Additional Side Effects: Muscle weakness, inability to move certain muscles.

NURSING CONSIDERATIONS

See also *Nursing Considerations* for *Cholinergic Blocking Agents,* Chapter 49.

Assessment
1. Note the client's age. Older clients

should receive lower doses of the medication.
2. Record other drugs the client is taking to prevent any unfavorable interactions.

Client/Family Teaching
1. Take drug after meals to avoid gastric irritation.
2. Do not use antacids or an antidiarrheal for 1–2 hr after taking medication.
3. Keep a record of stools. Encourage client to increase the intake of fluids, fruit juices, and fiber to avoid constipation.
4. Avoid overheating as drug decreases perspiration.
5. Maintain a record of I&O. Report any difficulty with urination.
6. Use sugarless gum or candies and rinse mouth often to control dry mouth effects.

Evaluate
• Control of drug-induced (phenothiazine) extrapyramidal manifestations (i.e.,↓ muscle rigidity and drooling)

Dicyclomine hydrochloride

(dye-**SYE**-kloh-meen)
Pregnancy Category: C
Antispas, A-Spas, Bentyl, Bentylol ✱, Byclomine, Dibent, Di-Cyclonex, Dilomine, Di-Spaz, Formulex ✱, Neoquess, Or-Tyl, Spasmoject **(Rx)**

See also *Cholinergic Blocking Agents,* Chapter 49.

How Supplied: *Capsule:* 10 mg; *Injection:* 10 mg/mL; *Syrup:* 10 mg/5 mL; *Tablet:* 20 mg

Action/Kinetics: t½, initial: 1.8 hr; **secondary:** 9–10 hr.

Uses: Hypermotility and spasms of GI tract associated with irritable colon and spastic colitis, mucous colitis.

Dosage

• **Capsules, Syrup, Tablets**

Hypermotility and spasms of GI tract.

Adults: 10–20 mg t.i.d.–q.i.d.; **then,** may increase to total daily dose of 160 mg if side effects do not limit this dosage. **Pediatric, 6 years and older, capsules or tablets:** 10 mg t.i.d.–q.i.d.; adjust dosage to need and incidence of side effects. **Pediatric, 6 months–2 years, syrup:** 5–10 mg t.i.d.–q.i.d.; **2 years and older:** 10 mg t.i.d.–q.i.d. The dose should be adjusted to need and incidence of side effects.

• **IM**

Hypermotility and spasms of GI tract.

Adults: 20 mg q 4–6 hr. **Not for IV use.**

Administration/Storage: Drug can be administered to clients with glaucoma.

Additional Contraindication: Use for peptic ulcer.

Special Concerns: Pediatric dosage of the injectable form has not been established. Use of capsules and tablets in children less than 6 years of age not recommended; use of the syrup in children less than 6 months of age not recommended.

Additional Side Effects: Brief euphoria, slight dizziness, feeling of abdominal distention. **Use of the syrup in infants less than 3 months of age:** ***Seizures,*** syncope, respiratory symptoms, fluctuations in pulse rate, ***asphyxia,*** muscular hypotonia, ***coma.***

NURSING CONSIDERATIONS

See also *Nursing Considerations* for *Cholinergic Blocking Agents,* Chapter 49.

Assessment
1. Document indications for therapy and onset of symptoms.
2. Determine any presence of peptic ulcer.

Special Concerns
1. Anticipate reduced dose in the elderly.
2. Elderly clients may be more inclined to develop confusion, agitation, excitement, or drowsiness.

Evaluate: Restoration of normal bowel function and GI motility.

Glycopyrrolate

(glye-koh-**PYE**-roh-layt)
Pregnancy Category: B

Robinul, Robinul Forte **(Rx)**

See also *Cholinergic Blocking Agents*

How Supplied: *Injection:* 0.2 mg/mL; *Tablet:* 1 mg, 2 mg

Action/Kinetics: Onset: PO, 1 hr; **IV,** 1 min; **IM, SC:** 15–30 min. **Duration: decrease salivation,** Up to 7 hr; **block vagal activity:** 2–3 hr. **t½:** 0.6–4.6 hr.

Uses: PO. Adjunct in treatment of peptic ulcer. Antidiarrheal. **IM, IV.** To reduce salivation, tracheobronchial and pharyngeal secretions during surgery. To decrease acidity and volume of gastric secretions; to block cardiac vagal inhibitory reflexes during induction of anesthesia and intubation. Prophylaxis of aspiration of gastric contents during anesthesia. Adjunct with neostigmine or pyridostigmine to reverse neuromuscular blockade due to nondepolarizing muscle relaxants.

Dosage

- **Tablets**

Peptic ulcer.

Adults, initial: 1–2 mg t.i.d. or 2 mg b.i.d.–t.i.d. (may also give 2 mg at bedtime); **maintenance:** 1 mg b.i.d. with dose adjusted as needed up to a maximum of 8 mg.

- **IM, IV**

Peptic ulcer.

Adults, IM, IV: 0.1–0.2 mg t.i.d.–q.i.d.

Prophylaxis of excessive salivation, respiratory tract secretions, gastric hypersecretion during anesthesia.

Adults, IM: 0.0044 mg/kg 30–60 min prior to anesthesia or at the time the preanesthetic sedative and/or narcotic are given; **pediatric, less than 12 years:** 0.0044–0.0088 mg/kg 30–60 min before anesthetic or at the time preanesthetic medication is given.

Prophylaxis of arrhythmias during anesthesia and surgery.

Adults, IV: 0.1 mg repeated, as needed, q 2–3 min; **pediatric, IV,** 0.0044 mg/kg not to exceed 0.1 mg/dose, repeated, as needed, q 2–3 min.

Reversal of neuromuscular blockade.

Adults and children, IV: 0.2 mg for each 1 mg neostigmine or 5 mg pyridostigmine. Give IV at the same time and in the same syringe.

Administration/Storage

1. Do not add to IV solution containing sodium chloride or bicarbonate.
2. Parenteral use may slow stomach emptying and cause pain at the injection site.
3. For direct IV administration, give undiluted at a rate of 0.2 mg over 1–2 min.

Additional Contraindication: Peptic ulcer in children under 12 years of age.

Special Concerns: Dosage has not been determined for injection in children with peptic ulcer.

Laboratory Test Interference: ↓ Serum uric acid in clients with gout or hyperuricemia.

NURSING CONSIDERATIONS

See also *Nursing Considerations* for *Cholinergic Blocking Agents,* Chapter 49.

Assessment

1. Document indications for therapy and onset of symptoms.
2. Note the age of the client. Elderly clients are more sensitive to the side effects of drug therapy than younger clients.

Client/Family Teaching

1. Caution that drug causes orthostatic hypotension.
2. Avoid temperature extremes as drug inhibits sweating.
3. Drug may cause dizziness and drowsiness.
4. Avoid activities that require mental alertness until drug effects realized.

Evaluate

- ↓ Secretion production and cholinergic effects during anesthesia
- ↓ Acidity and volume of gastric secretions
- Arrhythmia prophylaxis during surgery

Methantheline bromide

(meth-**AN**-theh-leen)
Pregnancy Category: C
Banthine Bromide **(Rx)**

See also *Cholinergic Blocking Agents*
How Supplied: *Tablet:* 50 mg
Action/Kinetics: PO: Onset, 30 min; **duration:** 6 hr. **IM: Duration,** 2–4 hr. Drug has some ganglionic blocking activity.
Uses: Adjunct in peptic ulcer therapy. Urinary incontinence.

Dosage

• **Tablets**
Adults: 50–100 mg q.i.d. **Pediatric, over 1 year:** 12.5–50 mg q.i.d. **Infants, 1–12 months:** 12.5 up to 25 mg q.i.d. **Newborns:** 12.5 mg b.i.d.; **then,** 12.5 mg t.i.d.
Additional Side Effects: Postural hypotension, impotence. ***Respiratory paralysis*** and tachycardia (overdosage).

NURSING CONSIDERATIONS

See also *Nursing Considerations* for *Cholinergic Blocking Agents,* Chapter 49.
Interventions
1. Initiate therapy for clients with duodenal ulcer while receiving a liquid diet.
2. If prescribed, anticholinergic agents may delay absorption of potassium. Report any client complaints that could indicate lesions in the GI mucosa.
3. Auscultate for bowel sounds and assess for abdominal distention, epigastric distress, and vomiting since the drug reduces gastric motility.
Client/Family Teaching
1. Rise slowly from a supine position to prevent postural hypotension.
2. Remind male clients that drug-induced impotence may occur and should be reported.
Evaluate
• ↓ GI pain and irritation
• Control of urinary incontinence

Procyclidine hydrochloride

(proh-**SYE**-klih-deen)
Pregnancy Category: C
Kemadrin, PMS-Procyclidine ✱, Procyclid ✱ **(Rx)**

See also *Cholinergic Blocking Agents,* Chapter 49.
How Supplied: *Tablet:* 5 mg
Action/Kinetics: Procyclidine, a synthetic anticholinergic, appears to be better tolerated by younger clients. It also possesses direct antispasmodic effects on smooth muscle. This drug is often more effective in relieving rigidity than tremor. **Onset:** 30–45 min. **Time to peak levels:** 1–2 hr. **Peak levels:** 80 mcg/L. **t½:** 11.5–12.6 hr. **Duration:** 4–6 hr.
Uses: Treatment of all types of parkinsonism. Drug-induced extrapyramidal symptoms. Control of sialorrhea following neuroleptic drug use.

Dosage

• **Elixir, Tablets**
Parkinsonism (for clients on no other therapy).
Initial: 2.5 mg t.i.d. after meals; dose may be increased slowly to 4–5 mg t.i.d. and, if necessary, before bedtime.
Parkinsonism (transferring from other therapy).
Initial: Substitute 2.5 mg t.i.d.; slowly increase dose of procyclidine and decrease dose of other drug to appropriate maintenance levels.
Drug-induced extrapyramidal symptoms.
Initial: 2.5 mg t.i.d.; increase to maintenance dose of 10–20 mg/day.
Additional Drug Interaction: ↑ Effectiveness of levodopa if used together; such combined use not recommended in clients with psychoses.

NURSING CONSIDERATIONS

See also *Nursing Considerations* for *Cholinergic Blocking Agents,* Chapter 49.
Evaluate
• ↓ Muscle spasm and rigidity

• Control of drug-induced extrapyramidal manifestations

Propantheline bromide

(proh-**PAN**-thih-leen)
Pregnancy Category: C
Norpanth, Pro-Banthine **(Rx)**

See also *Cholinergic Blocking Agents,* Chapter 49.
How Supplied: *Tablet:* 7.5 mg, 15 mg
Action/Kinetics: Duration: 6 hr. Metabolized in the liver and excreted through the urine.
Uses: Adjunct in peptic ulcer therapy. Spastic and inflammatory disease of GI and urinary tracts. Control of salivation and enuresis. Duodenography. Urinary incontinence.

Dosage

• **Tablets**

Adults: 15 mg 30 min before meals and 30 mg at bedtime. Reduce dose to 7.5 mg t.i.d. for mild symptoms, geriatric clients, or clients of small stature. **Pediatric:** 0.375 mg/kg (10 mg/m^2) q.i.d. with dose being adjusted as needed.
Special Concerns: Safety and effectiveness for use in children with peptic ulcer have not been established.

NURSING CONSIDERATIONS

See also *Nursing Considerations* for *Cholinergic Blocking Agents,*Chapter 49.

Assessment

1. Document indications for therapy and type and onset of symptoms.
2. A liquid diet is recommended during initiation of therapy in clients with edematous duodenal ulcer.

Client/Family Teaching

1. Drug may cause drowsiness or dizziness. Do not drive or operate equipment until drug effects are realized.
2. Visual acuity may be impaired; dark glasses may be necessary.
3. Increase dietary intake of fluids and fiber to minimize the constipating effects of drug therapy.
4. Report any symptoms of urinary retention and persistent constipation.

Evaluate

• Relief of GI pain R/T PUD
• Control of urinary incontinence

Scopolamine hydrobromide

(scoh-**POLL**-ah-meen)
Pregnancy Category: C
Hyoscine Hydrobromide, Isopto Hyoscine Ophthalmic **(Rx)**

Scopolamine transdermal therapeutic system

(scoh-**POLL**-ah-meen)
Pregnancy Category: C
Transderm-Scop, Transderm-V ✱ **(Rx)**

See also *Cholinergic Blocking Agents,* Chapter 49.
How Supplied: Scopolamine hydrobromide: *Injection:* 0.4 mg/mL, 1 mg/mL; *Ophthalmic Solution:* 0.25%. Scopolamine transdermal therapeutic system: *Film, extended release:* 0.5 mg/24 hr
Action/Kinetics: Scopolamine is an anticholinergic with CNS depressant effects. It produces amnesia when given with morphine or meperidine. In the presence of pain, delirium may be produced. Scopolamine dilates the pupil and paralyzes the muscle required to accommodate for close vision (cycloplegia). This enables the physician to examine the inner structure of the eye, including the retina, as well as to examine refractive errors of the lens without automatic accommodation by the client. Tolerance may develop if scopolamine is used alone. When used for refraction: **peak for mydriasis,** 20–30 min; **peak for cycloplegia:** 30–60 min; **duration:** 24 hr (residual cycloplegia and mydriasis may last for 3–7 days). Recovery time can be reduced by using 1–2 gtt pilocarpine

(1% or 2%). To reduce absorption, pressure should be applied over the nasolacrimal sac for 2–3 min.

The transdermal therapeutic system contains 1.5 mg scopolamine, which is slowly released from a mineral oil–polyisobutylene matrix. Approximately 0.5 mg is released from the system per day.

Uses: Ophthalmic: Cycloplegic refraction. Pre- and postoperative mydriasis during eye surgery. Dilate the pupil in treatment of uveitis, posterior synechiae, preoperative or postoperative iridocyclitis. *Investigational:* Prophylaxis of synechaie, treatment of iridocyclitis. **Parenteral:** Antiemetic, antivertigo. Preanesthetic sedation and obstetric amnesia. Antiarrhythmic during anesthesia and surgery. **Transdermal:** Antiemetic, antivertigo. Prevention of motion sickness.

Dosage

- **Ophthalmic Solution**

Cycloplegic refraction.

Adults: 1–2 gtt of the 0.25% solution in the conjunctiva 1 hr prior to refraction; **children:** 1 gtt of the 0.25% solution b.i.d. for 2 days prior to refraction.

Uveitis.

Adults and children: 1 gtt of the 0.25% solution in the conjunctiva 1–4 times/day, depending on the severity of the condition.

Treatment of posterior synechiae.

Adults and children: 1 gtt of the 0.25% solution q min for 5 min. (1 gtt of either a 2.5% or 10% solution of phenylephrine instilled q min for 3 min will enhance the effect of scopolamine.)

Mydriasis for diagnostic procedures.

Adults and children: 1 gtt of the 0.25% solution in the conjunctiva as needed to maintain mydriasis.

Postoperative mydriasis.

Adults: 1 gtt of the 0.25% solution once daily. For dark brown irides, administration 2 or 3 times/day may be required.

Pre- or Postoperative iridocyclitis.

Adults and children: 1 gtt of the 0.25% solution 1–4 times/day as required. The pediatric dose should be individualized based on age, weight, and severity of the inflammation.

- **Injection (IM, IV, SC)**

Anticholinergic, antiemetic.

Adults: 0.3–0.6 mg (single dose). **Pediatric:** 0.006 mg/kg (0.2 mg/m^2) as a single dose.

Prophylaxis of excessive salivation and respiratory tract secretions in anesthesia.

Adults: 0.2–0.6 mg 30–60 min before induction of anesthesia. **Pediatric (given IM): 8–12 years:** 0.3 mg; **3–8 years:** 0.2 mg; **7 months–3 years:** 0.15 mg; **4–7 months:** 0.1 mg. Not recommended for children less than 4 months of age.

Adjunct to anesthesia, sedative-hypnotic.

Adults: 0.6 mg t.i.d–q.i.d.

Adjunct to anesthesia, amnesia.

Adults: 0.32–0.65 mg.

- **Transdermal system**

Antiemetic, antivertigo.

Adults: 1 transdermal system placed on the postauricular skin to deliver 0.5 mg over 3 days (apply at least 4 hr before antiemetic effect is required). The Canadian product delivers 1 mg over a 3-day period; it should be applied about 12 hr before the antiemetic effect is desired.

Administration/Storage

1. Drops are instilled into the conjunctival sac followed by digital pressure for 2-3 min after instillation.
2. Scopolamine should not be administered alone for pain because it may cause delirium. Use an analgesic or sedative in this event.
3. The solution should be protected from light.
4. With the transdermal system:
   - wash hands before and after application
   - apply at least 4 hr before desired effect
   - apply to a clean, nonhairy site, behind the ear
   - use pressure to apply the patch to ensure contact with the skin
   - replace with a new system if patch becomes dislodged
   - system is water-proof so bathing and swimming are permitted

• system effects last for 3 days

Additional Contraindications: For transdermal therapeutic system: Children, lactating women. Ophthalmic use contraindicated in glaucoma, infants less than 3 months of age.

Special Concerns: Use with caution in children, infants, geriatric clients, diabetes, hypo- or hyperthyroidism, narrow anterior chamber angle. Use for prophylaxis of excess secretions is not recommended for children less than 4 months of age. The transdermal system is not recommended for children.

Additional Side Effects: Disorientation, delirium, increased HR, decreased respiratory rate. *Ophthalmologic:* Blurred vision, stinging, increased intraocular pressure. Long-term use may cause irritation, photophobia, conjunctivitis, hyperemia, or edema.

NURSING CONSIDERATIONS

See also *Nursing Considerations* for *Cholinergic Blocking Agents,* Chapter 49.

Assessment

1. Document indications for therapy and type and onset of symptoms. List other agents prescribed and the outcome.
2. Assess for additional side effects and for tolerance after a long course of therapy.
3. Before administering eyedrops, check whether client has a history of angle-closure glaucoma because the drug may precipitate an acute glaucoma crisis.
4. Observe closely during initial therapy. Some clients experience toxic delirium with therapeutic doses. Have physostigmine available to reverse drug effects.

Client/Family Teaching

1. Review appropriate method of administration and advise to take only as directed.
2. Advise not to drive a car or operate dangerous machinery because the drug may cause drowsiness, confusion, disorientation, and, when used ophthalmologically, blurred vision and dilated pupils.
3. Warn that scopolamine may temporarily impair vision when instilled in the eye. Advise to wear dark glasses if photosensitivity occurs.
4. Provide a printed list of side effects that should be reported.
5. Report any evidence of urinary retention and constipation. Increase fluids and bulk in diet to prevent constipation.
6. Use gum, sugarless candies, and frequent mouth rinses to alleviate symptoms of dry mouth.
7. Avoid alcohol and any other CNS depressants during drug therapy.

Evaluate

• Effective control of vomiting
• Preoperative sedation; postoperative amnesia
• Desired amount of mydriasis
• Prevention of motion sickness

Trihexyphenidyl hydrochloride

(try-hex-ee-**FEN**-ih-dill)

Pregnancy Category: C

Apo-Trihex ✱, Artane, Artane Sequels, PMS-Trihexyphenidyl ✱, Trihexy-2 and -5 **(Rx)**

See also *Cholinergic Blocking Agents,* Chapter 49, and *Antiparkinson Agents,* Chapter 46.

How Supplied: *Elixir:* 2 mg/5 mL; *Tablet:* 2 mg, 5 mg

Action/Kinetics: Synthetic anticholinergic, which relieves rigidity but has little effect on tremors. Causes a direct antispasmodic effect on smooth muscle. Has a high incidence of side effects. Small doses cause CNS depression, whereas larger doses may result in CNS excitation. **Onset, PO:** 60 min. **Duration, PO:** 6–12 hr.

Uses: Adjunct in the treatment of all types of parkinsonism (often used as adjunct with levodopa). Drug-induced extrapyramidal symptoms. Sustained-release medication is for maintenance dosage only.

Dosage

- **Elixir, Extended-Release Capsules, Tablets**

Parkinsonism.

Initial (day 1): 1–2 mg; **then,** increase by 2 mg q 3–5 days until daily dose is 6–10 mg given in divided doses. Some clients may require 12–15 mg/day (especially those with postencephalitic parkinsonism).

Adjunct with levodopa.

Adults: 3–6 mg/day in divided doses.

Drug-induced extrapyramidal reactions.

Initial: 1 mg/day; **then,** increase as needed to total daily dose of 5–15 mg. **Maintenance, Extended-Release Capsules:** 5–10 mg 1–2 times/day.

Additional Contraindications: Arteriosclerosis and hypersensitivity to drug.

Additional Side Effects: Serious CNS stimulation (restlessness, insomnia, delirium, agitation) and psychotic manifestations.

Additional Drug Interaction: ↑ Effectiveness of levodopa if used together; such combined use not recommended in clients with psychoses.

NURSING CONSIDERATIONS

See also *Nursing Considerations* for *Cholinergic Blocking Agents,* Chapter 49, and *Antiparkinson Agents,* Chapter 46.

Interventions

1. This drug has a high incidence of side effects; early detection and intervention are imperative.
2. Determine any added adverse CNS reactions to the drug. Note any evidence of extrapyramidal symptoms or an increase in restlessness, complaints of insomnia, agitation, or psychotic manifestations and report as drug dosage may need to be adjusted.
3. Monitor and record I&O, noting any urinary retention or constipation.

Client/Family Teaching

1. Take with or after meals to minimize GI upset.
2. Caution that drug may cause dizziness or drowsiness and othostatic effects.
3. Increase fluids and bulk in diet to prevent constipation.
4. May impair perspiration so avoid overheating and hot weather exposures.
5. Provide a printed list of adverse drug effects, stressing those that require immediate reporting.

Evaluate

- Control of symptoms of parkinsonism
- Prevention of drug-induced extrapyramidal symptoms

CHAPTER FIFTY

Sympathomimetic (Adrenergic) Drugs

See also the following individual entries:

Albuterol
Bitolterol Mesylate
Dobutamine Hydrochloride
Dopamine Hydrochloride
Ephedrine Sulfate
Epinephrine
Epinephrine Bitartrate
Epinephrine Borate
Epinephrine Hydrochloride
Ethylnorepinephrine Hydrochloride
Isoetharine Hydrochloride
Isoetharine Mesylate
Isoproterenol
Isoproterenol Hydrochloride
Isoproterenol Sulfate
Levarterenol Bitartrate
Mephentermine Sulfate
Metaproterenol Sulfate
Metaraminol Bitartrate
Oxymetazolone Hydrochloride - See Chapter 58
Phenylephrine Hydrochloride
Phenylpropanolamine Hydrochloride
Pirbuterol Acetate
Pseudoephedrine Hydrochloride
Pseudoephedrine Sulfate
Salmeterol Xinafoate
Terbutaline Sulfate
Xylometazoline Sulfate - See Chapter 58

General Statement: The adrenergic drugs supplement, mimic, and reinforce the messages transmitted by the natural neurohormones— norepinephrine and epinephrine. These hormones are responsible for transmitting nerve impulses at the postganglionic neurojunctions of the sympathetic nervous system. The adrenergic drugs work in two ways: (1) by mimicking the action of norepinephrine or epinephrine (directly acting sympathomimetics) or (2) by causing or regulating the release of the natural neurohormones from their storage sites at the nerve terminals (indirectly acting sympathomimetics). Some drugs exhibit a combination of effects 1 and 2.

The myoneural junction is equipped with special receptors for the neurohormones. These receptors have been classified into two types: alpha (α) and beta (β), according to whether they respond to norepinephrine, epinephrine, or isoproterenol and to certain blocking agents. Alpha-adrenergic receptors are blocked by phenoxybenzamine and phentolamine, whereas beta-adrenergic receptors are blocked by propranolol and similar drugs.

Both alpha and beta receptors have been divided into subtypes. Thus adrenergic stimulation of receptors will manifest the following general effects:

Alpha-1-adrenergic: / Vasoconstriction, decongestion, constriction of the pupil of the eye, contraction of splenic capsule, contraction of the trigone-sphincter muscle of the urinary bladder.

Alpha-2-adrenergic: / Presynaptic to regulate amount of transmitter released; decrease tone, motility, and secretory activity of the GI tract (possibly involved in hypersecretory response also); decrease insulin secretion.

Beta-1-adrenergic: / Myocardial contraction (inotropic), regulation of heartbeat (chronotropic), improved impulse conduction, ↑ lipolysis.
Beta-2-adrenergic: / Peripheral vasodilation, bronchial dilation; ↓ tone, motility, and secretory activity of the GI tract; ↑ renin secretion.

In addition, adrenergic agents affect the exocrine glands, the salivary glands, and the CNS. The adrenergic stimulants discussed in this section act preferentially on one or more of the above receptor subtypes; their pharmacologic effect must be carefully monitored and balanced.

Uses: The primary determinant of usefulness of sympathomimetics is their selectivity of action. Sympathomimetic agents are mainly used for the treatment of shock induced by sudden cardiac arrest, decompensation, MI, trauma, bronchodilation, acute renal failure, drug reactions, anaphylaxis. Adrenergic drugs are also used to reverse bronchospasm caused by bronchial asthma, emphysema, exercise-induced bronchospasm, chronic bronchitis, bronchiectasis, or other obstructive pulmonary disease. Drugs with beta-receptor activity are combined with an anti-inflammatory drug for moderate asthma and with an oral corticosteroid for severe asthma. Sympathomimetic drugs having predominantly alpha-receptor activity are used for the relief of nasal and nasopharyngeal congestion due to rhinitis, sinusitis, head colds. See individual drugs.

Contraindications: Tachycardia due to arrhythmias; tachycardia or heart block caused by digitalis toxicity.

Special Concerns: Use with caution in hyperthyroidism, diabetes, prostatic hypertrophy, seizures, degenerative heart disease, especially in geriatric clients or those with asthma, emphysema, or psychoneuroses. Also, use with caution in clients with coronary insufficiency, CAD, ischemic heart disease, CHF, cardiac arrhythmias, hypertension, or history of stroke. Asthma clients who rely heavily on inhaled beta-2-agonist bronchodilators may increase their chances of death. Thus, these agents should be used to "rescue" clients but should not be prescribed for regular long-term use. Beta-2 agonists may inhibit uterine contractions.

Side Effects: See individual drugs; side effects common to most sympathomimetics are listed. *CV:* Tachycardia, arrhythmias, palpitations, BP changes, anginal pain, precordial pain, pallor, skipped beats, chest tightness, hypertension. *GI:* N&V, heartburn, anorexia, altered taste or bad taste, GI distress, dry mouth, diarrhea. *CNS:* Restlessness, anxiety, tension, insomnia, hyperkinesis, drowsiness, weakness, vertigo, irritability, dizziness, headache, tremors, general CNS stimulation, nervousness, shakiness, hyperactivity. *Respiratory:* Cough, dyspnea, dry throat, pharyngitis, ***paradoxical bronchospasm,*** irritation. *Other:* Flushing, sweating, ***allergic reactions***.

Symptoms of Overdose: Following inhalation: Exaggeration of side effects resulting in anginal pain, hypertension, hypokalemia, ***seizures.*** Following systemic use: CV symptoms include bradycardia, tachycardia, palpitations, extrasystoles, ***heart block,*** elevated BP, chest pain, hypokalemia. CNS symptoms include anxiety, insomnia, tremor, delirium, ***convulsions, collapse, and coma.*** Also, fever, chills, cold perspiration, N&V, mydriasis, and blanching of the skin.

Drug Interactions

Beta-adrenergic blocking agents / Inhibit adrenergic stimulation of the heart and bronchial tree; cause bronchial constriction; hypertension, asthma, not relieved by adrenergic agents
Ammonium chloride / ↓ Effect of sympathomimetics due to ↑ excretion by kidney
Anesthetics / Halogenated anesthetics sensitize heart to adrenergics—causes cardiac arrhythmias
Anticholinergics / Concomitant use aggravates glaucoma

Antidiabetics / Hyperglycemic effect of epinephrine may necessitate ↑ dosage of insulin or oral hypoglycemic agents
Corticosteroids / Chronic use with sympathomimetics may result in or aggravate glaucoma; aerosols containing sympathomimetics and corticosteroids may be lethal in asthmatic children
Digitalis glycosides / Combination may cause cardiac arrhythmias
Furazolidone / Furazolidone ↑ effects of mixed-acting sympathomimetics
Guanethidine / Direct-acting sympathomimetics ↑ effects of guanethidine, while indirect-acting sympathomimetics ↓ effects of guanethidine; also reversal of hypotensive effects of guanethidine
Lithium / ↓ Pressor effect of direct-acting sympathomimetics
MAO inhibitors / All effects of sympathomimetics are potentiated; symptoms include hypertensive crisis with possible intracranial hemorrhage, hyperthermia, convulsions, coma; death may occur
Methyldopa / ↑ Pressor response
Methylphenidate / Potentiates pressor effect of sympathomimetics; combination hazardous in glaucoma
Oxytocics / ↑ Chance of severe hypertension
Phenothiazines / ↑ Risk of cardiac arrhythmias
Reserpine / ↑ Risk of hypertension following use of direct-acting sympathomimetics and ↓ effect of indirect-acting sympathomimetics
Sodium bicarbonate / ↑ Effect of sympathomimetics due to ↓ excretion by kidney
Theophylline / Enhanced toxicity (especially cardiotoxicity); also ↓ theophylline levels
Thyroxine / Potentiation of pressor response of sympathomimetics
Tricyclic antidepressants / ↑ Effect of direct-acting sympathomimetics and ↓ effect of indirect-acting sympathomimetics

Dosage

See individual drugs.

NURSING CONSIDERATIONS

Administration/Storage

1. Review the list of drugs with which adrenergic agents interact.
2. Discard colored solutions.
3. When administering IV infusions of adrenergic drugs, use an electronic infusion device, administer in a monitored environment, and assess IV site frequently to ensure patency.
4. *Treatment of Overdosage:*

- For overdosage due to inhalation: General supportive measures with sedatives given for restlessness. Cautious use of metoprolol or atenolol may be used but these drugs may induce an asthmatic attack in clients with asthma.
- For systemic overdosage: Discontinue or decrease dose. General supportive measures. For overdose due to PO agents, emesis, gastric lavage, or charcoal may be helpful. In severe cases, propranolol may be used but this may cause airway obstruction. Phentolamine may be given to block strong alpha-adrenergic effects.

Assessment

1. Determine if the client has any history of sensitivity to adrenergic drugs.
2. Document any previous experience with drugs in this class and the outcome.
3. In taking the nursing history, note especially if the client has a history of tachycardia, endocrine disturbances, or respiratory tract problems.
4. Obtain baseline data regarding the client's general physical condition and hemodynamic status including ECG, VS, and appropriate lab data.
5. Document indications for therapy, contributing factors, and anticipated response.

Interventions

1. During the period of dosage adjustment, closely monitor and record BP and pulse.

2. Monitor I&O and continue to assess VS throughout therapy.

Client/Family Teaching

1. Discuss prescribed drug therapy and provide printed material regarding potential drug side effects.
2. Explain the adverse side effects of the drugs and the importance of reporting these to the provider.
3. Instruct client not to increase the dosage of medication and not to take the medication more frequently than prescribed while on maintenance doses. If symptoms become more severe, client should consult the provider.
4. Advise client to take the medication early in the day because these drugs may cause insomnia.
5. Explain that symptoms of fear or anxiety may be evident because these drugs mimic the body's stress response.
6. Avoid all OTC preparations without provider approval.

SPECIAL NURSING CONSIDERATIONS FOR ADRENERGIC BRONCHODILATORS

Assessment

1. Obtain a full baseline client history prior to starting the drug therapy.
2. Review the contraindications for adrenergic bronchodilators.
3. Note any previous experience client may have had with this class of drugs.
4. Assess and record the client's VS prior to administering the medication.
5. Obtain ABGs (or O_2 saturation) as a baseline against which to measure the influence of medication once therapy begins.

Interventions

1. Monitor BP and pulse after therapy begins to assess client's CV response.
2. Observe the effects of the drug on the client's CNS and if pronounced, adjust the dosage of medication and the frequency of administration.
3. If the client has status asthmaticus and abnormal ABGs, continue to provide oxygen mixture and ventilating assistance even though the symptoms appear to be relieved by the bronchodilator.
4. To prevent depression of respiratory effort, administer oxygen on the basis of the evaluation of the client's clinical symptoms and the ABGs or O_2 saturations.
5. If three to five aerosol treatments of the same agent have been administered within the last 6–12 hr, with only minimal relief, further treatment is not advised.
6. If the client's dyspnea worsens after repeated excessive use of the inhaler, paradoxical airway resistance may occur. Be prepared to assist with alternative therapy and respiratory support.

Client/Family Teaching

1. To improve lung ventilation and reduce fatigue during eating, start inhalation therapy upon arising in the morning and before meals.
2. A single aerosol treatment is usually enough to control an asthma attack. Overuse of adrenergic bronchodilators may result in reduced effectiveness, possible paradoxical reaction, and death from cardiac arrest.
3. Stress that regular, consistent use of the medication is essential for maximum benefit, but overuse can be life-threatening.
4. Increased fluid intake will aid in liquefying secretions, facilitating removal.
5. If more than three aerosol treatments in a 24-hr period are required for relief, contact the provider.
6. If dizziness or chest pain occurs, or if there is no relief when the usual dose of medication is used, consult the provider.
7. Avoid OTC preparations and any other adrenergic medications unless expressly ordered.
8. Demonstrate how to accomplish postural drainage. Explain how to cough productively and show family how to clap and vibrate the chest to promote good respiratory hygiene.
9. Explain the appropriate technique for use and care of prescribed inhalers and respiratory equipment.
10. For clients using inhalable medications and bronchodilators, advise

to use the bronchodilator first and to wait 5 min before administering the other medication unless otherwise ordered.

11. Advise client to avoid crowds during "flu seasons," to dress warmly in cold weather, and to stay in air conditioning during hot, humid days to prevent exacerbations of illness.

12. Instruct family/significant other in CPR.

Evaluate

- Knowledge and understanding of illness and evidence of compliance with prescribed medication regimen
- A positive clinical response as evidenced by ↓ symptoms for which the therapy was originally prescribed

Albuterol (Salbutamol)

(al-**BYOU**-ter-ohl)

Pregnancy Category: C

Novo-Salmol ✦, Proventil, Proventil Repetabs, Ventodisk ✦, Ventolin, Ventolin Rotacaps, Volmax **(Rx)**

See also *Sympathomimetic Drugs,* Chapter 50.

How Supplied: *Aerosol solid w/adapter:* 0.09 mg/inh; *Aerosol solid:* 0.09 mg/inh; *Capsule:* 200 mcg; *Solution:* 0.083%, 0.5%; *Syrup:* 1 mg/2.5 mL, 2 mg/5 mL; *Tablet:* 2 mg, 4 mg; *Tablet, Extended Release:* 4 mg, 8 mg

Action/Kinetics: Albuterol stimulates beta-2 receptors of the bronchi, leading to bronchodilation. Causes less tachycardia and is longer-acting than isoproterenol. Has minimal beta-1 activity. **Onset, PO:** 15–30 min; **inhalation,** 5–15 min. **Peak effect, PO:** 2–3 hr; **inhalation,** 60–90 min (after 2 inhalations). **Duration, PO:** 8 hr (up to 12 hr for extended-release); **inhalation,** 3–6 hr. Metabolites and unchanged drug excreted in urine and feces. **Tablets not to be used in children less than 12 years of age.**

Uses: Bronchial asthma; bronchospasm due to bronchitis or emphysema; bronchitis; reversible obstructive pulmonary disease in those 4 years of age and older; exercise-induced bronchospasm. Prophylaxis of bronchial asthma or bronchospasms. Parenteral for treatment of status asthmaticus. *Investigational:* Nebulized albuterol may be useful as an adjunct to treat serious acute hyperkalemia in hemodialysis clients.

Dosage

- **Aerosol for Inhalation**

Bronchodilation.

Adults and children over 12 years of age: 180 mcg (2 inhalations) q 4–6 hr (Ventolin aerosol may be used in children over 4 years of age). In some clients 1 inhalation (90 mcg) q 4 hr may be sufficient.

Prophylaxis of exercise-induced bronchospasm.

Adults and children over 12 years of age: 180 mcg (2 inhalations) 15 min before exercise.

- **Solution for Inhalation**

Bronchodilation.

Adults and children over 12 years of age: 2.5 mg t.i.d.–q.i.d. by nebulization (dilute 0.5 mL of the 0.5% solution with 2.5 mL sterile NSS and deliver over 5–15 min).

- **Capsule for Inhalation**

Bronchodilation.

Adults and children over 4 years of age: 200 mcg q 4–6 hr using a Rotahaler inhalation device. In some clients, 400 mcg q 4–6 hr may be required.

Prophylaxis of exercise-induced bronchospasm.

Adults and children over 12 years: 200 mcg 15 min before exercise using a Rotahaler inhalation device.

- **Syrup**

Bronchodilation.

Adults and children over 14 years of age: 2–4 mg t.i.d.–q.i.d., up to a maximum of 8 mg q.i.d. **Children, 6–14 years, initial:** 2 mg (base) t.i.d.–q.i.d.; **then,** increase as necessary to a maximum of 24 mg/day in divided doses. **Children, 2–6 years, initial:** 0.1 mg/kg t.i.d.;

then, increase as necessary up to 0.2 mg/kg, not to exceed 4 mg t.i.d.

- **Tablets**

Bronchodilation.

Adults and children over 12 years of age, initial: 2–4 mg (of the base) t.i.d.–q.i.d.; **then,** increase dose as needed up to a maximum of 8 mg t.i.d.–q.i.d. In geriatric clients or those sensitive to beta-agonists, start with 2 mg t.i.d.–q.i.d. and then increase dose gradually, if needed, to a maximum of 8 mg t.i.d.–q.i.d. **Children, 6–12 years of age, usual, initial:** 2 mg t.i.d.–q.i.d.; **then,** if necessary increase the dose in a step-wise fashion to a maximum of 24 mg/day in divided doses.

- **Extended-Release Tablets**

Bronchodilation.

Adults and children over 12 years of age: 4 or 8 mg (of the base) q 12 hr up to a maximum of 32 mg/day. Clients on regular release albuterol can be switched to the Repetabs in that a 4-mg extended-release tablet q 12 hr is equivalent to a regular 2-mg tablet q 6 hr.

Administration/Storage

1. Do not exceed the recommended dose.
2. If the dose of drug used previously does not provide relief, contact the provider immediately.
3. When using albuterol inhalers, do not use other inhalation medication unless specifically prescribed.
4. The contents of the container are under pressure. Therefore, do not store near heat or open flames and do not puncture the container.
5. When given by nebulization, either a face mask or mouthpiece may be used. Compressed air or oxygen with a gas flow of 6–10 L/min should be used, with a single treatment lasting from 5–15 min.
6. When given by IPPB, the inspiratory pressure should be from 10 to 20 cm water with the duration of treatment ranging from 5 to 20 min depending on the client and instrument control.
7. The MDI may also be administered on a mechanical ventilator through an adapter.
8. Extended-release tablets should be taken whole with the aid of liquids. They should not be chewed or crushed. The outer coating of Volmax Extended-Release Tablets is not absorbed and is excreted in the feces; the empty outer coating may be observed in the stool.

Additional Contraindication: Use during lactation.

Special Concerns: Dosage has not been established for the syrup in children less than 2 years of age, for tablets in children less than 6 years of age, and for extended-release tablets in children less than 12 years of age. Aerosol for prevention of exercise-induced bronchospasm is not recommended for children less than 12 years of age. Albuterol may delay preterm labor.

Additional Side Effects: *GI:* Diarrhea, dry mouth, increased appetite, epigastric pain. *CNS:* CNS stimulation, malaise, emotional lability, fatigue, lightheadedness, nightmares, disturbed sleep, aggressive behavior, irritability. *Respiratory:* Bronchitis, epistaxis, hoarseness (especially in children), nasal congestion, increase in sputum. *Hypersensitivity (may be immediate):* Urticaria, ***angioedema,*** rash, ***bronchospasm.*** *Miscellaneous:* Muscle cramps, pallor, teeth discoloration, conjunctivitis, dilated pupils, difficulty in urination, muscle spasm, voice changes, oropharyngeal edema.

Symptoms of Overdose: Seizures, anginal pain, hypertension, hypokalemia, tachycardia (rate may increase to 200 beats/min).

NURSING CONSIDERATIONS

See also *Nursing Considerations* for *Sympathomimetic Drugs,* Chapter 50.

Assessment

1. Obtain a baseline nursing history and assess client's CNS status before initiating therapy.
2. Assess lung sounds. Note evidence of client anxiety because this may contribute to air hunger.
3. Determine if the client is able to self-administer the medication.

Interventions
1. Maintain a calm, reassuring approach. If the client is acutely short of breath, do not leave unattended.
2. Monitor pulmonary status for effects of the therapy, adjusting the dose or frequency of medication, if needed.
3. Observe for evidence of allergic responses and be prepared to intervene.
Client/Family Teaching
1. Advise to take only as directed.
2. Do not put lips around inhaler; go two fingerbreadths away before attempting to activate and inhale.
3. Provide a spacer (if over 12 years old) with the MDI to enhance drug administration. Always thoroughly rinse mouth and spacer with water following each use to prevent oral fungal infections.
4. Work with client to establish dosing regimens that fit lifestyle, i.e., 1–2 puffs every 6 hr or 4 puffs 4 times a day but stress that usual dosing is every 4–6 hr with a PRN order. Instruct client to call if requiring more puffs more frequently than prescribed.
Evaluate: Improved breathing patterns and improved airway exchange.

Bitolterol mesylate
(bye-**TOHL**-ter-ohl)
Pregnancy Category: C
Tornalate Aerosol **(Rx)**

See also *Sympathomimetic Drugs,* Chapter 50.
How Supplied: *Aerosol Liquid w/Adapter:* 0.37 mg/inh; *Solution:* 0.2%
Action/Kinetics: Bitolterol is considered a prodrug in that it is converted by esterases in the body to the active colterol. Colterol is said to combine with beta-2-adrenergic receptors, producing dilation of bronchioles. Minimal beta-1-adrenergic activity. **Onset following inhalation:** 3–4 min. **Time to peak effect:** 30–60 min. **Duration:** 5–8 hr.
Uses: Prophylaxis and treatment of bronchial asthma and bronchospasms. Treatment of bronchitis, emphysema, bronchiectasis, and COPD. May be used with theophylline and/or steroids.

Dosage
• **Inhalation Aerosol**
Bronchodilation.
Adults and children over 12 years: 2 inhalations at an interval of 1–3 min q 8 hr (if necessary, a third inhalation may be taken). The dose should not exceed 3 inhalations q 6 hr or 2 inhalations q 4 hr.
Prophylaxis of bronchospasm.
Adults and children over 12 years: 2 inhalations q 8 hr.
Administration/Storage
1. Bitolterol is available in an MDI. With the inhaler in an upright position, the client should breathe out completely in a normal fashion. As the client is breathing in slowly and deeply, the canister and mouthpiece should be squeezed between the thumb and forefinger, activating the medication. The breath should be held for 10 sec and then slowly exhaled. A spacer may facilitate administration.
2. The medication should not be stored above 120°F.
3. The inhaler delivers 0.37 mg bitolterol per actuation.
Special Concerns: Safety has not been established for use during lactation and in children less than 12 years of age. Use with caution in ischemic heart disease, hypertension, hyperthyroidism, diabetes mellitus, cardiac arrhythmias, seizure disorders, or in those who respond unusually to beta-adrenergic agonists. There may be decreased effectiveness in steroid-dependent asthmatic clients. Hypersensitivity reactions may occur.
Laboratory Test Interferences: ↑ AST. ↓ Platelets, WBCs. Proteinuria.
Additional Side Effects: *CNS:* Hyperactivity, hyperkinesia, lightheadedness. *CV:* Premature ventricular contractions. *Other:* Throat irritation.
Drug Interactions: Additive effects with other beta-adrenergic bronchodilators.

NURSING CONSIDERATIONS

See also *Nursing Considerations* for *Sympathomimetic Drugs,* Chapter 50.

Evaluate:

• Improved airway exchange with ↓ airway resistance

• Asthma and bronchospasm prophylaxis

Dobutamine hydrochloride

(doh-**BYOU**-tah-meen)
Dobutrex **(Rx)**

See also *Sympathomimetic Drugs,* Chapter 50.

How Supplied: *Injection:* 12.5 mg/mL

Action/Kinetics: Stimulates beta-1 receptors (in the heart), increasing cardiac function, CO, and SV, with minor effects on HR. The drug decreases after load reduction although SBP and pulse pressure may remain unchanged or increase (due to increased CO). Dobutamine also decreases elevated ventricular filling pressure and helps AV node conduction. **Onset:** 1–2 min. **Peak effect:** 10 min. **t½:** 2 min. **Therapeutic plasma levels:** 40–190 ng/mL. Metabolized by the liver and excreted in urine.

Uses: Short-term treatment of cardiac decompensation secondary to depressed contractility due to organic heart disease or cardiac surgical procedures.

Dosage

• **IV Infusion**

Adults, individualized, usual: 2.5–15 mcg/kg/min (up to 40 mcg/kg/min). Rate of administration and duration of therapy depend on response of client, as determined by HR, presence of ectopic activity, BP, and urine flow.

Administration/Storage

1. Reconstitute solution according to directions provided by manufacturer. Dilution process takes place in two stages.

2. The more concentrated solution may be stored in refrigerator for 48 hr and at room temperature for 6 hr.

3. Before administration, the solution is diluted further according to the fluid needs of the client. This more dilute solution should be used within 24 hr.

4. Dilute solutions of dobutamine may darken. This does not affect the potency of the drug when used within the time spans detailed above.

5. The drug is incompatible with alkaline solutions.

6. Have available IV equipment to infuse volume expanders before therapy with dobutamine is started.

7. Medication should be administered using an electronic infusion device. Carefully reconstitute and calculate dosage according to the client's weight and the desired response.

Contraindication: Idiopathic hypertrophic subaortic stenosis.

Special Concerns: Safe use during pregnancy, childhood, or after AMI not established.

Side Effects: *CV:* Marked increase in HR, BP, and ***ventricular ectopic activity.*** Anginal and nonspecific chest pain, palpitations. *Other:* Nausea, headache, and SOB.

Additional Drug Interactions: Concomitant use with nitroprusside causes ↑ CO and ↓ pulmonary wedge pressure.

NURSING CONSIDERATIONS

See also *Nursing Considerations* for *Sympathomimetic Drugs,* Chapter 50.

Assessment

1. Document indications for therapy and onset of symptoms.

2. Note other agents prescribed and the outcome.

3. Determine that client is adequately hydrated prior to infusion.

Interventions

1. Be prepared to monitor CVP to assess vascular volume and right-sided cardiac pumping efficiency.

The normal range is 5–10 cm water (1–7 mm Hg).
2. An elevated CVP generally indicates disruption of CO, as in pump failure or pulmonary edema. A low CVP may indicate hypovolemia.
3. Be prepared to monitor PACWP to assess the pressures in the left atrium and left ventricle and to measure the efficiency of CO. The usual PACWP range is 6–12 mm Hg.
4. Monitor ECG and BP continuously during drug administration.
5. Obtain written parameters for SBP and titrate infusion as ordered.
6. Monitor and record I&O.
7. Monitor blood sugar in clients with diabetes as an increased insulin dose may be necessary.

Evaluate

- Improved CO and coronary blood flow
- SBP > 90 mm Hg
- ↑ Urinary output

Dopamine hydrochloride

(**DOH**-pah-meen)
Pregnancy Category: C
Intropin, Revimine ✦ **(Rx)**

See also *Sympathomimetic Drugs,* Chapter 50.
How Supplied: 40 mg/mL, 80 mg/mL, 160 mg/mL
Action/Kinetics: Dopamine is the immediate precursor of epinephrine in the body. Exogenously administered, dopamine produces direct stimulation of beta-1 receptors and variable (dose-dependent) stimulation of beta-1 receptors and variable (dose-dependent) stimulation of alpha receptors (peripheral vasoconstriction). Also, dopamine will cause a release of norepinephrine from its storage sites. These actions result in increased myocardial contraction, CO, and SV, as well as increased renal blood flow and sodium excretion. Exerts little effect on DBP and induces fewer arrhythmias than are seen with isoproterenol. **Onset:** 5 min. **Duration:** 10 min. **t½:** 2 min. Metabolized in liver and excreted in urine.
Uses: Cardiogenic shock, especially in MIs associated with severe CHF. Also shock associated with trauma, septicemia, open heart surgery, renal failure, and CHF. Especially suitable for clients who react adversely to isoproterenol. Poor perfusion of vital organs; hypotension due to poor CO. CHF in clients refractory to digitalis and diuretics. CO may be increased if dopamine is combined with dobutamine, isoproterenol, or sodium nitroprusside.

Dosage

- **IV Infusion**

Shock.
Initial: 1–5 mcg/kg/min; **then,** increase in increments of 1–4 mcg/kg/min at 10–30- min intervals until desired response is obtained.
Severely ill clients.
Initial: 5 mcg/kg/min; **then,** increase rate in increments of 5–10 mcg/kg/min up to 20–50 mcg/kg/min as needed.

Administration/Storage

1. Drug must be diluted before use—see package insert.
2. For reconstitution use dextrose or saline solutions: 200 mg/250 mL for a concentration of 0.8 mg/mL or 800 mcg/mL; 400 mg/250 mL for a concentration of 1.6 mg/mL or 1,600 mcg/mL.
3. Dilute solution is stable for 24 hr. Protect from light.
4. To prevent overloading system with excess fluid, clients receiving high doses of dopamine may receive more concentrated solutions than average.
5. Medication should be administered using an electronic infusion device. Carefully reconstitute and calculate dosage according to the client's weight.
6. Check infusion site frequently for extravasation. Sloughing and necrosis may occur. If extravasation occurs, local SC administration of diluted

phentolamine may decrease the sloughing (see package insert).

Additional Contraindications: Pheochromocytoma, uncorrected tachycardia or arrhythmias. Pediatric clients.

Special Concerns: Dosage has not been established in children. Dosage may have to be adjusted in geriatric clients with occlusive vascular disease.

Additional Side Effects: *CV:* Ectopic heartbeats, tachycardia, anginal pain, palpitations, vasoconstriction, hypotension, hypertension. *Other:* Dyspnea, headache, mydriasis.

Additional Drug Interactions

Diuretics / Additive or potentiating effect

Phenytoin / Hypotension and bradycardia

Propranolol / ↓ Effect of dopamine

NURSING CONSIDERATIONS

See also *Nursing Considerations* for *Sympathomimetics,* Chapter 50.

Assessment

1. Document indications for therapy and onset of symptoms.
2. Determine that client is hydrated prior to initiating infusion.

Interventions

1. Monitor VS and ECG during drug administration.
2. Obtain written parameters for SBP and titrate the infusion as ordered.
3. Monitor I&O. If medication is being administered for renal perfusion, infuse as ordered, usually less than 5 mcg/kg/min.
4. Be prepared to monitor CVP and pulmonary artery wedge pressures.
5. Monitor for ectopic heart beats, palpitations, anginal pain, or vasoconstriction. If these side effects occur, document and report.

Evaluate

- SBP > 90 mm Hg
- Improved organ perfusion and hemodynamics (e.g., ↑ CO, ↑ SV)
- ↑ Urine output

Ephedrine sulfate

(eh-**FED**-rin)

Pregnancy Category: C

Nasal decongestants: Kondon's Nasal, Pretz-D, Vatronol Nose Drops **(OTC)**. **Systemic:** Ephed II (Rx: Injection; OTC: Oral dosage forms)

See also *Sympathomimetic Drugs,* Chapter 50, and *Nasal Decongestants,* Chapter 58.

How Supplied: *Capsule:* 24.3 mg, 25 mg, 50 mg; *Injection:* 50 mg/mL; *Spray:* 0.25%

Action/Kinetics: Releases norepinephrine from synaptic storage sites. Has direct effects on alpha, beta-1, and beta-2 receptors, causing increased BP due to arteriolar constriction and cardiac stimulation, bronchodilation, relaxation of GI tract smooth muscle, nasal decongestion, mydriasis, and increased tone of the bladder trigone and vesicle sphincter. It may also increase skeletal muscle strength, especially in myasthenia clients. Ephedrine is more stable and longer-lasting than epinephrine. **Onset, IM:** 10–20 min; **PO:** 15–60 min; **SC:** <20 min. **Duration, IM, SC:** 30–60 min; **PO:** 3–5 hr. Excreted mostly unchanged through the urine (rate dependent on urinary pH—increased in acid urine).

Uses: Bronchial asthma and reversible bronchospasms associated with obstructive pulmonary diseases. Nasal congestion in vasomotor rhinitis, acute sinusitis, hay fever, and acute coryza. Parenterally to treat narcolepsy and depression. Parenterally as a vasopressor to treat shock.

Dosage

- **Capsules**

Bronchodilator, systemic nasal decongestant, CNS stimulant.

Adults: 25–50 mg q 3–4 hr. **Pediatric:** 3 mg/kg (100 mg/m^2) daily in four to six divided doses.

- **SC, IM, Slow IV**

Bronchodilator.

Adults: 12.5–25 mg; subsequent doses determined by client response. **Pediatric:** 3 mg/kg (100 mg/m^2) daily divided into four to six doses SC or IV.

Vasopressor.

Adults: 25–50 mg (IM or SC) or 5–25 mg (IV) repeated in 5 min if necessary. **Pediatric (SC, IM, IV):** 3

mg/kg (100 mg/m²) daily in four to six divided doses.

- **Topical (0.5% Drops, 1% Jelly, 0.25% Spray)**

Nasal decongestant.

Adults and children over 6 years: 2–3 gtt of solution or small amount of jelly in each nostril q 4 hr. Should not be used topically for more than 3 or 4 consecutive days. Not to be used in children under 6 years of age unless so ordered by physician.

Administration/Storage

1. May administer 10 mg IV undiluted over at least 1 min.
2. Use only clear solutions and discard any unused solution with IV therapy.

Special Concerns: Geriatric clients may be at higher risk to develop prostatic hypertrophy. The drug may cause hypertension resulting in intracranial hemorrhage; it may also cause anginal pain in clients with coronary insufficiency or ischemic heart disease.

Additional Side Effects: *CNS:* Nervousness, shakiness, confusion, delirium, hallucinations. Anxiety and nervousness following prolonged use. *CV:* Precordial pain, ***excessive doses may cause hypertension sufficient to result in cerebral hemorrhage***. *GU:* Difficult and painful urination, urinary retention in males with prostatism, decrease in urine formation. *Miscellaneous:* Pallor, respiratory difficulty, hypersensitivity reactions. *Abuse:* Prolonged abuse can cause paranoid schizophrenia, tachycardia, poor nutrition and hygiene, dilated pupils, cold sweat, and fever.

Drug Interactions

Dexamethasone / Ephedrine ↓ effect of dexamethasone
Diuretics / Diuretics ↓ response to sympathomimetics
Guanethidine / ↓ Effect of guanethidine by displacement from its site of action
Methyldopa / Effect of ephedrine ↓ in methyldopa-treated clients

NURSING CONSIDERATIONS

See also *Nursing Considerations* for *Sympathomimetic Drugs,* Chapter 50, and *Nasal Decongestants,* Chapter 58.

Assessment

1. Document indications for therapy and onset and type of symptoms.
2. Assess mental status prior to beginning drug therapy.
3. Obtain baseline VS before initiating therapy. If the drug is being administered for hypotension, monitor BP frequently until stabilized.

Interventions

1. If the client has used ephedrine for prolonged periods of time, observe for drug resistance. Allow the client to rest without medication for 3–4 days, then resume therapy. The client will usually respond to the drug again. If there is no further response, document and report.
2. Monitor mental status regularly. Report any signs of depression, lack of interest in personal appearance, or complaints of insomnia or anorexia.
3. Monitor I&O. Elderly men may have difficulty and pain on urination. Be alert for urinary retention and report any difficulty in voiding.

Client/Family Teaching

1. Teach the client and family how to take and maintain a written record of radial pulse readings. Report an elevated or irregular pulse rate.
2. Notify provider if SOB is unrelieved by medication and accompanied by chest pain, dizziness, or palpitations.
3. Advise male clients to report any difficulty with voiding. This may be caused by drug-induced urinary retention.
4. Avoid any OTC drugs or alcohol.

Evaluate

- Improved airway exchange
- ↓ Nasal congestion and mucous production
- ↑ BP
- Control of narcolepsy

Epinephrine

(ep-ih-**NEF**-rin)
Pregnancy Category: C
Adrenalin Chloride Solution, Bronkaid Mist, Bronkaid Mistometer ✦, Epipen

✱, Epipen Jr. ✱, Primatene Mist Solution, Sus-Phrine (Both Rx and OTC)

Epinephrine bitartrate

(ep-ih-**NEF**-rin)
Pregnancy Category: C
Asthmahaler Mist, Bronitin Mist, Bronkaid Mist Suspension, Epitrate, Medihaler-Epi, Primatene Mist Suspension **(OTC)**

Epinephrine borate

(ep-ih-**NEF**-rin)
Pregnancy Category: C
Epinal Ophthalmic, EPPY/N 1/2%, 1%, 2% Ophthalmic Solutions **(Rx)**

Epinephrine hydrochloride

(ep-ih-**NEF**-rin)
Pregnancy Category: C
Adrenalin Chloride, AsthmaNefrin, Epifrin, Glaucon, microNefrin, Nephron, S-2 Inhalant, Vaponefrin (Both Rx and OTC)

See also *Sympathomimetic Drugs,* Chapter 50, and *Nasal Decongestants,* Chapter 58.

How Supplied: Epinephrine: *Aerosol Liquid:* 0.22 mg/inh, 0.25 mg/inh; *Aerosol Liquid w/Adapter:* 0.22 mg/inh; *Injection:* 1 mg/mL, 5 mg/mL; *Kit:* 0.5 mg/mL, 1 mg/mL; *Set.*
Epinephrine bitartrate: *Aerosol Liquid:* 0.3 mg/inh; *Aerosol Liquid w/Adapter:* 0.3 mg/inh
Epinephrine borate: *Opthalmic solution:* 0.5%, 1%, 2%
Epinephrine hydrochloride: *Injection:* 0.1 mg/mL, 1 mg/mL; *Solution:* 1:100, 1:1000; *Ophthalmic solution:* 0.5%, 1%, 2%

Action/Kinetics: Epinephrine, a natural hormone produced by the adrenal medulla, induces marked stimulation of alpha, beta-1, and beta-2 receptors, causing sympathomimetic stimulation, pressor effects, cardiac stimulation, bronchodilation, and decongestion. **Extreme caution must be taken never to inject 1:100 solution intended for inhalation—injection of this concentration has caused death. SC: Onset,** 6–15 min; **duration:** <1–4 hr. **Inhalation: Onset,** 1–5 min; **duration:** 1–3 hr. **IM, Onset:** variable; **duration:** <1–4 hr. Epinephrine is ineffective when given PO.

Uses: Cardiac arrest, Stokes-Adams syndrome, low CO following ECB. To prolong the action of local anesthetics. As a hemostatic during ocular surgery; treatment of conjunctival congestion during surgery; to induce mydriasis during surgery; treat ocular hypertension during surgery. Topically to control bleeding. Acute bronchial asthma, bronchospasms due to emphysema, chronic bronchitis, or other pulmonary diseases. Treatment of anaphylaxis, angioedema, anaphylactic shock, drug-induced allergic reactions, transfusion reactions, insect bites or stings. As an adjunct in the treatment of open-angle glaucoma. To produce mydriasis, to treat conjunctivitis.

Dosage

- **Inhalation Aerosol, Bitartrate Inhalation Aerosol**

Bronchodilation.

Adults and children over 4 years of age: 0.2–0.275 mg (1 inhalation) of the Aerosol or 0.16 mg (1 inhalation) of the Bitartrate Aerosol; may be repeated after 1–2 min if needed. At least 3 hr should elapse before subsequent doses. Dosage not established in children less than 4 years of age.

- **Inhalation Solution**

Bronchodilation.

Adults and children over 6 years of age: 1 inhalation of the 1% solution (of the base); may be repeated after 1–2 min.

- **IM, IV, SC**

Bronchodilation using the solution (1:1,000).

Adults: 0.3–0.5 mg SC or IM repeated q 20 min–4 hr as needed; dose may be increased to 1 mg/dose. **Infants and children (except premature infants and full-term newborns:** 0.01 mg/kg (0.3 mg/m^2) SC up to a maximum of 0.5 mg/dose; may be repeated q 15 min for two doses and then q 4 hr as needed.

Bronchodilation using the sterile suspension (1:200).

Adults: 0.5–1.5 mg SC. **Infants and children, 1 month–12 years:** 0.025 mg/kg SC; **children less than 30 kg:** 0.75 mg as a single dose.

Anaphylaxis.

Adults: 0.2–0.5 mg SC q 10–15 min as needed, up to a maximum of 1 mg/dose if needed. **Pediatric:** 0.01 mg/kg (0.3 mg/m²) up to a maximum of 0.5 mg/dose; may be repeated q 15 min for two doses and then q 4 hr as needed.

Vasopressor.

Adults, IM or SC, initial: 0.5 mg repeated q 5 min if needed; **then,** give 0.025–0.050 mg IV q 5–15 min as needed. **Adults, IV, initial:** 0.1–0.25 mg given slowly. May be repeated q 5–15 min as needed. Or, use IV infusion beginning with 0.001 mg/min and increasing the dose to 0.004 mg/min if needed. **Pediatric, IM, SC:** 0.01 mg/kg, up to a maximum of 0.3 mg repeated q 5 min if needed. **Pediatric, IV:** 0.01 mg/kg/5–15 min if an inadequate response to IM or SC administration is observed.

Cardiac stimulant.

Adults, intracardiac or IV: 0.1–1 mg repeated q 5 min if needed. **Pediatric, intracardiac or IV:** 0.005–0.01 mg/kg (0.15–0.3 mg/m²) repeated q 5 min if needed; this may be followed by IV infusion beginning at 0.0001 mg/kg/min and increased in increments of 0.0001 mg/kg/min up to a maximum of 0.0015 mg/kg/min.

Adjunct to local anesthesia.

Adults and children: 0.1–0.2 mg in a 1:200,000–1:20,000 solution.

Adjunct with intraspinal anesthetics.

Adults: 0.2–0.4 mg added to the anesthetic spinal fluid.

• **Solution**

Antihemorrhagic, mydriatic.

Adults and children, intracameral or subconjunctival: 0.01%–0.1% solution.

Topical antihemorrhagic.

Adults and children: 0.002%–0.1% solution.

Nasal decongestant.

Adults and children over 6 years of age: Apply 0.1% solution as drops or spray or with a sterile swab as needed.

• **Bitartrate Ophthalmic Solution, Borate Ophthalmic Solution, Hydrochloride Ophthalmic Solution**

Glaucoma.

Adults: 1–2 gtt into affected eye(s) 1–2 times/day. Dosage has not been established in children.

Administration/Storage

1. *Never administer* 1:100 solution IV. Use 1:1,000 solution for IV administration.
2. Preferably use a tuberculin syringe to measure epinephrine, as the parenteral doses are small and the drug is potent. An error in measurement may be disastrous.
3. For direct IV administration to adults, the drug must be well diluted as a 1:1,000 solution and quantities of 0.05–0.1 mL of solution should be injected cautiously and slowly, taking about 1 min for each injection, noting the response of the client (BP and pulse). Dose may be repeated several times if necessary.
4. May be further diluted in D5/W or NSS and infused with an electronic infusion device for safety and accuracy.
5. Briskly massage site of SC or IM injection to hasten the action of the drug. Do not expose epinephrine to heat, light, or air, as this causes deterioration of the drug.
6. Discard if solution is reddish brown and after expiration date.
7. Because of the presence of sodium bisulfite as a preservative in the topical preparation, there may be slight stinging after administration.
8. The topical preparation should not be used in children under 6 years of age.
9. Ophthalmic use may result in discomfort, which decreases over time.
10. The ophthalmic preparation is not for injection or intraocular use.

11. If the ophthalmic product for glaucoma is used with a miotic, the miotic should be instilled first.

Additional Contraindications: Narrow-angle glaucoma. Lactation.

Special Concerns: May cause anoxia in the fetus. Administer parenteral epinephrine to children with caution. Syncope may occur if epinephrine is given to asthmatic children. Administration of the SC injection by the IV route may cause severe or fatal hypertension or cerebrovascular hemorrhage. Epinephrine may temporarily increase the rigidity and tremor of parkinsonism. Use with caution and in small quantities in the toes, fingers, nose, ears, and genitals or in the presence of peripheral vascular disease as vasoconstriction-induced tissue sloughing may occur.

Laboratory Test Interferences: False + or ↑ BUN, fasting glucose, lactic acid, urinary catecholamines, glucose (Benedict's), ↓ coagulation time. The drug may affect electrolyte balance.

Additional Side Effects: *CV:* ***Fatal ventricular fibrillation, cerebral or subarachnoid hemorrhage,*** obstruction of central retinal artery. ***A rapid and large increase in BP may cause aortic rupture, cerebral hemorrhage, or angina pectoris.*** *GU:* Decreased urine formation, urinary retention, painful urination. *CNS:* Anxiety, fear, pallor. Parenteral use may cause or aggravate disorientation, memory impairment, psychomotor agitation, panic, hallucinations, ***suicidal or homicidal tendencies,*** schizophrenic-type behavior. *Miscellaneous:* Prolonged use or overdose may cause elevated serum lactic acid with severe metabolic acidosis. *At injection site:* Bleeding, urticaria, wheal formation, pain. Repeated injections at the same site may cause necrosis from vascular constriction. *Ophthalmic:* Transient stinging when administered, conjunctival hyperemia, brow ache, headache, blurred vision, photophobia, poor night vision, eye ache, eye pain. Prolonged ophthalmic use may cause deposits of pigment in the cornea, lids, or conjunctiva. When used for glaucoma, maculopathy with a decrease in visual acuity may occur in the aphakic eye.

Additional Drug Interactions

Beta-adrenergic blocking agents / Initial effectiveness in treating glaucoma of this combination may ↓ over time

Chymotrypsin / Epinephrine, 1:100, will inactivate chymotrypsin in 60 min

NURSING CONSIDERATIONS

See also *Nursing Considerations* for *Sympathomimetic Drugs,* Chapter 50, and *Nasal Decongestants,* Chapter 58.

Assessment

1. Note any history of sulfite sensitivity.
2. Document indications for therapy and describe type and onset of symptoms and anticipated results.
3. Assess cardiopulmonary status and document findings.

Interventions

1. Closely monitor the client receiving solutions of IV epinephrine. Keep the environment as peaceful as possible and monitor ECG continuously.
2. Monitor BP and pulse every minute until the desired effect from the drug has been achieved. Then take it every 2–5 min until condition has stabilized, Once stable, monitor BP q 15–30 min as indicated.
3. Note any symptoms of shock such as cold, clammy skin, cyanosis, and loss of consciousness. If the client goes into hypovolemic shock, be prepared to assist with administering additional IV fluids.

Client/Family Teaching

1. Review appropriate indications, methods, and time frames for medication administration.
2. Explain method for administration carefully. When prescribed for anaphylaxis, advise to administer immediately and then to seek further medical evaluation and follow-up.
3. Report any increased restlessness, chest pain, or insomnia as dosage adjustment may be necessary.

4. Do not take any OTC drugs without provider approval.
5. Advise that the ophthalmic solution may burn on administration but should subside.
6. Use caution when performing activities that require careful vision as ophthalmic solution may diminish visual fields, cause double vision, and alter night vision.

Evaluate

- Return of cardiac activity following cardiac arrest
- Improved CO following EC bypass
- ↓ Intraocular pressures
- Reversal of S&S of anaphylaxis
- Improved airway exchange
- Promotion of hemostasis

Ethylnorepinephrine hydrochloride

(eth-ill-nor-ep-ih-**NEF**-rin)
Pregnancy Category: C
Bronkephrine **(Rx)**

See also *Sympathomimetic Drugs,* Chapter 50.
How Supplied: *Injection:* 2 mg/mL
Action/Kinetics: Ethylnorepinephrine stimulates beta-1 and beta-2 receptors similarly to epinephrine with minor effects on alpha receptors. Has little effect on BP and may be safer than epinephrine. Especially suitable for children, for diabetic asthmatics, and for clients refractory to isoproterenol or epinephrine. **Onset, SC or IM:** 5–10 min. **Duration:** 1–2 hr.
Uses: Treatment of bronchial asthma, bronchospasms due to emphysema or bronchitis, bronchiectasis, obstructive pulmonary disease.

Dosage

- **IM, SC**

Adults: 1–2 mg (0.5–1 mL of 0.2% solution); **pediatric:** 0.2–1 mg (0.1–0.5 mL of 0.2% solution).
Contraindications: Intraneural or intravascular injection.
Additional Side Effect: Elevated pulse rate.

NURSING CONSIDERATIONS

See *Nursing Considerations* for *Sympathomimetic Drugs,* Chapter 50.
Evaluate: Improved airway exchange.

Isoetharine hydrochloride

(eye-so-**ETH**-ah-reen)
Pregnancy Category: C
Arm-a-Med Isoetharine HCl, Beta-2, Bronkosol **(Rx)**

Isoetharine mesylate

(eye-so-**ETH**-ah-reen)
Pregnancy Category: C
Bronkometer **(Rx)**

See also *Sympathomimetic Drugs,* Chapter 50.
How Supplied: Isoetharine hydrochloride: *Solution:* 0.02%, 0.062%, 0.08%, 0.1%, 0.125%, 0.167%, 0.17%, 0.2%, 0.25%, 1%.
Isoetharine mesylate: *Aerosol liquid:* 0.34 mg/inh; *Aerosol liquid w/adapter:* 0.34 mg/inh
Action/Kinetics: Isoetharine has a greater stimulating activity on beta-2 receptors of the bronchi than on beta-1 receptors of the heart. Causes relief of bronchospasms. **Inhalation: Onset,** 1–6 min; **peak effect:** 15–60 min; **duration:** 1–3 hr. Partially metabolized; excreted in urine.
Uses: Bronchial asthma, bronchospasms due to chronic bronchitis or emphysema, bronchiectasis, pulmonary obstructive disease.

Dosage

- **Inhalation Solution**

Hand nebulizer.
Adults: 3–7 inhalations (use undiluted) of the 0.5% or 1% solution.
Oxygen aerosolization or IPPB.
Adults: Dose depends on strength of solution used (range: 0.062%–1%) and whether the solution is used undiluted or diluted according to the following: **1%:** 0.25–1 mL by IPPB or 0.25–0.5 mL by oxygen aerosolization diluted 1:3 with saline or other diluent. **0.2–0.5%:** 2 mL used undiluted; **0.2%:** 1.25–2.5 mL used undilut-

ed; **0.167 or 0.17%:** 3 mL used undiluted; **0.125%:** 2–4 mL used undiluted; **0.1%:** 2.5-5 mL used undiluted; **0.08%:** 3 mL used undiluted; **0.062%:** 4 mL used undiluted.

• **Mesylate Inhalation Aerosol**

Adults: 0.34 mg (1 inhalation) repeated after 1–2 min if needed; **then,** dose may be repeated q 4 hr.

Administration/Storage

1. One or 2 inhalations are usually sufficient. Wait 1 min after giving initial dose to ensure necessity of another dose.
2. Treatment usually does not need to be repeated more than q 4 hr.
3. Do not use if solution contains a precipitate or is brown.

Special Concerns: Dosage has not been established in children less than 12 years of age.

NURSING CONSIDERATIONS

See *Special Nursing Considerations for Adrenergic Bronchodilators* under *Sympathomimetics*

Assessment

1. Note any allergy to sulfites.
2. Document indications for therapy and note pulmonary findings.

Evaluate: Evidence of improved airway exchange with ↓ airway resistance.

Isoproterenol

(eye-so-proh-**TER**-ih-nohl)
Pregnancy Category: C
Isuprel Glossets **(Rx)**

Isoproterenol hydrochloride

(eye-so-proh-**TER**-ih-nohl)
Pregnancy Category: C
Dispos-a-Med Isoproterenol HCl, Isuprel, Isuprel Mistometer, Norisodrine Aerotrol **(Rx)**

Isoproterenol sulfate

(eye-so-proh-**TER**-ih-nohl)
Pregnancy Category: C
Medihaler-Iso **(Rx)**
Classification: Sympathomimetic, direct-acting

See also *Sympathomimetic Drugs*

How Supplied: Isoproterenol Hydrochloride: *Aerosol liquid:* 0.131 mg/inh; *Aerosol liquid w/adapter:* 0.131 mg/inh; *Injection:* 0.02 mg/mL, 0.2 mg/mL; *Solution:* 0.25%, 0.5%, 1%; *Tablet:* 10 mg
Isoproterenol Sulfate: *Aerosol liquid:* 0.08 mg/inh; *Aerosol liquid w/adapter:* 0.08 mg/inh

Action/Kinetics: Isoproterenol produces pronounced stimulation of both beta-1 and beta-2 receptors of the heart, bronchi, skeletal muscle vasculature, and the GI tract. In contrast to other sympathomimetics, isoproterenol produces a drop in BP. It also causes less hyperglycemia than epinephrine, but produces bronchodilation and the same degree of CNS excitation. Inhalation: Onset, 2–5 min; peak effect: 3–5 min; duration: 30–120 min. IV: Onset, immediate; duration: less than 1 hr. Sublingual: Onset, 15–30 min; duration: 1–2 hr. Partially metabolized; excreted in urine.

Uses: Bronchodilator in asthma, chronic pulmonary emphysema, bronchiectasis, bronchitis, and other conditions involving bronchospasms. Treat bronchospasms during anesthesia. Cardiac arrest, heart block, syncope due to complete heart block, Adams-Stokes syndrome. Certain cardiac arrhythmias including ventricular tachycardia, ventricular arrhythmias; syncope due to carotid sinus hypersensitivity. Hypoperfusion shock syndrome.

Dosage

Isoproterenol hydrochloride

• **IV Infusion**

Shock.

0.5–5 mcg/min (0.25–2.5 mL of 1:500,000 diluted solution).

Cardiac standstill and cardiac arrhythmias.

Adults: 5 mcg/min (1.25 mL of 1:250,000 solution/min).

• **IV**

Cardiac standstill and cardiac arrhythmias.

1–3 mL (0.02–0.06 mg) of 1:50,000 solution (range: 0.01–0.2 mg).

Bronchospasm during anesthesia. **Adults:** Dilute 1 mL of the 1:5,000 solution to 10 mL with sodium chloride injection or 5% dextrose solution and given an initial dose of 0.01–0.02 mg IV; repeat when necessary.

• **IM, SC**

Cardiac standstill and cardiac arrhythmias.

Adults: 1 mL (0.2 mg) of 1:5,000 solution (range: 0.02–1 mg).

Intracardiac (in extreme emergencies): 0.1 mL of 1:5,000 solution.

• **Hand Bulb Nebulizer**

Acute bronchial asthma.

Adults and children: 5–15 deep inhalations of the 1:200 solution. In adults 3–7 inhalations of the 1:100 solution may be useful. If there is no relief after 5–10 min, the doses may be repeated one more time. Repeat treatment up to 5 times/day may be necessary if there are repeat attacks.

Bronchospasm in chronic obstructive lung disease.

Adults and children: 5–15 deep inhalations of the 1:200 solution (in clients with severe attacks, 3–7 inhalations of the 1:100 solution may be useful). An interval of 3–4 hr should elapse between uses.

• **Metered Dose Inhalation**

Acute bronchial asthma.

Adults, usual: 1–2 inhalations beginning with 1 inhalation, and if no relief occurs within 2–5 min, a second inhalation may be used. **Maintenance:** 1–2 inhalations 4–6 times/day. No more than 2 inhalations at any one time or more than 6 inhalations in 1 hr should be taken.

Bronchospasm in chronic obstructive lung disease.

Adults and children: 1–2 inhalations repeated at no less than 3–4 hr intervals (i.e., 4–6 times/day).

• **Nebulization by Compressed Air or Oxygen**

Bronchospasms in chronic obstructive lung disease.

Adults and children: 0.5 mL of the 1:200 solution is diluted to 2–2.5 mL (for a concentration of 1:800–1:1,000). The solution is delivered over 15–20 min and may be repeated up to 5 times/day.

• **IPPB**

Bronchospasms in chronic obstructive lung disease.

Adults and children: 0.5 mL of a 1:200 solution diluted to 2–2.5 mL with water or isotonic saline. The solution is delivered over 10–20 min and may be repeated up to 5 times/day.

• **Sublingual**

Bronchospasms.

Adults: 10–20 mg depending on response (not to exceed 60 mg/day). **Pediatric:** 5–10 mg up to a maximum of 30 mg/day. Should not be given more than t.i.d. or more often than every 3–4 hr.

Isoproterenol sulfate

Dispensed from metered aerosol inhaler for bronchospasms. See dosage above for *Hydrochloride.*

Administration/Storage

1. Administration to children, except where noted, is the same as that for adults, because a child's smaller ventilatory exchange capacity will permit a proportionally smaller aerosol intake. For acute bronchospasms in children, use 1:200 solution.
2. In children, no more than 0.25 mL of the 1:200 solution should be used for each 10–15 min of programmed treatment.
3. Elderly clients usually receive a lower dose.
4. The sublingual tablets should not be crushed or chewed; rather, they should be placed under the tongue and allowed to disintegrate. Clients should not swallow saliva until absorption has taken place.

Special Concerns: Use with caution in the presence of tuberculosis. Safety and effectiveness have not been determined in children less than 12 years of age.

Additional Side Effects: *CV:* ***Cardiac arrest,*** Adams-Stokes attack, hypotension, precordial pain or distress. *CNS:* Hyperactivity, hyperkinesia. *Respiratory:* Wheezing, bronchitis, increase in sputum, ***bronchial edema and inflammation, pulmonary edema, paradoxical airway resistance.*** Excessive inhalation causes refractory bronchial obstruction. *Miscellaneous:* Flushing, sweating, swelling of the parotid gland. Sublingual administration may cause buccal ulceration. Side effects of drug are less severe after inhalation.

Drug Interaction: Beta-adrenergic blocking agents reverse the effects of isoproterenol.

NURSING CONSIDERATIONS

See also *Special Nursing Considerations* for *Adrenergic Bronchodilators* under *Sympathomimetics*

Assessment

1. Document indications for therapy and type and onset of symptoms.
2. Perform a thorough pulmonary assessment. Observe and report respiratory problems that seem to worsen after the administration of isoproterenol. Refractory reactions may necessitate withdrawal of the drug.

Client/Family Teaching

1. Rinse mouth with water to remove any drug residue and to minimize dryness, after inhalation therapy.
2. Maintain an adequate fluid intake of 2-3 L/day to help liquefy secretions.
3. The sputum and saliva may appear pink after inhalation therapy. This is due to the drug and the client should not become alarmed.
4. When also taking inhalant glucocorticoids advise to take isoproterenol first and to wait 15 min before using the second inhaler.
5. Do not use inhaler therapy more frequently than prescribed. Excessive use can cause severe cardiac and respiratory problems.
6. Identify the parotid gland. Instruct client to withhold the drug and report immediately if the parotid gland becomes enlarged.

Evaluate

- Improved airway exchange
- ↓ Bronchoconstriction and bronchospasms
- Restoration of stable cardiac rhythm with ↑HR and ↑CO

Levarterenol bitartrate (Norepinephrine bitartrate)

(lee-var-**TER**-ih-nohl)
Levophed **(Rx)**

See also *Sympathomimetic Drugs,* Chapter 50.

How Supplied: *Injection:* 1 mg/mL

Action/Kinetics: Levarterenol produces vasoconstriction (increase in BP) by stimulating alpha-adrenergic receptors. Also causes a moderate increase in contraction of heart by stimulating beta-1 receptors. Minimal hyperglycemic effect. **Onset:** immediate; **duration:** 1–2 min. Metabolized in liver and other tissues by the enzymes MAO and catechol-O-methyltransferase; however, the pharmacologic activity is terminated by uptake and metabolism in sympathetic nerve endings. Metabolites excreted in urine.

Uses: Hypotensive states caused by trauma, septicemia, blood transfusions, drug reactions, spinal anesthesia, poliomyelitis, central vasomotor depression, and MIs. Adjunct to treatment of cardiac arrest and profound hypotension.

Dosage

- **IV Infusion Only**

Effect on BP determines dosage, initial: 8–12 mcg/min or 2–3 mL of a 4-mcg/mL solution/min; **maintenance,** 2–4 mcg/min with the dose determined by client response.

Administration/Storage

1. Discard solutions that are brown or that have a precipitate.
2. Do not administer through the same tube as blood products.
3. The infusion should be continued until BP is maintained without therapy. Abrupt withdrawal of levarterenol should be avoided.
4. Levarterenol should be diluted in either D5W or 5% dextrose in saline.
5. For IV administration, a large vein

should be used, preferably the antecubital or subclavian. Veins with poor circulation should be avoided.
6. Administer IV solutions with an electronic infusion device. Monitor the rate of flow constantly.
7. Have phentolamine available for use at the site of extravasation to dilate local blood vessels and to minimize local necrosis.

Additional Contraindications: Hypotension due to blood volume deficiency (except in emergencies), mesenteric or peripheral vascular thrombosis, in halothane or cyclopropane anesthesia (due to possibilities of fatal arrhythmias). Pregnancy (may cause fetal anoxia or hypoxia).
Special Concerns: Use with caution in clients taking MAO inhibitors or tricyclic antidepressants.
Additional Side Effect: Drug may cause bradycardia that can be abolished by atropine.

NURSING CONSIDERATIONS

See also *Nursing Considerations* for *Sympathomimetic Drugs,* Chapter 50.

Assessment
1. Document indications for therapy, onset of symptoms, and causative factors.
2. Determine that client is adequately hydrated.

Interventions
1. During administration of levarterenol, the client should be in a closely monitored environment.
2. Monitor BP frequently. An arterial line or *Dinemapp* for continuous BP determinations should be used. ECG tracings, CVP, and PA wedge pressure readings are useful.
3. Monitor the pulse frequently, noting any signs of bradycardia. Have atropine readily available.
4. Monitor I&O. Report if urine output is less than 30 cc/hr.
5. Observe infusion site frequently for evidence of extravasation because ischemia and sloughing may occur. Check the area for blanching along the course of the vein. This could indicate permeability of the vein wall, which could allow leakage to occur. As a result, the IV site would need to be changed and phentolamine administered to the site of the extravasation.
6. The drug should be gradually withdrawn. Avoid an abrupt withdrawal. Clients may experience an initial rebound drop in BP.
7. Extra fluids parenterally may diminish rebound hypotension and help stabilize BP during withdrawal of the drug.

Evaluate
- ↑ BP
- Evidence of improved tissue perfusion
- Adequate urinary output (>30 mL/hr)

Mephentermine sulfate

(meh-**FEN**-ter-meen)
Wyamine **(Rx)**

See also *Sympathomimetic Drugs,* Chapter 50.
How Supplied: *Injection:* 15 mg/mL, 30 mg/mL
Action/Kinetics: Mephentermine acts by releasing norepinephrine from its storage sites. It has slight effects on alpha and beta-1 receptors and moderate effects on beta-2 receptors mediating vasodilation. The drug causes increased CO; also elicits slight CNS effects. **IV: Onset,** immediate; **duration:** 15–30 min. **IM: Onset,** 5–15 min; **duration:** 1–4 hr. Metabolized in liver. Excreted in urine within 24 hr (rate increased in acidic urine).
Uses: Hypotension due to anesthesia, ganglionic blockade, or hemorrhage (only as emergency treatment until blood or blood substitutes can be given).

Dosage
- **IV, IM**

Hypotension during spinal anesthesia.

IV, Adults: 30–45 mg; 30-mg doses may be repeated as required; or, **IV infusion, Adults and children:** 0.1% (1 mg/mL) mephentermine in D5W with the rate of infusion and duration dependent on client response. **IV, Pediatric:** 0.4 mg/kg (12 mg/m^2) as a single dose.

Prophylaxis of hypotension in spinal anesthesia.

IM, Adults: 30–45 mg 10–20 min before anesthesia. **IM, Pediatric:** 0.4 mg/kg (12 mg/m^2) as a single dose.

Shock following hemorrhage.

Not recommended, but IV infusion of 0.1% in dextrose 5% in water may maintain BP until blood volume is replaced.

Additional Contraindications: Hypotension due to phenothiazines; in combination with MAO inhibitors.

Special Concern: Safe use during pregnancy has not been established.

Additional Drug Interaction: Mephentermine will potentiate hypotensive effects of phenothiazines.

NURSING CONSIDERATIONS

See also *Nursing Considerations* for *Sympathomimetics,* Chapter 50.

Interventions: Record BP every 5 min until stable. Once BP has stabilized, take a reading every 15–30 min beyond the duration of the drug's action (IM 1–4 hr; IV 5–15 min).

Evaluate: Stabilization of BP.

Metaproterenol sulfate (Orciprenaline sulfate)

(met-ah-proh-**TER**-ih-nohl)

Pregnancy Category: C

Alupent, Arm-A-Med Metaproterenol Sulfate, Metaprel **(Rx)**

See also *Sympathomimetic Drugs,* Chapter 50.

How Supplied: *Aerosol liquid:* 0.65 mg/inh; *Aerosol liquid w/adapter:* 0.65 mg/inh; *Solution:* 0.4%, 0.6%, 5%; *Syrup:* 10 mg/5 mL; *Tablet:* 10 mg, 20 mg

Action/Kinetics: Metaproterenol markedly stimulates beta-2 receptors, resulting in relaxation of smooth muscles of the bronchial tree, as well as peripheral vasodilation. It has minimal effects on beta-1 receptors. It is similar to isoproterenol, but it has a longer duration of action and fewer side effects. Has minimal beta-1 activity. **Onset: Inhalation aerosol,** within 1 min; **peak effect:** 1 hr; **duration:** 1–5 hr. **Onset, hand bulb nebulizer or IPPB:** 5–30 min; **duration:** 4–6 hr after repeated doses. **PO: Onset,** 15–30 min; **Peak effect:** 1 hr. **Duration:** 4 hr. PO administration produces a marked first-pass effect. Metabolized in the liver and excreted through the kidney.

Uses: Bronchodilator in asthma, bronchitis, emphysema, and other conditions associated with reversible bronchospasms. Treatment of acute asthmatic attacks in children over 6 years of age.

Dosage

- **Syrup, Tablets**

Bronchodilation.

Adults and children over 27.2 kg or 9 years: 20 mg t.i.d.–q.i.d.; **children under 27.2 kg or 6–9 years of age:** 10 mg t.i.d.–q.i.d.; **children less than 6 years of age:** 1.3–2.6 mg/kg/day of the syrup has been studied.

- **Inhalation. Hand nebulizer**

Bronchodilation.

Usual dose is 10 inhalations (range: 5–15 inhalations) of undiluted 5% solution.

- **IPPB**

Bronchodilation.

0.3 mL (range: 0.2–0.3 mL) of 5% solution diluted to 2.5 mL saline or other diluent.

- **MDI**

Bronchodilation.

2–3 inhalations (1.30–2.25 mg) q 3–4 hr. Total daily dose should not exceed 12 inhalations (9 mg).

Administration/Storage

1. Instruct client to shake the container.
2. Unit dose vials should be refrigerated at 2°C–8°C (35°F–46°F).
3. The inhalant solution can be stored at room temperature, but ex-

cessive heat and light should be avoided.
4. The solution should not be used if it is brown or shows a precipitate.
5. The inhalant solutions should not be used more often than q 4 hr to relieve acute bronchospasms. In chronic bronchospastic disease, the dose can be given t.i.d.–q.i.d. A single dose of the nebulized drug may not completely abort an attack of acute asthma.

Special Concerns: Dosage of syrup or tablets not determined in children less than 6 years of age.

Additional Side Effects: *GI:* Diarrhea, bad taste or taste changes. *Respiratory:* Worsening of asthma, nasal congestion, hoarseness. *Miscellaneous:* Hypersensitivity reactions, rash, fatigue, backache, skin reactions.

Drug Interactions: Possible potentiation of adrenergic effects if used before or after other sympathomimetic bronchodilators.

NURSING CONSIDERATIONS

See also *Special Nursing Considerations for Adrenergic Bronchodilators* under *Sympathomimetics,* Chapter 50.

Client/Family Teaching

1. Report loss of effectiveness with prescribed dosage.
2. Review drug side effects that should be reported if evident.

Evaluate: Reports of symptomatic relief and improved airway exchange.

Metaraminol bitartrate

(met-ah-**RAM**-ih-nohl)
Pregnancy Category: C
Aramine **(Rx)**

See also *Sympathomimetic Drugs,* Chapter 50.

How Supplied: *Injection:* 10 mg/mL

Action/Kinetics: Metaraminol indirectly releases norepinephrine from storage sites and directly stimulates primarily alpha receptors and, to a slight extent, beta-1 receptors. The drug causes marked increases in BP due primarily to vasoconstriction and to a slight increase in CO. Reflex bradycardia is also manifested. CNS stimulation usually does not occur. **Onset: IV:** 1–2 min; **IM:** 10 min; **SC:** 5–20 min. **Duration, IV:** 20 min; **IM, SC:** About 60 min. Metabolized in the liver and excreted through the urine and feces. Urinary excretion of unchanged drug can be enhanced by acidifying the urine.

Uses: Hypotension associated with surgery, spinal anesthesia, hemorrhage, trauma, infections, and adverse drug reactions. Adjunct to the treatment of either septicemia or cardiogenic shock. *Investigational:* Injected intracavernosally to treat priapism due to phentolamine, papaverine, or other causes.

Dosage

- **IM, SC, IV**

Prophylaxis of hypotension.

Adults: 2–10 mg given IM or SC; **pediatric:** 0.01 mg/kg (3 mg/m²) IM or SC.

Hypotension.

Adults: 15–100 mg in 500 mL of 0.9% sodium chloride injection or 5% dextrose injection by IV infusion at a rate to maintain desired BP (up to 500 mg/500 mL has been used). **Pediatric:** 0.4 mg/kg (12 mg/m²) by IV infusion in a solution containing 1 mg/25 mL 0.9% sodium chloride injection or 5% dextrose injection.

Severe shock.

Adults: 0.5–5.0 mg by direct IV followed by IV infusion of 15–100 mg in 500 mL fluid. **Pediatric:** 0.01 mg/kg (0.3 mg/m²) by direct IV.

Administration/Storage

1. Do not inject IM in areas that seem to have poor circulation because sloughing has occurred with extravasation.
2. Use an electronic infusion device when administering IV drug therapy for more adequate control and titration of drug.

Additional Contraindication: As a substitute for blood or fluid replacement.

Special Concerns: Use with caution in cirrhosis and malaria. Hypertension and ischemic ECG changes may occur when used to treat priapism.

NURSING CONSIDERATIONS

See also *Nursing Considerations* for *Sympathomimetic Drugs,* Chapter 50.

Assessment

1. Document indications for therapy and type and onset of symptoms as well as any precipitating factors.
2. Ensure that client is adequately hydrated.

Interventions

1. Take BP every 15 min. Obtain written parameters for maintaining the SBP. Monitor ECG, I&O, and VS.
2. Frequently assess administration site because extravasation may result in tissue necrosis.

Evaluate: Effective management of hypotension with desired ↑ SBP.

Phenylephrine hydrochloride

(fen-ill-**EF**-rin)

Pregnancy Category: C

Nasal: Alconefrin 12, 25, and 50, Children's Nostril, Doktors, Duration, Neo-Synephrine Solution, Nostril, Rhinall, Vicks Sinex. **Ophthalmic:** AK-Dilate, AK-Nefrin Ophthalmic, Dionephrine ✱, Isopto Frin, Mydfrin 2.5%, Neo-Synephrine, Neo-Synephrine Viscous, Phenoptic, Phenylephrine Minims ✱, Prefrin Liquifilm, Relief. **Systemic:** Neo-Synephrine. (Rx: Injection and Ophthalmic Solutions 2.5% or greater; OTC: Nasal products and ophthalmic solutions 0.12% or less)

See also *Sympathomimetic Drugs,* Chapter 50, and *Nasal Decongestants,* Chapter 58.

How Supplied: *Chew Tablet:* 10 mg; *Injection:* 10 mg/mL; *Liquid:* 5 mg/5 mL; *Nasal Solution:* 0.125%, 0.25%, 0.5%, 1%; *Ophthalmic Solution:* 0.12%, 2.5%, 10%; *Nasal Spray:* 0.25%, 0.5%, 1%; *Suppository:* 0.25%

Action/Kinetics: Phenylephrine stimulates alpha-adrenergic receptors, producing pronounced vasoconstriction and hence an increase in both SBP and DBP; reflex bradycardia results from increased vagal activity. The drug also acts on alpha receptors producing vasoconstriction in the skin, mucous membranes, and the mucosa as well as mydriasis by contracting the dilator muscle of the pupil. It resembles epinephrine, but it has more prolonged action and few cardiac effects. **IV: Onset,** immediate; **duration:** 15–20 min. **IM. SC: Onset,** 10–15 min; **duration:** 0.5–2 hr for IM and 50–60 min for SC. *Nasal decongestion (topical):* **Onset:** 15–20 min; **duration:** 30 min–4 hr. *Ophthalmic:* **Time to peak effect for mydriasis,** 15–60 min for 2.5% solution and 10–90 min for 10% solution. **Duration:** 0.5–1.5 hr for 0.12%, 3 hr for 2.5%, and 5–7 hr with 10% (when used for mydriasis). Excreted in urine.

Phenylephrine is also found in Chlor-Trimetron Expectorant, Naldecon, Dimetane, and Dimetapp.

Uses: Systemic: Acute hypotensive states caused by peripheral circulatory collapse. To maintain BP during spinal anesthesia; to prolong spinal anesthesia. Paroxysmal SVT. **Nasal:** Nasal congestion due to allergies, sinusitis, common cold, or hay fever. **Ophthalmologic: 0.12%:** Temporary relief of redness of the eye associated with colds, hay fever, wind, dust, sun, smog, smoke, contact lens. **2.5% and 10%:** Decongestant and vasoconstrictor, treatment of uveitis with posterior synechiae, open-angle glaucoma, refraction without cycloplegia, ophthalmoscopic examination, funduscopy, prior to surgery.

Dosage

- **IM, IV, SC**

Vasopressor, mild–moderate hypotension.

Adults: 2–5 mg IM or SC repeated no more often than q 10–15 min; or, 0.2 mg IV repeated no more often than q 10–15 min. **Pediatric:** 0.1 mg/kg (3 mg/m^2) IM or SC repeated in 1–2 hr if needed.

Vasopressor, severe hypotension and shock.

Adults: 10 mg by IV infusion using 500 mL 5% dextrose injection or 0.9% sodium chloride injection given at a rate of 0.1–0.18 mg/min initial; **then,** give at a rate of 0.04–0.06 mg/min.

Prophylaxis of hypotension during spinal anesthesia.

Adults: 2–3 mg IM or SC 3–4 min before anesthetic given; **pediatric:** 0.044–0.088 mg/kg IM or SC.

Hypotensive emergencies during spinal anesthesia.

Adults, initial: 0.2 mg IV; dose can be increased by no more than 0.2 mg for each subsequent dose not to exceed 0.5 mg/dose.

• **Nasal Solution**

Adults and children over 12 years of age: 2–3 gtt of the 0.25% or 0.5% solution into each nostril q 3–4 hr as needed. In resistant cases, the 1% solution can be used but no more often than q 4 hr. **Children, 6–12 years of age:** 2–3 gtt of the 0.25% solution q 3–4 hr as needed. **Infants, greater than 6 months of age:** 1–2 gtt of the 0.16% solution into each nostril q 3–4 hr.

• **Ophthalmic Solution, 0.12%, 2.5%, 10%**

Vasoconstriction, pupillary dilation.

1 gtt of the 2.5% or 10% solution on the upper limbus a few minutes following 1 gtt of topical anesthetic (prevents stinging and dilution of solution by lacrimation). An additional drop may be needed after 1 hr.

Uveitis.

1 gtt of the 2.5% or 10% solution with atropine. To free recently formed posterior synechiae, 1 gtt of the 2.5% or 10% solution to the upper surface of the cornea. Treatment should be continued the following day, if needed. In the interim, hot compresses should be applied for 5–10 min t.i.d. using 1 gtt of 1% or 2% atropine sulfate before and after each series of compresses.

Glaucoma.

1 gtt of 10% solution on the upper surface of the cornea as needed. Both the 2.5% and 10% solutions may be used with miotics in clients with open-angle glaucoma.

Surgery.

2.5% or 10% solution 30–60 min before surgery for wide dilation of the pupil.

Refraction.

Adults: 1 gtt of a cycloplegic (homatropine HBr, atropine sulfate, cyclopentolate, tropicamide HCl, or a combination of homatropine and cocaine HCl) in each eye followed in 5 min with 1 gtt of 2.5% phenylephrine solution and in 10 min with another drop of cycloplegic. The eyes are ready for refraction in 50–60 min. **Children:** 1 gtt of atropine sulfate, 1%, in each eye followed in 10–15 min with 1 gtt of phenylephrine solution, 2.5%, and in 5–10 min with a second drop of atropine sulfate, 1%. The eyes are ready for refraction in 1–2 hr.

Ophthalmoscopic examination.

1 gtt of 2.5% solution in each eye. The eyes are ready for examination in 15–30 min and the effect lasts for 1–3 hr.

Minor eye irritations.

1–2 gtt of the 0.12% solution in the eye(s) up to q.i.d. as needed.

Administration/Storage

1. Store drug in a brown bottle and away from light.
2. Anticipate that before administering the 10% ophthalmic solution, instillation of a drop of local anesthetic will be necessary.
3. When the drug is used as a nasal decongestant, instruct clients to blow their noses before administration.
4. For IV administration, dilute each 1 mg with 9 mL of sterile water and administer over 1 min. Further dilution of 10 mg in 500 mL of dextrose, Ringer's, or saline solution may be titrated to client response.

5. When drug is used parenterally, monitor infusion site closely to avoid extravasation. If evident, local SC administration of phentolamine should be performed to prevent tissue necrosis.
6. Prolonged exposure to air or strong light may result in oxidation and discoloration. Solution should not be used if it changes color, becomes cloudy, or contains a precipitate.

Special Concerns: Use with caution in geriatric clients, in severe arteriosclerosis, and during pregnancy and lactation. Nasal and ophthalmic use of phenylephrine may be systemically absorbed. Use of the 2.5% or 10% ophthalmic solutions in children may cause hypertension and irregular heart beat. In geriatric clients, chronic use of the 2.5% or 10% ophthalmic solutions may cause rebound miosis and a decreased mydriatic effect.

Side Effects: Reflex bradycardia. Overdosage may cause ventricular extrasystoles and short paroxysm or ***ventricular tachycardia,*** tingling of the extremities, and a sensation of heavy head. *Ophthalmologic:* Rebound miosis and decreased mydriatic response in geriatric clients, blurred vision.

NURSING CONSIDERATIONS

See also *Nursing Considerations* for *Sympathomimetic Drugs,* Chapter 50, and *Nasal Decongestants,* Chapter 58.

Assessment

1. Document indications for therapy and type and onset of symptoms.
2. During IV administration monitor cardiac rhythm and BP continuously until stabilized, noting any evidence of bradycardia or arrhythmias.

Client/Family Teaching

1. Demonstrate and review the appropriate method for drug administration.
2. Advise that ophthalmic instillations and nasal decongestants may produce systemic sympathomimetic effects. Stress that chronic excessive use may cause rebound congestion. Provide with printed material explaining how to identify these effects and instruct to report should they occur.
3. Wear sunglasses in bright light. Symptoms of photosensitivity and blurred vision should be reported if they persist after 12 hr.
4. When using ophthalmic solution, report if there is no relief of symptoms within 2 days.
5. When using the drug for nasal decongestion, report if there is no relief of symptoms within 3 days. Rebound nasal congestion may occur with longer therapy.

Evaluate

- ↑ BP
- Termination of PSVT
- Relief of nasal congestion
- ↓ Conjunctivitis and allergic manifestations
- Dilatation of pupils

Phenylpropanolamine hydrochloride

(fen-ill-**proh**-pah-**NOHL**-ah-meen)

Acutrim 16 Hour, Acutrim Late Day, Acutrim II Maximum Strength, Control, Dex-A-Diet Maximum Strength and Maximum Strength Caplets, Dexatrim, Dexatrim Maximum Strength and Maximum Strength Caplets, Dexatrim Maximum Strength Pre-Meal Caplets, Efed II Yellow, Maigret-50, Phenyldrine, Propagest, Rhindecon, Unitrol (OTC except Maigret-50 and Rhindecon)

See also *Stimulants,* Chapter 47, and *Sympathomimetic Drugs,* Chapter 50.

How Supplied: *Capsule:* 37.5 mg; *Capsule, Extended Release:* 75 mg; *Tablet:* 25 mg, 37.5 mg, 50 mg; *Tablet, Extended Release:* 75 mg

Action/Kinetics: Phenylpropanolamine is thought to stimulate both alpha and beta receptors as well as to act indirectly through release of norepinephrine from storage sites. Increases in BP are due mainly to increased CO rather than to vasoconstriction; has minimal CNS effects. The drug acts on alpha-adrenergic receptors to produce a decongestant effect in the nasal mucosa. **Onset, decongestant:** 15–30 min; **peak**

plasma levels: 1–2 hr; **duration, capsules and tablets:** 3 hr; **extended-release tablets:** 12–16 hr. **Peak plasma levels:** 100 ng. **t½:** 3–4 hr. Eighty percent to 90% excreted in the urine unchanged.

Uses: Nasal congestion due to colds, hay fever, allergies. Short-term (8–12 weeks) treatment of exogenous obesity in conjunction with a weight reduction program including reduced caloric intake, exercise, and behavior modification. *Investigational:* Mild to moderate stress incontinence in women.

Dosage

- **Capsules, Tablets**

Decongestant.

Adults: 25 mg/ q 4 hr or 50 mg/ q 6–8 hr (not to exceed 150 mg/day); **Children, 2–6 years:** 6.25 mg/ q 4 hr, not to exceed 37.5 mg in 24 hr; **6–12 years:** 12.5 mg/ q 4 hr, not to exceed 75 mg in 24 hr.

Anorexiant.

Adults: 25 mg t.i.d. 30 min before meals, not to exceed 75 mg in 24 hr.

- **Extended-Release Capsules, Extended-Release Tablets**

Decongestant.

Adults: 75 mg/ q 12 hr.

Anorexiant.

Adults: 75 mg once daily in the morning.

Contraindications: Arteriosclerosis, depression, glaucoma, hypertension, diabetes, kidney disease, hyperthyroidism, during or within 14 days of use of MAO inhibitors, hypersensitivity to sympathomimetics. Not recommended as an anorexiant for children less than 12 years of age. Sustained-release forms during lactation and in children less than 12 years of age.

Special Concerns: Safety and efficacy during pregnancy and lactation and for children not established. Children less than 6 years of age may be at greater risk for developing psychiatric disorders when using phenylpropanolamine. The anorexiant dose must be individualized for children 12–18 years of age.

Side Effects: *CNS:* Dizziness, headache, insomnia, restlessness, bizarre behavior. Serious effects due to abuse include: agitation, tremor, increased motor activity, hallucinations, ***seizures, stroke, and death.*** *CV:* Palpitations, ***hypertension (may be severe and lead to crisis),*** tachycardia. *Miscellaneous:* Dry mouth, dysuria, renal failure, nausea, nasal dryness.

Additional Drug Interactions

Bromocriptine / Worsening of side effects of bromocriptine; possibility of ventricular tachycardia and cardiac dysfunction

Caffeine / ↑ Serum caffeine levels, ↑ risk of pharmacologic and toxic effects

Indomethacin / Possibility of severe hypertensive episode

NURSING CONSIDERATIONS

See also *Nursing Considerations* for *Stimulants,* Chapter 47, and *Sympathomimetic Drugs,* Chapter 50.

Client/Family Teaching

1. Stress the importance of exercise, reduced caloric intake, and behavorial modification programs in the overall management of obesity.
2. Caution older men to report difficulties in voiding because they are more susceptible to drug-induced urinary retention.
3. Advise caution as drug may cause dizziness and tremors.
4. Avoid any caffeine-containing products or foods.

Evaluate

- ↓ Symptoms of nasal congestion
- ↓ Appetite and evidence of desired weight loss

Pirbuterol acetate

(peer-**BYOU**-ter-ohl)

Pregnancy Category: C

Maxair Autohaler **(Rx)**

See also *Sympathomimetic Drugs, Stimulants,* Chapter 50.

How Supplied: *Aerosol Solid w/Adapter:* 0.2 mg/inh

Action/Kinetics: Pirbuterol causes bronchodilation by stimulating beta-

2- adrenergic receptors. It has minimal effects on beta-1 receptors. The drug also inhibits histamine release from mast cells, causes vasodilation, and increases ciliary motility. It has minimal beta-1 activity. **Onset, inhalation:** Approximately 5 min. **Time to peak effect:** 30–60 min. **Duration:** 5 hr.
Uses: Alone or with theophylline or steroids, for prophylaxis and treatment of bronchospasm in asthma and other conditions with reversible bronchospasms, including bronchitis, emphysema, bronchiectasis, obstructive pulmonary disease. May be used with or without theophylline or steroids.

Dosage

- **Inhalation Aerosol**

Adults and children over 12 years: 0.2–0.4 mg (1–2 inhalations) q 4–6 hr, not to exceed 12 inhalations (2.4 mg) daily.
Contraindications: Cardiac arrhythmias due to tachycardia; tachycardia caused by digitalis toxicity.
Special Concerns: Safety and efficacy have not been determined in children less than 12 years of age.
Additional Side Effects: *CV:* PVCs, hypotension. *CNS:* Hyperactivity, hyperkinesia, anxiety, confusion, depression, fatigue, syncope. *GI:* Diarrhea, dry mouth, anorexia, loss of appetite, bad taste or taste change, abdominal pain, abdominal cramps, stomatitis, glossitis. *Dermatologic:* Rash, edema, pruritus, alopecia. *Miscellaneous:* Flushing, numbness in extremities, weight gain.

NURSING CONSIDERATIONS

See also *Nursing Considerations* for *Sympathomimetic Drugs* and *Adrenergic Bronchodilators,* Chapter 50.

Client/Family Teaching

1. Review appropriate methods, frequency, and indication for administration; observe self-administration to assess client technique.
2. Advise to seek medical intervention if condition deteriorates or if inhaler is ineffective in relieving symptoms at prescribed dosage.

Evaluate: Improved airway exchange and ↓ airway resistance.

Pseudoephedrine hydrochloride

(soo-doh-eh-**FED**-rin)
Pregnancy Category: B
Allermed, Balminil Decongestant Syrup 🍁, Benylin Decongestant Capsules 🍁, Cenafed, Children's Congestion Relief, Children's Sudafed Liquid, Congestion Relief, Decofed Syrup, DeFed-60, Dorcol Children's Decongestant Liquid, Efidac/24, Eltor 120 🍁, Genaphed, Halofed, Maxenal 🍁, Novafed, PediaCare Infants' Oral Decongestant Drops, PMS-Pseudoephedrine 🍁, Pseudo, Pseudo-Gest, Robidrine 🍁, Seudotabs, Sinustop Pro, Sudafed, Sudafed 12 Hour **(OTC)**

Pseudoephedrine sulfate

(soo-doh-eh-**FED**-rin)
Pregnancy Category: B
Afrin Extended-Release Tablets, Drixoral Non-Drowsy Formula **(OTC)**

See also *Sympathomimetic Drugs,* Chapter 50.
How Supplied: Pseudoephedrine hydrochloride: *Capsule, extended release:* 120 mg; *Liquid:* 7.5 mg/0.8 mL, 30 mg/5 mL; *Syrup:* 15 mg/5 mL, 30 mg/5 mL; *Tablet:* 30 mg, 60 mg; *Tablet, extended release:* 120 mg, 240 mg.
Pseudoephedrine sulfate: *Tablet:* 60 mg
Action/Kinetics: Pseudoephedrine produces direct stimulation of both alpha-(pronounced) and beta-adrenergic receptors, as well as indirect stimulation through release of norepinephrine from storage sites. These actions produce a decongestant effect on the nasal mucosa. Systemic administration eliminates possible damage to the nasal mucosa. **Onset:** 15–30 min. **Time to peak effect:** 30–60 min. **Duration:** 3–4 hr. **Extended-release: duration,** 8–12 hr. Urinary excretion slowed by alkalinization, causing reabsorption of drug.

Pseudoephedrine is also found in Actifed, Chlor-Trimeton, and Drixoral.

Uses: Nasal congestion associated with sinus conditions, otitis, allergies. Relief of eustachian tube congestion.

Dosage

HYDROCHLORIDE

• **Capsules, Oral Solution, Syrup, Tablets**

Decongestant.

Adults: 60 mg q 4–6 hr, not to exceed 240 mg in 24 hr. **Pediatric, 6–12 years:** 30 mg using the oral solution or syrup q 4–6 hr, not to exceed 120 mg in 24 hr; **2–6 years:** 15 mg using the oral solution or syrup q 4–6 hr, not to exceed 60 mg in 24 hr. For children less than 2 years of age, the dose must be individualized.

• **Extended-Release Capsules, Tablets**

Decongestant.

Adults and children over 12 years: 120 mg q 12 hr or 240 mg q 24 hr. Use is not recommended for children less than 12 years of age.

SULFATE

• **Extended-Release Tablets**

Decongestant.

Adults and children over 12 years: 120 mg q 12 hr. Use is not recommended for children less than 12 years of age.

Additional Contraindications: Lactation. Use of sustained-release products in children less than 12 years of age.

Special Concerns: Use with caution in newborn and premature infants due to a higher risk of side effects. Geriatric clients may be more prone to age-related prostatic hypertrophy.

NURSING CONSIDERATIONS

See also *Nursing Considerations* for *Sympathomimetic Drugs,* Chapter 50.

Client/Family Teaching

1. Avoid taking the drug at bedtime. Pseudoephedrine causes stimulation that can produce insomnia.
2. Advise clients with hypertension to report symptoms such as headache, dizziness, or increased BP readings.
3. Stress that extended-release products should not be crushed or chewed.

Evaluate: Symptomatic relief of nasal, sinus, or eustachian tube congestion and associated allergic manifestations.

Salmeterol xinafoate

(sal-**MET**-er-ole)

Pregnancy Category: C

Serevent **(Rx)**

See also *Sympathomimetic Drugs,* Chapter 50.

How Supplied: *Aerosol Solid w/Adapter*: 21 mcg/inh; *Aerosol Solid:* 21 mcg/inh

Action/Kinetics: Salmeterol is selective for beta-2 adrenergic receptors; these receptors are located in the bronchi and heart. The drug is thought to act by stimulating intracellular adenyl cyclase, the enzyme that converts ATP to cyclic AMP. Increased AMP levels cause relaxation of bronchial smooth muscle and inhibition of release of mediators of immediate hypersensitivity, especially from mast cells. Salmeterol is significantly bound to plasma proteins. The drug is cleared by hepatic metabolism.

Uses: Long-term maintenance treatment of asthma. Prevention of bronchospasms in clients over 12 years of age with reversible obstructive airway disease, including nocturnal asthma. Prevention of exercise-induced bronchospasms.

Dosage

• **Oral Inhalation Aerosol**

Maintenance of bronchodilation, prevention of symptoms of asthma, including nocturnal asthma.

Adults and children over 12 years of age: Two inhalations (42 mcg) b.i.d. (morning and evening, approximately 12 hr apart).

Prevention of exercise-induced bronchospasms.

Adults and children over 12 years of age: Two inhalations (42 mcg) at least 30–60 min before exercise. Additional doses should not be used for 12 hr.

Administration/Storage

1. The bronchodilator activity of salmeterol lasts for 12 hr; thus, doses should be spaced q 12 hr.
2. The safety of concomitant use of more than 8 inhalations per day of short-acting beta-2 agonists with salmeterol has not been established.
3. If a previously effective dose fails to provide the usual response, contact provider immediately.
4. Clients using salmeterol twice daily should not use additional doses to prevent exercise-induced bronchospasms.
5. Salmeterol should only be used with the actuator provided. The actuator should not be used with other aerosol medications.
6. The drug should be stored between 2°C and 30°C (36°F and 86°F). The canister should be stored nozzle end down and should be protected from freezing temperatures and direct sunlight.
7. Caution should be exercised so the drug is not sprayed in the eyes.
8. The canister should be shaken well before using and should be at room temperature, as the therapeutic effect may diminish if the canister is cold.
9. *Treatment of Overdose:* Supportive therapy. Consideration can be given to the judicious use of a beta-adrenergic blocking agent, although these drugs can cause bronchospasms. Cardiac monitoring is necessary. Dialysis is not an appropriate treatment of overdosage.

Contraindications: Use in clients who can be controlled by short-acting, inhaled beta-2 agonists. Use to treat acute symptoms of asthma. Lactation.

Special Concerns: Use with caution in clients with impaired hepatic function. The drug is not a substitute for PO or inhaled corticosteroids. The safety and efficacy of using salmeterol with a spacer or other devices has not been studied adequately. Use with caution in clients with cardiovascular disorders, including coronary insufficiency, cardiac arrhythmias, and hypertension; in clients with convulsive disorders or thyrotoxicosis; and in clients who respond unusually to sympathomimetic amines. Because of the potential of the drug interfering with uterine contractility, use of salmeterol during labor should be restricted to those in whom benefits clearly outweigh risks. Safety and efficacy in children less than 12 years of age have not been determined.

Laboratory Test Interference: ↓ Serum potassium.

Side Effects: *Respiratory:* Paradoxical bronchospasms, upper or lower respiratory tract infection, nasopharyngitis, disease of nasal cavity/sinus, cough, pharyngitis, allergic rhinitis, laryngitis, tracheitis, bronchitis. *Allergic:* ***Immediate hypersensitivity reactions,*** including urticaria, rash, and ***bronchospasm.*** *CV:* Palpitations, chest pain, increased BP, tachycardia. *CNS:* Headache, sinus headache, tremors, nervousness, malaise, fatigue, dizziness, giddiness. *GI:* Stomachache. *Musculoskeletal:* Joint pain, back pain, muscle cramps, muscle contractions, myalgia, myositis, muscle soreness. *Miscellaneous:* Flu, dental pain, rash, skin eruption, dysmenorrhea.

Symptoms of Overdose: Tachycardia, arrhythmia, tremors, headache, muscle cramps, hypokalemia, hyperglycemia.

Drug Interactions

MAO Inhibitors / Potentiation of the effect of salmeterol

Tricyclic antidepressants / Potentiation of the effect of salmeterol

---

NURSING CONSIDERATIONS

See also *Nursing Considerations* for *Sympathomimetic Drugs,* Chapter 50.

Assessment
1. Document onset of asthma, other agents prescribed, and the outcome.
2. Determine any evidence or history of cardiac or liver dysfunction, thyrotoxicosis, hypertension, or convulsive disorders.
3. Document pulmonary function status and lung sounds.
4. Obtain baseline VS, liver enzymes, peak expiratory flow rate (PEF), and forced expiratory volume at 1 sec (FEV-1) and assess periodically.

Client/Family Teaching
1. Demonstrate proper use (with actuator) and observe client self-administer.
2. Use only as prescribed and do not exceed prescribed dosage and administration frequency (drug effects last 12 hr).
3. Reinforce not to use this drug during an acute asthma attack.
4. Review the procedure for use of the short-acting beta-2 agonist prescribed to treat symptoms of asthma that occur between the salmeterol dosing schedule. Advise that increased utilization warrants medical evaluation (e.g., when used more than 4 times/day or more than one canister of 200 inhalations/8 weeks).
5. Client may experience palpitations, chest pain, headaches, tremors, and nervousness as side effects of drug therapy.
6. If client experiences chest pain, fast pounding irregular heart beat, hives, increased wheezing, or difficulty breathing, advise to notify provider immediately.
7. Instruct to take the drug 30–60 min before activity in order to prevent acute bronchospasms.
8. Stress that salmeterol does not replace inhaled or systemic steroids and to not stop prescribed steroid therapy abruptly without medical supervision.
9. Refer to appropriate support groups that may assist client to cope and live a normal life with this disorder.

Evaluate
- Prevention and control of asthmatic symptoms (e.g., decreased wheezing, dyspnea, orthopnea, and cough)
- Prevention of exercise-induced bronchospasms

Terbutaline sulfate
(ter-**BYOU**-tah-leen)
Pregnancy Category: B
Brethaire, Brethine, Bricanyl **(Rx)**

See also *Sympathomimetic Drugs,* Chapter 50.

How Supplied: *Aerosol Solid w/Adapter:* 0.2 mg/inh; *Aerosol Solid:* 0.2 mg/inh; *Injection:* 1 mg/mL; *Tablet:* 2.5 mg, 5 mg

Action/Kinetics: Terbutaline is specific for stimulating beta-2 receptors, resulting in bronchodilation and relaxation of peripheral vasculature. Minimum beta-1 activity. Drug action resembles that of isoproterenol. **PO: Onset:** 30 min; **maximum effect:** 2–3 hr; **duration:** 4–8 hr. **SC: Onset,** 5–15 min; **maximum effect:** 30 min—1 hr; **duration:** 1.5–4 hr. **Inhalation: Onset,** 5–30 min; **time to peak effect:** 1–2 hr; **duration:** 3–6 hr.

Uses: Bronchodilator in asthma, bronchitis, emphysema, bronchiectasis, pulmonary obstructive disease, and other conditions associated with reversible bronchospasms. *Investigational:* Inhibit premature labor.

Dosage
- **Tablets**

Bronchodilation.

Adults and children over 15 years: 5 mg t.i.d. q 6 hr during waking hours, not to exceed 15 mg q 24 hr. If disturbing side effects are observed, dose can be reduced to 2.5 mg t.i.d. without loss of beneficial effects. Anticipate use of other therapeutic measures if client fails to respond after second dose. **Children**

12–15 years: 2.5 mg t.i.d., not to exceed 7.5 mg q 24 hr.

Premature labor.

2.5 mg q 4–6 hr until term.

• **SC**

Bronchodilation.

Adults: 0.25 mg. May be repeated 1 time after 15–30 min if no significant clinical improvement is noted. If client does not respond to the second dose, other measures should be undertaken. Dose should not exceed 0.5 mg over 4 hr.

• **IV Infusion**

Premature labor.

10 mcg/min initially; **then,** increase rate by 0.005 mg/min q 10 min until contractions cease or a maximum dose of 80 mcg/min is reached. The minimum effective dose should be continued for 4–8 hr after contractions cease, Terbutaline may also be given SC for preterm labor.

• **Inhalation Aerosol**

Bronchodilation.

Adults and children over 12 years: 0.2–0.5 mg (1–2 inhalations) q 4–6 hr. Inhalations should be separated by 60-sec intervals. Dosage may be repeated q 4–6 hr.

Contraindication: Lactation.

Special Concerns: Safe use in children less than 12 years of age not established.

Laboratory Test Interference: ↑ Liver enzymes.

Additional Side Effects: *CV:* PVCs, ECG changes (e.g., atrial premature beats, AV block, sinus pause, ST-T wave depression, T-wave inversion, sinus bradycardia, atrial escape beat with aberrant conduction), tachycardia. *Respiratory:* Wheezing. *Miscellaneous:* Hypersensitivity reactions (including vasculitis), flushing, sweating, bad taste or taste change, muscle cramps, CNS stimulation, pain at injection site.

NURSING CONSIDERATIONS

See also *Nursing Considerations* for *Sympathomimetic Drugs,* Chapter 50.

Assessment

1. Document indications for therapy and type and onset of symptoms.
2. Auscultate and document baseline lung assessments with lung disorders.
3. Document frequency and duration of contractions and fetal HR with preterm labor.

Interventions

1. Observe respiratory client for evidence of drug tolerance and rebound bronchospasm.
2. Observe mother for evidence of headache, tremor, anxiety, palpitations, symptoms of pulmonary edema, and tachycardia. Monitor fetus for distress and report any increase in contractions.
3. Monitor mother and neonate for symptoms of hypoglycemia and mother for hypokalemia.

Client/Family Teaching

1. Take oral medication with meals to minimize GI upset.
2. Report any persistent or bothersome side effects. The drug dose and administration times may need to be adjusted.
3. Do not increase dose or frequency if symptoms are not relieved. Report so dose can be reevaluated.
4. Advise to increase fluid intake to help liquefy secretions.
5. In clients with preterm labor, advise to notify physician immediately if labor resumes or unusual side effects are noted.

Evaluate

• Improved airway exchange
• Inhibition of premature labor

CHAPTER FIFTY-ONE

Adrenergic Blocking Agents

See also the following individual entries:

Alpha-Adrenergic Blocking Agents - See Chapter 28

Dapiprazole Hydrochloride
Dihydroergotamine Meslyate
Methysergide Maleate
Phenoxybenzamine Hydrochloride
Phentolamine Mesylate

Beta-Adrenergic Blocking Agents

Acebutolol Hydrochloride
Atenolol
Betaxolol Hydrochloride
Bisoprolol Fumarate
Carteolol Hydrochloride
Esmolol Hydrochloride
Levobunolol Hydrochloride
Metipranolol Hydrochloride
Metoprolol Succinate
Metoprolol Tartrate
Nadolol
Penbutolol Sulfate
Pindolol
Propranolol Hydrochloride
Sotalol Hydrochloride
Timolol Maleate

General Statement: As their name implies, the adrenergic blocking agents (sympatholytics) reduce or prevent the action of the sympathomimetic agents. They do this by competing with norepinephrine or epinephrine (the neurotransmitters) for the various subtypes of either alpha-adrenergic or beta-adrenergic receptor sites. For example, alpha-adrenergic blocking agents prevent the smooth muscles surrounding the arterioles from contracting, whereas beta-adrenergic blocking agents prevent the excitatory effect of the neurotransmitters on the heart. It should also be noted that several antihypertensive agents act by blocking alpha (especially in the CNS) or beta receptors.

Some of the adrenergic blocking agents also have a direct systemic cardiac effect in addition to their peripheral vasodilating effect. The fall in BP accompanying their administration may trigger a compensatory tachycardia (reflex stimulation). The cardiac blood vessels of a client with arteriosclerosis may be unable to dilate rapidly enough to accommodate these changes in blood volume, and the client may experience an acute attack of angina pectoris or even cardiac failure.

Adrenergic blocking agents have many undesirable effects which, although not toxic, limit their use. Treatment should always be started at low doses and increased gradually.

ALPHA-ADRENERGIC BLOCKING AGENTS: These drugs reduce the tone of muscles surrounding peripheral blood vessels and consequently increase peripheral blood circulation and decrease BP.

BETA-ADRENERGIC BLOCKING AGENTS: These drugs block the nerve impulse transmission to the beta receptors of the sympathetic division of the ANS. These receptors are particularly numerous at the postjunctional terminals of the nerve fibers that control the heart muscle and reduce muscle tone. These drugs include atenolol, carteolol, metoprolol, nadolol, penbutolol, pindolol, propranolol, and timolol.

NURSING CONSIDERATIONS

Assessment

1. Obtain a thorough nursing history noting any evidence or history of PUD as drugs should be used cautiously in this setting.
2. Document indications for therapy, and type and onset of symptoms.
3. Determine baseline ECG, BP, and pulse; monitor throughout drug therapy.
4. Document any evidence of heart disease and note currently prescribed therapy. May cause vasospasm with Prinzmetal or vasospastic angina.

Client/Family Teaching

1. Take with milk or meals to minimize GI upset.
2. Advise client to rise slowly from a supine position and dangle legs and feet before standing to prevent orthostatic effects.
3. May transiently experience apprehension, fear, anxiety, and/or palpitations.

Evaluate

- Evidence of ↓ BP
- Reports of ↓ anxiety
- ECG evidence of control of ventricular arrhythmias

ALPHA-ADRENERGIC BLOCKING AGENTS

See Chapter 28

Dapiprazole Hydrochloride
Dihydroergotamine Meslyate
Methysergide Maleate
Phenoxybenzamine Hydrochloride
Phentolamine Mesylate

Dapiprazole hydrochloride

(dah-**PIP**-rah-zol)
Pregnancy Category: B
Rev-Eyes **(Rx)**

How Supplied: *Powder for Reconstitution:* 0.5%

Action/Kinetics: Dapiprazole produces miosis by blocking the alpha-adrenergic receptors on the dilator muscle of the iris. The drug does not have significant action on ciliary muscle contraction; thus, it does not cause changes in the depth of the anterior chamber of the thickness of the lens. Dapiprazole does not alter the intraocular pressure either in normal eyes or in eyes with elevated intraocular pressure. The rate of pupillary constriction may be slightly slower in clients with brown irides than in clients with blue or green irides.

Uses: To reverse diagnostic mydriasis induced by adrenergic (e.g., phenylephrine) or parasympatholytic (e.g., tropicamide) agents.

Dosage

- **Ophthalmic Solution**

Reverse mydriasis.

2 gtt followed in 5 min by 2 more gtt applied to the conjunctiva of the eye after ophthalmic examination.

Administration/Storage

1. The drug should not be used in the same client more frequently than once a week.
2. To prepare the solution, the aluminum seals and rubber plugs should be removed and discarded from both the drug and diluent vials. After pouring the diluent into the drug vial, the dropper assembly should be removed from its sterile wrapping and attached to the drug vial. The container should be shaken for several minutes to ensure adequate mixing.
3. Reconstituted eye drops may be stored at room temperature for 21 days.
4. Any solution that is not clear and colorless should be discarded.

Contraindications: Acute iritis or other conditions where miosis is not desirable. To reduce intraocular pressure or to treat open-angle glaucoma.

Special Concerns: Use with caution during lactation. Safety and effectiveness have not been determined in children. The drug may cause difficul-

ty in adaptation to dark and may reduce the field of vision.
Side Effects: *Ophthalmic:* Conjunctival injection lasting 20 min, burning on instillation, ptosis, lid erythema, itching, lid edema, chemosis, corneal edema, punctate keratitis, photophobia, tearing and blurring of vision, dryness of eyes. *Miscellaneous:* Headaches, browache.

NURSING CONSIDERATIONS

Assessment

1. Determine any hypersensitivity to alpha-adrenergic blocking agents.
2. Note eye color. Pupillary constriction may be slightly slower in clients with brown irides as opposed to those with blue or green irides.

Client/Family Teaching

1. Advise that medication may cause burning on instillation.
2. Instruct client to use care as medication may impair adaptation to dark and reduce visual fields.

Evaluate: Reversal of drug-induced mydriasis (constriction of pupils).

Dihydroergotamine mesylate

(dye-hy-droh-er-**GOT**-ah-meen)
Pregnancy Category: X
D.H.E. 45 **(Rx)**

How Supplied: *Injection:* 1 mg/mL
Action/Kinetics: Dihydroergotamine manifests alpha-adrenergic receptor blocking activity as well as a direct stimulatory action on vascular smooth muscle of peripheral and cranial blood vessels, resulting in vasoconstriction, thus preventing the onset of a migraine attack. Dihydroergotamine manifests greater adrenergic blocking activity, less pronounced vasoconstriction, less N&V, and less oxytocic properties than does ergotamine. It is more effective when given early in the course of a migraine attack. **Onset: IM,** 15–30 min; **IV,** <5 min. **Duration: IM,** 3–4 hr. **t½: initial,** 1.4 hr; **final,** 18–22 hr. Metabolized in liver and excreted in feces with less than 10% excreted through the urine.
Uses: To prevent or abort migraine, migraine variant, histaminic cephalalgia (cluster headaches). Especially useful when rapid effect is desired or when other routes of administration are not possible.

Dosage

• **IM**

Suppress vascular headache.

Adults, initial: 1 mg at first sign of headache; repeat q hr for a total of 3 mg (not to exceed 6 mg/week).

• **IV**

Suppress vascular headache.

Similar to IM but to a maximum of 2 mg/attack or 6 mg/week.

Administration/Storage

1. Adjust the dosage if the client complains of severe headaches. This dose should then be used when subsequent headaches begin.
2. *Treatment of Overdose:* Maintain adequate circulation. IV nitroglycerin and nitroprusside to treat vasospasm. IV heparin and low molecular weight dextran to minimize thrombosis.

Contraindications: Lactation. Pregnancy. Peripheral vascular disease, coronary heart disease, hypertension, impaired hepatic or renal function, sepsis, hypersensitivity, malnutrition, severe pruritus, presence of infection.
Special Concerns: Safety and efficacy have not been determined in children. Geriatric clients may be more affected by peripheral vasoconstriction that results in hypothermia. Prolonged administration may cause ergotism and gangrene.
Side Effects: *CV:* Precordial pain, transient tachycardia or bradycardia. Large doses may cause increased BP, vasoconstriction of coronary arteries, and bradycardia. *GI:* N&V, diarrhea. *Other:* Numbness and tingling of fingers and toes, muscle pain in extremities, weakness in legs, localized edema, and itching. *Prolonged use:* Gangrene, ergotism.

Symptoms of Overdose: N&V, pain in limb muscles, tachycardia or bradycardia, precordial pain, numbness and tingling of fingers and toes, weakness of the legs, hypertension or hypotension, localized edema, S&S of ischemia due to vasoconstriction of peripheral arteries and arterioles. Symptoms of ischemia include the feet and hands becoming cold, pale, and numb; muscle pain, gangrene. Occasionally confusion, depression, drowsiness, and ***seizures.***

Drug Interactions

Beta-adrenergic blockers / ↑ Peripheral ischemia resulting in cold extremities and possibly peripheral gangrene

Macrolide antibiotics / Acute ergotism resulting in peripheral ischemia

Nitrates / ↑ Bioavailability of hydroergotamine and ↓ anginal effects of nitrates

NURSING CONSIDERATIONS

Assessment

1. Obtain a thorough nursing, diet, and drug history.
2. Note any history of prior adverse reactions to ergotamine.
3. Determine if the client is taking nitrates as dihydroergotamine interacts and should be avoided.
4. Determine severity of headaches, how long they last, and what, if any, medications have been effective in relieving them in the past.
5. If female and of childbearing age note the possibility of pregnancy. Ergotamine has an oxytocic effect and therefore is contraindicated in this setting.
6. Note any history of liver or renal dysfunction, hypertension, PVD, or CAD.

Client/Family Teaching

1. Take the drug at the onset of a migraine headache. This drug is most effective when administered early in an attack.
2. Seek bed rest in a darkened room for 1–2 hr after drug ingestion.
3. Teach alternative methods for dealing with stress, such as relaxation techniques.
4. Report any bothersome side effects. Any evidence of cold extremities and numbness or tingling of the extremities should be reported immediately to avoid gangrene.
5. Take only as directed and do not stop abruptly without approval.

Evaluate: Relief of migraine headaches.

Methysergide maleate

(meth-ih-**SIR**-jyd)
Sansert **(Rx)**

How Supplied: *Tablet:* 2 mg

Action/Kinetics: Methysergide is an ergot alkaloid derivative structurally related to LSD. It is thought to act by directly stimulating smooth muscle leading to vasoconstriction. The drug blocks the effects of serotonin, a powerful vasodilator believed to play a role in vascular headaches; it also inhibits the release of histamine from mast cells and prevents the release of serotonin from platelets. It has weak emetic and oxytocic activity. **Onset:** 1–2 days. **Peak plasma levels:** 60 ng/mL. **Duration:** 1–2 days. Excreted through the urine as unchanged drugs and metabolites.

Uses: Prophylaxis of vascular headache (in clients having one or more per week or in cases where headaches are so severe preventive therapy is indicated). Clients should remain under supervision.

Dosage

• **Tablets**

Adults: Administer 4–8 mg/day in divided doses. Continuous administration should not exceed 6 months. Drug may be readministered after a 3–4-week rest period.

Administration/Storage

1. Administer the drug with meals or milk to minimize GI irritation due to increased hydrochloric acid production.
2. The drug must be discontinued gradually to avoid migraine headache rebound.

3. If the drug is not effective after 3 weeks, it is not likely to be beneficial and should be discontinued.

Contraindications: Severe renal or hepatic disease, severe hypertension, CAD, peripheral vascular disease, or tendency toward thromboembolic disease, cachexia (profound ill health or malnutrition), severe arteriosclerosis, phlebitis or cellulitis of lower limbs, collagen diseases, valvular heart disease, infectious disease, or peptic ulcer. Pregnancy, lactation, use in children.

Special Concerns: Geriatric clients may be more affected by peripheral vasoconstriction leading to the possibility of hypothermia.

Side Effects: The drug is associated with a high incidence of side effects. *Fibrosis:* ***Retroperitoneal fibrosis, cardiac fibrosis, pleuropulmonary fibrosis,*** Peyronie's-like disease. The fibrotic condition may result in vascular insufficiency in the lower legs. *CV:* Vasoconstriction of arteries leading to paresthesia, chest pain, abdominal pain, or extremities that are cold, numb, or painful. Tachycardia, postural hypotension. *CNS:* Dizziness, ataxia, drowsiness, vertigo, insomnia, euphoria, lightheadedness, and psychic reactions such as depersonalization, depression, and hallucinations. *GI:* N&V, diarrhea, heartburn, abdominal pain, increased gastric acid, constipation. *Hematologic:* Eosinophilia, neutropenia. *Other:* Peripheral edema, flushing of face, skin rashes, transient alopecia, myalgia, arthralgia, weakness, weight gain, telangiectasia.

Drug Interaction: Narcotic analgesics are inhibited by methysergide.

NURSING CONSIDERATIONS

Assessment

1. Note the frequency and severity of the client's headaches and efforts made in the past to control or prevent them.
2. Note any history of renal or hepatic disease. Obtain baseline liver and renal function studies.
3. Assess behavior prior to initiating therapy. Review diet, activity, and stress levels. Determine any recent ingestion of agents that may have precipitated event.
4. Obtain baseline eosinophil and neutrophil counts.

Client/Family Teaching

1. Take with meals or milk to minimize GI upset.
2. Report symptoms of nervousness, weakness, insomnia, rashes, alopecia, or peripheral edema.
3. Record weights daily and report any unusual weight gain. Check the extremities for edema and report if evident.
4. If the weight gain becomes excessive, instruct the client on how to adjust the caloric intake. Maintain a low-salt diet and refer to a dietitian for assistance.
5. Advise to keep a diary noting any events, foods, or activities that may relate to the onset of these headaches.
6. Administration of methysergide should not be continued on a regular basis for longer than 6 months.
7. Remind the client to remain under medical supervision. Stress that blood tests must be done at periodic intervals to detect complications of drug therapy.
8. General malaise, fatigue, weight loss, low-grade fever, or urinary tract problems may be symptoms of fibrosis (cardiac or pleuropulmonary), and the drug should be discontinued. Report any of these symptoms immediately.
9. Do not drive a car or engage in other hazardous tasks until drug effects are realized because drug may cause drowsiness.
10. If dizziness or lightheadedness occurs upon arising, rise slowly from a supine position and dangle the legs for a few minutes before standing erect.
11. If feeling faint, lie down with the legs elevated.
12. Avoid alcohol, caffeine, and canabalis, as these may precipitate vascular headaches.

13. Discuss with the family unusual psychologic changes that may occur, especially hallucinations that require reporting if evident.
14. Do not discontinue medication abruptly. Rebound migraine headaches may occur. Medication must be discontinued gradually.

Evaluate: ↓ Occurrence of severe vascular headaches.

Phenoxybenzamine hydrochloride

(fen-ox-ee-**BEN**-zah-meen)
Pregnancy Category: C
Dibenzyline **(Rx)**

How Supplied: *Capsule:* 10 mg

Action/Kinetics: Phenoxybenzamine is an irreversible alpha-adrenergic blocking agent. The drug increases blood flow to the skin, mucosa, and abdominal viscera and lowers BP. Beneficial effects may not be noted for 2–4 weeks. **Onset:** gradual. **Peak effect:** 4–6 hr. **Duration:** 3–4 days after one dose. **t½:** 24 hr. Metabolized slowly and excreted in urine and feces.

Uses: To control hypertension and sweating in pheochromocytoma before surgery, when surgery is contraindicated, or in malignant pheochromocytoma.

Dosage

- **Capsules**

Pheochromocytoma.

Adults, initial: 10 mg b.i.d.; may be increased every other day until desired effect is obtained. **Maintenance:** 20–40 mg b.i.d.–t.id. **Pediatric, initial:** 0.2 mg/kg (6 mg/m^2) up to a maximum of 10 mg/day; dose may be increased q 4 days until desired effect is reached. **Maintenance:** 0.4 mg (1.2 mg/m^2) daily in three to four divided doses.

Administration/Storage

1. Observe the client closely before increasing the dosage of drug.
2. Because phenoxybenzamine is irreversible, the drug is usually started in low doses and gradually increased.
3. It may take 2 weeks to titrate the medication to the optimum dosage.
4. *Treatment of Overdose:* Discontinue the drug and consider one or more of the following:

- Have client lie down with legs elevated to restore cerebral circulation.
- In severe overdose, institute measures to treat shock.
- Leg bandages and an abdominal binder may shorten the time the client needs to lie down.
- Severe hypotension may be helped by IV norepinephrine.

Contraindications: Conditions in which a decrease in BP is not desired. Essential hypertension.

Special Concerns: Geriatric clients may be more sensitive to the hypotensive hypothermic effects. Use with caution in coronary or cerebral arteriosclerosis, respiratory infections, and renal disease.

Side Effects: Due to adrenergic blockade and include miosis, postural hypotension, tachycardia, nasal congestion, and inhibition of ejaculation. Also, drowsiness, fatigue, GI upset.

Symptoms of Overdose: Dizziness or fainting due to postural hypotension. Also, tachycardia, GI irritation, drowsiness, fatigue, vomiting, lethargy, and shock.

NURSING CONSIDERATIONS

Interventions

1. Obtain renal function studies and monitor.
2. Take BP q 4 hr with the client in both supine and erect positions to check for excessive hypotension.
3. Note the quality of peripheral pulses, and assess the extremities for increased warmth for 4 days after a change in drug dosage. The results may help determine whether the client needs an adjustment in dosage.
4. If the client has a preexisting respiratory infection, it may be aggravated by the drug. Increased pulmonary supportive care may be required.

Client/Family Teaching

1. Rise slowly from a supine position to a sitting position and dangle feet for a few minutes before standing erect.

If feeling faint, lie down immediately and elevate the legs.
2. Avoid tasks that require mental alertness until drug effects are evident.
3. Take a radial pulse and report tachycardia as this is a sign of autonomic blockade and requires medical intervention. Concurrent use of a beta-adrenergic blocking agent may also be necessary.
4. Do not take any OTC drugs and avoid alcohol because this may enhance hypotensive effects.
5. It may take 1 month before the desired effects are obtained. Therefore, it is important to take medications as prescribed and if there are no changes after that time, report to the provider.
Evaluate: Control of hypertension and ↓ sweating in clients with pheochromocytoma.

Phentolamine mesylate

(fen-**TOLL**-ah-meen)
Pregnancy Category: C
Regitine, Rogitine ✱ **(Rx)**

How Supplied: *Powder for injection:* 5 mg
Action/Kinetics: Phentolamine competitively blocks both presynaptic (alpha-2) and postsynaptic (alpha-1) adrenergic receptors producing vasodilation and a decrease in peripheral resistance. The drug has little effect on BP. In CHF, phentolamine reduces afterload and pulmonary arterial pressure as well as increases CO. **Onset** (parenteral): Immediate. **Duration:** Short. Poorly absorbed from the GI tract. About 10% excreted unchanged in the urine after parenteral use.
Uses: Treatment of hypertension caused by pheochromocytoma prior to or during surgery. Dermal necrosis and sloughing following IV use or extravasation of norepinephrine. To test for pheochromocytoma (not the method of choice). *Investigational:* Treatment of CHF. In combination with papaverine as an intracavernous injection for impotence.

Dosage

- **IV, IM**

Prevent hypertension in pheochromocytoma, preoperative.
Adults, IV: 5 mg 1–2 hr before surgery; dose may be repeated if needed. **Pediatric, IV, IM:** 1 mg (or 0.1 mg/kg) 1–2 hr before surgery; dose may be repeated if needed.

Prevent or control hypertension during surgery.
Adults, IV: 5 mg. **IV infusion:** 0.5–1 mg/min. **Pediatric, IV:** 0.1 mg/kg (3 mg/m^2). May be repeated, if necessary. During surgery 5 mg for adults and 1 mg for children may be given to prevent or control symptoms of epinephrine intoxication (e.g., paroxysms of hypertension, respiratory depression, seizures, tachycardia).

Dermal necrosis/sloughing following IV or extravasation of norepinephrine.
Prevention: 10 mg/1,000 mL norepinephrine solution; *treatment:* 5–10 mg/10 mL saline injected into area of extravasation within 12 hr. **Pediatric:** 0.1–0.2 mg/kg to a maximum of 10 mg.

CHF.
Adults, IV infusion: 0.17–0.4 mg/min.

Diagnosis of pheochromocytoma.
Adults, rapid IV, initial: 2.5 mg (if response is negative, a 5-mg test should be undertaken before concluding the test is negative); **children, rapid IV:** 1 mg. **Adults, IM:** 5 mg; **children, IM:** 3 mg.

- **Intracavernosal**

Impotence.
Adults: Papaverine, 30 mg, and 0.5–1 mg phentolamine; adjust dose according to response.

Administration/Storage
1. For IV administration reconstitute 5 mg with 1 mL sterile water or 0.9% NaCl and inject over 1 min.
2. Drug may also be further diluted: 5–10 mg in 500 mL of D5W and titrated to desired response.

3. When the IV administration of norepinephrine or dopamine results in infiltration, administer solutions of phentolamine SC at the site and within 12 hr for beneficial effects. Use 5–10 mg of phentolamine in 10–15 mL of 0.9% NaCl.
4. *Treatment of Overdose:* Maintain BP by giving IV norepinephrine.

Contraindications: Coronary artery disease including angina, MI, or coronary insufficiency.

Special Concerns: Use during pregnancy and lactation only if benefits clearly outweigh risks. Geriatric clients may have a greater risk of developing hypothermia. Use with great caution in the presence of gastritis, ulcers, and clients with a history thereof.

Side Effects: *CV:* Acute and prolonged hypotension, tachycardia, and arrhythmias, especially after parenteral administration. Orthostatic hypotension, flushing. *GI:* N&V, diarrhea. *Other:* Dizziness, weakness, nasal stuffiness.

Symptoms of Overdose: ***Hypotension, shock.***

Drug Interactions

Ephedrine / Phentolamine antagonizes vasoconstrictor and hypertensive effect
Epinephrine / Phentolamine antagonizes vasoconstrictor and hypertensive effect
Norepinephrine / Suitable antagonist to treat overdosage induced by phentolamine
Propranolol / Concomitant use during surgery for pheochromocytoma is indicated

---

NURSING CONSIDERATIONS

Assessment

1. Note any history of CAD.
2. Determine any evidence of gastritis or PUD.

Interventions

1. Monitor the BP and pulse frequently during parenteral administration and until stabilized.
2. To avoid postural hypotension, keep clients supine for at least 30 min after injection. Then have clients dangle their legs over the side of the bed and rise slowly to avoid orthostatic hypotension.
3. If clients show signs of drug overdose, place them in the Trendelenburg position. Assist with the administration of parenteral fluids. Have levarterenol available to minimize hypotension. *Do not use epinephrine.*

For the diagnosis of pheochromocytoma:

1. The test for pheochromocytoma should not be undertaken on normotensive clients.
2. Sedatives, analgesics, and other nonessential medication should be withheld for 24 hr (and preferably 72 hr) prior to the test.
3. When testing for pheochromocytoma, the client should be kept in a supine position, preferably in a dark, quiet room.
4. If the IV test is used, BP should be measured immediately after the injection, at 30-sec intervals for the first 3 min and at 60-sec intervals for the next 7 min. If the IM test is used, BP should be measured every 5 min for 30–45 min.
5. The pheochromocytoma test is most reliable in clients with sustained hypertension and least reliable in clients with paroxysmal hypertension.
6. A positive response for pheochromocytoma is a drop in BP of more than 35 mm Hg systolic and 25 mm Hg diastolic pressure. Maximal decreases in BP usually occur within 2 min after injection of phentolamine and return to preinjection pressure within 15–30 min. A negative response is indicated when the BP is unchanged, elevated, or reduced less than 35 mm Hg systolic and 25 mm Hg diastolic pressure.

Evaluate

- Control of hypertension
- Prevention of local tissue necrosis following extravasation with norepinephrine or dopamine

BETA-ADRENERGIC BLOCKING AGENTS

See also the following individual agents:

Acebutolol Hydrochloride
Atenolol
Betaxolol Hydrochloride
Bisoprolol Fumarate
Carteolol Hydrochloride
Esmolol Hydrochloride
Levobunolol Hydrochloride
Metipranolol Hydrochloride
Metoprolol Tartrate
Nadolol
Penbutolol Sulfate
Pindolol
Propranolol Hydrochloride
Sotalol Hydrochloride
Timolol Maleate

Action/Kinetics: Beta-adrenergic blocking agents combine reversibly with beta-adrenergic receptors to block the response to sympathetic nerve impulses, circulating catecholamines, or adrenergic drugs. Beta-adrenergic receptors have been classified as beta-1 (predominantly in the cardiac muscle) and beta-2 (mainly in the bronchi and vascular musculature). Blockade of beta-1 receptors decreases HR, myocardial contractility, and CO; in addition, AV conduction is slowed. These effects lead to a decrease in BP, as well as a reversal of cardiac arrhythmias. Blockade of beta-2 receptors increases airway resistance in the bronchioles and inhibits the vasodilating effects of catecholamines on peripheral blood vessels. The various beta-blocking agents differ in their ability to block beta-1 and beta-2 receptors (see individual drugs); also, certain of these agents have intrinsic sympathomimetic action.

Certain of these drugs (betaxolol, carteolol, levobunolol, metipranolol, and timolol) are used for glaucoma. The drugs appear to act by reducing production of aqueous humor; metipranolol and timolol may also increase outflow of aqueous humor. These drugs have little or no effect on the pupil size or on accommodation.

Uses: Depending on the drug, these agents may be used to treat one or more of the following conditions: hypertension, angina pectoris (first-line agents for unstable angina), cardiac arrhythmias, MI, prophylaxis of migraine, tremors (essential, lithium-induced, parkinsonism), situational anxiety, aggressive behavior, antipsychotic-induced akathisia, esophageal varices rebleeding, and alcohol withdrawal syndrome. Propranolol is indicated for a number of other conditions (see information on propranolol).

Decrease intraocular pressure in chronic open-angle glaucoma. If intraocular pressure is not adequately controlled with a beta blocker, concomitant therapy with pilocarpine, other miotics, dipivefrin, or systemic carbonic anhydrase inhibitors may be instituted.

Contraindications: Sinus bradycardia, greater than first degree heart block, cardiogenic shock, CHF unless secondary to tachyarrhythmia treatable with beta blockers, overt cardiac failure. Most are contraindicated in chronic bronchitis, asthma, bronchospasm, emphysema.

Special Concerns: Use with caution in diabetes, thyrotoxicosis, and impaired hepatic and renal function. Safe use during pregnancy and lactation and in children has not been established. The drugs may be absorbed systemically when used for glaucoma; thus, there is the potential for an additive effect with beta blockers used systemically. Also, see individual agents.

Side Effects: *CV:* Bradycardia, hypotension (especially following IV use), CHF, cold extremities, claudication, worsening of angina, strokes, edema, syncope, arrhythmias, chest pain, peripheral ischemia, flushing, SOB, sinoatrial block, pulmonary edema, vasodilation, increased HR, palpitations, conduction disturbances,

first- and third-degree heart block, worsening of AV block, thrombosis of renal or mesenteric arteries, precipitation or worsening of Raynaud's phenomenon. Sudden withdrawal of large doses may cause angina, ventricular tachycardia, ***fatal MI, or sudden death.*** *GI:* N&V, diarrhea, flatulence, dry mouth, constipation, anorexia, cramps, bloating, gastric pain, dyspepsia, distortion of taste, weight gain or loss, retroperitoneal fibrosis, ischemic colitis. *Hepatic:* Hepatomegaly, acute pancreatitis, elevated liver enzymes. *Respiratory:* Asthma-like symptoms, ***bronchospasms, bronchial obstruction, laryngospasm with respiratory distress,*** wheeziness, worsening of chronic obstructive lung disease, dyspnea, cough, nasal stuffiness, rhinitis, pharyngitis, rales. *CNS:* Dizziness, fatigue, lethargy, vivid dreams, depression, hallucinations, delirium, psychoses, paresthesias, insomnia, nervousness, nightmares, headache, vertigo, disorientation of time and place, hypoesthesia or hyperesthesia, decreased concentration, short-term memory loss, change in behavior, emotional lability, slurred speech, lightheadedness. In the elderly, paranoia, disorientation, and combativeness have occurred. *Hematologic:* ***Agranulocytosis,*** thrombocytopenia. *Allergic:* Fever, sore throat, respiratory distress, rash, pharyngitis, ***laryngospasm, anaphylaxis.*** *Skin:* Pruritus, rashes, increased skin pigmentation, sweating, dry skin, alopecia, skin irritation, psoriasis (reversible). *Musculoskeletal:* Joint and muscle pain, arthritis, arthralgia, back pain, muscle cramps, muscle weakness when used in clients with myasthenic symptoms. *GU:* Impotence, decreased libido, dysuria, UTI, nocturia, urinary retention or frequency, pollakiuria. *Ophthalmic:* Visual disturbances, eye irritation, dry or burning eyes, blurred vision, conjunctivitis. When used ophthalmically: keratitis, blepharoptosis, diplopia, ptosis, and visual disturbances including refractive changes. *Other:* Hyperglycemia or hypoglycemia, lupus-like syndrome, Peyronie's disease, tinnitus, increase in symptoms of myasthenia gravis, facial swelling, decreased exercise tolerance, rigors, speech disorders.

Symptoms of Overdose: CV symptoms include bradycardia, hypotension, CHF, ***cardiogenic shock,*** intraventricular conduction disturbances, ***AV block, pulmonary edema, asystole,*** and tachycardia. Also, overdosage of pindolol may cause hypertension and overdosage of propranolol may result in systemic vascular resistance. CNS symptoms include respiratory depression, decreased consciousness, ***coma, and seizures.*** Miscellaneous symptoms include ***bronchospasm*** (especially in clients with obstructive pulmonary disease), hyperkalemia, and hypoglycemia.

Drug Interactions

Anesthetics, general / Additive depression of myocardium

Anticholinergic agents / Counteract bradycardia produced by beta-adrenergic blockers

Antihypertensives / Additive hypotensive effect

Chlorpromazine / Additive beta-adrenergic blocking action

Cimetidine / ↑ Effect of beta blockers due to ↓ breakdown by liver

Clonidine / Paradoxical hypertension; also, ↑ severity of rebound hypertension

Disopyramide / ↑ Effect of both drugs

Epinephrine / Beta blockers prevent beta-adrenergic action of epinephrine but not alpha-adrenergic action → ↑ systolic and diastolic BP and ↓ HR

Furosemide / ↑ Beta-adrenergic blockade

Hydralazine / ↑ Beta-adrenergic blockade

Indomethacin / ↓ Effect of beta blockers possibly due to inhibition of prostaglandin synthesis

Insulin / Beta blockers ↑ hypoglycemic effect of insulin

Lidocaine / ↑ Effect of lidocaine due to ↓ breakdown by liver

Methyldopa / Possible ↑ BP to alpha-adrenergic effect

NSAIDs / ↓ Effect of beta blockers, possibly due to inhibition of prostaglandin synthesis
Oral contraceptives / ↑ Effect of beta blockers due to ↓ breakdown by liver
Phenformin / ↑ Hypoglycemia
Phenobarbital / ↓ Effect of beta blockers due to ↑ breakdown by liver
Phenothiazines / ↑ Effect of both drugs
Phenytoin / Additive depression of myocardium; also phenytoin ↓ effect of beta blockers due to ↑ breakdown by liver
Prazosin / ↑ First-dose effect of prazosin (acute postural hypotension)
Reserpine / Additive hypotensive effect
Rifampin / ↓ Effect of beta blockers due to ↑ breakdown by liver
Ritodrine / Beta blockers ↓ effect of ritodrine
Salicylates / ↓ Effect of beta blockers, possibly due to inhibition of prostaglandin synthesis
Succinylcholine / Beta blockers ↑ effects of succinylcholine
Sympathomimetics / Reverse effects of beta blockers
Theophylline / Beta blockers reverse the effect of theophylline; also, beta blockers ↓ renal clearance of theophylline
Tubocurarine / Beta blockers ↑ effects of tubocurarine
Verapamil / Possible side effects since both drugs ↓ myocardial contractility or AV conduction; bradycardia and asystole when beta blockers are used ophthalmically

Laboratory Test Interference: ↓ Serum glucose.

Dosage

See individual drugs.

NURSING CONSIDERATIONS

Administration/Storage

1. Sudden cessation of beta blockers may precipitate or worsen angina.
2. The lowering of intraocular pressure may take a few weeks to stabilize when using betaxolol or timolol.
3. Due to diurnal variations in intraocular pressure, the response to b.i.d. therapy is best assessed by measuring intraocular pressure at different times during the day.
4. *Treatment of Overdosage:*

- To improve blood supply to the brain, place client in a supine position and raise the legs.
- Measure blood glucose and serum potassium. Monitor BP and ECG continuously.
- Provide general supportive treatment such as inducing emesis or gastric lavage and artificial respiration.
- *Seizures:* Give IV diazepam or phenytoin.
- *Excessive bradycardia:* If hypotensive, give atropine, 0.6 mg; if no response, give q 3 min for a total of 2–3 mg. Cautious administration of isoproterenol may be tried. Also, glucagon, 5–10 mg rapidly over 30 sec, followed by continuous IV infusion of 5 mg/hr may reverse bradycardia. Transvenous cardiac pacing may be needed for refractory cases.
- *Cardiac failure:* Digitalis, diuretic, and oxygen; if failure is refractory, IV aminophylline or glucagon may be helpful.
- *Hypotension:* Place client in Trendelenburg position. IV fluids unless pulmonary edema is present; also vasopressors such as norepinephrine (may be drug of choice), dobutamine, dopamine with monitoring of BP. If refractory, glucagon may be helpful. In intractable cardiogenic shock, intra-aortic balloon insertion may be required.
- *Premature ventricular contractions:* Lidocaine or phenytoin. Disopyramide, quinidine, and procainamide should be avoided as they depress myocardial function further.
- *Bronchospasms:* Give a beta-2-adrenergic agonist, epinephrine, or theophylline.

• *Heart block, second or third degree:* Isoproterenol or transvenous cardiac pacing.

Assessment

1. Note indications for therapy and carefully assess client's mental status.
2. Determine pulse and BP in both arms with client lying, sitting, and standing, before beginning therapy.
3. Obtain baseline EKG, serum glucose level, CBC, electrolytes, and liver and renal function studies.
4. Note any history of asthma, diabetes, or impaired renal function.
5. With any history of asthma, avoid nonselective beta antagonists due to B_2 receptor blockade which may lead to increased airway resistance.
6. Review drugs currently prescribed to ensure none interact unfavorably.

Interventions

1. Monitor pulse rate and BP; obtain written parameters for medication administration (e.g., hold for SBP < 90 or HR < 50).
2. When assessing the client's respirations note the rate and quality. Drugs in this category may cause dyspnea and bronchospasm.
3. Monitor I&O and daily weights. Observe for increasing dyspnea, coughing, client complaint of difficulty breathing or fatigue, or the presence of edema. These are symptoms of CHF and indicate that the client may require digitalization, diuretics, and/or discontinuation of drug therapy.
4. Assess any client complaints of "having a cold, easy fatigue, or feeling of lightheadedness." These side effects may indicate a need to have the medication changed.
5. If working with a client with diabetes be especially cognizant of symptoms of hypoglycemia, such as hypotension or tachycardia. Most beta-adrenergic blocking agents mask these signs.
6. During IV drug administration, monitor EKG (drug may slow AV conduction and increase PR interval) and activities closely until drug effects are realized.

Client/Family Teaching

1. Instruct in taking own BP and pulse rate. Assess client/family knowledge and understanding of illness and level of compliance based on responses to questions after teaching.
2. Develop a method to maintain accurate written records of BPs and pulse rates. Instruct client to maintain a written record for review by the health care provider so that medication can be adjusted as needed.
3. Provide written instructions as to when to call the provider, for example if the pulse rate goes below 50 beats/min or the BP is less than 90 mm Hg systolic.
4. Once dose is established, take and record BP at least twice a week and take pulse rate immediately prior to first dose each day unless otherwise directed.
5. Reinforce that when prescribed for BP control, medication controls hypertension but does not cure it. Stress the importance of continuing to take the medication despite feeling better and not to stop abruptly as rebound hypertension may occur.
6. Review alternative methods to assist in BP control and stress their importance: exercise, low-fat and reduced-calorie diet, decreased salt intake, and relaxation techniques.
7. Advise client to always consult provider before interrupting therapy because abrupt withdrawal of most beta-adrenergic blocking agents may precipitate angina, MI, or rebound hypertension.
8. Some drugs may cause blurred vision, dizziness or drowsiness; do not engage in activities that require mental alertness until drug effects become apparent.
9. Advise client to rise from a sitting or lying position slowly and to dangle legs before standing to avoid symptoms of orthostatic hypotension.
10. Dress warmly during cold weather because diminished blood supply to extremities may cause client to be more sensitive to the cold. Advise to check extremities for warmth.

11. Avoid excessive intake of alcohol, coffee, tea, or cola. Consult with provider before taking any OTC preparations.
12. Clients with diabetes should be attentive to symptoms of hypoglycemia and should perform finger sticks more often while on drug therapy. Document and report any overt changes.
13. Report any asthma-like symptoms, cough, or nasal stuffiness as these may be symptoms of CHF and require further medical evaluation.
14. Report any bothersome side effects or changes, especially new-onset depression.
15. Always keep all medications out of the reach of children.

Evaluate

- ↓ BP
- ↓ Intraocular pressure
- Reports of ↓ frequency and severity of anginal attacks and improved exercise tolerance
- ↓ Anxiety levels
- ↓ Tremors
- Effective migraine prophylaxis
- ECG confirmation of control of cardiac arrhythmias
- Any evidence of intolerance to drug therapy

Acebutolol hydrochloride

(ays-**BYOU**-toe-lohl)
Pregnancy Category: B
Monitan ✱, Rhotral ✱, Sectral **(Rx)**

See also *Beta-Adrenergic Blocking Agents,* Chapter 51.

How Supplied: *Capsule:* 200 mg, 400 mg

Action/Kinetics: Predominantly beta-1 blocking activity but will inhibit beta-2 receptors at higher doses. Acebutolol also has some intrinsic sympathomimetic activity. **t½:** 3–4 hr. Low lipid solubility. Metabolized in liver and excreted in urine and bile.

Uses: Hypertension (either alone or with other antihypertensive agents such as thiazide diuretics). Premature ventricular contractions.

Dosage

- **Capsules**

Hypertension.

Initial: 400 mg/day (although 200 mg b.i.d. may be needed for optimum control; **then,** 400–800 mg/day (range: 200–1,200 mg/day).

Premature ventricular contractions.

Initial: 200 mg b.i.d.; **then,** increase dose gradually to reach 600–1,200 mg/day.

Dosage should be decreased in geriatric clients (should not exceed 800 mg/day) and in those with impaired kidney or liver function (decrease dose by 50% when creatinine clearance is 50 mL/min/1.73 m^2 and by 75% when it is less than 25 mL/min/1.73 m^2).

Administration/Storage

1. When treatment is discontinued, the drug should be withdrawn gradually over a 2-week period.
2. The bioavailability increases in elderly clients; thus, such clients may require lower maintenance doses (no more than 800 mg/day).
3. Acebutolol may be combined with another antihypertensive agent.
4. Anticipate reduced dosage in clients with impaired liver and renal function.

Additional Contraindication: Severe, persistent bradycardia.

Special Concerns: Dosage has not been established in children.

NURSING CONSIDERATIONS

See also *Nursing Considerations* for *Beta-Adrenergic Blocking Agents,* Chapter 51, and *Antihypertensive Agents,* Chapter 28.

Client/Family Teaching

1. Drug may cause drowsiness; do not perform tasks that require mental alertness until drug effects realized.
2. Drug may cause an increased sensitivity to cold; dress appropriately.

Evaluate

- ↓ BP
- Resolution of PVCs

Atenolol

(ah-**TEN**-oh-lohl)
Pregnancy Category: C
Apo-Atenol ✱, Novo-Atenol ✱, Nu-Atenol ✱, Tenormin **(Rx)**

See also *Beta-Adrenergic Blocking Agents,* Chapter 51.
How Supplied: *Injection:* 0.5 mg/mL; *Tablet:* 25 mg, 50 mg, 100 mg
Action/Kinetics: Predominantly beta-1 blocking activity. Has no membrane stabilizing activity or intrinsic sympathomimetic activity. Low lipid solubility. **Peak blood levels:** 2–4 hr. **t½:** 6–9 hr. 50% eliminated unchanged in the feces.
Uses: Hypertension (either alone or with other antihypertensives such as thiazide diuretics). Angina pectoris due to hypertension, coronary atherosclerosis, and AMI. *Investigational:* Prophylaxis of migraine, alcohol withdrawal syndrome, situational anxiety, ventricular arrhythmias, prophylactically to reduce incidence of supraventricular arrhythmias in coronary artery bypass surgery.

Dosage

- **Tablets**

Hypertension.
Initial: 50 mg/day, either alone or with diuretics; if response is inadequate, 100 mg/day. Doses higher than 100 mg/day will not produce further beneficial effects. Maximum effects will usually be seen within 1–2 weeks.

Angina.
Initial: 50 mg/day; if maximum response is not seen in 1 week, increase dose to 100 mg/day (some clients require 200 mg/day).

Alcohol withdrawal syndrome.
50–100 mg/day.

Prophylaxis of migraine.
50–100 mg/day.

Ventricular arrhythmias.
50–100 mg/day.

Prior to coronary artery bypass surgery.
50 mg/day started 72 hr prior to surgery.

Adjust dosage in cases of renal failure to 50 mg/day if creatinine clearance is 15–35 mL/min/1.73 m² and to 50 mg every other day if creatinine clearance is less than 15 mL/min/1.73 m².

- **IV**

Acute myocardial infarction.
Initial: 5 mg over 5 min followed by a second 5-mg dose 10 min later. Treatment should begin as soon as possible after client arrives at the hospital. In clients who tolerate the full 10-mg dose, a 50-mg tablet should be given 10 min after the last IV dose followed by another 50-mg dose 12 hr later. **Then,** 100 mg/day or 50 mg b.i.d. for 6–9 days (or until discharge from the hospital).

Administration/Storage
1. For IV use, the drug may be diluted in sodium chloride injection, dextrose injection, or sodium chloride and dextrose injection.
2. For hemodialysis clients, 50 mg should be given in the hospital after each dialysis.

Special Concerns: Dosage has not been established in children.

NURSING CONSIDERATIONS

See also *Nursing Considerations* for *Antihypertensive Agents,* Chapter 28, and *Beta-Adrenergic Blocking Agents,* Chapter 51.

Assessment
1. Note any client history of diabetes mellitus, pulmonary disease, or cardiac failure.
2. Document indications for therapy, type, and onset of symptoms.

Client/Family Teaching
1. With angina, advise not to stop drug abruptly as this could precipitate an anginal attack.
2. Report any changes in mood or affect, especially severe depression.
3. Drug may enhance sensitivity to cold.

Evaluate
- ↓ BP to desired range
- ↓ Frequency of anginal attacks
- Prevention of reinfarction

Betaxolol hydrochloride

(beh-**TAX**-oh-lohl)
Pregnancy Category: C
Betoptic, Betoptic S, Kerlone **(Rx)**

See also *Beta-Adrenergic Blocking Agents,* Chapter 51.
How Supplied: *Ophthalmic Solution:* 0.5%; *Ophthalmic Suspension:* 0.25%; *Tablet:* 10 mg, 20 mg
Action/Kinetics: Inhibits beta-1-adrenergic receptors although beta-2 receptors will be inhibited at high doses. Has some membrane stabilizing activity but no intrinsic sympathomimetic activity. Low lipid solubility. When used in the eye, betaxolol reduces the production of aqueous humor, thus, reducing intraocular pressure. It has no effect on pupil size or accommodation. **t½:** 14–22 hr. Metabolized in the liver with most excreted through the urine; about 15% is excreted unchanged.
Uses: PO: Hypertension, alone or with other antihypertensive agents (especially diuretics). **Ophthalmic:** Ocular hypertension and chronic open-angle glaucoma (used alone or in combination with other drugs).

Dosage

- **Tablets**

  Hypertension.

Initial: 10 mg once daily either alone or with a diuretic. If the desired effect is not reached, the dose can be increased to 20 mg although doses higher than 20 mg will not increase the therapeutic effect. In geriatric clients the initial dose should be 5 mg/day.

- **Ophthalmic Solution**

Adults: One gtt b.i.d. If used to replace another drug, continue the drug being used and add 1 gtt of betaxolol b.i.d. The previous drug should be discontinued the following day. If transferring from several antiglaucoma drugs being used together, adjust one drug at a time at intervals of not less than 1 week. The antiglaucoma drug dosage can be decreased or discontinued depending on the response of the client.
Administration/Storage: PO
1. The full antihypertensive effect is usually observed within 7–14 days.
2. As the dose is increased, the HR decreases.
3. Drug therapy with betaxolol should be discontinued gradually over a 2-week period.

Special Concerns: Use with caution during lactation. Safety and effectiveness have not been determined in children. Geriatric clients are at greater risk of developing bradycardia.

NURSING CONSIDERATIONS

See also *Nursing Considerations* for *Beta-Adrenergic Blocking Agents,* Chapter 51, and *Antihypertensive Agents,* Chapter 28.
Evaluate
- ↓ BP (PO)
- ↓ Intraocular pressure (Ophth)

Bisoprolol fumarate

(**BUY**-soh-**proh**-lol)
Pregnancy Category: C
Zebeta **(Rx)**

See also *Beta-Adrenergic Blocking Agents,* Chapter 51.
How Supplied: *Tablet:* 5 mg, 10 mg
Action/Kinetics: At clinical doses, bisoprolol inhibits beta-1-adrenergic receptors; at higher doses beta-2 receptors are also inhibited. The drug has no intrinsic sympathomimetic activity and has no membrane stabilizing activity. **t½:** 9–12 hr. Over 90% of PO dose is absorbed. Approximately 50% is excreted unchanged through the urine and the remainder as inactive metabolites; a small amount (less than 2%) is excreted through the feces.
Uses: For hypertension alone or in combination with other antihypertensive agents. *Investigational:* Angina pectoris, SVTs, PVCs.

Dosage

- **Tablets**

  Antihypertensive.

Dose must be individualized. **Adults, initial:** 5 mg once daily (in some clients, 2.5 mg/day may be appropriate). **Maintenance:** If the 5-mg dose is inadequate, the dose may be increased to 10 mg/day and then, if needed, to 20 mg once daily. In clients with impaired renal or hepatic function, the initial daily dose should be 2.5 mg with caution used in titrating the dose upward.

Administration/Storage

1. Food does not affect the bioavailability of bisoprolol; thus, the drug may be given without regard to meals.
2. The half-life of bisoprolol is increased in clients with a creatinine clearance below 40 mL/min and in those with cirrhosis; thus, the dose must be adjusted.
3. Since bisoprolol is not dialyzable, dose adjustments are not necessary in clients undergoing hemodialysis.

Special Concerns: Use with caution during lactation. Safety and efficacy have not been determined in children. Since bisoprolol is rather selective for beta-1 receptors, it may be used with caution in clients with bronchospastic disease who do not respond to, or who cannot tolerate, other antihypertensive therapy.

Laboratory Test Interferences: ↑ AST, ALT, uric acid, creatinine, BUN, serum potassium, glucose, and phosphorus. ↓ WBCs and platelets.

NURSING CONSIDERATIONS

See also *Nursing Considerations* for *Beta-Adrenergic Blocking Agents,* Chapter 51.

Assessment

1. Document indications for therapy, previous agents used, and the outcome.
2. Obtain baseline CBC, electrolytes, and liver and renal function studies.
3. Once baseline parameters have been determined, continue to monitor BP in both arms with client lying, sitting, and standing.
4. Document cardiac rhythm and any evidence of arrhythmia by ECG.

Evaluate

- ↓ BP
- Relief of angina
- Restoration of stable cardiac rhythm

Carteolol hydrochloride

(kar-**TEE**-oh-lohl)

Pregnancy Category: C

Cartrol, Ocupress **(Rx)**

See also *Beta-Adrenergic Blocking Agents,* Chapter 51.

How Supplied: *Ophthalmic solution:* 1%; *Tablet:* 2.5 mg, 5 mg

Action/Kinetics: Carteolol has both beta-1 and beta-2 receptor blocking activity. The drug has no membrane-stabilizing activity but does have moderate intrinsic sympathomimetic effects. Low lipid solubility. **t½:** 6 hr. Approximately 50%–70% excreted unchanged in the urine.

Uses: PO. Hypertension. *Investigational:* Reduce frequency of anginal attacks. **Ophthalmic.** Chronic open-angle glaucoma and intraocular hypertension alone or in combination with other drugs.

Dosage

- **Tablets**

Hypertension.

Initial: 2.5 mg once daily either alone or with a diuretic. In the event of an inadequate response, the dose may be increased gradually to 5 mg and then 10 mg/day as a single dose. **Maintenance:** 2.5–5 mg once daily. Doses greater than 10 mg/day are not likely to increase the beneficial effect and may decrease the response. The dosage interval should be increased in clients with renal impairment.

Reduce frequency of anginal attacks.

10 mg/day.

- **Ophthalmic Solution**

Usual: 1 gtt in affected eye b.i.d.

Contraindications: Severe, persistent bradycardia. Bronchial asthma or bronchospasm, including severe COPD.

Special Concerns: Dosage has not been established in children.

NURSING CONSIDERATIONS

See also *Nursing Considerations* for *Beta-Adrenergic Blocking Agents,* Chapter 51, and *Antihypertensive Agents,* Chapter 28.

Assessment

1. Document indications for therapy and note baseline findings.
2. Assess renal function; anticipate reduced dose with impairment.

Client/Family Teaching

1. Do not exceed prescribed dose because desired response may be altered.
2. Drug may cause increased sensitivity to cold; dress appropriately.
3. Report any symptoms of bleeding, infection, dizziness, confusion, depression, or rash.

Evaluate

- ↓ BP
- ↓ Frequency of anginal attacks
- ↓ Intraocular pressure

Esmolol hydrochloride

(**EZ**-moh-lohl)
Pregnancy Category: C
Brevibloc **(Rx)**

See also *Beta-Adrenergic Blocking Agents,* Chapter 51.

How Supplied: *Injection:* 10 mg/mL, 250 mg/mL

Action/Kinetics: Esmolol preferentially inhibits beta-1 receptors. It has a rapid onset and a short duration of action. It has no membrane stabilizing or intrinsic sympathomimetic activity. Low lipid solubility. **t½:** 9 min. Is rapidly metabolized by esterases in RBCs.

Uses: Supraventricular tachycardia or arrhythmias, sinus tachycardia.

Dosage

- **IV infusion**

SVT.

Initial: 500 mcg/kg/min for 1 min; **then,** 50 mcg/kg/min for 4 min. If after 5 min an adequate effect is not achieved, repeat the loading dose followed by a maintenance infusion of 100 mcg/kg/min for 4 min. This procedure may be repeated, increasing the maintenance infusion by 50 mcg/kg/min increments (for 4 min) until the desired HR or lowered BP is approached. **Then,** omit the loading infusion and reduce incremental infusion rate from 50 to 25 mcg/kg/min or less. The interval between titrations may be increased from 5 to 10 min.

Once the HR has been controlled, the client may be transferred to another antiarrhythmic agent. The infusion rate of esmolol should be reduced by 50% 30 min after the first dose of the alternative antiarrhythmic agent. If satisfactory control is observed for 1 hr after the second dose of the alternative agent, the esmolol infusion may be stopped.

Administration/Storage

1. Infusions of esmolol may be necessary for 24–48 hr.
2. Esmolol HCl is not intended for direct IV push administration.
3. The concentrate should not be diluted with sodium bicarbonate.
4. To minimize venous irritation and thrombophlebitis, infusion concentrations should not be greater than 10 mg/mL.
5. Diluted esmolol (concentration of 10 mg/mL) is compatible with 5% dextrose injection, 5% dextrose in lactated Ringer's injection, 5% dextrose in Ringer's injection, 5% dextrose and 0.9% sodium chloride injection, 5% dextrose and 0.45% sodium chloride injection, 0.45% sodium chloride injection, lactated Ringer's injection, potassium chloride (40 mEq/L) in 5% dextrose injection, 0.9% sodium chloride injection, and 0.45% sodium chloride injection.

Special Concerns: Dosage has not been established in children.

Additional Side Effects: *Dermatologic:* Inflammation at site of infusion, flushing, pallor, induration, erythema, burning, skin discoloration, edema. *Other:* Urinary retention, midscapular pain, asthenia, changes in taste.

Additional Drug Interactions

Digoxin / Esmolol ↑ digoxin blood levels

Morphine / Morphine ↑ esmolol blood levels

NURSING CONSIDERATIONS

See also *Nursing Considerations* for *Beta-Adrenergic Blocking Agents,* Chapter 51.

Interventions

1. Monitor client closely for evidence of hypotension and/or bradycardia. Request written parameters for withholding drug.
2. Infusions should be administered in a monitored environment with an electronic infusion device. Wean according to guidelines.
3. Monitor VS. Ensure that BP and HR are within desired range.
4. Have emergency drugs and equipment readily available.

Evaluate

- Suppression of supraventricular tachyarrhythmias
- Restoration of stable cardiac rhythm

Levobunolol hydrochloride

(lee-voh-**BYOU**-no-lohl)

Pregnancy Category: C

AKBeta, Betagan ✱, Betagan Liquifilm **(Rx)**

See also *Beta-Adrenergic Blocking Agents,* Chapter 51.

How Supplied: *Solution:* 0.25%, 0.5%

Action/Kinetics: Levobunolol acts on both beta-1- and beta-2-adrenergic receptors. The drug may act by decreasing the formation of aqueous humor. **Onset:** <60 min. **Peak effect:** 2–6 hr. **Duration:** 24 hr.

Uses: To decrease intraocular pressure in chronic open-angle glaucoma or ocular hypertension.

Dosage

- **Ophthalmic Solution (0.25%, 0.5%)**

Adults, usual: 1 gtt of 0.25% or 0.5% solution in affected eye(s) 1–2 times/day (depending on variations in diurnal intraocular pressure).

Administration/Storage

1. If other eye drops are to be administered, wait at least 5 min before instillation of other eye drops.
2. Apply gentle pressure to the inside corner of the eye for approximately 60 sec following instillation.
3. If intraocular pressure is not decreased sufficiently, pilocarpine, epinephrine, or systemic carbonic anhydrase inhibitors may be used.

Special Concerns: Safety and effectiveness have not been determined in children. Significant absorption in geriatric clients may result in myocardial depression. Also, use with caution in angle-closure glaucoma (use with a miotic), in clients with muscle weaknesses, and in those with decreased pulmonary function.

Additional Side Effects: *Ophthalmic:* Stinging and burning (transient), decreased corneal sensitivity, blepharoconjunctivitis. *Dermatologic:* Urticaria, pruritus.

NURSING CONSIDERATIONS

See also *Nursing Considerations* for *Beta-Adrenergic Blocking Agents,* Chapter 51.

Client/Family Teaching

1. Review the method and frequency for instilling eye drops.
2. Instruct client not to close the eyes tightly or blink more frequently than usual after instillation of the drug.
3. Explain the reasons for the medication and the side effects that should be reported if they occur.
4. Stress the importance of return visits to evaluate intraocular pressure and the drug's effectiveness.

Evaluate: ↓ Intraocular pressure.

Metipranolol hydrochloride

(met-ih-**PRAN**-oh-lohl)

Pregnancy Category: C

OptiPranolol **(Rx)**

See also *Beta-Adrenergic Blocking Agents,* Chapter 51.

How Supplied: *Ophthalmic solution:* 0.3%

Action/Kinetics: Metipranolol blocks both beta-1- and beta-2-adrenergic receptors. The mechanism for causing a reduction in intraocular pressure is not known but may be related to a decrease in production of aqueous humor and a slight increase in the outflow of aqueous humor. A decrease from 20% to 26% in intraocular pressure may be seen if the intraocular pressure is greater than 24 mm Hg at baseline. The drug may be absorbed and exert systemic effects. When used topically, metipranolol does not have any local anesthetic effect and exerts no action on pupil size or accommodation. **Onset:** 30 min. **Maximum effect:** 1–2 hr. **Duration:** 12–24 hr.

Uses: To reduce intraocular pressure in clients with ocular hypertension and chronic open-angle glaucoma.

Dosage

- **Ophthalmic Solution**

Adults: 1 gtt in the affected eye(s) b.i.d. Increasing the dose or more frequent administration does not increase the beneficial effect.

Administration/Storage

1. Other drugs to lower intraocular pressure may be used concomitantly with metipranolol.
2. Due to diurnal variation in response, intraocular pressure should be measured at different times during the day.

Special Concerns: Use with caution during lactation. Safety and effectiveness have not been determined in children.

Side Effects: *Ophthalmologic:* Local discomfort, dermatitis of the eyelid, blepharitis, conjunctivitis, browache, tearing, blurred vision, abnormal vision, photophobia, edema. Due to absorption, the following systemic side effects have been reported. *CV:* Hypertension, MI, atrial fibrillation, angina, bradycardia, palpitation. *CNS:* Headache, dizziness, anxiety, depression, somnolence, nervousness. *Respiratory:* Dyspnea, rhinitis, bronchitis, coughing. *Miscellaneous:* Allergic reaction, asthenia, nausea, epistaxis, arthritis, myalgia, rash.

NURSING CONSIDERATIONS

See also *Nursing Considerations* for *Beta-Adrenergic Blocking Agents,* Chapter 51.

Assessment

1. Note ocular condition that requires drug therapy and record pretreatment intraocular pressures.
2. Document baseline ECG and VS.

Client/Family Teaching

1. Demonstrate and review appropriate method for administration.
2. Transient burning or stinging is common during administration but should be reported if severe.
3. Take only as directed and report any persistent bothersome side effects.
4. Stress the importance of reporting for follow-up visits to assess for systemic effects and to measure intraocular pressures to determine drug effectiveness.

Evaluate: A significant lowering of intraocular pressures.

Metoprolol succinate

(me-toe-**PROH**-lohl)

Pregnancy Category: C

Toprol XL **(Rx)**

Metoprolol tartrate

(me-toe-**PROH**-lohl)

Pregnancy Category: B

Apo-Metoprolol (Type L) ✱, Betaloc ✱, Betaloc Durules ✱, Lopressor, Novo–Metoprol ✱, Nu-Metop ✱ **(Rx)**

See also *Beta-Adrenergic Blocking Agents,* Chapter 51.

How Supplied: Metoprolol succinate: *Tablet, Extended Release:* 50 mg, 100 mg, 200 mg.

Metoprolol tartrate: *Injection:* 1 mg/mL; *Tablet:* 50 mg, 100 mg

Action/Kinetics: Exerts mainly beta-1-adrenergic blocking activity although beta-2 receptors are blocked at high doses. Has no membrane stabilizing or intrinsic sympathomimetic effects. Moderate lipid solubility. **Onset:** 15 min. **Peak plasma levels:** 90 min. **t½:** 3–7 hr. Effect of drug is cumulative. Food increases bioavailability. Exhibits significant first-pass effect. Metabolized in liver and excreted in urine.

Uses: Metoprolol Succinate: Alone or with other drugs to treat hypertension. Chronic management of angina pectoris.

Metoprolol Tartrate: Hypertension (either alone or with other antihypertensive agents, such as thiazide diuretics). Acute MI in hemodynamically stable clients. Angina pectoris. *Investigational:* IV to suppress atrial ectopy in COPD, aggressive behavior, prophylaxis of migraine, ventricular arrhythmias, enhancement of cognitive performance in geriatric clients, essential tremors.

Dosage

• **Metoprolol Succinate Tablets**

Angina pectoris.

Individualized. Initial: 100 mg/day in a single dose. Dose may be increased slowly, at weekly intervals, until optimum effect is reached or there is a pronounced slowing of HR. Doses above 400 mg/day have not been studied.

Hypertension.

Initial: 50–100 mg/day in a single dose with or without a diuretic. Dosage may be increased in weekly intervals until maximum effect is reached. Doses above 400 mg/day have not been studied.

• **Metoprolol Tartrate Tablets**

Hypertension.

Initial: 100 mg/day in single or divided doses; **then,** dose may be increased weekly to maintenance level of 100–450 mg/day. A diuretic may also be used.

Aggressive behavior.

200–300 mg/day.

Essential tremors.

50–300 mg/day.

Prophylaxis of migraine.

50–100 mg b.i.d.

Ventricular arrhythmias.

200 mg/day.

• **Metoprolol Tartrate Injection (IV) and Tablets**

Early treatment of MI.

3 IV bolus injections of 5 mg each at approximately 2-min intervals. If clients tolerate the full IV dose, give 50 mg q 6 hr PO beginning 15 min after the last IV dose (or as soon as client's condition allows). This dose is continued for 48 hr followed by **late treatment:** 100 mg b.i.d. as soon as feasible; continue for 1–3 months (although data suggest treatment should be continued for 1–3 years). In clients who do not tolerate the full IV dose, begin with 25–50 mg q 6 hr PO beginning 15 min after the last IV dose or as soon as the condition allows.

Additional Contraindications: Myocardial infarction in clients with a HR of less than 45 beats/min, in second- or third-degree heart block, or if SBP is less than 100 mm Hg. Moderate to severe cardiac failure.

Special Concerns: Safety and effectiveness have not been established in children. Use with caution in impaired hepatic function and during lactation.

Laboratory Test Interferences: ↑ Serum transaminase, LDH, alkaline phosphatase.

Additional Drug Interactions

Cimetidine / May ↑ plasma levels of metoprolol

Contraceptives, oral / May ↑ effects of metoprolol

Methimazole / May ↓ effects of metoprolol

Phenobarbital / ↓ Effect of metoprolol due to ↑ breakdown by liver

Propylthiouracil / May ↓ the effects of metoprolol

Quinidine / May ↑ effects of metoprolol

Rifampin / ↓ Effect of metoprolol due to ↑ breakdown by liver

NURSING CONSIDERATIONS

See also *Nursing Considerations* for *Beta-Adrenergic Blocking Agents,* Chapter 51, and *Antihypertensive Agents,* Chapter 28.

Assessment

1. Document indications for therapy and type and onset of symptoms.

2. Document any history of cardiac disease.
3. Obtain baseline ECG and VS prior to initiating therapy and monitor frequently during IV therapy.

Client/Family Teaching

1. Doses of metoprolol should be taken at the same time each day.
2. Review the importance of diet, regular exercise, and weight loss in the overall plan to control BP.
3. Report any symptoms of fluid overload such as sudden weight gain, edema, or dyspnea.
4. Advise to dress appropriately given that drug may cause increased sensitivity to cold.

Evaluate

- ↓ BP
- ↓ Frequency of anginal attacks
- Prevention of myocardial reinfarction and associated mortality

---

Nadolol

(**NAY**-doh-lohl)
Pregnancy Category: C
Apo-Nadol ✱, Corgard, Syn-Nadolol ✱ **(Rx)**

See also *Beta-Adrenergic Blocking Agents,* Chapter 51.

How Supplied: *Tablet:* 20 mg, 40 mg, 80 mg, 120 mg, 160 mg

Action/Kinetics: Manifests both beta-1- and beta-2-adrenergic blocking activity. Has no membrane stabilizing or intrinsic sympathomimetic activity. Low lipid solubility. **Peak serum concentration:** 3–4 hr. **t½:** 20–24 hr (permits once-daily dosage). **Duration:** 17–24 hr. Absorption variable, averaging 30%; steady plasma level achieved after 6–9 days of administration. Excreted unchanged by the kidney.

Uses: Hypertension, either alone or with other drugs (e.g., thiazide diuretic). Angina pectoris. *Investigational:* Prophylaxis of migraine, ventricular arrhythmias, aggressive behavior, essential tremor, tremors associated with lithium or parkinsonism, antipsychotic-induced akathisia, rebleeding of esophageal varices, situational anxiety, reduce intraocular pressure.

Dosage

- **Tablets**

Hypertension.

Initial: 40 mg/day; **then,** may be increased in 40–80-mg increments until optimum response obtained. **Maintenance:** 40–80 mg/day although up to 240–320 mg/day may be needed.

Angina.

Initial: 40 mg/day; **then,** increase dose in 40–80-mg increments q 3–7 days until optimum response obtained. **Maintenance:** 40–80 mg/day, although up to 160–240 mg/day may be needed.

Aggressive behavior.

40–160 mg/day.

Antipsychotic-induced akathisia.

40–80 mg/day.

Essential tremor.

120–240 mg/day.

Lithium-induced tremors.

20–40 mg/day.

Tremors associated with parkinsonism.

80–320 mg/day.

Prophylaxis of migraine.

40–80 mg/day.

Rebleeding from esophageal varices.

40–160 mg/day.

Situational anxiety.

20 mg.

Ventricular arrhythmias.

10–640 mg/day.

Reduction of intraocular pressure.

10–20 mg b.i.d.

NOTE: Dosage for all uses should be decreased in clients with renal failure.

Contraindications: Bronchial asthma or bronchospasm, including severe COPD.

Special Concerns: Dosage has not been established in children.

NURSING CONSIDERATIONS

See also *Nursing Considerations* for *Beta-Adrenergic Blocking Agents,*

Chapter 51, and *Antihypertensive Agents,* Chapter 28.

Client/Family Teaching

1. Report any evidence of rapid weight gain, increased SOB, or swelling of extremities.
2. Do not perform tasks that require mental alertness until drug effects realized. Nadolol may cause dizziness.
3. Drug may cause an increased sensitivity to cold; dress appropriately.

Evaluate

- ↓ BP
- ↓ Frequency and intensity of angina attacks

Penbutolol sulfate

(pen-**BYOU**-toe-lohl)
Pregnancy Category: C
Levatol **(Rx)**

See also *Beta-Adrenergic Blocking Agents,* Chapter 51.

How Supplied: *Tablet:* 20 mg

Action/Kinetics: Penbutolol has both beta-1- and beta-2-receptor blocking activity. It has no membrane-stabilizing activity but does possess minimal intrinsic sympathomimetic activity. High lipid solubility. **t½:** 5 hr. 80%–98% protein bound. Penbutolol is metabolized in the liver and excreted through the urine.

Uses: Mild to moderate arterial hypertension.

Dosage

- **Tablets**

Hypertension.

Initial: 20 mg/day either alone or with other antihypertensive agents. **Maintenance:** Same as initial dose. Doses greater than 40 mg/day do not result in a greater antihypertensive effect.

Administration/Storage

1. The full effect of a 20–40-mg dose may not be observed for 2 weeks.
2. Doses of 10 mg/day are effective but full effects are not evident for 4–6 weeks.

Contraindications: Bronchial asthma or bronchospasms, including severe COPD.

Special Concerns: Dosage has not been established in children. Geriatric clients may manifest increased or decreased sensitivity to the usual adult dose.

NURSING CONSIDERATIONS

See also *Nursing Considerations* for *Beta-Adrenergic Blocking Agents,* Chapter 51, and *Antihypertensive Agents,* Chapter 28.

Client/Family Teaching

1. Review the S&S associated with postural hypotension and instruct to rise slowly from a sitting or lying position.
2. Take medication only as prescribed because full effects may not be realized for a month or more.
3. Drug may cause an increased sensitivity to cold; dress appropriately.

Evaluate: ↓ BP with desired control of hypertension.

Pindolol

(**PIN**-doh-lohl)
Pregnancy Category: B
Apo-Pindol ✱, Novo–Pindol ✱, Nu-Pindol ✱, Syn-Pindolol ✱, Visken **(Rx)**

See also *Beta-Adrenergic Blocking Agents,* Chapter 51.

How Supplied: *Tablet:* 5 mg, 10 mg

Action/Kinetics: Manifests both beta-1 and beta-2 adrenergic blocking activity. Pindolol also has significant intrinsic sympathomimetic effects and minimal membrane-stabilizing activity. Moderate lipid solubility. **t½:** 3–4 hr; however, geriatric clients have a variable half-life ranging from 7 to 15 hr, even with normal renal function. The drug is metabolized by the liver, and the metabolites and unchanged (35%–40%) drug are excreted through the kidneys.

Uses: Hypertension (alone or in combination with other antihypertensive agents as thiazide diuretics). *Investigational:* Ventricular arrhythmias and tachycardias, antipsychotic-induced akathisia, situational anxiety.

Dosage

- **Tablets**

Hypertension.

Initial: 5 mg b.i.d. (alone or with other antihypertensive drugs). If no response in 3–4 weeks, increase by 10 mg/day/ q 3–4 weeks to a maximum of 60 mg/day.

Antipsychotic-induced akathisia. 5 mg/day.

Contraindications: Bronchial asthma or bronchospasm, including severe COPD.

Special Concerns: Dosage has not been established in children.

Laboratory Test Interferences: ↑ AST and ALT. Rarely, ↑ LDH, uric acid, alkaline phosphatase.

NURSING CONSIDERATIONS

See also *Nursing Considerations* for *Beta-Adrenergic Blocking Agents,* Chapter 51, and *Antihypertensive Agents,* Chapter 28.

Assessment

1. Document indications for therapy and type and onset of symptoms.
2. Assess diet, sodium consumption, weight, exercise regimens, and lifestyle.

Evaluate

- ↓ BP
- ↓ Agitation and anxiety

Propranolol hydrochloride

(proh-**PRAN**-oh-lohl)

Pregnancy Category: C

Apo-Propranolol ✱, Inderal, Inderal 10, 20, 40, 60, 80, and 90, Inderal LA, PMS Propranolol ✱, Propranolol Intensol **(Rx)**

See also *Beta-Adrenergic Blocking Agents,* Chapter 51.

How Supplied: *Capsule, extended release:* 60 mg, 80 mg, 120 mg, 160 mg; *Concentrate:* 80 mg/mL; *Injection:* 1 mg/mL; *Solution:* 20 mg/5 mL, 40 mg/5 mL; *Tablet:* 10 mg, 20 mg, 40 mg, 60 mg, 80 mg

Action/Kinetics: Propranolol manifests both beta-1- and beta-2-adrenergic blocking activity. The antiarrhythmic action results from both beta-adrenergic receptor blockade and a direct membrane-stabilizing action on the cardiac cell. Propranolol has no intrinsic sympathomimetic activity and has high lipid solubility. **PO: Onset,** 30 min. **Maximum effect:** 1–1.5 hr. **Duration:** 3–6 hr. **t½:** 3–5 hr (8–11 hr for long-acting). Onset after IV administration is almost immediate. Completely metabolized by liver and excreted in urine. Although food increases bioavailability of the drug, absorption may be decreased.

Uses: Hypertension (alone or in combination with other antihypertensive agents). Angina pectoris, hypertrophic subaortic stenosis, prophylaxis of MI, pheochromocytoma, prophylaxis of migraine, essential tremor. Cardiac arrhythmias including ventricular tachycardias and arrhythmias, tachycardias due to digitalis intoxication, supraventricular arrhythmias, PVCs, resistant tachyarrhythmias due to anesthesia/catecholamines.

Investigational: Schizophrenia, tremors due to parkinsonism, aggressive behavior, antipsychotic-induced akathisia, rebleeding due to esophageal varices, situational anxiety, acute panic attacks, gastric bleeding in portal hypertension, vaginal contraceptive, anxiety, alcohol withdrawal syndrome.

Dosage

- **Tablets, Sustained-Release Capsules, Oral Solution**

Hypertension.

Initial: 40 mg b.i.d. or 80 mg of sustained-release/day; **then,** increase dose to maintenance level of 120–240 mg/day given in two to three divided doses or 120–160 mg of sustained-release medication once daily. Maximum daily dose should not exceed 640 mg. **Pediatric, initial:** 0.5 mg/kg b.i.d.; dose may be increased at 3–5-day intervals to a maximum of 1 mg/kg b.i.d. The dosage range should be calculated by weight and not by body surface area.

Angina.
Initial: 80–320 mg b.i.d., t.i.d., or q.i.d.; or, 80 mg of sustained-release once daily; **then,** increase dose gradually to maintenance level of 160 mg/day of sustained-release capsule. The maximum daily dose should not exceed 320 mg.

Arrhythmias.
10–30 mg t.i.d.–q.i.d. given after meals and at bedtime.

Hypertrophic subaortic stenosis.
20–40 mg t.i.d.–q.i.d. before meals and at bedtime or 80–160 mg of sustained-release medication given once daily.

MI prophylaxis.
180–240 mg/day given in three to four divided doses. Total daily dose should not exceed 240 mg.

Pheochromocytoma, preoperatively.
60 mg/day for 3 days before surgery, given concomitantly with an alpha-adrenergic blocking agent.

Inoperable tumors.
30 mg/day in divided doses.

Migraine.
Initial: 80 mg sustained-release medication given once daily; **then,** increase dose gradually to maintenance of 160–240 mg/day in divided doses. If a satisfactory response has not been observed after 4–6 weeks, the drug should be discontinued and withdrawn gradually.

Essential tremor.
Initial: 40 mg b.i.d.; **then,** 120 mg/day up to a maximum of 320 mg/day.

Aggressive behavior.
80–300 mg/day.

Antipsychotic-induced akathisia.
20–80 mg/day.

Tremors associated with Parkinson's disease.
160 mg/day.

Rebleeding from esophageal varices.
20–180 mg b.i.d.

Schizophrenia.
300–5,000 mg/day.

Acute panic symptoms.
40–320 mg/day.

Anxiety.
80–320 mg/day.

Intermittent explosive disorder.
50–1,600 mg/day.

Nonvariceal gastric bleeding in portal hypertension.
24–480 mg/day.

• **IV**

Life-threatening arrhythmias or those occurring under anesthesia.
1–3 mg not to exceed 1 mg/min; a second dose may be given after 2 min, with subsequent doses q 4 hr. Clients should begin PO therapy as soon as possible. Although use in pediatrics is not recommended, investigational doses of 0.01–0.1 mg/kg/dose, up to a maximum of 1 mg/dose (by slow push), have been used for arrhythmias.

Administration/Storage

1. Do not administer for a minimum of 2 weeks after client has received MAO inhibitor drugs.
2. If signs of serious myocardial depression occur following propranolol administration, isoproterenol (Isuprel) should be slowly infused IV.
3. For IV use, dilute 1 mg in 10 mL of D5W and administer IV over at least 1 min. May be further reconstituted in 50 mL of dextrose or saline solution and infused IVPB over 10–15 min.
4. After IV administration, have available emergency drugs and equipment to combat hypotension or circulatory collapse.

Contraindications: Bronchial asthma, bronchospasms including severe COPD.

Special Concerns: It is dangerous to use propranolol for pheochromocytoma unless an alpha-adrenergic blocking agent is already in use.

Laboratory Test Interferences: ↑ Blood urea, serum transaminase, alkaline phosphatase, LDH. Interference with glaucoma screening test.

Additional Side Effects: Psoriasis-like eruptions, skin necrosis, SLE (rare).

Additional Drug Interactions

Haloperidol / Severe hypotension
Hydralazine / ↑ Effect of both agents

Methimazole / May ↑ effects of propranolol
Phenobarbital / ↓ Effect of propranolol due to ↑ breakdown by liver
Propylthiouracil / May ↑ the effects of propranolol
Rifampin / ↓ Effect of propranolol due to ↑ breakdown by liver
Smoking / ↓ Serum levels and ↑ clearance of propranolol

NURSING CONSIDERATIONS

See also *Nursing Considerations* for *Beta-Adrenergic Blocking Agents,* Chapter 51, and *Antihypertensive Agents,* Chapter 28.

Assessment

1. Document indications for therapy, other agents prescribed, and type and onset of symptoms.
2. Note any evidence of pulmonary disease or bronchospasms.

Interventions

1. Observe client for evidence of a rash, fever, and/or purpura. These may be symptoms of a hypersensitivity reaction.
2. Monitor I&O. Observe for S&S of CHF (e.g., SOB, rales, edema, and weight gain).

Client/Family Teaching

1. Caution that drug may cause drowsiness. Advise to assess drug response before performing activities that require mental alertness.
2. Do not smoke. Smoking decreases serum levels of the drug and interferes with drug clearance.
3. In clients with diabetes, drug may mask most symptoms of hypoglycemia. Monitor finger sticks carefully.
4. Instruct client to check BP and HR weekly and to report if any significant changes are noted.
5. Do not stop drug abruptly as this could precipitate hypertension, myocardial ischemia, or cardiac arrhythmias.
6. Dress appropriately; drug may cause increased sensitivity to cold.
7. Report any persistent side effects, e.g., skin rashes, abnormal bleeding, unusual crying, or feelings of depression.

Evaluate

- ↓ BP
- ↓ Frequency and intensity of angina episodes
- Effective migraine prophylaxis
- Control of tachyarrhythmias
- Desired behavioral changes
- Prevention of myocardial reinfarction
- Relief/control of chronic pain

Sotalol hydrochloride

(**SOH**-tah-lol)
Pregnancy Category: B
Betapace **(Rx)**

See also *Beta-Adrenergic Blocking Agents,* Chapter 51.

How Supplied: *Tablet:* 80 mg, 160 mg, 240 mg

Action/Kinetics: Sotalol blocks both beta-1 and beta-2 adrenergic receptors and has no membrane-stabilizing activity or intrinsic sympathomimetic activity. It has both Group II and Group III antiarrhythmic properties (dose dependent). Sotalol significantly increases the refractory period of the atria, His-Purkinje fibers, and ventricles. It also prolongs the QTc and JT intervals. **t½:** 12 hr. The drug is not metabolized and is excreted unchanged in the urine.

Uses: Treatment of documented ventricular arrhythmias such as life-threatening sustained ventricular tachycardia.

Dosage

- **Tablets**

Ventricular arrhythmias.

Adults, initial: 80 mg b.i.d. The dose may be increased to 240 or 320 mg/day after appropriate evaluation. **Usual:** 160–320 mg/day given in two or three divided doses. Clients with life-threatening refractory ventricular arrhythmias may require doses ranging from 480 to 640 mg/day (due to potential proarrhythmias, these doses should only be used if the potential benefit outweighs the increased risk of side effects).

Administration/Storage

1. Food decreases the absorption of sotalol; thus, the drug should be taken on an empty stomach.
2. Dosage should be adjusted gradually, allowing 2–3 days between increments in dosage. This allows steady-state plasma levels to be reached and QT intervals to be monitored.
3. Initiation of and increases in dosage should be undertaken in a hospital with facilities for cardiac rhythm monitoring and assessment. The dose for each client must be individualized only after appropriate clinical assessment.
4. Proarrhythmias can occur during initiation of therapy and with each increment in dosage.
5. In clients with impaired renal function, the dosing interval should be altered as follows: if creatinine clearance is 30–60 mL/min, the dosing interval is 24 hr; if creatinine clearance is 10–30 mL/min, the dosing interval should be 36–48 hr. The dose in clients with creatinine clearance less than 10 mL/min must be individualized. Dosage adjustments in clients with impaired renal function should only be undertaken after five to six doses at the intervals described.
6. Before initiating sotalol, previous antiarrhythmic therapy should be withdrawn with careful monitoring for a minimum of 2–3 plasma half-lives if the client's condition permits.
7. After amiodarone is discontinued, do not initiate sotalol until the QT interval is normalized.

Contraindications: Use in asymptomatic PVCs or supraventricular arrhythmias due to the proarrhythmic effects of sotalol. Congenital or acquired long QT syndromes. Use in clients with hypokalemia or hypomagnesemia until the imbalance is corrected, as these conditions aggravate the degree of QT prolongation and increase the risk for torsades de pointes.

Special Concerns: Clients with sustained ventricular tachycardia and a history of CHF appear to be at the highest risk for serious proarrhythmia. Dose, presence of sustained ventricular tachycardia, females, excessive prolongation of the QTc interval, and history of cardiomegaly or CHF are risk factors for torsades de pointes. Use with caution in clients with chronic bronchitis or emphysema and in those with asthma if an IV agent is required. Use with extreme caution in clients with sick sinus syndrome associated with symptomatic arrhythmias due to the increased risk of sinus bradycardia, sinus pauses, or sinus arrest. The dosage should be reduced in clients with impaired renal function. Safety and efficacy in children have not been established.

Additional Side Effects: *CV:* ***New or worsened ventricular arrhythmias, including sustained ventricular tachycardia or ventricular fibrillation that might be fatal. Torsades de pointes.***

NURSING CONSIDERATIONS

See also *Nursing Considerations* for *Beta-Adrenergic Blocking Agents,* Chapter 51.

Assessment

1. Perform a thorough nursing history. Document any evidence of cardiomegaly or CHF.
2. Obtain baseline electrolytes, magnesium level, and renal function studies.
3. List all medications used for treatment of arrhythmia and the outcome.
4. Document baseline ECG and note symptoms associated with the ventricular arrhythmia.

Interventions

1. Client should be in a closely monitored environment with VS and ECG monitored during initiation and adjustment of sotalol.
2. Monitor VS and I&O frequently and assess serum potassium and magnesium levels.
3. Document QT interval and report any prolongation or altered cardiac rhythm.
4. Report any symptoms of CHF (increased fatigue, dyspnea, or bradycardia).

Evaluate: ECG evidence of control or conversion of life-threatening ventricular arrhythmias to a stable cardiac rhythm.

Timolol maleate

(**TIE**-moh-lohl)

Pregnancy Category: C

Apo-Timol ✱, Apo-Timop ✱, Blocadren, Gen-Timolol ✱, Novo-Timol ✱, Timoptic, Timoptic in Acudose, Timoptic-XE **(Rx)**

See also *Beta-Adrenergic Blocking Agents,* Chapter 51.

How Supplied: *Gel forming solution:* 0.25%, 0.5%; *Ophthalmic solution:* 0.25%, 0.5%; *Tablet:* 5 mg, 10 mg, 20 mg

Action/Kinetics: Timolol exerts both beta-1- and beta-2-adrenergic blocking activity. Timolol has minimal sympathomimetic effects, direct myocardial depressant effects, and local anesthetic action. It does not cause pupillary constriction or night blindness. The mechanism of the protective effect in MI is not known. **Peak plasma levels:** 1–2 hr. **t½:** 4 hr. Metabolized in the liver. Metabolites and unchanged drug excreted through the kidney.

Timolol also reduces both elevated and normal intraocular pressure, whether or not glaucoma is present; it is thought to act by reducing aqueous humor formation and/or by slightly increasing outflow of aqueous humor. The drug does not affect pupil size or visual acuity. For use in eye: **Onset:** 30 min. **Maximum effect:** 1–2 hr. **Duration:** 24 hr.

Uses: Tablets: Hypertension (alone or in combination with other antihypertensives such as thiazide diuretics). Within 1–4 weeks of MI to reduce risk of reinfarction. Prophylaxis of migraine. *Investigational:* Ventricular arrhythmias and tachycardias, essential tremors.

Ophthalmic solution (Timoptic): Lower intraocular pressure in chronic open-angle glaucoma, selected cases of secondary glaucoma, ocular hypertension, aphakic (no lens) clients with glaucoma. *Ophthalmic gel forming solution (Timoptic-XE):* Reduce elevated intraocular pressure in glaucoma.

Dosage

• **Tablets**

Hypertension.

Initial: 10 mg b.i.d. alone or with a diuretic; **maintenance:** 20–40 mg/day (up to 80 mg/day in two doses may be required), depending on BP and HR. If dosage increase is necessary, wait 7 days.

MI prophylaxis in clients who have survived the acute phase.

10 mg b.i.d.

Migraine prophylaxis.

Initially: 10 mg b.i.d. **Maintenance:** 20 mg/day given as a single dose; total daily dose may be increased to 30 mg in divided doses or decreased to 10 mg, depending on the response and client tolerance. If a satisfactory response for migraine prophylaxis is not obtained within 6–8 weeks using the maximum daily dose, the drug should be discontinued.

Essential tremor.

10 mg/day.

• **Ophthalmic Solution (Timoptic)**

Glaucoma.

1 gtt of 0.25%–0.50% solution in each eye b.i.d.

• **Ophthalmic gel forming solution (0.25%, 0.5%)**

Glaucoma.

1 gtt once daily.

Administration/Storage

Ophthalmic Solution

1. When client is transferred from another antiglaucoma agent, continue old medication on day 1 of timolol therapy (1 gtt of 0.25% solution). Thereafter, discontinue former therapy. Initiate with 0.25% solution. Increase to 0.50% solution if response is insufficient. Further increases in dosage are ineffective.

2. When client is transferred from several antiglaucoma agents, the dose must be individualized. If one of the agents is a beta-adrenergic

blocking agent, it should be discontinued before starting timolol. Dosage adjustments should involve one drug at a time at 1-week intervals. The antiglaucoma drugs should be continued with the addition of timolol, 1 gtt of 0.25% solution b.i.d. (if response is inadequate, 1 gtt of 0.5% solution may be used b.i.d.). The following day, one of the other antiglaucoma agents should be discontinued while the remaining agents should be continued or discontinued based on client response.

Contraindications: Hypersensitivity to drug. Bronchial asthma or bronchospasm including severe COPD.

Special Concerns: Use ophthalmic preparation with caution in clients for whom systemic beta-adrenergic blocking agents are contraindicated. Safe use in children not established.

Laboratory Test Interferences: ↑ BUN, serum potassium, and uric acid. ↓ H&H.

Side Effects: *Systemic following use of tablets:* See *Beta-Adrenergic Blocking Agents,* Chapter 51.

Following use of ophthalmic product: Few. Occasionally, ocular irritation, local hypersensitivity reactions, slight decrease in resting HR.

Drug Interaction: When used ophthalmically, possible potentiation with systemically administered beta-adrenergic blocking agents.

NURSING CONSIDERATIONS

See also *Nursing Considerations* for *Beta-Adrenergic Blocking Agents,* Chapter 51, and *Antihypertensive Agents,* Chapter 28.

Client/Family Teaching

1. Review appropriate procedure for ophthalmic administration. Have client or person administering therapy return demonstrate.

• Instruct client to apply finger lightly to lacrimal sac for 1 min following administration.

• Stress the importance of continued regular intraocular measurements by an ophthalmologist because ocular hypertension may recur and/or progress without overt signs or symptoms.

2. When timolol tablets are used for long-term prophylaxis against MI, do not interrupt therapy without approval. Abrupt withdrawal may precipitate reinfarction.

3. Report any evidence of rash, dizziness, heart palpitations, or depression.

4. Drug may cause dizziness. Do not perform tasks such as driving or operating machinery until drug effects are realized.

5. Drug may cause increased sensitivity to cold; advise to dress appropriately.

6. Clients with diabetes should be advised that drug may mask some symptoms of hypoglycemia, so careful monitoring of glucose levels is imperative.

7. Remind to continue lifestyle modifications (i.e., weight reduction, regular exercise, reduced intake of sodium and alcohol, and no smoking) in the overall goal of BP control.

Evaluate

• Control of hypertension with ↓ BP

• Prevention of myocardial reinfarction

• Migraine prophylaxis

• ↓ Intraocular pressures

CHAPTER FIFTY-TWO

Skeletal Muscle Relaxants - Centrally Acting

See also the following individual entries:

Baclofen
Carisoprodol
Chlorzoxazone
Cyclobenzaprine Hydrochloride
Dantrolene Sodium
Diazepam - See Chapter 40
Metaxalone
Methocarbamol
Orphenadrine Citrate
Soma Compound
Soma Compound with Codeine

Action/Kinetics: The centrally acting skeletal muscle relaxants decrease muscle tone and involuntary movement. Many relieve anxiety and tension as well. Although the precise mechanism of action is unknown, most of these agents depress spinal polysynaptic reflexes. Their beneficial effects may also be attributable to their antianxiety activity. Several of the drugs in this group also manifest analgesic properties.

Uses: Musculoskeletal and neurologic disorders associated with muscle spasms, hyperreflexia, and hypertonia, including parkinsonism, tetanus, tension headaches, acute muscle spasms caused by trauma, and inflammation (e.g., low back syndrome, sprains, arthritis, bursitis). They also may be useful in the management of cerebral palsy and multiple sclerosis.

Side Effects: Side effects often involve the CNS, GI system, and urinary system. Symptoms of allergy may also be manifested. For specific side effects, see individual drugs.

Symptoms of Overdose: Often extensions of the side effects. Stupor, ***coma, shock-like syndrome, respiratory depression,*** loss of muscle tone, and impaired deep tendon reflexes may also occur.

Drug Interactions: Centrally acting muscle relaxants may increase the sedative and respiratory depressant effects of CNS depressants (e.g., alcohol, barbiturates, sedatives and hypnotics, and antianxiety agents).

Dosage

See individual agents.

NURSING CONSIDERATIONS

Administration

1. Crush tablets or empty capsules into a small amount of fruit juice if the client is unable to swallow.
2. If the skeletal muscle relaxant is to be discontinued after long-term use, the dose of drug should be tapered to prevent rebound spasticity, hallucinations, or other withdrawal symptoms.
3. Review list of drug interactions.
4. The lowest possible dosage of drug should be determined and used to treat the client's symptoms.
5. *Treatment of Overdose:* Symptomatic. Emesis or gastric lavage (followed by activated charcoal). If necessary, artificial respiration, oxygen administration, pressor agents, and IV fluids may be used. It may be possible to increase the rate of excretion of selected drugs by diuretics

(including mannitol); peritoneal dialysis, or hemodialysis.

Assessment

1. Document indications for therapy and type and onset of symptoms. Note other agents prescribed and the outcome.
2. Note any history of prior seizures. Some drugs in this category may cause loss of seizure control.
3. Assess the extent of the client's musculoskeletal and neurologic disorders associated with muscle spasm. Note muscle stiffness, pain, and extent of ROM.
4. Conduct a thorough baseline mental status examination and document findings.

Interventions

1. Monitor BP q 4 hr when therapy is initiated in a hospital setting.
2. Supervise ambulation and transfers and ensure a safe client environment. With these drugs, sedentary or immobilized clients are more prone to hypotension upon ambulation.
3. Note client complaints of nausea, anorexia, or changes in taste perception. Report if these symptoms persist, as nutritional state may become impaired.
4. Monitor the client's urinary output. Anticipate the need to use drugs to increase the rate of excretion if the output is too low.
5. Document the level of mobility (ROM) and comfort level (pain) prior to and following drug administration.
6. Check the client's muscle responses and deep tendon reflexes for symptoms of drug overdosage.

Client/Family Teaching

1. Take medication with meals to reduce GI irritation.
2. Review the goals of the medication therapy with the client and family and determine to what extent they have been met.
3. Do not operate dangerous machinery or drive a car when taking these drugs because they may impair mental alertness.
4. Advise not to stop medication abruptly as this may precipitate withdrawal symptoms.
5. Review additional therapies that may be prescribed for muscle spasm (heat, rest, exercise, physical therapy) and stress the importance of adhering to this regimen.
6. Advise to increase fluids and bulk in diet to prevent constipation.
7. Report if the urine becomes dark, the skin or sclera appears yellow, or pruritus develops, and discontinue using the medication.
8. Avoid using antihistamines because these drugs may produce an additive depressant effect.
9. Avoid the use of alcohol and any other CNS depressants.
10. Stress the importance of reporting for all scheduled lab and medical follow-up visits so therapy can be evaluated and drug dosage adjusted as needed.

Evaluate

- Reports of symptomatic improvement in extent and intensity of muscle spasm and pain
- Clinical evidence of ↑ ROM with measurable improvement in muscle tone, mobility, and involuntary movements
- Effective control of tension headaches

Baclofen

(**BAK**-low-fen)

Pregnancy Category: C

Alpha-Baclofen ✱, Lioresal **(Rx)**

See also *Skeletal Muscle Relaxants, Centrally Acting,* Chapter 52.

How Supplied: *Kit:* 0.5 mg/mL, 2 mg/mL; *Tablet:* 10 mg, 20 mg

Action/Kinetics: The mechanism of action of baclofen is not fully known, but the drug is known to inhibit both mono- and polysynaptic spinal reflexes perhaps by hyperpolarization of afferent terminals. It may also act at certain brain sites. **Peak serum levels PO:** 2–3 hr. **Therapeutic serum levels:** 80–400 ng/mL. **t½ PO:** 3–4 hr. **Onset after intrathecal bolus:** 30–60 min; **peak effect after intrathecal bolus:** 4 hr; **duration after intrathecal bolus:** 4–8 hr. **Onset after intrathecal**

continuous infusion: 6–8 hr; **peak effect after intrathecal continuous infusion:** 24–48 hr. Seventy percent to 80% of the drug is eliminated unchanged by the kidney.

Uses: PO. Multiple sclerosis (flexor spasms, pain, clonus, and muscular rigidity) and diseases and injuries of the spinal cord associated with spasticity. It is not effective for the treatment of cerebral palsy, stroke, parkinsonism, or rheumatic disorders. *Investigational:* Trigeminal neuralgia, tardive dyskinesia.

Intrathecal. Severe spasticity of spinal cord origin in clients unresponsive to PO baclofen therapy or who have intolerable CNS side effects. *Investigational:* Reduce spasticity in children with cerebral palsy.

Dosage

- **Tablets**

Muscle relaxant.

Adults, initial: 5 mg t.i.d. for 3 days; **then,** 10 mg t.i.d. for 3 days, 15 mg t.i.d. for 3 days, and 20 mg t.i.d. Additional increases in dose may be required but should not exceed 20 mg q.i.d.

- **Intrathecal**

Initial screening bolus.

50 mcg/mL given into the intrathecal space by barbotage over a period of not less than 1 min. The client is observed for 4–8 hr for a positive response consisting of a decrease in muscle tone, frequency, and/or severity of muscle spasms. If the response is not adequate, a second bolus dose of 75 mcg/1.5 mL, 24 hr after the first bolus dose, can be given with the client observed for 4–8 hr. If the response is still inadequate, a final bolus screening dose of 100 mcg/2 mL can be given 24 hr later.

Postimplant dose titration.

To determine the initial daily dose of baclofen following the implant for intrathecal use, the screening dose that gave a positive response should be doubled and given over a 24-hr period. However, if the effectiveness of the bolus dose lasted for more than 12 hr, the daily dose should be the same as the screening dose but delivered over a period of 24 hr. After the first 24 hr, the dose can be increased slowly by 10%–30% increments only once each 24 hr until the desired effect is reached.

Maintenance therapy.

The maintenance dose may need to be adjusted during the first few months of intrathecal therapy. The daily dose may be increased by 10% to no more than 40% daily. If side effects occur, the daily dose may be decreased by 10%–20%. Daily doses for long-term continuous infusion have ranged from 12 to 1,500 mcg (usual maintenance is 300-800 mcg/day). The lowest dose producing optimal control should be used.

Administration/Storage

1. If beneficial effects are not noted, the drug should be withdrawn slowly.
2. The manufacturer's manual should be checked for specific instructions and precautions as to how to program the implantable intrathecal infusion pump or how to refill the reservoir.
3. Prior to implantation of the pump for intrathecal use, clients must show a positive response to a bolus dose of baclofen in a screening trial.
4. If there is not a significant clinical response to increases in the daily dose given intrathecally, the pump should be checked for proper function and the catheter for patency.
5. During long-term intrathecal treatment, approximately 10% of clients become tolerant to increasing doses. If this occurs, a drug "holiday" consisting of a gradual decrease of intrathecal baclofen over a 2-week period can be considered. Alternate methods to treat spasticity must be undertaken. After a few days, sensitivity to baclofen may return. However, to avoid possible side effects or overdose, the alternative medication should be discontinued slowly.
6. Filling of the reservoir for intrathecal use must be performed only by

fully trained and qualified personnel. Refill intervals must be carefully calculated to avoid depletion of the reservoir.
7. Extreme caution should be used when filling an FDA-approved implantable pump equipped with an injection port (i.e., that allows direct access to the intrathecal catheter). Direct injection into the catheter through the access port may result in a life-threatening overdose of baclofen.
8. For screening purposes, intrathecal baclofen, either 10 mg/20 mL or 10 mg/5 mL, must be diluted with sterile preservative-free sodium chloride for injection, to a concentration of 50 mcg/mL for bolus administration. For maintenance, baclofen must be diluted with sterile preservative-free sodium chloride for injection USP for clients who require concentrations other than 500 mcg/mL (i.e., the 10 mg/20 mL product) or 2,000 mcg/mL (i.e., the 10 mg/5 mL product).
9. *Treatment of Overdose:*
• After PO use:
• Induce vomiting (only if the client is alert and conscious) followed by gastric lavage.
• If the client is not alert and conscious, undertake only gastric lavage making sure the airway is secured with a cuffed ET tube.
• Maintain an adequate airway.
• Atropine may be used to improve HR, BP, ventilation, and core body temperature.
• After intrathecal use:
• The residual solution is to be removed from the pump as soon as possible.
• Intubate the client with respiratory depression until the drug is eliminated.
• IV physostigmine (total dose of 1–2 mg given over 5–10 min) may be tried, with caution.
• Consideration can also be given to withdrawing 30–60 mL of CSF to decrease baclofen levels (provided that lumbar puncture is not contraindicated).

Contraindications: Hypersensitivity. Rheumatic disorders, spasm resulting from Parkinson's disease, stroke, cerebral palsy. Intrathecal product for IV, IM, SC, or epidural use.

Special Concerns: Safe use of the oral product for children under 12 years of age and of the intrathecal product for children under 18 years of age has not been established. Use with caution in impaired renal function. Geriatric clients may be at higher risk for developing CNS toxicity, including mental depression, confusion, hallucinations, and significant sedation. Due to serious, life-threatening side effects after intrathecal use, physicians must be trained and educated in chronic intrathecal infusion therapy.

Laboratory Test Interferences: ↑ AST, alkaline phosphatase, blood glucose.

Side Effects: *CNS:* Drowsiness, dizziness, weakness, fatigue, confusion, headaches, insomnia. Hallucinations following abrupt withdrawal. *CV:* Hypotension. Rarely, chest pain, syncope, palpitations. *GI:* Nausea, constipation. *GU:* Urinary frequency. *Other:* Rash, pruritus, ankle edema, increased perspiration, weight gain, dyspnea, nasal congestion. In addition, intrathecal use may cause weakness of the lower and upper extremities, numbness, itching, tingling, hypotonia, hypertension, and coma.

Symptoms of Overdose: Symptoms after PO use include vomiting, drowsiness, muscular hypotonia, muscle twitching, accommodation disorders, respiratory depression, seizures, coma. Symptoms after intrathecal use include drowsiness, dizziness, lightheadedness, somnolence, respiratory depression, rostral progression of hypotonia, ***seizures, loss of consciousness leading to coma (for up to 24 hr).***

Drug Interactions: Concomitant use with CNS depressants → additive CNS depression.

NURSING CONSIDERATIONS

See also *Nursing Considerations* for *Skeletal Muscle Relaxants, Centrally Acting,* Chapter 52.

Assessment

1. Document indications for therapy and include all pretreatment clinical assessment findings.
2. Assess clients with epilepsy for clinical S&S of their disease. Arrange for an EEG at regular intervals because baclofen has been associated with reduced seizure control.
3. Obtain liver and renal function studies before initiating therapy.
4. Note if the client has diabetes.
5. Clients must be closely monitored in a fully equipped and staffed facility during both the intrathecal screening phase and dose-titration period following the intrathecal implant. Resuscitative equipment should be readily available.
6. Ensure that client is free from S&S of infection. Systemic infection may alter response to screening trials and (during pump implantation) may lead to surgical complications and interfere with the pump dosing rate.
7. Assess client for level of useful spasticity (e.g., to aid in transfers or to maintain posture) as rigidity is important for gait in some clients.
8. In clients who require hypertonicity to stand upright, to maintain balance when walking, or to increase their function, baclofen may be contraindicated because it interferes with this coping mechanism.

Interventions

1. Note any evidence of hypersensitivity reaction and report.
2. If clients complain of constipation, increase fluid intake and increase roughage in the diet.
3. Monitor urinary output and test the urine for occult blood.
4. Monitor the client's weight. Report any evidence of edema.
5. If improvement in the client's condition does not occur within 6–8 weeks, the drug should be withdrawn gradually.
6. For clients with an intrathecal pump:
   - Calculate pump refill interval carefully to prevent an empty reservoir and the return of severe spasticity.
   - The pump reservoir should only be accessed percutaneously, refilled, and programmed by someone specifically trained in this procedure.
   - When filling pumps with injection ports that permit direct access to the catheter, use care as an injection directly into the catheter can cause a lethal overdose. In this event, immediately remove any residual drug from the pump and follow guidelines for Treatment of Overdose under Administration/Storage.
   - When the dose requirements suddenly escalate, assess for catheter kinks or dislodgement.
   - When programming for increased dosage, for example at bedtime, the flow rate should be programmed to change 2 hr before the desired effect.

Client/Family Teaching

1. Take oral medication with meals or a snack to avoid gastric irritation. Report if GI symptoms are severe or persistent.
2. Reassure that it may take several weeks of therapy before physical improvement occurs.
3. Instruct clients in how to monitor their own I&O and to keep a record of the frequency and amounts of each voiding.
4. Advise clients with diabetes mellitus that drug may alter insulin requirements.
5. Advise male clients of the potential for the drug to cause impotence and to report if this occurs as a change of drug or dosage may be required. Clients should be warned, however, not to discontinue taking the drug without approval.
6. For clients with an intrathecal pump:
   - Once the screening trials have been successfully completed, explain that the "baclofen pump" will be surgically placed in the abdominal

wall and attached to an implanted lumbar intrathecal catheter. Demonstrate proper postoperative site care and review S&S of infection that require immediate reporting.

- Advise client to maintain a log identifying when the spasms are greatest. This will facilitate the proper pump programming to ensure optimal control of spasticity and discomfort.
- Provide a printed list of the symptoms that require immediate medical intervention.
- Instruct clients to report for scheduled appointments (usually once a month with maintenance) to ensure proper levels of drug in the reservoir and to prevent air in the reservoir or loss of effect.
- Advise that drowsiness, dizziness, and lower extremity weakness may occur but should be reported if persistent or progressive as drug dose may require adjustment.
- Clients who become refractory to increasing doses may require hospitalization for a "drug holiday." This would consist of a *gradual reduction* of intrathecal baclofen over a 2-week period and alternative therapy with other agents. Sensitivity to baclofen usually returns after several days and may be resumed intrathecally at the initial continuous dose.

Evaluate

- ↓ Skeletal muscle spasticity and pain
- Improvement in muscle tone and involuntary movements
- A notable ↓ in painful or disabling symptoms permitting ↑ functioning level

Carisoprodol

(kar-eye-so-**PROH**-dohl)
Pregnancy Category: C
Soma **(Rx)**

See also *Skeletal Muscle Relaxants, Centrally Acting,* Chapter 52.

How Supplied: *Tablet:* 350 mg

Action/Kinetics: Carisoprodol does not directly relax skeletal muscles in humans. Sedative effects may be responsible for muscle relaxation. **Onset:** 30 min. **Duration:** 4–6 hr. **Peak serum levels:** 4–7 mcg/mL. **t½:** 8 hr. The drug is metabolized in the liver and excreted in the urine.

Uses: As an adjunct to rest, physical therapy, and other measures to treat skeletal muscle disorders including bursitis, low back disorders, contusions, fibrositis, spondylitis, sprains, muscle strains, and cerebral palsy.

Dosage

- **Tablets**

Skeletal muscle disorders.

Adults: 350 mg q.i.d. (take last dose at bedtime).

Administration/Storage

1. If the client is unable to swallow tablets, mix drug with syrup, chocolate, or a jelly mixture.
2. Administer the drug with food if gastric upset occurs.
3. *Treatment of Overdose:* Supportive measures. Diuresis, osmotic diuresis, peritoneal dialysis, hemodialysis. Urinary output should be monitored to avoid overhydration. Client should be observed for possible relapse due to incomplete gastric emptying and delayed absorption.

Contraindications: Acute intermittent porphyria. Hypersensitivity to carisoprodol or meprobamate. Children under 12 years of age.

Special Concerns: Use with caution during lactation. The drug may cause GI upset and sedation in the infant. Use with caution in impaired liver or kidney function.

Side Effects: *CNS:* Ataxia, dizziness, drowsiness, excitement, tremor, syncope, vertigo, insomnia, irritability, headache, depressive reactions. *GI:* N&V, gastric upset, hiccoughs. *CV:* Flushing of face, postural hypotension, tachycardia. *Allergic reactions:* Pruritus, skin rashes, erythema multiforme, eosinophilia, fever, dizziness, angioneurotic edema, asthmatic symptoms, "smarting" of the eyes, weakness, hypotension, ***anaphylaxis.***

Symptoms of Overdose: Stupor, coma, shock, respiratory depression, and rarely death.

Drug Interactions
Alcohol / Additive CNS depressant effects
Antidepressants, tricyclic / ↑ Effect of carisoprodol
Barbiturates / Possible ↑ effect of carisoprodol, followed by inhibition of carisoprodol
Chlorcyclizine / ↓ Effect of carisoprodol
CNS depressants / Additive CNS depression
MAO inhibitors / ↑ Effect of carisoprodol by ↓ breakdown by liver
Phenobarbital / ↓ Effect of carisoprodol by ↑ breakdown by liver
Phenothiazines / Additive depressant effects

NURSING CONSIDERATIONS

See also *Nursing Considerations* for *Skeletal Muscle Relaxants, Centrally Acting,* Chapter 52.

Assessment
1. Note any history of hypersensitivity to meprobamate or carisoprodol.
2. Record extent of skeletal muscular disorders noting baseline ROM and level of discomfort.
3. Review drugs currently prescribed to ensure no unfavorable interactions.

Interventions
1. Observe client for evidence of ataxia or tremors and report.
2. Report if the client develops postural hypotension or tachycardia. These may necessitate discontinuation of the medication.

Client/Family Teaching
1. Provide a printed list of side effects that require reporting should they occur.
2. Assist the client in establishing a drug schedule so that the last dose of drug is taken at bedtime.
3. Due to the possibility of drug-induced dizziness or drowsiness, caution should be used when driving or undertaking other tasks requiring mental alertness.
4. Advise that psychologic dependence may occur.

Evaluate: Improvement in skeletal muscle pain and spasticity with ↑ ROM.

Chlorzoxazone

(klor-**ZOX**-ah-zohn)
Paraflex, Parafon Forte DSC, Remular-S **(Rx)**

See also *Skeletal Muscle Relaxants, Centrally Acting,* Chapter 52.
How Supplied: *Capsule:* 500 mg; *Tablet:* 250 mg, 500 mg
Action/Kinetics: Chlorzoxazone inhibits polysynaptic reflexes at both the spinal cord and subcortical areas of the brain. Its effect may also be due to the sedative properties of the drug. **Onset:** 1 hr. **Time to peak blood levels:** 1–2 hr. **Peak serum levels:** 10–30 mcg/mL (after 750-mg dose). **Duration:** 3–4 hr. **t½:** 1 hr. The drug is metabolized in the liver and inactive metabolites excreted in the urine.
Uses: As adjunct to rest, physical therapy, and other approaches for treatment of acute, painful musculoskeletal conditions (e.g., muscle spasms, sprains, muscle strain).

Dosage

- **Tablets**

Skeletal muscle disorders.
Adults: 250–750 mg t.i.d.–q.i.d. with meals and at bedtime; **pediatric:** 125–500 mg t.i.d.–q.i.d. (or, 20 mg/kg in three to four divided doses daily).

Administration/Storage
1. The drug may be mixed with food or beverages for administration to children.
2. May be taken with food if GI upset occurs.
3. *Treatment of Overdose:* Supportive.

Special Concerns: Use during pregnancy only if benefits clearly outweigh risks. Use with caution in clients with known allergies or a history of allergic reactions to drugs.
Side Effects: *CNS:* Dizziness, drowsiness, malaise, lightheadedness,

overstimulation. *Dermatologic:* Allergic-type skin rashes, petechiae, ecchymoses (rare). *GI:* GI upset, GI bleeding (rare). *Allergic Reactions:* ***Angioneurotic edema, anaphylaxis*** (rare). *Miscellaneous:* Discoloration of urine, liver damage.

Symptoms of Overdose: N&V, diarrhea, drowsiness, dizziness, lightheadedness, headache, malaise, sluggishness. May be followed by marked loss of muscle tone (voluntary movement may be impossible), decreased or absent deep tendon reflexes, respiratory depression, decreased BP.

NURSING CONSIDERATIONS

See also *Nursing Considerations* for *Skeletal Muscle Relaxants, Centrally Acting,* Chapter 52.

Assessment

1. Determine that baseline liver and renal function studies have been performed and assess client for any evidence of dysfunction.
2. Document indications for therapy and note pretreatment findings.

Client/Family Teaching

1. Take with meals to minimize gastric irritation.
2. Drug may cause urine to have an orange or purple-red color when exposed to the air.
3. Do not operate dangerous machinery or drive a car until drug effects are evident because the drug causes drowsiness.
4. Review importance of RICE (rest, ice, compression, and elevation) in the setting of an acute injury.
5. Advise not to overuse extremity during therapy as drug may mask pathology.

Evaluate: Relief of musculoskeletal spasm and pain.

Cyclobenzaprine hydrochloride

(sye-kloh-**BENZ**-ah-preen)
Pregnancy Category: B
Flexeril **(Rx)**

See also *Skeletal Muscle Relaxants, Centrally Acting,* Chapter 52.

How Supplied: *Tablet:* 10 mg

Action/Kinetics: Structurally and pharmacologically, cyclobenzaprine is related to the tricyclic antidepressants and possesses both sedative and anticholinergic properties. In contrast to many skeletal muscle relaxants, cyclobenzaprine hydrochloride is thought to act mainly at the level of the brainstem (compared to the spinal cord) to inhibit reflexes by reducing tonic somatic motor activity. **Onset:** 1 hr. **Time to peak plasma levels:** 4–6 hr. **Therapeutic plasma levels:** 20–30 ng/mL. **Duration:** 12–24 hr. **t½:** 1–3 days. The drug is highly bound to plasma protein. Inactive metabolites are excreted in the urine.

Uses: Adjunct to rest and physical therapy for relief of muscle spasms associated with acute and/or painful musculoskeletal conditions. It is not indicated for the treatment of spastic diseases or for cerebral palsy. *Investigational:* Adjunct in the treatment of fibrositis syndrome.

Dosage

- **Tablets**

Skeletal muscle disorders.

Adults: 20–40 mg/day in three to four divided doses (usual: 10 mg t.i.d.), up to a maximum of 60 mg/day in divided doses.

Administration/Storage

1. Cyclobenzaprine should be used only for 2–3 weeks.
2. If the client has been taking an MAO inhibitor, do not administer cyclobenzaprine for at least 2 weeks after discontinuing the MAO inhibitor.
3. Review the list of drugs with which cyclobenzaprine interacts.
4. *Treatment of Overdose:* In addition to the treatment outlined on p. 198, physostigmine salicylate, 1–3 mg IV, may be used to reverse symptoms of severe cholinergic blockade.

Contraindications: Hypersensitivity. Arrhythmias, heart block or conduction disturbances, CHF, or during acute recovery phase of MI. Hyperthyroidism. Concomitant use of

MAO inhibitors or within 14 days of their discontinuation.

Special Concerns: Safe use during lactation and in children under age 15 has not been established. Due to atropine-like effects, use with caution in situations where cholinergic blockade is not desired (e.g., history of urinary retention, angle-closure glaucoma, increased intraocular pressure). Geriatric clients may be more sensitive to cholinergic blockade.

Side Effects: Since cyclobenzaprine resembles tricyclic antidepressants, side effects to these drugs should also be noted. *GI:* Dry mouth, N&V, constipation, dyspepsia, unpleasant taste, anorexia, diarrhea, GI pain, gastritis, thirst, flatulence, ageusia, paralytic ileus, discoloration of tongue, stomatitis, parotid swelling. *CNS:* Drowsiness, dizziness, fatigue, asthenia, blurred vision, nervousness, headache, ***convulsions,*** ataxia, vertigo, dysarthria, paresthesia, hypertonia, tremors, malaise, abnormal gait, delusions, Bell's palsy, alteration in EEG patterns, extrapyramidal symptoms. Psychiatric symptoms include: confusion, insomnia, disorientation, depressed mood, abnormal sensations, anxiety, agitation, abnormal thinking or dreaming, excitement, hallucinations. *CV:* Tachycardia, syncope, ***arrhythmias,*** vasodilation, palpitations, hypotension, edema, chest pain, hypertension, MI, heart block, stroke. *GU:* Urinary frequency or retention, impaired urination, dilation of urinary tract, impotence, decreased or increased libido, testicular swelling, gynecomastia, breast enlargement, galactorrhea. *Dermatologic:* Sweating, skin rashes, urticaria, pruritus, photosensitivity, alopecia. *Musculoskeletal:* Muscle twitching, weakness, myalgia. *Hematologic:* Purpura, bone marrow depression, leukopenia, eosinophilia, thrombocytopenia. *Hepatic:* Abnormal liver function, hepatitis, jaundice, cholestasis. *Miscellaneous:* Tinnitus, diplopia, peripheral neuropathy, increase and decrease of blood sugar, weight gain or loss, ***edema of the face and tongue,*** inappropriate ADH syndrome, dyspnea.

Symptoms of Overdose: Temporary confusion, disturbed concentration, transient visual hallucinations, agitation, hyperactive reflexes, muscle rigidity, vomiting, ***hyperpyrexia.*** Also, drowsiness, hypothermia, tachycardia, ***cardiac arrhythmias such as bundle branch block, ECG evidence of impaired conduction,*** CHF, dilated pupils, ***seizures, severe hypotension,*** stupor, ***coma,*** paradoxical diaphoresis.

Drug Interactions: *NOTE:* Because of the similarity of cyclobenzaprine to tricyclic antidepressants, the drug interactions for tricyclics should also be consulted.

Anticholinergics / Additive anticholinergic side effects
CNS depressants / Additive depressant effects
Guanethidine / Cyclobenzaprine may block effect
MAO inhibitors / Hypertensive crisis, severe convulsions
Tricyclic antidepressants / Additive side effects

NURSING CONSIDERATIONS

See also *Nursing Considerations* for *Skeletal Muscle Relaxants, Centrally Acting,* Chapter 52.

Assessment

1. Take a complete drug history, noting any evidence of hypersensitivity.
2. Check the client's CV system for evidence of cardiac arrhythmias. Note if the client has a history of recent MI.
3. Obtain baseline CBC and liver profile.
4. Document indications for therapy, the extent of the client's acute or painful musculoskeletal condition, and ROM. Review RICE (rest, ice, compression, and elevation) with an acute injury to reduce swelling and recovery time.
5. Determine if the client has any spasticity. This drug is contraindicat-

ed in the treatment of spastic diseases.

Client/Family Teaching

1. Report any unusual fatigue, sore throat, unexplained fever, easy bruising or bleeding. These symptoms could indicate a blood dyscrasia and require discontinuation of drug therapy.
2. Report nausea or abdominal pain, itchy skin, or evidence of yellow sclera or skin, because this could indicate hepatic toxicity and would require termination of therapy.
3. Symptoms such as dry mouth, blurred vision, dizziness, tachycardia, or urinary retention should also be reported so that therapy can be evaluated.
4. Due to drug-induced drowsiness, dizziness, and/or blurred vision, caution should be observed if driving or performing activities that require mental alertness.

Evaluate: Relief of musculoskeletal spasms and pain with evidence of ↑ ROM.

Dantrolene sodium

(**DAN**-troh-leen)
Pregnancy Category: C (parenteral use)
Dantrium, Dantrium IV **(Rx)**

See also *Skeletal Muscle Relaxants, Centrally Acting,* Chapter 52.

How Supplied: *Capsule:* 25 mg, 50 mg, 100 mg; *Powder for injection:* 20 mg

Action/Kinetics: Dantrolene is a hydantoin derivative and, as such, is chemically unrelated to other skeletal muscle relaxants. It acts directly on skeletal muscle, probably by dissociating the excitation-contraction coupling mechanism as a result of interference of release of calcium from the sarcoplasmic reticulum. This action results in a decreased force of reflex muscle contraction and a reduction of hyperreflexia, spasticity, involuntary movements, and clonus. Its effectiveness in malignant hyperthermia is due to an inhibition of release of calcium from the sarcoplasmic reticulum. This results in prevention or reduction of the increased myoplasmic calcium ion concentration that activates the acute catabolic processes associated with malignant hyperthermia. Absorption is slow and incomplete, but consistent. **Peak plasma levels:** 4–6 hr. **t½: PO,** 8.7 hr; **t½: IV,** 5 hr. There is significant plasma protein binding of the drug.

Uses: Muscle spasticity associated with severe chronic disorders, such as multiple sclerosis, cerebral palsy, spinal cord injury, and stroke. Muscle pain due to exercise. Malignant hyperthermia due to hypermetabolism of skeletal muscle. *Investigational:* Exercise-induced muscle pain, heat stroke, and neuroleptic malignant syndrome.

Dosage

- **Capsules**

Spastic conditions.

Adults, initial: 25 mg/day; **then,** increase to 25 mg b.i.d.–q.i.d.; dose may then be increased by 25-mg increments up to 100 mg b.i.d.–q.i.d. (doses in excess of 400 mg/day not recommended). **Pediatric: initial,** 0.5 mg/kg b.i.d.; **then,** increase to 0.5 mg/kg t.i.d.–q.i.d.; dose may then be increased by increments of 0.5 mg/kg to 3 mg/kg b.i.d.–q.i.d. (doses should not exceed 400 mg/day).

Malignant hyperthermia, preoperatively.

Adults and children: 4–8 mg/kg/day in three to four divided doses 1–2 days before surgery.

Postmalignant hyperthermic crisis.

Adults and children: 4–8 mg/kg/day in four divided doses for 1–3 days.

- **IV Infusion**

Malignant hyperthermia, crisis treatment.

Adults and children, initial: 2.5 mg/kg 60 min prior to surgery and infused over 1 hr.

- **IV Push**

Malignant hyperthermia, crisis treatment.

Initial: At least 1 mg/kg; continue administration until symptoms decrease or a cumulative dose of 10 mg/kg has been administered.

Administration/Storage

1. If the drug is to be administered IV, the powder should be reconstituted by adding 60 mL of sterile water for injection to each 20-mg vial.
2. Reconstituted solutions should be protected from light and used within 6 hr.
3. When administered PO, the drug can be mixed with fruit juice or other liquid vehicle.
4. If the drug is being administered to counteract spasticity, beneficial effects may not be noted for a week. The drug should be discontinued after 6 weeks if beneficial effects are not evident.
5. Due to potential hepatotoxicity, long-term benefits must be evaluated for each client.
6. *Treatment of Overdose:* Immediate gastric lavage. Maintain airway and have artificial resuscitation equipment available. Large quantities of IV fluids to prevent crystalluria. Monitor ECG.

Contraindications: Rheumatic diseases, pregnancy, lactation, or children under 5 years of age. Acute hepatitis and cirrhosis of the liver.

Special Concerns: Use with caution in clients with impaired pulmonary function.

Side Effects: Following PO use: Side effects are dose-related and decrease with usage. ***Fatal*** and nonfatal ***hepatotoxicity.*** *CNS:* Drowsiness, dizziness, weakness, malaise, lightheadedness, headaches, insomnia, seizures, speech disturbances, fatigue, confusion, depression, nervousness. *GI:* Diarrhea (common), anorexia, gastric upset, cramps, GI bleeding. *Musculoskeletal:* Backache, myalgia. *Dermatologic:* Rashes, photosensitivity, pruritus, urticaria, hair growth, sweating. *CV:* BP changes, phlebitis, tachycardia. *GU:* Urinary retention, hematuria, crystalluria, nocturia, impotence. *Miscellaneous:* Visual disturbances, chills, fever, tearing, feeling of suffocation, ***pleural effusion with pericarditis.***

Following IV use: Pulmonary edema, ***thrombophlebitis,*** urticaria, erythema.

NURSING CONSIDERATIONS

See also *Nursing Considerations* for *Skeletal Muscle Relaxants, Centrally Acting,* Chapter 52.

Assessment

1. Note the client's mental status and general appearance.
2. Obtain baseline CBC and liver and renal function studies and monitor throughout therapy. Impaired hepatic function is more likely to occur in women over 35 years of age.
3. Auscultate and document baseline lung and heart sounds prior to beginning therapy. Assess regularly during therapy and note any changes.
4. Note any evidence of impaired pulmonary function, cardiac disorders, or history of the client having either benign or malignant breast tumors. Dantrolene may increase the incidence of mammary tumors.
5. Note the extent of the client's muscle spasticity, involuntary movements, and clonus. Assess periodically to determine the response to drug therapy.
6. Inspect the skin integrity and periodically assess to detect any changes.
7. Obtain and monitor VS, I&O, electrolytes, and ECG during acute therapy.

Client/Family Teaching

1. Do not operate dangerous machinery or drive a car as drug causes drowsiness.
2. If client develops double vision, reassure that this and many of the other bothersome side effects associated with drug therapy may lessen with the continued use of the drug.
3. Report any increased muscle weakness or impaired physical ability.
4. Reassure client that several weeks of therapy may be required before improvements in condition will be

noted. Insomnia and depression should be reported.
5. Teach client how to monitor and take BP, check stools for the presence of occult blood, and keep a record of urinary output. Advise to report any marked changes in BP and any evidence of diarrhea or blood in the urine or stool.
6. If client develops slurred speech, drooling, inability to perform usual physical functions, or enuresis, the drug may require withdrawal.
7. Avoid alcohol and any other CNS depressants.
8. Use sunscreens, sunglasses, and protective clothing when sun exposure is necessary, to prevent photosensitivity reactions.
9. Encourage female clients to have mammograms and to perform BSE to detect any occurrence of lumps since this drug has the potential to cause these problems. This is especially important in women with a family history of malignant or benign breast tumors.
10. Explain to male clients the potential for impotence and advise to report if evident.
11. Advise clients with malignant hyperthermia to carry appropriate identification and to notify all providers.

Evaluate
- ↓ Muscle spasticity and/or pain
- Relief of exercise-induced muscle pain
- ↓ Temperature in malignant hyperthermia (due to hypermetabolism of skeletal muscle)

Metaxalone

(meh-**TAX**-ah-lohn)
Skelaxin **(Rx)**

See also *Skeletal Muscle Relaxants, Centrally Acting,* Chapter 52.
How Supplied: *Tablet:* 400 mg
Action/Kinetics: The beneficial effects of metaxalone may be due to its sedative effects. It has no direct effect on the contractile mechanism of striated muscle, the motor endplate, or the nerve fiber and it does not directly relax tense skeletal muscles. The drug resembles meprobamate. **Onset:** 1 hr. **t½:** 2–3 hr. **Peak serum levels:** 300 mcg/mL 2 hr after 800 mg. **Duration:** 4–6 hr. Metabolites are excreted in the urine.
Uses: As an adjunct for acute skeletal muscle spasm associated with acute, painful musculoskeletal conditions (e.g., sprains, strains, dislocation).

Dosage
- **Tablets**

Skeletal muscle disorders.
Adults and children over 12 years: 800 mg t.i.d.–q.i.d.
Contraindications: Liver disease, epilepsy, impaired renal function, history of drug-induced hemolytic or other anemias, pregnancy, children under 12 years.
Special Concern: Safe use during lactation has not been determined.
Side Effects: *CNS:* Drowsiness, dizziness, headache, nervousness, irritability. *GI:* N&V, gastric upset. *Miscellaneous:* Allergic reactions (light rash with or without pruritus), jaundice, leukopenia, ***hemolytic anemia.***

NURSING CONSIDERATIONS

See also *Nursing Considerations* for *Skeletal Muscle Relaxants, Centrally Acting,* Chapter 52.
Assessment
1. Obtain baseline CBC and liver and renal function studies.
2. Note any history of drug-induced hemolytic or other type anemias.
3. Determine if client has a history of epilepsy.

Client/Family Teaching
1. Drug causes drowsiness; do not operate dangerous machinery or drive a car until effects evident.
2. Complaints of sore throat, fever, and lassitude or of having a "cold" should be further explored because these may be symptoms of blood dyscrasias.
3. Clients with a history of grand mal epilepsy should be advised that metaxalone may precipitate seizures.
4. Complaints of high fever, nausea, abdominal pain, yellowing of skin

or sclera, or diarrhea should be reported. These are early symptoms of hepatotoxicity and require the withdrawal of metaxalone.
5. Avoid symptoms of a dry mouth by rinsing the mouth frequently and increasing the fluid intake. Sugarless gum and candy may also be of some benefit.
Evaluate: Control of skeletal muscle spasm and pain with improved mobility and ↑ ROM.

Methocarbamol

(meth-oh-**KAR**-bah-mohl)
Robaxin, Robaxin-750 **(Rx)**

See also *Skeletal Muscle Relaxants, Centrally Acting,* Chapter 52.
How Supplied: *Injection:* 100 mg/mL; *Tablet:* 500 mg, 750 mg
Action/Kinetics: The beneficial action of methocarbamol may be related to the sedative properties of the drug. It has no direct effect on the contractile mechanism of striated muscle, the motor endplate, or the nerve fiber and it does not directly relax tense skeletal muscles. Of limited usefulness. The drug may be given IM or IV in polyethylene glycol 300 (50% solution). PO therapy should be initiated as soon as possible. **Onset:** 30 min. **Peak plasma levels:** 2 hr after 2 g. **t½:** 1–2 hr. Inactive metabolites are excreted in the urine.
Uses: Adjunct for the relief of acute, painful musculoskeletal conditions (e.g., sprains, strains). Adjunct in tetanus.

Dosage

- **Tablets**

Skeletal muscle disorders.
Adults, initial: 1.5 g q.i.d. for the first 2–3 days (for severe conditions, 8 g/day may be given); **maintenance:** 1 g q.i.d., 0.75 g q 4 hr, or 1.5 g t.i.d.

- **IM, IV**

Skeletal muscle disorders.
Adults, usual initial: 1 g; in severe cases, up to 2–3 g may be necessary. **IV administration should not exceed 3 days.**

Tetanus.
Adults: 1–2 g IV, initially, into tube of previously inserted indwelling needle. An additional 1–2 g may be added to the infusion for a total initial dose of 3 g. May be given q 6 hr (up to 24 g/day may be needed) until **PO** administration is feasible. **Pediatric, initial:** 15 mg/kg given into tube of previously inserted indwelling needle. Dose may be repeated q 6 hr.
Administration/Storage
1. If the drug is to be administered IV, the rate should not exceed 3 mL/min.
2. For IV drip, one ampule may be added to no more than 250 mL of sodium chloride or 5% dextrose injection.
3. If the client is to receive the drug by IV, check frequently for infiltration. Extravasation of fluid may cause sloughing or thrombophlebitis.
4. Before removing IV, clamp off the tubing to prevent extravasation of the hypertonic solution, which may cause thrombophlebitis.
5. If the drug is to be administered IM, inject no more than 5 mL into each gluteal region.
6. When administering IM to an adult, select a large muscle mass. When administering the drug IM to a child, use the vastus lateralis. Document and rotate sites.
7. *Treatment of Overdose:* Supportive, depending on the symptoms.
Contraindications: Hypersensitivity, when muscle spasticity is required to maintain upright position, pregnancy, lactation, children under 12 years. Renal disease (parenteral dosage form only since it contains polyethylene glycol 300).
Special Concerns: Use with caution in epilepsy and during lactation. The injectable form should be used with caution in suspected or known epileptics.
Laboratory Test Interference: Color interference in 5-HIAA and VMA.

Side Effects: *Following PO use. CNS:* Dizziness, drowsiness, lightheadedness, vertigo, lassitude, headache. *GI:* Nausea. *Miscellaneous:* Allergic symptoms including rash, urticaria, pruritus, conjunctivitis, nasal congestion, blurred vision, fever. *Following IV use (in addition to above). CV:* Hypotension, bradycardia. *CNS:* Fainting, mild muscle incoordination. *Miscellaneous:* Metallic taste, GI upset, flushing, nystagmus, double vision, thrombophlebitis, pain at injection site, ***anaphylaxis.***

Symptoms of Overdose: CNS depression, including coma, is often seen when methocarbamol is used with alcohol or other CNS depressants.

Drug Interaction: Central nervous system depressants (including alcohol) may increase the effect of methocarbamol.

NURSING CONSIDERATIONS

See also *Nursing Considerations* for *Skeletal Muscle Relaxants, Centrally Acting,* Chapter 52.

Interventions

1. Monitor BP and pulse and report any overt changes.
2. Position the client in a recumbent position during IV administration. Have client maintain this position for 10–15 min after injection to minimize the side effects of postural hypotension.
3. Have side rails up and supervise ambulation of elderly clients or those who have been immobilized prior to drug therapy.
4. Observe seizure precautions.

Client/Family Teaching

1. Drug causes drowsiness; do not operate dangerous machinery and equipment or drive a car.
2. Rise slowly from a recumbent position and dangle legs before standing up to minimize hypotensive effects.
3. Diplopia, blurred vision, and nystagmus may occur. These side effects usually disappear with continued use of the medication. These symptoms should be reported if evident.
4. Report any urticaria, skin eruptions, rash, or pruritus. These are allergic responses and may necessitate withdrawal of the drug.
5. Nausea, anorexia, and a metallic taste may occur with drug therapy. Report if these symptoms become severe or interfere with nutrition.
6. Avoid the use of alcohol and any other CNS depressants.
7. Advise that urine may turn black, brown, or green. This side effect will disappear once the drug is discontinued.

Evaluate

- Improvement in muscle spasticity, pain, and mobility
- Control of tetanus-induced neuromuscular manifestations

Orphenadrine citrate

(or-**FEN**-ah-dreen)

Pregnancy Category: C

Banflex, Flexagin, Flexoject, Flexon, Myolin, Norflex **(Rx)**

See also *Skeletal Muscle Relaxants, Centrally Acting,* Chapter 52.

How Supplied: *Injection:* 30 mg/mL; *Tablet, Extended Release:* 100 mg

Action/Kinetics: Action may be related, in part, to its centrally mediated analgesic effects. It also possesses anticholinergic activity. **Onset, PO:** Within 1 hr; **IM:** 5 min; **IV:** immediate. **Peak effect:** 2 hr. **Peak serum levels:** 60–120 ng/mL (after 100 mg). **Duration:** 4–6 hr. **t½:** 14 hr. Excretion of a small amount of unchanged drug and metabolites is via both urine and feces.

Uses: Adjunct to the treatment of acute, painful musculoskeletal disorders. *Investigational:* Use at bedtime to treat quinine-resistant leg cramps.

Dosage

- **Extended-Release Tablets**

Skeletal muscle disorders.

Adults: 100 mg b.i.d. in the morning and evening.

Quinine-resistant leg cramps.

100 mg at bedtime.

- **IV or IM**

Skeletal muscle disorders.
Adults: 60 mg. May be repeated q 12 hr.

Administration/Storage

1. If the drug is to be administered IV, it should be given over a period of 5 min. The client should be in a supine position and should remain supine for 5–10 min following IV administration.
2. Sustained-release tablets should not be chewed or crushed .
3. *Treatment of Overdose:* Gastric lavage. Treat symptoms.

Contraindications: Angle-closure glaucoma, stenosing peptic ulcers, prostatic hypertrophy, obstruction of the bladder neck, cardiospasm, pyloric or duodenal obstruction, cardiospasm, and myasthenia gravis. Use in children. Some products contain sulfites; these products should not be used in sulfite-sensitive clients.

Special Concerns: Use with caution in cardiac disease and during lactation. Safety and efficacy have not been determined in children.

Side Effects: Most side effects are anticholinergic in nature. *GI:* Dry mouth (first to appear), N&V, constipation, gastric irritation. *CV:* Tachycardia, transient syncope, palpitation. *CNS:* Headache, dizziness, drowsiness, lightheadedness, agitation, tremor, hallucinations, weakness, confusion (in geriatric clients). *GU:* Urinary retention or hesitancy. *Ophthalmologic:* Dilated pupils, blurred vision, increased intraocular tension (especially in closed-angle glaucoma). *Miscellaneous:* Hypersensitivity reactions (e.g., urticaria, dermatoses, pruritus). ***Rarely, aplastic anemia or anaphylaxis.***

Symptoms of Overdose: Cardiac rhythm disturbances, ***seizures, shock, deep coma, respiratory arrest. Death can occur within 3–5 hr.***

Drug Interactions

Amantadine / ↑ Anticholinergic effects
Anticholinergics / Additive anticholinergic effects
Contraceptives, oral / Orphenadrine ↑ breakdown by liver
Griseofulvin / Orphenadrine ↑ breakdown by liver
Haloperidol / Worsening of schizophrenic symptoms, ↓ haloperidol levels, and development of tardive dyskinesia
Propoxyphene / Concomitant use may result in anxiety, tremors, and confusion

NURSING CONSIDERATIONS

See also *Nursing Considerations* for *Skeletal Muscle Relaxants, Centrally Acting* Chapter 52.

Assessment

1. Document indications for therapy and type and onset of symptoms.
2. Note evidence of impaired movement or mobility and ROM.
3. Determine any history of angle-closure glaucoma and sulfite sensitivity.
4. Review drugs and disorders listed that may preclude drug therapy.

Client/Family Teaching

1. Report any evidence of excess anticholinergic effects such as dry mouth, urinary retention or hesitancy. Presence of a dry mouth may be an indication to reduce the dosage of drug. Frequent rinsing of the mouth and more fluids in the diet may assist to relieve dry mouth symptoms.
2. Caution not to operate dangerous machinery or to drive a car because drug causes drowsiness.
3. Report any persistent adverse effects immediately.
4. Do not overuse area requiring treatment as medication may mask normal symptoms.
5. Follow other prescribed therapies such as elevation of extremity, application of ice and/or heat, and physical therapy program.
6. Avoid alcohol and any other CNS depressants.

Evaluate: Control of musculoskeletal pain and discomfort.

COMBINATION DRUG

Soma Compound

(**SO**-mah)
Pregnancy Category: C
(Rx)

Soma Compound with Codeine

(**SO**-mah, **KOH**-deen)
Pregnancy Category: C
(Rx) (C-III)

How Supplied: Soma compound: See Content
Soma compound with codeine: See Content

Content: Soma Compound contains: *Nonnarcotic analgesic:* Aspirin, 325 mg. *Centrally acting skeletal muscle relaxant:* Carisoprodol, 200 mg. In addition to the above, Soma Compound with Codeine contains: *Narcotic analgesic:* Codeine phosphate, 16 mg. See also information on individual components.

Uses: As an adjunct to rest and physical therapy for the relief of acute, painful musculoskeletal conditions including muscle spasm, pain, and conditions leading to limited mobility.

Dosage

- **Tablets: Soma Compound and Soma Compound with Codeine**

Analgesia.

Adults: 1–2 tablets q.i.d.

Contraindications: Acute intermittent porphyria, bleeding disorders, lactation. Use in children less than 12 years of age.

Special Concerns: Use with caution in clients with impaired hepatic or renal function, in elderly or debilitated clients, in clients with a history of gastritis or peptic ulcer, in those on anticoagulant therapy, and in individuals prone to addiction.

NURSING CONSIDERATIONS

See *Nursing Considerations* for *Acetylsalicylic Acid,* Chapter 41, and *Narcotic Analgesics,* Chapter 43.

Assessment: Document indications for therapy and onset of symptoms. List other agents prescribed and the outcome.

Evaluate: Reports of relief of musculoskeletal pain.

CHAPTER FIFTY-THREE

Neuromuscular Blocking Agents

See also the following individual entries:

Atracurium Besylate
Doxacurium Chloride
Mivacurium Chloride
Pancuronium Bromide
Pipecuronium Bromide
Succinylcholine Chloride
Tubocurarine Chloride
Vecuronium Bromide

General Statement: Upon stimulation, the muscles normally contract when acetylcholine is released from storage sites embedded in the motor end plate. The drugs considered in this section interfere with nerve impulse transmission between the motor end plate and the receptors of skeletal muscle (i.e., peripheral action).

The drugs fall into two groups: competitive (nondepolarizing) agents and depolarizing agents. Competitive agents—atracurium, doxacurium, gallamine, metocurine, mivacurium, pancuronium, tubocurarine, vecuronium—compete with acetylcholine for the receptor site in the muscle cells. These agents are also called *curariform* because their mode of action is similar to that of the poison curare. The depolarizing agent—succinylcholine—initially excites skeletal muscle and then prevents the muscle from contracting by prolonging the time during which the receptors at the end plate cannot respond to acetylcholine (depolarization during refractory time).

The muscle paralysis caused by the neuromuscular blocking agents is sequential. Therapeutic doses produce muscle depression in the following order: heaviness of eyelids, difficulty in swallowing and talking, diplopia, progressive weakening of the extremities and neck, followed by relaxation of the trunk and spine. The diaphragm (respiratory paralysis) is affected last. The drugs do not affect consciousness, and their use, in the absence of adequate levels of general anesthesia, may be frightening to the client. After IV infusion, flaccid paralysis occurs within a few minutes with maximum effects within about 6 min. Maximal effects last 35–60 min and effective muscle paralysis may last for 25–90 min with complete recovery taking several hours.

There is a narrow margin of safety between a therapeutically effective dose causing muscle relaxation and a toxic dose causing respiratory paralysis. **The neuromuscular blocking agents are always administered initially by a physician.** The nurse must be prepared to maintain and monitor respiration until the effect of the drug subsides.

Uses: See individual agents. General uses include as an adjunct to general anesthesia to cause muscle relaxation; to reduce the intensity of skeletal muscle contractions in either drug-induced or electrically induced convulsions; to assist in the management of mechanical ventilation.

Contraindications: Allergy or hypersensitivity to any of these drugs.

Special Concerns: The neuromuscular blocking agents should be used with caution in clients with myasthenia gravis; renal, hepatic, endocrine, or pulmonary impairment; respiratory depression; during lactation; and in elderly, pediatric, or debilitated clients. The action of these drugs may be altered in clients by electrolyte imbalances (especially hyperkalemia), some carcinomas, body temperature, dehydration, renal disease, and in those taking digitalis.

Side Effects: ***Respiratory paralysis. Severe and prolonged muscle relaxation.*** *CV:* Cardiac arrhythmias, bradycardia, hypotension, cardiac arrest. These side effects are more frequent in neonates and premature infants. *GI:* Excessive salivation during light anesthesia. *Miscellaneous:* ***Bronchospasms, hyperthermia,*** hypersensitivity (rare). See also individual agents.

Symptoms of Overdose: Decreased respiratory reserve, extended skeletal muscle weakness, prolonged apnea, low tidal volume, sudden release of histamine, ***CV collapse.***

Drug Interactions: The following drug interactions are for nondepolarizing skeletal muscle relaxants. For succinylcholine, see Chapter 53.

Aminoglycoside antibiotics / Additive muscle relaxation, including prolonged respiratory depression
Amphotericin B / ↑ Muscle relaxation
Anesthetics, inhalation / Additive muscle relaxation
Carbamazepine / ↓ Duration or effect of muscle relaxants
Clindamycin / Additive muscle relaxation, including prolonged respiratory depression
Colistin / ↑ Muscle relaxation
Corticosteroids / ↓ Effect of muscle relaxants
Furosemide / ↑ or ↓ Effect of skeletal muscle relaxants (may be dose-related)
Hydantoins / ↓ Duration or effect of muscle relaxants
Ketamine / ↑ Muscle relaxation, including prolonged respiratory depression
Lincomycin / ↑ Muscle relaxation, including prolonged respiratory depression
Lithium / ↑ Recovery time of muscle relaxants → prolonged respiratory depression
Magnesium salts / ↑ Muscle relaxation, including prolonged respiratory depression
Methotrimeprazine / ↑ Muscle relaxation
Narcotic analgesics / ↑ Respiratory depression and ↑ muscle relaxation
Nitrates / ↑ Muscle relaxation, including prolonged respiratory depression
Phenothiazines / ↑ Muscle relaxation
Pipercillin / ↑ Muscle relaxation, including prolonged respiratory depression
Polymyxin B / ↑ Muscle relaxation
Procainamide / ↑ Muscle relaxation
Procaine / ↑ Muscle relaxation by ↓ plasma protein binding
Quinidine / ↑ Muscle relaxation
Ranitidine / Significant ↓ effect of muscle relaxants
Theophyllines / Reversal of effects of muscle relaxant (dose-dependent)
Thiazide diuretics / ↑ Muscle relaxation due to hypokalemia
Verapamil / ↑ Muscle relaxation, including prolonged respiratory depression

Dosage

See individual drugs.

NURSING CONSIDERATIONS

Administration/Storage

1. When the drug is to be administered by a constant infusion, use a microdrip tubing administration set with an electronic infusion control device.
2. Generally, client should be sedated and intubated prior to use.
3. During drug administration, have a suction machine, oxygen, and resuscitation equipment immediately available for emergency use.
4. *Treatment of Overdose:* There are no known antidotes.

• Use a peripheral nerve stimulator to monitor and assess the client's response to the neuromuscular blocking medication.

• Have anticholinesterase drugs, such as edrophonium, pyridostigmine, or neostigmine available to counteract respiratory depression due to paralysis of skeletal muscles. These drugs increase the body's production of acetylcholine. To minimize the muscarinic cholinergic side effects, atropine should also be given.
• Correct BP, electrolyte imbalance, or circulating blood volume by fluid and electrolyte therapy. Vasopressors can be used to correct hypotension due to ganglionic blockade.

Assessment

1. Document indications for therapy, desired outcome, and anticipated length of use.
2. Note age and condition of the client. Elderly and debilitated clients should not receive drugs in this category.
3. Determine that baseline CBC, electrolytes, CXR, ECG, and liver and renal function studies have been performed.
4. Note all other drugs the client is receiving. Often, clients requiring neuromuscular blocking agents are also receiving other drugs that may have the effect of prolonging client response to the prescribed neuromuscular blocking agent.
5. Question the client concerning changes in vision, ability to chew or to move the fingers, and document findings.
6. Note initial selective paralysis followed by paralysis in the following sequence: levator muscles of the eyelids, mastication muscles, limb muscles, abdominal muscles, glottis muscles, intercostal muscles, and the diaphragm muscles. Of note is that neuromuscular recovery occurs in the reverse order.

Interventions

1. Drugs should only be administered in a closely monitored environment and generally are used only for intubated clients.
2. Prevent overdosage during infusions by frequent use (q 4 hr) of a peripheral nerve stimulator or by allowing partial return of muscle function.
3. Monitor the client's BP and pulse frequently. Respirations and pulmonary status should be monitored continuously. Ensure that cardiac monitor and ventilator alarms are set appropriately and checked at frequent intervals.
4. Observe for excessive bronchial secretions or respiratory wheezing, and suction to maintain patent airway (ET tube).
5. Perform frequent neurovascular assessments. Prolonged use of neuromuscular blocking agents may cause profound weakness and even paralysis once the drug has been discontinued. It may precipitate an acute myopathy in some individuals.
6. Observe the client closely for drug interactions. These can potentiate muscular relaxation and prove fatal. If interactions occur, report immediately to obtain orders for the appropriate medication to counteract the observed effects.
7. Consciousness and pain thresholds are not affected by neuromuscular blocking agents. Most clients can still hear, feel, and see while they are receiving blocking agents. Therefore, inappropriate talking and any discussions that should not be overheard should be avoided. Adequate anesthesia and analgesics should be administered for pain or when painful procedures are necessary.
8. Clients requiring prolonged ventilatory therapy should be adequately sedated with analgesics and benzodiazepines. Anxiety levels may be very high, but client cannot communicate this.
9. Administer eye drops and eye patches to protect corneas during prolonged therapy. Explain to client and family why this is done (i.e., because the blink reflex has been suppressed).
10. Avoid the use of corticosteroids during prolonged neuromuscular

blockade unless benefits outweigh the risks.

Evaluate

- Evidence of desired level of skeletal muscle paralysis
- Successful insertion of ET tube and tolerance of mechanical ventilation
- Adequate suppression of twitch response upon peripheral nerve stimulation tests

Atracurium besylate

(ah-trah-**KYOUR**-ee-um)

Pregnancy Category: C

Tracrium Injection **(Rx)**

See also *Neuromuscular Blocking Agents,* Chapter 53.

How Supplied: *Injection:* 10 mg/mL

Action/Kinetics: Atracurium prevents the action of acetylcholine by competing for the cholinergic receptor at the neuromuscular junction. It may also release histamine, leading to hypotension. **Onset:** Within 2 min. **Peak effect:** 1–2 min. **Duration:** 20–40 min with balanced anesthesia. Recovery occurs more quickly than with other nondepolarizing agents (e.g., *d*-tubocurarine). **t½:** 20 min. Drug is metabolized in the plasma.

Uses: Skeletal muscle relaxant during surgery; adjunct to general anesthesia; assist in ET intubation. *Investigational:* Treat seizures due to drugs or electrically induced.

Dosage

- **IV only**

General use.

Adults and children over 2 years, initial: 0.4–0.5 mg/kg as IV bolus; **maintenance:** 0.08–0.1 mg/kg.

Following use of succinylcholine for intubation under balanced anesthesia.

Initial: 0.3–0.4 mg/kg; if using potent inhalation anesthetics, further reductions may be required.

Use in CV disease or clients with history of asthma or anaphylaxis.

Initial: 0.3–0.4 mg/kg, given slowly over 1 min.

Use after steady-state enflurane or isoflurane anesthesia established.

0.25–0.35 mg/kg (about ⅓ less than the usual initial dose).

Use in infants 1 month to 2 years of age under halothane anesthesia.

0.3–0.4 mg/kg.

Supplemental use.

0.08–0.1 mg/kg 20–45 min after the initial dose; then q 15–25 min or as needed.

- **IV Infusion**

Balanced anesthesia.

IV infusion: 0.009–0.01 mg/kg until the level of neuromuscular blockade is reestablished; **then,** rate of infusion is adjusted according to client needs (usually 0.005–0.009 mg/kg/min although some clients may require as little as 0.002 mg/kg/min and others as much as 0.015 mg/kg/min).

For cardiopulmonary bypass surgery in which hypothermia is induced.

Reduce rate of infusion by 50%.

Administration/Storage

1. Initial dosage should be reduced to 0.25–0.35 mg/kg if drug is being used with steady-state enflurane or isoflurane (smaller reductions if halothane is being used).
2. Dosage should be reduced in clients with myasthenia gravis or other neuromuscular diseases, electrolyte disorders, or carcinomatosis.
3. Atracurium should *not* be mixed with alkaline solutions.
4. Maintenance doses can be given by continuous infusion of a diluted solution to clients 2 years of age to adulthood.
5. Solutions for infusion should be used within 24 hr.
6. To preserve potency, the drug should be refrigerated at 2°C–8°C (36°F–46°F).
7. IM administration may cause tissue irritation.
8. Drug does not affect consciousness or pain threshold. Concomitant antianxiety agents and analgesics should be employed.
9. IV atropine may be used to treat bradycardia due to atracurium.

Contraindications: In clients with myasthenia gravis, Eaton-Lambert syndrome, electrolyte disorders, bronchial asthma.

Special Concerns: Use with caution during labor and delivery. Safety and efficacy have not been determined during lactation. Children up to 1 month of age may be more sensitive to the effects of atracurium.

Additional Side Effects: *CV:* Bradycardia. Other side effects may be due to histamine release and include flushing, erythema, wheezing, urticaria, bronchial secretions, BP and HR changes.

Additional Drug Interactions

Enflurane / ↑ Muscle relaxation
Halothane / ↑ Muscle relaxation
Isoflurane / ↑ Muscle relaxation
Lithium / ↑ Muscle relaxation
Phenytoin / ↓ Effect of atracurium
Succinylcholine / ↑ Onset and depth of muscle relaxation
Theophylline / ↓ Effect of atracurium
Trimethaphan / ↑ Muscle relaxation
Verapamil / ↑ Muscle relaxation

NURSING CONSIDERATIONS

See also *Nursing Considerations* for *Neuromuscular Blocking Agents,* Chapter 53.

Evaluate

- Desired level of skeletal muscle relaxation
- Facilitation of ET intubation and tolerance of mechanical ventilation
- Control of electrically or pharmacologically induced seizures

Doxacurium chloride

(dox-ah-**KYOUR**-ee-um **KLOR**-ide)

Pregnancy Category: C

Neuromax **(Rx)**

See also *Neuromuscular Blocking Agents,* Chapter 53.

How Supplied: *Injection:* 1 mg/mL

Action/Kinetics: Doxacurium binds to cholinergic receptors on the motor end-plate to block the action of acetylcholine; this results in a blockade of neuromuscular transmission. Doxacurium is up to 3 times more potent than pancuronium and up to 12 times more potent than metocurine. The time to maximum neuromuscular blockade during balanced anesthesia is dose-dependent and ranges from 9.3 min (following doses of 0.025 mg/kg) to 3.5 min (following doses of 0.08 mg/kg). The time to 25% recovery from blockade following balanced anesthesia ranges from 55 min for doses of 0.025 mg/kg to 160 min for doses of 0.08 mg/kg. **t½, elimination:** Dose-dependent, ranging from 86 to 123 min. The half-life is prolonged in kidney transplant clients. Children require higher doses on a mg/kg basis than adults to achieve the same level of blockade. Also, the onset, time, and duration of block are shorter in children than adults. The blockade may be reversed by anticholinesterase agents. The drug is excreted unchanged through the urine and bile.

Uses: Adjunct to general anesthesia to provide skeletal muscle relaxation during surgery. Skeletal muscle relaxation for ET intubation.

Dosage

- **IV only**

As a component of thiopental/narcotic induction-intubation, to produce neuromuscular blockade of long duration.

Adults, initial: 0.05 mg/kg.

If administered during steady-state enflurane, halothane, or isoflurane anesthesia.

Reduce dose by one-third. **Children:** 0.03 mg/kg for blockade lasting about 30 min or 0.05 mg/kg for blockade lasting about 45 min when used during halothane anesthesia. Maintenance doses are required more frequently in children.

Used with succinylcholine to facilitate ET intubation.

Initial: 0.025 mg/kg will provide approximately 60 min of effective blockade. **Maintenance doses:** Required about 60 min after an initial dose of 0.025 mg/kg or 100 min after an initial dose of 0.05 mg/kg during balanced anesthesia. Maintenance doses between 0.005–0.01 mg/kg provide an average of 30 min and 45 min, respectively, of additional neuromuscular blockade.

Administration/Storage

1. The dose is individualized for each client.
2. The dose should be reduced in debilitated clients, in clients with neuromuscular disease, severe electrolyte abnormalities, and carcinomatosis.
3. The dose may need to be increased in burn clients.
4. The dose for obese clients is determined using the ideal body weight (IBW) calculated as follows:
• For men: IBW (kg) = (106 + [6 × inches in height above 5 feet])/2.2
• For women: IBW (kg) = (106 + [5 × inches in height above 5 feet])/2.2
5. Doxacurium may not be compatible with alkaline solutions with a pH more than 8 (e.g., barbiturates).
6. Doxacurium may be mixed with 5% dextrose injection, 5% dextrose and 0.9% sodium chloride injection, 0.9% sodium chloride injection, lactated Ringer's injection, and 5% dextrose and lactated Ringer's injection. The drug is also compatible with alfentanil, fentanyl, and sufentanil.
7. Doxacurium diluted 1:10 with 5% dextrose injection or 0.9% sodium chloride injection is stable for 24 hr if stored in polypropylene syringes at 5°C–25°C (41°F–77°F). However, immediate use of the drug, if diluted, is preferable.
8. Any unused portion of diluted doxacurium should be discarded after 8 hr at room temperature.
9. *Treatment of Overdose:* Maintain a patent airway and use controlled ventilation if necessary until recovery of normal neuromuscular function. Once recovery begins, it can be facilitated by giving neostigmine, 0.06 mg/kg.

Special Concerns: Use with caution during lactation. Safety and effectiveness have not been determined in children less than 2 years of age. The duration of action may be up to twice as long for clients over 60 years of age and those who are obese (more than 30% more than ideal body weight for height). Malignant hyperthermia may occur in any client receiving a general anesthetic.

Side Effects: *Neuromuscular:* Skeletal muscle weakness, ***profound and prolonged skeletal muscle paralysis causing respiratory insufficiency and apnea;*** difficulty in reversing the neuromuscular blockade. *CV:* Hypotension, flushing, ***ventricular fibrillation, MI.*** *Respiratory:* Wheezing, ***bronchospasm.*** *Dermatologic:* Urticaria, reaction at injection site. *Miscellaneous:* Fever, diplopia.

Symptoms of Overdose: Prolonged neuromuscular block.

Drug Interactions

Aminoglycosides / ↑ Duration of action of doxacurium
Bacitracin / ↑ Duration of action of doxacurium
Carbamazepine / ↑ Onset of effects and ↓ the duration of action of doxacurium
Clindamycin / ↑ Duration of action of doxacurium
Colistin / ↑ Duration of action of doxacurium
Enflurane / ↓ Amount of doxacurium necessary to cause blockade and ↑ the duration of action
Halothane / ↓ Amount of doxacurium necessary to cause blockade and ↑ the duration of action
Isoflurane / ↓ Amount of doxacurium necessary to cause blockade and ↑ the duration of action
Lincomycin / ↑ Duration of action of doxacurium
Lithium / ↑ Duration of action of doxacurium
Local anesthetics / ↑ Duration of action of doxacurium
Magnesium salts / ↑ Effects of doxacurium
Phenytoin / ↑ Onset of effects and ↓ the duration of action of doxacurium
Polymyxins / ↑ Duration of action of doxacurium
Procainamide / ↑ Duration of action of doxacurium
Quinidine / ↑ Duration of action of doxacurium

Tetracyclines / ↑ Duration of action of doxacurium

NURSING CONSIDERATIONS

See also *Nursing Considerations* for *Neuromuscular Blocking Agents,* Chapter 53.

Assessment

1. Determine any history of neuromuscular disease (e.g., myasthenia gravis) as doxacurium may have profound effects in these clients.
2. Note any drugs client is currently prescribed that may interact unfavorably with doxacurium.
3. Identify burn victims and anticipate altered requirements of drug as these clients tend to develop a resistance to doxacurium.
4. Obtain baseline weight and serum electrolyte levels.

Interventions

1. The drug should only be given if there are facilities for intubation, artificial respiration, and oxygen therapy, and the availability of an antagonist.
2. The drug should be administered only by those experienced with skeletal muscle relaxants.
3. A peripheral nerve stimulator should be used to monitor drug response.
4. Since doxacurium has no effect on consciousness, pain threshold, or cerebration, it generally should not be administered before unconsciousness (to avoid client stress).
5. Determine need for additional medication for anxiety and for sedation and administer as needed.
6. Explain all procedures and provide emotional support. Reassure clients that they will be able to talk and move once the drug effects are reversed.
7. Position the client for comfort and so that the body is in proper alignment. Turn client and perform mouth care and eye care frequently.
8. Provide continuous ventilatory support. Make certain that the ventilator alarms are set and on at all times. Assess airway at frequent intervals and have a suction machine readily available.
9. Monitor and record VS, I&O.

Evaluate

- Desired level of skeletal muscle relaxation/paralysis
- Suppression of the twitch response when tested with a peripheral nerve stimulator

Mivacurium chloride

(**mih**-vah-**KYOUR**-ee-um)

Pregnancy Category: C

Mivacron **(Rx)**

See also *Neuromuscular Blocking Agents,* Chapter 53.

How Supplied: *Injection:* 2 mg/mL, 50 mg/100 mL

Action/Kinetics: Mivacurium competitively inhibits the action of acetylcholine on the motor end plate, resulting in a block of neuromuscular transmission. The time to maximum neuromuscular blockade is similar to atracurium (2.3–4.9 min in adults depending on the dose and 1.6–2.8 min in children depending on the dose). **Clinically effective neuromuscular block, adults:** 15–20 min after 0.15 mg/kg; **children:** 6–15 min after 0.2 mg/kg. Spontaneous recovery may be 95% complete in 25–30 min after an initial dose of 0.15 mg/kg in adults during opioid/nitrous oxide/oxygen anesthesia. Repeated administration or continuous infusion (for up to 2.5 hr) does not cause tachyphylaxis or cumulative neuromuscular blockade. Higher doses may cause transient decreases in mean arterial BP (especially seen in obese clients) and increases in HR in some clients within 1–3 min following the dose (can be minimized by giving the drug over 30–60 sec). The product is actually a mixture of isomers with varying elimination half-lives. The drug is inactivated by plasma cholinesterase with metabolites excreted in the urine and bile.

Uses: Adjunct to general anesthesia to facilitate tracheal intubation and to provide relaxation of skeletal muscle during surgery or mechanical ventilation.

Dosage

- **IV Only**

Facilitation of tracheal intubation.

Adults: 0.15 mg/kg given over 5–15 sec. Maintenance doses of 0.1 mg/kg provide about 15 min of additional clinically effective blockade. **Children, 2–12 years:** The dosage requirements on a mg/kg basis are higher in children and onset and recovery occur more rapidly. **Initial:** 0.2 mg/kg given over 5–15 sec.

Facilitation of tracheal intubation using continuous IV infusion.

Continuous IV infusion may be used to maintain neuromuscular block. **Adults:** On evidence of spontaneous recovery from an initial dose, an initial infusion rate of 9–10 mcg/kg/min is recommended. If continuous infusion is started at the same time as the administration of an initial dose, a lower initial infusion rate (such as 4 mcg/kg/min) should be used. In either case, the initial infusion rate should be adjusted according to the response to peripheral nerve stimulation and to clinical criteria. An average infusion rate of 6–7 mcg/kg/min will maintain neuromuscular block within the range of 89%–99% for extended periods of time in adults receiving opioid/nitrous oxide/oxygen anesthesia. **Children:** Require higher infusion rates. During opioid/nitrous oxide/oxygen anesthesia, the infusion rate needed to maintain 89%–99% blockade averages 14 mcg/kg/min (range: 5–31 mcg/kg/min).

Tracheal intubation in clients with renal or hepatic impairment.

0.15 mg/kg. Infusion rates should be decreased by as much as 50% in these clients depending on the degree of renal or hepatic impairment.

Use in clients with reduced cholinesterase activity.

Initial doses greater than 0.03 mg/kg are not recommended.

Use in clients who are cachectic, are debilitated, or have carcinomatosis or neuromuscular disease.

A test dose of 0.015–0.02 mg/kg is recommended.

Use with isoflurane or enflurane anesthesia.

An initial dose of 0.15 mg/kg may be used for intubation prior to administration of the isoflurane or enflurane. If mivacurium is given after establishment of anesthesia, the initial dose should be reduced by as much as 25% and the infusion rate should be decreased by as much as 35%–40%. When used with halothane, no adjustment of the initial dose is necessary but the infusion rate should be decreased by as much as 20%.

Use in burn clients.

A test dose of not more than 0.015–0.02 mg/kg is recommended, followed by additional dosing guided by the use of a neuromuscular block monitor.

Use in obese clients weighing equal to or greater than 30% more than their ideal body weight (IBW).

The initial dose is calculated using the IBW according to the following formulas:

Men: IBW in kg = (106 + [6 × height in inches above 5 ft])/2.2

Women: IBW in kg = (100 + [5 × height in inches above 5 ft])/2.2

Use in clients with clinically significant CV disease or in those with any history of a greater sensitivity to the release of histamine or related mediators (asthma).

An initial dose less than or equal to 0.15 mg/kg given over 60 sec.

Administration/Storage

1. The drug should only be given in carefully adjusted dosage under the supervision of trained clinicians who know the action of the drug as well as possible complications from its use. The drug should only be given if personnel and facilities for resuscitation and life support are available immediately.
2. For adults and children, the amount of infusion solution required per hour depends on the clinical requirements, the concentration of mivacurium in the infusion solution, and the weight of the client. Tables

provided by the manufacturer should be consulted to determine the infusion rates using either the premixed infusion of 0.5 mg/mL or the injection containing 2 mg/mL.
3. Dosage adjustment may be necessary in the presence of significant liver, kidney, or CV disease; in obese clients weighing more than 30% of their ideal body weight for height; asthma; those with reduced plasma cholinesterase activity; and the use of inhalation general anesthetics.
4. Additives should not be introduced into mivacurium premixed infusion in flexible plastic containers.
5. Mivacurium premixed infusion should be clear and the container undamaged. It is intended for use in a single client only and any unused portion should be discarded.
6. Mivacurium in vials (2 mg/mL) may be diluted to 0.5 mg/mL with 5% dextrose injection, 5% dextrose and 0.9% sodium chloride injection, 0.9% sodium chloride injection, lactated Ringer's injection, or 5% dextrose in lactated Ringer's injection and then given by Y-site injection and titrated to desired response. The dilution is stable when stored in polyvinyl chloride bags at 5°C–25°C (41°F–77°F). The dilution should be used within 24 hr and is intended for use in a single client only with any unused portion discarded.
7. Mivacurium injection is compatible with sufentanil citrate injection, alfentanil hydrochloride injection, fentanyl citrate injection, midazolam hydrochloride injection, and droperidol injection. However, it may not be compatible with alkaline solutions having a pH greater than 8.5 (e.g., barbiturate solutions).
8. The injection and premixed infusion are stored at 15°C–25°C (59°F–77°F); exposure to direct ultraviolet light should be avoided and the products should not be frozen or exposed to excessive heat.
9. *Treatment of Overdose:*
• Primary treatment is maintenance of a patent airway and controlled ventilation until there is recovery of normal neuromuscular function
• Neostigmine (0.03–0.064 mg/kg) or edrophonium (0.5 mg/kg) can be given once there is evidence of recovery from neuromuscular blockade
• A peripheral nerve stimulator can be used to assess recovery and antagonism of neuromuscular block

Contraindications: Sensitivity to mivacurium or other similar agents. Use of multidose vials in clients with allergy to benzyl alcohol.

Special Concerns: Use with caution during lactation. Use with caution in clients with significant CV disease and in those with any history of a greater sensitivity to the release of histamine or related mediators such as asthma. Volatile anesthetics may decrease the dosing requirement and prolong the duration of action. The duration of action of mivacurium may be prolonged in clients with decreased plasma cholinesterase. Reduced clearance of one or more isomers is observed in clients with end-stage kidney or liver disease. Geriatric clients show a longer duration of neuromuscular blockade. Acid-base or serum electrolyte abnormalities may potentiate or antagonize the action of neuromuscular blocking agents. Antagonism of neuromuscular blockade may be delayed in the presence of debilitation, carcinomatosis, and concomitant use of certain broad-spectrum antibiotics, anesthetic agents, and other drugs that enhance neuromuscular blockade. In children 2–12 years of age, mivacurium has a faster onset, shorter duration, and a faster recovery following reversal than adults. The drug has not been studied in children less than 2 years of age.

Side Effects: *Neuromuscular:* Prolonged neuromuscular blockade, muscle spasms. *CV:* Flushing of face, neck, or chest; hypotension, tachycardia, bradycardia, cardiac arrhythmias, phlebitis. *Respiratory:* ***Bronchospasm,*** wheezing, hypoxemia. *Dermatolog-*

ic: Rash, urticaria, erythema, reaction at injection site. *CNS:* Dizziness.

Symptoms of Overdose: Neuromuscular blockade beyond the time needed for surgery and anesthesia. Increased risk of hemodynamic side effects such as hypotension.

Drug Interactions

See *Neuromuscular Blocking Agents,* Chapter 53.

Also, there is enhanced neuromuscular blockade when magnesium is given to pregnant women for toxemia.

NURSING CONSIDERATIONS

See also *Nursing Considerations* for *Neuromuscular Blocking Agents,* Chapter 53.

Assessment

1. Note indications for therapy. Review conditions and drugs that antagonize and enhance neuromuscular blockade and assess for their presence.
2. Note any history of CV disease or asthma.
3. Obtain baseline ABGs, electrolytes, and liver and renal function studies.
4. Multidose vials contain benzyl alcohol; assess for any client intolerance.
5. Clients homozygous for the atypical plasma cholinesterase gene are quite sensitive to mivacurium neuromuscular blocking effects.
6. Burn clients may show resistance depending on the time elapsed since the burn and the size of the burn; however, clients with burns may have decreased plasma cholinesterase, which offsets the resistance.

Interventions

1. Mivacurium should only be administered in a carefully monitored environment and by persons specially trained in the use of neuromuscular blocking agents.
2. Anticipate reduced dose with liver or renal dysfunction.
3. To avoid distress, ensure that client is unconscious or sedated before administering mivacurium.
4. Use a peripheral nerve stimulator to measure neuromuscular function (assess response), adjust dosage, and confirm recovery (5–sec head lift and grip strength).
5. Geriatric clients show a longer duration of neuromuscular blockade.
6. Monitor VS. Mivacurium will not counteract the bradycardia produced by many anesthetic agents or by vagal stimulation.
7. Advise that transient flushing, wheezing, and tachycardia may be experienced.

Evaluate

- Desired skeletal muscle relaxation
- Successful tracheal intubation
- Adequate suppression of twitch response on peripheral nerve stimulation tests

Pancuronium bromide

(pan-kyou-**ROH**-nee-um)

Pregnancy Category: C

Pavulon **(Rx)**

See also *Neuromuscular Blocking Agents,* Chapter 53.

How Supplied: *Injection:* 1 mg/mL, 2 mg/mL

Action/Kinetics: Effects similar to *d*-tubocurarine although pancuronium is 5 times as potent. Drug effects can be reversed by anticholinesterase agents. Pancuronium possesses vagolytic activity although it is not likely to cause histamine release. **Onset:** Within 45 sec. **Time to peak effect:** 3–4.5 min (depending on the dose). **Duration:** 35–45 min (increased with multiple doses). **t½, elimination:** 114–116 min. Ninety percent of the total dose is excreted through the urine either unchanged or as metabolites; 10% is excreted through the bile. In clients with renal failure, the t½ is doubled. Significantly bound to plasma protein.

Uses: Muscle relaxation during anesthesia, ET intubation, management of clients undergoing mechanical ventilation.

Dosage

- **IV Only**

Muscle relaxation during anesthesia.

Adults and children over 1 month of age, initial: 0.04–0.1 mg/

kg. Additional doses of 0.01 mg/kg may be administered as required (usually q 20–60 min). **Neonates:** A test dose of 0.02 mg/kg should be administered first to determine responsiveness.

When used with enflurane or isoflurane anesthesia and/or after succinylcholine-assisted ET intubation.

Initial: 0.05 mg/kg; **then,** adjust to client response.

ET intubation.

0.06–0.1 mg/kg as a bolus dose.

Administration/Storage

1. Additional doses of pancuronium significantly increase the duration of skeletal muscle relaxation.
2. The drug may be mixed with 5% dextrose, 5% dextrose and sodium chloride, lactated Ringer's injection, and 0.9% sodium chloride injection. When mixed with any of these solutions, the drug is stable for 2 days.
3. Anticipate the medication will act within 3 min upon administration and last 35–45 min.
4. Administer IV drug in a continuously monitored environment.
5. Have appropriate anticholinesterase agents available to reverse drug effects. These include pyridostigmine bromide, neostigmine, or edrophonium and are usually administered with atropine or glycopyrrolate.

Special Concerns: Children up to 1 month of age may be more sensitive to the effects of atracurium.

Additional Side Effects: *Respiratory:* ***Apnea, respiratory insufficiency.*** *CV:* Increased HR and MAP. *Miscellaneous:* Salivation, skin rashes, ***hypersensitivity reactions (e.g., bronchospasm,*** flushing, hypotension, redness, tachycardia).

Additional Drug Interactions

Azathioprine / Reverses effects of pancuronium

Bacitracin / Additive muscle relaxation

Enflurane / ↑ Muscle relaxation

Isoflurane / ↑ Muscle relaxation

Quinine / ↑ Effect of pancuronium

Succinylcholine / ↑ Intensity and duration of action of pancuronium

Tetracyclines / Additive muscle relaxation

Theophyllines / ↓ Effects of pancuronium; also, possible cardiac arrhythmias

NURSING CONSIDERATIONS

See also *Nursing Considerations* for *Neuromuscular Blocking Agents,* Chapter 53.

Interventions

1. Provide ventilatory support.
2. Monitor and record VS and I&O.
3. A peripheral nerve stimulator should be used to evaluate neuromuscular response.
4. Consciousness is not affected by pancuronium. Explain all procedures and provide emotional support. Do not discuss any topics that should not be overheard.
5. With short-term therapy, reassure clients that they will be able to talk and move once the drug effects are reversed.
6. Position the client for comfort and so that the body is in proper alignment. Turn and perform mouth care and eye care frequently (protect eyes; blink reflex is suppressed).
7. Assess the client's airway at frequent intervals. Have a suction machine at the bedside.
8. Check to be certain that the ventilator alarms are set and on at all times. *Never* leave client unmonitored.
9. Determine client need and administer medications for anxiety, pain, and/or sedation regularly.

Evaluate

- Muscle relaxation with desired level of paralysis
- Facilitation of intubation and tolerance of mechanical ventilation

Pipecuronium bromide

(pih-peh-kyour-**OHN**-ee-um)

Pregnancy Category: C

Arduan **(Rx)**

See also *Neuromuscular Blocking Agents,* Chapter 53.

How Supplied: *Powder for injection:* 10 mg

Action/Kinetics: Pipecuronium is similar to tubocurarine in that it competes for cholinergic receptors at the motor end-plate and is antagonized by acetylcholinesterase inhibitors. **Maximum time for blockade:** 5 min following single doses of 70–85 mcg/kg. **Time to recovery to 25% of control:** 30–175 min under balanced anesthesia following single doses of 70 mcg/kg. **t½, distribution:** 6.22 min; **t½, elimination:** 1.7 hr. Increased plasma levels are seen in clients with impaired renal function. The drug is metabolized in the liver and metabolites as well as unchanged drug are eliminated in the urine.

Uses: Adjunct to general anesthesia to provide relaxation of skeletal muscle during surgery. Skeletal muscle relaxation for ET intubation.

Dosage

- **IV Only**

Adjunct to general anesthesia.

Adults: Initial dose may be based on the creatinine clearance and the ideal body weight (see information provided by manufacturer). Dose is individualized. The dose range is 50–100 mcg/kg.

ET intubation using balanced anesthesia.

70–85 mcg/kg with halothane, isoflurane, or enflurane in clients with normal renal function who are not obese; duration of muscle relaxation is 1–2 hr using this dosage range.

Use following recovery from succinylcholine.

50 mcg/kg in clients with normal renal function who are not obese; duration of muscle relaxation using this dose is 45 min. *Maintenance.* **Adults:** 10–15 mcg/kg given at 25% recovery of control T_1 will provide muscle relaxation for an average of 50 min using balanced anesthesia; lower doses should be used in clients receiving inhalation anesthetics. **Pediatric:** The duration of action in infants following a dose of 40 mcg/kg ranged from 10 to 44 min while the duration in children following a dose of 57 mcg/kg ranged from 18 to 52 min.

Administration/Storage

1. Pipecuronium should be administered only under the supervision of individuals experienced with the use of neuromuscular blocking agents.
2. Pipecuronium can be reconstituted using 0.9% sodium chloride, 5% dextrose in saline, D5W, lactated Ringer's, sterile water for injection, and bacteriostatic water for injection.
3. If used in newborns, the drug should not be reconstituted with bacteriostatic water for injection because it contains benzyl alcohol.
4. When reconstituted with bacteriostatic water for injection, the solution may be stored at room temperature or in the refrigerator; it should be used within 5 days.
5. When reconstituted with sterile water for injection or other IV solutions, the vial should be refrigerated and used within 24 hr.
6. Pipecuronium should not be diluted with or administered from large volumes of IV solutions.
7. The drug should be stored at 2°C–30°C (35°F–86°F) and protected from light.
8. *Treatment of Overdose:* Artificial respiration until effects of drug have worn off. Antagonize neuromuscular blockade by administration of neostigmine, 0.04 mg/kg. Use of edrophonium is not recommended.

Contraindications: Use for procedures anticipated to last 90 min or longer. Due to the long duration of action, the drug should not be used in myasthenia gravis or Eaton-Lambert syndrome. Clients undergoing cesarean section. Use of pipecuronium before succinylcholine.

Special Concerns: Although the drug is used in infants and children, no information is available on maintenance dosing. Also, children 1–14 years of age under balanced or halothane anesthesia may be less sensitive to the drug than adults. Use with caution in clients with impaired renal function. The drug should be administered only if there are adequate facilities for intubation, artificial respiration, oxygen therapy, and administration of an antagonist. Obesity may prolong the duration of action. Conditions resulting in an increased volume of distribution (e.g., old age, edematous states, slower circulation time in CV disease) may cause a delay in the time of onset.

Side Effects: *Neuromuscular:* ***Prolongation of blockade including skeletal muscle paralysis resulting in respiratory insufficiency or apnea.*** Muscle atrophy, difficult intubation. *CV:* Hypotension, bradycardia, hypertension, CVA, thrombosis, myocardial ischemia, atrial fibrillation, ventricular extrasystole. *CNS:* Hypesthesia, CNS depression. *Respiratory:* Dyspnea, respiratory depression, laryngismus, atelectasis. *Metabolic:* Hypoglycemia, hyperkalemia, increased creatinine. *Miscellaneous:* Rash, urticaria, anuria.

Symptoms of Overdose: ***Skeletal muscle paralysis including depressed respiration.***

Drug Interactions

Aminoglycosides / ↑ Intensity and duration of neuromuscular blockade
Bacitracin / ↑ Intensity and duration of neuromuscular blockade
Colistin/Sodium colistimethate / ↑ Intensity and duration of neuromuscular blockade
Enflurane / ↑ Duration of action of pipecuronium
Halothane / ↑ Duration of action of pipecuronium
Isoflurane / ↑ Duration of action of pipecuronium
Magnesium salts / ↑ Intensity of neuromuscular blockade when used for toxemia of pregnancy
Polymyxin B / ↑ Intensity and duration of neuromuscular blockade
Quinidine / ↑ Risk of recurrent paralysis
Tetracyclines / ↑ Intensity and duration of neuromuscular blockade

NURSING CONSIDERATIONS

Assessment

1. Document height and weight and note any evidence of obesity because drug dose should be correlated for *ideal* body weight.
2. Review client history for evidence of myasthenia gravis or Eaton-Lambert syndrome because drug is not recommended with these conditions.
3. List drugs client currently prescribed because many interact unfavorably with pipecuronium.
4. Determine if diarrhea is present and the duration because this may alter desired neuromuscular blockade.
5. Obtain baseline electrolytes and renal function studies.

Interventions

1. The twitch response should be used to evaluate recovery from pipecuronium and to minimize overdosage potential. Individuals administering pipecuronium should use a peripheral nerve stimulator to assess the height of the twitch wave. This device will assist to monitor drug response, to assess the need for additional doses of the drug, and to evaluate the adequacy of spontaneous recovery or antagonism.
2. Allow more time for pipecuronium to achieve maximum effect in older clients with slowed circulation, CV diseases, and/or edematous states. *Do not* increase drug dose because this will produce a longer duration of action.
3. Monitor BP and pulse closely and observe postrecovery for adequate clinical evidence of antagonism:
• 5-sec head lift
• Adequate pronation
• Effective airway and ventilatory patterns

Evaluate

• Desired level of skeletal muscle relaxation
• Suppression of twitch response when tested with a peripheral nerve stimulator

Succinylcholine chloride

(suck-sin-ill-**KOH**-leen)
Pregnancy Category: C
Anectine, Anectine Flo-Pack, Quelicin, Succinylcholine Chloride Min-I-Mix, Sucostrin High Potency **(Rx)**

See also *Neuromuscular Blocking Agents,* Chapter 53.
How Supplied: *Injection:* 20 mg/mL, 50 mg/mL, 100 mg/mL; *Powder for injection:* 500 mg, 1 g
Action/Kinetics: Succinylcholine initially excites skeletal muscle by combining with cholinergic receptors preferentially to acetylcholine. Subsequently, it prevents the muscle from contracting by prolonging the time during which the receptors at the neuromuscular junction cannot respond to acetylcholine. Short-acting. It has no effect on pain threshold, cerebration, or consciousness; thus, it should be used with sufficient anesthesia. Effects are not blocked by anticholinesterase drugs and may even be enhanced by them. **IV: onset,** 1 min; **duration:** 4–6 min; **recovery:** 8–10 min. **IM: Onset,** 3 min; **duration:** 10–30 min. Metabolized by plasma pseudocholinesterase to succinylmonocholine, which is a nondepolarizing muscle relaxant. About 10% succinylcholine is excreted unchanged in the urine.
Uses: Muscle relaxant during surgery, ET intubation, endoscopy, and short manipulative procedures. *Investigational:* Reduce intensity of electrically induced seizures or seizures due to drugs.

Dosage

• **IM, IV**

Short or prolonged surgical procedures.

Adults, IV, initial: 0.3–1.1 mg/kg; **then,** repeated doses can be given based on client response. **Adults, IM:** 3–4 mg/kg, not to exceed a total dose of 150 mg.

Prolonged surgical procedures, IV infusion (preferred).

0.1%–0.2% solution in 5% dextrose, sodium chloride injection, or other diluent given at a rate of 0.5–10 mg/min depending on client response and degree of relaxation desired, for up to 1 hr.

Electroshock therapy.

Adults, IV: 10–30 mg given 1 min prior to the shock (individualize dosage). **IM:** Up to 2.5 mg/kg, not to exceed a total dose of 150 mg.

ET intubation.

Pediatric, IV: 1–2 mg/kg; if necessary, dose can be repeated. **IM:** Up to 2.5 mg/kg, not to exceed a total dose of 150 mg.

Administration/Storage

1. An initial test dose of 0.1 mg/kg should be given to assess sensitivity and recovery time.
2. Review the drugs with which succinylcholine interacts.
3. Do not mix with anesthetic.
4. For IV infusion, use 1 or 2 mg/mL solution of drug in 5% dextrose injection, 0.9% sodium chloride, or other suitable IV solution. Succinylcholine is not compatible with alkaline solutions.
5. Alter the degree of relaxation by altering the rate of flow.
6. To reduce salivation, premedication with atropine or scopolamine is recommended.
7. A low dose of a nondepolarizing agent (such as tubocurarine) may be given to reduce the severity of muscle fasciculations.
8. Store the drug in the refrigerator.
9. Have neostigmine or pyridostigmine available to reverse neuromuscular blockade.

Special Concerns: Use with caution during lactation. Pediatric clients may be especially prone to myoglobinemia, myoglobinuria, and cardiac effects. Use of IV infusion is not recommended in children due to the risk of malignant hyperpyrexia. Use with caution in clients with severe liver disease, severe anemia, malnutrition, impaired cholinesterase activity, genetic disorders of plasma pseudocholinesterase, myopathies associated with increased CPK, acute narrow-angle glaucoma, history of malignant hyperthermia, penetrating eye injuries, fractures. Also, in CV, pulmonary, renal, or metabolic diseases.

Side Effects: *Skeletal muscle:* May cause ***severe, persistent respiratory depression or apnea.*** Muscle fasciculations, postoperative muscle pain. *CV:* Bradycardia or tachycardia, BP changes, ***arrhythmias, cardiac arrest.*** *Respiratory:* ***Apnea, respiratory depression.*** *Other:* Fever, malignant hyperthermia, salivation, hyperkalemia, postoperative muscle pain, anaphylaxis, myoglobinemia, myoglobinuria, skin rashes, increased intraocular pressure. Repeated doses may cause tachyphylaxis.

Drug Interactions

Aminoglycoside antibiotics / Additive skeletal muscle blockade
Amphotericin B / ↑ Effect of succinylcholine
Antibiotics, nonpenicillin / Additive skeletal muscle blockade
Anticholinesterases / Additive skeletal muscle blockade
Beta-adrenergic blocking agents / Additive skeletal muscle blockade
Chloroquine / Additive skeletal muscle blockade
Clindamycin / Additive skeletal muscle blockade
Cyclophosphamide / ↑ Effect of succinylcholine by ↓ breakdown of drug in plasma by pseudocholinesterase
Diazepam / ↓ Effect of succinylcholine
Digitalis glycosides / ↑ Chance of cardiac arrhythmias
Echothiophate iodide / ↑ Effect of succinylcholine by ↓ breakdown of drug in plasma by pseudocholinesterase
Furosemide / ↑ Action of succinylcholine
Isoflurane / Additive skeletal muscle blockade
Lidocaine / Additive skeletal muscle blockade
Lincomycin / Additive skeletal muscle blockade
Lithium / ↑ Effect of succinylcholine
Magnesium salts / Additive skeletal muscle blockade
Narcotics / ↑ Risk of bradycardia and sinus arrest
Oxytocin / ↑ Effect of succinylcholine
Phenelzine / ↑ Effect of succinylcholine
Phenothiazines / ↑ Effect of succinylcholine
Polymyxin / Additive skeletal muscle blockade
Procainamide / ↑ Effect of succinylcholine
Procaine / ↑ Effect of succinylcholine by inhibiting plasma pseudocholinesterase activity
Promazine / ↑ Effect of succinylcholine
Quinidine / Additive skeletal muscle blockade
Quinine / Additive skeletal muscle blockade
Thiotepa / ↑ Effect of succinylcholine by ↓ breakdown of drug in plasma by pseudocholinesterase
Trimethaphan / ↑ Effect of succinylcholine by inhibiting plasma pseudocholinesterase activity

NURSING CONSIDERATIONS

See also *Nursing Considerations* for *Neuromuscular Blocking Agents,* Chapter 53.

Assessment

1. Note if the client is taking digitalis products. These clients are sensitive to the release of intracellular potassium.
2. Assess clients with low plasma pseudocholinesterase levels. They are sensitive to the effects of succinylcholine and require lower doses.
3. Document any evidence of a history of malignant hyperthermia.

Interventions

1. A peripheral nerve stimulator should be used to assess the client's neuromuscular response.
2. Monitor VS and ECG. Succinylcholine can cause vagal stimulation resulting in bradycardia, hypotension, and cardiac arrhythmias.
3. Observe for excessive, transient increase in intraocular pressure. Doc-

ument and report as this can be dangerous to the eye.
4. Muscle fasciculations may cause the client to be sore after recovery. Administer prescribed nondepolarizing agent (i.e., tubocurarine) and reassure that the soreness is likely caused by the unsynchronized contractions of adjacent muscle fibers just before the onset of paralysis.
5. Monitor closely for any evidence of malignant hyperthermia, unresponsive tachycardia, jaw spasm, or lack of laryngeal relaxation. Stop infusion and report. Temperature elevations are a late sign of this condition.
6. Document the length of time the client is taking the drug. It should be used only on a short-term basis and in a continuously monitored environment.
7. Remember that client is fully conscious and aware of surroundings and conversations.
8. Drug does not affect pain or anxiety so administer analgesics and antianxiety agents as indicated.
9. When used for seizures, ensure that serum level of anticonvulsant agent is therapeutic, as succinylcholine does not cross the blood-brain barrier and will only suppress peripheral manifestations of seizures, not the central process.

Evaluate

- Desired level of muscle relaxation/paralysis
- Suppression of the twitch response when tested with a peripheral nerve stimulator

Tubocurarine chloride

(too-boh-kyour-**AR**-een)
Pregnancy Category: C
Tubarine ✱ **(Rx)**

See also *Neuromuscular Blocking Agents,* Chapter 53.

How Supplied: *Injection:* 3 mg/mL

Action/Kinetics: Cumulative effects may occur. Most likely of the nondepolarizing drugs to cause histamine release. Narrow margin between therapeutic dose and toxic dose. Overdosage chiefly treated by artificial respiration, although neostigmine, atropine, and edrophonium chloride should also be on hand. **Onset, IV:** 1 min; **IM:** 15–25 min. **Time to peak effect, IV:** 2–5 min. **Duration, IV:** 20–40 min. **t½:** 1–3 hr. About 43% excreted unchanged in urine.

Uses: Muscle relaxant during surgery or setting of fractures and dislocations; spasticity caused by injury to or disease of CNS. Treat seizures electrically induced or induced by drugs. Diagnosis of myasthenia gravis.

Dosage

- **IV, IM**

Adjunct to surgical anesthesia.

Adults, IM, IV, initial: 6–9 mg (40–60 units); **then,** 3–4.5 mg (20–30 units) in 3–5 min if needed. Supplemental doses of 3 mg (20 units) can be given for prolonged procedures. Dosage can be calculated on the basis of 1.1 units/kg. **Pediatric, up to 4 weeks of age, IV, initial:** 0.3 mg/kg; **then,** give subsequent doses in increments of 1/5–1/6 the initial dose. **Infants and children, IV:** 0.6 mg/kg.

Electroshock therapy.

Adults, IV: 0.165 mg/kg (1.1 units/kg) given over 30–90 sec. It is recommended that the initial dose be 3 mg less than the calculated total dose.

Diagnosis of myasthenia gravis.

Adults, IV: 0.004–0.033 mg/kg. A test dose should be given within 2–3 min with IV neostigmine, 1.5 mg, to minimize prolonged respiratory paralysis.

Administration/Storage

1. The drug should be given IV as a sustained injection over 1–1.5 min. It may also be given IM.
2. Tubocurarine should be given in incremental doses until relaxation is reached.
3. The initial dose should be decreased if the inhalation anesthetic used enhances the action of curariform drugs or if the client has compromised renal function.
4. Review the drugs with which tubocurarine interacts.

5. Tubocurarine is incompatible with alkaline solutions and may form a precipitate when mixed with them (e.g., methohexital sodium or thiopental sodium).
6. After IV administration, expect the peak action to occur in 2–5 min and the effect to last 25–90 min.
7. Have neostigmine methylsulfate available as an antidote.

Additional Contraindications: Drug may cause excessive secretion and circulatory collapse. Clients in whom release of histamine is hazardous.

Special Concerns: Use with caution during pregnancy and lactation and in children. If repeated doses are used before delivery, the newborn may manifest decreased skeletal muscle activity. Children up to 1 month of age may be more sensitive to the effects of tubocurarine. Use with extreme caution in clients with renal dysfunction, liver disease, or obstructive states.

Additional Side Effects: ***Allergic reactions.***

Additional Drug Interactions

Acetylcholine / Acetylcholine antagonizes effect of tubocurarine
Anticholinesterases / Anticholinesterases antagonize effect of tubocurarine
Calcium salts / ↑ Effect of tubocurarine
Diazepam / Diazepam may cause malignant hyperthermia with tubocurarine
Potassium / Antagonizes effect of tubocurarine
Propranolol / ↑ Effect of tubocurarine
Quinine / ↑ Effect of tubocurarine
Succinylcholine chloride / ↑ Relaxant effect of both drugs
Trimethaphan / ↑ Effect of tubocurarine

NURSING CONSIDERATIONS

See also *Nursing Considerations* for *Neuromuscular Blocking Agents,* Chapter 53

Assessment: Document indications for therapy and onset of symptoms.

Interventions

1. Monitor VS and ECG. Drug can cause vagal stimulation resulting in bradycardia, hypotension, and cardiac arrhythmias.
2. Document length of time client is receiving the drug. It should be used only on a short-term basis and in a continuously monitored environment.
3. Remember that client may be fully conscious and aware of surroundings and conversations.
4. Drug does not affect pain or anxiety so administer analgesics and antianxiety agents as indicated.

Evaluate

- Desired level of skeletal muscle relaxation
- Control of drug or electrically induced seizures
- Diagnosis of myasthenia gravis

Vecuronium bromide

(vh-kyour-**OH**-nee-um)
Pregnancy Category: C
Norcuron **(Rx)**

See also *Neuromuscular Blocking Agents,* Chapter 53.

How Supplied: *Powder for injection:* 10 mg, 20 mg

Action/Kinetics: Less likely than other agents to cause histamine release. Effects can be antagonized by anticholinesterase drugs.

Onset: 2.5–3 min; **peak effect:** 3–5 min; **duration:** 25–30 min using balanced anesthesia. No cumulative effects noted after repeated administration. Metabolized in liver and excreted through the kidney and bile. Is bound to plasma protein.

Uses: To induce skeletal muscle relaxation during surgery or to assist in ET intubation. As an adjunct to general anesthesia. *Investigational:* To treat electrically induced seizures or seizures induced by drugs.

Dosage

- **IV Only**

Intubation.

Adults and children over 10 years of age. 0.08–0.1 mg/kg.

For use after succinylcholine-assisted ET intubation.

0.04–0.06 mg/kg for inhalation anesthesia and 0.05–0.06 mg/kg using balanced anesthesia. (*NOTE:* For halothane anesthesia, doses of 0.15–0.28 mg/kg may be given without adverse effects.)

For use during anesthesia with enflurane or isoflurane after steady state established.

0.06–0.085 mg/kg (about 15% less than the usual initial dose).

Supplemental use.

IV only: 0.01–0.015 mg/kg given 25–40 min following the initial dose; **then,** given q 12–15 min as needed. **IV infusion:** Initiated after recovery from effects of initial IV dose of 0.08–0.1 mg/kg has started. **Initial:** 0.001 mcg (1 mg)/kg; **then** adjust according to client response and requirements. Average infusion rate: 0.0008–0.0012 mg/kg/min (0.8–1.2 mcg/kg/min). After steady-state enflurane, isoflurane, and possibly halothane anesthesia has been established: IV infusion should be reduced by 25%–60%.

Administration/Storage

1. Dosage must be individualized and depends on prior or concomitant use of anesthetics or succinylcholine.
2. Vecuronium may be mixed with saline, 5% dextrose alone or with saline, lactated Ringer's solution, and sterile water for injection.
3. Vecuronium should be used within 8 hr of reconstitution.
4. Anticipate the onset of action to occur within 1–5 min and the effect to last 20–40 min.
5. The drug should be refrigerated after reconstitution.
6. Have neostigmine, pyridostigmine, or edrophonium available to reverse vecuronium; atropine helps counteract muscarinic effects.

Additional Contraindications: Use in neonates, obesity. Sensitivity to bromides.

Special Concerns: Pediatric clients from 7 weeks to 1 year of age are more sensitive to the effects of vecuronium leading to a recovery time up to 1½ times that for adults. The dose for children aged 1–10 years of age must be individualized and may, in fact, require a somewhat higher initial dose and a slightly more frequent supplemental dosing schedule than adults.

Additional Side Effects: Moderate to severe skeletal muscle weakness, which may require artificial respiration. ***Malignant hyperthermia.***

Additional Drug Interaction: Succinylcholine ↑ effect of vecuronium.

NURSING CONSIDERATIONS

See also *Nursing Considerations* for *Neuromuscular Blocking Agents,* Chapter 53.

Interventions:

1. A peripheral nerve stimulator should be used to assess the client's neuromuscular response.
2. Monitor VS and ECG. Drug can cause vagal stimulation resulting in bradycardia, hypotension, and cardiac arrhythmias.
3. Muscle fasciculations may cause the client to be sore after recovery. Administer prescribed nondepolarizing agent and reassure that the soreness is likely caused by the unsynchronized contractions of adjacent muscle fibers just before the onset of paralysis.
4. Monitor closely for any evidence of malignant hyperthermia, unresponsive tachycardia, jaw spasm, or lack of laryngeal relaxation. Stop infusion and report. Temperature elevations are a late sign of this condition.
5. Document length of time client is receiving the drug. It should be used only on a short-term basis and in a continuously monitored environment.
6. Remember client is fully conscious and aware of surroundings and conversations.
7. Drug does not affect pain or anxiety so administer analgesics and antianxiety agents as indicated.

8. Prolonged use, as in an ICU setting, may lead to skeletal muscle weakness and symptoms consistent with muscle disuse atrophy. This may complicate ventilator weaning and some clients may require extensive rehabilitation.

Evaluate

- Desired level of skeletal muscle relaxation
- Facilitation of intubation and tolerance of mechanical ventilation
- Suppression of the twitch response when tested with a peripheral nerve stimulator

Drugs Affecting the Respiratory Tract

CHAPTER FIFTY-FOUR

Antiasthmatic Drugs

See the following individual entries:

Cromolyn Sodium (Sodium Cromoglycate)
Nedocromil Sodium
Theophylline Derivatives
  Aminophylline
  Theophylline

Cromolyn sodium (Sodium cromoglycate)

(**CROH**-moh-lin)
Pregnancy Category: B
Gastrocrom, Intal, Nalcrom ✱, Nasalcrom, Opticrom 4%, Rynacrom ✱, Vistacrom ✱ **(Rx)**

How Supplied: *Aerosol Liquid w/Adapter:* 0.8 mg/inh; *Capsule:* 100 mg; *Ophthalmic solution:* 4%; *Solution:* 10 mg/mL, *Nasal spray:* 5.2 mg/inh

Action/Kinetics: Cromolyn sodium appears to act locally to inhibit the degranulation of sensitized mast cells that occurs after exposure to certain antigen. The effect prevents the release of histamine, slow-reacting substance of anaphylaxis, and other endogenous substances causing hypersensitivity reactions. The drug, when effective, reduces the number and intensity of asthmatic attacks as well as decreasing allergic reactions in the eye. The drug has no antihistaminic, anti-inflammatory, or bronchodilator effects and has no role in terminating an acute attack of asthma. After inhalation, some of the drug is absorbed systemically. It is excreted about equally in urine and bile (feces). **t½:** 81 min; from lungs: 60 min. About 50% excreted unchanged through the urine and 50% through the bile. When used in the eye, approximately 0.03% is absorbed. **Onset, ophthalmic:** Several days. **Onset, nasal:** Less than 1 week. **Time to peak effect, nasal:** Up to 4 weeks.

Uses: *Inhalation:* Prophylactic and adjunct in the management of severe bronchial asthma in selected clients. Prophylaxis of exercise-induced bronchospasms and bronchospasms due to allergens, cold dry air, or environmental pollutants. *Ophthalmologic:* Treat allergic ocular disorders, including allergic keratoconjunctivitis, giant papillary conjunctivitis, vernal keratoconjunctivitis, vernal conjunctivitis, and vernal keratitis. *Nasal:* Prophylaxis and treatment of allergic rhinitis. *PO:* Mastocytosis (improves symptoms including diarrhea, flushing, headaches, vomiting, urticaria, nausea, abdominal pain, and itching). *Investigational:* PO to treat food allergies.

Dosage

- **Capsules or Solution for Inhalation**

Prophylaxis of bronchial asthma.
Adults: 20 mg q.i.d. at regular intervals. Adjust dosage as required.

Prophylaxis of bronchospasm.
Adults: 20 mg as a single dose just prior to exposure to the precipitating factor. If used chronically, 20 mg q.i.d, up to a maximum of 160 mg/day.

- **Ophthalmic Solution**

Allergic ocular disorders.
Adults and children over 4 years: 1–2 gtt of the 4% solution 4–6 times/day at regular intervals.

- **Nasal Solution**

Allergic rhinitis.
Adults and children over 6 years: 2.6 mg in each nostril 6 times/day or 5.2 mg in each nostril 3–4 times/day at regular intervals.

- **Oral Capsules**

Mastocytosis.
Adults: 200 mg q.i.d. 30 min before meals and at bedtime. **Pediatric, term to 2 years:** 20 mg/kg/day in four divided doses; should be used in this age group only in severe incapacitating disease where benefits outweigh risks. **Pediatric, 2–12 years:** 100 mg q.i.d. 30 min before meals and at bedtime. If relief is not seen within 2–3 weeks, dose may be increased, but should not exceed 40 mg/kg/day for adults and children over 2 years of age and 30 mg/kg/day for children 6 months–2 years.

Administration/Storage

1. Institute only after acute episode is over, when airway is clear and client can inhale adequately.
2. Corticosteroid dosage should be continued when initiating cromolyn therapy. However, if improvement occurs, the steroid dosage may be tapered slowly. Steroid therapy may have to be reinstituted if cromolyn inhalation is impaired, in times of stress, or in adrenocortical insufficiency.
3. One drop of the ophthalmic solution contains 1.6 mg cromolyn sodium.
4. The ophthalmic solution should be protected from direct sunlight and, once opened, should be discarded after 4 weeks.

Contraindications: Hypersensitivity. Acute attacks and status asthmaticus. Due to the presence of benzalkonium chloride in the product, soft contact lenses should not be worn if the drug is used in the eye. For mastocytosis in premature infants.

Special Concerns: Dosage of the ophthalmic product has not been established in children less than 4 years of age; dosage of the nasal product has not been established in children less than 6 years of age. Use with caution for long periods of time, in the presence of renal or hepatic disease, and during lactation.

Side Effects: *Respiratory:* ***Bronchospasm, laryngeal edema (rare),*** cough, eosinophilic pneumonia. *CNS:* Dizziness, drowsiness, headache. *Allergic:* Urticaria, rash, angioedema, serum sickness, ***anaphylaxis.*** *Other:* Nausea, urinary frequency, dysuria, joint swelling and pain, lacrimation, swollen parotid gland.

Following nebulization: Sneezing, wheezing, itching, nose bleeds, burning, nasal congestion. **Following nasal solution:** Burning, stinging, irritation of nose; sneezing, nose bleeds, headache, bad taste in mouth, postnasal drip. **Following ophthalmic use:** Stinging and burning after use.

Following PO use: *GI:* Diarrhea, taste perversion, spasm of esophagus, flatulence, dysphagia, burning of mouth and throat. *CNS:* Headache, dizziness, fatigue, migraine, paresthesia, anxiety, depression, psychosis, behavior changes, insomnia, hallucinations, lethargy, lightheadedness after eating. *Dermatologic:* Flushing, angioedema, urticaria, skin burning, skin erythema.

Musculoskeletal: Arthralgia, stiffness and weakness in legs. *Miscellaneous:* Altered liver function test, dyspnea, dysuria, polycythemia, neutropenia.

NURSING CONSIDERATIONS

Client/Family Teaching

1. Provide written guidelines concerning the prescribed method of medication administration and anticipated results.
2. When the medication is administered by Spinhaler, the following guidelines should be used:
• Demonstrate how to puncture and load the capsule into the Spinhaler.
• Instruct the client to inhale and exhale fully and then to introduce the mouthpiece between the lips.
• Tilt head back and inhale deeply and rapidly through the inhaler. This causes the propeller to turn rapidly and to supply more medication in one breath.
• Remove inhaler, hold breath a few seconds, and exhale slowly.
• Repeat this procedure until the powder is completely administered.
• Do not wet powder with breath while exhaling.
• Taking a sip of water or rinsing the mouth immediately before and after using the Spinhaler will diminish the throat irritation and/or cough.
• The Spinhaler should be replaced every 6 months.
3. When used in the *eye*:
• Advise client not to wear soft contacts until medically cleared.
• Drug may sting on application, but this should subside.
4. Encourage the client to continue routine self-administration of medication as ordered. It may take up to 4 weeks for frequency of asthmatic attacks to decrease.
5. With exposure bronchoconstriction, advise client to use the inhaler within 10–15 min prior to exposure of precipitating agent (i.e., exercise, antigen, environmental pollutants) for best results.
6. If the client wishes to discontinue medication, stress the importance of notifying the provider. Rapid withdrawal of the drug may precipitate an asthmatic attack, and concomitant corticosteroid therapy may require adjustment.

Evaluate

• ↓ Frequency and intensity of asthmatic attacks
• Prevention of exposure-induced bronchoconstriction
• Control of symptoms of mastocytosis (↓ diarrhea, N&V, headache, flushing, and abdominal pain)
• Relief of ocular and/or nasal allergic manifestations

Nedocromil sodium

(neh-**DAH**-kroh-mill)
Pregnancy Category: B
Tilade **(Rx)**

How Supplied: *Aerosol Solid w/Adapter:* 1.75 mg/inh

Action/Kinetics: Nedocromil is an inhalation anti-inflammatory drug for the prophylaxis of asthma. It inhibits the release of various mediators, such as histamine, leukotriene C_4, and prostaglandin D_2, from a variety of cell types associated with asthma. The drug has no intrinsic bronchodilator, antihistamine, or glucocorticoid activity; also, systemic bioavailability is low. **t½:** 3.3 hr. Nedocromil is about 89% bound to plasma protein; it is excreted unchanged.

Use: Maintenance therapy in clients with mild to moderate bronchial asthma.

Dosage

• **Aerosol**

Bronchial asthma.

Adults and children over 12 years of age: two inhalations q.i.d. at regular intervals in order to provide 14 mg/day. If the client is under good control on q.i.d. dosing (i.e., requiring inhaled or oral beta agonist no more than twice a week or no worsening of symptoms occur with respiratory infections), a lower dose can be tried. In such instances, the dose should first be reduced to 10.5 mg/day (i.e., used t.i.d.); then, after several weeks with good control, the dose can be reduced to 7 mg/day (i.e., used b.i.d.).

Administration

1. Each actuation releases 1.75 mg.
2. Nedocromil must be used regularly, even during symptom-free period, in order to achieve beneficial effects.
3. Clients must be taught the proper method of use of the drug. An illustrated pamphlet is included in each pack of nedocromil.
4. Nedocromil should be added to the existing treatment (e.g., bronchodilators). When a clinical response is seen and if the asthma is under good control, a gradual decrease in the concomitant medication can be tried.
5. The drug should be stored between 2°C and 30°C (36°F and 86°F) and should not be frozen.

Contraindication: Use for the reversal of acute bronchospasms, especially status asthmaticus.

Special Concerns: Use with caution during lactation. Safety and efficacy have not been established in children less than 12 years of age. Nedocromil has not been shown to be able to substitute for the total dose of corticosteroids.

Laboratory Test Interference: ↑ ALT.

Side Effects: *Respiratory:* Coughing, pharyngitis, rhinitis, upper respiratory tract infection, increased sputum, bronchitis, dyspnea, ***bronchospasm.*** *GI tract:* N&V, dyspepsia, abdominal pain, dry mouth, diarrhea. *CNS:* Dizziness, dysphonia. *Skin:* Rash, sensation of warmth. *Body as a whole:* Headache, chest pain, fatigue, arthritis. *Miscellaneous:* Viral infection, unpleasant taste.

NURSING CONSIDERATIONS

Assessment

1. Assess respiratory status thoroughly; drug is not for use with status asthmaticus or for reversal of acute bronchospasm since drug is not a bronchodilator.
2. Document systemic and inhaled steroid therapy accurately. When a reduction is in progress, remind provider that nedocromil cannot substitute for total steroid dose/requirements.
3. Review drug usage and time between prescriptions to ensure proper use by client.

Client/Family Teaching

1. Review correct procedure for administration and observe client technique. Instruct client to use the step-by-step instructions provided with the medication to ensure proper administration.
2. Stress that beneficial effects will not be obtained if drug is not correctly administered by topical lung application.
3. Explain that drug is an inhaled anti-inflammatory that reduces lung inflammation.
4. Advise not to stop therapy during symptom-free periods. In order to achieve benefits, drug must be taken at regular intervals.
5. Instruct client to continue to use nedocromil inhaler along with other prescribed therapies unless otherwise specified.
6. Report any persistent headaches, unpleasant taste in mouth that interferes with nutrition, severe nausea, or chest pain.
7. Advise client to report any coughing or bronchospasm following use of nedocromil as drug should be discontinued and alternative therapy substituted.

Evaluate: ↓ Severity and frequency of asthmatic episodes.

THEOPHYLLINE DERIVATIVES

See also the following individual entries:

Aminophylline
Theophylline

General Statement: Asthma is a disease characterized by difficulty in breathing, resulting from smooth muscle contraction of the bronchi and bronchioles, edema of the mucosa of the respiratory tract, or mucous secretions that adhere to the walls of the bronchi and bronchioles. The cause of asthma is not known with certainty but, in some clients, allergy is the underlying reason.

The overall objectives of drug therapy for asthma are to open blocked airways and to alter the characteristics of respiratory tract fluid. The drugs and drug classes used to treat asthma are bronchodilators, such as theophyllines and sympathomimetic amines, mucolytics, corticosteroids, and cromolyn sodium.

Action/Kinetics: The theophylline derivatives are plant alkaloids, which, like caffeine, belong to the xanthine family. They stimulate the CNS, directly relax the smooth muscles of the bronchi and pulmonary blood vessels (relieve bronchospasms), produce diuresis, inhibit uterine contractions, stimulate gastric acid secretion, and increase the rate and force of contraction of the heart. The bronchodilator activity of theophyllines is due to direct relaxation of the bronchiolar smooth muscle and pulmonary blood vessels, which relieves bronchospasm. Theophylline was thought to act by inhibiting phosphodiesterase, which resulted in an increase in cyclic adenosine monophosphate (cAMP). cAMP increased the release of endogenous epinephrine resulting in bronchodilation. However, this effect is negligible at doses used clinically. Although the exact mechanism is not known, theophyllines may act by altering the calcium levels of smooth muscle, blocking adenosine receptors, inhibiting the effect of prostaglandins on smooth muscle, and inhibiting the release of slow-reacting substance of anaphylaxis and histamine. Aminophylline, oxtriphylline, and theophylline sodium glycinate release free theophylline in vivo. Response to the drugs is highly individualized. Theophylline is well absorbed from uncoated plain tablets and PO liquids. *Theophylline salts:* **Onset:** 1–5 hr, depending on route and formulation. **Therapeutic plasma levels:** 10–20 mcg/mL. **t½:** 3–15 hr in nonsmoking adults, 4–5 hr in adult heavy smokers, 1–9 hr in children, and 20–30 hr for premature neonates. An increased **t½** may be seen in individuals with CHF, alcoholism, liver dysfunction, or respiratory infections. Because of great variations in the rate of absorption (due to dosage form, food, dose level) as well as its extremely narrow therapeutic range, theophylline therapy is best monitored by determination of the serum levels. If these determinations cannot be obtained, saliva (contains 60% of corresponding theophylline serum levels) determinations can be used. 85%–90% metabolized in the liver and various metabolites, including the active 3-methylxanthine. Theophylline is metabolized partially to caffeine in the neonate. The premature neonate excretes 50% unchanged theophylline and may accumulate the caffeine metabolite. Excretion is through the kidneys (about 10% unchanged in adults).

Uses: Prophylaxis and treatment of bronchial asthma. Reversible bronchospasms associated with chronic bronchitis, emphysema, and COPD. *Investigational:* Treatment of neonatal apnea and Cheyne-Stokes respiration.

Contraindications: Hypersensitivity to any xanthine, peptic ulcer, seizure disorders (unless on medication), hypotension, CAD, angina pectoris.

Special Concerns: Use during lactation may result in irritability, insomnia, and fretfulness in the infant. Use with caution in premature infants due to the possible accumulation of caffeine. Xanthines are not usually tolerated by small children because of excessive CNS stimulation. Geriatric clients may manifest an increased risk of toxicity. Use with caution in the presence of gastritis, alcoholism, acute cardiac diseases, hypoxemia, severe renal and hepatic disease, severe hypertension, severe myocardial damage, hyperthyroidism, glaucoma.

Side Effects: Side effects are uncommon at serum theophylline levels less than 20 mcg/mL. At levels greater than 20 mcg/mL, 75% of individuals experience side effects including N&V, diarrhea, irritability, insomnia, and headache. At levels of 35 mcg/mL or greater, individuals may manifest ***cardiac arrhythmias,*** hypotension, tachycardia, hyperglycemia, ***seizures, brain damage, or death.*** *GI:* N&V, diarrhea, anorexia, epigastric pain, hematemesis, dyspepsia, rectal irritation (following use of suppositories), rectal bleeding, gastroesophageal reflux during sleep or while recumbent (theophylline). *CNS:* Headache, insomnia, irritability, fever, dizziness, lightheadedness, vertigo, reflex hyperexcitability, ***seizures,*** depression, speech abnormalities, alternating periods of mutism and hyperactivity, ***brain damage, death.*** *CV:* Hypotension, ***life-threatening ventricular arrhythmias,*** palpitations, tachycardia, ***peripheral vascular collapse,*** extrasystoles. *Renal:* Proteinuria, excretion of erythrocytes and renal tubular cells, dehydration due to diuresis, urinary retention (men with prostatic hypertrophy). *Other:* Tachypnea, ***respiratory arrest,*** fever, flushing, hyperglycemia, antidiuretic hormone syndrome, leukocytosis, rash, alopecia.

NOTE: Aminophylline given by rapid IV may produce hypotension, flushing, palpitations, precordial pain, headache, dizziness, or hyperventilation. Also, the ethylenediamine in aminophylline may cause allergic reactions, including urticaria and skin rashes.

Symptoms of Overdose: Agitation, headache, nervousness, insomnia, tachycardia, extrasystoles, anorexia, N&V, fasciculations, tachypnea, ***tonic-clonic seizures.*** The first signs of toxicity may be seizures or ventricular arrhythmias. Toxicity is usually associated with parenteral administration but can be observed after PO administration, especially in children.

Drug Interactions

Allopurinol / ↑ Theophylline levels
Aminoglutbethimide / ↓ Theophylline levels
Barbiturates / ↓ Theophylline levels
Benzodiazepines / Sedative effect may be antagonized by theophylline
Beta-adrenergic agonists / Additive effects
Beta-adrenergic blocking agents / ↑ Theophylline levels
Calcium channel blocking drugs / ↑ Theophylline levels
Carbamazepine / Either ↑ or ↓ theophylline levels
Charcoal / ↓ Theophylline levels
Cimetidine / ↑ Theophylline levels
Ciprofloxacin / ↑ Plasma levels of theophylline with ↑ possibility of side effects
Corticosteroids / ↑ Theophylline levels
Digitalis / Theophylline ↑ toxicity of digitalis
Disulfram / ↑ Theophylline levels
Ephedrine and other sympathomimetics / ↑ Theophylline levels
Erythromycin / ↑ Effect of theophylline due to ↓ breakdown by liver
Ethacrynic acid / Either ↑ or ↓ theophylline levels
Furosemide / Either ↑ or ↓ theophylline levels
Halothane / ↑ Risk of cardiac arrhythmias
Interferon / ↑ Theophylline levels
Isoniazid / Either ↑ or ↓ theophylline levels
Ketamine / Seizures of the extensor-type
Ketoconazole / ↓ Theophylline levels
Lithium / ↓ Effect of lithium due to ↑ rate of excretion
Loop diuretics / ↓ Theophylline levels
Mexiletine / ↑ Theophylline levels

Muscle relaxants, nondepolarizing / Theophylline ↓ effect of these drugs
Oral contraceptives / ↑ Effect of theophyllines due to ↓ breakdown by liver
Phenytoin / ↓ Theophylline levels
Propofol / Theophyllines ↓ sedative effect of propofol
Quinolones / ↑ Theophylline levels
Reserpine / ↑ Risk of tachycardia
Rifampin / ↓ Theophylline levels
Sulfinpyrazone / ↓ Theophylline levels
Sympathomimetics / ↓ Theophylline levels
Tetracyclines / ↑ Risk of theophylline toxicity
Thiabendazole / ↑ Theophylline levels
Thyroid hormones / ↓ Theophylline levels in hypothyroid clients
Tobacco smoking / ↓ Effect of theophylline due to ↑ breakdown by liver
Troleandomycin / ↑ Effect of theophylline due to ↓ breakdown by liver
Verapamil / ↑ Effect of theophyllines

Laboratory Test Interferences: ↑ Plasma free fatty acids, bilirubin, urinary catecholamines, erythrocyte sedimentation rate. Interference with uric acid tests and tests for furosemide, probenecid, theobromine, and phenylbutazone.

Dosage

Individualized. Initially, dosage should be adjusted according to plasma level of drug. Usual: 10–20 mcg theophylline/mL plasma. The dose of the various salts should be equivalent based on the content of anhydrous theophylline. See individual agents.

NURSING CONSIDERATIONS

Administration/Storage

1. Review the list of agents with which theophylline derivatives interact.
2. Dilute drugs and maintain proper infusion rates to minimize problems of overdosage. Use an infusion pump to regulate infusion rate of IV solutions.
3. Wait to initiate PO therapy for at least 4–6 hr after switching from IV therapy.
4. *Treatment of Overdose:*

- Have ipecac syrup, gastric lavage equipment, and cathartics available to treat overdose if the client is conscious and not having seizures. Otherwise a mechanical ventilator, oxygen, diazepam, and IV fluids may be necessary for the treatment of overdosage.
- For postseizure coma, an airway must be maintained and the client oxygenated. To remove the drug, perform only gastric lavage and give the cathartic and activated charcoal by a large bore gastric lavage tube. Charcoal hemoperfusion may be necessary.
- Atrial arrhythmias may be treated with verapamil and ventricular arrhythmias may be treated with lidocaine or procainamide.
- IV fluids are used to treat acid-base imbalance, hypotension, and dehydration. Hypotension may also be treated with vasopressors.
- Tepid water sponge baths or a hypothermic blanket are used to treat hyperpyrexia.
- Apnea is treated with artificial respiration.
- Serum levels of theophylline must be monitored until they fall below 20 mcg/mL as secondary rises of theophylline may occur, especially with sustained-release products.

Assessment

1. Assess the client for any history of hypersensitivity to xanthine compounds.
2. Document indications for therapy and type and onset of symptoms. List other agents prescribed and the outcome.
3. Note if the client has any history of hypotension, CAD, angina, PUD, or seizure disorders. These drugs should be avoided or used very cautiously in these conditions.
4. Determine if the client smokes cigarettes or has a history of smoking marijuana. These habits induce he-

patic metabolism of the drug. Smokers require an increase in the dosage of drug from 50%–100%.

5. Assess diet habits because these can influence the excretion of theophylline. A client eating a high-protein and/or low-carbohydrate diet will have an increased excretion of the drug. Clients eating a low-protein and/or high-carbohydrate diet will have a decrease in the excretion of theophylline. Therefore, dietary intake is an important part of the premedication assessment.

6. Obtain baseline BP and pulse prior to starting drug therapy.

7. Determine any previous experience with this class of drugs and the outcome.

8. Assess lung fields closely and describe findings. Note characteristics of the sputum.

Interventions

1. Monitor BP and pulse closely during therapy and report any significant changes.

2. Observe closely for signs of toxicity such as nausea, anorexia, insomnia, irritability, hyperexcitability, or cardiac arrhythmias and report if evident.

3. Observe small children in particular for excessive CNS stimulation; children often are unable to report side effects.

Client/Family Teaching

1. To avoid epigastric pain, take with a snack or with meals.

2. Take the medication ATC and only as prescribed, because more is *not* better.

3. Advise to report if nausea, vomiting, GI pain, or restlessness occurs. Avoid or minimize consumption of charbroiled foods (burgers).

4. Do not smoke because smoking may aggravate underlying medical conditions as well as interfere with drug absorption. Refer to a formal (behavior modification) smoking cessation program.

5. Explain to clients how to protect themselves from acute exacerbations of illness by avoiding crowds, dressing warmly in cold weather, covering their mouth and nose so that cold air is not directly inhaled, staying in air conditioning during excessively hot and humid weather, maintaining proper diet and nutrition and adequate fluid intake.

6. Provide written guidelines that identify the early S&S of infections, adverse side effects of drug therapy, and when to call the provider.

7. Reinforce that when secretions become thick and tacky, clients should increase their intake of fluids. This thins secretions and assists in their removal.

8. Advise client to pace activity and to avoid overexertion at all times.

9. Instruct to hold medication and report immediately any side effects or CNS depression in children and infants.

10. Review dietary restrictions and advise to limit intake of xanthine-containing products such as coffee, colas, and chocolate.

11. Identify support groups that may assist client to understand and cope with chronic respiratory dysfunction.

Evaluate

- Knowledge and understanding of illness and level of compliance with prescribed regimen
- Evidence of a positive clinical response characterized by improved airway exchange, ↓ wheezing, and reports of improved breathing patterns
- Laboratory confirmation that serum drug levels are within therapeutic range (10–20 mcg/mL)

Aminophylline

(am-in-**OFF**-ih-lin)

Pregnancy Category: C

Aminophyllin, Phyllocontin, Phyllocontin-350 ✱, Truphyllin **(Rx)**

See also *Theophylline Derivatives,* Chapter 54.

How Supplied: *Injection:* 25 mg/mL; *Solution:* 105 mg/5 mL; *Suppository:* 250 mg, 500 mg; *Tablet:*

100 mg, 200 mg; *Tablet, Extended Release:* 225 mg

Action/Kinetics: Aminophylline contains 79% theophylline.

Additional Uses: Neonatal apnea, respiratory stimulant in Cheyne-Stokes respiration. Parenteral form has been used for biliary colic, as a cardiac stimulant, diuretic, and an adjunct in treating CHF, although such uses have been replaced by more effective drugs.

Dosage

- **Oral Solution, Tablets**

Bronchodilator, acute attacks, in clients not currently on theophylline therapy.

Adults and children up to 16 years of age, loading dose: Equivalent of 5–6 mg of anhydrous theophylline/kg.

Bronchodilator, acute attacks, in clients currently receiving theophylline.

Adults and children up to 16 years of age: If possible, a serum theophylline level should be obtained first. Then, base loading dose on the premise that each 0.5 mg theophylline/kg lean body weight will result in a 0.5–1.6-mcg/mL increase in serum theophylline levels. If immediate therapy is needed and a serum level cannot be obtained, a single dose of the equivalent of 2.5 mg/kg of anhydrous theophylline can be given.

Maintenance in acute attack, based on equivalent of anhydrous theophylline.

Young adult smokers: 4 mg/kg q 6 hr; **healthy, nonsmoking adults:** 3 mg/kg q 8 hr; **geriatric clients or clients with cor pulmonale:** 2 mg/kg q 8 hr; **clients with CHF or liver failure:** 2 mg/kg q 8–12 hr. **Pediatric, 12–16 years:** 3 mg/kg q 6 hr; **9–12 years:** 4 mg/kg q 6 hr; **1–9 years:** 5 mg/kg q 6 hr; **6–12 months:** Use the formula: dose (mg/kg q 8 hr) = (0.05) (age in weeks) + 1.25; **up to 6 months:** Use the formula: dose (mg/kg q 8 hr) = (0.07) (age in weeks) + 1.7.

Chronic therapy, based on equivalent of anhydrous theophylline.

Adults, initial: 6–8 mg/kg up to a maximum of 400 mg/day in three to four divided doses at 6–8-hr intervals; **then,** dose can be increased in 25% increments at 2–3 day intervals up to a maximum of 13 mg/kg or 900 mg/day, whichever is less. **Pediatric, initial:** 16 mg/kg up to a maximum of 400 mg/day in three to four divided doses at 6–8 hr intervals; **then,** dose may be increased in 25% increments at 2–3 day intervals up to the following maximum doses (without measuring serum theophylline): **16 years and older:** 13 mg/kg or 900 mg/day, whichever is less; **12–16 years:** 18 mg/kg/day; **9–12 years:** 20 mg/kg/day; **1–9 years:** 24 mg/kg/day; **up to 12 months,** Use the following formula: dose (mg/kg/day) = (0.3) (age in weeks) + 8.0.

- **Enteric-Coated Tablets**

Bronchodilator, chronic therapy, based on equivalent of anhydrous theophylline.

Adults, initial: 6–8 mg/kg up to a maximum of 400 mg/day in three to four divided doses at 6–8-hr intervals; **then,** dose may be increased, if needed and tolerated, by increments of 25% at 2–3 day intervals up to a maximum of 13 mg/kg/day or 900 mg/day, whichever is less, without measuring serum theophylline. **Pediatric, over 12 years of age, initial:** 4 mg/kg q 8–12 hr; **then,** dose may be increased by 2–3 mg/kg/day at 3-day intervals up to the following maximum doses (without measuring serum levels): **16 years and older:** 13 mg/kg/day or 900 mg/day, whichever is less; **12–16 years:** 18 mg/kg/day.

- **Extended-Release Tablets**

Bronchodilator, chronic therapy, based on equivalent of anhydrous theophylline.

Adults, initial: 4 mg/kg q 8–12 hr; **then,** dose may be increased by 2–3 mg/kg/day at 3-day intervals to a maximum of 13 mg/kg or 900 mg/day, whichever is less. **Pediatric, initial:** Same as adults; **then,** dose may be increased by 2–3 mg/kg/day at 3-day intervals up to the following maximum doses: **16 years and older:** 13 mg/kg/day or 900 mg/day, whichever is less. **12–16 years:** 18 mg/kg/day.

• **Enema.**

For use as a bronchodilator for loading doses and for maintenance in acute attacks, see doses for oral solution and tablets.

• **IV Infusion**

Bronchodilator, acute attacks, for clients not currently on theophylline.

Adults and children up to 16 years, loading dose based on anhydrous theophylline: 5 mg/kg given over a period of 20 min.

Bronchodilator, acute attack, for clients currently on theophylline.

Adults and children up to 16 years, loading dose based on anhydrous theophylline: If possible, a serum theophylline level should be obtained first. Then, base loading dose on the premise that each 0.5 mg theophylline/kg lean body weight will result in a 0.5–1.6 mcg/mL increase in serum theophylline levels. If immediate therapy is needed and a serum level cannot be obtained, a single dose of the equivalent of 2.5 mg/kg of anhydrous theophylline can be given.

Maintenance for acute attacks, based on equivalent of anhydrous theophylline.

Young adult smokers: 0.7 mg/kg/hr; **nonsmoking, healthy adults:** 0.43 mg/kg/hr; **geriatric clients or clients with cor pulmonale:** 0.26 mg/kg/hr; **clients with CHF or liver failure:** 0.2 mg/kg/hr. **Pediatric, 12–16 years, nonsmokers:** 0.5 mg/kg/hr; **9–12 years,** 0.7 mg/kg/hr; **1–9 years,** 0.8 mg/kg/hr; **up to 1 year,** Based on the following formula: dose (mg/kg/hr) = (0.008) (age in weeks) + 0.21.

Administration/Storage

1. To avoid hypotension, administer IV doses of medication at a rate not to exceed 25 mg/min.
2. Only the 25 mg/mL injection (which should be further diluted) should be used for IV administration. Use an infusion pump or device to regulate infusion rates of IV solutions.
3. IM injection is not recommended due to severe, persistent pain at the site of injection.
4. A minimum of 4–6 hr should elapse when switching from IV infusion to the first dose of PO therapy.
5. Enteric-coated tablets may be incompletely and slowly absorbed.
6. Enteric-coated and extended-release tablets are not recommended for children less than 12 years of age.
7. Use of aminophylline suppositories is not recommended due to the possibility of slow and unreliable absorption.

Special Concerns: Use with caution when aminophylline and sodium chloride are used with corticosteroids or in clients with edema.

Additional Side Effects: The ethylenediamine in the product may cause exfoliative dermatitis or urticaria.

NURSING CONSIDERATIONS

See also *Nursing Considerations* for *Theophylline Derivatives,* Chapter 54.

Interventions

1. Monitor pulse and BP closely during IV administration. Aminophylline may cause a transitory lowering of the BP. If this occurs, the dosage of drug and rate of flow should be adjusted immediately.
2. Report serum levels greater than 20 mcg/mL.
3. Observe for symptoms of toxicity, i.e., N&V, restlessness, convulsions, and arrhythmias, and report.
4. Monitor clients with a history of CAD for chest pain and ECG changes.

Evaluate

• Improved airway exchange
• Termination of acute asthma attack
• ABGs within desired range
• Therapeutic serum drug levels (10–20 mcg/mL)

Theophylline

(thee-**OFF**-ih-lin)

Pregnancy Category: C

Immediate-release Capsules, Tablets. **Liquid Products:** Accurbron,

Aquaphyllin, Asmalix, Bronkodyl, Elixomin, Elixophyllin, Lanophyllin, Lixolin, Pulmophylline ✱, Quibron-T/SR ✱, Quibron-T Dividose, Slo-Phyllin, Solu-Phyllin, Somnophyllin-T, Theo, Theoclear-80, Theolair, Theomar, Theostat-80, Truxophyllin. **Timed-release Capsules and Tablets:** Aerolate III, Aerolate Jr., Aerolate Sr., Apo-Theo LA ✱, Quibron-T/SR Dividose, Respid, Slo-Bid Gyrocaps, Slo-Phyllin Gyrocaps, Somophyllin-12 ✱, Somophyllin-CRT, Sustaire, Theo-24, Theo 250, Theobid Duracaps, Theobid Jr Duracaps, Theoclear L.A.-130 Cenules, Theoclear L.A.-260 Cenules, Theocot, Theochron, Theo-Dur, Theo-Dur Sprinkle, Theo-SR ✱, Theolair-SR, Theospan-SR, Theo-Time, Theophylline SR, Theovent Long-Acting, Uniphyl **(Rx)**

See also *Theophylline Derivatives,* Chapter 54.

How Supplied: *Capsule:* 100 mg, 200 mg, 300 mg; *Capsule, extended release:* 50 mg, 65 mg, 75 mg, 100 mg, 125 mg, 130 mg, 200 mg, 250 mg, 260 mg, 300 mg, 400 mg; *Elixir:* 80 mg/15 mL; *Solution:* 80 mg/15 mL; *Syrup:* 80 mg/15 mL; *Tablet:* 100 mg, 125 mg, 200 mg, 250 mg, 300 mg; *Tablet, extended release:* 100 mg, 200 mg, 250 mg, 300 mg, 400 mg, 450 mg, 500 mg, 600 mg

Action/Kinetics: Time to peak serum levels, oral solution: 1 hr; **uncoated tablets:** 2 hr; **chewable tablets:** 1–1.5 hr; **enteric-coated tablets:** 5 hr; **extended-release capsules and tablets:** 4–7 hr. In healthy adults, about 60% is bound to plasma protein whereas in neonates 36% is bound to plasma protein.

Additional Uses: Oral liquid: Neonatal apnea as a respiratory stimulant. Theophylline and dextrose injection: Respiratory stimulant in neonatal apnea and Cheyne-Stokes respiration.

Dosage

• **Capsules, Tablets, Elixir, Oral Solution, Oral Suspension, Syrup**

See *Dosage* for *Oral Solution, Tablets,* under *Aminophylline,* Chapter 54.

• **Extended-Release Capsules, Extended-Release Tablets**

See *Dosage* for *Extended-Release Tablets,* under *Aminophylline,* Chapter 54.

• **Elixir, Oral Solution, Oral Suspension, Syrup**

Bronchodilator, chronic therapy.

9–12 years: 20 mg/kg/day; **6–9 years:** 24 mg/kg/day.

Neonatal apnea.

Loading dose: Using the equivalent of anhydrous theophylline administered by NGT, 5 mg/kg; **maintenance:** 2 mg/kg/day in two to three divided doses given by NGT.

Administration/Storage

1. Dosage is individualized to maintain serum levels of 10–20 mcg/mL.
2. Dosage should be calculated based on lean body weight (theophylline does not distribute to body fat).
3. Serum theophylline levels should be monitored in chronic therapy, especially if the maximum maintenance doses are used or exceeded.
4. The extended-release tablets or capsules are not recommended for children less than 6 years of age. Dosage for once-a-day products has not been established in children less than 12 years of age.

NURSING CONSIDERATIONS

See also *Nursing Considerations* for *Theophylline Derivatives,* Chapter 54.

Assessment

1. Document indications for therapy, onset of symptoms, and any other agents prescribed and the outcome.
2. Describe pulmonary assessment findings and note pulmonary function test and ABG results if available.
3. If switching from IV therapy, wait 4 hr before administering intermediate-release forms; may administer extended-release form at time of discontinuation of IV.

Client/Family Teaching

1. Take with food or milk to minimize GI upset.
2. Stress the importance of taking the drug only as prescribed; more is not better.
3. Do not crush or break slow-release forms of the drug.

4. Avoid cigarette smoking because this decreases drug's effectiveness.
5. Provide a printed list of side effects that require reporting if evident.
6. Caffeine- and xanthine-containing beverages and foods (chocolate, coffee, colas) and daily intake of charbroiled foods should be avoided because they tend to increase side effects of this drug.
7. Advise that fluid intake should be at least 2 L/day in order to decrease viscosity of secretions.
8. Do not take any OTC cough, cold, or breathing preparations without provider approval.
9. Report if symptoms do not improve or worsen with therapy.

Evaluate

- Improved airway exchange
- Reports of ease in secretion removal and breathing
- Stimulation of respirations in the neonate
- Therapeutic serum drug levels (10–20 mcg/mL)

CHAPTER FIFTY-FIVE

Antihistamines (H_1 Blockers)

See also the following individual entries:

Astemizole
Brompheniramine Maleate
Buclizine Hydrochloride
Chlorpheniramine Maleate
Cyclizine Hydrochloride
Cyproheptadine Hydrochloride
Dexchlorpheniramine Maleate
Dimenhydrinate
Diphenhydramine Hydrochloride
Levocabastine Hydrochloride
Loratidine
Meclizine Hydrochloride
Promethazine Hydrochloride
Terfenadine
Tripelennamine Hydrochloride
Triprolidine Hydrochloride

Action/Kinetics: The effects of histamine may be reversed either by drugs that block H_1-histamine receptors (antihistamines) or by drugs that have effects opposite to those of histamine (e.g., epinephrine). Antihistamines used for the treatment of allergic conditions are referred to as *H_1-receptor blockers* while antihistamines used for the treatment of GI disorders (e.g., peptic ulcer) are referred to as *H_2-receptor blockers* (see *Cimetidine, Famotidine, Nizatidine,* and *Ranitidine*).

Antihistamines do not prevent the release of histamine, antibody production, or antigen-antibody interactions. Rather, they compete with histamine for histamine receptors (competitive inhibition), thus preventing or reversing the effects of histamine. Antihistamines prevent or reduce increased capillary permeability (i.e., decrease edema, itching) and bronchospasms. Allergic reactions unrelated to histamine release are not affected by antihistamines.

The H_1 blockers manifest varying degrees of sedation, as well as anticholinergic, antiemetic, antipruritic, and antiserotonin effects. Although antihistamines may relieve symptoms of the common cold, they neither prevent or cure colds nor do they shorten the course of a cold. Clients unresponsive to a certain antihistamine may regain sensitivity by switching to a different antihistamine.

From a chemical point of view, the antihistamines can be divided into the following classes.

1. **Ethylenediamine Derivatives.** This group manifests low to moderate sedative effects and almost no anticholinergic or antiemetic activity. They frequently cause GI distress. Available agents: pyrilamine, tripelennamine.
2. **Ethanolamine Derivatives.** This group is most likely to cause CNS depression (drowsiness). There is a low incidence of GI side effects. There are significant anticholinergic and antiemetic effects. Available agents: carbinoxamine, clemastine, diphenhydramine.
3. **Alkylamines.** Members of this group are among the most potent antihistamines. They are effective at relatively low dosage and are most suitable agents for daytime use. This group manifests minimal sedation, moderate anticholinergic effects, and no antiemetic effects. Paradoxical excitation may also occur. Individual response to agents is variable. Available agents: brompheniramine, chlorpheniramine, dexchlorpheniramine, triprolidine.

4. **Phenothiazines.** These agents possess significant antihistaminic action, varying degrees of sedation, and a high degree of both anticholinergic and antiemetic effects. Available agents: methdilazine, promethazine, trimeprazine.
5. **Piperidines.** Members of this group have prolonged antihistaminic activity, with a comparatively low incidence of drowsiness, moderate anticholinergic activity, and no antiemetic effects. Available agents: azatadine, cyproheptadine, diphenylpyraline, phenindamine.
6. **Miscellaneous.** The drugs in this group are specific in that they bind to peripheral rather than central H_1-histamine receptors. They have no sedative, anticholinergic, or antiemetic effects. Available agents: astemizole, loratadine, terfenadine.

The kinetics of most antihistamines are similar. **Onset:** 15–30 min; **peak:** 1–2 hr; **duration:** 4–6 hr (piperidines have a longer duration). Many antihistamines are available as timed-release preparations. Most antihistamines are metabolized by the liver and excreted in the urine.

Uses: PO: Treatment of vasomotor, perennial, or seasonal allergic rhinitis and allergic conjunctivitis. Treatment of angioedema, urticarial transfusion reactions, urticaria, pruritus. Atopic dermatitis, contact dermatitis, pruritus ani, pruritus vulvae, insect bites. Sneezing and rhinorrhea due to the common cold. Treatment of anaphylaxis, parkinsonism, drug-induced extrapyramidal reactions, vertigo. Prophylaxis and treatment of motion sickness, including N&V. Nighttime sleep aid.

Parenteral: Relief of allergic reactions due to blood or plasma. As an adjunct to epinephrine in treating anaphylaxis. Uncomplication allergic conditions when PO therapy is not possible.

See also the individual drugs.

Contraindications: Hypersensitivity to the drug, narrow-angle glaucoma, prostatic hypertrophy, stenosing peptic ulcer, and pyloroduodenal or bladder neck obstruction. Use with MAO inhibitors. Pregnancy or possibility thereof (some agents), lactation, premature and newborn infants. The phenothiazine-type antihistamines are contraindicated in CNS depression from any cause, bone marrow depression, jaundice, dehydrated or acutely ill children, and in comatose clients. Use to treat lower respiratory tract symptoms such as asthma.

Special Concerns: Administer with caution to clients with convulsive disorders and in respiratory disease. Excess dosage may cause hallucinations, convulsions, and death in infants and children. Use in geriatric clients may result in dizziness, excessive sedation, syncope, toxic confusional states, and hypotension. Rare cases of serious CV side effects (including torsade de pointes, prolongation of the QT interval, other ventricular arrhythmias, cardiac arrest, and death) can occur with astemizole and terfenadine (see individual drugs). These effects do not appear to occur with loratadine.

Side Effects: *CNS:* Sedation ranging from mild drowsiness to deep sleep. Dizziness, incoordination, faintness, fatigue, confusion, lassitude, restlessnesss, excitation, nervousness, tremor, ***tonic-clonic seizures,*** headache, irritability, insomnia, euphoria, paresthesias, oculogyric crisis, torticollis, catatonic-like states, hallucinations, disorientation, tongue protrusion (usually with IV use or overdosage), disturbing dreams, nightmares, pseudoschizophrenia, weakness, diplopia, vertigo, hysteria, neuritis, paradoxical excitation, epileptiform seizures in clients with focal lesions. Extrapyramidal reactions include opisthotonus, dystonia, akathisia, dyskinesia, and parkinsonism. *CV:* Postural hypotension, palpitations, bradycardia, tachycardia, reflex tachycardia, extrasystoles, increased or decreased BP, ECG changes (including blunting of T waves and prolongation of the Q-T interval), ***cardiac arrest.*** *GI:* Epigastric distress, anorexia, increased appetite and weight gain, N&V, diarrhea, constipation, change in bowel habits, stomatitis. *GU:* Urinary frequency, dysuria, urinary retention, gynecomastia, inhibition of ejaculation, decreased libido, impotence, early menses, induction of lactation. *Hematologic:* Hypoplastic anemia, ***aplastic anemia, hemolytic anemia,*** thrombocytopenia, leukopenia, pancytopenia, ***agranulocytosis,*** thrombocytopenic purpura. *Respiratory:* Thickening of bronchial secretions, wheezing, nasal stuffiness, chest tightness, sore throat, ***respiratory depression;*** dry mouth, nose, and throat. *Ophthalmic:* Blurred vision, diplopia. *Miscellaneous:* Tinnitus, acute labyrinthitis, obstructive jaundice, erythema, high or prolonged glucose tolerance curves, glycosuria, elevated spinal fluid proteins, increased plasma cholesterol, increased perspiration, chills; tingling, heaviness, and weakness of the hands.

Topical use: Prolonged use may result in local irritation and allergic contact dermatitis.

Symptoms of Acute Toxicity: Although antihistamines have a wide therapeutic range, overdosage can nevertheless be fatal. Children are particularly susceptible. Early toxic effects may be seen within 30–120 min and include drowsiness, dizziness, blurred vision, tinnitus, ataxia, and hypotension. Symptoms range from CNS depression (sedation, ***coma,*** decreased mental alertness) to ***CV collapse*** and CNS stimulation (insomnia, hallucinations, tremors, or ***seizures***). Also, ***profound hypotension, respiratory depression, coma, and death*** may occur. Anticholinergic effects include flushing, dry mouth, hypotension, fever, ***hyperthermia*** (especially in children), and fixed, dilated pupils. Body temperature may be as high as 107°F. In children, symptoms include hallucinations, toxic psychosis, delirum tremens, ataxia, incoordination, muscle twitching, excitement, athetosis, ***hyperthermia, seizures,*** and hyperreflexia followed by postictal depression and ***cardiorespiratory arrest.***

Drug Interactions

Alcohol, ethyl / See *CNS depressants*
Anticoagulants / Antihistamines may ↓ the anticoagulant effects
Antidepressants, tricyclic / Additive anticholinergic side effects
CNS depressants, antianxiety agents, barbiturates, narcotics, phenothiazines, procarbazine, sedative-hypnotics / Potentiation or addition of CNS depressant effects. Concomitant use may lead to drowsiness, lethargy, stupor, respiratory depression, coma, and possibly death
Heparin / Antihistamines may ↓ the anticoagulant effects
MAO inhibitors / Intensification and prolongation of anticholinergic side effects; use with phenothiazine antihistamine → hypotension and extrapyramidal reactions

NOTE: Also see *Drug Interactions* for *Phenothiazines,* Chapter 38.

Laboratory Test Interference: Discontinue antihistamines 4 days before skin testing to avoid false – result.

Dosage

Usually PO. Parenteral administration is seldom used because of irritating nature of drugs. Topical usage is also limited because antihistamines often cause hypersensitivity reactions. When given for motion sickness, antihistamines are usually given 30–60 min before anticipated travel. See individual drugs.

NURSING CONSIDERATIONS

Administration/Storage

1. Inject IM preparations deep into the muscle. Preparations tend to be irritating to the tissues.
2. Sustained-release preparations should be swallowed whole. Scored tablets may be broken before swallowing. If the client has difficulty swallowing capsules, they can be opened and the contents put into soft food for ingestion.

3. Topical preparations should not be applied to raw, blistered, or oozing areas of the skin.
4. Do not apply to the eyes, around the genitalia, or to mucous membranes.
5. PO preparations may cause gastric irritation. Therefore, administer the medication with meals, milk, or a snack.
6. *Treatment of Overdose:*
• Treat symptoms and provide supportive care.
• Vomiting is induced with syrup of ipecac (do not use for phenothiazine overdosage) followed by activated charcoal and a cathartic. If vomiting has not been induced within 3 hr of ingestion, gastric lavage can be undertaken.
• Hypotension can be treated with a vasopressor such as norepinephrine, dopamine, or phenylephrine (do not use epinephrine).
• For convulsions, use only short-acting depressants (e.g., diazepam). IV physostigmine can be used to treat centrally mediated convulsions.
• Ice packs and a cool sponge bath are effective in reducing fever in children.
• Severe cases of overdose can be treated by hemoperfusion.

Assessment

1. Note any history of drug sensitivity to antihistamines and document known allergens.
2. Note if the client has any medical history of ulcers or glaucoma or if the client is pregnant. Antihistamines are contraindicated under these circumstances.
3. Document indications for therapy and the onset of symptoms. Assess the extent of the allergic response for which the antihistamine is being ordered.
4. Review the medications the client is currently taking, noting those which may interact unfavorably.
5. Determine if the client is to have skin testing conducted. Antihistamines generally should be *discontinued* 4 days prior to testing to avoid false negative results.
6. Obtain baseline BP, pulse, and respirations and document.
7. Assess lung sounds and note characteristics of secretions produced.
8. Assess skin condition. Note extent and describe any rash, if present.

Interventions

1. Note client complaints of severe CNS depression. This is a symptom of overdosage and may require the administration of syrup of ipecac. See Administration/Storage.
2. Monitor VS; document if the client develops hypotension or palpitations.
3. Monitor I&O and ensure adequate hydration. If clients experience difficulty in voiding, have them void prior to receiving the medication.
4. If the client complains of constipation, encourage at least 2 L/day of fluids unless restriction of fluids is necessary. Instruct client to increase the amount of exercise performed (if condition permits), and to consume more fruits, fruit juices, and dietary fiber. A stool softener may also be indicated if these measures are not successful.
5. Monitor lung sounds and secretion production. If bronchial secretions are thick, increase fluid intake to decrease the viscosity of secretions and advise to avoid milk temporarily.
6. If the client is hospitalized and sedated with antihistamines, put up the side rails, supervise ambulation and activities, and incorporate safety precautions.
7. If the client complains of dizziness, weakness, or lassitude, assist with ambulation and report these symptoms.
8. If clients complain of local irritation, they may have developed an adverse reaction to the drug which should be reported.
9. Recurrent reactions of a chronic nature should be referred to an allergist. Clients should be taught how to protect themselves from undue ex-

posure and how to create an allergen-free living area.

Client/Family Teaching

1. Explain that the medication should be taken before or at the onset of symptoms as antihistamines cannot reverse reactions but they may prevent them.
2. Review the appropriate steps to follow during an *acute* allergic reaction and how to differentiate, such as with a bee sting, and ensure the client has epinephrine available for self-administration.
3. Report all adverse effects immediately. Include onset of the side effects and duration, describing exactly what occurred. Another drug with fewer side effects may be indicated. The client should not discontinue taking the medication without first consulting the provider.
4. Provide a printed list of drugs to avoid. Advise the client to consult with the provider concerning any depressants that may be ordered since antihistamines tend to potentiate the effects of other CNS depressants.
5. Caution the client not to drive a car or operate other machinery until response to the medication (drowsiness) has worn off. Sedative effect may disappear spontaneously after several days of therapy.
6. If daytime sedation is a problem there are nondrowsy antihistamines available such as terfenadine and astemizole.
7. Report the development of sore throat, fever, unexplained bruising, bleeding, or petechiae. Laboratory studies (CBC and platelets) may be indicated to rule out a blood dyscrasia.
8. Advise that there is potential for developing a sensitivity to sun or ultraviolet light. Avoid any undue exposure to the sun, use a sunscreen, and wear a hat, sunglasses, and protective clothing when in the sun.
9. If the drug is being used for motion sickness, it should be taken 30 min before it is time to use the vehicle or board a plane.
10. Avoid alcohol and any OTC products unless prescribed.
11. Advise that symptoms of dry mouth may be reduced by frequent rinsing with water, good oral hygiene, and the use of sugarless gum or candies.
12. Explain that these products raise BP and should only be used for hypertensive clients under strict medical supervision.
13. Advise parents that children may manifest excitation rather than sedation at ordinary dosages.
14. The clinical effectiveness of one class may diminish with continued usage; switching to another class may restore drug effectiveness.
15. Encourage family/significant other to learn CPR and explain that survival is greatly increased when CPR is initiated immediately.

Evaluate

- Reports of ↓ frequency and intensity of allergic manifestations
- Control of severe itching and associated swelling
- Prevention of motion sickness
- Effective nighttime sedation

Astemizole

(ah-**STEM**-ih-zohl)
Pregnancy Category: C
Hismanil **(Rx)**

See also *Antihistamines,* Chapter 55.

How Supplied: *Tablet:* 10 mg

Action/Kinetics: Low to no sedative effect, antiemetic effect, or anticholinergic activity. The drug is metabolized in the liver to both active and inactive metabolites and is excreted through the feces. **$t^{1}/_{2}$:** About 1.6 days. **Onset:** 2–3 days. **Duration:** Up to several weeks. Over 95% is bound to plasma protein. Mainly excreted through the feces.

Dosage

• Tablets

Adults and children over 12 years: 10 mg once daily.

Administration/Storage

1. The recommended dose should not be exceeded in an attempt to increase the onset of action.
2. The drug should be taken on an empty stomach at least 2 hr after a

meal with no additional food taken for at least 1 hr postdosing.
Contraindication: Hepatic dysfunction.
Special Concerns: Safety and efficacy have not been established in children less than 12 years of age. Dose should not exceed 10 mg/day.
Additional Side Effects: ***Serious CV side effects, including death, cardiac arrest, QT interval prolongation, torsades de pointes and other ventricular arrhythmias*** have been observed in clients exceeding the recommended dose of astemizole. Syncope may precede severe arrhythmias. Overdose may be observed with doses as low as 20–30 mg/day.
Drug Interactions: Concomitant use of astemizole with erythromycin, itraconazole, or ketoconazole may cause serious CV effects, including death, cardiac arrest, torsades de pointes, and other ventricular arrhythmias (including QT interval prolongation).

NURSING CONSIDERATIONS

See also *Nursing Considerations* for *Antihistamines,* Chapter 55.
Client/Family Teaching
1. Take medication on an empty stomach.
2. Do not eat until at least 1 hr after medication administration because food interferes with the drug absorption.
3. Take medication only as directed because desired effects may not be noticeable immediately.
4. Report any persistent side effects, including depression or weight gain.
5. Advise all providers of drug therapy to prevent any potential adverse drug interactions (see above).
Evaluate: ↓ Allergic symptoms.

Brompheniramine maleate

(brohm-fen-**EAR**-ah-meen)
Pregnancy Category: B
Brombay, Bromphen, Chlorphed, Codimal-A, Conjec-B, Cophene-B, Dehist, Diamine T.D., Dimetane, Dimetane Extentabs, Dimetane-Ten, Histaject Modified, Nasahist B, ND Stat Revised, Oraminic II, Sinusol-B, Veltane (Rx; Dimetane and Dimetane Extentabs are OTC)

See also *Antihistamines,* Chapter 55.
How Supplied: *Elixer:* 2 mg/5 mL; *Injection:* 10 mg/mL; *Tablet:* 4 mg; *Tablet, Extended Release:* 8 mg, 12 mg
Action/Kinetics: Fewer sedative effects. **t½:** 25 hr. **Time to peak effect:** 3–9 hr. **Duration:** 4–25 hr.
Uses: Perennial and seasonal allergic rhinitis, allergic conjunctivitis, allergic and nonallergic pruritic symptoms.

Dosage

- **Elixir, Tablets**

Adults and children over 12 years: 4 mg q 4–6 hr, not to exceed 24 mg/day. **Pediatric, 6–12 years:** 2 mg q 4–6 hr, not to exceed 12 mg/day; **2–6 years:** 1 mg q 4–6 hr, not to exceed 6 mg/day.

- **Extended-Release Tablets**

Adults and children over 12 years: 8 mg q 8–12 hr or 12 mg q 12 hr; **pediatric, 6–12 years:** 8–12 mg q 12 hr.

- **IM, IV, SC**

Adults: usual, 10 mg (range: 5–20 mg) q 8–12 hr (maximum daily dose: 40 mg); **pediatric, under 12 years:** 0.125 mg/kg (3.75 mg/m^2) 3–4 times/day.
Administration/Storage
1. Do not use solutions containing preservatives for IV injection.
2. For children aged 6–12 years, sustained-release preparations require the supervision of a physician.
3. For IV administration, the 10-mg/mL preparations may be used undiluted or diluted 1:10 with sterile saline for injection. Administer over 1 min.
4. The 10-mg/mL preparations may also be added to 5% glucose, NSS, or whole blood for IV use.
5. The 100-mg/mL preparation is not recommended for IV use.
6. For IM or SC use, the drug may be used undiluted or diluted 1:10 with NSS.

Special Concerns: Use is not recommended for neonates. Geriatric clients may be more sensitive to the usual adult dose.

NURSING CONSIDERATIONS

See also *Nursing Considerations* for *Antihistamines,* Chapter 55.

Client/Family Teaching

1. Drug may cause drowsiness.
2. Consume 1.5–2 L of fluids per day to decrease viscosity of secretions.
3. Avoid alcohol.

Evaluate

- Relief of allergic manifestations
- ↓ Nasal congestion

Buclizine hydrochloride

(**BYOU**-klih-zeen)

Pregnancy Category: B

Bucladin-S Softabs **(Rx)**

See also *Antiemetics,* Chapter 62, and *Antihistamines,* Chapter 55.

How Supplied: *Tablet:* 50 mg

Action/Kinetics: Buclizine suppresses N&V through an action on the CNS to decrease vestibular stimulation and depress labyrinthine function. The drug may also act on the CTZ to decrease vomiting. **Duration:** 4–6 hr.

Uses: Nausea, vomiting, dizziness of motion sickness.

Dosage

- **Chewable Tablets**

Motion sickness.

Adults: 50 mg 30 min before travel; dosage may be repeated after 4–6 hr.

Severe nausea.

Up to 150 mg/day.

Administration/Storage

1. To prevent motion sickness, take medication 30 min before departure.
2. Tablets can be chewed, swallowed whole, or dissolved in the mouth.

Additional Contraindications: Hypersensitivity to drug, pregnancy, lactation.

Special Concerns: Safe use in children not established. Geriatric clients may be more susceptible to the usual adult dose.

Side Effects: Drowsiness, dry mouth, headache, nervousness.

NURSING CONSIDERATIONS

See also *Nursing Considerations* for *Antiemetics,* Chapter 62, and *Antihistamines,* Chapter 55.

Evaluate: Prevention of motion sickness and the associated symptoms.

Chlorpheniramine maleate

(klor-fen-**EAR**-ah-meen)

Pregnancy Category: B

Syrup, Tablets, Chewable Tablets: Aller-Chlor, Chlo-Amine, Chlorate, Chlor-Niramine, Chlortab 4, Chlor-Trimeton, Chlor-Tripolon ✱, Genallerate, Pfeiffer's Allergy, Phenetron, Trymegen. **Extended-release Capsules, Extended-release Tablets:** Chlorspan-12, Chlortab 8, Chlor-Trimeton Repetabs, Chlor-Tripolon ✱, Phenetron Telachlor, Teldrin. **Injectables:** Chlor-100, Chlor-Pro, Chlor-Pro 10, Chlor-Trimeton (OTC and Rx)

See also *Antihistamines,* Chapter 55.

How Supplied: *Capsule, Extended Release:* 8 mg, 12 mg; *Chew Tablet:* 2 mg; *Injection:* 10 mg/mL; *Syrup:* 2 mg/5 mL; *Tablet:* 4 mg; *Tablet, Extended Release:* 8 mg, 12 mg, 16 mg

Action/Kinetics: Sedation less pronounced. **t½:** 21–27 hr. **Time to peak effect:** 6 hr. **Duration:** 4–8 hr.

Dosage

- **Syrup, Tablets, Chewable Tablets**

Adults: 4 mg q 6 hr as needed. **Pediatric, 6–11 years:** 2 mg q 4–6 hr, not to exceed 12 mg/day; **2–5 years:** 1 mg q 4–6 hr.

- **Extended-Release Capsules, Extended-Release Tablets**

Adults: 8–12 mg q 8–12 hr as needed; **pediatric, 12 years and older:** 8 mg q 12 hr as needed.

- **IM, IV, SC**

Adults: 5–40 mg as a single dose as needed, up to 40 mg/day; **pediatric, SC:** 0.0875 mg/kg (2.5 mg/m²) q 6 hr as needed.

Administration/Storage
1. If administered with food, the absorption of drug is delayed.
2. The injection containing 10 mg/mL may be administered IV, IM, or SC. To administer IV, use 10 mg/mL and give over 1 min.
3. The injection containing 100 mg/mL should only be administered IM or SC.
4. Expect the onset of action to occur within 15–30 min and to last 3–6 hr.
Additional Contraindication: Not recommended for children under 6 years of age.
Special Concerns: Geriatric clients may be more sensitive to the adult dose. The parenteral route is not recommended for neonates.

NURSING CONSIDERATIONS

See also *Nursing Considerations* for *Antihistamines,* Chapter 55.
Client/Family Teaching
1. Drug may cause drowsiness; use caution.
2. Avoid alcohol in any form.
3. Anticipate dry mouth and use appropriate remedies.
Evaluate: ↓ Nasal congestion and associated allergic manifestations.

Cyclizine hydrochloride

(**SYE**-klih-zeen)
Marezine, Marzine ✱ **(OTC)**

See also *Antihistamines,* Chapter 55.
Action/Kinetics: The mechanism for the antiemetic effect is not known with certainty but may be due to central anticholinergic effects to cause reduced labyrinthine function and decreased vestibular stimulation. This action is thought to be mediated through pathways to the vomiting center from the CTZ or peripheral nerve pathways. **Onset:** 30–60 min. **Duration:** 4–6 hr.
Uses: Nausea and vomiting and dizziness of motion sickness.

Dosage
- **Tablets**

Motion sickness.
Adults: 50 mg 30 min before leaving and q 4–6 hr thereafter, not to exceed 200 mg/day; **pediatric, 6–12 years:** 1 mg/kg (33 mg/m²) t.i.d. or 25 mg 30 min before travel and repeated in 6–8 hr if needed, not to exceed 75 mg/day.
Contraindications: Pregnancy and lactation.
Special Concerns: Safety for use in children less than 12 years of age has not been determined; children may be more sensitive to the anticholinergic effects of the drug. Geriatric clients may experience a greater incidence of constipation, dry mouth, and urinary retention (i.e., due to the anticholinergic effects).
Side Effects: *CNS:* Drowsiness, excitation, nervousness, restlessness, insomnia, euphoria, vertigo, hallucinations (auditory or visual). *GI:* N&V, diarrhea, constipation, anorexia). *GU:* Urinary frequency or retention; difficulty in urination. *CV:* Hypotension, tachycardia, palpitations. *Miscellaneous:* Dry nose and throat, blurred or double vision, tinnitus, rash, urticaria.

NURSING CONSIDERATIONS

See also *Nursing Considerations* for *Antihistamines,* Chapter 55.
Client/Family Teaching
1. Take 30 min before travel.
2. Drug may cause dizziness so use caution.
3. Avoid alcohol.
4. Advise that older clients may experience more anticholinergic effects (e.g., dry mouth, constipation, and urinary retention).
Evaluate
- Prevention of N&V
- Control of dizziness R/T motion sickness

Cyproheptadine hydrochloride

(sye-proh-**HEP**-tah-deen)
Pregnancy Category: B
Periactin **(Rx)**

See also *Antihistamines,* Chapter 55.
How Supplied: *Syrup:* 2 mg/5 mL; *Tablet:* 4 mg
Action/Kinetics: Cyproheptadine also possesses antiserotonin activity.
Duration: 8 hr.
Additional Uses: Cold urticaria. *Investigational:* Cluster headaches, appetite stimulant in underweight clients and those with anorexia nervosa.

Dosage

- **Syrup, Tablets**

Antihistaminic.

Adults, initial: 4 mg q 8 hr; **then,** 4–20 mg/day, not to exceed 0.5 mg/kg/day. **Pediatric, 2–6 years:** 2 mg q 8–12 hr, not to exceed 12 mg/day; **6–14 years:** 4 mg q 8–12 hr, not to exceed 16 mg/day.

Appetite stimulant.

Adults: 4 mg t.i.d. with meals. **Pediatric, 6–14 years, initial:** 2 mg t.i.d.–q.i.d. with meals; **then,** reduce dose to 4 mg t.i.d. **Pediatric, 2–6 years, initial:** 2 mg t.i.d. with meals; **then,** dose may be increased to a total of 8 mg/day.

Administration/Storage

1. Drug should not be given more than 6 months to adults and 3 months to children for appetite stimulation.
2. Anticipate the onset of action to occur within 15–30 min and to last from 3 to 6 hr.

Additional Contraindications: Glaucoma, urinary retention.
Special Concerns: Geriatric clients may be more sensitive to the usual adult dose.
Laboratory Test Interferences: ↑ Serum amylase and prolactin if given with thyroid-releasing hormone.
Additional Side Effect: Increased appetite.

NURSING CONSIDERATIONS

See also *Nursing Considerations* for *Antihistamines,* Chapter 55.

Evaluate

- ↓ Allergic manifestations
- Weight gain
- Relief of cluster headaches

Dexchlorpheniramine maleate

(dex-klor-fen-**EAR**-ah-meen)
Pregnancy Category: B
Dexchlor, Poladex T.D., Polaramine, Polargen **(Rx)**

See also *Antihistamines,* Chapter 55.
How Supplied: *Syrup:* 2 mg/5 mL; *Tablet:* 2 mg; *Tablet, Extended Release:* 4 mg, 6 mg
Action/Kinetics: Less severe sedative effects. **Duration:** 8 hr.

Dosage

- **Syrup, Tablets**

Adults: 2 mg q 4–6 hr as needed. **Pediatric, 5–12 years:** 1 mg q 4–6 hr as needed; **2–5 years:** 0.5 mg q 4–6 hr as needed.

- **Extended-Release Tablets**

Adults: 4–6 mg q 8–12 hr as needed.
Special Concerns: Extended-release tablets should not be used in children. Geriatric clients may be more sensitive to the usual adult dose.

NURSING CONSIDERATIONS

See also *Nursing Considerations* for *Antihistamines,* Chapter 55.
Evaluate: Symptomatic relief and ↓ allergic manifestations.

Dimenhydrinate

(dye-men-**HY**-drih-nayt)
Pregnancy Category: B
Elixir, Syrup, Tablets, Chewable Tablets: Apo-Dimenhydrinate ✱, Calm-X, Dimentabs, Dramamine, Gravol ✱, Marmine, Motion-Aid, Nauseatol ✱, Travamine, Travel-Aid ✱, Travel Eze ✱, Travel Tabs ✱, Triptone **(OTC)**. **Injection:** Dimenhydrinate Injection ✱, Dinate, Dommanate, Dramamine, Dramanate, Dramilin, Dramocen, Dramoject, Dymenate, Gravol ✱, Hydrate, Marmine, Reidamine, Wehamine **(Rx)**

See also *Antihistamines,* Chapter 55, and *Antiemetics,* Chapter 62.
How Supplied: *Capsule:* 50 mg; *Chew Tablet:* 50 mg; *Injection:* 50 mg/mL; *Liquid:* 12.5 mg/4 mL, 12.5 mg/5 mL; *Tablet:* 25 mg, 50 mg

Action/Kinetics: Dimenhydrinate contains both diphenhydramine and chlorotheophylline. The precise mechanism for the antiemetic effect is not known but the drug does depress labyrinthine and vestibular function. The drug may mask ototoxicity due to aminoglycosides. Possesses anticholinergic activity. **Duration:** 3–6 hr.
Uses: Motion sickness, especially to relieve nausea, vomiting, or dizziness. Treat vertigo.

Dosage

• **Elixir, Syrup, Tablets, Chewable Tablets**

Motion sickness.

Adults: 50–100 mg q 4 hr, not to exceed 400 mg/day. **Pediatric, 6–12 years:** 25–50 mg q 6–8 hr, not to exceed 150 mg/day; **2–6 years:** 12.5–25 mg q 6–8 hr, not to exceed 75 mg/day.

• **Extended-Release Capsules**

Motion sickness.

Adults: 1 capsule q 12 hr. Use is not recommended in children.

• **IM, IV**

Adults: 50 mg as required. **Pediatric, over 2 years:** 1.25 mg/kg (37.5 mg/m^2) q.i.d., not to exceed 300 mg/day.

• **IV**

Adults: 50 mg in 10 mL sodium chloride injection given over 2 min; may be repeated q 4 hr as needed. **Pediatric:** 1.25 mg/kg (37.6 mg/m^2) in 10 mL of 0.9% sodium chloride injection given slowly over 2 min; may be repeated q 6 hr, not to exceed 300 mg/day.

• **Suppositories**

Adults: 50–100 mg q 6–8 hr. **Pediatric, 12 years and older:** 50 mg q 8–12 hr; **8–12 years:** 25–50 mg q 8–12 hr; **6–8 years:** 12.5–25 mg q 8–12 hr. Dosage not established in children less than 6 years of age.
Special Concerns: Use of the injectable form is not recommended in neonates. Geriatric clients may be more sensitive to the usual adult dose.

NURSING CONSIDERATIONS

See also *Nursing Considerations* for *Antihistamines,* Chapter 55, and *Antiemetics,* Chapter 62.

Assessment

1. Document indications for therapy and onset of symptoms.
2. Assess for any evidence of vestibular damage when administered with antihistamines.

Evaluate: Prevention of N&V and control of vertigo R/T motion sickness.

Diphenhydramine hydrochloride

(dye-fen-**HY**-drah-meen)

Pregnancy Category: B

Allerdryl ✱, AllerMax, Beldin Cough, Belix, Bena-D, Bena-D 50, Benadryl, Benadryl Complete Allergy, Benahist 10 and 50, Ben-Allergin-50, Benoject-10 and -50, Benylin Cough, Benaphen, Bydramine Cough, Clear Caladryl Spray ✱, Diahist, Dihydrex, Diphenacen-10 and -50, Diphenadryl, Diphen Cough, Fenylhist, Fynex, Hydramine, Hydramine Cough, Hydril, Hyrexin-50, Nauzene Maximum Strength, Noradryl, Nordryl, Nordryl Cough, PMS-Diphenhydramine ✱, Tusstat, Valdrene, Wehdryl (OTC and Rx). **Sleep-Aids:** Dormin, Miles Nervine, Nytol, Sleep-eze 3, Sleep-Eze D ✱, Sleepwell 2-nite, Sominex **(OTC)**

See also *Antihistamines,* Chapter 55, *Antiemetics,* Chapter 62, and *Antiparkinson Agents,* Chapter 46.
How Supplied: *Balm:* 2%; *Capsule:* 25 mg, 50 mg; *Chew Tablet:* 12.5 mg; *Cream:* 1%, 2%; *Elixir:* 12.5 mg/5 mL; *Gel/Jelly:* 1.25%; *Injection:* 10 mg/mL, 50 mg/mL; *Liquid:* 6.25 mg/5 mL, 12.5 mg/5 mL, 50 mg/15 mL; *Solution:* 1.25%; *Spray:* 1%, 2%; *Syrup:* 12.5 mg/5 mL; *Tablet:* 25 mg, 50 mg
Additional Uses: Treatment of parkinsonism in geriatric clients unable to tolerate more potent drugs. Also for mild parkinsonism in other age groups. Drug-induced extrapyramidal symptoms. Motion sickness, anti-

emetic, as a sleep-aid. Coughs, including those due to allergy.

Dosage

- **Capsules, Elixir, Syrup, Tablets**

Antihistamine, antiemetic, antimotion sickness, parkinsonism.

Adults: 25–50 mg t.i.d.–q.i.d.; **pediatric, over 9.1 kg:** 12.5–25 mg t.i.d.–q.i.d. (or 5 mg/kg/day not to exceed 300 mg/day or 150 mg/m^2/day).

Sleep aid.

Adults: 50 mg at bedtime.

Antitussive.

Adults: 25 mg q 4 hr, not to exceed 150 mg/day; **pediatric, 6–12 years:** 12.5–25 mg q 4–6 hr, not to exceed 75 mg/day; **pediatric, 2–6 years:** 6.25 mg q 4–6 hr, not to exceed 25 mg/day.

- **IV, Deep IM**

Parkinsonism.

Adults: 10–50 mg up to 100 mg if needed (not to exceed 400 mg/day); **pediatric:** 1.25 mg/kg (or 37.5 mg/m^2) q.i.d., not to exceed a total of 300 mg/day.

Administration/Storage

1. When using for motion sickness, the full prophylactic dose should be administered 30 min prior to travel and preferably 1–2 hr before exposures that precipitate sickness.
2. Similar doses should also be taken with meals and at bedtime.
3. Determine client symptoms that necessitate drug administration and note as drug has multiple indications.
4. Should not be used for more than 2 weeks to treat insomnia.
5. For IV administration, may give undiluted with each 25 mg over at least 1 min.

NURSING CONSIDERATIONS

See also *Nursing Considerations* for *Antihistamines,* Chapter 55, *Antiemetics,* Chapter 62, and *Antiparkinson Agents,* Chapter 46.

Client/Family Teaching

1. Drug may cause drowsiness; use caution until drug effects realized.
2. May cause photosensitivity reaction; avoid direct sun exposure and use protection.
3. Use sugarless gum and candy or frequent sips of water to diminish dry mouth effects.
4. Avoid alcohol and any other CNS depressants unless prescribed.

Evaluate

- ↓ Allergic manifestations
- Relief of nausea in motion sickness
- Control of cough
- Promotion of sleep
- Relief of dyskinesias and extrapyramidal symptoms with parkinsonism

Levocabastine hydrochloride

(**lee**-voh-kah-**BASS**-teen)

Pregnancy Category: C

Livostin Nasal Spray **(Rx)**

How Supplied: *Suspension:* 0.05%

Action/Kinetics: Levocabastine is a histamine H_1 receptor antagonist for ophthalmic use. **Duration:** 2 hr. A small amount of the drug is absorbed into the systemic circulation.

Uses: Temporary relief of seasonal allergic conjunctivitis.

Dosage

- **Ophthalmic suspension**

Allergic conjunctivitis.

1 gtt instilled in affected eye(s) q.i.d. for up to 2 weeks.

Administration/Storage

1. The suspension should be shaken well before using.
2. The dropper tip should not touch the eyelids or surrounding areas so that contamination to the dropper tip and suspension can be avoided.
3. The bottle should be kept tightly closed when not in use. The bottle is stored at room temperature (15°C–30°C, or 59°F– 86°F) and should not be frozen.
4. The suspension should not be used if it is discolored.

Contraindications: Use while soft contact lenses are being worn.

Special Concerns: The drug is only for ophthalmic use. Safety and efficacy have not been determined in children less than 12 years of age.

Side Effects: *Ophthalmologic:* Transient stinging and burning, visual disturbances, eye pain, eye dryness, red eyes, lacrimation, discharge from eyes, eyelid edema. *CNS:* Headache, fatigue, somnolence. *Miscellaneous:* Pharyngitis, cough, nausea, rash, erythema, dyspnea.

NURSING CONSIDERATIONS

Assessment

1. Document onset, type, and length of symptoms. Note other agents prescribed and the outcome.
2. Assess for any evidence of infection or abnormal drainage from the eye.
3. Determine if there have been any changes in or loss of vision.

Client/Family Teaching

1. Ensure that contents are thoroughly mixed before instillation.
2. Review the proper method and frequency for administration and observe client technique.
3. Stress that soft contact lens *cannot* be worn during this therapy.
4. Advise that some burning and stinging may be evident but should subside.
5. Remind client that if symptoms do not improve or if they become worse after 2–4 days of therapy to notify provider.

Evaluate: Relief of symptoms of ocular itching associated with seasonal allergic conjunctivitis.

Loratidine

(loh-**RAH**-tih-deen)
Pregnancy Category: B
Claritin **(Rx)**

See also *Antihistamines,* Chapter 55.
How Supplied: *Tablet:* 10 mg
Action/Kinetics: Loratidine is metabolized in the liver to an active metabolite (descarboethoxyloratidine). The drug has low to no sedative and anticholinergic effects. It has not been shown to alter cardiac repolarization and has not been linked to development of torsades de pointes as seen with astemizole and terfenadine. **Onset:** 1–3 hr. **Maximum effect:** 8–12 hr. **t½, loratidine:** 8.4 hr; **t½, descarboethoxyloratidine:** 28 hr. **Duration:** 24 hr. Excreted through both the urine and feces.
Uses: Relief of nasal and nonnasal symptoms of seasonal allergic rhinitis.

Dosage

- **Tablets**

Allergic rhinitis.

Adults: 10 mg once daily on an empty stomach. *In clients with impaired liver function:* 10 mg every other day.
Special Concerns: Use with caution, if at all, during lactation. Clients with liver impairment should be given a lower initial dose. Safety and efficacy have not been determined in children less than 12 years of age.
Side Effects: Most commonly, headache, somnolence, fatigue, and dry mouth. *GI:* Altered salivation, gastritis, dyspepsia, stomatitis, tooth ache, thirst, altered taste, flatulence. *CNS:* Hypoesthesia, hyperkinesia, migraine, anxiety, depression, agitation, paroniria, amnesia, impaired concentration. *Ophthalmologic:* Altered lacrimation, conjunctivitis, blurred vision, eye pain, blepharospasm. *Respiratory:* Upper respiratory infection, epistaxis, pharyngitis, dyspnea, coughing, rhinitis, sinusitis, sneezing, bronchitis, ***bronchospasm,*** hemoptysis, laryngitis. *Body as a whole:* Asthenia, increased sweating, flushing, malaise, rigors, fever, dry skin, aggravated allergy, pruritus, purpura. *Musculoskeletal:* Back/chest pain, leg cramps, arthralgia, myalgia. *GU:* Breast pain, menorrhagia, dysmenorrhea, vaginitis. *Miscellaneous:* Earache, dysphonia, dry hair, urinary discoloration.

NURSING CONSIDERATIONS

See also *Nursing Considerations* for *Antihistamines,* Chapter 55.

Assessment

1. Document any evidence or history of liver dysfunction. Obtain baseline liver function studies and anticipate reduced dosage with dysfunction.
2. Perform a drug profile. Cautiously

coadminister with drugs that inhibit hepatic metabolism (i.e., macrolide antibiotics, cimetidine, ranitidine, ketoconazole, or theophylline).
Intervention: The elderly and clients with hepatic and renal impairment warrant close observation for increasing somnolence.
Client/Family Teaching
1. Take on an empty stomach as food may delay absorption.
2. Do not perform activities that require mental alertness until drug effects are realized. Generally, drug does not cause drowsiness.
Evaluate: Subjective reports of relief of nasal congestion and seasonal allergic manifestations.

Meclizine hydrochloride

(**MEK**-lih-zeen)
Pregnancy Category: B
Antivert, Antivert/25 and /50, Antivert/25 Chewable, Antrizine, Bonamine ✦, Bonine, Dizmiss, Dramamine II, Meni-D, Ru-Vert-M (OTC and Rx)

See also *Antihistamines,* Chapter 55, and *Antiemetics,* Chapter 62.
How Supplied: *Capsule:* 25 mg, 30 mg; *Chew Tablet:* 25 mg; *Tablet:* 12.5 mg, 25 mg, 30 mg, 50 mg
Action/Kinetics: The mechanism for the antiemetic effect is not known but may be due to a central anticholinergic effect to decrease vestibular stimulation and depress labyrinthine activity. The drug may also act on the CTZ to decrease vomiting. **Onset:** 30–60 min; **Duration:** 8–24 hr. **t½:** 6 hr.
Uses: Nausea and vomiting, dizziness of motion sickness, vertigo associated with diseases of the vestibular system.

Dosage
- **Capsules, Tablets, Chewable Tablets**

Motion sickness.
Adults: 25–50 mg 1 hr before travel; may be repeated q 24 hr during travel.
Vertigo.
Adults: 25–100 mg/day in divided doses.
Special Concerns: Safety for use during lactation and in children less than 12 years of age has not been determined. Pediatric and geriatric clients may be more sensitive to the anticholinergic effects of meclizine.
Side Effects: *CNS:* Drowsiness, excitation, nervousness, restlessness, insomnia, euphoria, vertigo, hallucinations (auditory or visual). *GI:* N&V, diarrhea, constipation, anorexia. *GU:* Urinary frequency or retention; difficulty in urination. *CV:* Hypotension, tachycardia, palpitations. *Miscellaneous:* Dry nose and throat, blurred or double vision, tinnitus, rash, urticaria.

NURSING CONSIDERATIONS

See also *Nursing Considerations* for *Antihistamines,* Chapter 55, and *Antiemetics,* Chapter 62.
Assessment
1. Document indications for therapy and onset and type of symptoms.
2. Assess closely for other adverse symptoms in addition to nausea. An antiemetic drug may mask signs of drug overdose as well as signs of pathology such as increased ICP or intestinal obstruction.
Client/Family Teaching
1. Take only as directed and report if condition does not improve.
2. Antiemetics tend to cause drowsiness and dizziness. Caution against driving or performing other hazardous tasks until individual response to the drug has been evaluated.
Evaluate
- Prevention of motion sickness
- Control of vertigo

Promethazine hydrochloride

(proh-**METH**-ah-zeen)
Syrup, Tablets: Histanil ✦, Phenergan Fortis, Phenergan Plain, PMS Promethazine ✦, Prothazine Plain. **Parenteral:** Anergan 25 and 50, K-Phen, Mallergan, Pentazine, Phenazine 25 and 50, Phenergan, Phenoject-50, Pro-50, Prometh-25 and -50, Prorex-25 and -50, Prothazine, V-Gan-25 and -50. **Rectal:** Phenergan, Promethagan **(Rx)**

See also *Antihistamines,* Chapter 55, and *Antiemetics,* Chapter 62.

How Supplied: *Injection:* 25 mg/mL, 50 mg/mL; *Suppository:* 12.5 mg, 25 mg, 50 mg; *Syrup:* 6.25 mg/5 mL, 25 mg/5 mL; *Tablet:* 12.5 mg, 25 mg, 50 mg

Action/Kinetics: Promethazine is a potent antihistamine with prolonged action. It may cause severe drowsiness. The antiemetic effects are likely due to inhibition of the CTZ. The drug is effective in vertigo by its central anticholinergic effect which inhibits the vestibular apparatus and the integrative vomiting center as well as the CTZ. **Onset, PO, IM, PR:** 20 min; **IV:** 3–5 min. **Duration, antihistaminic:** 6–12 hr; **sedative:** 2–8 hr. Slowly eliminated through urine and feces.

Uses: Treatment and prophylaxis of motion sickness. N&V due to anesthesia or surgery. Pre- or postoperative sedative, obstetric sedative. Treatment of pruritus, urticaria, angioedema, dermographism, nasal and ophthalmic allergies. Adjunct in the treatment of anaphylaxis or anaphylactoid reactions. Adjunct to analgesics for postoperative pain. IV with meperidine or other narcotics in special surgical procedures as bronchoscopy, ophthalmic surgery, or in poor-risk clients.

Dosage

- **Syrup, Tablets**

Antihistaminic.

Adults: 12.5 mg q.i.d. before meals and at bedtime (or 25 mg at bedtime if needed). **Pediatric,** 0.125 mg/kg (3.75 mg/m^2) q 4–6 hr; 0.5 mg/kg (15 mg/m^2) at bedtime if needed; or, 6.26–12.6 mg t.i.d. (or 25 mg at bedtime if needed).

Vertigo.

Adults: 25 mg b.i.d.; **pediatric,** 0.5 mg/kg (15 mg/m^2) q 12 hr or 12.5–25 mg b.i.d.

Antiemetic.

Adults: 25 mg b.i.d. as needed; **pediatric,** 0.25–0.5 mg/kg (7.5–15 mg/m^2) q 4–6 hr as needed (or 12.5–25 mg q 4–6 hr).

Sedative-hypnotic.

Adults: 25–50 mg; **pediatric,** 0.5–1 mg/kg (15–30 mg/m^2) or 12.5–25 mg as needed.

- **IM, IV, Suppositories**

Antihistaminic.

Adults, IM, IV, Rectal: 25 mg repeated in 2 hr if needed; **pediatric, IM, Rectal:** 0.125 mg/kg q 4–6 hr (or 0.5 mg/kg at bedtime).

Antiemetic.

Adults, IM, IV, Rectal: 12.5–25 mg q 4 hr; **pediatric, IM, Rectal,** 0.25–0.5 mg/kg q 4–6 hr (or 12.5–25 mg q 4–6 hr).

Sedative-hypnotic.

Adults, IM, IV, Rectal: 25–50 mg; **pediatric, IM, Rectal,** 0.5–1 mg/kg (or 12.5–25 mg).

Vertigo.

Adults, Rectal: 25 mg b.i.d.; **pediatric, Rectal:** 0.5 mg/kg q 12 hr (or 12.5–25 mg b.i.d.)

Administration/Storage

1. Drug may be taken with food or milk to lessen GI irritation.
2. Dosage should be decreased in dehydrated clients or those with oliguria.
3. When used to prevent motion sickness, the medication should be taken 30 min, and preferably 1–2 hr, before travel.

Contraindications: Lactation. Children up to 2 years of age.

Special Concerns: Safe use during pregnancy has not been established. Use in children may cause paradoxical hyperexcitability and nightmares. Injection not recommended for children less than 2 years of age. Geriatric clients are more likely to experience confusion, dizziness, hypotension, and sedation.

Additional Side Effects: Leukopenia and ***agranulocytosis (especially if used with cytotoxic agents)***.

NURSING CONSIDERATIONS

See also *Nursing Considerations* for *Antihistamines,* Chapter 55, and *Antiemetics,* Chapter 62.

Assessment
1. Document indications for therapy and type and onset of symptoms.
2. Note age because older client may manifest more adverse side effects.

Evaluate
- Prevention of vertigo
- Control of N&V
- Promotion of sleep
- Control of allergic manifestations

Terfenadine
(ter-**FEN**-ah-deen)
Pregnancy Category: C
Apo-Terfenadine ✱, Seldane **(Rx)**

See also *Antihistamines,* Chapter 55.
How Supplied: *Tablet:* 60 mg
Action/Kinetics: Is said to manifest significantly less drowsiness and anticholinergic effects than other antihistamines. **Onset:** 1–2 hr; **peak effect:** 3–4 hr; **peak plasma levels:** 2 hr. **t½:** About 20 hr. **Duration:** Over 12 hr. Metabolized in the liver and excreted in the urine and feces.
Additional Uses: *Investigational:* Histamine-induced bronchoconstriction in asthmatics; exercise and hyperventilation-induced bronchospasm.

Dosage
- **Tablets**

Adults and children over 12 years: 60 mg q 8–12 hr as needed.
Contraindications: Significant hepatic dysfunction. Use with drugs that prolong the QT interval, such as disopyramide, procainamide, quinidine, most antidepressants, and most neuroleptics.
Special Concerns: Safety and efficacy in children less than 12 years of age have not been established. Hepatic insufficiency and any drug or food (e.g., grapefruit juice) that blocks the metabolism of terfenadine may cause serious CV effects (see *Additional Side Effects,* below).
Additional Side Effects: ***Doses of 360 mg or more may cause serious CV effects, including death, cardiac arrest, torsades de pointes, and other ventricular arrhythmias (including QT interval prolongation).*** Syncope may precede severe arrhythmias.

Drug Interactions
Erythromycins / ↑ Risk of serious CV effects, including death, cardiac arrest, torsades de pointes, and other ventricular arrhythmias
Itraconazole / See *Ketoconazole*
Ketoconazole / ↑ Risk of serious CV effects, including death, cardiac arrest, torsades de pointes, and other ventricular arrhythmias
Troleandomycin / ↑ Risk of serious CV effects, including death, cardiac arrest, torsades de pointes, and other ventricular arrhythmias

NURSING CONSIDERATIONS

See also *Nursing Considerations* for *Antihistamines,* Chapter 55.

Assessment
1. Document indications for therapy and type and onset of symptoms.
2. List any other agents prescribed and the outcome.
3. Describe pulmonary assessment findings.

Client/Family Teaching
1. Take with food or milk to minimize GI upset.
2. *Do not* exceed prescribed dosage as this increases the risk of side effects, especially those affecting the CV system.
3. Advise that with the H_1 antagonists, clinical effectiveness of one group may diminish with continuous use. Changing to another group may restore drug effectiveness.

Evaluate: Improved airway exchange and relief of allergic manifestations.

Tripelennamine hydrochloride
(try-pell-**EN**-ah-meen)
PBZ, PBZ-SR, Pelamine, Pyribenzamine ✱ **(Rx)**

See also *Antihistamines,* Chapter 55.
How Supplied: *Tablet:* 25 mg, 50 mg; *Tablet, extended release:* 100 mg
Action/Kinetics: GI effects more pronounced than other antihistamines. **Duration:** 4–6 hr.

Dosage

- **Elixir, Tablets**

Adults, usual: 25–50 mg q 4–6 hr; **pediatric:** 1.25 mg/kg (37.5 mg/m²) q 6 hr as needed, not to exceed 300 mg/day.

- **Extended-Release Tablets**

Adults: 100 mg q 8–12 hr as needed, up to a maximum of 600 mg/day. Do not use sustained-release form in children.

Special Concerns: Safe use during pregnancy has not been established. Use is not recommended in neonates. Geriatric clients may be more sensitive to the usual adult dose.

Side Effects: Low incidence. Moderate sedation, mild GI distress, paradoxical excitation, hyperirritability.

NURSING CONSIDERATIONS

See also *Nursing Considerations* for *Antihistamines,* Chapter 55.

Evaluate: Reports of ↓ allergic manifestations.

Triprolidine hydrochloride

(try-**PROH**-lih-deen)

Pregnancy Category: C

Alleract, Myidyl (OTC and Rx)

See also *Antihistamines,* Chapter 55.

How Supplied: *Syrup:* 1.25 mg/5mL

Action/Kinetics: Sedative effects less pronounced. **Time to peak effect:** 2–3 hr. **t½:** 3–3.3 hr. **Duration:** 4–25 hr. Also found in Actifed and Actifed-C.

Uses: See *Antihistamines,* Chapter 55.

Dosage

- **Syrup, Tablets**

Adults: 2.5 mg q 4–6 hr. **Pediatric 6–12 years:** 1.25 mg q 6–8 hr; **4–6 years:** 0.937 mg q 6–8 hr; **2–4 years:** 0.625 mg q 6–8 hr; **4 months–2 years:** 0.312 mg q 6–8 hr.

Special Concerns: Geriatric clients may be more susceptible to the usual adult dose.

Additional Side Effects: Low incidence of side effects. *CNS:* Drowsiness, dizziness, paradoxical excitement, hyperirritability. *GI:* GI distress.

NURSING CONSIDERATIONS

See also *Nursing Considerations* for *Antihistamines,* Chapter 55.

Evaluate: Relief of allergic manifestations.

CHAPTER FIFTY-SIX

Drugs Used for Respiratory Tract Disorders

See the following individual entries:

Acetylcysteine
Alpha-1-Proteinase Inhibitor
Beractant
Colfosceril Palmitate
Guaifenesin

Acetylcysteine

(ah-see-till-**SIS**-tay-een)
Pregnancy Category: B
Airbron ✱, Mucomyst, Mucosol, Parvolex **(Rx)**

How Supplied: *Solution:* 10%, 20%
Action/Kinetics: Acetylcysteine reduces the viscosity of purulent and nonpurulent pulmonary secretions and facilitates their removal by splitting disulfide bonds. Action increases with increasing pH (peak: pH 7–9). **Onset, inhalation:** Within 1 min; **by direct instillation:** immediate. **Time to peak effect:** 5–10 min.
Uses: Adjunct in the treatment of acute and chronic bronchitis, emphysema, tuberculosis, pneumonia, bronchiectasis, atelectasis. Routine care of clients with tracheostomy, pulmonary complications after thoracic or CV surgery, or in posttraumatic chest conditions. Pulmonary complications of cystic fibrosis. Diagnostic bronchial asthma. Antidote in acetaminophen poisoning to reduce hepatotoxicity. *Investigational:* As an ophthalmic solution for dry eye.

Dosage

• **Nebulization, Direct Application, or Direct Intratracheal Instillation Using 10% or 20% Solution**

Nebulization into face mask, tracheostomy, mouth piece.
1–10 mL of 20% solution or 2–10 mL of 10% solution 3–4 times/day.

Closed tent or croupette.
Up to 300 mL of 10% or 20% solution/treatment.

Direct instillation into tracheostomy.
1–2 mL of 10%–20% solution q 1–4 hr.

Percutaneous intratracheal catheter.
1–2 mL of 20% solution or 2–4 mL of 10% solution q 1–4 hr by syringe attached to catheter.

Instillation to particular portion of bronchopulmonary tree using small plastic catheter into the trachea.
2–5 mL of 20% solution instilled into the trachea by means of a syringe connected to a catheter.

Diagnostic procedures.
2–3 doses of 1–2 mL of 20% or 2–4 mL of 10% solution by nebulization or intratracheal instillation before the procedure.

Acetaminophen overdose.
Given PO, initial: 140 mg/kg; **then,** 70 mg/kg q 4 hr for a total of 17 doses.

Administration/Storage

1. Use nonreactive plastic, glass, or stainless steel equipment for administration.
2. The 10% solution may be used undiluted.
3. Use either water for injection or saline to dilute the 20% solution.
4. Administer the medication via face mask, face tent, oxygen tent, head tent, or by positive-pressure breathing apparatus as indicated.

5. Administer with compressed air for nebulization. Hand nebulizers are contraindicated.
6. After prolonged nebulization, dilute the last fourth of the medication with sterile water for injection to prevent concentration of the medication.
7. The solution may develop a light purple color. This does not affect the action of the medication.
8. Closed bottles of solution remain stable for 2 years when stored at 20°C (68°F). Open bottles should be stored at 2°C–8°C (35°F–46°F) and should be used within 96 hr. Once a bottle has been opened, record the time and date of opening so that the drug will not be used beyond the 96-hr period.
9. Acetylcysteine is incompatible with antibiotics and must be administered separately.
10. Have an ET tube available and a suction machine at the bedside for removal of increased bronchial secretions.

Contraindication: Sensitivity to drug.

Special Concerns: Use with caution during lactation, in the elderly, and in clients with asthma.

Side Effects: *Respiratory:* Acetylcysteine increases the incidence of bronchospasm in clients with asthma. The drug may also increase the amount of liquefied bronchial secretions, which must be removed by suction if cough is inadequate. Bronchial and tracheal irritation, tightness in chest, bronchoconstriction. *GI:* N&V, stomatitis. *Other:* Rashes, fever, drowsiness, rhinorrhea.

Drug Interactions: Acetylcysteine is incompatible with antibiotics and should be administered separately.

NURSING CONSIDERATIONS

Assessment

1. Determine from the client and history when bronchial spasms occur.
2. Discuss conditions likely to cause congestion and wheezing and document.
3. Identify the previous approaches (successful and unsuccessful) used in treating client conditions.
4. Determine if the client is currently taking any antibiotic medications.
5. Document time of acetaminophen overdose. Drug should be administered within 8–10 hr following overdose to protect from hepatoxicity and death. Monitor liver function tests and acetaminophen levels.

Interventions

1. If bronchospasm occurs, have a bronchodilator, such as isoproterenol for aerosol inhalation, readily available.
2. Position the client to facilitate the removal of secretions.
3. If the client is unable to cough up secretions, provide mechanical suction for their removal.
4. Monitor VS and I&O.
5. Wash the client's face following nebulization treatment. The medication may cause the face to become sticky.
6. Advise that the nauseous odor present when the treatment begins will likely become less noticeable as therapy continues.
7. The administration route for acetaminophen toxicity is oral and will consist of 17 doses.

Evaluate

- Improved airway exchange with mobilization and expectoration of secretions
- ↓ Acetaminophen levels and associated liver toxicity when used as an antidote with overdosage

Alpha-1-Proteinase Inhibitor (Human) (Alpha-1-PI)

(**AL**-fah-1-**PROH**-tee-in-ayz)

Pregnancy Category: C

Prolastin **(Rx)**

How Supplied: *Powder for injection*

Action/Kinetics: Alpha-1-PI is the enzyme that is deficient in alpha-1-antitrypsin disease. This disease causes a progressive breakdown of elastin tissues in the alveoli, resulting in emphysema. Often fatal, alpha-1-antitrypsin disease is usually manifested in the third and fourth decades of life. Prolastin is a sterile, lyophilized product obtained from pooled human plasma that is nonreactive for the HIV antibody and the hepatitis B surface antigen. **t½:** 4.5 days. **Therapeutic serum levels:** Approximately 80 mg/dL, although such levels may not reflect actual functional alpha-1-PI levels.

Use: Panacinar emphysema due to congenital alpha-1-proteinase deficiency.

Dosage

- **IV Only**

Panacinar emphysema.

Adults: 60 mg/kg each week at a rate of 0.08 mL/kg/min (or greater).

Administration/Storage

1. Administer within 3 hr after reconstitution. Do not refrigerate.
2. Administer only via IV. Follow recommended procedures for reconstitution.
3. When reconstituted, Prolastin is equal to or greater than 20 mg/mL and has a pH of 6.6–7.4.
4. Prolastin should be stored at 2°C–8°C (36°F–46°F) and should not be frozen.
5. The reconstituted drug should not be mixed with other diluents except for normal saline.
6. Clients should be immunized against hepatitis B prior to using Prolastin. If time does not permit adequate immunization, a single dose of Hepatitis B Immune Globulin (Human), 0.06 mL/kg IM, should be given at the time of the initial dose of Prolastin.
7. Equipment used and any unused reconstituted alpha-1-PI (human) should be appropriately discarded.

Contraindication: Clients with PiMZ or PiMS phenotypes of alpha-1-antitrypsin deficiency.

Special Concerns: Safety and efficacy for use in children not determined. Use with caution in clients at risk for circulatory overload.

Side Effects: Although precautions are taken during the manufacture of this product, it is possible that hepatitis and other infectious viruses may be present. *Miscellaneous:* Delayed fever up to 12 hr following treatment, dizziness, lightheadedness, mild transient leukocytosis.

NURSING CONSIDERATIONS

Assessment

1. Perform a complete nursing history and lung assessment.
2. Obtain a hepatitis profile. If the client has not received hepatitis B immunization, document and provide appropriate therapy.

Interventions

1. Observe client for delayed fever, which may occur within 12 hr. This is usually resolved in 24 hr.
2. Note any complaints of lightheadedness or dizziness and report.

Client/Family Teaching

1. Advise that cigarette smoking may accelerate and aggravate condition by causing an increase of elastin secretion.
2. Discuss familial tendency for alpha-1-antitrypsin deficiency, and explain the need for all blood relatives to be screened and provided appropriate counseling.
3. Stress the importance of reporting weekly for medication to maintain an adequate antielastase barrier.
4. Explain that therapy must continue throughout the client's lifetime.
5. Discuss that the product is prepared from human plasma and explain the potential associated risks.

Evaluate

- ↑ Serum prolastin levels (80 mg/dL)
- Slowing of destructive process on lung tissue
- Family members identified, screened, and counseled.

Beractant

(beh-**RACK**-tant)
Survanta **(Rx)**

How Supplied: *Injection:* 25 mg/mL

Action/Kinetics: Beractant, derived from natural bovine lung extract, contains phospholipids, fatty acids, neutral lipids, and surfactant-associated proteins (to which colfosceril palmitate, tripalmitin, and palmitic acid are added). The proteins in the product—SP-B and SP-C—are hydrophobic, low molecular weight, and surfactant associated. Beractant replenishes pulmonary surfactant and restores surface activity to the lungs of premature infants to reduce respiratory distress syndrome. The drug is intended for intratracheal use only. Significant improvement is observed in the arterial-alveolar oxygen ratio and mean airway pressure. Beractant significantly decreases the incidence of respiratory distress syndrome, mortality due to respiratory distress syndrome, and air leak complications.

Uses: Prevention and treatment ("rescue") of respiratory distress syndrome (hyaline membrane disease) in premature infants.

Dosage

- **Intratracheal Only**

4 mL/kg (100 mg phospholipids/kg birth weight).

Administration/Storage

1. For prevention of respiratory distress syndrome in premature infants weighing less than 1,250 g at birth or with evidence of surfactant deficiency, beractant should be given as soon as possible, preferably within 15 min of birth.
2. To treat infants with confirmed respiratory distress syndrome and who require mechanical ventilation, beractant should be given as soon as possible, preferably within 8 hr of birth.
3. Four doses can be given within the first 48 hr of life; doses should be given no sooner than q 6 hr.
4. Beractant should be refrigerated at 2°C–8°C (36°F–46°F) and warmed at room temperature for at least 20 min or in the hand for at least 8 min before administration. The drug does not have to be reconstituted or sonicated before use. If a prevention dose is required, preparation should begin before the infant is born. The drug should not be warmed and then returned to the refrigerator for future use more than once.
5. Before administration the vial should be visually inspected for discoloration (beractant is off-white to light brown). If settling occurs during storage, the vial should be swirled gently (not shaken) to redisperse although some foaming may occur at the surface during handling.
6. Each vial is for single use only; any residual drug should thus be discarded.
7. Instill beractant through a 5 French end-hole catheter that has been inserted into the ET tube of the infant with the tip of the catheter protruding just beyond the end of the ET tube above the infant's carina. The length of the catheter should be shortened before inserting it through the ET tube. The drug should not be given into a mainstem bronchus.
8. To ensure homogeneous distribution, each dose should be divided into four quarter-doses with each quarter-dose given with the infant in a different position—head and body inclined slightly down, head turned to the right; head and body inclined slightly down, head turned to the left; head and body inclined slightly up, head turned to the right; and head and body inclined slightly up, head turned to the left.
9. For the first dose, determine the total dose based on the infant's birth weight and withdraw the entire contents of the vial into the plastic syringe using at least a 20-gauge needle. The premeasured 5 French end-hole catheter is attached to the syringe and the catheter filled with beractant. Any excess should be discarded through the catheter so that only the total dose to be given remains in the syringe. Before giving the drug, proper placement and patency of the ET tube must be ensured (the tube may be suctioned before giving the drug). The infant should be al-

lowed to stabilize before proceeding with dosing.

10. If the first dose is to be used for prevention strategy, the dose should be administered to the stabilized infant as soon as possible after birth (preferably within 15 min). The infant is positioned appropriately and the first quarter-dose is gently injected through the catheter over 2–3 sec. After the first quarter-dose is given, the catheter is removed from the ET tube. To prevent cyanosis, manually ventilate with sufficient oxygen using a hand-bag (ambu type) at a rate of 60 breaths/min with sufficient positive pressure to provide adequate air exchange and chest wall excursion.

11. If rescue strategy is to be undertaken, the first dose should be given as soon as possible after the infant is placed on a ventilator for management of hyaline membrane disease. Studies have been undertaken in which the infant's ventilator settings were changed to a rate of 60/min (inspiratory time 0.5 sec and FiO_2 1) immediately before instilling the first quarter-dose. The infant is positioned appropriately and the first quarter-dose is gently injected through the catheter over 2–3 sec. The catheter is removed from the ET tube and the infant is returned to the mechanical ventilator.

12. When using both prevention and rescue strategies, the infant is ventilated for 20 sec or until stable. The infant is repositioned for instillation of the next quarter-dose. The remaining quarter-doses are given using the same procedures. After instillation of each quarter-dose, the catheter is removed and the infant is ventilated for 30 sec or until stabilized. After the final quarter-dose is instilled, the catheter is removed without flushing. The infant should not be suctioned for 1 hr after dosing unless signs of significant obstruction of the airway occur. After the dosing procedure is completed, usual ventilator management and clinical care should be resumed.

13. If repeat doses are necessary, the dose is also 100 mg phospholipids/kg with the dose based on the infant's birth weight (the infant should not be reweighed). Additional doses are determined by evidence of continuing respiratory distress. Repeat doses should not be given sooner than 6 hr after the preceding dose if the infant remains intubated and requires a FiO_2 of at least 30 to maintain a pO_2 of less than or equal to 80 torr. Radiographic confirmation of respiratory distress syndrome should be made before giving additional doses to infants who received a prevention dose.

14. Repeat doses are given by the same procedure as described for prevention strategy. However, studies have used different ventilator settings. For repeat doses, the FiO_2 was increased by 0.2 or an amount sufficient to prevent cyanosis. The ventilator delivered a rate of 30/min with an inspiratory time of less than 1 sec. If the infant's pretreatment rate was greater than or equal to 30, it was left unchanged during instillation. Manual hand-bag ventilation should *not* be used to give repeat doses.

15. Unopened vials should be stored in the refrigerator at 2°C–8°C (36°F–46°F) and protected from light. Vials should be stored in the carton until ready for use.

16. Ross Laboratories offers audiovisual instructional materials concerning administration procedures and dosing requirements.

Special Concerns: Beractant can quickly affect oxygenation and lung compliance; thus, it should only be used in a highly supervised setting with immediate availability of physicians experienced with intubation, ventilator management, and general care of premature infants.

Side Effects: Commonly, side effects are associated with the dosing procedure and include transient bradycardia, oxygen desaturation, ET tube reflux, vasoconstriction, pallor, hypotension, hypertension, ET tube blockage, hypocarbia, hypercarbia, and ***apnea***. Other symptoms include ***intracranial hemorrhage,*** rales, moist breath sounds, and nosocomial sepsis.

Symptom of Overdose: ***Acute airway obstruction.***

NURSING CONSIDERATIONS

Assessment

1. Note indications for medication therapy (prevention, rescue, or both).
2. The infant HR, color, chest expansion, facial expression, oximeter readings, and ET tube patency and position should be documented and monitored carefully before and during beractant therapy.
3. Ascertain that the ET tube tip is in the trachea and not in the esophagus or right or left mainstem bronchus, before inserting the 5 French end-hole catheter, to ensure appropriate drug dispersion to all lung areas.
4. Document baseline birth weight, ABGs, CXR, and physical assessment findings.

Interventions

1. Follow administration guidelines carefully. Beractant is for intratracheal administration only. It should only be administered by trained personnel in a highly supervised environment permitting continuous client observation.
2. Auscultate lung fields frequently and avoid suctioning for 1 hr after dosing unless symptoms of significant airway obstruction are evident.
3. Monitor ECG, arterial BP, and transcutaneous oxygen saturation continuously. After beractant treatment, frequent ABGs should be measured to prevent postdosing hyperoxia and hypocarbia.
4. Monitor (during dosing) for any evidence of transient bradycardia and decreased oxygen saturation. If evident, the dosing procedure should be stopped and the client treated symptomatically until stabilized; then the dosing procedure may be resumed.
5. Observe closely for air leaks and mucous plugs. If mucous plug is unrelieved by suctioning, the ET tube must be replaced immediately.

Evaluate

- Improved airway exchange with ↓ pulmonary air leaks
- Oxygen saturation readings between 90% and 95%; improved pulmonary parameters more consistent with survival
- Prevention or successful treatment of respiratory distress syndrome in premature infants

Colfosceril palmitate (Dipalmitoylphosphatidylcholine, DPPC)

(kohl-**FOSS**-sir-ill)
Exosurf Neonatal **(Rx)**

How Supplied: *Kit*

Action/Kinetics: Colfosceril contains dipalmitoylphosphatidylcholine (DPPC), which reduces surface tension in the lungs, as well as cetyl alcohol, which acts as a spreading agent for DPPC on the air–fluid surface. The product also contains tyloxapol, which is a nonionic surfactant that assists in dispersion of DPPC and cetyl alcohol, and sodium chloride to adjust osmolality. The drug can rapidly affect oxygenation and lung compliance. DPPC is reabsorbed from the alveoli into lung tissue where it is broken down and reutilized for further phospholipid synthesis and secretion.

Uses: Prophylaxis of respiratory distress syndrome in infants with birth weights of less than 1,350 g and in infants with birth weights greater than 1,350 g who manifest pulmonary immaturity. Treatment of infants who have developed respiratory distress syndrome. Such infants should be on mechanical ventilation and should have been diagnosed as having respiratory distress syndrome.

Dosage

- **Intratracheal**

Prophylaxis.
5 mL/kg (as two 2.5-mL/kg half-doses) as soon as possible after birth. A second and third dose should be given 12 and 24 hr later to infants who are still on mechanical ventilation.

Rescue treatment.
5 mL/kg (as two 2.5-mL/kg half-doses) as soon as possible after the diagnosis of respiratory distress syndrome is confirmed. A second 5-mL/kg dose is given after 12 hr to infants who are still on mechanical ventilation. The safety and effectiveness of additional doses are not known.

Administration/Storage

1. The drug should be reconstituted, according to the directions provided by the manufacturer, immediately prior to use with the diluent provided (preservative-free sterile water for injection). The reconstituted product is a milky white suspension.
2. The reconstituted suspension should be uniformly dispersed before administration. If the vial contains large flakes or particulate matter, it should not be used.
3. Five different-sized ET tube adapters are provided with each vial of colfosceril. The adapters are clean but not sterile. The adapters should be used according to the instructions provided by the manufacturer.
4. Colfosceril is administered directly into the trachea through the sideport on the special ET tube adapter without interruption of mechanical ventilation.
5. Each half-dose is given slowly over 1–2 min in small bursts timed with inspiration.
6. The first 2.5-mL/kg dose is given with the infant in the midline position; after the first half-dose is given, the infant's head and torso are first turned 45° to the right for 30 sec and then 45° to the left for 30 sec while continuing mechanical ventilation. This allows for gravity to help with lung distribution of the drug.
7. Refluxing of colfosceril into the ET tube may occur if the drug is given rapidly. If reflux is noted, administration of the drug should be stopped and the peak inspiratory pressure should be increased on the ventilator by 4–5 cm water until the ET tube clears.
8. Colfosceril administration should be undertaken only by experienced neonatologists and other individuals experienced at neonatal intubation and ventilatory management.

Special Concerns: Use of colfosceril should be undertaken only by medical personnel trained and experienced in airway and clinical management of unstable premature infants. Although colfosceril is effective in reducing mortality due to premature birth, infants may still develop severe complications resulting in either death or survival but with permanent handicaps. Benefits versus risks should be carefully assessed before using colfosceril in infants weighing 500–700 g.

Side Effects: *Respiratory:* ***Pulmonary hemorrhage, pulmonary air leak (pneumothorax, pneumomediastinum, pneumopericardium, pulmonary interstitial emphysema), mucous plugs in the ET tube, apnea,*** congenital pneumonia, nosocomial pneumonia. *CV:* ***Intraventricular hemorrhage,*** patent ductus arteriosus, hypotension, bradycardia, tachycardia, exchange transfusion, persistent fetal circulation. *Changes in blood gases:* Fall or rise in oxygen saturation, fall or rise in transcutaneous pO_2, fall or rise in transcutaneous pCO_2. *Miscellaneous:* ***Necrotizing enterocolitis,*** major anomalies, hyperbilirubinemia, gagging, thrombocytopenia, ***seizures.***

NURSING CONSIDERATIONS

Assessment

1. Review indications for drug therapy to ensure that infant meets criteria and document as rescue or prophylactic treatment.
2. The infant's color, chest expansion, facial expression, oximeter readings, HR, and ET tube patency and position should be documented and monitored carefully before and during colfosceril dosing.

3. Ascertain that the ET tube tip is in the trachea and not in the esophagus or right or left mainstem bronchus to ensure drug dispersion to all lung areas.
4. Document baseline weight, ABGs, CXR, and physical assessment findings.

Interventions

1. Confirm brisk and symmetrical chest movement and equal breath sounds in the two axillae with each mechanical inspiration prior to and at the conclusion of each dosing.
2. The infant should be suctioned before administration of the drug but not for 2 hr after colfosceril administration (unless clinically necessary).
3. It is essential that continuous monitoring of ECG, arterial BP, and transcutaneous oxygen saturation be undertaken during dosing. After either prophylactic or rescue treatment, frequent ABGs should be measured to prevent postdosing hyperoxia and hypocarbia.
4. The volume of the 5-mL/kg dose may cause a transient impairment of gas exchange due to physical blockage of the airway. Thus, infants may show a decrease in oxygen saturation during dosing, especially if they are on low ventilator settings prior to dosing. If this occurs, the peak inspiratory pressure on the ventilator should be increased by 4–5 cm water for 1–2 min. Also, the FiO_2 should be increased for 1–2 min.
5. If chest expansion improves significantly after dosing, the peak ventilator inspiratory pressure should be reduced immediately. Failure to do this may cause lung overdistention and fatal pulmonary air leak.
6. If the infant becomes pink and transcutaneous oxygen saturation is more than 95%, the FiO_2 should be reduced in small but repeated steps until saturation is 90%–95%. Failure to do this may cause hyperoxia.
7. If arterial or transcutaneous CO_2 levels are less than 30 mm Hg, the ventilator rate must be reduced immediately. Failure to do this can result in significant hypocarbia, which reduces cerebral blood flow.
8. After the dose has been administered, the position of the ET tube should be confirmed by listening for equal breath sounds in the two axillae. Particular attention should be paid to chest expansion, skin color, transcutaneous O_2 saturation, and ABGs (samples should be taken frequently). The nurse should remain at the bedside for at least 30 min after dosing.
9. Observe closely for air leaks and mucous plugs. If mucous plug is unrelieved by suctioning, the ET tube must be replaced immediately.

Evaluate

- Oxygen saturation between 90% and 95% and improved pulmonary parameters more consistent with survival
- ↓ Pulmonary air leaks and prevention of alveolar collapse

Guaifenesin (Glyceryl guaiacolate)

(gwye-**FEN**-eh-sin)

Pregnancy Category: C

Amonidrin, Anti-Tuss, Balminil Expectorant ✱, Benylin-E ✱, Breonesin, Calmylin Expectorant ✱, Fenesin, Gee-Gee, Genatuss, GG-Cen, Glyate, Glycotuss, Glytuss, Guiatuss, Halotussin, Humibid L.A. Humibid Sprinkle, Hytuss, Hytuss-2X, Mytussin, Naldecon Senior EX, Resyl ✱, Robitussin, Scottussin, Sinumist-SR Capsulets, Uni-tussin **(OTC)**

How Supplied: *Capsule:* 200 mg; *Capsule, Extended Release:* 300 mg; *Elixir:* 100 mg/5 mL; *Liquid:* 100 mg/5 mL, 200 mg/5 mL; *Syrup:* 100 mg/5 mL; *Tablet:* 100 mg, 200 mg; *Tablet, Extended Release:* 600 mg

Action/Kinetics: Guaifenesin is said to increase the output of fluid of the respiratory tract by reducing the viscosity and surface tension of respiratory secretions, thereby facilitating their expectoration. Data on efficacy are lacking; however, guaifenesin is an ingredient of many nonprescription cough preparations.

Uses: Dry, nonproductive cough due to colds and minor upper respiratory tract infections when there is mucus in the respiratory tract.

Dosage

• **Capsules, Tablets, Oral Liquid, Syrup**

Expectorant.

Adults and children over 12 years: 100–400 mg q 4 hr, not to exceed 2.4 g/day; **pediatric, 6–12 years:** 100–200 mg q 4 hr, not to exceed 1.2 g/day; **pediatric, 2–6 years:** 50–100 mg q 4 hr, not to exceed 600 mg/day. If less than 2 years of age, the dosage must be individualized by the physician.

• **Sustained-Release Capsules, Sustained-Release Tablets**

Expectorant.

Adults and children over 12 years: 600–1,200 mg q 12 hr, not to exceed 2.4 g/day; **pediatric, 6–12 years:** 600 mg q 12 hr, not to exceed 1.2 g/day; **pediatric, 2–6 years:** 300 mg q 12 hr, not to exceed 600 mg/day. *NOTE:* The liquid dosage forms may be more suitable for children less than 6 years of age.

Contraindications: Chronic cough (e.g., due to smoking, asthma, or emphysema), cough accompanied by excess secretions. Use in children under age 12 for persistent or chronic cough due to asthma or cough accompanied by excessive mucus (unless prescribed by a physician).

Special Concerns: Persistent cough may indicate a serious infection; thus, the provider should be consulted if cough lasts for more than 1 week, is recurring, or is accompanied by high fever, rash, or persistent headache.

Laboratory Test Interferences: False + urinary 5-hydroxyindoleacetic acid. Color interference with determination of urinary vanillylmandelic acid.

Side Effects: *GI:* N&V, GI upset. *CNS:* Dizziness, headache. *Dermatologic:* Rash, urticaria.

Symptoms of Overdose: N&V.

Drug Interaction: Inhibition of platelet adhesiveness by guaifenesin may result in bleeding tendencies.

NURSING CONSIDERATIONS

Client/Family Teaching

1. Take only as directed and do not exceed prescribed dosing guidelines.
2. If symptoms persist more than 1 week, recur, or are accompanied by a persistent headache, fever, or rash, medical intervention should be sought as cough may indicate a more serious condition.
3. Any evidence of increased bleeding tendencies or increased bruising should be reported.
4. Do not perform activities that require mental alertness because drug may cause drowsiness.

Evaluate

- Control of coughing episodes
- Mobilization and expectoration of pulmonary mucus

CHAPTER FIFTY-SEVEN

Cough, Cold, and Antiallergy Products

See the following individual entries:

Actifed Plus Caplets and Tablets
Actifed Sinus Daytime Caplets and Tablets
Actifed Sinus Nighttime Caplets and Tablets
Actifed Syrup
Actifed Tablets
Advil Cold and Sinus
Alka-Seltzer Plus Cold Medicine
Alka-Seltzer Plus Cold and Cough Medicine
Alka-Seltzer Plus Nighttime Cold Medicine
Alka-Seltzer Plus Sinus Allergy Medicine
Allerest 12 Hour Caplets
Allerest Children's Chewable Tablets
Allerest Headache Strength Tablets
Allerest Maximum Strength Tablets
Allerest No Drowsiness Tablets
Allerest Sinus Pain Formula Tablets
Allergy Sinus Comtrex
Chlor-Trimeton Allergy-Sinus Headache
Chlor-Trimeton Antihistamine and Decongestant Tablets
CoAdvil
Comtrex Multi-Symptom Cold Reliever
Contac Continuous Action
Contac Day & Night Cold & Flu
Contac Maximum Strength
Contac Severe Cold and Flu Formula
Contac Severe Cold and Flu Hot Medicine Drink
Contac Severe Cold and Flu Nighttime Liquid
Coricidin
Coricidin D
Cough Formula Comtrex
Day-Night Comtrex
Dextromethorphan Hydrobromide
Dimetane Decongestant Elixir and Tablets
Dimetapp Cold & Allergy Chewable Tablets
Dimetapp Cold & Flu Caplets
Dimetapp DM Elixir, Extentabs, Liquibels, Sinus Caplets, Tablets
Dristan Allergy Caplets
Dristan Cold Tablets
Dristan Menthol Nasal Spray and Nasal Decongestant Spray
Dristan Juice Mix-In
Dristan Sinus Caplets
Drixoral Cold & Allergy Sustained-Action Tablets
Drixoral Cold & Flu Extended-Release Tablets
Drixoral Non-Drowsy Formula
Drixoral Sinus
Entex LA
Hycodan Syrup and Tablets
Maximum Strength Dristan Cold Multi-Symptom Formula
Maximum Strength Dristan Cold No Drowsiness Formula
Medi-Flu
Medi-Flu without Drowsiness
Naldecon Syrup and Tablets
Non-Drowsy Comtrex
Novahistine DMX
Novahistine Elixir
Ornade
Phenergan with Codeine Syrup
Phenergan with Dextromethorphan Syrup

Phenergan VC with Codeine Syrup
Phenergan VC Syrup
Pseudoephedrine Hydrochloride and Guaifenesin
Robitussin-AC
Robitussin-CF
Robitussin-DM
Robitussin-PE
Robitussin Maximum Strength Cough and Cold
Robitussin Night Relief Cough/Cold/Flu Formula
Robitussin Pediatric Cough and Cold Formula
Rondec-DM Oral Drops
Rondec-DM Syrup
Rynatan
Tavist-D
Trinalin
Tussi-Organidin
Tussi-Organidin DM
Tussionex Capsules, Suspension, and Tablets

COMBINATION DRUG

Actifed Plus Caplets and Tablets

(OTC)
(**AK**-tih-fed)

Actifed Sinus Daytime Caplets and Tablets

(OTC)
(**AK**-tih-fed)

Actifed Sinus Nighttime Caplets and Tablets

(OTC)
(**AK**-tih-fed)

Actifed Syrup

(OTC)
(**AK**-tih-fed)

Actifed Tablets

(OTC)
(**AK**-tih-fed)

How Supplied: See Content
Content: Each Actifed Plus Caplet or Tablet contains: *Antihistamine:* Triprolidine HCl, 1.25 mg. *Decongestant:* Pseudoephedrine HCl, 30 mg. *Analgesic/Antipyretic:* Acetaminophen, 500 mg.

Each Actifed Sinus Daytime Caplet or Tablet contains: *Decongestant:* Pseudoephedrine HCl, 30 mg. *Analgesic/Antipyretic:* Acetaminophen, 325 mg.

Each Actifed Sinus Nighttime Caplet or Tablet contains: *Antihistamine:* Diphenhydramine HCl, 25 mg. *Decongestant:* Pseudoephedrine HCl, 30 mg. *Analgesic/Antipyretic:* Acetaminophen, 500 mg.

Each 5 mL of Actifed Syrup contains: *Antihistamine:* Triprolidine HCl, 1.25 mg. *Decongestant:* Pseudoephedrine HCl, 30 mg.

Each Actifed Tablet contains: *Antihistamine:* Triprolidine HCl, 2.5 mg. *Decongestant:* Pseudoephedrine HCl, 60 mg.

Uses: Relief of symptoms of the common cold, seasonal allergies (hay fever), and sinus congestion. Symptoms relieved include runny nose, sneezing, itching of the nose and throat, itchy and watery eyes, nasal congestion and stuffiness, sinus pressure. Products containing acetaminophen are used for the above symptoms as well as for minor aches, pains, headache, and fever due to the common cold.

Dosage

- **Actifed Plus Caplets or Tablets**

Adults and children over 12 years: 2 caplets q 6 hr, not to exceed 8 caplets or tablets in a 24-hr period. Not recommended for children under 12 years of age.

- **Actifed Sinus Daytime Caplets or Tablets**

Adults and children over 12 years: 2 caplets or tablets q 4–6 hr, not to exceed a total of 8 caplets or tablets in a 24-hr period. Not recommended for children under 12 years of age.

- **Actifed Sinus Nighttime Caplets or Tablets**

Adults and children over 12 years: 2 caplets or tablets at bedtime. Not to be taken during waking hours unless confined to a bed or resting at home; 2 caplets or tablets may then be taken q 6 hr, not to exceed a total of 8 caplets or tablets in a 24-hr period. Not recommended for children under 12 years of age.

• **Actifed Syrup**

Adults and children over 12 years: 10 mL (2 teaspoons) q 4–6 hr. **Children, 6–12 years of age:** 5 mL (1 teaspoon) q 4–6 hr. **Children under 6 years of age:** A physician should be consulted. No more than four doses should be taken in a 24-hr period.

• **Actifed Tablets**

Adults and children over 12 years of age: 1 tablet q 4–6 hr. **Children, 6–12 years of age:** ½ tablet q 4–6 hr. **Children under 6 years of age:** A physician should be consulted. No more than four doses should be taken in a 24-hr period.

Administration/Storage: Actifed Sinus Daytime products should not be taken within 4 hr of Actifed Sinus Nighttime products.

Contraindications: Use in hypertension, heart disease, diabetes, thyroid disease, asthma, glaucoma, chronic pulmonary disease, SOB, difficulty in breathing, difficulty in urination due to enlarged prostate gland. Actifed products containing pseudoephedrine should not be used in clients taking antihypertensive medications or products containing a MAO inhibitor, unless ordered by the physician.

Special Concerns: These products may cause excitability in children. If pregnant or nursing, a physician should be consulted before taking Actifed products.

NURSING CONSIDERATIONS

See *Nursing Considerations* for *Antihistamines,* Chapter 55.

Evaluate

• Relief of cold symptoms and nasal congestion

• ↓ Upper respiratory allergic manifestations

COMBINATION DRUG

Advil Cold and Sinus

(OTC)

How Supplied: See Content

Content: Each tablet contains: *Analgesic/Antipyretic:* Ibuprofen, 200 mg. *Decongestant:* Pseudoephedrine HCl, 30 mg. See also information on individual components.

Uses: Temporary relief of symptoms associated with the common cold, sinusitis, or flu, including nasal congestion, headache, fever, body aches, and pains.

Dosage

• **Tablets**

Adults and children over 12 years of age: 1 tablet q 4–6 hr; may be increased to 2 tablets if symptoms persist, up to a maximum of 6 tablets in a 24-hr period.

Administration/Storage: The product may be taken with food or milk if mild heartburn, stomach upset, or stomach pain occurs.

Contraindications: Clients sensitive to aspirin. Hypertension, heart disease, diabetes, thyroid disease, difficulty in urination due to enlarged prostate. During the last 3 months of pregnancy. Should not be taken for more than 7 days for a cold or more than 3 days for a fever.

Special Concerns: A physician should be consulted before using during pregnancy and lactation. Use in children less than 12 years of age only on the advice of a physician.

Side Effects: *Higher doses:* Nervousness, dizziness, sleeplessness.

NURSING CONSIDERATIONS

See *Nursing Considerations* for individual components.

Evaluate: Relief of cold and flu symptoms.

COMBINATION DRUG

Alka-Seltzer Plus Cold Medicine

(OTC)

Alka-Seltzer Plus Night-Time Cold Medicine

(OTC)

Alka-Seltzer Plus Sinus Allergy Medicine
(OTC)

Alka-Seltzer Plus Cold & Cough Medicine
(OTC)

How Supplied: See Content

Content: See also information on the individual components.

Each tablet of Alka-Seltzer Plus Cold Medicine contains: *Analgesic/antipyretic:* Aspirin, 325 mg. *Decongestant:* Phenylpropanolamine bitrate, 24.08 mg. *Antihistamine:* Chlorpheniramine maleate, 2 mg.

Each tablet of Alka-Seltzer Plus Night-Time Cold Medicine contains: *Analgesic/antipyretic:* Aspirin, 500 mg. *Decongestant:* Phenylpropanolamine bitartrate, 20 mg. *Antihistamine:* Brompheniramine maleate, 2 mg. *Antitussive:* Dextromethorphan HBr, 10 mg.

Each tablet of Alka-Seltzer Plus Sinus Allergy Medicine contains: *Analgesic/antipyretic:* Aspirin, 500 mg. *Decongestant:* Phenylpropanolamine bitartrate, 24.08 mg. *Antihistamine:* Brompheniramine maleate, 2 mg.

Each tablet of Alka-Seltzer Plus Cold and Cough Medicine contains: *Analgesic/antipyretic:* Aspirin, 500 mg. *Decongestant:* Phenylpropanolamine bitartrate, 24.08 mg. *Antihistamine:* Chlorpheniramine maleate, 2 mg. *Antitussive:* Dextromethorphan, 10 mg.

Uses: For temporary relief of the major symptoms of colds, flu, and allergy including nasal and sinus congestion, body aches and pains, runny nose, cough, headache, sore throat, sneezing, fever.

Dosage

- **Effervescent Tablets**

Adults: For all products, 2 tablets dissolved in 4 oz of water taken q 4 hr, up to a maximum of 8 tablets in a 24-hr period.

Administration/Storage: Additional fluid intake is encouraged for clients with colds.

Contraindications: Use during the last 3 months of pregnancy. Use in children and teenagers for chicken pox or flu symptoms, unless ordered by a physician. Use in aspirin allergy, asthma, glaucoma, bleeding problems, emphysema, chronic pulmonary disease, SOB, difficulty in breathing, heart disease, hypertension, thyroid disease, diabetes, or difficulty in urinating due to an enlarged prostate. Use if the client is taking anticoagulants or medication for gout, arthritis, hypertension, or depression, unless ordered by a physician. Dextromethorphan-containing products should not be taken for persistent or chronic cough due to smoking, asthma, or emphysema.

Special Concerns: These products may cause excitability, especially in children. Should not be taken for more than 7 days for cold symptoms or 3 days if fever is present.

Side Effects: *Higher doses:* Dizziness, nervousness, sleeplessness.

NURSING CONSIDERATIONS

See also *Nursing Considerations* for individual components.

Evaluate: Relief of cold and flu symptoms.

COMBINATION DRUG

Allerest 12 Hour Caplets
(OTC)

Allerest Children's Chewable Tablets
(OTC)

Allerest Headache Strength Tablets
(OTC)

Allerest Maximum Strength Tablets
(OTC)

Allerest No Drowsiness Tablets
(OTC)

Allerest Sinus Pain Formula Tablets
(OTC)

How Supplied: See Content

Content: Each Allerest 12 Hour Caplet contains: *Antihistamine:* Chlorpheniramine maleate, 12 mg. *Decontestant:* Phenylpropanolamine HCl, 75 mg.

Each Allerest Children's Chewable Tablet contains: *Antihistamine:* Chlorpheniramine maleate, 1 mg. *Decongestant:* Phenylpropanolamine HCl, 9.4 mg.

Each Allerest Headache Strength Tablet contains: *Analgesic/antipyretic:* Acetaminophen, 325 mg. *Antihistamine:* Chlorpheniramine maleate, 2 mg. *Decongestant:* Pseudoephedrine HCl, 30 mg.

Each Allerest Maximum Strength Tablet contains: *Antihistamine:* Chlorpheniramine maleate, 2 mg. *Decongestant:* Pseudoephedrine HCl, 30 mg.

Each Allerest No Drowsiness Tablet contains: *Analgesic/antipyretic:* Acetaminophen, 325 mg. *Decongestant:* Pseudoephedrine HCl, 30 mg.

Each Allerest Sinus Pain Formula Tablet contains: *Analgesic/antipyretic:* Acetaminophen, 500 mg. *Antihistamine:* Chlorpheniramine maleate, 2 mg. *Decongestant:* Pseudoephedrine HCl, 30 mg.

Uses: *12 Hour Caplets, Children's Chewable Tablets, Headache Strength, Maximum Strength, Sinus Pain Formula:* Relief of nasal congestion, runny nose, sneezing, itching of the nose or throat, and itchy, watery eyes due to hay fever or other upper respiratory tract allergies. 12 Hour Caplets are also used for relief of nasal congestion due to the common cold and associated with sinusitis. Headache Strength and Sinus Pain Formula are also used for relief of minor aches, pains, and headache. *No Drowsiness:* Relief of nasal congestion due to hay fever or other respiratory tract allergies and for relief of minor aches, pains, and headaches.

Dosage

- **12 Hour Caplets**

Adults and children over 12 years of age: 1 caplet q 12 hr, not to exceed 2 caplets in a 24-hr period.

- **Children's Chewable Tablets**

Children, 6–12 years of age: 2 tablets q 4 hr, not to exceed 8 tablets in a 24-hr period. **Children under 6 years of age:** A physician should be consulted.

- **Headache Strength Tablets, Maximum Strength Tablets, No Drowsiness Tablets**

Adults and children over 12 years of age: 2 tablets q 4 hr, not to exceed 8 tablets in a 24-hr period. **Children 6–12 years of age:** 1 tablet q 4 hr, not to exceed 4 tablets in a 24-hr period. **Children under 6 years of age:** A physician should be consulted.

- **Sinus Pain Formula Tablets**

Adults and children over 12 years of age: 2 tablets q 6 hr, not to exceed 8 tablets in a 24-hr period. **Children under 12 years of age:** A physician should be consulted.

Administration/Storage

1. The 12 Hour Caplets, Children's Chewable Tablets, and Maximum Strength Tablets should not be taken for more than 7 days. The Headache Strength, No Drowsiness Tablets, and Sinus Pain Formula should not be taken for more than 10 days by adults or 5 days by children.
2. If symptoms do not improve, fever lasts more than 3 days, or new symptoms appear, the provider should be notified.

Contraindications: Use in heart disease, hypertension, thyroid disease, diabetes, difficulty in urination due to an enlarged prostate. With the exception of the No Drowsiness Tablets, these products should not be taken by clients with asthma, glaucoma, emphysema, chronic pulmonary disease, SOB, difficulty in breathing.

Special Concerns: Use during pregnancy and lactation only if prescribed by a physician. May cause excitability, especially in children.

Side Effects: *Higher doses:* Dizziness, nervousness, sleeplessness.

Drug Interactions: Drowsiness may be increased by alcohol, sedative, and antianxiety agents.

NURSING CONSIDERATIONS

See also *Nursing Considerations* for individual components.

Evaluate

- Relief of nasal congestion
- ↓ Upper respiratory allergic manifestations

COMBINATION DRUG

Chlor-Trimeton Allergy-Sinus Headache
(OTC)

Chlor-Trimeton Antihistamine and Decongestant Tablets
(OTC)

See also information on individual components.

How Supplied: See Content

Content: Each Chlor-Trimeton Allergy-Sinus Headache caplet contains: *Analgesic/antipyretic:* Acetaminophen, 500 mg. *Antihistamine:* Chlorpheniramine maleate, 2 mg. *Decongestant:* Phenylpropanolamine HCl, 12.5 mg.

Each Chlor-Trimeton Antihistamine and Decongestant Tablet contains: *Antihistamine:* Chlorpheniramine maleate, 4 mg. *Decongestant:* Pseudoephedrine sulfate, 60 mg. The long- acting Repeatabs contain twice the amount of each component.

Uses: Relief of nasal congestion; sneezing, itchy, watery eyes; itchy throat and runny nose due to hay fever and other upper respiratory conditions. The Allergy-Sinus Headache caplets are also used for relief of sinus pain.

Dosage

- **Allergy-Sinus Headache Caplets**

Adults and children over 12 years of age: 2 caplets q 6 hr, not to exceed 8 caplets in a 24-hr period.

- **Antihistamine and Decongestant Tablets**

Adults and children over 12 years of age: 1 tablet q 4–6 hr, not to exceed 4 tablets in a 24-hr period. **Children, 6–11 years of age:** ½ tablet q 4–6 hr, not to exceed 2 whole tablets in a 24-hr period. **Children, less than 6 years of age:** Consult a physician. Commonly, ¼ tablet q 4 hr, not to exceed 1 whole tablet in a 24-hr period.

- **Antihistamine and Decongestant Long-Acting (Repeatabs)**

Adults and children over 12 years of age: 1 tablet q 12 hr, not to exceed 2 tablets in a 24-hr period.

Administration/Storage

1. These products should not be taken for more than 7 days for pain or congestion or more than 3 days for fever, unless directed by a physician.
2. Swallow only 1 caplet at a time.

Contraindications: Use of the Allergy-Sinus Headache product in children less than 12 years of age. Use in asthma, glaucoma, emphysema, chronic pulmonary disease, SOB, difficulty in breathing, heart disease, hypertension, thyroid disease, diabetes, or difficulty in urination due to prostate enlargement. Use of alcoholic beverages. Not to be used if the client is on medication for hypertension or depression or is taking a phenylpropanolamine-containing appetite suppressant.

Special Concerns: May cause excitability in children. A physician should be consulted before use in pregnancy and lactation.

Side Effects: *At higher doses:* Dizziness, nervousness, sleeplessness.

Drug Interactions: Alcohol, sedatives, and antianxiety agents enhance the effect of these products.

NURSING CONSIDERATIONS

See also *Nursing Considerations* for individual components.

Assessment

1. Document indications for therapy and type and onset of symptoms.
2. Determine any conditions that preclude the administration of this medication.

Evaluate: Relief of nasal congestion and symptoms of allergic manifestations.

—COMBINATION DRUG—

CoAdvil

(koh-**AD**-vil)
(OTC)

How Supplied: See Content
Content: Each tablet contains: *NSAID:* Ibuprofen, 200 mg. *Decongestant:* Pseudoephedrine HCl, 30 mg. See also information on individual components.
Uses: Temporary relief of symptoms associated with the common cold, flu, or sinusitis including fever, headache, nasal congestion, body aches, and pains.

Dosage
- **Tablets**

Adults: 1 tablet q 4–6 hr while symptoms persist. If no response, dose can be increased to 2 tablets but the total dose should not exceed 6 tablets in 24 hr, unless directed otherwise by a physician.
Administration/Storage: The drug can be taken with food or milk if mild heartburn, stomach upset, or stomach pain occurs.
Contraindications: Clients sensitive to aspirin. Hypertension, heart disease, diabetes, thyroid disease, difficulty in urination due to enlarged prostate. During the last 3 months of pregnancy. Should not be taken for more than 7 days for a cold or for more than 3 days for fever.
Special Concerns: Use with caution during lactation. Use in children under 12 years of age only on the advice of a physician.
Side Effects: *Higher doses:* Nervousness, dizziness, or sleeplessness. See also individual drugs.

NURSING CONSIDERATIONS

See also *Nursing Considerations* for individual components.
Assessment
1. Document any history of hypertension, CAD, diabetes, thyroid disease, or difficulty with urination as drug is contraindicated.
2. Determine indications for therapy and identify onset of symptoms.

Client/Family Teaching
1. Take only as directed.
2. Seek medical assistance if cold symptoms persist more than 7 days or if fever lasts more than 3 days.

Evaluate: Relief of cold and flu symptoms.

—COMBINATION DRUG—

Allergy-Sinus Comtrex
(OTC)

Comtrex Multi-Symptom Cold Reliever
(OTC)

Cough Formula Comtrex
(OTC)

Day-Night Comtrex
(OTC)

Non-Drowsy Comtrex
(OTC)

See also information on individual components.
How Supplied: See Content
Content: Each caplet or tablet of Allergy-Sinus Comtrex contains: *Analgesic/antipyretic:* Acetaminophen, 500 mg. *Antihistamine:* Chlorpheniramine maleate, 2 mg. *Decongestant:* Pseudoephedrine HCl, 30 mg.

Each caplet or tablet of Comtrex Multi-Symptom Cold Reliever contains: *Analgesic/antipyretic:* Acetaminophen, 325 mg. *Antihistamine:* Chlorpheniramine, 2 mg. *Decongestant:* Pseudoephedrine HCl, 30 mg. *Antitussive:* Dextromethorphan HBr, 10 mg. Each fluid ounce of the liquid contains twice the amount of each ingredient as is in the caplets or tablets. Comtrex Multi-Symptom Cold Reliever Liquid-Gel contains the same ingredients as the caplets or tablets except phenylpropanolamine HCl, 12.5 mg, is substituted for pseudoephedrine HCl.

Each ⅔ fluid ounce of Cough Formula Comtrex contains: *Expectorant:* Guaifenesin, 200 mg. *Antitussive:* Dextromethorphan HBr, 20 mg.

Analgesic/antipyretic: Acetaminophen, 500 mg. *Decongestant:* Pseudoephedrine HCl, 60 mg.

Each Daytime Comtrex Caplet contains: *Analgesic/antipyretic:* Acetaminophen, 325 mg. *Decongestant:* Pseudoephedrine HCl, 30 mg. *Antitussive:* Dextromethorphan HBr, 10 mg. In addition to the above, each Nighttime Tablet contains: *Antihistamine:* Chlorpheniramine maleate, 2 mg.

Each caplet of Non-Drowsy Comtrex contains: *Analgesic/antipyretic:* Acetaminophen, 325 mg. *Decongestant:* Pseudoephedrine HCl, 10 mg. *Antitussive:* Dextromethorphan HBr, 10 mg.

Uses: Relief of cold and flu symptoms, including nasal and sinus congestion, runny nose, sneezing, coughing, minor sore throat pain, headache, fever, body aches, and pain.

Dosage

• **Allergy-Sinus Comtrex Caplets or Tablets**

Adults and children over 12 years of age: 2 caplets or tablets q 6 hr while symptoms persist, not to exceed 8 caplets or tablets in a 24-hr period.

• **Comtrex Multi-Symptom Cold Reliever Caplets or Tablets**

Adults and children over 12 years of age: 2 caplets or tablets q 4 hr, not to exceed 8 caplets or tablets in a 24-hr period. **Children, 6–12 years of age:** 1 caplet or tablet q 4 hr, not to exceed 4 caplets or tablets in a 24-hr period.

• **Comtrex Multi-Symptom Cold Reliever Liqui-Gel**

Adults and children over 12 years of age: 2 liqui-gels q 4 hr, not to exceed 12 liqui-gels in a 24-hr period. **Children, 6–12 years of age:** 1 liqui-gel q 4 hr, not to exceed 5 liqui-gels in a 24-hr period.

• **Comtrex Multi-Symptom Cold Reliever Liquid**

Adults and children over 12 years of age: 30 mL (1 fluid oz or 2 tablespoons) q 4 hr, not to exceed four doses in a 24-hr period. **Children, 6–12 years of age:** 15 mL (½ fluid oz or 1 tablespoon) q 4 hr, not to exceed four doses in a 24-hr period.

• **Cough Formula Comtrex**

Adults and children over 12 years of age: 20 mL (⅔ oz or 4 teaspoons) q 4 hr, not to exceed four doses in a 24-hr period. **Children, 6–12 years of age:** 10 mL (⅓ fluid ounce or 2 teaspoons) q 4 hr, not to exeed four doses in a 24-hr period.

• **Day-Night Comtrex**

Adults and children over 12 years of age: 2 Daytime caplets q 4 hr, not to exceed 6 Daytime caplets in a 24-hr period. Two Night-time tablets at bedtime, if needed, to be taken no sooner than 4 hr after the last Daytime caplet dose.

• **Non-Drowsy Comtrex**

Adults and children over 12 years of age: 2 caplets q 4 hr, not to exceed 8 caplets in a 24-hr period. **Children, 6–12 years of age:** 1 caplet q 4 hr, not to exceed 4 caplets in a 24-hr period.

Administration/Storage

1. Products should not be used for more than 7 days in adults or 5 days in children.
2. Products should not be used for more than 3 days for fever.
3. Products should only be taken while symptoms persist.

Contraindications: Cough products should not be taken for persistent or chronic cough due to smoking, asthma, or emphysema or if cough is accompanied by excessive phlegm. These products should not be used by clients who have asthma, glaucoma, emphysema, chronic pulmonary disease, hypertension, heart disease, thyroid disease, diabetes, SOB, difficulty in breathing, or difficulty in urination due to an enlarged prostate. Should not be used by clients taking medications for hypertension or depression.

Special Concerns: A physician should be consulted before using these products during pregnancy or lactation. May cause excitability, especially in children.

Side Effects: *At higher doses:* Dizziness, nervousness, sleeplessness.

Drug Interactions: Use of alcohol, sedatives, or anti-anxiety agents will enhance the effects of products containing an antihistamine.

NURSING CONSIDERATIONS

See also *Nursing Considerations* for individual components.
Evaluate: Relief of cold and flu symptoms.

—COMBINATION DRUG—

Contac Continuous Action
(OTC)

Contac Day & Night Cold & Flu
(OTC)

Contac Maximum Strength
(OTC)

Contac Severe Cold and Flu Formula
(OTC)

Contac Severe Cold and Flu Hot Medicine Drink
(OTC)

Contac Severe Cold and Flu Nighttime Liquid
(OTC)

See also information on individual components.
How Supplied: See Content
Content: Each capsule of Contac Continuous Action contains: *Decongestant:* Phenylpropanolamine HCl, 75 mg. *Antihistamine:* Chlorpheniramine maleate, 8 mg. Contac Maximum Strength caplets contain the same amount of decongestant but 12 mg of the antihistamine.

Each caplet of Contac Day Cold & Flu contains: *Analgesic/antipyretic:* Acetaminophen, 650 mg. *Decongestant:* Pseudoephedrine HCl, 60 mg. *Antitussive:* Dextromethorphan HBr, 30 mg.

Each caplet of Contac Night Cold & Flu contains: *Analgesic/antipyretic:* Acetaminophen, 650 mg. *Decongestant:* Pseudoephedrine HCl, 60 mg. *Antihistamine:* Diphenhydramine HCl, 50 mg.

Each caplet of Contac Severe Cold & Flu Formula contains: *Analgesic/antipyretic:* Acetaminophen, 500 mg. *Decongestant:* Phenylpropanolamine HCl, 12.5 mg. *Antihistamine:* Chlorpheniramine maleate, 2 mg. *Antitussive:* Dextromethorphan HBr, 15 mg.

Each packet dose of Contac Severe Cold and Flu Hot Medicine Drink contains: *Analgesic/antipyretic:* Acetaminophen, 650 mg. *Decongestant:* Pseudoephedrine HCl, 60 mg. *Antihistamine:* Chlorpheniramine maleate, 4 mg. *Antitussive:* Dextromethorphan HBr, 20 mg.

Each 30 mL of Contac Severe Cold and Flu Nighttime Liquid contains: *Analgesic/antipyretic:* Acetaminophen, 1,000 mg. *Decongestant:* Pseudoephedrine HCl, 60 mg. *Antihistamine:* Chlorpheniramine maleate, 4 mg. *Antitussive:* Dextromethorphan HBr, 30 mg.
Uses: Relief of nasal congestion, fever, minor aches and pains, runny nose, sneezing due to the common cold and flu. Also, relief of nasal congestion due to sinusitis and upper respiratory allergies.

Dosage

- **Contac Continuous Action Capsules**

Adults and children over 12 years of age: 1 capsule q 12 hr, not to exceed 2 capsules in a 24-hr period.

- **Contac Day & Night Cold & Flu Caplets**

Adults and children over 12 years of age: 1 yellow day caplet q 6 hr. Or, 1 blue night caplet q 6 hr. A total of 4 caplets, whether day or night formula, should not be exceeded in a 24-hr period. Regardless of the caplet taken, they should be taken at least 6 hr apart.

• **Contac Maximum Strength Caplets**

Adults and children over 12 years of age: 1 caplet q 12 hr, not to exceed 2 caplets in a 24-hr period.

• **Contac Severe Cold & Flu Formula Caplets**

Adults and children over 12 years of age: 2 caplets q 6 hr, not to exceed 8 caplets in a 24-hr period.

• **Contac Severe Cold & Flu Nighttime Liquid**

Adults and children over 12 years of age: 30 mL (2 tablespoons) q 6 hr. May be repeated q 6 hr, not to exceed 120 mL (8 tablespoons) in a 24-hr period.

Administration/Storage

1. These products should not be taken for more than 7 days if cough or other symptoms do not improve and for more than 3 days for fever.
2. Medicine cups are provided for the liquid product.

Contraindications: Use in children less than 12 years of age. Use in hypertension, heart disease, diabetes, glaucoma, thyroid disease, difficulty in urinating due to an enlarged prostate. Use in persistent cough, as with smoking, asthma, and emphysema or if cough is accompanied by excessive phlegm. Use in clients taking medication for hypertension or depression. Products containing phenylpropanolamine should not be taken with other products containing this drug.

Special Concerns: May cause excitability, especially in children.

Side Effects: *At higher doses:* Dizziness, nervousness, sleeplessness.

Drug Interactions: The effect of products containing an antihistamine will be enhanced if taken with alcohol, sedatives, or anti-anxiety agents.

NURSING CONSIDERATIONS

See also *Nursing Considerations* for individual components.

Evaluate:

• ↓ Nasal congestion
• Relief of cold and flu symptoms

COMBINATION DRUG

Coricidin
(OTC)

Coricidin D
(OTC)

See also information on individual components.

How Supplied: See Content

Content: Each Coricidin tablet contains: *Analgesic/antipyretic:* Acetaminophen, 325 mg. *Antihistamine:* Chlorpheniramine maleate, 2 mg.

Each Coricidin D tablet contains: *Analgesic/antipyretic:* Acetaminophen, 325 mg. *Antihistamine:* Chlorpheniramine, 2 mg. *Decongestant:* Phenylpropanolamine HCl, 12.5 mg.

Uses: *Coricidin:* Relief of symptoms of cold, flu, and allergy.

Coricidin D: Relief of symptoms of congested cold, flu, and sinus.

Dosage

• **Coricidin or Coricidin D Tablets**

Adults and children over 12 years of age: 2 tablets q 4 hr, not to exceed 12 tablets in a 24-hr period. **Children, 6–11 years of age:** 1 tablet q 4 hr, not to exceed 5 tablets in a 24-hr period.

Administration/Storage: Coricidin should not be taken for more than 10 days for adults (7 days if using Coricidin D) and 5 days for children (6–11 years of age) and for fever for more than 3 days.

Contraindications: Use in hypertension, heart disease, diabetes, glaucoma, thyroid disease, difficulty in urinating due to an enlarged prostate. Use in persistent cough, as with smoking, asthma, and emphysema or if cough is accompanied by excessive phlegm. Use in clients taking medication for hypertension or depression. Products containing phenylpropanolamine should not be taken with other products containing this drug.

Special Concern: May cause excitability, especially in children.

Side Effects: *At higher doses:* Dizziness, nervousness, sleeplessness.

Drug Interactions: The effect of products containing an antihistamine will be enhanced if taken with alcohol, sedatives, or anti-anxiety agents.

NURSING CONSIDERATIONS

See also *Nursing Considerations* for individual components.

Evaluate

- Relief of cold and flu symptoms
- ↓ Allergic manifestations

Dextromethorphan hydrobromide

(dex-troh-meth-**OR**-fan)

Anti-Cough Syrup ✱, Balminil D.M. Syrup ✱, Benylin DM, Broncho-Grip-pol-DM ✱, Children's Hold, Delsym, D-M No Sugar ✱, Hold DM, Koffex Syrup ✱, Neo-DM ✱, Ornex-DM ✱, Pertussin CS, Pertussin ES, Robidex Syrup ✱, Robitussin Cough Calmers, Robitussin Pediatric, St. Joseph Cough Suppressant, Scot-Tussin DM Cough Chasers, Sedatuss ✱, Sucrets Cough Control, Suppress, Trocal, Vick's Children's Cough Syrup ✱, Vick's Formula 44, Vick's Formula 44 Pediatric Formula **(OTC)**

How Supplied: *Capsule*: 30mg; *Concentrate:* 40 mg/5 mL; *Liquid:* 3.5 mg/5 mL, 5 mg/5 mL, 7.5 mg/5 mL; *Lozenge/troche:* 2.5 mg, 5 mg, 15 mg; *Suspension, Extended Release:* 30 mg/5 mL; *Syrup:* 3.5 mg/5 mL, 7.5 mg/5 mL, 10 mg/5 mL, 15 mg/5 mL, 20 mg/15 mL; *Tablet:* 15 mg

Action/Kinetics: Dextromethorphan selectively depresses the cough center in the medulla. Dextromethorphan 15–30 mg is equal to 8–15 mg codeine as an antitussive. It is a common ingredient of nonprescription cough medications; it does not produce physical dependence or respiratory depression. Well absorbed from GI tract. **Onset:** 15–30 min. **Duration:** 3–6 hr. The sustained liquid contains dextromethorphan plistirex equivalent to 30 mg dextromethorphan hydrobromide per 5 mL.

Use: Symptomatic relief of nonproductive cough due to colds or inhaled irritants.

Dosage

- **Liquid, Lozenges, Syrup**

  Antitussive.

Adults and children over 12 years: 10–30 mg q 4–8 hr, not to exceed 120 mg/day; **pediatric, 6–12 years:** either 5–10 mg q 4 hr or 15 mg q 6–8 hr, not to exceed 60 mg/day; **pediatric, 2–6 years:** either 2.5–7.5 mg q 4 hr or 7.5 mg q 6–8 hr of the syrup, not to exceed 30 mg/day.

- **Sustained-Release Liquid**

  Antitussive.

Adults: 60 mg q 12 hr. **Pediatric, 6–12 years:** 30 mg q 12 hr, not to exceed 60 mg/day; **pediatric, 2–6 years:** 15 mg q 12 hr, not to exceed 30 mg/day.

Administration/Storage

1. Increasing the dose of dextromethorphan will not increase its effectiveness but will increase the duration of action.
2. The lozenges should not be given to children under 6 years of age.

Contraindications: Persistent or chronic cough or when cough is accompanied by excessive secretions. Use during first trimester of pregnancy unless directed otherwise by physician.

Special Concerns: Use is not recommended in children less than 2 years of age. Use with caution in clients with nausea, vomiting, high fever, rash, or persistent headache.

Side Effects: *CNS:* Dizziness, drowsiness. *GI:* N&V, stomach pain.

Symptoms of Overdose: **Adults:** Dysphoria, slurred speech, ataxia, altered sensory perception. **Children:** Ataxia, ***convulsions, respiratory depression.***

Drug Interaction: Use with MAO inhibitors may cause nausea, hypotension, hyperpyrexia, myoclonic leg jerks, and coma.

NURSING CONSIDERATIONS

Assessment

1. Note the length of time the client has had the cough. Document sputum production and characteristics. If the cough persists beyond a week, dextromethorphan should not be given.
2. Determine if the client has had nausea, vomiting, persistent headaches, or a high fever.
3. If the client is pregnant, determine if she is in the first trimester of pregnancy. The drug is contraindicated in this setting.

Client/Family Teaching

1. Do not perform any tasks that require mental alertness until drug effects realized.
2. Avoid alcohol in any form.
3. Humidity should be added to a dry environment.
4. Advise that smoke, dust, and chemical fumes are irritants that may aggravate underlying condition.
5. Symptoms that persist for more than a week require medical intervention; record onset and response to therapy.

Evaluate: Control of cough with improved sleep patterns.

—COMBINATION DRUG—

Dimetane Decongestant Elixir and Tablets

(**DYE**-meh-tayn)
(OTC)

See also information on individual components.

How Supplied: See Content

Content: *Antihistamine:* Brompheniramine maleate, 4 mg/tablet or 2 mg/5 mL elixir. *Decongestant:* Phenylephrine HCl, 10 mg/tablet or 5 mg/5 mL elixir. Also see information on individual components.

Uses: Relief of symptoms due to the common cold, hay fever, sinusitis, or other upper respiratory tract allergies including sneezing, itchy nose or throat, runny nose, itchy and watery eyes.

Dosage

- **Tablets**

Adults and children over 12 years: 1 tablet q 4 hr, not to exceed 6 tablets/day; **pediatric, 6–12 years:** ½ tablet q 4 hr, not to exceed 3 whole tablets/day.

- **Elixir**

Adults and children over 12 years: 10 mL q 4 hr, not to exceed 60 mL/day; **pediatric, 6–12 years:** 5 mL q 4 hr, not to exceed 30 mL/day.

Special Concern: May cause stimulation, especially in children.

NURSING CONSIDERATIONS

See *Nursing Considerations* for *Antihistamines,* Chapter 55.

Evaluate: Relief of nasal congestion and related allergic manifestations.

—COMBINATION DRUG—

Dimetapp Cold & Allergy Chewable Tablets

(**DYE**-meh-tap)
(OTC)

Dimetapp Cold & Flu Caplets

(OTC)

Dimetapp DM Elixir, Elixir, Extentabs, Liquigels, Sinus Caplets, Tablets

(OTC)

See also information on individual components.

How Supplied: See Content

Content: Each Dimetapp Cold & Allergy Chewable Tablet contains: *Decongestant:* Phenylpropanolamine HCl, 6.25 mg. *Antihistamine:* Brompheniramine maleate, 1 mg.

Each Dimetapp Cold & Flu Caplet contains: *Analgesic/antipyretic:* Acetaminophen, 500 mg. *Decongestant:* Phenylpropanolamine, 12.5 mg. *Antihistamine:* Brompheniramine maleate, 2 mg.

Each 5 mL of Dimetapp DM Elixir contains: *Decongestant:* Phenylpropanolamine HCl, 12.5 mg. *Antihistamine:* Brompheniramine maleate, 2 mg. *Antitussive:* Dextromethorphan

HBr, 10 mg. *NOTE:* Dimetapp Elixir contains the same amount of decongestant and antihistamine but does not contain an antitussive.

Each Dimetapp Extentab contains: *Decongestant:* Phenylpropanolamine HCl, 75 mg. *Antihistamine:* Brompheniramine maleate, 12 mg.

Each Dimetapp Sinus Caplet contains: *Analgesic/antipyretic:* Ibuprofen, 200 mg. *Decongestant:* Pseudoephedrine HCl, 30 mg.

Each Dimetapp Liquigel or Tablet contains: *Decongestant:* Phenylpropanolamine HCl, 25 mg. *Antihistamine:* Brompheniramine maleate, 4 mg.

Uses: Relief of nasal congestion, throat and bronchial irritation, runny nose, sneezing, itchy and watery eyes due to the common cold, hay fever, sinusitus, or other upper respiratory tract allergies. Products containing acetaminophen are also used for relief of minor aches and pains and headache acommpanying the common cold, sinusitis, or other upper respiratory tract conditions.

Dosage

• **Dimetapp Cold & Allergy Chewable Tablets**

Children, 6–12 years of age: Two chewable tablets q 4 hr, not to exceed six doses in a 24-hr period. **Children under 6 years of age:** A physician should be consulted.

• **Dimetapp Cold & Flu Caplets**

Adults and children over 12 years of age: 2 caplets q 6 hr, not to exceed 8 caplets in a 24-hr period. Not recommended for children under 12 years of age.

• **Dimetapp DM Elixir or Elixir**

Adults and children over 12 years of age: 10 mL (2 teaspooons) q 4 hr, not to exceed six doses in a 24-hr period. **Children, 6–12 years of age:** 5 mL (1 teaspoon) q 4 hr, not to exceed six doses in a 24-hr period.

• **Dimetapp Extentabs**

Adults and children over 12 years of age: 1 tablet q 12 hr, not to exceed 1 tablet q 12 hr or 2 tablets q 24 hr.

• **Dimetapp Sinus Caplets**

Adults and children over 12 years of age: 1 caplet q 4–6 hr. If symptoms persist, 2 caplets may be taken, but the total dose in a 24-hr period should not exceed 6 caplets.

• **Dimetapp Liquigel**

Adults and children over 12 years of age: 1 Liquigel q 4 hr, not to exceed 6 Liquigels in a 24-hr period.

• **Dimetapp Tablets**

Adults and children over 12 years of age: 1 tablet q 4 hr, not to exceed 6 tablets in a 24-hr period. **Children, 6–12 years of age:** ½ tablet q 4 hr, not to exceed 3 tablets in a 24-hr period.

Administration/Storage

1. Clients sensitive to aspirin should not take Dimetapp Sinus Caplets.
2. These products should not be taken for more than 7 days.
3. Dimetapp Sinus Caplets may be taken with food or milk if GI upset occurs.

Contraindications: Use in hypertension, heart disease, diabetes, glaucoma, thyroid disease, difficulty in urinating due to an enlarged prostate. Use in persistent cough, as with smoking, asthma, and emphysema, or if cough is accompanied by excessive phlegm. Use in clients taking medication for hypertension or depression. Products containing phenylpropanolamine or pseudoephedrine should not be taken with other products containing these drugs. Dimetapp Sinus Caplets should not be taken during the last 3 months of pregnancy.

Special Concerns: A physician should be consulted before using these products during pregnancy or lactation. May cause excitability, especially in children.

Side Effects: *At higher doses:* Dizziness, nervousness, sleeplessness.

Drug Interactions

CNS depressants (e.g., alcohol, sedatives, antianxiety agents) / ↑ Effect of products containing an antihistamine

MAO inhibitors / ↑ Risk of hypertensive crisis if taken with pseudoephedrine- or phenylpropanolamine-containing products
Sympathomimetic amines / Additive effects and ↑ risk of toxicity when taken with pseudoephedrine- or phenylpropanolamine-containing products

NURSING CONSIDERATIONS

See also *Nursing Considerations* for individual components.

Assessment

1. Document indications for therapy and type and onset of symptoms.
2. Determine any aspirin sensitivity.

Evaluate: Relief of cold symptoms and related allergic manifestations.

—COMBINATION DRUG—

Dristan Allergy Caplets
(OTC)

Dristan Cold Tablets
(OTC)

Dristan Menthol Nasal Spray and Nasal Decongestant Spray
(OTC)

Dristan Juice Mix-In
(OTC)

Dristan Sinus Caplets
(OTC)

Maximum Strength Dristan Cold Multi-Symptom Formula
(OTC)

Maximum Strength Dristan Cold No Drowsiness Formula
(OTC)

See also information on individual components.

How Supplied: See Content

Content: Each Dristan Allergy Caplet contains: *Decongestant:* Pseudoephedrine HCl, 60 mg. *Antihistamine:* Brompheniramine maleate, 4 mg.

Each Dristan Cold Tablet contains: *Analgesic/antipyretic:* Acetaminophen, 325 mg. *Decongestant:* Phenylephrine HCl, 5 mg. *Antihistamine:* Chlorpheniramine maleate, 2 mg.

Dristan Menthol Nasal Spray and Nasal Decongestant Spray: *Decongestant:* Phenylephrine HCl, 0.5%. *Antihistamine:* Pheniramine maleate, 0.2%

Each packet of Dristan Juice Mix-In contains: *Analgesic/antipyretic:* Acetaminophen, 500 mg. *Decongestant:* Pseudoephedrine HCl, 60 mg. *Antitussive:* Dextromethorphan HBr, 20 mg.

Each Dristan Sinus Caplet contains: *Analgesic/antipyretic:* Ibuprofen, 200 mg. *Decongestant:* Pseudoephedrine HCl, 30 mg.

Each Maximum Strength Dristan Cold Multi-Symptom Formula Gel Caplet contains: *Analgesic/antipyretic:* Acetaminophen, 500 mg. *Decongestant:* Pseudoephedrine HCl, 30 mg. *Antihistamine:* Brompheniramine maleate, 2 mg.

Each Maximum Strength Dristan Cold No Drowsiness Formula Caplet contains: *Analgesic/antipyretic:* Acetaminophen, 500 mg. *Decongestant:* Pseudoephedrine HCl, 30 mg.

Uses: *Oral products:* Relief of nasal congestion, runny nose, sore throat, sneezing, and itchy, watery eyes due to hay fever, colds, or other upper respiratory tract problems. Analgesic/antipyretic-containing products are also used to relieve headache, body aches, and fever.

Nasal Spray: Relief of nasal congestion due to colds, hay fever, or other upper respiratory tract allergies.

Dosage

- **Dristan Allergy Caplets**

Adults and children over 12 years of age: 1 caplet q 4–6 hr, not to exceed 4 caplets in a 24-hr period.

- **Dristan Cold Tablets**

Adults and children over 12 years of age: 2 tablets q 4 hr, not to exceed 12 tablets in a 24-hr period. **Children, 6–12 years of age:** 1 tablet q

4 hr, not to exceed 5 tablets in a 24-hr period.

• **Dristan Juice Mix-In Packets**

Adults and children over 12 years of age: Mix 1 packet in 6 oz of juice, stir briskly for 15 sec, and drink promptly. Dose may be repeated q 4 hr, not to exceed four doses in a 24-hr period. Not for use in children less than 12 years of age.

• **Dristan Sinus Caplets**

Adults and children over 12 years of age: 1 caplet q 4–6 hr. If symptoms persist, 2 caplets may be used, but the total dose in a 24-hr period should not exceed 6 caplets.

• **Maximum Strength Dristan Cold Multi-Symptom Formula Gel Caplets**

Adults and children over 12 years of age: 2 gel caplets q 6 hr, not to exceed 8 gel caplets in a 24-hr period.

• **Maximum Strength Dristan Cold No Drowsiness Formula Caplets**

Adults and children over 12 years of age: 2 caplets q 6 hr, not to exceed 8 caplets in a 24-hr period.

• **Dristan Menthol Nasal Spray or Nasal Decongestant Spray**

Adults and children over 12 years of age: With head held upright, spray 2–3 times in each nostril no more often than q 4 hr. **Children under 12 years of age:** A physician should be consulted.

Administration/Storage

1. Clients sensitive to aspirin should not take Dristan Sinus Caplets.
2. These products should not be taken for more than 7 days.
3. Dristan Sinus Caplets may be taken with food or milk if GI upset occurs.
4. The nasal spray should be administered quickly and firmly with the client inhaling deeply.

Contraindications: Use in hypertension, heart disease, diabetes, glaucoma, thyroid disease, difficulty in urinating due to an enlarged prostate. Use in persistent cough, as with smoking, asthma, and emphysema or if cough is accompanied by excessive phlegm. Use in clients taking medication for hypertension or depression. Products containing phenylephrine or pseudoephedrine should not be taken with other products containing these drugs. Dristan Sinus Caplets should not be taken during the last 3 months of pregnancy. Except for Dristan Cold Tablets, these products should not be used in children less than 12 years of age.

Special Concerns: A physician should be consulted before using these products during pregnancy or lactation. May cause excitability, especially in children.

Side Effects: *At higher doses:* Dizziness, nervousness, sleeplessness.

Drug Interactions

CNS depressants (e.g., alcohol, sedatives, antianxiety agents) / ↑ Effect of products containing an antihistamine

MAO inhibitors / ↑ Risk of hypertensive crisis if taken with pseudoephedrine- or phenylpropanolamine-containing products

Sympathomimetic amines / Additive effects and ↑ risk of toxicity when taken with pseudoephedrine- or phenylpropanolamine-containing products

NURSING CONSIDERATIONS

See also *Nursing Considerations* for individual components.

Assessment

1. Document indications for therapy and type and onset of symptoms.
2. Determine any aspirin sensitivity.

Evaluate: Relief of nasal congestion and allergic manifestations.

—COMBINATION DRUG—

Drixoral Cold & Allergy Sustained-Action Tablets

(OTC)

Drixoral Cold & Flu Extended-Release Tablets

(OTC)

Drixoral Non-Drowsy Formula
(OTC)

Drixoral Sinus
(OTC)

(drix-**OR**-al)

See also information on individual components.

How Supplied: See Content

Content: Each Drixoral Cold & Allergy Sustained-Action Tablet contains: *Decongestant:* Pseudoephedrine sulfate, 120 mg. *Antihistamine:* Dexbrompheniramine maleate, 6 mg.

Each Drixoral Cold & Flu Extended-Release Tablet and Drixoral Sinus Extended-Release Tablet contains: *Analgesic/antipyretic:* Acetaminophen, 500 mg. *Decongestant:* Pseudoephedrine sulfate, 60 mg. *Antihistamine:* Dexbrompheniramine maleate, 3 mg.

Each Drixoral Non-Drowsy Formula Long-Acting Tablet contains: *Decongestant:* Pseudoephedrine sulfate, 120 mg.

Uses: Relief of nasal congestion, runny nose, sore throat, sneezing, and itchy, watery eyes due to hay fever, colds, or other upper respiratory tract problems. Analgesic/antipyretic-containing products are also used to relieve headache, body aches, and fever.

Dosage

- **Drixoral Cold & Allergy Sustained-Action Tablets**

Adults and children over 12 years of age: 1 tablet q 12 hr, not to exceed 2 tablets in a 24-hr period.

- **Drixoral Cold & Flu Extended-Release Tablets and Drixoral Sinus**

Adults and children over 12 years of age: 2 tablets q 12 hr, not to exceed 4 tablets in a 24-hr period.

- **Drixoral Non-Drowsy Formula**

Adults and children over 12 years of age: 1 tablet q 12 hr, not to exceed 2 tablets in a 24-hr period.

Administration/Storage: These products should not be taken for more than 7 days.

Contraindications: Use in hypertension, heart disease, diabetes, glaucoma, thyroid disease, difficulty in urinating due to an enlarged prostate. Use in persistent cough, as with smoking, asthma, and emphysema or if cough is accompanied by excessive phlegm. Use in clients taking medication for hypertension or depression. Products containing pseudoephedrine should not be taken with other products containing this drug. Except for Drixoral Syrup, these products should not be used in children under 12 years of age.

Special Concerns: A physician should be consulted before using these products during pregnancy or lactation. May cause excitability, especially in children.

Side Effects: *At higher doses:* Dizziness, nervousness, sleeplessness.

Drug Interactions

CNS depressants (e.g., alcohol, sedatives, antianxiety agents) / ↑ Effect of products containing an antihistamine

MAO inhibitors / ↑ Risk of hypertensive crisis if taken with pseudoephedrine-containing products

Sympathomimetic amines / Additive effects and ↑ risk of toxicity when taken with pseudoephedrine-containing products

NURSING CONSIDERATIONS

See also *Nursing Considerations* for individual components.

Evaluate: Relief of nasal congestion and related allergic manifestations.

COMBINATION DRUG

Entex LA

(**EN**-tex)

Pregnancy Category: C

(Rx)

How Supplied: See Content

Content: *Expectorant:* Guaifenesin, 400 mg. *Decongestant:* Phenylpropanolamine HCl, 75 mg. See also information on individual components.

Uses: Nasal congestion and viscous mucus in the lower respiratory tract accompanying bronchitis, sinusitis, pharyngitis, coryza.

Dosage

• **Tablets**

Adults and children over 12 years: 1 tablet q 12 hr; **children, 6–12 years:** ½ tablet q 12 hr. Not recommended for children under 6 years of age.

Administration/Storage

1. Tablets should not be crushed or chewed before swallowing, although they may be broken in half for ease of administration.
2. Drug contains guaifenesin; prolonged use with high dosages may alter platelet function.

NURSING CONSIDERATIONS

See also *Nursing Considerations* for *Sympathomimetics,* Chapter 50.

Evaluate: Relief of nasal congestion with successful mobilization and expectoration of secretions.

COMBINATION DRUG

Hycodan Syrup and Tablets

(**HY**-koh-dan)

(Rx) (C-III)

Pregnancy Category: C

How Supplied: See Content

Content: Each tablet or 5 mL contains: *Antitussive, narcotic:* Hydrocodone bitartrate, 5 mg. *Anticholinergic:* Homatropine methylbromide, 1.5 mg.

See also information on narcotic analgesics and cholinergic blocking drugs.

Use: Relief of symptoms of cough.

Dosage

• **Tablets, Syrup**

Adults and children over 12 years: 1 tablet or 5 mL q 4–6 hr as needed, not to exceed 6 tablets or 30 mL in 24 hr. **Pediatric, 6–12 years:** ½ tablet or 2.5 mL q 4–6 hr as needed, not to exceed 3 tablets or 15 mL in 24 hr.

Administration/Storage

1. The single maximum dose of medication for adults is 3 tablets or 15 mL of syrup after meals and at bedtime.
2. For children over 12 years of age, the maximum dosage is 2 tablets or 10 mL of syrup after meals and at bedtime.
3. For children 2–12 years of age, the maximum dosage is 1 tablet or 5 mL of syrup after meals and at bedtime.
4. For children less than 2 years old, the maximum dosage is ¼ tablet or 1.25 mL of syrup after meals and at bedtime.
5. Doses should be taken at least 4 hr apart.

Special Concerns: May be habit-forming. Use with caution in children with croup, in geriatric or debilitated clients, impaired renal or hepatic function, hyperthyroidism, asthma, narrow-angle glaucoma, prostatic hypertrophy, urethral stricture, Addison's disease. Safety and effectiveness in children less than 6 years of age have not been determined.

NURSING CONSIDERATIONS

See also *Nursing Considerations* for *Cholinergic Blocking Agents,* Chapter 49, and *Narcotic Analgesics,* Chapter 43.

Client/Family Teaching

1. Drug may cause drowsiness and/or dizziness. Avoid tasks that require mental alertness, such as operating machinery or driving a car.
2. Report if symptoms persist, change, or intensify as medical intervention may be necessary.
3. Drug may be habit-forming if used over a prolonged period of time.
4. Safely store and keep out of reach of children.

Evaluate: Relief of cough permitting uninterrupted periods of sleep.

COMBINATION DRUG

Medi-Flu

Medi-Flu without Drowsiness

(OTC)

How Supplied: See Content

Content: Each caplet or ½ oz of Medi-Flu contains: *Decongestant:* Pseudoephedrine HCl, 30 mg. *Antihistamine:* Chlorpheniramine maleate,

2 mg. *Antitussive:* Dextromethorphan HBr, 15 mg. *Analgesic/antipyretic:* Acetaminophen, 500 mg.

Each caplet of Medi-Flu without Drowsiness contains the same formulation as Medi-Flu caplets with the exception of chlorpheniramine maleate. See also individual components.

Uses: Temporary relief of flu symptoms, including fever, body aches and pains, nasal and sinus congestion, minor sore throat pain, coughing, and headache. The antihistamine in Medi-Flu also provides relief of runny nose, sneezing, and watery eyes.

Dosage

MEDI-FLU CAPLETS OR MEDI-FLU WITHOUT DROWSINESS CAPLETS

Adults: 2 caplets q 6 hr, not to exceed 8 caplets in a 24- hr period.

MEDI-FLU LIQUID

Adults: 30 mL (2 tablespoons) q 6 hr as needed, not to exceed 120 mL (8 tablespoons) in a 24-hr period.

Administration/Storage: A physician should be consulted for use in children less than 12 years of age.

Contraindications: Hypertension, heart disease, diabetes, thyroid disease, or difficulty in urination due to an enlarged prostate gland. Antihistamine-containing products should not be taken with asthma, glaucoma, emphysema, chronic pulmonary disease, SOB, or difficulty in breathing. Should not be taken for persistent or chronic cough or if cough is due to excessive phlegm. Clients on antihypertensive or antidepressant medication.

Side Effects: *At higher doses:* Dizziness, nervousness, sleeplessness.

NURSING CONSIDERATIONS

See also *Nursing Considerations* for *Acetaminophen,* Chapter 41, *Antihistamines,* Chapter 55, *Sympathomimetics,* Chapter 50, and *Dextromethorphan,* Chapter 57.

Assessment

1. Document indications for therapy and type and onset of symptoms.
2. List any other agents used and the outcome.
3. Note any history of cardiac, respiratory, or endocrine disorders.
4. List agents currently prescribed to ensure that none interact unfavorably.

Client/Family Teaching

1. Advise to take only as directed and not to share medication.
2. Report if symptoms persist or intensify after 3 days of therapy.
3. Do not take without provider approval if also prescribed antihypertensive or antidepressant agents.

Evaluate: Reports of relief of flu symptoms.

—COMBINATION DRUG—

Naldecon Syrup and Tablets

(NAL-dek-on)

Pregnancy Category: C

(Rx)

How Supplied: See Content

Content: Each sustained action tablet contains the following (one-half for immediate release and one-half for delayed action): *Antihistamine:* Chlorpheniramine maleate, 5 mg. *Decongestant:* Phenylpropanolamine HCl, 40 mg. *Decongestant:* Phenylephrine HCl, 10 mg. *Antihistamine:* Phenyltoloxamine citrate, 15 mg.

NOTE: The syrup contains one-half the amount of the above components in each 5 mL, whereas the pediatric syrup (in each 5 mL) and pediatric drops (in each 1 mL) contain chlorpheniramine maleate, 0.5 mg; phenylpropanolamine HCl, 5 mg; phenylephrine HCl, 1.25 mg; and phenyltoloxamine citrate, 2 mg.

Uses: Nasal congestion and eustachian tube congestion observed with the common cold, acute upper respiratory tract infections, or sinusitis. Also, seasonal allergic rhinitis or vasomotor rhinitis. Also used to relieve eustachian tube congestion associated with serous otitis media, acute eustachian salpingitis, or aerotitis.

Dosage

- **Tablets, Syrup, Pediatric Drops and Syrup**

Adults and children over 12 years: 1 tablet on arising, in midafternoon, and at bedtime; or 5 mL syrup q 3–4 hr not to exceed four doses daily. **Pediatric, 6–12 years:** 10

mL pediatric syrup q 3–4 hr, not to exceed four doses daily; **1–6 years:** 5 mL pediatric syrup or 1 mL pediatric drops q 3–4 hr, not to exceed four doses daily; **6–12 months:** 2.5 mL pediatric syrup or 0.5 mL pediatric drops q 3–4 hr, not to exceed four doses daily; **3–6 months:** 0.25 mL pediatric drops q 3–4 hr, not to exceed four doses daily.

NURSING CONSIDERATIONS

See *Nursing Considerations* for *Antihistamines,* Chapter 55, and *Sympathomimetics,* Chapter 50.

Client/Family Teaching

1. Take only as directed.
2. Report if symptoms persist beyond 5 days or worsen.

Evaluate: Relief of congestion associated with respiratory infections and seasonal allergies.

—COMBINATION DRUG—

Novahistine DMX

Novahistine Elixir

(no-vah-**HISS**-teen)

Pregnancy Category: C

(OTC)

How Supplied: See Content

Content: Each 5 mL of Novahistine DMX contains: *Antitussive:* Dextromethorphan HBr, 10 mg. *Decongestant:* Pseudoephedrine HCl, 30 mg. *Expectorant:* Guaifenesin, 100 mg.

Each 5 mL of Novahistine Elixir contains: *Antihistamine:* Chlorpheniramine maleate, 2 mg. *Decongestant:* Phenylephrine HCl, 5 mg.

See also information on individual components.

Uses: *Novahistine DMX:* Relief of cough and nasal congestion; helps loosen phlegm and bronchial secretions. *Novahistine Elixir:* To treat congestion of the nose and eustachian tubes manifested by hay fever, the common cold, and sinusitis. Also useful for relief of other symptoms (e.g., runny nose, sneezing, itchy nose and throat, watery eyes) due to hay fever or the common cold.

Dosage

NOVAHISTINE DMX

Adults and children over 12 years of age: 10 mL q 4 hr. **Children, 6–12 years of age:** 5 mL q 4 hr.; **children, 2–6 years of age:** 2.5 mL q 4 hr. No more than four doses should be taken in a 24-hr period.

NOVAHISTINE ELIXIR

Adults and children over 12 years of age: 10 mL q 4 hr; **pediatric, 6–12 years:** 5 mL q 4 hr. No more than six doses should be taken in a 24-hr period.

Contraindications: Use in severe hypertension, in severe CAD, and in those taking MAO inhibitors. Pseudoephedrine is contraindicated during lactation. Use of Novahistine DMX for persistent cough due to smoking, emphysema, asthma, or chronic bronchitis. Use in clients taking medication for hypertension or depression. Use of Novahistine DMX in children less than 2 years of age or Novahistine Elixir in children less than 6 years of age, unless ordered by a physician.

Special Concerns: Sympathomimetic decongestants (pseudoephedrine or phenylephrine) should be used with caution in clients with hypertension, diabetes, ischemic heart disease, increased intraocular pressure, hyperthyroidism, and prostatic hypertrophy. Clients over 60 years of age are more likely to have side effects to sympathomimetics. Safety for use during pregnancy has not been established.

Side Effects: *Higher doses:* Dizziness, nervousness, sleeplessness.

NURSING CONSIDERATIONS

See also *Nursing Considerations* for *Antihistamines,* Chapter 55, *Sympathomimetics,* Chapter 50, and individual agents.

Assessment

1. Document indications for therapy and type and onset of symptoms.
2. List drugs currently prescribed to ensure none interact unfavorably.
3. Review list of conditions that preclude therapy with this medication.
4. Drug is for short-term therapy. Lack of response requires medical intervention.

Evaluate

- Mobilization of secretions
- Relief of congestion and allergic manifestations

COMBINATION DRUG

Ornade

(**OR**-nayd)
Pregnancy Category: B
(Rx)

See also information on individual components.
How Supplied: See Content
Content: Each capsule contains: *Antihistamine:* Chlorpheniramine maleate, 12 mg. *Decongestant:* Phenylpropanolamine HCl, 75 mg.
Uses: Symptoms of seasonal or perennial allergic rhinitis or the common cold including runny nose, nasal congestion, sneezing, itching throat or nose, itchy and watery eyes.

Dosage

- **Capsules**

Adults and children over 12 years: 1 capsule q 12 hr. Not to be used in children under 12 years of age.
Contraindication: Lactation.
Special Concerns: Safety and effectiveness in children less than 12 years of age have not been determined.

NURSING CONSIDERATIONS

See also *Nursing Considerations* for *Antihistamines,* Chapter 55, and *Sympathomimetics,* Chapter 50.
Evaluate: Relief of allergic manifestations and nasal congestion.

COMBINATION DRUG

Phenergan with Codeine syrup

(**FEN**-er-gan, **KOH**-deen)
Pregnancy Category: C
(C-V) (Rx)
How Supplied: See Content
Content: *Antihistamine:* Promethazine HCl, 6.25 mg/5 mL. *Antitussive, narcotic:* Codeine phosphate, 10 mg/5 mL. See also information on individual components.
Uses: Relief of coughs and other upper respiratory tract problems associated with the common cold or with allergy.

Dosage

- **Syrup**

Adults: 5 mL/ q 4–6 hr, not to exceed 30 mL/day; **pediatric, 6–12 years:** 2.5–5 mL/ q 4–6 hr, not to exceed 30 mL/day; **pediatric, 2–6 years:** 1.25–2.5 mL/4–6 hr.
Administration/Storage: The maximum daily dose of medication for children between 2 and 6 years of age depends on body weight. The amount of drug administered should not exceed:

- 9 mL for 18 kg of body weight, or
- 8 mL for 16 kg of body weight, or
- 7 mL for 14 kg of body weight, or
- 6 mL for 12 kg of body weight.

Contraindications: Clients with lower respiratory tract symptoms, including asthma. Use in children less than 2 years of age.
Special Concerns: Use with caution during lactation.

NURSING CONSIDERATIONS

See also *Nursing Considerations* for *Antihistamines,* Chapter 55.
Assessment: Take a thorough nursing history to determine how long the client has had the symptoms and assess whether or not the problem may be related to an allergy.
Client/Family Teaching
1. Report if symptoms persist or intensify.
2. Consume 2–3 L/day of fluids and include additional roughage in the diet to avoid constipation.
3. Drug may be habit-forming and is not for long-term indiscriminate use.
Evaluate: Control of cough and congestion.

COMBINATION DRUG

Phenergan with Dextromethorphan syrup

(**FEN**-er-gan, dex-troh-meth-**OR**-fan)
(Rx)
Pregnancy Category: C

How Supplied: See Content
Content: *Antihistamine:* Promethazine HCl, 6.25 mg/5 mL. *Nonnarcot-*

ic antitussive: Dextromethorphan HCl, 15 mg/5 mL. See also information on individual components.
Uses: To treat symptoms of cough and upper respiratory problems observed with the common cold and allergies.

Dosage

• **Syrup**
Adults: 5 mL q /4–6 hr, not to exceed 30 mL/day. **Pediatric, 6–12 years:** 2.5–5 mL/ q 4–6 hr, not to exceed 20 mL/day; **2–6 years:** 1.25–2.5 mL/ q 4–6 hr, not to exceed 10 mL/day.
Contraindication: Use in children less than 2 years of age.
Special Concerns: Use with caution during lactation.

NURSING CONSIDERATIONS

See also *Nursing Considerations* for *Antihistamines,* Chapter 55, and *Dextromethorphan,* Chapter 57.
Assessment
1. Determine type and onset of symptoms.
2. List any other agents used and the outcome.
3. Auscultate lungs and document respiratory findings.
Evaluate: Control of cough and relief of congestion.

—COMBINATION DRUG—

Phenergan VC with Codeine syrup

(**FEN**-er-gan, **KOH**-deen)
Pregnancy Category: C
(C-V) (Rx)

Phenergan VC syrup

(**FEN**-er-gan)
Pregnancy Category: C
(Rx)

How Supplied: See Content
Content: Phenergan VC contains the following: *Antihistamine:* Promethazine HCl, 6.25 mg/5 mL. *Decongestant:* Phenylephrine HCl, 5 mg/5 mL. Phenergan VC with Codeine contains the above plus: *Narcotic antitussive:* Codeine phosphate, 10 mg/5 mL.
Uses: Phenergan VC: Nasal congestion accompanying allergy or the common cold. Phenergan VC with Codeine: Cough and nasal congestion accompanying allergy or the common cold.

Dosage

• **Phenergan VC Syrup, Phenergan VC with Codeine Syrup**
Adults: 5 mL/ q 4–6 hr, not to exceed 30 mL/day. **Pediatric, 6–12 years:** 2.5–5 mL/ q 4–6 hr, not to exceed 30 mL/day; **2–6 years:** 1.25–2.5 mL/ q 4–6 hr (the maximum daily dose of Phenergan VC with Codeine ranges from 6 to 9 mL depending on the body weight).
Administration/Storage: The maximum daily dose of medication for children between 2 and 6 years of age depends on body weight. The amount of drug administered should not exceed:
• 9 mL for 18 kg of body weight, or
• 8 mL for 16 kg of body weight, or
• 7 mL for 14 kg of body weight, or
• 6 mL for 12 kg of body weight
Contraindications: Use for lower respiratory tract symptoms, including asthma. Use in children less than 2 years of age.
Special Concerns: Use with caution during lactation.

NURSING CONSIDERATIONS

See also *Nursing Considerations* for *Antihistamines,* Chapter 55, *Phenylephrine,* Chapter 50, and *Codeine,* Chapter 43.
Client/Family Teaching
1. Caution that medication may cause dizziness and drowsiness.
2. Avoid alcohol and any other CNS depressants.
3. Explain that drug is not for long-term use. Advise to report if symptoms do not subside or get worse over the next 5 days.
Evaluate: Control of cough and related congestion with fewer night time awakenings.

—COMBINATION DRUG—

Pseudoephedrine hydrochloride and Guaifenesin

(soo-doh-eh-**FED**-rin, gwye-**FEN**-eh-sin)

Duratuss HD Elixir, Duratuss Tablets

(OTC)

See also *Pseudoephedrine,* Chapter 50, *Guaifenesin,* Chapter 56, and *Narcotic Analgesics,* Chapter 43.

How Supplied: See Content

Content: Each 5 mL of Duratuss HD Elixir contains: *Antitussive:* Hydrocodone bitartrate, 2.5 mg. *Decongestant:* Pseudoephedrine HCl, 30 mg. *Expectorant:* Guaifenesin, 100 mg.

Each Duratuss Tablet contains: *Decongestant:* Pseudoephedrine HCl, 120 mg. *Expectorant:* Guaifenesin, 600 mg.

Uses: Relief of coughing (elixir) and congestion (tablet and elixir).

Dosage

- **Elixir**

Adults: 10 mL (2 teaspoons) q 4–6 hr. **Children, 6–12 years of age:** 5 mL (1 teaspoon) q 4–6 hr.

- **Tablets**

Adults: 1 tablet q 12 hr. **Children:** ½ tablet q 12 hr.

NURSING CONSIDERATIONS

See also *Nursing Considerations* for *Pseudoephedrine,* Chapter 50, *Guaifenesin,* Chapter 56, and *Narcotic Analgesics,* Chapter 43.

Assessment

1. Document indications for therapy and type and onset of symptoms.
2. List other agents used and the outcome.
3. Assess for impaired liver and clotting functions.

Evaluate

- Control of cough
- Mobilization of secretions with relief of congestion

—COMBINATION DRUG—

Robitussin-AC

(roh-bih-**TUS**-in)

(C-V) (Rx)

How Supplied: See Content

Content: *Expectorant:* Guaifenesin, 100 mg/5 mL. *Antitussive:* Codeine phosphate, 10 mg/5 mL. The product helps loosen mucus and thins bronchial secretions, making coughs more productive. See also information on individual components.

Uses: Coughs associated with bronchitis, the common cold, laryngitis, pharyngitis, pertussis, tracheitis, flu, and measles.

Dosage

- **Syrup**

Adults and children over 12 years: 10 mL q 4 hr, not to exceed 60 mL/day; **pediatric, 6–12 years:** 5 mL q 4 hr, not to exceed 30 mL/day; **pediatric, 2–6 years:** 2.5 mL q 4 hr, not to exceed 15 mL/day.

Contraindications: Chronic or persistent coughs. Children less than 2 years of age.

Laboratory Test Interferences: Guaifenesin may interfere with determination of 5-HIAA or VMA.

NURSING CONSIDERATIONS

See also *Nursing Considerations* for *Narcotic Analgesics,* Chapter 43.

Assessment: Review the client history. If the cough is chronic, the drug is contraindicated.

Client/Family Teaching

1. Take only as directed and report if symptoms persist after 5 days or intensify.
2. Consume 2–3 L/day of fluids and increase intake of fruits, grains, and other high-fiber foods to prevent constipation. A stool softener may be prescribed. Report if the stool softener is not effective as other reasons for the constipation may then need to be ruled out.
3. Report any unusual bruising or bleeding.
4. For short-term use, drug may be habit-forming.

Evaluate: Control of cough with mobilization and expectoration of secretions.

—*COMBINATION DRUG*—

Robitussin-CF

(roh-bih-**TUSS**-in)

(OTC)

Robitussin-DM

(roh-bih-**TUSS**-in)

(OTC)

Robitussin-PE

(roh-bih-**TUSS**-in)

(OTC)

How Supplied: See Content

Content: Robitussin-CF. *Expectorant:* Guaifenesin, 100 mg/5 mL; *Decongestant:* Phenylpropanolamine HCl, 12.5 mg/5 mL; and, *Antitussive:* Dextromethorphan HBr, 10 mg/5 mL.

Robitussin-DM. *Expectorant:* Guaifenesin, 100 mg/5 mL and *Antitussive:* Dextromethorphan HBr, 15 mg/5 mL.

Robitussin-PE. *Expectorant:* Guaifenesin, 100 mg/5 mL and *Decongestant:* Pseudoephedrine HCl, 30 mg/5 mL.

See also information on individual components.

Uses: Coughs associated with bronchitis, laryngitis, pharyngitis, the common cold, flu, pertussis, tracheitis, and measles. Robitussin-CF is indicated for coughs with congestion and irritating cough; Robitussin-DM is indicated for irritating coughs; and Robitussin-PE is indicated for coughs with congestion.

Dosage

ROBITUSSIN-CF SYRUP

Adults and children over 12 years: 10 mL q 4 hr, not to exceed 60 mL/day; **pediatric, 6–12 years:** 5 mL q 4 hr, not to exceed 30 mL/day; **pediatric, 2–6 years:** 2.5 mL q 4 hr, not to exceed 15 mL/day.

ROBITUSSIN-DM SYRUP

Adults and children over 12 years: 10 mL q 4 hr, not to exceed 60 mL/day; **pediatric, 6–12 years:** 5 mL q 4 hr, not to exceed 30 mL/day; **pediatric, 2–6 years:** 2.5 mL q 4 hr, not to exceed 15 mL/day.

ROBITUSSIN-PE SYRUP

Adults and children over 12 years: 10 mL q 4 hr, not to exceed 40 mL/day; **pediatric, 6–12 years:** 5 mL q 4 hr, not to exceed 20 mL/day; **pediatric, 2–6 years:** 2.5 mL q 4 hr, not to exceed 10 mL/day.

Administration/Storage: These products should not be taken for more than 7 days.

Contraindications: Products containing sympathomimetic decongestants should be used with caution in clients with hypertension, diabetes, cardiac disorders, peripheral vascular disease, glaucoma, prostatic hypertrophy.

Special Concerns: A physician should be consulted before giving to children less than 2 years of age.

Laboratory Test Interferences: Guaifenesin may interfere with determination of 5-HIAA and VMA.

Drug Interaction: Serious toxicity may occur if dextromethorphan is taken with MAO inhibitors.

NURSING CONSIDERATIONS

See also *Nursing Considerations* for *Sympathomimetic Drugs,* Chapter 50, *Dextromethorphan,* Chapter 57, and *Robitussin-AC,* Chapter 57.

Assessment

1. Document indications for therapy and type and onset of symptoms. List other agents used for this condition and the outcome.
2. Note any history of hypertension, cardiac disease, or peripheral vascular disorders that may preclude drug therapy.
3. Determine if the client has diabetes mellitus and document. Syrups and other drugs in this class may upset blood sugar levels and alter the amount of hypoglycemic agent required for adequate control.
4. When working with elderly male clients, discuss any possible problems they may have with urinary output or any knowledge the client

may have of prostatic hypertrophy and document.

Evaluate: Control of cough and reports of symptomatic improvement.

—COMBINATION DRUG—

Robitussin Maximum Strength Cough and Cold

(roh-bih-**TUSS**-in)

(OTC)

Robitussin Night Relief Cough/Cold/Flu Formula

(roh-bih-**TUSS**-in)

(OTC)

Robitussin Pediatric Cough and Cold Formula

(roh-bih-**TUSS**-in)

(OTC)

See also *Dextromethorphan,* Chapter 57, *Pseudoephedrine,* Chapter 50, and *Acetaminophen,* Chapter 41.

How Supplied: See Content

Content: Each 5 mL of Robitussin Maximum Strength Cough and Cold contains: *Antitussive:* Dextromethorphan, 15 mg. *Decongestant:* Pseudoephedrine, 30 mg.

Each fluid ounce of Robitussin Night Relief Cough/Cold/Flu Formula contains: *Analgesic/Antipyretic:* Acetaminophen, 650 mg. *Decongestant:* Pseudoephedrine HCl, 60 mg. *Antihistamine:* Pyrilamine maleate, 50 mg. *Antitussive:* Dextromethorphan HBr, 30 mg.

Each 5 mL of Robitussin Pediatric Cough and Cold Formula contains: *Antitussive:* Dextromethorphan, 7.5 mg. *Decongestant:* Pseudoephedrine HCl, 15 mg.

Uses: Maximum Strength Cough and Cold; Pediatric Cough and Cold Formula: Relief of cough due to minor throat and bronchial irritation and nasal congestion. **Night Relief Cough/Cold/Flu Formula:** Relief of minor aches, pains, headache, muscle aches, sore throat, and fever associated with a cold or flu; also relief of nasal congestion, cough, runny nose, and sneezing due to the common cold.

Dosage

MAXIMUM STRENGTH COUGH AND COLD

Adults and children over 12 years of age: 10 mL q 6 hr, not to exceed 40 mL in a 24-hr period.

NIGHT RELIEF COUGH/COLD/FLU FORMULA

30 mL (1 fluid ounce measured using a medicine cup) at bedtime. If cold or flu keeps the client confined to bed or at home, one dose may be taken q 6 hr, not to exceed four doses in a 24-hr period.

PEDIATRIC COUGH AND COLD FORMULA

Age 12 years and older: 20 mL q 6–8 hr, not to exceed four doses in a 24-hr period. **Children, 6–under 12 years of age:** 10 mL q 6–8 hr, not to exceed four doses in a 24-hr period. **Children, 2–6 years of age:** 5 mL q 6–8 hr, not to exceed four doses in a 24-hr period. Consult a physician if the child is under 2 years of age.

Contraindications: Use in clients with persistent or chronic cough (e.g., due to smoking, emphysema, asthma) or if cough is accompanied by excessive phlegm.

Special Concerns: Products containing sympathomimetic decongestants should be used with caution in clients with hypertension, diabetes, cardiac disorders, peripheral vascular disease, glaucoma, prostatic hypertrophy. Except for the Pediatric Cough and Cold Formula, these products should not be given to children under 12 years of age unless prescibed by a physician.

Drug Interaction: Serious toxicity may occur if dextromethorphan is taken with MAO inhibitors.

NURSING CONSIDERATIONS

See also *Nursing Considerations* for *Acetaminophen,* Chapter 41, *Pseudoephedrine,* Chapter 50, *Antihistamines,* Chapter 55, and *Dextromethorphan,* Chapter 57.

Evaluate

- Control of cough
- Relief of cold and flu symptoms

COMBINATION DRUG

Rondec-DM Oral Drops

(RON-deck)

(Rx)

Rondec-DM Syrup

(RON-deck)

(Rx)

How Supplied: See Content

Content: *Antitussive:* Dextromethorphan HBr, 4 mg/mL Oral Drops or 15 mg/5 mL Syrup. *Decongestant:* Pseudoephedrine HCl, 25 mg/mL Oral Drops or 60 mg/5 mL Syrup. *Antihistamine:* Carbinoxamine maleate, 2 mg/mL Oral Drops or 4 mg/5 mL Syrup. See also information on individual components.

Uses: Treatment of coughs, nasal congestion, and other upper respiratory tract symptoms due to the common cold or allergy.

Dosage

- **Syrup**

Adults and children over 6 years: 5 mL q.i.d.; **children 18 months–6 years:** 2.5 mL q.i.d.

- **Oral Drops**

Pediatric, 9–18 months: 1 mL q.i.d.; **6–9 months:** 0.75 mL q.i.d.; **3–6 months:** 0.5 mL q.i.d.; **1–3 months:** 0.25 mL q.i.d.

Special Concerns: Safe use during pregnancy has not been established. Use with caution in hypertension, ischemic heart disease, in clients over 60 years of age, and during lactation.

NURSING CONSIDERATIONS

See also *Nursing Considerations* for *Antihistamines,* Chapter 55, *Dextromethorphan,* Chapter 57, and *Sympathomimetics,* Chapter 50.

Assessment

1. Determine onset of symptoms and note other agents used and the outcome.
2. If female and of childbearing age determine if pregnant. Safe use of drug during pregnancy has not been established.

Evaluate: Control of cough and relief of nasal congestion with reports of symptomatic improvement.

COMBINATION DRUG

Rynatan

(RYE-nah-tan)

Pregnancy Category: C

(Rx)

How Supplied: See Content

Content: *Antihistamine:* Chlorpheniramine tannate, 8 mg (tablet) or 2 mg (per 5 mL suspension). *Antihistamine:* Pyrilamine tannate, 25 mg (tablet) or 12.5 mg (per 5 mL suspension). *Decongestant:* Phenylephrine tannate, 25 mg (tablet) or 5 mg (per 5 mL suspension). See also information on individual components.

Uses: Nasal congestion and runny nose due to upper respiratory tract conditions including the common cold, allergic rhinitis, sinusitis, and other respiratory tract conditions.

Dosage

- **Tablets, Oral Suspension**

Adults: 1–2 tablets q 12 hr. **Pediatric, over 6 years:** 5–10 mL of the suspension q 12 hr; **pediatric, 2–6 years:** 2.5–5 mL of the suspension q 12 hr. The dose should be carefully individualized in children under 2 years of age.

Contraindications: Use during lactation and in newborns.

Special Concerns: Use with caution in hypertension, hyperthyroidism, CV disease, narrow-angle glaucoma, diabetes, and prostatic hypertrophy. Use with caution (or avoid use) in clients taking MAO inhibitors.

Drug Interactions: Additive CNS depression if used with alcohol, sedative-hypnotics, antianxiety agents, or other drugs producing CNS depression.

NURSING CONSIDERATIONS

See also *Nursing Considerations* for *Antihistamines,* Chapter 55, and *Sympathomimetics,* Chapter 50.

Assessment: Document any history of diabetes, hypertension, or prostate enlargement.

Evaluate: Relief of nasal congestion and allergic respiratory manifestations.

COMBINATION DRUG

Tavist-D

(TAV-ist)

Pregnancy Category: B

(OTC)

See also *Antihistamines,* Chapter 55, and *Phenylpropanolamine,* Chapter 50.

How Supplied: See Content

Content: Each tablet contains: *Antihistamine:* Clemastine fumarate, 1.34 mg. *Decongestant:* Phenylpropanolamine HCl, 75 mg.

The clemastine is formulated in the outer shell of the tablet and is released immediately. The phenylpropanolamine component is incorporated into a sustained-release matrix, which releases the drug over a period of 12 hr; the slow release achieves blood levels equivalent to those achieved by giving 25 mg phenylpropanolamine q 4 hr for three doses.

Uses: To treat symptoms of upper respiratory allergies or sinusitus including nasal congestion; sneezing; itchy eyes, nose, or throat; runny nose or eyes.

Dosage

• **Tablets**

Adults and children over 12 years: 1 tablet (taken whole) q 12 hr, not to exceed 2 tablets in a 24-hr period.

Contraindications: Use in children less than 12 years of age and during lactation. To treat lower respiratory tract symptoms, including asthma. In clients taking MAO inhibitors or those with severe CAD or hypertension. Use in clients with asthma, diabetes, glaucoma, heart disease, emphysema, chronic pulmonary disease, SOB, difficulty in breathing, or prostatic hypertrophy. Not for use in clients taking medication for hypertension or depression, unless prescribed by a physician.

NURSING CONSIDERATIONS

See also *Nursing Considerations* for *Antihistamines,* Chapter 55, and *Sympathomimetics,* Chapter 50.

Client/Family Teaching

1. Instruct client not to break tablets or crush them but to take tablets whole. This permits the specially designed release system to remain intact.
2. Report if symptoms do not improve or worsen after 5 days of therapy.
3. Review conditions (i.e., hypertension, diabetes, CAD, asthma) in which drug should be avoided.

Evaluate: Relief of congestion and allergic manifestations.

COMBINATION DRUG

Trinalin

(TRIN-al-in)

Pregnancy Category: D

How Supplied: See Content

Content: *Antihistamine:* Azatadine maleate, 1 mg. *Decongestant:* Pseudoephedrine sulfate, 120 mg in a long-acting formulation. See also information on individual components.

Action/Kinetics: The tablet is formulated so that the azatadine and one-half of the pseudoephedrine are released immediately; the remaining one-half of the pseudoephedrine is released after several hours.

Uses: Symptoms of allergic rhinitis and perennial rhinitis, nasal and eustachian tube congestion.

Dosage

• **Tablets**

Adults: 1 tablet b.i.d.

Administration/Storage

1. Trinalin may be used in conjunction with other analgesics and/or antibiotics.
2. Do not administer to children under 12 years of age.

Contraindications: Lactation. Children under 12 years of age. Use to treat lower respiratory tract symptoms, including asthma. Narrow-angle glaucoma, urinary retention, clients taking MAO inhibitors, severe hy-

pertension, severe CAD, hyperthyroidism, clients hypersensitive to adrenergic agents.
Special Concerns: Use with caution in clients with stenosing peptic ulcer, pyloroduodenal obstruction, urinary bladder obstruction due to prostatic hypertrophy or narrowing of the bladder neck, hypertension, ischemic heart disease, increased intraocular pressure, and diabetes mellitus and in clients taking digitalis or oral anticoagulants.

NURSING CONSIDERATIONS

See also *Nursing Considerations* for *Antihistamines,* Chapter 55, and *Sympathomimetic Drugs,* Chapter 50.
Evaluate: Relief of congestion and improvement in allergic manifestations.

—COMBINATION DRUG—

Tussi-Organidin

(**TUSS**-ee-or-**GAN**-ih-din)
Pregnancy Category: X
(C-V) (Rx)

Tussi-Organidin DM

(**TUSS**-ee-or-**GAN**-ih-din)
Pregnancy Category: X
(Rx)

How Supplied: See Content
Content: Each 5 mL of Tussi-Organidin contains: *Mucolytic/expectorant:* Iodinated glycerol, 30 mg. *Narcotic antitussive:* Codeine phosphate, 10 mg. Each 5 mL of Tussi-Organidin DM contains: *Mucolytic/expectorant:* Iodinated glycerol, 30 mg. *Nonnarcotic antitussive:* Dextromethorphan, 10 mg. See also information on *Narcotic Analgesics,* Chapter 43, and *Dextromethorphan,* Chapter 57.
Uses: Relief of irritating, nonproductive cough due to a variety of respiratory tract problems including the common cold, chronic bronchitis, bronchial asthma, tracheobronchitis, laryngitis, pharyngitis, pertussis, emphysema, and croup.

Dosage

- **Tussi-Organidin Liquid or Tussi-Organidin DM Liquid**

Adults: 5–10 mL q 4 hr; **pediatric:** 2.5–5 mL q 4 hr.
Contraindications: History of hypersensitivity to inorganic iodides, pregnancy, lactation, use in newborns.
Special Concerns: Use with caution (or avoid use) in clients with a history of thyroid disease.

NURSING CONSIDERATIONS

See also *Nursing Considerations* for *Narcotic Analgesics,* Chapter 43, and *Dextromethorphan,*Chapter 57.

Assessment

1. Tussi-Organidin contains codeine. Assess for any history of drug addiction.
2. Determine how long the client has had the cough, the length of time the upper respiratory tract infection has been present, and what the client has done to correct the problems.
3. Note any history of thyroid dysfunction.

Client/Family Teaching

1. Report if the symptoms intensify or persist beyond a week.
2. Drug may be habit-forming and is not for long-term indiscriminate use.
3. Consume 2–3 L/day of fluids and increase intake of fruits, fruit juices, and grains to prevent constipation and liquify secretions.

Evaluate: Control of cough permitting uninterrupted periods of rest.

—COMBINATION DRUG—

Tussionex Capsules, Suspension, and Tablets

(**TUSS**-ee-oh-nex)
Pregnancy Category: C
(C-III) (Rx)

How Supplied: See Content
Content: Each capsule, tablet, or 5 mL of suspension contains: *Narcotic antitussive:* Hydrocodone, 5 mg. *Nonnarcotic antitussive:* Phenyltoloxamine, 10 mg. See also *Narcotic Analgesics,* Chapter 43.

Use: Antitussive.

Dosage

- **Capsules, Tablets, Suspension**

Adults: 1 capsule, tablet, or 5 mL of suspension q 8–12 hr. **Pediatric, over 5 years:** 5 mL q 12 hr; **pediatric, 1–5 years:** 2.5 mL of the suspension q 12 hr; **infants, less than 1 year:** 1.25 mL of the suspension q 12 hr.

NURSING CONSIDERATIONS

See also *Nursing Considerations* for *Narcotic Analgesics,* Chapter 43.

Client/Family Teaching

1. Report if the symptoms persist or intensify.
2. Drug may be habit-forming if it is used for long periods of time.

Evaluate:

- Relief of pulmonary congestion
- Control of cough

CHAPTER FIFTY-EIGHT

Nasal Decongestants

See also the following individual entries:

- Ephedrine Sulfate - See Chapter 50
- Epinephrine Hydrochloride - See Chapter 50
- Oxymetazoline Hydrochloride
- Phenylephrine Hydrochloride - See Chapter 50
- Pseudoephedrine Hydrochloride - See Chapter 50
- Xylometazoline Hydrochloride

Action/Kinetics: The most commonly used agents for relief of nasal congestion are the adrenergic drugs. They act by stimulating alpha-adrenergic receptors, thereby constricting the arterioles in the nasal mucosa; this reduces blood flow to the area, decreasing congestion. However, drugs such as ephedrine and pseudoephedrine also have beta-adrenergic effects. Both topical (sprays, drops) and oral agents may be used, although oral agents are not as effective.

Uses: PO. Nasal congestion due to hay fever, common cold, allergies, or sinusitis. To help sinus or nasal drainage. To relieve congestion of eustachian tubes. **Topical.** Nasal and nasopharyngeal mucosal congestion due to hay fever, common cold, allergies, or sinusitis. With other therapy to decrease congestion around the eustachian tubes. Relieve ear block and pressure pain during air travel.

Contraindications: Oral use in severe hypertension or CAD. Use with MAO inhibitors. Oral use of pseudoephedrine and phenylpropanolamine during lactation.

Special Concerns: Use with caution in hyperthyroidism, arteriosclerosis, increased intraocular pressure, prostatic hypertrophy, angina, diabetes, ischemic heart disease, hypertension. Also, clients receiving MAO inhibitors may manifest hypertensive crisis following the use of oral nasal decongestants. Use with caution in geriatric clients and during pregnancy and lactation. Rebound congestion may occur after topical use.

Side Effects: *Topical use:* Stinging and burning, mucosal dryness, sneezing, local irritation, rebound congestion (rhinitis medicamentosa). Systemic use may produce the following symptoms. *CV:* ***CV collapse with hypotension,*** arrhythmias, palpitations, precordial pain, tachycardia, transient hypertension, bradycardia. *CNS:* Anxiety, dizziness, headache, fear, restlessness, tremors, insomnia, tenseness, lightheadedness, drowsiness, psychologic disturbances, weakness, psychoses, hallucinations, ***seizures,*** depression. *GI:* N&V, anorexia. *Ophthalmologic:* Irritation, photophobia, tearing, blurred vision, blepharospasm. *Other:* Dysuria, sweating, pallor, breathing difficulties, orofacial dystonia.

NOTE: Ephedrine may also produce anorexia and urinary retention in men with prostatic hypertrophy.

Symptoms of Overdose: Somnolence, sedation, ***coma,*** profuse sweating, ***hypotension, shock. Severe hypertension,*** bradycardia, and rebound hypotension may occur with naphazoline and tetrahydrozoline.

Drug Interactions

Furazolidone / ↑ Pressor sensitivity to drugs with both alpha- and beta-adrenergic effects (e.g., ephedrine)

Guanethidine / ↑ Effect of direct-acting agents (e.g., epinephrine)

and ↓ effect of mixed-acting drugs; also, ↓ hypotensive effect of guanethidine
MAO inhibitors / Use with mixed-acting drugs (e.g., ephedrine) → severe headache, hypertension, hyperpyrexia, and possibly hypertensive crisis
Methyldopa / ↑ Risk of a pressor response
Phenothiazines / May ↓ or reverse action of nasal decongestants
Reserpine / ↑ Pressor effect of direct-acting drugs and ↓ effect of mixed-acting drugs
Theophyllines / Enhanced toxicity
Tricyclic antidepressants / ↑ Pressor effect of direct-acting agents → possibility of dysrhythmias; ↓ pressor effect of mixed-acting drugs
Urinary acidifiers / ↑ Excretion of nasal decongestants → ↓ effect
Urinary alkalinizers / ↓ Excretion of nasal decongestants → ↑ effect

Dosage

See individual drugs.

NURSING CONSIDERATIONS

Administration/Storage

1. Most nasal decongestants are used topically in the form of sprays, drops, or solutions.
2. Solutions of topical nasal decongestants may become contaminated with use. This may result in the growth of bacteria and fungi. Thus, the dropper or spray tip should be rinsed in hot water after each use and covered.
3. During administration, have facial tissues and a receptacle available for used tissues.
4. Topical decongestants should not be used longer than 3–5 days and should be used sparingly, especially in infants, children, and clients with CV disease.
5. *Treatment of Overdose:* Supportive therapy. IV phentolamine may be used in severe cases.

Interventions

1. Use separate equipment for each client to prevent the spread of infection. If only one container of medication is available, use an individual dropper for each client and rinse thoroughly with hot water after each use.
2. Instruct the client to blow the nose gently before administering therapy. If the client is unable to blow the nose, clear the nasal passages with a bulb-type aspirator as needed.
3. After completing the treatment, rinse the dropper or tip of spray container with hot water. Dry with a tissue and cover, using care not to introduce water into the spray container. Wipe the tip of the nasal jelly tube with a damp tissue and replace the cap.

Client/Family Teaching

1. Instruct in the appropriate technique for preparing the nasal passages.
2. Review the method of administration of the prescribed medication, whether drops, spray, or jelly.
3. Discuss and demonstrate the proper use and care of equipment.
4. Review the indications for therapy and the response that client should expect. Advise to seek medical assistance if symptoms worsen or do not improve after 3–5 days of therapy.
5. Caution that overuse or misuse of these agents may cause significant medical problems, i.e., a nasal spray used regularly for more than 3 or 4 days may precipitate rebound congestion.
6. Stress that many OTC agents contain sympathomimetics; these should be avoided in clients with hypertension, hyperthyroidism, angina, and insulin-dependent diabetes.

Evaluate

- Reports of ↓ nasal congestion
- Resolution of eustachian tube congestion and pain
- ↓ Duration and intensity of allergic manifestations

Oxymetazoline hydrochloride

(ox-ee-meh-**TAZ**-oh-leen)

Pregnancy Category: C

Nasal: 12-Hour Nasal, 12 Hour Sinarest Spray, 4-Way Long-Lasting Nasal, Afrin Children's Nose Drops, Afrin Menthol Nasal Spray, Afrin Nasal Spray (Cherry or Regular), Afrin Nose Drops, Allerest 12 Hour Nasal Spray, Chlorphed-LA Spray, Dristan Long Lasting Nasal Spray, Drixoral Nasal Solution, Duramist Plus, Duration Spray, Genasal, Nasal Relief Spray, Neo-Synephrine 12 Hour Spray and Drops, Nostrilla 12 Hour Nasal Decongestant, NTZ Long Acting Nasal Drops and Spray, Sinex Long-Acting Spray, Twice-A-Day **(OTC)**. **Ophthalmic:** Ocu-Clear, Visine L.R. **(OTC)**

See also *Nasal Decongestants,* Chapter 58.

How Supplied: *Solution:* 0.025%, 0.05%; *Spray:* 0.05%

Uses: Nasal: Treat congestion due to the common cold, hay fever, sinusitis, or other upper respiratory allergies. To decrease congestion around the eustachian ostia in middle ear infections. **Ophthalmic:** Relieve eye redness due to minor irritations.

Dosage

- **Nasal Drops, Spray**

Decongestant.

Adults and children over 6 years: 2–3 sprays or 2–3 gtt of 0.05% solution (regular or menthol) in each nostril in the morning and at night (or every 10–12 hr). **Pediatric, 2–5 years:** 2–3 gtt of the 0.025% solution in each nostril in the morning and at night.

- **Ophthalmic Solution**

Minor eye irritation. **Adults and children over 6 years:** 1–2 gtt of the 0.025% solution into affected eye(s) q 6 hr or longer.

Special Concerns: Use with caution during lactation.

NURSING CONSIDERATIONS

See *Nursing Considerations* for *Nasal Decongestants,* Chapter 58.

Client/Family Teaching

1. Review appropriate method for administration and observe self-administration technique.

2. Advise to report if symptoms worsen or do not improve with therapy.

Evaluate

- Reports of relief of nasal congestion
- Evidence of resolution of conjunctivitis

Xylometazoline hydrochloride

(zye-low-met-**AZ**-oh-leen)

Otrivin Nasal Drops or Spray, Otrivin Pediatric Nasal Drops **(OTC)**

See also *Nasal Decongestants,* Chapter 58.

How Supplied: *Nasal solution:* 0.05%, 0.1%; *Nasal spray:* 0.1%

Special Concerns: Use during pregnancy only if benefits clearly outweigh risks.

Dosage

- **Drops, Spray**

Nasal congestion.

Adults and children over 12 years: 2–3 gtt or 2–3 sprays of 0.1% product in each nostril q 8–10 hr; **pediatric, 2–12 years:** 2–3 gtt of 0.05% solution in each nostril q 8–10 hr.

Administration

1. Available as a 0.1% solution for drops and spray or as a 0.05% pediatric solution.

2. Should not be used in atomizers made of aluminum.

3. The nasal spray is more effective and is more likely to cause systemic side effects.

NURSING CONSIDERATIONS

See also *Nursing Considerations* for *Nasal Decongestants,* Chapter 58.

Assessment

1. Document indications for therapy, onset of symptoms, and any other agents used and the outcome.

2. Instruct client to report if symptoms intensify or do not resolve.

Evaluate: Reports of improvement in symptoms of nasal congestion.

Drugs Affecting the GI System

CHAPTER FIFTY-NINE

Antacids and Antiflatulents

See also the following individual entries:

- Aluminum Hydroxide Gel
- Aluminum Hydroxide Gel, Dried
- Basic Aluminum Carbonate Gel
- Calcium Carbonate
- Calcium Carbonate Precipitated
- Dihydroxyaluminum Sodium Carbonate
- Gelusil
- Gelusil-II
- Maalox Antacid Caplets
- Maalox HRP Suspension and Tablets
- Maalox Oral Suspension
- Maalox Plus Extra Strength Oral Suspension and Tablets
- Maalox Plus Tablets
- Magaldrate
- Magnesium Hydroxide
- Magnesium Oxide
- Mylanta Liquid and Tablets
- Mylanta Double Strength Liquid and Tablets
- Simethacone
- Sodium Bicarbonate - See Chapter 77

General Statement: Hydrochloric acid maintains the stomach at a pH (1–2) necessary for optimum activity of the digestive enzyme pepsin and for stimulating the release of secretin when the acid contents of the stomach pass into the duodenum. Under certain circumstances, however, people suffer adverse reactions due to gastric acidity ranging from heartburn to life-threatening peptic or duodenal ulcers. Although production of acid has an important role in the development of gastric and duodenal ulcers, other factors are also involved. These include endogenous histamine (which can stimulate gastric acid secretion), antigen-antibody reactions, and the psychologic makeup of the client. Acute and chronic GI disturbances are among the most common medical conditions requiring treatment. Various drugs and dietary measures are used for the treatment of hyperacidity states and ulcers, and the use of antacids is an important part of such regimens.

Action/Kinetics: Antacids act by neutralizing or reducing gastric acidity, thus increasing the pH of the stomach and relieving hyperacidity. If the pH is increased to 4, the activity of pepsin is inhibited. The ability of a specific antacid to neutralize acid is termed *acid-neutralizing capacity,* and antacids are selected on this basis. Acid-neutralizing capacity (ANC) is expressed as milliequivalents per milliliter and is defined by the HCl required to maintain an antacid suspension at pH 3.5 for 10 min in vitro. An antacid should neutralize at least 5 mEq/dose; also, to be considered an antacid, the compound should contribute to at least 25% of the ANC of a product.

Ideally, antacids should not be absorbed systemically, although substances such as sodium bicarbonate or calcium carbonate may produce significant systemic effects. The most effective dosage form for antacids is suspensions. Antacids also promote healing of peptic ulcers.

Antacids containing magnesium have a laxative effect, whereas those containing aluminum or calcium have a constipating effect. This is why clients are often given alternating doses of laxative and constipating antacids. Antacids containing aluminum bind with phosphate ions in the intestine forming the insoluble aluminum phosphate, which is excreted in the feces. This is of value in treating hyperphosphatemia of chronic renal failure. **Onset:** Depends on ability of the antacid to solubilize in the stomach and react with hydrochloric acid. The poorly soluble antacids (e.g., magnesium trisilicate) react slower with hydrochloric acid than do the more soluble compounds. **Duration of antacids:** 30 min if fasting; up to 3 hr if taken after meals.

Uses: Treatment of hyperacidity (heartburn, acid indigestion, sour stomach), gastric ulcer, duodenal ulcer, gastroesophageal reflux. Adjunct (with histamine H_2-receptor antagonists) in the treatment of hypersecretory conditions (e.g., Zollinger-Ellison syndrome), systemic mastocytosis, and multiple endocrine adenoma. Treatment of hypocalcemia, hypophosphatemia. Prophylaxis of renal calculi.

Contraindications: Sodium-containing products are contraindicated in CHF, hypertension, or conditions requiring a low-sodium diet. Pregnant or lactating women should not use antacids without physician approval. Children less than 6 years of age.

Special Concerns: Chronic use of aluminum-containing antacids may aggravate metabolic bone disease seen in geriatric clients; also, chronic use of aluminum-containing antacids may contribute to development of Alzheimer's disease. Taking too much of an antacid may result in an increased secretion of stomach acid.

Side Effects: *Aluminum-containing antacids:* Constipation, intestinal obstruction, aluminum intoxication, hypophosphatemia, osteomalacia. *Calcium carbonate, aluminum-magnesium hydroxide, magnesium oxide, soluble bismuth salts, sodium bicarbonate:* Milk-alkali syndrome (acute: headache, nausea, irritability, weakness; chronic: alkalosis, hypercalcemia, renal impairment). Rebound hyperacidity. *Magnesium-containing antacids:* Diarrhea, hypermagnesemia in clients with renal failure.

Drug Interactions

1. *Aluminum-containing antacids:* ↑ Effect of benzodiazepines. ↓ Effect of allopurinol, chloroquine, corticosteroids, diflunisal, digoxin, ethambutol, histamine H_2 antagonists, iron products, isoniazid, penicillamine, phenothiazines, tetracyclines, thyroid hormones, and ticlopidine by ↓ absorption from GI tract.

2. *Aluminum- and magnesium-containing antacids:* ↑ Effect of levodopa, quinidine, sulfonylureas, and valproic acid probably by ↓ excretion. ↓ Effect of benzodiazepines, captopril, corticosteroids, fluoroquinolones, histamine H_2 antagonists, hydantoins, iron products, ketoconazole, penicillamine, phenothiazines, salicylates, tetracyclines, and ticlopidine either by ↓ absorption from GI tract or ↑ excretion.

3. *Calcium-containing antacids:* ↑ Effect of quinidine by ↓ excretion. ↓ Effect of fluoroquinolones, hydantoins, iron products, salicylates, and tetracyclines either by ↓ absorption from GI tract or ↑ excretion.
4. *Magnesium-containing antacids:* ↑ Effect of dicumarol, quinidine, and sulfonylureas probably by ↓ excretion. ↓ Effect of benzodiazepines, corticosteroids, digoxin, histamine H_2 antagonists, hydantoins, iron products, nitrofurantoin, penicillamine, phenothiazines, tetracyclines, and ticlopidine either by ↓ absorption from GI tract or ↑ excretion.
5. *Sodium bicarbonate:* ↑ Effect of amphetamines, flecainide, quinidine, and sympathomimetics probably by ↑ excretion. ↓ Effect of benzodiazepines, hydantoins, ketoconazole, lithium, methenamine, methotrexate, salicylates, sulfonylureas, and tetracyclines either by ↓ absorption from GI tract or ↑ excretion.

Dosage

See individual drugs.

NURSING CONSIDERATIONS

Administration/Storage

1. Clients who have an active peptic ulcer should take antacids every hour during waking hours for the first 2 weeks.
2. For PUD, it is recommended that most antacids be taken 1 hr and 3 hr after meals and at bedtime.
3. Tablets should be thoroughly chewed before swallowing and followed by a glass of milk or water. Effervescent tablets should completely dissolve in water before ingestion.
4. Liquid preparations have a more rapid action time and greater activity than tablets. Refrigerate to improve palatability.
5. Shake liquid suspensions thoroughly before pouring the medication. After administering, follow with water to ensure passage to the stomach. When administering via feeding tube, flush with water.
6. The absorption rate of many drugs may be affected by antacids. Enteric-coated tablets may dissolve prematurely. Therefore, if other oral drugs are to be taken, it should be done at least 2 hr after ingestion of the antacid.
7. Administer laxative or cathartic dose at bedtime, as medication takes about 8 hr to be effective and the effect should not interfere with the client's rest.

Assessment

1. Document indications for therapy and type and onset of symptoms.
2. Note subjective reports of heartburn, indigestion, or epigastric pain. Document precipitating factors and foods as well as location, character, and duration of discomfort.
3. List other drugs the client may be taking to ascertain if any have an unfavorable interaction with the antacid ordered.
4. Note if the client has problems with diarrhea. Antacids containing magnesium may have a laxative effect, worsening this problem.
5. Determine if the client has a history of cardiac disease or hypertension. These clients often are on low-sodium diets, so prescribed antacids should also be low in sodium.

Interventions

1. Clients taking antacid preparations containing calcium or aluminum are prone to constipation. Encourage fluid intake of 2–3 L/day unless contraindicated and also increased consumption of foods high in bulk.
2. If the client has renal failure, increasing fluid intake to avoid constipation is not an option. Stool softeners may be necessary. Also, absorption of Na, Mg, Al, or Ca may precipitate alkalosis.
3. If constipation persists, determine if changing the antacid or using laxatives and/or enemas may be of some benefit.
4. Clients taking antacids that contain magnesium may report diarrhea. Document and report as a change in antacid or alternating a magnesium-based antacid with an aluminum- or calcium-based antacid may be indicated. Magnesium salts have a cathartic effect.

Client/Family Teaching

1. Take the tablets with water. The liquid acts as a vehicle, transporting the medication to the stomach, where the desired drug action occurs.
2. Take the drug at the prescribed times. Some may need to be taken on an empty stomach, whereas others, such as those used to bind phosphate, may need to be taken with meals.
3. Advise that refrigeration may improve taste.
4. Report any persistent constipation or diarrhea.
5. Advise that consumption of large amounts of TUMS can cause acid rebound.
6. Avoid taking OTC preparations unless specifically ordered.
7. Do not smoke or use alcoholic beverages.
8. Report any evidence of GI bleeding (dark black or tarry stools, coffee ground emesis).
9. Discuss the importance of following the specific dietary regime established as well as adhering to the medication protocol. Explain that antacids should be taken for 4–6 weeks after symptoms have disappeared as healing of the ulcer is not correlated with the disappearance of symptoms.
10. Instruct client to report if the symptoms for which they are being treated show little or no improvement after 2 weeks of therapy.

Evaluate

- Improvement in or resolution of pretreatment symptoms
- Reports of ↓ gastric pain and irritation
- Evacuation of a soft, formed stool
- ↑ Gastric pH
- Promotion of duodenal ulcer healing
- Prophylaxis of renal calculi

Aluminum hydroxide gel

(ah-**LOO**-mih-num)

AlternaGEL, Amphojel, Concentrated Aluminum Hydroxide, Gaviscon ✱ **(OTC)**

Aluminum hydroxide gel, dried

(ah-**LOO**-mih-num)

Alu-Cap, Alu-Tab, Amphojel Tablets, Basaljel ✱, Dialume **(OTC)**

See also *Antacids,* Chapter 59

How Supplied: Aluminum hydroxide gel: *Capsule:* 475 mg, 500 mg; *Concentrate:* 675 mg/5 mL; *Ointment*; *Suspension* 320 mg/5 mL, 450 mg/5 mL, 600 mg/5 mL; *Tablet:* 300 mg, 600 mg

Action/Kinetics: Aluminum hydroxide is nonsystemic, has demulcent activity, and is constipating. Aluminum hydroxide and phosphorus form insoluble phosphates that are eliminated in the feces. This yields a relatively phosphorus-free urine and prevents phosphate stone formation in susceptible clients. Acid-neutralizing capacity: 6.5–18 mEq/tablet, capsule, or 5 mL. Aluminum-containing antacids are believed to have a cytoprotective effect on the gastric mucosa (perhaps by stimulating prostaglandin synthesis), which protects against mucosal damage by aspirin and ethanol. Small amounts are absorbed from the intestine.

Additional Uses: Hyperphosphatemia, chronic renal failure.

Dosage

- **Capsules, Suspension, Tablets**

Antacid.

Adults, usual: 500–1,500 mg of capsules or tablets 3–6 times/day after meals, between meals, and at bedtime. For the suspension, 5–30 mL as needed between meals and at bedtime.

Hyperphosphatemia.

Children: 50–150 mg/kg/day in divided doses q 4–6 hr; adjust dosage until normal serum phosphate levels achieved.

Administration/Storage

1. Administer the gel in a half glass of water.

2. If administering the medication via stomach tube, dilute commercial solution 2 or 3 times with water. Administer this solution at a rate of 15–20 mL/min. The total daily dose should be approximately 1.5 L of the diluted suspension.

Contraindications: Sensitivity to aluminum. Peptic ulcer associated with pancreatic deficiency, diarrhea, or low-phosphorus diet. Aluminum hydroxide preparations contain sodium and thus should not be administered to clients on a low-sodium diet.

Side Effects: Chronic use may lead to bone pain, muscle weakness, or malaise due to chronic phosphate deficiency and osteomalacia. Constipation, intestinal obstruction. Decreased absorption of fluoride. Accumulation of aluminum in bone, CNS, and serum, which may be neurotoxic (e.g., encephalopathy has been reported).

Additional Drug Interactions: Aluminum hydroxide gel inhibits the absorption of barbiturates, digoxin, phenytoin, corticosteroids, quinidine, warfarin, and isoniazid, thereby decreasing their effect.

NURSING CONSIDERATIONS

See also *Nursing Considerations* for *Antacids,* Chapter 59.

Assessment

1. Note any history of hypersensitivity to aluminum products.
2. Determine if client is prescribed a low-sodium diet. Aluminum preparations may then be contraindicated.
3. Determine if the epigastric pain/discomfort is localized, burning, and gnawing, if it occurs 2–3 hr after a meal, and/or if it occurs during the early morning.
4. Test stools for occult blood.
5. Obtain baseline CBC and liver and renal function studies.
6. Assess and document bowel sounds, skin integrity, and neurologic status.
7. List any other drugs the client may be taking, either prescribed or OTC preparations.

Interventions

1. Monitor for relief of epigastric pain and describe any continued distress.
2. Assess bowel sounds and palpate abdomen. Note additive effects drug may have on GI motility.
3. Document and report acid rebound effects, evidenced by complaints of nocturnal pain.
4. With phosphatic urinary calculi, refer clients to a dietitian for a low-phosphate diet. The diet generally should consist of 1.3 g phosphorus, 700 mg calcium, 13 g nitrogen, and 2,500 cal/day for the duration of the therapy.
5. Determine urinary phosphate level monthly when used in the management of phosphatic urinary calculi.

Client/Family Teaching

1. Chew tablets before swallowing and take them with a glass of milk or water.
2. Report any changes in bowel elimination (drug may cause constipation).
3. These products are not indicated for prolonged, continual use except under medical supervision. Report if the symptoms persist so that further evaluation and therapy may be prescribed.

Evaluate

- ↓ Epigastric pain/discomfort
- Prevention of phosphatic urinary stones
- ↓ GI acidity
- ↓ Serum phosphate levels

Basic Aluminum Carbonate Gel

(ah-**LOO**-mih-num)
Basaljel **(OTC)**

See also *Antacids,* Chapter 59.

How Supplied: *Capsule:* 500 mg; *Suspension:* 400 mg/5 mL; *Tablet:* 500 mg

Action/Kinetics: The acid-neutralizing capacity of the capsules, suspension, or tablets is 12–13 mEq/capsule, tablet, or 5 mL. The acid-neutralizing capacity of the extra strength suspension is 22 mEq/5 mL.

Uses: Hyperacidity. With low-phosphorus diet to prevent phosphate urinary stones by reducing urinary phosphate levels.

NOTE: See *Aluminum Hydroxide Gel* for *Contraindications, Side Effects,* and *Additional Drug Interactions.*

Dosage

• **Tablets, Capsules, Suspension (Regular and Extra Strength)**

Antacid.

Adults: 2 tablets or capsules, 2 teaspoons of regular strength suspension, or 1 teaspoon of extra strength suspension q 2 hr, if necessary, up to 12 times/day.

Hyperphosphatemia.

Adults: 2 capsules or tablets, 12 mL suspension, or 5 mL extra strength suspension t.i.d.–q.i.d. after meals.

Administration/Storage

1. Dilute the liquid form in water or fruit juice.
2. Administer medication after meals and at bedtime.

NURSING CONSIDERATIONS

See also *Nursing Considerations* for *Aluminum Hydroxide Gel,* Chapter 59.

Assessment

1. Document indications for therapy, onset of symptoms, any other agents that were utilized, and the outcome.
2. Obtain and monitor appropriate laboratory data. Prolonged use may lead to hypophosphatemia, reabsorption of calcium, and bone demineralization.

Evaluate

• ↓ Gastric acidity
• ↓ Urinary phosphate levels

Calcium carbonate

(**KAL**-see-um **KAR**-bon-ayt)

Alka-Mints, Amitone, Antacid Tablets, Apo-Cal ✱, Cal Carb-HD, Calci-Chew, Calciday-667, Calci-Mix, Calcite 500, Calcium 500 ✱, Calcium 600, Cal-Plus, Calsan ✱, Caltrate 600, Caltrate Jr., Chooz, Dicarbosil, Equilet, Extra Strength Antacid, Extra Strength Tums, Florical, Gencalc 600, Maalox Antacid Caplets, Mallamint, Mylanta Lozenges, Nephro-Calci, Nu-Cal ✱, Os-Cal 500, Os-Cal 500 Chewable, Oysco 500 Chewable, Oyst-Cal 500, Oystercal 500, Oyster Shell Calcium-500, Tums, Tums Ultra **(OTC)**

See also *Calcium Salts,* Chapter 74, and *Antacids,* Chapter 59.

How Supplied: *Capsule:* 500 mg, 600 mg, 900 mg, 1250 mg; *Chew Tablet:* 200 mg, 300 mg, 420 mg, 500 mg, 600 mg, 650 mg, 750 mg, 1000 mg, 1250 mg, 1500 mg; *Lozenge/Troche:* 240 mg; *Suspension:* 500 mg/5 mL; *Tablet* 10 mg, 150 mg, 250 mg, 375 mg, 420 mg, 500 mg, 600 mg, 625 mg, 650 mg, 750 mg, 1000 mg, 1250 mg; *Tablet, Extended Release:* 500 mg; *Wafer:* 1250 mg

Uses: Mild hypocalcemia, antacid, antihyperphosphatemic.

Dosage

• **Chewable Tablets, Tablets, Suspension, Gum, Lozenges**

Adults: 0.5–1.5 g, as needed.

• **Capsules, Suspension, Tablets, Chewable Tablets**

Treat hypocalcemia, nutritional supplement.

Adults: 1.25–1.5 g 1–3 times/day with or after meals.

Antihyperphosphatemic.

Adults: 5–13 g/day in divided doses with meals.

NOTE: The preparation contains 40% elemental calcium and 400 mg elemental calcium/g (20 mEq/g).

• **Florical**

1 capsule or tablet daily (also contains 8.3 mg sodium fluoride per capsule or tablet).

Special Concerns: Dosage has not been established in children.

NURSING CONSIDERATIONS

See also *Nursing Considerations* for *Antacids,* Chapter 59, and *Calcium Salts,* Chapter 74.

Evaluate

• Serum calcium levels within desired range
• ↓ Gastric acidity

Calcium carbonate precipitated

(**KAL**-see-um **KAR**-bon-ayt)
Alka-Mints, Amitone, Calcilac, Calglycine, Chooz, Dicarbosil, Equilet, Genalac, Glycate, Gustalac, Mallamint, Pama No. 1, Rolaids Calcium Rich, Titralac, Tums, Tums E-X Extra Strength, Tums Liquid Extra Strength **(OTC)**

See also *Antacids,* Chapter 59.
Action/Kinetics: Nonsystemic antacid regarded by some as the antacid of choice. Since calcium carbonate is constipating, it is often alternated or even mixed with magnesium salts. Acid-neutralizing capacity: 8.25–10 mEq/tablet. Contains 40% calcium. Chronic use may lead to systemic effects. Rapid onset of action and relatively prolonged activity.
Uses: Antacid; adjunct in peptic ulcer therapy. Calcium deficiency.

Dosage

- **Chewing Gum, Oral Suspension, Tablets, Chewable Tablets**

Antacid.

Adults, individualize, usual: 0.5–1 g as necessary (or 0.5–1.5 g/2–4 hr).
Administration/Storage: Tablets should be chewed before being swallowed.
Side Effects: *GI:* Constipation, rebound hyperacidity, flatulence, eructation, intestinal obstruction. *Milk-alkali syndrome:* Hypercalcemia, metabolic alkalosis, renal dysfunction.

NURSING CONSIDERATIONS

See also *Nursing Considerations* for *Antacids,* Chapter 59.
Evaluate

- ↓ Gastric acidity
- Return of desired serum calcium levels

Dihydroxyaluminum sodium carbonate

(dye-hy-**drox**-ee-ah-**LOO**-mih-num)
Rolaids Antacid **(OTC)**

See also *Antacids,* Chapter 59.
Action/Kinetics: Nonsystemic antacid with adsorbent and protective properties similar to those of aluminum hydroxide but reported to act more rapidly. Acid-neutralizing capacity: 7 mEq/tablet. *NOTE:* See *Aluminum Hydroxide Gel* for Uses, Contraindications, Side Effects, and Drug Interactions.

Dosage

- **Chewable Tablets**

Antacid.

Adults: 1–2 tablets chewed after meals and at bedtime; 1–2 tablets chewed q 2–4 hr may be required to alleviate severe discomfort.

NURSING CONSIDERATIONS

See also *Nursing Considerations* for *Antacids,* Chapter 59.
Evaluate: Relief of abdominal discomfort R/T acid neutralization.

COMBINATION DRUG

Gelusil and Gelusil-II

(**JELL**-you-sill)
(OTC)

See also *Antacids,* Chapter 59.
How Supplied: See Content
Content: Gelusil contains the following in each tablet or 5 mL:

Antacid: Aluminum hydroxide, 200 mg.

Antacid: Magnesium hydroxide, 200 mg.

Antiflatulent: Simethicone, 25 mg.

Gelusil-II contains aluminum hydroxide and magnesium hydroxide, each 400 mg, and simethicone, 30 mg. See also information on individual components.
Action/Kinetics: Gelusil has a high capacity to neutralize acid and has a low sodium content.
Uses: To treat acid indigestion, heartburn, sour stomach; relieve symptoms of gas. Also as an adjunct in the treatment of peptic ulcer.

Dosage

- **Oral Chewable Tablets, Suspension**

Gelusil or Gelusil-II. Two or more tablets or teaspoonfuls 1 hr after meals and at bedtime.

Administration/Storage

1. Tablets should be chewed before being swallowed.
2. The maximum daily dosage of Gelusil should be 12 tablets or teaspoons, and the maximum daily dosage for Gelusil-II should be 8 tablets or teaspoonsful. Maximum dosage should not be taken for more than 2 weeks.

Additional Contraindication: Kidney disease.

Special Concerns: Prolonged use of aluminum-containing antacids in clients with renal failure may result in or worsen osteomalacia.

Drug Interaction: Antacids ↓ the absorption of tetracyclines from the GI tract.

NURSING CONSIDERATIONS

See also *Nursing Considerations* for *Antacids,* Chapter 59.

Assessment

1. Document indications for therapy and type and onset of symptoms.
2. Note any other agents previously used for this condition and the outcome.
3. Determine any evidence of renal dysfunction; ensure adequate calcium levels and vitamin D replacement with extended therapy.

Evaluate: ↓ GI upset and relief of abdominal discomfort R/T gas.

Maalox Antacid Caplets

(MAY-lox)
(OTC)

See also *Calcium carbonate,* Chapter 74, and *Antacids,* Chapter 59.

How Supplied: See Content

Content: Each caplet contains *Antacid:* calcium carbonate, 1,000 mg. The acid-neutralizing capacity is 20 mEq.

Uses: Symptomatic relief of hyperacidity associated with peptic ulcer, gastritis, peptic esophagitis, gastric hyperacidity, and hiatal hernia.

Dosage

- **Caplet**

  Antacid.

1 caplet as needed, not to exceed 8 caplets in a 24-hr period.

Administration/Storage

1. Caplets should not be chewed.
2. The maximum daily dosage should not be used for more than 2 weeks, unless authorized by a physician.

Special Concerns: Clients with a history of calcium stones or decreased renal function should consult a physician before use.

Drug Interactions

Beta-adrenergic blocking agents / ↓ Absorption of beta blockers from the GI tract

Phenytoin / ↓ Absorption of phenytoin from the GI tract

Thiazide diuretics / Hypercalcemia due to ↓ renal excretion of calcium carbonate

NURSING CONSIDERATIONS

See also *Nursing Considerations* for *Antacids,* Chapter 59.

Client/Family Teaching: Do not take 1 hr before or 1 hr after other prescribed medications unless specifically ordered.

Evaluate: ↓ Gastric acidity.

—COMBINATION DRUG—

Maalox HRF Suspension and Tablets

(MAY-lox)
(OTC)

See also *Antacids,* Chapter 59, and individual agents.

How Supplied: See Content

Content: Each 10 mL of the suspension contains: *Antacid:* Aluminum hydroxide–magnesium carbonate codried gel, 280 mg. *Antacid:* Magnesium carbonate, 350 mg. The acid-neutralizing capacity of 10 mL is 19 mEq.

Each tablet contains: *Antacid:* Aluminum hydroxide–magnesium carbonate codried gel, 180 mg. *Antacid:* Magnesium carbonate, 160 mg. The acid-neutralizing capacity of 2 tablets is 14.7 mEq.
Use: Relief of heartburn.

Dosage

- **Suspension**

Heartburn.

10–20 mL after meals and at bedtime.

- **Tablets**

Heartburn.

2–4 tablets chewed thoroughly after meals and at bedtime and followed with 4 oz of water or other liquid.

Administration/Storage

1. Dosage should not exceed 80 mL of the suspension or 16 of the tablets in a 24-hr period.
2. The maximum dosage should not be used more than 2 weeks or in those with kidney disease, unless authorized by a physician.
3. Both the suspension and tablets are mint flavored.

Contraindication: Use with tetracycline antibiotics.
Additional Side Effects: Prolonged use of antacids containing aluminum may cause or worsen dialysis osteomalacia and may cause hypophosphatemia. Elevated tissue aluminum levels may also cause development of dialysis encephalopathy.

NURSING CONSIDERATIONS

See also *Nursing Considerations* for *Antacids,* Chapter 59.
Evaluate: Reports of symptomatic relief.

COMBINATION DRUG

Maalox Oral Suspension

(MAY-lox)
(OTC)

See also *Antacids,* and *Maalox HRF,* Chapter 59, and individual agents.
How Supplied: See Content
Content: Each 5 mL of the oral suspension contains: *Antacid:* Aluminum hydroxide, 225 mg. *Antacid:* Magnesium hydroxide, 200 mg. The acid-neutralizing capacity of each 5 mL is 13.3 mEq.
Uses: Symptomatic relief of hyperacidity due to peptic ulcer, gastritis, peptic esophagitis, gastric hyperacidity, heartburn, or hiatal hernia.

Dosage

- **Oral Suspension**

Hyperacidity.

10–20 mL q.i.d. 20–60 min after meals and at bedtime.

Administration/Storage

1. Dosage should not exceed 80 mL of the suspension in a 24-hr period.
2. The maximum dosage should not be used for more than 2 weeks or in those with kidney disease, unless authorized by a physician.
3. The suspension is supplied as mint flavored or cherry creme flavored.

NURSING CONSIDERATIONS

See also *Nursing Considerations* for *Antacids,* Chapter 59.
Evaluate: Reports of symptomatic improvement.

COMBINATION DRUG

Maalox Plus Tablets

(MAY-lox)
(OTC)

See also *Antacids,* and *Maalox HRF,* Chapter 59, and individual agents.
How Supplied: See Content
Content: Each Maalox Plus Tablet contains: *Antacid:* Aluminum hydroxide dried gel, 200 mg. *Antacid:* Magnesium hydroxide, 200 mg. *Antiflatulent:* Simethicone, 25 mg. The acid-neutralizing capacity of each tablet is 10.65 mEq.
Uses: Symptomatic relief of hyperacidity due to peptic ulcer, gastritis, peptic esophagitis, gastric hyperacidity, heartburn, or hiatal hernia. Also as an antiflatulent to relieve symptoms of gas, including postoperative gas pain.

Dosage

- **Tablets**

Antacid/antiflatulent.

1–4 tablets q.i.d. taken 20–60 min after meals and at bedtime.

Administration/Storage

1. Tablets should be well chewed before swallowing.
2. No more than 16 tablets should be taken in a 24-hr period.
3. The maximum dosage should not be used for more than 2 weeks or in those with kidney disease, unless authorized by a physician.
4. Tablets are supplied in Lemon Swiss Creme or Cherry Creme flavors.

NURSING CONSIDERATIONS

See also *Nursing Considerations* for *Antacids,* Chapter 59.

Evaluate:

- ↓ Gastric acidity
- Relief of abdominal discomfort postoperatively R/T ↑ flatus

—COMBINATION DRUG—

Maalox Plus Extra Strength Oral Suspension

(MAY-lox)
(OTC)

Maalox Plus Extra Strength Tablets

(MAY-lox)
(OTC)

See also *Antacids,* and *Maalox HRF,* Chapter 59, and individual components.

How Supplied: See Content

Content: Each 5 mL of Maalox Plus Extra Strength Oral Suspension contains: *Antacid:* Magnesium hydroxide, 450 mg. *Antacid:* Aluminum hydroxide, 500 mg. *Antiflatulent:* Simethicone, 40 mg.

Each Maalox Plus Extra Strength Tablet contains: *Antacid:* Magnesium hydroxide, 350 mg. *Antacid:* Aluminum hydroxide, 350 mg. *Antiflatulent:* Simethicone, 40 mg. The acid-neutralizing capacity is 18.6 mEq for each extra strength tablet and 58.1 mEq/10 mL of the extra strength oral suspension.

Uses: Relief of hyperacidity due to peptic ulcer, peptic esophagitis, gastric hyperacidity, gastritis, hiatal hernia, or heartburn. Also, to relieve symptoms of gas, including postoperative gas pain.

Dosage

- **Extra Strength Oral Suspension**

Adults: 10–20 mL q.i.d. 20–60 min after meals and at bedtime.

- **Extra Strength Tablets**

Adults: 1–3 tablets q.i.d. 20–60 min after meals and at bedtime.

Administration/Storage

1. The tablets should be chewed well before swallowing.
2. No more than 60 mL of the suspension or 16 tablets should be taken within a 24-hr period.
3. The maximum dosage should not be used for more than 2 weeks or in those with kidney disease, unless authorized by provider.
4. The suspension is available in three flavors—lemon swiss creme, cherry creme, and mint creme—and the tablets are available in the mint creme flavor.

NURSING CONSIDERATIONS

See also *Nursing Considerations* for *Antacids,* Chapter 59.

Evaluate:

- ↓ Gastric acidity
- Relief of abdominal discomfort postoperatively R/T ↑ flatus

Magaldrate (Hydroxymagnesium aluminate)

(MAG-al-drayt)
Lowsium, Riopan, Riopan Extra Strength ✱ (OTC)

See also *Antacids,* Chapter 59.

How Supplied: *Suspension*

Action/Kinetics: Chemical combination of aluminum hydroxide and magnesium hydroxide. This compound is an effective nonsystemic antacid. It buffers

(pH 3.0–5.5) without causing alkalosis. Acid-neutralizing capacity: 13.5 mEq/tablet or 15 mEq/5 mL suspension.
Use: Antacid.

Dosage

- **Oral Suspension, Tablets**

Antacid.

Adults: 480–1,080 mg q.i.d. between meals and at bedtime. Frequency of administration may have to be increased initially to every hour to control severe symptoms. The suspension contains 540 mg/5 mL.
Contraindications: Sensitivity to aluminum. Use with caution in clients with impaired renal function.
Side Effects: Mild constipation and hypermagnesemia. Rebound hyperacidity, milk-alkali syndrome.

NURSING CONSIDERATIONS

See also *Nursing Considerations* for *Antacids,* Chapter 59.
Assessment: Obtain baseline renal function studies to determine any dysfunction.
Evaluate: ↓ Gastric acidity and relief of associated GI pain.

Magnesium hydroxide (magnesia)

(mag-**NEE**-see-um hy-**DROX**-eyed)

Concentrated Phillips' Milk of Magnesia, Phillips' Chewable, Phillips' Milk of Magnesia, M.O.M. **(OTC)**

See also *Antacids,* Chapter 59, and *Laxatives,* Chapter 60.
How Supplied: *Capsule; Concentrate; Liquid; Tablet*
Action/Kinetics: Depending on dosage, drug acts as an antacid or as a laxative. Neutralizes hydrochloric acid. Does not produce alkalosis and has a demulcent effect. A dose of 1 mL neutralizes 2.7 mEq of acid. As an antacid, often alternated with aluminum hydroxide to counteract laxative effect.

As a laxative, magnesium hydroxide increases the bulk of the stools by attracting and holding large amounts of fluids. The increased bulk results in the mechanical stimulation of peristalsis. **Onset:** 2–6 hr.
Uses: Antacid. As a laxative to empty the bowel prior to diagnostic or surgical procedures, to eliminate parasites following anthelmintic therapy, to remove toxic materials following poisoning, and to collect a stool specimen for parasite examination.

Dosage

- **Oral Suspension, Tablets, Chewable Tablets**

Antacid.

Adults and children over 12 years: 5–15 mL liquid, 2.5–7.5 mL of the concentrated liquid (with water) or 622–1,244 mg tablets q.i.d. **Children, 6–12 years:** 2.5–5 mL liquid with water.

Laxative.

Adults and children over 12 years: 15–40 mL liquid once daily with water. **Children, 6–12 years:** 15–30 mL (depending on age) once daily with water. **Children, 2–6 years:** 5–15 mL of the liquid once daily with water.

Administration/Storage

1. Suspensions should be administered with water.
2. Administer combined magnesia magma and aluminum hydroxide gel with one-half glass of water.
3. To minimize the unpleasant aftertaste provide a slice of orange or glass of orange juice after administration as a laxative.
4. Administer laxative dose at bedtime because medication takes about 8 hr to be effective and, therefore, will not interfere with client's rest.

Contraindication: Poor renal function.
Side Effects: Diarrhea, abdominal pain, N&V. Hypermagnesemia and CNS depression (especially in clients with renal failure). Magnesium intoxication is manifested by drowsiness, dizziness, other signs of CNS depression, and thirst.

Additional Drug Interactions

Procainamide / Procainamide ↑ muscle relaxation produced by Mg salts
Skeletal muscle relaxants (surgical), succinylcholine, tubocurarine / ↑ Muscle relaxation

NURSING CONSIDERATIONS

See also *Nursing Considerations* for *Antacids,* Chapter 59, and *Laxatives,* Chapter 60.

Evaluate

- ↓ Gastric acidity
- Successful bowel evacuation

Magnesium oxide

(mag-**NEE**-see-um **OX**-eyed)

Mag-Ox 400, Maox, Uro-Mag **(OTC)**

See also *Antacids,* Chapter 59, and *Laxatives,* Chapter 60.

How Supplied: *Capsule:* 140 mg; *Tablet:* 200 mg, 250 mg, 400 mg, 420 mg, 500 mg

Action/Kinetics: Magnesium oxide is a nonsystemic antacid with a laxative effect. The compound has a rather high neutralizing capacity (1.0 g neutralizes 50 mEq acid). Magnesium oxide is slower acting than sodium bicarbonate but has a more prolonged activity.

Use: Antacid.

Dosage

- **Capsules**

  Antacid.

140 mg with water or milk t.i.d.–q.i.d.

- **Tablets**

  Antacid.

400–840 mg/day.

Contraindication: Poor renal function.

Side Effects: Abdominal pain, nausea, diarrhea. Hypermagnesemia and CNS depression in clients with poor renal function. Symptoms of magnesium intoxication include drowsiness, dizziness, other signs of CNS depression, and thirst. Rebound hyperacidity, milk-alkali syndrome.

Drug Interactions: See *Magnesium Hydroxide,* Chapter 59.

NURSING CONSIDERATIONS

See *Nursing Considerations* for *Antacids,* Chapter 59, and *Laxatives,* Chapter 60.

Evaluate: Reports of symptomatic relief.

—COMBINATION DRUG—

Mylanta Liquid and Tablets

(my-**LAN**-tah)

(OTXC)

Mylanta Double Strength Liquid and Tablets

(my-**LAN**-tah)

(OTC)

See also *Antacids,* Chapter 59.

How Supplied: See Content

Content: Mylanta. Each tablet or 5 mL of the liquid contains: *Antacid:* Aluminum hydroxide dried gel, 200 mg; *Antacid:* Magnesium hydroxide, 200 mg; and, *Antiflatulent:* Simethicone, 20 mg. The acid-neutralizing capacity is 25.4 mEq/10 mL of the liquid and 23.0 mEq/2 tablets.

Mylanta Double Strength. Each tablet or 5 mL of the liquid contains: *Antacid:* Aluminum hydroxide dried gel, 400 mg; *Antacid:* Magnesium hydroxide, 400 mg; *Antiflatulent:* Simethicone, 40 mg. The acid-neutralizing capacity is 50.8 mEq/10 mL of the liquid and 46 mEq/2 tablets. See also information on individual components.

Uses: Antacid for relief of hyperacidity due to peptic ulcer, gastritis, peptic esophagitis, heartburn, and hiatal hernia.

The product also relieves accompanying distress due to mucus- entrapped gas, including postoperative gas pain.

Dosage

- **Oral Suspension, Chewable Tablets**

Mylanta or Mylanta Double Strength. **Adults:** 10–20 mL of the liquid or 2–4 tablets between meals and at bedtime.

Administration/Storage

1. The gastric acid output and gastric emptying time vary greatly; thus, the dosage schedule should be individualized.
2. For Mylanta, no more than 120 mL

or 24 tablets should be taken within a 24-hr period. For Mylanta Double Strength, no more than 60 mL or 12 tablets should be taken within a 24-hr period.
3. The maximum doses of these products should not be used for more than 2 weeks, unless ordered by the provider.
Contraindications: Use with kidney disease or in clients receiving any form of tetracycline.
Special Concerns: Chronic use of aluminum-containing antacids in clients with renal failure may cause or worsen dialysis osteomalacia. Hypophosphatemia may result following prolonged use of aluminum- containing antacids.

NURSING CONSIDERATIONS

See also *Nursing Considerations* for *Antacids,* Chapter 59.
Client/Family Teaching
1. Chew tablets well before swallowing.
2. If a suspension is to be used, shake the container well before pouring the medication.
3. Report if symptoms persist or intensify.
4. Avoid antacids during tetracycline therapy.
Evaluate: ↓ Gastric acidity and relief of abdominal discomfort R/T gas.

Simethicone

(sye-**METH**-ih-kohn)
Extra-Strength Gas-X, Flatulex, Gas Relief, Gas-X, Major-Con, Maximum Strength Mylanta Gas, Maximum Strength Phazyme 125 Softgels, Mylanta Gas-40 and -80, Mylicon, Ovol ✱, Ovol-40 and -80 ✱, Phazyme, Phazyme 55 ✱, Phazyme 95 **(OTC)**

How Supplied: *Capsule:* 125 mg; *Chew Tablet:* 40 mg, 62.5 mg, 80 mg, 125 mg, 150 mg; *Liquid:* 40 mg/0.6 mL; *Tablet:* 60 mg, 95 mg
Action/Kinetics: Simethicone acts as a defoamant, which decreases surface tension of gas bubbles, thus facilitating their coalescence and expulsion as flatus or belching. It also prevents the accumulation of mucus-enclosed pockets of gas. Excreted in feces unchanged.
Uses: Relief of pain caused by excess gas in digestive tract. Adjunct in the treatment of postoperative gaseous distention and pain, air swallowing, endoscopic examination, functional dyspepsia, peptic ulcer, spastic or irritable colon, diverticulitis. *Investigational:* Treat symptoms of infant colic (given with meals).

Dosage
- **Chewable Tablets, Tablets**

Adults: 40–125 mg after each meal and at bedtime (up to a maximum of 480 mg/day if used OTC).
- **Capsules**

Adults: 125 mg after each meal and at bedtime.
- **Drops**

Adults: 40–80 mg q.i.d., up to 500 mg/day. **Pediatric, 2–12 years old:** 40 mg q.i.d. after meals and at bedtime; **pediatric, less than 2 years old:** 20 mg q.i.d. (up to 240 mg/day total dose) taken after meals and at bedtime.
Administration/Storage
1. Tablets should be chewed thoroughly or dissolved in mouth.
2. Use calibrated dropper to administer medication.
3. In children less than 2 years old, the drops may be mixed with 30 mL cool water, infant formula, or other liquids.

NURSING CONSIDERATIONS

Interventions
1. Document indications for therapy, onset of symptoms, other agents used, and the outcome.
2. Assess bowel sounds periodically during therapy.
3. Question client concerning the effectiveness of prescribed therapy because dosage may need to be adjusted.
Evaluate
- ↓ Tympany and ↓ abdominal distention
- ↓ Abdominal pain with relief of flatus

CHAPTER SIXTY

Laxatives

See also the following individual entries:

Bisacodyl
Bisacodyl Tannex
Cascara Sagrada
Castor Oil
Castor Oil, Emulsified
Docusate Calcium
Docusate Potassium
Docusate Sodium
Glycerin
Lactulose
Magnesium Hydroxide - See Chapter 59
Magnesium Oxide - See Chapter 59
Magnesium Sulfate
Methylcellulose
Mineral Oil
Phenolphthalein
Psyllium Hydrophilic Muciloid
Senna
Sennosides A and B, Calcium Salts

General Statement: Difficult or infrequent passage of stools (constipation) is a symptom of many conditions ranging from purely organic causes (obstruction, megacolon) to common functional disorders. Clients confined to bed may often develop constipation. Constipation may also be of psychologic origin. The underlying cause of constipation should be elucidated by a physician, especially since a marked change in bowel habits may be a symptom of a pathologic condition.

Laxatives are effective because they act locally, either by specifically stimulating the smooth muscles of the bowel or by changing the bulk or consistency of the stools. Laxatives can be divided into five categories.

1. *Stimulant laxatives:* Substances that chemically stimulate the smooth muscles of the bowel to increase contractions. Drugs include bisacodyl, cascara, danthron, phenolphthalein, and senna.
2. *Saline laxatives:* Substances that increase the bulk of the stools by retaining water. Includes magnesium salts and sodium phosphate.
3. *Bulk-forming laxatives:* Nondigestible substances that pass through the stomach and then increase the bulk of the stools. Examples are methylcellulose, psyllium, and polycarbophil.
4. *Emollient and lubricant laxatives:* Agents that soften hardened feces and facilitate their passage through the lower intestine. Examples include docusate and mineral oil.
5. *Miscellaneous:* Includes glycerin suppositories and lactulose.

Chronic use of laxatives may cause chronic constipation and other intestinal disorders because the client may start to depend on the psychologic effect and physical stimulus of the drug rather than on the body's own natural reflexes. Prevention of constipation should include adequate fluid intake and diet, as well as daily exercise.

Uses: Short-term treatment of constipation. Prophylaxis in clients who should not strain during defecation, i.e., following anorectal surgery or after MI (fecal softeners or lubricant laxatives). To evacuate the colon for rectal and bowel examinations (certain lubricant, saline, and stimulant laxatives). In conjunction with surgery or anthelmintic therapy. See also individual agents.

Contraindications: Severe abdominal pain that *might* be caused by appendicitis, enteritis, ulcerative colitis, diverticulitis, intestinal obstruction. The administration of laxatives in such cases might cause rupture of the abdomen or intestinal hemorrhage. Undiagnosed abdominal pain. Children under the age of 2. Castor oil is contraindicated during pregnancy as the irritant effects may result in premature labor.

Special Concerns: Chronic use may lead to laxative dependency.

Side Effects: *GI:* Excess activity of the colon resulting in nausea, diarrhea, griping, or vomiting. Perianal irritation, bloating, flatulence. *Electrolyte Balance:* Dehydration, disturbance of the electrolyte balance. *Miscellaneous:* Dizziness, fainting, weakness, sweating, palpitations.

Bulk laxatives: Obstruction in the esophagus, stomach, small intestine, or rectum. *Stimulant laxatives:* Chronic abuse may lead to malfunctioning colon. *Mineral Oil:* Large doses may cause anal seepage resulting in itching, irritation, hemorrhoids, and perianal discomfort.

Drug Interactions

Anticoagulants, oral / ↓ Absorption of vitamin K from GI tract induced by laxatives may ↑ effects of anticoagulants and result in bleeding

Digitalis / Cathartics may ↓ absorption of digitalis

Tetracyclines / Laxatives containing Al, Ca, or Mg may ↓ effect of tetracyclines due to ↓ absorption from GI tract

NURSING CONSIDERATIONS

Administration

1. When administering a laxative, note the length of time it takes for the laxative to take effect and give it so that the result of the laxative will not interfere with the client's rest.
2. Administer laxatives at a temperature that makes them more agreeable to the client.
3. If the laxative is to be administered in a liquid, try to select one that the client finds palatable.
4. Administer laxatives at a time that will not interfere with the client's digestion and absorption of nutrients.
5. If the laxative is ordered to prepare the client for a diagnostic study, check the directions carefully to ensure accurate administration in preparation for the study.

Assessment

1. Determine the extent of the client's problem with constipation. Note how long the client has had to rely on laxatives and the underlying causes.
2. Note the type of laxative the client has been taking and the relative effectiveness associated with this laxative.
3. Note if the client has abdominal pain and discomfort, its exact location, and the type of discomfort the client is experiencing. The symptoms may indicate appendicitis or some other intestinal disorder and laxatives would be contraindicated.
4. Determine the character of the stool and assess the frequency of bowel movements expected by the client. The client's definition of constipation may determine if, in fact, constipation exists.
5. Note the age of the client, state of health, and general nutritional status.
6. Identify any special restriction or limitation due to illness. This may include fluid restriction as well as a sodium-restricted diet.
7. List other prescribed medications the client is taking that may contribute to a constipation problem (i.e., diuretics, anticholinergics, antihistamines, antidepressants, and some antihypertensive agents).
8. Identify if the client has had any recent changes in life-style that may contribute to the current problem.

Interventions

1. If the client is hospitalized or is ill at home, provide a commode at the bedside. This will promote better bowel function by encouraging the client to move about and ensure privacy.
2. Encourage the client to alter dietary habits to include bulk foods and sufficient fluid in the daily diet to enhance elimination.

3. Discuss with clients the need for regular exercise, as well as a need for a reduction of their dependence on laxatives.

Client/Family Teaching

1. Discuss the need to have a regular schedule for defecation.
2. Instruct the client to keep a record of bowel function and response to all laxatives taken.
3. Advise that laxatives reduce the amount of time other drugs remain in the intestine and may diminish their intended effectiveness.
4. If the laxative is to be taken in preparation for a diagnostic study, review the directions with the client and provide a printed set of instructions to follow. If the client is unable to read, try to ensure that someone in the family or a friend can review the directions with the client so that an accurate result of the test can be obtained.
5. Instruct the client in techniques that facilitate elimination. Sitting with the legs slightly elevated and leaning forward to increase abdominal pressure often encourages elimination.
6. Discuss the dangers of relying on laxatives for bowel movements and laxative dependence. Stress the use of diet to achieve the same purpose. Two or three prunes a day are preferable to laxatives.
7. Advise that frequent use of any type of enemas may cause damage to the rectum and small bowel as well as inhibit bowel tone and may cause electrolyte abnormalities.
8. Review the importance of a diet high in fiber foods (and juices such as prune) and daily exercise and their benefits in maintaining proper bowel function. Refer to a dietitian if assistance is needed in meal planning and preparation and food selections.
9. Consult the provider if constipation persists because there could be a physiologic problem that requires attention.
10. If the client is pregnant, advise her to consult with the provider before taking any laxatives to treat constipation.
11. Advise nursing mothers to avoid using laxatives unless prescribed as many are excreted in breast milk and can cause the infant to develop diarrhea.

Evaluate

- Relief of constipation as evidenced by evacuation of a soft, formed stool
- Reports that bowel movements occur regularly with a minimum of difficulty and without having to resort to the chronic use of laxatives, enemas, or suppositories
- Evidence of effective colon preparation for diagnostic procedures (no stool in bowel)

Bisacodyl

(bis-ah-**KOH**-dill)
Apo-Bisacodyl ✱, Bisacodyl Uniserts, Bisacolax ✱, Dulcagen, Dulcolax, Fleet Bisacodyl, Fleet Bisacodyl Prep, PMS-Bisacodyl ✱ **(OTC)**

Bisacodyl tannex

(bis-ah-**KOH**-dill)
Clysodrast **(Rx)**

See also *Laxatives,* Chapter 60.

How Supplied: Bisacodyl: *Enteric Coated Tablet:* 5 mg; *Enema:* 10 mg; *Suppository:* 10 mg.
Bisacodyl tannex: *Packet:* 1.5 mg bisacodyl with 2.5 g tannic acid

Action/Kinetics: Bisacodyl is a local chemical stimulant that acts by increasing the contraction of the muscles of the colon by stimulating the myenteric plexus; this results in an alteration of water and electrolyte secretion. Bisacodyl is not absorbed systemically and can be administered PO or as a rectal suppository or solution. It produces a gentle bowel movement with soft, formed stools. It usually acts within 6–10 hr after PO administration and 15–60 min after rectal administration.

Uses: Cleansing of colon preoperatively and postoperatively and for diagnostic procedures (radiology, barium enemas, proctoscopy), colostomies. Short-term treatment of constipation.

May be used during pregnancy or in the presence of CV, renal, or hepatic disease.

Dosage

- **Bisacodyl Tablets**

Laxative.

Adults: 10–15 mg at bedtime or before breakfast.

Preparation of lower GI tract.

Adults: Up to 30 mg; **Pediatric, over 6 years:** 5–10 mg at bedtime or before breakfast.

- **Bisacodyl Rectal Suppository**

Laxative.

Adults and children over 2 years: 10 mg; **under 2 years:** 5 mg.

- **Bisacodyl Tannex Enema**

Cleansing enema.

2.5 g (1 packet) in 1 L warm water.

Barium enema.

2.5 or 5 g in 1 L barium suspension. *NOTE:* No more than 10 g should be given within a 3-day period. Also, the total dose for one examination of the colon should not exceed 7.5 g.

Administration/Storage

1. Bisacodyl tablets should be swallowed whole and should not be taken within 1 hr of milk or antacids.
2. Bisacodyl tablets should be taken either at bedtime for effectiveness in the morning or before breakfast so as not to interfere with the client's rest at night. The tablets should be effective within 6 hr.
3. If the tablets are being given to prepare the client for surgery, radiography, or sigmoidoscopy, the drug should be taken PO the night before the procedure and by rectal suppository early that morning.
4. Bisacodyl tablets should be refrigerated at temperatures not to exceed 30°C (86°F).
5. Lubricate suppositories with warm water prior to administration.

Contraindications: Acute surgical abdomen or acute abdominal pain. Children less than 6 years of age. Use of bisacodyl tannex in clients with ulcerative lesions of the colon or in children less than 10 years of age.

Special Concern: Use bisacodyl tannex with caution when multiple enemas are given.

Additional Side Effects: Suppositories may cause burning sensation, proctitis, and inflammation.

Drug Interaction: Use of bisacodyl with antacids, milk, or cimetidine may result in premature dissolution of the enteric coating, leading to cramping and vomiting.

NURSING CONSIDERATIONS

See also *Nursing Considerations* for *Laxatives,* Chapter 60.

Client/Family Teaching

1. Swallow the tablet whole. Do not crush or chew the tablets.
2. Children who cannot swallow tablets will be unable to take the laxative by mouth.
3. Advise the client not to take the laxative within 1 hr of ingesting milk, an antacid, or cimetidine.
4. Review the appropriate method for rectal administration when prescribed.

Evaluate

- Relief of constipation
- Effective colon cleansing for bowel preps

Cascara sagrada

(kas-**KAR**-ah sah-**GRAD**-ah)

Cascara Sagrada Fluid Extract, Cascara Sagrada Aromatic Fluid Extract, Cascara Tablets **(OTC)**

See also *Laxatives,* Chapter 60.

How Supplied: *Liquid*; *Tablet:* 325 mg

Action/Kinetics: Cascara sagrada directly stimulates the intestinal mucosa and the myenteric plexus. The drug alters secretion of water and electrolytes. It produces stools within 6–10 hr. The drug is available in tablet form as well as an aromatic fluid extract.

Use: Short-term treatment of constipation.

Dosage

- **Aromatic Fluid Extract**

Laxative.

Adults: 5 mL at bedtime; **pediatric, over 2 years of age:** 1–3 mL.

- **Fluid Extract**
  Laxative.

Adults: 1 mL at bedtime.

- **Tablets**
  Laxative.

Adults: 1 tablet at bedtime.
Additional Contraindication: The drug gets into breast milk and may cause diarrhea in the infant.
Additional Side Effects: Dark pigmentation of the mucosa of the colon (called melanosis coli), which is slowly reversed after the drug is discontinued. Acid urine may be colored yellowish brown while an alkaline urine may be colored pink, red, or violet.

NURSING CONSIDERATIONS

See also *Nursing Considerations* for *Laxatives,* Chapter 60.
Assessment
1. Review client's elimination patterns and determine any precipitating factors that may be causing constipation.
2. Determine how long and how often the client has been using cascara. If the client has taken cascara over an extended period of time, monitor serum electrolyte levels (especially K^+).
Client/Family Teaching
1. Cascara sagrada may discolor urine and stool yellow-brown, violet, or reddish.
2. Read the bottle carefully to distinguish between the aromatic fluid extract and the fluid extract because the dosage is different.
3. Advise nursing mothers that breast milk may appear brownish. Additionally, infant may experience diarrhea.
4. Use cascara for a short time only. Cascara sagrada can cause electrolyte imbalance, especially hypokalemia and laxative dependence. This can be particularly dangerous for elderly clients.
5. Explain the importance of diet, increased liquids, and exercise in the management of constipation and focus on areas that are deficient.
Evaluate: Relief of constipation.

Castor oil

(**KAS**-tor)
Kellogg's Castor Oil, Purge **(OTC)**

Castor oil, emulsified

(**KAS**-tor)
Alphamul, Emulsoil, Fleet Flavored Castor Oil, Neoloid, Ricifruit ✱ **(OTC)**

See also *Laxatives,* Chapter 60.
How Supplied: Castor oil: *Liquid.* Castor oil, emulsified: *Liquid*
Action/Kinetics: The active ingredient is ricinoleic acid, which is liberated in the small intestine. This substance inhibits water and electrolyte absorption, leading to fluid accumulation and increased peristalsis. Prompt (within 2–6 hr) and complete evacuation of the bowel occurs, often with a watery stool.
Uses: Preparation of bowel for diagnostic procedures. Short-term relief of constipation.

Dosage

- **Castor Oil**
  Preparation of bowel.

Adults: 15–60 mL before diagnostic procedures; **infants:** 1–5 mL; **children over 2 years:** 5–15 mL.

- **Castor Oil Emulsified**
  Preparation of bowel, laxative.

Adults: 15–60 mL; **infants less than 2 years:** 1.25–7.5 mL; **children over 2 years:** 5–30 mL. Dose depends on strength of preparation.
Administration/Storage
1. Shake emulsions well prior to administering. They may be further diluted in water, juice or cola before administering unless otherwise indicated.
2. Regular castor oil does not mix well with water-based materials. Adding a small amount of sodium bicarbonate to castor oil immediately before administering it will cause the mixture to fizz, particularly suspending the castor oil for a few

minutes in the diluent. Discuss prior to administering the laxative, unless the client's condition does not permit.
Contraindications: Pregnancy, menstruation, abdominal pain, and intestinal obstruction. Common constipation. Concomitantly with fat-soluble anthelmintics.
Side Effects: Severe diarrhea, abdominal pain and colic, altered mucosal permeability in the small intestine, dehydration, and changes in electrolyte balance, including hyperkalemia, acidosis, or alkalosis.

NURSING CONSIDERATIONS

See also *Nursing Considerations* for *Laxatives,* Chapter 60.
Client/Family Teaching
1. Clients usually prefer the more palatable oil-in-water emulsions that have been aromatized with flavoring agents.
2. Disguise the taste of plain castor oil by mixing with a glass of orange juice.
Evaluate
- Relief of constipation
- Desired bowel prep for diagnostic procedures

Docusate calcium (Dioctyl calcium sulfosuccinate)

(**DEW**-kyou-sayt)
Pregnancy Category: C
Calax ✱, DC Softgels, Doxate-C ✱, PMS Docusate Calcium ✱, Pro-Cal-Sof, Sulfalax Calcium, Surfak ✱, Surfak Liquigels **(OTC)**

Docusate potassium (Dioctyl potassium sulfosuccinate)

(**DEW**-kyou-sayt)
Pregnancy Category: C
Dialose, Diocto-K **(OTC)**

Docusate sodium (Dioctyl sodium sulfosuccinate)

(**DEW**-kyou-sayt)
Pregnancy Category: C
Colace, Diocto, Dioeze, Disonate, DOK, DOS Softgel, Doxate-S ✱, Doxinate, D-S-S, Modane Soft, PMS-Docusate Sodium ✱, Pro-Sof, Regulax SS, Regulex ✱, Regutol, Selax ✱ **(OTC)**

See also *Laxatives,* Chapter 60.
How Supplied: Docusate calcium: *Capsule:* 100 mg, 240 mg, 250 mg.
Docusate potassium: *Capsule:* 100 mg, 240 mg
Docusate sodium: *Capsule:* 50 mg, 100 mg, 240 mg, 250 mg; *Liquid:* 150 mg/15 mL; *Powder for Reconstitution:* 283 mg; *Solution:* 100 mg/15 mL; *Syrup:* 50 mg/15 mL, 60 mg/15 mL; *Tablet:* 100 mg
Action/Kinetics: These laxatives promote defecation by softening the feces. Useful when it is desirable to keep the feces soft or when straining at stool is undesirable. They act by lowering the surface tension of the feces and promoting their penetration by water and fat, thus increasing the softness of the fecal mass. Docusate is not absorbed systemically and does not seem to interfere with the absorption of nutrients. **Onset:** 24–72 hr.
Uses: To lessen strain of defecation in persons with hernia or CV diseases or other diseases in which straining at stool should be avoided. Megacolon or bedridden clients. Constipation associated with dry, hard stools.

Dosage
DOCUSATE CALCIUM
- **Capsules**

Adults: 240 mg/day until bowel movements are normal; **pediatric, over 6 years:** 50–150 mg/day.
DOCUSATE POTASSIUM
- **Capsules**

Adults: 100–300 mg/day; **pediatric, over 6 years:** 100 mg at bedtime.
DOCUSATE SODIUM
- **Capsules, Oral Solution, Syrup, Tablets**

Adults and children over 12 years: 50–500 mg; **pediatric, under 3 years:** 10–40 mg; **3–6 years:** 20–60 mg; **6–12 years:** 40–120 mg.
- **Rectal Solution**

Flushing or retention enema.
Adults: 50–100 mg.

Administration/Storage
1. Administer PO solutions of docusate sodium with milk or fruit juices to help mask the bitter taste.
2. If docusate sodium is to be used in enemas, add 50–100 mg (5–10 mL) to a retention or flushing enema.
3. A glass of water should be consumed with each PO dose of docusate sodium.
4. Because docusate salts are minimally absorbed, it may require 1–3 days to soften fecal matter.

Contraindications: Nausea, vomiting, abdominal pain, and intestinal obstruction.

Drug Interaction: Docusate may ↑ absorption of mineral oil from the GI tract.

NURSING CONSIDERATIONS

See also *Nursing Considerations* for *Laxatives,* Chapter 60.

Evaluate: Elimination of a soft, formed stool with a minimum of effort.

Glycerin

(**GLIH**-sir-in)
Pregnancy Category: C (oral use)
Fleet Babylax, Osmoglyn, Sani-Supp
(OTC)

How Supplied: *Suppository*

Action/Kinetics: Glycerin suppositories promote defecation by irritating the rectal mucosa as well as by a hyperosmotic action. Glycerin may also soften and lubricate fecal material. The suppository does not have to melt to be effective. **Onset:** 15–60 min. Glycerin also acts as an osmotic diuretic to reduce intraocular pressure. **Peak effect:** 1 hr. **Duration:** 5 hr.

Uses: To establish normal bowel function in clients dependent on laxatives. To evacuate the colon prior to rectal and bowel examinations as well as colon surgery. Acute glaucoma attacks. Prior to or after ocular surgery to decrease intraocular pressure. *Investigational:* IV to lower intraocular and intracranial pressure.

Dosage

• **Suppository**

Insert one adult or pediatric suppository high in the rectum and hold for 15 min.

• **Liquid**

The contents of one unit (4 mL) inserted gently with the tip of the applicator pointed toward the navel.

• **Oral Solution**

1–2 g/kg 1–1.5 hr prior to surgery.

Administration/Storage
1. Store in a tight container in the refrigerator below 25°C (77°F).
2. A small amount of liquid glycerin will remain in the applicator unit.
3. Anticipate onset of action within 1 hr.
4. The suppository does not need to melt in order to produce a laxative effect.

Contraindications: *Rectally:* Should not be used in the presence of anal fissures, fistulas, ulcerative hemorrhoids, or proctitis. *Orally:* Anura, severe dehydration, frank or impending acute pulmonary edema, severe cardiac decompensation.

Special Concerns: Use with caution (orally) in hypervolemia, confused mental states, CHF, diabetes, severely dehydrated clients, and cardiac, renal, or hepatic disease.

Side Effects: *Rectally.* Mucous membrane irritation. *Orally. GI:* Nausea, vomiting. *CNS:* Headache, confusion, disorientation. *Miscellaneous:* Weight gain following continuous oral use. Severe dehydration, cardiac arrhythmias, ***hyperosmolar nonketotic coma (may be fatal).*** Mucous membrane irritation.

NURSING CONSIDERATIONS

See also *Nursing Considerations* for *Laxatives,* Chapter 60.

Evaluate
- Restoration of normal bowel function
- Evacuation of a soft, formed stool
- ↓ Intraocular pressure
- ↓ Intracranial pressure

Lactulose

(**LAK**-tyou-lohs)

Pregnancy Category: B
Acilac ✦, Cephulac, Cholac, Chronulac, Comalose-R ✦, Constilac, Constulose, Duphalac, Enulose, Lactulax ✦, PMS Lactulose ✦ **(Rx)**

How Supplied: *Syrup:* 10 g/15 mL
Action/Kinetics: Lactulose, a disaccharide containing both lactose and galactose, causes a decrease in the blood concentration of ammonia in clients suffering from portal-systemic encephalopathy. The mechanism involved is attributed to the bacteria-induced degradation of lactulose in the colon, resulting in an acid medium. Ammonia will then migrate from the blood to the colon to form ammonium ion, which is trapped and cannot be absorbed. A laxative action due to increased osmotic pressure from lactic, formic, and acetic acids then expels the trapped ammonium. The decrease in blood ammonia concentration improves the mental state, EEG tracing, and diet protein tolerance of clients. The increased osmotic pressure also results in a laxative effect, which may take up to 24 hr. The drug is partly absorbed from the GI tract. **Onset:** 24–48 hr.
Uses: Prevention and treatment of portal-systemic encephalopathy, including hepatic and prehepatic coma (Cephylac, Cholac, Enulose are used). Chronic constipation (Chronulac, Constilac, Duphalac are used).

Dosage

- **Syrup**

Encephalopathy.

Adults, initial: 30–45 mL (20–30 g) t.i.d.–q.i.d.; adjust q 2–3 days to obtain two or three soft stools daily. Long-term therapy may be required in portal-systemic encephalopathy; **infants:** 2.5–10 mL/day (1.6–6.6 g/day) in divided doses; **older children and adolescents:** 40–90 mL/day (26.6–60 g/day) in divided doses.

During acute episodes of constipation.

30–45 mL (20–30 g) q 1–2 hr to induce rapid initial laxation.

Chronic constipation.

Adults and children: 15–30 mL/day (10–20 g/day) as a single dose after breakfast (up to 60 mL/day may be required).

- **Retention Enema**

300 mL (200 g), diluted to 1,000 mL with water or saline and retained for 30–60 min; may be repeated q 4–6 hr.

Administration/Storage

1. To minimize sweet taste, dilute with water or fruit juice or add to desserts.
2. When given by gastric tube, dilute well to prevent vomiting and the possibility of aspiration pneumonia.
3. When administered by enema use a rectal balloon catheter to assist with retention.
4. Store below 30°C (86°F). Avoid freezing.
5. Other laxatives should not be taken with lactulose.

Contraindication: Clients on galactose-restricted diets.
Special Concerns: Safe use during lactation and in children has not been established. Infants who have been given lactulose have developed hyponatremia and dehydration. Use with caution in presence of diabetes mellitus.
Side Effects: *GI:* N&V, diarrhea, cramps, flatulence, gaseous distention, belching.

Drug Interactions

Antacids / May inhibit the drop in pH of the colon required for lactulose activity
Neomycin / May cause ↓ degradation of lactulose due to neomycin-induced ↑ in elimination of certain bacteria in the colon

---

NURSING CONSIDERATIONS

Interventions

1. Document mental status and monitor serum ammonia levels during therapy.
2. Report any client complaint of GI distress. The problem may subside as the therapy continues or the dose of medication may need to be reduced.
3. Monitor serum potassium levels of clients who have portal-systemic encephalopathy. This is to determine

whether the drug is causing further potassium loss that will intensify symptoms of the disease.
4. The medication contains carbohydrate. Therefore, observe clients for flushed, dry skin, complaints of dry mouth and intense thirst, a fruity odor to the breath, abdominal pain, and low BP. These are symptoms of hyperglycemia that are more likely to occur in clients with diabetes.
5. Keep the client clean and dry. Assess skin condition and reposition frequently because skin breakdown may occur rapidly.

Evaluate

- Improvement in level of consciousness and mental status
- ↓ Serum ammonia levels
- Relief of constipation

Magnesium sulfate

(mag-**NEE**-see-um **SUL**-fayt)
Pregnancy Category: A
Epsom Salts (OTC and Rx)

See also *Anticonvulsants,* Chapter 36, and *Laxatives,* Chapter 60.

How Supplied: *Injection:* 100 mg/mL, 125 mg/mL, 500 mg/mL; *Ointment:* 80%

Action/Kinetics: Magnesium is an important cation present in the extracellular fluid at a concentration of 1.5–2.5 mEq/L. Magnesium is an essential element for muscle contraction, certain enzyme systems, and nerve transmission.

Magnesium depresses the CNS and controls convulsions by blocking release of acetylcholine at the myoneural junction. Also, the drug decreases the sensitivity of the motor end plate to acetylcholine and decreases the excitability of the motor membrane. **Therapeutic serum levels:** 4–6 mEq/L (normal Mg levels: 1.5–3.0 mEq/L). **Onset: IM,** 1 hr; **IV,** immediate. **Duration: IM,** 3–4 hr; **IV,** 30 min. Magnesium is excreted by the kidneys.

Uses: Seizures associated with toxemia of pregnancy, epilepsy, or when abnormally low levels of magnesium may be a contributing factor in convulsions, such as in hypothyroidism or glomerulonephritis. For eclampsia, IV use is restricted to control of life-threatening seizures. Acute nephritis in children to control hypertension, encephalopathy, and seizures. Replacement therapy in magnesium deficiency. Adjunct in TPN. Laxative. *Investigational:* Inhibit premature labor (not a first-line agent). IV use as an adjunct to treat acute exacerbations of moderate to severe asthma in clients who respond poorly to beta agonists. IV use to reduce early mortality in clients with acute MI (is given as soon as possible and continued for 24–48 hr).

Dosage

- **IM**

Anticonvulsant.

Adults: 1–5 g of a 25%–50% solution up to 6 times/day. **Pediatric:** 20–40 mg/kg using the 20% solution (may be repeated if necessary).

- **IV**

Anticonvulsant.

Adults: 1–4 g using 10%–20% solution, not to exceed 1.5 mL/min of the 10% solution.

Hypomagnesemia, mild.

Adults: 1 g as a 50% solution q 6 hr for 4 times (or total of 32.5 mEq/24 hr).

Hypomagnesemia, severe.

Adults: Up to 2 mEq/kg over 4 hr.

- **IV Infusion**

Anticonvulsant.

Adults: 4–5 g in 250 mL 5% dextrose at a rate not to exceed 3 mL/min.

Hypomagnesemia, severe.

Adults: 5 g (40 mEq) in 1,000 mL dextrose 5% or sodium chloride solution by **slow** infusion over period of 3 hr.

Hyperalimentation.

Adults: 8–24 mEq/day; **infants:** 2–10 mEq/day.

- **Oral Solution**

Laxative.

Adults: 10–15 g; **pediatric:** 5–10 g.

Administration/Storage

1. For IV injections, administer undiluted only 1.5 mL of 10% solution per minute. Discontinue administration when convulsions cease.

2. For IV infusion, dilute 4 g in 250 mL of D5W or NSS; administration should not exceed 3 mL/min.
3. Dilutions for IM: deep injection of 50% concentrate is appropriate for adults. A 20% solution should be used for children. IV: dilute as specified by manufacturer.
4. When used as a laxative, dissolve in a glassful of ice water or other chilled fluid to lessen the disagreeable taste.
5. *Treatment of Overdose:*
• Use artificial ventilation immediately.
• Have 5–10 mEq of calcium (e.g., 10–20 mL of 10% calcium gluconate) readily available for IV injection to reverse heart block and respiratory depression.
• Hemodialysis and peritoneal dialysis are effective.

Contraindications: In the presence of heart block or myocardial damage. In toxemia of pregnancy during the 2 hr prior to delivery.

Special Concerns: Use with caution in clients with renal disease because magnesium is removed from the body solely by the kidneys.

Side Effects: Magnesium intoxication. *CNS:* Depression. *CV:* Flushing, hypotension, ***circulatory collapse, depression of the myocardium.*** *Other:* Sweating, hypothermia, muscle paralysis, CNS depression, ***respiratory paralysis.*** Suppression of knee jerk reflex can be used to determine toxicity. ***Respiratory failure may occur if given after knee jerk reflex disappears.*** Hypocalcemia with signs of tetany secondary to magnesium sulfate when used for eclampsia.

Symptoms of Overdose: Serum levels can predict symptoms of toxicity. Symptoms include ***sharp decrease in BP and respiratory paralysis,*** changes in ECG (increased PR interval, increased QRS complex, prolonged QT interval), ***asystole, heart block.*** At serum levels of 7–10 mEq/L there is hypotension, narcosis, and loss of deep tendon reflexes. ***Levels of 12–15 mEq/L result in respiratory paralysis; greater than 15 mEq/L cause cardiac conduction problems. Levels greater than 25 mEq/L cause cardiac arrest.***

Drug Interactions
CNS depressants (general anesthetics, sedative-hypnotics, narcotics) / Additive CNS depression
Digitalis / Heart block when Mg intoxication is treated with calcium in digitalized clients
Neuromuscular blocking agents / Possible additive neuromuscular blockade

NURSING CONSIDERATIONS

See also *Nursing Considerations* for *Anticonvulsants,* Chapter 36, and *Laxatives,* Chapter 60.

Assessment
1. Document indications for therapy and onset of symptoms.
2. Determine any history of kidney disease.
3. Assess ECG for evidence of any abnormality prior to administering drug IV.
4. Obtain baseline serum magnesium levels and renal function.

Interventions
1. Before administering magnesium check if any of the following conditions exist:
• Absent patellar reflexes or knee jerk reflex
• Respirations below 16/min
• Urinary output less than 100 mL during the past 4 hr
• Early signs of hypermagnesemia: flushing, sweating, hypotension, or hypothermia
• Past history of heart block or myocardial damage; prolonged PR and widened QRS intervals
2. Anticipate an adjustment in the dose of CNS depressants.
3. If receiving digitalis preparations monitor closely. Toxicity treated with calcium is extremely dangerous and may result in heart block.
4. When used in the setting of AMI, drug should be administered immediately and continued for 24-48 hr.
5. Do not administer magnesium sulfate for 2 hr preceding the delivery of a baby.
6. If a mother has received continuous IV therapy of magnesium sulfate

during 24 hr prior to delivery, assess the newborn for neurologic and respiratory depression.
Evaluate
• Control of toxemia-induced seizures
• Serum magnesium levels within desired range (1.8–3 mg/dL)
• ↓ Mortality with AMI
• Successful evacuation of stool (when used as a laxative)

Methylcellulose

(meth-ill-**SELL**-you-lohs)
Citrucel, Cologel, Murocel ✱ **(OTC)**

How Supplied: *Ointment*; *Powder for reconstitution*; *Tablet*
Action/Kinetics: Methylcellulose is composed of indigestible fibers that form a colloidal, bulky gelatinous mass on contact with water. The fibers pass through the stomach and increase the bulk of the feces, stimulating peristalsis. The drug is usually effective within 12–24 hr.
Uses: Prophylaxis of constipation in clients who should not strain during defecation. Short-term treatment of constipation; useful in geriatric clients with diminished colonic motor response and during pregnancy and postpartum to reestablish normal bowel function. To soften feces during fecal impaction.

Dosage

• **Capsules, Tablets**
Adults: 2–3 capsules or tablets t.i.d.; **pediatric, over 6 years:** 1–2 capsules or tablets b.i.d.
• **Powder**
Adults: 1–1.5 g t.i.d. **pediatric:** 1–1.5 g/day.
• **Citrucel Granules**
Adults and pediatric over 12 years: one 19-g packet in 8 oz water 1–3 times/day; **pediatric, 6–12 years:** 1 level teaspoon in 4 oz water t.i.d.–q.i.d.
• **Cologel Oral Solution**
Adults: 5–20 mL t.i.d. with a glass of water; **pediatric, over 6 years:** 5 mL b.i.d.

Administration/Storage: Follow each dose of medication with a full glass of water or milk to prevent impaction.
Contraindications: Intestinal obstruction, ulceration, and severe abdominal pain.

NURSING CONSIDERATIONS

See also *Nursing Considerations* for *Laxatives*, Chapter 60.
Evaluate: Prevention and/or relief of constipation.

Mineral oil

Agoral Plain, Fleet Mineral Oil, Kondremul Plain, Lansoyl ✱, Milkinol, Neo-Cultrol **(OTC)**

How Supplied: *Liquid*
Action/Kinetics: This mixture of liquid hydrocarbons obtained from petroleum lubricates the intestine; it also decreases absorption of fecal water from the colon. **Onset: PO,** 6–8 hr; **Enema,** 2–15 min.
Uses: Constipation, to avoid straining under certain conditions, such as rectal surgery, hemorrhoidectomy, and certain CV conditions. Short-term treatment of constipation; useful in geriatric clients with diminished colonic motor response and during pregnancy and postpartum to reestablish normal bowel function. To soften feces during fecal impaction.

Dosage

• **Emulsion, Gel, Oral Suspension**
Adults: 15–45 mL at bedtime; **children:** 5–20 mL at bedtime.
Administration/Storage
1. Administer mineral oil at bedtime and cautiously as there is the possibility of lipid pneumonitis. Unless contraindicated, give the client orange juice or a piece of orange to suck on after taking the mineral oil.
2. The emulsion form is pleasant tasting and does not require anything to make it more palatable. However, when taken at bedtime,

there is an increased risk of developing lipid pneumonia.
3. Store in the refrigerator to make the medication more palatable.
4. Administer mineral oil slowly to elderly, debilitated clients to prevent aspiration. Aspiration could result in lipid pneumonia.
5. Administer mineral oil carefully and slowly to children to prevent aspiration.
6. Do not administer mineral oil with food or vitamin preparations. The medication may delay digestion and prevent absorption of fat-soluble vitamins, A, D, E, and K.

Contraindications: Nausea and vomiting, abdominal pain, or intestinal obstruction.

Special Concerns: Mineral oil may decrease absorption of fat-soluble vitamins (vitamins A, D, E, K).

Side Effects: Acute or chronic lipid pneumonia due to aspiration of mineral oil; young, elderly, and dysphagic clients are at greatest risk. Pruritus ani, which may interfere with healing following anorectal surgery. Use during pregnancy may decrease vitamin K absorption sufficiently to cause hypoprothrombinemia in the newborn.

Drug Interactions

Anticoagulants, oral / ↑ Hypoprothrombinemia by ↓ absorption of vitamin K from GI tract; also, mineral oil could ↓ absorption of anticoagulant from GI tract
Sulfonamides / ↓ Effect of nonabsorbable sulfonamide in GI tract
Surface-active laxatives / ↑ Absorption of mineral oil
Vitamins A, D, E, K / ↓ Absorption following prolonged use of mineral oil

NURSING CONSIDERATIONS

See also *Nursing Considerations* for *Laxatives,* Chapter 60.

Assessment

1. Document indications for therapy, onset of symptoms, and any other agents used and the outcome.
2. Note if the client is of childbearing age and likely to be pregnant. Mineral oil may cause hypoprothrombinemia in the newborn and therefore should be avoided.
3. If the client is taking more than 30 mL of mineral oil, check the perianal area for leakage of feces. These clients require more frequent cleansing and a perianal pad to prevent soiling of clothes and linens.

Client/Family Teaching

1. Sit upright when taking mineral oil to avoid the possibility of aspiration.
2. If taking mineral oil in large amounts and over extended periods of time, caution client of the potential problem of leakage of fecal matter.
3. Warn pregnant women not to take the medication to relieve constipation, but rather, to check with their provider for suitable alternatives.

Evaluate: Relief of constipation with evidence of successful evacuation of a soft, formed stool.

Phenolphthalein

(fee-nohl-**THAY**-leen)
Alophen Pills No. 973, Espotabs, Evac-U-Gen, Evac-U-Lax, Ex-Lax, Feen-A-Mint Chocolated, Feen-A-Mint Gum, Feen-A-Mint Tablets, Lax Pills, Laxative Pills, Medilax, Modane, Phenolax, Prulet **(OTC)**

See also *Laxatives,* Chapter 60.

How Supplied: *Chew tablet,* 90 mg; *Gum:* 97.2 mg; *Liquid*; *Powder for reconstitution*; *Tablet:* 60 mg, 90 mg, 97.2 mg, 130 mg, 135 mg

Action/Kinetics: Phenolphthalein acts directly on the intestinal mucosa. It also stimulates the myenteric plexus and alters water and electrolyte absorption. It produces a semifluid stool with little or no accompanying colic. Available products contain either white or yellow phenolphthalein with yellow phenolphthalein being 2–3 times more potent than the white. **Onset:** 6–10 hr. **Duration:** May be 3–4 days due to residual effect.

Use: Short-term use for constipation.

Dosage

• **Gum, Tablets, Chewable Tablets, Wafers**

Adults: 60–194 mg/day; **pediatric, over 6 years:** 30–60 mg/day; **2–5 years:** 15–20 mg/day. Usually taken at bedtime.
Administration/Storage: Oral doses take 6–10 hr to be effective.
Additional Side Effects: Hypersensitivity reactions: Dermatitis, pruritus; rarely, nonthrombocytopenic purpura or ***anaphylaxis.*** Phenolphthalein may color alkaline urine pink-red and acidic urine yellow-brown.

NURSING CONSIDERATIONS

See also *Nursing Considerations* for *Laxatives,* Chapter 60.
Client/Family Teaching
1. Phenolphthalein colors alkaline stools and urine a reddish-pink color and acidic urine a brownish-yellow color.
2. Store medication out of the reach of children. This is particularly important when the laxative looks like chocolate and may be accidentally ingested as candy.
3. Remind clients that Ex-Lax is a medication and to use only as directed.
Evaluate: Relief of constipation.

Psyllium hydrophilic muciloid

(**SILL**-ee-um hi-droh-**FILL**-ik)
Effer-syllium, Fiberall Natural Flavor, Fiberall Orange Flavor, Fiberall Wafers, Fibrepur ✱, Hydrocil Instant, Konsyl, Konsyl-D, Metamucil, Metamucil Lemon-Lime Flavor, Metamucil Orange Flavor, Metamucil Sugar Free, Metamucil Sugar Free Orange Flavor, Modane Bulk, Natural Vegetable, Novo-Mucilax ✱, Perdiem Fiber, Prodiem Plain ✱, Reguloid Natural, Reguloid Orange, Reguloid Sugar Free Orange, Reguloid Sugar Free Regular, Serutan, Siblin, Syllact, V-Lax **(OTC)**

See also *Laxatives,* Chapter 60.
How Supplied: *Capsule*; *Granule*; *Granule for reconstitution*; *Powder for reconstitution:* 3.4 g/15 mL; *Tablet:* 500 mg; *Wafer*
Action/Kinetics: This drug is obtained from the fruit of various species of plantago. The powder forms a gelatinous mass with water, which adds bulk to the stools and stimulates peristalsis. It also has a demulcent effect on an inflamed intestinal mucosa. These preparations may also contain dextrose, sodium bicarbonate, monobasic potassium phosphate, citric acid, and benzyl benzoate. Dependence may occur.
Uses: Prophylaxis of constipation in clients who should not strain during defecation. Short-term treatment of constipation; useful in geriatric clients with diminished colonic motor response and during pregnancy and postpartum to reestablish normal bowel function. To soften feces during fecal impaction.

Dosage

Dose depends on the product. General information on adult dosage follows.

- **Granules/Flakes**

Adults: 1–2 teaspoons 1–3 times/day spread on food or with a glass of water.

- **Powder**

Adults: 1 rounded teaspoon in 8 oz of liquid 1–3 times/day.

- **Effervescent Powder**

Adults: 1 packet in water 1–3 times/day.

- **Chewable Pieces**

Adults: 2 pieces followed by a glass of water 1–3 times/day.
Administration/Storage
1. Laxative effects usually occur in 12–24 hr. The full effect may take 2–3 days.
2. The powder may be noxious and irritating to some personnel when removing from the packets or canister. Perform in a well-ventilated area and avoid inhaling particulate matter.
3. Mix powder with liquid just prior to administering; otherwise, the mix-

ture may become thick and difficult to drink.
Contraindications: Severe abdominal pain or intestinal obstruction.
Side Effects: Obstruction of the esophagus, stomach, small intestine, and rectum.
Drug Interactions: Psyllium should not be used concomitantly with salicylates, nitrofurantoin, or cardiac glycosides (e.g., digitalis).

NURSING CONSIDERATIONS

See *Nursing Considerations* for *Laxatives,* Chapter 60.
Evaluate: Prophylaxis and/or relief of constipation with evacuation of a soft, formed stool.

Senna

(**SEN**-nah)
Black-Draught Lax-Senna, Dr. Caldwell Senna Laxative, Fletcher's Castoria for Children, Senexon, Senokot, Senolax, X-Prep Liquid **(OTC)**

Sennosides A and B, Calcium Salts

(**SEN**-noh-syd)
Gentle Nature, Glysennid ✸, Nytilax, PMS-Sennosides ✸ **(OTC)**

How Supplied: Senna: *Granule*; *Granule for reconstitution*; *Kit*; *Liquid*; *Powder for reconstitution*; *Suppository*; *Syrup*; *Tablet*
Sennosides A and B: *Tablet*
Action/Kinetics: Senna is prepared from the dried leaf or fruit of the *Cassia acutifolia* or *C. angustifolia* tree. Senna is similar to cascara although it is more potent. It increases peristalsis of the colon by stimulating the intestinal mucosa and the myenteric plexus; it also alters electrolyte secretion. **Onset:** 6–10 hr.
Uses: Constipation, preoperative and prediagnostic procedures involving the GI tract.

Dosage

SENNA TABLETS
Adults: 2 at bedtime; **pediatric, over 27.3 kg:** 1 tablet at bedtime.
SENNA SUPPOSITORIES
Adults: 1 at bedtime; **pediatric, over 27.3 kg:** ½ suppository at bedtime.
BLACK-DRAUGHT GRANULES
Adults: ¼–½ level teaspoon with water (not recommended for children).
SENOKOT GRANULES
Adults: 1 teaspoon; **pediatric, over 27.3 kg:** ½ teaspoon. Taken at bedtime.
SENOKOT SYRUP
Adults: 10–15 mL at bedtime; **pediatric, 1–12 months:** 1.25–2.5 mL at bedtime; **pediatric, 1–5 years:** 2.5–5 mL; **5–15 years:** 5–10 mL.
DR. CALDWELL SENNA LAXATIVE
Adults: 15–30 mL with or after meals or at bedtime; **pediatric, 6–15 years:** 10–15 mL at bedtime; **1–5 years:** 5–10 mL at bedtime.
FLETCHER'S CASTORIA FOR CHILDREN
Children, 6–12 years: 10–15 mL; **1–5 years:** 5–10 mL; **7–12 months:** 2.5–5 mL; **1–6 months:** 1.25–2.5 mL.
GENTLE NATURE (SENNOSIDES A AND B)
Adults: 1–2 tablets at bedtime taken with water; **children 6 years and older:** 1 tablet at bedtime.
NYTILAX
Adults: 12–36 mg (1–3 tablets) at bedtime.
Contraindications: Irritable colon, N&V, abdominal pain, and appendicitis or possibility thereof.
Special Concern: Administer with caution to nursing mothers.
Side Effects: Abdominal pain, colic, and diarrhea. Senna colors alkaline urine pink, red, or violet and acid urine yellow-brown.

NURSING CONSIDERATIONS

See also *Nursing Considerations* for *Laxatives,* Chapter 60.
Client/Family Teaching
1. Gripping pain may be a symptom of overdosage. Omit drug when this occurs and report.
2. Drug causes acid urine to have a yellow-brown color. Alkaline urine will develop a reddish color.
3. Review foods that may diminish constipation, such as increased bulk, more fruits and juices, less cheese, etc.

4. Advise that long-term use may cause chronic stimulation of the colon, which may lead to chronic colonic distension and a perceived need for laxatives.

Evaluate: Relief of constipation with evacuation of a soft, formed stool.

CHAPTER SIXTY-ONE

Antidiarrheals

See the following individual entries:

Difenoxin Hydrochloride with Atropine Sulfate
Diphenoxylate Hydrochloride with Atropine Sulfate
Loperamide Hydrochloride

—COMBINATION DRUG—

Difenoxin hydrochloride with Atropine sulfate

(dye-fen-**OX**-in, **AH**-troh-peen)
Pregnancy Category: C
Motofen **(Rx)**

See also *Cholinergic Blocking Agents,* Chapter 49.
How Supplied: See Content
Content: Each tablet contains: 1 mg difenoxin hydrochloride, 0.025 mg atropine sulfate.
Action/Kinetics: Difenoxin is related chemically to meperidine; thus, atropine sulfate is incorporated to prevent deliberate overdosage. Difenoxin is the active metabolite of diphenoxylate and is effective at one-fifth the dosage of diphenoxylate. Difenoxin slows intestinal motility by a local effect on the GI wall. **Peak plasma levels:** 40–60 min. The drug and its inactive metabolites are excreted through both the urine and feces.
Uses: Management of acute nonspecific diarrhea and acute episodes of chronic functional diarrhea.

Dosage

• Tablets

Adults, initial: 2 tablets (2 mg difenoxin); **then,** 1 tablet (1 mg difenoxin) after each loose stool or 1 tablet q 3–4 hr as needed. Total dose during a 24-hr period should not exceed 8 mg (i.e., 8 tablets).

Administration/Storage

1. Continued administration beyond 48 hr is not recommended, if clinical improvement is not noted.
2. Treatment beyond 48 hr is usually not necessary for acute diarrhea or acute exacerbation of functional diarrhea.
3. *Treatment of Overdose:* Naloxone may be used to treat respiratory depression.

Contraindications: Diarrhea caused by *Escherichia coli, Salmonella,* or *Shigella;* pseudomembranous colitis caused by broad-spectrum antibiotics; jaundice; children less than 2 years of age.
Special Concerns: Use with caution in ulcerative colitis, liver and kidney disease, lactation, and in clients receiving dependence-producing drugs or in those who are addiction prone. Safety and effectiveness in children less than 12 years of age have not been determined.
Side Effects: *GI:* N&V, dry mouth, epigastric distress, constipation. *CNS:* Lightheadedness, dizziness, drowsiness, headache, tiredness, nervousness, confusion, insomnia. *Ophthalmic:* Blurred vision, burning eyes.

Symptoms of Overdose: Initially include dry skin and mucous membranes, hyperthermia, flushing, and tachycardia. These are followed by hypotonic reflexes, nystagmus, miosis, lethargy, coma, and ***respiratory depression*** (may occur up to 30 hr after overdose taken).

Drug Interactions

Antianxiety agents / Potentiation or addition of CNS depressant effects
Barbiturates / Potentiation or addition of CNS depressant effects

Ethanol / Potentiation or addition of CNS depressant effects
MAO inhibitors / Precipitation of hypertensive crisis
Narcotics / Potentiation or addition of CNS depressant effects

NURSING CONSIDERATIONS

Assessment

1. Note the onset, characteristics, and frequency of diarrhea.
2. Discuss the possible precipitating factors, e.g., travel, stress, food, medication regimens.
3. Note evidence of dehydration such as weakness, weight loss, poor skin turgor, elevated temperature, rapid weak pulse, or decreased urinary output.
4. Monitor levels and assess for evidence of electrolyte imbalance such as weakness, irritability, anorexia, nausea, and dysrhythmias.
5. Monitor liver function studies as drug may precipitate hepatic coma in clients with abnormal liver function.

Interventions

1. If the client has a history of heart disease, monitor closely and report any adverse effects immediately.
2. Monitor I&O. Keep a record of the number, frequency, and characteristics of the stools.
3. Check the client's gums for swelling and the extremities for numbness.
4. If also prescribed Lomotil and other narcotics or barbiturates, observe closely for the potentiation of CNS depression.
5. If the client has a history of liver disease, observe for signs of impending coma, such as increased drowsiness, mental aberrations, motor disturbances, or a flapping tremor of the hands.
6. Difenoxin contains atropine sulfate as an active ingredient; closely observe Down syndrome children receiving this drug for symptoms of atropinism.
7. Do not administer to clients receiving MAO inhibitors as concomitant use may precipitate hypertensive crisis.
8. Difenoxin has the potential to become addictive; monitor usage accordingly.
9. Overdosed clients should be hospitalized for observation since latent (12–30 hr later) respiratory depression may occur.
10. Stool cultures may be indicated to determine if therapy is appropriate.

Client/Family Teaching

1. Provide printed instructions concerning the recommended dosage schedule and side effects to report.
2. Do not perform tasks that require mental alertness until drug effects are realized.
3. Take only as directed and do not share medications with anyone, no matter what the symptoms.
4. Chew sugarless gum, or suck on hard, sugarless candy or ice chips if dry mouth is a problem.
5. Keep out of reach of children as drug may be fatal if ingested.
6. Drug should *not* be taken by mothers who are breast-feeding.
7. Avoid alcohol or any other unprescribed CNS depressants.
8. Advise that treatment may take 24–36 hr before effects are evident.

Evaluate: ↓ Frequency and number of diarrheal stools.

—COMBINATION DRUG—

Diphenoxylate hydrochloride with Atropine Sulfate

(dye-fen-**OX**-ih-layt, **AH**-troh-peen)

Pregnancy Category: C

Lofene, Logen, Lomanate, Lomodix, Lomotil, Lonox, Low-Quel **(C-V) (Rx)**

See also *Cholinergic Blocking Agents,* Chapter 49.

How Supplied: See Content

Content: Each tablet contains: 2.5 mg diphenoxylate hydrochloride, 0.025 mg atropine sulfate.

Each 5 mL of liquid contains: 2.5 mg diphenoxylate hydrochloride, 0.025 mg atropine sulfate.

Action/Kinetics: Diphenoxylate is a systemic constipating agent chemically related to the narcotic analgesic drug meperidine but without the analgesic properties. Diphenoxylate inhibits GI motility and has a constipating effect. This product may aggravate diarrhea due to organisms that penetrate the intestinal mucosa (e.g., *Escherichia coli, Salmonella, Shigella)* or in antibiotic-induced pseudomembranous colitis. High doses over prolonged periods can, however, cause euphoria and physical dependence. The preparation also contains small amounts of atropine sulfate, which is not present in sufficient quantities to decrease GI motility. However, the atropine will prevent abuse by deliberate overdosage. **Onset:** 45–60 min. **t½, diphenoxylate:** 2.5 hr; **diphenoxylic acid:** 12–24 hr. **Duration:** 2–4 hr. Diphenoxylate is metabolized in the liver to the active diphenoxylic acid and excreted through the urine.

Uses: Symptomatic treatment of chronic and functional diarrhea. Also, diarrhea associated with gastroenteritis, irritable bowel, regional enteritis, malabsorption syndrome, ulcerative colitis, acute infections, food poisoning, postgastrectomy, and drug-induced diarrhea. Therapeutic results for control of acute diarrhea are inconsistent. Also used in the control of intestinal passage time in clients with ileostomies and colostomies.

Dosage

- **Oral Solution, Tablets**

Adults, initial: 2.5–5 mg (of diphenoxylate) t.i.d.–q.i.d.; **maintenance:** 2.5 mg b.i.d.–t.i.d. **Pediatric, 2–12 years:** 0.3–0.4 mg/kg/day (of diphenoxylate) in divided doses. Contraindicated in children under 2 years of age. See also below.

Pediatric / Dose

2–3 years / 0.75–1.5 mg q.i.d.
3–4 years / 1–1.5 mg q.i.d.
4–5 years / 1–2 mg q.i.d.
5–6 years / 1.25–2.25 mg q.i.d.
6–9 years / 1.25–2.5 mg q.i.d.
9–12 years / 1.75–2.5 mg q.i.d.

Based on 4 mL/tsp or 2 mg of diphenoxylate. Each tablet or 5 mL of liquid preparation contains 2.5 mg diphenoxylate hydrochloride and 25 mcg of atropine sulfate. Dosage should be maintained at initial levels until symptoms are under control; then reduce to maintenance levels.

Administration/Storage

1. For liquid preparations, use only the plastic dropper supplied by the manufacturer to measure the dosage of drug.
2. If clinical improvement is not evident after 10 days with a maximum dose of 20 mg/day, further use will not likely control symptoms.
3. *Treatment of Overdose:* Gastric lavage, induce vomiting, establish a patent airway, and assist respiration. Activated charcoal (100 g) given as a slurry. IV administration of a narcotic antagonist. Administration may be repeated after 10–15 min. Observe client and readminister antagonist if respiratory depression returns.

Contraindications: Obstructive jaundice, liver disease, diarrhea associated with pseudomembranous enterocolitis after antibiotic therapy or enterotoxin-producing bacteria, children under the age of 2.

Special Concerns: Use with caution during lactation and in clients in whom anticholinergics may be contraindicated. Use with caution in those with advanced hepatic-renal disease or abnormal renal functions. Children (especially those with Down syndrome) are susceptible to atropine toxicity. Children and geriatric clients may be more sensitive to the respiratory depressant effects of diphenoxylate. Dehydration, especially in young children, may cause a delayed diphenoxylate toxicity.

Side Effects: *GI:* N&V, anorexia, abdominal discomfort, paralytic ileus, megacolon. *Allergic:* Pruritus, ***angioneurotic edema,*** swelling of gums. *CNS:* Dizziness, drowsiness, malaise, restlessness, headache, depression, numbness of extremities, ***respiratory depression, coma.*** *Topical:* Dry skin and mucous membranes, flushing.

Other: Tachycardia, urinary retention, hyperthermia.

Symptoms of Overdose: Dry skin and mucous membranes, flushing, ***hyperthermia,*** mydriasis, restlessness, tachycardia followed by miosis, lethargy, hypotonic reflexes, nystagmus, ***coma, severe (and possibly fatal) respiratory depression.***

Drug Interactions

Alcohol / Additive CNS depression
Antianxiety agents / Additive CNS depression
Barbiturates / Additive CNS depression
MAO inhibitors / ↑ Chance of hypertensive crisis
Narcotics / ↑ Effect of narcotics

NURSING CONSIDERATIONS

See also *Nursing Considerations* for *Difenoxin Hydrochloride with Atropine sulfate,* Chapter 61.

Assessment

1. Document indications for therapy, onset of symptoms, and other agents used without success.
2. Determine fluid and electrolyte status. Dehydration in young children may cause a delayed diphenoxylate toxicity.
3. Review laboratory culture reports to determine if drug is appropriate therapy for diarrhea especially if it is not effective within 24–36 hr after administration.
4. Note any evidence of hepatic or renal dysfunction.

Evaluate: ↓ Number and frequency of diarrheal stools.

Loperamide hydrochloride

(loh-**PER**-ah-myd)

Pregnancy Category: B

Imodium, Imodium A-D Caplets, Kaopectate II Caplets, Maalox Anti-Diarrheal Caplets, Pepto Diarrhea Control, PMS-Loperamide Hydrochloride (Imodium is Rx, all others are OTC)

How Supplied: *Capsule:* 2 mg; *Liquid:* 1 mg/5 mL; *Tablet:* 2 mg

Action/Kinetics: Loperamide is a piperidine derivative that slows intestinal motility by acting on the nerve endings and/or intramural ganglia embedded in the intestinal wall. The prolonged retention of the feces in the intestine results in reducing the volume of the stools, increasing viscosity, and decreasing fluid and electrolyte loss. The drug is reported to be more effective than diphenoxylate. **Time to peak effect, capsules:** 5 hr; **PO solution:** 2.5 hr. **t½:** 9.1–14.4 hr. Twenty-five percent excreted unchanged in the feces.

Uses: Rx: Symptomatic relief of acute nonspecific diarrhea and of chronic diarrhea associated with inflammatory bowel disease. Decrease the volume of discharge from ileostomies.

OTC: Control symptoms of diarrhea, including traveler's diarrhea. *Investigational:* With trimethoprim-sulfamethoxazole to treat traveler's diarrhea.

Dosage

- **Rx Capsules, Liquid**

Acute diarrhea.

Adults, initial: 4 mg, followed by 2 mg after each unformed stool, up to maximum of 16 mg/day. **Pediatric:** *Day 1 doses:* **8–12 years:** 2 mg t.i.d.; **6–8 years:** 2 mg b.i.d.; **2–5 years:** 1 mg t.i.d. using only the liquid. *After day 1:* 1 mg/10 kg after a loose stool (total daily dosage should not exceed day 1 recommended doses).

Chronic diarrhea.

Adults: 4–8 mg/day as a single or divided dose. Dosage not established for chronic diarrhea in children.

- **OTC Oral Solution, Tablets**

Acute diarrhea.

Adults: 4 mg after the first loose bowel movement followed by 2 mg after each subsequent bowel movement to a maximum of 8 mg/day for no more than 2 days. **Pediatric, 9–11 years:** 2 mg after the first loose bowel movement followed by

1 mg after each subsequent loose bowel movement, not to exceed 6 mg/day for no more than 2 days. **Pediatric, 6–8 years:** 1 mg after the first bowel movement followed by 1 mg after each subsequent loose bowel movement, not to exceed 4 mg/day for no more than 2 days.

Administration/Storage

1. OTC products are not intended for use in children less than 6 years of age unless the physician prescribes.
2. If improvement is not seen within 10 days after using up to 16 mg/day for *chronic diarrhea,* symptoms are not likely to improve with further use. Seek medical intervention.
3. In *acute diarrhea,* discontinue drug after 48 hr if ineffective.
4. *Treatment of Overdose:* Give activated charcoal (it will reduce absorption up to ninefold). If vomiting has not occurred, perform gastric lavage followed by activated charcoal, 100 g, through a gastric tube. Give naloxone for respiratory depression.

Contraindications: Discontinue drug promptly if abdominal distention develops in clients with acute ulcerative colitis. In clients in whom constipation should be avoided. OTC if body temperature is over 101°F and in presence of bloody diarrhea. Use in acute diarrhea associated with organisms that penetrate the intestinal mucosa, such as *E. coli, Salmonella,* and *Shigella.*

Special Concerns: Safe use in children under 2 years of age and during lactation has not been established. Fluid and electrolyte depletion may occur in clients with diarrhea. Children less than 3 years of age are more sensitive to the narcotic effects of loperamide.

Side Effects: *GI:* Abdominal pain, distention, or discomfort. Constipation, dry mouth, N&V, epigastric distress. Toxic megacolon in clients with acute colitis. *CNS:* Drowsiness, dizziness, fatigue. *Other:* Allergic skin rashes.

Symptoms of Overdose: Constipation, CNS depression, GI irritation.

NURSING CONSIDERATIONS

Assessment

1. Note any history of allergy to piperidine derivatives prior to administering drug.
2. Document indications for therapy and frequency and onset of symptoms.
3. Attempt to identify any causative factors contributing to symptoms.

Client/Family Teaching

1. Since loperamide may cause a dry mouth, provide instructions suggesting methods (ice, sugarless gum, and candy) to alleviate.
2. Use caution while driving or performing tasks requiring alertness because the drug may cause dizziness and drowsiness.
3. Record the number, frequency, and consistency of stools per day and the amount of medication consumed.
4. Report if diarrhea lasts up to 10 days without relief.
5. If fever, nausea, abdominal pain, or abdominal distention occurs, report because dosage may require adjustment or drug may need to be discontinued.
6. Remind parents that dietary treatment of diarrhea is preferred, if possible, in children (avoid apple juices, high-fat foods, and highly spiced foods).

Evaluate: ↓ Amount and frequency of diarrheal stools.

CHAPTER SIXTY-TWO

Antiemetics/ Antinauseants

See also the following individual entries:

Buclizine Hydrochloride - See Chapter 55
Cyclizine Hydrochloride - See Chapter 55
Dimenhydrinate - See Chapter 55
Diphenhydramine Hydrochloride - See Chapter 55
Dronabinol (Delta-9-Tetrahydrocannabinol)
Granisetron Hydrochloride
Hydroxyzine Hydrochloride - See Chapter 40
Hydroxyzine Pamoate - See Chapter 40
Meclizine Hydrochloride
Ondansetron Hydrochloride
Phosphorated Carbohydrate Solution
Prochlorperazine - See Chapter 38
Prochlorperazine Edisylate - See Chapter 38
Prochlorperazine Maleate - See Chapter 38
Scopolamine Hydrobromide - See Chapter 49
Trimethobenzamide Hydrochloride

General Statement: Nausea and vomiting can be caused by a variety of conditions, such as infections, drugs, radiation, motion, organic disease, or psychologic factors. The underlying cause of the symptoms must be elicited before emesis is corrected.

The act of vomiting is complex. The chemoreceptor trigger zone in the medulla responds to stimulation from many peripheral areas, as well as to stimuli from the CNS itself, the CTZ in the medulla, the vestibular apparatus of the ear, and the cerebral cortex.

The selection of an antiemetic depends on the cause of the symptoms, as well as on the manner in which the vomiting is triggered.

Many drugs used for other conditions, such as the antihistamines, phenothiazines, barbiturates, and scopolamine, have antiemetic properties and can be so used. (For details see appropriate sections.) These agents often have serious side effects (mostly CNS depression) that make their routine use undesirable.

Drug Interaction: Because of their antiemetic and antinauseant activity, the antiemetics may mask overdosage caused by other drugs.

NURSING CONSIDERATIONS

Assessment

1. Take a complete client history, determining if nausea is an unusual occurrence or if it is a recurring phenomenon. Attempt to establish causative factors.
2. Determine the onset and extent of the nausea and what event seems to have triggered it.
3. Note the number of times the client has had to take an antiemetic in the past, under what conditions and the response.
4. Ensure that client has no evidence of intestinal obstruction, drug overdose, or increased ICP.
5. Attempt to determine physiologic mechanism triggering client's N&V. Generally, if it is centrally mediated to the CTZ, one would see nausea

without vomiting, whereas if the vomiting center were triggered directly, then one may see retching with vomiting.

Interventions

1. Assess for other side effects as antiemetic drugs may mask signs of underlying pathology or overdosage of other drugs.
2. Monitor fluid status (I&O) and observe for symptoms of dehydration.
3. Supervise ambulation until drug effects are resolved.
4. Offer ice chips initially, if tolerated, then water and then clear liquids, and then full liquids, gradually advancing to regular food.

Client/Family Teaching

1. Caution client that the drug tends to cause drowsiness and dizziness. Avoid driving or performing other hazardous tasks until individual response to the drug has been evaluated.
2. Review measures to decrease nausea such as ice chips, sips of water, nongreasy foods, removal of noxious stimuli from the environment (odors or materials), and frequent oral hygiene. Stress the importance of advancing diet slowly.
3. Advise client to dangle legs before standing and to rise slowly to prevent symptoms of orthostatic hypotension.
4. Instruct client to report any unresponsive N&V or abdominal pain.
5. Avoid alcohol and any other nonprescribed CNS depressants.

Evaluate

- Reports of effective control of N&V
- Prevention of dehydration related to N&V
- Improved nutritional status once N&V have been controlled as evidenced by weight gain and/or ↑ caloric intake

Dronabinol (Delta-9-tetrahydro-cannabinol)

(droh-**NAB**-ih-nohl)

Pregnancy Category: C
Marinol **(C-II) (Rx)**

How Supplied: *Capsule:* 2.5 mg, 5 mg, 10 mg

Action/Kinetics: Dronabinol is the active component in marijuana and, as such, will manifest significant psychoactive effects. These include euphoria, anxiety, panic, depression, paranoia, decrement in memory and cognitive performance, decreased ability to control drives and impulses, and distortion in perception including time. In therapeutic doses, the drug also causes conjunctival injection and an increased HR. The antiemetic effect is thought to be due to inhibition of the vomiting center in the medulla. **Peak plasma levels:** 2–3 hr. Significant first-pass effect. The 11-hydroxytetrahydrocannabinol metabolite is active. **t1/2, biphasic:** 4 hr and 25–36 hr. **t1/2, 11-hydroxy-THC:** 15–18 hr. Metabolized in the liver and mainly excreted in the feces. Cumulative toxicity using clinical doses may occur. The drug is highly bound to plasma proteins and may thus displace other protein-bound drugs.

Uses: Nausea and vomiting associated with cancer chemotherapy, especially in clients who have not responded to other antiemetic treatment. To stimulate appetite and prevent weight loss in AIDS clients.

Dosage

- **Capsules**

Antiemetic.

Adults and children, initial: 5 mg/m^2 1–3 hr before chemotherapy; **then,** 5 mg/m^2 q 2–4 hr for a total of four to six doses/day. If ineffective, this dose may be increased by 2.5 mg/m^2 to a maximum of 15 mg/m^2/dose. However, the incidence of serious psychoactive side effects increases dramatically at these higher dose levels.

Appetite stimulation.

Initial: 2.5 mg b.i.d. before lunch and dinner. If the client cannot tolerate 5 mg/day, the dose should be reduced to 2.5 mg/day as a single evening or bedtime dose. If side effects are absent or minimal and an increased effect is desired, the dose may be increased to 2.5 mg before lunch and 5 mg before dinner (or 5 mg at lunch and 5 mg after dinner). The dose may be increased to 20 mg/day in divided doses. The incidence of side effects increases at higher doses.

Administration/Storage

1. Due to its CNS effects, dronabinol should be used only when the client can be under close supervision.
2. Dronabinol has the potential for abuse. Therefore, prescriptions should be limited to one course of chemotherapy (i.e., several days) and reordered as needed to ensure that the client receives the benefit of therapy.
3. *Treatment of Overdose:* Clients with depressive, hallucinatory, or psychotic reactions should be placed in a quiet environment and provided supportive treatment, including reassurance. Diazepam (5–10 mg PO) may be used for extreme agitation. Hypotension usually responds to IV fluids and Trendelenburg position. In unconscious clients with a secure airway, administer activated charcoal (30–100 g in adults and 1–2 g/kg in children); this may be followed by a saline cathartic.

Contraindications: Nausea and vomiting from any cause other than cancer chemotherapy. Lactation. Hypersensitivity to sesame oil.

Special Concerns: Pediatric and geriatric clients should be monitored carefully due to an increased risk of psychoactive effects. Use with caution in clients with hypertension, occasional hypotension, syncope, tachycardia; those with a history of substance abuse, including alcohol abuse or dependence; clients with mania, depression, or schizophrenia (the drug may exacerbate these illnesses); clients receiving sedatives, hypnotics, or other psychoactive drugs (due to the potential for additive or synergistic CNS effects).

Side Effects: *CNS:* Side effects are due mainly to the psychoactive effects of the drug and, in addition to those listed above, include dizziness, muddled thinking, coordination difficulties, irritability, weakness, headache, ataxia, cannabinoid "high," paresthesia, hallucinations, visual distortions, depersonalization, confusion, nightmares, disorientation, and confusion. *CV:* Palpitations, tachycardia, vasodilation, facial flush, hypotension. *GI:* Abdominal pain, N&V, diarrhea, dry mouth, fecal incontinence, anorexia. *Respiratory:* Cough, rhinitis, sinusitis. *Other:* Asthenia, conjunctivitis, myalgias, tinnitus, speech difficulty, vision difficulties, chills, headache, malaise, sweating, elevated hepatic enzymes.

Symptoms of Overdose: Extension of the pharmacologic effects. Symptoms of mild overdose include: drowsiness, euphoria, heightened sensory awareness, altered time perception, reddened conjunctiva, dry mouth, and tachycardia. Symptoms of moderate toxicity include impaired memory, depersonalization, mood alteration, urinary retention, and reduced bowel motility. Severe intoxication includes decreased motor coodination, lethargy, slurred speech, and postural hypotension. Seizures may occur in clients with existing seizure disorders. Hallucinations, psychotic episodes, ***respiratory depression***, and ***coma*** have been reported.

Symptoms of Abstinence Syndrome: An abstinence syndrome has been reported following discontinuation of doses greater than 210 mg/day for 12–16 days. Symptoms include irritability, insomnia, and restlessness within 12 hr; within 24 hr, symptoms include "hot flashes," sweating, rhinorrhea, loose stools, hiccoughs, and anorexia. Disturbed sleep may occur for several weeks.

Drug Interactions

Amphetamine / Additive hypertension, tachycardia, possibly cardiotoxicity
Anticholinergics / Additive or super-additive tachycardia; drowsiness
CNS depressants / Additive CNS depressant effects
Cocaine / See *Amphetamine*

Antidepressants, tricyclic / Additive tachycardia, hypertension, drowsiness
Ethanol / During subchronic dronabinol use, lower and delayed peak alcohol blood levels
Sympathomimetics / See *Amphetamine*
Theophylline / Possible increased metabolism of theophylline

NURSING CONSIDERATIONS

Assessment

1. Note if the client has any history of allergic responses to sesame oil or seeds.
2. Document onset of symptoms and determine if N&V are caused by anything other than cancer chemotherapy agents.
3. If clients develop serious psychoactive side effects, they should be placed in a quiet environment and provided supportive nursing care.

Client/Family Teaching

1. Discuss the anticipated benefits to be derived from the therapy.
2. Take the medication 1–3 hr before the scheduled cancer chemotherapy.
3. Use caution when sitting or standing suddenly because dizziness may occur.
4. Do not drive or perform hazardous tasks requiring mental acuity.
5. Discuss the potential for psychoactive symptoms, visual distortions, and mental confusion. Advise the family that these symptoms may be minimized by providing a quiet, supportive environment.
6. Keep medication out of reach of children and do not share medications with anyone, no matter what their symptoms.

Evaluate

- Relief of N&V associated with cancer chemotherapy
- Improved appetite and prevention of weight loss in clients with AIDS

Granisetron hydrochloride

(gran-**ISS**-eh-tron)
Pregnancy Category: B
Kytril **(Rx)**

How Supplied: *Injection:* 1 mg/mL; *Tablet:* 1 mg

Action/Kinetics: Granisetron is a selective 5-HT_3 (serotonin) receptor antagonist with little or no affinity for other 5-HT, beta-adrenergic, dopamine, or histamine receptors. During chemotherapy-induced vomiting, mucosal enterochromaffin cells release serotonin, which stimulates 5-HT_3 receptors. The stimulation of 5-HT_3 receptors by serotonin causes vagal discharge resulting in vomiting. Granisetron blocks serotonin stimulation and subsequent vomiting. In adult cancer clients undergoing chemotherapy, infusion of a single 40-mcg/kg dose over 5 min produced the following data. **Peak plasma level:** 63.8 ng/mL. **Plasma t½, terminal:** 8.95 hr. The drug is metabolized in the liver with about 12% excreted unchanged in the urine. Metabolites are excreted through both the urine and feces.

Use: Prevention of nausea and vomiting associated with initial and repeat cancer chemotherapy, including high-dose cisplatin.

Dosage

- **IV**

Antiemetic.

Adults and children over 2 years of age: 10 mcg/kg infused over 5 min beginning 30 min before initiation of chemotherapy.

Administration/Storage

1. The drug is given only on the day chemotherapy is given.
2. Dosage adjustment is not necessary for geriatric clients.
3. The infusion should be prepared at the time of administration by diluting in either NSS or D5W to a total volume of 20–50 mL. However, the drug is stable for at least 24 hr when diluted in NSS or D5W and stored at room temperature under normal lighting.
4. The drug should not be mixed in solution with other drugs.

Contraindication: Known hypersensitivity to the drug.

Special Concerns: Use with caution during lactation. Safety and effi-

cacy in children less than 2 years of age have not been established.
Laboratory Test Interferences: ↑ AST, ALT.
Side Effects: *CNS:* Headache, somnolence, agitation, anxiety, CNS stimulation, insomnia, extrapyramidal syndrome. *GI:* Diarrhea, constipation, taste disorder. *CV:* Hypertension, hypotension, arrhythmias (e.g., sinus bradycardia, atrial fibrillation, ***AV block,*** ventricular ectopy including nonsustained tachycardia, ECG abnormalities). *Allergic:* ***Hypersensitivity reactions,*** skin rashes. *Miscellaneous:* Asthenia, fever.
Drug Interactions: Because granisetron is metabolized by hepatic cytochrome P-450 drug-metabolizing enzymes, agents that induce or inhibit these enzymes may alter the clearance (and thus the half-life) of granisetron.

NURSING CONSIDERATIONS

Assessment

1. Identify condition requiring treatment and list the chemotherapy prescribed.
2. Anticipate administration of granisetron 20 min before the start of emetogenic cancer chemotherapy.

Evaluate: Prevention of chemotherapy-induced N&V.

Meclizine hydrochloride

(MEK-lih-zeen)
Pregnancy Category: B
Antivert, Antivert/25 and /50, Antivert/25 Chewable, Antrizine, Bonamine ✦, Bonine, Dizmiss, Dramamine II, Meni-D, Ru-Vert-M (OTC and Rx)

See also *Antihistamines,* Chapter 55, and *Antiemetics/Antinauseants,* Chapter 62.
How Supplied: *Capsule:* 25 mg, 30 mg; *Chew Tablet:* 25 mg; *Tablet:* 12.5 mg, 25 mg, 30 mg, 50 mg
Action/Kinetics: The mechanism for the antiemetic effect is not known but may be due to a central anticholinergic effect to decrease vestibular stimulation and depress labyrinthine activity. The drug may also act on the CTZ to decrease vomiting. **Onset:** 30–60 min; **Duration:** 8–24 hr. **$t^{1/2}$:** 6 hr.
Uses: Nausea and vomiting, dizziness of motion sickness, vertigo associated with diseases of the vestibular system.

Dosage

• **Capsules, Tablets, Chewable Tablets**

Motion sickness.

Adults: 25–50 mg 1 hr before travel; may be repeated q 24 hr during travel.

Vertigo.

Adults: 25–100 mg/day in divided doses.
Special Concerns: Safety for use during lactation and in children less than 12 years of age has not been determined. Pediatric and geriatric clients may be more sensitive to the anticholinergic effects of meclizine.
Side Effects: *CNS:* Drowsiness, excitation, nervousness, restlessness, insomnia, euphoria, vertigo, hallucinations (auditory or visual). *GI:* N&V, diarrhea, constipation, anorexia. *GU:* Urinary frequency or retention; difficulty in urination. *CV:* Hypotension, tachycardia, palpitations. *Miscellaneous:* Dry nose and throat, blurred or double vision, tinnitus, rash, urticaria.

NURSING CONSIDERATIONS

See also *Nursing Considerations* for *Antihistamines,* Chapter 55, and *Antiemetics/Antinauseants,* Chapter 62.

Assessment

1. Document indications for therapy and onset and type of symptoms.
2. Assess closely for other adverse symptoms in addition to nausea. An antiemetic drug may mask signs of drug overdose as well as signs of pathology such as increased ICP or intestinal obstruction.

Client/Family Teaching

1. Take only as directed and report if condition does not improve.
2. Antiemetics tend to cause drowsiness and dizziness. Caution against driving or performing other hazardous

tasks until individual response to the drug has been evaluated.

Evaluate

- Prevention of motion sickness
- Control of vertigo

Ondansetron hydrochloride

(on-**DAN**-sih-tron)

Pregnancy Category: B

Zofran **(Rx)**

How Supplied: *Injection:* 2 mg/mL, 32 mg/50 mL, *Tablet:* 4 mg, 8 mg

Action/Kinetics: Ondansetron is a 5-HT_3 (serotonin) antagonist. Serotonin receptors of the 5-HT_3 type are found centrally in the CTZ and peripherally on vagal nerve terminals. It is believed that cytotoxic chemotherapy results in the release of serotonin from enterochromoffin cells of the small intestine. The released serotonin may stimulate the vagal afferent nerves through the 5-HT_3 receptors, thus stimulating the vomiting reflex. It is not known, however, whether the drug acts centrally and/or peripherally to antagonize the effect of serotonin. **Time to peak plasma levels, after PO:** 1.7–2.1 hr. **t¹/₂, after IV use:** 3.5–4.7 hr; **after PO use:** 3.1–6.2 hr, depending on the age. A decrease in clearance and increase in half-life are observed in clients over 75 years of age, although no dosage adjustment is recommended. Clients less than 15 years of age show a shortened plasma half-life after IV use (2.4 hr). The drug is significantly metabolized with 5% of a dose excreted unchanged in the urine.

Uses: Parenteral: Prevent N&V resulting from initial and repeated courses of cancer chemotherapy, including high-dose cisplatin. Prophylaxis and treatment of selected cases of postoperative N&V, especially situations where there is multiple retching and long periods of N&V. **Oral:** Prevention of N&V due to initial and repeated courses of cancer chemotherapy.

Dosage

- **IV**

N&V due to chemotherapy.

Adults and children, 4–18 years: Three doses of 0.15 mg/kg each. The first dose is infused over 15 min starting 30 min before the start of chemotherapy; the second and third doses are given 4 hr and 8 hr, respectively, after the first dose. Alternatively, a single 32-mg dose may be given over 15 min beginning 30 min before the start of chemotherapy.

N&V postoperatively.

Adults: 4 mg over 2–5 min immediately before induction of anesthesia or postoperatively as needed.

- **Tablets**

In clients receiving moderately emetogenic chemotherapy agents.

Adults and children over 12 years of age: 8 mg 30 min before treatment followed by 8 mg at both 4 hr and 8 hr after the first dose; **then** 8 mg q 8 hr for 1–2 days after chemotherapy. **Children, 4–12 years:** 4 mg administered on same schedule as adults.

Administration/Storage

1. In clients with impaired hepatic function, the PO dose should not exceed 8 mg and the IV daily dose should not exceed 8 mg infused over 15 min beginning 30 min prior to the start of chemotherapy.
2. The injection (containing 2 mg/mL) should be diluted in 50 mL of 5% dextrose injection or 0.9% sodium chloride injection before administration and infused over 15 min.
3. The diluted drug is stable at room temperature, with normal lighting, for 48 hr after dilution with 0.9% sodium chloride injection, 5% dextrose injection, 5% dextrose and 0.9% sodium chloride injection, 5% dextrose and 0.45% sodium chloride injection, and 3% sodium chloride injection.

Special Concerns: Use with caution during lactation. Data on safety and effectiveness in children 3 years of age and younger are not available.

Laboratory Test Alteration: ↑ AST, ALT.

Side Effects: *GI:* Diarrhea (most common), constipation, xerostomia, abdominal pain. *CNS:* Headache, dizziness, drowsiness, sedation, fatigue, anxiety, agitation, ***clonic-tonic seizures.*** *CV:* Tachycardia, chest pain, hypotension, ECG alterations. *Miscellaneous:* Rash, ***bronchospasm,*** hypokalemia, weakness, fever, musculoskeletal pain, shivers, urinary retention, dysuria, cold sensation, pruritus, paresthesia, reaction at injection site, postoperative carbon dioxide-related pain.

NURSING CONSIDERATIONS

See also *Nursing Considerations* for *Antiemetics/Antinauseants,* Chapter 62.

Assessment

1. Document indications for therapy, onset of symptoms, any other agent prescribed, and the outcome.
2. Document any evidence of liver dysfunction, obtain baseline liver function tests and monitor during therapy.
3. Determine that the initial dose of drug has been administered 30 min before the start of cancer chemotherapy and at 4- and 8-hr intervals following the first dose. Anticipate continuation of PO antiemetics for several days following a course of ondansetron therapy.

Evaluate

- Prevention of chemotherapy-induced N&V
- Control of refractory N&V R/T chemotherapy
- Prophylaxis and/or relief of prolonged and excessive postoperative N&V

Phosphorated carbohydrate solution

(**FOS**-for-**ay**-ted **kar**-boh-**HIGH**-drayt)

Emetrol, Naus-A-Way, Nausetrol

(OTC)

How Supplied: *Solution; Syrup; Tablet*

Action/Kinetics: Phosphorated carbohydrate solution contains fructose, dextrose, and orthophosphoric acid with controlled hydrogen ion concentration. It relieves N&V due to a direct action on the wall of the GI tract that decreases smooth muscle contraction and delays gastric emptying time; the effect is directly related to the amount used. There is some question as to the effectiveness of this product.

Use: Symptomatic relief of N&V.

Dosage

- **Oral Solution**

N&V due to psychogenic factors, functional vomiting.

Adults: 15–30 mL at 15-min intervals until vomiting ceases; if the first dose is rejected, the same dosage should be given in 5 min. Should not be taken for more than five doses (1 hr). **Infants and children:** 5–10 mL at 15-min intervals in the same manner as adults.

Regurgitation in infants.

5 or 10 mL, 10–15 min before each feeding; in refractory cases, 10 or 15 mL, 30 min before feeding.

Morning sickness.

15–30 mL on arising; repeat q 3 hr or when nausea threatens.

N&V due to drug therapy or inhalation anesthesia, motion sickness.

Adults and older children: 15 mL; **young children:** 5 mL.

Administration/Storage

1. Should not be diluted.
2. Oral fluids should not be taken immediately before a dose or for at least 15 min after a dose.

Contraindications: Diabetic clients due to the presence of carbohydrates. Individuals with hereditary fructose intolerance.

Special Concerns: Since nausea may be a symptom of a serious condition, a physician should be consulted if symptoms are not relieved or recur often.

Side Effects: *GI:* Abdominal pain and diarrhea due to large doses of fructose.

NURSING CONSIDERATIONS

See also *Nursing Considerations* for *Antiemetics/Antinauseants,* Chapter 62.

Assessment

1. Document indications for therapy, onset of symptoms, other agents utilized, and the outcome.

2. Note any history of diabetes or hereditary fructose intolerance as drug is contraindicated.

Client/Family Teaching

1. Provide printed guidelines for the frequency and method of administration.
2. Advise client to report if symptoms persist, recur often, or become worse.
3. Stress the importance of increasing the intake of fluids to prevent the development of dehydration but not immediately before or for 15 min following administration.

Evaluate: Relief of N&V.

Trimethobenzamide hydrochloride

(try-meth-oh-**BENZ**-ah-myd)

Arrestin, Hymetic, Tebamide, T-Gen, Ticon, Tigan **(Rx)**

How Supplied: *Capsule:* 100 mg, 250 mg; *Injection:* 100 mg/mL; *Suppository:* 100 mg, 200 mg

Action/Kinetics: Trimethobenzamide is an antiemetic related to the antihistamines but with weak antihistaminic properties. The drug is less effective than the phenothiazines but has fewer side effects. Not suitable as sole agent for severe emesis. Can be used PR. Trimethobenzamide appears to control vomiting by depressing the CTZ of the medulla. **Onset: PO and IM,** 10–40 min. **Duration:** 3–4 hr. 30%–50% of drug excreted unchanged in urine in 48–72 hr.

Uses: Nausea and vomiting.

Dosage

• **Capsules**

Adults: 250 mg t.i.d.–q.i.d.; **pediatric, 13.6–40.9 kg:** 100–200 mg t.i.d.–q.i.d.

• **Suppositories**

Adults: 200 mg t.i.d.–q.i.d.; **pediatric, under 13.6 kg:** 100 mg t.i.d.–q.i.d.; **13.6–40.9 kg:** 100–200 mg t.i.d.–q.i.d.

• **IM**

Adults only: 200 mg t.i.d.–q.i.d. *IM route not to be used in children.*

Administration/Storage

1. Inject drug IM deeply into the upper, outer quadrant of the gluteus muscle. Be careful to avoid escape of fluid from the needle so as to minimize local reaction.
2. Expect the onset of action to occur in 10–40 min after PO administration and to last 3–4 hr.
3. After IM injection, the action of the drug lasts 2–3 hr.
4. Do not administer suppositories to clients allergic to benzocaine or similar anesthetics.

Contraindications: Hypersensitivity to drug, benzocaine, or similar local anesthetics. Do not use suppositories for neonates; do not use IM in children.

Special Concerns: Use during pregnancy only if benefits outweigh risks. Use with caution during lactation.

Side Effects: *CNS:* Depression of mood, disorientation, headache, drowsiness, dizziness, ***seizures, coma,*** Parkinson-like symptoms. *Other:* Hypersensitivity reactions, hypotension, blood dyscrasias, jaundice, muscle cramps, opisthotonos, blurred vision, diarrhea, allergic skin reactions. *After IM injection:* Pain, burning, stinging, redness at injection site.

Drug Interactions: Concomitant use with atropine-like drugs and CNS depressants including alcohol should be avoided.

NURSING CONSIDERATIONS

See also *Nursing Considerations* for *Antiemetics/Antinauseants,* Chapter 62.

Assessment

1. Identify cause for N&V.
2. Document any history of sensitivity to benzocaine.
3. Assess for any evidence of skin reaction. This is the first sign of hypersensitivity to the drug.
4. Note any local reaction to the suppositories.

Client/Family Teaching

1. Provide a printed list of adverse drug effects that require reporting should they occur.
2. Do not drive or operate machinery until drug effects are realized. Drug may cause drowsiness and dizziness.
3. Avoid the use of alcohol and any other CNS depressants.

Evaluate: Prevention and control of N&V.

CHAPTER SIXTY-THREE

Antiulcer and Other GI Drugs

See also the following individual entries:

Histamine H_2 Antagonists

Cimetidine
Famotidine
Nizatidine
Ranitidine Hydrochloride

Other GI Drugs

Cisapride
Donnatal Capsules, Elixir, Tablets
Librax
Metoclopramide
Misoprostol
Omeprazole
Pancrelipase (Lipancreatin)
Sucralfate

(HISTAMINE H_2 ANTAGONISTS)

Action/Kinetics: Histamine H_2 antagonists are competitive blockers of histamine. As such they inhibit all phases of gastric acid secretion including that caused by histamine, gastrin, and muscarinic agents. Both fasting and nocturnal acid secretion are inhibited. In addition, the volume and hydrogen ion concentration of gastric juice are decreased. Cimetidine, famotidine, and ranitidine have no effect on gastric emptying; cimetidine and famitidine have no effect on lower esophageal pressure. Fasting or postprandial serum gastrin is not affected by famotidine, nizatidine, or ranitidine. Cimetidine is known to affect the cytochrome P-450 drug metabolizing system for other drugs. Ranitidine also affects the P-450 enzyme system, but its effect on elimination of other drugs is not significant. Neither famotidine nor nizatidine affects the P-450 enzyme system.

Uses: See individual drugs. Treatment of duodenal ulcer and maintenance therapy after healing of the active ulcer. Benign gastric ulcer (use of nizatidine is investigational). Pathologic hypersecretory conditions (except nizatidine) including Zollinger-Ellison syndrome, systemic mastocytosis, and multiple endocrine adenomas. Cimetidine, famotidine, and ranitidine are approved for use in gastroesophageal reflex disease, including erosive esophagitis. *Investigational:* All drugs except nizatidine are used experimentally for prevention of aspiration pneumonitis, prophylaxis of stress ulcers, and acute upper GI bleeding (cimetidine is approved for this use).

Contraindications: Hypersensitivity to H_2-receptor antagonists.

Special Concerns: Use with caution in impaired hepatic and renal function. Symptomatic response to these drugs does not preclude gastric malignancy. Cimetidine, famotidine, and nizatidine should not be used during lactation; ranitidine should be used with caution. Safety and effectiveness have not been established for use in children; use of cimetidine is not recommended in children less than 16 years of age unless benefits outweigh risks.

Side Effects: The following side effects are common to all or most of the H_2-histamine antagonists. See individual drugs for complete listing. *GI:* N&V, abdominal discomfort, diarrhea, constipation, hepatocellular effects. *CNS:* Headache, fatigue, somnolence, dizziness, confusion, hallucinations. *Dermatologic:* Rash, urticaria, pruritus, alopecia (rare), erythema multiforme (rare). *Other:* Thrombocytopenia, gynecomastia, impotence, loss of libido, cardiac arrhythmias following rapid IV use (rare), arthralgia (rare), ***anaphylaxis*** (rare).

Symptoms of Overdose: No experience is available for deliberate overdose.

Dosage

See individual drugs.

NURSING CONSIDERATIONS

Administration/Storage

1. These drugs may be taken without regard for meals.
2. Doses of antacids should be staggered if used with cimetidine or ranitidine.
3. *Treatment of Overdose:* Induce vomiting or perform gastric lavage to remove any unabsorbed drug. Monitor the client and undertake supportive therapy.

Assessment

1. Document indications for therapy. Assess client symptoms of epigastric or abdominal pain/discomfort, noting onset, duration, intensity, and any previous treatment and the results.
2. Obtain baseline CBC and liver and renal function studies.
3. Perform baseline CNS assessment noting level of orientation.
4. List other agents prescribed to ensure that none interact unfavorably.
5. Assess for number of occurrences. Chronic treatment is usually not initiated until two to three recurrences are documented.

Client/Family Teaching

1. Explain that antacids must be taken as prescribed but not to take within 1 hr of the histamine H_2 antagonist.
2. Stress the importance of taking the medication as prescribed and not to stop if pain subsides or if "feeling better" as drug is necessary to inhibit gastric acid secretion.
3. Explain that these agents reduce the secretion of gastric acid. They are usually prescribed for 4–8 weeks initially to control symptoms and to promote healing.
4. Any evidence of confusion or disorientation should be reported immediately. This has been noted more often in the elderly and severely ill.
5. Avoid alcohol, caffeine, aspirin-containing products, and foods that may cause GI irritation.
6. Instruct client to inform provider of drug therapy when undergoing skin testing. These drugs generally should be discontinued 24 hr before testing begins as a false negative response may be evident in tests with allergen extracts.
7. Smoking may interfere with drug's action. Advise client to stop smoking and most especially not to smoke following the last prescribed dose of the day. Offer referrals and assistance in accessing formal smoking cessation programs.
8. Advise that any new evidence of bleeding, such as blood-tinged emesis or dark tarry stools as well as dizziness or rash, require immediate reporting.
9. Stress the importance of reporting for all scheduled follow-up studies and advise that a response to these agents does not preclude gastric malignancy.

Evaluate

- Radiographic or endoscopic evidence of duodenal ulcer healing
- Clinical evidence of ↓ gastric irritation and bleeding
- Reports of ↓ abdominal pain and discomfort
- Laboratory confirmation of ↓ gastric acid secretion
- Stabilization of H&H
- GI secretions and stool, negative for occult blood

Cimetidine

(sye-**MET**-ih-deen)
Pregnancy Category: B
Apo-Cimetidine ✱, Novo-Cimetidine ✱, Nu-Cimet ✱, Peptol ✱, Tagamet
(Rx)

See also *Histamine H_2 Antagonists,* Chapter 63.

How Supplied: *Injection:* 150 mg/mL, 300 mg/50 mL; *Solution:* 300 mg/5 mL; *Tablet:* 200 mg, 300 mg, 400 mg, 800 mg

Action/Kinetics: Cimetidine reduces postprandial daytime and nighttime gastric acid secretion by about 50%–80%. It is well absorbed from GI tract. The drug may increase gastromucosal defense and healing in acid-related disorders (e.g., stress-induced ulcers) by increasing production of gastric mucus, increasing mucosal secretion of bicarbonate and gastric mucosal blood flow as well as increasing endogenous mucosal synthesis of prostaglandins. It also inhibits cytochrome P-450 and P-448, which will affect metabolism of drugs. Cimetidine also possesses antiandrogenic activity and will increase prolactin levels following an IV bolus injection. **Peak plasma level, PO:** 45–90 min. **Time to peak effect, after PO:** 1–2 hr. **Duration, nocturnal:** 6–8 hr; **basal:** 4–5 hr. **t½:** 2 hr, longer in presence of renal impairment. After PO use, most metabolized in liver; after parenteral use, about 75% of drug excreted unchanged in the urine.

Uses: Short-term (up to 8 weeks) and maintenance treatment of active duodenal ulcers; short-term (6 weeks) treatment of benign gastric ulcers. Management of gastric acid hypersecretory states (Zollinger-Ellison syndrome, systemic mastocytosis). Gastroesophageal reflux disease, including erosive esophagitis. Prophylaxis of upper GI bleeding in critically ill hospitalized clients. *Investigational:* Prior to surgery to prevent aspiration pneumonitis, secondary hyperparathyroidism in chronic hemodialysis clients, prophylaxis of stress-induced ulcers, hyperparathyroidism, dyspepsia, herpes virus infections, tinea capitis, hirsute women, chronic idiopathic urticaria, dermatologic anaphylaxis, acetaminophen overdosage.

Dosage

- **Tablets, Oral Solution**

Duodenal ulcers, short-term.

Adults: 800 mg at bedtime. Alternate dosage: 300 mg q.i.d. with meals and at bedtime for 4–6 weeks (administer with antacids, staggering the dose of antacids) or 400 mg b.i.d. (in the morning and evening). **Maintenance:** 400 mg at bedtime.

Active benign peptic ulcers.

Adults: 800 mg at bedtime (preferred regimen) or 300 mg q.i.d. with meals and at bedtime for no more than 8 weeks.

Pathologic hypersecretory conditions.

Adults: 300 mg q.i.d. with meals and at bedtime up to a maximum of 2,400 mg/day for as long as needed.

Erosive gastroesophageal reflux disease.

Adults: 800 mg b.i.d. or 400 mg q.i.d. for 12 weeks.

Dyspepsia.

Adults: 400 mg b.i.d.

Prophylaxis of aspiration pneumonitis.

Adults: 400–600 mg 60–90 min before anesthesia.

Primary hyperparathyroidism, secondary hyperparathyroidism in chronic hemodialysis clients.

Up to 1 g/day.

- **IM, IV, IV Infusion**

Hospitalized clients with pathologic hypersecretory conditions, intractable ulcers, or those unable to take PO medication.

Adults: 300 mg IM or IV q 6-8 hr. If an increased dose is necessary, administer 300 mg more frequently than q 6–8 hr, not to exceed 2,400 mg/day.

Prophylaxis of upper GI bleeding.

Adults: 50 mg/hr by continuous IV infusion. If creatinine clearance is less than 30 mL/min, use one-half the recommended dose.

Prophylaxis of aspiration pneumonitis.

Adults: 300 mg IV 60–90 min before induction of anesthetic.

Administration/Storage

1. For IV injections, dilute 300 mg in 0.9% sodium chloride injection (or other compatible solution) to a total volume of 20 mL. Inject over at least 2 min.
2. For intermittent IV infusion, dilute 300 mg in at least 50 mL of dextrose or saline solution and infuse over 15–20 min.
3. For continuous IV infusion, give a loading dose of 150 mg (by intermittent IV infusion); then, administer 37.5 mg/hr (900 mg/day) in 0.9% sodium chloride injection, 5% or 10% dextrose injection, 5% sodium bicarbonate injection, lactated Ringer's solution, or as part of TPN. Is stable for 24 hr at room temperature if mixed with these diluents.
4. Drugs or additives should *not* be introduced to cimetidine solutions in plastic containers.
5. The premixed single-dose product should not be exposed to excessive heat; store at 15°C–30°C (59°F–86°F).
6. Cimetidine may be diluted in 100–1000 mL; however, if the volume for a 24-hr infusion is less than 250 mL, a volumetric pump should be used.
7. Cimetidine is incompatible with aminophylline and barbiturates in IV solutions. Also, it is incompatible in the same syringe with pentobarbital sodium and a pentobarbital sodium/atropine sulfate combination.
8. For IM use, cimetidine can be given undiluted.
9. Administer PO medication with meals and with a snack at bedtime.
10. If antacids are to be used, stagger the dose with that of cimetidine.
11. In impaired renal function, a dose of 300 mg PO or IV q 12 hr may be necessary. If necessary the dose may be given, with caution, q 8 hr.

Contraindications: Children under 16, lactation. Cirrhosis, impaired liver and renal function.

Special Concerns: In geriatric clients with impaired renal or hepatic function, confusion is more likely to occur. Not recommended for children less than 16 years of age.

Side Effects: *GI:* Diarrhea, pancreatitis, hepatitis, hepatic fibrosis. *CNS:* Dizziness, sleepiness, headache, confusion, delirium, hallucinations, double vision, dysarthria, ataxia. Severely ill clients may manifest agitation, anxiety, depression, disorientation, hallucinations, mental confusion, and psychosis. *CV:* Hypotension and arrhythmias following rapid IV administration. *Hematologic:* Agranulocytosis, thrombocytopenia, ***hemolytic or aplastic anemia,*** granulocytopenia. *GU:* Impotence (high doses for prolonged periods of time), gynecomastia (long-term treatment). *Other:* Arthralgia, myalgia, rash, vasculitis, galactorrhea, alopecia, bronchoconstriction.

Drug Interactions

Antacids / ↓ Effect of cimetidine due to ↓ absorption from GI tract

Anticholinergics / ↓ Effect of cimetidine due to ↓ absorption from GI tract

Benzodiazepines / ↑ Effect of benzodiazepines due to ↓ breakdown by liver

Beta-adrenergic blocking drugs / ↑ Effect of beta blockers due to ↓ breakdown by liver

Caffeine / ↑ Effect of caffeine due to ↓ breakdown by liver

Calcium channel blockers / ↑ Effect of calcium channel blockers due to ↓ breakdown by liver

Carbamazepine / ↑ Effect of carbamazepine due to ↓ breakdown by liver

Carmustine / Additive bone marrow depression

Chloroquine / ↑ Effect of iron due to ↓ breakdown by liver

Chlorpromazine / ↓ Effect of chlorpromazine due to ↓ absorption from GI tract

Digoxin / ↓ Serum levels of digoxin

Flecainide / ↑ Effect of flecainide

Fluconazole / ↓ Effect of fluconazole due to ↓ absorption from GI tract
Fluorouracil / ↓ Serum levels of fluorouracil
Indomethacin / ↓ Effect of indomethacin due to ↓ absorption from GI tract
Iron salts / ↓ Effect of iron due to ↓ absorption from GI tract
Ketoconazole / ↓ Effect of ketoconazole due to ↓ absorption from GI tract
Lidocaine / ↑ Effect of lidocaine due to ↓ breakdown by liver
Metoclopramide / ↓ Effect of cimetidine due to ↓ absorption from GI tract
Metronidazole / ↑ Effect of metronidazole due to ↓ breakdown by liver
Moricizine / ↑ Effect of moricizine due to ↓ breakdown by liver
Narcotics / Possible ↑ toxic effects (respiratory depression) of narcotics
Pentoxifylline / ↑ Effect of pentoxifylline due to ↓ breakdown by liver
Phenytoin / ↑ Effect of phenytoin due to ↓ breakdown by liver
Procainamide / ↑ Effect of procainamide due to ↓ excretion by kidney
Propafenone / ↑ Effect of propafenone due to ↓ breakdown by liver
Quinidine / ↑ Effect of quinidine due to ↓ breakdown by liver
Quinine / ↑ Effect of quinine due to ↓ breakdown by liver
Succinylcholine / ↑ Neuromuscular blockade → respiratory depression and extended apnea
Sulfonylureas / ↑ Effect of sulfonylureas due to ↓ breakdown by liver
Tetracyclines / ↓ Effect of tetracyclines due to ↓ absorption from GI tract
Theophyllines / ↑ Effect of theophyllines due to ↓ breakdown by liver
Tocainide / ↓ Effect of tocainide
Triamterene / ↑ Effect of triamterene due to ↓ breakdown by liver
Tricyclic antidepressants / ↑ Effect of tricyclic antidepressants due to ↓ breakdown by liver
Warfarin / ↑ Effect of anticoagulant due to ↓ breakdown by liver

NURSING CONSIDERATIONS

See also *Nursing Considerations* for *Histamine H_2 Antagonists,* Chapter 63.

Assessment

1. Note the general overall client condition. Those receiving radiation therapy or myelosuppressive drugs may have their actions potentiated by cimetidine.
2. Review the long list of drug interactions prior to administering the drug. Determine if any of the drugs the client is taking may interact unfavorably with cimetidine.
3. Document indications for therapy, type and onset of symptoms, and the expected time frame for therapy.
4. Assess location, characteristics, and extent of abdominal pain. Note any blood in emesis, stool, or gastric aspirate.
5. Obtain baseline CBC, electrolytes, and liver and renal function studies.

Interventions

1. Be alert to mood swings and report any new symptoms of confusion. These are more common among the elderly than among people in other age groups.
2. Note any increased susceptibility to infections. Clients taking cimetidine may develop agranulocytosis, thrombocytopenia, or anemia and should receive periodic hematologic evaluations.
3. For the elderly, severely ill client or one who has renal impairment, monitor renal function, and I&O during therapy.
4. If diarrhea develops, monitor the frequency and severity and report if persistent. Maintain adequate hydration and monitor serum electrolytes.
5. Inspect the skin routinely for rashes or other skin changes; report any abnormalities.
6. Drug may alter response to skin tests with allergenic extracts. Discontinue drug 24 hr prior to skin testing.

Client/Family Teaching

1. Take tablets with meals and a snack at bedtime. Avoid antacids 1 hr before or after dose.
2. Review goals of prescribed therapy and explain the need to continue taking the drug even though the symptoms may have disappeared.
3. Discuss other drugs that have been ordered and establish an appropriate schedule to assure compliance with drug therapy.
4. Discuss any required dietary modifications, especially if the client is being treated for GI problems. Evaluate carefully because it may be necessary for a dietitian to work with the client.
5. Do not perform tasks that require mental alertness until drug effects are realized.
6. Instruct clients about the symptoms of gynecomastia or galactorrhea and advise to report these side effects should they occur.
7. Report immediately if abdominal pain, bloody stools, or other indications that the ulcer has been reactivated are evident.
8. Avoid alcohol, caffeine, spicy foods, and aspirin-containing products, all of which may enhance GI irritation.
9. Smoking may alter the drug's response. Do not smoke after the last dose of cimetidine to ensure optimal suppression of nocturnal gastric acid secretion. If necessary, refer client to a formal smoking cessation program.

Evaluate

- ↓ GI pain and promotion of ulcer healing
- Control of hypersecretion of acid
- Prophylaxis of GI bleeding
- Prophylaxis of aspiration pneumonia
- GI secretions and stool negative for occult blood

Famotidine

(fah-**MOH**-tih-deen)

Pregnancy Category: B

Apo-Famotidine ✦, Novo-Famotidine ✦, Pepcid, Pepcid IV **(Rx)**

See also *Histamine H_2 Antagonists,* Chapter 63.

How Supplied: *Injection:* 10 mg/mL; *Powder for Reconstitution:* 40 mg/5 mL; *Tablet:* 10 mg, 20 mg, 40 mg

Action/Kinetics: Famotidine is a competitive inhibitor of histamine H_2 receptors, thus leading to inhibition of gastric acid secretion. Both basal and nocturnal gastric acid secretion, as well as secretion stimulated by food or pentagastrin, are inhibited. **Peak plasma levels:** 1–3 hr. **t½:** 2.5–3.5 hr. **Onset:** 1 hr. **Duration:** 10–12 hr. Famotidine does not inhibit the cytochrome P-450 system in the liver; thus, drug interactions, as a result of inhibition of liver metabolism, are not expected to occur. From 25% to 30% of a PO dose is eliminated through the kidney unchanged.

Uses: Short-term treatment of active duodenal ulcer (up to 8 weeks). Maintenance therapy for duodenal ulcer, at reduced dosage, after active ulcer has healed. Pathologic hypersecretory conditions such as Zollinger-Ellison syndrome or multiple endocrine adenomas. Gastroesophageal reflux disease, including erosive esophagitis. Benign gastric ulcer. *Investigational:* Prevent aspiration pneumonitis, prophylaxis of stress ulcers, prevent acute upper GI bleeding.

Dosage

- **Oral Suspension, Tablets**

Duodenal ulcer, acute therapy.

Adults: 40 mg once daily at bedtime or 20 mg b.i.d. for up to 8 weeks.

Duodenal ulcer, maintenance therapy.

Adults: 20 mg once daily at bedtime.

Benign gastric ulcers, acute therapy.

Adults: 40 mg at bedtime.

Hypersecretory conditions.

Adults, individualized, initial: 20 mg q 6 hr; **then,** adjust dose to response, although doses of up to 160 mg q 6 hr may be required for severe cases.

Gastroesophageal reflux disease.
Adults: 20 mg b.i.d. for 6 weeks. For esophagitis with erosions and ulcerations, give 20 or 40 mg b.i.d. for up to 12 weeks.

Prophylaxis of upper GI bleeding.
Adults: 20 mg b.i.d.

Prophylaxis of stress ulcers.
Adults: 40 mg/day.

• **IM, IV, IV Infusion**

Hospitalized clients with hypersecretory conditions, duodenal ulcers, gastric ulcers, clients unable to take PO medication.
Adults: 20 mg IV q 12 hr.

Before anesthesia to prevent aspiration of gastric acid.
Adults: 40 mg IM or PO.

Administration/Storage

1. Antacids may be used concomitantly if required.
2. In clients with a creatinine clearance less than 10 mL/min, the dose may be reduced to 20 mg at bedtime or the interval between doses may be increased to 36–48 hr.
3. For IV injection, dilute 2 mL (containing 10 mg/mL) with 0.9% sodium chloride injection to a total volume of 5–10 mL and give over at least a 2-min period.
4. For IV infusion, dilute 2 mL (20 mg) with 100 mL of 5% dextrose and infuse over 15–30 min.
5. A solution is stable for 48 hr at room temperature when added to or diluted with water for injection, 0.9% sodium chloride injection, 5% or 10% dextrose injection, lactated Ringer's injection, or 5% sodium bicarbonate injection.
6. Famotidine is stable when mixed with various TPN solutions. Length of stability depends on the solution.

Contraindications: Cirrhosis of the liver, impaired renal or hepatic function, lactation.

Special Concerns: Safety and efficacy in children have not been established.

Side Effects: *GI:* Constipation, diarrhea, N&V, anorexia, dry mouth, abdominal discomfort. *CNS:* Dizziness, headache, paresthesias, depression, anxiety, confusion, hallucinations, insomnia, fatigue, sleepiness, agitation, ***grand mal seizure,*** psychic disturbances. *Skin:* Rash, acne, pruritus, alopecia, urticaria, dry skin, flushing. *CV:* Palpitations, AV block, arrhythmia. *Musculoskeletal:* Arthralgia, asthenia, musculoskeletal pain. *Hematologic:* Rarely, ***agranulocytosis,*** pancytopenia, leukopenia, thrombocytopenia. *Other:* Fever, liver enzyme abnormalities, orbital or facial edema, conjunctival injection, bronchospasm, tinnitus, taste disorders, cholestatic jaundice, ***anaphylaxis,*** angioedema, decreased libido, impotence, pain at injection site (transient).

Drug Interactions

Antacids / ↓ Absorption of famotidine from the GI tract
Diazepam / ↓ Absorption of diazepam from the GI tract

NURSING CONSIDERATIONS

See also *Nursing Considerations* for *Histamine H_2 Antagonists,* Chapter 63.

Assessment

1. Document indications for therapy and onset of symptoms.
2. Note location, extent, and characteristics of abdominal pain.
3. Perform a baseline assessment of the client's mental status.
4. Assess for occult blood in stools and gastric secretions.
5. Determine if the client has a history of seizures.
6. If the client is pregnant, discuss the benefits versus risks of drug therapy.
7. Note any evidence of hepatic or renal dysfunction.

Client/Family Teaching

1. Drug may cause dizziness, headaches, and anxiety; use caution and report if symptoms persist.
2. Changes in client attitude such as increasing lack of concern for personal appearance, depression, or sleeplessness warrant medical assessment.
3. Report any GI side effects, such as diarrhea, constipation, or loss of appetite.
4. Avoid alcohol, aspirin-containing products, smoking, and foods that increase GI irritation.
5. Any reduction in urinary output should be reported because a reduction in drug dosage may be indicated.

Evaluate

• ↓ Abdominal pain

- Prophylaxis of stress ulcers
- Control of hypersecretion of acid
- Evidence (x-ray or endoscopic) of duodenal ulcer healing

Nizatidine

(nye-**ZAY**-tih-deen)
Pregnancy Category: C
Axid **(Rx)**

See also *Histamine H_2 Antagonists,* Chapter 63.

How Supplied: *Capsule:* 150 mg, 300 mg

Action/Kinetics: Nizatidine decreases gastric acid secretion by blocking the effect of histamine on histamine H_2 receptors. Does not affect the P-450 and P-448 drug metabolizing enzymes. **Peak plasma levels:** 0.5–3 hr after a PO dose. **Time to peak effect:** 0.5–3 hr. **Duration, nocturnal:** Up to 12 hr; **basal:** Up to 8 hr. **$t^1/_2$:** 1–2 hr. Antacids containing aluminum and magnesium hydroxides and simethicone decrease the absorption by about 10%. Approximately 60% of a PO dose is excreted unchanged in the urine. Clients with moderate to severe renal impairment manifest a significant prolongation of $t^1/_2$ with decreased clearance.

Uses: Treatment of acute duodenal ulcer and maintenance following healing of a duodenal ulcer. Gastroesophageal reflux disease, including erosive and ulcerative esophagitis. Short-term treatment of benign gastric ulcer.

Dosage

- **Capsules**

Active duodenal ulcer.

Adults: Either 300 mg once daily at bedtime or 150 mg b.i.d. The dose should be 150 mg/day if the creatinine clearance is 20–50 mL/min and 150 mg every other day if creatinine clearance is less than 20 mL/min.

Prophylaxis following healing of duodenal ulcer.

Adults: 150 mg/day at bedtime. The dose should be 150 mg every other day if creatinine clearance is 20–50 mL/min and 150 mg every 3 days if creatinine clearance is less than 20 mL/min.

Treatment of benign gastric ulcer.

Adults: 150 mg b.i.d. or 300 mg at bedtime

Gastroesophageal reflux disease, incldùing erosive and ulcerative esophagitis.

Adults: 150 mg b.i.d.

Administration/Storage

1. Treatment for active duodenal ulcer should be maintained for up to 8 weeks.
2. Gastric malignancy may be present even though a clinical response to nizatidine has occurred.
3. Doses of 150 and 300 mg can be mixed with commercial juices (apple juice, *Gatorade, Ocean Spray,* and others); such preparations are stable for 48 hr when refrigerated. However, a 10% loss in potency is seen if mixed with *V8* or *Cran-Grape* juices.

Contraindications: Hypersensitivity to H_2 receptor antagonists. Cirrhosis of the liver, impaired renal or hepatic function. Lactation.

Special Concerns: Safety and efficacy have not been determined in children.

Laboratory Test Interference: False + test for urobilinogen.

Side Effects: *CNS:* Headache, fatigue, somnolence, insomnia, dizziness, abnormal dreams, anxiety, nervousness, confusion (rare). *GI:* N&V, diarrhea, pancreatitis, constipation, abdominal discomfort, flatulence, dyspepsia, anorexia, dry mouth. *Dermatologic:* Exfoliative dermatitis, erythroderma, pruritus, urticaria, erythema multiforme. *CV:* Asymptomatic ventricular tachycardia; ***rarely, cardiac arrhythmias or arrest following rapid IV use.*** *Respiratory:* Rhinitis, pharyngitis, sinusitis, cough. *Body as a whole:* Asthenia, back pain, chest pain, infection, fever, myalgia. *Miscellaneous:* Impotence, loss of libido, thrombocytopenia, sweating, gynecomastia, hyperuricemia, eosinophilia, gout, and cholestatic or hepatocellular effects (resulting in increased AST, ALT, or alkaline phosphatase).

Drug Interaction: Following high doses of aspirin, nizatidine → ↑ salicylate serum levels.

NURSING CONSIDERATIONS

See also *Nursing Considerations* for *Histamine H_2 Antagonists,* Chapter 63.

Assessment

1. Take a drug history to determine if the client has any allergies to H_2 receptor antagonists.
2. Obtain baseline hepatic and renal function studies.

Interventions

1. Anticipate reduced dosage in clients with renal insufficiency.
2. Drug may cause a false positive test for urobilinogen. Notify the lab that client is taking nizatidine if this test is ordered.

Client/Family Teaching

1. Report any side effects, such as rashes, flaking of skin, or extreme sleepiness.
2. Take the medication at bedtime due to potential sedative effects.
3. Use caution when performing tasks that require mental alertness until drug effects realized.
4. Continue to take the medication as ordered even if symptoms subside.
5. Avoid alcohol, caffeine, spicy foods, and aspirin-containing products.
6. Do not smoke as this interferes with drug effects.

Evaluate: Reports of symptomatic improvement in gastric ulcer pain and irritation.

Ranitidine hydrochloride

(rah-**NIH**-tih-deen)

Pregnancy Category: B

Apo-Ranitidine ✱, Novo-Ranidine ✱, Nu-Ranit ✱, Zantac, Zantac-C ✱, Zantac Efferdose, Zantac GELdose Capsules **(Rx)**

See also *Histamine H_2 Antagonists,* Chapter 63.

How Supplied: *Capsule:* 150 mg, 300 mg; *Granule for reconstitution:* 150 mg; *Injection:* 1 mg/mL, 25 mg/mL; *Syrup:* 15 mg/mL; *Tablet:* 150 mg, 300 mg; *Tablet, effervescent:* 150 mg

Action/Kinetics: Ranitidine competitively inhibits gastric acid secretion by blocking the effect of histamine on histamine H_2 receptors. Both daytime and nocturnal basal gastric acid secretion, as well as food- and pentagastrin-stimulated gastric acid are inhibited. It is a weak inhibitor of cytochrome P-450 (drug-metabolizing enzymes); thus, drug interactions involving inhibition of hepatic metabolism are not expected to occur. Food increases the bioavailability. **Peak effect: PO,** 1–3 hr; **IM, IV,** 15 min. **t½:** 2.5–3 hr. **Duration, nocturnal:** 13 hr; **basal:** 4 hr. **Serum level to inhibit 50% stimulated gastric acid secretion:** 36–94 ng/mL. Excreted in urine.

Uses: Short-term (4–8 weeks) and maintenance treatment of duodenal ulcer. Pathologic hypersecretory conditions such as Zollinger-Ellison syndrome and systemic mastocytosis. Short-term treatment of active, benign gastric ulcers. Gastroesophageal reflux disease, including erosive esophagitis. Maintenance of healing of erosive esophagitis. *Investigational:* Prophylaxis of pulmonary aspiration of acid during anesthesia, prevent gastric damage from NSAIDs, prevent stress ulcers, prevent acute upper GI bleeding.

Dosage

- **Capsules (soft gelatin), Effervescent Tablets and Granules, Syrup, Tablets**

Duodenal ulcer, short-term.

Adults: 150 mg b.i.d. or 300 mg at bedtime to heal ulcer, although 100 mg b.i.d. will inhibit acid secretion and may be as effective as the higher dose. **Maintenance:** 150 mg at bedtime.

Hypersecretory conditions.

Adults: 150 mg b.i.d. (up to 6 g/day has been used in severe cases).

Gastroesophageal reflux, benign gastric ulcer.

Adults: 150 mg b.i.d.

Erosive esophagitis.

Adults: 150 mg q.i.d.

Maintenenace of healing of erosive esophagitis.

Adults: 150 mg b.i.d.

• **IM, IV**

Treatment and maintenance for duodenal ulcer, hypersecretory conditions, gastroesophageal reflux.

Adults, IM: 50 mg q 6–8 hr. **Intermittent IV injection or infusion:** 50 mg q 6–8 hr, not to exceed 400 mg/day. **Continuous IV infusion:** 6.25 mg/hr.

Zollinger-Ellison clients.

Continuous IV infusion: Dilute ranitidine in 5% dextrose injection to a concentration no greater than 2.5 mg/mL with an initial infusion rate of 1 mg/kg/hr. If after 4 hr the client shows a gastric acid output of greater than 10 mEq/hr or if symptoms appear, the dose should be increased by 0.5-mg/kg/hr increments and the acid output measured. Doses up to 2.5 mg/kg/hr may be necessary.

Administration/Storage

1. In clients with a creatinine clearance of less than 50 mL/min, the dose should be 150 mg PO every 24 hr or 50 mg parenterally q 18–24 hr.
2. Antacids should be given concomitantly for gastric pain although they may interfere with absorption of ranitidine.
3. About one-half of clients may heal completely within 2 weeks; thus, endoscopy may show no need for further treatment.
4. No dilution is required for IM use. For IV injection, 50 mg should be diluted with 0.9% sodium chloride injection to a total volume of 20 mL. The diluted solution should be given over 5 min or more. For intermittent IV infusion, dilute 50 mg in 100 mL 5% dextrose injection and give over 15–20 min.
5. May also be used for continuous infusions.
6. The premixed injection does not require dilution and should be given only by slow IV drip over 15–20 min. Additives should not be introduced into the solution. If used with a primary IV fluid system, the primary solution should be discontinued during infusion of the drug.
7. For continuous IV infusion, ranitidine injection should be added to 5% dextrose injection
8. The drug is stable for 48 hr at room temperature when mixed with 0.9% sodium chloride, 5% or 10% dextrose injection, lactated Ringer's injection, or 5% sodium bicarbonate injection.

Contraindications: Cirrhosis of the liver, impaired renal or hepatic function.

Special Concerns: Use with caution during lactation and in clients with decreased hepatic or renal function. Safety and efficacy not established in children.

Laboratory Test Interference: False + test for urine protein using Multistix.

Side Effects: *GI:* Constipation, N&V, diarrhea, abdominal pain, pancreatitis (rare). *CNS:* Headache, dizziness, malaise, insomnia, vertigo, confusion, anxiety, agitation, depression, fatigue, somnolence, hallucinations. *CV:* Bradycardia or tachycardia, premature ventricular beats following rapid IV use (especially in clients predisposed to cardiac rhythm disturbances). *Hematologic:* Thrombocytopenia, granulocytopenia, leukopenia, pancytopenia, ***agranulocytosis, aplastic anemia, autoimmune hemolytic anemia.*** *Hepatic:* Hepatotoxicity, jaundice, hepatitis, increase in ALT. *Dermatologic:* Pruritus, urticaria, erythema multiforme, rash, alopecia. *Allergic:* ***Bronchospasm,*** rashes, fever, eosinophilia. *Other:* Arthralgia, gynecomastia, impotence, loss of libido, blurred vision, angioneurotic edema, pain at injection site, local burning or itching following IV use.

Drug Interactions

Antacids / Antacids may ↓ the absorption of ranitidine

Glipizide / Ranitidine ↑ effect of glipizide

Procainamide / Ranitidine ↓ excretion of procainamide → possible ↑ effect
Theophylline / Possible ↑ effect of theophylline
Warfarin / Ranitidine may ↑ hypoprothrombinemic effects of warfarin

NURSING CONSIDERATIONS

See also *Nursing Considerations* for *Histamine H_2 Antagonists,* Chapter 63.

Assessment

1. Document indications for therapy, onset of symptoms, and anticipated treatment period.
2. Assess for any evidence of infections. Obtain a CBC with differential to detect any potential increased risk of infection.
3. Note any evidence of renal or liver disease and obtain baseline studies.
4. When working with sexually active female clients, determine if pregnant. The drug should be used cautiously in this setting.
5. Skin tests using allergens may elicit false negative results. Discontinue drug 24 hr prior to testing.

Client/Family Teaching

1. Take with or immediately following meals. Wait 1 hr before taking an antacid.
2. Do not drive a car or operate machinery until drug effects are realized; dizziness or drowsiness may occur.
3. Avoid alcohol, aspirin-containing products, and beverages that contain caffeine (tea, cola, coffee) because these tend to increase stomach acid.
4. Do not smoke because smoking may interfere with the healing of duodenal ulcers and decreases the drug's effectiveness.
5. Report any evidence of diarrhea and maintain adequate hydration.
6. Any confusion or disorientation should be reported immediately.
7. Symptoms of breast tenderness will usually disappear after several weeks. Report if persistent because the drug therapy may need to be discontinued.
8. Report for scheduled visits to determine the extent of healing and when the drug can be safely discontinued.

Evaluate

- ↓ Gastric acid production
- Improvement in abdominal pain and discomfort
- Endoscopic or radiographic evidence of duodenal ulcer healing

OTHER GI DRUGS

See the following individual entries:

Cisapride
Donnatal Capsules, Elixir, Tablets
Librax
Metoclopramide
Misoprostol
Omeprazole
Pancrelipase (Lipancreatin)
Sucralfate

Cisapride

(SISS-ah-pryd)
Pregnancy Category: C
Propulsid **(Rx)**

How Supplied: *Tablet:* 10 mg, 20 mg

Action/Kinetics: The drug acts by enhancing release of acetylcholine at the myenteric plexus, resulting in increased strength of esophageal peristalsis and an increase in lower esophageal sphincter pressure. The drug also increases gastric emptying time. **Onset:** 30–60 min. **Peak plasma levels:** 1–1.5 hr. **Terminal t½:** 6–12 hr (up to 20 hr following IV use). The drug is metabolized in the liver with less than 10% excreted unchanged through the urine and feces.

Use: Symptomatic treatment of clients with nocturnal heartburn due to gastroesophageal reflux disease (GERD).

Dosage

- **Tablets**

GERD.

Adults, initial: 10 mg q.i.d. at least 15 min before meals and at bedtime. Dosage may need to be increased in some clients to 20 mg q.i.d. 15 min before meals and at bedtime.

Administration/Storage: *Treatment of Overdose:* Gastric lavage or activated charcoal. Observe client closely. Provide general supportive treatment.

Contraindications: Use in clients in whom an increase in GI motility could be harmful (i.e., in the presence of GI hemorrhage, mechanical obstruction, perforation).

Special Concerns: Use with caution during lactation. Safety and efficacy have not been demonstrated in children. Steady-state plasma levels are generally higher in older clients as a result of increased elimination half-life although doses used are similar to those in younger adults. The increased rate of gastric emptying time due to cisapride could affect the rate of absorption of other drugs.

Side Effects: *GI:* Diarrhea, abdominal pain, nausea, constipation, flatulence, dyspepsia, vomiting, dry mouth. *CNS:* Headache, insomnia, anxiety, nervousness, dizziness, depression, tremor, ***seizures,*** extrapyramidal effects, somnolence, migraine. *CV:* Palpitation, sinus tachycardia, tachycardia. *Respiratory:* Rhinitis, sinusitis, coughing, pharyngitis, upper respiratory tract infection. *GU:* UTI, increased frequency of urination, vaginitis. *Hepatic:* Hepatitis, elevated liver enzymes. *Musculoskeletal:* Arthralgia, back pain, myalgia. *Hematologic:* Thrombocytopenia, leukopenia, aplastic anemia, pancytopenia, granulocytopenia (rare). *Miscellaneous:* Pain, fever, viral infection, rash, pruritus, abnormal vision, chest pain, fatigue, dehydration, edema.

Symptoms of Overdose: One case of overdose included symptoms of retching, borborygmi, flatulence, stool and urinary frequency.

Drug Interactions

Alcohol / Possible ↑ sedative effect
Anticholinergics / ↓ Effect of cisapride
Anticoagulants / ↑ Coagulation times
Benzodiazepines / Possible ↑ sedative effect
Cimetidine / ↑ Peak plasma levels of cisapride; also ↑ GI absorption of cimetidine
Ranitidine / ↑ GI absorption of ranitidine

NURSING CONSIDERATIONS

Assessment

1. Document indications for therapy and type and onset of symptoms.
2. List drugs currently prescribed. Drug causes increased gastric emptying. Note any conditions or prescribed drugs that may preclude this therapy.
3. Monitor coagulation times closely in clients receiving oral anticoagulants and adjust dosage accordingly.

Client/Family Teaching

1. Advise to take at least 15 min before meals and at bedtime.
2. Explain that in addition to relieving symptoms of esophageal reflux, the drug also increases gastric emptying time. Therefore plan administration of additional prescribed medications accordingly.
3. Avoid alcohol and benzodiazepines since drug may potentiate sedative effects.
4. Review most frequently experienced symptoms (e.g., headaches, abdominal pain, nausea, rhinitis, and constipation), advising to report any persistent or intolerable symptoms.

Evaluate: Symptomatic relief of esophageal reflux and associated symptoms.

—COMBINATION DRUG—

Donnatal Capsules, Elixir, Tablets

(DON-nah-tal)

Pregnancy Category: C

(Rx)

How Supplied: See Content

Content: Each tablet, capsule, or 5 mL elixir contains: *Anticholinergic:* Atropine sulfate, 0.0194 mg. *Anticholinergic:* Hyoscyamine sulfate, 0.1037 mg. *Anticholinergic:* Scopolamine hydrobromide, 0.0065 mg. *Sedative:* Phenobarbital, 16.2 mg. *NOTE:* The Extentabs contain three times the amount of drugs found in tablets.

Uses: Possibly effective as an adjunct in the treatment of irritable colon, spastic colon, mucous colitis, and acute enterocolitis. Has also been used in the treatment of duodenal ulcer.

Dosage

• **Tablets, Capsules, Extentabs, Elixir**

Adults, usual: 1–2 tablets or capsules t.i.d.–q.i.d. (or one Extentab q 12 hr). If the elixir is used, **adult, usual:** 5–10 mL t.i.d.–q.i.d. **Pediatric:** Use elixir as follows: **4.5–9.0 kg:** 0.5 mL q 4 hr or 0.75 mL q 6 hr; **9.1–13.5 kg:** 1.0 mL q 4 hr or 1.5 mL q 6hr; **13.6–22.6 kg:** 1.5 mL q 4 hr or 2.0 mL q 6 hr; **22.7–33.9 kg:** 2.5 mL q 4 hr or 3.75 mL q 6 hr. **34.0–45.3 kg:** 3.75 mL q 4 hr or 5 mL q 6 hr; **45.4 kg:** 5 mL q 4 hr or 7.5 mL q 6 hr.

Special Concerns: It is not known with certainty whether or not anticholinergic drugs aid in the healing in duodenal ulcer or decrease the rate of recurrence or prevent complications.

NURSING CONSIDERATIONS

See also *Nursing Considerations* for *Cholinergic Blocking Agents,* Chapter 49, and *Barbiturates,* Chapter 39.

Evaluate: Relief of abdominal pain with restoration of normal bowel motility.

—COMBINATION DRUG—

Librax

(**LIB**-rax)

(Rx)

How Supplied: *Capsule:* 5 mg-2.5 mg

Content: *Antianxiety agent:* Chlordiazepoxide, 5 mg. *Anticholinergic agent:* Clidinium bromide, 2.5 mg. See also information on individual components.

Uses: Possibly effective as an adjunct in the treatment of irritable colon, spastic colon, mucous colitis, and acute enterocolitis.

Dosage

• **Capsules**

Individualized. Adults, usual: 1–2 capsules t.i.d.–q.i.d. before meals and at bedtime.

Contraindications: Pregnancy, glaucoma, prostatic hypertrophy.

NURSING CONSIDERATIONS

See *Nursing Considerations* for *Anti-Anxiety/Antimanic Drugs,* Chapter 40, and *Cholinergic Blocking Agents,* Chapter 49.

Evaluate: Restoration of normal bowel motility and relief of pain.

Metoclopramide

(meh-toe-kloh-**PRAH**-myd)

Pregnancy Category: B

Apo-Metoclop ✱, Maxeran ✱, Maxolon, Octamide PFS, Reglan **(Rx)**

How Supplied: *Concentrate:* 10 mg/mL; *Injection:* 5 mg/mL; *Syrup:* 1 mg/mL, 5 mg/5 mL; *Tablet:* 5 mg, 10 mg

Action/Kinetics: Metoclopramide, considered a dopamine agonist, acts by increasing sensitivity to acetylcholine; this results in increased motility of the upper GI tract and relaxation of the pyloric sphincter and duodenal bulb. Thus gastric emptying time and GI transit time are shortened. It has no effect on gastric, biliary, or pancreatic secretions. The drug facilitates intubation of the small bowel and speeds transit of a barium meal. The drug also produces sedation, induces release of prolactin, increases circulating aldosterone levels (is transient), and is an antiemetic. **Onset, IV:** 1–3 min; **IM,** 10–15 min; **PO,** 30–60 min. **Duration:** 1–2 hr. **t½:** 5–6 hr. Significant first-pass effect following PO use; unchanged drug and metabolites excreted in urine. Renal impairment decreases clearance of the drug.

Uses: PO: Acute and recurrent diabetic gastroparesis, gastroesophageal reflux.

Parenteral: Facilitate small bowel intubation, stimulate gastric emptying, and increase intestinal transit of barium to aid in radiologic examination of stomach and small intestine. Prophylaxis of N&V in cancer chemotherapy and following surgery (when nasogastric suction is not desired). *Investigational:* To improve lactation. N&V due to various causes, including vomiting during pregnancy and labor, gastric ulcer, anorexia nervosa. Improve client response to ergotamine, analgesics, and sedatives when used to treat migraine (may increase absorption). Postoperative gastric bezoars. Atonic bladder. Esophageal variceal bleeding.

Dosage

- **Tablets, Syrup**

Diabetic gastroparesis.

Adults: 10 mg 30 min before meals and at bedtime for 2–8 weeks (therapy should be reinstituted if symptoms recur).

Gastroesophageal reflux.

Adults: 10–15 mg q.i.d. 30 min before meals and at bedtime. If symptoms occur only intermittently, single doses up to 20 mg prior to the provoking situation may be used.

To enhance lactation.

Adults: 30–45 mg/day.

- **IM, IV**

Prophylaxis of vomiting due to chemotherapy.

Initial: 1–2 mg/kg IV q 2 hr for two doses, with the first dose 30 min before chemotherapy; **then,** 10 mg or more q 3 hr for three doses. Inject slowly IV over 15 min.

Prophylaxis of postoperative N&V.

Adults: 10–20 mg IM near the end of surgery.

Facilitate small bowel intubation.

Adults: 10 mg given over 1–2 min; **pediatric, 6–14 years:** 2.5–5 mg; **pediatric, less than 6 years:** 0.1 mg/kg.

Radiologic examinations to increase intestinal transit time.

Adults: 10 mg as a single dose given IV over 1–2 min.

- **Rectal Suppositories**

If PO dosing is not possible, suppositories can be made by incorporating 25 mg metoclopramide (5 pulverized PO tablets) in polyethylene glycol. Give 1 suppository 30–60 min before meals and at bedtime.

Administration/Storage

1. Inject slowly IV over 1–2 min to prevent transient feelings of anxiety and restlessness.
2. After PO use, absorption of certain drugs from the GI tract may be affected (see *Drug Interactions*).
3. Metoclopramide is physically and/or chemically incompatible with a number of drugs; check package insert if drug is to be admixed.
4. For IV use, doses greater than 10 mg should be diluted in 50 mL of D5W, dextrose 5% in 0.45% sodium chloride, lactated Ringer's injection, Ringer's injection, or sodium chloride injection and infused over 15 min.
5. *Treatment of Overdose:* Treat extrapyramidal effects by giving anticholinergic drugs, antiparkinson drugs, or antihistamines with anticholinergic effects. General supportive treatment. Reverse methemoglobinemia by giving methylene blue.

Contraindications: Gastrointestinal hemorrhage, obstruction, or perforation; epilepsy; clients taking drugs likely to cause extrapyramidal symptoms, such as phenothiazines. Pheochromocytoma.

Special Concerns: Use with caution during lactation. Extrapyramidal effects are more likely to occur in children and geriatric clients. Use with caution in hypertension.

Side Effects: *CNS:* Restlessness, drowsiness, fatigue, lassitude, akathisia, anxiety, insomnia, confusion. Headaches, dizziness, extrapyramidal symptoms (especially acute dystonic reactions), Parkinson-like symptoms (including cogwheel rigidity, mask-like facies, bradykinesia, tremor), dystonia, myoclonus, ***depression (with suicidal ideation),*** tardive dyskinesia (including involuntary movements of the tongue, face, mouth, or jaw), seizures, hallucinations. *GI:* Nausea, bowel disturbances (usually diarrhea). *CV:* Hypertension (transient), hypotension, SVT, bradycardia. *Hematologic:* ***Agranulocytosis,*** leukopenia, neutropenia. Methemoglobinemia in premature and full-term infants at doses of 1–4 mg/kg/ day IM, IV, or PO for 1–3 or more days. *Endocrine:* Galactorrhea, amenorrhea, gynecomastia, impotence (due to hyperprolactinemia), fluid retention (due to transient elevation of aldosterone). ***Neuroleptic malignant syndrome: Hyperthermia, altered consciousness, autonomic dysfunction, muscle rigidity, death.*** *Miscellaneous:* Incontinence, urinary frequency, porphyria, visual disturbances, flushing of the face and upper body, hepatotoxicity.

Symptoms of Overdose: Agitation, irritability, hypertonia of muscles, drowsiness, disorientation, extrapyramidal symptoms.

Drug Interactions

Acetaminophen / ↑ GI absorption of acetaminophen
Anticholinergics / ↓ Effect of metoclopramide
Cimetidine / ↓ Effect of cimetidine due to ↓ absorption from GI tract
CNS depressants / Additive sedative effects
Cyclosporine / ↓ Absorption of cyclosporine → ↑ immunosuppressive and toxic effects
Digoxin / ↓ Effect of digoxin due to ↓ absorption from GI tract
Ethanol / ↑ GI absorption of ethanol
Levodopa / ↑ GI absorption of levodopa and levodopa ↓ effects of metoclopramide on gastric emptying and lower esophageal pressure
MAO inhibitors / ↑ Release of catecholamines → toxicity
Narcotic analgesics / ↓ Effect of metoclopramide
Succinylcholine / ↑ Effect of succinylcholine due to inhibition of plasma cholinesterase
Tetracyclines / ↑ GI absorption of tetracyclines

NURSING CONSIDERATIONS

Assessment

1. Document indications for therapy and type and onset of symptoms.
2. List drugs currently prescribed, noting any that may interact unfavorably.
3. Assess abdomen for bowel sounds and distention, and note any reports of N&V.

Client/Family Teaching

1. Operating a car or hazardous machinery should not be attempted because medication has a sedative effect.
2. Report any persistent side effects so they can be properly evaluated and counteracted.
3. Avoid alcohol and any other CNS depressants. Metoclopramide will have an added sedative effect.
4. Extrapyramidal effects (trembling hands, facial grimacing) should be reported. These may be treated by the provider with IM diphenhydramine.

Evaluate

- Prevention of N&V
- Enhanced gastric motility
- Promotion of gastric emptying
- Prophylaxis of gastric bezoars

Misoprostol

(my-soh-**PROST**-ohl)
Pregnancy Category: X
Cytotec **(Rx)**

How Supplied: *Tablet:* 100 mcg, 200 mcg

Action/Kinetics: Misoprostol is a synthetic prostaglandin E_1 analog that inhibits gastric acid secretion, protects the gastric mucosa by increasing bicarbonate and mucous production, and decreases pepsin levels during basal conditions. The drug may also stimulate uterine contractions that may endanger pregnancy. Misoprostol is rapidly converted to the active misoprostol acid. **Time for peak levels of misoprostol acid:** 12 min. **t½, misoprostol acid:** 20–40 min. Misoprostol acid is less than 90% bound to plasma protein. *NOTE:* Misoprostol does not prevent development of duodenal ulcers in clients on NSAIDs.

Uses: Prevention of aspirin and other nonsteroidal anti-inflammatory-induced gastric ulcers in clients with a high risk of gastric ulcer complications (e.g., geriatric clients with debilitating disease) or in those with a history of ulcer. *Investigational:* Treat duodenal ulcers including those unresponsive to histamine H_2 antagonists. With cyclosporine and prednisone to decrease the incidence of acute graft rejection in renal transplant clients (the drug improves renal function).

Dosage

• **Tablets**

Adults: 200 mcg q.i.d. with food. Dose can be reduced to 100 mcg if the larger dose cannot be tolerated. In renal impairment, the 200-mcg dose can be reduced if necessary.

Administration/Storage

1. The incidence of diarrhea can be reduced by giving the drug after meals and at bedtime as well as by avoiding magnesium-containing antacids. Diarrhea is usually self-limiting, however.
2. Maximum plasma levels of misoprostol are decreased if the drug is taken with food.
3. Misoprostol should be taken for the duration of nonsteroidal anti-inflammatory therapy.
4. Drug may increase gastric bicarbonate and mucous production.
5. Available in both 100-mcg and 200-mcg tablets.
6. *Treatment of Overdose:* Use supportive therapy.

Contraindications: Allergy to prostaglandins, pregnancy, during lactation (may cause diarrhea in nursing infants).

Special Concerns: Use with caution in clients with renal impairment and in clients older than 64 years of age. Safety and efficacy have not been established in children less than 18 years of age. Misoprostol may cause miscarriage with potentially serious bleeding.

Side Effects: *GI:* Diarrhea, abdominal pain, nausea, dyspepsia, flatulence, vomiting, constipation. *Gynecologic:* Spotting, cramps, dysmenorrhea, hypermenorrhea, menstrual disorders, postmenopausal vaginal bleeding. *Miscellaneous:* Headache.

Symptoms of Overdose: Abdominal pain, diarrhea, dyspnea, sedation, tremor, fever, palpitations, bradycardia, hypotension, ***seizures.***

NURSING CONSIDERATIONS

Assessment

1. Obtain a negative pregnancy test on females of childbearing age prior to initiating drug therapy.
2. Document any history of ulcer disease.

Client/Family Teaching

1. Provide both oral and written warnings of adverse drug effects. Instruct to keep a record of events to share so that side effects and drug therapy can be evaluated.
2. Do not share medications.
3. Take misoprostol exactly as prescribed for the duration of aspirin or NSAID therapy.
4. Clients may experience abdominal discomfort and/or diarrhea. Instruct to take misoprostol after meals and at bedtime to minimize these side effects.
5. Persistent diarrhea or increased menstrual bleeding should be reported.
6. Stress that all women of childbearing age must practice effective contraceptive measures because drug has abortifacient properties.

Evaluate: Prevention of drug-induced gastric ulcers during therapy with NSAIDs or acetylsalicylic acid.

Omeprazole

(oh-**MEH**-prah-zohl)

Pregnancy Category: C

Losec ✱ Prilosec **(Rx)**

How Supplied: *Enteric Coated Capsule:* 20 mg

Action/Kinetics: Omeprazole does not possess either anticholinergic or histamine H_2 receptor antagonist effects. Rather, the drug is thought to be a gastric pump inhibitor in that it blocks the final step of acid production by inhibiting the H^+–K^+ ATPase system at the secretory surface of the gastric parietal cell. Both basal and stimulated acid secretions are inhibited. Serum gastrin levels are increased during the first 1 or 2 weeks of therapy and are maintained at such levels during the course of therapy. Because omeprazole is acid-labile, the product contains an enteric-coated granule formulation; however, absorption is rapid. **Peak plasma levels:** 0.5–3.5 hr. **Onset:** Within 1 hr. **$t^{1/2}$:** 0.5–1 hr. **Duration:** Up to 72 hr (due to prolonged binding of the drug to the parietal H^+–K^+ ATPase enzyme). The drug is significantly bound (95%) to plasma protein. Omeprazole is metabolized in the liver and inactive metabolites are excreted through the urine. Although plasma levels of omeprazole are increased in clients with chronic hepatic disease and in the elderly, dosage adjustment is not necessary.

Uses: Short-term (4–8-week) treatment of duodenal ulcer, severe erosive esophagitis, and poorly responsive gastroesophageal reflux disease. Long-term treatment of pathologic hypersecretory conditions such as Zollinger-Ellison syndrome, multiple endocrine adenomas, and systemic mastocytosis. Long-term maintenance treatment of healed erosive esophagitis. *Investigational:* Gastric ulcers, including healing gastric ulcers in clients receiving NSAIDs.

Dosage

- **Capsules, Sustained-Release**

Active duodenal ulcer, severe erosive esophagitis, poorly responsive gastroesophageal reflux disease.

Adults, 20 mg/day for 4–8 weeks.

Pathologic hypersecretory conditions.

Adults, initial: 60 mg/day; **then,** dose individualized although doses up to 120 mg t.i.d. have been used. Daily doses greater than 80 mg should be divided.

Gastric ulcers.

Adults: 20–40 mg/day.

Administration/Storage

1. Antacids can be administered with omeprazole.
2. The capsule should be taken before eating and is to be swallowed whole; it should not be opened, chewed, or crushed.

Contraindications: Lactation.

Special Concerns: Safety and effectiveness have not been determined in children.

Side Effects: *CNS:* Headache, dizziness. Possibly, anxiety disorders, abnormal dreams, vertigo, insomnia, nervousness, apathy, paresthesia, somnolence, hemifacial dysesthesia. *GI:* Diarrhea, nausea, abdominal pain, vomiting, constipation, flatulence, acid regurgitation, abdominal swelling. Possibly, anorexia, fecal discoloration, esophageal candidiasis, mucosal atrophy of the tongue, dry mouth, irritable colon. *CV:* Angina, chest pain, tachycardia, bradycardia, palpitation, peripheral edema. *Respiratory:* Upper respiratory infection, pharyngeal pain, epistaxis. *Skin:* Inflammation, alopecia, urticaria, pruritus, dry skin, hyperhidrosis. *GU:* UTI, urinary frequency, hematuria, proteinuria, glycosuria, testicular pain, microscopic pyuria. *Hematologic:* Pancytopenia, thrombocytopenia, anemia, leukocytosis, neutropenia. *Musculoskeletal:* Asthenia, back pain, myalgia, joint pain, muscle cramps, leg pain. *Miscellaneous:* Rash, cough, fever, pain, fatigue, malaise, hypoglycemia, weight gain, tinnitus, abdominal swelling, alteration in taste.

NOTE: Data are lacking on the effect of long-term hypochlorhydria and hypergastrinemia on the risk of developing tumors.

Drug Interactions

Ampicillin (esters) / Possible ↓ absorption of ampicillin esters due to ↑ pH of stomach

Diazepam / ↑ Plasma levels of diazepam due to ↓ rate of metabolism by the liver

Iron salts / Possible ↓ absorption of iron salts due to ↑ pH of stomach

Ketoconazole / Possible ↓ absorption of ketoconazole due to ↑ pH of stomach

Phenytoin / ↑ Plasma levels of phenytoin due to ↓ rate of metabolism of the liver

Warfarin / Prolonged rate of elimination of warfarin due to ↓ rate of metabolism by the liver

NURSING CONSIDERATIONS

Assessment

1. Document indications for therapy and type and onset of symptoms.
2. Note any history of hepatic dysfunction.
3. Assess females of childbearing age to determine if pregnant.
4. Obtain baseline CBC, prior to initiating therapy.

Client/Family Teaching

1. Take medication only as prescribed and before meals. Do not open, crush, or chew drug.
2. Review the list of side effects associated with drug therapy and instruct client to report persistent symptoms.
3. Report any changes in urinary elimination or pain and discomfort associated with voiding.
4. Explain that the drug inhibits total gastric acid secretion and is for short-term use only. Side effects of prolonged therapy and suppression of acid secretion alter bacterial colonization and lead to hypochlorhydria and hypergastrinemia which may cause an increased risk for the development of gastric tumors.

Evaluate

- ↓ Gastric acid production
- Promotion of ulcer healing and relief of pain

Pancrelipase (Lipancreatin)

(pan-kree-**LY**-payz)

Pregnancy Category: C

Cotazym, Cotazym-S, Creon ✱, Ilozyme, Ku-Zyme HP, Pancrease, Pancrease MT 4, Pancrease MT 10, Pancrease MT 16, Pancrease MT 20, Protilase, Viokase, Ultrase MT12, Ultrase MT20, Ultrase MT24, Viokase ✱, Zymase **(Rx)**

How Supplied: *Capsule; Capsule, Extended Release; Enteric Coated capsule; Enteric Coated tablet; Powder; Tablet*

Action/Kinetics: Enzyme concentrate from hog pancreas, which contains lipase, amylase, and protease, enzymes that replace or supplement naturally occurring enzymes. The product is more active at neutral or slightly alkaline pH. Pancrelipase has 12 times the lipolytic activity and 4 times both the proteolytic and amylolytic activity of pancreatin. Certain products have an enteric coating that protects the enzymes from deactivation in the stomach.

Uses: Pancreatic deficiency diseases such as chronic pancreatitis, cystic fibrosis of the pancreas, pancreatectomy, ductal obstructions caused by cancer of the pancreas or common bile duct, steatorrhea of malabsorption syndrome or postgastrectomy or postgastrointestinal surgery. Presumptive test for pancreatic function, especially in insufficiency due to chronic pancreatitis.

Dosage

- **Capsules; Enteric-Coated Microspheres, Microtablets, Spheres, Pellets; Powder; Tablets**

Pancreatic insufficiency.

Adults and children over 12 years of age: 4,000–48,000 units of lipase with each meal and with snacks. **Children, 7–12 years:** 4,000–12,000 units of lipase with each meal and snacks; **1–6 years:** 4,000–8,000 units of lipase with each meal and 4,000 units lipase with snacks. **6–12 months:** 2,000 units lipase with each meal. Dosage has not been established in children less than 6 months of age. Severe deficiencies may require up to 64,000–88,000 units of lipase with meals (or the frequency of administration can be increased if side effects are not manifested).

Pancreatectomy or obstruction of pancreatic ducts.

Adults: 8,000–16,000 units of lipase at 2 hr intervals or as directed by a physician.

Cystic fibrosis.

Use 0.7 g of the powder with meals.

Administration/Storage

1. When administering to young children, the contents of the capsule can be sprinkled on food.
2. After several weeks of use, the dosage should be adjusted according to the therapeutic response.

3. Unopened preparations should be stored in tight containers at a temperature not to exceed 25°C (77°F).
4. Enteric-coated products (i.e., microspheres, microtablets) should not be crushed or chewed. If the client cannot swallow the capsule, it may be opened and shaken on a small amount of soft, cold food (e.g., applesauce, gelatin) that does not require chewing. This should be swallowed immediately without chewing (the enzymes may irritate the mucosa). Follow with a glass of juice or water to ensure complete swallowing of the product. Enteric-coated products that come in contact with foods with a pH greater than 5.5 will dissolve.
5. Generally, 300 mg of pancrelipase is required to digest every 17 g of dietary fat.
6. Products are not bioequivalent and thus should not be interchanged without approval.

Contraindications: Hog protein sensitivity. Acute pancreatitis, acute exacerbation of chronic pancreatic disease.

Special Concerns: Safety for use during lactation and in children less than 6 months of age not established.

Side Effects: *GI:* Nausea, diarrhea, abdominal cramps following high doses. *Other:* Inhalation of the powder is irritating to the skin and mucous membranes and may result in an asthma attack. High doses cause hyperuricemia and hyperuricosuria.

Symptoms of Overdose: Diarrhea, intestinal upset.

Drug Interactions

Calcium carbonate / ↓ Effect of pancreatic enzymes
Iron / Response to oral iron may ↓ if given with pancreatic enzymes
Magnesium hydroxide / ↓ Effect of pancreatic enzymes

NURSING CONSIDERATIONS

Assessment

1. Obtain a thorough nursing history and document indications for therapy.
2. Determine any sensitivity or allergy to hog protein, since this is the main constituent of pancrelipase.

Client/Family Teaching

1. Review the appropriate dietary recommendations (usually low fat, high calorie, high protein) and refer to a dietitian for appropriate dietary counseling and assistance in meal planning.
2. The medication should be taken just before or with meals and snacks and with plenty of liquids to prevent oral mucosal irritation.
3. Report any nausea, cramping, or diarrhea. The dosage of medication may need to be adjusted to control steatorrhea.
4. Discuss the importance of reporting for follow-up lab studies as scheduled.

Evaluate

- Improved nutritional status following replacement in deficiency states
- Control of diarrhea in clients with steatorrhea

Sucralfate

(sue-**KRAL**-fayt)

Pregnancy Category: B

Carafate, Novo-Sucralate ✱, Sulcrate ✱, Sulcrate Suspension Plus ✱

(Rx)

How Supplied: *Suspension:* 1 g/10 mL; *Tablet:* 1 g

Action/Kinetics: Sucralfate is the aluminum salt of a sulfurated disaccharide. It is thought to form an ulcer-adherent complex with albumin and fibrinogen at the site of the ulcer, protecting it from further damage by gastric acid. It may also form a viscous, adhesive barrier on the surface of the gastric mucosa and duodenum. The drug adsorbs pepsin, thus inhibiting its activity. May be used in conjunction with antacids. Approximately 90% excreted in the feces. **Duration:** 5 hr.

Uses: Short-term treatment (up to 8 weeks) of active duodenal ulcers. Maintenance for duodenal ulcer at decreased dosage after healing of acute ulcers. *Investigational:* Hasten healing of gastric ulcers, chronic treatment of gastric ulcers. Treatment of reflux and peptic esophagitis. Treatment of aspirin- and NSAID-induced GI symptoms; prevention of stress ulcers and GI bleeding in critically ill clients. The suspension has been used to treat oral and esophageal ulcers due to chemotherapy, radiation, or sclerotherapy (suspension used).

Dosage

- **Suspension, Tablets**

Adults: usual: 1 g q.i.d. (10 mL of the suspension) 1 hr before meals and at bedtime (it may also be taken 2 hr after meals). The drug should be taken for 4–8 weeks unless X-ray films or endoscopy have indicated significant healing. **Maintenance (tablets only):** 1 g b.i.d.

Administration/Storage

1. If antacids are used, they should be taken 30 min before or after sucralfate.
2. Even though healing of ulcers may result, the frequency or severity of subsequent attacks is not altered.
3. Do not crush or chew tablets. If NGT administration is necessary, consult with pharmacist for a diluent as sucralfate is fairly insoluble and may form a bezoar.

Special Concerns: Safety for use in children and during lactation has not been fully established. A successful course resulting in healing of ulcers will not alter posthealing frequency or severity of duodenal ulceration.

Side Effects: *GI:* Constipation (most common); also, N&V, diarrhea, indigestion, flatulence, dry mouth, gastric discomfort. *Hypersensitivity:* Urticaria, angioedema, ***respiratory difficulty,*** rhinitis. *Miscellaneous:* Back pain, dizziness, sleepiness, vertigo, rash, pruritus, facial swelling, laryngospasm.

Drug Interactions

Antacids containing aluminum / ↑ Total body burden of aluminum
Anticoagulants / ↓ Hypoprothrombinemic effect of warfarin
Cimetidine / ↓ Absorption of cimetidine due to binding to sucralfate
Ciprofloxacin / ↓ Absorption of ciprofloxacin due to binding to sucralfate
Digoxin / ↓ Absorption of digoxin due to binding to sucralfate
Ketoconazole / ↓ Bioavailability of ketoconazole
Norfloxacin / ↓ Absorption of norfloxacin due to binding to sucralfate
Phenytoin / ↓ Absorption of phenytoin due to binding to sucralfate
Quinidine / ↓ Quinidine levels → ↓ effect
Ranitidine / ↓ Absorption of ranitidine due to binding to sucralfate
Tetracycline / ↓ Absorption of tetracycline due to binding to sucralfate
Theophylline / ↓ Absorption of theophylline due to binding to sucralfate

NURSING CONSIDERATIONS

Assessment

1. Document indications for therapy and type and onset of symptoms.
2. List other agents prescribed and the outcome.
3. Ensure that tablets are reconstituted prior to administering through the NGT. Generally when placed in a medicine cup with a small amount of water and left for 10–15 min, the tablets will dissolve completely.
4. Monitor CBC and serum phosphate levels. Drug binds phosphate and may lead to hypophosphatemia.

Client/Family Teaching

1. Take on an empty stomach 1 hr before or 2 hr after meals. Wait 30 min before or after dose when taking antacids.
2. Stress the importance of taking the medication exactly as prescribed. Explain that it binds to proteins at the site of the lesions to create a protective barrier that prevents diffusion of hydrogen ions at a normal gastric pH.
3. Review side effects and advise to report if persistent or bothersome.
4. Drug may cause constipation. Advise to increase fluids and bulk in the diet and to exercise regularly.

5. Avoid smoking as this may assist to prevent a recurrence of duodenal ulcers.

Evaluate

- Abdominal pain and discomfort
- Prophylaxis of GI bleeding
- Endoscopic or radiographic evidence of healing of duodenal ulcers

CHAPTER SIXTY-FOUR

Drugs Used for Gallbladder Disease

See the following individual entries:

Chenodiol (Chenodeoxycholic Acid)
Monoctanoin
Ursodiol

Chenodiol (Chenodeoxycholic acid)

(kee-noh-**DYE**-ohl)
Pregnancy Category: X
Chenix **(Rx)**

How Supplied: *Tablet:* 250 mg
Action/Kinetics: Chenodiol, by reducing hepatic synthesis of cholesterol and cholic acid, replaces both cholic and deoxycholic acids in the bile acid pool. This effect helps desaturation of biliary cholesterol and leads to dissolution of radiolucent cholesterol gallstones. The drug is ineffective on calcified gallstones or on radiolucent bile pigment stones. Fifty percent of clients have stone recurrence within 5 years. The drug also increases LDLs and inhibits absorption of fluid from the colon. Chenodiol is well absorbed following PO administration. It is metabolized by bacteria in the colon to lithocholic acid, most of which is excreted in the feces.
Uses: Clients with radiolucent cholesterol gallstones in whom surgery is a risk due to age or systemic disease. The drug is ineffective in some clients and has potential liver toxicity. The best results have been seen in thin females with a serum cholesterol not higher than 227 mg/dL and who have a small number of radiolucent cholesterol gallstones.

Dosage

- **Tablets**

Radiolucent cholesterol gallstones.
Adults, initial: 250 mg b.i.d. for 2 weeks; **then,** increase by 250 mg/week until maximum tolerated or recommended dose is reached (13–16 mg/kg/day in two divided doses morning and night with milk or food). *NOTE:* Doses less than 10 mg/kg are usually ineffective and may result in increased risk of cholecystectomy.
Contraindications: Known hepatic dysfunction or bile ductal abnormalities. Colon cancer. Pregnancy or in those who may become pregnant.
Special Concerns: Safety and efficacy in lactation and in children have not been established.
Side Effects: Hepatotoxicity including increased ALT in one-third of clients, intrahepatic cholestasis. *GI:* Diarrhea (common), anorexia, constipation, dyspepsia, flatulence, heartburn, cramps, epigastric distress, N&V, abdominal pain. *Hematologic:* Decreased white cell count. ***Chenodiol may contribute to colon cancer in susceptible clients.***

Drug Interactions

Antacids, aluminum / ↓ Effect of chenodiol due to ↓ absorption from GI tract
Cholestyramine / See *Antacids*
Clofibrate / ↓ Effect of chenodiol due to ↑ biliary cholesterol secretion
Colestipol / See *Antacids*

Estrogens, oral contraceptives / ↓ Effect of chenodiol due to ↑ biliary cholesterol secretion

NURSING CONSIDERATIONS

Assessment

1. Obtain baseline liver and renal function studies.
2. Obtain a complete drug history, listing those currently prescribed and note any potential drug interactions.
3. Test women of childbearing years for pregnancy.
4. Document indications for therapy, onset of symptoms, and any previous therapy utilized.

Interventions

1. Obtain periodic liver function tests such as serum aminotransferase level and serum cholesterols. Monitor for stone dissolution.
2. Note any client complaint of severe, sudden upper quadrant pain that radiates to the shoulder, nonspecific abdominal pain, nausea, or vomiting. Report these symptoms immediately since these may indicate that the client has developed gallstone complications.
3. If the client develops diarrhea, the dose of medication may be reduced temporarily and antidiarrheal agents may be administered.

Client/Family Teaching

1. Advise that the drug may need to be taken for 24 months before gallstones are dissolved.
2. Discuss the likelihood that gallstones may recur even after successful treatment.
3. Pregnancy should be avoided during drug therapy. Oral contraceptives may decrease the effectiveness of chenodiol. Therefore, advise women of childbearing age to practice alternative methods of birth control.
4. Advise women to report if there is any possibility that conception has occurred.
5. Stress the importance of having periodic liver function tests and cholecystograms or gallbladder ultrasonography to evaluate the effectiveness of the drug therapy.
6. Consult with the provider if there is a need to use antacids. Most antacids have an aluminum base that absorbs the drug.
7. Report any incidence of diarrhea. This may be related to the dose of drug and can be relieved by appropriate changes in the dosage.
8. Discuss drug relationship to colon cancer and potential risks.

Evaluate: Dissolution of radiolucent cholesterol gallstones.

Monoctanoin

(mahn-**OCK**-tah-noyn)
Pregnancy Category: C
Moctanin **(Rx)**

How Supplied: *Solution*

Action/Kinetics: Monoctanoin is a semisynthetic esterified glycerol that causes complete dissolution of gallstones in approximately one-third of treated clients, with an additional one-third manifesting a decrease in the size of stones. The decreased size may allow the stone to pass spontaneously.

Uses: To solubilize cholesterol gallstones located in the biliary tract, especially when other treatments have failed or cannot be undertaken. Most effective if the stones are radiolucent.

Dosage

• **Infusion via Catheter Inserted into Common Bile Duct**

Cholesterol gallstones.

Perfuse at rate not to exceed 3–5 mL/hr at a pressure of 10 cm water (to minimize irritation) for 7–21 days.

Administration/Storage

1. The drug should not be administered IM or IV.
2. The drug should be maintained at a temperature of 37°C (98.6°F) for maximum effects.
3. To reduce viscosity and enhance the bathing effect on the stones, the drug should be diluted with 120 mL sterile water for injection.
4. Perfusion pressure should never exceed 15 cm water (use overflow manometer or peristaltic pump).

5. The perfusion should be continued for approximately 9–10 days after which X-ray or endoscopy studies should be conducted. If tests do not show a reduction in size or dissolution of stones, the drug should be discontinued.
6. Irritation of the GI and biliary tracts may occur. These usually disappear within 2–7 days after the termination of therapy.
7. The drug is intended only for direct biliary duct infusion.

Contraindications: Biliary tract infection, recent duodenal ulcer or jejunitis, clinical jaundice, impaired hepatic function, acute pancreatitis, portosystemic shunting.

Special Concerns: Use with caution during lactation. Safety and effectiveness in children have not been established.

Laboratory Test Interference: ↑ Serum Amylase.

Side Effects: *GI:* Irritation of GI and biliary tracts, ascending cholangitis, erythema in antral and duodenal mucosa, ulceration or irritation of the mucosa of the common bile duct, increased fistula drainage, duodenal erosion, abdominal pain or discomfort, N&V, diarrhea, indigestion, anorexia, burning epigastrium, bile shock. *CNS:* Fever, fatigue, lethargy, depression, headache. *Other:* Leukopenia, pruritus, chills, diaphoresis, hypokalemia, intolerance, allergic symptoms.

NURSING CONSIDERATIONS

Assessment

1. Note if the client has a history of biliary tract infection or recent duodenal ulcer.
2. If client has a history of hepatic dysfunction, obtain baseline liver function studies.

Interventions

1. Note any client complaint of GI irritation.
2. Test stools for occult blood.
3. Report any evidence of fever, lethargy, depression, pruritus, diaphoresis, and hypokalemia.

Evaluate

- Dissolution or a marked ↓ size of gallstones
- Freedom from complication of prolonged direct bile duct infusion

Ursodiol

(ur-so-**DYE**-ohl)
Pregnancy Category: B
Actigall, Ursofalk ✦ **(Rx)**

How Supplied: *Capsule:* 300 mg

Action/Kinetics: Ursodiol is a naturally occurring bile acid that inhibits the hepatic synthesis and secretion of cholesterol; it also inhibits intestinal absorption of cholesterol. The drug acts to solubilize cholesterol in micelles and to cause dispersion of cholesterol as liquid crystals in aqueous media. The drug undergoes a significant first-pass effect where it is conjugated with either glycine or taurine and then secreted into hepatic bile ducts.

Uses: In clients with radiolucent, noncalcified gallstones (<20 mm) in whom elective surgery would be risky.

Dosage

- **Capsules**

  Gallstones.

Adults: 8–10 mg/kg/day in two or three divided doses, usually with meals.

Administration/Storage

1. If partial stone dissolution is not observed within 12 months, the drug will probably not be effective.
2. For the first year of therapy, ultrasound of the gallbladder should be performed every 6 months to determine the response.
3. *Treatment of Overdose:* Treat with supportive measures.

Contraindications: Clients with calcified cholesterol stones, radioopaque stones, or radiolucent bile pigment stones. Acute cholecystitis, cholangitis, biliary obstruction, gallstone pancreatitis, biliary-gastrointestinal fistula, allergy to bile acids, chronic liver disease.

Special Concerns: Use with caution during lactation. Safety and efficacy have not been determined in children. Safety for use beyond 24 months is not known.

Side Effects: *GI:* Diarrhea, N&V, dyspepsia, metallic taste, abdominal pain, biliary pain, cholecystitis, constipation, stomatitis, flatulence. *Skin:* Pruritus, rash, dry skin, urticaria. *CNS:* Headache, fatigue, anxiety, depression, sleep disorders. *Other:* Sweating, thinning of hair, back pain, arthralgia, myalgia, rhinitis, cough.

Symptom of Overdose: Diarrhea.

Drug Interactions

Antacids, aluminum-containing / ↓ Effect of ursodiol due to ↓ absorption from GI tract
Cholestyramine / ↓ Effect of ursodiol due to ↓ absorption from GI tract
Clofibrate / ↓ Effect of ursodiol by ↑ hepatic cholesterol secretion
Colestipol / ↓ Effect of ursodiol due to ↓ absorption from GI tract
Contraceptives, oral / ↓ Effect of ursodiol by ↑ hepatic cholesterol secretion
Estrogens / ↓ Effect of ursodiol by ↑ hepatic cholesterol secretion

NURSING CONSIDERATIONS

Assessment

1. Obtain a baseline ultrasound of the gallbladder and order liver function studies to serve as a baseline against which to measure subsequent studies and evaluate response throughout drug therapy.
2. List drugs the client is taking, noting those with which ursodiol interacts unfavorably.
3. If the client is female, determine the possibility of pregnancy.
4. The drug is not indicated for calcified cholesterol stones, radiopaque stones, or radiolucent bile pigment stones.

Interventions

1. Document and report any complaints of N&V, diarrhea, abdominal pain, or the presence of a metallic taste in the mouth.
2. Observe and report complaints of any new onset of headache, anxiety, depression, and sleep disorders.

Client/Family Teaching

1. Explain that the ursodiol therapy may take up to 24 months and that the drug will need to be taken 2–3 times/day.
2. Avoid taking antacids unless prescribed. Many antacids have an aluminum base, which adsorbs the drug.
3. Discuss with the client the fact that stones may recur after the dissolution of the current stones.
4. Provide a printed list of drug side effects. Explain the importance of reporting symptoms such as persistent N&V, abdominal pain, headaches, itching, rash, or altered bowel function.
5. For women of childbearing age, discuss the need to practice birth control because pregnancy should be avoided during drug therapy. The use of estrogens and oral contraceptives may decrease the effectiveness of the drug; therefore, other forms of birth control are advisable.
6. Stress the importance of reporting for follow-up medical visits and for routine lab studies and ultrasonography to evaluate the effectiveness of the drug therapy.
7. Explain that ursodiol therapy will be continued for 1–3 months following stone dissolution and then reconfirmed with another ultrasound.

Evaluate

- Radiographic evidence of a reduction or complete dissolution of radiolucent, noncalcified gallstones.
- Reversal of intracellular accumulation of toxic bile acids

Hormone and Hormone Antagonists

CHAPTER SIXTY-FIVE

Antidiabetic Agents and Hyperglycemic Agents

See also the following individual entries:

Hypoglycemic Agents

Acetohexamide
Chlorpropamide
Glipizide
Glyburide
Tolazamide
Tolbutamide
Tolbutamide Sodium

Insulins

Insulin, Human
Insulin Injection (Crystalline Zinc Insulin, Unmodified Insulin, Regular Insulin)
Insulin Injection, Concentrated
Insulin Zinc Suspension (Lente)
Insulin Zinc Suspension, Extended
Insulin Zinc Suspension, Prompt (Semilente)
Isophane Insulin Suspension (NPH)
Isophane Insulin Suspension and Insulin Injection

Hyperglycemic Agents

Diazoxide Oral
Glucagon

General Statement: Tne American Diabetes Association has recently developed new standards for treating clients with diabetes. If followed, the new standards will enable clients to decrease their blood glucose levels closer to normal; this will reduce the risk of complications, including blindness, kidney disease, heart disease, and amputations. The goals of the new standards include establishing specific targets for control of blood glucose (usually between 80 and 120 mg/dL before meals and between 100 and 140 mg/dL at bedtime) and increased emphasis on educating clients for self-management of their disease. Targets for BP and lipid levels are also provided. If the guidelines are followed, it is estimated that the risk of development or progression of retinopathy, nephropathy, and neuropathy can be reduced by

50%–75% in clients with insulin-dependent (type I) diabetes. The guidelines suggest the following treatment modalities:

- Frequent monitoring of blood glucose.
- Regular exercise.
- Close attention to meal planning; a registered dietitian should be consulted.
- For type I diabetics, either continuous SC insulin infusion or multiple daily insulin injections; for type II diabetics, insulin administration should be considered in certain situations (although dietary modification, exercise, and weight reduction are the cornerstone of treatment).
- Instruction of the client in the prevention and treatment of hypoglycemia and other complications (both acute and chronic) of diabetes.
- Development of a process for ongoing support and continuing education for the client.
- Routine assessment of treatment goals.

HYPOGLYCEMIC AGENTS

See also the following individual entries:

Acetohexamide
Chlorpropamide
Glipizide
Glyburide
Tolazamide
Tolbutamide
Tolbutamide Sodium

Action/Kinetics: The sulfonylureas are related chemically to sulfonamides; however, they are devoid of antibacterial activity. Oral hypoglycemic drugs are classified as either first or second generation. *Generation* refers to structural changes in the basic molecule. Second-generation oral hypoglycemic drugs are more lipophilic and, as such, have greater hypoglycemic potency. Also, second-generation drugs are bound to plasma protein by covalent bonds, whereas first-generation drugs are bound to plasma protein by ionic bonds. The implication is that the second-generation drugs are potentially less susceptible to displacement from plasma protein by drugs such as salicylates and oral anticoagulants.

Sulfonylureas are believed to act by one or more of the following mechanisms: (1) stimulating insulin release from pancreatic beta cells, possibly due to increased intracellular cyclic AMP; (2) the peripheral tissues become more sensitive to insulin due to an increase in the number of insulin receptors or an increased ability of circulating insulin to combine with receptors; or (3) extrapancreatic effects, including decreased glucagon release and hepatic glucose production. To be effective, the client must have some ability for endogenous insulin production. All of the oral hypoglycemic drugs are significantly bound (90%) to plasma protein. Differences in sulfonylureas are mainly duration of action.

Clients whose condition is to be controlled by oral antidiabetics should undergo a 7-day therapeutic trial. A drop in blood sugar level, a decrease in glucosuria, and disappearance of pruritus, polyuria, polydipsia, and polyphagia indicate that the client can probably be managed on oral antidiabetic agents. These drugs should not be used in clients with ketosis. If the client is transferred from insulin to an oral antidiabetic drug, the hormone should be discontinued gradually over a period of several days. The sulfonylureas have similar pharmacologic actions but differ in their pharmacokinetic properties (see individual agents).

Uses: Non–insulin-dependent diabetes mellitus (type II) that does not respond to diet management alone. Concurrent use of insulin and an oral sulfonylurea (usually glipizide or glyburide) for type II diabetics who are difficult to control with diet and sulfonylurea therapy alone. One method used is the BIDS system: bedtime insulin (usually NPH) with daytime (morning only or morning and evening) sulfonylurea.

Guidelines for oral hypoglycemic therapy include onset of diabetes in clients over 40 years of age, duration of diabetes less than 5 years, absence of ketoacidosis, client is obese or has normal body weight, fasting serum glucose of 200 mg/dL or less, has a daily insulin requirement of 40 units or less, and hepatic and renal function is normal.

Contraindications: Stress before and during surgery, severe trauma, fever, infections, pregnancy, diabetes complicated by recurrent episodes of ketoacidosis or coma; juvenile, growth-onset, insulin-dependent, or brittle diabetes; impaired endocrine, renal, or liver function. Not indicated for clients whose diabetes can be controlled by diet alone. Relapse may occur with the sulfonylureas in undernourished clients. Long-acting products in geriatric clients.

Special Concerns: Use with caution during lactation since hypoglycemia may occur in the infant. Safety and effectiveness in children have not been established. Geriatric clients may be more sensitive to oral hypoglycemics and hypoglycemia may be more difficult to recognize in these clients. Use with caution in debilitated and malnourished clients. Use of sulfonylureas has been associated with an increased risk of CV mortality compared to treatment with either diet alone or diet plus insulin. There may be loss of blood glucose control if the client experiences stress such as infection, fever, surgery, or trauma.

Side Effects: Hypoglycemia is the most common side effect. *GI:* Nausea, heartburn, full feeling. *CNS:* Fatigue, dizziness, fever, headache, weakness, malaise, vertigo. *Hepatic:* Cholestatic jaundice, aggravation of hepatic porphyria. *Dermatologic:* Skin rashes, urticaria, erythema, pruritus, eczema, photophobia, morbilliform or maculopapular eruptions, lichenoid reactions, porphyria cutanea tardia. *Hematologic:* Thrombocytopenia, leukopenia, ***agranulocytosis, aplastic anemia,*** pancytopenia, ***hemolytic anemia.*** *Endocrine:* Inappropriate secretion of ADH resulting in excessive water retention, hyponatremia, low serum osmolality, and high urine osmolality. *Miscellaneous:* Paresthesia, tinnitus, resistance to drug action develops in a small percentage of clients.

Symptoms of Overdose: Hypoglycemia. The following symptoms of hypoglycemia are listed in their general order of appearance: tingling of lips and tongue, hunger, nausea, decreased cerebral function (lethargy, yawning, confusion, agitation, nervousness), increased sympathetic activity (tachycardia, sweating, tremor), seizures, stupor, coma.

Drug Interactions

Acetazolamide / ↑ Blood sugar in prediabetics and diabetics on oral hypoglycemics

Alcohol / Possible Antabuse-like syndrome, especially flushing of face and SOB. Also, ↓ effect of oral hypoglycemic due to ↑ breakdown by liver

Androgens/anabolic steroids / ↑ Hypoglycemic effect

Anticoagulants, oral / ↑ Effect of oral hypoglycemics by ↓ breakdown by liver and ↓ plasma protein binding

Beta-adrenergic blocking agents / ↓ Hypoglycemic effect; also, symptoms of hypoglycemia may be masked

Charcoal / ↓ Hypoglycemic effect due to ↓ absorption from GI tract

Chloramphenicol / ↑ Effect due to ↓ breakdown by liver and ↓ renal excretion

Cholestyramine / ↓ Hypoglycemic effect

Clofibrate / ↑ Hypoglycemic effect due to ↓ plasma protein binding

Diazoxide / ↓ Effects of both drugs

Digitoxin / ↑ Digitoxin serum levels

Fenfluramine / ↑ Hypoglycemic effect

Fluconazole / ↑ Hypoglycemic effect
Gemfibrozil / ↑ Hypoglycemic effect
Histamine H_2 antagonists / ↑ Hypoglycemic effect to ↓ breakdown by liver
Hydantoins / ↓ Effect of sulfonylureas due to ↓ insulin release
Isoniazid / ↑ Requirements for sulfonylureas
Magnesium salts / ↑ Hypoglycemic effect
MAO inhibitors / ↑ Hypoglycemic effect due to ↓ breakdown by liver
Methyldopa / ↑ Hypoglycemic effect due to ↓ breakdown by liver
Miconazole / ↑ Effect of oral hypoglycemics
Nicotinic acid / ↓ Effect of oral hypoglycemics
NSAIDs / ↑ Hypoglycemic effect of oral antidiabetics
Oral contraceptives / ↓ Hypoglycemic effect of oral antidiabetics
Phenobarbital / ↓ Effect of oral hypoglycemics due to ↑ breakdown by liver
Phenothiazines / ↑ Requirements for sulfonylureas due to ↓ release of insulin
Phenylbutazone / ↑ Effect of oral hypoglycemics due to ↓ breakdown by liver, ↓ plasma protein binding, and ↓ renal excretion
Probenecid / ↑ Hypoglycemic effect
Rifampin / ↓ Effect of sulfonylureas due to ↑ breakdown by liver
Salicylates / ↑ Effect of oral hypoglycemics by ↓ plasma protein binding
Sulfinpyrazone / ↑ Hypoglycemic effect
Sulfonamides / ↑ Effect of oral hypoglycemics by ↓ plasma protein binding and ↓ breakdown by liver
Sympathomimetics / ↑ Requirements for sulfonylureas
Thiazides / ↑ Requirements for sulfonylureas
Thyroid hormone / ↑ Requirements for sulfonylureas
Tricyclic antidepressants / ↑ Hypoglycemic effect
Urinary acidifiers / ↑ Hypoglycemic effect due to ↓ renal excretion
Urinary alkalinizers / ↓ Hypoglycemic effect due to ↑ renal excretion

Laboratory Test Interferences: ↑ BUN and serum creatinine.

Dosage

PO. See individual preparations. Adjust dosage according to needs of client. Exercise and diet are of primary importance in the control of diabetes.

NURSING CONSIDERATIONS

See also *Nursing Considerations* for *Insulins* Chapter 65.

Administration/Storage

1. PO drugs may be taken with food to decrease the incidence of gastric upset.
2. If ketonuria, acidosis, increased glycosuria, or serious side effects occur, withdraw the medication.
3. *Treatment of Overdose:* Mild hypoglycemia is treated with PO glucose and adjusting the dose of the drug or meal patterns. Severe hypoglycemia requires hospitalization. Concentrated (50%) dextrose is given by rapid IV and is followed by continuous infusion of 10% dextrose at a rate that will maintain blood glucose above 100 mg/dL. Client should be monitored for at least 24–48 hr as hypoglycemia may recur (clients with chlorpropamide toxicity should be monitored for 3–5 days due to the long duration of action of this drug).

TRANSFER FROM INSULIN

1. If the client has been receiving 20 units or less of insulin daily, initiate oral hypoglycemic therapy and discontinue insulin abruptly.
2. For clients receiving 20–40 units of insulin daily, initiate oral hypoglycemic therapy and reduce insulin dose by 25%–50%. Insulin should be discontinued gradually, using the absence of glucose in the urine as a guide. With glyburide, insulin may be discontinued abruptly.
3. For clients receiving more than 40 units of insulin daily, initiate PO therapy and reduce insulin by 20%. Discontinue insulin gradually, using glucose in the urine or finger sticks as

a guide. It may be advisable to hospitalize clients on such high doses of insulin while they are being transferred to oral hypoglycemic agents.
4. Be prepared to begin treatment with IV dextrose solution if the client develops severe hypoglycemia.
5. Review the drugs with which oral hypoglycemic agents interact and determine if the client is taking any of them.

TRANSFER FROM ONE ORAL ANTIDIABETIC AGENT TO ANOTHER
1. Except for chlorpropamide, no conversion period is necessary. When transferring clients from chlorpropamide, caution should be exercised for 1–2 weeks due to the long half-life of chlorpropamide.
2. Mild symptoms of hyperglycemia may appear during the transfer period. Clients should perform finger sticks or test their urine for glucose and ketone bodies regularly (1–3 times daily) during the transfer period. Positive results must be reported.
3. No transition period is needed when a client is transferred from one sulfonylurea to another. However, if a client is to be transferred from chlorpropamide, caution should be exercised due to the prolonged duration of action of this drug.

THERAPEUTIC FAILURE OF HYPOGLYCEMIC AGENTS: Type II diabetic clients who do not respond to the sulfonylureas are said to be *primary failures*. Clients may respond to the sulfonylureas during the initial months of therapy, yet fail to respond thereafter. These clients are referred to as *secondary failures*.

Assessment
1. Obtain a thorough nursing history.
2. Document any stress the client may be experiencing. Clients about to undergo surgical procedures, who have suffered severe trauma, who have a fever and infection, or who are pregnant should not be placed on oral hypoglycemic agents.
3. Assess mental functions and note the potential of the client to understand the complexities of the transfer process. Also, assess client's ability to adhere to the established protocol.
4. If the client is female, sexually active, and of childbearing age, note if she is taking oral contraceptives. The effectiveness of oral contraceptive agents is lessened by oral hypoglycemic agents.
5. Determine that baseline lab studies have been drawn prior to initiation of therapy.

Interventions
1. Assess clients taking a sulfonylurea closely during the first 7 days of treatment to determine their therapeutic response.
2. Closely supervise and observe the client during the 3–5 days after the transfer.

Client/Family Teaching
1. Instruct the client in testing blood or urine at home for glucose and in maintaining a written record of glucose levels for review by the health care provider. (Urine testing is not an accurate reflection of true serum glucose levels and should not be used to modify treatment).
2. Review the symptoms of hypoglycemia and hyperglycemia. Advise client with hypoglycemic episodes to check finger stick at the time of the reaction. Then drink 4 oz of juice, eat a carbohydrate (CHO) such as bread or graham crackers, and recheck finger stick in 15 min. If glucose is less than 100, repeat the process, i.e., juice and a CHO and another finger stick. Request written guidelines from the provider if this occurs often.
3. Instruct that the medication helps to control hyperglycemia but does not cure diabetes. Stress that the therapy is usually long term.
4. Explain the need to adhere to the prescribed diet if sulfonylurea is to be effective. Remind clients that most secondary failures are due to poor dietary compliance and refer to dietitian as needed.
5. Stress the importance of regular exercise. Advise client to check

weight at least weekly, to maintain a written record for review, and to report any overt changes.
6. Advise that self-administering insulin may be necessary if complications occur. Instruct the client in self-administration of insulin and how to maintain a record of site rotations.
7. Explain the importance of not changing brands of insulin or syringes. Review equipment, methods of storage, and proper method for safely discarding used syringes.
8. Advise clients to report when not feeling as well as usual, or if they develop pruritus, skin rash, jaundice, dark urine, fever, sore throat, nausea or vomiting, or diarrhea.
9. If scheduled for a thyroid test, advise client to report to the lab that they are taking a sulfonylurea, as the drug interferes with the uptake of radioactive iodine.
10. Avoid alcohol when taking oral hypoglycemic agents as a disulfuram-like reaction may occur.
11. Do not take any OTC medications without approval.
12. Stress the need for close medical supervision for the first 6 weeks of therapy.
13. Explain the need for periodic lab tests, as oral hypoglycemic agents may cause blood dyscrasias.
14. Remind the client to carry identification, a list of the medications currently prescribed, juice, and hard candy (such as Lifesavers) or a fast-acting carbohydrate (raisins) at all times.

Evaluate

- An understanding of diabetes and evidence of compliance with prescribed treatment and dietary regime
- Reports of ↓ frequency of hypo- or hyperglycemic episodes
- Laboratory confirmation that serum glucose levels are within desired range

Acetohexamide

(ah-seat-oh-**HEX**-ah-myd)
Pregnancy Category: C
Dimelor ✱, Dymelor **(Rx)**

See also *Hypoglycemic Agents,* Chapter 65.
How Supplied: *Tablet:* 250 mg, 500 mg
Action/Kinetics: Onset: 1 hr. **t½:** 1.3 hr for acetohexamide and 6–8 hr for active metabolite. **Duration:** 12–24 hr. Metabolized in the liver to a potent active metabolite. Excreted through the kidney (80%) and feces (10%).

Dosage

- **Tablets**
  Diabetes.

Adults, initial: 250–1,500 mg/day; **maintenance:** 500 mg/day, adjusting dosage thereafter until optimum control is achieved. Doses in excess of 1.5 g/day are not recommended. **Geriatric clients, initial:** 125–250 mg/day; **then,** adjust dosage gradually until desired effect is achieved.
Administration/Storage: Doses of 1 g or over should be divided, usually before the morning and evening meals.
Additional Side Effect: Hair loss.

NURSING CONSIDERATIONS

See *Nursing Considerations* for *Hypoglycemic Agents* and *Insulins,* Chapter 65.
Evaluate: Control of serum glucose levels to within desired range.

Chlorpropamide

(klor-**PROH**-pah-myd)
Pregnancy Category: C
Apo-Chlorpropamide ✱, Diabinese
(Rx)

See also *Hypoglycemic Agents,* Chapter 65.
How Supplied: *Tablet:* 100 mg, 250 mg
Action/Kinetics: Chlorpropamide may be effective in clients who do not respond well to other antidiabetic agents. **Onset:** 1 hr. **t½:** 35 hr. **Time to peak levels:** 2–4 hr. **Duration:** Up to 60 hr (due to slow excretion). Eighty percent metabolized in liver; 80%–90% excreted in the urine.
Additional Use: *Investigational:* Neurogenic diabetes insipidus.

Dosage

- **Tablets**

Diabetes.

Adults, middle-aged clients, mild to moderate diabetes, initial: 250 mg/day as a single or divided dose; **geriatric, initial:** 100–125 mg/day. **All clients, maintenance:** 100–250 mg/day as single or divided doses. Severe diabetics may require 500 mg/day; doses greater than 750 mg/day are not recommended.

Neurogenic diabetes insipidus.

Adults: 200–500 mg/day.

Special Concerns: If the client is susceptible to fluid retention or has impaired cardiac function, frequent monitoring is necessary.

Additional Side Effects: Occur frequently with chlorpropamide. Severe diarrhea is occasionally accompanied by bleeding in the lower bowel. Severe GI distress may be relieved by dividing total daily dose in half. In older clients, hypoglycemia may be severe. May cause inappropriate ADH secretion, leading to hyponatremia, water retention, low serum osmolality, and high urine osmolality.

Additional Drug Interactions

Ammonium chloride / ↑ Effect of chlorpropamide due to ↓ excretion by kidney

Disulfiram / More likely to interact with chlorpropamide than other oral antidiabetics

Probenecid / ↑ Effect of chlorpropamide

Sodium bicarbonate / ↓ Effect of chlorpropamide due to ↑ excretion by kidney

NURSING CONSIDERATIONS

See also *Nursing Considerations* for *Hypoglycemic Agents and Insulin,* Chapter 65.

Assessment

1. Note age of client. Elderly clients tend to be more sensitive to hypoglycemic agents and exhibit more side effects.
2. Determine if pregnant. The drug is contraindicated in pregnancy.
3. Document any allergy to sulfa drugs.
4. Assess for any history of cardiac dysfunction or fluid retention.

Interventions

1. Monitor weight and BP and assess for evidence of the inappropriate secretion of ADH. Clients may appear confused, complain of feeling dizzy, depressed, and complain of nausea.
2. Monitor I&O, serum electrolytes, and urine osmolality.

Evaluate: Normalization of serum glucose levels.

Glipizide

(**GLIP**-ih-zyd)

Pregnancy Category: C

Glucotrol, Glucotrol XL **(Rx)**

See also *Hypoglycemic Agents,* Chapter 65.

How Supplied: *Tablet:* 5 mg, 10 mg; *Tablet, Extended Release:* 5 mg, 10 mg

Action/Kinetics: Glipizide also has mild diuretic effects. **Onset:** 1–1.5 hr. **t½:** 2–4 hr. **Time to peak levels:** 1–3 hr. **Duration:** 10–16 hr. Metabolized in liver to inactive metabolites, which are excreted through the kidneys.

Additional Drug Interaction: Cimetidine may ↑ effect of glipizide due to ↓ breakdown by liver.

Use: Adjunct to diet for control of hyperglycemia in clients with non-insulin-dependent diabetes.

Dosage

- **Tablets, Extended Release Tablets**

Diabetes.

Adults, initial: 5 mg before breakfast; **then,** adjust dosage by 2.5–5 mg every few days until adequate control is achieved. **Maintenance:** 15–40 mg/day. Older clients should begin with 2.5 mg. The Extended Release Tablets are taken once daily (usually at breakfast) in doses of either 5 or 10 mg.

Administration/Storage

1. Some clients are better controlled on once daily dosing while others are better controlled with divided dosing.

2. Maintenance doses greater than 15 mg/day should be divided and given before the morning and evening meals. Total daily doses of 30 mg or more may be given safely on twice daily dosing.
3. For greatest effect, give 30 min before meals.

NURSING CONSIDERATIONS

See also *Nursing Considerations* for *Hypoglycemic Agents* and *Insulins,* Chapter 65.

Client/Family Teaching

1. Report any complaints of CNS side effects such as drowsiness or headache.
2. Some clients may suffer from anorexia, constipation or diarrhea, vomiting, and gastralgia. If the symptoms are severe, advise client to record weight and I&O.
3. Skin reactions may occur and skin changes should be reported. Avoid exposure to the sun; when in the sun, use a sunscreen and wear sunglasses and protective clothing.
4. Avoid alcohol in any form.
5. Practice barrier form of contraception.

Evaluate: Restoration of serum glucose levels to within desired range.

Glyburide

(**GLYE**-byou-ryd)
Pregnancy Category: B
Albert Glyburide ✱, Apo-Glyburide ✱, Diabeta, Euglucon ✱, Gen-Glybe ✱, Glynase PresTab, Micronase, Novo-Glyburide ✱ **(Rx)**

See also *Hypoglycemic Agents,* Chapter 65.

How Supplied: *Tablet:* 1.25 mg, 1.5 mg, 2.5 mg, 3 mg, 5 mg, 6 mg

Action/Kinetics: Glyburide has a mild diuretic effect. **Onset, nonmicronized:** 2–4 hr; **micronized:** 1 hr. **t½, nonmicronized:** 10 hr; **micronized:** Approximately 4 hr. **Time to peak levels:** 4 hr. **Duration, both forms:** 24 hr. Metabolized in liver to weakly active metabolites. Excreted in bile (50%) and through the kidneys (50%).

Dosage

- **Tablets, Nonmicronized (DiaBeta/Micronase)**

Diabetes.

Adults, initial: 2.5–5 mg/day given with breakfast (or the first main meal); **then,** increase by 2.5 mg at weekly intervals to achieve the desired response. **Maintenance:** 1.25–20 mg/day. Clients sensitive to sulfonylureas should start with 1.25 mg/day.

- **Tablets, Micronized (Glynase)**

Diabetes.

Adults, initial: 1.5–3 mg/day given with breakfast (or the first main meal); **then,** increase by no more than 1.5 mg at weekly intervals to achieve the desired response. **Maintenance:** 0.75–12 mg/day.

Administration/Storage

1. For best results, administer prior to meals.
2. Daily doses of the nonmicronized products should not exceed 20 mg; daily doses of the micronized product should not exceed 12 mg.
3. If daily dosage of the nonmicronized product exceeds 15 mg or the micronized product exceeds 6 mg, the dose should be divided and given before the morning and evening meals.

NURSING CONSIDERATIONS

See also *Nursing Considerations* for *Hypoglycemic Agents* and *Insulins,* Chapter 65.

Evaluate: ↓Serum glucose levels to within desired range.

Tolazamide

(toll-**AZ**-ah-myd)
Pregnancy Category: C
Tolinase **(Rx)**

See also *Hypoglycemic Agents,* Chapter 65.

How Supplied: *Tablet:* 100 mg, 250 mg, 500 mg

Action/Kinetics: Drug is effective in some clients with a history of coma or ketoacidosis. Also, it may be effective in clients who do not respond well to other oral antidiabetic agents. Use with insulin is not recommended for maintenance. **Onset:** 4–6 hr. **t½:** 7 hr. **Time to peak levels:** 3–4 hr. **Duration:** 12–24 hr. Metabolized in liver to metabolites with minor hypoglycemic activity. Excreted through the kidneys (85%) and feces (7%).

Dosage

- **Tablets**

Diabetes.

Adults, initial: 100 mg/day if fasting blood sugar is less than 200 mg/100 mL, or 250 mg/day if fasting blood sugar is greater than 200 mg/100 mL. Adjust dose to response not to exceed 1 g/day. If more than 500 mg/day is required, it should be given in two divided doses, usually before the morning and evening meals. **Elderly or debilitated clients:** 100 mg once daily with breakfast, adjusting dose by increments of 50 mg/day each week. Doses greater than 1 g/day will probably not improve control.

Additional Contraindication: Renal glycosuria.

Additional Drug Interaction: Concomitant use of alcohol and tolazamide may → photosensitivity.

NURSING CONSIDERATIONS

See also *Nursing Considerations* for *Hypoglycemic Agents* and *Insulins,* Chapter 65.

Client/Family Teaching

1. Take 30 min before meals for best results; do not take if vomiting or unable to eat.
2. Avoid alcohol as a disulfiram-like reaction may occur.
3. Use caution as drug may cause dizziness.
4. Use a nonhormonal form of contraception.
5. Wear protective clothing and a sunscreen to prevent a photosensitivity reaction.

Evaluate: Normalization of serum glucose levels.

Tolbutamide

(toll-**BYOU**-tah-myd)

Pregnancy Category: C

APO-Tolbutamide ✱, Mobenol ✱, Orinase **(Rx)**

Tolbutamide sodium

(toll-**BYOU**-tah-myd)

Pregnancy Category: C

Orinase Diagnostic **(Rx)**

See also *Hypoglycemic Agents,* Chapter 65.

How Supplied: Tolbutamide: *Tablet:* 250 mg, 500 mg

Tolbutamide sodium: *Powder for injection:* 1 g

Action/Kinetics: Onset: 1 hr. **t½:** 4.5–6.5 hr. **Time to peak levels:** 3–4 hr. **Duration:** 6–12 hr. Changed in liver to inactive metabolites. Excreted through the kidney (75%) and feces (9%).

Additional Uses: Most useful for clients with poor general physical status who should receive a short-acting compound.

Tolbutamide sodium is used to diagnose pancreatic islet cell tumors. It causes blood glucose, in the presence of a tumor, to drop quickly after IV administration and remain low for 3 hr.

Dosage

- **Tablets**

Diabetes.

Adults, initial: 0.25–3 g/day (usually 1–2 g); adjust dosage depending on response (usual maintenance: 0.25–2 g/day). Maximum daily dose should not exceed 3 g.

Administration/Storage: Administered as a single dose before breakfast or as divided doses before the morning and evening meals. Divided doses may improve GI tolerance.

Additional Side Effects: Melena (dark, bloody stools) in some clients with a history of peptic ulcer. Relapse or secondary failure may occur a few months after therapy has been started. May cause hyponatremia and a mild goiter.

Additional Drug Interactions

Alcohol / Photosensitivity reactions

Sulfinpyrazone / ↑ Effect of tolbutamide due to ↓ breakdown by liver

NURSING CONSIDERATIONS

See also *Nursing Considerations* for *Hypoglycemic Agents* and *Insulins,* Chapter 65

Client/Family Teaching

1. Take 30 min before meals for best results.
2. Caution that drug may cause dizziness.
3. Provide a printed list of adverse drug effects that require immediate reporting.
4. Avoid alcohol and any OTC medications without approval.
5. Drug may cause a photosensitivity reaction. Wear protective clothing and sunscreen when exposure to sunlight is necessary.
6. Use a nonhormonal form of birth control.

Evaluate:

- Serum glucose levels within desired range
- Evidence to support pancreatic islet cell tumor presence

INSULINS

See the following individual entries:

Insulin, Human
Insulin Injection (Crystalline Zinc Insulin, Unmodified Insulin, Regular Insulin)
Insulin Injection, Concentrated
Insulin Zinc Suspension (Lente)
Insulin Zinc Suspension, Extended
Insulin Zinc Suspension, Prompt (Semilente)
Isophane Insulin Suspension (NPH)
Isophane Insulin Suspension and Insulin Injection

General Statement: Diabetes mellitus is a disease in which the islets of Langerhans in the pancreas produce either no insulin or insufficient quantities of insulin. Diabetes mellitus is classified as insulin-dependent (type I; formerly referred to as *juvenile-onset*) and non-insulin-dependent (type II; formerly referred to as *maturity-onset*). Diabetes mellitus can be treated successfully by the administration of insulin isolated from the pancreas of cattle or hogs or of human insulin made either semisynthetically or derived from recombinant DNA technology.

The structure of insulin from pork sources more closely resembles human insulin than that from beef sources.

Proinsulin still remains the major impurity in insulin products. Such impurities may lead to local or systemic allergic reactions as well as antibody-mediated insulin resistance. In recent years, however, technology has improved so that insulin preparations currently marketed in the United States do not contain more than 25 ppm of proinsulin. Insulin products that contain less than 20 ppm of proinsulin are referred to as *improved single peak* insulins; those products that contain 10 ppm or less of proinsulin are referred to as *purified insulins.* In reality, purified pork insulins have approximately 1 ppm of proinsulin and human insulins made semisynthetically or from recombinant DNA have 1 and 0 ppm, respectively.

Insulin preparations with different times of onset, peak activity, and duration of action have been developed. Such products are prepared by precipitating insulin in the presence of zinc chloride to form zinc insulin crystals and/or by combining insulin with a protein such as protamine. Based on these modifications, insulin products are classified as fast-acting, intermediate-acting, and long-acting. These preparations permit the physician to select the preparation best suited to the life-style of the client.

RAPID-ACTING INSULIN

1. Insulin injection (Regular Insulin, Crystalline Zinc Insulin, Unmodified Insulin)
2. Prompt insulin zinc suspension (Semilente)

INTERMEDIATE-ACTING INSULIN

1. Isophane insulin suspension (NPH)
2. Insulin zinc suspension (Lente)

LONG-ACTING INSULIN: Extended insulin zinc suspension (Ultralente)

NOTE: Insulin preparations with various times of onset and duration of action are often mixed to obtain optimum control in diabetic clients.

Action/Kinetics: Insulin, following combination with insulin receptors on cell plasma membranes, facilitates the transport of glucose into cardiac and skeletal muscle and adipose tissue. It also increases synthesis of glycogen in the liver. Insulin stimulates protein synthesis and lipogenesis and inhibits lipolysis and release of free fatty acids from fat cells.

This latter effect prevents or reverses the ketoacidosis sometimes observed in the type I diabetic. Insulin also causes intracellular shifts in magnesium and potassium.

Since insulin is a protein, it is destroyed in the GI tract. Thus, it must be administered subcutaneously so that it is readily absorbed into the bloodstream and distributed throughout the extracellular fluid. Insulin is metabolized mainly by the liver.

Uses: Replacement therapy in type I diabetes. Diabetic ketoacidosis or diabetic coma (use regular insulin). Insulin is also indicated in type II diabetes when other measures have failed (e.g., diet, exercise, weight reduction) or with surgery, trauma, infection, fever, endocrine dysfunction, pregnancy, gangrene, Raynaud's disease, or kidney or liver dysfunction.

Purified or human insulins are used for local insulin allergy, lipodystrophy at the injection site, immunologic insulin resistance, temporary insulin use (e.g., surgery, acute stress, gestational diabetes), and newly diagnosed diabetes.

Regular insulin is used in IV hyperalimentation solutions, in IV dextrose to treat severe hyperkalemia, and IV as a provocative test for growth hormone secretion.

Insulin and oral hypoglycemic drugs have been used in type II diabetics who are difficult to control with diet and PO therapy alone.

Diet: The dietary control of diabetes is as important as medication with appropriate drugs. The role of the nurse and dietitian in teaching the client how to eat properly cannot be underestimated.

As a first step, the provider must determine the individual client's dietary requirements. Since there is a close relationship between carbohydrate (CHO), fat (F), and protein (P), intake of each of these nutrients must be regulated. The prescribed amount of CHO, P, and F eaten at each meal must remain constant.

The nurse and/or dietitian must teach the client how to calculate exchange values of various foods. Food lists and food-exchange values published by the American Diabetes Association and the American Dietetic Association are valuable teaching aids.

Diabetic clients should adhere to a regular meal schedule. The frequency of meals and the overall caloric intake vary with the type of drug taken and individual client needs. Close attention to meal frequency and meal planning is imperative and a registered dietitian should be consulted. Diabetic children may be on a less restricted diet, adjusting the insulin dosage according to blood and urine glucose readings. Children with negative urine glucose tend to become hypoglycemic rapidly with exercise or decrease in appetite, and many physicians allow for glucose spilling.

Contraindication: Hypersensitivity to insulin.

Special Concerns: Pregnant diabetic clients often manifest decreased insulin requirements during the first half of pregnancy and increased requirements during the latter half. Lactation may decrease insulin requirements.

Side Effects: *Hypoglycemia:* Due to insulin overdose, delayed or decreased food intake, too much exercise in relationship to insulin dose, or when transferring from one preparation to another. Even carefully controlled clients occasionally develop signs of insulin overdosage characterized by one or more of the following: hunger, weakness, fatigue, nervousness, pallor or flushing, profuse sweating, headache, palpitations, numbness of mouth, tingling in the fingers, tremors, blurred and double vision, hypothermia, excess yawning, mental confusion, incoordination, tachycardia, loss of sensitivity, and loss of consciousness. Level of awareness is markedly diminished after an attack.

Symptoms of hypoglycemia may mimic those of psychic disturbances. Severe prolonged hypoglycemia may cause brain damage, and in the elderly, may mimic stroke.

Allergic: Urticaria, angioedema, lymphadenopathy, bullae, anaphylaxis. Occurs mostly following intermittent insulin therapy or IV administration of large doses to insulin-resistant clients. Antihistamines or corticosteroids may be used to treat these symptoms. Clients who are highly allergic to insulin and cannot be treated with oral hypoglycemics may respond to human insulin products.

At site of injection: Swelling, stinging, redness, itching, warmth. These symptoms often disappear with continued use. Lipoatrophy or hypertrophy of subcutaneous fat tissue (minimize by rotating site of injection).

Insulin resistance: Usual cause is obesity. Acute resistance may occur following infections, trauma, surgery, emotional disturbances, or other endocrine disorders.

Ophthalmologic: Blurred vision, transient presbyopia. Occurs mainly during initiation of therapy or in clients who have been uncontrolled for a long period of time.

Hyperglycemic rebound (Somogyi effect): Usually in clients who receive chronic overdosage.

DIFFERENTIATION BETWEEN DIABETIC COMA AND HYPOGLYCEMIC REACTION (INSULIN SHOCK): Coma in diabetes may be caused by uncontrolled diabetes (high sugar content in blood or urine, ketoacidosis) or by too much insulin (insulin shock, hypoglycemia).

Diabetic coma and insulin shock can be differentiated in the following manner:

Hyperglycemia (Diabetic Coma)
Onset / Gradual (days)
Medication / Insufficient insulin
Food intake / Normal or excess
Overall appearance / Extremely ill
Skin / Dry and flushed
Infection / Frequent
Fever / Frequent
Mouth / Dry
Thirst / Intense
Hunger / Absent
Vomiting / Common
Abdominal pain / Frequent
Respiration / Increased, air hunger
Breath / Acetone odor
BP / Low
Pulse / Weak and rapid
Vision / Dim
Tremor / Absent
Convulsions / None
Urine sugar / High
Ketone bodies / High (type I only)
Blood sugar / High

Hypoglycemia (Insulin Shock)
Onset / Sudden (24–48 hr)
Medication / Excess insulin
Food intake / Probably too little
Overall appearance / Very weak
Skin / Moist and pale
Infection / Absent
Fever / Absent
Mouth / Drooling
Thirst / Absent
Hunger / Occasional
Vomiting / Absent
Abdominal pain / Rare
Respiration / Normal
Breath / Normal
BP / Normal
Pulse / Full and bounding
Vision / Diplopia
Tremor / Frequent
Convulsions / In late stages
Urine sugar / Absent in second specimen

Ketone bodies / Absent in second specimen
Blood sugar / Less than 60 mg/100 mL

Source: Adapted with permission from *The Merck Manual,* 11th ed.

Diabetic coma is usually precipitated by the client's failure to take insulin. Hypoglycemia is often precipitated by the client's unpredictable response, excess exertion, stress due to illness or surgery, errors in calculating dosage, or failure to eat.

TREATMENT OF DIABETIC COMA OR SEVERE ACIDOSIS: Administer 30–60 units regular insulin. This is followed by doses of 20 units or more q 30 min. To avoid a hypoglycemic state, 1 g dextrose is administered for each unit of insulin given. Treatment is often supplemented by electrolytes and fluids. Urine samples are collected for analysis, and VS are monitored as ordered.

TREATMENT OF HYPOGLYCEMIA (INSULIN SHOCK): Mild hypoglycemia can be relieved by PO administration of CHOs such as orange juice, candy, or a lump of sugar. If the client is comatose, adults may be given 10–30 mL of 50% dextrose solution IV; children should receive 0.5–1 mL/kg of 50% dextrose solution. Epinephrine, hydrocortisone, or glucagon may be used in severe cases to cause an increase in blood glucose.

Drug Interactions

Alcohol, ethyl / ↑ Hypoglycemia → low blood sugar and shock
Anabolic steroids / ↑ Hypoglycemic effect of insulin
Beta-adrenergic blocking agents / ↑ Hypoglycemic effect of insulin
Chlorthalidone / ↓ Hypoglycemic effect of antidiabetics
Clofibrate / ↑ Hypoglycemic effects of insulin
Contraceptives, oral / ↑ Dosage of antidiabetic due to impairment of glucose tolerance
Corticosteroids / ↓ Effect of insulin due to corticosteroid-induced hyperglycemia
Dextrothyroxine / ↓ Effect of insulin due to dextrothyroxine-induced hyperglycemia
Diazoxide / Diazoxide-induced hyperglycemia ↓ diabetic control
Digitalis glycosides / Use with caution, as insulin affects serum potassium levels
Diltiazen / ↓ Effect of insulin
Dobutamine / ↓ Effect of insulin
Epinephrine / ↓ Effect of insulin due to epinephrine-induced hyperglycemia
Estrogens / ↓ Effect of insulin due to impairment of glucose tolerance
Ethacrynic acid / ↓ Hypoglycemic effect of antidiabetics
Fenfluramine / Additive hypoglycemic effects
Furosemide / ↓ Hypoglycemic effect of antidiabetics
Glucagon / Glucagon-induced hyperglycemia ↓ effect of antidiabetics
Guanethidine / ↑ Hypoglycemic effect of insulin
MAO inhibitors / MAO inhibitors ↑ and prolong hypoglycemic effect of antidiabetics
Oxytetracycline / ↑ Effect of insulin
Phenothiazines / ↑ Dosage of antidiabetic due to phenothiazine-induced hyperglycemia
Phenytoin / Phenytoin-induced hyperglycemia ↓ diabetic control
Propranolol / Inhibits rebound of blood glucose after insulin-induced hypoglycemia
Salicylates / ↑ Effect of hypoglycemic effect of insulin
Sulfinpyrazone / ↑ Hypoglycemic effect of insulin
Tetracyclines / May ↑ hypoglycemic effect of insulin
Thiazide diuretics / ↓ Hypoglycemic effect of antidiabetics
Thyroid preparations / ↓ Effect of antidiabetic due to thyroid-induced hyperglycemia
Triamterene / ↓ Hypoglycemic effect of antidiabetic

Laboratory Test Interferences: Alters liver function tests and thyroid function tests. False + Coombs' test, ↑ serum protein, ↓ serum amino acids, calcium, cholesterol, potassium, and urine amino acids.

Dosage

Insulin is usually administered SC. Insulin injection (regular insulin) is the **only** preparation that may be administered IV. This route should be used only for clients with severe ketoacidosis or diabetic coma.

Dosage for insulin is always expressed in USP units.

Dosage is established and monitored by blood glucose (often using glucose monitoring machines in the home), urine glucose, and acetone tests. Dosage is highly individualized. Furthermore, since the requirements of clients may change with time, dosage must be checked at regular intervals. It may be advisable to hospitalize some clients while their daily insulin and caloric requirements are being established. The main goal is to control the blood sugar and send the client home to fine tune as generally the home environment is more reliable for determining drug requirements.

In pregnancy, insulin requirements may increase suddenly during the last trimester. After delivery, requirements may suddenly drop to prepregnancy levels. To prevent the development of hypoglycemia, insulin is often discontinued on the day of delivery and glucose is administered IV.

The various insulin preparations can be mixed to obtain the combination best suited for the individual client. However, mixing must be done according to the directions received from the physician and/or pharmacist.

NURSING CONSIDERATIONS

Also includes general applications for all clients with diabetes controlled by medication (whether it be insulin or an oral hypoglycemic agent).

Administration/Storage

1. Read the product information brochure and any important notes inserted into the package of prescribed insulin.
2. Discard open vials that have not been used for several weeks or any whose expiration date has passed.
3. Refrigerate stock supply of insulin but avoid freezing. Freezing destroys the manner in which insulin is suspended in the formulation.
4. Store insulin vial in a cool place, avoiding extremes of temperature or exposure to sunlight.
5. The following guidelines should be followed with respect to mixing the various insulins.

- Regular insulin may be mixed with NPH or Lente insulins. However, to avoid transfer of the longer-acting insulin into the regular insulin vial, regular insulin should be drawn into the syringe first.
- A mixture of regular insulin with NPH or Lente insulin should be administered within 15 min of mixing due to binding of regular insulin by excess protamine and/or zinc in the longer-acting preparations.
- Lente, Semilente, or Ultralente insulins may be mixed with each other in any proportion; however, these insulins should not be mixed with NPH insulins.
- When used in an insulin infusion pump, insulin may be mixed in any proportion with either 0.9% sodium

Figure 1 Each injection area is divided into squares; each square is an injection site. Start in a corner of an injection area and move down or across the injection sites in order. Jumping from site to site will make it more difficult to remember where the last shot was administered. Keep track of the rotation pattern to assist in maintaining site rotation. A grid may be developed from this figure and numbered to keep track of injections. Systematically use all the sites in one area before moving to another (for example, use all the sites in both arms before moving to the legs). This will help keep the blood sugar more even from day to day. An important consideration when choosing injection sites is that insulin is absorbed into the bloodstream faster from some areas than from others; it enters the bloodstream most quickly from the abdomen (stomach), a little more slowly from the arms, even more slowly from the legs, and most slowly from the buttocks. (Courtesy Eli Lilly & Company.)

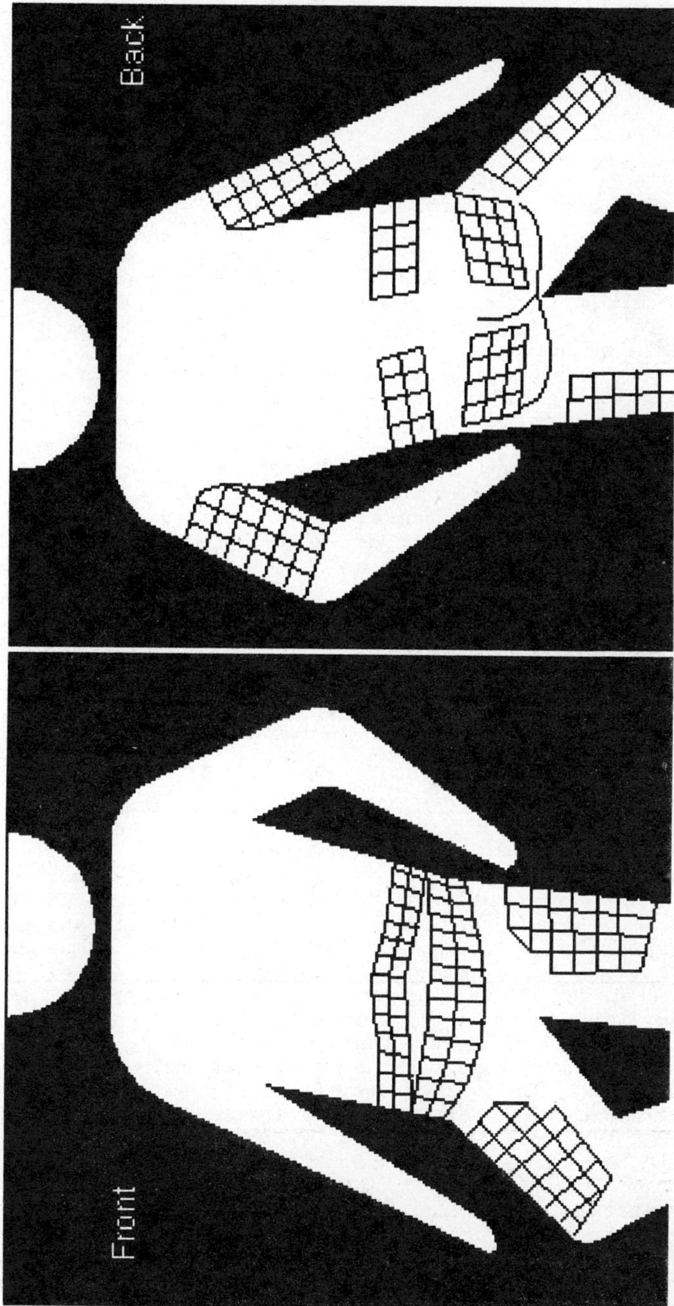
Back
Front

chloride injection or water for injection. Due to stability changes, such mixtures should be used within 24 hr of their preparation. Buffered insulin is usually the form prescribed and utilized with the insulin pump.

6. Store compatible mixtures of insulin for no longer than 1 month at room temperature or 3 months at 2°C–8°C (36°F–46°F). However, bacterial contamination may occur.

7. To ensure a constant amount of precipitate in each dose, invert the vial several times to mix before the material is withdrawn. Avoid vigorous shaking and frothing of the material. (Regular and globin insulin are the only two insulins that do not have a precipitate.)

8. Discard any vial in which the precipitate is clumped or granular in appearance or which has formed a solid deposit of particles on the side of the vial.

9. To prevent dosage error, do not alter the order of mixing insulins or change the model or brand of syringe or needle.

10. Administer at a 90° angle with a 28- or 29-gauge needle. Syringes come in 3/10-cc (30-U), 5/10-cc (50-U) and 1-cc (100-U) sizes. Encourage client to get the smallest syringe with the smallest needles to enhance dosage validity (e.g., if client is prescribed less than 30 U insulin, advise to obtain the 3/10-cc syringe).

11. Provide an automatic injector for clients who are fearful of injecting themselves.

12. Assist the visually impaired client with diabetes to obtain information and devices for self-administration of insulin by consulting their local diabetes association or by writing to the American Diabetes Association, 149 Madison Avenue, New York, NY 10016 (telephone: 212-725-4925), for their buyer's guide, which lists numerous available products for diabetics. Clients may also contact The Lighthouse, Inc., 800 Second Avenue, New York, NY 10017 (telephone: 212-808-0077) for additional information on visual impairments.

13. Lipoatrophy may occur. This may appear as mild dimpling of the skin or as deep pits in young girls and women, and lipodystrophy, appearing as well-developed muscle on the anterior and lateral thighs of young boys and men. To prevent this problem, rotate the sites of SC injections of insulin.

- Make a chart indicating the injection sites (see Figure 1, page 59).
- Allow 3–4 cm between injection sites.
- Do not inject in the same site for at least 1–2 weeks.
- Avoid injecting within 1 cm around the umbilicus because of the high vascularity in this area.
- Avoid injections around the waistline because of the sensitive nerve supply to this area.
- Use insulin at room temperature to prevent lipodystrophy.

14. Note that rotation of injection sites may lead to differences in blood levels of insulin. The abdomen is considered the best site due to constant insulin peak times with better gradual absorption.

15. If the insulin has been refrigerated, allow it to remain at room temperature for at least 1 hr before using.

16. Apply gentle pressure after injection but do not massage since this may interfere with the rate of absorption.

17. If breakfast must be delayed because of lab tests, check with the provider for adjustment in dosage.

18. Care of reusable syringes and needles.

- Do not use heavily chlorinated water or water with a high chemical content for sterilizing syringes. To sterilize, boil the syringe and needle for 5 min.
- Needle and syringe can be sterilized by soaking in isopropyl alcohol for at least 5 min. The alcohol must evaporate from the equipment before use to prevent reduction in the strength (dilution) of the insulin.
- Clean syringes covered by a precipitate with a cotton-tipped swab soaked in vinegar; then thoroughly rinse syringe in water and sterilize it.

Clean needles with a wire and sharpen with a pumice stone.

• Alcohol should be avoided when reusing disposable syringes, as it removes silicone (which facilitates the ease of insertion) from the needle.

• Disposable syringes may be reused by the same individual and are generally usable for several sticks. Client will be the judge depending on comfort and experienced "dullness."

Assessment

1. Obtain a thorough nursing history from the client and/or family.
2. Assess the client for symptoms of hyperglycemia: thirst, polydypsia, polyuria, drowsiness, blurred vision, loss of appetite, fruity odor to the breath, and flushed dry skin. Note state of consciousness.
3. Assess the client for symptoms of hypoglycemia: drowsiness, chills, confusion, anxiety, cold sweats and cool pale skin, excessive hunger, nausea, headache, irritability, shakiness, rapid pulse, and unusual weakness or tiredness.
4. Determine when clients first noticed changes in their physical condition and what these changes were.
5. Note if the client and/or family has noticed any psychologic changes and list what they consisted of.
6. Identify and list other medications the client may be taking.
7. Weigh the client. This is especially important when working with elderly clients because the amount of hypoglycemic agent prescribed is determined by their weight.
8. Obtain baseline serum electrolytes, blood sugar, phosphate, magnesium, and glycosolated hemoglobin levels as indicated.
9. Assess psychologic state including client's acceptance of disease, readiness to learn, family support and understanding, any evidence of depression, or need for client/family counseling.
10. Identify and document as type I or type II diabetes.

Interventions

1. If the client has symptoms of a ***hyperglycemic reaction,*** obtain medical supervision as rapidly as possible.

• Have regular insulin available for administration.

• Immediately obtain a blood sample for glucose or perform a finger stick before administering medication.

• After administering the insulin, monitor the client closely.

• Observe the client for further signs of hyperglycemia such as SOB, facial flushing, air hunger, and acetone on the breath.

• Check serum glucose and acetone level, urine acetone, serum pH, and any other relevant lab data.

2. Check the client for early symptoms of ***hypoglycemia,*** such as easy fatigue, hunger, headache, drowsiness, nausea, lassitude, and tremulousness.

• More marked symptoms such as weakness, sweating, tremors, and/or nervousness may occur later.

• Observe the client at night for excessive restlessness and profuse sweating.

• Obtain a blood sugar level and/or finger stick and promptly administer 4 oz of juice and a carbohydrate, if the client is conscious, and report.

• If the client is conscious and has been taking long-acting insulin, also administer a slowly digestible carbohydrate, such as bread with corn syrup or honey. Provide additional carbohydrates such as crackers and milk for the next 2 hr.

• If the client is unconscious, apply honey or Karo syrup to the buccal membrane or administer glucagon if available.

• If the client is in the hospital, minimally responsive or unconscious, have available 10%–20% dextrose solution for IV fluid therapy and D 50% bristojets for IV push.

3. Some clients experience a Somogyi effect and are often mistaken for clients who do not follow the prescribed methods of therapy. The Somogyi effect occurs when hypo-

glycemia triggers the release of epinephrine, glucocorticoids, and growth hormone, which stimulates glycogenesis and results in a higher blood glucose level. Reduction in the dosage of insulin is necessary to stabilize the client. This should be anticipated in the client who has originally been treated for hypoglycemia.

4. Juveniles with diabetes demand closer attention and observation for hypoglycemia. They are more susceptible to insulin shock than clients with diabetes in other age groups and have a more limited response to glucagon. Determine if client is being managed with intensive or conventional insulin therapy.

5. Assess juvenile diabetics more closely for infection or emotional disturbances that may increase their insulin requirements.

6. For the elderly client who has been newly diagnosed as having diabetes, the initial doses of insulin should be low, gradually increasing the dose until the desired effects have been achieved.

- Be alert for signs of hypoglycemia, such as slurred speech and mental confusion.
- If the client is to be on NPO status for whatever reason, consult the provider about the dosage adjustment that will be required.

7. Review the client's entire medication regimen for drugs that may enhance or antagonize antidiabetic agents being used. A dosage adjustment of antidiabetic agents may be necessary.

Client/Family Teaching

1. Review with the client and family the nature of diabetes mellitus and its S&S. Advise that medications assist to control diabetes but do not cure it. Explain simply until client can grasp. Type I diabetes is usually early onset and the pancreas makes little or no insulin; so individuals with type I diabetes must take insulin injections or they will die. Type II diabetes is usually later onset and the pancreas still makes insulin, but the body cannot use it; so individuals with type II diabetes can use either oral hypoglycemic agents or insulin to lower their blood sugar and to help them utilize their own insulin better.

2. Explain the necessity for close, regular medical supervision. Explain the relationship of diabetes to BP (reduced blood flow) and the importance of careful monitoring. Encourage client to learn how to take own BP.

3. Urine testing is not considered an accurate reflection of what the blood sugar is doing and is not generally used to adjust the treatment plan. If the client is testing urine, explain how to test the urine for sugar, and demonstrate how this test should be conducted. When testing the urine for glycosuria with Clinitest Tablets, Tes-Tape, Diastix, or Clinistix, as prescribed, give the client printed instructions.

- Test a fresh second-voided specimen.
- Empty the bladder by voiding about 1 hr before mealtime.
- As soon as the client can void again, obtain the specimen and test.
- If the client is taking other medications, note what they are and determine if they may interfere with the test. Notify the lab and use appropriate tests if interference may be a problem.

4. In type I diabetics, ketones in the urine indicate that there is not enough insulin present to get the body's sugar into the cells so it is burning body fat as an alternative and producing ketones as waste products. This may lead to ketoacidosis, a life-threatening condition. Advise client with diabetes to test urine for ketones with a "dip-and-read" product when:

- Finger sticks greater than 240 mg/dL
- Pregnant
- Experiencing severe stress
- Vomiting or sick to stomach
- Sick with flu or cold or virus infection
- Experiencing symptoms of hyperglycemia (unusual fatigue, vision difficulty, increased thirst and/or

hunger, polydipsia, unusually tired or sleepy, stomach pain, increased nausea, fruity odor to breath, rapid respirations, weight loss without altering food intake or activity patterns) and report results to provider

5. If the client is performing finger sticks to monitor glucose levels, demonstrate how this test should be conducted. If using a glucose monitoring machine, have clients perform a return demonstration to ensure they know the proper technique, proper calibration, method of operation, and maintenance for the device. Some general principles may be followed.

- Rotate sites.
- Cleanse area with soap and water or alcohol prior to stabbing.
- Stab finger and let a bead of blood form.
- Wipe off with a cotton ball.
- Then, let the bead of blood reform and apply to the test strip.
- Follow specific guidelines for the specific device in use.

6. Discuss the fact that regimens are specific to the individual client, based on age, the severity of the diabetes, weight, any other medical problems the client may have, as well as the philosophy of the health care team.

7. Instruct clients in administering insulin and have them perform a return demonstration. Administer at a 90° angle with a 28- or 29-gauge needle. Syringes come in 3⁄10-cc (30-U), 5⁄10-cc (50-U) and 1-cc (100-U) sizes. Encourage client to purchase the smallest syringe with the smallest needles to enhance dosage validity (e.g., if client is prescribed less than 30 U insulin, advise to obtain the 3⁄10-cc syringe). Advise clients they may reuse their disposable insulin syringes; they will be the judges based on comfort and perceived dullness.

8. Provide a chart and instruct clients in how to document the injection sites and how to avoid either lipoatrophy or lipodystrophy of injection sites.

- For self-injection, instruct the client to brace the arm against a hard surface such as the wall or a chair.
- Cleanse the area thoroughly, allow the area to dry, then, depending on the condition of the skin, either pinch the skin between the thumb and forefingers of one hand, or spread the skin using the thumb and fingers of one hand.
- Insert into the subcutaneous tissue and aspirate to be sure that the needle is not in a blood vessel.
- Inject the insulin and withdraw the needle.

9. Explain the use and care of equipment, the proper way to dispose of needles and syringes, as well as the provision and storage of medication.

10. *Always* check expiration dates. Advise to have an extra vial of insulin and extra equipment on hand for administration when traveling, at home, or when hospitalized.

11. Have regular insulin available for emergency use.

12. Explain the importance of exercise and the effect of exercise on the utilization of carbohydrates and increasing carbohydrate needs. Have a snack available at all times; five lifesavers is the usual recommendation.

13. Stress the importance of adhering to the prescribed diet. Emphasize weight control and ingestion of food relative to the peak action of the insulin being used. Record weekly weights and report any major variations. Stress the importance of reducing intake of animal fats and salt while selecting a variety of foods to meet starch and sugar, protein, and fat requirements. Review the kinds of fiber that should be consumed and that can help lower blood sugar and fat levels (breads, cereals, and crackers made from whole grains, such as whole wheat and brown rice, fresh vegetables and fruits, dried beans, and peas).

14. Provide a food exchange list, explain it, and answer questions. Refer the client to a dietitian for assistance

in shopping, food selection, and meal planning.

15. Explain the importance of carrying juice or hard candy at all times to counteract hypoglycemia, should it occur.

16. Discuss the possibility of allergic responses. Itching, redness, swelling, stinging, or warmth may occur at the injection site. These will usually disappear after a few weeks of therapy. However, they should be reported because the type of insulin may need to be changed. Purified or human insulins are used for local insulin allergy and lipodystrophy at the injection site.

17. Provide a printed chart explaining symptoms of hypoglycemia and hyperglycemia (see Interventions) and instructions concerning what to do for each. Also, instruct the client to report when either event occurs, explaining as specifically as possible what happened and what activity the client was engaged in. The dosage of insulin may need to be adjusted.

18. The client may experience blurred vision at the beginning of insulin therapy. Advise that the condition should subside in 6–8 weeks. The effect is caused by the fluctuation of blood glucose levels, which produce osmotic changes in the lens of the eye and within the ocular fluids. If the condition does not clear up in 8 weeks, the client should be advised to have an eye examination and evaluation.

19. If the client feels ill and omits a meal because of fever, nausea, or vomiting, advise to replace solid foods that contain starch and sugar, such as bread and fruit, with liquids that contain sugar (fruit juice, regular sodas) and follow designated sliding scale for "sick days." Do not omit insulin or hypoglycemic agents unless advised to do so by the provider. Perform finger sticks q 4 hr, and with type I, also test urine for ketones and report if moderate or high.

20. If client becomes ill, the provider should be notified immediately. Explain that to prevent coma, the client should maintain adequate hydration by drinking 1 cup or more of noncaloric fluids such as coffee, tea, water, or broth every hour. The client or family member should conduct finger sticks and urine testing more frequently under these circumstances.

21. If the supply of insulin is exhausted or the equipment to administer is not available, decrease the food intake by one-third and drink plenty of fluids. Obtain the necessary supplies as soon as possible in order to return to the prescribed diet and insulin dosage.

22. Explain the importance of good hygienic practices to prevent infection. Bathe daily with mild soap and lukewarm water. Use lotion to prevent skin dryness. Avoid injury from punctures. Avoid scratches; wear gloves when working with the hands. Use sunscreen and protective clothing to avoid sunburn, and dress appropriately for the weather, taking care to prevent frostbite.

23. Advise a daily routine of checking and caring for the feet. Review appropiate comfortable shoes (leather or canvas), stockings (no garters or elastic tops), and exercises that should be followed. Review how to clip the toenails (straight across) and stress not to undertake any self-treatment for ingrown toenails, corns, or calluses. Do not use any heat treatments, hot water bottles, or heating pads, and do not smoke, as this decreases the blood flow to the feet.

24. Review dental care and explain that hyperglycemia compounds the risk for tooth and gum problems. Advise to brush after meals, to floss daily, and to see a dentist q 6 months.

25. Since diabetes can damage the small blood vessels to the eye, advise complete yearly eye exams that include assessing the small blood vessels at the back of the eye. Stress that eye damage has no symptoms when it is in the early, treatable stage. Also, advise to seek eye care if client experiences blurred or double vision, narrowed visual fields, in-

creased difficulty seeing in dim light, pressure or pain in the eye, or seeing dark spots.

26. Advise the client to wear a Medic Alert bracelet or carry a card identifying the client as having diabetes, currently prescribed medications, who to notify and what to do in the event the client is unable to respond.

27. Avoid alcoholic beverages because alcohol can cause hypoglycemia. Excessive intake of alcohol may require a reduction in the dosage of insulin because alcohol potentiates the hypoglycemic effect of insulin. It also causes a disulfiram-type reaction with oral hypoglycemic agents.

28. Advise clients to carry all medications, syringes, glucagon, and blood testing equipment in their carry-on luggage when traveling. Always carry diabetes identification and know where to obtain emergency medical help when traveling. Keep to the usual meal, exercise, and medication routines as closely as possible. Keep food and fast-acting sugar handy in the event meals are delayed. Request medication from provider in the event of vomiting or diarrhea and plan ahead for mealtimes when crossing two or more time zones. Take care to protect insulin and test strips from extremes in heat or cold (keeping between 59°F and 86°F).

29. Caution clients to use only the insulin prescribed and to check carefully each time they purchase insulin to be certain it is the correct species (human, beef, pork, or mixed beef-pork), brand name (Humulin, Iletin I, Iletin II, etc.), and type (Regular, Lente, NPH, etc.). If there is any change in insulin purity, strength, type, source of the insulin, or manufacturer, there may be a need to adjust the dosage of insulin.

30. Check vials of insulin carefully before each dose is taken. Regular insulin and Buffered Regular insulin (for pumps) should be clear and colorless, whereas other forms may be cloudy.

31. Two kinds of insulin can be mixed in the same syringe if the following guidelines are followed:

- Regular insulin can be mixed with any other insulin.
- Lente forms can be mixed with other Lente insulins but cannot be mixed with other insulins with the exception of regular insulin.
- A single form of insulin in a syringe can be stable for weeks or a month.
- Except for the commercially prepared mixtures, mixtures of insulin are not stable and should be administered within 5 min of preparation.
- When insulins are mixed, regular (unmodified) insulin should always be drawn up in the syringe first. Instruct the client to use the same procedure at all times when drawing up two insulins to avoid contamination of the two vials of insulin.

32. Explain that impotence may be caused by damaged nerves and reduced blood flow related to diabetes but should be evaluated by the provider in order to find the true cause and the best treatment.

33. A dietitian referral should be made for assistance with dietary modification. Support groups may assist clients and families to understand and learn to cope with this disease. Refer the client and family to the American Diabetes Association, 1660 Duke Street, Alexandria, VA 22314 (telephone: 703-549-1500 or 1-800-ADA-DISC), and local diabetes support groups for additional information and support.

34. Stress the importance of follow-up visits and lab studies to evaluate the effectiveness of therapy.

Evaluate

- Evidence of an understanding and effective management of their diabetes
- Development of positive coping strategies
- Laboratory confirmation that serum glucose and acetone levels are within desired range
- Evidence of healthy and intact skin at injection sites
- Prevention of target organ disease

Insulin, human

Buffered Human Insulin: Humulin BR. **Insulin Injection:** Humulin R, Novolin R, Novolin R PenFill, Velosulin Human. **Insulin Zinc Suspension:** Humulin L, Novolin L. **Insulin Zinc Suspension and Insulin Injection:** Humulin 70/30, Novolin 70/30, Novolin 70/30 PenFill. **Insulin Zinc Suspension Extended:** Humulin U Ultralente. **Isophane Insulin Suspension:** Humulin N, Novolin N, Novolin N PenFill.

See also *Insulins,* Chapter 65.

Insulin injection (crystalline zinc insulin, unmodified insulin, regular insulin)

(**IN**-sue-lin)

Pork: Insulin-Toronto ✱, Pork Regular Iletin II, Regular Insulin, Regular Purified Pork Insulin. **Beef/Pork:** Regular Iletin I. **Human:** Humulin R, Novolin R, Novolin R PenFill, Velosulin Human **(OTC)**

See also *Insulins,* Chapter 65.

How Supplied: Insulin, human: *Injection:* 100 U/mL.

Insulin injection: *Injection:* 100 U/mL

Action/Kinetics: This product is rarely administered as the sole agent due to its short duration of action. Injections of 100 units/mL are clear; cloudy, colored solutions should not be used. Regular insulin is the only preparation suitable for IV administration. Is available only as 100 units/mL. **Onset, SC:** 30–60 min; **IV:** 10–30 min. **Peak, SC:** 2–4 hr; **IV:** 15–30 min. **Duration, SC:** 6–8 hr; **IV:** 30–60 min.

Uses: Suitable for treatment of diabetic coma, diabetic acidosis, or other emergency situations. Especially suitable for the client suffering from labile diabetes. During acute phase of diabetic acidosis or for the client in diabetic crisis, client is monitored by serum glucose and serum ketone levels.

Dosage

• **SC**

Diabetes.

Adults, individualized, usual, initial: 5–10 units; **pediatric:** 2–4 units. Injection is given 15–30 min before meals and at bedtime.

Diabetic ketoacidosis.

Adults: 0.1 unit/kg/hr given by continuous IV infusion.

Administration/Storage

1. When used IV, the rate of insulin infusion should be decreased when plasma glucose levels reach 250 mg/dL.
2. Due to the short half-life of regular insulin, large single IV doses should not be administered.

NURSING CONSIDERATIONS

See also *Nursing Considerations* for *Insulins,* Chapter 65.

Evaluate: Restoration of serum glucose levels to within desired range.

Insulin injection, concentrated

(**IN**-sue-lin)

Regular (Concentrated) Iletin II U-500 **(Rx)**

See also *Insulins,* Chapter 65.

How Supplied: *Injection:* 100 U/mL, 500 U/mL

Action/Kinetics: This concentrated preparation (500 units/mL) of insulin injection (see above) is indicated for clients with a marked resistance to insulin who require more than 200 units/day. Clients must be kept under close observation until dosage is established. Depending on response, dosage may be given SC or IM as a single or as two or three divided doses.

Not suitable for IV administration because of possible allergic or anaphylactoid reactions.

Use: Diabetic clients requiring more than 200 units insulin/day.

Dosage

• **SC, IM**

Individualized, depending on severity of condition.

Administration/Storage

1. Administer only water clear solu-

tions (concentrated insulin may appear straw-colored).
2. Use a tuberculin type or insulin syringe for accuracy of measurement.
3. Deep secondary hypoglycemia may occur 18–24 hr after administration. Therefore, have 10%–20% dextrose solution or 50% dextrose available.
4. Keep insulin cool or refrigerated.
Contraindication: Allergy to pork or mixed pork/beef insulin (unless client has been desensitized).
Additional Side Effect: Deep secondary hypoglycemia 18–24 hr after administration.

NURSING CONSIDERATIONS

See also *Nursing Considerations* for *Insulins,* Chapter 65.
Interventions
1. Observe closely for S&S of hyper- or hypoglycemia during the period when the dosage is being established.
2. Monitor blood glucose levels frequently.
Client/Family Teaching
1. Review and observe client technique for self-administration.
2. Teach the client to be alert for signs of hypoglycemia, which may indicate that responsiveness to insulin has been regained and that a reduction in dosage is warranted.
Evaluate: Serum glucose levels within desired range.

Insulin zinc suspension (Lente)

(**IN**-sue-lin)
Beef: Lente Insulin. **Pork:** Lente Iletin II, Lente L. **Beef/Pork:** Lentin Iletin I. **Human:** Humulin L, Novolin L **(OTC)**

See also *Insulins,* Chapter 65.
How Supplied: *Injection:* 100 U/mL
Action/Kinetics: Contains 70% crystalline and 30% amorphous insulin suspension. Considered intermediate-acting. Principal advantage is the absence of a sensitizing agent such as protamine. **Onset:** 1–2.5 hr. **Peak:** 7–15 hr. **Duration:** About 22 hr.
Uses: Useful in clients allergic to other types of insulin and in clients disposed to thrombotic phenomena in which protamine may be a factor. Zinc insulin is not a replacement for regular insulin and is not suitable for emergency use.

Dosage
- **SC**

Diabetes.

Adults, initial: 7–26 units 30–60 min before breakfast. Dosage is then increased by daily or weekly increments of 2–10 units until satisfactory readjustment is established. A second smaller dose may be given prior to the evening meal or at bedtime. Clients on NPH can be transferred to insulin zinc suspension on a unit-for-unit basis. Clients being transferred from regular insulin should begin zinc insulin at two-thirds to three-fourths the regular insulin dosage. If the client is being transferred from protamine zinc insulin, the dose of zinc insulin should be about 50% of that required for protamine zinc insulin.

NURSING CONSIDERATIONS

See *Nursing Considerations* for *Insulins,* Chapter 65.
Evaluate: Normalization of serum glucose levels.

Insulin zinc suspension, extended

Beef: Ultralente U. **Human:** Humulin U Ultralente. **(OTC)**

See also *Insulins,* Chapter 65.
How Supplied: *Injection:* 100 U/mL
Action/Kinetics: Large crystals of insulin and a high content of zinc are responsible for the slow-acting properties of this preparation. Products containing both 40 units/mL and 100 units/mL are available. **Onset:** 4–8 hr. **Peak:** 10–30 hr. **Duration:** 36 hr or longer.

Uses: Mild to moderate hyperglycemia in stabilized diabetics. Not suitable for the treatment of diabetic coma or emergency situations.

Dosage

- **SC**

  Individualized.

Usual, initial: 7–26 units as a single dose 30–60 min before breakfast. **Do not administer IV.**

NURSING CONSIDERATIONS

See *Nursing Considerations* for *Insulins,* Chapter 65.
Evaluate: Normalization of serum glucose levels and control of symptoms of diabetes.

Insulin zinc suspension, prompt (Semilente)

(**IN**-sue-lin)
Beef: Semilente Insulin (Beef). **Beef/Pork:** Iletin I Semilente. **(OTC)**

See also *Insulins,* Chapter 65.
Action/Kinetics: Contains small particles of zinc insulin in a nearly colorless suspension. Not suitable for emergency use. Cannot be injected IV. **Onset:** 1–1.5 hr. **Peak:** 5–10 hr. **Duration:** 12–16 hr.
Uses: In combination with insulin zinc or extended insulin zinc suspensions to control diabetes. May also be used alone for rapid control when initiating therapy.

Dosage

- **SC**

  Diabetes.

Adults, individualized, initial: 10–20 units 30 min before breakfast. A second daily dose is usually required.

NURSING CONSIDERATIONS

See *Nursing Considerations* for *Insulins,* Chapter 65.
Evaluate: Restoration of serum blood sugars to within desired range.

Isophane insulin suspension (NPH)

(**EYE**-so-fayn **IN**-sue-lin)
Beef: NPH Insulin. **Pork:** NPH-N, Pork NPH Iletin II. **Beef/Pork:** NPH Iletin I. **Human:** Humulin N, Novolin N, Novolin N PenFill. **(OTC)**

See also *Insulins,* Chapter 65.
How Supplied: *Injection:* 100 U/mL
Action/Kinetics: Contains zinc insulin crystals modified by protamine, appearing as a cloudy or milky suspension. Not recommended for emergency use. Not suitable for IV administration. Not useful in the presence of ketosis. **Onset:** 1–1.5 hr. **Peak:** 4–12 hr. **Duration:** Up to 24 hr.

Dosage

- **SC**

  Diabetes.

Adult, individualized, usual, initial: 7–26 units as a single dose 30–60 min before breakfast. A second smaller dose may be given, if needed, prior to the evening meal or at bedtime. If necessary, the daily dose may be increased in increments of 2–10 units at daily or weekly intervals until desired control is achieved.

Clients on insulin zinc may be transferred directly to isophane insulin on a unit-for-unit basis. If client is being transferred from regular insulin, the initial dose of isophane should be from two-thirds to three-fourths the dose of regular insulin.

NURSING CONSIDERATIONS

See *Nursing Considerations* for *Insulins,* Chapter 65.
Evaluate

- Normalization of serum glucose
- Control of symptoms of diabetes

—COMBINATION DRUG—

Isophane insulin suspension and insulin injection

(**EYE**-so-fayn **IN**-sue-lin)
Human: Humulin 70/30, Humulin 50/50, Novolin 70/30, Novolin 70/30 PenFill **(OTC)**

See also *Insulins,* Chapter 65.
How Supplied: See Content
Content: Humulin 50/50 (100 units/mL) contains: 50% isophane insulin and 50% insulin injection.
Action/Kinetics: Contains either 30% insulin injection and 70% isophane insulin (Humulin 70/30, Novolin 70/30) or 50% insulin injection and 50% isophane insulin (Humulin 50/50). This combination allows for a rapid onset (30–60 min) due to insulin injection and a long duration (24 hr) due to isophane insulin. **Peak effect:** 4–8 hr.

Dosage

- **SC**
  Diabetes.

Adults: Individualized and given once daily 15–30 min before breakfast, or as directed. **Children:** Individualized according to client size.

NURSING CONSIDERATIONS

See *Nursing Considerations* for *Insulins,* Chapter 65.
Evaluate: Normalization of serum glucose levels.

HYPERGLYCEMIC AGENTS

See the following individual entries:

Diazoxide Oral
Glucagon

Diazoxide oral

(dye-az-**OX**-eyed)
Pregnancy Category: C
Proglycem **(Rx)**

How Supplied: *Capsule*: 50 mg; *Suspension:* 50 mg/mL
Action/Kinetics: Diazoxide inhibits the release of insulin from beta islet cells of the pancreas, leading to an increase in blood glucose levels. Effect is dose related. Diazoxide causes sodium, potassium, uric acid, and water retention. **Onset:** 1 hr. **t½:** 28 hr (up to 53 hr in clients with anuria). **Duration:** 8 hr. Metabolized in the liver although 50% is excreted through the kidneys unchanged.
Uses: Hypoglycemia caused by insulin overdosage or overproduction of insulin by malignant beta cells. The drug is used parenterally as an antihypertensive agent (see *Diazoxide,* Chapter 28).

Dosage

- **Capsules, Oral Suspension**
  Diabetes.

Dosage is individualized on the basis of blood glucose level and response of client. **Adults and children, usual, initial:** 1 mg/kg q 8 hr (adjust according to response); **maintenance:** 3–8 mg/kg/day divided into two or three equal doses q 8–12 hr. **Infants and newborns, initial:** 3.3 mg/kg q 8 hr (adjust according to response); **maintenance:** 8–15 mg/kg/day divided into two or three equal doses q 8–12 hr.

Administration/Storage

1. Blood glucose levels and urinary glucose and ketones must be monitored carefully until stabilized, which usually takes 1 week. The drug is discontinued if a satisfactory effect has not been established within 2–3 weeks.
2. Have available insulin and IV fluids to counteract possible ketoacidosis.
3. *Treatment of Overdose:* Insulin to treat hyperglycemia; use Trendelenburg maneuver to reverse hypotension.

Contraindications: Functional hypoglycemia, hypersensitivity to diazoxide or thiazides.
Special Concerns: Infants are particularly prone to development of edema. Use with extreme caution in clients with history of gout and in those in whom edema presents a risk (cardiac disease).
Laboratory Test Interferences: ↑ Serum uric acid, AST, alkaline phosphatase; ↓ creatinine clearance.
Side Effects: *CV:* Sodium and fluid retention (common), palpitations, in-

creased HR, hypotension, transient hypertension. *Metabolic:* Hyperglycemia, glycosuria, ***diabetic ketoacidosis, hyperosmolar nonketotic coma.*** *GI:* N&V, diarrhea, transient taste loss, anorexia, ileus, abdominal pain. *CNS:* Weakness, headache, insomnia, extrapyramidal symptoms, dizziness, paresthesia, fever. *Hematologic:* Thrombocytopenia, purpura, eosinophilia, neutropenia, decreased hemoglobin. *Dermatologic:* Skin rashes, hirsutism, herpes, loss of hair from scalp, monilial dermatitis. *GU:* Hematuria, proteinuria, decrease in urine production, nephrotic syndrome (reversible). *Ophthalmologic:* Blurred or double vision, lacrimation, transient cataracts, ring scotoma, subconjunctival hemorrhage. *Other:* Pancreatitis, ***pancreatic necrosis,*** galactorrhea, gout, premature aging of bone, polyneuritis, enlargement of lump in breast.

Symptoms of Overdose: Hypotension; excessive hyperglycemia.

Drug Interactions

Alpha-adrenergic blocking agents / ↓ Effect of diazoxide

Anticoagulants, oral / ↑ Effect of anticoagulant due to ↓ plasma protein binding

Antihypertensives / Excessive ↓ BP due to additive effects

Phenytoin / ↓ Effect of phenytoin due to ↑ breakdown by liver

Sulfonylureas / ↓ Effect of both drugs

Thiazide diuretics / ↑ Hypoglycemic and hyperuricemic effects

NURSING CONSIDERATIONS

Assessment

1. Note any sensitivity to thiazides.
2. Determine any history of gout or CAD.
3. Document indications for therapy and time frame for anticipated results.

Interventions

1. If the client has a history of CHF, observe carefully for fluid retention, which could precipitate heart failure.
2. If currently taking an antihypertensive agent, monitor BP for potentiation of antihypertensive effect.
3. Observe for ecchymosis, petechiae, or frank bleeding. These symptoms should be reported as they may require discontinuation of the drug.
4. If the client has had an overdosage of drug, observe closely for the first 7 days until blood sugar level is again within normal limits (80–120 mg/100 mL).
5. If hirsutism develops, reassure that the condition should subside once the drug is discontinued.
6. Review list of drug side effects to determine if clinical presentations may be drug related.

Evaluate: Restoration of serum glucose levels.

Glucagon

(GLOO-kah-gon)

Pregnancy Category: B

(Rx)

How Supplied: *Powder for injection:* 1 mg, 10 mg

Action/Kinetics: Glucagon is a hormone produced by the alpha islet cells of the pancreas. The hormone increases blood glucose by increasing breakdown of glycogen to glucose, stimulating gluconeogenesis from amino acids and fatty acids, and inhibiting conversion of glucose to glycogen. Also, lipolysis is increased, resulting in free fatty acids and glycerol for gluconeogenesis. The drug is effective in overcoming hypoglycemia only if the liver has a glycogen reserve. **Onset, hypoglycemia:** 5–20 min. **Maximum effect:** 30 min. **Duration:** 1–2 hr. **$t^{1}/_{2}$:** 3–6 min. Metabolized in the liver, kidney, plasma membrane receptor sites, and plasma.

Uses: Used to terminate insulin-induced shock in diabetic or psychiatric clients. Client usually regains consciousness 5–20 min after the parenteral administration of glucagon. The drug should only be used under medical supervision or in accordance with strict instructions received from the physician. Failure to respond may be an indication for IV administration of glucose—especially true in juvenile diabetics. As a diagnostic aid in radiologic examination of the GI tract when a hypotonic state is desirable. *Investigational:* Inhibit bowel peristalsis in abdominal digital vascular imaging and in abdominal CT scanning to prevent misregistration artifact. Adjunct in diagnosis of GI bleeding. Treatment of toxicity due to beta-adrenergic blocking agents, quinidine, or tricyclic antidepressants.

Dosage

- **IM, IV, SC**

Hypoglycemia.

Adults: 0.5–1 mg; one to two additional doses may be given at 20-min intervals, if necessary. **Pediatric:** 0.025 mg/kg, up to a maximum of 1 mg; may be repeated in 20 min if needed.

Insulin shock therapy.

IM, IV, SC: 0.5–1 mg after 1 hr of coma; if no response, dose may be repeated.

Diagnostic aid for GI tract.

Dose dependent on desired onset of action and duration of effect necessary for the examination. **IV:** 0.25–0.5 mg (onset: 1 min; duration: 9–17 min); 2 mg (onset: 1 min; duration 22–25 min). **IM:** 1 mg (onset: 8–10 min; duration: 12–27 min); 2 mg (onset: 4–7 min; duration: 21–32 min).

For colon examination.

IM: 2 mg 10 min prior to procedure.

Treatment of toxicity of beta-adrenergic blocking agents.

Adults, IV, initial: 2–3 mg given over 30 sec; may be repeated at the rate of 5 mg/hr until client is stabilized.

Administration/Storage

1. Once the client with hypoglycemia responds, supplemental carbohydrates should be given to prevent secondary hypoglycemia.
2. Before reconstituting, the powder should be stored at room temperature.
3. Following reconstitution, the solution should be used immediately. However, if necessary, the solution may be stored at 5°C (41°F) for up to 2 days.
4. Doses higher than 2 mg should be reconstituted with sterile water for injection and used immediately.
5. With direct IV administration, inject at a rate not exceeding 1 mg/min.
6. Administer with dextrose solutions. A precipitate may form if saline solutions are used.
7. *Treatment of Overdose:* Symptomatic.

Special Concerns: Use with caution in clients with renal or hepatic disease, in those who are undernourished and emaciated, and in clients with a history of pheochromocytoma or insulinoma.

Side Effects: *GI:* N&V. *Allergy:* Respiratory distress, urticaria, hypotension. ***Stevens-Johnson syndrome when used as diagnostic aid.***

Symptoms of Overdose: N&V, hypokalemia.

Drug Interactions

Anticoagulants, oral / ↑ Effect of anticoagulants by ↑ hypoprothrombinemia

Antidiabetic agents / Hyperglycemic effect of glucagon antagonizes hypoglycemic effect of antidiabetics

Corticosteroids, Epinephrine, Estrogens, Phenytoin / Additive hyperglycemic effect of drugs listed

NURSING CONSIDERATIONS

Client/Family Teaching

1. Instruct family in the administration of glucagon SC or IM in the event the client has a hypoglycemic reaction, loses consciousness, and is unable to swallow.
2. Following the administration of glucagon, advise family to keep clients on their side and to administer a carbohydrate once they awaken.
3. Have rapidly available sugar, such as orange juice and Karo syrup in water, to administer. If the shock was caused by a long-acting medication, administer slowly digestible carbohydrates, such as bread with honey.
4. Advise family not to try to administer fluids by mouth if the client has a reaction and is not fully conscious. The client could easily aspirate these fluids into the lungs.
5. Discuss the need to record and re-

port all hypoglycemic reactions so that the dosage of insulin can be properly adjusted.

Evaluate

- Reversal of S&S of hypoglycemia
- Termination of insulin-induced shock
- Inhibition of bowel peristalsis with small muscle relaxation during radiologic imaging of the GI tract

CHAPTER SIXTY-SIX

Thyroid and Antithyroid Drugs

See also the following individual entries:

Thyroid Drugs

Levothyroxine Sodium (T_4)
Liothyronine Sodium (T_3)
Liotrix
Thyroid, Desiccated
Thyrotropin

Antithyroid Drugs

Methimazole (Thiamazole)
Propylthiouracil

THYROID DRUGS

General Statement: The thyroid manufactures two active hormones: thyroxine and triiodothyronine, both of which contain iodine. These thyroid hormones are released into the bloodstream, where they are bound to protein. Synthetic derivatives include liothyronine (T_3), levothyronine (T_4), and liotrix (a 4:1 mixture of T_4 and T_3).

Thyroid abnormalities are classified as follows:

1. Hypothyroidism or diseases in which little or no hormone is produced. These can be subdivided into cretinism, resulting from a deficiency of thyroid hormone during fetal and early life, and myxedema, a deficiency of thyroid hormone in the adult. Cretinism is characterized by arrested physical and mental development, with dystrophy of the bones and soft parts and lowered basal metabolism. Myxedema is characterized by a dry, waxy swelling, with abnormal deposits of mucin in the skin. The edema is nonpitting and the facial changes are distinctive, with swollen lips and a thickened nose. Primary myxedema results from atrophy of the thyroid gland. Secondary myxedema may result from hypofunction of the pituitary gland or prolonged administration of antithyroid drugs.
2. Hyperthyroidism or conditions associated with an overproduction of hormones, as in Graves' or Basedow's disease (diffuse enlargement of the thyroid gland; often characterized by protruding eyes) and Plummer's disease, in which extra thyroid hormone is produced by a single "hot" thyroid nodule. These conditions are usually characterized by hypertrophy and hyperplasia of the thyroid and a state of extreme nervousness.
3. Euthyroid or simple, nontoxic goiter (endemic goiter) in which a normal or near-normal amount of hormone is produced by an enlarged thyroid gland. This condition can occur when the dietary intake of iodine is below normal. Today the disease is much rarer because iodine is added as a matter of routine to cooking salt. In these individuals, the thyroid tends to become enlarged, especially during adolescent growth and pregnancy. Surgery may be necessary to alleviate the pressure on the trachea caused by the enlarged thyroid and to prevent the oxygen supply from being diminished. Drugs used in the treatment of thyroid disease fall into two groups: (1) thyroid preparations used to correct thyroid deficiency

diseases and (2) antithyroid drugs that reduce production of hormones by an overactive gland. The external supply of thyroid hormones usually results in a reduction in the amount of natural hormone produced by the thyroid gland. The accurate determination of thyroid function is crucial for the treatment of thyroid disease. Thyroid function can be evaluated by (1) total levothyroxine (T_4), (2) free levothyroxine, (3) serum liothyronine (T_3), (4) liothyronine resin uptake (RT_3U), (5) free thyroxine index, and (6) thyroid-stimulating hormone (TSH). The results of some of the tests are at times skewed by medications the client is taking, so that the effect of these drugs must be considered when evaluating the test.

Action/Kinetics: The thyroid hormones regulate growth by controlling protein synthesis and regulating energy metabolism by increasing the resting or basal metabolic rate. This results in increases in respiratory rate; body temperature; CO; oxygen consumption; HR; blood volume; enzyme system activity; rate of fat, carbohydrate, and protein metabolism; and growth and maturation. Thyroid hormones have a significant effect on every organ system and are particularly important for growth and differentiation of tissues, CNS development, and maturation of the skeletal system. The thyroid gland is under the control of the hypothalamus and the pituitary gland, which produce TSH-releasing factor and thyrotropin (TSH), respectively. Like other hormone systems, the thyroid, pituitary, and hypothalamus work together in a feedback mechanism. Excess thyroid hormone causes a decrease in TSH, and a lack of thyroid hormone causes an increase in the production and secretion of TSH. Normally, the ratio of T_4 to T_3 released from the thyroid gland is 20:1 with about 35% of T_4 being converted in the periphery (e.g., kidney, liver) to T_3.

Uses: Replacement or supplemental therapy in hypothyroidism due to all causes except transient hypothyroidism during the recovery phase of subacute thyroiditis. Causes include cretinism, myxedema, nontoxic goiter, primary hypothyroidism (i.e., resulting from functional deficiency, partial or total absence of the thyroid gland, primary atrophy, surgery, radiation, or drugs). Secondary (pituitary) or tertiary (hypothalamic) hypothyroidism. To treat or prevent euthyroid goiters. With antithyroid drugs for thyrotoxicosis (to prevent goiter or hypothyroidism). Diagnostically to differentiate suspected hyperthyroidism from euthyroidism. The treatment of choice for hypothyroidism is usually T_4 because of its consistent potency and its prolonged duration of action although it does have a slow onset and its effects are cumulative over several weeks.

Contraindications: Uncorrected adrenal insufficiency, acute MI, hyperthyroidism, and thyrotoxicosis. When hypothyroidism and adrenal insufficiency coexist unless treatment with adrenocortical steroids is initiated first. Not to be used to treat obesity or infertility.

Special Concerns: Geriatric clients may be more sensitive to the usual adult dosage of these hormones. Use with extreme caution in the presence of angina pectoris, hypertension, and other CV diseases, renal insufficiency, and ischemic states. Use with caution during lactation.

Side Effects: Thyroid preparations have cumulative effects, and overdosage (e.g., symptoms of hyperthyroidism) may occur. *CV:* Arrhythmias, palpitations, angina, increased HR and pulse pressure, ***cardiac arrest,*** aggravation of CHF. *GI:* Cramps, diarrhea, N&V, appetite changes. *CNS:* Headache, nervousness, mental agitation, irritability, insomnia, tremors. *Miscellaneous:* Weight loss, hyperhidrosis, excessive warmth, irregular menses, heat intolerance, fever, dyspnea, allergic skin reactions (rare). Decreased bone density in pre- and postmenopausal women following long-term use of levothyroxine.

Symptoms of Overdose: Signs and

symptoms of hyperthyroidism including headache, irritability, sweating, tachycardia, nervousness, increased bowel motility, palpitations, vomiting, psychosis, menstrual irregularities, ***seizures,*** fever. Production or aggravation of angina or CHF, ***shock, arrhythmias, cardiac failure.***

Drug Interactions

Anticoagulants / ↑ Effect of anticoagulants by ↑ hypoprothrombinemia
Antidepressants, tricyclic / ↑ Effect of antidepressants and ↑ effect of thyroid
Antidiabetic agents / Hyperglycemic effect of thyroid preparations may necessitate ↑ in dose of antidiabetic agent
Beta-adrenergic blockers / ↓ Effect of beta blockers when the hypothyroid state is converted to the euthyroid state
Cholestyramine / ↓ Effect of thyroid hormone due to ↓ absorption from GI tract
Colestipol / ↓ Effect of thyroid hormone due to ↓ absorption from GI tract
Corticosteroids / Thyroid preparations ↑ tissue demands for corticosteroids. Adrenal insufficiency must be corrected with corticosteroids before administering thyroid hormones. In clients already treated for adrenal insufficiency, dosage of corticosteroids must be increased when initiating therapy with thyroid drug
Digitalis compounds / ↓ Effect of digitalis, with worsening of arrhythmias or CHF
Epinephrine / CV effects ↑ by thyroid preparations
Estrogens / May ↑ requirements for thyroid hormone
Ketamine / Concomitant use may result in severe hypertension and tachycardia
Levarterenol / CV effects ↑ by thyroid preparations
Phenytoin / ↑ Effect of thyroid hormone by ↓ plasma protein binding
Salicylates / Salicylates compete for thyroid-binding sites on protein
Theophylline / ↓ Theophylline clearance in hypothyroid client is returned to normal when euthyroid state is reached

Laboratory Test Interferences: Alter thyroid function tests. ↑ PT. ↓ Serum cholesterol. A large number of drugs alter thyroid function tests.

Dosage

Thyroid drugs are started with a low dose that is gradually increased until a satisfactory response is achieved within safe dose limits. When necessary, a decrease in dosage and a more gradual upward adjustment relieve severe side effects.

NURSING CONSIDERATIONS

Administration/Storage

1. The treatment is initiated with small doses that are gradually increased.
2. The dose of medication for a child may be the same as the dosage for an adult.
3. When changing from one thyroid drug to another, follow the specific instructions to prevent overdosage or relapse.
4. Store thyroid preparations in a cool, dark place away from moisture and light.
5. Due to differences from one brand of drug to another, brand interchange is not recommended without consulting with the provider or pharmacist.

Assessment

1. Perform a thorough nursing history, documenting onset and noting symptoms that warrant drug therapy.
2. Review all medications the client is currently receiving to be sure none interacts unfavorably with the antithyroid medication.
3. Note if the client is taking antidiabetic agents or is on anticoagulant therapy.
4. Assess clinical presentation noting any symptoms consistent with hypothyroidism (i.e., fatigue, lethargy, weight gain, puffy face and eyelids,

large tongue, cold intolerance, hair loss, and cardiomegaly).
5. Assess the client's general physical condition (age, severity and duration of disease) and note any history of angina, cardiac problems, or any other health problems.
6. Take a baseline ECG against which to compare subsequent ECG tracings once therapy has been instituted.
7. Ensure that all lab studies and thyroid function levels have been performed before initiating therapy.

Interventions

1. Monitor the client's thyroid function studies closely.
2. Observe for any side effects of the drug. Complaints of headache, insomnia, and tremors should be documented and reported.
3. Observe the client on anticoagulant therapy for bleeding from any orifice or for purpura. Monitor PT and PTT closely because the action of anticoagulants is potentiated by thyroid preparations.
4. Report any symptoms of CAD. Clients with a history of angina or other CV disorders need to have their BP, HR, and cardiac rhythms monitored. If the HR exceeds 100 beats/min, withhold drug and report, unless otherwise directed.
5. Note the client's general response to the therapy. Complaints of abdominal cramps, weight gain, edema, dyspnea, palpitations, angina, fatigue, or increased pallor may indicate that the client is experiencing cardiac problems and further assessment is indicated.
6. Monitor weights. Observe for evidence of heat intolerance and excessive weight loss and report if evident.
7. Note agent prescribed and monitor client. Thyroid extracts from hog or sheep do not have as predictable a response as the synthetic agents and you may see more reactions with these. Also, animal derivatives are less stable and will degrade with exposure to moisture.

Client/Family Teaching

1. Stress that the drug must be taken only while the client is under medical supervision and that it must be taken for life.
2. Side effects of the medication may not appear for 4–6 weeks after the start of therapy. Therefore, explain to clients that they should report any new signs or symptoms. The same is true if the dosage of drug is increased.
3. Instruct client to maintain a record of BP, pulse, and weight for review at each visit, to evaluate effectiveness of drug therapy.
4. Any excessive weight loss, palpitations, leg cramps, nervousness, or insomnia requires immediate reporting, as dosage may be too high. Provide a printed list of the symptoms that require immediate medical attention and a number to call to report these events.
5. If the client has diabetes, explain that thyroid preparations may require adjustment of the dosage of insulin. Therefore, it is important to monitor the finger sticks closely and to report any significant changes in glucose levels.
6. Note that certain foods, such as cabbage, turnips, pears, and peaches, are goitrogenic and may alter the requirements for thyroid hormone. Provide a list of such foods and have the dietitian discuss diet and assist with meal planning.
7. Thyroid hormones increase the client's toxicity to iodine. Therefore explain the need to avoid foods high in iodine (dried kelp, iodized salt, saltwater fish/shellfish), multivitamins, dentifrices, and other nonprescription medications containing iodine.
8. Have the dietitian counsel clients regarding diet so they will select foods according to the increased energy demands resulting from the medication therapy.
9. Thyroid preparations potentiate the action of anticoagulants; therefore, if the client is also receiving anticoagulant therapy, explain the importance of reporting any excessive bruising or bleeding.

10. Female clients should keep a record of their menstrual periods and report any significant changes.
11. Take the thyroid medication in a single morning dose to reduce the likelihood of insomnia.
12. Do not substitute or change brands of medication without approval.
13. Advise that children may experience temporary hair loss.
14. Report for all scheduled follow-up visits and lab tests.

Evaluate

- Evidence that appropriate weight and normal sleep patterns are maintained
- Laboratory confirmation that thyroid function studies are within desired range
- Promotion of normal metabolism as evidenced by ↑ mental alertness, improvement in hair and skin condition, normal growth and development, normal HR, and bowel function

Levothyroxine sodium (t_4)

Pregnancy Category: A

Eltroxin ✱, Levo-T, Levothroid, Levoxyl, PMS-Levothyroxine Sodium, Synthroid, L-Thyroxine Sodium **(Rx)**

See also *Thyroid Drugs,* Chapter 66.

How Supplied: *Powder for injection:* 0.2 mg, 0.5 mg; *Tablet:* 0.025 mg, 0.05 mg, 0.075 mg, 0.088 mg, 0.1 mg, 0.112 mg, 0.125 mg, 0.137 mg, 0.15 mg, 0.175 mg, 0.2 mg, 0.3 mg, 0.5 mg

Action/Kinetics: Levothyroxine is the synthetic sodium salt of the levoisomer of T_4 (tetraiodothyronine). Levothyroxine from the GI tract is incomplete and variable, especially when taken with food. This hormone has a slower onset but a longer duration than sodium liothyronine. It is more active on a weight basis than thyroid. Is usually the drug of choice. Effect is predictable as thyroid content is standard. **Time to peak therapeutic effect:** 3–4 weeks. **t½:** 6–7 days in a euthyroid person, 9–10 days in a hypothyroid client, and 3–4 days in a hyperthyroid client. Is 99% protein bound. **Duration:** 1–3 weeks after withdrawal of chronic therapy. *NOTE:* All levothyroxine products are not bioequivalent; thus, changing brands is not recommended.

Dosage

- **Tablets**

Mild hypothyroidism.

Adults, initial: 50 mcg once daily; **then,** increase by 25–50 mcg q 2–3 weeks until desired clinical response is attained; **maintenance, usual:** 75–125 mcg/day (although doses up to 200 mcg/day may be required in some clients).

Severe hypothyroidism.

Adults, initial: 12.5–25 mcg once daily; **then,** increase dose, as necessary, in increments of 25 mcg at 2–3-week intervals.

Hypothyroidism.

Pediatric, 10 years and older: 2–3 mcg/kg once daily until the adult daily dose (usually 150 mcg) is reached. **6–10 years of age:** 4–5 mcg/kg/day or 100–150 mcg once daily. **1–5 years of age:** 3–5 mcg/kg/day or 75–100 mcg once daily. **6–23 months of age:** 5–6 mcg/kg/day or 50–75 mcg once daily. **Less than 6 months of age:** 5–6 mcg/kg/day or 25–50 mcg once daily.

- **IM, IV**

Myxedematous coma without heart disease.

Adults, initial: 200–500 mcg IV, even in geriatric clients. If there is no response in 24 hr, 100–300 mcg may be given on the second day. Smaller daily doses should be given until client can tolerate PO medication.

Hypothyroidism.

Adults: 50–100 mcg once daily; **pediatric, IV, IM:** A dose of 75% of the usual PO pediatric dose should be given.

Administration/Storage

1. Transfer from liothyronine to levothyroxine: administer replacement

drug for several days before discontinuing liothyronine. Transfer from levothyroxine to liothyronine: discontinue levothyroxine before starting client on low daily dose of liothyronine.
2. Prepare the solution for injection immediately before administration.
3. Add the prescribed amount of NSS to the powder and shake the solution until it is clear (usually 500 mcg in 5 mL NSS). Administer at a rate of 100 mcg over 1 min.
4. Discard any unused portion of the IV medication.
5. Do not mix with other IV infusion solutions.

NURSING CONSIDERATIONS

See also *Nursing Considerations* for *Thyroid Drugs,* Chapter 66.

Assessment

1. Note age of the client. Elderly clients are likely to have undetected cardiac problems. Therefore, a baseline ECG should be taken prior to initiating drug therapy.
2. If the client is pregnant, she must continue taking thyroid preparations throughout the pregnancy.
3. Document height, weight, and psychomotor development in children.

Client/Family Teaching

1. Advise not to switch brands because bioavailability may change.
2. Do not take with food since this may interfere with absorption.
3. Report any persistent headaches, increased HR (hold if resting HR is greater than 100), chest pain, diarrhea, more than 2 lb/week weight loss, and excessive sweating.
4. Stress that the drug is not a cure for hypothyroidism and will have to be taken for client's lifetime.

Evaluate

- Promotion of normal metabolism
- ↑ Levels of T_3 and T_4

Liothyronine sodium (T_3)

(lye-oh-**THIGH**-roh-neen)

Pregnancy Category: A
Cytomel, Sodium-L-Triiodothyronine, Triostat **(Rx)**

See also *Thyroid Drugs,* Chapter 66.

How Supplied: *Injection:* 10 mcg/mL; *Tablet:* 5 mcg, 25 mcg, 50 mcg

Action/Kinetics: Synthetic sodium salt of levoisomer of T_3. Liothyronine has more predictable effects due to standard hormone content. From 15 to 37.5 mcg is equivalent to about 60 mg of desiccated thyroid. It may be preferred when a rapid effect or rapidly reversible effect is required. Drug has a rapid onset, which may result in difficulty in controlling the dosage as well as the possibility of cardiac side effects and changes in metabolic demands. However, its short duration allows quick adjustment of dosage and helps control overdosage. **t½:** 24 hr for euthyroid clients, approximately 34 hr in hypothyroid clients, and approximately 14 hr in hyperthyroid clients. **Duration:** Up to 72 hr. Is 99% protein bound.

Dosage

- **Tablets**

Mild hypothyroidism.

Adults, individualized, initial: 25 mcg/day. Increase by 12.5–25 mcg q 1–2 weeks until satisfactory response has been obtained. **Usual maintenance:** 25–75 mcg/day (100 mcg may be required in some clients). Use lower initial dosage (5 mcg/day) for the elderly, children, and clients with CV disease. Increase only by 5-mcg increments.

Myxedema.

Adults, initial: 5 mcg/day increased by 5–10 mcg/day q 1–2 weeks until 25 mcg/day is reached; **then,** increase q 1–2 weeks by 12.5–50 mcg. **Usual maintenance:** 50–100 mcg/day.

Simple (nontoxic) goiter.

Adults, initial: 5 mcg/day; **then,** increase q 1–2 weeks by 5–10 mcg until 25 mcg/day is reached; **then,** dose can be increased by 12.5–25 mcg/week until the maintenance dose of 50–100 mcg/day is reached (usual is 75 mcg/day).

T_3 suppression test.
75–100 mcg/day for 7 days followed by a repeat of the I^{131} thyroid uptake test (a 50% or greater suppression of uptake indicates a normal thyroid-pituitary axis).

Congenital hypothyroidism.
Adults and children, initial: 5 mcg/day; **then,** increase by 5 mcg/day q 3–4 days until the desired effect is achieved. Approximately 20 mcg/day may be sufficient for infants a few months of age while children 1 year of age may require 50 mcg/day. Children above 3 years may require the full adult dose.

- **IV Only**

Myxedema coma, precoma.
Adults, initial: 25–50 mcg. Base subsequent doses on continuous monitoring of client's clinical status and response. Doses should be given at least 4 hr, and no more than 12 hr, apart. Total daily doses of 65 mcg in initial days of therapy are associated with a lower incidence of mortality. In cases of known CV disease, an initial dose of 10–20 mcg should be given.

Administration/Storage
1. *Transfer from other thyroid preparations to liothyronine:* Discontinue old preparation before starting on low daily dose of liothyronine. *Transfer from liothyronine to another thyroid preparation:* Start therapy with replacement drug several days prior to complete withdrawal of sodium liothyronine.
2. If symptoms of hyperthyroidism are noted, the drug can be withdrawn for 2–3 days after which therapy can be reinstituted, but at a lower dose.
3. A *Cytomel* injection kit is available for the emergency treatment of myxedema coma.

Additional Contraindications: Use of liothyronine is not recommended in children with cretinism because there is some question about whether the hormone crosses the blood-brain barrier.

NURSING CONSIDERATIONS

See also *Nursing Considerations* for *Thyroid Drugs,* Chapter 66.
Evaluate: Desired thyroid hormone replacement.

Liotrix

(LYE-oh-trix)
Pregnancy Category: A
Thyrolar **(Rx)**

See also *Thyroid Drugs,* Chapter 66.
How Supplied: *Tablet:* 15 mg, 30 mg, 60 mg, 120 mg, 180 mg
General Statement: Mixture of synthetic levothyroxine sodium (T_4) and liothyronine (T_3). The mixture contains the products in a 4:1 ratio by weight and in a 1:1 ratio by biologic activity. The two commercial preparations contain slightly different amounts of each component. Because of this discrepancy, a switch from one preparation to the other must be made cautiously. Liotrix has standard hormone content; thus, the effect is predictable.

Dosage

- **Tablets**

Hypothyroidism.
Adults and children, initial: 50 mcg levothyroxine and 12.5 mcg liothyronine (Thyrolar) or 60 mcg levothyroxine and 15 mcg liothyronine (Euthroid) daily; **then,** at monthly intervals, increments of like amounts can be made until the desired effect is achieved. **Usual maintenance:** 50–100 mcg of levothyroxine and 12.5–25 mcg liothyronine daily.

Congenital hypothyroidism.
Children, 0–6 months: 8–10 mcg T_4/kg/day (25–50 mcg/day); **6–12 months:** 6–8 mcg T_4/kg/day (50–75 mcg/day); **1–5 years:** 5–6 mcg T_4/kg/day (75–100 mcg/day); **6–12 years:** 4–5 mcg T_4/kg/day (100–150 mcg/day); **over 12 years:** 2–3 mcg T_4/kg/day (over 150 mcg/day).

Administration/Storage
1. The initial dose for geriatric clients should be ¼–½ the usual

adult dose; this dose can be doubled q 6–8 weeks until the desired effect is attained.
2. In children, dosing increments should be made q 2 weeks until the desired response has been attained.
3. Thyroid function tests should always be done before initiating dosage changes.
4. Administer as a single dose before breakfast.
5. Protect tablets from light, heat, and moisture.
6. Due to differences in the amounts of hormones between Euthroid and Thyrolar, once started on a particular brand, the client should not be switched.

NURSING CONSIDERATIONS

See also *Nursing Considerations* for *Thyroid Drugs,* Chapter 66.
Evaluate: ↑ T_3 and T_4 levels during thyroid hormone replacement therapy.

Thyroid, desiccated

(THIGH-royd)
Pregnancy Category: A
Armour Thyroid, S-P-T, Thyrar, Thyroid Strong **(Rx)**

See also *Thyroid Drugs,* Chapter 66.
How Supplied: *Capsule:* 60 mg, 120 mg, 180 mg, 300 mg; *Tablet:* 15 mg, 30 mg, 60 mg, 65 mg, 90 mg, 120 mg, 130 mg, 180 mg, 240 mg, 300 mg
Action/Kinetics: These products are comprised of desiccated thyroid glands from bovine and porcine sources. Due to variable content of both levothyroxine and liothyronine in the product, fluctuations in plasma levels of these hormones will be observed. The drug has a slow onset of action that makes it unsuitable for the treatment of myxedematous coma. *NOTE:* Thyroid Strong is 50% stronger than thyroid USP (each grain is equivalent to 1.5 grains of thyroid USP).

Dosage

• **Tablets**

Hypothyroidism without myxedema, pediatric hypothyroidism.

Adults, children, initial: 30 mg/day; **then,** increase by 15 mg q 2–3 weeks until the desired effect is reached. **Usual maintenance:** 60–120 mg/day.

Myxedema, hypothyroidism with CV disease, cretinism or severe hypothyroidism.

Adults, children, initial: 15 mg/day; **then,** increase to 30 mg after 2 weeks and to 60 mg/day after an additional 2 weeks. The client should be evaluated carefully after 30 and 60 days of treatment. If required, the dose can be further increased to 120 mg/day. **Usual maintenance:** 50–120 mg/day.

Congenital hypothyroidism.

Over 12 years of age: Over 90 mg/day (1.2–1.8 mg/kg/day); **6-12 years:** 60–90 mg/day (2.4–3 mg/kg/day); **1–5 years:** 45–60 mg/day (3–3.6 mg/kg/day); **6–12 months:** 30–45 mg/day (3.6–4.8 mg/kg/day); **up to 6 months:** 15–30 mg/day (4.8–6 mg/kg/day).

Administration/Storage
1. Store protected from moisture and light.
2. In geriatric clients, the initial dose should be 7.5–15 mg/day, which can then be doubled q 6–8 weeks until desired effect has been attained.
3. Transfer from liothyronine: Start thyroid several days before withdrawal. When transferring from thyroid, discontinue thyroid before starting with low daily dose of replacement drug.

NURSING CONSIDERATIONS

See also *Nursing Considerations* for *Thyroid Drugs,* Chapter 66.

Client/Family Teaching
1. Take in the morning (at the same time) in order to prevent insomnia.
2. Explain that drug does not cure disease and that drug must be taken lifelong as a replacement.
3. Advise parents that children may experience hair loss; this is usually only temporary.
4. Stress the importance of scheduled appointments to assess child for proper development.

5. Do not substitute medications without approval as response may vary.

Evaluate

- ↓ S&S of hypothyroidism evidenced by weight loss, ↑ HR, ↑ energy levels, and improved texture of skin and hair
- T_3 and T_4 levels within desired range

Thyrotropin

(thigh-roh-**TROH**-pin)
Pregnancy Category: C
Thytropar, Thyroid Stimulating Hormone, TSH **(Rx)**

How Supplied: *Injection:* 10 IU/vial
Action/Kinetics: Highly purified TSH from bovine pituitary glands. Thyrotropin administration results in increased iodine uptake by the thyroid gland and increased formation and release of thyroid hormone. **Onset:** Within a few minutes. **Peak effect:** 1–2 days. **Duration:** Drug effects are terminated after the drug is withdrawn.
Use: Diagnostic agent to evaluate thyroid function.

Dosage

- **IM, SC**

Administer 10 IU/day for 1–3 days followed by radioiodine uptake study within 24 hr. *NOTE:* No response will occur if there is thyroid failure; however, a significant response will occur in pituitary failure.
Administration/Storage: The reconstituted solution may be stored in the refrigerator but for no longer than 2 weeks.
Contraindications: Untreated Addison's disease, coronary thrombosis.
Special Concerns: Safe use during lactation or in children has not been established. Use with caution in clients with cardiac disease who cannot withstand stress.
Side Effects: *CV:* Tachycardia, hypotension. *GI:* N&V. *Miscellaneous:* Swelling of thyroid gland, urticaria, headache, ***anaphylaxis.***

NURSING CONSIDERATIONS

See also *Nursing Considerations* for *Thyroid Drugs,* Chapter 66.

Assessment

1. Document any history or evidence of CAD.
2. Assess for any evidence of hypopituitarism or untreated Addison's disease, which would preclude drug therapy.

Interventions

1. Monitor VS and observe closely for evidence of allergic reactions.
2. Document and report immediately any evidence of urticaria, swelling of the thyroid gland, headaches, and symptoms of anaphylaxis.
3. Normal thyroid tissue responds to thyrotropin by ↑ uptake of iodine and by releasing T_3 and T_4. This drug therefore tests the ability of the thyroid to respond to appropriate stimulation.

Evaluate: Desired thyroid function evaluation and the diagnosis of hypothyroidism (if present).

ANTITHYROID DRUGS

See also the following individual entries:

Methimazole (Thiamazole)
Propylthiouracil

Action/Kinetics: Antithyroid drugs include thiouracil derivatives and large doses of iodide. These drugs inhibit (partially or completely) the production of thyroid hormones by the thyroid gland. The drugs act by preventing the incorporation of iodide into tyrosine and coupling of iodotyrosines. Since these agents do not affect release or activity of preformed hormone, it may take several weeks for the therapeutic effect to become established.
Uses: Hyperthyroidism; prior to surgery or radiotherapy. Adjunct in treatment of thyrotoxicosis or thyroid storm. Propylthiouracil is also used to reduce mortality due to alcoholic liver disease.

Contraindication: Lactation (may cause hypothyroidism in the infant).
Special Concerns: Use with caution in the presence of CV disease. PT should be monitored during therapy as propylthiouracil may cause hypoprothrombinemia and bleeding.
Side Effects: *Hematologic:* ***Agranulocytosis,*** thrombocytopenia, granulocytopenia, hypoprothrombinemia, ***aplastic anemia,*** leukopenia. *GI:* N&V, taste loss, epigastric pain, sialadenopathy. *CNS:* Headache, paresthesia, drowsiness, vertigo, depression, CNS stimulation. *Dermatologic:* Skin rash, urticaria, alopecia, skin pigmentation, pruritus, exfoliative dermatitis, erythema nodosum. *Miscellaneous:* Jaundice, arthralgia, myalgia, neuritis, edema, lymphadenopathy, vasculitis, lupus-like syndrome, drug fever, periarteritis, hepatitis, nephritis, interstitial pneumonitis, insulin autoimmune syndrome resulting in hypoglycemic coma.

Symptoms of Overdose: N&V, headache, fever, pruritus, epigastric distress, arthralgia, pancytopenia, ***agranulocytosis*** (most serious). Rarely, exfoliative dermatitis, hepatitis, neuropathies, CNS stimulation or depression.

NURSING CONSIDERATIONS

Administration/Storage

1. The medication should be taken q 8 hr around the clock.
2. *Treatment of Overdose:* Maintain a patent airway and support ventilation and perfusion. Very carefully monitor and maintain VS, blood gases, and serum electrolytes. Monitor bone marrow function.

Assessment

1. Document onset of illness, symptoms experienced, and the underlying cause.
2. Note if the client is taking any medications that may interact unfavorably with the antithyroid drug and document.
3. If the client is female and of childbearing age, determine if pregnant.
4. Ensure that baseline PT, CBC, and thyroid function studies have been performed and monitor.
5. Assess the thyroid gland and note any enlargement, pain, asymmetry, or nodules.

Interventions

1. Monitor VS, I&O, and weights during initial drug therapy.
2. Note any client complaint of unusual bleeding, nausea, loss of taste, or epigastric pain as these symptoms should be reported.
3. Document the presence of skin rashes, urticaria, alopecia, changes in skin pigmentation, or pruritus and report.

Client/Family Teaching

1. Advise that it takes 6–12 weeks for the drug to produce the full effect. Stress that the drug must be taken regularly and exactly as directed. Hyperthyroidism may recur if the drug is not taken properly.
2. Review the symptoms of hyperthyroidism or thyrotoxicosis (palpitations, increased HR, nervousness, sleeplessness, sweating, diarrhea, weight loss, fever) and advise client to report if symptoms resurface or are persistent.
3. Review the symptoms of hypothyroidism (weak, listless, tired, headache, dry skin, cold intolerance, constipation) and advise client to report as dosage may require adjustment.
4. Report any sore throat, enlargement of the cervical lymph nodes, GI disturbances, fever, rash, or jaundice as these symptoms may necessitate either a reduction of the dosage or withdrawal of the drug.
5. Discuss the potential loss of taste perception. If this occurs, advise clients to increase the use of herbs and nonsodium seasonings.
6. Review symptoms of iodism (cold symptoms, skin lesions, stomatitis, GI upset, metallic taste) and advise client to report.
7. Identify the dietary sources of iodine (iodized salt, shellfish, turnips, cabbage, kale) that may need to be omitted from the diet.
8. Explain that if the drug is taken as ordered for 1 or more years, more than half the clients achieve a permanent remission.

9. Stress the importance of reporting for follow-up lab studies and medical evaluations to determine the response to drug therapy.
10. Advise client to carry identification at all times, listing medical problems and medications currently prescribed.

Special Concerns: Children must be checked every 6 months for appropriate growth and development. This should be plotted on a graph.

Evaluate

- Laboratory confirmation that thyroid function studies are within desired range
- Clinical evidence of the control of symptoms associated with hyperthyroidism
- ↓ Vascularity and friability of the thyroid gland in preparation for surgery
- ↓ Mortality in clients with alcoholic liver disease

Methimazole (Thiamazole)

(meth-**IM**-ah-zohl)
Pregnancy Category: D
Tapazole **(Rx)**

See also *Antithyroid Drugs,* Chapter 66.

How Supplied: *Tablet:* 5 mg, 10 mg

Action/Kinetics: Onset is more rapid but effect is less consistent than that of propylthiouracil. Bioavailability may be affected by food. **t½:** 4–14 hr. **Onset:** 10–20 days. **Time to peak effect:** 2–10 weeks. **t½:** 6–13 hr. Crosses the placenta; high levels appear in breast milk. Metabolized in the liver and excreted through the kidneys (7% unchanged).

Dosage

- **Tablets**

Mild hyperthyroidism.

Adults, initial: 15 mg/day.

Moderately severe hyperthyroidism.

Adults, initial: 30–40 mg/day.

Severe hyperthyroidism.

Adults, initial: 60 mg/day. For hyperthyroidism, the daily dose is usually given in three equal doses 8 hr apart. **Maintenance:** 5–15 mg/day as a single dose or divided into two doses. **Pediatric:** 0.4 mg/kg given once daily or divided into two doses; **maintenance:** 0.2 mg/kg. Alternatively, **initial:** 0.5–0.7 mg/kg/day (15–20 mg/m²/day in three divided doses; **maintenance:** ⅓–⅔ initial dose when client is euthyroid up to a maximum of 30 mg/day.

Thyrotoxic crisis.

Adults, 15–20 mg/4 hr during the first day as an adjunct to other treatments.

Special Concerns: Incidence of hepatic toxicity may be greater than for propylthiouracil.

NURSING CONSIDERATIONS

See also *Nursing Considerations* for *Antithyroid Drugs,* Chapter 66.

Assessment

1. Document indications for therapy and type and onset of symptoms.
2. Obtain baseline CBC and thyroid function studies.

Interventions

1. Assess for changes in sensation of the extremities. For example, determine if the client has any strange, tingling sensations of the fingers and toes as some clients develop paresthesias.
2. If 40 years of age, monitor for agranulocytosis. Question client about sore throats, fever, chills, and unexplained bleeding.
3. Report any evidence of hair loss.

Client/Family Teaching

1. May take the medication with a snack to reduce gastric irritation. Report if GI upset persists.
2. Take the medication as prescribed at evenly spaced intervals and with evenly spaced doses throughout the day.
3. Report any unexpected symptoms immediately. The effects of the medication may not be evident for weeks after the therapy begins, and

the dosage of drug may require adjusting.

Evaluate

• Suppression of thyroid hormone secretion with the promotion of normal metabolism

• Serum thyroid levels within desired range

Propylthiouracil

(proh-pill-thigh-oh-**YOUR**-ah-sill)

Pregnancy Category: D

Propyl-Thyracil ✱ **(Rx)**

See also *Antithyroid Drugs,* Chapter 66.

How Supplied: *Tablet:* 50 mg

Action/Kinetics: May be preferred for treatment of thyroid storm as the drug inhibits peripheral conversion of thyroxine to triiodothyronine. Rapidly absorbed from the GI tract. **Duration:** 2–3 hr. **t½:** 1–2 hr. **Onset:** 10–20 days. **Time to peak effect:** 2–10 weeks. Eighty percent is protein bound. Metabolized by the liver and excreted through the kidneys.

Dosage

• **Tablets**

Hyperthyroidism.

Adults, initial: 300 mg/day (up to 900 mg/day may be required in some clients with severe hyperthyroidism) given as one to four divided doses; **maintenance, usual:** 100–150 mg/day. **Pediatric, 6–10 years, initial:** 50–150 mg/day in one to four divided doses; **over 10 years, initial:** 150–300 mg/day in one to four divided doses. Maintenance for all pediatric use is based on response. **Alternative dose for children, initial:** 5–7 mg/kg/day (150–200 mg/m^2/day) in divided doses q 8 hr; **maintenance:** ⅓–⅔ the initial dose when the client is euthyroid.

Thyrotoxic crisis.

Adults: 200–400 mg q 4 hr during the first day as an adjunct to other treatments.

Neonatal thyrotoxicosis.

10 mg/kg daily in divided doses.

Special Concern: Incidence of vasculitis is increased.

Drug Interactions: Propylthiouracil may produce hypoprothrombinemia, adding to the effect of anticoagulants.

NURSING CONSIDERATIONS

See also *Nursing Considerations* for *Antithyroid Drugs,* Chapter 66.

Client/Family Teaching

1. Take only as directed. May take with meals to decrease GI upset.
2. Review dietary sources of iodine (shellfish, iodized salt) that should be avoided.
3. Any fever, sore throat, enlarged cervical lymph nodes, or rash should be reported immediately.
4. Alert provider to any evidence of unusual bruising or bleeding and report for periodic CBC as scheduled.
5. Review S&S of hypothyroidism (cold intolerance, increased fatigue, mental depression) and advise to report if evident.

Evaluate

• Promotion of normal metabolism with evidence of ↑ weight, ↓ sweating, and ↓ HR

• Suppression of thyroid hormones with ↓ thyroid levels after 3 weeks of therapy

CHAPTER SIXTY-SEVEN

Corticosteroids

See also the following individual entries:

Beclomethasone Dipropionate
Betamethasone
Betamethasone Benzoate
Betamethasone Dipropionate
Betamethasone Sodium Phosphate
Betamethasone Sodium Phosphate and Betamethasone Acetate
Betamethasone Valerate
Corticotropin Injection
Corticotropin Repository Injection
Cortisone Acetate
Cosyntropin
Dexamethasone
Dexamethasone Acetate
Dexamethasone Sodium Phosphate
Fludrocortisone Acetate
Flunisolide
Hydrocortisone
Hydrocortisone Acetate
Hydrocortisone Butyrate
Hydrocortisone Cypionate
Hydrocortisone Sodium Phosphate
Hydrocortisone Sodium Succinate
Hydrocortisone Valerate
Methylprednisolone
Methylprednisolone Acetate
Methylprednisolone Sodium Succinate
Prednisolone
Prednisolone Acetate
Prednisolone Acetate and Prednisolone Sodium Phosphate
Prednisolone Sodium Phosphate
Prednisolone Tebutate
Prednisone
Triamcinolone
Triamcinolone Acetonide
Triamcinolone Diacetate
Triamcinolone Hexacetonide

Action/Kinetics: The hormones of the adrenal gland influence many metabolic pathways and all organ systems and are essential for survival.

The release of corticosteroids is controlled by hormones such as corticotropin-releasing factor, produced by the hypothalamus, and ACTH (corticotropin), produced by the anterior pituitary.

The natural corticosteroids play an important role in most major metabolic processes. They have the following effects:

1. **Carbohydrate metabolism.** Deposition of glucose as glycogen in the liver and the conversion of glycogen to glucose when needed. Gluconeogenesis (i.e., the transformation of protein into glucose).
2. **Protein metabolism.** The stimulation of protein loss from many organs (catabolism). This is characterized by a negative nitrogen balance.
3. **Fat metabolism.** The deposition of fatty tissue in facial, abdominal, and shoulder regions.
4. **Water and electrolyte balance.** Alteration of glomerular filtration rate; increased sodium and consequently fluid retention. Also affects the excretion rate of potassium, calcium, and phosphorus. Urinary excretion rate of creatine and uric acid increases.

According to their chemical structure and chief physiologic effect, the corticosteroids fall into two subgroups, which have considerable functional overlap.

1. Those, like cortisone and hydrocortisone, that mainly regulate the metabolic pathways involving protein, carbohydrate, and fat. This

group is often referred to as *glucocorticoids*. Glucocorticoids are qualitatively similar. Differences between these agents are due to duration of action and half-life (see individual agents).

2. Those, like aldosterone and desoxycorticosterone, that are more specifically involved in electrolyte and water balance. These are often referred to as *mineralocorticoids*. Hormones with mineralocorticoid activity result in reabsorption of sodium (and therefore water retention) and enhanced potassium and hydrogen excretion. Substances such as cortisone and hydrocortisone, although classified as glucocorticoids, possess significant mineralocorticoid activity.

Therapeutically, the corticosteroids are used for a variety of purposes; a distinction must be made between physiologic doses used for replacement therapy and pharmacologic doses used to treat inflammatory and other disease states. Many slightly modified synthetic variants are available today that possess glucocorticoid but minimal or no mineralocorticoid activity.

The hormones have a marked anti-inflammatory effect because of their ability to inhibit prostaglandin synthesis. These agents also inhibit accumulation of macrophages and leukocytes at sites of inflammation as well as inhibit phagocytosis and lysosomal enzyme release. They aid the organism in coping with various stressful situations (trauma, severe illness). The immunosuppressant effect is thought to be due to a reduction of the number of T lymphocytes, monocytes, and eosinophils. Corticosteroids also decrease binding of immunoglobulin to receptors on the cell surface and inhibit the synthesis and/or release of interleukins which, in turn, decrease T-lymphocyte blastogenesis and reduce the primary immune response.

Uses: When used for anti-inflammatory or immunosuppressant therapy, the corticosteroid should possess minimal mineralocorticoid activity. Therapy with glucocorticoids is not curative and in many situations should be considered as adjunctive rather than primary therapy.

1. **Replacement therapy.** Acute and chronic adrenal insufficiency, including Addison's disease, congenital adrenal hyperplasia, adrenal insufficiency secondary to anterior pituitary insufficiency. However, not all drugs can be used for replacement therapy; some lack glucocorticoid effects, whereas others lack mineralocorticoid effects. For replacement therapy, drugs must possess both effects.

2. **Rheumatic disorders.** Rheumatoid arthritis (including juveniles), ankylosing spondylitis, acute and subacute bursitis, acute nonspecific tenosynovitis, acute gouty arthritis, psoriatic arthritis, posttraumatic osteoarthritis, synovitis of osteoarthritis, epicondylitis.

3. **Collagen diseases.** Including SLE, acute rheumatic carditis, polymyositis.

4. **Allergic diseases.** Control of severe allergic conditions refractory to conventional treatment as serum sickness, drug hypersensitivity reactions, anaphylaxis, urticarial transfusion reactions, acute noninfectious laryngeal edema.

5. **Respiratory diseases.** Including bronchial asthma (and status asthmaticus), symptomatic sarcoidosis, seasonal or perennial rhinitis, berylliosis, aspiration pneumonitis, fulminating or disseminated pulmonary tuberculosis (with appropriate antitubercular therapy), Loeffler's syndrome refractory to other treatment.

6. **Ocular diseases.** Severe acute and chronic allergic and inflammatory conditions including conjunctivitis, keratitis, herpes zoster ophthalmicus, iritis, iridocyclitis, chorioretinitis, diffuse posterior uveitis and choroiditis, optic neuritis, allergic corneal marginal ulcers, sympathetic ophthalmia, and anterior segment inflammation.

7. **Dermatologic diseases.** Including severe erythema multiforme (Stevens-Johnson syndrome), exfolia-

tive dermatitis, mycosis fungoides, severe seborrheic dermatitis, bullous dermatitis herpetiformis, severe psoriasis, angioedema or urticaria, contact dermatitis, atopic dermatitis, pemphigus.

8. **Diseases of the intestinal tract.** To assist client through crises of chronic ulcerative colitis, regional enteritis, intractable sprue.

9. **Nervous system.** Acute exacerbations of multiple sclerosis. Short-term treatment with high doses of methylprednisolone and prednisone in clients with optic neuritis (often the first sign of multiple sclerosis) may prevent full-blown multiple sclerosis for 2 years.

10. **Malignancies.** Including leukemias and lymphomas in adults and acute leukemia in children.

11. **Nephrotic syndrome.** To induce diuresis or remission of proteinuria due to lupus erythematosus or of the idiopathic type.

12. **Hematologic diseases.** Including acquired hemolytic anemia, RBC anemia, idiopathic and secondary thrombocytopenic purpura in adults, congenital hypoplastic anemia.

13. **Intra-articular or soft tissue administration.** To treat acute episodes of synovitis of osteoarthritis, rheumatoid arthritis, acute gouty arthritis, epicondylitis, acute nonspecific tenosynovitis, posttraumatic osteoarthritis.

14. **Intralesional administration.** To treat keloids, psoriatic plaques, granuloma annulare, lichen simplex chronicus, discoid lupus erythematosus, cystic tumors of an aponeurosis or ganglia, lesions of lichen planus, necrobiosis lipoidica diabeticorum, alopecia areata.

15. **Miscellaneous.** Septic shock (use controversial), trichinosis with neurologic or myocardial involvement, tuberculosis meningitis with subarachnoid block or impending block (with appropriate antitubercular therapy).

Contraindications: Corticosteroids are contraindicated if infection is suspected because these drugs may mask infections. Also peptic ulcer, psychoses, acute glomerulonephritis, herpes simplex infections of the eye, vaccinia or varicella, the exanthematous diseases, Cushing's syndrome, active tuberculosis, myasthenia gravis. Recent intestinal anastomoses, CHF or other cardiac disease, hypertension, systemic fungal infections, open-angle glaucoma. Also, hyperlipidemia, hyperthyroidism or hypothyroidism, osteoporosis, myasthenia gravis, tuberculosis. Lactation (if high doses are used).

Topical application in the treatment of eye disorders is contraindicated in dendritic keratitis, vaccinia, chickenpox, or other viral disease that may involve the conjunctiva or cornea. Also tuberculosis and fungal or acute purulent infections of the eye. Topical treatment of the ear is contraindicated in aural fungal infections and perforated eardrum. Topical use in dermatology is contraindicated in tuberculosis of the skin, herpes simplex, vaccinia, varicella, and infectious conditions in the absence of anti-infective agents.

Special Concerns: Glucocorticoids should be used with caution in the presence of diabetes mellitus, hypertension, chronic nephritis, thrombophlebitis, convulsive disorders, infectious diseases, renal or hepatic insufficiency, pregnancy. Chronic use of corticosteroids may inhibit the growth and development of children or adolescents. Pediatric clients are also at greater risk for developing cataracts, osteoporosis, avascular necrosis of the femoral heads, and glaucoma. Geriatric clients are more likely to develop hypertension and osteoporosis (especially postmenopausal women).

Side Effects: Small physiologic doses given as replacement therapy or short-term high-dosage therapy during emergencies rarely cause side effects. Prolonged therapy may cause a Cushing-like syndrome with atrophy of the adrenal cortex and subsequent adrenocortical insufficiency. A steroid withdrawal syndrome may occur following prolonged use; symptoms include anorexia, N&V, lethargy, headache, fever, joint pain, desquamation, myalgia, weight loss, hypotension.

Fluid and electrolyte: Edema, hypokalemic alkalosis, hypokalemia, hypocalcemia, hypotension or shock-like reaction, hypertension, CHF. *Musculoskeletal:* Muscle wasting, muscle pain or weakness, osteoporosis, spontaneous fractures including vertebral compression fractures and fractures of long bones, tendon rupture, aseptic necrosis of femoral and humeral heads. *GI:* N&V, anorexia or increased appetite, diarrhea or constipation, abdominal distention, pancreatitis, gastric irritation, ulcerative esophagitis. ***Development or exacerbation of peptic ulcers with the possibility of perforation and hemorrhage; perforation of the small and large bowel,*** especially in inflammatory bowel disease. *Endocrine:* Cushing's syndrome (e.g., central obesity, moonface, buffalo hump, enlargement of supraclavicular fat pads), amenorrhea, postmenopausal bleeding, menstrual irregularities, decreased glucose tolerance, hyperglycemia, glycosuria, increased insulin or sulfonylurea requirement in diabetics, development of diabetes mellitus, negative nitrogen balance due to protein catabolism, suppression of growth in children, secondary adrenocortical and pituitary unresponsiveness (especially during periods of stress). *CNS/Neurologic:* Headache, vertigo, insomnia, restlessness, increased motor activity, ischemic neuropathy, EEG abnormalities, ***seizures,*** pseudotumor cerebri. Also, euphoria, mood swings, depression, anxiety, personality changes, psychoses. *CV:* Thromboembolism, thrombophlebitis, ECG changes (due to potassium deficiency), fat embolism, necrotizing angiitis, cardiac arrhythmias, ***myocardial rupture following recent MI,*** syncopal episodes. *Dermatologic:* Impaired wound healing, skin atrophy and thinning, petechiae, ecchymoses, erythema, purpura, striae, hirsutism, urticaria, ***angioneurotic edema,*** acneiform eruptions, allergic dermatitis, lupus erythematosus-like lesions, suppression of skin test reactions, perineal irritation. *Ophthalmic:* Glaucoma, posterior subcapsular cataracts, increased intraocular pressure, exophthalmos. *Miscellaneous:* Hypercholesterolemia, atherosclerosis, aggravation or masking of infections, leukocytosis, increased or decreased motility and number of spermatozoa.

In children: Suppression of linear growth; reversible pseudobrain tumor syndrome characterized by papilledema, oculomotor or abducens nerve paralysis, visual loss, or headache.

PARENTERAL USE: Sterile abscesses, Charcot-like arthropathy, subcutaneous and cutaneous atrophy, burning or tingling (especially in the perineal area following IV use), scarring, inflammation, paresthesia, induration, hyperpigmentation or hypopigmentation, blindness when used intralesionally around the face and head (rare), transient or delayed pain or soreness, nystagmus, ataxia, muscle twitching, hiccoughs, ***anaphylaxis with or without circulatory collapse, cardiac arrest, bronchospasm,*** arachnoiditis after intrathecal use, foreign body granulomatous reactions.

INTRA-ARTICULAR: Postinjection flare, Charcot-like arthropathy, tendon rupture, skin atrophy, facial flushing, osteonecrosis. Due to reduction in inflammation and pain, clients may overuse the joint.

INTRASPINAL: Aseptic, bacterial, chemical, cryptococcal, or tubercular meningitis; adhesive arachnoiditis, conus medullaris syndrome.

INTRAOCULAR: Application of corticosteroid preparations to the eye may reduce aqueous outflow and increase ocular pressure, thereby inducing or aggravating simple glaucoma. Ocular pressure therefore should be checked frequently in the elderly or in clients with glaucoma.

Stinging, burning, dendritic keratitis (herpes simplex), corneal perforation (especially when the drugs are used for diseases that cause corneal thinning). Posterior subcapsular cataracts, especially in children. Exophthalmos, secondary fungal or viral eye infections.

TOPICAL USE: Except when used over large areas, when the skin is broken, or with occlusive dressings, topically applied corticosteroids are not absorbed systemically in sufficiently large quantities to cause the side effects noted in the previous paragraphs. Topically applied corticosteroids, however, may cause atrophy of the epidermis, drying of the skin, or atrophy of the dermal collagen. When used on the face, the agents may cause diffuse thinning and homogenization of the collagen, epidermal thinning, and striae formation. Topical corticosteroids should be used cautiously, or not at all, for infected lesions, and in that case, the use of occlusive dressings is contraindicated. Occasionally, topical corticosteroids may cause a sensitization reaction, which necessitates discontinuation of the drug.

Symptoms of Overdose (continued use of large doses)–Cushing's syndrome: Acne, hypertension, moonface, striae, hirsutism, central obesity, ecchymoses, myopathy, sexual dysfunction, osteoporosis, diabetes, hyperlipidemia, increased susceptibility to infection, peptic ulcer, electrolyte and fluid imbalance. Acute toxicity or death is rare.

Drug Interactions

Acetaminophen / ↑ Risk of hepatotoxicity due to ↑ rate of formation of hepatotoxic acetaminophen metabolite

Alcohol / ↑ Risk of GI ulceration or hemorrhage

Amphotericin B / Corticosteroids ↑ K depletion caused by amphotericin B

Aminoglutethimide / ↓ Adrenal response to corticotropin

Anabolic steroids / ↑ Risk of edema

Antacids / ↓ Effect of corticosteroids due to ↓ absorption from GI tract

Antibiotics, broad-spectrum / Concomitant use may result in emergence of resistant strains, leading to severe infection

Anticholinergics / Combination ↑ intraocular pressure; will aggravate glaucoma

Anticoagulants, oral / ↓ Effect of anticoagulants by ↓ hypoprothrombinemia; also ↑ risk of hemorrhage due to vascular effects of corticosteroids

Anticholinesterases / Corticosteroids may ↓ effect of anticholinesterases when used in myasthenia gravis

Antidiabetic agents / Hyperglycemic effect of corticosteroids may necessitate an ↑ dose of antidiabetic agent

Asparaginase / ↑ Hyperglycemic effect of asparaginase and the risk of neuropathy and disturbances in erythropoiesis

Barbiturates / ↓ Effect of corticosteroids due to ↑ breakdown by liver

Bumetanide / Enhanced potassium loss due to potassium-losing properties of both drugs

Carbonic anhydrase inhibitors / Corticosteroids ↑ K depletion caused by carbonic anhydrase inhibitors

Cholestyramine / ↓ Effect of corticosteroids due to ↓ absorption from GI tract

Colestipol / ↓ Effect of corticosteroids due to ↓ absorption from GI tract

Contraceptives, oral / Estrogen ↑ anti-inflammatory effect of hydrocortisone by ↓ breakdown by liver

Cyclophosphoramide / ↑ Effect of cyclophosphoramide due to ↓ breakdown by liver

Cyclosporine / ↑ Effect of both drugs due to ↓ breakdown by liver

Digitalis glycosides / ↑ Chance of digitalis toxicity (arrhythmias) due to hypokalemia

Ephedrine / ↓ Effect of corticosteroids due to ↑ breakdown by liver

Estrogens / ↑ Anti-inflammatory effect of hydrocortisone by ↓ breakdown by liver
Ethacrynic acid / Enhanced potassium loss due to potassium-losing properties of both drugs
Folic acid / Requirements may ↑
Furosemide / Enhanced potassium loss due to potassium-losing properties of both drugs
Heparin / Ulcerogenic effects of corticosteroids may ↑ risk of hemorrhage
Immunosuppressant drugs / ↑ Risk of infection
Indomethacin / ↑ Chance of GI ulceration
Insulin / Hyperglycemic effect of corticosteroids may necessitate ↑ dose of antidiabetic agent
Isoniazid / ↓ Effect of isoniazid due to ↑ breakdown by liver and ↑ excretion
Ketoconazole / ↓ Effect of corticosteroids due to ↑ rate of clearance
Mexiletine / ↓ Effect of mexiletine due to ↑ breakdown by liver
Mitotane / ↓ Response of adrenal gland to corticotropin
Muscle relaxants, nondepolarizing / ↓ Effect of muscle relaxants
Neuromuscular blocking agents / ↑ Risk of prolonged respiratory depression or paralysis
NSAIDs / ↑ Risk of GI hemorrhage or ulceration
Phenobarbital / ↓ Effect of corticosteroids due to ↑ breakdown by liver
Phenytoin / ↓ Effect of corticosteroids due to ↑ breakdown by liver
Potassium supplements / ↓ Plasma levels of potassium
Rifampin / ↓ Effect of corticosteroids due to ↑ breakdown by liver
Ritodrine / ↑ Risk of maternal edema
Salicylates / Both are ulcerogenic; also, corticosteroids may ↓ blood salicylate levels
Somatrem, Somatropin / Glucocorticoids may inhibit effect of somatrem
Streptozocin / ↑ Risk of hyperglycemia
Theophyllines / Corticosteroids ↑ effect of theophyllines
Thiazide diuretics / Enhanced potassium loss due to potassium-losing properties of both drugs
Tricyclic antidepressants / ↑ Risk of mental disturbances
Vitamin A / Topical vitamin A can reverse impaired wound healing in clients receiving corticosteroids

Laboratory Test Interferences: ↑ Urine glucose, serum cholesterol, serum amylase. ↓ Serum potassium, triiodothyronine, serum uric acid. Alteration of electrolyte balance.

Dosage

Dosage is highly individualized, according to both the condition being treated and the client's response. Although the various corticosteroids are similar in their actions, clients may respond better to one type of drug than to another. It is most important that therapy not be discontinued abruptly. Except for replacement therapy, treatment should always involve the minimum effective dose and the shortest period of time. Long-term use often causes severe side effects. If corticosteroids are used for replacement therapy or high doses are used for prolonged periods of time, the dose must be *increased* if surgery is required.

For topical use, ointment, cream, lotion, solution, plastic tape, aerosol suspension, and aerosol cream are selected, depending on dermatologic condition to be treated.

Lotions are considered best for weeping eruptions, especially in areas subject to chafing (axilla, feet, and groin). Creams are suitable for most inflammations; ointments are preferred for dry, scaly lesions.

NURSING CONSIDERATIONS

Administration of Oral Corticosteroids

1. Administer PO forms of drug with food to minimize ulcerogenic effect.
2. When corticosteroids are given chronically, use the smallest dose possible that will achieve the desired effect.
3. At frequent intervals, the dose of medication should be gradually de-

creased to determine if symptoms of the disease can be effectively controlled by the smaller amount of drug.

4. When treating clients with conditions such as asthma, ulcerative colitis, and rheumatoid arthritis, corticosteroids, given every other day, may maintain therapeutic effects while reducing or eliminating undesirable side effects. When ordered every other day, administer in the morning to coincide with the normal body secretion of cortisol.

5. Local administration of corticosteroids is preferred over systemic therapy to minimize systemic side effects.

6. Corticosteroids should be discontinued gradually if used chronically.

7. Alternate day therapy may be beneficial in selected clients requiring chronic steroid therapy. With this therapy, twice the usual daily dose of an intermediate-acting steroid is given every other morning. This regimen provides the beneficial effect of the steroid while minimizing pituitary-adrenal suppression.

8. *Treatment of Chronic Overdose:* Gradually taper the dose of the steroid and frequently monitor lab tests. During periods of stress, steroid supplementation is necessary. Dose should be reduced to the lowest one that will control the symptoms (or discontinue the steroid completely). Recovery of normal adrenal and pituitary function may take up to 9 months. Large, acute overdoses may be treated with gastric lavage, emesis, and general supportive measures.

Administration of Topical Corticosteroids

1. Cleanse the area before applying the medication.

2. Wear gloves to apply the agent; apply sparingly and rub gently into the area.

3. When prescribed, apply an occlusive dressing to promote hydration of the stratum corneum and increase the absorption of the medication.

4. The following are two methods of applying an occlusive type dressing (do not apply an occlusive dressing if infection is present):

• Apply a large amount of medication to the cleansed area. Cover with a thin, pliable, nonflammable plastic film (film enhances absorption), which is then sealed to the surrounding tissue with skin tape or held in place with gauze. Change the dressing q 3–4 days.

• Apply a small amount of medication to the area and cover with a damp cloth. Then cover with a thin, pliable, nonflammable plastic film and seal to the surrounding tissue with tape, or hold in place with gauze. Change dressing b.i.d.

Assessment: (General)

1. Document indications for therapy, type and onset of symptoms, and underlying cause: adrenal or nonadrenal disorder.

2. Record baseline data concerning the client's mental status and neurologic function.

3. Check medication history for evidence of allergic reactions to corticosteroids or tartrazine, a coloring agent used in certain preparations.

4. Obtain baseline ECG, electrolytes, and liver and renal function studies.

5. Document baseline VS and weight. Obtain CXR and purified protein derivative (PPD) if prolonged therapy is anticipated.

6. List any medication the client is taking and identify those that may interact with corticosteroids. These include antidiabetic agents, cardiac glycosides, oral contraceptives, anticoagulants, and drugs influenced by liver enzymes.

7. If the client is female, of childbearing age, and sexually active, discuss the possibility of pregnancy and notify the provider if pregnancy is determined.

8. With specific conditions, carefully assess and describe the affected area requiring treatment. This may be useful as a baseline against which to

evaluate the effectiveness of prescribed therapy.

Interventions

TOPICAL CORTICOSTEROIDS

1. Assess for local sensitivity reaction at the site of application. Withhold the medication and report any sensitivity response.
2. Absorption varies regionally with the highest absorption in scrotal skin and the lowest on the foot. Inflamed skin enhances absorption severalfold.
3. Better action has been noted with the ointment bases than with the lotion or cream vehicles.
4. Observe the client closely for signs of infections since corticosteroids tend to mask the problem. Do not apply an occlusive dressing when an infection is present. Document the site of the infection, the nature of the infection, and if there is any redness, swelling, odor, or drainage present.
5. If the client has a large occlusive dressing, take temperatures q 4 hr. Report if the temperature is elevated and remove the dressing unless otherwise specified.
6. Routinely assess the client for evidence of systemic absorption of the medication. Protracted use of large quantities of potent topical corticosteroids to large BSAs may precipitate iatrogenic Cushing's syndrome. Symptoms may include edema and transient inhibition of pituitary-adrenal cortical function as manifested by muscular pain, lassitude, depression, hypotension, and weight loss.
7. If family members are to apply the topical ointment, advise them to wash their hands and to wear gloves or to apply the medication with a sterile applicator. Instruct them concerning what to expect in response to the prescribed therapy.
8. Review adverse side effects that should be reported, some of which are erythema, telangiectases, purpura, bruising, pustules, and depressed shiny, wrinkled skin. Prolonged use of potent topical corticosteroids may increase incidence of systemic side effects.

Interventions

ORAL CORTICOSTEROIDS

1. When the client is first placed on corticosteroids, take the BP at least b.i.d. until a maintenance dose has been established. Document and report any significant increases in BP.
2. Short-term oral therapy (e.g., 60 mg PO for 5 days) does not require divided doses or titration. With long-term therapy, continuously monitor for symptoms of adrenal insufficiency, which include hypotension, confusion, restlessness, lethargy, weakness, N&V, anorexia, and weight loss.
3. Repeatedly evaluate the client for increased sodium and fluid retention. Monitor the client's weight and observe for other evidences of edema. If fluid and salt retention are noted, adjust the client's diet to one that is low in sodium and high in potassium. Weigh daily under standard conditions. Anticipate a small weight gain due to increased appetite, but sudden increases are probably due to edema and must be reported. Edema occurs most frequently with cortisone or desoxycorticosterone acetate and occurs less frequently with the new synthetic agents.
4. Assess the client for SOB, distended neck veins, edema, and easy fatigue. The client may be in CHF. Obtain a CXR and ECG and compare with the baseline studies.
5. Conduct periodic blood glucose determinations and monitor serum electrolytes and platelet counts for clients on long-term therapy. Report any unusual bleeding, bruising, the presence of petechiae and any other skin changes.
6. Assess the client's muscles for weakness and wasting as these are signs of a negative nitrogen balance.
7. Report changes in the client's appearance, especially those resembling Cushing's syndrome (such as rounding of the face, hirsutism, presence of acne, and thinning of

the hair and nails) so that dosage can be adjusted.

8. If the client has diabetes, monitor the blood glucose levels frequently while on corticosteroid therapy. The client may develop hyperglycemia and a change in diet and insulin dosage may be necessary.

9. Assess the client for signs of depression, lack of interest in personal appearance, complaints of insomnia and anorexia. Document on the client's record, compare with initial clinical presentation, and report findings.

10. Discuss with female clients the potential for menstrual difficulties and amenorrhea that may be caused by long-term therapy with corticosteroids.

11. Observe the client for S&S of other illnesses during therapy with corticosteroids as these drugs tend to mask the severity of most illnesses.

12. GI bleeding may occur. Therefore, when the client is on long-term therapy, periodically test the stools for the presence of occult blood and monitor hematologic profile.

Client/Family Teaching

1. Take the oral medication with food and report any symptoms of gastric distress. To prevent the problem of gastric irritation, discuss the use of antacids and special diets. Suggest eating frequent small meals. If the symptoms persist, diagnostic X rays may be ordered.

2. Review the appropriate method for administration or application and the prescribed dosing intervals.

3. Explain that these agents generally work by inhibiting or decreasing the inflammatory response.

4. Review the symptoms of adrenal insufficiency (see #2 under Interventions) and provide a printed list of adverse drug reactions that should be reported if they occur.

5. Caution clients and family members to report any changes in mood or affect immediately.

6. Instruct clients to monitor and record their weight, BP, temperature, and pulse for evidence of physiologic changes that should be further evaluated. Advise clients to weigh themselves daily at the same time, wearing clothing of approximately the same weight, and using the same scales. Consistent weight gain may be evidence of fluid retention but caloric management should be instituted to prevent obesity.

7. Assist in identifying foods high in potassium and low in sodium content to prevent electrolyte disturbances. Explain how to supplement the diet with potassium-rich foods such as citrus juices and bananas. Instruct in what to look for on labels of canned or processed foods and refer to dietician for assistance in shopping, meal planning, and preparation.

8. Encourage clients to eat a diet high in protein to compensate for the loss due to protein breakdown from gluconeogenesis.

9. To decrease the possibility of osteoporosis (due to catabolic bone effects), explain the need to exercise daily and review foods high in calcium that should be included in the diet. Stress the importance of adequate intake of protein, calcium, and vitamin D to minimize bone loss and for short-term drug use. On-going bone resorption with depressed bone formation is the cause of osteoporosis.

10. High doses of glucocorticoids stimulate the stomach to produce excess acid and pepsin and may cause peptic ulcers. Advise that antacids 3–4 times/day may relieve epigastric distress.

11. Be especially careful to avoid falls and other accidents. Steroids may cause osteoporosis, which makes the bones more susceptible to fractures. To reduce the possibility of falling and subsequent injury, advise clients to use a night light and to have a hand rail or other device for support if they get up at night.

12. Women using oral contraceptives need to be warned that corticosteroids can cause a loss of contraceptive action. Teach the client how to keep an accurate record of her menstrual periods and to consider alternative methods of birth control, and advise to report immediately if pregnancy is suspected.
13. Warn males that corticosteroids may have an adverse effect on the sperm production and count.
14. Review the possible effects on body image (weight gain, acne, excess hair growth, etc.) and explore coping mechanisms and identify support persons and groups.
15. Explain that there is a need to withdraw the medication when therapy has exceeded 7 consecutive days. The process should proceed slowly so that the client's own adrenal cortex will gradually be reactivated and take over the production of hormones. Sudden withdrawal may be life-threatening. If adverse side effects occur, remind the client not to discontinue therapy with the idea that the changes will be reversed. Any sudden change will provoke symptoms of adrenal insufficiency.
16. If dosage of drug is reduced, provide supportive measures and reassurance to clients who are having flare-ups. Explain that these symptoms are caused by the reduction of drug dosage.
17. Explain to clients with arthritis that they should not overuse the joint once it has become painless. Permanent joint damage may result from overuse, because underlying pathology is still present.
18. If the client has diabetes, discuss the need to monitor glucose levels frequently while taking steroids. Any changes should be reported as alterations in insulin dose and diet may be necessary.
19. Explain that wounds may heal slowly because steroid therapy causes a delay in development of granulation tissue. The potential for infection also increases. Therefore, clients should observe any healing process carefully for signs of infection and report any injury so that appropriate medical supervision can be implemented. Postoperative clients should report any separation of wound or suture line.
20. These drugs mask symptoms of infection and cause immunosuppression. Because antibody production is decreased by corticosteroids, clients are at risk for infection. Explain the need to maintain general hygiene and scrupulous cleanliness to avoid infection. Advise clients to report if they have a sore throat, cough, fever, malaise, or an injury that does not heal. Avoid contact with persons with known contagious diseases.
21. Advise the client to delay any vaccinations, immunizations, or skin testing while receiving corticosteroid therapy because there is limited immune response during therapy with steroids.
22. Clients on long-term ophthalmic therapy are prone to developing cataracts, exophthalmus, and increased intraocular pressure. Advise these clients to have routine visits to the ophthalmologist for eye examinations.
23. Assist the client in establishing a means of maintaining a supply of medication on hand to avoid running out of the drug.
24. Avoid any OTC medications, including aspirin and ibuprofen compounds, as well as alcohol, since these may aggravate gastric irritation and bleeding.
25. Stress the need for regular medical supervision to have the dosage of medication checked and periodically adjusted.
26. Remind the client to wear a Medic Alert tag and/or to carry identification listing the drug being used, the dosage, the condition being treated, and who to contact in the event of an emergency.

Evaluate

- Clinical response to date and the need for modifications in diet, drug dosage, or length of therapy
- Effective wound healing

• Suppression of inflammatory and immune responses or disease manifestation in allergic reactions, autoimmune diseases, and organ transplant recipients
• Laboratory confirmation that serum cortisol levels are within desired range in adrenal deficiency states

Special Concerns

1. Check the height and weight of children regularly and maintain a graph because growth suppression is a hazard of corticosteroid therapy and is not prevented by growth hormone administration.
2. Advise parents that large doses of glucocorticoids in children may increase intracranial pressure (pseudotumor cerebri). Symptoms of this disorder include vertigo, headache, and convulsions. This should be reported immediately and advise that these symptoms should disappear once the therapy is discontinued (under medical supervision).

Beclomethasone dipropionate

(be-kloh-**METH**-ah-zohn)

Pregnancy Category: C

Becloforte Inhaler ✱, **Aerosol:** Beclovent, Vanceril **(Rx)**. **Intranasal:** Beclodisk ✱, Beconase AQ, Beconase Nasal Inhaler, Vancenase AQ, Vancenase Nasal Inhaler **(Rx)**. **Topical:** Propaderm ✱

See also *Corticosteroids,* Chapter 67.

How Supplied: *Aerosol Solid w/Adapter:* 0.042 mg/inh; *Aerosol Solid:* 0.042 mg/inh

Action/Kinetics: Rapidly inactivated, thereby resulting in few systemic effects.

NOTE: If a client is on systemic steroids, transfer to beclomethasone may be difficult because recovery from impaired renal function may be slow.

Uses: Inhalation therapy for chronic use in bronchial asthma. In glucocorticoid-dependent clients, beclomethasone often permits a decrease in the dosage of the systemic agent. Withdrawal of systemic corticosteroids must be carried out gradually.

Dosage

• **Inhalation Aerosol**

Asthma.

Adults: 2 inhalations (total of 84 mcg beclomethasone) t.i.d.–q.i.d. In some clients, 2–4 inhalations (84–168 mcg) b.i.d. have been effective. **Pediatric, 6–12 years:** 1–2 inhalations (42–84 mcg) t.i.d.–q.i.d., not to exceed 10 inhalations (420 mcg) daily. Dosage has not been determined in children less than 6 years of age.

Severe asthma.

Adults, initial: 12–16 inhalations (504–672 mcg beclomethasone) daily; **then,** decrease dose according to response. **Maximum daily dose:** 20 inhalations (840 mcg beclomethasone).

• **Nasal Aerosol or Spray**

Rhinitis.

Adults and children over 12 years: 1 inhalation (42 mcg) in each nostril b.i.d.–q.i.d. (i.e., total daily dose: 168–336 mcg). If no response after 3 weeks, discontinue therapy.

In clients also receiving systemic glucocorticosteroids, beclomethasone should be started when client's condition is relatively stable.

Contraindications: Status asthmaticus, acute episodes of asthma, hypersensitivity to drug or aerosol ingredients.

Special Concerns: Safe use during lactation and in children under 6 years of age not established.

Administration/Storage

1. To administer beclomethasone with an inhaler, use the following procedure and instruct clients to:
• Shake metal canister thoroughly immediately prior to use.
• Exhale as completely as possible.
• Place the mouthpiece of the inhaler into the mouth and tighten their lips around it.
• Inhale deeply through the mouth while pressing the metal canister down with their forefinger.
• Hold their breath for as long as possible.
• Remove mouthpiece.

• Exhale slowly.
2. A minimum of 60 sec must elapse between inhalations.
3. To prevent explosion of contents under pressure, do not store or use near heat or open flame, or throw into a fire or incinerator. Keep secure from children.

NURSING CONSIDERATIONS

See also *Nursing Considerations* for *Corticosteroids,* Chapter 67.

Assessment

1. Note any history of sensitivity to corticosteroids or fluorocarbon propellants.
2. Document indications for therapy and pretreatment pulmonary assessments and findings.

Interventions

1. For clients who are receiving systemic steroid therapy, initiate beclomethasone therapy *very* slowly, withdrawing the systemic steroids as ordered. The benefit of inhaled steroids is that it requires a much lower dose since it goes to the target organ and does not require weaning.
2. Report any subjective signs of adrenal insufficiency (such as muscular pain, lassitude, and depression) even if the client's respiratory function has improved.
3. Symptoms of adrenal insufficiency, such as hypotension and weight loss, are indications that the dosage of systemic steroid should be boosted temporarily, and then withdrawn more gradually.

Client/Family Teaching

1. Instruct in the use, care, and storage of the inhaler. Caution the client to wash the mouth piece, spacer, and sprayer and to dry it after each use.
2. Observe client technique to ensure proper administration. A spacer may facilitate administration. With nasal administration advise to aim toward the eye and not the septum to decrease nasal irritation.
3. Explain that the inhaler is not to be used for acute asthma attacks but should be used regularly as prescribed to prevent the occurrence of these attacks.
4. Stress the importance of complying with the prescribed drug therapy even though it may take 1–4 weeks for any improvement in respiratory function to be realized.
5. More than 1 mg in adults or more than 500 mcg in children may precipitate hypothalamic-pituitary axis depression, resulting in adrenal insufficiency. Therefore, advise clients not to overuse the inhaler.
6. Report any symptoms of localized fungal infections in the mouth. Gargling and rinsing after treatments and rinsing of the spacer and/or administration port may help prevent these infections. These must be reported immediately and will require antifungal medication and possibly discontinuation of the drug.
7. Advise clients also receiving bronchodilators by inhalation that they should use the bronchodilator first to open the airways and then use beclomethasone. This increases the penetration of steroid and reduces the potential toxicity from inhaled fluorocarbon propellants of both inhalers.
8. Once clients have had a systemic steroid withdrawn, they should be provided with a supply of PO glucocorticoids. These are to be taken immediately if subjected to unusual stress. All usage should be noted and reported.
9. Carry a card indicating the diagnosis, treatment, and possible need for systemic glucocorticoids, in the event of exposure to unusual stress.
10. Instruct in several relaxation techniques to perform during stressful situations.

Evaluate

• Control of the symptoms of asthma
• Successful ↓ in or withdrawal of systemic steroids
• Relief of rhinitis

Betamethasone

(bay-tah-**METH**-ah-zohn)
Celestone **(Rx)**

Betamethasone benzoate

(bay-tah-**METH**-ah-zohn)

Topical: Beben ✱, Uticort **(Rx)**

Betamethasone dipropionate

(bay-tah-**METH**-ah-zohn)

Topical: Alphatrex, Diprolene, Diprosone, Maxivate, Occlucort ✱ **(Rx)**

Betamethasone sodium phosphate

(bay-tah-**METH**-ah-zohn)

Betnesol ✱, Celestone Phosphate, Cel-U-Jec, Selestoject **(Rx)**

Betamethasone sodium phosphate and Betamethasone acetate

(bay-tah-**METH**-ah-zohn)

Celestone Soluspan **(Rx)**

Betamethasone valerate

(bay-tah-**METH**-ah-zohn)

Topical: Betacort ✱, Betaderm ✱, Betagel ✱, Betatrex, Beta-Val, Betnovate ✱, Betnovate-1/2 ✱, Celestoderm-V ✱, Celestoderm-V/2 ✱, Dermabet, Ectosone Regular, Prevex B ✱, Rholosone ✱, Valisone, Valisone Reduced Strength, Valnac **(Rx)**

See also *Corticosteroids,* Chapter 67.

How Supplied: Betamethasone: *Syrup:* 0.6 mg/5 mL; *Tablet:* 0.6 mg.
Betamethasone benzoate: *Cream:* 0.025%.
Betamethasone dipropionate: *Cream:* 0.05%; *Lotion:* 0.05%; *Ointment:* 0.05%; *Spray:* 0.1%.
Betamethasone sodium phosphate: *Injection:* 4 mg/mL.
Betamethasone sodium phosphate and betamethasone acetate: *Injection:* 3 mg-3 mg/mL.
Betamethasone valerate: *Cream:* 0.01%, 0.1%; *Lotion:* 0.1%; *Ointment:* 0.1%

Action/Kinetics: Causes low degree of sodium and water retention, as well as potassium depletion. The injectable form contains both rapid-acting and repository forms of betamethasone (mixture of betamethasone sodium phosphate and betamethasone acetate). Not recommended for replacement therapy in any acute or chronic adrenal cortical insufficiency because it does not have strong sodium-retaining effects. Long-acting. **t½:** over 300 min.

Additional Use: Prevention of respiratory distress syndrome in premature infants.

Dosage

BETAMETHASONE

• **Syrup, Tablets**

0.6–7.2 mg/day.

BETAMETHASONE SODIUM PHOSPHATE

• **IV, Intra-articular, Intralesional, Soft Tissue Injection**

Initial: up to 9 mg/day; **then,** adjust dosage at minimal level to reduce symptoms.

BETAMETHASONE SODIUM PHOSPHATE AND BETAMETHASONE ACETATE (contains 3 mg each of the acetate and sodium phosphate per mL)

• **IM**

Initial: 0.5–9 mg/day (dose ranges are ⅓–½ the PO dose given q 12 hr.)

• **Intra-articular, Intrabursal, Intradermal, Intralesional**

Bursitis, peritendinitis, tenosynovitis.
1 mL.

Rheumatoid arthritis and osteoarthritis.
0.25–2 mL, depending on size of the joint.

Foot disorders, bursitis.
0.25–0.5 mL under heloma durum or heloma molle; 0.5 mL under calcaneal spur or over hallux rigidus or digiti quinti varus. Tenosynovitis or periostitis of cuboid: 0.5 mL.

Acute gouty arthritis.
0.5–1 mL.

• **Intradermally**

0.2 mL/cm^2 not to exceed 1 mL/week.

BETAMETHASONE BENZOATE, BETAMETHASONE DIPROPIONATE, BETAMETHASONE VALERATE

• **Topical Aerosol, Cream, Gel,**

Lotion, Ointment
Apply sparingly to affected areas and rub in lightly.
Administration/Storage: Avoid injection into deltoid muscle because SC atrophy of tissue may occur.
Special Concern: Safe use during pregnancy and lactation has not been established.

NURSING CONSIDERATIONS

See *Nursing Considerations* for *Corticosteroids,* Chapter 67.
Evaluate
- ↓ Pain and inflammation with improved mobility of extremity
- Prevention of respiratory distress syndrome in premies
- Evidence of improved skin integrity and healing of lesions

Corticotropin injection (ACTH, Adrenocorticotropic hormone)

(kor-tih-koh-**TROH**-pin)
Pregnancy Category: C
ACTH, Acthar **(Rx)**

Corticotropin repository injection (ACTH gel, Corticotropin gel)

(kor-tih-koh-**TROH**-pin)
Pregnancy Category: C
ACTH-40 and -80 Acthar Gel (H.P.) ✱, H.P. Acthar Gel **(Rx)**

See also *Corticosteroids,* Chapter 67.
How Supplied: Corticotropin injection: *Powder for injection:* 25 U, 40 U. Corticotropin repository injection: *Injection:* 40 U/mL, 80 U/mL.
Action/Kinetics: Corticotropin is extracted from the anterior pituitary gland. The hormone stimulates the functional adrenal cortex to secrete its entire spectrum of hormones, including the corticosteroids.

Thus, the overall physiologic effects of corticotropin are similar to those of cortisone. Since the latter is more easily obtainable, is more predictable, and has more prolonged activity, it is usually used for therapeutic purposes. Corticotropin is, however, useful for the diagnosis of Addison's disease and other conditions in which the functionality of the adrenal cortex is to be determined. *Corticotropin cannot elicit a hormonal response from a nonfunctioning adrenal gland.* **Peak plasma levels (corticotropin injection):** 1 hr. **t½:** 15 min. The repository injection contains ACTH in a gelatin base to delay the rate of absorption and increase the duration. Corticotropin zinc hydroxide also has a slow absorption rate and increased duration. **Duration** (repository and zinc hydroxide forms): Up to 3 days.
Uses: Diagnosis of adrenal insufficiency syndromes, nonsuppurative thyroiditis, hypercalcemia associated with cancer, tuberculous meningitis with subarachnoid block or impending block (with tuberculostatic drugs). *Investigational:* Infant spasm, multiple sclerosis. For same diseases as glucocorticosteroids.

Dosage
- **SC, IM, or Slow IV Drip**

Most uses.
Highly individualized. Usual, using aqueous solution IM or SC: 20 units q.i.d. **IV:** 10–25 units of aqueous solution in 500 mL 5% dextrose injection over period of 8 hr. Infants and young children require larger dose per body weight than do older children or adults.

Acute exacerbation of multiple sclerosis.
IM: 80–120 units/day for 2–3 weeks.

Infantile spasms.
IM: 20–40 units/day or 80 units every other day for 3 months (or 1 month after cessations of seizures).
- **Repository Gel (IM, SC)**

40–80 units q 24–72 hr. A dose of 12.5 units q.i.d. causes little metabolic disturbance; 25 units q.i.d. causes definite metabolic alterations.

As a general rule, clients are started on 10–12.5 units q.i.d. If no clinical effect is noted in 72–96 hr, dosage is increased by 5 units every few days to a final maximum of 25 units q.i.d.

Administration/Storage

1. Check label carefully for IV administration. **The label must say that the product is for IV use.** IV administration should be slow, taking 8 hr.
2. Corticotropin zinc products should be injected deeply into the gluteal muscle.

Additional Contraindications: Cushing's syndrome, psychotic or psychopathic clients, active tuberculosis, active peptic ulcers. Lactation.

Special Concerns: Use with caution in clients who have diabetes and hypotension.

Laboratory Test Interferences: ↓ I^{131} uptake and suppress skin test reactions. False ↓ levels of estradiol and estriol using the Brown method. False – estrogens using colorimetric or fluorometric tests.

Additional Side Effects: In the treatment of myasthenia gravis, corticotropin may cause severe muscle weakness 2–3 days after initiation of therapy. Equipment for respiratory assistance must be on hand for such emergencies. Muscle strength returns and increases 2–7 days after cessation of treatment, and improvement lasts for about 3 months.

NURSING CONSIDERATIONS

See also *Nursing Considerations* for *Corticosteroids,* Chapter 67.

Assessment

1. Before administering IV corticotropin, make sure that the client allergic to porcine proteins has been tested for any sensitivity to the brand of corticotropin to be used.
2. Document indications for therapy, noting type and onset of symptoms.

Interventions

1. Anticipate that the potassium requirements will be increased during IV administration of ACTH. Therefore, monitor serum potassium and sodium levels.
2. Observe client for exaggerated euphoria and nervousness or complaints of insomnia and depression. Report as these are indications that the dosage should be reduced or discontinued.
3. Sedatives may be ordered as necessary.
4. Monitor BP, I&O, and weight for any marked changes and report.

Client/Family Teaching

1. Drug may mask S&S of infection.
2. Avoid vaccinations during therapy.
3. Report any unusual bruising or bleeding.

Evaluate

- Adrenal cortex function (ability to respond to stimulation and differentiate primary versus secondary adrenal cortical insufficiency)
- ↓ Serum calcium levels
- Control of infantile seizures
- Remission of symptoms in MS

Cortisone acetate (Compound E)

(**KOR**-tih-zohn)

Cortone ✦, Cortone Acetate, Cortone Acetate Sterile Suspension **(Rx)**

See also *Corticosteroids,* Chapter 67.

How Supplied: *Injection:* 50 mg/mL; *Tablet:* 5 mg, 10 mg, 25 mg

Action/Kinetics: Possesses both glucocorticoid and mineralocorticoid activity. Short-acting. **t½, plasma:** 30 min; **t½, biologic:** 8–12 hr.

Uses: Primarily used for replacement therapy in chronic cortical insufficiency. Also inflammatory or allergic disorders, but only for short-term use because the drug has a strong mineralocorticoid effect. The sterile suspension is used to treat children suffering from congenital adrenal hyperplasia.

Dosage

- **Tablets**

Initial or during crisis.

25–300 mg/day. Decrease gradually to lowest effective dose.

Anti-inflammatory.

25–150 mg/day, depending on severity of the disease.

Acute rheumatic fever.
200 mg b.i.d. day 1, thereafter, 200 mg/day.

Addison's disease.
Maintenance: 0.5–0.75 mg/kg/day.
Administration/Storage: Single course of therapy should not exceed 6 weeks. Rest periods of 2–3 weeks are indicated between treatments.
Special Concerns: Use during pregnancy only if benefits outweigh risks.

NURSING CONSIDERATIONS

See also *Nursing Considerations* for *Corticosteroids,* Chapter 67.
Evaluate
- Replacement therapy in cortical insufficiency
- Relief of allergic manifestations

Cosyntropin

(koh-**SIN**-troh-pin)
Pregnancy Category: C
Cortrosyn, Synacthen ✱ **(Rx)**

See also *Corticosteroids,* Chapter 67.
How Supplied: *Powder for injection:* 0.25 mg
Action/Kinetics: Cosyntropin is a synthetic ACTH derivative that causes effects similar to those of ACTH although fewer hypersensitivity reactions have been noted. The activity of 0.25 mg cosyntropin is equal to 25 units of ACTH.
Use: Diagnosis of adrenocortical insufficiency.

Dosage
- **IM, SC**

Adults, usual: 0.25 mg dissolved in sterile saline. Range: 0.25–0.75 mg. **Pediatric, under 2 years:** 0.125 mg IM.
- **IV**

Adults: 0.25 mg given over a 2-min period.
- **IV Infusion**

Adults: 0.25 mg given at a rate of 0.04 mg/hr over a 6-hr period.
Administration/Storage
1. When given by IV infusion, 0.25 mg cosyntropin is added to dextrose or NSS, and 40 mcg/hr is administered over 6 hr.
2. For IM use, the drug (usually 0.25 mg) should be dissolved in sterile saline.

NURSING CONSIDERATIONS

See also *Nursing Considerations* for *Corticosteroids,* Chapter 67.
Evaluate: Determination of adrenal gland function.

Dexamethasone

(dex-ah-**METH**-ah-zohn)
Oral: Decadron, Deronil ✱, Dexameth, Dexamethasone Intensol, Dexasone ✱, Dexone, Hexadrol **(Rx)**. **Topical:** Aeroseb-Dex, Decaderm, Decaspray **(Rx)**. **Ophthalmic:** Maxidex Ophthalmic **(Rx)**

See also *Corticosteroids,* Chapter 67.
How Supplied: *Concentrate:* 1 mg/mL; *Elixir:* 0.5 mg/5 mL; *Ointment:* 0.05%; *Spray:* 0.01%, 0.04%; *Ophthalmic suspension:* 0.1%; *Tablet:* 0.25 mg, 0.5 mg, 0.75 mg, 1 mg, 1.5 mg, 2 mg, 4 mg, 6 mg
Action/Kinetics: Long-acting. Low degree of sodium and water retention. Diuresis may ensue when clients are transferred from other corticosteroids to dexamethasone. Not recommended for replacement therapy in adrenal cortical insufficiency. **t½:** 110–210 min.
Additional Uses: In acute allergic disorders, PO dexamethasone may be combined with dexamethasone sodium phosphate injection. This combination is used for 6 days. Used to test for adrenal cortical hyperfunction. Cerebral edema due to brain tumor, craniotomy, or head injury. *Investigational:* Diagnosis of depression. Antiemetic in cisplatin-induced vomiting. Prophylaxis or treatment of acute mountain sickness. Decrease hearing loss in bacterial meningitis. Bronchopulmonary dysplasia in preterm infants. Hirsutism.

Dosage
- **Oral Solution, Tablets**

Most uses.
Initial: 0.75–9 mg/day; **maintenance:** gradually reduce to minimum effective dose (0.5–3 mg/day).

Suppression test for Cushing's syndrome.
0.5 mg q 6 hr for 2 days for 24-hr urine collection (or 1 mg at 11 p.m. with blood withdrawn at 8 a.m. for blood cortisol determination).

Suppression test to determine cause of pituitary ACTH excess.
2 mg q 6 hr for 2 days (for 24-hr urine collection).

Acute allergic disorders or acute worsening of chronic allergic disorders.
Day 1: Dexamethasone sodium phosphate injection, 4–8 mg IM. **Days 2 and 3:** Two 0.75-mg dexamethasone tablets b.i.d. **Day 4:** One 0.75-mg dexamethasone tablet b.i.d. **Days 5 and 6:** One 0.75-mg dexamethasone tablet. **Day 7:** No treatment. **Day 8:** Follow-up visit to physician.

- **Topical Aerosol, Cream, Gel**

Apply sparingly as a light film to affected area b.i.d.–t.i.d.

- **Ophthalmic Suspension**

1–2 gtt in the conjunctival sac q hr during day and q 2 hr during night until a satisfactory response obtained; **then,** 1 gtt q 4 hr and finally 1 gtt q 6–8 hr.

Special Concerns: Use during pregnancy only if benefits outweigh risks.
Additional Drug Interaction: Ephedrine ↓ effect of dexamethasone due to ↑ breakdown by the liver.

NURSING CONSIDERATIONS

See also *Nursing Considerations* for *Corticosteroids,* Chapter 67.

Evaluate
- Status of adrenal cortical function
- ↓ Symptoms of allergic response
- ↓ Cerebral edema
- Control of cisplatin-induced vomiting
- Prevention of mountain sickness

Dexamethasone acetate

(dex-ah-**METH**-ah-zohn)
Dalalone D.P., Dalalone L.A., Decadron-LA, Decaject-L.A., Dexacen LA-8, Dexasone L.A., Dexone LA, Solurex LA **(Rx)**

See also *Corticosteroids,* Chapter 67.
How Supplied: *Injection:* 8 mg/mL, 16 mg/mL
Action/Kinetics: This ester of dexamethasone is practically insoluble and provides the prolonged activity suitable for repository injections, although it has a prompt onset of action. Not for IV use.

Dosage

- **Repository Injection**
- **IM**

8–16 mg q 1–3 weeks, if necessary.

- **Intralesional**

0.8–1.6 mg.

- **Soft Tissue and Intra-articular**

4–16 mg repeated at 1–3-week intervals.

Special Concern: Use during pregnancy only if benefits outweigh risks.

NURSING CONSIDERATIONS

See *Nursing Considerations* for *Corticosteroids,* Chapter 67.

Evaluate
- ↓ Inflammation
- Reports of symptomatic improvement

Dexamethasone sodium phosphate

(dex-ah-**METH**-ah-zohn)
Systemic: Dalalone, Decadron Phosphate, Decaject, Dexacen-4, Dexasone, Dexone, Hexadrol Phosphate, Oradexon ✦, Solurex **(Rx)**. **Inhaler:** Decadron Phosphate Respihaler **(Rx)**. **Nasal:** Decadron Phosphate Turbinaire **(Rx)**. **Ophthalmic:** AK-Dex, Baldex, Decadron Phosphate Ophthalmic, Dexotic, I-Methasone, Maxidex, PMS-Dexamethasone Sodium Phosphate ✦, Spersadex ✦ **(Rx)**. **Otic:** AK-Dex, Decadron, I-Methasone

(Rx). **Topical:** Decadron Phosphate **(Rx)**

See also *Corticosteroids,* Chapter 67.

How Supplied: *Aerosol Solid w/Adapter:* 0.1 mg/inh; *Cream:* 0.1%; *Injection:* 4 mg/mL, 8 mg/mL, 10 mg/mL, 24 mg/mL; *Ophthalmic ointment:* 0.05%; *Ophthalmic solution:* 0.1%

Additional Uses: For IV or IM use in emergency situations when dexamethasone cannot be given PO. Has a rapid onset and a short duration of action. Routes of administration include inhalation (especially for bronchial asthma), ophthalmic, topical, intrasynovial, and intra-articular. Intranasally for nasal polyps, allergic or inflammatory nasal conditions.

Dosage

• **IM, IV**

Most uses.

Range: 0.5–9 mg/day (1/3–1/2 the PO dose q 12 hr).

Cerebral edema.

Adults, initial: 10 mg IV; **then,** 4 mg IM q 6 hr until maximum effect obtained (usually within 12–24 hr). Switch to PO therapy (1–3 mg t.i.d.) as soon as feasible and then slowly withdraw over 5–7 days.

Shock, unresponsive.

Initial: either 1–6 mg/kg IV or 40 mg IV; **then,** repeat IV dose q 2–6 hr as long as necessary.

• **Intralesional, Intra-articular, Soft Tissue Injections**

0.4–6 mg, depending on the site (e.g., small joints: 0.8–1 mg; large joints: 2–4 mg; soft tissue infiltration: 2–6 mg; ganglia: 1–2 mg; bursae: 2–3 mg; tendon sheaths: 0.4–1 mg.

• **Inhalation**

Bronchial asthma.

Adults, initial: 3 inhalations (84 mcg dexamethasone/inhalation) t.i.d.–q.i.d.; **maximum:** 3 inhalations/dose; 12 inhalations/day. **Pediatric: initial,** 2 inhalations t.i.d.–q.i.d.; **maximum:** 2 inhalations/dose; 8 inhalations/day.

• **Intranasal**

Allergies, nasal polyps.

Adults: 2 sprays (total of 168 mcg dexamethasone) in each nostril b.i.d.–t.i.d. (maximum: 12 sprays/day); **pediatric, 6–12 years:** 1–2 sprays (total of 84–168 mcg dexamethasone) in each nostril b.i.d. (maximum: 8 sprays/day).

• **Ophthalmic Ointment**

Instill a small amount of the ointment into the conjunctival sac t.i.d.–q.i.d. As response is obtained, reduce the number of applications.

• **Ophthalmic Solution**

Instill 1–2 gtt into the conjunctival sac q hr during the day and q 2 hr at night until response obtained; **then,** reduce to 1 gtt q 4 hr and later 1 gtt t.i.d.–q.i.d. may control symptoms.

• **Otic Solution**

3–4 gtt into the ear canal b.i.d.–t.i.d.

• **Topical Cream**

Apply sparingly to affected areas and rub in.

Administration/Storage

1. Do not use preparation containing lidocaine IV.
2. For IV administration may give undiluted over 1 min.
3. For intranasal use, some clients are controlled using 1 spray in each nostril b.i.d.

Contraindications: Acute infections, persistent positive sputum cultures of *Candida albicans.* Lactation.

Special Concerns: Use during pregnancy only if benefits outweigh risks.

Side Effects: *Following inhalation:* Nasal and nasopharyngeal irritation, burning, dryness, stinging, headache.

NURSING CONSIDERATIONS

See also *Nursing Considerations* for *Corticosteroids,* Chapter 67.

Evaluate

• Improved airway exchange
• Relief of allergic manifestations
• Suppression of inflammatory and immune response
• Reversal of symptoms of shock; enhanced tissue perfusion

Fludrocortisone acetate

(flew-droh-**KOR**-tih-sohn)
Pregnancy Category: C
Florinef **(Rx)**

See also *Corticosteroids,* Chapter 67.
How Supplied: *Tablet:* 0.1 mg
Action/Kinetics: Produces marked sodium retention and inhibits excess adrenocortical secretion. Should not be used systemically for its anti-inflammatory effects. Supplementary potassium may be indicated.
Uses: Addison's disease and adrenal hyperplasia.

Dosage

- **Tablets**

Addison's disease.
0.1–0.2 mg/day to 0.1 mg 3 times/week, usually in conjunction with hydrocortisone or cortisone.
Salt-losing adrenogenital syndrome.
0.1–0.2 mg/day.

NURSING CONSIDERATIONS

See *Nursing Considerations* for *Corticosteroids,* Chapter 67.
Assessment
1. Document clinical presentation and onset of symptoms.
2. Obtain baseline lab studies including serum cortisol, Na, and K levels.
3. Explain that this condition (Addison's disease) will require lifetime replacement therapy.

Evaluate: Relief of symptoms during adrenal cortical hypofunction.

Flunisolide

(flew-**NISS**-oh-lyd)
Pregnancy Category: C
Inhalation: AeroBid, Bronalide Aerosol ✱ **(Rx)**. **Intranasal:** Nasalide, Rhinalar ✱ **(Rx)**

See also *Corticosteroids,* Chapter 67.
How Supplied: *Aerosol Solid w/Adapter:* 0.25 mg/inh; *Spray:* 0.025 mg/inh
Action/Kinetics: Produces anti-inflammatory effects intranasally with minimal systemic effects. Several days may be required for full beneficial effects. After inhalation, there is a significant first-pass effect through the liver and the drug is rapidly metabolized. **t½:** 1.8 hr.
Uses: Inhalation: Bronchial asthma in combination with other therapy. Not used when asthma can be relieved by other drugs, in clients where systemic corticosteroid treatment is infrequent, and in nonasthmatic bronchitis. **Intranasal:** Seasonal or perennial rhinitis, especially if other treatment has proven unsatisfactory.

Dosage

- **Inhalation**

Bronchial asthma.
Adults: 2 inhalations (total of 500 mcg flunisolide) in a.m. and p.m., not to exceed 4 inhalations b.i.d. (i.e., total daily dose of 2 mg). **Pediatric, 6–15 years:** 2 inhalations in the morning and evening, with total daily dose not to exceed 1 mg.

- **Intranasal**

Rhinitis.
Adults, initial: 50 mcg (2 sprays) in each nostril b.i.d.; may be increased to 2 sprays t.i.d. up to maximum daily dose of 400 mcg (i.e., 8 sprays in each nostril). **Pediatric, 6–14 years, initial:** 25 mcg (1 spray) in each nostril t.i.d. or 50 mcg (2 sprays) in each nostril b.i.d. Up to maximum daily dose of 200 mcg (i.e., 4 sprays in each nostril). **Maintenance, adults, children:** Smallest dose necessary to control symptoms. Some clients (approximately 15%) are controlled on 1 spray in each nostril daily.
Administration/Storage
1. When initiating the inhalant in clients receiving corticosteroids systemically, the aerosol should be used concomitantly with the systemic steroid for 1 week. Then, slowly withdraw the systemic corticosteroid over several weeks.

2. If nasal congestion is present, use a decongestant before administration to ensure the drug reaches the site of action.
3. If beneficial effects do not occur within 3 weeks, discontinue therapy.

Contraindications: Active or quiescent tuberculosis, especially of the respiratory tract. Untreated fungal, bacterial, systemic viral infections. Ocular herpes simplex. Do not use until healing occurs following recent ulceration of nasal septum, nasal surgery, or trauma. Lactation.

Special Concerns: Safety and effectiveness in children less than 6 years of age have not been determined.

Additional Side Effects: *Respiratory:* Hoarseness, coughing, throat irritation; *Candida* infections of nose, larynx, and pharynx. *After intranasal use:* Nasopharyngeal irritation, stinging, burning, dryness, headache. *GI:* Dry mouth. Systemic corticosteroid effects, especially if recommended dose is exceeded.

NURSING CONSIDERATIONS

See also *Nursing Considerations* for *Corticosteroids,* Chapter 67.

Client/Family Teaching

1. Instruct client and family how to administer nasal spray or inhalant.
2. Remind clients to gargle and rinse their mouth with water after inhalation to prevent alterations in taste and to maintain adequate oral hygiene. Report any symptoms of fungal infections.
3. Provide a printed list of drug side effects. Identify those that require immediate reporting.

Evaluate

- Improved airway exchange
- ↓ Allergic manifestations

Hydrocortisone (Cortisol)

(hy-droh-**KOR**-tih-zohn)

Pregnancy Category: C (topical and dental products)

Parenteral: Sterile Hydrocortisone Suspension. **Rectal:** Dermolate Anal-Itch, Cortenema 🍁, Proctocort, ProctoCream.HC 2.5%, Rectocort 🍁. **Retention Enema:** Cortenema, Hycort 🍁, Rectocort 🍁. **Tablets:** Cortef, Hydrocortone. **Topical Aerosol Solution:** Aeroseb-HC, CaldeCORT Anti-Itch. **Topical Cream:** Ala-Cort, Allercort, Alphaderm, Bactine, Cortate 🍁, Cort-Dome, Cortifair, Dermacort, DermiCort, Dermolate Anti-Itch, Dermtex HC, Emo-Cort 🍁, H_2Cort, Hi-Cor 1.0 and 2.5, Hydro-Tex, Hytone Lemoderm, Nutracort, Penecort, Prevex HC 🍁, Synacort. **Topical Lotion:** Acticort 100, Ala-Cort, Ala-Scalp HP, Allercort, Cetacort, Cortate 🍁, Cort-Dome, Delacort, Dermacort, Dermolate Scalp-Itch, Emo-Cort 🍁, Gly-Cort, Hytone, LactiCare-HC, Lemoderm, Lexocort Forte, My Cort, Nutracort, Pentacort, Rederm, S-T Cort. **Suppository:** Cortiment 🍁. **Topical Ointment:** Allercort, Cortril, Dermolate Anal-Itch, Hytone, Lemoderm, Penecort. **Topical Solution:** Penecort, Emo-Cort Scalp Solution, Texacort Scalp Solution. **Topical Spray:** Cortaid, Dermolate Anti-Itch **(OTC) (Rx)**

Hydrocortisone acetate

(hy-droh-**KOR**-tih-zohn)

Pregnancy Category: C (topical and dental products)

Dental Paste: Orabase-HCA. **Intrarectal Foam:** Cortifoam. **Ophthalmic/Otic:** Cortamed 🍁. **Parenteral:** Hydrocortone Acetate. **Rectal:** Anusol HC, Cort-Dome High Potency, Cortenema, Corticaine, Cortifoam. **Suppository:** Cortiment 🍁. **Topical Aerosol Foam:** Epifoam. **Topical Cream:** Allocort 🍁, Anusol-HC, CaldeCORT Anti-Itch, CaldeCORT Light, Carmol-HC, Cortacet 🍁, Cortaid, Cortef Feminine Itch, Corticaine, Corticreme 🍁, FoilleCort, Gynecort, Hyderm 🍁, Lanacort, Pharma-Cort, Rhulicort. **Topical Lotion:** Cortaid, Rhulicort. **Topical Ointment:** Cortaid, Cortef Acetate, Cortoderm 🍁, Dermaflex HC 1% 🍁, Lanacort, Nov–Hydrocort. **(OTC) (Rx)**

Hydrocortisone butyrate

(hy-droh-**KOR**-tih-zohn)

Pregnancy Category: C (topical products)

Topical Cream: Locoid **(Rx)**

Hydrocortisone cypionate

(hy-droh-**KOR**-tih-zohn)

Oral Suspension: Cortef **(Rx)**

Hydrocortisone sodium phosphate

(hy-droh-**KOR**-tih-zohn)

Parenteral: Hydrocortone Phosphate **(Rx)**

Hydrocortisone sodium succinate

(hy-droh-**KOR**-tih-zohn)

Parenteral: A-hydroCort, Solu-Cortef **(Rx)**

Hydrocortisone valerate

(hy-droh-**KOR**-tih-zohn)

Pregnancy Category: C (topical products)

Topical Cream/Ointment: Westcort **(Rx)**

See also *Corticosteroids,* Chapter 67.

How Supplied: Hydrocortisone Cortisol: *Balm:* 1%; *Cream:* 0.5%, 1%, 2.5%; *Enema:* 100 mg/60 mL; *Gel/jelly:* 1%; *Liquid:* 1%; *Lotion:* 0.25%, O.5%, 1%, 2%, 2.5%; *Ointment:* 0.5%, 1%, 2.5%; *Pad:* 0.5%, *Solution:* 1%, 2.5%; *Spray:* 0.5%, 1%; *Tablet:* 5 mg, 10 mg, 20 mg.
Hydrocortisone acetate: *Cream:* 0.5%, 1%; *Foam:* 10%; *Injection:* 25 mg/mL, 50 mg/mL; *Lotion:* 1%; *Ointment:* 0.5%, 1%; *Paste:* 0.5%; *Spray:* 0.5%; *Suppository:* 25 mg.
Hydrocortisone butyrate: *Cream:* 0.1%; *Ointment:* 0.1%; *Solution:* 0.1%.
Hydrocortisone cypionate: *Suspension:* 10 mg/5 mL.
Hydrocortisone sodium phosphate: *Injection:* 50 mg/mL.
Hydrocortisone sodium succinate: *Powder for injection:* 100 mg, 250 mg, 500 mg, 1 g.
Hydrocortisone valerate: *Cream:* 0.2%; *Ointment:* 0.2%.

Action/Kinetics: Short-acting. **t½:** 80–118 min. Topical products are available without a prescription in strengths of 0.5% and 1%.

Dosage

HYDROCORTISONE

• **Tablets**

20–240 mg/day, depending on disease.

• **IM Only**

One-third to one-half the PO dose q 12 hr.

• **Rectal**

100 mg in retention enema nightly for 21 days (up to 2 months of therapy may be needed; discontinue gradually if therapy exceeds 3 weeks).

• **Topical Ointment, Cream, Gel, Lotion, Solution, Spray**

Apply sparingly to affected area and rub in lightly t.i.d.–q.i.d.

HYDROCORTISONE ACETATE

• **Intralesional, Intra-articular, Soft Tissue**

5–50 mg, depending on condition.

• **Intrarectal Foam**

1 applicatorful (90 mg) 1–2 times/day for 2–3 weeks; **then** every second day.

• **Topical**

See *Hydrocortisone.*

HYDROCORTISONE BUTYRATE

• **Topical**

See *Hydrocortisone.*

HYDROCORTISONE CYPIONATE

• **Suspension**

20–240 mg/day, depending on the severity of the disease.

HYDROCORTISONE SODIUM PHOSPHATE

• **IV, IM, SC**

General uses.

Initial: 15–240 mg/day depending on use and on severity of the disease. Usually, one-half to one-third of the PO dose is given q 12 hr.

Adrenal insufficiency, acute.

Adults, initial: 100 mg IV; **then,** 100 mg q 8 hr in an IV fluid; **older children, initial:** 1–2 mg/kg by IV bolus; **then,** 150–250 mg/kg/day **IV** in divided doses; **infants, initial:** 1–2 mg/kg by IV bolus; **then,** 25–150 mg/kg/day in divided doses.

HYDROCORTISONE SODIUM SUCCINATE

• **IM, IV**

Initial: 100–500 mg; **then,** may be repeated at 2-, 4-, and 6-hr intervals depending on response and severity of condition.

HYDROCORTISONE VALERATE

• **Topical Cream**

See *Hydrocortisone.*

Administration/Storage

1. Check label of parenteral hydrocortisone to verify route that can be used for a particular preparation, because IM and IV preparations are not necessarily interchangeable.
2. Reconstituted direct IV solution may be administered at a rate of 100 mg over 30 sec. Doses larger than 500 mg should be infused over 10 min. Drug may be further diluted in 50–100 mL of dextrose or saline solutions and administered as ordered within 24 hr.
3. No part of the hydrocortisone acetate intrarectal foam aerosol container should be inserted into the anus.
4. When using topical products, washing the area prior to application may increase the penetration of the drug.
5. Topical products should not come in contact with the eyes.
6. Prolonged use of topical products should be avoided near the genital/rectal areas and eyes, on the face, and in creases of the skin.

NURSING CONSIDERATIONS

See also *Nursing Considerations* for *Corticosteroids,* Chapter 67.

Assessment

1. Document indications for therapy and type and onset of symptoms.
2. List other agents previously prescribed and the outcome.

Evaluate

- Replacement therapy with adrenocortical deficiency
- Restoration of skin integrity
- Relief of allergic manifestations

Methylprednisolone

(meth-ill-pred-**NISS**-oh-lohn)

Tablets: Medrol, Meprolone **(Rx)**

Methylprednisolone acetate

(meth-ill-pred-**NISS**-oh-lohn)

Cream: Medrol Veriderm Cream ✱. **Enema:** Medrol Enpak **(Rx)**. **Parenteral:** depMedalone-40 and -80, Depoject 40 and 80, Depo-Medrol, D-Med 80, Duralone-40 and -80, Medralone-40 and -80, M-Prednisol-40 and -80, **Topical Ointment:** Medrol **(Rx)**

Methylprednisolone sodium succinate

(meth-ill-pred-**NISS**-oh-lohn)

Parenteral: A-methaPred, Solu-Medrol **(Rx)**

See also *Corticosteroids,* Chapter 67.

How Supplied: Methylprednisolone: *Tablet:* 2 mg, 4 mg, 8 mg, 16 mg, 24 mg, 32 mg.

Methylprednisolone acetate: *Injection:* 20 mg/mL, 40 mg/mL, 80 mg/mL.

Methylprednisolone sodium succinate: *Powder for injection:* 40 mg, 125 mg, 500 mg, 1 g, 2 g

Action/Kinetics: Low incidence of increased appetite, peptic ulcer, and psychic stimulation. Also, low degree of sodium and water retention. May mask negative nitrogen balance. **Onset:** Slow, 12–24 hr. **t½, plasma:** 78–188 min. **Duration:** Long, up to 1 week. The sodium succinate product has a rapid onset by both the IM and IV routes. Methylprednisolone acetate has a long duration of action.

Additional Uses: Severe hepatitis due to alcoholism. Within 8 hr of severe spinal cord injury (to improve neurologic function). Septic shock (controversial).

Dosage

METHYLPREDNISOLONE

• **Tablets**

Rheumatoid arthritis.

Adults: 6–16 mg/day. Decrease gradually when condition is under control. **Pediatric:** 6–10 mg/day.

SLE.

Adults, acute: 20–96 mg/day; **maintenance:** 8–20 mg/day.

Acute rheumatic fever.
1 mg/kg body weight daily. Drug is always given in four equally divided doses after meals and at bedtime.
METHYLPREDNISOLONE ACETATE
• **IM**
Adrenogenital syndrome.
40 mg q 2 weeks.
Rheumatoid arthritis.
40–120 mg/week.
Dermatologic lesions, dermatitis.
40–120 mg/week for 1–4 weeks; for severe cases, a single dose of 80–120 mg should provide relief.
Seborrheic dermatitis.
80 mg/week.
Asthma, rhinitis.
80–120 mg.
• **Intra-articular, Soft Tissue and Intralesional Injection**
4–80 mg, depending on site.
• **Retention Enema**
40 mg 3–7 times/week for 2 or more weeks.
• **Topical Ointment**
0.25%–1% applied sparingly b.i.d.–q.i.d.
METHYLPREDNISOLONE SODIUM SUCCINATE
• **IM, IV**
Most conditions.
Adults, initial: 10–40 mg, depending on the disease; **then,** adjust dose depending on response, with subsequent doses given either **IM, IV.**
Severe conditions.
Adults: 30 mg/kg infused IV over 10–20 min; may be repeated q 4–6 hr for 2–3 days only. **Pediatric:** not less than 0.5 mg/kg/day.
Administration/Storage
1. Dosage must be highly individualized.
2. Methylprednisolone acetate is not for IV use.
3. Solutions of methylprednisolone sodium succinate should be used within 48 hr after preparation.
4. For alternate day therapy using methylprednisolone, twice the usual PO dose is given every other morning (the client receives the beneficial effect while minimizing side effects).
Special Concerns: Use during pregnancy only if benefits outweigh risks.
Laboratory Test Interference: ↓ Immunoglobulins A, G, M.
Additional Drug Interactions
Erythromycin / ↑ Effect of methylprednisolone due to ↓ breakdown by liver
Troleandomycin / ↑ Effect of methylprednisolone due to ↓ breakdown by liver

---

NURSING CONSIDERATIONS

See also *Nursing Considerations* for *Corticosteroids,* Chapter 67.
Assessment
1. Document indications for treatment and describe clinical presentation.
2. Obtain baseline CBC and electrolytes and monitor with long-term therapy.
Evaluate
• Relief of allergic manifestations
• Control of pain and inflammation with improved mobility
• ↓ Destruction of nerve fibers in spinal cord injury

Prednisolone
(pred-**NISS**-oh-lohn)
Syrup: Prelone, **Tablets:** Delta-Cortef
(Rx)

Prednisolone acetate
(pred-**NISS**-oh-lohn)
Parenteral: Articulose-50, Key-Pred 25 and 50, Predaject-50, Predalone 50, Predcor-50, **Ophthalmic Suspension:** Econopred Ophthalmic, Econopred Plus, Ophtho-Tate ✱, Pred Forte Ophthalmic, Pred Mild Ophthalmic **(Rx)**

Prednisolone acetate and Prednisolone sodium phosphate
(pred-**NISS**-oh-lohn)
(Rx)

Prednisolone sodium phosphate
(pred-**NISS**-oh-lohn)
Pregnancy Category: C

Oral Solution: Pediapred **(Rx)**, **Ophthalmic Solution:** AK-Pred Ophthalmic, Inflamase Forte Ophthalmic, Inflamase Mild Ophthalmic, Metreton Ophthalmic **(Rx)**, **Parenteral:** Hydeltrasol, Key-Pred-SP **(Rx)**

Prednisolone tebutate

(pred-**NISS**-oh-lohn)
Hydeltra-T.B.A., Prednisol TPA **(Rx)**

See also *Corticosteroids,* Chapter 67.
How Supplied: Prednisolone: *Syrup:* 15 mg/5 mL; *Tablet:* 5 mg.
Prednisolone acetate: *Injection:* 25 mg/mL, 40 mg/mL, 50 mg/mL, 80 mg/mL; *Ophthalmic Suspension:* 0.12%, 0.125%, 1%.
Prednisolone sodium phosphate: *Injection:* 20 mg/mL; *Liquid:* 5 mg/5 mL; *Ophthalmic Solution:* 0.125%, 1%.
Prednisolone tebutate: *Injection:* 20 mg/mL
Action/Kinetics: Intermediate-acting. Prednisolone is five times more potent than hydrocortisone and cortisone. Side effects are minimal except for GI distress. Has moderate mineralocorticoid activity. **Plasma t½:** over 200 min.

Dosage

PREDNISOLONE
- **Tablets**

Most uses.
5–60 mg/day, depending on disease being treated.
Multiple sclerosis (exacerbation).
200 mg/day for 1 week; **then,** 80 mg on alternate days for 1 month.
Pleurisy of tuberculosis.
0.75 mg/kg/day (then taper) given concurrently with antituberculosis therapy.

PREDNISOLONE ACETATE
- **IM**

4–60 mg/day. **Not for IV use.**
Multiple sclerosis (exacerbation).
See *Prednisolone.*
- **Intralesional, Intra-articular, Soft Tissue Injection**

4–100 mg (larger doses for large joints).
- **Ophthalmic Suspension (0.12%–1%)**

1–2 gtt in the conjunctival sac q hr during the day and q 2 hr during the night; **then,** after response obtained, decrease dose to 1 gtt/ q 4 hr and then later 1 gtt t.i.d.–q.i.d.

PREDNISOLONE ACETATE AND PREDNISOLONE SODIUM PHOSPHATE
- **IM Only**

20–80 mg acetate and 5–20 mg sodium phosphate every few days for 3–4 weeks.
- **Intra-articular, Intrasynovial**

20–40 mg prednisolone acetate and 5–10 mg prednisolone sodium phosphate.

PREDNISOLONE SODIUM PHOSPHATE
- **PO Solution**

Most uses.
5–60 mg/day in single or divided doses.
Adrenocortical insufficiency.
Pediatric: 0.14 mg/kg (4 mg/m²) daily in three to four divided doses.
Other pediatric uses.
0.5–2 mg/kg (15–60 mg/m²) daily in three to four divided doses.
- **IM, IV**

4–60 mg/day.
Multiple sclerosis (exacerbation).
See *Prednisolone.*
- **Intralesional, Intra-articular, Soft Tissue Injection**

2–30 mg, depending on site and severity of disease.
- **Ophthalmic (0.125%–1% Solution)**

See *Prednisolone acetate.*

PREDNISOLONE TEBUTATE
- **Intra-articular, Intralesional, Soft Tissue Injection**

4–30 mg, depending on site and severity of disease. Doses higher than 40 mg are not recommended.

Administration/Storage
1. Before administering prednisolone, check spelling and dose carefully; this drug is frequently confused with prednisone.
2. Check to see if provider wants PO form of drug administered with an antacid.
3. Prednisolone sodium phosphate oral solution produces a 20% higher peak plasma level of prednisolone than is seen with tablets.

4. The IV form (sodium phosphate) may be administered at a rate not to exceed 10 mg/min.
Contraindication: Lactation.
Special Concerns: Use during pregnancy only if benefits outweigh risks. Use with particular caution in diabetes.

NURSING CONSIDERATIONS

See also *Nursing Considerations* for *Corticosteroids,* Chapter 67.
Assessment
1. Document indications for therapy and type and onset of symptoms.
2. Note any previous experiences with this drug and the outcome.
Evaluate
- Desired replacement therapy during adrenocortical hypofunction
- Symptomatic relief of allergic, immune, and inflammatory manifestations

Prednisone

(**PRED**-nih-sohn)
Oral Solution: Prednisone Intensol Concentrate **(Rx)**. **Syrup:** Liquid Pred **(Rx)**. **Tablets:** Apo-Prednisone ✦, Deltasone, Meticorten, Orasone 1, 5, 10, 20, and 50, Panasol-S, Prednicen-M, Sterapred, Sterapred DS, Winpred ✦ **(Rx)**

See also *Corticosteroids,* Chapter 67.
How Supplied: *Concentrate:* 5 mg/mL; *Solution:* 5 mg/5 mL; *Syrup:* 5 mg/5 mL; *Tablet:* 1 mg, 2.5 mg, 5 mg, 10 mg, 20 mg, 50 mg
Action/Kinetics: Drug is three to five times as potent as cortisone or hydrocortisone. May cause moderate fluid retention. Prednisone is metabolized in the liver to prednisolone, the active form.

Dosage
- **Oral Solution, Syrup, Tablets**

Acute, severe conditions.
Initial: 5–60 mg/day in four equally divided doses after meals and at bedtime. Decrease gradually by 5–10 mg q 4–5 days to establish minimum maintenance dosage (5–10 mg) or discontinue altogether until symptoms recur.

Replacement.
Pediatric: 0.1–0.15 mg/kg/day.

COPD.
30–60 mg/day for 1–2 weeks; then taper.

Ophthalmopathy due to Graves' disease.
60 mg/day; **then,** taper to 20 mg/day.

Duchenne's muscular dystrophy.
0.75–1.5 mg/kg/day (used to improve strength).
Special Concerns: Use during pregnancy only if benefits outweigh risks. Dose must be highly individualized.

NURSING CONSIDERATIONS

See also *Nursing Considerations* for *Corticosteroids,* Chapter 67.
Assessment
1. Document indications for therapy and type and onset of symptoms.
2. List other agents prescribed and the outcome.
Evaluate: Symptomatic relief of allergic, immune, and inflammatory manifestations.

Triamcinolone

(try-am-**SIN**-oh-lohn)
Dental Paste: Kenalog in Orabase, Oracort, Oralone **(Rx)**. **Tablets:** Aristocort, Atolone, Kenacort **(Rx)**

Triamcinolone acetonide

(try-am-**SIN**-oh-lohn)
Inhalation Aerosol: Azmacort, Nasacort **(Rx)**. **Parenteral:** Kenaject-40, Kenalog-10 and -40, Tac-3 and -40, Triam-A, Triamonide 40, Tri-Kort, Trilog **(Rx)**. **Topical Aerosol:** Kenalog **(Rx)**. **Topical Cream:** Aristocort, Aristocort A, Delta-Tritex, Flutex, Kenac, Kenalog, Kenalog-H, Kenonel, Triacet, Triaderm ✦, Trianide Mild, Trianide Regular, Triderm, Trymex **(Rx)**. **Topical Lotion:** Kenalog, Kenonel **(Rx)**. **Topical Ointment:** Aristocort, Aristocort A, Ke-

nac, Kenalog, Kenonel, Triaderm ✱, Trymex **(Rx)**

Triamcinolone diacetate

(try-am-**SIN**-oh-lohn)
Parenteral: Amcort, Aristocort Forte, Aristocort Intralesional, Articulose L.A., Triam-Forte, Triamolone 40, Trilone, Tristoject **(Rx)**. Kenacort Diacetate **(Rx)**

Triamcinolone hexacetonide

(try-am-**SIN**-oh-lohn)
Aristospan Intra-Articular, Aristospan Intralesional **(Rx)**

See also *Corticosteroids,* Chapter 67.
How Supplied: Triamcinolone: *Tablet:* 1 mg, 2 mg, 4 mg, 8 mg.
Triamcinolone acetonide: *Aerosol Solid w/Adapter:* 55 mcg/inh, 100 mcg/inh; *Cream:* 0.025%, 0.1%, 0.5%; *Injection:* 3 mg/mL, 10 mg/mL, 40 mg/mL; *Lotion:* 0.025%, 0.1%; *Ointment:* 0.025%, 0.1%, 0.5%; *Paste:* 0.1%; *Spray:* 0.147 mg/g.
Triamcinolone diacetate: *Injection:* 25 mg/mL, 40 mg/mL.
Triamcinolone hexacetonide: *Injection:* 5 mg/mL, 20 mg/mL.
Action/Kinetics: More potent than prednisone. Intermediate-acting. Has no mineralocorticoid activity. **Onset:** several hours. **Duration:** 1 or more weeks. **t½:** Over 200 min.
Additional Uses: Pulmonary emphysema accompanied by bronchospasm or bronchial edema. Diffuse interstitial pulmonary fibrosis. With diuretics to treat refractory CHF or cirrhosis of the liver with ascites. Multiple sclerosis. Inflammation following dental procedures. Triamcinolone hexacetonide is restricted to intra-articular or intralesional treatment of rheumatoid arthritis and osteoarthritis.

Dosage

Triamcinolone

• **Tablets**

Adrenocortical insufficiency (with mineralocorticoid therapy).
4–12 mg/day.

Acute leukemias (children).
1–2 mg/kg.

Acute leukemia or lymphoma (adults).
16–40 mg/day (up to 100 mg/day may be necessary for leukemia).

Edema.
16–20 mg (up to 48 mg may be required until diuresis occurs).

Tuberculosis meningitis.
32–48 mg/day.

Rheumatic disease, dermatologic disorders, bronchial asthma.
8–16 mg/day.

SLE.
20–32 mg/day.

Allergies.
8–12 mg/day.

Hematologic disorders.
16–60 mg/day.

Ophthalmologic diseases.
12–40 mg daily.

Respiratory diseases.
16–48 mg/day.

Triamcinolone acetonide.

• **IM Only (Not for IV Use)**

2.5–60 mg/day, depending on the disease and its severity.

• **Intra-articular, Intrabursal, Tendon Sheaths**

2.5–5 mg for smaller joints and 5–15 mg for larger joints, although up to 40 mg has been used.

• **Intradermal**

1 mg/injection site (use 3 mg/mL or 10 mg/mL suspension only).

• **Topical: 0.025%, 0.1%, 0.5% Ointment or Cream; 0.025%, 0.1% Lotion; Aerosol—to deliver 0.2 mg)**

Apply sparingly to affected area b.i.d.–q.i.d. and rub in lightly.

• **Respiratory Inhalant**

Adults, usual: 2 inhalations (about 200 mcg) t.i.d.–q.i.d., not to exceed 1,600 mcg/day. High initial doses (1,200–1,600 mcg/day) may be needed in some clients with severe asthma. **Pediatric, 6–12 years:** 1–2 inhalations (100–200 mcg) t.i.d.–q.i.d., not to exceed 1,200 mcg/day. Use in children less than 6 years of age has not been determined.

• **Respiratory Spray**

Seasonal and perennial allergic rhinitis.

Adults and children over 12 years of age: 2 sprays (110 mcg) into each nostril once a day (i.e., for a total dose of 220 mcg/day). The dose may be increased to 440 mcg/day given either once daily or q.i.d. (1 spray/nostril).

Triamcinolone diacetate.

- **IM Only**

40 mg/week.

- **Intra-articular, Intrasynovial**

5–40 mg.

- **Intralesional, Sublesional**

5–48 mg (no more than 12.5 mg/injection site and 25 mg/lesion).

Triamcinolone hexacetonide. **Not for IV use.**

- **Intra-articular**

2–6 mg for small joints and 10–20 mg for large joints.

- **Intralesional/Sublesional**

Up to 0.5 mg/sq. in. of affected area.

Administration/Storage

1. Initially the aerosol should be used concomitantly with systemic steroid. After 1 week, a gradual withdrawal of systemic steroid should be initiated. The next reduction should be made after 1–2 weeks, depending on the response. If symptoms of insufficiency occur, the dose of systemic steroid can be increased temporarily. Also, the dose of systemic steroid may need to be increased in times of stress or a severe asthmatic attack.
2. The acetonide products should not be used if they clump due to exposure to freezing temperatures.
3. A single IM dose of the diacetate provides control from 4–7 days up to 3–4 weeks.
4. Triamcinolone acetonide nasal spray for allergic rhinitis may be effective as soon as 12 hr after initiation of therapy. If improvement is not seen within 2–3 weeks, the client should be reevaluated.

Special Concerns: Use during pregnancy only if benefits clearly outweigh risks. Use with special caution in clients who have decreased renal function or renal disease. Dose must be highly individualized.

Additional Side Effects: Intra-articular, intrasynovial, or intrabursal administration may cause transient flushing, dizziness, local depigmentation, and rarely, local irritation. Exacerbation of symptoms has also been reported. A marked increase in swelling and pain and further restricted joint movement may indicate septic arthritis. Intradermal injection may cause local vesicular ulceration and persistent scarring.

Syncope and anaphylactoid reactions have been reported with triamcinolone regardless of route of administration.

NURSING CONSIDERATIONS

See also *Nursing Considerations* for *Corticosteroids,* Chapter 67.

Assessment

1. Document indications for therapy and type and onset of symptoms.
2. Assess area requiring treatment and describe findings.

Client/Family Teaching

1. Take at the same time each morning.
2. Ingest a liberal amount of protein because with this drug clients experience gradual weight loss, associated with anorexia, muscle wasting, and weakness. Refer to dietitian for assistance in meal planning and preparation.
3. Remind client to lie down if feeling faint. Report if syncopal episodes persist and interfere with daily activities.
4. Report any evidence of abnormal bruising, bleeding, weight gain, edema, or dyspnea.
5. Advise that drug may suppress reactions to skin allergy testing.
6. With topical application, apply to clean, slightly moist skin. Report if area does not improve with therapy or symptoms worsen.
7. Report immediately any new onset of symptoms of depression as well as aggravation of existing symptoms.

Evaluate

- ↓ Immune and inflammatory responses in autoimmune disorders and allergic reactions
- Improved airway exchange
- Restoration of skin integrity
- Relief of pain and inflammation with improved joint mobility

CHAPTER SIXTY-EIGHT

Estrogens, Progestins, and Oral Contraceptives

See also the following individual entries:

Estrogens

- Chlorotrianisene
- Diethylstilbestrol Diphosphate
- Esterified Estrogens
- Estradiol Transdermal System
- Estrogens Conjugated, Oral
- Estrogens Conjugated, Parenteral
- Estrogens Conjugated, Vaginal
- Estropipate

Progestins

- Levonorgestrel Implants
- Medroxyprogesterone Acetate
- Megestrol Acetate

Oral Contraceptives

ESTROGENS

General Statement: Estrogens are first produced in large quantities during puberty and are responsible for the development of primary and secondary female sex characteristics. From puberty on, estrogens are secreted primarily by the ovarian follicles during the early phase of the menstrual cycle. Their production decreases sharply at menopause, but small quantities continue to be produced. Men also produce some estrogens. During each menstrual cycle, estrogens trigger the proliferative phase of the endometrium, affect the vaginal tract mucosa and breast tissue, and increase uterine tone. During adolescence, estrogens cause closure of the epiphyseal junction. Large doses inhibit the development of the long bones by causing premature closure and inhibiting endochondral bone formation. In adult women, estrogens participate in bone maintenance by aiding the deposition of calcium in the protein matrix of bones. They increase elastic elements in the skin, tend to cause sodium and fluid retention, and produce an anabolic effect by enhancing the turnover of dietary nitrogen and other elements into protein. Furthermore, they tend to keep plasma cholesterol at relatively low levels. All natural estrogens, including estradiol, estrone, and estriol, are steroids. These compounds are either obtained from the urine of pregnant mares or prepared synthetically. Nonsteroidal estrogens, including diethylstilbestrol and chlorotrianisene, are prepared synthetically.

Action/Kinetics: Estrogens combine with receptors in the cytoplasm of the cell, resulting in an increase in protein synthesis. For example, estrogens are required for development of secondary sex characteristics, development and maintenance of the female genital system and breasts. They also produce effects in the pituitary and hypothalamus. Natural estrogens are generally administered parenterally because they are either destroyed in the GI tract or have a significant first-pass effect; hence, adequate plasma levels are never reached. Synthetic derivatives can be given PO and are rapidly absorbed, distributed, and excreted. Estrogens are metabolized in the liver and excreted in urine (major portion) and feces.

Uses: Systemic. Primary ovarian failure, female hypogonadism or castration, menopausal symptoms (especially flushing, sweating, chills), atrophic vaginitis, kraurosis vulvae, abnormal uterine bleeding (progestins are preferred), postpartum breast engorgement. Adjunct to diet and calcium for prophylaxis of osteoporosis. Palliative treatment in advanced, inoperable, metastatic breast carcinoma in postmenopausal women and in men. Advanced inoperable carcinoma of the prostate. Certain estrogens are used as postcoital contraceptives. Mestranol or ethinyl estradiol in combination with a progestin are components of oral contraceptives. **Vaginal.** Atrophic vaginitis, atrophic dystrophy of the vulva due to menopause or ovariectomy.

Contraindications: Cancerous or precancerous lesions of the breast (until 5 years after menopause) and of the genital tract. Administer with caution, if at all, to clients with a history of thrombophlebitis, thromboembolism, asthma, epilepsy, migraine, cardiac failure, renal insufficiency, diseases involving calcium or phosphorous metabolism, or a family history of mammary or genital tract cancer. Estrogen therapy may be contraindicated in clients with blood dyscrasias, hepatic disease, or thyroid dysfunction. Prolonged therapy is inadvisable in women who plan to become pregnant. Undiagnosed abnormal genital bleeding. Estrogens are also contraindicated in clients who have not yet completed bone growth. Estrogens should not be used during pregnancy because they may damage the fetus (pregnancy category: X). Use during lactation.

Special Concerns: Safety and effectiveness have not been determined in children and should be used with caution in adolescents in whom bone growth is incomplete.

Side Effects: Systemic use. Side effects to estrogens are dose dependent. *CV:* Potentially, the most serious side effects involve the CV system. ***Thromboembolism,*** thrombophlebitis, ***MI, pulmonary embolism,*** retinal thrombosis, ***mesenteric thrombosis, subarachnoid hemorrhage, postsurgical thromboembolism.*** Hypertension, edema, ***stroke.*** *GI:* N&V, abdominal cramps, bloating, diarrhea, changes in appetite. *Dermatologic:* Most common are chloasma or melasma. Also, erythema multiforme, erythema nodosum, hirsutism, alopecia, hemorrhagic eruptions. *Hepatic:* Cholestatic jaundice, aggravation of porphyria, benign (most common) or malignant liver tumors. *GU:* Breakthrough bleeding, spotting, changes in amount and/or duration of menstrual flow, amenorrhea (following use), dysmenorrhea, premenstrual-like syndrome. Increased incidence of *Candida* vaginitis. *CNS:* Mental depression, dizziness, changes in libido, chorea, headache, aggravation of migraine headaches, fatigue, nervousness. *Ocular:* Steepening of corneal curvature resulting in intolerance of contact lenses. Optic neuritis or retinal thrombosis, resulting in sudden or gradual, partial or complete loss of vision, double vision, papilledema. *Hematologic:* Increase in prothrombin and blood coagulation factors VII, VIII, IX, and X. Decrease in antithrombin III. *Miscellaneous:* Breast tenderness, enlargement, or secretions. Increased risk of gallbladder disease. Premature closure of epiphyses in children. Increased frequency of benign or malignant tumors of the cervix, uterus, vagina, and other organs. Weight gain. Increased risk of congenital abnormalities. Hypercalcemia in clients with metastatic breast carcinoma. In males, estrogens may cause gynecomastia, loss of libido, decreased spermatogenesis, testicular atrophy, and feminization. Prolonged use of high doses may inhibit the function of the anterior pituitary.

Estrogen therapy affects many laboratory tests. **Vaginal use.** *GU:* Vaginal bleeding, vaginal discharge, endometrial withdrawal bleeding, serious bleeding in ovariectomized women with endometriosis. *Miscellaneous:* Breast tenderness.

Drug Interactions

Anticoagulants, oral / ↓ Anticoagulant response by ↑ activity of certain clotting factors

Anticonvulsants / Estrogen-induced fluid retention may precipitate seizures. Also, contraceptive steroids ↑ effect of anticonvulsants by ↓ breakdown in liver and ↓ plasma protein binding

Antidiabetic agents / Estrogens may impair glucose tolerance and thus change requirements for antidiabetic agent

Barbiturates / ↓ Effect of estrogen by ↑ breakdown by liver

Phenytoin / See *Anticonvulsants*

Rifampin / ↓ Effect of estrogen due to ↑ breakdown by liver

Succinylcholine / Estrogens may ↑ effects of succinylcholine

Tricyclic antidepressants / Possible ↑ effects of tricyclic antidepressants

Laboratory Test Interferences: Alter liver function tests and thyroid function tests. False + urine glucose test. ↓ Serum cholesterol, total serum lipids, pregnanediol excretion, serum folate. ↑ Serum triglyceride levels, thyroxine-binding globulin, sulfobromophthalein retention, prothrombin; factors VII, VIII, IX, X. Impaired glucose tolerance, reduced response to metyrapone.

Dosage

PO, IM, SC, vaginal, topical, or by implantation. The dosage of estrogens is highly individualized and is aimed at the minimal effective amount.

NURSING CONSIDERATIONS

Administration/Storage

1. Estrogens may be administered PO, parenterally, topically, intravaginally, or by implanting pellets.
2. The dose is highly individualized and is aimed at the minimal amount that will be effective.
3. Most PO administered estrogens are metabolized rapidly and, with the exception of chlorotrianisene, must be administered daily.
4. Parenterally administered estrogens are released more slowly from their aqueous suspensions or oily solutions. When administered by injection, the drug should be administered slowly and deeply.
5. To avoid continuous stimulation of reproductive tissue, cyclic therapy consisting of 3 weeks on and 1 week off is usually recommended.
6. To reduce postpartum breast engorgement, doses are administered during the first few days after delivery.

Assessment

1. Obtain a thorough health history and report any history of thromboembolic problems before administering the drug as estrogens enhance blood coagulability.
2. Document indications for therapy and type and onset of symptoms. List other agents prescribed and the outcome.
3. Note if the client has diabetes. Obtain baseline serum glucose level if client is diabetic and liver function studies if long-term therapy is anticipated.
4. Assess mental status. Document and report any history of depression, migraine headaches, or suicide attempts.
5. Assess for any undiagnosed genital bleeding, liver disease, or cancer of the endometrium or breast (estrogen-dependent neoplasms), as these preclude drug therapy.

Interventions

1. Observe for alterations in mental attitude, signs of depression or withdrawal, complaints of insomnia or anorexia, or a lack of attention to personal appearance.
2. Monitor BP and liver function studies during therapy.

3. Monitor serum glucose and triglyceride levels and report any significant elevations.
4. If the client has a history of problems with blood coagulation factors, monitor these and the PT routinely and report any increases.

Client/Family Teaching

1. Review the prescribed therapy and ensure that client understands the dose, form, and frequency of the prescribed agent.
2. Taking oral medications with meals or a light snack will prevent gastric irritation and usually eliminate the nausea. If the medication is to be taken once a day, taking it at bedtime may eliminate the problem. Warn that nausea, bloating, abdominal cramping, changes in appetite, and vomiting may occur. These usually disappear with the continuation of therapy.
3. Medical supervision is essential during prolonged estrogen therapy. Report any new or unusual changes that occur during drug therapy.
4. Advise those receiving cyclical therapy to take the medication for 3 weeks and then to omit it for 1 week. Menstruation may then occur, but pregnancy will not occur because ovulation is suppressed. Instruct the client to keep a record for the provider of menstruation and any problem encountered, such as missed menses, spotting, or irregularity.
5. Notify the provider immediately if pregnancy is suspected.
6. Explain that breast tenderness, enlargement, or secretion may occur. Instruct in BSE and encourage client to perform BSE monthly (usually 2 weeks after menses). Any continued problems or changes in the breasts should be reported.
7. If the client has a history of thromboembolic problems, review reportable warning S&S, instruct in how to take BP and pulse, and advise to keep an accurate written record to share at each visit.
8. Report immediately if there are leg pains, sudden onset of chest pain, dizziness, SOB, weakness of the arms or legs, or any evidence of numbness.
9. Report any unusual vaginal bleeding. This may be caused by excessive amounts of estrogen and the dosage may need to be reduced.
10. Some clients may develop changes in the curvature of the cornea, making it difficult to wear contact lenses. The client who wears contact lenses needs to be made aware of this potential problem and advised to consult an ophthalmologist if evidenced.
11. Report any skin changes such as alopecia or melasma. The dose of drug may need to be changed or the provider may elect to use a different drug.
12. If the client has diabetes, estrogen can alter glucose tolerance. Advise particularly close monitoring of blood and urine to detect hyperglycemia and glycosuria, and to report any significant increases immediately as the dose of antidiabetic medication may need to be changed.
13. Discuss with male clients who are receiving estrogen therapy the fact that they may develop feminine characteristics or suffer from impotence. Reassure that these symptoms usually disappear once the course of therapy has been completed.
14. If the treatment demands the use of vaginal suppositories, teach the client how to correctly insert the suppository. Advise to wear a perineal pad if there is an increase in vaginal discharge during the treatment. Store suppositories in the refrigerator.
15. If the client is to apply a vaginal preparation, it is best done at bedtime. Advise to wear a sanitary napkin when vaginal preparations are being used and to avoid the use of tampons.
16. Estrogen ointments may cause systemic reactions. Advise client to report these findings if evident.
17. If the client is pregnant and is planning to breast-feed her baby, advise that while breast-feeding, she should not take estrogens and should consult with her provider for alternative forms of contraception.

Stress that breast-feeding does not provide any degree of protection or contraception.
18. If the client smokes, explain the added dangers in combination with this drug therapy and assist client in efforts to stop smoking. Refer to a formal smoking cessation program if necessary.
19. Explain that some potential risks, related to endometrial cancer, have been associated with estrogen therapy. Stress the importance of close medical follow-up.

Evaluate

- Control of symptoms of estrogen imbalance
- Effective contraceptive agent
- Adjunct in slowing postmenopausal osteoporosis
- Reports of symptomatic relief of postmenopausal symptoms
- Evidence of control of tumor size and spread in metastatic breast and prostate cancers

Chlorotrianisene

(klor-oh-try-**AN**-ih-seen)
Tace **(Rx)**

See also *Estrogens,* Chapter 68.
How Supplied: *Capsule:* 12 mg
Action/Kinetics: The long-lasting effect of this synthetic estrogen is attributed to its storage in adipose tissue, which then acts as a reservoir. The long duration of action makes cyclic therapy difficult.
Uses: Female hypogonadism, atrophic vaginitis, menopausal symptoms, vulvar squamous hyperplasia. Prostatic carcinoma.

Dosage

- **Capsules**

Female hypogonadism.
12–25 mg/day cyclically for 21 days; give oral progestin for last 5 days of therapy or IM progesterone (100 mg). Begin next course on day 5 of menstrual flow.

Atrophic vaginitis, kraurosis vulvae.
12–25 mg/day given cyclically for 30–60 days.

Vasomotor symptoms associated with menopause.
12–25 mg/day given cyclically for 30 days; additional courses of treatment may be necessary.

Prostatic cancer.
12–25 mg/day (given chronically).

NURSING CONSIDERATIONS

See *Nursing Considerations* for *Estrogens,* Chapter 68.

Assessment

1. Document indications for therapy and onset of symptoms.
2. Determine last menstrual cycle.

Evaluate

- Stimulation of menses
- Relief of menopausal symptoms
- Suppression of prostatic cancer growth and spread

Diethylstilbestrol diphosphate

(dye-eth-ill-still-**BESS**-trohl)
Pregnancy Category: X
Honvol ✤, Stilbestrol ✤, Stilphostrol (Abbreviation: DES) **(Rx)**

See also *Estrogens,* Chapter 68.
How Supplied: *Injection:* 250 mg/5 mL; *Tablet:* 50 mg
Action/Kinetics: Synthetic estrogen, which competes with androgen receptors, thereby preventing androgen from inducing further growth of the neoplasm. Diethylstilbestrol also binds to cytoplasmic receptor protein. The estrogen-receptor complex translocates to the nucleus, where metabolic alterations ensue. Metabolized in the liver.
Uses: Palliative treatment of inoperable, progressive prostatic cancer. Postcoital contraceptive (emergency use only).

Dosage

- **Tablets**

Palliative treatment of prostatic carcinoma.
50 mg t.i.d. up to 200 mg t.i.d., not to exceed 1 g/day.

• **IV**

Palliative treatment of prostatic carcinoma.

500 mg (in 250 mL 5% dextrose or saline) on day 1 followed by 1 g (in 250–500 mL 5% dextrose or saline) daily for 5 days. **Maintenance, IV:** 250–500 mg 1–2 times/week. Maintenance dose may also be given PO.

Administration/Storage

1. Administer the diphosphate slowly by drip (20–30 gtt/min for first 10–15 min); then adjust flow for a total administration period of 1 hr.
2. The diphosphate solution is stable for 5 days at room temperature if stored away from direct light. Do not use if solution appears cloudy or if a precipitate has formed.

Contraindications: Known or suspected breast cancer, estrogen-dependent neoplasia, active thrombophlebitis, thromboembolic disease, markedly impaired liver function. **Not to be used during pregnancy because of the possibility of vaginal cancer in female offspring.** The diphosphate is not to be used to treat any disorder in women.

Special Concerns: Use with caution in presence of hypercalcemia, epilepsy, migraine, asthma, cardiac and renal disease. Use with caution in children in whom bone growth is incomplete.

Side Effects: *CV:* ***Thrombophlebitis, pulmonary embolism, cerebral thrombosis,*** neuro-ocular lesions. *GI:* N&V, anorexia. *CNS:* Headaches, malaise, irritability. *Skin:* Allergic rash, itching. *GU:* Gynecomastia, changes in libido. *Other:* Porphyria, backache, pain and sterile abscess at injection site, postinjection flare.

NURSING CONSIDERATIONS

See also *Nursing Considerations* for *Estrogens,* Chapter 68.

Assessment

1. Perform a thorough nursing history. Note any past occurrences of thrombophlebitis, thromboembolic conditions, or impaired liver function.
2. Document indications for therapy and onset of symptoms.
3. Assess client with poor cardiac function for edema and ensure that baseline ECG is done.
4. If female, determine if pregnant. The drug is not administered during pregnancy because of the high incidence of genital tumors in offspring.

Interventions

1. Withhold drug and report high serum calcium levels. The effect of the steroid and osteolytic metastases may result in hypercalcemia. Assess for symptoms of hypercalcemia: insomnia, lethargy, anorexia, N&V, coma, and vascular collapse.
2. Be prepared to assist with administration of IV fluids, diuretics, corticosteroids, and phosphate supplements for severe hypercalcemia.
3. Monitor VS, weights, and I&O. Encourage high fluid intake to minimize hypercalcemia.
4. Closely monitor clients who resume therapy after drug-induced hypercalcemia is corrected.
5. Gynecomastia in men may be prevented by administering low doses of radiation prior to initiating diethylstilbestrol therapy.
6. The diphosphate should not be used to treat any disorder in women.
7. Observe closely for any evidence of thrombic disorders or visual changes.

Client/Family Teaching

1. Take with food as solid foods often relieve nausea.
2. Monitor weights. Report any N&V, abdominal pain, and painful swelling of breasts. Provide a printed list identifying symptoms that require immediate reporting.
3. In clients with poor cardiac function explain the importance of daily weights and of reporting increases as this could be a symptom of edema. Demonstrate how to check the extremities and sacral region for edema.
4. Avoid smoking cigarettes; refer to formal smoking cessation group as needed.
5. Advise females that withdrawal bleeding may occur if drug suddenly stopped.

6. Clients with diabetes should monitor glucose levels closely as drug may alter amount of antidiabetic agent required.
7. May cause photosensitivity reaction; use sunscreen, sunglasses, and appropriate clothing when exposed.

Evaluate

- ↓ Tumor size and spread with metastatic prostate cancer
- Inhibition of malignant cell proliferation

Esterified estrogens

(es-**TER**-ih-fyd **ES**-troh-jens)
Pregnancy Category: X
Estratab, Menest, Neo-Estrone ✱ **(Rx)**

See also *Estrogens,* Chapter 68.
How Supplied: *Tablet:* 0.3 mg, 0.625 mg, 1.25 mg, 2.5 mg
Action/Kinetics: This product is a mixture of sodium salts of sulfate esters of natural estrogenic substances: 75%–85% estrone sodium sulfate and 6%–15% equilin sodium sulfate. Less potent than estrone.
Uses: Replacement therapy in primary ovarian failure, following castration, or hypogonadism. Inoperable, progressing prostatic or breast carcinoma (in postmenopausal women and selected men). Moderate to severe vasomotor symptoms, atrophic vaginitis, and kraurosis vulvae due to menopause.

Dosage

- **Tablets**

Moderate to severe vasomotor symptoms, atrophic vaginitis, or kraurosis vulvae due to menopause.
0.3–1.25 mg/day given cyclically for short-term use. The dose should be adjusted to the lowest effective level and discontinued as soon as possible.

Hypogonadism.
2.5–7.5 mg/day in divided doses for 20 days, followed by a 10-day rest period. If menses does not occur by the end of this period of time, the dosage schedule should be repeated. The number of courses of estrogen required to produce bleeding varies, depending on the responsiveness of the endometrium. If bleeding occurs before the end of the 10-day period, a 20-day estrogen-progestin cycle should be started with 2.5–7.5 mg/day of estrogen with a progestin added the last 5 days. If bleeding occurs before the end of this regimen, therapy is discontinued and resumed on day 5 of bleeding.

Primary ovarian failure, castration.
1.25 mg/day given cyclically.

Prostatic carcinoma, inoperable and progressing.
1.25–2.5 mg t.i.d. Effectiveness can be determined using phosphatase determinations and symptomatic improvement.

Breast carcinoma, inoperable and progressing, in selected men and postmenopausal women.
10 mg t.i.d. for at least 3 months.

NURSING CONSIDERATIONS

See *Nursing Considerations* for *Estrogens,* Chapter 68.
Assessment: Document indications for therapy, and note onset and type of symptoms.

Evaluate

- Adjunct in slowing postmenopausal osteoporosis
- Stimulation of menses
- Relief of postmenopausal symptoms
- Suppression of tumor growth and spread in metastatic breast and prostate cancers
- Osteoporosis prophylaxis

Estradiol transdermal system

(ess-trah-**DYE**-ohl)
Pregnancy Category: X
Estraderm, Vivelle **(Rx)**

See also *Estrogens,* Chapter 68.
How Supplied: *Film, Extended Release:* 0.05 mg/24 hr, 0.1 mg/24 hr
Action/Kinetics: This transdermal system allows a constant low dose of estradiol to reach the systemic circulation directly. It is believed that this system overcomes certain of the problems associated with PO use,

including first-pass hepatic metabolism, GI upset, and induction of liver enzymes. The system is available in surface areas of 10 cm^2 (4 mg estradiol with a release rate of 0.05 mg/24 hr) and 20 cm^2 (8 mg estradiol with a release rate of 0.1 mg/24 hr).
Uses: Vasomotor symptoms due to menopause; female hypogonadism or castration; atrophic vaginitis or kraurosis vulvae due to menopause; primary ovarian failure; prevention of osteoporosis.

Dosage

• **Dermal System**

Menopausal symptoms.

Initial: One patch (0.0375 mg/day; 0.05 mg/day; 0.075 mg/day; or 0.1 mg/day) applied to the skin (abdomen or buttocks) 2 times/week; **then,** dose is adjusted to control symptoms. Attempts should be made to decrease the dose or withdraw the medication q 3–6 months.

Prevention of osteoporosis.

Initial: 0.05 mg/day as soon as possible after menopause. Adjust dosage to control concurrent menopausal symptoms.

Administration/Storage

1. If the client has been taking oral estrogens, withdraw the PO therapy and wait 1 week before applying the system.
2. For clients who have not undergone a hysterectomy, the system is usually used for 3 weeks, followed by 1 week of rest.
3. Place the system on a clean, dry area of the skin on the trunk of the body (preferably the abdomen).
4. The system should not be applied to the breasts or the waistline.
5. The application site should be rotated. Allow at least a 1-week interval between reapplication to a particular site.
6. The system is to be applied immediately after the pouch is opened and the protective liner is removed. The patch is pressed firmly in place with the palm for approximately 10 sec. Ensure there is good contact, especially around the edges. If the system should fall off, the same system is to be reapplied.
7. Addition of a progestin for 7 or more days may reduce the incidence of endometrial hyperplasia.

NURSING CONSIDERATIONS

See also *Nursing Considerations* for *Estrogens,* Chapter 68.

Client/Family Teaching

1. If client is to use a transdermal patch, instruct to cleanse the area first (usually on the abdomen) and then to apply the patch as directed.
2. Avoid using areas of the body with excessive amounts of hair.
3. Apply the system immediately after opening the pouch and removing the protective liner. Press the system firmly in place by holding for 10 sec.
4. If the patch falls off, it should be replaced by a new one and the days of dosage administration should be readjusted. If the client has difficulty following the instructions, stress the importance of contacting the provider to review the instructions.
5. The drug is usually prescribed to be used twice a week. Discuss the importance of administering the drug only as prescribed.
6. Explain the importance of rotating the patch sites, dating the patches on application, and teach the client how to record so that one area is not overused.

Evaluate

- Relief of menopausal symptoms
- Therapeutic serum levels of estrogen

Estrogens conjugated, oral (conjugated estrogenic substances)

(**ES**-troh-jens)
Pregnancy Category: X
C.E.S. ✱, Congest ✱, Premarin **(Rx)**

Estrogens conjugated, parenteral

Pregnancy Category: X
(**ES**-troh-jens)
Premarin IV **(Rx)**

Estrogens conjugated, vaginal

(ES-troh-jens)
Pregnancy Category: X
Premarin **(Rx)**

See also *Estrogens,* p. 155, and *Esterified Estrogens,* Chapter 68.

How Supplied: Estrogens conjugated, oral: *Tablet:* 0.3 mg, 0.625 mg, 0.9 mg, 1.25 mg, 2.5 mg.
Estrogens conjugated, parenteral: *Powder for injection:* 25 mg.
Estrogens conjugated, vaginal: *Cream:* 0.625 mg/g

Action/Kinetics: This preparation contains 50%–65% sodium estrone sulfate and 20%–35% sodium equilin sulfate.

Uses: PO: Moderate to severe vasomotor symptoms due to menopause, atrophic vaginitis, kraurosis vulvae, female hypogonadism, primary ovarian failure, female castration. Palliation in mammary cancer in men or postmenopausal women; prostatic carcinoma (inoperable and progressive). Prophylaxis of osteoporosis. Prevention of postpartum breast engorgement.

Parenteral: Abnormal bleeding due to imbalance of hormones and in the absence of disease.

Vaginal: Atrophic vaginitis and kraurosis vulvae associated with menopause.

Dosage

- **Tablets**

Moderate to severe vasomotor symptoms due to menopause.
1.25 mg/day given cyclically. If the client has not menstruated in 2 or more months, begin therapy on any day; if, however, the client is menstruating, begin therapy on day 5 of bleeding.

Primary ovarian failure, female castration.
1.25 mg/day given cyclically. Adjust dose to lowest effective level.

Atrophic vaginitis, kraurosis vulvae.
0.3–1.25 mg/day (higher doses may be necessary, depending on the response) given cyclically.

Hypogonadism in females.
2.5–7.5 mg/day in divided doses for 20 days, followed by a 10-day rest period. If menses does not occur by the end of this period of time, the dosage schedule should be repeated. The number of courses of estrogen required to produce bleeding varies, depending on the responsiveness of the endometrium. If bleeding occurs before the end of the 10-day period, a 20-day estrogen-progestin cycle should be started with 2.5–7.5 mg/day of estrogen with a progestin added the last 5 days. If bleeding occurs before the end of this regimènt, therapy is discontinued and resumed on day 5 of bleeding.

Palliation of mammary carcinoma in men or postmenopausal women.
10 mg t.i.d. for at least 90 days.

Palliation of prostatic carcinoma.
1.25–2.5 mg t.i.d. Effectiveness can be measured by phosphatase determinations and symptomatic improvement.

Prophylaxis of osteoporosis.
0.625 mg/day given cyclically.

Prevention of postpartum breast engorgement.
3.75 mg q 4 hr for 5 doses or 1.25 mg q 4 hr for 5 days.

- **IM, IV**

Abnormal bleeding.
25 mg, which may be repeated after 6–12 hr if necessary.

- **Vaginal Cream**

2–4 g (containing 1.25–2.5 mg conjugated estrogens) daily given for 3 weeks on and 1 week off. Regimen can be repeated as needed.

Administration/Storage

1. For all uses, except palliation of mammary and prostatic carcinoma and prevention of postpartum breast engorgement, oral conjugated estrogens are best administered cyclically—3 weeks of hormone therapy and 1 week off.

2. Parenteral solutions of conjugated estrogens are compatible with normal NSS, invert sugar solutions, and dextrose solutions.
3. Parenteral solutions are incompatible with acid solutions, ascorbic acid solutions, and protein hydrolysates.
4. Reconstituted parenteral solutions should be used within a few hours after mixing if kept at room temperatures. Put the date and time of reconstitution on the solution label.
5. If the solution is refrigerated, it will remain stable for 60 days.
6. IV use is preferred over IM as it induces a more rapid response.
7. IV premarin should be administered slowly to prevent flushing.
8. When used vaginally, the cream should be inserted high into the vagina (two-thirds the length of the applicator).

NURSING CONSIDERATIONS

See also *Nursing Considerations* for *Estrogens,* Chapter 68.

Assessment

1. Document indications for therapy and type and onset of symptoms.
2. Determine baseline serum phosphatase levels to evaluate the effectiveness in palliation of prostatic carcinoma.

Evaluate

- Control of mammary and prostatic cancer growth
- Control of abnormal uterine bleeding R/T hormonal imbalance
- Osteoporosis prophylaxis
- Relief of menopausal symptoms

Estropipate (Piperazine estrone sulfate)

(es-troh-**PIE**-payt)
Pregnancy Category: X
Ogen, Ortho-Est **(Rx)**

See also *Estrogens,* Chapter 68.

How Supplied: *Vaginal cream:* 1.5 mg/g; *Tablet:* 0.625 mg, 1.25 mg, 2.5 mg, 3 mg, 5 mg

Action/Kinetics: This product contains solubilized crystalline estrone stabilized with piperazine.

Uses: PO: Vasomotor symptoms, atrophic vaginitis, or kraurosis vulvae associated with menopause. Primary ovarian failure, female castration, female hypogonadism. Prevention of osteoporosis.

Vaginal: Atrophic vaginitis and kraurosis vulvae associated with menopause.

Dosage

- **Tablets**

Vasomotor symptoms, atrophic vaginitis, kraurosis vulvae.
0.625–5 mg/day for short-term therapy (give cyclically). May also be used continuously.

Hypogonadism, primary ovarian failure, castration.
1.25–7.5 mg/day for first 3 weeks; **then,** rest period of 8–10 days. A PO progestin can be given during the third week if withdrawal bleeding does not occur.

Prevention of osteoporosis.
0.625 mg/day for 25 days of a 31-day cycle per month.

- **Vaginal Cream**

2–4 g (containing 3–6 mg estropipate) daily (depending on severity of condition) for 3 weeks followed by a 1-week rest period.

Administration/Storage

1. Administration should be cyclic—3 weeks on the medication and 1 week off.
2. Attempts should be made to taper or discontinue the medication at 3–6-month intervals.
3. When used to relieve vasomotor symptoms, cyclic administration is initiated on day 5 of bleeding if the client is menstruating. If the client has not menstruated within the last 2 months (or more), cyclic administration may be initiated at any time.
4. To deliver the vaginal cream, the end of the applicator (after the appropriate amount is introduced) should be inserted into the vagina and the plunger pushed all the way down.
5. Between uses the plunger of the applicator should be pulled out of

the barrel and washed in warm, soapy water. The applicator should not be put in hot or boiling water.
Contraindication: Use during pregnancy.

NURSING CONSIDERATIONS

See also *Nursing Considerations* for *Estrogens,* Chapter 68.

Client/Family Teaching

1. Review appropriate method and frequency of administration, advising client to take medications at the same time each day.
2. Nausea may be relieved during PO therapy by consuming solid foods.
3. Review side effects of drug therapy stressing those symptoms requiring immediate reporting such as thromboembolic S&S (headache, blurred vision, pain, swelling or tenderness in the extremities); fluid retention (weight gain, swelling of extremities); hepatic dysfunction (yellowing of skin or eyes, itching, dark urine, clay-colored stools); changes in mental status or any unusual bleeding.
4. During treatment with vaginal preparations advise client to administer at bedtime remaining recumbent for 30 min. Protect clothing and bed linens by using a sanitary pad.
5. Avoid cigarette smoking; review added risks and refer to a formal smoking cessation program as needed.
6. Drug may cause increased pigmentation of skin. Wear protective clothing and sunscreens when sunlight exposure is necessary; otherwise avoid prolonged exposure.
7. Stop therapy and report if pregnancy is suspected.
8. Stress the importance of reporting for all follow-up lab studies and exams to assess drug effectiveness and to determine the need to continue therapy.

Evaluate

- Relief of menopausal symptoms
- Stimulation of menses
- Restoration of hormonal balance in deficiency states

PROGESTINS

See also the following individual entries:

Levonorgestrel Implants
Medroxyprogesterone Acetate
Megestrol Acetate

General Statement: Progesterone is a natural female ovarian steroid hormone produced in large amounts during pregnancy. It is chiefly secreted by the corpus luteum during the second half of the menstrual cycle and is produced by the placenta during pregnancy.

The hormone acts on the thick muscles of the uterus (myometrium) and on its lining (endometrium). It prepares the lining for the implantation of the fertilized ovum. Under the influence of progesterone, the estrogen-primed endometrium enters its "secretory phase" during which it thickens and secretes large quantities of mucus and glycogen. The myometrium relaxes under the effect of progesterone. During puberty, progesterone participates in the maturation of the female body, acting on the breasts and the vaginal mucosa.

Progesterone interacts, by a feedback mechanism, with FSH and LH, produced by the anterior pituitary. When progesterone and estrogen are high, there is a decrease in the production of FSH and LH. This inhibits ovulation and accounts for the fact that progesterone is an effective contraceptive. Natural progesterone has to be injected, but a whole series of compounds with progesterone-type activity (collectively called *progestins*) can be taken PO. These substances are now routinely substituted for natural progesterone. Progesterone is essential for the maintenance of pregnancy.

Although progesterone stimulates the development of alveolar mammary tissue during pregnancy, it does not initiate lactation. On the contrary, it suppresses the lactogenic hormone; lactation starts postpartum only when progesterone and estrogen levels have decreased.

Action/Kinetics: Physiologic doses are used for replacement therapy and to suppress gonadotropin production, which inhibits ovulation. Pharmacologic doses have several uses (see below). Progesterone must be administered parenterally because of major inactivation in the liver (first-pass effect). The hormones are metabolized in the liver and a major portion is excreted in the urine (urinalysis is used to monitor progesterone levels).

Uses: Abnormal uterine bleeding, primary or secondary amenorrhea (used with an estrogen), endometriosis, premenstrual tension. Alone or with an estrogen for contraception. May also be used in combination with an estrogen for endometriosis and hypermenorrhea. Certain types of cancer. *NOTE:* Not to be used to prevent habitual abortion or to treat threatened abortion.

Contraindications: Genital malignancies, thromboembolic disease, vaginal bleeding of unknown origin, impaired liver function. Pregnancy, especially during the first 4 months. Cancer of the breast, missed abortion, as a diagnostic test for pregnancy. Lactation.

Special Concerns: Use with caution in case of asthma, epilepsy, depression, and migraine.

Side Effects: Occasionally noted with short-term dosage, frequently observed with prolonged high dosage. *GU:* Spotting, irregular periods, amenorrhea, changes in amount and/or duration of menstrual flow, changes in cervical secretions and cervical erosion, breast tenderness or secretions. *Dermatologic:* Allergic rashes, pruritus, acne, melasma, chloasma, alopecia, hirsutism. *CNS:* Depression, pyrexia, insomnia. *Miscellaneous:* Weight gain or loss, cholestatic jaundice, masculinization of the female fetus, nausea, edema, precipitation of acute intermittent porphyria, photosensitivity.

Drug Interactions: Rifampin and possibly phenobarbital ↓ the effect of progesterone by ↑ breakdown by the liver.

Dosage

Progesterone must be administered parenterally. Other progestins can be administered PO and parenterally. The usual schedule of administration for *functional uterine bleeding, amenorrhea, infertility, dysmenorrhea, premenstrual tension, and contraception* is days 5 through 25 of the menstrual cycle, with day 1 being the first day of menstrual flow.

NURSING CONSIDERATIONS

Assessment

1. Identify indications for therapy. Assess client's clinical history for any evidence of thrombophlebitis, pulmonary embolism, or cerebrovascular accidents.
2. Document baseline BP, pulse, and weight and monitor at each visit.
3. Determine if the client has any history of psychic depression.
4. Note if the client has diabetes mellitus.
5. Determine that baseline lab studies have been performed.
6. Document last menstrual period and absence of pregnancy.

Client/Family Teaching

1. To avoid gastric irritation and nausea, take medication with a light snack, in the evening. Establish a schedule and take medication at the same time each day.
2. Explain that gastric distress usually subsides after the first few cycles of the drug. However, if these symptoms persist, they should be reported.
3. Review the symptoms of thrombic disorders such as pains in the legs, sudden onset of chest pain, SOB, and coughing for no apparent reason. Instruct the client to report these symptoms immediately.
4. Advise clients to weigh themselves at least twice a week and to report any unusual weight gain. Rapid weight gain may indicate the presence of edema.

5. Discuss the need to report any yellowing of the skin or sclera. This indicates jaundice and may necessitate the discontinuation of the medication, lab evaluation of liver function, and possibly a change in the dosage.
6. Report any episodes of unusual bleeding.
7. Discuss the fact that progestins may reactivate or worsen a psychic depression. Advise family to take particular note of any psychic changes the client may undergo, the circumstance of the depression, and to report these findings.
8. Advise clients with diabetes that progesterone may alter glucose tolerance. Instruct them to report positive urine tests and abnormal finger stick results promptly because the dosage of antidiabetic medication may need to be adjusted.
9. Early symptoms of ophthalmic pathology, such as headaches, dizziness, blurred vision, or partial loss of vision, should be reported when noted so that a thorough eye exam can be performed.
10. Advise clients to stop smoking. If they express difficulty, offer assistance and suggest enrollment in a formal smoking cessation program.
11. With birth control, stress that injections must be administered every 3 months to ensure adequate protection.
12. Emphasize the need to report for regular medical follow-up.

Evaluate

- Control of abnormal menstrual bleeding
- Effective hormone replacement therapy
- Establishment of menstrual regularity
- Effective contraceptive agent
- Reports of symptomatic improvement in menstrual pain and flow
- Radiographic evidence of ↓ size or resolution of ovarian cyst(s)

Levonorgestrel Implants

(**lee**-voh-nor-**JES**-trel)

Norplant System **(Rx)**

See also *Progesterone and Progestins,* Chapter 68.

How Supplied: *Kit:* 36 mg/implant

Action/Kinetics: Levonorgestrel implants are marketed in a set of six flexible Silastic capsules each containing 36 mg of levonorgestrel; an insertion kit is provided to the physician to assist with implantation. Small amounts of the drug slowly diffuse through the wall of each capsule resulting in blood levels of levonorgestrel that are lower than those seen when levonorgestrel or norgestrel is taken as oral contraceptive. The dose released is initially 85 mcg/day, followed by a decrease to approximately 50 mcg/day after 9 months, to 35 mcg/day after 18 months, and then leveling off to 30 mcg/day thereafter. Blood levels of levonorgestrel vary over a wide range and cannot be used as the sole measure of the risk of pregnancy. If used properly, the risk of pregnancy is less than 1 for every 100 users. Levonorgestrel does not have any estrogenic effects. The implant system lasts up to 5 years and the contraceptive effect is rapidly reversed if the system is removed from the body.

Use: Prevention of pregnancy (system lasts for up to 5 years). New capsules may be inserted after 5 years if continuing contraception is desired.

Dosage

- **Silastic capsules**

Six levonorgestrel-containing (36 mg each) Silastic capsules implanted subdermally in the midportion of the upper arm (8–10 cm above the elbow crease). Capsules are distributed in a fan-like pattern 15° apart (total of 75°).

Administration/Storage

1. To ensure effectiveness and to be sure the woman is not pregnant at the time of capsule implantation, the capsules should be implanted during the first 7 days of the cycle or immediately after an abortion.

2. Capsules should be inserted only by individuals instructed on the proper procedure for insertion. If capsules are placed too deeply, they may be more difficult to remove.
3. If all capsules cannot be removed at the first attempt, the site should be healed before another attempt is made.
4. Expulsion is not common but may occur if the capsules are placed too shallow or too close to the incision or if infection occurs.
5. If infection occurs, it should be treated and cured before replacing capsules.
6. After 5 years, capsules should be removed; if the woman desires additional contraception, a new set of capsules can be inserted.
7. *Treatment of Overdose:* All capsules should be removed.

Contraindications: Active thrombophlebitis, thromboembolic disorders, undiagnosed abnormal genital bleeding, acute liver disease, benign or malignant liver tumors, known or suspected breast carcinoma, confirmed or suspected pregnancy.

Special Concerns: Menstrual bleeding irregularities are commonly observed. Women who have a family history of breast cancer or who have breast nodules should be monitored carefully. Use with caution in individuals in whom fluid retention might be dangerous and in those with a history of depression. Women being treated for hyperlipidemias should be monitored closely because an increase in LDL levels may occur. Capsules should not be inserted until 6 weeks after parturition in women who are breast-feeding.

Laboratory Test Interferences: ↓ Sex hormone binding globulin levels, T_4 levels (slight). ↑ Uptake of T_3.

Side Effects: *Menstrual irregularities:* Prolonged menses, spotting, irregular onset of menses, frequent menses, amenorrhea, scanty bleeding, cervicitis, vaginitis. *At implant site:* Pain or itching, infection, bruising following insertion or removal, hyperpigmentation (reversible upon removal). *GI:* Abdominal discomfort, nausea, change of appetite, weight gain. *CNS:* Headache, nervousness, dizziness. *Dermatologic:* Dermatitis, acne, hirsutism, scalp hair loss, excess hair growth. *Miscellaneous:* Breast discharge, breast pain, leukorrhea, musculoskeletal pain, fluid retention, possibility of ectopic pregnancy in long-term users, delayed follicular atresia.

Symptoms of Overdose: Overdosage can result if more than six capsules are inserted. Symptoms include fluid retention and uterine bleeding irregularities.

Drug Interactions

Carbamazepine / ↓ Effectiveness → ↑ risk of pregnancy
Phenytoin / ↓ Effectiveness → ↑ risk of pregnancy

NURSING CONSIDERATIONS

See also *Nursing Considerations* for *Progestins,* Chapter 68.

Assessment

1. A complete medical history, physical, and gynecologic examination should be performed prior to implantation or reimplantation and annually during use.
2. Ensure that the woman is not pregnant at the time the capsules are implanted.
3. Determine if client is breast-feeding. Capsules should not be inserted until 6 weeks after delivery.
4. Note any history of thromboembolic disorders or depression.
5. Assess liver function and note any evidence of hyperlipidemia and associated treatment.
6. Note any family history of breast cancer. Document the presence of breast nodules because these require careful monitoring.
7. Obtain baseline weight. Be aware that the effectiveness of levonorgestrel may be slightly decreased with weights exceeding 70.5 kg.

Client/Family Teaching

1. Review appropriate procedure for wound care postinsertion and identify symptoms of infection and rejection that should be reported. Advise that

a scar may be evident at the insertion site.
2. Provide a printed list of side effects associated with drug therapy and instruct clients in what requires immediate reporting.
3. Advise client to expect some irregularity with the menstrual cycle such as longer periods, missed periods, and spotting in between during the first year of implantation.
4. Stress the importance of reporting for regularly scheduled follow-up visits so that therapy can be carefully evaluated.
5. Advise that the capsules may be removed at any time for any reason and that pregnancy can occur after the next menstrual cycle.

Evaluate
- Effective contraception
- Freedom from complications and side effects of drug therapy

Medroxyprogesterone acetate

(meh-**drox**-see-proh-**JESS**-ter-ohn)

Pregnancy Category: X

Amen, Curretab, Cycrin, Depo-Provera, Depo-Provera C-150, Provera **(Rx)**

See also *Progestins,* Chapter 68.

How Supplied: *Injection:* 150 mg/mL, 400 mg/mL; *Tablet:* 2.5 mg, 5 mg, 10 mg

Action/Kinetics: Medroxyprogesterone acetate, a synthetic progestin, is devoid of estrogenic and androgenic activity. The drug prevents stimulation of endometrium by pituitary gonadotropins. Also available in depot form. Priming with estrogen is necessary before response is noted.

Uses: Secondary amenorrhea, abnormal uterine bleeding due to hormonal imbalance (no organic pathology). Adjunct in palliative treatment of inoperable, recurrent, or metastatic endometrial or renal carcinoma. Long-acting contraceptive (injectable form). *Investigational:* Polycystic ovary syndrome, precocious puberty. With estrogen to treat menopausal symptoms and hypermenorrhea. To stimulate respiration in obesity-hypoventilation syndrome (oral).

Dosage

- **Tablets**

Secondary amenorrhea.

5–10 mg/day for 5–10 days, with therapy beginning at any time during the menstrual cycle. If endometrium has been estrogen primed: 10 mg medroxyprogesterone/day for 10–13 days (beginning on day 13 through day 16, respectively).

Abnormal uterine bleeding with no pathology.

5–10 mg/day for 5–10 days, with therapy beginning on day 16 or 21 of the menstrual cycle. If endometrium has been estrogen primed: 10 mg/day for 10 days, beginning on day 16 of the menstrual cycle. Bleeding usually begins within 3–7 days.

- **IM**

Endometrial or renal carcinoma.

Initial: 400–1,000 mg/week; **then, if improvement noted,** 400 mg/month. Medroxyprogesterone is not intended to be the primary therapy.

Long-acting contraceptive.

150 mg of depot form q 3 months by deep IM injection given only during the first 5 days after the onset of a normal menstrual period, within 5 days postpartum if not breastfeeding, or 6 weeks postpartum if breastfeeding.

Contraindications: Clients with or a history of thrombophlebitis, thromboembolic disease, cerebral apoplexy. Liver dysfunction. Known or suspected malignancy of the breasts or genital organs. Missed abortion; as a diagnostic for pregnancy. Undiagnosed vaginal bleeding. Use during the first 4 months of pregnancy.

Special Concerns: The overall risk of breast, liver, ovarian, endometrial, and cervical cancer is not thought to increase with use of the injectable long-acting contraceptive preparation. There is the possibility of ectopic pregnancy. Use with caution in clients with a history of depression. Due to the possibility of fluid retention, use with caution in cli-

ents with epilepsy, migraine, asthma, or cardiac or renal dysfunction.
Side Effects: *GU:* Amenorrhea or infertility for up to 18 months. *CV:* Thrombophlebitis, ***pulmonary embolism.*** *GI:* Nausea (rare), jaundice. *CNS:* Nervousness, drowsiness, insomnia, fatigue, dizziness, headache (rare). *Dermatologic:* Pruritus, urticaria, rash, acne, hirsutism, alopecia, angioneurotic edema. *Miscellaneous:* ***Hyperpyrexia, anaphylaxis,*** decrease in glucose tolerance, weight gain, fluid retention.

NURSING CONSIDERATIONS

See also *Nursing Considerations* for *Progestins,* Chapter 68.

Assessment

1. Document indications for therapy and type and onset of symptoms.
2. Note any history of thromboembolic disease.
3. Obtain baseline calcium levels and liver function studies.

Interventions

1. The combined effect of the drug and osteolytic metastases may result in hypercalcemia. Therefore, note especially client complaints of insomnia, lethargy, anorexia, and N&V. Withhold the drug, obtain serum calcium levels, and report if elevated.
2. In the event the client develops severe hypercalcemia, have IV fluids, diuretics, corticosteroids, and phosphate supplements available.
3. Monitor I&O. Encourage a high fluid intake to minimize hypercalcemia.
4. Closely monitor the client who has resumed therapy after drug-induced hypercalcemia has been corrected.
5. Set up a regular schedule for clients utilizing this drug as a contraceptive agent. May see improved compliance in younger clients with this form of contraception. Stress that additional protection is necessary to prevent STDs and HIV transmission.

Evaluate

- Prevention of pregnancy
- Control of tumor size and spread
- Reestablishment of regular menses with evidence of normal hormone levels

Megestrol acetate

(meh-**JESS**-trohl)
Pregnancy Category: D
Megace **(Rx)**

See also *Progestins,* Chapter 68.
How Supplied: *Suspension:* 40 mg/mL; *Tablet:* 20 mg, 40 mg
Action/Kinetics: The antineoplastic activity is due to suppression of gonadotropins (antiluteinizing effect). The drug, through an unknown mechanism, has appetite-enhancing properties. The product contains tartrazine, which can cause allergic-type reactions, including asthma, often occurring in clients sensitive to aspirin.
Uses: *Tablets:* Palliative treatment of advanced endometrial or breast cancer. Should not be used instead of chemotherapy, radiation, or surgery. *Oral suspension:* Treatment of anorexia, cachexia, or an unexplained, significant weight loss in clients with a diagnosis of AIDS.

Dosage

- **Oral Suspension**

Appetite stimulant in AIDS clients.
Adults, initial: 800 mg/day (20 mL/day). The dose should be adjusted to 400 mg/day (10 mL/day) after 1 month.

- **Tablets**

Breast cancer.
40 mg q.i.d.
Endometrial cancer.
40–320 mg/day in divided doses. To determine efficacy, treatment should be continued for at least 2 months.

Administration/Storage

1. The oral suspension should be shaken well before using.
2. The oral suspension is available in a lemon-lime flavor that contains 40 mg of micronized megestrol acetate/mL.

Additional Contraindications: Not to be used for diagnosis of pregnancy. Use during the first 4 months of pregnancy. Prophylactically to avoid weight loss.
Special Concerns: Use with caution in clients with a history of thromboembolic disease. Use in HIV-infected

women with endometrial or breast cancer has not been widely studied. Safety and efficacy in children have not been determined.
Laboratory Test Interferences: Hyperglycemia, ↑ LDH.
Side Effects: *GI:* Diarrhea, flatulence, nausea, dyspepsia, vomiting, constipation, dry mouth, hepatomegaly, increased salivation, abdominal pain, oral moniliasis. *CV:* Hypertension, ***cardiomyopathy,*** palpitation. *CNS:* Insomnia, headache, paresthesia, confusion, ***seizures,*** depression, neuropathy, hypesthesia, abnormal thought process. *Respiratory:* Pneumonia, dyspnea, cough, pharyngitis, chest pain, lung disorder, increased risk of respiratory infection with chronic use. *Dermatologic:* Rash, alopecia, herpes, pruritus, vesiculobullous rash, sweating, skin disorder. *GU:* Impotence, decreased libido, urinary frequency, albuminuria, urinary incontinence, UTI, gynecomastia. *Body as a whole:* Asthenia, anemia, fever, pain, moniliasis, infection, sarcoma. *Miscellaneous:* Leukopenia, edema, peripheral edema, amblyopia.

NURSING CONSIDERATIONS

See also *Nursing Considerations* for *Progestins,* and *Medroxyprogesterone Acetate,* Chapter 68.

Assessment

1. Document indications for therapy and onset of symptoms.
2. Note any history of thromboembolic disease.
3. If female and of childbearing age, determine if pregnant.
4. Document any client history or sensitivity to tartrazines.

Client/Family Teaching

1. Take with meals if GI upset occurs.
2. Take exactly as prescribed and do not skip or double up doses.
3. Report any vaginal bleeding, edema, swelling or pain in leg veins, and pain and weakness in thumb (carpal tunnel syndrome).
4. Females of childbearing age should practice birth control if sexually active.

Evaluate

- Regression or control of tumor size and spread
- Prevention of further weight loss in clients with AIDS

ORAL CONTRACEPTIVES

See Table 1, Chapter 68.

Pregnancy Category: X

General Statement: The majority of oral contraceptives contain both an estrogen and a progestin in each tablet; such products are referred to as *combination oral contraceptives.* There are three types of combination products: (1) monophasic—contain the same amount of estrogen and progestin in each tablet; (2) biphasic—contain the same amount of estrogen in each tablet but the progestin content is lower for the first part of the cycle and higher for the last part of the cycle; (3) triphasic—the estrogen content may be the same or may vary throughout the medication cycle; the progestin content varies, depending on the part of the cycle. The purpose of the biphasic and triphasic products is to provide hormones in a manner similar to that occurring physiologically. This is said to decrease breakthrough bleeding during the medication cycle.

The other type of oral contraceptive is the progestin-only ("mini-pill") product, which contains small amounts of a progestin in each tablet.
Action/Kinetics: The combination oral contraceptives are thought to act by inhibiting ovulation due to an inhibition (through negative-feedback mechanism) of LH and FSH, which are required for development of ova. These products also alter the cervical mucus so that it is not conducive to sperm penetration, and render the endometrium less suitable for implantation of the blastocyst should fertilization occur.

The estrogen used in combination oral contraceptives is either ethinyl estradiol or mestranol. Mestranol is demethylated to ethinyl estradiol in the liver. **t½:** 6–20 hr. The progestin used in combination oral contraceptives is either desogestrel, ethynodiol diacetate, levonorgestrel, norethindrone, norethindrone acetate, norgestimate, or norgestrel.

The progestin-only products do not consistently inhibit ovulation. However, these products also alter the cervical mucus and render the endometrium unsuitable for implantation. These products contain either norethindrone or norgestrel. This method of contraception is less reliable than combination therapy.

Although oral contraceptives may be associated with serious side effects, a number of noncontraceptive health benefits have been confirmed. These include increased regularity of the menstrual cycle, decreased incidence of dysmenorrhea, decreased blood loss, decreased incidence of functional ovarian cysts and ectopic pregnancies, and decreased incidence of diseases such as fibroadenomas, fibrocystic disease, acute pelvic inflammatory disease, endometrial cancer, and ovarian cancer.

Uses: Contraception, menstrual irregularities, menopausal symptoms. High doses are used for endometriosis and hypermenorrhea. *Investigational:* High doses of Ovral (ethinyl estradiol and norgestrel) have been used as a postcoital contraceptive.

Contraindications: Thrombophlebitis, history of deep-vein thrombophlebitis, thromboembolic disorders, cerebral vascular disease, CAD, MI, current or past angina, known or suspected breast cancer or estrogen-dependent neoplasm, endometrial carcinoma, hepatic adenoma or carcinoma, undiagnosed abnormal genital bleeding, known or suspected pregnancy, cholestatic jaundice of pregnancy. Smoking.

Special Concerns: Cigarette smoking increases the risk of cardiovascular side effects from use of oral contraceptives. Use with caution in clients with a history of hypertension, preexisting renal disease, hypertension-related diseases during pregnancy, familial tendency to hypertension or its consequences, a history of excessive weight gain or fluid retention during the menstrual cycle; these individuals are more likely to develop elevated BP. Use with caution in clients with asthma, epilepsy, migraine, diabetes, metabolic bone disease, renal or cardiac disease, and a history of mental depression. Use with drugs (e.g., barbiturates, hydantoins, rifampin) that increase the hepatic metabolism of oral contraceptives may result in breakthrough bleeding and an increased risk of pregnancy. Use during lactation only if absolutely necessary.

Side Effects: The oral contraceptives have wide-ranging effects. These are particularly important, since the drugs may be given for several years to healthy women. Many authorities have voiced concern about the long-term safety of these agents. Some advise discontinuing therapy after 18–24 months of continuous use. The majority of side effects of oral contraceptives are due to the estrogen component. *CV:* ***MI, thrombophlebitis, venous thrombosis with or without embolism, pulmonary embolism, coronary thrombosis, cerebral thrombosis, arterial thromboembolism, mesenteric thrombosis, thrombotic and hemorrhagic strokes, postsurgical thromboembolism, subarachnoid hemorrhage,*** elevated BP, hypertension. *CNS:* Onset or exacerbation of migraine headaches, depression. *GI:* N&V, bloating, abdominal cramps. *Ophthalmic:* Optic neuritis, retinal thrombosis, steepening of the corneal curvature, contact lens intolerance. *Hepatic:* ***Benign and malignant hepatic adenomas,*** focal nodular hyperplasia, ***hepatocellular carcinoma,*** gallbladder disease, cholestatic jaundice. *GU:* Breakthrough bleeding, spotting, amenorrhea, change in menstrual flow, change in cervical erosion and cervical secretions, ***invasive cervical cancer,*** bleeding irregularities (more common with progestin-only products), vaginal candidiasis, ***ectopic pregnancies in contraceptive failures***, breast tenderness, breast enlargement. *Miscellaneous:* Acute intermittent porphyria, photosensitivity, congenital anomalies, melasma, skin rash, edema, increase or decrease in weight, decreased carbohydrate tolerance, increased incidence of cervical *Chlamydia trachomatis,* decrease in the quantity and quality of breast milk.

Drug Interactions

Acetaminophen / Onset of the effect of acetaminophen may be delayed or ↓ slightly
Anticoagulants, oral / ↓ Effect of anticoagulants by ↑ levels of certain clotting factors (however, an ↑ effect of anticoagulants has also been noted in some clients)
Tricyclic antidepressants / ↑ Effect of antidepressants due to ↓ breakdown by liver
Barbiturates / ↓ Effect of oral contraceptives due to ↑ breakdown by liver
Benzodiazepines / ↑ or ↓ Effect of benzodiazepines due to changes in breakdown by liver
Beta-adrenergic blockers / ↑ Effect of beta blockers due to ↓ breakdown by liver
Caffeine / ↑ Effect of caffeine due to ↓ breakdown by liver
Carbamazepine / ↓ Effect of oral contraceptives due to ↑ breakdown by liver
Clofibrate / ↑ Excretion of the active form of clofibrate (clofibric acid) → ↓ effect
Corticosteroids / ↑ Effect of corticosteroids due to ↓ breakdown by liver
Griseofulvin / May ↓ effect of oral contraceptives due to altered steroid gut metabolism
Hypoglycemics / Oral contraceptives ↓ effect of hypoglycemics due to their effect on carbohydrate metabolism
Insulin / Oral contraceptives may ↑ insulin requirements
Isoniazid / ↓ Effect of oral contraceptives due to ↑ breakdown by liver
Lorazepam / ↓ Effect of lorazepam due to ↑ breakdown by liver
Neomycin / ↓ Effect of oral contraceptives due to ↑ breakdown by liver
Oxazepam / ↓ Effect of oxazepam due to ↑ breakdown by liver
Penicillins / May ↓ effect of oral contraceptives due to altered steroid gut metabolism
Phenylbutazone / ↓ Effect of contraceptives due to ↑ breakdown by liver
Phenytoin / ↓ Effect of oral contraceptives due to ↑ breakdown by liver
Rifampin / ↓ Effect of contraceptives due to ↑ breakdown by liver
Salicylates / ↓ Effect of salicylates due to ↑ metabolic clearance
Temazepam / ↓ Effect of temazepam due to ↑ breakdown by liver
Tetracyclines / ↓ Effect of contraceptives due to tetracycline-induced inhibition of gut bacteria that hydrolyze steroid conjugates
Theophyllines / ↑ Effect of theophyllines due to ↓ breakdown by liver
Troleandomycin / ↑ Chance of jaundice

Laboratory Test Interferences: Altered liver and thyroid function tests. ↓ PT, 17-hydroxycorticosteroids, 17-ketosteroids, and 17-ketogenic steroids. ↑ Factors I (prothrombin), VII, VIII, IX, and X. (Therapy with ovarian hormones should be discontinued 60 days before performance of laboratory tests.) ↑ Gamma globulins.

Dosage

See *Administration/Storage.*

NURSING CONSIDERATIONS

See also *Nursing Considerations* for *Estrogens and Progestins,* Chapter 68.

Administration/Storage

1. Tablets should be taken at approximately the same time each day (e.g., with a meal or at bedtime).
2. Spotting or breakthrough bleeding may occur for the first 1–2 cycles; if it continues past this time, consult the physician.
3. For the initial cycle, an **additional** form of contraception should be used for the first week.
4. The type of oral contraceptive preparation will determine the precise manner in which the drug is taken:
• For the 21-day regimen, 1 tablet is taken daily beginning on day 5 of menses (day 1 is the first day of menstrual flow). No tablets are taken for 7 days.
• For a 28-day regimen, hormone-containing tablets are taken for the first 21 days, followed by 7 days of inert or iron-containing tablets.
• Certain products, including the biphasic and selected triphasic oral contraceptives, are termed *Sunday start*. The first tablet should be taken the Sunday following the beginning of menses (if menses begins on Sunday, the first tablet should be taken that day). *NOTE:* The biphasic and triphasic products have varying amounts of estrogen and/or progestin, depending on the stage of the cycle; the client should understand fully how these preparations are to be taken and which tablets are to be taken at various times during the medication cycle.
• For progestin-only products, the first tablet is taken on the first day of menses; thereafter, 1 tablet is taken every day of the year.
5. It is recommended that for a woman beginning combination oral contraceptive therapy a product be chosen that contains the least amount of estrogen for that particular client.
6. If a woman fails to take 1 or more tablets, the following recommendations should be followed:
• If 1 tablet is missed, it should be taken as soon as it is remembered. Alternatively, 2 tablets can be taken the following day.
• If 2 tablets are missed, 2 tablets can be taken each day for 2 days; alternatively, 2 tablets can be taken on the day the missed tablets are remembered, with the second missed tablet being discarded.
• If 3 tablets are missed, a new medication cycle should be initiated 7 days after the last tablet was taken, and an additional form of contraception should be used until the start of the next menstrual period. *NOTE:* With each succeeding tablet missed, the possibility increases that ovulation will occur.
7. If it is necessary to switch brands of oral contraceptives, the client should wait 7 days to start the new pack if on a 21-day regimen or the day after the last tablet if on a 28-day regimen.
8. Non-nursing mothers may begin oral contraceptive therapy at the first postpartum exam (i.e., 4–6 weeks), regardless of whether spontaneous menstruation has occurred. Nursing mothers should not take oral contraceptives until the infant has been weaned.

Assessment

1. Women should have annual physical and internal examinations and Pap smears performed, especially when taking oral contraceptives.
2. Note any previous experience with these medications and their results.
3. Determine the client's beliefs and needs concerning contraception and instruct accordingly.
4. Note any existing medical condition that may preclude this drug therapy. Assist clients to explore other forms of birth control that suit their life-style and beliefs.

Client/Family Teaching

1. Advise client to take the tablets exactly as prescribed to prevent pregnancy.
2. Remind client that if 1 tablet is missed, she should take the tablet as soon as the oversight has been detected.
3. If 2 consecutive tablets have been missed, the dosage must be doubled for the next 2 consecutive days. The

regular schedule may then be resumed. However, the client or her partner should use additional contraceptive measures for the remainder of the cycle.

4. If 3 tablets are missed, discontinue the therapy and start a new course as indicated by the type of medication. Alternative contraceptive measures should be used when the tablets are not taken and should be continued for 7 days after a new course has been started.

5. Provide a written list of symptoms that require immediate reporting. Reinforce that if the client develops pain in the legs or chest, respiratory distress, an unexplained cough, severe headaches, dizziness, or blurred vision, the therapy should be discontinued and the provider notified immediately.

6. Symptoms of eye pathology, such as headaches, dizziness, blurred vision, or partial loss of sight, should also be reported immediately.

7. Oral contraceptives decrease the viscosity of cervical mucus, increasing the susceptibility to vaginal infections. These are difficult to treat successfully; therefore, good hygienic practice is essential.

8. If the client has persistent nausea, edema, and skin eruptions beyond the four cycles, she should consult with the provider for a possible adjustment of drug dosage or for a different combination.

9. Alterations in thought processes, depression, or fatigue should be reported because a medication preparation with less progesterone activity may be indicated.

10. Androgenic effects, such as weight gain, increased oiliness of the skin, acne, or hirsutism, should be reported because a change in medication or dosage may also be in order.

11. Report any missed menstrual periods. If two consecutive periods are missed, discontinue the therapy until pregnancy has been ruled out.

12. Advise the client not to take the tablets longer than 18 months without medical consultation. Stress the importance for the client to report for a yearly Pap smear and physical examination. Teach how and when to perform BSE.

13. Explain the need to practice another form of contraception if receiving ampicillin, anticonvulsants, phenylbutazone, rifampin, or tetracycline. These drugs may cause intermittent bleeding and the drug interactions could result in an unwanted pregnancy.

14. Contraceptives interfere with the elimination of caffeine. Therefore, advise clients to limit their caffeine consumption to prevent insomnia, irritability, tremors, and cardiac irregularities.

15. If the woman is breast-feeding her infant, another form of contraception should be used until lactation is well established.

16. **Do not smoke.** Offer encouragement and assist the client to quit. Suggest participation in a formal smoking cessation program.

17. Be certain that the client and significant other are made aware of all potential inherent risks prior to initiating drug therapy.

Evaluate

- Effective contraception
- Menstrual regularity
- ↓ Menstrual blood loss resulting from hormone imbalances

Table 1 Combination Oral Contraceptive Preparations Available in the United States

Trade Name	Estrogen	Progestin
	MONOPHASIC	
Brevicon 21-Day and 28-Day	Ethinyl estradiol (35 mcg)	Norethindrone (0.5 mg)
Demulen 1/35–21 and 1/35–28	Ethinyl estradiol (35 mcg)	Ethynodiol diacetate (1 mg)
Demulen 1/50–21 and 1/50–28	Ethinyl estradiol (50 mcg)	Ethynodiol diacetate (1 mg)
Desogen (28 day)	Ethinyl estradiol (30 mcg)	Desogestrel (0.15 mg)
Genora 0.5/35 21 Day and 28 Day	Ethinyl estradiol (35 mcg)	Norethindrone (0.5 mg)
Genora 1/35 21 Day and 28 Day	Ethinyl estradiol (35 mcg)	Norethindrone (1 mg)
Genora 1/50 21 Day and 28 Day	Mestranol (50 mcg)	Norethindrone (1 mg)
Levlen 21 and 28	Ethinyl estradiol (30 mcg)	Levonorgestrel (0.15 mg)
Levora 0.15/30-21 and -28	Ethinyl estradiol (30 mcg)	Levonorgestrel (0.15 mg)
Loestrin 21 1/20	Ethinyl estradiol (20 mcg)	Norethindrone acetate (1 mg)
Loestrin 21 1.5/30	Ethinyl estradiol (30 mcg)	Norethindrone acetate (1.5 mg)
Loestrin Fe 1/20 (28 day)	Ethinyl estradiol (20 mcg)	Norethindrone acetate (1 mg)
Loestrin Fe 1.5/30 (28 day)	Ethinyl estradiol (30 mcg)	Norethindrone acetate (1.5 mg)
Lo/Ovral-21 and -28	Ethinyl estradiol (30 mcg)	Norgestrel (0.3 mg)
Modicon 21 and 28	Ethinyl estradiol (35 mcg)	Norethindrone (0.5 mg)
N.E.E. 1/35 21 Day and 28 Day	Ethinyl estradiol (35 mcg)	Norethindrone (1 mg)
Nelova 0.5/35E 21 Day and 28 Day	Ethinyl estradiol (35 mcg)	Norethindrone (0.5 mg)
Nelova 1/35E 21 Day and 28 Day	Ethinyl estradiol (35 mcg)	Norethindrone (1 mg)
Nelova 1/50M 21 Day and 28 Day	Mestranol (50 mcg)	Norethindrone (1 mg)
Nordette-21 and -28	Ethinyl estradiol (35 mcg)	Levonorgestrel (0.15 mg)
Norethin 1/35E 21 Day and 28 Day	Ethinyl estradiol (35 mcg)	Norethindrone (1 mg)
Norethin 1/50M 21 Day and 28 Day	Mestranol (50 mcg)	Norethindrone (1 mg)
Norinyl 1 + 35 21-Day and 28-Day	Ethinyl estradiol (35 mcg)	Norethindrone (1 mg)
Norinyl 1 + 50 21-Day and 28-Day	Mestranol (50 mcg)	Norethindrone (1 mg)
Ortho-Cept 21 Day and 28 Day	Ethinyl estradiol (30 mcg)	Desogestrel (0.15 mg)
Ortho-Cyclen-21 and -28	Ethinyl estradiol (35 mcg)	Norgestimate (0.25 mg)

Trade Name	Estrogen	Progestin
	MONOPHASIC	
Ortho Novum 1/35–21 and –28	Ethinyl estradiol (35 mcg)	Norethindrone (1 mg)
Ortho Novum 1/50–21 and –28	Mestranol (50 mcg)	Norethindrone (1 mg)
Ovcon-35 21 Day and 28 Day	Ethinyl estradiol (35 mcg)	Norethindrone (0.4 mg)
Ovcon-50 21 Day and 28 Day	Ethinyl estradiol (50 mcg)	Norethindrone (1 mg)
Ovral 21 Day and 28 Day	Ethinyl estradiol (50 mcg)	Norgestrel (0.5 mg)
	BIPHASIC	
Jenest-28	Ethinyl estradiol (35 mcg in each tablet)	Norethindrone (10 tablets of 0.5 mg followed by 11 tablets of 1 mg)
Nelova 10/11–21 and –28	Ethinyl estradiol (35 mcg in each tablet)	Norethindrone (10 tablets of 0.5 mg followed by 11 tablets of 1 mg)
Ortho-Novum 10/11–21 and –28	Ethinyl estradiol (35 mcg in each tablet)	Norethindrone (10 tablets of 0.5 mg followed by 11 tablets of 1 mg)
	TRIPHASIC	
Ortho-Novum 7/7/7 (21 or 28 days)	Ethinyl estradiol (35 mcg in each tablet)	Norethindrone (0.5 mg the first 7 days, 0.75 the next 7 days, and 1 mg the last 7 days)
Ortho-Tri-Cyclen (21 or 28 days)	Ethinyl estradiol (35 mcg in each tablet)	Norgestimate (0.18 mg the first 7 days, 0.215 mg the next 7 days, and 0.25 mg the last seven days)
Tri-Levlen 21 Day and	First 6 days: Ethinyl estradiol (30 mcg)	Levonogestrel (0.05 mg)
Tri-Levlen 28 Day	Next 5 days: Ethinyl estradiol (40 mcg)	Levonorgestrel (0.075 mg)
	Last 10 days: Ethinyl estradiol (30 mcg)	Levonorgestrel (0.125 mg)
Tri-Norinyl (21 or 28 day)	Ethinyl estradiol (35 mcg in each tablet)	Norethindrone (0.5 mg the first 7 days, 1 mg the next 9 days, and 0.5 mg the last 5 days)
Triphasil 21 (21 or 28 day)	First 6 days: Ethinyl estradiol (30 mcg)	Levonorgestrel (0.05 mg)
	Next 5 days: Ethinyl estradiol (40 mcg)	Levonorgestrel (0.075 mg)
	Last 10 days: Ethinyl estradiol (30 mcg)	Levonorgestrel (0.125 mg)

All combination oral contraceptives are Rx and Pregnancy category: X.

CHAPTER SIXTY-NINE

Gonadotropic Hormones/Ovarian Stimulants and Inhibitors

See the following individual entries:

Chorionic Gonadotropin
Clomiphene Citrate
Danazol
Gonadorelin Acetate
Histrelin Acetate
Menotropins
Nafarelin Acetate
Urofollitin for Injection

Chorionic gonadotropin (HCG)

(kor-ee-**ON**-ik go-**NAD**-oh-troh-pin)

Pregnancy Category: C

A.P.L., Chorex-5 and -10, Chorigon, Choron 10, Corgonject-5, Follutein, Glukor, Gonic, Pregnyl, Profasi HP **(Rx)**

How Supplied: *Powder for injection:* 5,000 U, 10,000 U, 20,000 U

Action/Kinetics: The actions of HCG, produced by the trophoblasts of the fertilized ovum and then by the placenta, resemble those of LH. In males, HCG stimulates androgen production by the testes, the development of secondary sex characteristics, and testicular descent when no anatomic impediment is present. In women, HCG stimulates progesterone production by the corpus luteum and completes expulsion of the ovum from a mature follicle.

Uses: *Males:* Prepubertal cryptorchidism, hypogonadism due to pituitary insufficiency. *Females:* Infertility (together with menotropins).

Dosage

- **IM Only**

Prepubertal cryptorchidism, not due to anatomic obstruction.

Various regimens including (1) 4,000 USP units 3 times/week for 3 weeks; (2) 5,000 USP units every other day for 4 injections; (3) 15 injections over a period of 6 weeks of 500–1,000 USP units/injection; (4) 500 USP units 3 times/week for 4–6 weeks; may be repeated after 1 month using 1,000 USP units.

Hypogonadism in males.

The following regimens may be used: (1) 500–1,000 USP units 3 times/week for 3 weeks; **then,** same dose twice weekly for 3 weeks; (2) 4,000 USP units 3 times/week for 6–9 months; then, 2,000 USP units 3 times/week for 3 more months; (3) 1,000–2,000 USP units 3 times/week.

Stimulation of spermatogenesis (used with menotropins).

5,000 USP units 3 times/week for 4–6 weeks; reduce dose of 2,000 USP units twice weekly when menotropin therapy is begun.

Induction of ovulation (used with menotropins).

5,000–10,000 USP units 1 day after the last dose of menotropins.

Administration/Storage

1. Reconstituted solutions are stable for 1–3 months, depending on manufacturer, when stored at 2°C–8°C (35.6°F–46.4°F).
2. Have emergency drugs and equipment available in the event of an acute allergic response.

Contraindications: Precocious puberty, prostatic cancer or other androgen-dependent neoplasm, hypersensitivity to drug. Development of precocious puberty is cause for discontinuance of therapy.

Special Concerns: Since HCG increases androgen production, drug should be used with caution in clients in whom androgen-induced edema may be harmful (epilepsy, migraines, asthma, cardiac or renal diseases).

Side Effects: *CNS:* Headache, irritability, restlessness, depression, fatigue. *Miscellaneous:* Edema, precocious puberty, gynecomastia, pain at injection site.

NURSING CONSIDERATIONS

Assessment

1. Note any client history of hypersensitivity to the drug.
2. Assess the prepubescent male client for the appearance of secondary sex characteristics. The drug is contraindicated in this instance.
3. Document indications for therapy, onset of symptoms, and pretreatment assessment.

Interventions

1. Once started on the therapy, periodically examine the client for the beginning of secondary sex characteristics. This is an indication of sexual precocity and the drug should be withdrawn.
2. Report complaints of headache, easy fatigue, and restlessness, or if the family complains that the client has become increasingly irritable and depressed. Note if there is any change in the client's attention to physical appearance as the drug may have to be withdrawn.
3. When treating clients for cryptorchidism, examine once a week for testicular descent to evaluate the response to therapy.
4. Monitor weight and extent of edema at regular intervals and report because edema is common.
5. Observe client for gynecomastia and offer emotional support. This is especially important for young male clients.
6. In female clients being treated for corpus luteum deficiency, question about the occurrence of bleeding after day 15 of therapy. If bleeding occurs, hold the drug and report.

Client/Family Teaching

1. Review indications for therapy and the anticipated results.
2. Warn that medication may cause pain at the site of injection.
3. Record daily weights. Teach how to assess for and advise to report evidence of edema.
4. Explain that delayed menses, excessive menstrual bleeding, pain in the pelvic region, weakness, and fatigue are S&S of ectopic pregnancy and should be reported immediately.
5. Discuss the possibility of multiple births when the drug is used with menotropins.
6. Encourage client to return for scheduled follow-up visits to monitor the effectiveness of drug therapy.

Evaluate

- Testicular descent
- Formation of functional spermatozoa
- ↑ Progesterone production resulting in release of egg in females

Clomiphene citrate

(**KLOH**-mih-feen)

Clomid, Milophene, Serophene **(Rx)**

How Supplied: *Tablet:* 50 mg

Action/Kinetics: The drug acts by combining with estrogen receptors, thus decreasing the number of available receptor sites. Through negative feedback, the hypothalamus and pituitary are thus stimulated to increase secretion of LH and FSH. Under the influence of increased levels of these hormones, an ovarian follicle develops, followed by ovulation and corpus luteum development. Most women ovulate after the first course of therapy. Further treatment may be inadvisable if pregnancy fails to occur after ovulatory responses. It is readily absorbed from the GI tract and is excreted in the feces. **t½:** 5–7 days. **Time to peak effect:** 4–10 days after the last day of treatment for ovulation. **Uses:** Selected cases of female infertility in which normal endogenous estrogen levels have been observed. *Investigational:* Male infertility, insufficiency of the corpus luteum, diagnosis of hypothalamic-pituitary-gonadal axis function in males and in ovarian function studies.

Dosage

- **Tablets**

  First course.

25–50 mg/day for 5 days.

  Second course.

Same dosage if ovulation has occurred. In absence of ovulation, dose may be increased to 100 mg/day for 5 days (some clients may require up to 250 mg/day to induce ovulation).

Administration

1. Therapy may be started any time in clients who have had no recent incidence of uterine bleeding.
2. If the client has had recent uterine bleeding, start the therapy on the fifth day of the cycle.
3. If the client has had a previous course of therapy to which she did not respond, start the new therapy after 30 days have elapsed.

NOTE: Most clients will respond following the first course of therapy. Further therapy is not recommended if pregnancy does not result following three or four ovulatory responses.

Contraindications: Pregnancy, liver disease or history thereof, abnormal bleeding of undetermined origin. Ovarian cysts. The absence of neoplastic disease should be established before treatment is initiated. Therapy is ineffective in clients with ovarian or pituitary failure.

Laboratory Test Interferences: ↑ Serum thyroxine and thyroxine-binding globulin.

Side Effects: *Ovarian:* Ovarian overstimulation and/or enlargement and subsequent symptoms resembling those of PMS. *Ophthalmologic:* Blurred vision, spots, or flashes, probably due to intensification of after images. *GI:* Abdominal distention, pain, or soreness; N&V. *GU:* Abnormal uterine bleeding, breast tenderness. *CNS:* Insomnia, nervousness, headache, depression, fatigue, lightheadedness, dizziness. *Other:* Hot flashes, increased urination, allergic symptoms, weight gain, alopecia (reversible).

NURSING CONSIDERATIONS

Assessment

1. Obtain menstrual history and note any previous therapy.
2. Determine any history of abnormal bleeding of undetermined origin.
3. Note if the client has a history of hepatic dysfunction; document LFTs.
4. If sexually active, determine the possibility of pregnancy.

Client/Family Teaching

1. Teach client to take basal body temperature and chart temperature on a graph to determine if ovulation has occurred.
2. Discontinue the drug and report if pain in the pelvic area or abdominal distention occur. These symptoms indicate ovarian enlargement and the possible presence of an ovarian cyst.
3. If client develops blurred vision or has spots or flashes in the eyes, the retina of the eye may be affected. Discontinue taking the medication and report as an ophthalmologic examination is needed.
4. Avoid performing hazardous tasks involving body coordination or mental alertness because the drug may cause lightheadedness, dizziness, or visual disturbances.
5. Discontinue taking the medication and check with the provider if pregnancy is suspected because the drug may have teratogenic effects.
6. Advise of the potential risks related to ovarian cancer.

Evaluate

- ↑ Levels of FSH and LH
- Desired ovulation resulting in pregnancy

Danazol

(**DAN**-ah-zohl)

Cyclomen ✱, Danocrine **(Rx)**

How Supplied: *Capsule:* 50 mg, 100 mg, 200 mg

Action/Kinetics: This synthetic androgen inhibits the release of gonadotropins (FSH and LH) by the anterior pituitary. The drug inhibits synthesis of sex steroids and competitively inhibits binding of steroids to their cytoplasmic receptors in target tissues. In women this action arrests ovarian function, induces amenorrhea, and causes atrophy of normal and ectopic endometrial tissue. Has weak androgenic effects. **Onset, fibrocystic disease:** 4 weeks. **Time to peak effect, amenorrhea and anovulation:** 6–8 weeks; **fibrocystic disease:** 2–3 months to eliminate breast pain and tenderness and 4–6 months for elimination of nodules. **t½:** 4.5 hr. **Duration:** Ovulation and cyclic bleeding usually resume 60–90 days after cessation of therapy.

Uses: Endometriosis amenable to hormonal management in clients who cannot tolerate or who have not responded to other drug therapy. Fibrocystic breast disease. Hereditary angioedema in males and females. *Investigational:* Gynecomastia, menorrhagia, precocious puberty, idiopathic immune thrombocytopenia, lupus-associated thrombocytopenia, and autoimmune hemolytic anemia.

Dosage

- **Capsules**

Endometriosis.

400 mg b.i.d. (moderate to severe) or 100–200 mg b.i.d. (mild) for 3–6 months (up to 9 months may be required in some clients). Begin therapy during menses, if possible, to be sure that client is not pregnant.

Fibrocystic breast disease.

50–200 mg b.i.d. beginning on day 2 of menses.

Hereditary angioedema.

Initial: 200 mg b.i.d.–t.i.d.; after desired response, decrease dosage by 50% (or less) at 1–3-month intervals. Subsequent attacks can be treated by giving up to 200 mg/day. No more than 800 mg/day should be given to adults.

Administration/Storage

1. For fibrocystic disease, therapy should begin during menses to ensure the client is not pregnant.
2. Breast pain and tenderness in fibrocystic disease are usually relieved within 30 days and eliminated in 2–3 months; elimination of nodularity requires 4–6 months of uninterrupted therapy. Treatment may be reinstituted if symptoms recur (50% of clients have recurring symptoms within 6 months).

Contraindications: Undiagnosed genital bleeding; markedly impaired hepatic, renal, and cardiac function; pregnancy and lactation.

Special Concerns: Use with caution in children treated for hereditary angioedema due to the possibility of virilization in females and precocious sexual development in males. Geriatric clients may have an increased risk of prostatic hypertrophy or prostatic carcinoma. Use with caution in conditions aggravated by fluid retention (e.g., epilepsy, migraine, cardiac, or renal dysfunction).

Side Effects: *Androgenic:* Acne, decrease in breast size, oily hair and skin, weight gain, deepening of voice and hair growth, clitoral hypertrophy, testicular atrophy. *Estrogen deficiency:* Flushing, sweating, vaginitis, nervousness, changes in emotions. *GI:* N&V, constipation, gastroenteritis. *Hepatic:* Jaundice, dysfunction. *CNS:* Fatigue, tremor, headache, dizziness, sleep problems, paresthesia of extremities, anxiety, depression, appetite changes. *Musculoskeletal:* Muscle cramps or spasms, joint swelling or lock-up, pain in back, legs, or neck. *Miscellaneous:* Allergic reactions (skin rashes and rarely nasal congestion), hematuria, increased BP, chills, pelvic pain, carpal tunnel syndrome, hair loss, change in libido.

Drug Interactions

Insulin / Danazol ↑ insulin requirements

Warfarin / Danazol ↑ PT in warfarin-stabilized clients

NURSING CONSIDERATIONS

Assessment

1. Document indications for therapy, treatment time frames, and expected outcomes.
2. Determine the presence of any undiagnosed genital bleeding. Note the onset, frequency, extent, and any precipitating factors.
3. Obtain baseline renal and liver function studies.
4. If sexually active and of childbearing age, determine if pregnant.
5. Note any evidence or history of cardiac dysfunction.
6. Document subjective reports of endometrial pain. Note breast pain, tenderness, and the presence of any nodules.
7. Attempt to identify factors that precipitate angioedema (usually C-1 inhibitor deficiency; determine what triggers response).

Interventions

1. Observe the client closely for signs of virilization such as hirsutism, reduced breast size, deepening of the voice, acne, increased oiliness of the skin, and clitoral enlargement. Some androgenic side effects may not be reversible and may require a change in drug dosage or discontinuation of the drug.
2. Observe clients with a history of epilepsy, migraines, and cardiac or renal dysfunction for fluid retention. Danazol may cause fluid retention with resultant edema and require discontinuation of drug therapy.

Client/Family Teaching

1. Take with meals to decrease GI upset.
2. Describe the signs of virilization that may occur with drug therapy (e.g., abnormal hair growth, deepening of the voice). Advise to report these symptoms so that the dosage of drug can be adjusted.
3. Explain that the hypoestrogenic side effects usually disappear after the therapy is discontinued.
4. Ovulation will resume 60–90 days after the drug has been discontinued.
5. Wearing cotton underwear and paying careful attention to hygiene may diminish the incidence of vaginitis associated with danazol therapy.
6. Stress the importance of practicing birth control.
7. Advise that several months of therapy may be required before any improvements may be noted.
8. Continue to perform breast self-exams and report any changes.

Evaluate

- Relief of endometrial pain (usually requires 3–6 months of therapy)
- ↓ Breast tenderness and pain (usually after 2–3 months)
- Control of allergic manifestations of hereditary angioedema

---

Gonadorelin acetate

(go-nad-oh-**RELL**-in)

Pregnancy Category: B

Factrel ★, Lutrepulse **(Rx)**

How Supplied: *Kit:* 0.8 mg, 3.2 mg; *Powder for injection:* 0.8 mg, 3.2 mg

Action/Kinetics: Gonadorelin is a synthetic hormone identical in amino acid sequence to the naturally occurring gonadotropin-releasing hormone. Thus, gonadorelin stimulates the synthesis and release of FSH and LH from the adenohypophysis. FSH and LH then stimulate the ovaries to synthesize estrogen and progesterone, which are necessary for development and release of an ovum. **t½, initial:** 2–10 min; **final:** 10–40 min. Gonadorelin is metabolized to inactive peptide fragments, which are excreted in the urine.

Use: Primary hypothalamic amenorrhea.

Dosage

- **IV**

Primary hypothalamic amenorrhea.

5 mcg q 90 min (range: 1–20 mcg) delivered by Lutrepulse pump using

the 0.8-mg solution at 50 mcL/pulse. The recommended treatment interval is 21 days. If there is no response after three treatment intervals, the dose should be increased cautiously and in stepwise fashion.

Administration/Storage

1. The kit contains the lyophilized powder for injection, diluent, catheter and tubing, alcohol swabs, IV cannula units, syringe and needle, elastic belt, batteries, the Lutrepulse pump, physician pump manual, and package insert.
2. Gonadorelin is reconstituted with 8 mL of diluent immediately before use and then transferred to the plastic reservoir.
3. The presterilized bag with the supplied infusion catheter set is filled with the reconstituted solution for IV administration.
4. The drug is then administered IV using the Lutrepulse pump, which can deliver 25 or 50 mcL of solution over a period of 1 min and at a pulse frequency of 90 min. Depending on the concentration of the solution and the volume/pulse, the pump can deliver 2.5, 5, 10, or 20 mcg of gonadorelin.
5. The 8 mL of solution will last for approximately 7 consecutive days.
6. The cannula and peripheral IV site should be changed every 48 hr.
7. Have emergency drugs and equipment available in the event of an anaphylactic reaction.

Contraindications: Sensitivity to gonadorelin acetate or gonadorelin HCl (used for determining gonadotropic function of the pituitary). Pituitary prolactinoma, causes of anovulation other than those of hypothalamic origin (e.g., ovarian cysts), hormone-dependent tumors.

Special Concerns: There is no indication for use of gonadorelin acetate during lactation. Safety and efficacy have not been determined in children less than 18 years of age.

Side Effects: *Ovarian hyperstimulation:* Ovarian enlargement, ascites with or without pain, pleural effusion. *Local, due to use of infusion pump:* Inflammation, infection, mild phlebitis, hematoma at site of catheter. *Anaphylaxis:* ***Bronchospasm,*** flushing, tachycardia, urticaria, induration at injection site. *Miscellaneous:* Multiple pregnancy.

Drug Interaction: Gonadorelin should not be used with ovarian stimulators.

NURSING CONSIDERATIONS

Assessment

1. Perform a thorough nursing history. Proper diagnosis is critical for treatment to be successful.
2. Determine that hypothalamic amenorrhea or hypogonadism is due to a deficiency in quantity or pulsing of endogenous gonadotropin-releasing hormone.
3. Note any history of ovarian cysts or pituitary tumors because drug is contraindicated under these circumstances.
4. Obtain baseline ovarian ultrasound, pelvic exam, and mid-luteal phase serum progesterone level prior to initiating therapy.

Client/Family Teaching

1. Demonstrate the appropriate method for drug administration. Provide detailed instructions both orally and in writing regarding the proper use and care of the Lutrepulse infusion pump.
2. Have client return demonstrate so that any problems or questions may be identified prior to leaving the office. Provide client with a phone number where assistance may be found 24 hr a day.
3. Stress the importance of using aseptic technique.
4. Instruct in how to assess the infusion site for evidence of inflammation, phlebitis, erythema, infection, or hematoma and to report these findings because the site will need to be changed.
5. Provide a list of symptoms of hyperstimulation of the ovaries and advise client to avoid having intercourse if these symptoms are evident. A rupture

of an ovarian cyst could occur, resulting in hemoperitoneum.
6. Explain the importance of careful recordkeeping in relation to menses, basal temperatures and graph recordings, medication administration, and any side effects that may be noted. All side effects should always be reported.
7. Explain that if ovulation occurs with the pump in place, notify provider because the therapy should be continued for 2 more weeks to maintain the corpus luteum.
8. Explain that clinical response to gonadorelin acetate therapy is generally monitored by ovarian ultrasound, mid-luteal phase serum progesterone levels, and regularly scheduled physical exams including a pelvic. Additionally, the peripheral infusion site will be examined and changed every 48 hr. Stress the importance of complying with these frequently scheduled tests. This therapy may require a relatively long-term commitment by the client.
Evaluate: Restoration of menstrual cycle with evidence of ovum production (response to gonadorelin usually occurs within 2–3 weeks after initiation of therapy).

Histrelin acetate

(hiss-**TREL**-in)
Pregnancy Category: X
Supprelin, Synarel **(Rx)**

How Supplied: *Kit:* 0.2 mg/mL, 0.5 mg/mL, 1 mg/mL
Action/Kinetics: Histrelin contains a synthetic nonapeptide agonist of the naturally occurring GnRH. Initially the drug stimulates release of GnRH; however, chronic use desensitizes responsiveness of the pituitary gonadotropin, causing a reduction in ovarian and testicular steroidogenesis. Decreases in LH, FSH, and sex steroid levels are observed within 3 months of initiation of therapy.
Uses: To control the biochemical and clinical symptoms of central precocious puberty (either idiopathic or neurogenic) occurring before 8 years of age in girls or 9.5 years of age in boys.

Dosage

- **SC**

Central precocious puberty.
10 mcg/kg given as a single, daily SC injection. Doses greater than 10 mcg/kg/day have not been evaluated.
Administration/Storage
1. If prepubertal levels of sex hormones or a prepubertal gonadotropin response to GnRH administration are not achieved within the first 3 months of therapy, the client should be reevaluated.
2. The injection site should be varied daily.
3. Histrelin contains no preservative. Vials should be stored at 2°C–8°C (36°F–46°F) and protected from light.
4. Vials are to be used only once and any unused solution should be discarded.
5. The vial should be removed from the packaging only at the time of use. The vial should reach room temperature before using the contents.
Contraindications: Hypersensitivity to the product or any of its components. Lactation.
Special Concerns: Acute, serious hypersensitivity reactions may occur that require emergency medical treatment. Safety and efficacy in children less than 2 years of age have not been determined.
Side Effects: *Acute hypersensitivity reaction:* Angioedema, urticaria, ***CV collapse,*** hypotension, tachycardia, loss of consciousness, ***bronchospasm,*** dyspnea, flushing, pruritus. *CV:* Vasodilation (common), edema, palpitations, tachycardia, epistaxis, hypertension, migraine headache, pallor. *GI:* GI or abdominal pain, N&V, diarrhea, flatulence, decrease appetite, dyspepsia, GI cramps or distress, constipation, decreased appetite, thirst, gastritis. *CNS:* Headache (common), nervousness, dizziness, depression, changes in libido, mood changes, insomnia, anxiety, paresthesia, syncope, somnolence, cognitive changes, lethargy, impaired consciousness, tremor, hyperkinesia,

convulsions (increased frequency), hot flashes or flushes, conduct disorder. *Endocrine:* Vaginal dryness, leukorrhea, metrorrhagia, breast pain, breast edema, decreased breast size, breast discharge, tenderness of female genitalia, anemia, goiter, hyperlipidemia, glycosuria. *Musculoskeletal:* Arthralgia, joint stiffness, muscle cramp or stiffness, myalgia, hypotonia, pain. *Respiratory:* Cough, upper respiratory infection, pharyngitis, respiratory congestion, asthma, breathing disorder, rhinorrhea, bronchitis, sinusitis, hyperventilation. *Dermatologic:* Commonly, redness, itching, and swelling at the injection site. Also, urticaria, sweating, keratoderma, pruritus, pain, dyschromia, alopecia, erythema. *Ophthalmologic:* Visual disturbances, abnormal pupillary function, polyopia, photophobia. *Otic:* Otalgia, hearing loss. *GU:* Vaginal bleeding (most often one episode within 1–3 weeks after starting therapy and lasting several days). Also, vaginitis, dysmenorrhea, and problems of the female genitalia including pruritus, irritation, odor, pain, infections, and hypertrophy. Dyspareunia, polyuria, dysuria, incontinence, urinary frequency, hematuria, nocturia. *Miscellaneous:* Pyrexia (common), weight gain, fatigue, viral infection, chills, various body pains, malaise, purpura.

NURSING CONSIDERATIONS

Assessment

1. Assess for any histrelin-related hypersensitivity reactions.
2. Ensure that a thorough physical and endocrinologic evaluation has been performed. This should include:
• Baseline height and weight
• Baseline hand and wrist X rays to determine bone age
• Sex steroid level (estradiol or testosterone)
• Adrenal steroid level (to R/O congenital hyperplasia)
• Beta-human chorionic gonadotropin level (to R/O chorionic gonadotropin-secreting tumor)
• GnRH stimulation test (to document activation of HPG [hypothalamic-pituitary-gonadal] axis)
• Pelvic ultrasound (adrenal, testicular) to R/O steroid-secreting tumor and to obtain baseline gonadal size
• CT of head (to R/O any undiagnosed intracranial tumor)

Client/Family Teaching

1. Review administration instructions provided with client 7-day kit. Observe client/family in administration and offer guidance and assistance as needed.
2. Remind client that drug contains no preservative and that once vials are entered any unused solution is to be discarded.
3. Administer drug at room temperature.
4. Assist client to develop a method for establishing a daily administration schedule and record of injection sites.
5. Stress that if the medication is not administered daily, the pubertal process may be reactivated.
6. Report any persistent swelling, irritation or erythema at the injection sites.
7. Explain the importance of compliance with prescribed therapy and of reporting for scheduled serial clinical evaluations to assess progress and perform height measurements. Yearly bone growth determinations and serial GnRH testing will be done to document that gonadotropin responsiveness of the pituitary remains prepubertal during drug therapy.
8. Provide a printed list of drug side effects. Identify symptoms that require immediate medical intervention such as sudden swelling, dyspnea, dysphagia, rash, itching, and/or rapid heartbeat.
9. Advise that hypogonadism may result if HPG axis reactivation fails after discontinuation of drug therapy.
10. Drug should be discontinued when onset of puberty is desired. Clients require F/O to assess menstrual cyclicity, reproductive function, and adult height attained.

Evaluate: Control of the biochemical and physical manifestations of puberty.

Menotropins

(men-oh-**TROH**-pinz)
Pregnancy Category: X
Humegon, Pergonal **(Rx)**

How Supplied: *Powder for injection:* 75 IU, 150 IU

Action/Kinetics: Menotropins is a mixture of FSH and LH, which cause growth and maturation of ovarian follicles. For ovulation to occur, HCG is administered the day following menotropins. **Time to peak effect, females:** 18 hr. In men, menotropins with HCG given for a minimum of 3 months induce spermatogenesis. Eliminated through the kidneys.

Uses: *Females:* In combination with HCG to induce ovulation in clients with anovulatory cycles not due to primary ovarian failure. *Males:* In combination with HCG to induce spermatogenesis in clients with primary or secondary hypogonadotrophic hypogonadism.

Dosage

• **IM**

Induction of ovulation.

Individualized, initial: 75 IU of FSH and 75 IU of LH for 9–12 days, followed by 5,000–10,000 USP units of HCG 1 day after last dose of menotropins. *Subsequent courses:* Same dosage schedule for two more courses, if ovulation has occurred. **Then,** dose may be increased to 150 IU of FSH and 150 IU of LH for 9–12 days, followed by HCG as above for two or more courses.

Induction of spermatogenesis.

It may be necessary to give HCG alone, 5,000 IU 3 times/week, for 4–6 months prior to menotropins; **then,** 75 IU FSH and 75 IU LH **IM** 3 times/week and HCG 2,000 IU 2 times/week for at least 4 months. If no response after 4 months, double each dose of menotropins with the HCG dose unchanged.

Administration/Storage

1. Menotropins are destroyed in the GI tract, therefore, they must be administered parenterally.
2. Reconstituted solutions must be used immediately.
3. Discard any unused portions of the reconstituted drug.
4. Have emergency drugs and equipment available to treat allergic reactions should they occur.

Contraindications: *Women:* Pregnancy. Primary ovarian failure as indicated by high levels of urinary gonadotropins, ovarian cysts, intracranial lesions, including pituitary tumors. *Men:* Normal gonadotropin levels, primary testicular failure, disorders of fertility other than hypogonadotrophic hypogonadism. Thyroid or adrenal dysfunction. Absence of neoplastic disease should be established before treatment is initiated.

Side Effects: *Women:* Ovarian overstimulation, hyperstimulation syndrome (maximal 7–10 days after discontinuation of drug), ovarian enlargement (20% of clients), ***ruptured ovarian cysts, hemoperitoneum, thromboembolism,*** multiple births (20%). Fever, hypersensitivity. *Men:* Gynecomastia.

NURSING CONSIDERATIONS

Assessment

1. Document indications for therapy, onset of symptoms, and other therapy or drugs used.
2. Determine if the client has been tested for high levels of urinary gonadotropins or evaluated for the presence of ovarian cysts. The drug is contraindicated in these instances.
3. Obtain baseline lab studies (CBC, electrolytes, gonadotropin levels, thyroid and adrenal function studies) and document neurovascular assessments (especially peripheral pulses).

Interventions

1. Obtain urinary estrogen excretion levels daily. If greater than 100 mcg or if the daily estriol excretion exceeds 50 mcg, *withhold HCG* and notify the provider. These elevated levels are signs of an impending hyperstimulation syndrome.

2. Monitor CBC on a routine basis; an occasional client will develop erythrocytosis.
3. Observe for unexplained fever or complaints of abdominal pain. Withhold medication and report if evident.
4. If the client requires hospitalization for hyperstimulation, the following interventions should be performed:
• Place the client on bed rest.
• Monitor I&O; weigh daily.
• Monitor the specific gravity of the urine as well as serum and urinary electrolytes.
• Assess for hemoconcentration. If the hematocrit rises to critical levels, have sodium heparin on hand for administration.
• Increase fluid intake and anticipate electrolyte replacement therapy.
• Provide analgesics as needed for comfort.

Client/Family Teaching
1. Report any pain in the extremities, if an extremity is cool to the touch, or if an extremity becomes pale blue. This is a sign of arterial thromboembolism and must be reported immediately.
2. Explain that fever or the development of lower abdominal pain may be the result of overstimulation of the ovaries that has caused cysts to form, a loss of fluid into the peritoneum, or bleeding and must be reported immediately. Discuss the need for examination for this phenomenon at least every other day during drug therapy and for 2 weeks thereafter. If overstimulation occurs, hospitalization is necessary for close monitoring.
3. Explain the need to collect a 24-hr urine daily to be analyzed for estrogen and provide a suitable container for collection. Provide printed instructions concerning the collection and the delivery of a 24-hr urine sample to the appropriate lab facility.
4. Instruct client in taking her basal body temperature and charting it on a graph.
5. Describe the signs that indicate ovulation, such as an increase in the basal body temperature, and an increase in the appearance and volume of cervical mucus. Also, discuss the significance of the urinary excretion of estriol.
6. Client should engage in daily intercourse from the day before chorionic gonadotropin is administered and until ovulation occurs.
7. If symptoms indicate overstimulation of the ovaries, a significant ovarian enlargement may have occurred. Instruct client to abstain from intercourse because of the increased possibility of rupturing the ovarian cysts and to report.
8. Advise client and family that with this therapy the possibility of multiple births is increased.
9. Explain that pregnancy usually occurs 4–6 weeks after the completion of therapy.

Evaluate
• Ovulation in females as evidenced by ↑ estrogen levels
• Spermatogenesis in males as evidenced by ↑ testosterone levels

Nafarelin acetate

(**NAF**-ah-rel-in)
Pregnancy Category: X
Synarel **(Rx)**

How Supplied: *Spray:* 0.2 mg/inh
Action/Kinetics: Nafarelin is a hormone produced through biotechnology; it differs by only one amino acid from naturally occurring GnRH. The drug stimulates the release of LH and FSH from the adenohypophysis. These hormones cause estrogen and progesterone synthesis in the ovary, resulting in the maturation and subsequent release of an ovum. With repeated use of the drug, however, the pituitary becomes desensitized and no longer produces endogenous LH and FSH; thus endogenous estrogen is not produced, leading to a regression of endometrial tissue, cessation of menstruation, and a menopausal-like state. The drug is broken down by the enzyme peptidase. **Peak serum**

levels: 10–40 min. **t½:** 3 hr; 80% is bound to plasma proteins.
Uses: Endometriosis (including reduction of endometriotic lesions) in clients aged 18 or older; use restricted to no more than 6 months. Central precocious puberty in children of both sexes.

Dosage

- **Nasal Spray**

Endometriosis.

200 mcg into one nostril in the morning and 200 mcg into the other nostril at night (400 mcg b.i.d. may be required by some women).

Central precocious puberty.

400 mcg (2 sprays) into each nostril in the morning (i.e., 4 sprays) and in the evening (total of 8 sprays/day). If adequate suppression is not achieved, 3 sprays (600 mcg) into alternating nostrils t.i.d. (i.e., a total of 9 sprays/day).

Administration/Storage

1. Treatment with nafarelin should be initiated between days 2 and 4 of the menstrual cycle.
2. Use for longer than 6 months is not recommended due to the lack of safety data.
3. The product should be stored at room temperature in an upright position protected from light.

Contraindications: Hypersensitivity to GnRH or analogs. Abnormal vaginal bleeding of unknown origin. Pregnancy or possibility of becoming pregnant. Lactation.
Special Concerns: Use of nafarelin in pregnancy is not recommended; pregnancy should be ruled out before initiating therapy. Safety and effectiveness in children have not been established.
Laboratory Test Interferences: ↑ Cholesterol and triglyceride levels, plasma phosphorus, eosinophils. ↓ Serum calcium, WBCs.
Side Effects: *Due to hypoestrogenic effects:* Hot flashes (common), decreased libido, vaginal dryness, headaches, emotional lability, insomnia. *Due to androgenic effects:* Acne, myalgia, reduced breast size, edema, seborrhea, weight gain, increased libido, hirsutism. *Musculoskeletal:* Decrease in vertebral trabecular bone density and total vertebral bone mass. *Miscellaneous:* Nasal irritation, depression, weight loss.

NURSING CONSIDERATIONS

Assessment

1. Perform a complete client history and note any evidence of chronic alcohol, tobacco, or corticosteroid use. Query about any family history of osteoporosis. Conditions such as these are major risk factors for loss of bone mineral content and would deter repeated courses of treatment with this drug.
2. Note client description of menstrual cycles. Document any incidence of abnormal vaginal bleeding of unknown origin because drug is contraindicated in this event.
3. Determine if client is pregnant before administering therapy because drug is teratogenic.
4. Review the method of contraception being practiced. A nonhormonal method should be advised and practiced during drug therapy.

Client/Family Teaching

1. Treatment should begin between the second and fourth day of the menstrual cycle. Stress the importance of accurate record keeping in relation to menstrual patterns and cycles.
2. Teach the client how to administer the nasal spray and remind to use only as directed. The client should be encouraged to take the spray upon arising and just before bedtime. Stress the importance of alternating the nostrils to decrease mucosal irritation.
3. Explain that menses should cease while on nafarelin therapy. If regular menses continues, the provider should be notified.
4. Remind client that breakthrough bleeding may occur if successive doses are missed.
5. Stress the importance of using a nonhormonal form of contraception. Explain the potential hazards to the fetus should one become pregnant during therapy with nafarelin acetate.
6. If a topical nasal decongestant is required during treatment, the decongestant should be used at least 30 min af-

ter nafarelin to decrease the chances of reducing the absorption of nafarelin.
7. Provide a printed list of the hypoestrogenic and androgenic side effects that may occur with this drug therapy. Report these symptoms if evident because a change in drug dosage or drug therapy may be indicated.

Evaluate

- Restoration of normal function of the pituitary-gonadal system in 4–8 weeks
- ↓ Number and size of endometriotic lesions

Urofollitropin for injection

(**YOUR**-oh-foll-ee-**troh**-pin)
Pregnancy Category: X
Metrodin **(Rx)**

How Supplied: *Powder for injection:* 75 IU, 150 IU

Action/Kinetics: Urofollitropin is prepared from the urine of postmenopausal women. The drug is a gonadotropin that stimulates follicular growth in the ovaries of women without primary ovarian failure. Because treatment with urofollitropin only causes growth and maturation of a follicle, HCG must also be given to effect ovulation. **Time to peak effect:** 32–36 hr after HCG.

Uses: To cause ovulation in women with polycystic ovarian disease; such clients should have an elevated LH/FSH ratio and should have failed to respond to therapy with clomiphene. In conjunction with HCG to stimulate development of several ova in clients undergoing in vitro fertilization.

Dosage

- **IM**

Polycystic ovary syndrome.

Adults, initial: 75 IU urofollitropin daily for 7–12 days followed by 5,000–10,000 IU HCG 24 hr after the last dose of urofollitropin. If ovulation has occurred but pregnancy has not resulted, this dosage regimen may be repeated for two more courses of therapy. If pregnancy still has not resulted, the dose of urofollitropin may be increased to 150 IU/day for 7–12 days followed by 5,000–10,000 IU HCG 24 hr after the last dose of urofollitropin. This regimen may be repeated for two additional courses if pregnancy has not occurred.

In vitro fertilization.

Adults: 150 IU/day beginning on day 2 or 3 of the cycle followed by 5,000–10,000 IU of HCG 1 day after the last dose of urofollitropin. Treatment is usually limited to 10 days.

Administration/Storage

1. The powder for injection should be reconstituted by dissolving in 1–2 mL of sterile saline immediately before use.
2. Any unused drug should be discarded.
3. Urofollitropin should be protected from light and stored at 3°C–25°C (37°F–77°F).

Contraindications: Primary ovarian failure (as indicated by high levels of both LH and FSH), renal dysfunction, thyroid dysfunction, pituitary tumor, abnormal uterine bleeding of unknown cause, ovarian cysts, enlarged ovaries (not as a result of polycystic disease), infertility due to causes other than failure to ovulate. Pregnancy.

Special Concerns: Use with caution in lactation.

Side Effects: *Ovarian:* Hyperstimulation resulting in ovarian enlargement, abdominal distention or pain, ascites, pleural effusion. *GI:* N&V, diarrhea, bloating, abdominal cramps. *Pyrogenic or allergic reaction:* Chills, fever, muscle aches or pains, fatigue, malaise. *Dermatologic:* Hives, dry skin, loss of hair, rash. *Other:* Headache, ***ectopic pregnancy,*** breast tenderness.

Symptoms of Overdose: Hyperstimulation of the ovary, multiple gestations.

NURSING CONSIDERATIONS

Assessment

1. A thorough gynecologic and endocrinologic evaluation and examination should be completed before initiating urofollitropin therapy.
2. Note any history of renal dysfunction, thyroid dysfunction, or abnormal uterine bleeding from an unknown cause.

Client/Family Teaching

1. Report any sudden abdominal pain or tenderness.
2. Explain that the treatment usually consists of daily injections for 7–12 days.
3. Advise the couple to engage in daily intercourse, beginning 1 day prior to the administration of HCG until ovulation occurs.
4. During the treatment and for 2 weeks thereafter, the client should be examined at least every other day for hyperstimulation of the ovaries. Explain that if evidence of hyperstimulation occurs, the drug will be stopped immediately.
5. Provide a list of symptoms of hyperstimulation (of the ovaries) and advise client to avoid having intercourse if these symptoms occur. A rupture of an ovarian cyst could occur resulting in hemoperitoneum.
6. Explain that the use of this drug enhances the risk of multiple births.
7. Stress the importance of reporting all side effects to the provider and reporting for all examinations as scheduled.

Evaluate: Stimulation of ovulation to enhance fertility. (In combination with HCG therapy, drug will stimulate ova development.)

CHAPTER SEVENTY

Androgens and Androgen Inhibitor

See the following individual entries:

Finasteride
Testosterone Aqueous Suspension
Testosterone Cypionate (in Oil)
Testosterone Enanthate (in Oil)
Testosterone Propionate (in Oil)
Testosterone Transdermal System

Finasteride

(fin-**AS**-teh-ride)
Pregnancy Category: X
Proscar **(Rx)**

How Supplied: *Tablet:* 5 mg
Action/Kinetics: Finasteride is a specific inhibitor of steroid 5-alpha-reductase, the enzyme that converts testosterone to the active 5-alpha-dihydrotestosterone (DHT). The reduced plasma level of DHT results in regression of prostate tissue. **Elimination $t^{1}/_{2}$:** 6 hr in clients 45–60 years of age and 8 hr in clients over 70 years of age. There is slow accumulation after multiple dosing. Metabolized in the liver and excreted through both the urine and feces.
Uses: Treatment of symptomatic benign prostatic hyperplasia. There is rapid regression of the enlarged prostate gland in most clients; however, less than 50% of clients show an increase in urine flow and improvement of symptoms of benign prostatic hyperplasia when treated for 12 months. *Investigational:* Adjuvant monotherapy following radical prostatectomy, prevention of the progression of first-stage prostate cancer, treatment of male pattern baldness, acne, and hirsutism.

Dosage

- **Tablets**

Benign prostatic hyperplasia.
5 mg/day, with or without meals.

Administration/Storage

1. At least 6–12 months of therapy may be required in some clients to determine whether a beneficial response has been achieved.
2. Crushed finasteride tablets should not be handled by a woman who is pregnant or who may become pregnant; there is potential for absorption of the drug and subsequent potential risk to the male fetus. Also, when the male client's sexual partner is or may become pregnant, the client should either avoid exposure of his partner to semen or finasteride use should be discontinued.
3. No dosage adjustment is required in elderly clients or in those with impaired renal function.

Contraindications: Hypersensitivity to finasteride or any excipient in the product. Use during pregnancy, during lactation, and in children.
Special Concerns: Use with caution in clients with impaired liver function.
Laboratory Test Interference: ↓ Serum PSA levels.
Side Effects: *GU:* Impotence, decreased libido, decreased volume of ejaculate.

NURSING CONSIDERATIONS

Assessment

1. Determine that a complete urologic exam has been performed to ensure that other conditions similar to BPH have been ruled out (e.g., prostate cancer, infection, stricture, hy-

potonic bladder, neurogenic disorders).
2. Drug may cause a decrease in serum PSA levels (prostate-specific antigen: a screening study to detect prostate cancer) in clients with benign prostatic hyperplasia even in the presence of prostate cancer.
3. Digital rectal exams should be performed before and periodically during drug therapy to assess the prostate gland.
4. Not for use in females.
5. Note any history or evidence of liver dysfunction. Monitor clients with liver impairment closely as drug is metabolized by the liver.
6. Not all clients show a response to finasteride. Therefore, carefully monitor clients with a large residual urinary volume or severely diminished urinary flow for obstructive uropathy. Such clients may not be candidates for finasteride therapy.

Client/Family Teaching

1. Explain that 6–12 months of continued therapy may be necessary before a beneficial effect is evident.
2. Advise client that the following symptoms should show improvement with continued drug therapy: hesitance, feeling of incomplete bladder emptying, interruption of urinary stream, impairment of size and force of urinary stream, and terminal urinary dribbling.
3. Instruct client to use barrier contraception as drug may cause male fetal abnormalities.
4. If partner becomes pregnant, advise client to either discontinue finasteride or avoid exposure of partner to semen.
5. Explain that decreased libido, decreased volume of ejaculate, and impotence may occur.
6. Advise that symptoms return upon discontinuation of the drug.

Evaluate

- ↓ Size of enlarged prostate gland
- ↑ Maximum urinary flow rate
- Improvement in symptoms of BPH

Testosterone aqueous suspension

(tess-**TOSS**-ter-ohn)
Pregnancy Category: X
Histerone 100, Malogen ✱, Tesamone 100, Testandro **(Rx) (C-III)**

Testosterone cypionate (in oil)

(tess-**TOSS**-ter-ohn)
Pregnancy Category: X
depAndro 100 and 200, Depotest 100 and 200, Depo-Testosterone, Depo-Testosterone Cypionate ✱, Duratest-100 and -200 **(Rx) (C-III)**

Testosterone enanthate (in oil)

(tess-**TOSS**-ter-ohn)
Pregnancy Category: X
Andro L.A. 200, Andropository-200, Delatestryl, Depo-Testosterone Enanthate ✱, Durathate-200, Everone 200 **(Rx) (C-III)**

Testosterone propionate (in oil)

(tess-**TOSS**-ter-ohn)
Pregnancy Category: X
(Rx) (C-III)

Testosterone transdermal system

(tess-**TOSS**-ter-ohn)
Pregnancy Category: X
Testoderm **(Rx) (C-III)**

How Supplied: Testosterone aqueous suspension: *Injection:* 50 mg/mL, 100 mg/mL.
Testosterone cypionate: *Injection:* 100 mg/mL, 200 mg/mL.
Testosterone enanthate: *Injection:* 100 mg/mL, 200 mg/mL.
Testosterone propionate: *Injection:* 100 mg/mL.
Testosterone transdermal system: *Film, extended release:* 4 mg/24 hr, 6 mg/24 hr

Action/Kinetics: Testosterone, its degradation products, and synthetic substitutes are collectively referred to as the *androgens* (from the Greek *andros,* man). Like the primary female hormones, estrogen and progesterone, the production of testosterone is controlled by the gonadotropins: FSH and the interstitial cell-stimulating hormone, both of which are produced by the anterior pituitary.

At puberty, these gonadotropins initiate the production of testosterone, which in turn stimulates the development of primary sex organs and secondary sexual characteristics. Testosterone also stimulates bone and skeletal muscle growth, increases the retention of dietary protein nitrogen (anabolism), and slows down the breakdown of body tissues (catabolism). The anabolic effect is due to stimulation of RNA polymerase activity and specific RNA synthesis, resulting in increased protein production. Androgens promote retention of sodium, potassium, nitrogen, and phosphorus and the excretion of calcium. Toward the end of puberty, testosterone hastens the conversion of cartilage into bone, thereby terminating linear growth.

Treatment with testosterone and its congeners is complicated by the fact that the exogenous supply of the hormone may depress secretion of the natural hormone through inhibitory effects on the pituitary. Too large a dose may cause permanent damage. Treatment is usually associated with a feeling of well-being. In addition to testosterone and its various esters, several synthetic variants are available commercially.

Following PO use, 44% of testosterone is cleared by the liver in the first pass. Thus, the parenteral forms are used. **t½, testosterone cypionate after IM:** 8 days. Ninety percent is excreted through the urine as metabolites and 6% is excreted through the feces. Testosterone and testosterone propionate are considered short-acting; testosterone enanthate and testosterone cypionate are long-acting.

Uses: Replacement therapy in males for congenital or acquired primary hypogonadism, congenital or acquired hypogonadotropic hypogonadism, delayed puberty. In postmenopausal women to treat inoperable metastatic breast carcinoma or in premenopausal women following oophorectomy. Postpartum breast engorgement (evidence for effectiveness is lacking). *Investigational:* Male contraceptive (testosterone enanthate).

Dosage

Testosterone aqueous suspension and testosterone propionate in oil

- **IM Only**

Replacement therapy.

25–50 mg 2–3 times/week.

Breast cancer.

50–100 mg 3 times/week.

Growth stimulation in Turner syndrome or constitutional delay of puberty.

40–50 mg/m²/dose given monthly for 6 months.

Male hypogonadism, initiation of pubertal growth.

40–50 mg/m²/month until growth rate falls to prepubertal levels (about 5 cm/year).

Male hypogonadism, during terminal growth phase.

100 mg/m²/month until growth ceases.

Male hypogonadism, maintain virilization.

100 mg/m² twice monthly or 50–400 mg/dose q 2–4 weeks.

Postpartum breast engorgement.

25–50 mg of testostrone propionate for 3–4 days.

Testosterone enanthate and cypionate

- **IM Only**

Hypogonadism, replacement therapy.

50–400 mg q 2–4 weeks.

Delayed puberty.

50–200 mg q 2–4 weeks for no more than 4–6 months.

Palliation of inoperable breast cancer in women.

200–400 mg q 2–4 weeks.

- **Patch**

Replacement therapy (congenital or acquired primary hypogonadism, congenital or acquired hypogonadotropic hypogonadism).

One 6-mg patch applied daily on clean, dry scrotal skin that has been dry-shaved to remove hair. Clients with a smaller scrotum can use a 4-mg patch. The patch should be worn for 22–24 hr/day for 6–8 weeks.

Administration/Storage

1. Crystals of testosterone enanthate or cypionate may be redissolved by warming and shaking the vial.
2. If the needle or syringe is wet, the product may become cloudy; this does not affect potency.
3. For IM oil-based suspensions, warm the unopened vial in warm water to decrease the viscosity of the oil. Vigorously rotate the vial to resuspend the medication in the oil. A film may appear on the sides of the vial. When no more suspended particles are observed on the bottom or sides of the vial, the drug has been suspended appropriately. Administer the needle deep into the muscle, and administer the medication slowly.
4. When parenteral injection is to be used, testosterone propionate is more effective than testosterone because it is released more slowly.
5. Continue the therapy for at least 2 months for a satisfactory response and for 5 months for an objective response.
6. When used for delayed puberty, the chronological and skeletal ages should be considered when determining initial and subsequent doses. Use is usually for a limited time (e.g., 4–6 months).
7. The patch is made of a cloth and co-polymer that sticks to the skin without a sticky adhesive. The patch should be warmed in the hands before application. Clients should wear loose clothing to keep the patch in place.
8. Prior to sexual activity, the patch should be removed from the scrotum, and the scrotal area should be washed to remove residue.

Contraindications: Serious renal, hepatic, or cardiac disease due to edema formation. Prostatic or breast (males) carcinoma. Pregnancy (masculinization of female fetus) and lactation. Discontinue if hypercalcemia occurs.

Special Concerns: Use with caution in young males and females who have not completed their growth (because of premature epiphyseal closure). Androgens may also cause virilization in females or precocious sexual development in males. Geriatric clients may manifest an increased risk of prostatic hypertrophy or prostatic carcinoma. Androgen therapy occasionally seems to accelerate metastatic breast carcinoma in women.

Laboratory Test Interferences: Alter thyroid function tests. False + or ↑ BSP, alkaline phosphatase, bilirubin, cholesterol, and acid phosphatase (in women). Alteration of glucose tolerance tests.

Side Effects: *Hepatic:* Liver toxicity is the most serious side effect. Jaundice, cholestasis, alterations in BSP retention, AST, and ALT. Rarely, ***hepatic necrosis, hepatocellular neoplasms,*** peliosis hepatis, acute intermittent porphyria in clients with this disease. *GI:* N&V, diarrhea, anorexia, symptoms of peptic ulcer. *CNS:* Headache, anxiety, increased or decreased libido, insomnia, excitation, paresthesias, sleep apnea syndrome, ***CNS hemorrhage,*** chills, choreiform movements, habituation, confusion (toxic doses). *GU:* Testicular atrophy with inhibition of testicular function (e.g., oligospermia), impotence, epididymitis, irritable bladder, prepubertal phallic enlargement, gynecomastia. *Electrolyte:* Retention of sodium, chloride, calcium, potassium, phosphates. Edema. *Miscellaneous:* Acne, flushing, suppression of clotting factors (II, V, VII, X), polycythemia, leukopenia, rashes, dermatitis, ***anaphylaxis (rare),*** muscle cramps, hypercholesterolemia, male-pattern baldness, acne, seborrhea, hirsutism. Hypercalcemia, especially in immobilized clients or those with metastatic breast carcinoma. Virilization in women.

In females, menstrual irregularities (including amenorrhea), virilization, clitoral enlargement, hirsutism, increased libido, baldness (male pattern), virilization of external genitalia of female fetus.

In males, decreased ejaculatory volume, oligospermia (high doses), gynecomastia, increased frequency and duration of penile erections.

In children, disturbances of growth, premature closure of epiphyses, precocious sexual development.

Buccal preparations may cause stomatitis. Inflammation and pain at site of IM or SC injection.

NOTE: Side effects of the cypionate and enanthate products are not readily reversible due to the long duration of action of these dosage forms.

The patch may cause itching, irritation, or discomfort of the scrotum. Potentially, small amounts of testosterone may be transferred to a sex partner.

Drug Interactions

Anticoagulants, oral / Anabolic steroids ↑ effect of anticoagulants
Antidiabetic agents / Additive hypoglycemia
Barbiturates / ↓ Effect of androgens due to ↑ breakdown by liver
Corticosteroids / ↑ Chance of edema
Phenylbutazone / Certain androgens ↑ effect of phenylbutazone

NURSING CONSIDERATIONS

Assessment

1. Document indications for therapy and type and onset of symptoms.
2. Review the client's general health history for evidence of existing cardiac, renal, or hepatic dysfunction.
3. Obtain baseline data concerning client's neurologic status, BP, respirations, heart sounds, and GU function.
4. Note hair distribution and skin texture.
5. Check prescribed medications for any drugs that may interact unfavorably (i.e., anticoagulants, hypoglycemic agents, and mineralocorticoids).
6. If female, of childbearing age, and sexually active, note the potential for pregnancy.
7. Obtain baseline CBC, serum glucose, calcium, electrolytes, cholesterol, and liver and renal function studies. Treatment of clients with aplastic anemia has resulted in several cases of hepatocellular carcinoma.

Interventions

1. Monitor for signs of mental depression such as insomnia, lack of interest in personal appearance, and a general withdrawal from social contacts.
2. Document and report any complaints of tingling of the fingers and toes or loss of appetite.
3. Monitor client's weight, BP, pulse, and serum electrolytes. Auscultate lung sounds and note any distention of the jugular veins. Report any signs of edema, as sodium retention and edema can be easily treated with diuretics.
4. Assess for relaxation of the skeletal muscles and note if client complains of pain deep in the bones. The discomfort in the bones is caused by a honeycombing of the bones. These complaints are often a first indication of an increased calcium level and must be further investigated.
5. Complaints of flank pain may be caused by kidney stones, which may result from excessively high serum calcium levels.
6. Normal serum calcium levels are 8.8–10.4 mg/dL. Withdraw the drug and report if the client has a high serum calcium level. Administer large amounts of fluids to prevent renal calculi. If the hypercalcemia is the result of metastases, other appropriate therapy should be instituted.
7. Observe for jaundice, malaise, complaints of right upper quadrant pain, pruritus, or a change in the color or consistency of the stools. Obtain liver function studies and document and report.
8. Observe client for easy bruising, reports of bleeding, or complaints of

sore throat or the development of a fever. Obtain a CBC to rule out polycythemia and leukopenia.
9. If the client is a child, monitor closely for growth retardation and development of precocious puberty. Use with caution as the effect on the CNS in developing children is still being explored.
• Review the program of therapy with the parents. Often therapy will be intermittent to allow for periods of normal bone growth.
• Regular X rays to monitor the maturation of bone and effects on epiphyseal centers should be obtained every 6 months.
• Monitor and routinely record the child's height and weight..
10. If the client is female, report the onset of signs of virilization, such as deepening of the voice, hirsuitism, acne, menstrual irregularity, and clitoral enlargement. Usually only evident with doses exceeding 200–300 mg/month.
11. Discuss with female clients any changes in libido. Provide emotional support and report if evident as increased libido may be an early sign of serious drug toxicity.
12. Note the presence of acne and other skin changes. Report if the acne is severe since it may be necessary to change the dose of medication.
13. May alter serum lipid levels enhancing susceptibility to arteriosclerotic heart disease in women; monitor cholesterol levels periodically.

Client/Family Teaching

1. Report any unusual incidents of bleeding or bruising. Androgens suppress clotting factors (II, V, VII, and X) and polycythemia and leukopenia may also occur.
2. If the client has received the drug via pellets, sloughing can occur. Report immediately if this occurs.
3. Discuss the potential for bladder irritation. In older males, urinary obstruction may occur as a result of prostate hyperplasia.
4. Instruct parents of children receiving testosterone to weigh the child at least twice a week and to measure the child's height at least every 2–3 months. These measurements should be recorded graphically and maintained for provider review. Advise that X rays will be performed periodically on prepubertal children to assess effect on bone growth.
5. Advise women with metastatic breast cancer of the importance of lab tests of serum and urine calcium levels, alkaline phosphatase, and serum cholesterol. If the serum cholesterol level is high, the dosage of drug may need to be changed. Also, discuss the need to follow a low-cholesterol diet and refer to a dietitian for further assistance in meal planning and preparation.
6. Reassure female clients that any growth in facial hair and the development of acne are reversible once the drug is withdrawn.
7. Explain to premenopausal female clients that the medication may cause irregularities in the menstrual cycle. In postmenopausal women the medication may cause withdrawal bleeding.
• Advise women to keep a written record of their menstrual periods.
• For sexually active women, discuss the importance of reliable birth control measures during the first few weeks of androgen therapy and for several weeks after the androgen therapy has been withdrawn.
• Advise women to report immediately if pregnancy is suspected. There is an increased risk of fetal abnormalities with this drug.
8. Instruct male clients to report gynecomastia or priapism as this may necessitate withdrawal of the drug (at least temporarily).
9. Unless contraindicated, recommend that the client follow a diet high in calories, proteins, vitamins, minerals, and other nutrients. Restricting sodium intake may assist to reduce edema if this is evident.
10. Advise clients with diabetes that hypoglycemia may occur as a result of drug therapy. Monitor finger sticks frequently and report extreme variations because diet and/or dose of antidiabetic agents may require modification.

11. Discuss with young clients and their parents, if possible, the potential for drug abuse. High doses of androgens for enhancement of athletic performance can result in serious irreversible side effects. Explain the long-term effects and the permanent physical damage that is caused by indiscriminate use of these agents.

Evaluate

- Replacement therapy with control and prevention of S&S of androgen deficiency
- Effective male contraceptive agent
- Suppression of breast tumor size and spread

CHAPTER SEVENTY-ONE

Posterior Pituitary Hormones

See the following individual entries:

Desmopressin Acetate
Lypressin

Desmopressin acetate

(des-moh-**PRESS**-in)
Pregnancy Category: B
Concentraid, DDAVP, Stimate **(Rx)**

How Supplied: *Injection:* 4 mcg/mL; *Solution:* 0.01%; *Spray:* 0.01 mg/inh

Action/Kinetics: Desmopressin is a synthetic antidiuretic devoid of vasopressor and oxytocic effects. The drug acts to increase absorption of water in the kidney by increasing permeability of cells in the collecting ducts. **Onset:** 1 hr. **Peak:** 1–5 hr. **Duration:** 8–20 hr. **t½:** initial, 8 min; final: 75 min. Effect ceases abruptly. It also increases factor VIII levels (**onset:** 30 min; **peak:** 1.5–2 hr) and von Willebrand's factor activity.

Uses: *Parenteral:* Neurogenic diabetes insipidus, hemophilia A with factor VIII levels more than 5%, Type I von Willebrand's disease with factor VIII levels greater than 5%. Concentraid is used for renal concentration capacity testing.

Intranasal: Central diabetes insipidus (drug of choice due to low incidence of side effects, ease of administration, effectiveness, and long duration of action). To manage temporary polydipsia and polyuria due to trauma or surgery in the pituitary area. Primary nocturnal enuresis. Treatment of hemophilia A with factor VIII coagulant activity levels greater than 5%. Type I von Willebrand's disease with factor VIII levels greater than 5%. *Investigational:* Chronic autonomic failure resulting in nocturnal polyuria, overnight weight loss, morning postural hypotension.

Dosage

- **SC, Direct IV**

Neurogenic diabetes insipidus.

Adults, usual: 0.002–0.004 mg/day (0.5–1 mL/day) in two doses given in the morning and evening. Then, adjust dosage depending on response. If switching from the intranasal to the IV route, the IV dose is about 1/10 the intranasal dose.

Hemophilia A, von Willebrand's disease.

Adults: 0.0003 mg/kg diluted in 50 mL 0.9% sodium chloride injection infused IV over 15–30 min; dose may be repeated, if necessary. **Pediatric, 3 months or older, weighing 10 kg or less, IV:** 0.0003 mg/kg diluted in 10 mL of 0.9% sodium chloride injection and given over 15–30 min; repeat if necessary. **Pediatric, 3 months or older, weighing 10 kg or more, IV:** 0.0003 mg/kg diluted in 50 mL of 0.9% sodium chloride injection and given over 15–30 min; repeat if necessary.

- **Intranasal**

Neurogenic diabetes insipidus.

Adults, initial: 0.01 mg at bedtime; dose may be increased 0.0025 mg/night until a satisfactory response is obtained. If urine volume is still large, 0.01 mg can be given in the morning. **Maintenance:** 0.01–0.04 mg/day in one to three doses. **Pediatric, 3 months–12 years:** 0.005 mg at bedtime; dose may be increased by 0.0025 mg/night until a satisfactory response is obtained. A 0.005-mg morning dose may be added if the urine volume remains large.

Nocturnal enuresis.

Age 6 years and older, initial: 0.02 mg (0.2 mL) at bedtime with one-half the dose in each nostril; if no response, the dose may be increased to 0.04 mg.

Hemophilia A and type I von Willenbrand's disease.

In clients weighing 50 kg or more: One spray per nostril (total dose of 300 mcg). **In clients weighing less than 50 kg:** Given as a single spray of 150 mcg. The drug may be given 2 hr prior to minor surgery in the same doses as described above.

Renal concentration capacity test.

Adults: 0.040 mg (0.020 mg in each nostril) given any time during the day. **Children, 3–12 years:** 0.020 mg given in the morning.

Administration/Storage

1. Measure the dosage exactly because the drug is potent.
2. For direct IV administration (with neurogenic DI) give each dose over 1 min. With hemophilia, may dilute drug in 50 mL of NSS and infuse over 15–30 min.
3. Note the three graduation marks on the soft flexible plastic nasal tube: 0.2, 0.1, and 0.05 mL. The 0.05-level is not designated by number. Cleanse and dry the tube appropriately.
4. Stimate nasal spray pump can only deliver 0.1 mL (150 mcg). The pump must be primed prior to the first use by pressing down four times. The bottle should be discarded after 25 (150 mcg) doses since the amount delivered thereafter may be significantly less than 150 mcg.
5. Refrigerate the solution and injection at 4°C (39.2°F).
6. Stimate nasal spray should be kept refrigerated although the product will be stable for up to 3 weeks when stored at room temperature.
7. If the drug is used for hemophilia A or von Willebrand's disease, do not use it more often than q 2 days. Tachyphylaxis may occur if used more often.
8. To determine the renal concentration capacity in adults, the urine voided within 1 hr after drug administration is discarded; the two subsequent urines collected within 8 hr are saved and tested for osmolality. In children, osmolality is measured on urine voided during 3–5 hr after drug administration. Clients should drink only small amounts of fluid during the test day.
9. *Treatment of Overdose:* Reduce dose, decrease frequency of administration, or withdraw the drug depending on the severity of the condition.

Contraindications: Hypersensitivity to drug. Children under 3 months for hemophilia A or severe classic von Willebrand's disease (type III). Parenteral administration for diabetes insipidus in children under 12 years and intranasal administration in children less than 3 months. Nephrogenic diabetes insipidus, polyuria due to psychogenic diabetes insipidus, renal disease, hypercalcemia, hyperkalemia, or administration of demeclocycline or lithium.

Special Concerns: Safety for use during lactation not established. Use with caution and with restricted fluid intake in infants due to an increased risk of hyponatremia and water intoxication. Geriatric clients may have a greater risk of developing hyponatremia and water intoxication. Use with caution in clients with coronary artery insufficiency and/or hypertensive cardiovascular disease.

Side Effects: *DDAVP Injection:* High doses may cause dose-dependent transient headaches, nausea, nasal congestion, rhinitis, facial flushing, mild abdominal cramps, vulval pain, slight increase in BP, nosebleed, sore throat, cough, upper respiratory infections. Local erythema, swelling, or burning pain at injection site. *CV:* ***Rarely, thrombosis, acute cerebrovascular thrombosis,***

acute MI in clients predisposed to thrombus formation.

Concentraid: ***Symmetrical convulsions*** due to water retention and resultant hyponatremia in infants in whom the drug was given without restricted fluid intake. Headache, N&V, SOB, palpitations, yawning.

Stimate Nasal Spray: CNS: Somnolence, dizziness, insomnia, agitation. *CV:* Chest pain, palpitations, tachycardia. *Miscellaneous:* Itchy or light-sensitive eyes, chills, warm feeling, pain, dyspepsia, edema, vomiting, balanitis.

Symptoms of Overdose: Headache, abdominal cramps, nausea, facial flushing.

Drug Interactions: Chlorpropamide, clofibrate, and carbamazepine may potentiate the effects of desmopressin.

NURSING CONSIDERATIONS

Assessment

1. Note any client history of hypersensitivity to the drug.
2. Determine if client is taking any medications that could be potentiated by the use of desmopressin acetate.
3. Document indications for therapy and onset of symptoms.
4. Obtain baseline CBC, calcium, blood sugar, electrolytes, and appropriate factor levels.

Interventions

1. Monitor I&O. Observe for early S&S of water intoxication, such as drowsiness, headache, and vomiting, coupled with reports of excessive fluid consumption, weight gain, and/or seizures.
2. Adjust the client's fluid intake to avoid water intoxication and hyponatremia.
3. If there is excessive fluid retention, this may be treated with a diuretic such as furosemide.
4. With hemophilia therapy, during IV administration, closely monitor BP and HR.
5. With neurogenic diabetes insipidus, monitor urine osmolarity and volume. Weigh daily and assess for edema and any evidence of dehydration.
6. Monitor the duration of sleep. The amount of sleep, together with the client's daily I&O provide parameters to estimate the clinical response to drug therapy.

Client/Family Teaching

1. If a spray is used, instruct client in the appropriate administration technique and observe. Advise to use the special catheter provided. To administer, insert tip of the catheter into nose and blow on the other end of the catheter to deliver the medication deep into the nasal cavity. (A syringe filled with air may be used in children and comatose persons).
2. Provide recommendations concerning fluid intake.
3. Explain how to measure I&O and stress the importance of keeping an accurate record of fluid status. Provide the client with printed instructions indicating the symptoms of water intoxication and hyponatremia.
4. Stress the importance of notifying the provider at the earliest signs of trouble, such as a decrease in urinary output, the development of headaches, or severe nasal congestion. The latter two can be mistaken for an upper respiratory infection.
5. Avoid alcohol in any form.
6. Tolerance may develop over time and response may be diminished.

Evaluate

- Prevention and control of dehydration
- Prevention of hemorrhage due to improved factor VIII levels and ↑ clotting activity
- Control of nocturnal enuresis
- Desired antidiuretic effects (↓urine volume, ↑urine osmolarity, and relief of polydipsia)

Lypressin

(lye-**PRESS**-in)

Pregnancy Category: C

Diapid **(Rx)**

How Supplied: *Nasal Spray:* 0.185 mg/mL

Action/Kinetics: Lypressin is a synthetic antidiuretic, similar to vasopressin, for intranasal use only. This drug increases reabsorption of water from kidney by increasing the permeability of the collecting ducts. It has minimal vasopressor and oxytocic effects. **Onset:** Within 1 hr. **Time to peak effect:** 30–120 min. **Duration:** 3–8 hr. **t½:** 15 min. The drug is metabolized in the kidney and liver and excreted in urine.

Uses: Diabetes insipidus of neurohypophyseal origin; symptoms benefited include polydipsia, polyuria, and dehydration. Particularly suitable for clients allergic or refractory to vasopressin of animal origin.

Dosage

- **Nasal Spray**

Neurogenic diabetes insipidus.

Adults and children: 1–2 sprays (2–4 USP units) 3–4 times/day. Two or three sprays in each nostril is maximum that can be absorbed at any one time. (Each spray contains approximately 7 mcg lypressin.)

Administration/Storage

1. Encourage client to clear nasal passages before use.
2. Hold the bottle upright and insert the nozzle into the client's nostril with the head in a vertical position.
3. Apply gentle pressure to the bottle, spraying medication into the nostril while client is inhaling.
4. If more than 2 sprays per nostril are required q 4–6 hr, the time between doses should be reduced rather than increasing the number of sprays per dose.

Special Concerns: Safety for use during pregnancy has not been established. Clients with known sensitivity to ADH should be tested prior to use. Use with caution in clients with CAD. Due to decreased absorption by the nasal mucosa, effectiveness may be decreased in nasal congestion, allergic rhinitis, and upper respiratory infections.

Side Effects: *Nasal:* Congestion, pruritus, irritation, or ulceration of nasal passages. Rhinorrhea. *GI:* Increased bowel movements, abdominal cramps. *Miscellaneous:* Periorbital edema with itching. Heartburn (due to dripping into pharynx). Headache, conjunctivitis, hypersensitivity. Inhalation has resulted in coughing, transient dyspnea, substernal tightness.

Symptom of Overdose: Fluid retention.

Drug Interactions: Chlorpropamide, clofibrate, or carbamazepine may potentiate the effects of lypressin.

NURSING CONSIDERATIONS

Interventions

1. Check skin turgor and the condition of the mucous membranes for evidence of dehydration.
2. Observe for early signs of water intoxication, such as drowsiness, headaches, and vomiting and document. Monitor serum electrolyte profile.

Client/Family Teaching

1. Explain and demonstrate the appropriate technique for drug administration. Have client return demonstrate.
2. Discuss the need to take the medication only as directed and not to increase the number of sprays. If a change is indicated, the frequency of administration is usually increased, rather than increasing the number of sprays administered at one time.
3. Report feelings of drowsiness, listlessness, headaches, SOB, heartburn, nausea, abdominal cramps, or severe nasal congestion. These are symptoms of water intoxication and demand immediate attention.
4. Provide client with printed instructions including recommended fluid intake levels. Explain how to measure I&O and instruct client to keep a written record for review at each follow-up visit.
5. If increased thirst occurs or frequency of urination increases, 1 or 2 sprays may be administered to control the symptoms. This occurrence should be noted and reported so that the frequency of administration may be determined.

Evaluate: Prevention and control of dehydration R/T deficiency of ADH.

CHAPTER SEVENTY-TWO

Drugs Used for Inducing Labor

See the following individual entries:

Dinoprostone
Methylergonovine Maleate
Oxytocin, Parenteral
Oxytocin, Synthetic, Nasal

Dinoprostone

(**die**-noh-**PROS**-tohn)
Pregnancy Category: C
Prepidil Gel **(Rx)**

How Supplied: *Vaginal Gel/Jelly:* 0.5 mg/3 g; *Vaginal suppository:* 20 mg; *Vaginal insert, controlled release:* 0.3 mg/hr

Action/Kinetics: Dinoprostone, a prostaglandin E_2 derivative, is a cervical ripener.

Use: Ripening of an unfavorable cervix in pregnant women at or near term with a medical or obstetric need for induction of labor.

Dosage

• **Gel**

Initial: 0.5 mg. If there is no cervical/uterine response, repeat doses of 0.5 mg may given q 6 hr. The maximum cumulative dose for 24 hr is 1.5 mg dinoprostone.

Administration/Storage

1. The gel should be brought to room temperature just prior to administration.
2. Caution should be used to prevent contact with the skin. The hands should be washed thoroughly with soap and water after administration.
3. The gel is intended for endocervical placement. The degree of cervical effacement will regulate shielded catheter size to be used (20-mm catheter for no effacement and 10-mm catheter for 50% effacement).
4. The gel should be administered by sterile technique and introduced just below the level of the internal os.
5. The client should be kept supine for at least 15–30 min after administration.
6. If the desired response is obtained from the initial dose of dinoprostone, the recommended interval before giving oxytocin is 6–12 hr.
7. *Treatment of Overdose:* Symptoms may be relieved by changing maternal position, giving oxygen to the mother, or the use of beta-adrenergic drugs to treat hyperstimulation.

Contraindications: Use when oxytocic drugs are contraindicated or when prolonged uterine contractions are inappropriate (e.g., history of cesarean section or major uterine surgery), presence of cephalopelvic disproportion, history of difficult labor and/or traumatic delivery, grand multiparae with six or more previous term pregnancies, non–vertex presentation, hyperactive or hypertonic uterine patterns, fetal distress where delivery is not imminent, obstetric emergencies when surgical intervention may be favored. Also, use is contraindicated in ruptured membranes, hypersensitivity to prostaglandins or constituents of the gel, placenta previa or unexplained vaginal bleeding during current pregnancy, or when vaginal delivery is contraindicated (e.g., vasa previa or active herpes genitalis). Use in conjunction with oxytocic agents.

Special Concerns: Uterine rupture is possible when high-tone uterine contractions are sustained. Use with caution in clients with asthma or a history thereof, glaucoma, increased intraocular pressure, or impaired hepatic or renal function.

Side Effects: *Maternal:* Uterine contractile abnormality, GI effects, back pain, warm feeling in vagina, fever, premature rupture of membranes, uterine rupture. *Fetal:* Abnormality in fetal heart rate, bradycardia, deceleration, ***fetal depression.*** Extra-amniotic administration has resulted in amnionitis and ***intrauterine fetal sepsis.***

Symptoms of Overdose: Uterine hypercontractility, hypertonus.

NURSING CONSIDERATIONS

Assessment

1. Perform a thorough nursing history to determine any contraindication to oxytocic drugs; see *Contraindications.*
2. Document client's calculated and ultrasound-derived due date.
3. Fetopelvic relationships should be evaluated before the drug is used.
4. The cervix should be carefully examined to determine the degree of effacement (shortening of cervical canal) which will regulate the size of the shielded endocervical catheter used.

Interventions

1. Handle product carefully to avoid any contact of gel with skin. Wash hands thoroughly with soap and water immediately after administration.
2. Carefully monitor uterine activity, fetal status, and cervical dilation and effacement by visual assessment and auscultation and electronic fetal monitoring to detect undesired effects during dinoprostone use.
3. Continuous monitoring of uterine activity and fetal status should be undertaken when there is a history of hypertonic uterine contractility or tetanic uterine contractions.
4. Monitor for uterine rupture when high-tone myometrial contractions are sustained.

Evaluate: Desired cervical presentation to facilitate induction of labor.

Methylergonovine maleate

(meth-ill-er-**GON**-oh-veen)
Pregnancy Category: C
Methergine **(Rx)**

How Supplied: *Injection:* 0.2 mg /mL; *Tablet:* 0.2 mg

Action/Kinetics: Methylergonovine is a closely related synthetic drug of ergonovine, a natural alkaloid obtained from ergot. Methylergonovine stimulates the rate, tone, and amplitude of uterine contractions. The uterus becomes more sensitive to the drug toward the end of pregnancy. **Onset** (uterine contractions): **PO,** 5–10 min; **IM,** 2–5 min; **IV,** immediate. **$t^{1/2}$, IV:** 2–3 min (initial) and 20–30 min (final). **Duration, PO, IM:** 3 hr; **IV:** 45 min.

Uses: Management and prevention of postpartum and postabortal hemorrhage by producing firm uterine contractions and decreasing uterine bleeding. Incomplete abortion. *Investigational:* Ergonovine has been used to diagnose Prinzmetal's angina (variant angina).

Dosage

- **IM, IV (Emergencies Only)**

0.2 mg q 2–4 hr following delivery of placenta, of the anterior shoulder, or during the puerperium.

- **Tablets**

0.2–0.4 mg b.i.d.–q.i.d. until danger of hemorrhage and uterine atony is over (usually within 2 days, although treatment for up to 7 days may be necessary).

Administration/Storage

1. IV methylergonovine should be administered slowly over 1 min. After IV administration, check VS for evidence of shock or hypertension. Have emergency drugs available.
2. Ampules of discolored methylergonovine should be discarded.
3. *Treatment of Overdose:* Induce vomiting or perform gastric lavage. Admin-

ister a cathartic; institute diuresis. Maintain respiration, especially if seizures or coma occur. Treat seizures with anticonvulsant drugs. Warm extremities to control peripheral vasospasm.
Contraindications: Pregnancy, toxemia, hypertension. Ergot hypersensitivity. Should be given with caution in sepsis, obliterative vascular disease, impaired renal or hepatic function. To induce labor or threatened spontaneous abortions. Administration before delivery of the placenta.
Side Effects: *GI:* N&V. *CNS:* Dizziness, headache, tinnitus. *Miscellaneous:* Sweating, chest pain, dyspnea, palpitations, transient hypertension.

NOTE: ***Use of methylergonovine during labor may result in uterine tetany with rupture, cervical and perineal lacerations, embolism of amniotic fluid as well as hypoxia and intracranial hemorrhage in the infant.***

Symptoms of Overdose: Initially, N&V, abdominal pain, increase in BP, tingling of extremities, numbness. Symptoms of severe overdose include hypotension, hypothermia, ***respiratory depression, seizures, coma.***

NURSING CONSIDERATIONS

Assessment

1. Document indications for therapy and onset of symptoms.
2. Avoid smoking as nicotine constricts blood vessels.
3. Assess for S&S or ergotism (cold and numb fingers and toes; N&V; headache; muscle pain; chest pain; weakness).

Evaluate: Improved uterine tone with control of postpartum bleeding.

Oxytocin, parenteral

(ox-eh-**TOE**-sin)
Pitocin, Toesen ✱ **(Rx)**

Oxytocin, synthetic, nasal

(ox-eh-**TOE**-sin)
Pregnancy Category: X
Syntocinon **(Rx)**

How Supplied: Oxytocin, parenteral: *Injection:* 10 IU/mL.
Oxytocin, synthetic, nasal: *Spray:* 40 IU/mL
Action/Kinetics: These products are synthetic compounds identical to the natural hormone isolated from the posterior pituitary. Oxytocin has uterine stimulant, vasopressor, and antidiuretic properties. It acts by an indirect effect to mimic contractions of normal labor. Uterine sensitivity to oxytocin, as well as amplitude and duration of uterine contractions, increases gradually during gestation and just before parturition increases rapidly. The hormone facilitates ejection of milk from the breasts by stimulating smooth muscle. **Onset, IV:** immediate; **IM,** 3–5 min; **Nasal,** several minutes. **Peak effects:** 40 min. **t$^{1}/_{2}$:** 1–6 min (decreased in late pregnancy and lactation). **Duration, IV:** 20 min after infusion is stopped; **IM:** 30–60 min; **nasal:** 20 min. Eliminated through the urine, liver, and functional mammary gland.
Uses: *Antepartum:* Induction or stimulation of labor at term. Used to overcome true primary or secondary uterine inertia. Induction of labor with oxytocin is indicated only under certain *specific* conditions and is not usual because serious toxic effects can occur.

Oxytocin is indicated:

1. For uterine inertia.
2. For induction of labor in cases of erythroblastosis fetalis, maternal diabetes mellitus, preeclampsia, and eclampsia.
3. For induction of labor after premature rupture of membranes in last month of pregnancy when labor fails to develop spontaneously within 12 hr.
4. For routine control of postpartum hemorrhage and uterine atony.
5. To hasten uterine involution.
6. To complete inevitable abortions after the 20th week of pregnancy.
7. Intranasally for initial letdown of milk.

Investigational: Breast engorgement, oxytocin challenge test for determining antepartum fetal HR.

Dosage

• **IV Infusion, IM**

Induction or stimulation of labor. Dilute 10 units (1 mL) to 1,000 mL isotonic saline or 5% dextrose for IV infusion. **Initial:** 0.001–0.002 unit/min (0.1–0.2 mL/min); dose can be gradually increased at 15–30-min intervals by 0.001 unit/min (0.1 mL/min) to maximum of 0.02 unit/min (2 mL/min).

Reduction of postpartum bleeding. Dilute 10–40 units (1–4 mL) to 1,000 mL with isotonic saline or 5% dextrose for IV infusion. Administer at a rate to control uterine atony, usually at a rate of 0.02–0.1 unit/min.

Incomplete or therapeutic abortion.

10 units at a rate of 0.02–0.04 unit/min by IV infusion or 10 units IM after placental delivery.

• **Synthetic, Nasal**

For milk letdown.

One spray into one or both nostrils 2–3 min before nursing or pumping breasts.

Administration/Storage

1. For *IV* use: Use Y-tubing system, with one bottle containing IV solution and oxytocin, and the other containing only the IV solution. This allows for the discontinuation of the drug while maintaining the patency of the vein when it is decided to change to the drug-free infusion bottle. Parenteral oxytocin infusions should be administered only with an electronic infusion device.

2. As a *nasal spray:* Have the client sit upright and hold the bottle upright. Apply gentle pressure while spraying medication into the nostril. The nasal spray may be administered in drop form by applying gentle pressure to the bottle.

3. Oxytocin is rapidly broken down by sodium bisulfite. Have magnesium sulfate immediately available to relax the uterus in case of tetanic uterine contractions.

4. The physician should be immediately available during the administration of the drug.

5. *Treatment of Overdose:* Discontinue the drug and restrict fluid intake. Diuresis should be initiated and a hypertonic saline solution administered IV. Electrolyte imbalance should be corrected and seizures controlled with a barbiturate. If the client is comatose, special nursing care should be provided.

Contraindications: Hypersensitivity to drug, cephalopelvic disproportion, malpresentation of the fetus, undilated cervix, overdistention of the uterus, hypotonic uterine contractions, and history of cesarean section or other uterine surgery. Also, predisposition to thromboplastin and amniotic fluid embolism (dead fetus, abruptio placentae), history of previous traumatic deliveries, or women with four or more deliveries. Oxytocin should never be given IV undiluted or in high concentrations. Oxytocin citrate is contraindicated in severe toxemia, CV or renal disease. Intranasal oxytocin is contraindicated during pregnancy.

Side Effects: *Mother:* Tetanic uterine contractions, ***rupture of the uterus,*** hypertension, tachycardia, and ECG changes after IV administration of concentrated solutions. Also, rarely, anxiety, dyspnea, precordial pain, edema, cyanosis or reddening of the skin, and CV spasm. Water intoxication from prolonged IV infusion, ***maternal deaths due to hypertensive episodes, subarachnoid hemorrhage, or uterine rupture.***

Fetus: ***Death,*** PVCs, bradycardia, tachycardia, hypoxia, ***intracranial hemorrhage due to overstimulation of the uterus during labor leads to uterine tetany with marked impairment of uteroplacental blood flow.***

NOTE: Hypersensitivity reactions occur rarely. When they do, they occur most often with natural oxytocin administered IM or in concentrated IV doses and least frequently after IV infusion or diluted doses. Accidental swallowing of buccal tablets is not harmful.

Symptoms of Overdose: ***Hyperstim-***

ulation of the uterus resulting in hypertonic or tetanic contractions. Or, a resting tone of 15–20 cm water between contractions can result in uterine rupture, cervical and vaginal lacerations, tumultuous labor, uteroplacental hypoperfusion, postpartum hemorrhage, and a variable deceleration of fetal heart, fetal hypoxia, hypercapnia, or death. Water intoxication with seizures can occur if large doses (40–50 mL/min) of the drug are infused for long periods of time.

Drug Interactions: Severe hypertension and possible stroke when used with sympathomimetic pressor amines.

NURSING CONSIDERATIONS

Assessment

1. Note any history of hypersensitivity to the drug.
2. Document indications for therapy and onset of symptoms.
3. Determine fetal maturity, pelvic adequacy, and fetal presentation prior to initiating drug.
4. Check for dilation, assess resting uterine tone, and time the duration and frequency of uterine contractions. Note fetal HR and intrauterine pressure.
5. Carefully review the client's history for any contraindications prior to administering oxytocin.

For induction and stimulation of labor and/or oxytocin challenge test:

Interventions

1. Before initiating therapy, inform client of the rationale for using oxytocic agents and reassure that the procedure is not unusual. Prepare client by explaining that the medication will induce contractions. Advise that these may feel like cramps initially but can be very painful and that analgesics can be used when necessary.
2. Remain with the client during the induction period and throughout the stimulation of labor. The client must be attended by a qualified registered nurse.
3. Record VS and check I&O q 15 min.
4. Note resting uterine tone and assess the uterine contractions for frequency, duration, and strength of the contraction.
5. Monitor the fetal HR and rhythm at least every 10 min. Document and immediately report any alterations from the normal pattern.
6. Prevent uterine rupture and fetal damage by clamping off IV oxytocin, starting medication-free IV fluids, turning client on her left side, providing oxygen, and reporting when the following events occur:
   - If the contractions occur more frequently than every 2 min and last longer than 60–90 sec with no period of uterine relaxation between contractions.
   - If the contractions are excessively strong and/or exceed 50 mm Hg, as measured either on an external monitor or by an internal uterine catheter with an electronic monitor.
   - If resting uterine tone is 15–20 mm Hg or more.
   - If the fetal HR indicates bradycardia, tachycardia, or irregularities of rhythm, as measured by the fetoscope, Dopptone, or other type of electronic monitor.
7. Assess for water intoxication following prolonged administration of oxytocin. Monitor I&O and serum electrolytes closely.
8. Observe client for lethargy, confusion, and stupor. Note if the client has developed neuromuscular hyperexcitability with increased reflexes and muscular twitching. These symptoms should be reported immediately since convulsions and coma may occur if left untreated. Magnesium sulfate should be readily available for IV administration.

During the fourth stage of labor when oxytocin is administered for prevention or control of hemorrhage:

Interventions

1. Describe the location, size, and firmness of the uterus. Report if the uterus is displaced or boggy and follow designated hospital protocol.

2. In clients with spinal anesthesia, visually inspect for any evidence of bleeding. Sensation is diminished and hemorrhage may occur insidiously.
3. Note the amount and color of the lochia. Report any bright red lochia, excessive bleeding, or the passage of clots.
4. Monitor the client's VS until they remain stable.
5. Closely monitor I&O. Observe client for S&S of water intoxication; document and report immediately.

Evaluate

- Induction of labor with effective uterine contractions
- ↑ Uterine tone with ↓ bleeding
- Promotion of milk letdown

CHAPTER SEVENTY-THREE

Growth Hormone

See the following individual entries:

Somatrem
Somatropin

Somatrem

(**SO**-mah-trem)
Pregnancy Category: C
Protropin **(Rx)**

Somatropin

(so-mah-**TROH**-pin)
Pregnancy Category: C
Humatrope, Nutropin **(Rx)**

How Supplied: Somatrem: *Powder for injection:* 5 mg, 10 mg.
Somatropin: *Powder for injection:* 5 mg, 10 mg

Action/Kinetics: Both somatrem and somatropin are derived from recombinant DNA technology. Somatrem contains the same sequence of amino acids (191) as human growth hormone derived from the pituitary gland plus one additional amino acid (methionine). Somatropin, on the other hand, has the identical sequence of amino acids as does human growth hormone of pituitary origin. These agents stimulate linear growth by increasing somatomedin-C serum levels, which, in turn, increases the incorporation of sulfate into proteoglycans, thereby stimulating skeletal growth. These hormones also increase the number and size of muscle cells, increase synthesis of collagen, increase protein synthesis, and increase internal organ size. Serum insulin levels increase (indicative of insulin resistance), and there is acute mobilization of lipid.

Use: Stimulate linear growth of children who suffer from lack of adequate levels of endogenous growth hormone. Nutropin is used up to the time of transplantation in children who have growth failure associated with chronic renal insufficiency; also used in conjunction with other approaches in chronic renal insufficiency.

Dosage

SOMATREM

• **IM**

Individualized. Usual: Up to 0.1 mg/kg (0.2 IU/kg) 3 times/week. The incidence of side effects increases if the dose is greater than 0.1 mg/kg.

SOMATROPIN (HUMATROPE)

• **IM, SC**

Individualized. Usual: Up to 0.06 mg/kg (0.16 IU/kg) 3 times/week. Side effects increase if the dose exceeds 0.06 mg/kg.

SOMATROPIN (NUTROPIN)

• **SC**

Growth hormone inadequacy.

Individualized. Usual: A weekly dose of 0.3 mg/kg (about 0.78 IU/kg) given by daily injection.

Chronic renal insufficiency.

Individualized. Usual: A weekly dose of 0.35 mg/kg (about 0.91 IU/kg) given by daily injection.

Administration/Storage

1. Somatrem should be administered only by a physician experienced in the diagnosis and treatment of pituitary disorders.
2. Due to the development of insulin resistance, clients should be evaluated for possible glucose intolerance.
3. The powder for injection for somatrem should be reconstituted *only* with bacteriostatic water for injection (benzyl alcohol preserved).
4. If somatrem is to be used in newborns, it should be reconstituted with water for injection because

benzyl alcohol can be toxic to newborns.

5. Somatropin should be reconstituted only with the diluent provided; if sensitivity occurs, sterile water for injection can be used.

6. If somatropin (Humatrope) is reconstituted with sterile water for injection, the following guidelines must be followed.

- Use only one dose per reconstituted vial.
- The solutions should be refrigerated if not used immediately after reconstitution.
- The reconstituted dose should be used within 24 hr.
- After the dose is administered, any unused portion should be discarded.
- The solution should not be injected if it is cloudy or contains particulate material.

7. When reconstituting somatrem or somatropin, the vial should not be shaken. Rather, it should be swirled with a gentle rotary motion.

8. Only reconstituted somatrem solution that is clear and without particulate matter should be injected.

9. The needle used for injection should be at least 1 in. or greater in length to ensure that the injection reaches the muscle layer.

10. Reconstituted somatrem should be used within 7 days and should not be frozen.

11. The following guidelines should be used when giving Nutropin for clients who require dialysis:

- Hemodialysis clients should receive Nutropin at night just prior to going to sleep or at least 3–4 hr after dialysis in order to prevent hematoma formation due to heparin.
- Chronic cycling peritoneal dialysis clients should receive Nutropin in the morning after they have completed dialysis.
- Chronic ambulatory peritoneal dialysis clients should receive Nutropin in the evening at the time of the overnight exchange.

12. To reconstitute the 5-mg vial of Nutropin, use 1–5 mL of bacteriostatic water for injection (benzyl alcohol preserved), and to reconstitute the 10-mg vial, use 1–10 mL bacteriostatic water for injection. After introducing the diluent, gently swirl the vial using a gentle rotary motion (do not shake). Solutions that are cloudy immediately after reconstitution or refrigeration must not be used.

13. Before reconstitution, vials should be stored at 2°C–8°C (36°F–46°F). After reconstitution, solutions are stable for 14 days stored at the same temperature as the unreconstituted vials.

Contraindications: In clients in whom epiphyses have closed. Active intracranial lesions, sensitivity to benzyl alcohol (somatrem); sensitivity to m-cresol or glycerin (somatropin). *NOTE:* Hypothyroidism (which may be induced by the drug) decreases the response to somatrem.

Special Concerns: Use with caution during lactation. Concomitant use of glucocorticoids may decrease the response to growth hormone.

Side Effects: Development of persistent antibodies to growth hormone (30%–40% of clients taking somatrem and 2% of clients taking somatropin). Development of insulin resistance. Development of hypothyroidism. Sodium retention and mild edema (especially in adults). Slipped capital femoral epiphysis or avascular necrosis of the femoral head in children with advanced renal osteodystrophy. Intracranial hypertension manifested by papilledema, visual changes, headache, N&V. *In adults:* Hyperglycemia, glucosuria; mild, transient edema; headache, weakness, muscle pain. *In children:* Injection site pain, leukemia.

Symptoms of Overdose: Acute overdose can cause hypoglycemia followed by hyperglycemia. Long-term overdose can result in S&S of acromegaly or gigantism.

Drug Interaction: Glucocorticoids inhibit the effect of somatrem on growth.

NURSING CONSIDERATIONS

Assessment

1. Determine that X-ray evidence of bone growth (wrists, hands) has been conducted.
2. Note if the client is receiving glucocorticoids. These inhibit the effect of somatrem on growth.
3. If growth is slow in the absence of rising antibody titers, hypopituitarism should be ruled out; untreated hypothyroidism or excessive glucocorticoid replacement can impair growth.

Interventions

1. Measure the client's height and weight monthly and record. Advise that generally a growth increase of 2 cm/year should be attained in order for treatment to be continued.
2. Monitor blood sugar and thyroid function studies routinely for any evidence of diabetes or hypothyroidism.
3. Routinely assess clients with diabetes for evidence of hyperglycemia and acidosis.
4. Note any limps or knee/hip pain because a slipped capital epiphysis may occur.
5. Advise that the cost per year is based on client's weight and typically runs $10,000–30,000.

Evaluate: Evidence of desired skeletal growth.

CHAPTER SEVENTY-FOUR

Calcium Salts and Calcium Regulators

See also the following drug classes and individual drugs:

Calcium Salts

- Calcium Carbonate
- Calcium Carbonate, Precipitated - See Chapter 59
- Calcium Chloride
- Calcium Citrate
- Calcium Glubionate
- Calcium Gluceptate (Calcium Glucoheptonate)
- Calcium Gluconate
- Calcium Lactate
- Dibasic Calcium Phosphate Dihydrate

Calcium Regulators

- Calcitonin, Human
- Calcitonin, Salmon
- Etidronate Disodium (Oral)
- Etidronate Disodium (Parenteral)
- Gallium Nitrate
- Pamidronate Disodium

CALCIUM SALTS

Action/Kinetics: Calcium is essential for maintaining normal function of nerves, muscles, the skeletal system, and permeability of cell membranes and capillaries. For example, calcium is necessary for activation of many enzyme reactions and is required for nerve impulses; contraction of cardiac, smooth, and skeletal muscle, renal function, respiration, and blood coagulation. It has a role in the release of neurotransmitters and hormones, in the uptake and binding of amino acids, in vitamin B_{12} absorption, and in gastrin secretion. The normal serum calcium concentration is 9–10.4 mg/dL (4.5–5.2 mEq/L). When the calcium level of the extracellular fluid falls below this level, calcium is first mobilized from bone. However, eventually blood calcium depletion may be significant. Hypocalcemia is characterized by muscular fibrillation, twitching, skeletal muscle spasms, leg cramps, tetanic spasms, cardiac arrhythmias, smooth muscle hyperexcitability, mental depression, and anxiety states. Excessive, chronic hypocalcemia is characterized by brittle, defective nails, poor dentition, and brittle hair. The daily RDA for elemental calcium is 0.8 g/day for adults over 25 years of age and children 1–10 years of age, 1.2 g for pregnant or lactating women and both males and females 11–24 years of age, 0.6 g for children 6–12 months of age, and 0.4 g for infants less than 6 months of age. Calcium deficiency can be corrected by the administration of various calcium salts. Calcium is well absorbed from the upper GI tract. However, severe low-calcium tetany is best treated by IV administration of calcium gluconate. The presence of vitamin D is necessary for maximum calcium utilization. The hormone of the parathyroid gland is necessary for the regulation of the calcium level.

Uses: IV: Acute hypocalcemic tetany secondary to renal failure, hypoparathyroidism, premature delivery, maternal diabetes mellitus in infants, and poisoning due to magnesium, oxalic acid, radiophosphorus, carbon tetrachloride, fluoride, phosphate, strontium, and radium. To treat depletion of electrolytes. Also during cardiac resuscitation when epinephrine or isoproterenol has not improved myocardial contraction (may also be given into the ventricular cavity for this purpose). To reverse cardiotoxicity or hyperkalemia. **IM or IV:** Reduce spasms in renal, biliary, intestinal, or lead colic. To relieve muscle cramps due to insect bites and to decrease capillary permeability in various sensitivity reactions. **PO:** Osteoporosis, osteomalacia, chronic hypoparathyroidism, rickets, latent tetany, hypocalcemia secondary to use of anticonvulsant drugs. Myasthenia gravis, Eaton-Lambert syndrome, supplement for pregnant, postmenopausal, or nursing women. Also, prophylactically for primary osteoporosis. *Investigational:* As an infusion to diagnose Zollinger-Ellison syndrome and medullary thyroid carcinoma. To antagonize neuromuscular blockade due to aminoglycosides.

Contraindications: Digitalized clients, sarcoidosis, renal or cardiac disease, ventricular fibrillation. Cancer clients with bone metastases. Renal calculi, hypophosphatemia, hypercalcemia.

Special Concerns: Calcium requirements decrease in geriatric clients; thus, dose may have to be adjusted. Also, low levels of active vitamin D metabolites may impair calcium absorption in older clients. Use with caution in cor pulmonale, respiratory acidosis, renal disease or failure, ventricular fibrillation, hypercalcemia.

Side Effects: Following PO use: GI irritation, constipation. **Following IV use:** Venous irritation, tingling sensation, feeling of oppression or heat, chalky taste. Rapid IV administration may result in vasodilation, decreased BP and HR, ***cardiac arrhythmias,*** syncope, or ***cardiac arrest.*** **Following IM use:** Burning feeling, necrosis, tissue sloughing, cellulitis, soft tissue calcification. *NOTE:* If calcium is injected into the myocardium rather than into the ventricle, ***laceration of coronary arteries, cardiac tamponade, pneumothorax, and ventricular fibrillation*** may occur. *Symptoms due to excess calcium (hypercalcemia):* Lassitude, fatigue, GI symptoms (anorexia, N&V, abdominal pain, dry mouth, thirst), polyuria, depression of nervous and neuromuscular function (emotional disturbances, confusion, skeletal muscle weakness, and constipation), confusion, delirium, stupor, ***coma,*** impairment of renal function (polyuria, polydipsia, and azotemia), renal calculi, arrhythmias, and bradycardia.

Symptoms of Overdose: Systemic overloading from parenteral administration can result in an acute hypercalcemic syndrome with symptoms including markedly increased plasma calcium levels, lethargy, intractable N&V, weakness, ***coma, and sudden death.***

Drug Interactions

Atenolol / ↓ Effect of atenolol due to ↓ bioavailability and plasma levels

Cephalocin / Incompatible with calcium salts

Corticosteroids / Interfere with absorption of calcium from GI tract

Digitalis / ↑ Digitalis arrhythmias and toxicity. Death has resulted from combination of digitalis and IV calcium salts

Iron salts / ↓ Absorption of iron from the GI tract

Milk / Excess of either may cause hypercalcemia, renal insufficiency with azotemia, alkalosis, and ocular lesions

Norfloxacin / ↓ Bioavailability of norfloxacin

Sodium polystyrene sulfonate / Metabolic alkalosis and ↓ binding of resin to potassium in clients with renal impairment

Tetracyclines / ↓ Effect of tetracyclines due to ↓ absorption from GI tract

Thiazide diuretics / Hypercalcemia due to thiazide-induced renal tubular reabsorption of calcium and bone release of calcium

Verapamil / Calcium antagonizes the effect of verapamil

Vitamin D / Enhances intestinal absorption of dietary calcium

Dosage
See individual agents.

NURSING CONSIDERATIONS

Administration/Storage

ORAL

1. Administer 1–1.5 hr after meals. Alkalis and large amounts of fat decrease the absorption of calcium.
2. If the client has difficulty swallowing large tablets, obtain a calcium in water suspension. Because calcium goes into suspension six times more readily in hot water than in cold water, the solution can be prepared by diluting the medication with *hot* water. Solution may then be cooled before administering to the client.

IV

1. Warm solutions to body temperature and give slowly (0.5–2 mL/min), stopping administration if client complains of discomfort.
2. Administer slowly, observing VS closely for evidence of bradycardia, hypotension, and cardiac arrhythmias.
3. Prevent leakage of medication into the tissues. These salts are extremely irritating.
4. Client should remain recumbent for a short time following the injection.
5. Calcium salts should not be mixed with carbonates, phosphates, sulfates, or tartrates in parenteral admixtures.

IM

1. Rotate the injection sites because this medication may cause sloughing of tissue.
2. Do not administer IM calcium gluconate to children.

Treatment of Overdose: Discontinue therapy and lower serum calcium levels by giving an IV infusion of sodium chloride plus a potent diuretic such as furosemide. Consider hemodialysis.

Assessment

1. Perform a thorough nursing history, noting indications for therapy and underlying cause.
2. Note if the client is receiving digitalis products. Document and report as the drug is generally contraindicated.
3. Obtain baseline serum calcium level and renal function studies to determine if renal disease is present.

Interventions

1. Monitor serum calcium levels.
2. If the client goes into hypocalcemic tetany, provide appropriate safety precautions to protect the client from injury.
3. Observe for symptoms of hypercalcemia, such as fatigue and CNS depression.

Client/Family Teaching

1. Explain that calcium requirements are best met by dietary sources (including milk in the diet). Supplements need vitamin D.
2. Stress that multivitamin and mineral preparations are expensive and do not contain sufficient calcium to meet the daily calcium requirements.
3. Provide printed instructions concerning prescribed diet. Have a dietitian work with client to assist with proper selection of foods and meal planning and preparation.
4. Review the prescribed replacement regimen. Advise close follow-up for dosage adjustments to prevent hypercalcemia and hypercalciuria.

Evaluate

- Evidence of resolution of clinical symptoms of hypocalcemia
- Reports of relief of muscle cramps
- Osteoporosis prophylaxis
- Laboratory confirmation that serum calcium level is within desired range (8.8–10.4 mg/dL)

Calcium carbonate

(**KAL**-see-um **KAR**-bon-ayt)

Alka-Mints, Amitone, Antacid Tablets, Apo-Cal ✱, Cal Carb-HD, Calci-Chew, Calciday-667, Calci-Mix, Calcite 500, Calcium 500 ✱, Calcium 600, Cal-Plus, Calsan ✱, Caltrate 600, Caltrate Jr., Chooz, Dicarbosil, Equilet, Extra Strength Antacid, Extra Strength Tums, Florical, Gencalc 600,

Maalox Antacid Caplets, Mallamint, Mylanta Lozenges, Nephro-Calci, Nu-Cal ✱, Os-Cal 500, Os-Cal 500 Chewable, Oysco 500 Chewable, Oyst-Cal 500, Oystercal 500, Oyster Shell Calcium-500, Tums, Tums Ultra **(OTC)**

See also *Calcium Salts,* Chapter 74, and *Antacids and Antiflatulents,* Chapter 59.

How Supplied: *Capsule:* 500 mg, 600 mg, 900 mg, 1250 mg; *Chew Tablet:* 200 mg, 300 mg, 420 mg, 500 mg, 600 mg, 650 mg, 750 mg, 1000 mg, 1250 mg, 1500 mg; *Lozenge/Troche:* 240 mg; *Suspension:* 500 mg/5 mL; *Tablet* 10 mg, 150 mg, 250 mg, 375 mg, 420 mg, 500 mg, 600 mg, 625 mg, 650 mg, 750 mg, 1000 mg, 1250 mg; *Tablet, Extended Release:* 500 mg; *Wafer:* 1250 mg

Uses: Mild hypocalcemia, antacid, antihyperphosphatemic.

Dosage

• **Chewable Tablets, Tablets, Suspension, Gum, Lozenges**

Adults: 0.5–1.5 g, as needed.

• **Capsules, Suspension, Tablets, Chewable Tablets**

Treat hypocalcemia, nutritional supplement.

Adults: 1.25–1.5 g 1–3 times/day with or after meals.

Antihyperphosphatemic.

Adults: 5–13 g/day in divided doses with meals.

NOTE: The preparation contains 40% elemental calcium and 400 mg elemental calcium/g (20 mEq/g).

• **Florical**

1 capsule or tablet daily (also contains 8.3 mg sodium fluoride per capsule or tablet).

Special Concerns: Dosage has not been established in children.

NURSING CONSIDERATIONS

See also *Nursing Considerations* for *Antacids and Antiflatulents,* Chapter 59, and *Calcium Salts,* Chapter 74.

Evaluate

• Serum calcium levels within desired range

• ↓ Gastric acidity

Calcium chloride

(**KAL**-see-um **KLOH**-ryd)

Pregnancy Category: C

Calciject ✱ **(Rx)**

See also *Calcium Salts,* Chapter 74.

How Supplied: *Injection:* 100 mg /mL

Uses: Mild hypocalcemia due to neonatal tetany, tetany due to parathyroid deficiency or vitamin D deficiency, and alkalosis. Prophylaxis of hypocalcemia during exchange transfusions. Intestinal malabsorption. Treat effects of serious hyperkalemia as measured by ECG. Cardiac resuscitation after open heart surgery when epinephrine fails to improve weak or ineffective myocardial contractions. Adjunct to treat insect bites or stings to relieve muscle cramping. Depression due to magnesium overdosage. Acute symptoms of lead colic. Rickets, osteomalacia. Reverse symptoms of verapamil overdosage.

Dosage

• **IV Only**

Hypocalcemia, replenish electrolytes.

Adults: 0.5–1 g q 1–3 days (given at a rate not to exceed 13.6–27.3 mg/min). **Pediatric:** 25 mg/kg (0.2 mL/kg up to 1–10 mL/kg) given slowly.

Magnesium intoxication.

0.5 g promptly; observe for recovery before other doses given.

Cardiac resuscitation.

0.5–1 g IV or 0.2–0.8 g injected into the ventricular cavity as a single dose. **Pediatric:** 0.2 mL/kg.

Hyperkalemia.

Sufficient amount to return ECG to normal.

NOTE: The preparation contains 27.2% calcium and 272 mg calcium/g (13.6 mEq/g).

Administration/Storage

1. *Never administer IM.*

2. May administer undiluted IV push.

Contraindication: Use to treat hypocalcemia of renal insufficiency.

Special Concerns: Use usually restricted in children due to significant irritation and possible tissue necrosis and sloughing caused by IV calcium chloride.
Additional Side Effects: Peripheral vasodilation with moderate decreases in BP. Extravasation can cause severe necrosis, sloughing, or abscess formation following IM or SC use.

NURSING CONSIDERATIONS

See also *Nursing Considerations* for *Calcium Salts,* Chapter 74.
Evaluate
- Serum calcium level within desired range
- ↓ Serum magnesium level

Calcium citrate

(**KAL**-see-um **CIH**-trayt)
Citracal, Citracal Liquitab **(OTC)**

See also *Calcium Salts,* Chapter 74.
How Supplied: *Syrup; Tablet:* 200 mg, 950 mg; *Tablet, Effervescent:* 1000 mg
Additional Use: Renal osteodystrophy.

Dosage
- **Tablets**

Hypocalcemia.
Adults: 0.9–1.9 g t.i.d.–q.i.d. after meals.
Nutritional supplement.
3.8–7.1 g/day in three to four divided doses.
NOTE: Contains 21.1% elemental calcium and 211 mg calcium/g (10.5 mEq/g).
Special Concerns: Dosage has not been established in children.

NURSING CONSIDERATIONS

See *Nursing Considerations* for *Calcium Salts,* Chapter 74.
Evaluate: Restoration of serum calcium levels.

Calcium glubionate

(**KAL**-see-um glue-**BYE**-oh-nayt)
Pregnancy Category: C
Neo-Calglucon, Calcium-Sandoz **(OTC)**

See also *Calcium Salts,* Chapter 74.
How Supplied: *Syrup; Tablet*
Uses: Hypocalcemia, calcium deficiency, tetany of newborn, hypoparathyroidism, pseudohypoparathyroidism, osteoporosis, rickets, osteomalacia.

Dosage
- **Syrup**

Dietary supplement.
Adults and children over 4 years: 15 mL t.i.d.–q.i.d. **Pediatric (under 4 years):** 10 mL t.i.d. **Infants:** 5 mL 5 times/day.
Tetany of newborn.
On the basis of laboratory tests, usually 50–150 mg/kg/day in three or more divided doses.
Other calcium deficiencies.
Adults: 15–45 mL 1–3 times/day.
NOTE: The preparation contains 115 mg calcium ion/5 mL.

NURSING CONSIDERATIONS

See *Nursing Considerations* for *Calcium Salts,* Chapter 74.
Evaluate: Desired calcium replacement in deficiency states.

Calcium gluceptate (Calcium glucoheptonate)

(**KAL**-see-um **GLUE**-sep-tayt)
Pregnancy Category: C
Calcium Zurich ✱ **(Rx)**

See also *Calcium Salts,* Chapter 74.
How Supplied: *Injection:* 220 mg /mL
Uses: Mild hypocalcemia due to neonatal tetany, tetany due to parathyroid deficiency or vitamin D deficiency, and alkalosis. Prophylaxis of hypocalcemia during exchange transfusions. Intestinal malabsorption. To replenish electrolytes. Antihypermagnesemic.

Dosage
- **IM**

Hypocalcemia.
Adults and children: 0.44–1.1 g.
- **IV**

Hypocalcemia.
Adults: 1.1–4.4 g given slowly at a rate not exceeding 36 mg calcium ion/min (2 mL/min). **Pediatric, IV:** 0.44–1.1 g; give as a single dose at a rate not to exceed 36 mg calcium ion/min.

Antihypermagnesemic.
Adults: 1.2–2.4 g given slowly at a rate not to exceed 36 mg calcium ion/min.

Exchange transfusions in newborns.
0.11 g after every 100 mL blood exchanged.

NOTE: The elemental calcium content is 8.2% and there is 82 mg calcium/g (4.1 mEq/g).
Administration/Storage: In adults if more than 5 mL must be used IM, the IM dose should be given in the gluteal area. For infants, the dose should be given in the lateral thigh.
Special Concerns: Should only be given IM to infants and children in emergency situations when the IV route is not possible.

NURSING CONSIDERATIONS

See also *Nursing Considerations* for *Calcium Salts,* Chapter 74.
Evaluate: ↑ Serum calcium and ↓ serum magnesium levels.

Calcium gluconate

(**KAL**-see-um **GLUE**-koh-nayt)
H-F Antidote Gel ✦, Kalcinate (Rx, injection; OTC, tablets)

See also *Calcium Salts,* Chapter 74.
How Supplied: *Injection:* 100 mg /mL; *Tablet:* 325 mg, 486 mg, 500 mg, 650 mg, 975 mg
Uses: Mild hypocalcemia due to neonatal tetany, tetany due to parathyroid deficiency or vitamin D deficiency, and alkalosis. Prophylaxis of hypocalcemia during exchange transfusions. Intestinal malabsorption. Adjunct to treat insect bites or stings to relieve muscle cramping. Depression due to magnesium overdosage. Acute symptoms of lead colic. Rickets, osteomalacia. Reverse symptoms of verapamil overdosage. Decrease capillary permeability in allergic conditions, nonthrombocytopenic purpura, and exudative dermatoses (e.g., dermatitis herpetiformis). Pruritus due to certain drugs. Hyperkalemia to antagonize cardiac toxicity (as long as client is not receiving digitalis).

Dosage
- **Tablets**

Treatment of hypocalcemia.
Adults: 8.8–16.5 g/day in divided doses; **pediatric,** 0.5–0.72 g/kg/day in divided doses.

Nutritional supplement.
Adults, 8.8–16.5 g/day in divided doses.
- **IV Only**

Treatment of hypocalcemia.
Adults: 2.3–9.3 mEq (5–20 mL of the 10% solution) as needed (range: 4.65–70 mEq/day). **Children:** 2.3 mEq/kg/day (or 56 mEq/m^2/day) given well diluted and slowly in divided doses. **Infants:** No more than 0.93 mEq (2 mL of the 10% solution).

Emergency elevation of serum calcium.
Adults: 7–14 mEq (15–30.1 mL). **Children:** 1–7 mEq (2.2–15 mL). **Infants:** Less than 1 mEq (2.2 mL). Depending on client response, the dose may be repeated q 1–3 days.

Hypocalcemic tetany.
Children: 0.5–0.7 mEq/kg (1.1–1.5 mL/kg) t.i.d.–q.i.d. until tetany is controlled. **Infants:** 2.4 mEq/kg/day (5.2 mL/kg/day) in divided doses.

Hyperkalemia with cardiac toxicity.
2.25–14 mEq (4.8–30.1 mL) while monitoring the ECG. If needed, the dose can be repeated after 1–2 min.

Magnesium intoxication.
Initial: 4.5–9 mEq (9.7–19.4 mL). Subsequent dosage based on client response.

Exchange transfusion.

Adults: 1.35 mEq (2.9 mL) concurrent with each 100 mL citrated blood. **Neonates:** 0.45 mEq (1 mL)/100 mL citrated blood.

• **IM**

Hypocalcemic tetany.

Adults: 4.5–16 mEq (9.7–34.4 mL) until a therapeutic response is noted.

Magnesium intoxication.

If IV administration is not possible: 2–5 mEq (4.3–10.8 mL) in divided doses as needed.

NOTE: The preparation contains 9% calcium and 90 mg calcium/g (4.5 mEq/g).

Administration/Storage

1. IV rate should not exceed 0.5–2 mL/min.
2. Can also be given by intermittent IV infusion at a rate not exceeding 200 mg (19.5 mg calcium ion)/min. Can also be used by continuous IV infusion.
3. If a precipitate is noted in the syringe, do not use.
4. If a precipitate is noted in the vials or ampules, heat to 80°C (146°F) in a dry heat oven for 1 hr to dissolve. Shake vigorously and allow to cool to room temperature. Do not use if precipitate remains.

Contraindications: Intramuscular, intramyocardial, or SC use due to severe tissue necrosis, sloughing, and abscess formation.

NURSING CONSIDERATIONS

See also *Nursing Considerations* for *Calcium Salts,* Chapter 74.

Evaluate

• Restoration of serum calcium levels
• ↓ Serum magnesium level

Calcium lactate

(**KAL**-see-um **LACK**-tayt)
(OTC)

See also *Calcium Salts,* Chapter 74.

How Supplied: *Tablet:* 325 mg, 500 mg, 648 mg, 650 mg

Uses: Latent hypocalcemic tetany, hyperphosphatemia.

Dosage

• **Tablets**

Treatment of hypocalcemia.

Adults: 7.7 g/day in divided doses with meals. **Pediatric:** 0.34–0.5 g/kg/day in divided doses.

NOTE: The preparation contains 13% calcium and 130 mg calcium/g (6.5 mEq/g).

NURSING CONSIDERATIONS

See *Nursing Considerations* for *Calcium Salts,* Chapter 74.

Evaluate: Restoration of serum calcium levels.

Dibasic calcium phosphate dihydrate

(OTC)

See also *Calcium Salts,* Chapter 74.

How Supplied: *Tablet:* 600 mg

Uses: Calcium deficiency states, dietary supplement.

Dosage

• **Tablets**

Treatment of hypocalcemia.

Adults: 4.4 g/day in divided doses with or after meals; **pediatric:** 0.2–0.28 g/kg/day in divided doses with or after meals. *NOTE:* This preparation contains 23% calcium and 230 mg calcium/g (11.5 mEq/g).

Administration/Storage

1. A full glass of water should be consumed with each dose.
2. Should be taken with meals in clients with achlorhydria or hypochlorhydria.

Special Concerns: Increased risk of hypoparathyroidism or hyperphosphatemia in clients with renal insufficiency.

NURSING CONSIDERATIONS

See also *Nursing Considerations* for *Calcium Salts,* Chapter 74.

Evaluate: Restoration of serum calcium levels.

CALCIUM REGULATORS

See the following individual entries:

Calcitonin, Human
Calcitonin, Salmon
Etidronate Disodium (Oral)
Etidronate Disodium (Parenteral)
Gallium Nitrate
Pamidronate Disodium

Calcitonin-human

(kal-sih-**TOH**-nin)
Pregnancy Category: C
Cibacalcin **(Rx)**

Calcitonin-salmon

(kal-sih-**TOH**-nin)
Pregnancy Category: C
Calcimar, Miacalcin, Osteocalcin **(Rx)**

How Supplied: Calcitonin-human: *Powder for injection:* 0.5 mg. Calcitonin-salmon: *Injection:* 200 IU /mL.

Action/Kinetics: Calcitonins are polypeptide hormones produced in mammals by the parafollicular cells of the thyroid gland. Calcitonin isolated from salmon has the same therapeutic effect as the human hormone, except for a greater potency per milligram and a somewhat longer duration of action. Calcitonin-human is a synthetic product that has the same sequence of amino acids as the naturally occurring calcitonin found in human beings. Calcitonin is ineffective when administered PO. Calcitonin is beneficial in Paget's disease of bone by reducing the rate of turnover of bone; the drug acts to both block initial bone resorption, decreasing alkaline phosphatase levels in the serum and urinary hydroxyproline excretion. Its effectiveness in treating osteoporosis or hypercalcemia is due to decreased serum calcium levels from direct inhibition of bone resorption. **Time to peak effect, calcitonin-salmon:** 2 hr for hypercalcemia. **Duration, calcitonin-salmon:** 6–8 hr for hypercalcemia. **t½:** 60 min for calcitonin-human and 70–90 min for calcitonin-salmon. The onset of calcitonin-human in reducing serum alkaline phosphatase level and urinary hydroxyproline excretion in Paget's disease may take 6–24 months. Calcitonin is metabolized to inactive compounds in the kidneys, blood, and peripheral tissues.

Uses: Moderate to severe Paget's disease characterized by polyostotic involvement with elevation of serum alkaline phosphatase and urinary excretion of hydroxyproline. For the early treatment of hypercalcemia. Calcitonin-salmon is used concomitantly with calcium and vitamin D to treat postmenopausal osteoporosis.

Dosage

- **SC. Calcitonin-Human**

Paget's disease.

Adults, initial: 0.5 mg/day; **then,** depending on severity of disease, dosage may range from 0.5 mg 2–3 times/week to 0.25 mg/day.

- **IM, SC. Calcitonin-Salmon**

Paget's disease.

Adults, initial: 100 IU/day; **maintenance, usual:** 50 IU/day, every other day, or 3 times/week.

Hypercalcemia.

Adults, initial: 4 IU/kg q 12 hr; **then,** increase the dose, if necessary, to 8 IU/kg q 12 hr up to a maximum of 8 IU/kg q 6 hr.

Postmenopausal osteoporosis.

Adults: 100 IU/day, once every other day, or 3 times/week given with calcium and vitamin D.

Administration/Storage

1. Before initiating therapy, determine serum alkaline phosphatase level and urinary hydroxyproline excretion.
2. Repeat the above studies at the end of 3 months and q 3–6 months thereafter.
3. Store calcitonin-salmon at a temperature between 2°C and 6°C (36°F and 43°F).
4. Store calcitonin-human below 25°C (77°F).
5. When being used to treat Paget's disease, more than 1 year of therapy may be required to treat neurologic lesions.
6. Check for hypersensitivity reactions before administering either

medication. Administer 1 IU intracutaneously in the inner forearm and observe for 15 min to ensure test is negative.
7. Have emergency drugs on hand for immediate use in the event of a hypersensitivity reaction.

Contraindication: Allergy to calcitonin-salmon or its gelatin diluent.

Special Concerns: Use with caution during lactation. Safe use in children not established.

Laboratory Test Interferences: Reduction of alkaline phosphatase and 24-hr urinary excretion of hydroxyproline are indicative of successful therapy. Monitor urine for casts (indicative of kidney damage).

Side Effects: *Allergic:* Due to foreign protein reaction to calcitonin or gelatin diluent. Skin rashes, systemic allergic reactions. *GI:* N&V, abdominal pain, diarrhea, anorexia, abdominal pain, salty taste. *Dermatologic:* Flushing of hands or face, inflammation at site of injection (salmon), foot edema. *CNS:* Headache, dizziness. *Other:* Antibody formation rendering the drug ineffective, increased urinary frequency, nocturia, eye pain, sensation of fever, chills, weakness, nasal congestion, SOB, paresthesia.

Symptoms of Overdose: N&V.

NURSING CONSIDERATIONS

Assessment

1. Note any history of client hypersensitivity to calcitonin-salmon or its gelatin diluent.
2. Document indications for therapy, noting baseline assessments and appropriate laboratory results.

Interventions

1. Perform a test dose. Note any local inflammatory reactions at the site of injection. Assess for systemic allergic reactions.
2. Observe for hypocalcemic tetany. Clients will exhibit muscular fibrillation, twitching, tetanic spasms, and may go into convulsions. Have calcium available for emergency use and check clients at least q 10 min for the next 30 min following the injection.
3. Check for evidence of hypercalcemia. Complaints of increased thirst, anorexia, polyuria, and N&V should be reported.
4. Observe for facial flushing, and report if evident. Assess for abdominal distress, anorexia, diarrhea, epigastric distress, or changes in taste perception. Monitor and record weights, I&O, and report if symptoms persist.
5. If the client has a good initial clinical response and then has a relapse, evaluate for antibody formation in response to serum calcitonin.

Client/Family Teaching

1. Explain how to make appropriate assessments of the disorder and how to assess the response to therapy.
2. Review aseptic methods of reconstituting the solution, proper injection technique, and the importance of alternating and documenting injection sites.
3. Explain that N&V may occur at the onset of therapy. The problem should subside as the treatment continues; report if it persists.
4. Stress the importance of returning for periodic urine sedimentation tests to be sure there is no kidney damage.
5. Suggest taking the doses of medication in the evening to minimize the problem of flushing.
6. Refer to a dietitian for counselling concerning possible adjustments in the diet.

Evaluate

- Laboratory evidence of ↓ serum calcium, ↓ serum alkaline phosphatase, and ↓ 24-hr urinary excretion of hydroxyproline
- Promotion of bone formation
- ↓ Bone pain
- Halt in the progression of postmenopausal osteoporosis

Etidronate disodium (oral)

(eh-tih-**DROH**-nayt)

Pregnancy Category: B
Didronel **(Rx)**

Etidronate disodium (parenteral)

(eh-tih-**DROH**-nayt)
Pregnancy Category: C
Didronel, Didronel IV **(Rx)**

How Supplied: *Injection:* 50 mg /mL

Action/Kinetics: Paget's disease is characterized by bone resorption, compensatory new bone formation, and increased vascularization of the bone. Etidronate disodium slows bone metabolism, thereby decreasing bone resorption, bone turnover, and new bone formation; it also reduces bone vascularization. Renal tubular reabsorption of calcium is not affected. **Absorption:** Dose-dependent; after 24 hr, one-half of absorbed drug is excreted unchanged. Absorption is affected by food or preparations containing divalent ions. **Onset:** 1 month for Paget's disease and within 24 hr for hypercalcemia. The drug remaining in the body is adsorbed to bone, where therapeutic effects for Paget's disease persist 3–12 months after discontinuation of the drug. **Plasma t½:** 6 hr. Approximately 50% excreted unchanged in the urine; unabsorbed drug is excreted through the feces.

Uses: *PO:* Paget's disease (osteitis deformans), especially of the polyostotic type accompanied by pain and increased urine levels of hydroxyproline and serum alkaline phosphatase. Heterotopic ossification due to spinal cord injury or total hip replacement. *Parenteral:* Hypercalcemia due to malignancy, which is not responsive to hydration or dietary control. *Investigational:* Postmenopausal osteoporosis.

Dosage

- **Tablets**

Paget's disease.

Adults, initial: 5–10 mg/kg/day for 6 months or less; 11 mg/kg up to a maximum of 20 mg/kg/day for clients when bone metabolism suppression is highly advisable; treatment at this dose level should not exceed 3 months. Another course of therapy may be instituted after rest period of 3 months if there is evidence of active disease process.

Heterotopic ossification due to spinal cord injury.

Adults: 20 mg/kg/day for 2 weeks; **then** 10 mg/kg/day for 10 weeks. Treatment should be initiated as soon as possible after the injury, preferably before evidence of heterotopic ossification.

Heterotopic ossification complicating total hip replacement.

Adults: 20 mg/kg/day for 30 days preoperatively; **then,** 20 mg/kg/day for 90 days postoperatively.

- **IV Infusion**

Hypercalcemia due to malignancy.

7.5 mg/kg/day for 3 successive days. If necessary, a second course of treatment may be instituted after a 7-day rest period. The safety and effectiveness of more than two courses of therapy has not been determined. Etidronate tablets may be started the day after the last infusion at a dose of 20 mg/kg/day for 30 days (treatment may be extended to 90 days if serum calcium levels are normal). Use for more than 90 days is not recommended.

Administration/Storage

1. Administer as a single dose of medication with juice or water 2 hr before meals.
2. Urinary hydroxyproline excretion and/or serum alkaline phosphatase levels should be determined periodically when the drug is given for Paget's disease.
3. There are no indications to date that etidronate will affect mature heterotopic bone.
4. The IV dose must be diluted in at least 250 mL of sterile NSS and should be administered over a period of 2 hr.
5. A metallic taste may be experienced during IV administration.
6. *Treatment of Overdose:* Gastric lavage following PO ingestion. Treat hypocalcemia by giving calcium IV.

Contraindications: Enterocolitis, fracture of long bones, hypercalcemia of hyperparathyroidism. In clients with a serum creatinine greater than 5 mg/dL.

Special Concerns: Use with caution in the presence of renal dysfunction and during lactation. Safety and efficacy have not been established in children.

Side Effects: *GI:* Nausea, diarrhea, loose bowel movements, ulcerative stomatitis. *Bones:* Increased incidence of bone fractures and increased or recurrent bone pain. Drug should be discontinued if fracture occurs and not restarted until healing takes place. *Allergy:* Angioedema, rash, pruritus, urticaria. *Electrolytes:* Hypophosphatemia, hypomagnesemia. *Miscellaneous:* Metallic taste, abnormalities in renal function, fever, fluid overload. Symptoms of rachitic syndrome have been reported in children receiving 10 mg or more/kg daily for long periods (up to 1 year) to treat heterotopic ossification or soft tissue calcification.

Symptoms of Overdose: Following PO ingestion, hypocalcemia may occur. Rapid IV administration may cause renal insufficiency.

NURSING CONSIDERATIONS

Assessment

1. Document indications for therapy and presenting symptoms.
2. Note any evidence of renal dysfunction. Obtain baseline serum calcium and renal function studies and monitor during drug therapy.
3. If female and of childbearing age, determine the possibility of pregnancy.

Client/Family Teaching

1. Assist the client and family in understanding the importance of maintaining a well-balanced diet with adequate intake of calcium and vitamin D. Refer to dietitian as needed.
2. Do not eat for 2 hr after taking medication because foods particularly high in calcium may reduce the absorption of the drug.
3. Review S&S of hypercalcemia that require immediate reporting, i.e., lethargy, N&V, anorexia, tremors, and bone pain.
4. Stress the importance of reporting for lab studies as scheduled. During treatment of Paget's disease, levels of urinary hydroxyproline excretion and serum alkaline phosphatase must be determined because reduction in these levels is the first indication of a beneficial therapeutic response. Levels usually decrease 1–3 months after initiation of therapy.
5. In clients with hypercalcemia, serum calcium levels are necessary to assess drug response and the need for continued therapy. Desired reduction usually occurs in 2–8 days in hypercalcemia R/T bone metastasis. Therapy may be repeated only after 7 days of rest. The risk for hypocalcemia is greatest 3 days after IV therapy.

Evaluate

- Suppression of bone metabolism in Paget's disease
- ↓ Serum calcium levels in hypercalcemia

Gallium nitrate

(**Gal**-ee-um **NIGH**-trayt)
Pregnancy Category: C
Ganite **(Rx)**

How Supplied: *Injection:* 25 mg /mL

Action/Kinetics: Gallium nitrate produces a hypocalcemic effect by inhibiting calcium resorption from bone; it may reduce increased bone turnover. After infusion, steady state is reached in 24–48 hr. **Plasma levels:** 1134–2399 ng/mL. The drug is not metabolized by the liver or kidney and is excreted through the kidneys.

Uses: Cancer-related hypercalcemia that is not responsive to adequate hydration and where there are symptoms of hypercalcemia.

Dosage

- **IV Infusion**

Serious hypercalcemia.

Adults: 200 mg/m²/day for 5 consecutive days.

Mild hypercalcemia.
Adults: 100 mg/m²/day for 5 consecutive days.
Administration/Storage
1. The daily dose must be given as an IV infusion over 24 hr.
2. The daily dose should be diluted in 1 L of 0.9% sodium chloride injection or 5% dextrose injection. When diluted as such, it is stable for 48 hr at room temperature and for 7 days if refrigerated.
3. If serum calcium levels are brought into the normal range in less than 5 days, treatment may be discontinued early.
4. Since the product contains no preservative, any unused portion should be discarded.
5. *Treatment of Overdose:* Discontinue administration of the drug and monitor serum calcium. Give fluids IV, with or without diuretics, for 2–3 days. Carefully monitor renal function and urinary output.
Contraindications: Severe renal impairment (serum creatinine > 2.5 mg/dL). Lactation.
Special Concerns: Safety and effectiveness have not been determined in children.
Side Effects: *Metabolic:* Hypocalcemia, transient hypophosphatemia, decreased serum bicarbonate (possibly secondary to mild respiratory alkalosis). *GU:* Increased BUN and creatinine. *Hematologic:* Anemia (relationship to drug itself not certain), leukopenia. *GI:* N&V, diarrhea, constipation. *CV:* Tachycardia, edema of lower extremities, decrease in mean SBP and DBP. *Respiratory:* Dyspnea, rales and rhonchi, pulmonary infiltrates, pleural effusion. *Miscellaneous:* Acute optic neuritis, visual impairment, decreased hearing, hypothermia, fever, skin rash, lethargy, confusion.

Symptoms of Overdose: N&V, increased risk of renal insufficiency.
Drug Interactions: Use of gallium nitrate with nephrotoxic drugs (e.g., aminoglycosides, amphotericin B) may increase the incidence of renal insufficiency in clients with hypercalcemia due to cancer.

NURSING CONSIDERATIONS
Assessment
1. Determine that cancer-related hypercalcemia was previously unresponsive to saline hydration. In treating hypercalcemia due to carcinoma, it is important to first establish adequate hydration to increase renal excretion of calcium and to correct for dehydration caused by hypercalcemia.
2. Obtain baseline CBC, serum calcium, phosphorus, and renal function studies and monitor throughout therapy.
Interventions
1. Monitor serum calcium levels closely and observe client for symptoms of hypocalcemia. If hypocalcemia occurs, stop gallium infusion and report.
2. Monitor I&O. Hypercalcemia is frequently associated with impaired renal function; thus, monitor serum creatinine and BUN closely and discontinue therapy if serum creatinine levels exceed 2.5 mg/dL.
3. A satisfactory urine output (2 L/day) should be established before gallium nitrate therapy is initiated. Adequate hydration should be maintained throughout therapy with care taken to avoid overhydration in clients with compromised CV function.
4. Diuretic therapy should *not* be used prior to correction of hypovolemia.
5. Encourage client to immediately report any visual or hearing disturbances as these may be drug related.
Evaluate: ↓ Serum calcium levels to within desired range (8.8–10.4 mg/dL).

Pamidronate disodium

(pah-**MIH**-droh-nayt)
Pregnancy Category: C
Aredia **(Rx)**

How Supplied: *Powder for injection:* 30 mg, 60 mg, 90 mg
Action/Kinetics: Pamidronate inhibits both normal and abnormal bone resorption without inhibiting bone formation and mineralization.

The precise mechanism is not known, but the drug may inhibit dissolution of hydroxyapatite crystal or have an effect on bone reabsorbing cells. The drug causes decreased serum phosphate levels probably due to a decreased release of phosphate from bone and increased renal excretion as parathyroid levels return to normal. Urinary calcium/creatinine and urinary hydroxyproline/creatinine ratios decrease and usually return to normal or below normal after treatment. **t½:** Biphasic, 1.6 hr (alpha) and 27.3 hr (beta). Approximately 50% of an IV infused dose is excreted unchanged in the urine within 72 hr.

Uses: In conjunction with hydration to treat moderate to severe hypercalcemia associated with malignancy (with or without bone metastases). Moderate to severe Paget's disease. *Investigational:* Postmenopausal osteoporosis; bone metastases from breast cancer to prevent further development of tumor-related hypercalcemia and to reduce the incidence of pathologic fractures and severe bone pain; hyperparathyroidism; prophylaxis of glucocorticoid-induced osteoporosis; reduce bone pain in clients with prostatic carcinoma and multiple myeloma osteolytic lesions; treat immobilization-induced hypercalcemia.

Dosage

• **IV Infusion**

Moderate hypercalcemia (corrected serum calcium of about 12–13.5 mg/dL).

Initial therapy: 60–90 mg.

Severe hypercalcemia (corrected serum calcium greater than 13.5 mg/dL).

Initial therapy: 90 mg. If retreatment is necessary, use the same dose as for initial therapy.

Moderate to severe Paget's disease. 30 mg/day given as a 4-hr infusion on 3 consecutive days (total dose: 90 mg). If retreatment is necessary, the same dosage schedule is used.

Administration/Storage

1. Initially, give as a single dose IV infusion over 24 hr.
2. If hypercalcemia recurs, retreatment can be instituted provided a minimum of 7 days has elapsed to allow full response to the initial dose.
3. The drug is reconstituted by adding 10 mL sterile water for injection, which results in a concentration of 30 mg/10 mL with a pH of 6–7.4.
4. The drug is given over a 24-hr period by diluting in 1,000 mL of sterile 0.45% or 0.9% sodium chloride or 5% dextrose injection.
5. The solution for infusion is stable for up to 24 hr at room temperature. If reconstituted with sterile water for injection, the drug may be stored in the refrigerator for up to 24 hr at 2°C–8°C (36°F–46°F).
6. The drug should not be mixed with calcium-containing infusion solutions such as Ringer's solution.

Contraindication: Hypersensitivity to biphosphonates.

Special Concerns: Use with caution during lactation. Safety and effectiveness have not been determined in children. Pamidronate has not been tested in clients who have creatinine levels greater than 5 mg/dL.

Side Effects: *Metabolic/Electrolytes:* Hypocalcemia, hypokalemia, hypomagnesemia, hypophosphatemia. *Body as a whole:* Slight increase in body temperature, fluid overload, generalized pain, fatigue, moniliasis. *GI:* N&V, constipation, abdominal pain, anorexia, ***GI hemorrhage,*** ulcerative stomatitis. *CNS:* Somnolence, insomnia, abnormal vision, slight possibility of ***seizures.*** *CV:* Hypertension, atrial fibrillation, syncope, tachycardia. *Respiratory:* Rales, rhinitis, upper respiratory tract infection. *GU:* UTI. *Musculoskeletal:* Bone pain. *At site of administration:* Redness, swelling or induration, pain on palpation. *Miscellaneous:* Anemia, hypothyroidism.

NURSING CONSIDERATIONS

Assessment

1. Note indications for therapy, i.e., hypercalcemia of malignancy, symptomatic Paget's disease, postmenopausal osteoporosis, bone pain.
2. Document any history of biphosphonate hypersensitivity.
3. Note any evidence of cardiac disease.
4. Obtain baseline serum calcium, magnesium, potassium, and phosphorous levels.
5. Determine that CBC with differential and renal function studies have been performed.

Interventions

1. Monitor I&O. Ensure adequate administration of fluids to correct hypovolemia and correct any volume deficits before administering diuretics.
2. At the time of drug administration, vigorous saline hydration should be undertaken for moderate to severe hypercalcemia to restore the urine output to about 2 L/day. For less severe hypercalcemia, more conservative approaches can be taken including saline hydration with or without loop diuretics. Overhydration should be avoided, however, especially in clients with heart failure.
3. Weigh client and observe for any evidence of edema.
4. Observe for any evidence of seizure activity and incorporate seizure precautions.
5. Monitor the following lab parameters carefully: serum calcium, phosphate, magnesium, electrolytes, and creatinine as well as CBC and differential. Clients with preexisting anemia, leukopenia, or thrombocytopenia should be carefully monitored during the first 2 weeks following treatment.

Client/Family Teaching

1. Review dietary sources of calcium (dark green vegetables, yogurt, cheese, milk, etc.) that should be avoided unless otherwise prescribed.
2. Advise clients they may experience transient mild temperature elevations for up to 48 hr following therapy.
3. Stress the importance of maintaining adequate hydration. A daily log of I&O may assist to ensure compliance.

Evaluate: Restoration of serum calcium levels to within desired range

Agents Affecting Water and Electrolytes

CHAPTER SEVENTY-FIVE

Diuretics

See also the following drug classes and individual drugs:

Thiazide Diuretics

Chlorothiazide
Chlorothiazide Sodium
Chlorthalidone
Hydrochlorothiazide
Indapamide

Loop Diuretics

Bumetanide
Ethacrynate Sodium
Ethyacrynic Acid
Furosemide
Torsemide

Potassium-Sparing Diuretics

Amiloride Hydrochloride
Spironolactone
Triamterene

Miscellaneous Diuretic

Mannitol

THIAZIDE DIURETICS

General Statement: The kidney is a complex organ with three main functions:
1. Elimination of waste materials and return of useful metabolites to the blood.
2. Maintenance of the acid-base balance.
3. Maintenance of an adequate electrolyte balance, which in turn governs the amount of fluid retained in the body.

Malfunction of one or more of these regulatory processes may result in the retention of excessive fluid by various tissues (edema). The latter can be an important manifestation of many conditions (e.g., CHF, pregnancy, and premenstrual tension).
Action/Kinetics: Diuretic drugs increase the urinary output of water and sodium (prevention or correction of edema), mostly through one of the following mechanisms:
1. Increasing the glomerular filtration rate.
2. Decreasing the rate at which sodium is reabsorbed from the glomerular filtrate by the renal tubules; therefore, water is excreted along with sodium.
3. Promoting the excretion of sodium, and therefore water, by the kidney.

Some of the commonly used diuretics, especially the thiazides, also have an antihypertensive effect. Diuretic drugs can enhance the normal function of the kidney but cannot stimulate a failing kidney into functioning. According to their mode of action and chemical structure, the diuretics fall into the following classes: thiazides (benzothiadiazides which are related chemically to the sulfonamides); carbonic anhydrase inhibitors (used mainly for glaucoma); osmotic diuretics; loop diuretics; and potassium-sparing drugs.

The thiazide diuretics are related chemically to the sulfonamides. Although devoid of anti-infective activity, the thiazides can cause the same hypersensitivity reactions as the sulfonamides.

The thiazides and related diuretics promote diuresis by decreasing the rate at which sodium and chloride are reabsorbed by the distal renal tubules of the kidney. By increasing the excretion of sodium and chloride, they force excretion of additional water. They also increase the excretion of potassium and, to a lesser extent, bicarbonate, as well as decrease the excretion of calcium and uric acid. Sodium and chloride are excreted in approximately equal amounts. The thiazides do not affect the glomerular filtration rate.

The antihypertensive mechanism of action of the thiazides is attributed to direct dilation of the arterioles, as well as to a reduction in the total fluid volume of the body and altered sodium balance. *Diuretic effect:* Usual, **Onset:** 1–2 hr. **Peak:** 4–6 hr. **Duration:** 6–24 hr. *Antihypertensive effect:* **Onset:** several days. *Optimal therapeutic effect:* 3–4 weeks.

Most thiazides are absorbed from the GI tract; a large fraction is excreted unchanged in urine.

Uses: Edema, CHF, hypertension, pregnancy, and premenstrual tension. Thiazides are used for edema due to CHF, nephrosis, nephritis, renal failure, PMS, hepatic cirrhosis, corticosteroid or estrogen therapy. Hypertension. *Investigational:* Thiazides are used alone or in combination with allopurinol (or amiloride) for prophylaxis of calcium nephrolithiasis. Nephrogenic diabetes insipidus.

Contraindications: Hypersensitivity to drug, anuria, renal decompensation. Impaired renal function and advanced hepatic cirrhosis.

Drugs should not be used indiscriminately in clients with edema and toxemia of pregnancy, even though they may be therapeutically useful, because the thiazides may have adverse effects on the newborn (thrombocytopenia and jaundice).

Thiazides and related diuretics may precipitate MIs in elderly clients with advanced arteriosclerosis, especially if the client is also receiving therapy with other antihypertensive agents.

Clients with advanced heart failure, renal disease, or hepatic cirrhosis are most likely to develop hypokalemia.

Thiazides may activate or worsen SLE.

Special Concerns: Geriatric clients may manifest an increased risk of hypotension and changes in electrolyte levels. Administer with caution to debilitated clients or to those with a history of hepatic coma or precoma, gout, diabetes mellitus, or during pregnancy and lactation. Particular care must be exercised when thiazides are administered concomitantly with drugs that also cause potassium loss, such as digitalis, corticosteroids, and some estrogens.

Side Effects: The following side effects may be observed with most thiazides. See also individual drugs. *Electrolyte imbalance:* Hypokalemia (most frequent) characterized by cardiac arrhythmias. Hyponatremia characterized by weakness, lethargy, epigastric distress, N&V. Hypokalemic alkalosis. *GI:* Anorexia, epigastric distress or irritation, N&V, cramping, bloating, abdominal pain, diarrhea, constipation, jaundice, pancreatitis. *CNS:* Dizziness, lightheadedness, headache, vertigo, xanthopsia, paresthesias, weakness, insomnia, restlessness. *CV:* Orthostatic hypotension. *Hematologic:* ***Agranulocytosis, aplastic or hypoplastic anemia, hemolytic anemia,*** leukopenia, thrombocytopenia. *Dermatologic:* Purpura, photosensitivity, photosensitivity dermatitis, rash, urticaria, necrotizing angiitis, vasculitis, cutaneous vasculitis. *Metabolic:* neutropenia, hemolytic anemia. *Endocrine:* Hyperglycemia, glycosuria, hyperuricemia. *Miscellaneous:* Blurred vision, impotence, reduced libido, fever, muscle cramps, muscle spasm, respiratory distress.

Symptoms of Overdose: Symptoms of plasma volume depletion, including orthostatic hypotension, dizziness, drowsiness, syncope, electrolyte abnormalities, hemoconcentration, hemodynamic changes. Signs of potassium depletion, including confusion, dizziness, muscle weakness, and GI disturbances. Also, N&V, GI irritation, GI hypermotility, CNS effects, cardiac abnormalities, ***seizures, hypotension, decreased respiration, and coma.***

Drug Interactions

Allopurinol / ↑ Risk of hypersensitivity reactions to allopurinol
Amphotericin B / Enhanced loss of electrolytes, especially potassium
Anesthetics / Thiazides may ↑ effects of anesthetics
Anticholinergic agents / ↑ Effect of thiazides due to ↑ amount absorbed from GI tract
Anticoagulants, oral / Anticoagulant effects may be decreased
Antidiabetic agents / Thiazides antagonize hypoglycemic effect of antidiabetic agents
Antigout agents / Thiazides may ↑ uric acid levels; thus, ↑ dose of antigout drug may be necessary
Antihypertensive agents / Thiazides potentiate the effect of antihypertensive agents
Antineoplastic agents / Thiazides may prolong leukopenia induced by antineoplastic agents
Calcium salts / Hypercalcemia due to renal tubular reabsorption or bone release may be ↑ by exogenous calcium
Cholestyramine / ↓ Effect of thiazides due to ↓ absorption from GI tract
Colestipol / ↓ Effect of thiazides due to ↓ absorption from GI tract
Corticosteroids / Enhanced potassium loss due to potassium-losing properties of both drugs
Diazoxide / Enhanced hypotensive effect. Also, ↑ hyperglycemic response
Digitalis glycosides / Thiazides produce ↑ potassium and magnesium loss with ↑ chance of digitalis-induced arrhythmias
Ethanol / Additive orthostatic hypotension
Fenfluramine / ↑ Antihypertensive effect of thiazides
Furosemide / Profound diuresis and electrolyte loss
Guanethidine / Additive hypotensive effect
Indomethacin / ↓ Effect of thiazides, possibly by inhibition of prostaglandins
Insulin / ↓ Effect due to thiazide-induced hyperglycemia
Lithium / ↑ Risk of lithium toxicity due to ↓ renal excretion; may be used together but use should be carefully monitored
Loop diuretics / Additive effect to cause profound diuresis and serious electrolyte losses
Methenamine / ↓ Effect of thiazides due to alkalinization of urine by methenamine
Methyldopa / ↑ Risk of hemolytic anemia (rare)
Muscle relaxants, nondepolarizing / ↑ Effect of muscle relaxants due to hypokalemia
Norepinephrine / Thiazides ↓ arterial response to norepinephrine
Quinidine / ↑ Effect of quinidine due to ↑ renal tubular reabsorption
Reserpine / Additive hypotensive effect
Sulfonamides / ↑ Effect of thiazides due to ↓ plasma protein binding
Sulfonylureas / ↓ Effect due to thiazide-induced hyperglycemia

Tetracyclines / ↑ Risk of azotemia
Tubocurarine / ↑ Muscle relaxation and ↑ hypokalemia
Vasopressors (sympathomimetics) / Thiazides ↓ responsiveness of arterioles to vasopressors
Vitamin D / ↑ Effect of vitamin D due to thiazide-induced hypercalcemia

Laboratory Test Interferences: Hypokalemia, hypercalcemia, hyponatremia, hypomagnesemia, hypochloremia, hypophosphatemia, hyperuricemia. ↑ BUN, creatinine, glucose in blood and urine. ↓ Serum PBI levels (no signs of thyroid disturbance). Initial ↑ total cholesterol, LDL cholesterol, and triglycerides.

Dosage

Drugs are preferentially given **PO,** but some preparations can be given parenterally. They are usually given in the morning, so the peak effect occurs during the day.

NURSING CONSIDERATIONS

Administration/Storage

1. If a diuretic is to be taken daily, administer it in the morning so that the major diuretic effect will occur before bedtime.
2. Liquid potassium preparations are bitter. Therefore, when they are to be used, administer with fruit juice or milk to make them more palatable.
3. Thiazides may be taken with food or milk if GI upset occurs.
4. Clients resistant to one type of thiazide may respond to another.
5. Thiazides should not be taken with any other medication (including OTC drugs for asthma, cough and colds, hay fever, weight control) unless approved by the provider.
6. To minimize electrolyte imbalance, thiazides may be taken every other day or on a 3–5-day basis for treatment of edema.
7. To prevent excess hypotension, the dose of other antihypertensive agents should be reduced when beginning thiazide therapy.
8. *Treatment of Overdose:*

- Induce emesis or perform gastric lavage followed by activated charcoal. Undertake measures to prevent aspiration.
- Electrolyte balance, hydration, respiration, CV, and renal function must be maintained. Cathartics should be avoided, as use may enhance fluid loss.
- Although GI effects are usually of short duration, treatment may be required.

Assessment

1. Note if the client has any history of hypersensitivity to the drug. Document indications for therapy and any previous experience with this class of drugs.
2. Obtain baseline electrolytes, Ca, Mg, and liver and renal function tests prior to initiating therapy.
3. Note any history of heart disease, an indication that the client will require close monitoring once the drug has been administered.
4. Determine if client has a history of gout and check baseline uric acid level.
5. Determine the extent of the client's edema and assess skin turgor, mucous membranes, and lung fields.
6. Review drugs the client has been taking to identify those with which diuretics interact so that appropriate adjustments and/or changes can be made.
7. Note any history of hepatic cirrhosis and if evident, closely monitor serum K to avoid depletion and hepatic encephalopathy.

Interventions

1. Weigh each morning after the client has voided and before the client has eaten or taken fluids. Record the weight and report any sudden increase.
2. Monitor I&O and keep bedpan or urinal within reach. Report any absence of or decrease in diuresis and note any changes in lung sounds.
3. Check ambulatory clients for edema in the extremities. Check clients on bed rest for edema in the sacral area. Measure daily, document the extent of edema or ascites, and report.
4. Monitor for serum electrolyte levels, pH, and the following *signs of electrolyte imbalance:*

- *Hyponatremia* (low-salt syndrome)—characterized by muscle weakness, leg cramps, dryness of mouth, dizziness, and GI disturbances.
- *Hypernatremia* (excessive sodium retention in relation to body water)—characterized by CNS disturbances such as confusion, loss of sensorium, stupor, and coma. Poor skin turgor or postural hypotension are not as prominent as when there are combined deficits of sodium and water.
- *Water intoxication* (caused by defective water diuresis)—characterized by lethargy, confusion, stupor, and coma. Neuromuscular hyperexcitability with increased reflexes, muscular twitching, and convulsions if water intoxication is acute.
- *Metabolic acidosis*—characterized by weakness, headache, malaise, abdominal pain, and N&V. Hyperpnea occurs in severe metabolic acidosis. Signs of volume depletion, such as poor skin turgor, soft eyeballs, and a dry tongue may also be observed.
- *Metabolic alkalosis*—characterized by irritability, neuromuscular hyperexcitability, and, in severe cases, tetany.
- *Hypokalemia* (deficiency of potassium in the blood)—characterized by muscular weakness, failure of peristalsis, postural hypotension, respiratory embarrassment, and cardiac arrhythmias.
- *Hyperkalemia* (excess of potassium in the blood)—characterized by early signs of irritability, nausea, intestinal colic, and diarrhea; and by later signs of weakness, flaccid paralysis, dyspnea, difficulty in speaking, and arrhythmias.

5. All signs of electrolyte imbalance should be reported and documented in the chart. Electrolyte levels should be monitored and the physical safety of the client should be safeguarded.
6. With high doses monitor for hyperlipidemia and hyperuricemia. Increased serum uric acid levels may precipitate a gout attack.
7. If the client is receiving enteric-coated potassium tablets, monitor for the presence of abdominal pain, distention, or GI bleeding. These tablets can cause small bowel ulceration. If these symptoms occur, discontinue the tablets. Also, monitor the client's stool to ensure that the tablets have not passed through intact.
8. If the client is also receiving antihypertensive drugs, monitor for excessively low BP. Diuretics potentiate the effects of antihypertensive agents.
9. Diuretics may precipitate symptoms of diabetes mellitus in clients with latent or mild diabetes. Therefore, test the urine or perform finger sticks routinely in clients with diabetes and observe for signs of hyperglycemia.
10. If the client is taking digitalis, check the apical pulse. Hyper- or hypokalemia associated with diuretic therapy may potentiate the toxic effects of digitalis and precipitate cardiac arrhythmias.
11. Assess the client for complaints of sore throat, the presence of a skin rash, and yellowing of the skin or sclera, and report. These may be signs of blood dyscrasias due to drug hypersensitivity.
12. If the client has a history of liver disease, be alert for electrolyte imbalances, which could cause stupor, coma, and death.
13. If the client has a history of gout, note any increase in the frequency of acute attacks that may be precipitated by diuretics and report.

Interventions

1. If the client is to undergo surgery, anticipate that the drug will be stopped at least 48 hr before the procedure. Thiazide inhibits the pressor effects of epinephrine.
2. Evaluate dietary potassium intake. Potassium chloride supplements should be given only when dietary measures are inadequate.
3. If potassium supplements are required, use liquid preparations to avoid ulcerations that may be

produced by potassium salts in the solid dosage form. Exceptions include slow-K forms (potassium salt imbedded in a wax matrix) and micro-K forms (microencapsulated potassium salt).

4. If the client has diabetes, monitor blood glucose levels more frequently after beginning thiazide therapy. It may be necessary to change the dose of insulin or oral hypoglycemic agent.

Client/Family Teaching

1. Instruct clients in taking their BP and pulse and in recording the measurements. Provide written guidelines to assist clients in determining what needs to be reported. These measurements may assist to determine if symptoms are drug related and if the dosage of drug is appropriate.
2. Maintain a written record of weight. Explain that there may be some weight loss from the diuresis related to the drug therapy.
3. Advise that the drug may cause frequent, copious voiding and to take in the morning to prevent disruption of sleep. Assist the client in planning activities to accommodate this occurrence. Assure the client that there is no need to be alarmed by the diuresis and that it is expected.
4. Advise clients who need additional potassium intake to include foods in the diet that are high in potassium. Eating such foods is preferable to taking potassium chloride supplements. Provide the client with a list of foods high in potassium such as citrus, grape, cranberry, apple, pear, and apricot juices; bananas; meat, fish, or fowl; cereals; and tea and cola beverages. Refer the client to a dietitian, as needed, for assistance in shopping, planning, and preparing appropriate menus.
5. Unless the client has a preexisting condition such as gastric ulcer or diabetes, clients who are taking diuretics and who require potassium supplements should be encouraged to drink a large glass of orange juice daily.
6. Use caution in driving a car or operating other hazardous machinery until drug effects become apparent. Weakness and/or dizziness may occur with diuresis.
7. Rise slowly from bed and sit down or lie down if feeling faint or dizzy.
8. Advise that the use of alcohol, standing for prolonged periods, and exercise in hot weather may enhance effects of orthostatic hypotension.
9. Instruct clients to report immediately if they experience dizziness, nausea, muscle weakness, cramps, or tingling of the extremities.
10. Advise client to wear protective clothing, sunscreens, and sunglasses while in the sun, to prevent photosensitivity reactions.
11. Do not take any OTC preparations without approval.

Client/Family Teaching

1. Avoid alcoholic beverages because alcohol, in combination with thiazides, causes severe hypotension.
2. Avoid eating licorice; it may precipitate severe hypokalemia.
3. Eat a diet high in potassium. Encourage clients to include orange juice, bananas, citrus fruits, broccoli, spinach, tomato juice, cucumbers, beets, dried fruits, or apricots.
4. Take thiazide diuretic in the morning to avoid interrupting sleep with the frequent need to void.
5. If clients have a history of gout, advise them to reduce their intake of purines. Provide a printed list of foods to avoid.
6. Advise the client to maintain a written record of weight. Explain that there may be some weight loss from the diuresis related to the drug therapy. Weights should be performed at the same time of day in the same weight clothing.
7. Caution client to rise slowly and to dangle legs before standing to minimize orthostatic effects. Sit or lie down if feeling faint or dizzy.
8. If the client has diabetes, discuss the importance of more careful monitoring of urine and finger sticks for glu-

cose determinations. Advise the client how to adjust the hypoglycemic agent in accordance with the prescribed orders and to keep the provider informed of any changes in blood glucose levels or the effectiveness of the hypoglycemic agent being used.
9. Explain the importance of taking thiazides as directed and stress the importance of reporting for scheduled follow-up visits to evaluate the effectiveness of drug therapy.
10. Provide a printed list of side effects that should be reported should they occur. Occasionally skin rashes may occur but severe symptoms R/T allergic reactions include acute pulmonary edema, acute pancreatitis, thrombocytopenia, cholestatic jaundice, and hemolytic anemia.

Evaluate

- Control of hypertension with ↓ BP to within desired range
- Reports of ↑ urine output
- Evidence of ↓ edema with resultant ↓ weight
- Adequate tissue perfusion as evidenced by warm dry skin and good pulses
- Freedom from complications of drug therapy
- Laboratory confirmation of normal electrolyte levels and fluid balance

Chlorothiazide

(klor-oh-**THIGH**-ah-zyd)
Pregnancy Category: C
Diurigen, Diuril **(Rx)**

Chlorothiazide sodium

(klor-oh-**THIGH**-ah-zyd)
Pregnancy Category: C
Sodium Diuril **(Rx)**

See also *Thiazide Diuretics,* Chapter 75.

How Supplied: Chlorothiazide: *Suspension:* 250 mg/5 mL; *Tablet:* 250 mg, 500 mg.
Chlorothiazide sodium: *Powder for injection:* 0.5 g

Action/Kinetics: Onset: 2 hr for PO, 15 min for IV; **Peak effect:** 4 hr for PO, 30 min for IV; **Duration:** 6–12 hr. **t½:** 45–120 min. Incompletely absorbed from the GI tract. Produces a greater diuretic effect if given in divided doses. Also found in Diupres.

Dosage

- **Oral Suspension, Tablets, IV**

Diuretic.

Adults: 0.5–2 g 1–2 times/day either PO or IV (reserved for clients unable to take PO medication or in emergencies). Some clients may respond to the drug given 3–5 days each week.

Antihypertensive.

Adults, IV, PO: 0.5–1 g/day in one or more divided doses. **Pediatric, 6 months and older, PO:** 22 mg/kg/day (10 mg/lb/day) in two divided doses; **6 months and younger, PO:** 33 mg/kg/day (15 mg/lb/day) in two divided doses. Thus, children up to 2 years of age may be given 125–375 mg/day in two doses while children 2–12 years of age may be given 375 mg–1 g/day in two doses. IV use in children is not recommended.

Administration/Storage

1. To obtain an isotonic solution for injection, add 18 mL sterile water for injection to 500 mg powder and administer over 5 min.
2. IV use is not recommended for children and should be reserved for those adults unable to take medication PO or in emergency situations.
3. Unused reconstituted solutions should be discarded after 24 hr.
4. Simultaneous administration of whole blood or derivatives with chlorothiazide should be avoided.
5. The IV solution is compatible with sodium chloride or dextrose solutions.
6. Should not be given SC or IM.

Special Concerns: Geriatric clients may be more sensitive to the usual adult dose.

Additional Side Effects: Hypotension, renal failure, renal dysfunction, interstitial nephritis. Following IV use: Alopecia, hematuria, exfoliative dermatitis, toxic epidermal necrolysis, erythema multiforme, ***Stevens-Johnson syndrome.***

NURSING CONSIDERATIONS

See also *Nursing Considerations* for *Thiazide Diuretics,* Chapter 75, and *Antihypertensive Agents,* Chapter 28.

Assessment

1. List drugs currently prescribed.
2. Note any sulfa allergy.

Client/Family Teaching

1. Drug may cause orthostatic hypotension; use caution when rising or changing positions.
2. Follow high-potassium diet, if prescribed.
3. Use sun screens (avoid ones with PABA), sunglasses, and protective clothing during sun exposure to diminish drug's photosensitivity effects.

Evaluate

- ↓ BP
- Enhanced diuresis with ↓ edema

Chlorthalidone

(klor-**THAL**-ih-dohn)

Pregnancy Category: B

Apo-Chlorthalidone ✱, Hygroton, Thalitone **(Rx)**

See also *Thiazide Diuretics,* Chapter 75.

How Supplied: *Tablet:* 15 mg, 25 mg, 50 mg, 100 mg

Action/Kinetics: Onset: 2–3 hr. **Peak effect:** 2–6 hr. **Duration:** 24–72 hr. **t½:** 40 hr. Bioavailability may be dose-dependent.

Dosage

- **Tablets**

Diuretic.

Adults: 50–100 mg/day or 100–200 mg 3 times/week. **Maximum daily dose:** 200 mg. **Pediatric:** All uses, 2 mg/kg (60 mg/m^2) 3 times/week.

Hypertension.

Adults, initial: 25 mg/day; if response is not sufficient, dose may be increased to 50 mg. For additional control, increase the dose to 100 mg/day or a second antihypertensive drug may be added to the regimen. **Maintenance:** Determined by client response.

Administration/Storage

1. Administer in the morning with food.
2. Doses higher than 25 mg/day will increase potassium excretion but will not cause further benefit in sodium excretion or reduction of BP.

Additional Uses: Particularly good for potentiating and reducing dosage of other antihypertensive agents.

Special Concerns: Geriatric clients may be more sensitive to the usual adult dose.

Additional Side Effects: Exfoliative dermatitis, toxic epidermal necrolysis.

NURSING CONSIDERATIONS

See *Nursing Considerations* for *Thiazide Diuretics,* Chapter 75, and *Antihypertensive Agents,* Chapter 28.

Evaluate

- Enhanced diuresis
- ↓ Edema
- ↓ BP

Hydrochlorothiazide

(**hy**-droh-klor-oh-**THIGH**-ah-zyd)

Pregnancy Category: B

Apo-Hydro ✱, Esidrex, Ezide, HydroDIURIL, Hydro-Par, Oretic **(Rx)**

See also *Thiazide Diuretics,* Chapter 75.

How Supplied: *Solution:* 50 mg/5 mL; *Tablet:* 25 mg, 50 mg, 100 mg

Action/Kinetics: Onset: 2 hr. **Peak effect:** 4–6 hr. **Duration:** 6–12 hr. **t½:** 5.6–14.8 hr. Hydrochlorothiazide is also found in Aldactazide, Aldoril, Apresazide, Dyazide, Hydropres, and Ser-Ap-Es.

Dosage

- **Oral Solution, Tablets**

Diuretic.

Adults, initial: 25–200 mg/day for several days until dry weight is reached; **then,** 25–100 mg/day or intermittently. Some clients may require up to 200 mg/day.

Antihypertensive.

Adults, initial: 25 mg/day as a single dose. The dose may be increased to 50 mg/day in one to two doses. Doses greater than 50 mg are associat-

ed with significant reductions in serum potassium. **Pediatric, under 6 months:** 3.3 mg/kg/day in two doses; **up to 2 years of age:** 12.5–37.5 mg/day in two doses; **2–12 years of age:** 37.5–100 mg/day in two doses.
Administration/Storage
1. Divide daily doses in excess of 100 mg.
2. Give b.i.d. at 6–12-hr intervals.
3. When used with other antihypertensives, clients usually do not require the dose of hydrochlorothiazide to be greater than 50 mg.
Special Concerns: Geriatric clients may be more sensitive to the usual adult dose.
Additional Side Effects: *CV:* Allergic myocarditis, hypotension. *Dermatologic:* Alopecia, exfoliative dermatitis, ***toxic epidermal necrolysis,*** erythema multiforme, ***Stevens-Johnson syndrome.*** *Miscellaneous:* ***Anaphylactic reactions, respiratory distress including pneumonitis and pulmonary edema.***

NURSING CONSIDERATIONS

See also *Nursing Considerations* for *Thiazide Diuretics,* Chapter 75.
Evaluate
- ↓ BP
- ↑ Urine output with a reduction in refractory edema

Indapamide

(in-**DAP**-ah-myd)
Pregnancy Category: B
Lozide ✱, Lozol **(Rx)**

See also *Thiazide Diuretics,* Chapter 75.
How Supplied: *Tablet:* 1.25 mg, 2.5 mg
Action/Kinetics: Onset: 1–2 weeks after multiple doses. **Peak levels:** 2 hr. **Duration:** Up to 8 weeks with multiple doses. **t½:** 14 hr. Nearly 100% is absorbed from the GI tract. Excreted through the kidneys (70% with 7% unchanged) and the GI tract (23%).
Uses: Alone or in combination with other drugs for treatment of hypertension. Edema in CHF.
Dosage
- **Tablets**

Edema of CHF.
Adults: 2.5 mg as a single dose in the morning. If necessary, may be increased to 5 mg/day after 1 week.
Hypertension.
Adults: 1.25 mg as a single dose in the morning. If the response is not satisfactory after 4 weeks, the dose may be increased to 2.5 mg taken once daily. If the response to 2.5 mg is not satisfactory after 4 weeks, the dose may be increased to 5 mg taken once daily (however, consideration should be given to adding another antihypertensive).
Administration/Storage
1. May be combined with other antihypertensive agents if the response is inadequate. Initially, the dose of other agents should be reduced by 50%.
2. Doses greater than 5 mg/day do not increase effectiveness but may increase hypokalemia.
Special Concerns: Dosage has not been established in children. Geriatric clients may be more sensitive to the hypotensive and electrolyte effects.

NURSING CONSIDERATIONS

See also *Nursing Considerations* for *Thiazide Diuretics,* Chapter 75, and *Antihypertensive Agents,* Chapter 28.
Assessment
1. Document indications for therapy and onset and type of symptoms.
2. List other drugs prescribed for these symptoms and the outcome.
Evaluate
- ↓ BP
- ↑ Urinary output with ↓ edema
- Improvement in S&S of CHF

LOOP DIURETICS

See the following individual entries:

Bumetanide
Ethacrynate Sodium
Ethyacrynic Acid

Furosemide
Torsemide

See also *Thiazide Diuretics,* Chapter 75.

Action/Kinetics: Loop diuretics inhibit reabsorption of sodium and chloride in the proximal and distal tubules and the loop of Henle. These diuretics are metabolized in the liver and excreted primarily through the urine. They are significantly bound to plasma protein.

Uses: Are potent diuretics and are used when a significant diuretic effect is required. Edema associated with CHF, hepatic cirrhosis, and renal disease (including nephrotic syndrome). Furosemide and torsemide are used alone or in combination with antihypertensive drugs to treat hypertension. Ethacrynic acid is used for short-term management of ascites due to malignancy, idiopathic edema, and lymphedema; it is also used for nephrotic syndrome and congenital heart disease in hospitalized pediatric clients (but not infants). Ethacrynic acid is used as adjunctive therapy in acute, pulmonary edema.

Dosage

See individual drugs.

Administration/Storage

1. Since these drugs increase urination, they should be taken early in the day.
2. Take with food or milk to decrease GI upset.
3. *Treatment of Overdose:* Replace fluid and electrolyte loss. Carefully monitor urine and plasma electrolyte levels. Emesis and gastric lavage may be useful. Supportive measures may include oxygen or artificial respiration.

Contraindications: Hypersensitivity to loop diruetics or to sulfonylureas. In hepatic coma or severe electrolyte depletion (until condition improves or is corrected). Use during lactation.

Special Concerns: Sudden alterations of electrolytes in hepatic cirrhosis and ascites may precipitate hepatic encephalopathy and coma. SLE may be activated or worsened. Ototoxicity is most common with rapid injection, in severe renal impairment, with doses several times the usual dose, and with concurrent use of other ototoxic drugs. Safety and efficacy of most loop diuretics have not been determined in children or infants.

Side Effects: See individual drugs. Excessive diuresis may cause dehydration with the possibility of ***circulatory collapse and vascular thrombosis or embolism.*** Ototoxicity including tinnitus, hearing impairment, deafness (usually reversible), and vertigo with a sense of fullness are possible. Electrolyte imbalance, especially in clients with restricted salt intake. Photosensitivity. Changes include hypokalemia, hypomagnesemia, and hypocalcemia.

Symptoms of Overdose: Acute profound water loss, volume and electrolyte depletion, dehydration, decreased blood volume, and ***circulatory collapse with possibility of fascicular thrombosis and embolism.***

Drug Interactions

Aminoglycosides / ↑ Ototoxicity with hearing loss
Anticoagulants / ↑ Anticoagulant activity
Chloral hydrate / Transient diaphoresis, hot flashes, hypertension, tachycardia, weakness and nausea
Cisplatin / Additive ototoxicity
Digitalis glycosides / ↑ Risk of arrhythmias due to diuretic- induced electrolyte disturbances
Lithium / ↑ Plasma levels of lithium → toxicity
Muscle relaxants, nondepolarizing / Effect of muscle relaxants may be either ↑ or ↓ , depending on the dose of diuretic
Nonsteroidal anti-inflammatory drugs / ↓ Effect of loop diuretics
Probenecid / ↓ Effect of loop diuretics
Salicylates / Diuretic effect may be ↓ in clients with cirrhosis and ascites
Sulfonylureas/ Loop diuretics may ↓ glucose tolerance

Theophyllines / Action of theophyllines may be ↑ or ↓
Thiazide diuretics / Additive effects with loop diuretics → profound diuresis and serious electrolyte abnormalities

NURSING CONSIDERATIONS

See also *Thiazides Diuretics,* Chapter 75.

Assessment

1. Document indications for therapy and type and onset of symptoms. Note other agents prescribed and the outcome.
2. Obtain baseline electrolytes, Mg, Ca, and liver and renal function studies.
3. List other agents prescribed to ensure that none interact unfavorably.
4. Note any history of sensitivity to sulfonamides. Furosemide is a derivative and client may exhibit cross-reactivity.
5. Determine any evidence or history of SLE, as drug may worsen condition.
6. Assess auditory function carefully especially when large doses are anticipated or when used concurrently with other ototoxic agents. Ototoxicity is dose related and generally reversible.

Client/Family Teaching

1. Advise clients to get up slowly as orthostatic hypotension may occur.
2. Use sunscreens or protective clothing when exposed to ultraviolet light or sunlight.
3. Notify provider if cramps, muscle weakness, nausea, or dizziness occurs.
4. Stress the importance of close medical supervison and periodic lab tests to enhance safety margin.

Evaluate

- ↓ Edema
- Reports of symptomatic relief (↓ swelling, ↑ diuresis)
- Clinical improvement in S&S associated with CHF and renal failure

Bumetanide

(byou-**MET**-ah-nyd)

Pregnancy Category: C
Bumex **(Rx)**

See also *Loop Diuretics,* Chapter 75.
How Supplied: *Injection:* 0.25 mg /mL; *Tablet:* 0.5 mg, 1 mg, 2 mg
Action/Kinetics: Bumetanide inhibits reabsorption of both sodium and chloride in the proximal tubule as well as the ascending loop of Henle. It may also have some activity in the proximal tubule to promote phosphate excretion. **Onset, PO:** 30–60 min. **Peak effect, PO:** 1–2 hr. **Duration, PO:** 4–6 hr (dose-dependent). **Onset, IV:** Several minutes. **Peak effect, IV:** 15–30 min. **Duration, IV:** 3.5–4 hr. **t½:** 1–1.5 hr. Metabolized in the liver although 45% excreted unchanged in the urine.
Uses: Edema associated with CHF, nephrotic syndrome, hepatic disease. Adjunct to treat acute pulmonary edema. Especially useful in clients refractory to other diuretics. *Investigational:* Treatment of adult nocturia. The drug is not effective in males with prostatic hypertrophy.

Dosage

- **Tablets**

Adults: 0.5–2 mg once daily; if response is inadequate, a second or third dose may be given at 4–5-hr intervals up to a maximum of 10 mg/day.

- **IV, IM**

Adults: 0.5–1 mg; if response is inadequate, a second or third dose may be given at 2–3-hr intervals up to a maximum of 10 mg/day. PO dosing should be started as soon as possible.

Administration/Storage

1. Solutions for IM or IV use should be freshly prepared and used within 24 hr.
2. Ampules may be reconstituted with 5% dextrose in water, 0.9% sodium chloride, or lactated Ringer's solution.
3. IV solutions should be administered slowly over 1–2 min.
4. IV or IM administration should be reserved for clients in whom PO use

is not practical or in whom absorption from the GI tract is impaired.
5. The recommended PO medication schedule is on alternate days or for 3–4 days with a 1–2-day rest period in between.
6. Bumetanide, at a 1:40 ratio of bumetanide:furosemide, may be ordered for clients allergic to furosemide.
7. In severe chronic renal insufficiency, a continuous infusion of bumetanide, 12 mg over 12 hr, may be more effective and cause fewer side effects than intermittent bolus therapy.
8. *Treatment of Overdose:* Replace electrolyte and fluid losses and monitor urinary electrolyte levels as well as serum electrolytes. Emesis or gastric lavage. Oxygen or artificial respiration may be necessary. General supportive measures.

Contraindications: Anuria. Hepatic coma or severe electrolyte depletion until the condition is improved or corrected. Hypersensitivity to the drug. Lactation.

Special Concerns: Safety and efficacy in children under 18 have not been established. Geriatric clients may be more sensitive to the hypotensive and electrolyte effects and are at greater risk in developing thromboembolic problems and circulatory collapse. SLE may be activated or made worse. Clients allergic to sulfonamides may show cross sensitivity to bumetanide. Sudden changes in electrolyte balance may cause hepatic encephalopathy and coma in clients with hepatic cirrhosis and ascites.

Laboratory Test Interferences: Alterations in LDH, AST, ALT, alkaline phosphatase, creatinine clearance, total serum bilirubin, serum proteins, cholesterol. Changes in hemoglobin, PT, hematocrit, WBCs, platelet and differential counts, phosphorus, carbon dioxide content, bicarbonate, and calcium. ↑ Urinary glucose and protein, serum creatinine. Also, hyperuricemia, hypochloremia, hypokalemia, azotemia, hyponatremia, hyperglycemia.

Side Effects: *Electrolyte and fluid changes:* Excess water loss, ***dehydration,*** electrolyte depletion including hypokalemia, hypochloremia, hyponatremia; hypovolemia, thromboembolism, ***circulatory collapse.*** *Otic:* Tinnitus, reversible and irreversible hearing impairment, deafness, vertigo (with a sense of fullness in the ears). *CV:* ***Reduction in blood volume may cause circulatory collapse and vascular thrombosis and embolism, especially in geriatric clients.*** Hypotension, ECG changes, chest pain. *CNS:* Asterixis, encephalopathy with preexisting liver disease, vertigo, headache, dizziness. *GI:* Upset stomach, dry mouth, N&V, diarrhea, GI pain. *GU:* Premature ejaculation, difficulty maintaining erection, renal failure. *Musculoskeletal:* Arthritic pain, weakness, muscle cramps, fatigue. *Hematologic:* Agranulocytosis, thrombocytopenia. *Allergic:* Pruritus, urticaria, rashes. *Miscellaneous:* Sweating, hyperventilation, rash, nipple tenderness, photosensitivity, pain following parenteral use.

Symptoms of Overdose: ***Profound loss of water, electrolyte depletion, dehydration, decreased blood volume, circulatory collapse (possibility of vascular thrombosis and embolism).*** Symptoms of electrolyte depletion include: anorexia, cramps, weakness, dizziness, vomiting, and mental confusion.

NURSING CONSIDERATIONS

See also *Nursing Considerations* for *Loop Diuretics,* Chapter 75.

Assessment

1. Document indications for therapy and pretreatment findings.
2. Note any sulfonamide allergy as there may be cross sensitivity.
3. Obtain hepatic and renal function studies as well as serum electrolyte levels and monitor throughout therapy; assess for hypokalemia.
4. Review history and note any evidence of lupus, hearing impairment, or thromboembolic events.
5. *NOTE:* 1 mg of bumetanide is essentially equivalent to 40 mg of furosemide.

Interventions
1. Monitor BP and pulse regularly. Rapid diuresis may cause dehydration and circulatory collapse (especially in the elderly). Hypotension may also occur when drug is administered with antihypertensive drugs.
2. Observe for ototoxicity, especially if the client is receiving other ototoxic drugs and assess hearing periodically.

Client/Family Teaching
1. Take medication early in the day to prevent nocturnal diuresis.
2. Do not perform activities that require mental alertness until drug effects are realized.
3. Provide instructions concerning dietary requirements such as reduced sodium and high potassium. Refer to dietitian as needed.
4. Record weights and report any sudden weight gain or evidence of swelling in the hands or feet.
5. Review the list of drug side effects and advise which require immediate attention.

Evaluate
- ↓ Peripheral and sacral edema
- Enhanced diuresis

Ethacrynate sodium
(eth-ah-**KRIH**-nayt)
Pregnancy Category: B
Sodium Edecrin **(Rx)**

Ethacrynic acid
(eth-ah-**KRIH**-nik **AH**-sid)
Pregnancy Category: B
Edecrin **(Rx)**

See also *Loop Diuretics,* Chapter 75.
How Supplied: Ethacrynate Sodium: *Powder for injection:* 50 mg. Ethacrynic Acid: *Tablet:* 25 mg, 50 mg
Action/Kinetics: Ethacrynic acid inhibits the reabsorption of sodium and chloride in the loop of Henle; the drug also decreases reabsorption of sodium and chloride and increases potassium excretion in the distal tubule. It also acts directly on the proximal tubule to enhance excretion of electrolytes. Large quantities of sodium and chloride and smaller amounts of potassium and bicarbonate ion are excreted during diuresis. **Onset: PO,** 30 min; **IV,** Within 5 min. **Peak: PO,** 2 hr; **IV,** 15–30 min. **Duration: PO,** 6–8 hr. **IV,** 2 hr. **t½, after PO:** 60 min. Metabolites are excreted through the urine. Diuresis and electrolyte loss are more pronounced with ethacrynic acid than with thiazide diuretics. Ethacrynic acid is often effective in clients refractory to other diuretics. Careful monitoring of the diuretic effects is necessary.
Uses: Of value in clients resistant to less potent diuretics. CHF, acute pulmonary edema, edema associated with nephrotic syndrome, ascites due to idiopathic edema, lymphedema, malignancy. Short-term use for ascites as a result of malignancy, lymphedema, or idiopathic edema; also, for short-term use in pediatric clients (except infants) with congenital heart disease. *Investigational.* **Ethacrynic acid:** Single injection into the eye to treat glaucoma (effective for a week or more). **Ethacrynate sodium:** Hypercalcemia, bromide intoxication, and with mannitol in ethylene glycol poisoning.

Dosage

ETHACRYNATE SODIUM
- **IV**

Adults: 50 mg (base) (or 0.5–1 mg/kg); may be repeated in 2–4 hr, although only one dose is usually needed. A single 100-mg dose IV has also been used.

ETHACRYNIC ACID
- **Tablets**

Adults, initial: 50–200 mg/day in single or divided doses to produce a gradual weight loss of 2.2–4.4 kg/day (1–2 lb/day). The dose can be increased by 25–50 mg/day if needed. **Maintenance:** Usually 50–200 mg (up to a maximum of 400 mg) daily may be required in severe, refractory edema. If used with other diuretics, the initial dose should be 25 mg with increments of 25 mg. **Pediatric, initial:** 25 mg/day; can increase by 25 mg/day if needed. **Maintenance:** Adjust dose to needs of client. Dosage for infants has not been determined.

Administration/Storage

1. When used PO, administer after meals.
2. Due to local pain and irritation, the drug should not be given SC or IM.
3. Reconstitute the powder for injection by adding 50 mL of 5% dextrose injection or sodium chloride injection.
4. Intermittent IV administration should be at a slow rate over a 30-min period given either directly or through IV tubing. For direct IV, may give at a rate of 10 mg/min.
5. When reconstituted with 5% dextrose injection, the resulting solution may be hazy or opalescent. Such solutions should not be used. Also, this solution should not be mixed with whole blood or its derivatives.
6. If a second IV injection is necessary, a different site should be used to prevent thrombophlebitis.
7. Use reconstituted solutions within 24 hr after which any unused solution should be discarded.
8. Ammonium chloride or arginine chloride may be prescribed for clients who are at a higher risk of developing metabolic acidosis.
9. *Treatment of Overdose:* Replace electrolytes and fluid and monitor urine output and serum electrolyte levels. Induce emesis or perform gastric lavage. Artificial respiration and oxygen may be needed. Treat other symptoms.

Contraindications: Usually not recommended during pregnancy. Lactation. Not recommended for use in neonates. Anuria and severe renal damage. Clients with history of gout should be watched closely.

Special Concerns: Geriatric clients may be more sensitive to the usual adult dose. To be used with caution in diabetic clients and those with hepatic cirrhosis (who are particularly susceptible to electrolyte imbalance). Safety and efficacy of oral use in infants and IV use in children have not been established.

Side Effects: *Electrolyte imbalance:* Hypokalemia, hyponatremia, hypochloremic alkalosis, hypomagnesemia, hypocalcemia. *GI:* Anorexia, nausea, vomiting, diarrhea (may be sudden watery, profuse diarrhea), acute pancreatitis, abdominal discomfort or pain, jaundice, ***GI bleeding or hemorrhage,*** dysphagia. *Hematologic:* Severe neutropenia, thrombocytopenia, ***agranulocytosis,*** rarely Henoch-Schoenlein purpura in clients with rheumatic heart disease. *CNS:* Apprehension, confusion, vertigo, headache. *Body as a whole:* Fever, chills, fatigue, malaise. *Otic:* Sense of fullness in the ears, tinnitus, irreversible hearing loss. *Miscellaneous:* Hematuria, acute gout, abnormal liver function tests in seriously ill clients on multiple drug therapy including ethacrynic acid, blurred vision, rash, local irritation and pain following parenteral use, hyperuricemia, hyperglycemia.

Ethacrynic acid may cause death in critically ill clients refractory to other diuretics. These include (a) clients with severe myocardial disease who also received digitalis and who developed acute hypokalemia with fatal arrhythmias and (b) those with severely decompensated hepatic cirrhosis with ascites, with or without encephalopathy, who had electrolyte imbalances with death due to intensification of the electrolyte effect.

Symptoms of Overdose: Profound water loss, electrolyte depletion (causes dizziness, weakness, mental confusion, vomiting, anorexia, lethargy, cramps), dehydration, reduction of blood volume, ***circulatory collapse (possibility of vascular thrombosis and embolism).***

NURSING CONSIDERATIONS

See also *Nursing Considerations* for *Loop Diuretics,* Chapter 75.

Assessment

1. Note any history of diabetes or cirrhosis.

2. Determine that anuria is not present.
3. List drugs the client is taking to identify any with which the drug may interact unfavorably.
4. Obtain baseline electrolytes, CBC, and liver function studies.
5. If prolonged therapy is anticipated, obtain audiometric assessment.

Interventions

1. Monitor VS, I&O, and weight. Observe for excessive diuresis or weight loss because electrolyte imbalance may develop quickly.
2. Assess clients with rapid excessive diuresis for pain in their calves, in the pelvic area, or in the chest. Rapid hemoconcentration may cause thromboembolic effects.
3. Observe for GI effects that may necessitate discontinuing the drug. The drug should be withdrawn if the client manifests severe, watery diarrhea.
4. Test for occult blood in the urine and the stools.
5. Observe the client for vestibular disturbances. Do not administer the drug IV concomitantly with any other ototoxic agent. Hearing loss is most common following high dosing or rapid IV administration.
6. Monitor serum potassium levels and determine the need for supplementary potassium.
7. Since ethacrynic acid has such a profound effect on sodium excretion, dietary salt restriction is not necessary; if sodium is restricted, hyponatremia may result.

Evaluate

- Enhanced diuresis
- ↓ Edema (↑ weight loss R/T edema)
- ↓ Abdominal girth R/T ascites

Furosemide

(fur-**OH**-seh-myd)
Pregnancy Category: C
Apo-Furosemide ✱, Lasix, Myrosemide **(Rx)**

See also *Loop Diuretics,* Chapter 75.

How Supplied: *Injection:* 10 mg/mL; *Solution:* 10 mg/ mL, 40 mg/5 mL; *Tablet:* 20 mg, 40 mg, 80 mg

Action/Kinetics: Furosemide inhibits the reabsorption of sodium and chloride in the proximal and distal tubules as well as the ascending loop of Henle; this results in the excretion of sodium, chloride, and, to a lesser degree, potassium and bicarbonate ions. The resulting urine is more acid. Diuretic action is independent of changes in clients' acid-base balance. Furosemide has a slight antihypertensive effect. **Onset: PO, IM:** 30–60 min; **IV:** 5 min. **Peak: PO, IM:** 1–2 hr; **IV:** 20–60 min. **t½:** About 2 hr after PO use. **Duration: PO, IM:** 6–8 hr; **IV:** 2 hr. Metabolized in the liver and excreted through the urine. The drug may be effective for clients resistant to thiazides and for those with reduced GFRs.

Uses: Edema associated with CHF, nephrotic syndrome, hepatic cirrhosis, and ascites. IV for acute pulmonary edema. Furosemide can be used orally to treat hypertension in conjunction with spironolactone, triamterene, and other diuretics *except* ethacrynic acid. *Investigational:* Hypercalcemia.

Dosage

- **Oral Solution, Tablets**

Edema.

Adults, initial: 20–80 mg/day as a single dose. For resistant cases, dosage can be increased by 20–40 mg q 6–8 hr until desired diuretic response is attained. Maximum daily dose should not exceed 600 mg. **Pediatric, initial:** 2 mg/kg as a single dose; **then,** dose can be increased by 1–2 mg/kg q 6–8 hr until desired response is attained (up to 5 mg/kg may be required in children with nephrotic syndrome; maximum dose should not exceed 6 mg/kg). A dose range of 0.5–2 mg/kg b.i.d. has also been recommended.

Hypertension.

Adults, initial: 40 mg b.i.d. Adjust dosage depending on response.

CHF and chronic renal failure.

Adults: 2–2.5 g/day.

Antihypercalcemic.

Adults: 120 mg/day in one to three doses.

• **IV, IM**

Edema.

Adults, initial: 20–40 mg; if response inadequate after 2 hr, increase dose in 20-mg increments. **Pediatric, initial:** 1 mg/kg given slowly; if response inadequate after 2 hr, increase dose by 1 mg/kg. Doses greater than 6 mg/kg should not be given.

Antihypercalcemic.

Adults: 80–100 mg for severe cases; dose may be repeated q 1–2 hr if needed.

• **IV**

Acute pulmonary edema.

Adults: 40 mg slowly over 1–2 min; if response inadequate after 1 hr, give 80 mg slowly over 1–2 min. Concomitant oxygen and digitalis may be used.

CHF, chronic renal failure.

Adults: 2–2.5 g/day. For IV bolus injections, the maximum should not exceed 1 g/day given over 30 min.

Hypertensive crisis, normal renal function.

Adults: 40–80 mg.

Hypertensive crisis with pulmonary edema or acute renal failure.

Adults: 100–200 mg.

Administration/Storage

1. The drug should be given 2–4 days/week.
2. IV injections are given slowly over 1–2 min.
3. If used IV, furosemide should not be mixed with solutions with a pH below 5.5. After pH adjustment, furosemide can be mixed with sodium chloride injection, lactated Ringer's injection, and 5% dextrose injection and infused at a rate not to exceed 4 mg/min to prevent ototoxicity.
4. A precipitate may form if furosemide is mixed with gentamicin, netilmicin, or milrinone in either 5% dextrose or 0.9% sodium chloride.
5. Food decreases the bioavailability of furosemide and ultimately the degree of diuresis.
6. Slight discoloration resulting from light does not affect potency. However, discolored tablets or injection should not be dispensed.
7. If used with other antihypertensives, the dose of other agents reduced by at least 50% when furosemide is added in order to prevent an excessive drop in BP.
8. Store in light-resistant containers at room temperature (15°C–30°C or 59°F–86°F).
9. In CHF or chronic renal failure oral and parenteral doses as high as 2–2.5 g/day (or higher) are well tolerated.
10. *Treatment of Overdose:* Replace fluid and electrolytes. Monitor urine electrolyte output and serum electrolytes. Induce emesis or perform gastric lavage. Oxygen or artificial respiration may be needed. Treat symptoms.

Contraindications: Never use with ethacrynic acid. Anuria, hypersensitivity to drug, severe renal disease associated with azotemia and oliguria, hepatic coma associated with electrolyte depletion. Lactation.

Special Concerns: Use with caution in premature infants and neonates due to prolonged half-life in these clients (dosing interval must be extended). Geriatric clients may be more sensitive to the usual adult dose. Allergic reactions may be seen in clients who show hypersensitivity to sulfonamides.

Side Effects: *Electrolyte and fluid effects:* Fluid and electrolyte depletion leading to dehydration, hypovolemia, thromboembolism. Hypokalemia and hypochloremia may cause metabolic alkalosis. Hyperuricemia, azotemia, hyponatremia. *GI:* Nausea, oral and gastric irritation, vomiting, anorexia, diarrhea (especially in children) or constipation, cramps, pancreatitis, jaundice, ischemic hepatitis. *Otic:* Tinnitus, hearing impairment (may be reversible or permanent), reversible deafness. Usually following rapid IV or IM administration of high doses. *CNS:* Vertigo, headache, dizziness, blurred vision, restlessness, paresthesias, xanthopsia. *CV:* Orthostatic hypotension, thrombophlebitis, chronic aortitis. *Hematologic:* Anemia, thrombocytopenia, neutropenia, leukopenia, ***agranulocytosis,*** purpura. ***Rarely, aplastic anemia.*** *Allergic:* Rashes, pruritus, urticaria, photosensitivity, exfoliative dermatitis, vasculitis, erythema multiforme. *Miscellaneous:* Interstitial nephritis, fever, weakness, hyperglycemia, glycosuria, exacerbation of, aggravation of or worsening of SLE, increased perspiration, muscle spasms, urinary bladder spasm, urinary frequency.

Following IV use: Thrombophlebitis, ***cardiac arrest.*** *Following IM use:* Pain and irritation at injection site, ***cardiac arrest.***

Because this drug is resistant to the effects of pressor amines and potentiates the effects of muscle relaxants, it is recommended that the PO drug be discontinued 1 week before surgery and the IV drug 2 days before surgery.

Symptoms of Overdose: Profound water loss, electrolyte depletion (manifested by weakness, anorexia, vomiting, lethargy, cramps, mental confusion, dizziness), decreased blood volume, ***circulatory collapse (possibly vascular thrombosis and embolism).***

Additional Drug Interactions

Charcoal / ↓ Absorption of furosemide from the GI tract

Clofibrate / Enhanced diuretic effect

Hydantoins / Hydantoins ↓ the diuretic effect of furosemide

Propranolol / Furosemide may cause ↑ plasma levels of propranolol

NURSING CONSIDERATIONS

See also *Nursing Considerations* for *Loop Diuretics,* Chapter 75.

Interventions

1. Monitor serum electrolytes and observe for S&S of hypokalemia.
2. In clients with rapid diuresis, observe for dehydration and circulatory collapse. Monitor BP and pulse and document.
3. When the client has renal impairment or is receiving other ototoxic drugs, observe for ototoxicity.
4. Assess closely for signs of vascular thrombosis and embolism, particularly in the elderly.
5. With chronic use, assess for thiamine deficiency.

Client/Family Teaching

1. Assure client that any pain after IM injection will be transitory.
2. Take medication in the morning to avoid interruption of sleep.
3. Provide a printed list of adverse side effects of drug therapy. Stress those that require immediate reporting, i.e., muscle weakness, dizziness, numbness, or tingling.
4. Assist clients to establish the timing of the diuretic so that they can participate in social activities and not have to get up during the night to void frequently.
5. Caution that drug may cause orthostatic hypotension.
6. Advise to consult with the provider before taking aspirin for any reason. Salicylate intoxication occurs at lower levels than normal because of competition at the renal excretory sites.
7. Use sunscreens and protective clothing when exposed to the sun to minimize the effects of drug-induced photosensitivity.
8. Discuss the need for a diet high in potassium. Instruct in how to supplement diet with vegetables and fruits high in potassium if oral supplements are not prescribed.
9. Advise that the sorbitol in the solution vehicle may result in diarrhea, especially in children.

Evaluate

- Enhanced diuresis
- Resolution of pulmonary edema
- ↓ Dependent edema
- ↓ BP
- ↓ Serum calcium levels

Torsemide

(TOR-seh-myd)
Pregnancy Category: B
Demadex **(Rx)**

See also *Loop Diuretics,* Chapter 75.

How Supplied: *Injection:* 10 mg /mL; *Tablet:* 5 mg, 10 mg, 20 mg, 100 mg

Action/Kinetics: Onset, IV: Within 10 min; **PO:** within 60 min. **Peak effect, IV:** Within 60 min; **PO:** 60–120 min. **Duration:** 6–8 hr. **t½:** 210 min. Metabolized by the liver and excreted through the urine. Food intake delays the time to peak effect by about 30 min, but the overall bioavailability and the diuretic activity are not affected.

Uses: Congestive heart failure, chronic renal failure, hepatic cirrhosis, hypertension.

Dosage

- **Tablets, IV**

Congestive heart failure.

Adults, initial: 10 or 20 mg once daily.

Chronic renal failure.

Adults, initial: 20 mg once daily.

Hepatic cirrhosis.

Adults, initial: 5 or 10 mg once daily given with an aldosterone antagonist or a potassium-sparing diuretic.

Hypertension.

Adults, initial: 5 mg once daily. If this dose does not lead to an adequate decrease in BP within 4–6 weeks, the dose may be increased to 10 mg once daily. If the 10-mg dose is not adequate, an additional antihypertensive agent is added to the treatment regimen.

Administration/Storage

1. Oral and IV doses are therapeutically equivalent, and clients may be switched to and from the IV form with no change in dose.
2. If the response is inadequate for the initial dose used for CHF, chronic renal failure, or hepatic cirrhosis, the dose can be doubled until the desired diuretic response is obtained. Doses greater than 200 mg for CHF or chronic renal failure and greater than 40 mg for hepatic cirrhosis have not been adequately studied.
3. Torsemide may be given at any time in relation to a meal.
4. The IV dose is given slowly over a period of 2 min.
5. The dose does not need to be adjusted for geriatric clients.

Contraindication: Lactation.

Special Concerns: Clients sensitive to sulfonamides may show allergic reactions to torsemide. Safety and efficacy in children have not been determined.

Laboratory Test Interferences: Hyperglycemia, hyperuricemia, hypokalemia, hypovolemia.

Side Effects: *CNS:* Headache, dizziness, asthenia, insomnia, nervousness, syncope. *GI:* Diarrhea, constipation, nausea, dyspepsia, edema, ***GI hemorrhage,*** rectal bleeding. *CV:* ECG abnormality, chest pain, atrial fibrillation, hypotension, ventricular tachycardia, shunt thrombosis. *Respiratory:* Rhinitis, increase in cough. *Musculoskeletal:* Arthralgia, myalgia. *Miscellaneous:* Sore throat, excessive urination, rash.

NURSING CONSIDERATIONS

See also *Nursing Considerations* for *Loop Diuretics,* Chapter 75.

Assessment

1. Document indications for therapy and type and onset of symptoms.
2. List other agents prescribed and the outcome.
3. Query client and note any sensitivity to sulfonamides.
4. List drugs currently prescribed to ensure none interact unfavorably.
5. Obtain baseline VS, serum blood sugar, uric acid, and potassium levels and monitor periodically. Drug may increase blood sugar and uric acid levels.
6. Assess and document baseline pulmonary, renal, and CV data.
7. Initially monitor VS, daily weight, and I&O.

Client/Family Teaching

1. Take only as directed. May take with food to decrease GI upset.

2. With hypertension, instruct how to take BP and to keep a written record for review at each visit.
3. Advise to report immediately any chest pain, increased SOB, or sudden weight gain with evidence of extremity edema.
4. Caution that drug may cause dizziness, lightheadedness, and fatigue.
5. Advise to rise slowly from a sitting or lying position to minimize orthostatic drug effects.
6. May experience blurred vision, yellowing of vision, or sensitivity to sunlight. Report any unusual or persistent symptoms.
7. Report as scheduled for labs and follow-up exams so provider can evaluate drug effectiveness.

Evaluate

- Promotion of diuresis
- Reduction of edema in furosemide refractory clients
- ↓BP
- Reduction of interdialysis weight gain and promotion of Na, Cl, and water excretion

POTASSIUM-SPARING DIURETICS

See the following individual entries:

Amiloride Hydrochloride
Spironolactone
Triamterene

Amiloride hydrochloride

(ah-**MILL**-oh-ryd)
Pregnancy Category: B
Midamor **(Rx)**

How Supplied: *Tablet:* 5 mg
Action/Kinetics: Amiloride acts on the distal tubule to inhibit Na^+, K^+-ATPase, thereby inhibiting sodium exchange for potassium; this results in increased secretion of sodium and water and conservation of potassium. In the proximal tubule, amiloride inhibits the Na^+/H^+ exchange mechanism. The drug also has weak diuretic and antihypertensive activity. **Onset:** 2 hr. **Peak effect:** 6–10 hr. **Peak plasma levels:** 3–4 hr. **Duration:** 24 hr. **t½:** 6–9 hr. Twenty-three percent is bound to plasma protein. Approximately 50% is excreted unchanged by kidney and 40% by the feces unchanged.
Uses: Adjunct with thiazides or loop diuretics in the treatment of hypertension or edema due to CHF, hepatic cirrhosis, and nephrotic syndrome to help restore normal serum potassium or prevent hypokalemia. Prophylaxis of hypokalemia in clients who would be at risk if hypokalemia developed (e.g., digitalized clients or clients with significant cardiac arrhythmias). *Investigational:* To reduce lithium-induced polyuria. Aerosolized amiloride may slow the progression of pulmonary function reduction in adults with cystic fibrosis.

Dosage

- **Tablets**

As single agent or with other diuretics.

Adults, initial: 5 mg/day; 10 mg/day may be necessary in some clients. Doses as high as 20 mg/day may be used, if needed, with careful monitoring of electrolytes.

Reduce lithium-induced polyuria. 10–20 mg/day.

Slow progression of pulmonary function development in cystic fibrosis.

Adults: Drug is dissolved in 0.3% saline and delivered by nebulizer.

Administration/Storage

1. Administer with food to reduce chance of GI upset.
2. *Treatment of Overdose:* Induce emesis or gastric lavage. Treat hyperkalemia by IV sodium bicarbonate or oral or parenteral glucose with a rapid-acting insulin. Sodium polystyrene sulfonate, oral or by enema, may also be used.

Contraindications: Hyperkalemia (>5.5 mEq potassium/L). In clients receiving other potassium-sparing diuretics or potassium supplements. Impaired renal function. Diabetes mellitus. Use during lactation.

Special Concerns: Use with caution in metabolic or respiratory acidosis; during lactation. Geriatric clients may have a greater risk of developing hyperkalemia. Safety and efficacy have not been determined in children.

Side Effects: *Electrolyte:* Hyperkalemia, hyponatremia, and hypochloremia if used with other diuretics. *CNS:* Headache, dizziness, encephalopathy, tremors, paresthesias, mental confusion, insomnia, decreased libido, depression, sleepiness, vertigo, nervousness. *GI:* Nausea, anorexia, vomiting, diarrhea, changes in appetite, gas and abdominal pain, dry mouth, flatulence, abdominal fullness, GI bleeding, GI disturbance, thirst, dyspepsia, heartburn, jaundice, constipation, activation of preexisting peptic ulcer. *Respiratory:* Dyspnea, cough, SOB. *Musculoskeletal:* Weakness; muscle cramps; fatigue; joint, chest and back pain; neck or shoulder ache; pain in extremities. *GU:* Impotence, polyuria, dysuria, bladder spasms, urinary frequency. *CV:* Angina, palpitations, ***arrhythmias,*** orthostatic hypotension. *Hematologic:* ***Aplastic anemia,*** neutropenia. *Dermatologic:* Skin rash, itching, pruritus, alopecia. *Miscellaneous:* Visual disturbances, nasal congestion, tinnitus, increased intraocular pressure, abnormal liver function.

Symptoms of Overdose: Electrolyte imbalance, ***dehydration.***

Drug Interactions

ACE inhibitors / ↑ Risk of significant hyperkalemia
Digoxin / Possible ↑ renal clearance and ↓ nonrenal clearance of digoxin. Possible ↑ inotropic effect of digoxin
Lithium / ↓ Renal excretion of lithium → ↑ chance of toxicity
NSAIDs / ↓ Therapeutic effect of amiloride
Potassium products / Hyperkalemia with possibility of cardiac arrhythmias or cardiac arrest
Spironolactone, Triamterene / Hyperkalemia, hyponatremia, hypochloremia

NURSING CONSIDERATIONS

See also *Nursing Considerations* for *Thiazide Diuretics,* Chapter 75.

Interventions

1. Monitor renal function studies, I&O, and weights.
2. Monitor serum electrolytes. Assess for hyperkalemia and for indications to withdraw the drug. Cardiac irregularities may be precipitated.
3. Do not encourage potassium supplementation or foods rich in potassium because drug does not promote potassium excretion.
4. Do not administer with other potassium-sparing diuretics.

Evaluate

- ↓ BP and enhanced diuresis
- Conservation of potassium; serum levels within desired range
- ↓ Lithium-induced polyuria
- Maintenance of pulmonary function with cystic fibrosis

Spironolactone

(speer-oh-no-**LAK**-tohn)
Aldactone, Novo-Spiroton ✱ **(Rx)**

See also *Thiazide Diuretics,* Chapter 75.

How Supplied: *Tablet:* 25 mg, 50 mg, 100 mg

Action/Kinetics: Spironolactone is a mild diuretic that acts on the distal tubule to inhibit sodium exchange for potassium, which results in increased secretion of sodium and water and conservation of potassium. It is also an aldosterone antagonist. The drug manifests a slight antihypertensive effect. It also interferes with synthesis of testosterone and may increase formation of estradiol from testosterone, thus leading to endocrine abnormalities. **Onset:** Urine output increases over 1–2 days. **Peak:** 2–3 days. **Duration:** 2–3 days, and declines thereafter. It is metabolized to an active metabolite (canrenone). **t½:** 13–24 hr for canrenone. Canrenone is excreted through the urine (primary) and the bile. The drug is almost completely bound to plasma protein. Spironolactone is also found in Aldactazide.

Uses: Primary hyperaldosteronism, including diagnosis, short-term preoperative treatment, long-term maintenance therapy for those who are poor surgical risks and those with bilateral micronodular or macronodular adrenal hyperplasia. To treat edema when other approaches are inadequate or ineffective (e.g., CHF, cirrhosis of the liver, nephrotic syndrome). Essential hypertension (usually in combination with other drugs). Prophylaxis of hypokalemia in clients taking digitalis. *Investigational:* Hirsutism, treat symptoms of PMS, with testolactone to treat familial male precocious puberty (short-term treatment), acne vulgaris.

Dosage

• **Tablets**

Treat edema.

Adults, initial: 100 mg/day (range: 25–200 mg/day) in two to four divided doses for at least 5 days; **maintenance:** 75–400 mg/day in two to four divided doses. **Pediatric:** 3.3 mg/kg/day as a single dose or as two to four divided doses.

Antihypertensive.

Adults, initial: 50–100 mg/day as a single dose or as two to four divided doses—give for at least 2 weeks; **maintenance:** adjust to individual response. **Pediatric:** 1–2 mg/kg in a single dose or in two to four divided doses.

Treat hypokalemia.

Adults: 25–100 mg/day as a single dose or two to four divided doses.

Diagnosis of primary hyperaldosteronism.

Adults: 400 mg/day for either 4 days (short-test) or 3–4 weeks (long-test).

Hyperaldosteronism, prior to surgery.

Adults: 100–400 mg/day in two to four doses prior to surgery.

Hyperaldosteronism, chronic-therapy.

Use lowest possible dose.

Hirsutim.

50–200 mg/day.

Symptoms of PMS.

25 mg q.i.d. beginning on day 14 of the menstrual cycle.

Familial male precocious puberty, short-term.

Spironolactone, 2 mg/kg/day, and testolactone, 20–40 mg/kg/day, for at least 6 months.

Acne vulgaris.

100 mg/day.

Administration/Storage

1. When used as the sole drug to treat edema, the initial dose should continue for at least 5 days. After that, adjustments may be made. If the dosage is not effective, a second diuretic may be added, especially one that acts in the proximal tubules.
2. When administered to small children, the tablets may be crushed and given as a suspension in cherry syrup.
3. Food may increase the absorption of spironolactone.
4. Protect the drug from light.

Contraindications: Acute renal insufficiency, progressive renal failure, hyperkalemia, and anuria. Clients receiving potassium supplements, amiloride, or triamterene.

Special Concerns: Use during pregnancy only if benefits clearly outweigh risks. Use with caution in impaired renal function. Geriatric clients may be more sensitive to the usual adult dose.

Laboratory Test Interferences: Interference with radioimmunoassay for digoxin. False + plasma cortisol (as determined by fluorometric assay of Mattingly).

Side Effects: *Electrolyte:* Hyperkalemia, hyponatremia (characterized by lethargy, dry mouth, thirst, tiredness). *GI:* Diarrhea, cramps, ulcers, gastritis, gastric bleeding, vomiting. *CNS:* Drowsiness, ataxia, lethargy, mental confusion, headache. *Endocrine:* Gynecomastia, menstrual irregularities, impotence, bleeding in postmenopausal women, deepening of voice, hirsutism. *Dermatologic:* Maculopapular or erythematous cutaneous eruptions, urticaria. *Miscellane-*

ous: Drug fever, breast carcinoma, gynecomastia, hyperchloremic metabolic acidosis in hepatic cirrhosis (decompensated), ***agranulocytosis.*** *NOTE:* Spironolactone has been shown to be tumorigenic in chronic rodent studies.

Drug Interactions

Anesthetics, general / Additive hypotension

ACE inhibitors / Significant hyperkalemia

Anticoagulants, oral / Inhibited by spironolactone

Antihypertensives / Potentiation of hypotensive effect of both agents. Reduce dosage, especially of ganglionic blockers, by one-half

Captopril / ↑ Risk of significant hyperkalemia

Digitalis / ↑ Half-life of digoxin → ↓ clearance. Spironolactone may ↓ inotropic effect of digoxin. Spironolactone both ↑ and ↓ elimination t½ of digitoxin

Diuretics, others / Often administered concurrently because of potassium-sparing effect of spironolactone. Severe hyponatremia may occur. Monitor closely

Lithium / ↑ Chance of lithium toxicity due to ↓ renal clearance

Norepinephrine / ↓ Responsiveness to norepinephrine

Potassium salts / Since spironolactone conserves potassium excessively, hyperkalemia may result. Rarely used together

Salicylates / Large doses may ↓ effects of spironolactone

Triamterene / Hazardous hyperkalemia may result from combination

NURSING CONSIDERATIONS

See also *Nursing Considerations* for *Thiazide Diuretics,* Chapter 75.

Assessment

1. Document indications for therapy, type and onset of symptoms, other agents prescribed, and the outcome.
2. Obtain baseline ECG, ABGs, and serum electrolyte levels prior to starting therapy. If the serum potassium level is greater than 5.5 mEq/L, withhold the medication and report.
3. If the client has a history of cardiac disease, be alert for cardiac irregularities R/T hypokalemia.

Interventions

1. Monitor ABGs, serum electrolytes, and liver and renal function studies. Compare with the baseline data and report any abnormalities.
2. If the client develops deep, rapid respirations, complains of headaches, or appears to be slower mentally, document and report as this may indicate hyperchloremic metabolic acidosis.
3. Record VS, I&O, and weights.
4. Note if the client develops dysuria, urinary frequency, or renal spasm. Take a urine culture, check for sensitivity, request a urinalysis, and report.
5. Assess client for tolerance to the drug, which may be characterized by edema and reduced urine output.
6. Report if the client develops jaundice or tremors or appears mentally confused. If hepatic disease already exists, clients may develop hepatic encephalopathy. Drug is metabolized in the liver.
7. Administer the drug with a snack or meals to relieve the symptoms of gastric distress. Report if nausea, bloating, anorexia, vomiting, or diarrhea persist. The dosage of drug may need to be changed or the drug may need to be discontinued.

Client/Family Teaching

1. Take with food to minimize GI upset.
2. Instruct client in how to take BP and assist to develop a method to maintain a written record for review by the provider.
3. Avoid foods or salt substitutes high in potassium because spironolactone is potassium-sparing.
4. Record weight twice a week. Report any evidence of edema or weight gain of more than 3 lb (6.6 kg) weekly.
5. Caution clients taking large doses of medication not to drive a car and not to operate dangerous machinery until drug effects become apparent because drowsiness or ataxia may occur.

6. Advise that drug may cause gynecomastia and diminished libido by reducing testosterone levels.

Evaluate

- Enhanced diuresis with ↓ edema
- ↓ BP
- Antagonism of high levels of aldosterone
- Prevention of hypokalemia in those taking digitalis and/or other diuretics

Triamterene

(try-**AM**-ter-een)

Pregnancy Category: B

Dyrenium **(Rx)**

See also *Thiazide Diuretics,* Chapter 75.

How Supplied: *Capsule:* 50 mg, 100 mg

Action/Kinetics: Triamterene is a mild diuretic that acts directly on the distal tubule. It promotes the excretion of sodium—which is exchanged for potassium or hydrogen ions—bicarbonate, chloride, and fluid. The drug increases urinary pH. It is also a weak folic acid antagonist. **Onset:** 2–4 hr. **Peak effect:** 6–8 hr. **Duration:** 7–9 hr. **t½:** 3 hr. From one-half to two-thirds of the drug is bound to plasma protein. Triamterene is metabolized to hydroxytriamterene sulfate, which is also active. About 20% is excreted unchanged through the urine. Triamterene is also found in Dyazide.

Uses: Edema due to CHF, hepatic cirrhosis, nephrotic syndrome, steroid therapy, secondary hyperaldosteronism, and idiopathic edema. May be used alone or with other diuretics. *Investigational:* Prophylaxis and treatment of hypokalemia, adjunct in the treatment of hypertension.

Dosage

Capsules.

Diuretic. **Adults, initial:** 100 mg b.i.d. after meals; **maximum daily dose:** 300 mg.

Administration/Storage

1. Minimize nausea by giving the drug after meals.
2. Triamterene dosage is usually reduced by one-half when another diuretic is added to the regimen.
3. *Treatment of Overdose:* Immediately induce vomiting or perform gastric lavage. Electrolyte levels and fluid balance should be evaluated and treated if necessary. Dialysis may be beneficial.

Contraindications: Hypersensitivity to drug, severe or progressive renal insufficiency, severe hepatic disease, anuria, hyperkalemia, hyperuricemia, gout, history of nephrolithiasis. Lactation.

Special Concerns: Safety and efficacy have not been determined in children.

Laboratory Test Interferences: Triamterene may impart blue fluorescence to urine, interfering with fluorometric assays (e.g., lactic dehydrogenase, quinidine). ↑ BUN, creatinine. ↑ Serum uric acid in clients predisposed to gouty arthritis.

Side Effects: *Electrolyte:* Hyperkalemia, electrolyte imbalance. *GI:* Nausea, vomiting (may also be indicative of electrolyte imbalance), diarrhea, dry mouth. *CNS:* Dizziness, drowsiness, fatigue, weakness, headache. *Hematologic:* Megaloblastic anemia, thrombocytopenia. *Renal:* Azotemia, interstitial nephritis. *Miscellaneous:* ***Anaphylaxis,*** photosensitivity, hypokalemia, jaundice, muscle cramps, rash.

Symptoms of Overdose: Electrolyte imbalance, especially hyperkalemia. Also, nausea, vomiting, other GI disturbances, weakness, hypotension, reversible acute renal failure.

Drug Interactions

Amantadine / ↑ Toxic effects of amantadine due to ↓ renal excretion

Angiotensin-converting enzyme inhibitors / Significant hyperkalemia

Antihypertensives / Potentiated by triamterene

Captopril / ↑ Risk of significant hyperkalemia
Cimetidine / ↑ Bioavailability and ↓ clearance of triamterene
Digitalis / Inhibited by triamterene
Indomethacin / ↑ Risk of nephrotoxicity and acute renal failure
Lithium / ↑ Chance of lithium toxicity due to ↓ renal clearance
Potassium salts / Additive hyperkalemia
Spironolactone / Additive hyperkalemia

NURSING CONSIDERATIONS

See also *Nursing Considerations* for *Thiazide Diuretics,* Chapter 75.

Assessment

1. Take a complete drug history, noting drugs with which triamterene interacts.
2. Obtain baseline serum electrolytes, renal function studies, and uric acid levels before administering the drug.
3. Determine that a CBC with differential and an ECG have been performed prior to initiating therapy.

Interventions

1. Monitor serum electrolytes, BUN, uric acid, and CBC and report any variations.
2. If the client has a history of heart disease, obtain an ECG and be alert to the development of cardiac arrhythmias.
3. If the client has a history of alcoholism, megaloblastic anemia may occur because triamterene is a weak antagonist of folic acid. Monitor the CBC and WBC differential periodically.
4. Observe for hyperkalemia; this is an indication to withdraw the drug because cardiac irregularities may result.

Client/Family Teaching

1. Take drug with food to minimize GI upset.
2. Report any symptoms of sore throat, rash, or fever. These may be signs of blood dyscrasias and may require withdrawal of the drug.
3. Report persistent headaches, drowsiness, vomiting, restlessness, mental wandering, lethargy, and foul breath since these may be signs of uremia.
4. Caution that drug may cause dizziness.
5. Avoid using any OTC agents, potassium supplements, salt substitutes that contain potassium, and foods high in potassium without approval, because the drug is potassium-sparing.
6. Advise that urine may appear pale fluorescent blue and not to be alarmed.
7. Avoid direct sunlight for prolonged periods because drug may cause a photosensitivity reaction. Use appropriate precautions (e.g., sunscreens, sunglasses, hat, and long sleeves and pants).

Evaluate

- ↓ Edema
- Reports of ↑ diuresis

MISCELLANEOUS DIURETIC

Mannitol

(**MAN**-nih-tol)
Pregnancy Category: C
Osmitrol **(Rx)**

How Supplied: *Injection:* 5%, 10%, 15%, 20%, 25%; *Irrigation solution:* 5%

Action/Kinetics: Mannitol increases the osmolarity of the glomerular filtrate, which decreases the reabsorption of water while increasing excretion of sodium and chloride. It also increases the osmolarity of the plasma, which causes enhanced flow of water from tissues into the interstitial fluid and plasma. Thus, cerebral edema, increased ICP, and CSF volume and pressure are decreased. **Onset, IV:** 30–60 min for diuresis and within 15 min for reduction of cerebrospinal and intraocular pressures. **Peak:** 30–60 min. **Duration:** 6–8 hr diuresis and 4–8 hr for reduction of intraocular pressure. **t½:** 15–100 min. Over 90% excreted through the urine unchanged. A test dose is given in clients with impaired renal function or oliguria.

Uses: Diuretic to prevent or treat the oliguric phase of acute renal failure before irreversible renal failure occurs. Decrease ICP and cerebral edema by decreasing brain mass. Decrease elevated intraocular pressure when the pressure cannot be lowered by other means. To promote urinary excretion of toxic substances. As a urinary irrigant to prevent hemolysis and hemoglobin buildup during transurethral prostatic resection or other transurethral surgical procedures. *Investigational:* Prevent hemolysis during cardiopulmonary bypass surgery.

Dosage

- **IV infusion only**

Test dose (oliguria or reduced renal function).

Either 50 mL of a 25% solution, 75 mL of a 20% solution, or 100 mL of a 15% solution infused over 3–5 min. If urine flow is 30–50 mL/hr, therapeutic dose can be given. If urine flow does not increase, give a second test dose; if still no response, client must be reevaluated.

Prevention of acute renal failure (oliguria).

Adults: 50–100 g, as a 5%–25% solution, given at a rate to maintain urine flow of at least 30–50 mL/hr.

Treatment of oliguria.

Adults: 50–100 g of a 15%–25% solution.

Reduction of intracranial pressure and brain mass.

Adults: 1.5–2 g/kg as a 15%–25% solution, infused over 30–60 min.

Reduction of intraocular pressure.

Adults: 1.5–2 g/kg as a 20% solution (7.5–10 mL/kg) or as a 15% solution (10–13 mL/kg) given over 30–60 min. When used preoperatively, the dose should be given 1–1.5 hr before surgery to maintain the maximum effect.

Antidote to remove toxic substances.

Adults: Dose depends on the fluid requirement and urinary output. IV fluids and electrolytes are given to replace losses. If a beneficial effect is not seen after 200 g mannitol, the infusion should be discontinued.

Urologic irrigation.

Adults: Use as a 2.5% irrigating solution for the bladder (this concentration minimizes the hemolytic effect of water alone).

Administration/Storage

1. If concentrated mannitol is used (15%, 20%, and 25%), a filter should be used.
2. If the concentration of mannitol is greater than 15%, it may crystallize. To redissolve, warm the bottle in a hot water bath or autoclave. Then cool to body temperature before administering to the client.
3. IV administration can reduce cerebrospinal and intraocular pressures within 15 min. Onset of diuresis occurs in about 1–3 hr.
4. Mannitol should not be added to other IV solutions nor should it be mixed with other medications.
5. If blood is to be administered at the same time, add 20 mEq of sodium chloride to each liter of mannitol to prevent pseudoagglutination.
6. *Treatment of Overdose:* Discontinue the infusion immediately and begin supportive measures to correct fluid and electrolyte imbalances. Hemodialysis is effective.

Contraindications: Anuria, pulmonary edema, severe dehydration, active intracranial bleeding except during craniotomy, progressive heart failure or pulmonary congestion after mannitol therapy, progressive renal damage following mannitol therapy.

Special Concerns: Use with caution during lactation. If blood is given simultaneously with mannitol, add at least 20 mEq of sodium chloride to each liter of mannitol solution to avoid pseudoagglutination. Sudden expansion of the extracellular volume that occurs after rapid IV mannitol may lead to fulminating CHF. Mannitol may obscure and intensify inadequate hydration or hypovolemia.

Laboratory Test Interferences: ↑ or ↓ Inorganic phosphorus. ↑ Ethylene glycol values because mannitol also is oxidized to an aldehyde during test.

Side Effects: *Electrolyte:* Fluid and electrolyte imbalance, acidosis, loss of electrolytes, dehydration. *GI:* Nausea, vomiting, dry mouth, thirst, diarrhea. *CV:* Edema, hypotension or hypertension, increase in heart rate, angina-like chest pain, CHF, thrombophlebitis. *CNS:* Dizziness, headaches, blurred vision, ***seizures.*** *Miscellaneous:* Pulmonary congestion, marked diuresis, rhinitis, chills, fever, urticaria, pain in arms, skin necrosis.

Symptoms of Overdose: Increased electrolyte excretion, especially sodium, chloride, and potassium. Sodium depletion results in orthostatic tachycardia or hypotension and decreased CVP. Potassium loss can impair neuromuscular function and cause intestinal dilation and ileus. If urine flow is inadequate, pulmonary edema or water intoxication may occur. Other symptoms include hypotension, polyuria that rapidly becomes oliguria, stupor, ***seizures,*** hyperosmolality, and hyponatremia.

Drug Interaction: May cause deafness when used in combination with kanamycin.

NURSING CONSIDERATIONS

See also *Nursing Considerations* for *Thiazide Diuretics,* Chapter 75

Assessment

1. Document indications for therapy and type and onset of symptoms.
2. List other medications prescribed that can be affected by mannitol. Lithium, for example, can be excreted more rapidly than normal, thereby impairing the therapeutic effects of the drug.
3. When used to reduce ICP and brain mass, evaluate the circulatory and renal reserve, fluid and electrolyte balance, body weight, and total I&O before and after mannitol infusion.
4. Ensure that appropriate baseline lab data have been performed. Note any evidence of renal failure.
5. Determine that client is not dehydrated as drug may mask clinical presentation.

Interventions

1. Monitor carefully and record VS and I&O.
2. If renal failure or oliguria is present, ensure that test dose is performed.
3. Observe the client for S&S of electrolyte imbalances and dehydration.
4. Monitor serum electrolytes and renal function throughout the drug therapy.
5. Observe for S&S of pulmonary edema manifested by dyspnea, cyanosis, rales, and frothy sputum. Slow the rate of infusion, and notify the provider immediately.

Evaluate

- Desired diuresis
- ↓ ICP
- ↓ Intraocular pressures

CHAPTER SEVENTY-SIX

Intravenous Nutritional Therapy and Electrolytes

See also the following individual entries:

Amino Acid Formulation for Hepatic Failure or Hepatic Encephalopathy
Amino Acid Formulation for High Metabolic Stress
Amino Acid Formulations for Renal Failure
Crystalline Amino Acid Infusion
Dextrose and Electrolytes
Intravenous Fat Emulsion
Sodium Chloride

Action/Kinetics: Intravenous nutrition is an important treatment regimen for clients in whom oral feeding is not possible or is inadequate. A large number of products provide one or more of the following nutrients: dextrose (source of calories; to decrease protein and nitrogen loss; promote glycogen deposition; prevent ketosis), electrolytes (to compensate for normal sensible and insensible losses), amino acids (promote anabolism; reduce catabolism; promote wound healing; act as buffer in extracellular and intracellular fluids), fat emulsion (source of energy and to prevent deficiency of essential fatty acids), vitamins, minerals, and fluids. These preparations are administered IV either peripherally or via a central venous catheter. Such regimens are often referred to as total parenteral nutrition (TPN). The success of TPN is gauged by weight gain and positive nitrogen balance.

The proper administration of TPN products requires a thorough knowledge of the nutritional needs of the clients, as well as of their fluid and electrolyte balance. Central administration, via a central venous catheter, is used in clients requiring long-term parenteral nutrition or in those who are severely debilitated. Peripheral parenteral administration is used for short-term parenteral nutrition (up to 12 days), in situations where the caloric requirements are not excessive, or as a supplement to oral feeding. Clients receiving TPN must be frequently evaluated by means of complete laboratory tests.

Uses: Parenteral nutrition would be indicated in the following situations: (a) the alimentary tract cannot or should not be used; (b) absorption of protein is impaired due to inflammatory disease, obstruction, or during cancer chemotherapy; (c) rest of the GI tract is necessary due to GI surgery or complications such as anastomotic leaks, fistulae, or ileus; (d) increased requirements for protein such as with extensive burns, infections, trauma, or hypermetabolic states; (e) acute renal failure when it is necessary to replace amino acids lost from tissue breakdown; and (f) feeding by tube alone cannot provide adequate nutrition.

Special preparations are available for use in renal failure, hepatic failure or encephalopathy, or in acute metabolic stress.

Contraindications: Hypersensitivity to specific proteins or inborn errors of amino acid metabolism. Anuria. General amino acid formulations should not be used in severe kidney or liver disease, hepatic coma, or encephalopathy, or metabolic disorders involving impaired nitrogen utilization. Renal failure formulations should not be used in severe electrolyte and acid-base imbalance or in hyperammonemia. Formulations for hepatic failure or hepatic encephalopathy should not be used in anuria. High metabolic stress formulations are contraindicated in hepatic coma, anuria, hyperammonemia, and severe electrolyte or acid-base imbalance.

Special Concerns: Use with caution in children with acute renal failure (especially low-birth-weight infants). Sodium-containing products should be used with caution in clients with CHF, renal insufficiency, or edema. Potassium-containing products should be used cautiously in clients with severe renal failure or hyperkalemia. Products containing acetate should be used with care in alkalosis and hepatic insufficiency.

Side Effects: *Metabolic:* Metabolic acidosis or alkalosis, hyperammonemia, dehydration, hypo- or hypervitaminosis, elevated hepatic enzymes, electrolyte imbalances, hypophosphatemia, hypocalcemia, osteoporosis, glycosuria, hypervolemia, osmotic diuresis, hyperglycemia, hypo- or hypermagnesemia, rebound hypoglycemia (due to rapid withdrawal of concentrated dextrose solutions). Essential fatty acid deficiency following long-term use of fat-free products (symptoms include dry, scaly skin, rash resembling eczema, alopecia, slow wound healing, and fatty infiltration of the liver). *Dermatologic:* Skin rashes, flushing, sweating. *Other:* Nausea, vertigo, fever, headache, dizziness. *At site of catheter:* Venous thrombosis, phlebitis. *Due to central venous catheter:* Pneumothorax, hydrothorax, hemothorax, artery puncture and transection, brachial plexus injury, formation of arteriovenous fistula, phlebitis, thrombosis, and air and catheter embolus.

Drug Interactions

Folic acid / Precipitation of calcium as calcium folate

Sodium bicarbonate / Precipitation of calcium and magnesium carbonate; ↓ effect of insulin and vitamin B complex with C

Tetracyclines / ↓ Effect of amino acids to conserve protein

Dosage

The dose, route of administration, and content of the infusion are determined individually for each client depending on the nutritional need, physical state, and length of therapy anticipated. However, the recommended dietary allowances for protein are approximately 0.9 g/kg for a healthy adult and 1.4–2.2 g/kg for healthy growing infants and children. Protein and caloric requirements may be significantly increased in traumatized or malnourished clients. For example, daily doses of 1–1.5 g/kg protein for adults and 2–3 g/kg protein for infants are usually sufficient to promote a positive nitrogen balance. In adults, from 60–180 mEq potassium, 10–30 mEq magnesium, and 10–40 mM phosphate daily should achieve an optimum metabolic response. Daily adult fluid requirements range from 2500 to 3000 mL but may be significantly higher in burn clients or with fistula drainage.

NURSING CONSIDERATIONS

Administration/Storage

1. Appropriate lab monitoring with baseline values and evaluation are required before and during administration.
2. Dextrose, 12.5% or greater, should not be used in peripheral venous infusions.
3. Blood should not be administered through the same infusion site. An exception would be a multilumen catheter in the subclavian (or large central) vein. Maintain one port of a multilumen catheter exclusively for nutritional therapy.

4. Solutions must be freshly prepared, aseptically, under a laminar flow hood in the pharmacy.
5. Solutions should be used as soon as possible after preparation. No more than 24 hr should elapse for administration of a single bottle.
6. The IV administration set, bottles/bags, and filters should be replaced daily.
7. Appropriate guidelines must be followed for clients in whom indwelling catheters will be in place for a long period of time.
8. Administer TPN solutions using an electronic infusion device and an in-line filter whenever possible.
9. If the infusion must be discontinued, do not stop the infusion abruptly. Infuse dextrose 10% at the TPN rate until the next bag/bottle is available.
10. Antibiotics, pressor agents, and steroids should not be added to these solutions.

Assessment

1. Obtain a thorough nursing history, documenting indications for therapy and clinical presentation.
2. Determine that a full nutritional assessment has been performed by the dietitian (including height, weight, anthropometric measurements, caloric needs, lab values, and evaluation of nitrogen balance, as well as GI tract function) prior to initiating therapy.
3. Obtain baseline lab data including hepatic and renal function studies, blood glucose level, electrolyte levels, serum pH, and protein and albumin levels.
4. Consult the nutritional support team, if available, for a more thorough evaluation of client needs.
5. Determine if the client has a history of allergic responses to protein hydrolysate. This is characterized by pruritus, urticaria, and wheals. Report positive responses and observations to the provider and nutritional support team.

Interventions

1. Monitor blood glucose levels at least q 6 hr initially; use finger sticks or serum determinations. Generally blood glucose levels over 200 mg/100 mL indicate the need for insulin to be added to the TPN solution or administered to the client.
2. Obtain written parameters and guidelines (sliding scale) from the provider for insulin administration to control hyperglycemia.
3. If the blood glucose level exceeds 1,000 mg/100 mL, immediately discontinue TPN and substitute a hypo-osmolar solution (e.g., 0.45% NSS) to prevent neurologic dysfunction and coma.
4. Monitor and record VS, I&O, and weights throughout TPN therapy.
5. Auscultate chest and report any evidence of rales and peripheral edema (as symptoms of fluid overload).
6. Clients with impaired liver or renal function should have blood ammonia levels monitored closely.
7. Inspect infusion site noting any evidence of inflammation, extravasation, or infection.
8. Report chills, fever, and diaphoresis and follow nutritional support team guidelines for managing infections.
9. Assess oral cavity frequently and if client is unable to eat perform frequent mouth care.
10. Review lab data to determine if the prescribed therapy is meeting the client's nutritional and metabolic needs.

Client/Family Teaching

1. For clients receiving IV nutritional therapy at home, review the appropriate procedure for site care, accessing the site, spiking and hanging the fluids, inserting the tubing, and operating the infusion pump, as well as removing and capping the site and discarding used equipment properly. Observe client performing procedure on several occasions and offer support and encouragement as needed. Generally, clients find that if

the therapy is run during their sleep time, less barriers to their normal routines are encountered. Provide printed, easy-to-follow steps and guidelines and stress the importance of using aseptic technique.
2. List symptoms that require immediate reporting: fever, chills, sweating, pain, bleeding, blockage, drainage, and leaking at infusion site.
3. Advise that most therapy may be administered during the night so as not to interfere with client's daily routine.
4. Coordinate discharge with home health care agency to facilitate adjustment of client and to provide appropriately prescribed equipment as well as support to client and family. Provide a number to call if client has questions or requires help or more supplies.

Evaluate

- Appropriate nutrient replacement as evidenced by ↑ weight, proper healing, positive nitrogen balance, and improved parameters as compared to baseline nutritional assessment data
- Freedom from complications of IV nutritional therapy

Amino Acid Formulation for Hepatic Failure or Hepatic Encephalopathy

(ah-**ME**-no **AH**-sid)

Pregnancy Category: C

HepatAmine **(Rx)**

How Supplied: *Injection*

Action/Kinetics: This product contains both essential and nonessential amino acids with high levels of branched chain amino acids as leucine, isoleucine, and valine. The branched chain amino acids improve mental status and EEG patterns. HepatAmine also contains electrolytes (sodium, chloride, acetate, and phosphate). Fat emulsion, dextrose, and vitamins may be added if required.

Uses: To normalize amino acid levels and improve nitrogen balance in clients with cirrhosis and hepatitis who manifest hepatic encephalopathy and who are intolerant of amino acid injections (which are contraindicated in clients with hepatic coma).

Dosage

- **IV**

80–120 g amino acids (equivalent to 12–18 g nitrogen) daily. Usually, 500 mL HepatAmine is mixed with about 500 mL of 50% dextrose supplemented with electrolytes and vitamins.

Additional Contraindication: Anuria.

Administration/Storage

1. The total daily fluid (500 mL HepatAmine mixed with 500 mL 50% dextrose supplemented with electrolytes and vitamins) intake is usually 2–3 L given over a period of 8–12 hr. Clients with restrictions on fluid intake may only tolerate 1–2 L.
2. Infusion rates should be slow to start and gradually increased from 60–125 mL/hr.
3. The product may be given either peripherally or by central venous indwelling catheter.
4. Isotonic or slightly hypertonic solutions are prepared by mixing HepatAmine with sterile water for injection or 5% or 10% dextrose.
5. Administration through a peripheral vein is indicated for clients in whom the central venous route is not indicated and who can take adequate calories enterally.

NURSING CONSIDERATIONS

See also *Nursing Considerations* for *Intravenous Nutritional Therapy,* Chapter 76.

Evaluate

- Desired nutritional replacement
- Improved nitrogen balance

Amino Acid Formulation for High Metabolic Stress

(ah-**ME**-noh **AH**-sid)

Pregnancy Category: C
Aminosyn-HBC 7%, 4% BranchAmin, FreAmine HBC 6.9% **(Rx)**

How Supplied: *Injection:* 7%
Action/Kinetics: The products contain mixtures of essential and nonessential amino acids with high amounts of branched chain amino acids, isoleucine, leucine, and valine. Acute metabolic stress is manifested by increased urinary nitrogen excretion and hyperglycemia; fat store mobilization and utilization of glucose are impaired. The products reverse negative nitrogen balance or prevent nitrogen losses and meet energy requirements.
Uses: Prophylaxis of nitrogen loss or treatment of negative nitrogen balance in individuals if adequate protein intake is not possible by the oral, gastronomy, or jejunostomy routes, when GI protein absorption is impaired, or there is impairment of nitrogen homeostasis due to sepsis or severe trauma.

Dosage

- **IV**

Adults with adequate calories.
1.5 g/kg (approximate). Higher doses are required in severely catabolic conditions.
Administration/Storage: This product may be administered either peripherally or by central venous indwelling catheter.
Additional Contraindications: Anuria, electrolyte imbalance, acid-base imbalance, hepatic coma.

NURSING CONSIDERATIONS

See also *Nursing Considerations* for *Intravenous Nutritional Therapy,* Chapter 76.
Evaluate: Prevention or reversal of negative nitrogen balance.

Amino Acid Formulations for Renal Failure

(ah-**ME**-noh **AH**-sid)

Pregnancy Category: C
Aminess 5.2%, Aminosyn-RF 5.2%, 5.4% NephrAmine, RenAmin **(Rx)**

How Supplied: *Injection* 5.2%
Action/Kinetics: The nutritional requirements for clients with renal disease are different from those for clients with normal renal function. Administration of minimal amounts of essential amino acids enhances utilization of urea, promotes protein synthesis, improves cellular metabolic balance, decreases the rate of rise of BUN, and minimizes deterioration of serum magnesium, phosphorus, and potassium balance. Administration of nonessential amino acids should be restricted.
Use: Treatment of uremia when PO nutrition is not practical or feasible. *NOTE:* Injection of essential amino acids does not replace dialysis or other conventional therapy for clients with renal failure.

Dosage

- **IV**

Aminess 5.2%.
Adults: 400 mL mixed with 500 mL of 70% dextrose (solution contains 2.3% essential amino acids and 30% dextrose; calorie:nitrogen ratio is 450:1).
Aminosyn-RF 5.2%.
Adults: 300 mL (up to 600 mL may be used) mixed with 500 mL of 70% dextrose (solution contains 1.96% essential amino acids and 44% dextrose; calorie:nitrogen ratio is 504:1).
5.4% NephrAmine.
Adults: 250 mL (up to 500 mL may be used) mixed with 500 mL of 70% dextrose (solution contains 1.8% essential amino acids and 47% dextrose; calorie:nitrogen ratio is 744:1).
RenAmin.
Adults: 250–500 mL. **Pediatric.** *Individualized.* **Usual:** 0.5–1 g/kg/day (initial doses should be lower and then slowly increased). Doses over 1 g/kg/day are not recommended.
Administration/Storage
1. These products should be given through a central venous catheter at

an initial rate not to exceed 20–30 mL/hr for the first 6–8 hr. Then the rate can be increased by 10 mL/hr/24 hr to a maximum of 60–100 mL/hr.
2. Use of Aminess or NephrAmine in infants may increase the chance of hyperammonemia because these products do not contain arginine.
3. If the hypertonic dextrose solution is discontinued, rebound hypoglycemia may be prevented by giving 5% or 10% dextrose solutions.
4. Adequate calories must be provided simultaneously.
Contraindications: Acid-base imbalance, electrolyte imbalance, hyperammonemia.
Special Concerns: Use with caution in children with acute renal failure and in infants with low birth weight. The risk of hyperammonemia may be increased in infants due to the absence of arginine in Aminess and NephrAmine (Aminosyn-RF and RenAmin contain arginine).

NURSING CONSIDERATIONS

See also *Nursing Considerations* for *Intravenous Nutritional Therapy,* Chapter 76.
Evaluate: Enhanced utilization of urea in clients with renal failure.

Crystalline Amino Acid Infusion

(ah-**ME**-no **AH**-sid)
Pregnancy Category: C
Aminosyn 3.5%, 3.5%M, 5%, 7%, 8.5%, and 10%; Aminosyn (pH 6) 7% and 8.5%, 10%; Aminosyn 7% and 8.5% with Electrolytes; Aminosyn II 3.5%, 3.5%M, 5%, 7%, 8.5%, 10%; Aminosyn II 7%, 8.5%, or 10% with Electrolytes; Aminosyn II 3.5% with 5% Dextrose; Aminosyn II 4.25% in 10% or 20% Dextrose; Aminosyn II 3.5%, 4.25%, or 5% in 25% Dextrose; Aminosyn II 3.5% or 4.25% with Electrolytes in 25% Dextrose; Aminosyn-PF 7% and 10%; Freamine III 8.5% and 10%; Freamine III 3% or 8.5% with Electrolytes; Novamine 11.4% or 15%; Procalamine; Travasol 10%; Travasol 5.5% with Electrolytes; Travasol 5.5% and 8.5% without Electrolytes; 3.5% and 5.5% Travasol with Electrolytes; TrophAmine 6%, 10% **(Rx)**

See information on *Intravenous Nutritional Therapy,* Chapter 76.
How Supplied: *Injection:* 3.5%, 5%, 5.5 %, 11.4%, 15%
Action/Kinetics: These products are hypertonic solutions containing both essential and nonessential amino acids as well as various electrolytes. Dextrose, IV fat emulsion, vitamins, and minerals may be added as required. Percentage refers to the amino acid concentration. The amino acids present in the products either conserve protein or induce protein synthesis by providing the necessary amino acids.

Dosage

- **IV**

Peripheral protein sparing.
1–1.7 g/kg/day through a peripheral vein.

Peripheral vein administration.
Mix with low concentrations of dextrose solutions (5% or 10%) and give with fat emulsions.

Central vein administration.
500 mL mixed with 500 mL concentrated dextrose injection, vitamins, or electrolytes given over 8 hr.
Administration/Storage: The initial rate of infusion should not exceed 2 mL/min. The rate may then be increased slowly depending on laboratory values of urinary and blood glucose and client response.

NURSING CONSIDERATIONS

See also *Nursing Considerations* for *Intravenous Nutritional Therapy,* Chapter 76.
Assessment
1. Document indications for therapy and presenting symptoms, including weights and laboratory studies.
2. Obtain baseline nutritional assessment and TPN team evaluation.
Evaluate: Improved nutritional state and maintenance of positive nitrogen balance.

Dextrose and electrolytes

(DEX-trohs)
Pedialyte, Rehydralyte, Resol **(Rx)**

How Supplied: *Injection*; *Kit*; *Solution*

Action/Kinetics: These oral products contain varying amounts of sodium, potassium, chloride, citrate, and dextrose (Lytren and Resol contain 20 g/L whereas Pedialyte and Rehydralyte contain 25 g/L). In addition, Resol contains magnesium, calcium, and phosphate. **Time to peak effect:** 8–12 hr.

Uses: Diarrhea. Prophylaxis and treatment of electrolyte depletion in diarrhea or in continuing fluid loss. Maintenance of hydration.

Dosage

- **Oral Solution**

Mild dehydration.

Adults and children over 10 years, initial: 50 mL/kg over 4–6 hr; **maintenance:** 100–200 mL/kg over 24 hr until diarrhea stops.

Moderate dehydration.

Adults and children over 10 years, initial: 100 mL/kg over 6 hr; **maintenance:** 15 mL/kg q hr until diarrhea stops.

Moderate to severe dehydration.

Pediatric, 2–10 years, initial: 50 mL/kg over the first 4–6 hr followed by 100 mL/kg over the next 18–24 hr; **less than 2 years, initial:** 75 mL/kg during the first 8 hr and 75 mL/kg during the next 16 hr.

Administration/Storage

1. No more than 1,000 mL/hr should be given to adults and no more than 100 mL of fluid should be given to children over a 20-min period.
2. The amount and rate of solution should be adjusted depending on need, thirst, and response.
3. Infants and small children should be assisted in drinking the solution slowly and frequently in small quantities and, if necessary, being fed by a spoon.
4. Rehydration solutions should not be diluted with water.

Contraindications: Anuria, oliguria. Severe dehydration including severe diarrhea (IV therapy is necessary for prompt replacement of fluids and electrolytes). Malabsorption of glucose. Severe and sustained vomiting when the client is unable to drink. Intestinal obstruction, perforated bowel, paralytic ileus.

Special Concern: Use with caution in premature infants.

Side Effects: Overhydration indicated by puffy eyelids. Hypernatremia, vomiting (usually shortly after treatment has started).

NURSING CONSIDERATIONS

Client/Family Teaching

1. Soft foods such as bananas, cereal, cooked peas, beans, and potatoes should be given to maintain nutrition.
2. Explain that if output of fluid exceeds intake, if there is no weight gain, or if clinical symptoms of dehydration persist, bring client to be seen immediately.
3. If vomiting occurs after PO therapy is initiated, continue therapy but use small amounts of solution administered frequently and slowly.
4. If dehydration is severe, instruct parents and client to seek medical attention immediately. IV fluids and electrolytes should be started since the onset of action of PO solution is too slow. Explain that the PO solution should not be discarded because it can be used for maintenance.
5. Dextrose calorie content: D5%/W is 170 cal/L and D10%/W is 340 cal/L.

Evaluate

- Maintenance of adequate hydration
- Prevention of electrolyte depletion

Intravenous Fat Emulsion

Pregnancy Category: B (Soyacal); C (all other products)

Intralipid 10% and 20%, Liposyn II 10% and 20%, Liposyn III 10% and 20%, Nutrilipid 10% and 20%, Soyacal 10% and 20% **(Rx)**

See also *Intravenous Nutritional Therapy,* Chapter 76.

How Supplied: *Injection:* 10%, 20%, 30%

Action/Kinetics: These products contain either soybean oil or safflower oil in a concentration of 10% or 20%, egg yolk phospholipids (1.2%), glycerin (2.21%–2.5%), and water for injection. The fatty acids present in these preparations (linoleic, linolenic, oleic, palmitic, and stearic) provide essential fatty acids to maintain normal cellular membrane function. The products provide from 1.1 cal/mL (10% oil) to 2.0 cal/mL (20% oil). Since it is isotonic, it can be administered into a peripheral vein. The preparations increase heat production and oxygen consumption and decrease the respiratory quotient (ratio of CO_2/O_2; normal: 0.77–0.90).

Uses: Source of calories and essential fatty acids for prolonged parenteral nutrition (longer than 5 days). Fatty acid deficiency.

Dosage

- **IV**

TPN.

Maximum: 3 g/kg/day. **Pediatric maximum:** 4 g/kg/day. The product should not exceed 60% of daily caloric intake.

Fatty acid deficiency.

Approximately 8%–10% of caloric intake.

Administration/Storage

1. Discard if oiling out occurs before administration.
2. May be given parenterally or centrally using a separate line, though it can be administered into same peripheral vein as carbohydrate–amino acid solutions using a Y-connection located near the infusion site. Flow rate of each solution should be controlled separately by an infusion pump. Do not use filters.
3. May be mixed with certain nutrient solutions (check package insert).
4. The rate of infusion should be: **Adults: 10% products, initial,** 1 mL/min for first 15–30 min; **then,** if no adverse effects, increase to 83–125 mL/hr up to 500 mL the first day. Amount may be increased the second day. **Adults: 20% products, initial,** 0.5 mL/min for first 15–30 min; **then,** if no adverse side effects, increase to 62.5 mL/hr up to 250–500 mL (depending on product) the first day. Amount may be increased the second day. Total daily dose should not exceed 3 g/kg. **Pediatric: 10% products, initial,** 0.1 mL/min for first 10–15 min; **then,** if no adverse effects, increase to maximum of 1 g/kg/4 hr (100 mL/hr). **Pediatric: 20% products, initial,** 0.05 mL/min over the first 10–15 min; **then,** if no adverse effects, increase to maximum of 1 g/4 hr (50 mL/hr). Total daily dose should not exceed 4 g/kg.
5. The addition of 1 or 2 units/mL heparin to fat emulsion may minimize risks associated with hypercoagulability, cause a more rapid clearance of lipemia, and prevent thrombosis of the catheter; however, such use is generally not recommended.
6. Carefully review and follow institutional IV fluid administration guidelines for IV fats.
7. Store in refrigerator at 4°C–8°C (39.2°F–46.4°F) if so designated on product literature.

Contraindications: Disturbances of fat metabolism (e.g., lipoid nephrosis, pathologic hyperlipidemia, acute pancreatitis with hyperlipemia). Sensitivity to egg yolk.

Special Concerns: Extreme caution should be exercised when used in premature or jaundiced premature infants. Use with caution in clients with hepatic damage, anemia, respiratory disease, coagulation problems, or possibility of fat embolism. Clients sensitive to eggs, soybeans, or legumes may be sensitive to fat emulsions.

Side Effects: ***Premature infants: Deaths due to intravascular fat accumulation in the lungs.*** **Acute side effects.** *GI:* N&V. *CNS:* Headache, fever, drowsiness, dizziness. *Other:* Hyperlipemia, dyspnea, increased coagulation, flushing, sweating, cyanosis, back and chest pain, pressure over eyes, hypersensitivity reactions with urticaria, increases in liver enzymes (transient). Neonates may manifest thrombocytopenia. **Long-term side effects.** *Hepatic:* Jaundice, hepatomegaly, alterations in liver function tests. *Overloading syndrome:* Splenomegaly, ***focal seizures,*** fever, leukocytosis, ***shock.*** *Other:* Deposition of pigment (brown) in reticuloendothelial system.

Sepsis and thrombophlebitis due to contamination or procedure.

NURSING CONSIDERATIONS

See also *Nursing Considerations* for *Intravenous Nutritional Therapy,* Chapter 76.

Assessment

1. Perform baseline nutritional assessment, noting lab parameters, and document weights.
2. Note any allergy to egg; may precipitate an acute hypersensitivity reaction.
3. Observe client closely for the first 10–15 min of administration for signs of allergic reaction to the parenteral product. Stop the infusion, document, and report immediately.

Evaluate

- Laboratory evidence that serum triglyceride and fatty acid levels within desired range
- Evidence of ↑ weight

Sodium chloride

(**SO**-dee-um **KLOR**-eyed)

Pregnancy Category: C

Tablets: Slo-Salt. **Topical:** Ayr Saline, HuMIST Saline Nasal, NaSal Saline Nasal, Ocean Mist, Otrivin Saline ✤, Salinex Nasal Mist. **Ophthalmic:** Adsorbonac Ophthalmic, AK-NaCl, Cordema ✤, Hypersal 5%, Muro-128 Ophthalmic. **Parenteral:** Sodium Chloride IV Infusions (0.45%, 0.9%, 3%, 5%), Sodium Chloride Injection for Admixtures (50, 100, 625 mEq/vial), Sodium Chloride Diluent (0.9%), Concentrated Sodium Chloride Injection (14.6%, 23.4%) (Parenteral is Rx; topical and ophthalmic are OTC)

How Supplied: *Dressing*; *Injection:* 0.45%, 0.9%, 2.5%, 3%, 5%, 14.6%, 23.4%; *Inhalation solution:* 0.45%, 0.9%, 3%, 10%; *Irrigation solution:* 0.45%, 0.9%; *Nasal solution:* 0.4%, 0.65%, 0.75%; *Ophthalmic ointment:* 5%; *Ophthalmic solution:* 0.44%, 2%, 5%; *Powder for reconstitution*; *Tablet:* 250 mg, 1 g

Action/Kinetics: Sodium is the major cation of the body's extracellular fluid. It plays a crucial role in maintaining the fluid and electrolyte balance. Excess retention of sodium results in overhydration (edema, hypervolemia), which is often treated with diuretics. Abnormally low levels of sodium result in dehydration. Normally, the plasma contains 136–145 mEq sodium/L and 98–106 mEq chloride/L. The average daily requirement of salt is approximately 5 g.

Uses: PO: Prophylaxis of heat prostration or muscle cramps, chloride deficiency due to diuresis or salt restriction, prevention or treatment of extracellular volume depletion.

Parenteral:

0.9% (Isotonic) Sodium Chloride. To restore sodium and chloride losses; to dilute or dissolve drugs for IV, IM, or SC use; flushing of IV catheters; extracellular fluid replacement; priming solution for hemodialysis; initiate and terminate blood transfusions so RBCs will not hemolyze; metabolic alkalosis when there is fluid loss and mild sodium depletion.

0.45% (Hypotonic) Sodium Chloride. Fluid replacement when fluid loss exceeds depletion of electrolytes; hyperosmolar diabetes when dextrose should not be used (need for large volume of fluid but without excess sodium ions).

3% or 5% (Hypertonic) Sodium Chloride. Hyponatremia and hypochloremia due to electrolyte losses; to dilute body water significantly following excessive fluid intake; emergency treatment of severe salt depletion.

Concentrated Sodium Chloride. Additive in parenteral therapy for clients with special needs for sodium intake.

Bacteriostatic Sodium Chloride. Used only to dilute or dissolve drugs for IM, IV, or SC injection.

Topical: Relief of inflamed, dry, or crusted nasal membranes; irrigating solution. **Ophthalmic:** Use hypertonic solutions to decrease corneal edema due to bullous keratitis; as an aid to facilitate ophthalmoscopic examination in gonioscopy, biomicroscopy, and funduscopy.

Dosage

• **Tablets (Including Extended-Release and Enteric-Coated)**

Heat cramps/dehydration.

0.5–1 g with 8 oz water up to 10 times/day; total daily dose should not exceed 4.8 g.

• **IV**

Individualized. Daily requirements of sodium and chloride can be met by administering 1 L of 0.9% sodium chloride.

To calculate sodium deficit. Amount of sodium to be given to raise serum sodium to the desired level:

Total body water (TBW): sodium deficit (mEq) = TBW × (desired plasma Na – observed plasma Na).

• **Ophthalmic Solution**

1–2 gtt in eye q 3–4 hr.

• **Ophthalmic Ointment**

Instill once (or more often, if necessary) daily.

Administration/Storage

1. Hypertonic injections of NaCl must be given slowly through a small-bore needle placed well within the lumen of a large vein (to minimize irritation). Infiltration should be avoided.
2. Concentrated NaCl injection must be diluted before use.
3. If the fluid is given using a pumping device, it should be disconnected before the container runs dry or an air embolism may occur.
4. IV catheters should be flushed before and after the medication is given using 0.9% NaCl for injection.
5. Incompatibilities may occur when mixing NaCl injection with other additives; the final product should be inspected for cloudiness or a precipitate immediately after mixing, before administration, and periodically during administration. These mixtures should not be stored.
6. *Treatment of Overdose:* Supportive measures, including gastric lavage, induction of vomiting, provide adequate airway and ventilation, maintain vascular volume and tissue perfusion. Magnesium sulfate given as a cathartic.

Contraindications: Congestive heart failure, severely impaired renal function, hypernatremia, fluid retention. The 3% or 5% solutions are contraindicated in elevated, normal, or only slightly depressed levels of plasma sodium and chloride. Use of bacteriostatic sodium chloride injection in newborns.

Special Concerns: Administer with caution to clients with CV, cirrhotic, or renal disease; in presence of hyperproteinemia, hypervolemia, urinary tract obstruction, and CHF; in those with concurrent edema and sodium retention and in clients receiving corticosteroids or corticotropin; and during lactation. Use with caution in geriatric or postoperative clients with renal or CV insufficiency with or without CHF.

Side Effects: Hypernatremia. Excessive sodium chloride may lead to hypopotassemia and acidosis. Fluid and solute overload leading to dilution of serum electrolyte levels, CHF, overhydration, ***acute pulmonary edema*** (especially in clients with CV disease or in those receiving corticosteroids or other drugs that cause sodium retention). Too rapid administration may cause local pain and venous irritation.

Postoperative intolerance of sodium chloride: Cellular dehydration, weakness, asthenia, disorientation, anorexia, nausea, oliguria, increased BUN levels, distention, deep respiration.

Symptoms due to solution or administration technique: Fever, abscess, tissue necrosis, infection at injection site, venous thrombosis or phlebitis extending from injection site, local tenderness, extravasation, hypervolemia.

Inadvertent administration of concentrated sodium chloride (i.e., without dilution) will cause sudden hypernatremia with the possibility of CV shock, extensive hemolysis, CNS problems, necrosis of the cortex of the kidneys, local tissue necrosis (if given extravascularly).

Symptoms of Overdose: Irritation of GI mucosa, N&V, abdominal cramps, diarrhea, edema. Hypernatremia symptoms include irritability, restlessness, weakness, seizures, coma, tachycardia, hypertension, fluid accumulation, ***pulmonary edema, respiratory arrest.***

NURSING CONSIDERATIONS

Interventions

1. Observe client for S&S of hypernatremia including flushed skin, elevated temperature, rough dry tongue, and edema.
2. Symptoms of hyponatremia may include N&V, muscle cramps, dry mucous membranes, increased HR, and headaches.
3. Monitor VS and I&O. Assess urine specific gravity and serum sodium levels. If the urine specific gravity is above 1.020 and serum sodium level is above 146 mEq/L, report and anticipate that the drug will be discontinued.
4. Monitor electrolyte levels and hepatic and renal function studies.
5. Note level of consciousness and periodically assess heart and lung sounds.
6. When administering IV the 0.45% NaCl is hypotonic, the 0.9% NaCl is isotonic, and the 3% and 5% NaCl solutions are hypertonic.

Evaluate

- Prophylaxis of heat prostration during exposure to high temperatures or during increased activity
- Prevention of chloride deficiency R/T excessive diuresis or salt restriction or excessive sweating
- Correction of sodium and/or chloride deficiency

CHAPTER SEVENTY-SEVEN

Alkalinizing Agents

See the following individual entries:

Sodium Bicarbonate
Tromethamine

Sodium bicarbonate

(**SO**-dee-um bye-**KAR**-bon-ayt)
Pregnancy Category: C
Arm and Hammer Pure Baking Soda, Bell/ans, Citrocarbonate, Neut, Soda Mint (Rx and OTC)

How Supplied: *Granule, effervescent; Injection:* 4%, 4.2%, 5%, 7.5%, 8.4%; *Powder, Tablet:* 325 mg, 520 mg, 648 mg, 650 mg

Action/Kinetics: The antacid action is due to neutralization of hydrochloric acid by forming sodium chloride and carbon dioxide (1 g of sodium bicarbonate neutralizes 12 mEq of acid). Provides temporary relief of peptic ulcer pain and of discomfort associated with indigestion. Although widely used by the public, sodium bicarbonate is rarely prescribed as an antacid because of its high sodium content, short duration of action, and ability to cause alkalosis (sometimes desired). Sodium bicarbonate is also a systemic and urinary alkalinizer by increasing plasma and urinary bicarbonate, respectively.

Uses: Treatment of hyperacidity, severe diarrhea (where there is loss of bicarbonate). Alkalization of the urine to treat drug toxicity (e.g., due to barbiturates, salicylates, methanol). Treatment of acute mild to moderate metabolic acidosis due to shock, severe dehydration, anoxia, uncontrolled diabetes, renal disease, cardiac arrest, extracorporeal circulation of blood, severe primary lactic acidosis. Prophylaxis of renal calculi in gout. During sulfonamide therapy to prevent renal calculi and nephrotoxicity. Neutralizing additive solution to decrease chemical phlebitis and client discomfort due to vein irritation at or near the site of infusion of IV acid solutions. *Investigational:* Sickle cell anemia.

Dosage

- **Effervescent Powder**

  Antacid.

Adults: 3.9–10 g in a glass of cold water after meals. **Geriatric and pediatric, 6–12 years:** 1.9–3.9 g after meals.

- **Oral Powder**

  Antacid.

Adults: ½ teaspoon in a glass of water q 2 hr; adjust dosage as required.

Urinary alkalinizer.

Adults: 1 teaspoon in a glass of water q 4 hr; adjust dosage as required. Dosage not established for this form for children.

- **Tablets**

  Antacid.

Adults: 0.325–2 g 1–4 times/day; **pediatric, 6–12 years:** 520 mg; may be repeated once after 30 min.

Urinary alkalinizer.

Adults, initial: 4 g; **then,** 1–2 g q 4 hr. **Pediatric:** 23–230 mg/kg/day; adjust dosage as needed.

- **IV**

  Cardiac arrest.

Adults: 200–300 mEq given rapidly as a 7.5% or 8.4% solution. In emergencies, 300–500 mL of a 5% solution given as rapidly as possible without overalkalinizing the client. **Infants, less than 2 years of age, initial:** 1–2 mEq/kg/min given over 1–2 min; **then,** 1 mEq/kg q 10 min of arrest. Do not exceed 8 mEq/kg/day.

Severe metabolic acidosis.

90–180 mEq/L (about 7.5–15 g) at a rate of 1–1.5 L during the first hour. Adjust to needs of client.

Less severe metabolic acidosis.

Add to other IV fluids. **Adults and older children:** 2–5 mEq/kg given over a 4–8-hr period.

Neutralizing additive solution. One vial of neutralizing additive solution added to 1 L of commonly used parenteral solutions, including dextrose, sodium chloride, and Ringer's.

Administration/Storage

1. Hypertonic solutions must be administered by trained personnel. Avoid extravasation as tissue irritation or cellulitis may result.
2. IV dose should be determined by arterial blood pH, pCO_2, and base deficit and may be given IV push in an arrest situation or may be diluted in dextrose or saline solution and administered over 4–8 hr.
3. Isotonic solutions should be administered slowly as ordered. Too-rapid administration may result in death due to cellular acidity. Therefore, check rate of flow frequently.
4. If only the 7.5% or 8.4% solution is available, it should be diluted 1:1 with 5% dextrose in water when used in infants for cardiac arrest.
5. The rate of administration in infants with cardiac arrest should not exceed 8 mEq/kg/day to guard against hypernatremia, induction of intracranial hemorrhage, and decreasing CSF pressure.
6. Have available a parenteral solution of calcium gluconate and 2.14% solution of ammonium chloride in the event of severe alkalosis or tetany.
7. Sodium bicarbonate should not be added to calcium-containing solutions, except where the compatibility has been established.
8. Norepinephrine and dobutamine are incompatible with sodium bicarbonate.
9. *Treatment of Overdose:* Discontinue sodium bicarbonate. Symptoms of alkalosis can be reversed by rebreathing expired air from a paper bag or using a rebreathing mask. An IV infusion of ammonium chloride solution, 2.14%, can be used to control severe cases. Hypokalemia may be treated by IV sodium chloride or potassium chloride. Calcium gluconate will control tetany.

Contraindications: Chloride loss due to vomiting or from continuous GI suction. With diuretics known to produce a hypochloremic alkalosis. Metabolic and respiratory alkalosis. Hypocalcemia in which alkalosis may cause tetany. Hypertension, convulsions, CHF, and other situations where administration of sodium can be dangerous. As a systemic alkalinizer when used as a neutralizing additive solution. Do not use as an antidote for strong mineral acids because carbon dioxide is formed, which may cause discomfort and even perforation.

Special Concerns: Use with caution in impaired renal function, in clients with oliguria or anuria, and during lactation. Also use with caution in geriatric or postoperative clients with renal or CV insufficiency with or without CHF.

Side Effects: *GI:* Acid rebound, gastric distention. *Milk-alkali syndrome:* Hypercalcemia, metabolic alkalosis (dizziness, cramps, thirst, anorexia, N&V, hyperexcitability, tetany, diminished breathing, ***seizures***), renal dysfunction. *Following rapid infusion:* Hypernatremia, alkalosis, hyperirritability, tetany, fluid or solute overload. Extravasation following IV use may manifest ulceration, sloughing, cellulitis, or tissue necrosis at the site of injection.

Symptoms of Overdose: Severe alkalosis that may be accompanied by tetany or hyperirritability.

Drug Interactions

Amphetamines / ↑ Effect of amphetamines by ↑ renal tubular reabsorption
Antidepressants, tricyclic / ↑ Effect of tricyclics by ↑ renal tubular reabsorption
Benzodiazepines / ↓ Effect due to ↑ alkalinity of urine
Chlorpropamide / ↑ Rate of excretion due to alkalinization of the urine

Ephedrine / ↑ Effect of ephedrine by ↑ renal tubular reabsorption
Erythromycin / ↑ Effect of erythromycin in urine due to ↑ alkalinity of urine
Flecainide / ↑ Effect due to ↑ alkalinity of urine
Iron products / ↓ Effect due to ↑ alkalinity of urine
Ketoconazole / ↓ Effect due to ↑ alkalinity of urine
Lithium carbonate / Excretion of lithium is proportional to amount of sodium ingested. If client on sodium-free diet, may develop lithium toxicity because less lithium is excreted
Mecamylamine / ↓ Excretion due to alkalinization of the urine
Methenamine compounds / ↓ Effect of methenamine due to ↑ alkalinity of urine
Methotrexate / ↑ Renal excretion due to alkalinization of the urine
Nitrofurantoin / ↓ Effect of nitrofurantoin due to ↑ alkalinity of urine
Procainamide / ↑ Effect of procainamide due to ↓ excretion by kidney
Pseudoephedrine / ↑ Effect of pseudoephedrine due to ↑ tubular reabsorption
Quinidine / ↑ Effect of quinidine by ↑ renal tubular reabsorption
Salicylates / ↑ Rate of excretion due to alkalinization of the urine
Sulfonylureas / ↓ Effect due to ↑ alkalinity of urine
Sympathomimetics / ↓ Renal excretion due to alkalinization of the urine
Tetracyclines / ↓ Effect of tetracyclines due to ↑ excretion by kidney

NURSING CONSIDERATIONS

Assessment

1. Note any history of renal impairment, CHF, or if prescribed a sodium-restricted diet.
2. Assess for evidence of edema that may indicate the inability to utilize sodium bicarbonate.
3. If the client is on low continuous or intermittent NG suctioning or is vomiting, assess for evidence of excessive loss of chloride.
4. List other medications prescribed and determine any potential interactive effects.
5. If prescribed to counteract metabolic acidosis, obtain baseline serum electrolytes and ABGs (pH, pCO_2, and HCO_3).

Interventions

1. Record I&O. Observe the client for dry skin and mucous membranes, polydipsia, polyuria, and air hunger. These are indications of a reversal of symptoms of metabolic acidosis and need to be documented and reported.
2. Monitor serum pH and electrolyte values to ensure that the client is not developing an alkalosis. Report if there is evidence of alkalosis and be prepared to have the client breathe in and out of a paper bag.
3. Observe acidotic clients for the relief of dyspnea and hyperpnea. Relief of these symptoms indicates that sodium bicarbonate may be discontinued.
4. Report if edema develops and anticipate the order will be changed to potassium bicarbonate since the sodium content of the drug is 27%.
5. Test urine periodically with nitrazine paper to determine if the urine is becoming alkaline. Adjust the dosage of sodium bicarbonate accordingly.

Client/Family Teaching

1. Warn clients routinely taking excessive PO preparations of sodium bicarbonate to relieve gastric distress that a rebound reaction may occur, resulting either in an increased acid secretion or systemic alkalosis. Persistent symptoms of gastric distress require medical intervention.
2. Continuous, routine ingestion of sodium bicarbonate may cause the formation of phosphate crystals in the kidney and fluid retention.
3. Consuming sodium bicarbonate with milk or calcium may result in a milk-alkali syndrome. Clients may develop anorexia, nausea, and vomiting or become mentally confused. Report immediately if these symptoms occur.

4. Avoid OTC preparations that contain sodium bicarbonate, such as Alka-Seltzer or Fizrin.

Evaluate

- Reversal of metabolic acidosis
- ↑ Urinary and serum pH
- ↓ Gastric discomfort

Tromethamine

(troh-**METH**-ah-meen)
Pregnancy Category: C
Tham, Tham-E **(Rx)**

How Supplied: *Injection:* 3.6 g/100 mL

Action/Kinetics: Tromethamine, an organic amine, is a buffering and systemic alkalizing agent. It actively binds hydrogen ions, thereby decreasing and correcting acidosis. It promotes the excretion of acids, carbon dioxide, and electrolytes and is thought to be able to neutralize some intracellular acid. It acts as an osmotic diuretic, increasing urine flow. Seventy-five percent of the drug is eliminated within 8 hr, the remainder within 3 days.

Uses: Prevention and correction of systemic acidosis, especially that accompanying cardiac bypass surgery, correction of acidity of acid citrate dextrose (ACD) blood in cardiac bypass surgery, and cardiac arrest.

Dosage

Minimum amount to correct acid-base imbalance. The amount of tromethamine can be estimated using the buffer base deficit of the extracellular fluid: mL of 0.3 M tromethamine solution required=body weight (kg) × base deficit (mEq/L) × 1.1.

- **Slow IV Infusion**

Acidosis in cardiac bypass surgery.

Adults: 500 mL (150 mEq or 18 g) as a single dose. Severe cases may require 1,000 mL. The dose should not exceed 500 mg/kg over a period of not less than 1 hr.

- **Injection into Ventricular Cavity or Large Peripheral Vein**

Acidosis in cardiac arrest (given at the same time as other standard procedures are being applied).

If chest is open. Adults: 62–185 mL (2–6 g) into the ventricular cavity (not into the cardiac muscle). **If chest closed. Adults:** 111–333 mL (3.6–10.8 g) into a large peripheral vein.

- **Addition to Pump Oxygenator Acid Citrate Dextrose Blood**

For acidity in ACD blood.

15–77 mL (0.5–2.5 g) added to each 500 mL of ACD blood. Usually 62 mL (2 g) added to 500 mL of ACD blood is adequate.

Administration/Storage

1. Tests on blood pH, pCO_2, bicarbonate, glucose, and electrolytes should be determined before, during, and after administration of tromethamine.
2. Concentration of solution administered *must not* exceed 0.3 M.
3. Prepare a 0.3-M solution of tromethamine by adding 1,000 mL of sterile water for injection to 36 g of lyophilized tromethamine.
4. Infuse slowly.
5. Administer into the largest antecubital vein through a large needle or indwelling catheter and elevate limb.
6. For treatment of cardiac arrest, the drug may be injected into the ventricular cavity if the chest is open. If the chest is not open, the drug may be injected into a large peripheral vein.
7. Do not administer longer than 1 day unless acute life-threatening situation exists.
8. Discontinue administration *immediately,* if extravasation occurs:
   - Administer 1% procaine hydrochloride with hyaluronidase to reduce venospasm and to dilute the drug in the tissues.
   - Phentolamine mesylate (Regitine) has been used for local infiltration for its adrenergic blocking properties.
   - If necessary, a nerve block of the autonomic fibers may be done.
9. *Treatment of Overdose:* Discontinue the infusion and treat symptoms.

Contraindications: Uremia and anuria.

Special Concerns: Use with caution in newborns and infants. Administer with caution to clients with renal disorders.

Side Effects: *Respiratory:* Respiratory depression, especially in those with chronic hypoventilation or getting drugs that depress respiration. *Other:* Fever, hypervolemia, transient decrease of blood glucose. *At injection site:* Extravasation may cause inflammation, vascular spasms, and tissue damage (e.g., chemical phlebitis, thrombosis, necrosis, sloughing). *In newborn:* ***Hemorrhagic liver necrosis when given by umbilical vein.***

Symptoms of Overdose: Alkalosis, overhydration, hypoglycemia (severe and prolonged), solute overload.

NURSING CONSIDERATIONS

Assessment

1. Note if the client has any history of urinary or bladder problems.
2. Obtain baseline renal and hepatic function studies.
3. Determine that pH, pCO_2, bicarbonate, glucose, and electrolytes have been analyzed before administering drug.
4. If the client is female and of childbearing age, check to determine if pregnant.

Interventions

1. Observe for respiratory depression and have mechanical ventilation equipment readily available.
2. Document and report any complaints of weakness, presence of moist pale skin, tremors, and a full bounding pulse. These are symptoms of hypoglycemia, which can occur after a rapid or high dose of the drug has been administered.
3. Maintain an accurate record of I&O.
4. Assess for nausea, diarrhea, tachycardia, oliguria, weakness, numbness, or tingling sensations. These are symptoms of hyperkalemia and are more likely to occur in clients with impaired renal function.
5. Monitor serum electrolytes, blood glucose levels, pH, and hepatic and renal function studies periodically throughout drug therapy. Report any abnormal findings.
6. Observe closely for extravasation as the drug is extremely irritating to the vein.

Evaluate

- Neutralization of ACD blood in pump oxygenator
- Correction of systemic acidosis with serum pH within desired range

CHAPTER SEVENTY-EIGHT

Potassium Salts

Potassium acetate, parenteral

Pregnancy Category: C
(Rx)

Potassium acetate, Potassium bicarbonate, and Potassium citrate (Trikates)

Oral Solution: Tri-K **(Rx)**

Potassium bicarbonate

K + Care ET **(Rx)**

Potassium bicarbonate and citric acid

Effervescent Tablets: K+ Care ET, Klor-Con/EF **(Rx)**

Potassium bicarbonate and Potassium chloride

Effervescent Granules: Neo-K ✱ **(Rx)**. **Effervescent Tablets:** Klorvess, K-Lyte/Cl, K-Lyte/Cl 50, Potassium-Sandoz ✱ **(Rx)**

Potassium bicarbonate and Potassium citrate

Effervescent Tablets: Effer-K, Effervescent Potassium, K-Lyte **(Rx)**

Potassium chloride

Extended-Release Capsules: K-Lease, K-Norm, Micro-K Extencaps, Micro-K 10 Extencaps **(Rx)**. **Injection:** Potassium Chloride for Injection Concentrate **(Rx)**. **Oral Solution:** Cena-K 10% and 20%, K-10 ✱, Kaochlor-10 and -20 ✱, Kaochlor 10%, Kaochlor S-F 10%, Kaon-Cl 20% Liquid, Kay Ciel, KCl 5% ✱, Klorvess 10% Liquid, Potasalan, Rum-K **(Rx)**. **Powder for Oral Solution:** Gen-K, Kato, Kay Ciel, K+ Care, K-Lor, Klor-Con Powder, Klor-Con/25 Powder, K-Lyte/Cl Powder, Micro-K LS **(Rx)**. **Extended-Release Tablets:** Apo-K ✱, K+ 10, Kalium Durules ✱, Kaon-Cl, Kaon-Cl-10, K-Dur 10 and 20, K-Long ✱, Klor-Con 8 and 10, Klotrix, K-Tab, Novolente-K ✱, Slow-K, Slo-Pot 600 ✱, Slow-K ✱, Ten-K **(Rx)**

Potassium chloride, Potassium bicarbonate, and Potassium citrate

Effervescent Granules: Klorvess Effervescent Granules **(Rx)**

Potassium gluconate

Elixir: Kaon, Kaylixir, K-G Elixir, Potassium-Rougier ✱, Royonate ✱ **(Rx)**. **Tablets:** Kaon ✱ **(Rx)**

Potassium gluconate and Potassium chloride

Oral Solution and Powder for Oral Solution: Kolyum **(Rx)**

Potassium gluconate and Potassium citrate

Oral Solution: Twin-K **(Rx)**
Classification: Electrolyte

General Statement: Potassium is the major cation of the body's intracellular fluid. It is essential for the maintenance of important physiologic processes, including cardiac, smooth, and skeletal muscle function, acid-base balance, gastric secretions, renal function, protein and carbohydrate metabolism. Symptoms of hypokalemia include weakness, cardiac arrhythmias, fatigue, ileus, hyporeflexia or areflexia, tetany, polydipsia, and, in severe cases, flaccid paralysis and inability to concentrate urine. Loss of potassium is usually accompanied by a loss of chloride resulting in hypochloremic metabolic alkalosis.

The usual adult daily requirement of potassium is 40–80 mg. In adults, the normal extracellular concentration of potassium ranges from 3.5 to 5 mEq/L with the intracellular levels being 150–160 mEq/L. Extracellular concentrations of up to 5.6 mEq/L are normal in children.

Both hypokalemia and hyperkalemia, if uncorrected, can be fatal; thus, potassium must always be administered cautiously.

Potassium is readily and rapidly absorbed from the GI tract. Though a number of salts can be used to supply the potassium cation, potassium chloride is the agent of choice since hypochloremia frequently accompanies potassium deficiency. Dietary measures can often prevent and even correct potassium deficiencies. Potassium-rich foods include most meats (beef, chicken, ham, turkey, veal), fish, beans, broccoli, brussels sprouts, lentils, spinach, potatoes, milk, bananas, dates, prunes, raisins, avocados, watermelon, cantaloupe, apricots, and molasses.

From 80% to 90% of potassium intake is excreted by the kidney and is partially reabsorbed from the glomerular filtrate.

How Supplied: Potassium acetate, parenteral: *Injection:* 2 mEq/mL, 4 mEq/mL
Potassium acetate, potassium bicarbonate, and potassium citrate: *Liquid:* 45 mEq/15 mL
Potassium bicarbonate: *Tablet, effervescent:* 25 mEq, 650 mg
Potassium bicarbonate and citric acid, Potassium bicarbonate and Potassium chloride, and Potassium bicarbonate and Potassium citrate: information not available at time of printing.
Potassium chloride: *Capsule, extended release:* 8 mEq, 10 mEq; *Granule for reconstitution:* 20 mEq; *Injection:* 1.5 mEq/mL, 2 mEq/mL, 3 mEq/mL, 10 mEq/50 mL, 10 mEq/100 mL, 20 mEq/50 mL, 20 mEq/100 mL, 30 mEq/100 mL, 40 mEq/100 mL, 100 mEq/L, 200 mEq/L; *Liquid:* 20 mEq/15 mL, 30 mEq/15 mL, 40 mEq/15 mL, 40 mEq/mL; *Powder for reconstitution:* 15 mEq, 20 mEq, 25 mEq, 200 mEq; *Tablet:* 99 mg, 180 mg; *Tablet, extended release:* 6.7 mEq, 8 mEq, 10 mEq, 20 mEq
Potassium chloride, Potassium bicarbonate, and Potassium citrate: information not available at time of printing.
Potassium gluconate: *Liquid:* 20 mEq/15 mL; *Tablet:* 500 mg, 550 mg, 595 mg, 620 mg; *Tablet, extended release:* 595 mg
Potassium gluconate and Potassium chloride: information not available at time of printing.
Potassium gluconate and potassium citrate: *Liquid:* 20 mEq/15 mL

Uses: PO. Treat hypokalemia due to digitalis intoxication, diabetic acidosis, diarrhea and vomiting, familial periodic paralysis, certain cases of uremia, hyperadrenalism, starvation and debilitation, and corticosteroid or diuretic therapy. Also, hypokalemia with or without metabolic acidosis and following surgical conditions accompanied by nitrogen loss, vomiting and diarrhea, suction drainage, and increased urinary excretion of potassium. Prophylaxis of potassium depletion when dietary intake is not adequate in the following conditions: clients on digitalis and diuretics for CHF, hepatic cirrhosis with ascites, excess aldosterone with normal renal function, significant cardiac arrhythmias, potassium-losing nephropathy, and certain states accompanied by diarrhea. *Investigational:* Mild hypertension.

NOTE: Potassium chloride should be used when hypokalemia is associated with alkalosis; potassium bicarbonate, citrate, acetate, or gluconate should be used when hypokalemia is associated with acidosis.

IV. Prophylaxis and treatment of moderate to severe potassium loss when PO therapy is not feasible. Potassium acetate is used as an additive for preparing specific IV formulas when client needs cannot be met by usual nutrient or electrolyte preparations. Potassium acetate is also used in the following conditions: marked loss of GI secretions due to vomiting, diarrhea, GI intubation, or fistulas; prolonged parenteral use of potassium-free fluids (e.g., dextrose or NSS); diabetic acidosis, especially during treatment with insulin and dextrose infusions; prolonged diuresis; metabolic alkalosis; hyperadrenocorticism; primary aldosteronism; overdose of adrenocortical steroids, testosterone, or corticotropin; attacks of hereditary or familial periodic paralysis; during the healing phase of burns or scalds; and cardiac arrhythmias, especially due to digitalis glycosides.

Dosage

Highly individualized. Oral administration is preferred because the slow absorption from the GI tract prevents sudden, large increases in plasma potassium levels. Dosage is usually expressed as mEq/L of potassium. The bicarbonate, chloride, citrate, and gluconate salts are usually administered PO. The chloride, acetate, and phosphate may be administered by **slow IV** infusion.

• **IV Infusion**

Serum K less than 2.0 mEq/L.
400 mEq/day at a rate not to exceed 40 mEq/hr. A maximum concentration of 80 mEq/L should be used.

Serum K more than 2.5 mEq/L.
200 mEq/day at a rate not to exceed 20 mEq/hr. A maximum concentration of 40 mEq/L should be used.

Pediatric: Up to 3 mEq potassium/kg (or 40 mEq/m^2) daily. The volume administered should be adjusted depending on the body size.

• **Effervescent Granules, Effervescent Tablets, Elixir, Extended-Release Capsules, Extended-Release Tablets, Oral Solution, Powder for Oral Solution, Tablets**

Prophylaxis of hypokalemia.
16–24 mEq/day.

Potassium depletion.
40–100 mEq/day.

NOTE: Usual dietary intake of potassium is 40–250 mEq/day.

For clients with accompanying metabolic acidosis, an alkalizing potassium salt (potassium bicarbonate, potassium citrate, or potassium acetate) should be selected.

Administration/Storage

Oral

1. Dilute or dissolve PO liquids, effervescent tablets, or soluble powders in 3–8 oz of cold water, fruit or vegetable juice, or other suitable liquid and drink slowly.
2. Chill to increase palatability.
3. Instruct client to swallow enteric-coated tablets and extended-release capsules and tablets and not to dissolve them in the mouth.
4. Give PO doses 2–4 times/day. Hypokalemia should be corrected slowly over a period of 3–7 days to minimize the development of hyperkalemia.
5. Salt substitutes should not be used concomitantly with potassium preparations.
6. Administer dilute liquid solutions of potassium rather than tablets to clients with esophageal compression.
7. If GI upset occurs, products can be taken after meals or with food with a full glass of water.

Parenteral

1. All parenteral products must be diluted with a suitable large volume of parenteral solution, mixed well, and given by slow IV infusion. The usual concentration of potassium chloride is 40 mEq/L of IV fluid (up to a maximum of 80 mEq/L).
2. "Layering" of potassium should be avoided by properly agitating the prepared IV solution. Potassium should never be added to an IV bottle that is hanging.
3. Potassium should not be administered IV undiluted. Usual method is to administer by slow IV infusion in dextrose solution at a concentration of

40–80 mEq/L and at a rate not to exceed 10–20 mEq/hr.
4. Ensure uniform distribution of potassium by inverting container during addition of potassium solution and then by agitating container. Squeezing the plastic container will not prevent potassium chloride from settling to the bottom.
5. Check site of administration frequently for pain and redness because drug is extremely irritating.
6. In critical clients, potassium chloride may be given slow IV in a solution of saline (unless contraindicated) since dextrose may lower serum potassium levels by producing an intracellular shift.
7. Administer all concentrated potassium infusions and riders with an infusion control device.
8. Have sodium polystyrene sulfonate (Kayexalate) available for PO/PR administration in the event of hyperkalemia.
9. *Treatment of Overdose (plasma potassium levels greater than 6.5 mEq/L.):* All measures must be monitored by ECG. Measures consist of actions taken to shift potassium ions from plasma into cells by:
- **Sodium bicarbonate:** IV infusion of 50–100 mEq over period of 5 min. May be repeated after 10–15 minutes if ECG abnormalities persist.
- **Glucose and insulin:** IV infusion of 3 g glucose to 1 unit regular insulin to shift potassium into cells.
- **Calcium gluconate—or other calcium salt** (only for clients not on digitalis or other cardiotonic glycosides): IV infusion of 0.5–1 g (5–10 mL of a 10% solution) over period of 2 min. Dosage may be repeated after 1–2 min if ECG remains abnormal. When ECG is approximately normal, the excess potassium should be removed from the body by administration of polystyrene sulfonate, hemodialysis or peritoneal dialysis (clients with renal insufficiency), or other means.
- **Sodium polystyrene sulfonate, hemodialysis, peritoneal dialysis:** To remove potassium from the body.

Contraindications: Severe renal function impairment with azotemia or oliguria, postoperatively before urine flow has been reestablished. Crush syndrome, Addison's disease, hyperkalemia from any cause, anuria, heat cramps, acute dehydration, severe hemolytic reactions, adynamia episodica hereditaria, clients receiving potassium-sparing diuretics or aldosterone-inhibiting drugs. Solid dosage forms in clients in whom there is a reason for delay or arrest in passage of tablets through the GI tract.

Special Concerns: Safety during lactation and in children has not been established. Geriatric clients are at greater risk of developing hyperkalemia due to age-related changes in renal function. Administer with caution in the presence of cardiac and renal disease. Potassium loss is often accompanied by an obligatory loss of chloride resulting in hypochloremic metabolic alkalosis; thus, the underlying cause of the potassium loss should be treated.

Side Effects: Hypokalemia. *CNS:* Dizziness, mental confusion. *CV:* Arrhythmias; weak, irregular pulse; hypotension, ***heart block,*** ECG abnormalities, ***cardiac arrest.*** *GI:* Abdominal distention, anorexia, N&V, *Neuromuscular:* Weakness, paresthesia of extremities, flaccid paralysis, areflexia, muscle or ***respiratory paralysis,*** weakness and heaviness of legs. *Other:* Malaise.

Hyperkalemia. *CV:* Bradycardia, then tachycardia, ***cardiac arrest.*** *GI:* N&V, diarrhea, abdominal cramps, GI bleeding or obstruction. Ulceration or perforation of the small bowel from enteric-coated potassium chloride tablets. *GU:* Oliguria, anuria. *Neuromuscular:* Weakness, tingling, paralysis. *Other:* Skin rashes, hyperkalemia.

Effects due to solution or IV technique used. Fever, infection at injection site, venous thrombosis, phlebitis extending from injection site, extravasation, venospasm, hypervolemia, hyperkalemia.

Symptoms of Overdose: Mild (5.5–6.5 mEq/L) to moderate (6.5–8 mEq/L) hyperkalemia (may be asymptomatic except for ECG changes). ECG changes include progression in height and peak of T waves, lowering of the R wave, decreased amplitude and eventually disappearance of P waves, prolonged PR interval and QRS complex, shortening of the QT interval, ***ventricular fibrillation, death. Muscle weakness that may progress to flaccid quadriplegia and respiratory failure,*** although dangerous cardiac arrhythmias usually occur before onset of complete paralysis.

Drug Interactions

ACE inhibitors / May cause potassium retention → hyperkalemia
Digitalis glycosides / Cardiac arrhythmias
Potassium-sparing diuretics / Severe hyperkalemia with possibility of cardiac arrhythmias or arrest

NURSING CONSIDERATIONS

Assessment

1. Obtain baseline serum electrolytes and ECG.
2. Note any prior history of impaired renal function.
3. Assess for adequate urinary flow before administering potassium. Impaired renal function can lead to hyperkalemia.

Interventions

1. Once parenteral potassium administration is initiated, discontinue administering potassium-rich foods and potassium supplements.
2. If the client develops abdominal pain, distention, or GI bleeding, withhold PO potassium medication and report.
3. Note any complaints of weakness, fatigue, or the presence of cardiac arrhythmias. These may be symptoms of hypokalemia indicating a low *intracellular* potassium level, although the serum potassium level may appear to be within normal limits.
4. Monitor I&O. If the client develops oliguria, anuria, or azoturia, withhold the drug and report.
5. Observe carefully for symptoms of adrenal insufficiency or extensive tissue breakdown.
6. Report complaints of weakness or heaviness of the legs, the presence of a gray pallor, cold skin, listlessness, mental confusion, flaccid paralysis, hypotension, or cardiac arrhythmias. These are symptoms of hyperkalemia and the medication should be stopped immediately as the client may go into CV collapse.
7. Monitor serum potassium levels while the client is receiving parenteral potassium. The normal level is 3.5–5.0 mEq/L; any variation should be reported.

Client/Family Teaching

1. Clients receiving potassium-sparing diuretics, such as spironolactone or triamterene, should not take potassium supplements or eat foods high in potassium unless specifically ordered.
2. Provide printed information explaining the symptoms of hypo- and hyperkalemia; identify what should be reported.
3. Review the importance of potassium in the diet and its importance to other medications prescribed for the client.
4. Explain that once the parenteral potassium is discontinued, it is important to ingest potassium-rich foods such as citrus juices, bananas, apricots, raisins, and nuts. The daily adult requirement is usually 40–80 mg. Have a dietitian work with the client to ensure a proper dietary regimen and to assist with meal planning.

Evaluate

- Correction of potassium deficiency
- Serum potassium levels within desired range

Immunomodulating Drugs

CHAPTER SEVENTY-NINE

Immunosuppressants

See the following individual entries:

Azathioprine
Cyclosporine
Cytomegalovirus Immune Globulin Intravenous (Human)
Interferon Gamma-1b
Muromonab-CD3

Azathioprine

(ay-zah-**THIGH**-oh-preen)
Pregnancy Category: D
Imuran **(Rx)**

How Supplied: *Powder For Injection:* 100 mg; *Tablet:* 50 mg
Action/Kinetics: Antimetabolite that is quickly split to form mercaptopurine. To be effective, the drug must be given during the induction period of the antibody response. The precise mechanism in depressing the immune response is unknown, but it suppresses cell-mediated hypersensitivities and alters antibody production. The drug inhibits synthesis of DNA, RNA, and proteins and may interfere with miosis and cellular metabolism. The mechanism for its effect on autoimmune diseases is not known. Is readily absorbed from the GI tract. The anuric client manifests increased effectiveness and toxicity (up to twofold). **Onset:** 6–8 weeks for rheumatoid arthritis. **t$^1/_2$:** 3 hr.

Uses: As an adjunct to prevent rejection in renal homotransplantation. In adult clients meeting criteria for classic or definite rheumatoid arthritis as defined by the American Rheumatism Association. Use should be restricted to clients with severe, active, and erosive disease that is not responsive to conventional therapy. *Investigational:* Chronic ulcerative colitis, generalized myasthenia gravis, to control the progression of Behçet's syndrome (especially eye disease), Crohn's disease (low doses).

Dosage

- **Tablets, IV**

Use in renal homotransplantation.

Adults and children, initial: 3–5 mg/kg (120 mg/m^2), 1–3 days before or on the day of transplantation; **maintenance:** 1–3 mg/kg (45 mg/m^2) daily.

Rheumatoid arthritis, SLE.

Adults and children, tablets, initial: 1 mg/kg (50–100 mg); **then,** increase dose by 0.5 mg/kg/day after 6–8 weeks and thereafter q 4 weeks up to maximum of 2.5 mg/kg/day; **maintenance:** lowest effective dose. Dosage should be reduced in clients with renal dysfunction.

Myasthenia gravis.

2–3 mg/kg/day. However, side effects occur in more than 35% of clients.

To control progression of Behçet's syndrome.
2.5 mg/kg/day.

To treat Crohn's disease.
75–100 mg/day.

Administration/Storage

1. Reconstitute the drug (100 mg) with 10 mL of sterile water for injection and use within 24 hr. Further dilution into sterile saline or dextrose is usually made for infusion. The infusion time ranges from 5 min to 8 hr.
2. If GI upset occurs, the drug may be given in divided doses or taken with food.
3. When used for rheumatoid arthritis, a therapeutic response may not be observed for 6–8 weeks.
4. Azathioprine may be discontinued abruptly, but delayed effects are possible.
5. When used with allopurinol, the dose of azathioprine should be reduced by 25%–33% of the usual dose.
6. *Treatment of Overdose:* Approximately 45% can be removed from the body following 8 hr of hemodialysis.

Contraindications: Treatment of rheumatoid arthritis in pregnancy or in clients previously treated with alkylating agents. Pregnancy and lactation.

Special Concerns: Hematologic toxicity is dose-related and may occur late in the course of therapy; may be more severe in renal transplant clients undergoing rejection. Although used in children, safety and efficacy have not been established.

Side Effects: *Hematologic:* Leukopenia, thrombocytopenia, macrocytic anemia, ***severe bone marrow depression,*** selective erythrocyte aplasia. *GI:* N&V, diarrhea, abdominal pain, steatorrhea. *CNS:* Fever, malaise. *Other:* ***Increased risk of carcinoma,*** severe infections (fungal, viral, bacterial, and protozoal), and ***hepatotoxicity*** are major side effects. Also, skin rashes, alopecia, myalgias, increase in liver enzymes, hypotension, negative nitrogen balance.

Symptoms of Overdose: Large doses may result in ***bone marrow hypoplasia,*** bleeding, infection, and death.

Drug Interactions

ACE inhibitors / ↑ Risk of severe leukopenia
Allopurinol / ↑ Pharmacologic effect of azathioprine due to ↓ breakdown in liver
Anticoagulants / ↓ Effect of anticoagulants
Corticosteroids / With azathioprine, it may cause muscle wasting after prolonged therapy
Cyclosporine / ↑ Plasma levels of cyclosporine
Methotrexate / ↑ Plasma levels of the active metabolite, 6-mercaptopurine
Tubocurarine / Azathioprine ↓ effect of tubocurarine and other nondepolarizing neuromuscular blocking agents

---

NURSING CONSIDERATIONS

Assessment

1. Perform a drug profile to determine if the client is taking any drugs with which azathioprine interacts unfavorably.
2. Determine that baseline CBC and liver and renal function studies have been performed.
3. Document indications for therapy and include preassessment data.

Interventions

1. Observe client for symptoms of hepatic dysfunction. Discontinue the drug and report if the client develops jaundice.
2. Monitor I&O and weigh client daily.
3. Observe for any decreases in urine volume and creatinine clearance; report oliguria. These are symptoms of kidney transplant rejection.
4. Encourage client to increase fluid intake.

Client/Family Teaching

1. Advise to take only as directed

and not to skip or stop medication without approval.
2. Women of childbearing age should practice contraceptive methods during and for 4 months following therapy.
3. Provide a printed list of side effects that should be reported immediately such as bruising, bleeding, S&S of infection, abdominal pain, itching, and/or clay-colored stools.
4. With organ transplant, explain that in order to prevent transplant rejection the client must take this medication for life.
5. Avoid contact with any person who has taken oral poliovirus vaccine recently or persons with active infections.
6. When used for rheumatoid arthritis, advise that improvement in joint pain, swelling, and stiffness may take 6–8 weeks. The client should be considered refractory if no beneficial effect is noted after 12 weeks of therapy.

Evaluate

- Prevention of transplant rejection
- Suppression of cell-mediated immunity
- ↓ Joint pain and inflammation with improved mobility

Cyclosporine

(sye-kloh-**SPOR**-een)
Pregnancy Category: C
Sandimmune **(Rx)**

How Supplied: *Capsule:* 25 mg, 50 mg, 100 mg, 250 mg; *Injection:* 50 mg/mL; *Solution:* 100 mg/mL

Action/Kinetics: Cyclosporine is an immunosuppressant thought to act by inhibiting the immunocompetent lymphocytes in the G_0 or G_1 phase of the cell cycle. T-lymphocytes are specifically inhibited; both the T-helper cell and the T-suppressor cell may be affected. Cyclosporine also inhibits interleukin 2 or T-cell growth factor production and release. **Peak plasma levels:** 3.5 hr. Food may both delay and impair absorption of the drug. **t½:** Approximately 19 hr for adults and 7 hr in children. Metabolized by the liver. Inactive metabolites are excreted mainly through the bile.

Uses: In combination with corticosteroids for prophylaxis of rejection in kidney, liver, and heart transplants. Treatment of chronic rejection in clients previously treated with other immunosuppressants.

A number of other diseases have been treated with cyclosporine including aplastic anemia, myasthenia gravis, atopic dermatitis, Crohn's disease, Graves ophthalmology, severe psoriasis, multiple sclerosis, polymyositis, dermatomyositis, uveitis, biliary cirrhosis, and others.

Dosage

- **Capsules, Oral Solution**

Immunosuppressant.

Adults and children, initial: 15 mg/kg/day given 4–12 hr before transplantation; **then,** 15 mg/kg/day postoperatively for 1–2 weeks followed by 5% decrease in dose per week to maintenance dose of 5–10 mg/kg/day (some have used a dose of 3 mg/kg/day successfully).

- **IV (Only in Clients Unable to Take PO Medication)**

Immunosuppressant.

Adults: 5–6 mg/kg/day 4–12 hr prior to transplantation and postoperatively until client can be switched to PO dosage. *NOTE:* Steroid therapy must be used concomitantly.

Administration/Storage

1. The oral solution may be diluted with milk, chocolate milk, or juice immediately before being administered. The oral solutions should not be stored in the refrigerator; contents should be used within 2 months after being opened.
2. Due to variable absorption of the oral solution, blood levels of cyclosporine should be monitored.
3. The IV concentration should be diluted 1 mL (50 mg) in 20–100 mL 0.9% sodium chloride injection or 5% dextrose injection. The IV solution is given by slow IV infusion over 2–6 hr.
4. The polyoxyethylated castor oil found in the concentrate for IV infu-

sion may cause phthalate stripping from PVC.
5. The IV solution should be protected from light.
6. Clients with malabsorption from the GI tract may not achieve appropriate blood levels.
7. Due to the possibility of anaphylaxis, clients receiving IV cyclosporine should be closely monitored for 30 min following the initiation of the infusion. Epinephrine (1:1,000) should be available at the bedside for treating anaphylaxis.
8. *Treatment of Overdose:* Induction of vomiting (up to 2 hr after ingestion). General supportive measures.

Contraindications: Hypersensitivity to cyclosporine or polyoxyethylated castor oil. Lactation. Use of potassium-sparing diuretics.

Special Concerns: Use with caution in clients with impaired renal or hepatic function. Safety and efficacy have not been established in children. Clients with malabsorption may not achieve therapeutic levels following PO use.

Laboratory Test Interferences: ↑ Serum creatinine, BUN, total bilirubin, alkaline phosphatase, serum potassium. Possibly ↑ cholesterol, LDL, and apolipoprotein B.

Side Effects: *GI:* N&V, diarrhea, gum hyperplasia, anorexia, gastritis, hiccoughs, peptic ulcer, abdominal discomfort, upper GI bleeding, pancreatitis, constipation, mouth sores, difficulty in swallowing. *Hematologic:* Leukopenia, lymphoma, thrombocytopenia, microangiopathic hemolytic anemia syndrome. *Allergic:* ***Anaphylaxis (rare).*** *CV:* Hypertension, edema, MI. *CNS:* Headache, tremor, confusion, fever, ***seizures,*** anxiety, depression, weakness, lethargy, ataxia, hallucinations, mania, encephalopathy, sleep disturbances. *GU:* Renal dysfunction, glomerular capillary thrombosis. *Miscellaneous:* Hepatotoxicity, acne, hirsutism, flushing, paresthesia, sinusitis, gynecomastia, conjunctivitis, brittle fingernails, hearing loss, tinnitus, hyperglycemia, hyperkalemia, hyperuricemia, muscle pain, infections (including fungal, viral), pneumonia, hematuria, blurred vision, cramps, weight loss, chest and joint pain, conjunctivitis, night sweats, hair breaking, pruritus, tingling, hypomagnesemia in some clients with seizures.

Symptoms of Overdose: Transient hepatotoxicity and nephrotoxicity.

Drug Interactions

Aminoglycosides / ↑ Risk of nephrotoxicity
Amphotericin B / ↑ Risk of nephrotoxicity
Azathioprine / ↑ Immunosuppression due to suppression of lymphocytes → possible infection and malignancy
Bromocriptine / ↑ Plasma level of cyclosporine due to ↓ breakdown by liver
Carbamazepine / ↓ Plasma level of cyclosporine due to ↑ breakdown by liver
Cimetidine / ↑ Risk of nephrotoxicity
Corticosteroids / ↑ Immunosuppression due to suppression of lymphocytes → possible infection and malignancy
Cyclophosphamide / ↑ Immunosuppression due to suppression of lymphocytes → possible infection and malignancy
Danazol / ↑ Plasma level of cyclosporine due to ↓ breakdown by liver
Diclofenac / ↑ Risk of nephrotoxicity
Digoxin / ↑ Digoxin levels due to ↓ clearance; also, ↓ volume of distribution of digoxin → toxicity
Diltiazem / ↑ Plasma level of cyclosporine due to ↓ breakdown by liver
Diuretics, potassium-sparing / ↑ Risk of hyperkalemia
Erythromycin / ↑ Plasma level of cyclosporine due to ↓ breakdown by liver and ↓ biliary excretion
Fluconazole / ↑ Plasma level of cyclosporine due to ↓ breakdown by liver

Imipenem-cilastatin / ↑ Plasma level of cyclosporine due to ↓ breakdown by liver
Isoniazid / ↓ Plasma level of cyclosporine due to ↑ breakdown by liver
Itraconazole / ↑ Plasma level of cyclosporine due to ↓ breakdown by liver
Ketoconazole / ↑ Plasma level of cyclosporine due to ↓ breakdown by liver; also, ↑ risk of nephrotoxicity
Lovastatin / ↑ Plasma levels of lovastatin due to ↓ clearance; also, ↑ risk of myositis
Melphalan / ↑ Risk of nephrotoxicity
Methylprednisolone / ↑ Plasma levels of cyclosporine
Metoclopramide / ↑ Plasma level of cyclosporine due to ↑ absorption from GI tract
Nephrotoxic drugs / Additive nephrotoxicity
Nicardipine / ↑ Plasma level of cyclosporine due to ↓ breakdown by liver
Nifedipine / ↑ Risk of gingival hyperplasia
Nondepolarizing muscle relaxants / ↑ Neuromuscular blockade
NSAIDs / ↑ Risk of nephrotoxicity
Oral contraceptives / ↑ Plasma level of cyclosporine due to ↓ breakdown by liver
Phenobarbital / ↓ Plasma level of cyclosporine due to ↑ breakdown by liver
Phenytoin / ↓ Plasma level of cyclosporine due to ↑ breakdown by liver
Prednisolone / ↑ Plasma level of cyclosporine due to ↓ breakdown by liver
Ranitidine / ↑ Risk of nephrotoxicity
Rifampin / ↓ Plasma level of cyclosporine due to ↑ breakdown by liver
Sulfamethoxazole and/or trimethoprim / ↑ Risk of nephrotoxicity; also, ↓ serum levels of cyclosporine → possible rejection
Trimethoprim with sulfamethoxazole / ↑ Risk of nephrotoxicity
Vancomycin / ↑ Risk of nephrotoxicity
Verapamil / ↑ Plasma level of cyclosporine

NURSING CONSIDERATIONS

Assessment

1. List all drugs the client is currently taking and note the potential for any drug interactions.
2. Obtain baseline CBC, liver profile, BUN, and creatinine levels.
3. Document indications for therapy and note any previous treatment with immunosuppressants.
4. Anticipate that clients will receive concomitant administration of adrenal corticosteroids.
5. Obtain baseline VS and monitor, reporting any baseline variations. Drug may increase serum potassium, lipid, and uric acid levels.

Client/Family Teaching

1. Demonstrate and explain how to measure the dose of medication accurately.
2. Explain the importance of following the written guidelines for medication therapy explicitly. Call with questions or if problems arise. Reinforce that the drug must be taken throughout one's lifetime to prevent transplant rejection.
3. Review the side effects of drug therapy. Because this drug is so important to transplant clients in preventing rejection, the client and family should be provided a written list of all possible side effects of drugs and know which side effects need to be reported.
4. Teach how to monitor BP. Keep an account of daily weight. Discuss the importance of reporting any persistent diarrhea and N&V and of recording I&O.
5. Advise client that taking the drug with food may reduce nausea and associated GI upset. If client finds the PO medication unpalatable, mix with milk or juice in a glass container to minimize adherence to the container. The medication should be taken immediately after mixing.

6. Do not stop the drug abruptly. If the drug must be discontinued, it should be done gradually.
7. Stress the importance of using nystatin swish and swab as directed to prevent the development of thrush. Frequent oral care and dental exams should be routine. Note any signs of changes in dentition.
8. Warn clients that they may develop acne and hirsutism as a side effect. This should be reported because a dermatology referral may be necessary.
9. Yellow discoloration of eyes, skin, or stools; fever; other signs of hepatotoxicity require immediate medical intervention. Report for scheduled liver and renal function studies throughout drug therapy.
10. Note any complaints of fatigue, malaise, unexplained bleeding or bruising, bleeding from the gums, nosebleeds, or hematuria. Hematologic parameters will also be monitored.

Evaluate: Prevention of transplant rejection with improved organ function.

Cytomegalovirus Immune Globulin Intravenous (Human)

(**sigh**-toh-**meg**-ah-loh-**VIGH**-rus im-**MYOUN GLOB**-you-lin)

Pregnancy Category: C

CytoGam **(Rx)**

How Supplied: *Injection*

Action/Kinetics: This purified product is obtained from pooled adult human plasma that has been selected for high titers of antibody for cytomegalovirus (CMV). When reconstituted, each milliliter contains 50 mg of immunoglobulin that is primarily IgG with trace amounts of IgA and IgM; albumin is also present. In individuals exposed to CMV, the immune globulin can increase the relevant antibodies to levels that prevent or reduce the incidence of serious CMV disease.

Uses: Attenuation of primary CMV disease for kidney transplant recipients who are seronegative for CMV and who receive a kidney from a CMV seropositive donor. (*NOTE:* There is a 50% decrease in primary CMV disease in renal transplant clients given this product.)

Dosage

- **IV**

Prevention of rejection of kidney transplants.

The maximum total dose/infusion is 150 mg/kg given according to the following schedule:

Within:	
72 hr of transplant:	150 mg/kg
2–8 weeks of transplant:	100 mg/kg
12–16 weeks of transplant:	50 mg/kg

The rate of infusion for the initial dose is 15 mg/kg/hr. If no side effects occur after 30 min, the rate may be increased to 30 mg/kg/hr. If no side effects occur after a subsequent 30-min period, the dose may be increased to 60 mg/kg/hr at a volume not to exceed 7.5 mL/hr. **This rate of infusion must not be exceeded.** For subsequent doses, the rate of infusion is 15 mg/kg/hr for 15 min. If no side effects occur, increase the rate to 30 mg/kg/hr for 15 min and then increase to a maximum rate of 60 mg/kg/hr at a volume not to exceed 7.5 mL/hr. **This rate of infusion must not be exceeded.**

Administration/Storage

1. The reconstituted solution should be colorless and translucent. The solution should not be used if it is turbid.
2. After removing the tab portion of the vial cap, the rubber stopper is cleaned with 70% alcohol or equivalent. The lyophilized powder is reconstituted with 50 mL of sterile water for injection using a double-ended transfer needle or large syringe. When using a double-ended transfer needle, insert one end first into the vial of water. The lyophilized powder

is supplied in an evacuated vial; thus, the water should transfer by suction. To avoid foaming, the vial should not be shaken. After the water is transferred into the evacuated vial, the residual vacuum should be released to hasten dissolution. The container should be rotated gently to wet all the undissolved powder. Thirty minutes should be allowed for complete dissolution of the powder.

3. This product does not contain a preservative. Thus, after reconstitution, the vial should be entered only once and the infusion should begin within 6 hr and be completed within 12 hr of reconstitution.

4. The drug should be administered through a separate IV line using a constant infusion pump. If this is not possible, the drug may be "piggy-backed" into a preexisting line that contains either sodium chloride injection or one of the following dextrose solutions (with or without NaCl added): 2.5%, 5%, 10%, or 20% dextrose in water. If used with a preexisting line, the drug should not be diluted more than 1:2 with any of the solutions. See *Dosage* for administration guidelines.

5. *Treatment of Overdose:* Discontinue the infusion immediately and have epinephrine and diphenhydramine available for treatment of acute allergic symptoms.

Contraindications: Use in clients with a history of a prior severe reaction to this product or other human immunoglobulin preparations.

Special Concerns: Individuals with selective immunoglobulin (Ig) A deficiency may develop antibodies to IgA and could develop anaphylactic reactions to subsequent administration of blood products that contain IgA.

Side Effects: Usually minor and often due to the rate of infusion; the infusion schedule should be adhered to closely. *GI:* N&V. *Body as a whole:* Flushing, chills, fever. *Musculoskeletal:* Muscle cramps, back pain. *Respiratory:* Wheezing. Hypotension and allergic reactions such as ***angioneurotic edema*** and ***anaphylactic shock*** are possible but have not been observed.

Symptoms of Overdose: Major effects would be those related to volume overload.

Drug Interactions: The antibodies present in this product may interfere with the immune response to live virus vaccines, including measles, mumps, and rubella. Thus, such vaccinations should be deferred until at least 3 months after administration of CMV immune globulin or revaccination may be required.

NURSING CONSIDERATIONS

Assessment

1. Determine any previous experience with human immunoglobulin preparations.
2. Document any IgA deficiency as these clients may experience anaphylactic reactions to subsequent exposure to IgA products.

Interventions

1. Follow the infusion dosing schedules carefully to minimize side effects.
2. Monitor VS continuously and observe closely for adverse symptoms. If side effects develop, slow the infusion rate or interrupt it and notify provider.
3. Monitor client closely during each rate change.

Client/Family Teaching

1. Explain the reasons for this therapy. If client is seronegative for CMV and receives a seropositive donor kidney, CMV disease may develop.
2. Review anticipated side effects and identify those that would indicate an acute allergic reaction and warrant immediate medical attention.
3. Advise not to receive any vaccinations for a least 3 months following therapy as revaccination may be necessary. Explain that antibodies in suspension may interfere with the immune response to live virus vaccines.
4. Review the source of drug and the potential associated effects. Advise that in order to prevent transmission of infectious agents/hepatitis virus from one client to another, sterile

disposable syringes and needles should be used; the syringes and needles should not be reused.
5. Identify appropriate support groups that may assist family to cope with chronic disease condition.
Evaluate: CMV prophylaxis (postoperatively) in renal transplant recipients.

Interferon gamma-1b

(in-ter-**FEER**-on **GAM**-uh)
Pregnancy Category: C
Actimmune **(Rx)**

How Supplied: *Injection:* 3 million U/0.5 mL
Action/Kinetics: Interferon gamma-1b consists of a single-chain polypeptide of 140 amino acids. It is produced by fermentation of a genetically engineered *Escherichia coli* bacterium containing the DNA that encodes for the human protein. Interferon gamma manifests potent phagocyte-activating effects including generation of toxic oxygen metabolites within phagocytes. Such metabolites result in the death of microorganisms such as *Staphylococcus aureus, Toxoplasma gondii, Leishmania donovani, Listeria monocytogenes,* and *Mycobacterium avium intracellulare.* Since interferon gamma regulates activity of immune cells, it is characterized as a lymphokine of the interleukin type. Data indicate that interferon gamma interacts functionally with other interleukin molecules (e.g., interleukin-2) and that all interleukins form part of a complex, lymphokine regulatory network. As an example, interferon gamma and interleukin-4 may interact reciprocally to regulate murine IgE levels; interferon gamma can suppress IgE levels and inhibit the production of collagen at the transcription level in humans.

Interferon gamma is slowly absorbed after SC injection. **t½, elimination: SC,** 5.9 hr. **Peak plasma levels:** 7 hr after SC dosing.

Uses: Decrease the frequency and severity of serious infections associated with chronic granulomatous disease.

Dosage

- **SC**

Chronic granulomatous disease.
50 mcg/m² (1.5 million units/m²) for clients whose body surface is greater than 0.5 m². If the body surface is less than 0.5 m², the dose of interferon gamma should be 1.5 mcg/kg/dose. The drug is given 3 times/week (e.g., Monday, Wednesday, Friday).

Administration/Storage

1. The preferred sites of injection are the right and left deltoid and anterior thigh.
2. The product does not contain a preservative. Thus, the vial is to be used only for a single dose with any unused portion discarded.
3. Safety and effectiveness have not been determined for doses greater or less than 50 mcg/m².
4. If severe side effects occur, the dose can be reduced by 50% or therapy can be discontinued until the side effects subside.
5. The drug may be administered using either sterilized glass or plastic disposable syringes.
6. Vials must be stored at 2°C–8°C (36°F–46°F) to assure optimal retention of activity. The vial should not be frozen.
7. The vial should not be shaken and vigorous agitation should be avoided.
8. Vials stored at room temperature for more than 12 hr should be discarded.
9. Although not approved by the FDA, the drug has been given by continuous (10 days to 8 weeks) or intermittent (at 1, 6, or 24 hr) IV infusion as well as by IM injection.
10. Undiluted drug should not be stored in syringes due to adhesion to syringe surfaces.

Contraindications: Hypersensitivity to interferon gamma or *E. coli*-derived products. Use during lactation.

Special Concerns: Safety and effectiveness have not been determined in children less than 1 year of age. Use with caution in clients with preexisting cardiac disease, including symptoms of ischemia, arrhythmia, or CHF, and in clients with myelosuppression, seizure disorders, or compromised CNS function.

Side Effects: The following side effects were noted in clients with chronic granulomatous disease receiving the drug SC. *GI:* Diarrhea, vomiting, nausea, abdominal pain, anorexia. *CNS:* Fever (over 50%), headache, fatigue, depression. *Miscellaneous:* Rash, chills, erythema or tenderness at injection site, pain at injection site, weight loss, myalgia, arthralgia, back pain.

When used in clients other than those with chronic granulomatous disease, in addition to above, the following side effects were reported. *GI:* ***GI bleeding,*** pancreatitis, hepatic insufficiency. *CV:* Hypotension, heart block, ***heart failure,*** syncope, ***tachyarrhythmia, MI.*** *CNS:* Confusion, disorientation, symptoms of parkinsonism, gait disturbance, ***seizures,*** hallucinations, transient ischemic attacks. *Hematologic:* ***Deep venous thrombosis, pulmonary embolism.*** *Respiratory:* ***Bronchospasm,*** tachypnea, interstitial pneumonitis. *Metabolic:* Hyperglycemia, hyponatremia. *Miscellaneous:* Reversible renal insufficiency, worsening of dermatomyositis.

NURSING CONSIDERATIONS

Assessment

1. Note any history or evidence of CAD or CNS disorders.
2. Obtain baseline urinalysis, CBC, and liver and renal function studies, and monitor every 3 months during drug therapy.
3. Determine client age when symptoms presented (onset of chronic granulomatous disease) and what if any treatments in the past were used to reduce the frequency and severity of infections.

Client/Family Teaching

1. Review the appropriate method for medication administration and observe the client in self-administration.
2. Stress the importance of keeping the drug in the refrigerator and **not** to shake the container.
3. Advise client to take medication at bedtime with acetaminophen, unless contraindicated, to minimize flu-like symptoms (fever and headaches) associated with this drug therapy.
4. Consume 2–3 L/day of fluids.
5. Avoid alcohol and any other CNS depressants.
6. Provide a printed list of drug side effects stressing those that should be reported immediately.
7. Remind client that close medical supervision is imperative with this disease and genetically engineered medication therapy as the dosage may require frequent adjustments. All concerns and any adverse effects should be reported immediately.

Evaluate: Suppression of infective microorganisms associated with chronic granulomatous disease.

Muromonab-CD3

(myour-oh-**MON**-ab)
Pregnancy Category: C
Orthoclone OKT 3 **(Rx)**

How Supplied: *Injection:* 1 mg/mL

Action/Kinetics: Muromonab-CD3 is a murine monoclonal antibody; the antibody is a purified IgG_{2a} immunoglobulin. The antibody acts to prevent rejection of transplanted kidney tissue by blocking the action of T cells, which play a significant role in acute rejection. Specifically, the CD3 molecule in the membrane of T cells is blocked; this molecule is necessary for signal transduction. The drug does not cause myelosuppression. Antibodies to muromonab-CD3 have been observed after approximately 20 days. **Average serum levels after 3 days:** 0.9 mcg/mL. **Time to steady-state trough levels:** 3 days. **Duration:** 1 week for return of circulating CD3 positive T cells to pretreatment levels.

Uses: To reverse acute allograft rejection in kidney transplant clients;

used in combination with azathioprine, cyclosporine, corticosteroids. Treatment of steroid-resistant acute allograft rejection in cardiac and hepatic transplant clients.

Dosage

- **IV Bolus**

Reverse acute allograft rejection in kidney transplants.

Adults: 5 mg/day for 10–14 days.

Cardiac/hepatic allograft rejection, steroid-resistant.

5 mg/day for 10–14 days with treatment beginning after determination that corticosteroids will not reverse the rejection.

Administration/Storage

1. Methylprednisolone sodium succinate, 8 mg/kg IV, should be given 1–4 hr before muromonab-CD3 to decrease the incidence of reactions to the first dose. Acetaminophen and antihistamines, given together, may reduce early reactions.
2. Treatment should be initiated as soon as acute renal rejection is diagnosed.
3. The dose should be given in less than 1 min.
4. The drug is not to be given by IV infusion or with any other drug solutions.
5. If the body temperature of the client is 37.8°C (100°F), drug therapy should not be initiated.
6. The solution (which is a protein) should be drawn into a syringe through a 0.2- or 0.22-µm filter; the filter is then discarded and a 20-gauge needle is attached.
7. Other drugs should not be added or infused through the same IV line. If the same IV line is used for sequential infusion of different drugs, the line should be flushed with saline before and after infusion of muromonab-CD3.
8. The appearance of a few translucent particles of protein does not affect the potency of the preparation.
9. The ampule should be used immediately after opening as there is no bacteriostatic agent in the product. Any unused drug should be discarded.
10. The dose of other immunosuppressant drugs should be decreased as follows during muromonab-CD3 use: prednisone, 0.5 mg/kg/day; azathioprine, 25 mg/day. Cyclosporine should be discontinued. Maintenance doses of these drugs can be resumed approximately 3 days prior to termination of muromonab-CD3 therapy.
11. The drug should be stored at 2°C–8°C (36°F–46°F) and should not be frozen or shaken.

Contraindications: Hypersensitivity to drug (or any product of murine origin), clients with anti-mouse titers greater than or equal to 1:1,000. Clients with fluid overload or uncompensated CHF. History of seizures or predisposition to seizures. Use during pregnancy and lactation.

Special Concerns: Should not be used in pregnancy as it is an IgG antibody with potential hazard to the fetus. Although used in children, safety and effectiveness have not been assessed. Following the first two to three doses, a cytokine release syndrome due to the release of cytokines by activated lymphocytes or monocytes may occur. Clients at greatest risk for cytokine release syndrome are those with unstable angina, recent MI, symptomatic ischemic heart disease, heart failure, pulmonary edema, COPD, intravascular volume overload or depletion, cerebrovascular disease, advanced symptomatic vascular disease or neuropathy, history of seizures, or septic shock.

Laboratory Test Interferences: ↑ AST, ALT.

Side Effects: *Cytokine release syndrome (CRS):* Flu-like symptoms, such as pyrexia, chills, dyspnea, N&V, chest pain, diarrhea, tremor, wheezing, headache, tachycardia, rigor, and hypertension. ***Rarely, severe, life-threatening shock-like syndrome including serious CV and CNS effects.***

Within the first 45 days of therapy for renal transplants: ***Infections (which may be life-threatening) due to CMV, HSV, Staphylococcus epidermidis, Pneumocystis carinii, Legionella, Cryptococcus, Serratia, and other gram-negative bacteria***.

Within the first 45 days of therapy for liver transplants: ***CMV, fungal infections, HSV, Legionella, and other severe, life-threatening gram-positive, gram-negative, and viral infections.***

Within the first 45 days of therapy for heart transplants: Most commonly herpes simplex, fungal, and cytomegaloviral infections. *Hypersensitivity reactions:* ***Cardiovascular collapse, cardiorespiratory arrest, shock,*** loss of consciousness, hypotension, tachycardia, tingling, angioedema, ***airway obstruction, bronchospasm,*** dyspnea, urticaria, pruritus. *Neuro-psychiatric:* ***Seizures,*** encephalopathy, cerebral edema, ***aseptic meningitis,*** headaches. *CV:* ***Cardiac arrest, shock, heart failure, CV collapse, MI,*** hypotension, angina, tachycardia, bradycardia, hemodynamic instability, hypertension, LV dysfunction, arrhythmias, chest pain or tightness. *Respiratory:* ***Respiratory arrest, ARDS, respiratory failure, cardiogenic or noncardiogenic pulmonary edema, apnea,*** dyspnea, ***bronchospasm,*** wheezing, SOB, hypoxemia, tachypnea, hyperventilation, abnormal chest sounds, pneumonia, pneumonitis. *Dermatologic:* Rash, urticaria, pruritus, erythema, flushing, diaphoresis. *GI:* Nausea, vomiting, abdominal pain, ***bowel infarction.*** *Hematologic:* Pancytopenia, ***aplastic anemia,*** neutropenia, leukopenia, thrombocytopenia, lymphopenia, leukocytosis, lymphadenopathy, ***arterial and venous thrombosis of allografts and other vascular beds (heart, lung, brain, bowel), disturbances of coagulation.*** *Musculoskeletal:* Arthralgia, arthritis, myalgia, stiffness, aches and pain. *Hepatic:* Hepatomegaly, splenomegaly, hepatitis (usually secondary to viral infection or lymphoma). *Ophthalmic:* Blindness, blurred vision, diplopia, photophobia, conjunctivitis. *Otic:* Hearing loss, otitis media, tinnitus, vertigo, nasal and ear stuffiness. *Body as a whole:* Fever, chills, rigors, flu-like syndrome, fatigue, malaise, generalized weakness, anorexia. *Miscellaneous:* Palsy of cranial nerve VI, ***increased risk of developing neoplasms.***

Drug Interactions

Azathioprine, corticosteroids, cyclosporine / Psychosis, infections, malignancies, seizures, encephalopathy, and thrombosis when taken with muromonab-CD3

Indomethacin / Encephalopathy and other CNS effects

NURSING CONSIDERATIONS

Assessment

1. Determine if client has received this drug therapy in the past and assess closely for evidence of antibodies. Drug is usually only given for one course of therapy.
2. Note any history of sensitivity to murine derivatives.
3. Obtain baseline CBC and T-cell assays with CD_3 antigen daily.

Interventions

1. Anticipate pretreatment administration of an antihistamine, antipyretic, and methylprednisolone sodium succinate and hydrocortisone sodium succinate posttreatment to minimize intensity of side effects.
2. Monitor I&O; assess for a positive fluid balance, and report.
3. Obtain CXR, assess lung sounds, and report any evidence of congestion.
4. Document daily weights and report any evidence of rapid weight gain.
5. Take the temperature q 4 hr. If the temperature goes above 37.7°C (100°F), withhold the drug until the temperature drops. Monitor CBC with differential and circulating T cells.
6. Monitor the client's renal status for a decrease in urine volume and a decrease in creatinine clearance. These are signs of transplant rejection and should be reported immediately.
7. Administer acetaminophen for flu-like symptoms and febrile reaction. This is usually noted after the first dose.

8. Symptoms of aseptic meningitis are usually evident within 3 days. Fever, headache, nuchal rigidity, and photophobia characterize this condition.

Client/Family Teaching

1. Explain that chills, fever, SOB, and malaise are first-dose symptoms that will diminish on consecutive treatment days.
2. Any symptoms of dyspnea, edema, weight gain, chest pain, N&V, or infection require immediate reporting.
3. Perform frequent, careful oral care to minimize occurrence of oral inflammation.
4. Avoid vaccinia and crowds.
5. Advise women of childbearing age to continue to practice birth control for 12 weeks following therapy.

Evaluate: Reversal of kidney transplant rejection and improved organ function.

CHAPTER EIGHTY

Drugs Used In Immunocompromised Clients

See the following individual entries:

Epoetin Alfa Recombinant
Filgrastim
Immune Globulin IV (Human)
Pegademase Bovine
Sargramostim

Epoetin alfa recombinant

(ee-**POH**-ee-tin)
Pregnancy Category: C
Epogen, Procrit **(Rx)**

How Supplied: *Injection:* 2,000 U/mL, 3,000 U/mL, 4,000 U/mL, 10,000 U/mL

Action/Kinetics: Epoetin alfa is a 165-amino-acid glycoprotein made by recombinant DNA technology; it has the identical amino acid sequence and same biologic effects as endogenous erythropoietin (which is normally synthesized in the kidney and stimulates RBC production). Epoetin alfa will elevate or maintain the RBC level, decreasing the need for blood transfusions. **$t^{1}/_{2}$:** 4–13 hr in clients with chronic renal failure. **Peak serum levels after SC:** 5–24 hr.

Uses: Treatment of anemia associated with chronic renal failure, including clients on dialysis (end-stage renal disease) or not on dialysis. AZT-induced anemia in HIV-infected clients. Treatment of anemia in clients with nonmyeloid malignancies (Procrit only). *Investigational:* To increase the procurement of autologous blood in clients undergoing elective surgery (i.e., to decrease the need for homologous blood transfusions).

Dosage

- **IV, SC**

Chronic renal failure.

IV, initial (dialysis or nondialysis clients), SC (nondialysis clients), initial: 50–100 U/kg 3 times/week. The rate of increase of hematocrit depends on both dosage and client variation. **Maintenance:** Individualize (usual: 25 U/kg 3 times/week).

AZT-treated, HIV-infections.

IV, SC, initial: 100 U/kg 3 times/week for 8 weeks (in clients with serum erythropoietin levels less than or equal to 500 mU/mL who are receiving less than or equal to 4,200 mg/week of AZT). If a satisfactory response is obtained, the dose can be increased by 50–100 U/kg 3 times/week. The response should be evaluated q 4–8 weeks thereafter with dosage adjusted by 50–100 U/kg increments 3 times/week. If clients have not responded to 300 U/kg 3 times/week, it is likely they will not respond to higher doses.

Cancer clients on chemotherapy (Procrit only).

Initial, SC: 150 units/kg 3 times/week. Treatment of clients with highly elevated erythropoetin levels (> 200 mU/mL) is not recommended. If response is not satisfactory after 8 wks, the dose may be increased up to 300 units/kg 3 times/week. Clients not responding at this level are not likely to respond at higher levels. If the hematocrit exceeds 40%, the dose should be withheld until the hematocrit falls to 36%. When treatment is resumed, reduce the dose by 25%.

Administration/Storage

1. During hemodialysis, clients treated with epoetin alfa may require increased anticoagulation with heparin to prevent clotting of the artificial kidney.
2. The hematocrit should be determined twice weekly until it has stabilized in the target range and the maintenance dose of epoetin alfa has been determined. Also, after any dosage adjustment, the hematocrit should be monitored twice weekly for 2–6 weeks.
3. The dose of epoetin alfa should be reduced by about 25 U/kg 3 times/week when the target range (30%–33%) is reached. Maintenance doses must then be individually determined.
4. If the hematocrit exceeds 36%, the drug should be withheld temporarily until the hematocrit decreases to 30%–33%. Upon reinitiation of therapy, the dose should be reduced by about 25 U/kg 3 times/week.
5. The dose of epoetin alfa should be reduced immediately if the hematocrit increases more than 4 points in any 2-week period. After reduction, the hematocrit should be monitored twice a week for 2–6 weeks with maintenance doses individually determined.
6. The dose of epoetin alfa should be increased in increments of 25 U/kg 3 times/week if the hematocrit does not increase by 5–6 points after 8 weeks of therapy. Further increases of 25 U/kg 3 times/week may be made at 4–6-week intervals until a desired response is observed.
7. The preparation should not be shaken because shaking will denature the glycoprotein, making it biologically inactive.
8. Vials showing particulate matter or discoloration should not be used.
9. Only one dose per vial should be withdrawn and any unused portion should be discarded. The product contains no preservative.
10. The drug should be stored at 2°C–8°C (36°F–46°F).
11. Epoetin alfa should not be given with any other drug solutions.

Contraindications: Uncontrolled hypertension, hypersensitivity to mammalian cell-derived products, hypersensitivity to human albumin. Use in clients with chronic renal failure who need severe anemia corrected. Use in treating anemia in HIV-infected or cancer clients due to factors such as iron or folate deficiences, hemolysis, or GI bleeding.

Special Concerns: Safety and efficacy have not been established in children. The safety and efficacy of epoetin alfa are not known in clients with a history of seizures or underlying hematologic disease (e.g., hypercoagulable disorders, myelodysplastic syndromes, sickle cell anemia). Use with caution in clients with porphyria, during lactation, and preexisting vascular disease. Increased anticoagulation with heparin may be required in clients on epoetin alfa undergoing hemodialysis.

Side Effects: In Chronic Renal Failure Clients (symptoms may be due to the disease). *CV:* Hypertension, tachycardia, edema, ***MI, CV accident,*** transient ischemic attack, clotted vascular access. *CNS:* Headache, fatigue, dizziness, ***seizures.*** *GI:* Nausea, diarrhea, vomiting, worsening of porphyria. *Allergic reactions:* Skin rashes, urticaria, ***anaphylaxis.*** *Miscellaneous:* SOB, hyperkalemia, arthralgias, chest pain, skin reaction at administration site, asthenia.

In AZT-Treated HIV-Infected Clients. *CNS:* Pyrexia, fatigue, headache, dizziness, ***seizures.*** *Respiratory:* Cough, respiratory congestion, SOB. *GI:* Diarrhea, nausea. *Miscellaneous:* Rash, asthenia, reaction at injection site, allergic reactions.

In Cancer Clients. *CNS:* Pyrexia, fatigue, dizziness. *GI:* Diarrhea, nausea, vomiting. *Musculoskeletal:* Asthenia, paresthesia, trunk pain. *Miscellaneous:* Edema, SOB, upper respiratory infection.

Symptom of Overdose: Polycythemia.

NURSING CONSIDERATIONS

Assessment

1. During the nursing history, note if client has any history of hypersensitivity to mammalian cell-derived products or human albumin.
2. Determine client iron stores prior to initiating therapy. Transferrin saturation should be at least 20% and serum ferritin should be at least 200 ng/mL. It may be necessary to provide supplemental iron to increase or maintain transferrin saturation to levels required to support stimulation of erythropoiesis by epoetin alfa. Carefully assess the client's iron stores (including transferrin saturation and serum ferritin) prior to and during therapy.
3. Obtain baseline CBC and platelet count before starting therapy.
4. Note history of hypertension and perform baseline BP readings.
5. In clients infected with HIV, note when AZT therapy was instituted and the onset and cause of anemia.

Interventions

1. Monitor CBC and platelet count throughout therapy and report as drug dose may need to be adjusted frequently.
2. Assess BP and monitor throughout epoetin alfa therapy. Hypertension should be controlled prior to initiation of drug therapy.
3. Monitor renal function studies, electrolytes, and phosphorous and uric acid levels especially in clients with chronic renal failure.
4. Supplemental iron should be administered to enhance the effects of epoetin alfa.

Client/Family Teaching

1. Advise clients and family that over 95% of clients with chronic renal failure manifested significant increases in hematocrit and nearly all clients were transfusion-independent within 2 months after beginning epoetin alfa therapy. Stress that drug does not cure renal disease.
2. Explain that the desired drug response may take as long as 6 weeks.
3. Stress the importance of reporting for scheduled lab studies because drug dose must be adjusted based on these results.
4. Provide a printed list of drug side effects. Instruct client to report any persistent and/or bothersome side effects and to practice contraception during therapy.
5. Explain the importance of continuing to follow the prescribed dietary and dialysis recommendations.
6. Caution client not to perform any tasks that require mental alertness during the first 90 days of therapy with epoetin alfa.

Evaluate

- ↑ Hematocrit (↑ RBCs)
- Relief of symptoms of anemia

Filgrastim

(fill-**GRASS**-tim)
Pregnancy Category: C
Neupogen **(Rx)**

How Supplied: *Injection:* 300 mcg/mL

Action/Kinetics: Filgrastim is a human granulocyte colony stimulating factor (G-CSF). It is produced by recombinant DNA technology by *Escherichia coli* that has been inserted with the human G-CSF gene. Endogenous G-CSF is a glycoprotein that is produced by monocytes, fibroblasts, and other endothelial cells and that regulates the production of neutrophils in the bone marrow. It has minimal effects, either in vivo or in vitro, on the production of other hematopoietic cell types. Filgrastim has an amino acid sequence that is identical to the natural sequence predicted from human DNA sequence analysis except there is an N-terminal methionine that is required for expression in *E. coli*. IV infusion of 20 mcg/kg over 24 hr resulted in a mean serum level of 48 ng/mL, whereas SC administration of 11.5 mcg/kg resulted in a maximum serum level of 49 ng/mL within 2–8 hr. **$t^{1/2}$, elimination:** 3.5 hr.

Uses: To decrease the incidence of infection, as manifested by febrile neutropenia, in clients with nonmyeloid malignancies who are receiving myelosuppressive anticancer drugs, which are associated with severe neutropenia with fever. To reduce the duration of neutropenia in clients with nonmyeloid malignancies undergoing myeloablative chemotherapy followed by bone marrow transplantation. To reduce infection in severe chronic neutropenia (e.g., congenital, cyclical, or idiopathic neutropenia).

Dosage

- **SC, IV**

Myelosuppressive chemotherapy.

Initial: 5 mcg/kg/day as a single injection, either as a SC bolus, by short IV infusion (15–30 min), or by continuous SC or IV infusion (over a 24-hr period). The dose may be increased in increments of 5 mcg/kg for each chemotherapy cycle depending on the duration and severity of the absolute neutrophil count (ANC) nadir.

Severe chronic neutropenia.

5 mcg/kg/day SC for idiopathic and cyclic disease; 6 mcg/kg/day SC for congenital disease.

Bone marrow transplantation.

10 mcg/kg/day given as an IV infusion of 4 or 24 hr or as a continuous 24-hr SC infusion.

NOTE: During the period of neutrophil recovery, the daily dose should be titrated against the neutrophil response as follows:

1. When ANC is greater than 1,000/mm^3 for 3 consecutive days, reduce the dose of filgrastim to 5 mcg/kg/day. If ANC decreases to less than 1,000/mm^3 at any time during the 5-mcg/kg/day dosage, increase filgrastim to 10 mcg/kg/day.
2. If ANC remains greater than 1,000/mm^3 for 3 more consecutive days, discontinue filgrastim.
3. If ANC decreases to less than 1,000/mm^3, resume filgrastim at 5 mcg/kg/day.

Administration/Storage

1. Filgrastim is given daily for up to 2 weeks until the ANC has reached 10,000/m^3 following the expected chemotherapy-induced neutrophil nadir.
2. Therapy should be discontinued if the ANC is greater than 10,000/mm^3 after the expected chemotherapy-induced neutrophil nadir.
3. For myelosuppressive therapy or bone marrow transplantation, give no earlier than 24 hr after cytotoxic chemotherapy and in the 24 hr before administration of chemotherapy.
4. Discontinuing therapy usually results in a 50% decrease in circulating neutrophils within 1–2 days with a return to pretreatment levels in 1–7 days.
5. The product should not be frozen but stored in the refrigerator at 2°C–8°C (36°F–46°F). Prior to use, filgrastim can be at room temperature for a maximum of 24 hr. Any product left at room temperature for more than 24 hr should be discarded.
6. Filgrastim solution should be clear and colorless.
7. The product should not be shaken.
8. Only one dose should be used for each vial; the vial should not be reentered.
9. The drug is compatible with glass, PVC, or plastic syringes.
10. Filgrastim may be diluted in 5% dextrose. When diluted to concentrations between 5 and 15 mcg/mL, the product should be protected from adsorption to plastic materials by adding human albumin to a final concentration of 2 mg/mL.

Contraindications: Hypersensitivity to proteins derived from *E. coli*. The safety and effectiveness of filgrastim given simultaneously with cytotoxic chemotherapy have not been determined; thus, filgrastim should not be given 24 hr before to 24 hr after cytotoxic chemotherapy.

Special Concerns: Use with caution during lactation. Use with caution in any malignancy with myeloid characteristics since the drug may act as a growth factor for any tumor type. Filgrastim does not cause any greater incidence of toxicity in children than in adults. The safety and effectiveness of chronic filgrastim therapy have not been determined. Hypersensitivity reactions usually occur within 30 min after administration and are more frequent in clients receiving the drug IV.

Laboratory Test Interferences: ↑ Uric acid, LDH, alkaline phosphatase.

Side Effects: *Musculoskeletal:* Medullary bone pain, skeletal pain. *GI:* N&V, diarrhea, anorexia, stomatitis, constipation, peritonitis. *Hypersensitivity:* skin rash, urticaria, facial edema, wheezing, dyspnea, hypotension, tachycardia. *Hematologic:* Leukocytosis; greater risk of thrombocytopenia and anemia. *Respiratory:* Dyspnea, cough, chest pain, sore throat. *Body as a whole:* Alopecia, neutropenic fever, fever, fatigue, headache, skin rash, mucositis, generalized weakness, unspecified pain. *CV:* Decreased BP (transient), cutaneous vasculitis, hypertension, ***arrhythmias, MI.***

NURSING CONSIDERATIONS

Assessment

1. Determine any client hypersensitivity to *E. coli*-derived products.
2. Obtain baseline CBC and platelet counts and perform twice weekly during therapy.
3. Document last dose of cytotoxic agent and determine ANC nadir. Drug should not be administered 24 hr before to 24 hr after cytotoxic chemotherapy.

Client/Family Teaching

1. Review the appropriate technique for administration of prescribed drug therapy and have client return demonstrate. Provide written guidelines concerning dose, administration time, drug storage, and the proper method for storing, handling, and discarding of syringes.
2. Ensure that the client has the appropriate materials for drug administration and for proper disposal of equipment.
3. Remind client not to shake the container and to only enter the vial once.
4. Advise that "flu-like" symptoms (N&V and aching) may be side effects of drug therapy. Also, bone pain has occurred; advise client to take at bedtime, to take prescribed analgesics, and to report if persistent.
5. Encourage client to maintain a record of daily temperatures.
6. Advise to report for scheduled lab follow-up to evaluate the effectiveness of drug therapy.

Evaluate

- Prevention of infection during therapy with myelosuppressive anticancer drugs
- Decreased duration of neutropenia during chemotherapy
- Improved neutrophil counts

Immune globulin IV (Human)

(im-**MYOUN GLOH**-byou-lin)
Pregnancy Category: C
Gamimune N 5% and 10%, Gammabulin Immuno ✱, Gammagard S/D, Gammar I.V., Iveegam ✱, Sandoglobulin, Venoglobulin-I, Venoglobulin-S **(Rx)**

How Supplied: *Injection:* 50 mg/mL, 100 mg/mL; *Powder for injection:* 2.5 g, 0.5 g, 1 g, 2.5 g, 3 g, 5 g, 6 g, 10 g, 12 g

Action/Kinetics: Immune globulin IV is a polyvalent antibody product derived from a human volunteer pool. It contains the various IgG antibodies normally occurring in humans. The products may also contain traces of IgA and IgM. Plasma in the manufacturing pool has been found nonreactive for hepatitis B antigen. Also, there have been no documented cases of viral transmission. The antibodies present in the products will cause both opsonization and neutralization of microbes and toxins. The reconstituted products may contain sucrose, maltose, protein, and/or small amounts of sodium chloride. Doses of immune globulin IV will restore abnormally low IgG levels to within the normal range with equilibrium reached between the intra- and extravascular compartments within 6 days. The percentage of IgG in the products is over 90%. **t½:** Gamimune N and Sandoglobulin, 3 weeks; Venoglobulin-I, 29 days.

Uses: Severe combined immunodeficiency and primary immunoglobulin deficiency syndromes, including congenital agammaglobulinemia, X-linked agammaglobulinemia, and Wiskott-Aldrich syndrome. Acute and chronic idiopathic thrombocytopenic purpura in both children and adults. B-cell chronic lymphocytic leukemia (Gammagard). Prophylactic use to decrease infections and the incidence of graft-versus-host-disease in bone marrow clients and in HIV-infected children to prevent bacterial infections (Gamimune).

Dosage

• **IV Only for All Products**

GAMIMUNE N

Immunodeficiency syndrome.

100–200 mg/kg given once a month; if response is satisfactory, dose can be increased to 400 mg/kg or infusion may be repeated more frequently than once a month. Rate of infusion: 0.01–0.02 mL/kg/min for 30 min; if no discomfort is experienced, the rate can be increased up to 0.08 mL/kg/min.

Idiopathic thrombocytopenic purpura.

400 mg/kg for 5 consecutive days.

GAMMAGARD

Immunodeficiency syndrome.

200–400 mg/kg (minimum of 100 mg/kg/month).

B-cell lymphocytic leukemia.

400 mg/kg q 3–4 weeks.

Idiopathic thrombocytopenic purpura.

1,000 mg/kg; additional doses depend on platelet count (up to three doses can be given on alternate days). Rate of infusion: 0.5 mL/kg initially; may be increased gradually to 4 mL/kg/hr if there is no client distress.

SANDOGLOBULIN

Immunodeficiency syndrome.

200 mg/kg/month; increase to 300 mg/kg if client response satisfactory (i.e., IgG serum level of 300 mg/dL). Rate of administration: 3% solution at an initial rate of 0.5–1 mL/min; after 15–30 min can increase to 1.5–2.5 mL/min (subsequent infusions at a rate of 2–2.5 mL/min). If the 6% solution is used, the initial infusion rate should be 1–1.5 mL/min and increased after 15–30 min to a maximum of 2.5 mL/min.

Idiopathic thrombocytopenic purpura.

400 mg/kg for 2–5 consecutive days.

VENOGLOBULIN-I

Immunodeficiency disease.

200 mg/kg/month; can increase to 300–400 mg/kg if response is insufficient or can repeat infusion more frequently than once monthly.

Idiopathic thrombocytopenic purpura.

Induction: 500 mg/kg for 2–7 consecutive days; **maintenance:** 500–2,000 mg/kg as a single infusion q 2 weeks or less if platelet count falls to below 30,000/μL.

VENOGLOBULIN-S

Immunodeficiency disease.

200 mg/kg/month by IV infusion; can increase to 300–400 mg/kg if response is insufficient or can repeat infusion more frequently than once monthly.

Idiopathic thrombocytopenic purpura.

Induction: Maximum cumulative dose of 2,000 mg/kg (40 mL/kg) over a maximum of 5 days; **maintenance:** 1,000 mg/kg/infusion (20 mL/kg/infusion) as needed to maintain a platelet count of 30,000/mm^3 in children and 20,000/mm^3 in adults or to prevent bleeding episodes between infusions.

Administration/Storage

1. Follow the administration guidelines explicitly and follow the manufacturer's directions carefully for reconstitution of either the 3% or 6% solution.

2. In agamma- or hypogammaglobulinemic clients, the 3% solution should be used. Initially, administer at a rate of 10–20 gtt/min (0.5–1 mL/min). After 15–30 min the rate may be increased to 30–50 gtt/min (1.5–2.5 mL/min). Subsequent infusions may be given at a rate of 40–50 gtt/min (2–2.5 mL/min). If the first bottle of the 3% solution is given in these clients with good tolerance, subsequent infusions may be given using the 6% solution.

3. The solutions should not be shak-

en because excessive foaming will occur.
4. The solution should be infused only if it is clear and at room temperature.
5. These products should be given only IV because the IM or SC routes have not been evaluated.
6. These products should be given by a separate IV line without mixing with other IV fluids or medications.
7. A rapid decrease in serum IgG level in the first week postinfusion will be observed; this is expected and is due to the equilibration of IgG between the plasma and extravascular space.
8. Utilize an electronic infusion device for administration.
9. Epinephrine should be readily available in the event of an acute anaphylactic reaction.

Contraindications: Clients with selective IgA deficiency who have antibodies to IgA (the products contain IgA). Sensitivity to human immune globulin.

Special Concerns: The various products are used for different conditions and at different doses; thus, check information carefully.

Side Effects: *CNS:* Headache, malaise, feeling of faintness, headache. *Allergic:* Hypersensitivity or ***anaphylactic reactions.*** *Body as a whole:* Fever, chills. *GI:* Headache, nausea, vomiting. *Miscellaneous:* Chest tightness, dyspnea; chest, back, or hip pain; mild erythema following infiltration; burning sensation in the head; tachycardia.

Agammaglobulinemic and hypogammaglobulinemic clients never having received immunoglobulin therapy or where the time from the last treatment is more than 8 weeks may manifest side effects if the infusion rate exceeds 1 mL/min. Symptoms include flushing of the face, hypotension, tightness in chest, chills, fever, dizziness, diaphoresis, and nausea.

NURSING CONSIDERATIONS

Assessment

1. Document indications for therapy.
2. For passive immunization note date and type of exposure and assess closely for anaphylaxis.
3. Immune globulin should be administered within 2 weeks of exposure to hepatitis A, within 6 days after measles exposure, and within 7 days after hepatitis B exposure.
4. Any past history of idiopathic thrombocytopenia purpura warrants close hematologic monitoring.

Interventions

1. Monitor VS throughout the infusion.
2. If the client develops hypotension, decrease or interrupt the rate of infusion until the hypotension subsides.
3. Administer drug therapy in a closely monitored environment and away from persons with active infections if immunocompromised.
4. Monitor liver function studies, hematologic parameters, IgG levels, and appropriate blood and urine chemistries.

Client/Family Teaching

1. Explain that drug may cause N&V, fever, chills, flushing, lightheadedness, and tightness in the chest. These symptoms should be reported immediately because they may be related to the dosage and rate of drug administration.
2. Explain that immunoglobulin helps to prevent and/or reduce the intensity of various infectious diseases. With thrombocytopenia, increased platelets and enhanced clotting should occur.
3. Discuss the need to have drug therapy once a month to maintain appropriate IgG serum levels.
4. Advise that warm soaks to injection site and Tylenol may assist to relieve discomfort.
5. Explain that the drug is derived from human plasma and discuss the associated potential risks.

Evaluate

- Serum IgG levels within normal range
- ↑ Antibody titer with evidence of passive immunity
- ↑ Platelet counts in clients with idiopathic thrombocytopenia purpura

Pegademase bovine

(peg-**AD**-eh-mace **BOH**-veen)
Pregnancy Category: C
Adagen **(Rx)**

How Supplied: *Injection:* 250 U/mL

Action/Kinetics: Pegademase is derived from bovine intestine and is the conjugate of numerous strands of monomethoxypolyethylene glycol, which is attached covalently to the enzyme ADA. In deficiency clients, adenosine, 2'-deoxyadenosine, and their metabolites are toxic to lymphocytes. Replacement with pegademase bovine improves immune function and decreases the frequency of opportunistic infections. The time required to correct the metabolic abnormalities may range from a few weeks to 6 months. Adequate dosage may be evaluated by measuring ADA levels and by monitoring the level of dATP in erythrocytes. **Peak plasma levels, after IM:** 2–3 days. **t½:** 3 to more than 6 days. After initiation of therapy, the trough level should be between 15 and 35 micromol/hr/mL before a maintenance injection is given.

Uses: Enzyme replacement for the treatment of SCID in which there is a deficiency of ADA. Pegademase bovine may be used in infants from birth and in children of any age at the time of diagnosis of deficiency. The drug is ineffective in clients with immunodeficiency due to other causes.

Dosage

- **IM**

Individualized. Dose is given q 7 days. *First dose:* 10 units/kg. *Second dose:* 15 units/kg. *Third dose:* 20 units/kg. *Maintenance doses:* 20 units/kg/week. If necessary, the weekly dose may be increased by 5 units/kg but the maximum single dose should not exceed 30 units/kg.

Administration/Storage

1. Pegademase bovine should not be mixed with any other drug prior to administration.
2. Pegademase should be stored in the refrigerator between 2°C and 8°C (36°F–46°F). It should not be stored frozen or at room temperature.
3. Drug is for IM use only.
4. Pegademase should not be used if there is any chance the vial has been frozen.

Contraindications: Severe thrombocytopenia. IV use.

Special Concerns: Use with caution during lactation. There is no evidence to support the safety and effectiveness of pegademase bovine either before or as support therapy for bone marrow transplantation. Use with caution in mild to moderate thrombocytopenia.

Side Effects: Data are limited but pain at the injection site and headache have been reported.

Drug Interactions: Since vidarabine is a substrate for ADA, use of vidarabine with pegademase bovine may alter the activities of both drugs.

NURSING CONSIDERATIONS

Assessment

1. Document onset of SCID with ADA deficiency. Record baseline level of ADA activity in plasma and erythrocyte dATP.
2. Note if client has a failed bone marrow transplant or if client is not suitable for transplant because this is the usual cure for ADA deficiency.
3. Obtain baseline CBC to determine if thrombocytopenia is present.

Interventions

1. Antibodies to pegademase bovine may develop and should be suspected if the preinjection level of ADA is less than 10 micromol/hr/mL and if other causes for the decrease have been ruled out (e.g., improper storage of vials, improper handling of plasma samples).
2. Protect client from opportunistic infections until immune response/function has returned.
3. Monitor plasma ADA activity and RBC dATP levels to determine drug response and adequate dosing levels of pegademase bovine.

Client/Family Teaching

1. Review early S&S of infection. Instruct client to report any such symptoms immediately.
2. Explain that after initial therapy, ADA activity should be measured every 1–2 weeks during the first 8–12 weeks of therapy. Between 3 and 9 months, activity should be measured twice a month and then monthly until after 18–24 months of therapy. ADA activity can then be monitored every 2–4 months.
3. Advise that lab studies of dATP, once it has decreased to acceptable levels, should be measured 2–4 times during the remainder of the first year of therapy and 2–3 times yearly thereafter provided that therapy has not been interrupted.

Evaluate

• Desired enzyme replacement as evidenced by plasma ADA activity in the range of 15–35 micromol/hr/mL
• ↓ Erythrocyte dATP to less than or equal to 0.005–0.015 micromol/mL packed erythrocytes or less than or equal to 1% of the total erythrocyte adenine nucleotide (ATP + dATP) content, with a normal ATP level (as measured in a preinjection sample)

Sargramostim

(sar-**GRAM**-oh-stim)
Pregnancy Category: C
Leukine **(Rx)**

How Supplied: *Powder for injection:* 250 mcg, 500 mcg

Action/Kinetics: Sargramostim is a granulocyte-macrophage colony-stimulating factor (rhu GM-CSF) that is produced by recombinant DNA technology in a yeast expression system. GM-CSF stimulates the proliferation and differentiation of hematopoietic progenitor cells. It stimulates partially committed progenitor cells to divide and differentiate in the granulocyte-macrophage pathways. Division, maturation, and activation are induced through GM-CSF binding to specific receptors located on the surface of target cells. GM-CSF can also activate mature granulocytes and macrophages. Sargramostim increases the cytotoxicity of monocytes toward certain neoplastic cell lines as well as activates polymorphonuclear neutrophils, thus inhibiting the growth of tumor cells. Sargramostim differs from the naturally occurring GM-CSF by one amino acid and by a different carbohydrate moiety. **Peak levels:** 2 hr. **t½, alpha half-life:** 12–17 min; **beta half-life:** 2 hr. Neutralizing antibodies have been detected in a small number of clients.

Uses: Increased myeloid recovery in clients with non-Hodgkin's lymphoma, acute lymphoblastic leukemia, and Hodgkin's disease undergoing autologous bone marrow transplantation. Bone marrow transplantation failure or engraftment delay. *Investigational:* To increase WBC counts in clients with myelodysplastic syndrome and in AIDS clients taking AZT; to correct neutropenia in clients with aplastic anemia; to decrease the nadir of leukopenia secondary to myelosuppressive chemotherapy and to decrease myelosuppression in preleukemic clients; and to decrease organ system damage following transplantation, especially in the liver and kidney.

Dosage

• **IV infusion**

Myeloid reconstitution after autologous bone marrow transplantation.
250 mcg/m²/day for 21 days as a 2-hr infusion beginning 2–4 hr after the autologous bone marrow infusion.

Bone marrow transplantation failure or engraftment delay.
250 mcg/m²/day for 14 days as a 2-hr IV infusion. If engraftment has not occurred, therapy may be repeated after 7 days off therapy. A third course of 250 mcg/m²/day may be undertaken after another 7 days off therapy. However, if no response occurs after three courses, it is unlikely the drug will be beneficial.

Administration/Storage

1. Daily dosage should be given as a 2-hr IV infusion beginning 2–4 hr after the autologous bone marrow infusion making sure at least 24 hr have elapsed after the last dose of chemo-

therapy and 12 hr have elapsed since the last dose of radiotherapy.
2. The dose should be reduced or temporarily terminated if severe adverse reactions occur; therapy may be continued once the reactions abate.
3. The lyophilized powder is reconstituted with 1 mL of sterile water for injection without preservatives. The sterile water should be directed at the side of the vial, followed by a gentle swirling of the contents to avoid foaming. Excessive or vigorous agitation should be avoided.
4. Reconstituted solutions are clear, colorless, and isotonic with a pH of 7.4.
5. The vial should not be reentered or reused, and any unused portion should be discarded.
6. Dilution for IV infusion should be with 0.9% sodium chloride injection. If the final concentration is less than 10 mcg/mL, human albumin should be added at a final concentration of 0.1% to the saline before sargramostim is added, to prevent adsorption to the components of the drug delivery system.
7. Since sargramostim contains no preservatives, it should be given as soon as possible, but within 6 hr, following reconstitution or dilution for IV infusion. Solutions can be stored in the refrigerator at 2°C–6°C (36°F–46°F).
8. Other drugs should not be added to infusion solutions containing sargramostim.
9. *Treatment of Overdose:* Discontinue therapy. Monitor for increases in WBCs and for respiratory symptoms.

Contraindications: More than 10% leukemic myeloid blasts in the bone marrow or peripheral blood. Known hypersensitivity to GM-CSF, yeast-derived products, or any component of the product. Use within 24 hr preceding or following chemotherapy or within 12 hr preceding or following radiotherapy.

Special Concerns: Use with caution in clients with preexisting cardiac disease and hypoxia and during lactation. Safety and effectiveness have not been determined in children although it appears the drug is no more toxic in children than in adults. The drug may aggravate fluid retention in clients with preexisting peripheral edema, or pleural or pericardial effusion. Insufficient data are available to support the effectiveness of sargramostim in increasing myeloid recovery after peripheral blood stem cell transplantation. It is possible that sargramostim can act as a growth factor for any tumor type, especially myeloid malignancies; thus, use with caution in any malignancy with myeloid characteristics.

Side Effects: *Body as a whole:* Fever (most common), mucous membrane disorder, asthenia, malaise, edema, peripheral edema, sepsis, headache. *GI:* Most commonly nausea, diarrhea, vomiting. Also, anorexia, GI disorder, ***GI hemorrhage,*** stomatitis. *Dermatologic:* Alopecia, rashes. *Respiratory:* Dyspnea, lung disorder. *GU:* Urinary tract disorder, abnormal kidney function. *Miscellanous:* Liver damage, blood dyscrasias, ***hemorrhage,*** CNS disorders, myalgia, arthralgia.

Symptoms of Overdose: Dyspnea, malaise, nausea, fever, rash, sinus tachycardia, chills, headache.

Drug Interactions: Drugs such as corticosteroids and lithium may ↑ the myeloproliferative effects of sargramostim.

NURSING CONSIDERATIONS

Assessment

1. Determine any sensitivity to yeast-derived products or cardiac history.
2. Document indications for therapy and type and onset of symptoms.
3. Obtain baseline CBC and liver and renal function studies.
4. Document any therapy with drugs or radiation. Drug should *not* be administered 24 hr preceding or following chemotherapy or within 12

hr preceding or following radiation therapy.

Interventions

1. Monitor I&O, VS, and weight. Observe for evidence of fluid retention or edema.
2. Carefully monitor for respiratory symptoms during or immediately following infusion, especially in clients with preexisting lung disease. In the event of dyspnea during administration, the rate of infusion should be reduced by one-half.
3. Monitor CBC and platelet count. The hematologic response to sargramostim can be detected by a CBC performed twice weekly. If the absolute neutrophil count exceeds 20,000/mm^3 or if the platelet count exceeds 500,000/mm^3, therapy should be stopped and the dose reduced by one-half. The decision to reduce the dose should be based on the clinical condition of the client. Excessive blood counts have returned to normal levels within 3–7 days following termination of therapy.
4. Renal and hepatic function should be monitored every 2 weeks in clients who have hepatic or renal dysfunction.
5. Drug effectiveness may be limited in clients who, before autologous bone marrow transplantation, received extensive radiotherapy in the chest or abdomen to treat the primary disease; effectiveness is also limited in clients who have received multiple myelotoxic agents such as antimetabolites, alkylating agents, or anthracycline antibiotics.

Evaluate

- Inhibition of tumor cell growth
- Improved hematologic parameters with ↑granulocytes, monocytes, and macrophages

CHAPTER EIGHTY-ONE

Vaccines

General Statement: Vaccines have played an important role in the health and life span of our population. They have been in use over 200 years, but since World War II, once the importance of disease prevention became evident, research into the area of vaccine development exploded.

Use of a vaccine (or actually contracting the disease) usually renders one temporary or permanent resistance to an infectious disease. Vaccines and toxoids promote the type of antibody production one would see if they had experienced the natural infection. This active immunization involves the direct administration of antigens to the host to cause them to produce the desired antibodies and cell-mediated immunity. These agents may consist of live attenuated agents or killed (inactivated) agents. Immunizations confer this resistance without actually producing the disease.

Passive immunization occurs when immunologic agents are administered. Immunoglobulins and antivenins only offer passive short-term immunity and are usually administered for a specific exposure.

Aggressive pediatric immunization programs have helped reduce preventable infections and death in children worldwide. This focus should continue and be expanded to the adult population, many of whom have missed the natural infection and their past immunizations. A careful immunization history should be documented for every client, regardless of age. Table 2, pp. 1232-1233, lists some of the more common diseases, the general recommended schedule to confer immunization, and the length of immunity conferred; Table 3, pp. 1234, outlines the active childhood immunization schedule.

Table 2 Common Diseases, General Recommended Immunization Schedule, and Length of Immunity

DISEASE	IMMUNIZATION SCHEDULE	LENGTH OF IMMUNITY
Cholera	Two doses 1 week to 1 month apart	6 months
Diphtheria	Given as DPT; four doses at ages 2, 4, 6, and 15–18 months	10 years
Haemophilus influenzae (Hib)	Four doses at ages 2, 4, 6, and 15 months	Unknown
Hepatitis B	Three doses: at birth (or initial dose), 1 month, and 6 months or more after second dose	10 years
Influenza	One dose (or two doses of split virus if under 13 years)	1–3 years
Measles	Given as MMR at ages 12–15 months and 4–6 years	Lifetime
Meningococcal meningitis	One dose (antibody response requires 5 days); antibiotic prophylaxis (Rifampin 600 mg or 10 mg/kg q 12 hr for four doses should be given to all contacts)	?Lifetime; not consistently effective in those < 2 years of age
Mumps	Given as MMR at ages 12–15 months and 4–6 years	Lifetime
Pertussis	Given as DPT; four doses at ages 2, 4, 6, and 15–18 months	10 years
Pneumococcus	One dose (0.5 mL)	Approx. 5 years
Poliomyelitis	Four doses at ages 2, 4, and 6 months, then at age 4–6 years	Lifetime

(continued)

Table 2 *(continued)*

DISEASE	IMMUNIZATION SCHEDULE	LENGTH OF IMMUNITY
Rabies	Postexposure: five doses on days 0, 3, 7, 14, and 28 with the rabies immuneglobulin; pre-exposure: two doses 1 week apart, third dose 2–3 weeks later	Approx. 2 years
Rubella	Given as MMR at ages 12–15 months and 4–6 years	Lifetime
Smallpox	One dose; this disease has been eradicated and vaccine is used only with military personnel and lab workers using pox viruses	3 years
Tetanus	Given initially as DPT; four doses at ages 2, 4, 6, and 15–18 months	10 years; a tetanus booster is required q 10 years
VZV (varicellazoster virus; chicken pox)	One dose (0.5 mL) age 12 months to 12 years; two injections of 0.5 mL 4–8 weeks apart in age 13 and older	?Lifetime
Yellow fever	One dose	10 years

Table 3 Active Childhood Immunization Schedule

	#1	#2	#3	#4
DPT	2 months	4 months	6 months	15–18 months
OPV	2 months	4 months	6 months	4–6 years
Hib	2 months	4 months	6 months	15–18 months
MMR	12 months	4 years		
Hep B	birth	1 month	6 months or more after second dose	

Miscellaneous Drug Categories

CHAPTER EIGHTY-TWO

Antigout Drugs

See the following individual entries:

Allopurinol
Probenecid
Sulfinpyrazone

Allopurinol

(al-oh-**PYOUR**-ih-nohl)
Pregnancy Category: C
Apo-Allopurinol ✱, Purinol ✱, Zyloprim **(Rx)**

How Supplied: *Tablet:* 100 mg, 300 mg

Action/Kinetics: Allopurinol and its major metabolite, oxipurinol, are potent inhibitors of xanthine oxidase, an enzyme involved in the synthesis of uric acid, without disrupting the biosynthesis of essential purine. This results in decreased levels of uric acid. The drug also increases reutilization of xanthine and hypoxanthine for synthesis of nucleotide and nucleic acid synthesis by acting on the enzyme hypoxanthine-guanine phosphoribosyltransferase. The resultant increases in nucleotides cause a negative feedback to inhibit synthesis of purines and a decrease in uric acid levels. **Peak plasma levels:** 1.5 hr for allopurinol and 4.5 hr for oxipurinol. **Onset:** 2–3 days. **t½** (allopurinol); 1–3 hr; **t½** (oxipurinol): 12–30 hr. **Peak serum levels, allopurinol:** 2–3 mcg/mL; **oxipurinol:** 5–6.5 mcg/mL (up to 50 mcg/mL in clients with impaired renal function). **Maximum therapeutic effect:** 1–3 weeks. Well absorbed from GI tract, metabolized in liver, excreted in urine and feces (20%).

Uses: Primary or secondary gout (acute attacks, tophi, joint destruction, nephropathy, uric acid lithiasis). Clients with leukemia, lymphoma, or other malignancies in whom drug therapy causes elevations of serum and urinary uric acid. Recurrent calcium oxalate calculi. *Investigational:* Mixed with methylcellulose as a mouthwash to prevent stomatitis following fluorouracil administration.

Dosage

- **Tablets**

Gout/hyperuricemia.

Adults: 200–600 mg/day, depending on severity (minimum effective dose: 100–200 mg/day). Maximum daily dose should not exceed 800 mg.

Prevention of uric acid nephropathy during treatment of neoplasms.

Adults: 600–800 mg/day for 2–3 days (with high fluid intake).

Prophylaxis of acute gout.

Initial: 100 mg/day; increase by 100 mg at weekly intervals until serum uric acid level of 6 mg/100 mL or less is reached.

Hyperuricemia associated with malignancy.

Pediatric, 6–10 years of age: 300 mg/day either as a single dose of 100 mg t.i.d.; **under 6 years of age:** 150 mg/day in three divided doses.

Recurrent calcium oxalate calculi.

200–300 mg/day in one or more doses (dose may be adjusted according to urinary levels of uric acid).

Administration/Storage

1. Administer with food or immediately after meals to lessen potential gastric irritation.
2. At least 10–12 8-oz glasses of fluid should be taken each day.
3. To prevent the formation of uric acid stones, the urine should be kept slightly alkaline.
4. Transfer from colchicine, uricosuric agents, and/or anti-inflammatory agents to allopurinol should be made gradually by decreasing the dosage of the above agents and increasing the dosage of allopurinol until a normal serum uric acid level is achieved.

Contraindications: Hypersensitivity to drug. Clients with idiopathic hemochromatosis or relatives of clients suffering from this condition. Children except as an adjunct in treatment of neoplastic disease. Severe skin reactions on previous exposure.

Special Concerns: Use with caution during lactation. Use with caution in clients with liver or renal disease. In children use has been limited to rare inborn errors of purine metabolism or hyperuricemia as a result of malignancy or cancer therapy.

Laboratory Test Interferences: ↑ ALT, AST, alkaline phosphatase. ↑ Serum cholesterol. ↓ Serum glucose levels.

Side Effects: *Dermatologic* (most frequent): Pruritic maculopapular skin rash (may be accompanied by fever and malaise). Exfoliative urticarial, purpura-type dermatitis and alopecia. ***Stevens-Johnson syndrome.*** Skin rash has been accompanied by hypertension and cataract development. *Allergy:* Fever, chills, leukopenia, eosinophilia, arthralgia, skin rash, pruritus, N&V, nephritis. *GI:* N&V, diarrhea, gastritis, dyspepsia, abdominal pain (intermittent). *Hematologic:* Leukopenia, eosinophilia, thrombocytopenia, leukocytosis. *Hepatic:* Hepatomegaly, cholestatic jaundice, ***hepatic necrosis,*** granulomatous hepatitis. *Neurologic:* Headache, peripheral neuropathy, paresthesia, somnolence, neuritis. *CV:* Necrotizing angiitis, hypersensitivity vasculitis. *Miscellaneous:* Ecchymosis, epistaxis, taste loss, arthralgia, acute attacks of gout, fever, myopathy, renal failure, uremia, alopecia.

Drug Interactions

ACE inhibitors / ↑ Risk of hypersensitivity reactions

Aluminum salts / ↓ Effect of allopurinol

Ampicillin / ↑ Risk of ampicillin-induced skin rashes

Anticoagulants, oral / ↑ Effect of anticoagulant due to ↓ breakdown by liver

Azathioprine / ↑ Effect of azathioprine due to ↓ breakdown by liver

Cyclophosphamide / ↑ Risk of bleeding or infection due to ↑ myelosuppressive effects of cyclophosphamide

Iron preparations / Allopurinol ↑ hepatic iron concentrations

Mercaptopurine / ↑ Effect of mercaptopurine due to ↓ breakdown by liver

Theophylline / Allopurinol ↑ plasma theophylline levels → possible toxicity

Thiazide diuretics / ↑ Risk of hypersensitivity reactions to allopurinol

Uricosuric agents / ↓ Effect of oxipurinol due to ↑ rate of excretion

NURSING CONSIDERATIONS

Assessment

1. Take a complete drug history, noting any medications that may interact unfavorably.
2. Document indications for therapy and type and onset of symptoms.

3. If female and of childbearing age, or if the woman is nursing, allopurinol is contraindicated.
4. Determine any history of idiopathic hemochromatosis as drug is contraindicated.

Interventions

1. Assess for changes in vision. If changes occur, schedule an ophthalmologic exam.
2. Monitor CBC, platelet count, liver and renal function studies, and serum uric acid on a routine basis during therapy.
3. Dosage should be decreased with renal impairment.

Client/Family Teaching

1. Take medication at or following meal time to decrease GI upset.
2. Advise client to monitor weight if experiencing N&V or other signs of gastric irritation. Report if persistent and weight loss is evident.
3. Skin rashes may start after months of drug therapy. Report because if they are caused by allopurinol, the drug needs to be discontinued.
4. Unless contraindicated, advise to maintain a fluid intake that will result in a minimum excretion of 2 L of urine daily. This will assist to prevent stone formation.
5. Do not take iron salts while taking allopurinol as high concentrations of iron may occur in the liver.
6. Avoid excessive intake of vitamin C, which may lead to increased potential for the formation of kidney stones.
7. Avoid alcoholic beverages. These decrease the effect of allopurinol.
8. Provide a printed list of foods high in purine to avoid. These may include sardines, roe, scallops, anchovies, organ meats, and mincemeat.
9. Minimize exposure to ultraviolet light because of the increased risk of cataracts.

Evaluate

- ↓ Serum and urinary uric acid levels
- ↓ Frequency of gout attacks
- Inhibition of stomatitis following fluorouracil therapy

Probenecid

(proh-**BEN**-ih-sid)
Benemid, Probalan **(Rx)**

How Supplied: *Tablet:* 500 mg
Action/Kinetics: Probenecid, a uricosuric agent, increases the excretion of uric acid by inhibiting the tubular reabsorption of uric acid; this action results in a decreased serum level of uric acid. Probenecid also inhibits the renal secretion of penicillins and cephalosporins; this effect is often taken advantage of in the treatment of infections because concomitant administration of probenecid will increase plasma levels of antibiotics. **Peak plasma levels:** 2–4 hr. **Time to peak effect, uricosuric:** 0.5 hr; **for suppression of penicillin excretion:** 2 hr. **Therapeutic plasma levels for inhibition of antibiotic secretion:** 40–60 mcg/mL; **therapeutic plasma levels for uricosuric effect:** 100–200 mcg/mL. **t½:** approximately 5–8 hr. **Duration for inhibition of penicillin excretion:** 8 hr. Probenecid is metabolized in the liver to active metabolites and is excreted in urine (5%–10% unchanged). Excretion is increased in alkaline urine.
Uses: Hyperuricemia in chronic gout and gouty arthritis. Adjunct in therapy with penicillins or cephalosporins to elevate and prolong plasma antibiotic levels.

Dosage

- **Tablets**

Gout.

Adults, initial: 250 mg b.i.d. for 1 week. **Maintenance:** 500 mg b.i.d. Dosage may have to be increased further (by 500 mg/day/ q 4 weeks to maximum of 2 g) until urate excretion is less than 700 mg in 24 hr. Colbenemid, a combination tablet containing colchicine (0.5 mg) and probenecid (500 mg), is available.

Adjunct to penicillin or cephalosporin therapy.

Adults: 500 mg q.i.d. Dosage is decreased for elderly clients with renal damage. **Pediatric, 2–14 years, in-**

itial: 25 mg/kg (or 700 mg/m²); **maintenance,** 10 mg/kg q.i.d. (or 300 mg/m² q.i.d.). **For children 50 kg or more:** give adult dosage.

Gonorrhea.

Adults: 1 g (as a single dose) 30 min before 4.8 million units of penicillin G procaine aqueous; **pediatric, less than 45 kg:** 25 mg/kg (up to a maximum of 1 g) with appropriate antibiotic therapy.

Contraindications: Hypersensitivity to drug, blood dyscrasias, uric acid, and kidney stones. Use for hyperuricemia in neoplastic disease or its treatment. Not recommended for use in children less than 2 years of age.

Special Concerns: Use during pregnancy only if benefits clearly outweigh risks. Administer with caution to clients with renal disease. Use with caution in porphyria, G6PD deficiency, and peptic ulcer.

Side Effects: *CNS:* Headaches, dizziness. *GI:* Anorexia, N&V, diarrhea, constipation, and abdominal discomfort. *Allergic:* Skin rash or drug fever and ***rarely anaphylaxis.*** *GU:* Nephrotic syndrome, uric acid stones with or without hematuria, urinary frequency, renal colic. *Miscellaneous:* Hypersensitivity reactions (dermatitis, pruritus, fever, ***anaphylaxis***), flushing, ***hemolytic anemia,*** sore gums, ***hepatic necrosis, aplastic anemia,*** costovertebral pain.

Initially, the drug may increase frequency of acute gout attacks due to mobilization of uric acid.

Drug Interactions

Acyclovir / Probenecid ↓ renal excretion of acyclovir
Allopurinol / Additive effects to ↓ uric acid serum levels
AZT / ↑ Bioavailability of AZT
Captopril / ↑ Effect of captopril due to ↓ excretion by kidney
Cephalosporins / ↑ Effect of cephalosporins due to ↓ excretion by kidney
Ciprofloxacin / 50% ↑ in systemic levels of ciprofloxacin
Clofibrate / ↑ Effect of clofibrate due to ↓ excretion and ↓ plasma protein binding
Dapsone / ↑ Effect of dapsone
Dyphylline / ↑ Effect of dyphylline due to ↓ excretion by kidney
Indomethacin / ↑ Effect of indomethacin due to ↓ excretion by kidney
Methotrexate / ↑ Effect of methotrexate due to ↓ excretion by kidney
NSAIDs / ↑ Effect of NSAIDs due to ↓ excretion by kidney
PAS / ↑ Effects of PAS due to ↓ excretion by kidney
Penicillins / ↑ Effect of penicillins due to ↓ excretion by kidney
Pyrazinamide / Probenecid inhibits hyperuricemia produced by pyrazinamide
Rifampin / ↑ Effect of rifampin due to ↓ excretion by kidney
Salicylates / Salicylates inhibit uricosuric activity of probenecid
Sulfinpyrazone / ↑ Effect of sulfinpyrazone due to ↓ excretion by kidney
Sulfonamides / ↑ Effect of sulfonamides due to ↓ plasma protein binding
Sulfonylureas, oral / ↑ Action of sulfonylureas → hypoglycemia
Thiopental / ↑ Effect of thiopental

NURSING CONSIDERATIONS

Assessment

1. Document indications for therapy and type and onset of symptoms.
2. Determine any evidence of PUD, G6PD deficiency, uricemia R/T neoplastic disease, kidney stones, or blood dyscrasia.

Interventions

1. Anticipate that sodium bicarbonate may be used to maintain an alkaline urine to prevent urates from crystallizing and forming kidney stones.
2. Use a glucose oxidase method (Tes-Tape or Keto-Diastix) for urine glucose determinations in clients with diabetes mellitus; finger sticks may be more accurate. Drug may increase hypoglycemic effects of oral antidiabetic agents.
3. Promptly report any gastric intolerance so that dosage may be corrected without loss of therapeutic effect.

4. Be alert to hypersensitivity reactions that occur more frequently with intermittent therapy.
5. Assess for toxic plasma antibiotic levels if excretion is inhibited by probenecid. Make appropriate dosage adjustments.
6. Observe client for skin rash, flushing, or complaints of increased sweating, headaches, or dizziness and report if evident.
7. Monitor CBC and liver and renal function studies on a regular basis and report any abnormal findings.

Client/Family Teaching

1. Take with food or milk to minimize gastric irritation.
2. Take a liberal amount of fluid (2.5–3 L/day) to prevent the formation of sodium urate stones. Avoid cranberry juice or vitamin C preparations, which acidify urine.
3. Advise that acute gout attacks may initially be more frequent due to mobilization of uric acid. Instruct client to report any increase in the number of acute attacks of gout at the initiation of therapy since colchicine may need to be added to the regimen.
4. Continue to take probenecid during acute attacks along with colchicine unless otherwise specified.
5. Report any unexplained fever, fatigue, skin rash, or persistent GI upset.
6. Do not take salicylates or use caffeine or alcohol during uricosuric therapy. Acetaminophen preparations may be used for analgesic purposes.

Evaluate

- ↓ Serum uric acid level
- ↓ Joint pain and swelling
- ↓ Frequency of acute gout attacks
- Evidence of elevated and prolonged plasma antibiotic (penicillins or cephalosporins) levels
- Therapeutic serum drug levels for designated effect

Sulfinpyrazone

(sul-fin-**PEER**-ah-zohn)
Anturane, Apo-Sulfinpyrazone ✱, Novo-Pyrazone ✱ **(Rx)**

How Supplied: *Capsule:* 200 mg; *Tablet:* 100 mg

Action/Kinetics: Sulfinpyrazone inhibits the tubular reabsorption of uric acid, thereby increasing its excretion. Sulfinpyrazone also manifests antithrombotic and platelet inhibitory actions. **Peak plasma levels:** 1–2 hr. **Therapeutic plasma levels:** Up to 160 mcg/mL following 800 mg/day for uricosuria. **Duration:** 4–6 hr (up to 10 hr in some). **t½:** 3–8 hr. Sulfinpyrazone is metabolized by the liver. Approximately 45% of the drug is excreted unchanged by the kidney, and a small amount is excreted in the feces.

Uses: Chronic gouty arthritis to reduce frequency and intensity of acute attacks of gout; hyperuricemia. Sulfinpyrazone is not effective during acute attacks of gout and may even increase the frequency of acute episodes during the initiation of therapy. However, the drug should not be discontinued during acute attacks. Concomitant administration of colchicine during initiation of therapy is recommended. *Investigational:* To decrease sudden death during first year after MI.

Dosage

- **Capsules, Tablets**

Gout.

Adults, initial: 200–400 mg/day in two divided doses with meals or milk. Clients who are transferred from other uricosuric agents can receive full dose at once. **Maintenance:** 100–400 mg b.i.d. Maintain full dosage without interruption even during acute attacks of gout.

Following MI.

Adults: 300 mg q.i.d. or 400 mg b.i.d.

Administration/Storage

1. At least ten to twelve 8-oz glasses of fluid should be taken daily.
2. If GI upset occurs, medication should be taken with food, milk, or antacids.
3. Acidification of the urine may cause formation of uric acid stones.

4. *Treatment of Overdose:* Supportive measures.
Contraindications: Active peptic ulcer. Blood dyscrasias. Sensitivity to phenylbutazone or other pyrazoles.
Special Concerns: Use with caution in pregnant women. Dosage has not been established in children. Use with extreme caution in clients with impaired renal function and in those with a history of peptic ulcers.
Side Effects: *GI:* N&V, abdominal discomfort. May reactivate peptic ulcer. *Hematologic:* Leukopenia, ***agranulocytosis,*** anemia, thrombocytopenia, ***aplastic anemia.*** *Miscellaneous:* Skin rash (which usually disappears with usage), ***bronchoconstriction in aspirin-induced asthma.*** Acute attacks of gout may become more frequent during initial therapy. Give concomitantly with colchicine at this time.

Symptoms of Overdose: N&V, diarrhea, epigastric pain, labored respiration, ataxia, seizures, coma.

Drug Interactions
Acetaminophen / ↑ Risk of acetaminophen hepatotoxicity; ↓ effect of acetaminophen
Anticoagulants / ↑ Effect of anticoagulants due to ↓ plasma protein binding
Insulin / Potentiation of hypoglycemic effect
Niacin / ↓ Uricosuric effect of sulfinpyrazone
Probenecid / ↑ Effect of sulfinpyrazone due to ↓ excretion by kidney
Salicylates / Inhibit uricosuric effect of sulfinpyrazone
Sulfonamides / ↑ Effect of sulfonamides by ↓ plasma protein binding
Sulfonylureas, oral / Potentiation of hypoglycemic effect
Theophylline / ↓ Effect of theophylline due to ↑ plasma clearance
Verapamil / ↓ Effect of verapamil due to ↑ plasma clearance

NURSING CONSIDERATIONS

Client/Family Teaching
1. Take with meals, milk, or an antacid to minimize gastric irritation.
2. Take a liberal amount of fluid (2.5–3 L/day) to prevent the formation of uric acid stones. Avoid cranberry juice or vitamin C preparations as these acidify urine.
3. Explain that sodium bicarbonate may be ordered to alkalinize the urine. This is to prevent urates from crystallizing in acid urine and forming kidney stones.
4. Avoid alcohol and aspirin because they interfere with drug effectiveness.
5. Advise that during *acute* attacks of gout concomitant administration of colchicine is indicated.

Evaluate
- ↓ Frequency and intensity of gout attacks
- ↓ Serum uric acid levels

CHAPTER EIGHTY-THREE

Drugs Used For Topical Conditions

See the following individual entries:

Capsaicin
Collagenase
Etretinate
Isotretinoin
Masoprocol
Minoxidil, Topical Solution
Podofilox
Tretinoin (Retinoic acid, Vitamin A acid)

Capsaicin

(kap-**SAY**-ih-sin)
Axsain ✱, Zostrix, Zostrix-HP **(Rx)**

How Supplied: *Cream* 0.025%, 0.075%; *Lotion:* 0.025%, 0.075%
Action/Kinetics: Capsaicin is derived from natural sources from plants of the Solanaceae family. It is believed the drug depletes and prevents the reaccumulation of substance P, thought to be the main mediator of pain impulses from the periphery to the CNS.
Uses: Temporary relief of pain due to rheumatoid arthritis and osteoarthritis. Pain following herpes zoster (shingles), painful diabetic neuropathy. *Investigational:* Possible use in psoriasis, vitiligo, intractable pruritus, reflex sympathetic dystrophy, postmastectomy, vulvar vestibulitis, apocrine chromhidrosis, and post-amputation and postmastectomy neuroma.

Dosage

- **Cream, 0.025% or 0.075%**

Adults and children over 2 years of age: Apply to affected area no more than 3–4 times/day.

Special Concern: The drug is for external use only.
Side Effects: *Skin:* Transient burning following application, stinging, erythema. *Respiratory:* Cough, respiratory irritation.

NURSING CONSIDERATIONS
Client/Family Teaching
1. Advise that the drug is for external use only.
2. Avoid getting the medication in the eyes or on broken or irritated skin.
3. If applying the medication with the fingers, wash hands immediately after application.
4. Do not bandage the affected area tightly.
5. Report if the condition worsens, if symptoms persist more than 14–28 days, or if the symptoms clear but then recur within a few days.
Evaluate: Relief of pain.

Collagenase

(koh-**LAJ**-eh-nace)
Biozyme-C, Santyl **(Rx)**

How Supplied: *Ointment:* 250 U/g
Action/Kinetics: Collagenase digests collagen, which accounts for 75% of the dry weight of skin; thus, it is effective to remove tissue debris. Collagenase assists in the formation of granulation tissue and subsequent epithelialization of dermal ulcers and severely burned areas. The drug may also reduce the incidence of hypertrophic scarring. Collagen in healthy tissue or newly formed granulation is not affected.

Uses: Reduces pus, odor, necrosis, and inflammation in chronic dermal ulcers and severely burned areas.

Dosage

- **Ointment**

Chronic dermal ulcers, burns.

Apply once daily (more frequently if the dressing becomes soiled).

Administration/Storage

1. If any of the agents listed under drug interactions have been used, the area should be cleaned thoroughly with repeated washings using NSS before collagenase ointment is applied.
2. Before applying the ointment, the site should be cleansed of debris and other material by gently rubbing with a gauze pad saturated with hydrogen peroxide or Dakin's solution followed by sterile NSS.
3. If infection is present, a topical antibiotic powder should be applied to the lesion before collagenase is applied. If the infection does not respond, collagenase therapy should be discontinued until the infection is in remission.
4. Apply collagenase ointment to deep lesions using a wooden tongue depressor or spatula; for shallow lesions, a sterile gauze pad may be applied to the area and then properly secured.
5. Crosshatching thick eschar with a #10 blade allows more surface area for the collagenase to come in contact with necrotic tissue. Remove as much loosened debris as possible with forceps and scissors.
6. All excess ointment should be removed each time the dressing is changed.
7. Collagenase ointment therapy should be terminated when debridement of necrotic tissue is complete and granulation tissue is well established.
8. The action of the enzyme may be stopped by applying Burrow's solution (pH 3.6–4.4) to the lesion.

Contraindications: Local or systemic hypersensitivity to collagenase.

Side Effects: No allergic sensitivity or toxic reactions have been noted.

Drug Interactions: Detergents, benzalkonium chloride, hexachlorophene, nitrofurazone, tincture of iodine, and certain heavy metal ions used in some antiseptics (e.g., mercury, silver) inhibit the activity of collagenase.

NURSING CONSIDERATIONS

Assessment

1. Document underlying cause and describe area of tissue disruption.
2. Assess area to be treated noting wound size, depth, color, presence of eschar, any evidence of drainage, swelling, or odor and document.

Client/Family Teaching

1. Review the appropriate method for tissue preparation (described under *Administration*) and demonstrate collagenase application. Observe a return demonstration to generate questions and to assess for problems in administration.
2. Explain the importance of frequent position changes, methods to reduce pressure to bony prominences, proper body alignment, proper skin care, adequate nutrition, and clean, dry linens in the overall goal to reduce the size and spread of the disrupted tissue, whether from an ulcer or from a burn.
3. Stress the importance of returning for follow-up evaluations to determine the effectiveness of prescribed therapy.

Evaluate

- Formation of new granulation tissue
- Wound reepithelialization

Etretinate

(eh-**TRET**-ih-nayt)
Pregnancy Category: X
Tegison **(Rx)**

How Supplied: *Capsule:* 10 mg, 25 mg

Action/Kinetics: Etretinate is related to vitamin A; it acts to decrease the thickness, erythema, and scale of lesions in individuals with psoriasis. The drug may act to reduce cell proliferation by inhibiting ornithine decarboxylase; this is the rate-limiting enzyme in polyamine production which is responsible for regulating cell growth, proliferation, and differentiation. The drug may also inhibit migration of neutrophils into the epidermis. Significant first-pass metabolism occurs to the active acid form of the drug. The ingestion of milk or a high-lipid diet increases the absorption of etretinate. Has a long half-life due to storage in adipose tissue. The drug has been found in the blood of certain clients up to 3 years after therapy was terminated. Etretinate itself is bound more than 99% to plasma lipoproteins, whereas the active acid metabolite is bound to albumin.

Uses: Severe recalcitrant psoriasis (including erythrodermic and generalized pustular types) unresponsive to psoralens plus UVA light, systemic corticosteroids, methotrexate, or topical tar plus UVB light. *Investigational:* Mycosis fungoides, actinic keratoses, arsenical keratoses, basal cell carcinoma, bronchial metaplasia, genodermatosis, pustular bacterids, cutaneous lupus erythematosus, and hyperkeratotic eczemas of the palms and soles.

Dosage

- **Capsules**

  Psoriasis.

Adults, initial: 0.75–1 mg/kg/day in divided doses, not to exceed 1.5 mg/kg/day. **Maintenance:** 0.5–0.75 mg/kg/day, usually after 8–16 weeks of therapy.

Erythrodermic psoriasis.

Initial: 0.25 mg/kg/day; **then,** increase by 0.25 mg/kg/day each week until optimum response has been obtained.

Administration/Storage

1. Individualization of dosage is required to achieve maximal therapeutic effects with a tolerable degree of side effects.
2. Lesions may require up to 9 months of therapy to be completely cleared.
3. The drug should be administered with food.
4. Most clients have relapses within 2 months after therapy is terminated. Subsequent courses of therapy, up to 9 months, result in a response similar to that achieved during the initial course of therapy.

Contraindications: Individuals who are pregnant, intend to become pregnant, or who are not using effective contraceptive measures while taking the drug. Lactation. Use in children unless other alternatives have been exhausted.

Laboratory Test Interferences: ↑ Triglycerides, AST, ALT, globulin, cholesterol, alkaline phosphatase, gamma-glutamyl transpeptidase, bilirubin, BUN, creatinine. ↑ or ↓ Total protein or albumin.

Side Effects: The toxic effects of etretinate resemble those of hypervitaminosis A. They include benign intracranial hypertension (pseudotumor cerebri); the symptoms include headache, N&V, papilledema, and visual disturbances. *CNS:* Fatigue, headache, fever, lethargy, pain, dizziness, rigors, amnesia, anxiety, abnormal thought processes, depression, emotional lability, faint feeling. *CV:* Edema, ***thrombotic or obstructive events,*** fainting, postural hypotension, chest pain, atrial fibrillation, phlebitis, ***coagulation disorder***. *GI:* GI pain, changes in appetite, nausea, constipation, flatulence, melena, diarrhea, alteration in taste, ulcers of mouth, tooth caries. *Hepatic:* Hepatitis. *Ophthalmic:* Eye irritation, eyeball pain, eyelid abnormalities, conjunctivitis, decreased visual acuity, double vision, abnormalities of the conjunctiva, cornea, lens, and retina; abnormalities of lacrimation, vision, extraocular musculature, ocular tension, pupil, and vitreous; decreased night vision, photophobia, vision change, scotoma; corneal erosion, abrasion, irregularity, and punctate staining. *Dermatologic:* Peeling of soles, palms, fingertips; loss of hair, itching, rash, dry skin, skin fragility, red scaly face, bruising, sunburn, cold clammy skin, bullous eruptions, onycholysis, changes in perspiration, paronychia, pyogenic granuloma, impaired healing, herpes simplex, hirsutism, abnormal skin odor, urticaria, granulation tissue, increased pore size, skin peeling, nail disorder. Skin atrophy, infection, fissures, nodules or ulceration. *Mucocutaneous:* Dry nose, chapped lips, thirst, sore mouth, nosebleed, cheilitis, sore tongue, dry eyes, mucous membrane abnormalities, dry mouth, gingival bleeding or inflammation, decreased mucous secretion, rhinorrhea. *Musculoskeletal:* Joint and bone pain, myalgia, muscle cramps, gout, ossification of interosseous ligaments and tendons of extremities, hyperkinesia, hypertonia. *Hematologic:* Significant alterations of platelets, reticulocytes, hemoglobin, WBCs, or PT. *GU:* Kidney stones; WBCs, proteins, glucose, acetone, blood, casts, or hemoglobin in the urine; dysuria, urinary retention, polyuria. Microscopic hematuria, abnormal menses, atrophic vaginitis. *Respiratory:* Dyspnea, coughing, increased sputum, dysphonia, pharyngitis. *Electrolyte disturbances:* Increased or decreased calcium, potassium, or phosphorus; increased or decreased venous CO_2, sodium, or chloride. *Otic:* Earache, otitis externa, changes in equilibrium, drainage or infection of ear, hearing change. *Other:* Increased CPK and malignant neoplasms, flu-like symptoms. Increased or decreased fasting blood sugar.

Drug Interaction: Not to be used with vitamin A as there may be additive toxic effects.

NURSING CONSIDERATIONS

Assessment

1. Document indications for therapy, other agents used, and the outcome.
2. Determine if female clients are sexually active and likely to become pregnant, prior to initiating therapy.
3. Ensure that women of childbearing age, who are to receive this medication, are using reliable forms of birth control.
4. Obtain pretreatment lipid profile under fasting conditions.

Client/Family Teaching

1. Take the medication with meals to avoid GI upset.
2. The ingestion of milk or a high-lipid diet increases the absorption of drug. Review dietary recommendations.
3. Clients may experience a worsening of psoriasis at the beginning of therapy.
4. Discuss with clients who wear contact lenses the fact that they may experience a decreased tolerance to contact lenses during and following therapy.
5. Provide a printed list of drug side effects. Report any symptoms that may indicate toxicity, such as headaches, N&V, dizziness, and visual disturbances.
6. Do not take vitamin A supplements during therapy since etretinate is similar to vitamin A.
7. Stress the importance of reporting for all lab tests.
8. Advise client not to donate blood during therapy and for several years thereafter due to the possible risks to a developing fetus if a pregnant client receives such blood.

Evaluate: Improvement in resistant psoriatic skin lesions.

Isotretinoin

(eye-so-**TRET**-ih-noyn)
Pregnancy Category: X
Accutane, Accutane Roche ✱, Isotrex ✱ **(Rx)**

How Supplied: *Capsule:* 10 mg, 20 mg, 40 mg

Action/Kinetics: Isotretinoin reduces sebaceous gland size, decreases sebum secretion, and inhibits abnormal keratinization. Approximately 25% of the PO dosage form is bioavailable. **Peak plasma levels:** 3 hr. **Steady-state blood levels following 80 mg/day:** 160 ng/mL. The drug is nearly 100% bound to plasma protein. **t½:** 10–20 hr. **Time to peak**

levels: 3 hr. Metabolized in the liver to 4-oxo-isotretinoin, which is also active. Approximately equal amounts are excreted through the urine and in the feces.

Uses: Severe recalcitrant nodular acne unresponsive to other therapy. *Investigational:* Cutaneous disorders of keratinization, leukoplakia, mycosis fungoides, prophylaxis of skin cancers in xeroderma pigmentosum, to prevent second primary tumors in clients treated for squamous-cell carcinoma.

Dosage

- **Capsules**

Recalcitrant cystic acne.

Adults, individualized, initial: 0.5–1 mg/kg/day (range: 0.5–2 mg/kg/day) divided in two doses for 15–20 weeks. Dose should be adjusted based on toxicity and clinical response; if cyst count decreases by 70% or more, drug may be discontinued. If necessary, a second course of therapy may be instituted after a rest period of 2 months. Doses of 0.05–0.5 mg/kg/day are effective but result in higher frequency of relapses.

Keratinization disorders.

Doses up to 4 mg/kg/day have been used.

Prophylaxis of skin cancer in xeroderma pigmentosum.

2 mg/kg/day.

Prevent second tumors in squamous-cell carcinoma of the head and neck.

50–100 mg/m^2.

Administration/Storage

1. Do not crush the drug.
2. To enhance absorption, administer the drug with meals.
3. Before using the drug, the client should complete a client consent form included with the package insert. Follow appropriate institutional guidelines for obtaining client consent.
4. If a second course of drug therapy is needed, the client should have a rest period of 2 months before it begins.

Contraindications: Due to the possibility of fetal abnormalities or spontaneous abortion, women who are pregnant or intend to become pregnant should not use the drug. Certain conditions for use should be met in women with childbearing potential (see package insert). Use during lactation and in children.

Special Concern: Intolerance to contact lenses may develop.

Laboratory Test Interferences: ↑ Plasma triglycerides, sedimentation rate, platelet counts, alkaline phosphatase, AST, ALT, GGTP, LDH, fasting serum glucose, uric acid in blood, cholesterol, CPK levels in clients who exercise vigorously. ↓ HDL, RBC parameters, WBC counts.

Side Effects: *Skin:* Cheilitis, skin fragility, pruritus, dry skin, desquamation of facial skin, drying of mucous membranes, brittle nails, photosensitivity, rash, hypo- or hyperpigmentation, urticaria, erythema nodosum, hirsutism, excess granulation of tissues as a result of healing, pruritus, petechiae, peeling of palms and soles, skin infections, paronychia, thinning of hair, nail dystrophy, pyogenic granuloma, bruising. *CNS:* Headache, fatigue, pseudotumor cerebri (i.e., headaches, papilledema, disturbances in vision), depression. *Ocular:* Conjunctivitis, optic neuritis, corneal opacities, dry eyes, decrease in acuity of night vision, photophobia, eyelid inflammation, cataracts, visual disturbances. *GI:* Dry mouth, N&V, abdominal pain, inflammatory bowel disease (including regional enteritis), anorexia, weight loss, inflammation and bleeding of gums. *Neuromuscular:* Arthralgia, muscle pain, bone and joint pain and stiffness, skeletal hyperostosis. *CV:* Flushing, palpitation, tachycardia. *GU:* White cells in urine, proteinuria, nonspecific urogenital findings, microscopic or gross hematuria, abnormal menses. *Other:* Epistaxis, dry nose and mouth, respiratory infections, disseminated herpes simplex, edema, transient chest pain, development of diabetes, hepatitis, vasculitis, anemia, lymphadenopathy.

Symptoms of Overdose: Abdominal pain, ataxia, cheilosis, dizziness, facial flushing, headache, vomiting. Symptoms are transient.

Drug Interactions

Alcohol / Potentiation of ↑ in serum triglycerides

Benzoyl peroxide / ↑ Drying effects of isotretinoin

Minocycline / ↑ Risk of development of pseudotumor cerebri or papilledema

Tetracycline / ↑ Risk of development of pseudotumor cerebri or papilledema

Tretinoin / ↑ Drying effects of isotretinoin

Vitamin A / ↑ Risk of toxicity

NURSING CONSIDERATIONS

Assessment

1. Note if the client is female and of childbearing age. Perform a pregnancy test on all sexually active women of childbearing age.
2. Take a complete drug history, noting those medications with which the drug interacts unfavorably.
3. Determine any other agents used for this condition and the outcome.
4. Obtain baseline serum glucose levels and liver function studies, especially lipoprotein, cholesterol, and triglycerides, and monitor throughout drug therapy.

Client/Family Teaching

1. Advise clients who receive isotretinoin to avoid donating blood for 30 days after the drug therapy has been discontinued.
2. Instruct females of childbearing age to practice some reliable form of birth control 1 month before, during, and 1 month following this drug therapy because severe fetal damage may occur.
3. Advise sexually active women that a pregnancy test will be performed monthly because drug is teratogenic.
4. Advise that only a 30-day prescription will be dispensed to ensure compliance.
5. Report immediately if a persistent headache, N&V, or visual disturbances develop.
6. Instruct clients who wear contact lenses that they may develop sensitivity to contacts during and after therapy. Excessively dry eyes may require an eye lubricant.
7. Explain that the condition may become worse before healing starts.
8. Avoid taking any OTC medications, especially vitamin A, without approval.
9. Eliminate or markedly reduce consumption of alcohol as it may increase triglyceride levels.
10. Avoid prolonged exposure to sunlight as the drug may cause photosensitivity. Wear protective clothing, sunscreen, and sunglasses when exposure is necessary.
11. Lubricants may assist to diminish symptoms of dry, chapped skin and lips.

Evaluate: ↓ Severity and number of cystic acne lesions.

Masoprocol

(mah-**SOH**-proh-kol)
Pregnancy Category: B
Actinex **(Rx)**

How Supplied: *Cream:* 10%

Action/Kinetics: Mechanism of action is unknown. Less than 1% is absorbed through the skin over a 4-day period following application.

Use: Actinic (solar) keratoses.

Dosage

- **Cream**

Following washing and drying areas where actinic keratoses are located, the drug should be gently massaged into the area, until it is evenly distributed, morning and evening for 28 days.

Administration/Storage

1. The drug is for external use only. Contact with the eyes should be avoided. Special care should be exercised if the drug must be applied near the eyes, nose, or mouth. If the drug comes in contact with the eyes, wash the eye promptly with water.
2. The client may experience a tran-

sient local burning sensation immediately after applying masoprocol.
3. If applied with the fingers, hands should be washed immediately after use.
4. Occlusive dressings should not be used.
5. Masoprocol cream may stain clothing or fabrics.
Contraindications: Hypersensitivity to masoprocol or other ingredients in the formulation. Use with an occlusive dressing.
Special Concerns: Use with caution during lactation. Safety and efficacy have not been determined in children. The presence or absence of local skin reactions does not correlate with effectiveness of the drug.
Side Effects: *Dermatologic:* Commonly, erythema, flaking, itching, dryness, edema, burning, soreness. Also, bleeding, crusting, eye irritation, oozing, rash, soreness, skin irritation, stinging, tightness, tingling, blistering, eczema, fissuring, leathery feeling to the skin, skin roughness, wrinkling, excoriation.

NURSING CONSIDERATIONS

Assessment

1. Determine any sulfite sensitivity as product contains sulfites. These may cause allergic-type reactions, especially in asthmatics or in atopic nonasthmatic clients.
2. Document symptoms and onset of skin disorder; list other treatments used and the outcome.

Client/Family Teaching

1. Review the proper method and frequency for administration using the following guidelines:
- Wash hands.
- Wash and dry involved area thoroughly.
- Apply masoprocol evenly and gently.
- Massage into area with actinic keratoses.
- Wash hands immediately after application.
- Avoid contact with eyes, nose, and mouth.
- Apply each morning and each evening for 28 days as directed.
- Do not cover treated areas with any type of occlusive dressing.
- Protect linens and clothing as cream may stain fabrics and clothing.
- Avoid all other skin products and makeup during therapy with masoprocol.

2. Advise that a local transient burning sensation may be experienced following topical application.
3. Local skin reactions are frequent; however, they usually resolve within 2 weeks of discontinuing therapy.
4. Discontinue drug and immediately report any evidence of a severe sensitivity reaction or severe external skin reaction characterized by blistering or oozing lesions.
5. Avoid undue sun exposure, especially since solar keratoses may be related to sun exposure.

Evaluate: ↓ Number and size of actinic lesions.

Minoxidil, topical solution

(mih-**NOX**-ih-dill)
Pregnancy Category: C
Rogaine **(Rx)**

How Supplied: *Solution:* 2%
Action/Kinetics: Minoxidil topical solution stimulates vertex hair growth in clients with male pattern baldness. The mechanism is unknown, but may be related to the fact that minoxidil dilates arterioles and stimulates resting hair follicles into active growth. PO minoxidil is used to treat hypertension and, when used systemically, is associated with a significant number of potential side effects. Following topical administration, approximately 1.4% is absorbed into the systemic circulation. **Onset:** 4 months but is variable. **Duration:** New hair growth may be lost 3–4 months after withdrawal of therapy. Minoxidil and its inactive metabolites are excreted in the urine.

Uses: To treat male and female pattern baldness (alopecia androgenetica). In males this is manifested by baldness of the vertex of the scalp and in females as thinning of the frontoparietal areas or diffuse hair loss. *Investigational:* Alopecia areata.

Dosage

- **Topical Solution**

Stimulate hair growth.

Adults: 1 mL of the 2% solution is applied to the affected area of the scalp in the morning and before bedtime. The total daily dose should not exceed 2 mL.

Administration/Storage

1. Only clients with normal, healthy scalps should use topical minoxidil. Dermatitis, scalp abrasions, scalp psoriasis, or severe sunburn may increase the absorption of topical minoxidil and lead to systemic side effects (See *Minoxidil, oral*).
2. Hair may be shampooed before treatment, but the hair and scalp should be dry prior to application of topical minoxidil.
3. The product comes with a metered spray attachment (for application to large areas of the scalp), extender spray attachment (for application to small scalp areas or under the hair), and a rub-on applicator tip (to spread the solution on the scalp). The directions on the package insert should be followed carefully for each of these methods of application.
4. If the fingertips are used to apply the drug, the hands should be washed thoroughly after application.
5. At least 4 months of continuous therapy is necessary before evidence of hair growth can be expected. Further hair growth continues through 1 year of treatment.
6. The alcohol base in topical minoxidil will cause irritation and burning of the eyes, abraded skin, or mucous membranes. If there is contact with any of these areas, wash the site with copious amounts of water.
7. The client should avoid inhaling the spray mist.

Contraindication: Lactation.

Special Concerns: Use with caution in clients with hypertension, coronary heart disease, or predisposition to heart failure. Safety and efficacy in clients under 18 years of age have not been determined. Increased systemic absorption may occur if the scalp is irritated or there are abrasions.

Side Effects: *Dermatologic:* Allergic contact dermatitis, irritant dermatitis, pruritus, dry skin, flaking of scalp, alopecia, hypertrichosis, erythema, worsening of hair loss. *Allergic:* Hives, facial swelling, allergic rhinitis. *CNS:* Dizziness, lightheadedness, headache, faintness, anxiety, depression, fatigue. *Respiratory:* Sinusitis, bronchitis, respiratory infection. *Miscellaneous:* Conjunctivitis, vertigo, decreased visual acuity, vertigo. *NOTE:* The incidence of side effects due to placebos is often similar to the incidence of side effects due to the drug itself.

Drug Interactions

Corticosteroids, topical / Enhance absorption of topical minoxidil
Guanethidine / Possible ↑ risk of orthostatic hypotension
Petrolatum / Enhances absorption of topical minoxidil
Retinoids / Enhance absorption of topical minoxidil

NURSING CONSIDERATIONS

Client/Family Teaching

1. Review appropriate method and frequency for application. Advise that solution may dry and leave a residue on the hair; this is harmless.
2. Advise that more frequent than prescribed applications will not enhance hair growth but will increase systemic side effects.
3. Advise the client that the new hair growth is not permanent. Stress that drug is a treatment, not a cure, and that cessation of therapy will lead to hair loss within a few months. Thus, the topical minoxidil must be used for an indefinite period of time.
4. Discuss the fact that the treatment has positive benefits for only ap-

proximately one-half the population. Assist the client to set realistic goals.
5. Explain that it may take up to 4 months of continuous therapy before any response is noted.
6. Report any evidence of irritation or rash at the site of treatment.
7. Do not apply any other topical products to the scalp without approval.
8. Stress that clients should be monitored 1 month after starting therapy and every 6 months thereafter for any systemic drug effects.
Evaluate: Evidence of hair regrowth in a previously bald scalp area.

Podofilox

(poh-**DAHF**-ih-lox)
Pregnancy Category: C
Condyline ✱, Condylox **(Rx)**

How Supplied: *Solution:* 0.5%
Action/Kinetics: Podofilox is either derived from species of *Juniperus* or *Podophyllum* or chemically synthesized. It is an antimitotic agent that causes necrosis of visible wart tissue when applied topically. Small amounts are absorbed into the system 1–2 hr after application. **t½:** 1–4.5 hr. The drug does not accumulate following multiple treatments.
Uses: Topical treatment of *Condyloma acuminatum* (external genital warts). *Investigational:* Systemically for treatment of cancer.

Dosage

- **Topical Solution**
  External genital warts.

Adults, initial: Apply b.i.d. in the morning and evening (i.e., q 12 hr) for 3 consecutive days; **then,** withhold use for 4 consecutive days. The 1-week cycle of treatment may be repeated up to 4 times until there is no visible sign of wart tissue. Alternative treatment should be considered if the response is incomplete after four treatments.
Administration/Storage
1. Apply podofilox to the warts with the cotton-tipped applicator supplied with the drug.
2. Apply only the minimum amount of solution required to cover the lesion. Treatment should be limited to less than 10 cm^2 of wart tissue and to 0.5 mL or less of the solution daily. Higher amounts do not increase efficacy but may increase the incidence of side effects.
3. The solution should be allowed to dry before allowing the return of opposing skin surfaces to their normal positions.
4. After each treatment, the used applicator should be disposed of properly and the individual instructed to wash hands thoroughly.
5. The solution should not be frozen or exposed to excessive heat.
6. *Treatment of Overdose:* General supportive therapy to treat symptoms.
Contraindications: Use for perianal or mucous membrane warts. Lactation.
Special Concerns: It is essential that genital warts be distinguished from squamous cell carcinoma prior to initiation of treatment. Safety and effectiveness have not been demonstrated in children. Avoid contact with the eyes.
Side Effects: Topical Use. *Dermatologic:* Commonly, burning, pain, inflammation, erosion, and itching. Also, tenderness, chafing, scarring, vesicle formation, dryness and peeling, tingling, bleeding, ulceration, malodor, crusting edema, foreskin irretraction. *Miscellaneous:* Pain with intercourse, insomnia, dizziness, hematuria, vomiting.

Systemic Use. *GI:* N&V, diarrhea, oral ulcers. *Hematologic:* Bone marrow depression, leukocytosis, pancytosis. *CNS:* Altered mental status, lethargy, ***coma, seizures.*** *Miscellaneous:* Peripheral neuropathy, tachypnea, ***respiratory failure,*** hematuria, renal failure.

Symptoms of Overdose: N&V, diarrhea, fever, altered mental status, hematologic toxicity, peripheral neuropathy, lethargy, tachypnea, ***respiratory failure,*** hematuria, leukocytosis, pancytosis, renal failure, ***seizures, coma.***

NURSING CONSIDERATIONS

Assessment

1. Note histologic confirmation of differentiation of lesion from squamous cell carcinoma.
2. Document the number and size of condyloma, location, and condition of pretreatment area(s) as this will determine further treatment needs.

Client/Family Teaching

1. Demonstrate the appropriate method for topical administration and have client return demonstrate procedure.
2. Stress the importance of adhering to the exact dosing instructions (on for 3 days, off for 4 days) because the incidence of side effects may otherwise increase.
3. Avoid contact of the solution with the eyes. If contact does occur, instruct to immediately flush the eye with large amounts of water and to report.
4. Review the appropriate procedure for handling the medication and for the disposal of applicators.
5. Provide a printed list of side effects that should be reported should they occur.

Evaluate: Absence or ↓ number and size of condylomas.

Tretinoin (Retinoic acid, Vitamin A acid)

(**TRET**-ih-noyn)

Pregnancy Category: C

Retin-A, Retisol-A ✦, StieVAA ✦ **(Rx)**

How Supplied: *Cream:* 0.025%, 0.05%, 0.1%; *Gel/jelly:* 0.01%, 0.025%; *Liquid:* 0.05%

Action/Kinetics: Topical tretinoin is believed to decrease microcomedo formation by decreasing the cohesiveness of follicular epithelial cells. The drug is also believed to increase mitotic activity and increase turnover of follicular epithelial cells as well as decrease keratin synthesis. Some systemic absorption occurs (approximately 5% is recovered in the urine).

Uses: Acne vulgaris. *Investigational:* Treat various forms of skin cancer. Dermatologic conditions including lamellar ichthyosis, mollusca contagiosa, verrucae plantaris, verrucae planae juveniles, ichthyosis vulgaris, bullous congenital ichthyosiform, and pityriasis rubra pilaris. To enhance the percutaneous absorption of topical minoxidil. To improve photoaged skin, especially wrinkling and liver spots.

Dosage

- **Cream, Gel, or Liquid**

  Acne vulgaris.

Apply lightly over the affected areas once daily at bedtime. Beneficial effects many not be seen for 2–6 weeks.

Administration/Storage

1. The liquid should be applied carefully with the fingertip, cotton swab, or gauze pad only to affected areas.
2. Excessive amounts of the gel will cause a "pilling" effect.
3. The hands should be washed thoroughly immediately after applying tretinoin.

Contraindications: Eczema, sunburn.

Special Concerns: Use with caution during lactation. Safety and effectiveness have not been determined in children. The drug should not be used around the eyes, mouth, angles of the nose, and mucous membranes. Excessive sunlight and weather extremes (e.g., wind and cold) may be irritating.

Side Effects: *Dermatologic:* Red, edematous, crusted, or blistered skin; hyperpigmentation or hypopigmentation, increased susceptibility to sunlight. Excessive application will cause redness, peeling, or discomfort with no increase in results.

Drug Interactions: Concomitant use with sulfur, resorcinol, benzoyl peroxide, or salicylic acid may cause significant skin irritation.

NURSING CONSIDERATIONS

Assessment

1. Thoroughly describe pretreatment

skin condition and obtain photographs, if possible, to compare after completion of therapy.
2. Document other medications and agents previously used and the outcome.
3. Note if the client is of childbearing age and sexually active. Determine if pregnant prior to initiating therapy.

Client/Family Teaching

1. Keep the medication away from mucous membranes, eyes, mouth, and the angles of the nose.
2. Instruct client to wash with mild soap and warm water and to pat skin dry. Wait 20–30 min before applying tretinoin.
3. On application there will be a transitory feeling of warmth and stinging.
4. Wash hands thoroughly before and immediately after applying tretinoin.
5. Client may be more sensitive to wind and cold during therapy.
6. Expect dryness and peeling of skin from the affected areas.
7. Do not apply to wind or sunburned skin or to open wounds.
8. Avoid alcohol-containing preparations such as shaving lotions and creams, perfumes, cosmetics with drying effects, skin cleansers, and medicated soaps.
9. During the early weeks of therapy, the lesions may worsen. This is caused by the effect of the drug on deep lesions that had been previously undetected. Report if the lesions become severe and anticipate that the drug will be discontinued until the integrity of the skin has been restored.
10. Improvement should be evident in 6 weeks but therapy should be continued for at least 3 months.
11. Advise women of childbearing age to practice a reliable form of birth control while they are receiving drug therapy.
12. Avoid excessive exposure to sunlamps and to the sun. Persons who must be in sunlight while using the medication should be instructed to use a sunscreen or protective clothing over affected areas.

Evaluate

- ↓ Size and number of acne vulgaris eruptions
- Clearing of skin condition and reports of symptomatic improvement

CHAPTER EIGHTY-FOUR

Antidotes

See the following individual entries:

Deferoxamine Mesylate
Digoxin Immune Fab (Ovine)
Dimercaprol
Edetate Disodium
Flumazenil
Penicillamine
Protamine Sulfate
Sodium Benzoate and Sodium Phenylacetate
Sodium Polystyrene Sulfonate
Trientine Hydrochloride

Deferoxamine mesylate

(deh-fer-**OX**-ah-meen)
Desferal **(Rx)**

How Supplied: *Powder for injection:* 500 mg

Action/Kinetics: Deferoxamine, a complex organic molecule, binds to trivalent iron forming ferrioxamine, which is a water-soluble chelate excreted by the kidneys (urine is a reddish color) as well as in the feces via the bile. Iron is removed from ferritin, hemosiderin, and to a lesser extent from transferrin, but iron is not removed from hemoglobin, myoglobin, or cytochromes. The drug must be given parenterally for systemic activity. Adequate renal function is necessary for effectiveness. **t½, IV:** 60 min. The drug may be quickly eliminated by the kidneys without binding to iron.

Uses: Adjunct in treatment of acute iron intoxication. Chronic iron overload including thalassemia. *Investigational:* Accumulation of aluminum in renal failure and in encephalopathy due to aluminum.

Dosage

- **IM, IV, SC**

Acute iron intoxication.

Adults and children over 3 years of age, IM (preferred), initial: 1 g; **then,** 0.5 g q 4 hr for two doses; if necessary, then give 0.5 g q 4–12 hr, not to exceed 6 g/day. **IV infusion** (*only in emergencies such as CV collapse:*) Same as IM at a rate not to exceed 15 mg/kg/hr. Begin IM therapy as soon as possible.

Chronic iron overload.

IM: 0.5–1.0 g/day; **SC:** 1–2 g (20–40 mg/kg/day) given by mini-infusion pump over an 8–24-hr period; **IV:** 2 g (given separately but at same time as each unit of blood and in addition to IM administration); IV rate not to exceed 15 mg/kg/hr.

Administration/Storage

1. Dissolve deferoxamine mesylate by adding 2 mL of sterile water to each ampule.
2. For IV administration use physiologic saline, glucose in water, or Ringer's lactate solution and administer *slowly* at a rate not exceeding 15 mg/kg/hr.
3. Discard dissolved drug if not used within 1 week.
4. Pain and induration may occur at IM injection site.
5. Have epinephrine available to treat allergic reactions.
6. In the event of iron intoxication and/or acidosis, have gastric lavage equipment, suction, IV fluids, blood, and respiratory equipment to maintain a patent airway, readily available.

Contraindications: Severe renal disease, anuria. Should *not* be used to treat primary hemochromatosis.

Special Concerns: Use in pregnancy only if clearly necessary. Use with caution for clients with pyelonephritis. Should not be used in children under the age of 3 years unless mobilization of 1 mg iron/day or more can be shown. Deferoxamine and ascorbic acid should be used with caution in geriatric clients due to a greater risk of cardiac decompensation.

Side Effects: *Allergic:* Rash, itching, wheal formation, ***anaphylaxis.*** *GI:* Abdominal discomfort, diarrhea. *Other:* Dysuria, blurred vision, leg cramps, fever, tachycardia, high-frequency hearing loss. *Ophthalmologic:* Rarely, impaired peripheral, night, or color vision; cataracts, decreased visual acuity. *Following rapid IV use:* Hypotension, urticaria, erythema. *Following SC use:* Local pain, erythema, swelling, pruritus, skin irritation.

NURSING CONSIDERATIONS

Assessment

1. Perform a nursing history and note any evidence of pyelonephritis.
2. Document indications for therapy and onset of symptoms.
3. In poisoning, note amount ingested and type of preparation.
4. Obtain baseline serum iron, total iron-binding capacity, transferrin, and urinary iron excretion levels.
5. Conduct renal function studies and determine if the client has an adequate flow of urine before initiating therapy.
6. Obtain baseline ophthalmologic and audiometric exams. Drug is oto and ocular toxic.
7. If the client is female and of childbearing age, determine if pregnant.

Interventions

1. Monitor VS and I&O. If anuric, report as chelated iron is excreted by the kidneys.
2. Observe for early S&S of iron toxicity: abdominal pain, emesis, and bloody diarrhea; and late S&S: decreased level of consciousness, metabolic acidosis, and shock.

Client/Family Teaching

1. Explain the likelihood of pain and induration occurring at the site of administration.
2. Advise that the drug may give the urine a reddish color due to the chelated iron.
3. In clients with a history of pyelonephritis, report the development of hematuria or pain. These may be caused by deferoxamine, which may induce an exacerbation of the disease.
4. Report any complaints of visual disturbances such as changes in color vision or altered visual acuity as these may be drug induced.
5. Instruct client to report for periodic ophthalmologic and audiometric exams.
6. Report any sudden hearing loss as these may be drug related.
7. Advise women of childbearing age to practice reliable birth control.

Evaluate

- Relief of symptoms of iron toxicity
- ↓ Serum iron levels to 50–150 mcg/100 mL

Digoxin Immune Fab (Ovine)

(dih-**JOX**-in)
Pregnancy Category: C
Digibind **(Rx)**

How Supplied: *Injection:* 10 mg/mL

Action/Kinetics: Digoxin immune Fab are antibodies that bind to digoxin. The antibody is produced in sheep by immunization with digoxin bound to human albumin. In cases of digoxin toxicity, the antibodies can bind to digoxin and the complex is excreted through the kidneys. As serum levels of digoxin decrease, digoxin bound to tissue is released into the serum to maintain equilibrium and this is then bound and excreted. The net result is a decrease in both tissue and serum digoxin. **Onset:** Less than 1 min. **t½:** 15–20 hr (after IV administration). Each vial contains 40 mg of pure digoxin immune Fab, which will bind approximately 0.6 mg digoxin or digitoxin.

Uses: Life-threatening digoxin or digitoxin toxicity or overdosage. Symptoms of toxicity include severe sinus bradycardia, second- or third-degree heart block which does not respond to atropine, ventricular tachycardia, ventricular fibrillation.

NOTE: Cardiac arrest can be expected if a healthy adult ingests more than 10 mg digoxin or a healthy child ingests more than 4 mg. Also, steady-state serum concentrations of digoxin greater than 10 ng/mL or potassium concentrations greater than 5 mEq/L as a result of digoxin therapy require use of digoxin immune Fab.

Dosage

• IV

Dosage depends on the serum digoxin concentration. A large dose has a faster onset but there is an increased risk of allergic or febrile reactions. The package insert should be carefully consulted.

Administration/Storage

1. The lyophilized material should be reconstituted with 4 mL of sterile water for injection to give a concentration of 10 mg/mL. If small doses are required (e.g., in infants), reconstituted antibody can be further diluted with 36 mL sterile isotonic saline to obtain a concentration of 1 mg/mL.
2. The reconstituted antibody should be used immediately. However, it may be stored for up to 4 hr at 2°C–8°C (36°F–46°F).
3. The dose should be administered over a 30-min period through a 0.22-µm membrane filter. A bolus injection may be used if there is immediate danger of cardiac arrest.
4. The total number of vials of antibody needed can be determined by dividing the total body load (in mg) by the amount of digoxin bound by each vial (0.6 mg).
5. If acute digoxin ingestion results in severe symptoms and a serum concentration is not known, 800 mg (20 vials) of digoxin immune Fab may be given. However, volume overload must be monitored in small children.
6. The dosage in infants should be administered with a tuberculin syringe.

Special Concerns: Use with caution during lactation. Use in infants only if benefits outweigh risks. Clients sensitive to products of sheep origin may also be sensitive to digoxin immune Fab.

Side Effects: *CV:* Worsening of CHF or low CO, atrial fibrillation (all due to withdrawal of the effects of digoxin). *Other:* Hypokalemia.

NURSING CONSIDERATIONS

Assessment

1. Evaluate laboratory data for electrolyte imbalance and correct. Note the presence of hypokalemia or evidence of increased CHF and document.
2. Clients with known allergy to sheep proteins should be appropriately identified and this information should be documented in their records. Do not administer digoxin immune Fab to these persons.
3. If previous reaction suspected, consider performing skin testing. Prepare a 10-mL solution (0.1 mL of drug in 9.9 mL NSS) and perform an intradermal injection or scratch test. Administer 0.1 mL intradermally or a scratch test may be performed by placing 1 drop of solution on the skin and making a scratch through the drop with a sterile needle; assess site in 20 min. A positive reaction would consist of a urticarial wheal with erythematous surrounding skin. *Do not* use if reaction is positive.
4. Document pretreatment digoxin or digitoxin levels.
5. Determine amount of drug ingested and time of overdose to ensure appropriate dosing (generally a 40-mg vial will bind 0.6 mg of digoxin).

Interventions

1. Monitor VS and cardiac rhythm. Have epinephrine (1:1,000) available in the event of a hypersensitivity reaction.
2. Wait several days if redigitalization is anticipated to ensure complete elimination of digibind.
3. Anticipate that serum digoxin levels will take 5–7 days to stabilize following treatment.

Evaluate

• Resolution of digoxin toxicity with serum levels to within desired range

• Restoration of baseline cardiac rhythm

Dimercaprol

(dye-mer-**KAP**-rohl)
Pregnancy Category: C
BAL In Oil **(Rx)**

How Supplied: *Injection:* 10%
Action/Kinetics: Dimercaprol forms a chelate by binding sulfhydryl groups with arsenic, mercury, lead, and gold, thus increasing both urinary and fecal excretion of the metals. Thus, because the drug has a higher affinity for the metal than it does for sulfhydryl groups on protein in the body, BAL reverses enzyme inhibition by regenerating free sulfhydryl groups. To be fully effective, the drug should be administered 1–2 hr after exposure. **Peak plasma concentration: IM,** 30–60 min. Mostly distributed to extracellular fluid. **Time to peak levels:** 30–60 min.

Rapidly metabolized to inactive product and completely excreted in urine and feces in 4 hr.
Uses: Acute arsenic, mercury, and gold poisoning. With EDTA in acute lead poisoning. Not effective for chronic mercury poisoning.

Dosage

• **Deep IM Only**

Mild arsenic and gold poisoning.
Adults: 2.5 mg/kg q 4 hr for day 1; 2.5 mg/kg q 6 hr on day 2; b.i.d. on day 3; once daily for 10 days thereafter or until recovery is complete.

Severe arsenic or gold poisoning.
Adults: 3 mg/kg q 4 hr for days 1 and 2; q.i.d. on day 3; b.i.d. for 10 more days.

Mercury poisoning, mild.
Adults, initial: 5 mg/kg; **then,** 2.5 mg/kg 1 or 2 times/day for 10 days. Alternate dosing regimen: 2.5 mg/kg q 4 hr on day 1, q 6 hr on day 2, q 12 hr on day 3, and thereafter, once daily for the next 10 days or until recovery occurs.

Mercury poisoning, severe.
Adults: 5 mg/kg for the first dose followed by 2.5 mg/kg q 3 hr for the first 24 hr; **then,** 2 mg/kg q 4 hr on day 2; 3 mg/kg q 6 hr on day 3; and 3 mg/kg q 12 hr for the next 10 days or until recovery.

Mild lead encephalopathy.
Adults: 4 mg/kg alone initially; **then,** 3 mg/kg q 4 hr in combination with calcium EDTA administered in a separate site. Treatment should be continued for 2–7 days only if the blood level at the end of the first course of combined BAL-CaEDTA therapy exceeds 80–90 mcg/dL.

Severe lead encephalopathy.
Adults: 4 mg/kg alone initially; **then,** 4 mg/kg q 4 hr in combination with calcium EDTA administered in a separate site. Treatment should be continued for 2–7 days and repeated after an interval of 2 days for 5 additional days only if the blood lead level at the end of the first course of combined BAL-CaEDTA therapy exceeds 80–90 mcg/dL.

Lead toxicity in symptomatic children, acute encephalopathy.
75 mg/m^2 q 4 hr (up to 450 mg/m^2 in 24 hr). After the first dose, give calcium EDTA, 1,500 mg/m^2 over a 24-hr period in divided doses q 4 hr at a separate IM site; maintain treatment for 5 days and after an interval of 2 days, the treatment may be repeated for 5 additional days.

Lead toxicity in children, other symptoms.
50 mg/m^2 q 4 hr. After the first dose, give calcium EDTA, 1,000 mg/m^2 over a 24-hr period in divided doses q 4 hr at a separate IM site; maintain treatment for 5 days and after an interval of 2 days, the treatment may be repeated for 5 more days if the lead levels are still high.

Administration/Storage

1. Check with the provider whether a local anesthetic may be given with IM injection to minimize pain at the injection site.
2. Inject IM deeply into muscle and massage after injection. Do not allow the fluid to come in contact with

the skin as it may cause a skin reaction.

3. Have ephedrine and/or an antihistamine available for premedication or for later use if the client should experience any adverse effects from the drug.

4. Do not administer iron therapy until at least 24 hr after the last dose of dimercaprol.

Contraindications: Iron, cadmium, silver, uranium, or selenium poisoning. Hepatic insufficiency. Poisoning from arsine gas.

Special Concerns: Use during pregnancy only if poisoning is life-threatening. Use with caution in the presence of renal insufficiency and in clients with G6PD deficiency. The drug is of questionable value in poisoning by bismuth or antimony.

Laboratory Test Interference: Iodine-131 thyroidal uptake ↓ during and immediately after dimercaprol therapy.

Side Effects: *CV:* Most common including hypertension and tachycardia. *GI:* N&V, salivation, abdominal pain, burning feeling of the lips, mouth and throat. *CNS:* Anxiety, weakness, restlessness, headache. *Other:* Constriction and pain in the throat, chest, or hands; sweating of the hands and forehead, conjunctivitis, blepharal spasm, lacrimation, rhinorrhea, tingling of hands, burning feeling in the penis, sterile abscesses. Children may also develop fever. ***At high doses dimercaprol may cause coma or convulsions*** and metabolic acidosis.

Drug Interactions: Dimercaprol may increase the toxicity of cadmium, iron, selenium, or uranium salts.

NURSING CONSIDERATIONS

Assessment

1. Document exposure or when agent ingested, in what form, and what quantity.

2. Assess client for adequate flow of urine prior to initiating therapy.

3. Determine if women of childbearing age are pregnant.

4. Obtain baseline liver and renal function studies.

5. Request serum levels of toxic substance.

Interventions

1. Increase fluid intake and monitor urinary pH throughout drug therapy. Urine should be kept alkaline to protect the kidneys during drug therapy.

2. Record VS and monitor readings to assist in evaluating the client's response to the medication.

3. If the client develops adverse GI or CNS symptoms during drug therapy, reassure that these symptoms will pass within 30–90 min; provide emotional support.

4. The drug imparts a strong, unpleasant garlic-like odor to the client's breath. Offer mouth rinses as needed.

Evaluate: Enhanced excretion of arsenic, mercury, gold, or lead with relief of toxic symptoms during acute poisonings.

Edetate disodium (EDTA)

(**ED**-eh-tayt)

Chealamide, Disotate, Endrate **(Rx)**

How Supplied: *Injection:* 150 mg/mL

Action/Kinetics: Edetate disodium has a great affinity for calcium, forming a soluble chelate in the blood. The chelate is then excreted through the urine. This leads to a lowering of serum calcium and a mobilization of calcium stores, especially from bone. When used to treat digitalis toxicity, edetate disodium exerts a negative inotropic effect on the heart and thus the chronotropic and inotropic effects of digitalis on the heart are antagonized. The drug also forms chelates with magnesium, zinc, and other trace elements. When used ophthalmically, calcified corneal deposits are dissolved from the conjunctiva, corneal epithelium, and anterior layers of the stroma.

Uses: *Systemic:* Treatment of hypercalcemia, digitalis glycoside toxicity. Anticoagulant for blood drawn for hematologic studies. *Investigational:*

Ophthalmically to treat corneal calcium deposits, eye burns from calcium hydroxide, and eye injury by zinc chloride.

Dosage

- **IV**

Hypercalcemia, digitalis toxicity.
Individualized and depending on degree of hypercalcemia. **Adults, usual:** 50 mg/kg over 24 hr (up to 3 g/day may be prescribed); dose may be repeated for 5 consecutive days followed by a 2-day rest period with repeated courses, if needed, up to 15 doses. **Pediatric:** 40 mg/kg over 24 hr up to a maximum of 70 mg/kg/day.

- **Ophthalmic**

Calcium deposits, calcium hydroxide burns.
Adults and children: 0.35%–1.85% solution as an irrigation for 15–20 min.

Zinc chloride injury.
Adults and children: 1.7% solution as an irrigation for 15 min.

Administration/Storage

1. Administer to client while in a Fowler's position.
2. Check label on vial carefully to determine that drug is disodium edetate and not calcium disodium edetate.
3. For use in adults, dilute medication in 500 mL of 5% dextrose solution or isotonic saline solution as ordered. For pediatric use, the drug can be dissolved in either 5% dextrose injection or 0.9% sodium chloride injection; the final concentration should not exceed 3%.
4. Record which vein is used for site of administration because repeated use of the same vein is likely to result in thrombophlebitis. Greater dilution of the solution and slower administration reduce the incidence of thrombophlebitis if the same vein must be used.
5. Infuse slowly over 3–4 hours, being careful not to exceed the cardiac reserve of the client.
6. Do not exceed the recommended dose, concentration, or rate of administration.
7. There is no ophthalmic product available in the U.S.; however, the injection can be used to prepare the ophthalmic dosage form.
8. *Treatment of Overdose:* IV calcium gluconate.

Contraindications: Use with caution in clients with heart disease (e.g., CHF) or hypokalemia. Anuric clients; clients with ventricular arrhythmias. Not to be used to treat arteriosclerosis, atherosclerotic vascular disease, lead poisoning, or renal calculi by retrograde irrigation.

Special Concerns: Use during pregnancy only if the benefits clearly outweigh the risks. Use with extreme caution in digitalized clients as EDTA and calcium may reverse the desired effect of digitalis.

Laboratory Test Interference: ↓ Alkaline phosphatase levels.

Side Effects: *Metabolic:* Electrolyte imbalance including hypocalcemia, hypokalemia, hypomagnesemia, hyperuricemia may occur during treatment. *CV:* Decrease in both systolic and diastolic pressure, thrombophlebitis, anemia. *GI:* N&V, diarrhea. *CNS:* Headache, numbness, circumoral paresthesia, fever. *Other:* Exfoliative dermatitis, nephrotoxicity, ***reticuloendothelial system damage with hemorrhagic tendencies.***

Rapid injection may produce hypocalcemic tetany and convulsions, respiratory arrest, and severe arrhythmias.

Symptoms of Overdose: Precipitous drop in calcium.

NURSING CONSIDERATIONS

Assessment

1. Document indications for therapy and anticipated results.
2. Review history and use cautiously in clients who have heart disease, seizures, and/or TB.

Interventions

1. Monitor serum calcium, magnesium, and electrolyte levels and renal function studies. Assess urinalysis before and during drug therapy.

2. Monitor BP during infusion because a transitory hypotension may occur. This would necessitate lowering the client from a Fowler's position until hypotension has passed and BP has stabilized.
3. Be alert to a generalized systemic reaction that may occur from 4 to 8 hr after infusion of the drug and that usually subsides within 12 hr. Report such a reaction and provide supportive care for fever, chills, back pain, vomiting, muscle cramps, or urinary urgency should these symptoms occur.
4. With lead toxicity, notify local health department, noting source if known.

Client/Family Teaching

1. Advise clients with diabetes mellitus that the drug may cause hypoglycemia. The client should consult with the provider concerning whether to reduce insulin dosage or increase food intake in the event of hypoglycemia.
2. Clients with diabetes should be instructed to test the urine or finger sticks regularly. If urine is negative for glucose or if the finger sticks reveal low glucose levels, the clients should consult with the provider concerning management of their diabetes.

Evaluate

- ↓ Serum calcium levels
- Relief of symptoms of digitalis toxicity
- Dissolution of corneal deposits

Flumazenil

(floo-**MAZ**-eh-nill)
Pregnancy Category: C
Anexate ✱, Romazicon I.V. **(Rx)**

How Supplied: *Injection:* 0.1 mg/mL

Action/Kinetics: Flumazenil antagonizes the effects of benzodiazepines on the CNS by competitively inhibiting their action at the benzodiazepine recognition site on the GABA/benzodiazepine receptor complex. The drug does not antagonize the CNS effects of ethanol, general anesthetics, barbiturates, or opiates. Depending on the dose of flumazenil, there will be partial or complete antagonism of sedation, impaired recall, and psychomotor impairment. **Onset of reversal:** 1–2 min. **Peak effect:** 6–10 min. The duration of reversal is related to the plasma levels of the benzodiazepine and the dose of flumazenil. **Distribution t½, initial:** 7–15 min; **terminal t½:** 41–79 min. The drug is metabolized in the liver with 90%–95% excreted through the urine and 5%–10% excreted in the feces. Hepatic impairment prolongs the half-life of the drug.

Uses: Complete or partial reversal of the sedative effects of benzodiazepines in cases where general anesthesia has been induced or maintained by benzodiazepines, where sedation has been produced by benzodiazepines for diagnostic and therapeutic procedures, and for the management of benzodiazepine overdosage.

Dosage

- **IV Only**

To reverse conscious sedation or in general anesthesia.

Adults, initial: 0.2 mg (2 mL) given IV over 15 sec. If the desired level of consciousness is not reached after waiting an additional 45 sec, a second dose of 0.2 mg (2 mL) can be given and repeated at 60-sec intervals, up to a maximum total dose of 1 mg (10 mL). Most clients will respond to doses of 0.6–1 mg. To treat resedation, give no more than 1 mg (given as 0.2 mg/min) at any one time and give no more than 3 mg in any 1 hr.

Management of suspected benzodiazepine overdose.

Adults, initial: 0.2 mg (2 mL) given IV over 30 sec; a second dose of 0.3 mg (3 mL) can be given over another 30 sec. Further doses of 0.5 mg (5 mL) can be given over 30 sec at 1-min intervals up to a total dose of 3 mg (although some clients may require up to 5 mg given slowly as described). If the client has not responded 5 min after receiving a cumulative dose of 5 mg, the major cause of sedation is probably not due to benzodiazepines and additional doses of flumazenil are likely to have no effect. For resedation, repeated doses may be given at 20-min intervals; no more than 1 mg (given as 0.5 mg/min) at any one time and no more than 3 mg in any 1 hr should be administered.

Administration/Storage

1. The dosage must be individualized. It is important to give only the smallest amount of flumazenil that is effective. The 1-min wait between individual doses in the dose-titration recommended for general uses may be too short for high-risk clients as it takes 6–10 min for any single dose of flumazenil to reach full effects. Thus, the rate of administration should be slowed in high-risk clients.
2. A major risk is resedation because the duration of effect of a long-acting or a large dose of a short-acting benzodiazepine may exceed that of flumazenil. If there is resedation, repeated doses may be given at 20-min intervals as needed.
3. Flumazenil is best given as a series of small injections to allow the physician to control the reversal of sedation to the end point desired and to decrease the possibility of side effects.
4. The dose of flumazenil should be reduced to 40%–60% of normal in clients with severe hepatic dysfunction.
5. Flumazenil should be given through a freely running IV infusion into a large vein to minimize pain at the injection site.
6. Doses larger than a total of 3 mg do not reliably produce additional effects.
7. Flumazenil is compatible with 5% dextrose in water, lactated Ringer's, and NSS solutions. If flumazenil is drawn into a syringe or mixed with any of these solutions, it should be discarded after 24 hr.
8. For optimum sterility, flumazenil should remain in the vial until just before use.

Contraindications: Use in clients given a benzodiazepine for control of intracranial pressure or status epilepticus. In clients manifesting signs of serious cyclic antidepressant overdose. Use during labor and delivery or in children as the risks and benefits are not known. To treat benzodiazepine dependence or for the management of protracted benzodiazepine abstinence syndrome.

Special Concerns: The reversal of benzodiazepine effects may be associated with the onset of seizures in certain high-risk clients (e.g., concurrent major sedative-hypnotic drug withdrawal, recent therapy with repeated doses of parenteral benzodiazepines, myoclonic jerking or seizure activity prior to administration of flumazenil in cases of overdose, and concurrent cyclic antidepressant overdosage). Use with caution in clients with head injury as the drug may precipitate seizures or alter cerebral blood flow in clients receiving benzodiazepines. Use with caution in clients with alcoholism and other drug dependencies due to the increased frequency of benzodiazepine tolerance and dependence.

Flumazenil may precipitate a withdrawal syndrome if the client is dependent on benzodiazepines. Flumazenil may cause panic attacks in clients with a history of panic disorder.

Side Effects: ***Deaths*** have occurred in clients receiving flumazenil, especially in those with serious underlying disease or in those who have ingested large amounts of nonbenzodiazepine drugs (usually cyclic antidepressants) as part of an overdose. ***Seizures are the most common serious side effect noted.***

CNS: Dizziness, vertigo, ataxia, anxiety, nervousness, tremor, palpitations, insomnia, dyspnea, hyperventilation, abnormal crying, depersonalization, euphoria, increased tears, depression, dysphoria, paranoia, delirium, difficulty concentrating, ***seizures,*** somnolence, stupor, speech disorder. *GI:* N&V, hiccoughs, dry mouth. *CV:* Sweating, flushing, hot flushes, ***arrhythmias (atrial, nodal, ventricular extrasystoles),*** bradycardia, tachycardia, hypertension, chest pain. *At injection site:* Pain, thrombophlebitis, rash, skin abnormality. *Body as a whole:* Headache, increased sweating, asthenia, malaise, rigors, shivering, paresthesia. *Ophthalmologic:* Abnormal vision including visual field defect and diplopia; blurred vision. *Otic:* Transient hearing impairment, tinnitus, hyperacusis.

NURSING CONSIDERATIONS

Assessment

1. Review client history, noting any evidence of seizure disorder or panic attacks.
2. Determine type and amount of drug ingested; especially note any overdose of cyclic antidepressant.
3. Document any liver dysfunction as subsequent doses require adjustment.
4. Assess for any evidence of head injury or increased ICP.
5. Note any evidence of sedative or benzodiazepine dependence, alcohol abuse, or recent use as drug may precipitate withdrawal symptoms.

Interventions

1. The effects of flumazenil usually wear off before the effects of many benzodiazepines. Observe client closely for resedation, depressed respirations, or other residual benzodiazepine effects for up to 120 min after flumazenil administration. The availability of flumazenil does not decrease the need for prompt detection of hypoventilation and the need to establish an airway and assist with ventilation.
2. Flumazenil is intended as an adjunct to, not a substitute for, proper management of the airway, assisted breathing, circulatory access and support, use of lavage and charcoal, and adequate clinical evaluation. Prior to giving flumazenil, proper measures should be undertaken to secure an airway for ventilation and IV access. Be prepared for clients attempting to withdraw ET tubes or IV lines due to confusion and agitation following awakening.
3. The drug should be used with caution in the intensive care unit (ICU) due to the increased risk of unrecognized benzodiazepine dependence in such settings. Drug may produce convulsions in benzodiazepine-dependent clients.
4. Flumazenil is not intended to be used to diagnose benzodiazepine-induced sedation in the ICU. Failure to respond may be masked by metabolic disorders, traumatic injury, or other drugs.
5. Incorporate seizure precautions. There is an increased risk for seizures with large overdoses of cyclic antidepressants and in clients on long-term sedation with benzodiazepines.
6. Convulsions associated with administration of flumazenil may be treated with benzodiazepines, phenytoin, or barbiturates. Higher than usual doses of benzodiazepines may be needed.
7. Flumazenil should not be used until the effects of neuromuscular blockade have been fully reversed.
8. Flumazenil does not consistently reverse amnesia. Therefore, clients cannot be expected to remember what is told to them in the postprocedure period. Instructions should be given in writing to the client or family member.

Client/Family Teaching

1. After the procedure, review instructions and postoperative teaching to reinforce client understanding and provide written instructions for reference.
2. Do not undertake any activities requiring complete alertness and do not operate hazardous machinery or a motor vehicle until at least 18–24 hr after discharge and until it has been determined that no residual sedative effects of benzodiazepines remain. Memory and judgment may be impaired.
3. Instruct clients not to take any alcohol or nonprescription drugs for 18–24 hr after administration of flu-

mazenil or if the effects of the benzodiazepines persist.
Evaluate: Reversal of benzodiazepine sedative and psychomotor effects.

Penicillamine

(pen-ih-**SILL**-ah-meen)
Cuprimine, Depen **(Rx)**

How Supplied: *Capsule:* 125 mg, 250 mg; *Tablet:* 250 mg
Action/Kinetics: Penicillamine, a degradation product of penicillin, is a chelating agent for mercury, lead, iron, and copper, thus decreasing toxic levels of the metal (e.g., copper in Wilson's disease). The anti-inflammatory activity of penicillamine may be due to its ability to inhibit T-lymphocyte function and therefore decrease cell-mediated immune response. It may also protect lymphocytes from hydrogen peroxide generated at the site of inflammation by inhibiting release of lysosomal enzymes and oxygen radicals. In cystinuria, penicillamine is able to reduce excess cystine excretion, probably by disulfide interchange between penicillamine and cystine. This results in penicillamine-cysteine disulfide, which is a complex that is more soluble than cystine and is thus readily excreted. Penicillamine is well absorbed from the GI tract and is excreted in urine. **Peak plasma levels:** 1–3 hr. About 80% is bound to plasma albumin. **t½:** Approximately 2 hr. Metabolites are excreted through the urine. **It may take 2–3 months for positive responses to become apparent when treating rheumatoid arthritis.**
Uses: Wilson's disease, cystinuria, and rheumatoid arthritis—severe active disease unresponsive to conventional therapy. Heavy metal antagonist. *Investigational:* Primary biliary cirrhosis. Rheumatoid vasculitis, Felty's syndrome.

Dosage

- **Capsules, Tablets**

Rheumatoid arthritis.
Adults, individualized, initial: 125–250 mg/day. Dosage may be increased at 1–3-month intervals by 125–250-mg increments until adequate response is attained. **Maximum:** 500–750 mg/day. Up to 500 mg/day can be given as a single dose; higher dosages should be divided. **Maintenance, individualized. Range:** 500–750 mg/day.

Wilson's disease.
Dosage is usually calculated on the basis of the urinary excretion of copper. One gram of penicillamine promotes excretion of 2 mg of copper. **Adults and adolescents, usual, initial:** 250 mg q.i.d. Dosage may have to be increased to 2 g/day. A further increase does not produce additional excretion. **Pediatric, 6 months—young children:** 250 mg as a single dose given in fruit juice.

Antidote for heavy metals.
Adults: 0.5–1.5 g/day for 1–2 months; **pediatric:** 30–40 mg/kg/day (600–750 mg/m²/day) for 1–6 months.

Cystinuria.
Individualized and based on excretion rate of cystine (100–200 mg/day in clients with no history of stones, below 100 mg with clients with history of stones or pain). Initiate at low dosage (250 mg/day) and increase gradually to minimum effective dosage. **Adult, usual:** 2 g/day (range: 1–4 g/day); **pediatric:** 7.5 mg/kg q.i.d. If divided in fewer than four doses, give larger dose at night.

Primary biliary cirrhosis.
Adults: 600–900 mg/day.

Administration/Storage

1. Give penicillamine on an empty stomach 1 hr before or 2 hr after meals. Also wait 1 hr after ingestion of any other food, milk, or drug.
2. If client cannot tolerate dosage for cystinuria, the bedtime dosage should be larger and should be continued.
3. Administer the contents of the capsule in 15–30 mL of chilled juice or pureed fruit if client is unable to swallow capsules or tablets.

4. The drug should be discontinued if doses of penicillamine up to 1.5 g/day for 2–3 months do not produce improvement when treating rheumatoid arthritis.

Contraindications: Pregnancy, lactation, penicillinase-related aplastic anemia or agranulocytosis, hypersensitivity to drug. Clients allergic to penicillin may cross-react with penicillamine. Renal insufficiency or history thereof.

Special Concerns: The use of penicillamine for juvenile rheumatoid arthritis has not been established. Clients older than 65 years may be at greater risk of developing hematologic side effects.

Laboratory Test Interferences: ↑ Serum alkaline phosphatase, LDH. Positive thymol turbidity test and cephalin flocculation test.

Side Effects: This drug manifests a large number of potentially serious side effects. Clients should be carefully monitored. *GI:* Altered taste perception (common), N&V, diarrhea, anorexia, GI pain, stomatitis, oral ulcerations, reactivation of peptic ulcer, glossitis, cheilosis, colitis. *Hematologic:* Thrombocytopenia, leukopenia, ***agranulocytosis, aplastic anemia,*** eosinophilia, monocytosis, red cell aplasia, thrombocytopenia, ***hemolytic anemia,*** leukocytosis, thrombocytosis. *Renal:* Proteinuria, hematuria, nephrotic syndrome, ***Goodpasture's syndrome*** (a severe and ultimately fatal glomerulonephritis). *Allergic:* Rashes (common), lupus-like syndrome, pruritus, pemphigoid-type symptoms (e.g., bullous lesions), drug fever, arthralgia, lymphadenopathy, dermatoses, urticaria, obliterative bronchiolitis, thyroiditis, hypoglycemia, migratory polyarthralgia, polymyositis, allergic alveolitis. *Other:* Tinnitus, optic neuritis, neuropathy, thrombophlebitis, alopecia, precipitation of myasthenia gravis, increased body temperature, pulmonary fibrosis, pneumonitis, bronchial asthma, renal vasculitis (may be fatal), hot flashes, increased skin friability, pancreatitis, hepatic dysfunction, intrahepatic cholestasis.

Drug Interactions
Antacids / ↓ Effect of penicillamine due to ↓ absorption from GI tract
Digoxin / Penicillamine ↓ effect of digoxin
Iron salts / ↓ Effect of penicillamine due to ↓ absorption from GI tract
Antimalarials, cytotoxic drugs, gold therapy, oxyphenbutazone, phenylbutazone / ↑ Risk of blood dyscrasias and adverse renal effects

---

NURSING CONSIDERATIONS

Assessment

1. Determine indications for therapy, presenting symptoms, other therapies prescribed and the outcome.
2. Note if the client is taking any medication with which penicillamine will interact unfavorably. Also, it impedes absorption of many drugs.
3. Assess hearing to detect any evidence of hearing loss and to serve as a baseline for further auditory testing throughout drug therapy.
4. Women of childbearing age who are sexually active should be tested for pregnancy. Penicillamine is contraindicated during pregnancy because it can cause fetal damage.
5. Ensure that liver function tests are conducted prior to the start of therapy.
6. Obtain baseline CBC, platelet count, and urinalysis.

Interventions

1. Note client complaints of N&V or diarrhea. Check for any alterations in taste. Monitor weight and I&O, and report any significant changes.
2. Inspect mucosal surfaces at regular intervals. If ulcers appear and are severe or persistent, it may be necessary to reduce the dose of drug as it may interfere with wound healing.
3. Routinely monitor the client's WBC and platelet counts. If the WBC falls below 3,500/mm^3 or the platelet count falls below 100,000/mm^3, withhold the penicillamine and report. If the counts are low for three successive lab tests, a temporary interruption of therapy is indicated.
4. Monitor liver function studies, especially if the client develops jaundice

or demonstrates other signs of hepatic dysfunction.
5. White papules appearing at the site of venipuncture or at surgical sites may indicate sensitivity to penicillamine or the presence of infection.
6. If the client is to undergo surgery, anticipate that the dosage of medication will be reduced to 250 mg/day until wound healing is complete. Anticipate that vitamin B_6 may be ordered prophylactically prior to and following surgery.
7. Penicillamine increases the body's need for pyridoxine. Therefore, pyridoxine (25 mg/day) should be ordered as a supplement.
8. A positive ANA test indicates that the client may develop a lupus-like syndrome in the future. The drug need not be discontinued. Rather, the practitioner needs to be aware of the potential and to report any symptoms should they occur.
9. If the client develops cystinuria, encourage a high fluid intake throughout the day and at bedtime.
10. For clients being treated for Wilson's disease, avoid multivitamin preparations containing copper.

Client/Family Teaching

1. Review the goals of the therapy and the anticipated benefits, and provide clients with a printed list of possible side effects.
2. Instruct clients to take their temperature nightly during the first few months of therapy. A fever may indicate a hypersensitivity reaction and should be reported.
3. Any evidence of fever, sore throat, chills, bruising, or bleeding need to be reported immediately. These are early symptoms of granulocytopenia.
4. If stomatitis occurs, it needs to be reported immediately and the drug discontinued. Instruct the client on oral hygiene such as brushing the teeth with a soft toothbrush, flossing daily, and using mouth rinses free of alcohol.
5. A loss of taste perception or a metallic taste may develop. This relates to zinc chelation and may last for 2 months or more. Encourage the client to maintain adequate nutrition, noting that nutrition is important and that the condition is usually self-limiting.
6. If the client is to receive an oral iron preparation, at least 2 hr should elapse between ingestion of penicillamine and the dose of therapeutic iron. Iron decreases the cupruretic effects of penicillamine.
7. The skin of clients taking penicillamine tends to become friable and susceptible to injury. Caution clients to avoid activities that could injure the skin. When working with elderly clients teach them how to avoid excessive pressure on the shoulders, elbows, knees, toes, and buttocks. Document and report all skin changes.
8. Report cloudy urine or urine that is smoky brown. These are signs of proteinuria and hematuria and may require withdrawal of the drug.
9. Women of childbearing age should be instructed to practice a safe form of birth control. If the client misses a menstrual period or has other symptoms of pregnancy, advise to report.
10. If the drug is used to treat clients with Wilson's disease, they should be advised as follows:

- Eat a diet low in copper. Exclude foods such as chocolate, nuts, shellfish, mushrooms, liver, molasses, broccoli, and copper-enriched cereals.
- Use distilled or demineralized water if the drinking water contains more than 0.1 mg/L copper.
- Unless the client is taking iron supplements, take sulfurated potash or Carbo-Resin with meals to minimize the absorption of copper.
- It may take 1–3 months for neurologic improvements to occur. Therefore, continue the therapy even if no improvements seem evident.
- Check any vitamin preparations being used to ensure that they do not contain copper.

11. If a client develops cystinuria, advise the following:

• Drink large amounts of fluid to prevent the formation of renal calculi. Drink 500 mL of fluid at bedtime and another pint during the night, when the urine tends to be the most concentrated and most acidic.

• Teach client how to measure specific gravity and determine pH. The urine specific gravity should be maintained at less than 1.010 and the pH maintained at 7.5–8.0.

• Advise clients to have a yearly X ray of the kidneys to detect the presence of renal calculi.

• Eat a diet low in methionine, a major precursor of cystine. Exclude from the diet foods high in cystine such as rich meat, soups and broths, milk, eggs, cheeses, and peas.

• If the client is pregnant or is a child, a diet low in methionine is also low in calcium. Therefore, such a diet is contraindicated in these instances unless calcium supplemented.

12. If clients have rheumatoid arthritis, advise them to continue using other approaches and medications to achieve relief from their symptoms because penicillamine may take 4–6 months to have a therapeutic effect.

Evaluate

• ↑ Urinary excretion of copper with control of symptoms of copper toxicity

• ↓ Cystine excretion and prevention of renal calculi in cystinuria

• ↓ Joint pain, swelling, and stiffness with ↑ mobility

Protamine sulfate

(**PROH**-tah-meen)
Pregnancy Category: C
(Rx)

How Supplied: *Injection:* 10 mg/mL

Action/Kinetics: Protamine sulfate is a strongly basic polypeptide that complexes with strongly acidic heparin to form an inactive stable salt. The complex has no anticoagulant activity. **Onset:** 30–60 sec. **Duration:** 2 hr (but depends on body temperature). Upon metabolism, the complex may liberate heparin (heparin rebound).

Use: Only for treatment of heparin overdose resulting in hemorrhage. Administration of whole blood or fresh frozen plasma may also be needed if hemorrhage is severe.

Dosage

• **Slow IV**

No more than 50 mg of protamine sulfate should be given in any 10-min period. One milligram of protamine sulfate can neutralize about 90 USP units of heparin derived from lung tissue or about 115 USP units of heparin derived from intestinal mucosa. *NOTE:* The dose of protamine sulfate depends on the amount of time that has elapsed since IV heparin administration. For example, if 30 min has elapsed, one-half the usual dose of protamine sulfate may be sufficient because heparin is cleared rapidly from the circulation.

Administration/Storage

1. Protamine sulfate is incompatible with several penicillins and with cephalosporins.

2. If dilution of the product is required, use either dextrose 5% or NSS. Diluted solutions should not be stored.

3. To minimize side effects, give protamine sulfate slowly over 1–3 min. May also be diluted in 50 mL of dextrose or saline solution and administered at a rate of 50 mg over 10–15 min.

4. Protamine should be refrigerated at 2°C–8°C (36°F–46°F).

5. *Treatment of Overdose:* Replace blood loss with blood transfusions or fresh frozen plasma. Fluids, epinephrine, dobutamine, or dopamine to treat hypotension.

Contraindications: Previous intolerance to protamine. Not suitable for treating spontaneous hemorrhage, postpartum hemorrhage, menorrhagia, or uterine bleeding. Administration of over 100 mg over a short period.

Special Concerns: Use with caution during lactation. Safety and efficacy have not been determined in children. Rapid administration may cause severe hypotension and anaphylaxis.

Side Effects: *CV:* Sudden fall in BP, bradycardia, transitory flushing, warm feeling, ***acute pulmonary hypertension, circulatory collapse (possibly irreversible) with myocardial failure*** and decreased CO. Pulmonary edema in clients on cardiopulmonary bypass undergoing CV surgery. *GI:* N&V. *CNS:* Lassitude. *Other:* ***Anaphylaxis,*** dyspnea, back pain in clients undergoing cardiac catheterization.

Symptoms of Overdose: Bleeding. Rapid administration may cause dyspnea, bradycardia, flushing, warm feeling, severe hypotension, hypertension. In assessing overdose, there may be the possibility of multiple drug overdoses leading to drug interactions and unusual pharmacokinetics.

NURSING CONSIDERATIONS

Assessment

1. Determine amount and time of overdose and source of heparin to ensure appropriate dosing of antidote.
2. Request type and crossmatch; assess need for fresh frozen plasma or whole blood.
3. Note any history of previous intolerance to protamine.
4. Coagulation studies should be performed 5–15 min after protamine sulfate has been administered to evaluate its effectiveness. Repeat in 2–8 hr to assess for heparin rebound.

Interventions

1. Observe client in a monitored environment. Record VS and I&O, assessing closely for sudden variations. Note any sudden fall in BP, bradycardia, dyspnea, transitory flushing, or client complaint of a sensation of warmth.
2. Observe for increased bleeding, lowered BP, and/or shock. These are signs of heparin rebound and should be reported immediately as repeated doses of protamine sulfate may be indicated.

Evaluate

- Stable H&H with control of heparin-induced hemorrhage
- Restoration of clotting factors

Sodium benzoate and Sodium phenylacetate

(**SO**-dee-um **BEN**-zoh-ayt, fen-ill-**AH**-seh-tayt)
Pregnancy Category: C
Ucephan **(Rx)**

How Supplied: *Solution:* 10%-10%

Action/Kinetics: In clients with urea cycle enzymopathies, there is a deficiency (either partial or complete) of argininosuccinate synthetase, carbamoylphosphate synthetase, and ornithine transcarbamylase. This leads to elevated blood ammonia levels, which is fatal in nearly 80% of clients. Sodium benzoate and sodium phenylacetate lower elevated blood ammonia levels by decreasing ammonia formation, thus substituting for the defective enzymes in these individuals.

Uses: Prophylaxis and chronic treatment of hyperammonemia in clients with urea cycle enzymopathies.

Dosage

- **Oral Solution**

Hyperammonemia.

Adults: 2.5 mL/kg/day (250 mg each of sodium benzoate and sodium phenylacetate) in three to six equally divided doses. Total daily dose should not exceed 100 mL (i.e., 10 g each of sodium benzoate and sodium phenylacetate).

Administration/Storage

1. This product must be diluted in 4–8 oz of milk (or infant formula) and given with meals. Acidic liquids should not be used since the drug may precipitate in an acid medium. The mixture should be visually inspected for compatibility before it is administered.
2. Sodium benzoate and sodium phenylacetate should be considered

as adjunctive therapy for urea cycle enzymopathies.
3. For optimum results, combine with a low-protein diet and amino acid supplements.
4. Care should be exercised when mixing and administering sodium phenylacetate since contact with the skin and clothing will result in a lingering odor.
5. The product should be stored at room temperature; excess heat should be avoided.
6. *Treatment of Overdose:* Discontinue the drug and treat symptoms. It may be necessary to treat for metabolic acidosis and circulatory collapse. Hemodialysis or peritoneal dialysis may be helpful.

Contraindications: Hypersensitivity to sodium benzoate or sodium phenylacetate. The sodium ions in this product should be used with care (if at all) in CHF, edema due to sodium retention, and renal insufficiency.

Special Concerns: Use with caution during lactation and in neonates with hyperbilirubinemia.

Side Effects: *GI:* N&V, worsening of peptic ulcers. *Respiratory:* Respiratory alkalosis and hyperventilation.

Symptoms of Overdose: Vomiting, irritability, metabolic acidosis, circulatory collapse.

Drug Interactions

Penicillin / ↑ Renal tubular secretion due to competition from sodium benzoate and sodium phenylacetate

Probenecid / ↓ Renal excretion of conjugation products of sodium benzoate and sodium phenylacetate

NURSING CONSIDERATIONS

Assessment

1. Document indications for therapy and onset of symptoms.
2. Obtain serum electrolytes, pH, and ammonia levels and monitor throughout therapy.

Client/Family Teaching

1. Follow a low-protein diet. Refer to a dietitian for assistance with the diet and meal planning.
2. Provide written guidelines for the correct dilution and administration of the drug.
3. Instruct client in keeping an accurate record of weight and advise to report any significant changes.
4. Teach how to assess for edema and to report any unusual weight gain, swollen ankles, or dyspnea.
5. Provide a printed list of adverse side effects. Discuss the importance of reporting any adverse effects and/or changes in mental attitude.
6. Explain the importance of reporting for medical follow-up visits and for scheduled lab studies so that the effectiveness of the drug therapy can be evaluated.

Evaluate: Reduction of elevated serum ammonia levels.

Sodium polystyrene sulfonate

(**SO**-dee-um pol-ee-**STY**-reen **SUL**-fon-ayt)

Kayexalate, PMS Sodium Polystyrene Sulfonate ★, SPS **(Rx)**

How Supplied: *Powder for reconstitution; Suspension:* 15 g/60 mL, 50 g/200 mL

Action/Kinetics: Sodium polystyrene sulfonate is a resin that exchanges sodium ions for potassium ions primarily in the large intestine. Thus, excess amounts of potassium (as well as calcium and magnesium) may be removed. Therapy is governed by daily monitoring of serum potassium levels. Discontinue therapy when serum potassium levels have reached 4–5 mEq/L. Clients should also be monitored for serum calcium and magnesium levels. **Onset, PO:** 2–12 hr.

Uses: Hyperkalemia.

Dosage

• **Powder for Suspension, Suspension**

Hyperkalemia.

Adults: 15 g resin suspended in 20–100 mL water or syrup (to increase palatability) 1–4 times/day. Up to 40 g/day has been used. **Pediatric:** To calculate dose, use an exchange ratio of 1 mEq potassium/g resin (usually, 1 g/kg dose).

- **Enema**

Hyperkalemia.

25–100 g suspended in 100 mL sorbitol or 20% dextrose in water q 6 hr.

Administration/Storage

1. To treat or to prevent constipation, 10–20 mL of 70% sorbitol may be given PO q 2 hr (or as necessary) to produce 1–2 watery stools each day.
2. For PO administration, give the resin suspended in water or sorbitol syrup (3–4 mL/g resin). If necessary, the resin can be administered through a NGT, either as an aqueous suspension, mixed with dextrose, or as a peanut or olive oil emulsion.
3. Rectal administration:

- First, administer a cleansing enema.
- To administer medication, insert a large-size rubber tube (e.g., French 28) into the rectum for a distance of 20 cm until it is well into the sigmoid colon and tape in place.
- Suspend resin in appropriate vehicle (see *Dosage*) at body temperature. Administer by gravity while stirring suspension.
- Flush suspension that remains in the container with 50–100 mL fluid, clamp the tube, and leave in place.
- Elevate client's hips or ask the client to assume a knee-chest position for a short time if there is back leakage.
- The enema should be kept in the colon as long as possible (3–4 hr).
- Resin is removed by colonic irrigation with 2 quarts of a *non-sodium*-containing solution warmed to body temperature. Returns are drained constantly through a Y tube.

4. Retention enemas of the resin are less effective than PO administration.
5. Use freshly prepared solutions within 24 hr. Do not heat resin.
6. Oral suspension products contain sorbitol and sodium.
7. Orders for the drug should designate the grams of powder and the percent sorbitol and volume to be used or the amount of premixed suspension. The frequency and route of administration should also be specified.
8. Avoid inhaling the powder for suspension when admixing.

Special Concerns: Use with caution in geriatric clients because they are more likely to develop fecal impaction. Use with caution in clients sensitive to sodium overload (e.g., in CV disease) or for those receiving digitalis preparations because the action of these agents is potentiated by hypokalemia.

Side Effects: *GI:* N&V, constipation, anorexia, gastric irritation, diarrhea (rarely). Fecal impaction in geriatric clients. *Electrolyte:* Sodium retention, hypokalemia, hypocalcemia, hypomagnesemia. *Other:* Overhydration, ***pulmonary edema.***

Drug Interactions

Aluminum hydroxide / ↑ Risk of intestinal obstruction

Calcium- or magnesium-containing antacids or laxatives / ↑ Risk of metabolic alkalosis

NURSING CONSIDERATIONS

Assessment

1. Document serum potassium levels. Attempt to identify cause for increased levels.
2. Determine if the client has a history of CV disease and/or is taking any digitalis preparations.

Interventions

1. Monitor renal function studies and the level of serum potassium, sodium, magnesium, and calcium. Observe for symptoms of electrolyte imbalance.
2. Assess clients on sodium restrictions closely; drug contains 100 mg Na/g.
3. The administration of calcium- or magnesium-containing antacids during PO administration of sodium polystyrene sulfonate may predispose the client to metabolic alkalosis. Therefore, administer antacids cautiously.
4. Monitor VS and I&O. Report any increase in urinary output or constipation.

5. Encourage clients receiving the medication PR to retain the solution for several hours to ensure effectiveness of drug therapy.
Evaluate: Reduction of high serum potassium levels to within desired range (4.0–5.0 mEq/L).

Trientine hydrochloride

(**TRY**-en-teen)
Pregnancy Category: C
Syprine **(Rx)**

How Supplied: *Capsule:* 250 mg
Action/Kinetics: Trientine is a chelating agent that binds copper, thus facilitating its excretion from the body.
Use: Individuals with Wilson's disease (a metabolic defect resulting in excess copper accumulation) who are intolerant of penicillamine.

Dosage

- **Capsules**

Wilson's disease.

Adults, initial: 750 mg/day–1.25 g/day in divided doses b.i.d., t.i.d., or q.i.d.; **then,** may increase to a maximum of 2 g/day. **Children less than 12 years of age, initial:** 500–750 mg/day in divided doses b.i.d., t.i.d., or q.i.d.; **then,** may increase to a maximum of 1.5 g/day.
Administration/Storage
1. Trientine should be taken on an empty stomach at least 1 hr before meals or 2 hr after meals and at least 1 hr apart from any other drug, food, or milk.
2. Capsules should be swallowed whole with water; they should not be chewed or opened.
3. The daily dose should be increased only if the response is not adequate or the serum copper level is consistently greater than 20 mcg/dL.
4. At 6–12-month intervals, the optimal long-term maintenance dosage should be determined.
5. If the contents of the capsule come in contact with any site on the body, it should be promptly washed with water to avoid contact dermatitis.
6. Capsules should be stored at 2°C–8°C (36°F–46°F).
Contraindications: Use in cystinuria, rheumatoid arthritis, biliary cirrhosis.
Special Concerns: Use with caution during lactation. Safety and effectiveness in children have not been determined although the drug has been used in children as young as 6 years of age.
Side Effects: Iron deficiency anemia, SLE.

NURSING CONSIDERATIONS

Assessment
1. Obtain baseline CBC and serum copper levels.
2. Note previous treatment regimens and their results.
Client/Family Teaching
1. Take only as directed and on an empty stomach.
2. Advise to avoid mineral supplements as they may interfere with the absorption of trientine.
3. Emphasize that iron deficiency anemia may develop in children, in menstruating or pregnant women, or as a result of the low-copper diet necessary to treat Wilson's disease. Iron may be given in such cases but allow 2 hr between administration of iron and trientine.
4. Instruct that body temperature should be taken and recorded nightly for the first month of treatment and any symptoms such as fever or skin eruption should be reported.
5. Report for all scheduled lab studies so that effectiveness of drug therapy can be assessed. Serum copper levels will be followed, and periodically, clients may be monitored with a 24-hr urinary copper analysis (i.e., q 6–12 months).
6. Determination of free serum copper is the most reliable way to monitor the effectiveness of therapy. Clients who are responsive to therapy will have less than 10 mcg/dL of free copper in the serum.
Evaluate: ↓ Serum copper levels and relief of symptoms of copper toxicity.

CHAPTER EIGHTY-FIVE

Vitamins

See the following individual entries:

Cyanocobalamin
Cyanocobalamin Crystalline
Folic Acid
Leucovorin Calcium
Niacin
Niacinamide
Pantothenic Acid
Pyridoxine Hydrochloride
Riboflavin
Thiamine Hydrochloride
Vitamin K
Phytonadione

Cyanocobalamin (Vitamin B_{12})

(sye-**an**-oh-koh-**BAL**-ah-min)
Pregnancy Category: C
Nasal gel: Ener-B **(OTC)**. **Parenteral:** Anacobin ✱, Berubigen, Kaybovite-1000, Redisol, Rubion ✱, Rubramin ✱, Rubramin PC **(OTC) (Rx)**

Cyanocobalamin crystalline

(sye-**an**-oh-koh-**BAL**-ah-min)
Pregnancy Category: C
Crystamine, Crysti 1000, Cyanoject, Cyomin, Rubesol-1000, Vitamin B_{12}

How Supplied: Cyanocobalamin: *Tablet:* 25 mcg, 50 mcg, 100 mcg, 250 mcg, 500 mcg, 1,000 mcg, 2,500 mcg; *Tablet, Extended Release:* 1,000 mcg, 1,500 mcg
cyanocobalamin crystalline: *Injection:* 100 mcg/mL, 1,000 mcg/mL

Action/Kinetics: Cyanocobalamin (vitamin B_{12}) is a cobalt-containing vitamin essential to growth. The vitamin can also be isolated from liver and is identical to that of the antianemic factor of liver. This vitamin is required for hematopoiesis, cell reproduction, nucleoprotein and myelin synthesis. Plasma vitamin B_{12} levels: 150–750 pg/mL.

Intrinsic factor is required for adequate absorption of PO vitamin B_{12} and in pernicious anemia and malabsorption diseases intrinsic factor is administered simultaneously. This vitamin is rapidly absorbed following IM or SC administration. Following absorption, vitamin B_{12} is carried by plasma proteins to the liver where it is stored until required for various metabolic functions.

Products containing less than 500 mcg vitamin B_{12} are nutritional supplements and are not to be used for the treatment of pernicious anemia. **t½:** 6 days (400 days in the liver). **Time to peak levels, after PO:** 8–12 hr.

Uses: Nutritional vitamin B_{12} deficiency, including cancer of the bowel or pancreas, sprue, total or partial gastrectomy, accompanying folic acid deficiency, GI surgery or pathology, gluten enteropathy, fish tapeworm infestation, bacterial overgrowth of the small intestine. Oral products should not be used to treat pernicious anemia. Also, in conditions with an increased need for vitamin B_{12} such as thyrotoxicosis, hemorrhage, malignancy, pregnancy, and in liver and kidney disease. Vitamin B_{12} is particularly suitable for the treatment of clients allergic to liver extract.

Investigational: Diagnosis of vitamin B_{12} deficiency.

NOTE: Folic acid is not a substitute for vitamin B_{12} although concurrent folic acid therapy may be required.

Dosage

- **Tablets, Nasal Gel**
  Nutritional supplement.

Adults: 1 mcg/day (up to 25 mcg for increased requirements). The RDA is 2 mcg/day. **Pediatric, up to 1 year:** 0.3 mcg/day; **over 1 year:** 1 mcg/day.

Nutritional deficiency.

25–250 mcg/day.

• **IM, Deep SC**

Addisonian pernicious anemia.

Adults: 100 mcg/day for 6–7 days; **then,** 100 mcg every other day for seven doses. If improvement is noted along with a reticulocyte response, 100 mcg q 3–4 days for 2–3 weeks; **maintenance, IM:** 100 mcg once a month for life. Give folic acid if necessary.

Vitamin B_{12} deficiency.

Adults: 30 mcg daily for 5–10 days; **then,** 100–200 mcg/month. Doses up to 1,000 mcg have been recommended. **Pediatric, for hematologic signs:** 10–50 mcg/day for 5–10 days followed by 100–250 mcg/dose q 2–4 weeks. **Pediatric, for neurologic signs:** 100 mcg/day for 10–15 days; **then,** 1–2 times/week for several months (can possibly be tapered to 250–1,000 mcg/month by 1 year).

Diagnosis of vitamin B_{12} deficiency.

Adults: 1 mcg/day IM for 10 days plus low dietary folic acid and vitamin B_{12}. Loading dose for the Schilling test is 1,000 mcg given IM.

Administration/Storage

1. Protect cyanocobalamin crystalline injection from light.
2. The medication should not be frozen.
3. Note that if the client is being treated for pernicious anemia, the drug cannot be administered PO.
4. Have epinephrine, antihistamines, and steroids available in the event of an adverse drug reaction.

Contraindications: Hypersensitivity to cobalt, Leber's disease.

Special Concern: Use with caution in clients with gout.

Laboratory Test Interferences: Antibiotics may interfere with the microbiologic assay for serum and erythrocyte vitamin B_{12}.

Side Effects: Manifested following parenteral use. *Allergic:* Urticaria, itching, exanthema, ***anaphylaxis, shock, death.*** *CV:* ***Peripheral vascular thrombosis,*** CHF, ***pulmonary edema.*** *Other:* Polycythemia vera, optic nerve atrophy in clients with hereditary optic nerve atrophy, diarrhea, hypokalemia, body feels swollen.

NOTE: Benzyl alcohol, which is present in certain products, may cause ***a fatal "gasping syndrome"*** in premature infants.

Drug Interactions

Alcohol / ↓ Vitamin B_{12} absorption
Chloramphenicol / ↓ Response to vitamin B_{12} therapy
Cholestyramine / ↓ Vitamin B_{12} absorption
Cimetidine / ↓ Digestion and release of vitamin B_{12}
Colchicine / ↓ Vitamin B_{12} absorption
Neomycin / ↓ Vitamin B_{12} absorption
PAS / ↓ Vitamin B_{12} absorption
Potassium, timed-release / ↓ Vitamin B_{12} absorption

NURSING CONSIDERATIONS

Assessment

1. Determine if client is allergic to cobalt.
2. Note if client has been taking chloramphenicol. This drug antagonizes the hematopoietic response to vitamin B_{12}.
3. Determine any other prescribed drugs that could cause an unfavorable response to vitamin B_{12}.
4. Perform a baseline assessment of peripheral pulses.
5. Document indications for therapy and onset of symptoms.
6. Obtain and monitor serum potassium levels if client is being treated for megaloblastic anemia.
7. With pernicious anemia and malabsorption syndromes, note that intrinsic factor should be administered simultaneously.

Client/Family Teaching

1. If the client is being treated for pernicious anemia, stress that vitamin B_{12} replacement *must* be taken for life.

2. When repository vitamin B_{12} is used, it will provide medication for at least 4 weeks.
3. Explain that the stinging, burning sensation that may occur after injection is transitory. However, remind the client that if the burning sensation occurs anywhere except where the needle is, to call it to the nurse's attention immediately. The needle should be withdrawn and a different site selected for injection.
4. If vitamin B_{12} therapy is the result of dietary deficiency, discuss diet with the client. Provide printed material concerning appropriate foods (such as meats, especially liver, fermented cheeses, egg yolks, and seafood) and review with clients methods of achieving a balance in their diet. Refer to a dietitian for additional assistance as needed.
5. Avoid alcohol while taking vitamin B_{12} because it will interfere with the absorption of the medication.
6. Report any symptoms of urticaria, complaints of itching, and evidence of anaphylaxis immediately.
7. If clients complain of diarrhea, monitor the frequency and consistency of their stools. If the diarrhea is severe or persists, a change in drug may be required.

Evaluate

- Client understanding of the underlying cause and associated symptoms of vitamin B_{12} deficiency state
- Improvement in symptoms of vitamin B_{12} deficiency following replacement therapy
- Plasma vitamin B_{12} levels of 150–750 pg/mL

Folic acid

(**FOH**-lik **AH**-sid)

Pregnancy Category: A

Apo-Folic ✱, Folvite (Rx and OTC)

How Supplied: *Injection:* 5 mg/mL; *Tablet:* 0.4 mg, 0.8 mg, 1 mg

Action/Kinetics: Folic acid (which is converted to tetrahydrofolic acid) is necessary for normal production of RBCs and for synthesis of nucleoproteins. Tetrahydrofolic acid is a cofactor in the biosynthesis of purines and thymidylates of nucleic acids. Megaloblastic and macrocytic anemias in folic acid deficiency are believed to be due to impairment of thymidylate synthesis. Natural sources of folic acid include liver, dried beans, peas, lentils, whole-wheat products, asparagus, beets, broccoli, brussels sprouts, spinach, and oranges. Synthetic folic acid is absorbed from the GI tract even if the client suffers from malabsorption syndrome. **Peak plasma levels after an oral dose:** 1 hr. It is stored in the liver.

Uses: Treatment of megaloblastic anemias due to folic acid deficiency (e.g., tropical and nontropical sprue, pregnancy, infancy or childhood, nutritional causes). Diagnosis of folate deficiency.

Dosage

- **Tablets**

Dietary supplement.

Adults and children: 100 mcg/day (up to 1 mg in pregnancy); may be increased to 500–1,000 mcg if requirements increase.

Treatment of deficiency.

Adults, initial: 250–1,000 mcg/day until a hematologic response occurs; **maintenance:** 400 mcg/day (800 mcg during pregnancy and lactation). **Pediatric, initial:** 250–1,000 mcg/day until a hematologic response occurs. **Maintenance, infants:** 100 mcg/day; **children up to 4 years:** 300 mcg/day; **children 4 years and older:** 400 mcg/day.

- **IM, IV, Deep SC**

Treatment of deficiency.

Adults and children: 250–1,000 mcg/day until a hematologic response occurs.

Diagnosis of folate deficiency.

Adults, IM: 100–200 mcg/day for 10 days plus low dietary folic acid and vitamin B_{12}.

Administration/Storage

1. Folic acid is given PO unless there

is severe malabsorption in which case it can be given either IV or SC.
2. Regardless of age, the dosage should never be less than 0.1 mg/day.
3. Folic acid will remain stable in solution if the pH is kept above 5.
4. The drug may be administered IM or by direct IV push or added to infusions. However, if administered by IV, the rate should not exceed 5 mcg/min.
5. When parenteral forms are used, have drugs and equipment available to treat potential allergic drug reactions.

Contraindications: Use in aplastic, normocytic, or pernicious anemias (is ineffective). Folic acid injection that contains benzyl alcohol should not be used in neonates or immature infants.

Special Concerns: Daily folic acid doses of 0.1 mg or greater may obscure pernicious anemia. Prolonged folic acid therapy may cause decreased vitamin B_{12} levels.

Side Effect: *Allergic:* Skin rash, itching, erythema, general malaise, respiratory difficulty due to bronchospasm. *GI:* Nausea, anorexia, abdominal distention, flatulence, bitter or bad taste (in those taking 15 mg/day for 1 month). *CNS:*In doses of 15 mg daily, altered sleep patterns, irritability, excitement, difficulty in concentration, overactivity, depression, impaired judgment, confusion.

Drug Interactions

Aminosalicylic acid / ↓ Serum folate levels
Corticosteroids (chronic use) / ↑ Folic acid requirements
Methotrexate / Is a folic acid antagonist
Oral contraceptives / ↑ Risk of folate deficiency
Phenytoin / Folic acid ↑ seizure frequency; also, phenytoin ↓ serum folic acid levels.
Pyrimethamine / Folic acid ↓ effect of pyrimethamine in toxoplasmosis; also, pyrimethamine is a folic acid antagonist
Sulfonamides / ↓ Absorption of folic acid
Triamterene / ↓ Utilization of folic acid as it is a folic acid antagonist
Trimethoprim / ↓ Utilization of folic acid as it is a folic acid antagonist

NURSING CONSIDERATIONS

Client/Family Teaching

1. Take only as directed.
2. Review dietary sources of folic acid such as dark green leafy vegetables, beans, fortified breads, and cereals. Prolonged cooking destroys folate in vegetables.
3. Advise that drug may discolor urine a deep yellow.
4. The U.S. Public Health Service recommends that all women of childbearing age consume 0.4 mg of folic acid to reduce the risk of neural tube birth defects. The consumption of folic acid may prevent the development of spina bifida or anencephaly, which occur during the first month of pregnancy.

Evaluate

• Desired hematologic response (↑ RBCs, WBCs, and platelet counts)
• Reversal in symptoms of folic acid deficiency and megaloblastic anemia
• Prophylaxis of neural tube defects

Leucovorin calcium (citrovorum factor, folinic acid)

(loo-koh-**VOR**-in)
Pregnancy Category: C
Lederle Leucovorin Calcium ✱, Wellcovorin **(Rx)**

How Supplied: *Powder for injection:* 50 mg, 100 mg, 350 mg; *Tablet:* 5 mg, 10 mg, 15 mg, 25 mg

Action/Kinetics: Leucovorin is a derivative of folic acid and is a mixture of the diasterioisomers of the 5-formyl derivative of tetrahydrofolic acid. It does not require reduction by dihydrofolate reductase to be active in intracellular metabolism; thus, it is not affected by dihydrofolate inhibitors. Leucovorin is rapidly absorbed following PO administration. It is quickly metabolized to 1,5-methyltetrahydrofolate, which is then metabolized by other pathways back to 5,10-methylene-tetrahydrofolate and then converted to 5-methyltetrahydrofolate using the cofactors $FADH_2$ and NADPH. Leucovorin can counteract the therapeutic and toxic effects of methotrexate (acts by inhibiting dihydrofolate reductase) but can enhance the effects of 5-fluorouracil (5-FU). Is rapdily absorbed. **Peak serum levels, PO:** Approximately 2.3 hr; **after IM:** 52 min; **after IV:** 10 min. **Onset, PO:** 20–30 min; **IM:** 10–20 min; **IV:** <5 min. **Terminal t½:** 5.7 hr (PO), 6.2 hr (IM and IV). **Duration:** 3–6 hr. The drug is excreted by the kidney.

Uses: PO and Parenteral: Prophylaxis and treatment of toxicity due to methotrexate and folic acid antagonists (e.g., pyrimethamine and trimethoprim). Leucovorin rescue following high doses of methotrexate for osteosarcoma. **Parenteral:** Megaloblastic anemias due to nutritional deficiency, sprue, pregnancy, and infancy when oral folic acid is not appropriate. Adjunct with 5-FU to treat metastatic colorectal carcinoma.

Dosage

- **IM, IV, Tablets**

Advanced colorectal cancer.

Either leucovorin, 200 mg/m² by slow IV over a minimum of 3 min followed by 5-FU, 370 mg/m² IV **or** leucovorin 20 mg/m² IV followed by 5-FU, 425 mg/m² IV. Treatment is repeated daily for 5 days with the 5-day treatment course repeated at 28-day intervals for two courses and then repeated at 4–5-week intervals as long as the client has recovered from the toxic effects.

Leucovorin rescue after high-dose methotrexate therapy.

The dose of leucovorin is based on a methotrexate dose of 12–15 mg/m² given by IV infusion over 4 hr. The dose of leucovorin is 15 mg (10 mg/m²) PO, IM, or IV q 6 hr for 10 doses starting 24 hr after the start of the methotrexate infusion. Give leucovorin parenterally if there is nausea, vomiting, or GI toxicity. If serum methotrexate levels are greater than 0.2 μM at 72 hr and greater than 0.05 μM at 96 hr after administration, leucovorin should be continued at a dose of 15 mg PO, IM, or IV q 6 hr until methotrexate levels are less than 0.05 μM. If serum methotrexate levels are equal to or greater than 50 μM at 24 hr or equal to or greater than 5 μM at 48 hr after administration or if there is a 100% or greater increase in serum creatinine levels at 24 hr after methotrexate administration, the dose of leucovorin should be 150 mg IV q 3 hr until methotrexate levels are less than 1 μM; **then,** give leucovorin, 15 mg IV q 3 hr until methotrexate levels are less than 0.05 μM. If significant clinical toxicity is seen following methotrexate, leucovorin rescue should total 14 doses over 84 hr in subsequent courses of methotrexate therapy.

Impaired methotrexate elimination or accidental overdose.

Start leucovorin rescue as soon as the overdose is discovered and within 24 hr of methotrexate administration when excretion is impaired. Give leucovorin, 10 mg/m² PO, IM, or IV q 6 hr until serum methotrexate levels are less than 10^{-8} M. If the 24-hr serum creatinine has increased 50% over baseline or if the 24- or 48-hr methotrexate level is more than 5×10^{-6} M or greater than 9×10^{-7} M, respectively, the dose of leucovorin should be increased to 100 mg/m² IV q 3 hr until the methotrexate level is less than 10^{-8} M. Urinary alkalinization with sodium bicarbonate solution (to maintain urine pH at 7 or greater) and hydration with 3 L/day should be undertaken at the same time.

Overdosage of folic acid antagonists.

5–15 mg/day.

Megaloblastic anemia due to folic acid deficiency.

Adults and children: Up to 1 mg/day.

Administration/Storage

1. If leucovorin is used for methotrexate rescue purposes, the client should be well hydrated and the urine should be alkalinized to reduce nephrotoxicity.
2. Leucovorin calcium injection should be diluted with 5 mL bacteriostatic water for injection and used within 1 week. If sterile water for injection is added, the solution should be used immediately.
3. The oral solution is stable for 14 days if refrigerated or for 7 days if stored at room temperature.
4. Doses higher than 25 mg should be given parenterally because oral absorption is saturated.
5. Leucovorin calcium injection containing benzyl alcohol should not be used for doses greater than 10 mg/m^2.
6. Parenteral use is preferred if there is a possibility that the client may vomit or not absorb leucovorin.
7. In treating overdosage due to folic acid antagonists, leucovorin should be given as soon as possible. As the time interval between the overdosage and administration of leucovorin increases, the effectiveness of leucovorin decreases.
8. The drug should be protected from light.

Contraindications: Pernicious anemia or megaloblastic anemia due to vitamin B_{12} deficiency.

Special Concerns: It is recommended for megaloblastic anemia caused by pregnancy even though the drug is pregnancy category C. Use with caution during lactation. May increase the frequency of seizures in susceptible children. When leucovorin is used with 5-FU for advanced colorectal cancer, the dosage of 5-FU must be lower than usual as leucovorin enhances the toxicity of 5-FU. The benzyl alcohol in the parenteral form may caues a fatal gasping syndrome in premature infants.

Side Effects: Leucovorin alone. Allergic reactions, including urticaria and ***anaphylaxis.***

Leucovorin and 5-FU. *GI:* N&V, diarrhea, stomatitis, constipation, anorexia. *Hematologic:* Leukopenia, thrombocytopenia. *CNS:* Fatigue, lethargy, malaise. *Miscellaneous:* Infection, alopecia, dermatitis.

Drug Interactions

5-FU / ↑ Toxicity of 5-FU
Methotrexate / High doses of leucovorin ↓ effect of intrathecally administered methotrexate
PAS / ↓ Serum folate levels → folic acid deficiency
Phenobarbital / ↓ Effect of phenobarbital → ↑ frequency of seizures, especially in children
Phenytoin / ↓ Effect of phenytoin due to ↑ rate of breakdown by liver; also, phenytoin may ↓ plasma folate levels
Primidone / ↓ Effect of primidone → ↑ frequency of seizures, especially in children
Sulfasalazine / ↓ Serum folate levels → folic acid deficiency

NURSING CONSIDERATIONS

Assessment

1. Document indications for therapy as replacement or rescue. If the client is receiving the drug for rescue therapy, it should be administered promptly (first dose within 1 hr) following a high dose of folic acid antagonists. The prescribed dosage must be followed exactly to be effective.
2. Note if the client has a history of vitamin B_{12} deficiency that has resulted in pernicious anemia or megaloblastic anemia. Leucovorin may obscure the diagnosis of pernicious anemia if previously undiagnosed.
3. Determine any history of seizure disorders and assess for a recurrence.
4. Obtain baseline renal, folic acid, and hematologic values and monitor throughout therapy. Creatinine increases of 50% over pretreatment levels indicate severe renal toxicity.

Interventions

1. Anticipate that leucovorin rescue is used in conjunction with methotrexate therapy.
2. Document and report any client complaints of skin rash, itching,

malaise, or difficulty breathing immediately.
3. Parenteral therapy generally is used following chemotherapy because N&V may prevent oral absorption.
4. Urine pH should be greater than 7.0; monitor q 6 hr during therapy. Urine alkalinization with $NaHCO_3$ or acetazolamide may be necessary to prevent nephrotoxic effects.
5. When high-dose therapy is used, be alert for mental confusion and impaired judgment. Provide appropriate safety measures and supervision to ensure client safety and protection.
6. Monitor I&O; encourage fluid intake of 3 L/day with rescue therapy.

Evaluate
- Improved symptomatology (↓ fatigue, weight gain)
- Laboratory evidence of an ↑ production of normoblasts (with megaloblastic anemias)
- Prevention and reversal of GI, renal, and bone marrow toxicity in methotrexate therapy or during overdosage of folic acid antagonists

Niacin (Nicotinic acid)

(**NYE**-ah-sin, nih-koh-**TIN**-ick **AH**-sid)
Pregnancy Category: C
Nia-Bid, Niacels, Nico-400, Nicobid, Nicolar, Nicotinex, Slo-Niacin, Span-Niacin, Tega-Span (Rx and OTC)

Niacinamide

(nye-ah-**SIN**-ah-myd)
Pregnancy Category: C
Papulex ✱ (Rx: Injection; OTC: Tablets)

How Supplied: Niacin: *Capsule:* 100 mg; *Capsule, Extended Release:* 125 mg, 250 mg, 400 mg, 500 mg, 750 mg; *Elixir:* 50 mg/5 mL; *Tablet:* 50 mg, 100 mg, 500 mg; *Tablet, Extended Release:* 250 mg, 500 mg, 750 mg, 1,000 mg.
Niacinamide: *Tablet:* 50 mg, 100 mg, 500 mg

Action/Kinetics: Niacin (nicotinic acid) and niacinamide are water-soluble, heat-resistant vitamins prepared synthetically. Niacin (after conversion to the active niacinamide) is a component of the coenzymes nicotinamide-adenine dinucleotide and nicotinamide-adenine dinucleotide phosphate, which are essential for oxidation-reduction reactions involved in lipid metabolism, glycogenolysis, and tissue respiration. Deficiency of niacin results in pellagra, the most common symptoms of which are dermatitis, diarrhea, and dementia. In high doses niacin also produces vasodilation and a reduction in serum lipids. **Peak serum levels:** 45 min; **t½:** 45 min.

Uses: Prophylaxis and treatment of pellagra; niacin deficiency. Niacin is also used to treat hyperlipidemia in clients not responding to either diet or weight loss.

Dosage

NIACIN
- **Extended-Release Capsules, Oral Solution, Tablets, Extended-Release Tablets**

Vitamin.

Adults: Up to 500 mg/day; **pediatric:** Up to 300 mg/day.

Antihyperlipidemic.

Adults, initial: 1 g t.i.d.; **then:** increase dose in increments of 500 mg/day q 2–4 weeks as needed. **Maintenance:** 1–2 g t.i.d. (up to a maximum of 6 g/day).
- **IM, IV**

Pellagra.

Adults, IM: 50–100 mg 5 or more times/day. **IV, slow:** 25–100 mg 2 or more times/day. **Pediatric, IV slow:** Up to 300 mg/day.

NIACINAMIDE
- **Capsules, Tablets**

Vitamin.

Adults: Up to 500 mg/day. **Pediatric:** Up to 300 mg/day. Capsules not recommended for use in children.

Administration/Storage
1. Nicotinic acid should be taken PO only with cold water (no hot beverages).

2. Can be taken with meals if GI upset occurs.
3. May administer IV form diluted (to 2 mg/mL solution concentration) at a rate not exceeding 2 mg/min.

Contraindications: Hypotension, hemorrhage, liver dysfunction, peptic ulcer. Use with caution in diabetics, gall bladder disease, and clients with gout.

Special Concerns: The extended-release tablets and capsules are not recommended for use in children. Extended-release niacin may be hepatotoxic.

Side Effects: *GI:* N&V, diarrhea, peptic ulcer activation, abdominal pain. *Dermatologic:* Flushing, warm feeling, skin rash, pruritus, dry skin, itching and tingling feeling, keratosis nigricans. *Other:* Hypotension, headache, macular cystoid edema, amblyopia. *NOTE:* Megadoses are accompanied by serious toxicity including the symptoms listed above as well as liver damage, hyperglycemia, hyperuricemia, arrhythmias, tachycardia, and dermatoses.

Drug Interactions

Chenodiol / ↓ Effect of chenodiol
Probenecid / Niacin may ↓ uricosuric effect of probenecid
Sulfinpyrazone / Niacin ↓ uricosuric effect of sulfinpyrazone
Sympathetic blocking agents / Additive vasodilating effects → postural hypotension

---

NURSING CONSIDERATIONS

Assessment

1. Obtain baseline plasma lipid levels and monitor periodically throughout therapy.
2. Note any history of peptic ulcer disease or liver or gallbladder dysfunction.

Client/Family Teaching

1. Client may experience a warm flushing in the face and ears within 2 hr after taking the medication. One aspirin may reduce effect. Alcohol may increase these effects.
2. Lie down if feeling weak and dizzy after taking niacin (until this feeling passes) and inform provider.
3. Identify foods sources high in niacin (dairy products, meats, tuna, and eggs) and determine levels of consumption.
4. Clients with diabetes mellitus should not take niacin unless specifically ordered and then the blood glucose levels must be closely monitored for hyperglycemia; also monitor for ketonuria and glucosuria. Clients taking antidiabetic agents may require an increase in dosage of these agents.
5. Clients with hepatic dysfunction should report any skin color changes or yellowing of the sclera.
6. Clients predisposed to gout may experience flank, joint, or stomach pains, which should be reported immediately.
7. If blurred vision occurs, advise to remain out of direct sunlight.
8. Advise against unsupervised excessive vitamin ingestion. Caution that high doses may impair liver function.
9. Report for all scheduled lab studies.

Evaluate

- ↓ Serum cholesterol and triglyceride levels
- Relief of symptoms of pellagra and niacin deficiency

Pantothenic acid (Vitamin B_5)

(pan-toe-**THEHN**-ick **AH**-sid)
Calcium Pantothenate **(OTC)**

How Supplied: *Tablet:* 100 mg, 200 mg, 250 mg, 500 mg, 1,000 mg; *Tablet, Extended Release:* 1,000 mg

Action/Kinetics: Pantothenic acid is a precursor of coenzyme A, which is a cofactor required for oxidative metabolism of carbohydrates, synthesis and breakdown of fatty acids, sterol synthesis, gluconeogenesis, and steroid synthesis. Pantothenic acid is found in many foods; thus, deficiency in human beings has not been observed.

Uses: There is no therapeutic indication for pantothenic acid alone because deficiency has not been observed. However, it is included in vitamin preparations for the prophylaxis and treatment of vitamin deficiency.

Dosage

• **Tablets**

Adults and children: Up to 100 mg/day has been used.

Contraindications: Hemophilia. Should not be used to treat diabetic neuropathy, increasing GI peristalsis, Addison's disease, allergies, respiratory disorders, improvement of mental processes, prevention of birth defects, or treatment of toxicity due to salicylate or streptomycin.

Side Effects: Allergic symptoms have occurred occasionally.

NURSING CONSIDERATIONS

Assessment

1. Review client history to determine any evidence of conditions for which drug is contraindicated.
2. Assess for any allergic manifestations such as rash, erythema, or itching as this is an indication to discontinue drug therapy.

Evaluate: Desired vitamin B5 replacement therapy.

Pyridoxine hydrochloride (Vitamin B_6)

(peer-ih-**DOX**-een)

Pregnancy Category: A

Hexa-Betalin ✦, Nestrex (Rx: Injection; OTC: Tablets)

How Supplied: *Capsule:* 150 mg; *Enteric coated tablet:* 20 mg; *Injection:* 100 mg/mL; *Tablet:* 10 mg, 25 mg, 32.5 mg, 50 mg, 100 mg, 200 mg, 250 mg, 500 mg; *Tablet, extended release:* 100 mg, 200 mg

Action/Kinetics: Pyridoxine hydrochloride is a water-soluble, heat-resistant vitamin that is destroyed by light. It is prepared synthetically. It acts as a coenzyme in the metabolism of protein, carbohydrates, and fat. As the amount of protein increases in the diet, the pyridoxine requirement increases. However, pyridoxine deficiency alone is rare. **t½:** 2–3 weeks. Metabolized in the liver and excreted through the urine.

Uses: Pyridoxine deficiency including poor diet, drug-induced (e.g., oral contraceptives, isoniazid), and inborn errors of metabolism. *Investigational:* Hydrazine poisoning, PMS, high urine oxalate levels, N&V due to pregnancy.

Dosage

• **Extended-Release Capsules, Tablets**

Dietary supplement.

Adults: 10–20 mg/day for 2 weeks; **then,** 2–5 mg/day as part of a multivitamin preparation for several weeks. **Pediatric,** 2.5–10 mg/day for 3 weeks; **then,** 2–5 mg/day as part of a multivitamin preparation for several weeks.

Pyridoxine dependency syndrome.

Adults and children, initial: 30–600 mg/day; **maintenance,** 30 mg/day for life. **Infants, maintenance:** 2–10 mg/day for life.

Drug-induced deficiency.

Adults, prophylaxis: 10–50 mg/day for penicillamine or 100–300 mg/day for cycloserine, hydralazine, or isoniazid. **Adults, treatment:** 50–200 mg/day for 3 weeks followed by 25–100 mg/day to prevent relapse. **Adults, alcoholism:** 50 mg/day for 2–4 weeks; if anemia responds, continue pyridoxine indefinitely.

Hereditary sideroblastic anemia.

Adults: 200–600 mg/day for 1–2 months; **then,** 30–50 mg/day for life.

• **IM, IV**

Pyridoxine dependency syndrome.

Adults: 30–600 mg/day. **Pediatric:** 10–100 mg initially.

Drug-induced deficiency.

Adults: 50–200 mg/day for 3 weeks followed by 25–100 mg/day as needed.

Cycloserine poisoning.

Adults: 300 mg/day.

Isoniazid poisoning.
Adults: 1 g for each gram of isoniazid taken.
Administration/Storage
1. If client also receiving levodopa, preparations of vitamins containing vitamin B_6 should be avoided because vitamin B_6 decreases the availability of levodopa to the brain.
2. May be administered direct IV or placed in infusion solutions.
3. *Treatment of Overdose:* Discontinue pyridoxine; allow up to 6 months for CNS sensation to return.
Special Concerns: Safety and effectiveness have not been established in children.
Side Effects: *CNS:* Unstable gait; decreased sensation to touch, temperature, and vibration; paresthesia, sleepiness; numbness of feet; awkwardness of hands; perioral numbness. *NOTE:* Abuse and dependence have been noted in adults administered 200 mg/day.
Symptoms of Overdose: Ataxia, severe sensory neuropathy.
Drug Interactions
Chloramphenicol / ↑ Pyridoxine requirements
Contraceptives, oral / ↑ Pyridoxine requirements
Cycloserine / ↑ Pyridoxine requirements
Ethionamide / ↑ Pyridoxine requirements
Hydralazine / ↑ Pyridoxine requirements
Immunosuppressants / ↑ Pyridoxine requirements
Isoniazid / ↑ Pyridoxine requirements
Levodopa / Daily doses exceeding 5 mg pyridoxine antagonize the therapeutic effect of levodopa
Penicillamine / ↑ Pyridoxine requirements
Phenobarbital / Pyridoxine ↓ serum levels of phenobarbital
Phenytoin / Pyridoxine ↓ serum levels of phenytoin

NURSING CONSIDERATIONS

Assessment
1. Document indications for therapy and type and onset of symptoms.
2. Take a complete drug history. If the client is taking cycloserine, isoniazid, or oral contraceptives, report before administering vitamin B_6. These drugs increase pyridoxine requirements.
Client/Family Teaching
1. Provide a printed list of foods high in vitamin B_6 (e.g., potatoes, lima beans, broccoli, bananas, chicken breast, liver, whole-grain cereals). Explain that well-balanced diets are the best source of vitamins and refer to dietitian as needed.
2. If client is prescribed levodopa, avoid vitamin supplements containing vitamin B_6. More than 5 mg of the vitamin antagonizes the effect of levodopa. At the same time, concomitant administration of carbidopa will prevent the effect of vitamin B_6 on levodopa.
3. Clients taking phenobarbital and/or phenytoin should be scheduled for serum drug levels on a routine basis since pyridoxine alters serum concentrations.
4. If client is a nursing mother, advise that pyridoxine may inhibit lactation.
5. Explain reasons for drug therapy, e.g., to prevent toxicity (peripheral neuropathy) with long term isoniazid or contraceptive therapy, to replace vitamin B_6 with inborn errors of metabolism or with poor nutrition, etc.
Evaluate
- Relief of symptoms of pyridoxine deficiency
- Prophylaxis of drug-induced deficiency
- Reduction in certain toxic drug side effects
- Relief of pregnancy-associated N&V

Riboflavin (Vitamin B_2)

(**RYE**-boh-flay-vin)
(OTC)

How Supplied: *Enteric Coated Tablet:* 5 mg; *Tablet:* 10 mg, 25 mg, 50 mg, 100 mg, 250 mg

Action/Kinetics: Riboflavin is a water-soluble, heat-resistant substance that is sensitive to light. Riboflavin acts as a coenzyme as flavin adenine dinucleotide and flavin mononucleotide, which are required for various respiration systems in tissues. Riboflavin deficiency is characterized by characteristic lesions of the tongue, lips, and face, photophobia, itching, burning and keratosis of the eyes. Riboflavin deficiency often accompanies pellagra.
Uses: Prophylaxis or treatment of riboflavin deficiency. Adjunct, with niacin, in the treatment of pellagra.

Dosage

- **Tablets**

Deficiency states.
5–25 mg/day for several days; **then,** 1–4 mg/day.

Recommended dietary allowances.
Adults, males: 1.4–1.8 mg/day; **females:** 1.2–1.3 mg/day.
Side Effect: Large doses may cause urine to have a yellow discoloration.
Drug Interactions
Alcohol / Impairs absorption of riboflavin
Antidepressants, tricyclic / ↑ Requirements of riboflavin
Chloramphenicol / Riboflavin may counteract bone marrow depression and optic neuritis due to chloramphenicol
Phenothiazines / ↑ Requirements for riboflavin
Probenecid / ↑ Requirements for riboflavin
Tetracyclines / Antibiotic activity ↓ by riboflavin

NURSING CONSIDERATIONS

Client/Family Teaching
1. Take with meals or food to enhance absorption.
2. Review dietary sources of riboflavin (dairy products, green leafy vegetables, nuts, veal, beef and chicken livers, and enriched flours) and refer client to dietitian for assistance in meal planning and preparation.
3. Drug may cause urine to appear bright yellow; this is harmless.
4. Avoid alcohol as this impairs riboflavin absorption.
Evaluate: Relief of symptoms and/or desired prophylaxis with riboflavin deficiency.

Thiamine hydrochloride (Vitamin B_1)

(**THIGH**-ah-min)
Pregnancy Category: A (parenteral use)
Betaxin ✱, Bewon ✱, Thiamilate (Rx: Injection; OTC: Tablets)

How Supplied: *Enteric Coated Tablet:* 20 mg; *Injection:* 100 mg/mL; *Tablet:* 25 mg, 50 mg, 100 mg, 250 mg, 500 mg
Action/Kinetics: Water-soluble vitamin, stable in acid solution. The vitamin is decomposed in neutral or acid solutions. Thiamine is required for the synthesis of thiamine pyrophosphate, a coenzyme required in carbohydrate metabolism. The maximum amount absorbed PO is 8–15 mg/day although absorption may be increased by giving in divided doses with food.
Uses: Prophylaxis and treatment of thiamine deficiency states and associated neurologic and CV symptoms. Prophylaxis and treatment of beriberi. Alcoholic neuritis, neuritis of pellagra, and neuritis of pregnancy. To correct anorexia due to thiamine insufficiency. *Investigational:* Treatment of subacute necrotizing encephalomyelopathy, maple syrup urine disease, pyruvate carboxylase deficiency, hyperalaninemia.

Dosage

- **Tablets**

Mild beriberi or maintenance following severe beriberi.
Adults: 5–10 mg/day (as part of a multivitamin product); **infants:** 10 mg/day.

Treatment of deficiency.

Adults: 5–10 mg/day; **pediatric:** 10–50 mg/day.

Alcohol-induced deficiency.

Adults: 40 mg/day.

Dietary supplement.

Adults: 1–2 mg/day; **pediatric:** 0.3–0.5 mg/day for infants and 0.5 mg/day for children.

Genetic enzyme deficiency disease.

10–20 mg/day (up to 4 g/day has been used in some clients).

• **Slow IV**

Wet beriberi with myocardial failure.

Adults: 10–30 mg t.i.d.

• **IM**

Beriberi.

10–20 mg t.i.d. for 2 weeks. A PO multivitamin product containing 5–10 mg/day thiamine should be given for 1 month to cause body saturation.

Recommended dietary allowance.

Adult males: 1.2–1.5 mg; **adult females:** 1.1 mg.

Administration/Storage

1. May administer direct IV undiluted over at least 5 min or may be reconstituted in dextrose or saline solution and administered with daily solution therapy.
2. The drug may enhance the effects of neuromuscular blocking agents. Have epinephrine available to treat clients for anaphylactic shock if a large parenteral dose of thiamine is ordered.

Special Concerns: Use with caution during lactation.

Side Effects: ***Serious hypersensitivity reactions;*** thus, intradermal testing is recommended if sensitivity is suspected. *Dermatologic:* Pruritus, urticaria, sweating, feeling of warmth. *CNS:* Weakness, restlessness. *Other:* Nausea, tightness in throat, ***angioneurotic edema,*** cyanosis, ***hemorrhage into the GI tract, pulmonary edema, CV collapse. Death has been reported.*** *Following IM use:* Induration, tenderness.

Drug Interactions: Because vitamin B_1 is unstable in neutral or alkaline solutions, the vitamin should not be used with substances that yield alkaline solutions, such as citrates, barbiturates, carbonates, or erythromycin lactobionate IV.

NURSING CONSIDERATIONS

Assessment

1. Document indications for therapy and type and onset of symptoms.
2. List any other agents prescribed to ensure none interact unfavorably.

Client/Family Teaching

1. Review dietary sources high in thiamine (enriched and whole grain cereals, meats, especially pork, and fresh vegetables) and refer to a dietitian for assistance in meal planning and preparation.
2. Provide a printed list of side effects that require reporting if evident.

Evaluate

• Prophylaxis and/or relief of symptoms of thiamine deficiency

• Prevention or reduction of symptoms of neuritis

VITAMIN K

See also the following individual entries:

Phytonadione

Action/Kinetics: Vitamin K is essential for the hepatic synthesis of factors II, VII, IX, and X, all of which are essential for blood clotting. The chief manifestation of vitamin K deficiency is an increase in bleeding tendency, demonstrated by ecchymoses, epistaxis, hematuria, GI bleeding, postoperative and intracranial hemorrhage.

Vitamin K is available as phytonadione (vitamin K_1), a synthetic lipid-soluble analog and menadiol sodium diphosphate (vitamin K_4), a water-soluble synthetic analog.

Uses: Primary and drug-induced hypoprothrombinemia, especially that caused by anticoagulants of the coumarin and phenindione type. Vitamin K cannot reverse the anticoagulant activity of heparin.

Parenteral use for vitamin K malabsorption syndromes. Adjunct during whole blood transfusions. Preoperatively to prevent the danger of hemorrhages in surgical clients who may require anticoagulant therapy.

Certain forms of liver disease. Hemorrhagic states associated with obstructive jaundice, celiac disease, ulcerative colitis, sprue, biliary fistula, cystic fibrosis of the pancreas, regional enteritis, resection of intestine.

Contraindications: Severe liver disease.

Special Concerns: Use in infants. Use with caution during lactation. Use with caution in clients with sulfite sensitivity.

Side Effects: *Allergic:* Rash, urticaria, ***anaphylaxis.*** *After PO use:* N&V, stomach upset, headache. *After parenteral use:* Flushing, alteration of taste, sweating, hypotension, dizziness, rapid and weak pulse, dyspnea, cyanosis, delayed skin reactions. Pain, swelling, and tenderness at injection site. *Newborns:* Hyperbilirubinemia and ***fatal kernicterus.***

Drug Interactions

Antibiotics / May inhibit the body's production of vitamin K and may lead to bleeding. Vitamin K supplements should be given

Anticoagulants, oral / Vitamin K antagonizes anticoagulant effect

Cholestyramine / ↓ Effect of phytonadione and menadione due to ↓ absorption from GI tract

Colestipol / ↓ Effect of phytonadione and menadione due to ↓ absorption from GI tract

Hemolytics / ↑ Potential for toxicity (especially with menadione)

Mineral oil / ↓ Effect of phytonadione and menadione due to ↓ absorption from GI tract

Quinidine, Quinine / ↑ Requirement for vitamin K

Salicylates / High doses of salicylates → ↑ requirements for vitamin K

Sulfonamides / ↑ Requirements for vitamin K

Sucralfate / ↓ Effect of phytonadione and menadione due to ↓ absorption from GI tract

Dosage

See individual drugs.

NURSING CONSIDERATIONS

Assessment

1. Document any sensitivity to sulfites.
2. Note drugs the client is taking to determine how they may interact with vitamin K
3. Obtain baseline PT and PTT and liver and hematologic values prior to initiating therapy.
4. Determine if client has any history or lab evidence of advanced liver disease. This condition results in loss of protein synthesis and is not responsive to vitamin K.
5. Note indications for drug therapy and any associated symptoms.

Interventions

1. Monitor liver function studies and hematologic values during drug therapy.
2. Note any evidence of frank bleeding. Test stools, urine, and GI drainage for occult blood.
3. Observe hospitalized clients with poor nutrition (receiving TPN), uremia, recent surgery, and multiple antibiotic therapy for vitamin K deficiency.

Client/Family Teaching

1. Advise client to take vitamin K only as directed.
2. Identify dietary sources high in vitamin K (dairy products, meats, and green leafy vegetables). Explain that generally the dietary requirement is low since it is also synthesized by colonized bacteria in the intestine.
3. Report any evidence of unusual bruising or bleeding immediately.
4. Avoid alcohol, aspirin, and ibuprofen compounds (NSAIDs) as well as any other OTC preparations without medical approval.

Evaluate

- Prevention or control of bleeding
- PT within desired range (usually 1.5–2 times the control)

Phytonadione (Vitamin K_1)

(fye-toe-nah-**DYE**-ohn)

Pregnancy Category: C
Aqua-Mephyton, Konakion, Mephyton **(Rx)**

See also *Vitamin K,* Chapter 85.
How Supplied: *Injection:* 1 mg/0.5 mL, 10 mg /mL; *Tablet:* 5 mg
Action/Kinetics: Phytonadione is similar to natural vitamin K. It has a more rapid and more prolonged effect than menadiol sodium diphosphate and is generally more effective. GI absorption occurs only via intestinal lymphatics and requires the presence of bile salts. Vitamin K is not effective in reversing the anticoagulant effect of heparin. Frequent determinations of PT are indicated during therapy. **IM: Onset,** 1–2 hr. *Control of bleeding:* Parenteral, 3–6 hr. *Normal PT:* 12–14 hr. **PO: Onset,** 6–12 hr.
Additional Use: Prophylaxis of hemorrhagic disease of the newborn.

Dosage

- **Tablets**

Hypoprothrombinemia, drug-induced.

Adults: 2.5–10 mg (up to 25 mg); dose may be repeated after 12–48 hr if needed.

Vitamin supplement, prothrombogenic, drug-induced hypoprothrombinemia.

Pediatric: 5–10 mg.

- **IM, SC**

Vitamin supplement, prothrombogenic, drug-induced hypoprothrombinemia.

Adults: 2.5–10 mg (up to 25 mg) which may be repeated after 6–8 hr if needed. **Infants:** 1–2 mg; **children:** 5–10 mg.

Prophylaxis of hypoprothrombinemia during prolonged TPN.

Adults, IM: 5–10 mg once weekly; **pediatric:** 2–5 mg IM once weekly.

Infants receiving milk substitutes or who are breastfed.

1 mg/month if vitamin K in diet is less than 0.1 mg/L.

Prevention of hemorrhagic disease in the newborn.

0.5–1 mg IM within 1 hr after delivery. The dose may be repeated in 2–3 weeks if the mother took anticoagulant, anticonvulsant, antituberculosis, or recent antibiotic therapy during pregnancy. Alternatively, 1–5 mg given to the mother 12–12 hr before delivery.

Treatment of hemorrhagic disease in the newborn.

1 mg SC or IM (higher doses may be needed if the mother has been taking oral anticoagulants).

Administration/Storage

1. Store injectable emulsion or colloidal solutions in cool, 5°C–15°C (41°F–59°F), dark place.
2. Do not freeze.
3. Protect vitamin K from light.
4. Mix emulsion only with water or D5W.
5. Mix colloidal solution with D5W, isotonic sodium chloride injection, or dextrose and sodium chloride injection.
6. Heparin may be used to reverse effects from overdosage.

Special Concerns: Use with caution during lactation as phytonadione is excreted in breast milk. Safety and efficacy have not been determined in children. Benzyl alcohol, contained in some preparations, may cause toxicity in newborns.
Additional Side Effects: ***Intravenous administration may cause severe reactions (e.g., shock, cardiac or respiratory arrest, anaphylaxis) leading to death.*** These effects may occur when receiving vitamin K for the first time.

May be transient flushing of the face, sweating, a sense of constriction of the chest, and weakness. Cramp-like pain, weak and rapid pulse, convulsive movements, chills and fever, hypotension, cyanosis, or hemoglobinuria have been reported occasionally. ***Shock and cardiac and respiratory failure*** may be observed.

In newborns: ***Hemolysis, jaundice, hyperbilirubinemia (especially in premature infants).***

NURSING CONSIDERATIONS

See also *Nursing Considerations* for *Vitamin K,* Chapter 85.

Interventions

1. Monitor liver function studies and PT during drug therapy.
2. Administer slowly. Rapid parenteral administration can produce dyspnea, chest and back pain, and even death.
3. If the client has decreased bile secretion, administer bile salts to ensure the absorption of PO phytonadione.
4. If the client is receiving bile acid-binding resins such as colestipol or cholestyramine monitor PT and assess carefully for malabsorption of vitamin K.

Evaluate

- Control of bleeding in hypoprothrombinemia
- Prophylaxis of hypoprothrombinemia during prolonged TPN
- Prevention of hemorrhagic disease in the newborn

CHAPTER EIGHTY-SIX

Miscellaneous

See the following individual entries:

- Albumin, Normal Human Serum, 5% and 25%
- Alglucerase
- Alprostadil
- Chymopapain for Injection
- Disulfiram
- Dornase Alfa Recombinant
- Etomidate
- Hetastarch
- Hyaluronidase
- Hydroxypropyl Cellulose Ophthalmic Insert
- Interferon Beta-1b
- Ketamine Hydrochloride
- Lodoxamide Tromethamine
- Nicotine Polacrilex
- Nicotine Transdermal System
- Ritodrine Hydrochloride
- Sermorelin Acetate
- Tacrine Hydrochloride
- Teriparatide Acetate
- Tiopronin

Albumin, Normal Human Serum, 5%

(al-**BYOU**-min)

Pregnancy Category: C

Albuminar-5, Albutein 5%, Buminate 5%, Normal Serum Albumin (Human) 5% Solution, Plasbumin-5 **(Rx)**

Albumin, Normal Human Serum, 25%

(al-**BYOU**-min)

Pregnancy Category: C

Albuminar-25, Albutein 25%, Buminate 25%, Normal Serum Albumin (Human) 25% Solution, Plasbumin-25 **(Rx)**

How Supplied: *Injection:* 5%, 25%

Action/Kinetics: Prepared from whole blood, serum, plasma, or placentas from healthy human donors. It is supplied as a 5% (isotonic and isosmotic with normal human plasma) and 25% (salt-poor solution of which each 50 mL is osmotically equivalent to 250 mL of citrated plasma) strength. It contains sodium, 130–160 mEq/L.

Uses: Blood volume expander in shock, following surgery, hemorrhage, burns, or other trauma. Hypoproteinemia due to toxemia of pregnancy, anuria, acute hepatic cirrhosis or coma, acute nephrotic syndrome, tuberculosis, and premature infants. As an adjunct to exchange transfusions in hyperbilirubinemia and erythroblastosis fetalis. ARDS, cardiopulmonary bypass (presurgically to dilute blood), acute liver failure (with or without coma), renal dialysis, acute nephrosis. Sequestration of protein-rich fluids as in extensive cellulitis, mediastinitis, pancreatitis, and acute peritonitis. To avoid excessive hypoproteinemia in exchange transfusions or where large volumes of washed or previously frozen RBCs have been used.

Dosage

- **5% IV infusion**

  Hypoproteinemia.

Rate not to exceed 5–10 mL/min.

Burns.

Sufficient solution to establish and maintain a plasma albumin level of 2–3 g/100 mL (total serum protein of approximately 5.2 g/100 mL).

Shock.

Adults and children, initial: 500 mL as rapidly as tolerated; repeat after 30 min if response inadequate. **Infants and neonates:** 10–20 mL/kg.

- **25% IV infusion**

  Hypoproteinemia with or without edema.

Adults: 50–75 g/day; **pediatric:** 25 g/day. Rate should not exceed 2 mL/min.

Nephrosis.
100 mL/day for 7–10 days, given with a loop diuretic.
Burns.
Determined by extent; dose must be sufficient to maintain plasma albumin levels of 2–3 g/100 mL with a plasma oncotic pressure of 20 mm Hg.
Shock.
Dose determined by client's condition. For significantly reduced blood volume, give as rapidly as desired; for normal or slightly low blood volume, give 1 mL/min.
Hyperbilirubinemia and erythroblastosis fetalis.
4 mL/kg (1 g/kg) 1–2 hr before transfusion of blood.
Erythrocyte resuspension.
Usually, 25 g/L of erythrocytes.
Renal dialysis.
100 mL (avoid fluid overload).

Administration/Storage

1. Do not use turbid or sedimented solution.
2. Preparation does not contain preservatives. Use each opened bottle at once.
3. Use the accompanying vented IV administration sets when administering commercial vials of blood volume expanders.
4. May be given as rapidly as needed initially. However, as plasma volume approaches normal, the 5% solution should not be given faster than 2–4 mL/min and the 25% solution should not be given faster than 1 mL/min.
5. In hypoproteinemia, the 5% solution should not be given faster than 5–10 mL/min and the 25% solution should not be given faster than 2–3 mL/min to minimize the possibility of circulatory overload and pulmonary edema.
6. Albumin should not be considered as a nutrient.
7. These products should be stored at room temperature, not to exceed 30°C (86°F).

Contraindications: Severe anemia, cardiac failure, allergy to albumin, renal insufficiency, presence of increased intravascular volume, chronic nephrosis, clients on cardiopulmonary bypass.

Special Concerns: This product is not a substitute for whole blood.

Laboratory Test Interference: ↑ Serum alkaline phosphatase.

Side Effects: *Allergic:* Chills, fever, headache, rash, N&V, flushing, urticaria, tachycardia, hypotension, respiratory and BP changes, increased salivation. *CV:* Hypotension in clients on cardiopulmonary bypass. ***Rapid administration may cause pulmonary edema, dyspnea, and vascular overload.***

NURSING CONSIDERATIONS

Assessment

1. Note laboratory reports that may indicate the presence of any contraindications to therapy (e.g., anemia, renal insufficiency).
2. Document baseline VS, lung sounds, and invasive pressure readings, when available, to assess for volume overload.
3. Weigh client, if possible, before the start of therapy.

Interventions

1. Take BP and pulse q 15 min during infusion.
2. Note symptoms of pulmonary edema, demonstrated by cough, dyspnea, rales, and cyanosis. **Stop** the administration of albumin and report immediately. Obtain CXR.
3. Observe client for diuresis (record output q 1–2 hr) and for reduction of edema. Monitor I&O and weights.
4. Check for evidence of dehydration such as dry, cracked lips, flushed, dry skin, reduced urinary output, unusually dark colored urine, or loss of skin turgor; replace fluids as needed.
5. Note evidence of hemorrhage or shock, which may occur following surgery or trauma. A rapid increase in BP causes bleeding in severed blood vessels that had not been noted previously.

Evaluate

- ↑ BP and circulating blood volume with adequate tissue perfusion
- Mobilization of extravascular tissue fluids back into the intravascular space

Alglucerase

(al-**GLOO**-sir-ace)

Pregnancy Category: C

Ceredase **(Rx)**

How Supplied: *Injection:* 10 U/mL, 80 U/mL

Action/Kinetics: Gaucher's disease is a rare congenital disorder of lipid metabolism where there is a deficiency in beta-glucocerebrosidase leading to an accumulation of lipid glucocerebroside in the liver, spleen, and bone marrow. Symptoms of the disease include an enlarged spleen, increased skin pigmentation, bone lesions, severe anemia, and thrombocytopenia. Alglucerase, which is a modified form of beta-glucocerebrosidase, is derived from human placental tissue; it catalyzes the hydrolysis of the glycolipid glucocerebroside to glucose and ceramide, which is part of the normal degradation pathway for membrane lipids. Following IV infusion, steady state enzyme levels were observed in 60 min. **t½:** 3.6–10.4 min.

Uses: Chronic enzyme replacement in clients with confirmed diagnosis of type I Gaucher's disease who meet the following criteria: moderate-to-severe anemia, thrombocytopenia with bleeding tendency, significant hepatomegaly or splenomegaly, and bone disease.

Dosage

- **IV Infusion**

Gaucher's disease.

Initial: Up to 60 units/kg/infusion with infusions usually given q 2 weeks. Dose is then adjusted downward for maintenance therapy; dosage can be lowered q 3–6 months with some clients responding to doses as low as 1 unit/kg.

Administration/Storage

1. Although the dose is usually given every 2 weeks, the severity of the disease (and client convenience) may require administration as frequently as every other day or as infrequently as every 4 weeks.
2. Response parameters should be closely monitored as the dose is progressively lowered.
3. Prior to administration, the drug is diluted with normal saline to a final volume not to exceed 100 mL. An in-line particulate filter is recommended for the infusion apparatus.
4. The product should not be shaken as shaking may denature the glycoprotein, making it inactive.
5. The product should be stored at 4°C (39°F). If the bottle shows any discoloration or particulate matter, it should not be used.
6. Since the product does not contain any preservative, it should not be stored for subsequent use after being opened.
7. Small dosage adjustments (either increased or decreased) may be made to avoid discarding partially used bottles provided that the monthly administered dosage is not altered.

Special Concerns: Use with caution during lactation. Since alglucerase is derived from human placental tissue, there is always the risk of some viral contamination; however, the drug product has been found to be free from hepatitis B surface antigen and for antigens of HIV (HIV-1).

Side Effects: Nausea, vomiting, chills, abdominal discomfort, slight fever.

NURSING CONSIDERATIONS

Assessment

1. Note onset and list symptoms of disease requiring treatment.
2. Obtain baseline CBC and determine laboratory confirmation of type I Gaucher's disease noting the presence of anemia, thrombocytopenia with bleeding tendency, enlarged liver and spleen, and any evidence of bone disease (potential for pathologic fractures due to demineralization).

3. Perform a full client assessment to use as baseline data to determine the effectiveness of drug therapy.

Client/Family Teaching

1. Explain that the client may experience "flu-like" symptoms (N&V, fever, chills, and abdominal discomfort) but that this is usually only temporary.
2. Advise that the drug has been derived from pooled human placental tissue and review the potential risks.
3. Stress the importance of reporting for scheduled visits as the dose is progressively lowered based on response parameters.

Evaluate

- ↓ Splenomegaly and hepatomegaly within 6 months of continued alglucerase therapy
- Improved hematologic parameters (e.g., ↑ H&H, erythrocyte, and platelet counts)

Alprostadil (PGE1)

(al-**PROSS**-tah-dill)
Prostin VR ✱, Prostin VR Pediatric **(Rx)**

How Supplied: *Injection:* 0.5 mg/mL

Action/Kinetics: Alprostadil is one of the prostaglandins that is a naturally occurring acidic lipid. Alprostadil relaxes smooth muscle of the ductus arteriosus leading to increased pulmonary blood flow with increased blood oxygenation and lower body perfusion. Clients with low pO_2 values respond best. The drug may also cause vasodilation, inhibit platelet aggregation, and stimulate both intestinal and uterine smooth muscle. When injected intracavernosally, alprostadil relaxes the trabecular cavernous smooth muscles and causes dilation of penile arteries. This results in increased arterial blood flow to the corpus cavernosa and thus swelling and elongation of the penis. **Onset, systemic:** 1.5–3 hr for acyanotic congenital heart disease and 15–30 min for cyanotic congenital heart disease. **Time to peak effect:** 3 hr for coarctation of the aorta and 1.5 hr for interruption of aortic arch. **Duration:** Closure of the ductus arteriosus usually begins 1–2 hr after infusion discontinued. Alprostadil is rapidly metabolized (80% in one pass) by oxidation in the lung, and metabolites are excreted by the kidney.

Uses: For temporary maintenance of patency of the ductus arteriosus (until surgery can be performed) in neonates with congenital heart defects. *Investigational:* Diagnosis and treatment of impotence.

Dosage

- **Continuous IV Infusion or Umbilical Artery**

Maintain patency of ductus arteriosus.

Initial: 0.05–0.1 mcg/kg/min; **then,** after response achieved, decrease infusion rate to lowest dose that will maintain response (e.g., 0.1–0.05 to 0.025–0.01 mcg/kg/min). *NOTE:* If 0.1 mcg/kg/min is insufficient, dosage can be increased up to 0.4 mcg/kg/min.

- **Intracavernosal**

Impotence.

2.5–20 mcg (up to 40 mcg) with dose adjusted according to response; should not be given more than 3 times/week or for 2 days in succession.

Administration/Storage

1. Administer infusions only in pediatric intensive care facilities.
2. Dilute 500 mcg with either sodium chloride injection or dextrose injection in volumes appropriate for the infant's fluid intake and suitable for the type of infusion pump available.
3. Use a Y set-up.
4. Discard any unused solutions and prepare a fresh infusion solution q 24 hr.
5. Sterile solutions should be infused for the shortest time and at the lowest dose that will produce the desired effect.
6. Have a respirator available at the cribside.
7. Store ampules at 2°C–8°C (36°F–46°F).

8. *Treatment of Overdose:* Reduce rate of infusion if symptoms of hypotension or pyrexia occur; discontinue infusion if symptoms of apnea or bradycardia occur.

Contraindications: Respiratory distress syndrome (hyaline membrane disease). Use with caution in neonates with bleeding tendencies. History of priapism, sickle cell disease.

Laboratory Test Interferences: ↑ Bilirubin. ↓ Glucose, serum calcium. ↑ or ↓ Potassium.

Side Effects: *Respiratory:* ***Apnea (in 10%–12% of neonates), especially in neonates less than 2 kg at birth;*** bronchial wheezing, bradypnea, hypercapnia, respiratory depression. *CNS:* Fever, ***seizures,*** hypothermia, jitteriness, lethargy, ***cerebral bleeding,*** stiffness, hyperextension of the neck, irritability. *CV:* Flushing, especially after intra-arterial dosage, bradycardia, hypotension, tachycardia, edema, ***cardiac arrest, CHF, shock, arrhythmias.*** *GI:* Diarrhea, hyperbilirubinemia, gastric regurgitation. *Renal:* Hematuria, anuria. *Skeletal:* Cortical proliferation of long bones. *Hematologic:* ***Disseminated intravascular coagulation,*** thrombocytopenia, anemia, bleeding. *Miscellaneous:* ***Sepsis, peritonitis,*** hypoglycemia, hypokalemia or hyperkalemia.

Symptoms of Overdose: ***Apnea,*** bradycardia, flushing, hypotension, pyrexia.

NURSING CONSIDERATIONS

Assessment

1. Assess client's VS and cardiac and respiratory function and document before administering the medication.
2. Determine if the neonate has restricted pulmonary blood flow.
3. Note any evidence of bleeding tendencies or sickle cell anemia as these are contraindications to drug therapy.

Interventions

1. Monitor arterial pressure intermittently by umbilical artery catheter, auscultation, Dinemapp or with a Doppler transducer. Obtain written guidelines for arterial pressures; if the arterial pressure falls significantly, decrease the rate of flow immediately and report.
2. Observe the infant for apnea, bradycardia, pyrexia, flushing, and hypotension. These are symptoms of *overdose.* The following guidelines are appropriate.
   - If the infant develops apnea or bradycardia, stop the administration of drug, change to the unmedicated solution, start resuscitation, and report.
   - If the infant develops pyrexia or hypotension, reduce the rate of IV flow and report. The rate of IV flow will likely be reduced until the temperature and BP return to baseline values.
   - Report if flushing occurs. This symptom indicates an incorrect intra-arterial placement of the catheter and it requires repositioning.
3. If the infant has restricted pulmonary blood flow, monitor ABGs. A positive response to alprostadil is indicated by at least a 10 mm Hg increase in blood pO_2.
4. If the infant has restricted systemic blood flow, monitor the systemic BP and serum pH. If the infant has acidosis, a positive response to alprostadil would be indicated by an increased pH, an increase in BP, and a decreased ratio of PA pressure to aortic pressure.

Evaluate

- Improved pulmonary blood flow with a resultant ↑ blood oxygenation level
- Closure of ductus arteriosus 1–2 hr following infusion
- Promotion of penile erection with intracavernosal therapy

Chymopapain for injection

(**KYE**-moh-pah-payn)
Pregnancy Category: C
Chymodiactin **(Rx)**

How Supplied: *Powder for injection:* 4000 U

Action/Kinetics: Chymopapain is a proteolytic enzyme derived from the crude latex of *Carica papaya.* The nanoKatal (nKat) is used as the unit of chymopapain activity (1 mg of chymopapain is equivalent to at least 0.52 nKat units). The preparation also contains sodium L-cysteinate hydrochloride as a reducing agent to keep the sulfur in the sulfhydryl form. Chymopapain is injected into the herniated lumbar intervertebral disc (nucleus pulposus), where it hydrolyzes the noncollagenous proteins or polypeptides that maintain the structure of the chondromucoprotein of the nucleus pulposus. As a result of hydrolysis, the osmotic activity is decreased, leading to a decreased fluid absorption, thus reducing intradiscal pressure. Although chymopapain acts locally in the disc, it does appear in the plasma, where it is inactivated. Small amounts are excreted in the urine.

Uses: Chymopapain should be used only in a hospital setting by physicians and supportive personnel trained in the diagnosis and treatment of herniated lumbar intervertebral disc disease that has not responded to more conservative therapy.

Dosage

- **Disc Injection**

Herniated lumbar intervertebral disc disease.

A single injection of 2–4 nKat units/disc (usual is 3 nKat units/disc in a volume of 1.5 mL). Maximum dose with multiple disc herniation is 10 nKat units.

Administration/Storage

1. An open IV line must always be available in the event of anaphylaxis. Epinephrine is the drug of choice to treat anaphylaxis.
2. Sterile water for injection should be used for reconstitution, as bacteriostatic water for injection inactivates the enzyme. The reconstituted drug must be used within 2 hr. Any unused, reconstituted drug should be discarded promptly.
3. Automatic filling syringes should not be used since a residual vacuum is present in the vial.
4. Alcohol should be used to cleanse the vial stopper before inserting the needle; since alcohol inactivates the enzyme, it should be allowed to *dry* before continuing with reconstitution.
5. The package literature should be consulted for the specific procedures for administration.
6. Prior to use, the client should be treated with histamine receptor H_1 and H_2 antagonists to decrease the severity of an anaphylactic reaction (e.g., cimetidine, 300 mg PO, q 6 hr, and diphenhydramine, 50 mg PO, q 6 hr, both for 24 hr prior to therapy).

Contraindications: Sensitivity to chymopapain, papaya, or its derivatives. Severe spondylolisthesis, significant spinal stenosis, spinal cord tumor or a cauda equina lesion, or in progressing paralysis manifested by rapidly progressing neurologic dysfunction. Clients previously treated with chymopapain. Injection into any location other than lumbar area.

Special Concerns: Safety and efficacy have not been established for use in children.

Side Effects: *Neuromuscular:* Back pain, stiffness, soreness, back spasm, paraplegia, acute transverse myelitis or myelopathy characterized by onset of paraplegia or paraparesis (without prior symptoms) within 2–3 weeks. Also, sacral burning, leg pain, hyperalgesia, leg weakness, tingling/numbness in legs/toes, cramping in both calves, paresthesia, pain in opposite leg, postinjection pain, bacterial and aseptic discitis. *Allergic:* ***Anaphylaxis (more common in females).*** Complications secondary to anaphylaxis including staphylococcal meningitis with disc abscess. Rash, itching, urticaria, pilomotor erection, vasomotor rhinitis, conjunctivitis, angioedema, GI disturbances. *Other:* ***Cerebral hemorrhage,*** nausea, itching, paralytic ileus, urinary retention, headache, dizziness.

Drug Interactions: Possible arrhythmias if used with halothane or epinephrine.

NURSING CONSIDERATIONS

Assessment

1. Document indications for therapy and any prior treatments that were not effective.
2. Note onset of injury and pain and lumbar discs involved.
3. Determine if therapy with chymopapain has been used previously because additional treatments are contraindicated.

Interventions

1. Monitor VS and neurologic (level of consciousness) and respiratory status. The drug can cause hypotension and bronchospasms.
2. Perform neurovascular checks postprocedure (extremity checks q 15 min for 2 hr) and document; report any progressive dysfunction.
3. Observe for hypersensitivity reaction (reduced BP, rash, itching) and advise client to check contact lens cleaner and meat tenderizer labels as these may also contain papaya derivatives (papain) that may enhance the reaction.
4. Supervise ambulation and activities until response evident.

Client/Family Teaching

1. Back pain and muscle spasms may occur within several days to several weeks following treatment. Residual soreness and stiffness may be evident for several months.
2. Discuss the possibility of paraplegia and paresis occurring suddenly, several weeks after treatment. This should be reported immediately.
3. If leg weakness, tingling or numbness of the legs and/or toes, or cramping in the calves of the legs occurs, report immediately.
4. Advise client that responses are not immediately evident. Prepare them for a lack of or poor response as surgery may be necessary in this event.

Evaluate

- ↓ Intradiscal pressure
- Relief of pain and discomfort with ↑ ROM

Disulfiram

(dye-**SUL**-fih-ram)
Antabuse **(Rx)**

How Supplied: *Tablet:* 250 mg, 500 mg

Action/Kinetics: Disulfiram produces severe hypersensitivity to alcohol. It is used as an adjunct in the treatment of alcoholism. The toxic reaction to disulfiram appears to be due to the inhibition of liver enzymes that participate in the normal degradation of alcohol. When alcohol and disulfiram are both present, acetaldehyde accumulates in the blood. High levels of acetaldehyde produce a series of symptoms referred to as the disulfiram-alcohol reaction or syndrome. The specific symptoms are listed under *Side Effects*. The symptoms vary individually, are dose-dependent with respect to both alcohol and disulfiram, and persist for periods ranging from 30 min to several hours. A single dose of disulfiram may be effective for 1–2 weeks. **Onset:** May be delayed up to 12 hr because disulfiram is initially localized in fat stores.

Uses: To prevent further ingestion of alcohol in chronic alcoholics. Disulfiram should be given only to cooperating clients fully aware of the consequences of alcohol ingestion.

Dosage

- **Tablets**

  Alcoholism.

Adults, initial (after alcohol-free interval of 12–48 hr): 500 mg/day for 1–2 weeks; **maintenance: usual,** 250 mg/day (range: 120–500 mg/day). Dose should not exceed 500 mg/day.

Administration/Storage

1. Tablets can be crushed or mixed with liquid.
2. Clients should always carry appropriate identification indicating disulfiram is being taken.
3. Have oxygen, pressor agents, and antihistamines available to treat disulfiram-alcohol reactions.

Contraindications: Alcohol intoxication. Severe myocardial or occlusive coronary disease. Use of paraldehyde or alcohol-containing products such as cough syrups. If client is exposed to ethylene dibromide.
Special Concerns: Use in pregnancy only if benefits outweigh risks. Use with caution in narcotic addicts or clients with diabetes, goiter, epilepsy, psychosis, hypothyroidism, hepatic cirrhosis, or nephritis.
Side Effects: In the absence of alcohol, the following symptoms have been reported: Drowsiness (most common), headache, restlessness, fatigue, psychoses, peripheral neuropathy, dermatoses, hepatotoxicity, metallic or garlic taste, arthropathy, impotence. **In the presence of alcohol,** the following symptoms may be manifested. *CV:* Flushing, chest pain, palpitations, tachycardia, hypotension, syncope, arrhythmias, ***CV collapse, MI, acute CHF.*** *CNS:* Throbbing headaches, vertigo, weakness, uneasiness, confusion, unconsciousness, ***seizures, death.*** *GI:* Nausea, severe vomiting, thirst. *Respiratory:* Respiratory difficulties, dyspnea, hyperventilation, ***respiratory depression.*** *Other:* Throbbing in head and neck, sweating. In the event of an Antabuse-alcohol interaction, measures should be undertaken to maintain BP and treat shock. Oxygen, antihistamines, ephedrine, and/or vitamin C may also be used.

Drug Interactions

Anticoagulants, oral / ↑ Effect of anticoagulants by ↑ hypoprothrombinemia
Barbiturates / ↑ Effect of barbiturates due to ↓ breakdown by liver
Chlordiazepoxide, diazepam / ↑ Effect of chlordiazepoxide or diazepam due to ↓ plasma clearance
Isoniazid / ↑ Side effects of isoniazid (especially CNS)
Metronidazole / Acute toxic psychosis or confusional state
Paraldehyde / Concomitant use produces Antabuse-like effect
Phenytoin / ↑ Effect of phenytoin due to ↓ breakdown by liver
Tricyclic antidepressants / Acute organic brain syndrome

NURSING CONSIDERATIONS

Client/Family Teaching

1. Emphasize to the family that disulfiram should never be given to the client without client's knowledge.
2. Explain the effects of disulfiram and emphasize the need for close medical and psychiatric supervision.
3. If the client experiences CNS side effects, explain that these will lessen as the drug is continued.
4. Ingesting as little as 30 mL of 100-proof alcohol (e.g., one shot) while on disulfiram therapy may cause severe symptoms and possibly death.
5. Avoid alcohol in any form, in foods, sauces, or other medications, such as cough syrups or tonics. Clients should also be advised to avoid vinegar, paregoric, liniments, or lotions containing alcohol.
6. Instruct to read carefully all labels on foods before consuming them to avoid those that may contain some form of alcohol.
7. Discuss with clients the fact that they may feel tired, experience drowsiness and headaches, and develop a metallic or garlic-like taste. These side effects tend to subside after about 2 weeks of therapy.
8. Explain to male clients that they may have occasional impotence. This is usually transient. Remind clients that they should discuss this problem with the provider before discontinuing the medication.
9. If skin eruptions occur, advise client to report since an antihistamine may be prescribed.
10. Advise clients to carry an identification card stating that they are taking disulfiram and describing the symptoms and treatment if clients have a disulfiram reaction. Included should be the name of the person treating the client and a telephone number where the provider may be

reached. (Cards may be obtained from the Wyeth-Ayerst Laboratories, P.O. Box 8299, Philadelphia, PA 19101-1245; attention: Professional Services.)

11. Advise client and family to attend meetings of local support groups such as Alcoholics Anonymous (AA) and Al-Anon to gain a better understanding of the disease. These groups offer the support, structure, referral, and encouragement that may help the client in the quest for an alcohol-free life.

Evaluate: Freedom from alcohol and its effects with resultant sobriety.

Dornase alfa recombinant

(**DOR**-nace **AL**-fah)
Pregnancy Category: B
Pulmozyme **(Rx)**

How Supplied: *Solution:* 2.5 mg/2.5 mL

Action/Kinetics: This drug is a highly purified solution of recombinant human deoxyribonuclease I (rhDNase), an enzyme that selectively cleaves DNA. It is produced by genetically engineered Chinese hamster ovary cells that contain DNA encoded for the native human protein, deoxyribonuclease (DNase). The amino acid sequence is identical to that of the native human enzyme. Cystic fibrosis clients have viscous purulent secretions in the airways that contribute to reduced pulmonary function and worsening of infection. These secretions contain high concentrations of extracellular DNA released by degenerating leukocytes that accumulate as a result of infection. Dornase alfa hydrolyzes the DNA in sputum of cystic fibrosis clients, thereby reducing sputum viscoelasticity and reducing infections.

Uses: In cystic fibrosis clients in conjunction with standard therapy to decrease the frequency of respiratory infections that require parenteral antibiotics and to improve pulmonary function.

Dosage

- **Inhalation Solution**

Cystic fibrosis.

One 2.5-mg single-dose ampule inhaled once daily using a recommended nebulizer (see below). Older clients and clients with baseline FVC above 85% may benefit from twice daily dosing.

Administration/Storage

1. Approved nebulizers include the disposable jet nebulizer Hudson T U-draft II, disposable jet nebulizer Marquest Acorn II in conjunction with a Pulmo-Aide compressor, and the reusable PARI LC Jet+ nebulizer in conjunction with the PARI PRONEB compressor. Safety and efficacy have been demonstrated with only these nebulizers.
2. The drug should not be diluted or mixed with other drugs in the nebulizer. Mixing with other drugs could lead to adverse physicochemical or functional changes in dornase alfa.
3. The drug must be stored in the refrigerator at 2°C–8°C (36°F–46°F) in the protective foil pouch and protected from strong light.
4. The product should be refrigerated when transported and should not be exposed to room temperature for a total time of 24 hr.
5. The solution should be discarded if it is cloudy or discolored.
6. The product does not contain a preservative; thus, once opened, the entire ampule must be used or discarded.

Contraindications: Use in clients with known sensitivity to dornase alfa or products from Chinese hamster ovary cells.

Special Concerns: Safety and effectiveness of daily use have not been demonstrated in clients less than 5 years of age, in clients with forced vital capacity (FVC) of less than 40% of predicted or for longer than 12 months. Use with caution during lactation.

Side Effects: *Respiratory:* Pharyngitis, voice alteration, and laryngitis are the most common. Also, ***apnea,*** bronchiectasis, bronchitis, change in sputum, cough increase, dyspnea, hemoptysis, lung function decrease, nasal polyps, pneumonia, pneumothorax, rhinitis, sinusitis, sputum increase, wheezing. *Body as a whole:* Abdominal pain, asthenia, fever, flu syndrome, malaise, sepsis, weight loss. *GI:* Intestinal obstruction, gall bladder disease, liver disease, pancreatic disease. *Miscellaneous:* Rash, urticaria, chest pain, conjunctivitis, diabetes mellitus, hypoxia.

NURSING CONSIDERATIONS

Assessment

1. Document age of symptom onset of cystic fibrosis, other therapies prescribed, and the outcome.
2. Drug is produced by genetically engineered Chinese hamster ovary cells; assess for any known sensitivity.
3. Obtain baseline pulmonary function parameters. Drug is for children over 5 years old with baseline FVC above 40%.

Client/Family Teaching

1. Review the dose, frequency, and proper method for inhalation administration. Explain that drug is administered by inhalation of an aerosol mist generated by a compressed air-driven nebulizer system.
2. Ensure that client/family are familiar with the use, care, and storage of inhalation equipment and provide written guidelines to guide them. Observe their technique.
3. Stress that treatments must be performed on a daily schedule to obtain full pharmacologic benefits.
4. Advise that standard prescribed therapies for cystic fibrosis such as chest PT, antibiotics, bronchodilators, oral and inhaled corticosteroids, enzyme supplements, vitamins, and analgesics should be continued during treatment with dornase alfa.
5. Review symptoms that require immediate medical intervention: severe rashes, itching, respiratory distress, fever, etc.
6. Advise family members caring for client with cystic fibrosis to learn CPR.
7. Identify support groups that may assist family to adjust and cope with this chronic disease.

Evaluate:

- ↓ Frequency of respiratory tract infectious exacerbations in clients with cystic fibrosis
- Clinical evidence of improved pulmonary function studies

Etomidate

(eh-**TOM**-ih-dayt)
Pregnancy Category: C
Amidate **(Rx)**

How Supplied: *Injection:* 2 mg/mL
Action/Kinetics: Etomidate is actually a hypnotic without any analgesic activity. The drug seems to act like GABA and is thought to exert its mechanism by depressing the activity of the brain stem reticular system. It has minimal CV and respiratory depressant effects. **Onset:** 1 min. **Duration:** 3–5 min. **t½:** 75 min. Rapidly metabolized in the liver with inactive metabolites excreted mainly through the urine.
Uses: Induction of general anesthesia. As a supplement to nitrous oxide during short surgical procedures.

Dosage

- **IV Only**

Induction of anesthesia.

Adults and children over 10 years of age: 0.2–0.6 mg/kg (usual: 0.3 mg/kg) injected over 30–60 sec.

Administration/Storage

1. Lower doses of etomidate may be used as adjuncts to supplement less potent general anesthetics such as nitrous oxide.
2. Etomidate may be used following preanesthetic medications.
3. The drug should be protected from extreme heat and freezing.

Special Concerns: Use with caution during lactation. Safety and efficacy have not been established in children less than 10 years of age.
Side Effects: *Skeletal muscle:* Myoclonic skeletal muscle movements, tonic movements. *Respiratory:* Apnea, hyperventilation or hypoventila-

tion, ***laryngospasm.*** *CV:* Either hypertension or hypotension; tachycardia or bradycardia; arrhythmias. *GI:* N&V. *Miscellaneous:* Eye movements (common), hiccoughs, snoring.

NURSING CONSIDERATIONS

Interventions

1. Nausea and vomiting are likely to occur postoperatively. Have essential equipment (suction, emesis basins, washcloths, etc.) available to manage this problem.
2. Monitor client during the immediate postoperative period for hypotension, hypertension, tachycardia, and/or bradycardia and treat symptomatically.

Evaluate: Desired anesthetic level.

Hetastarch (HES)

(**HEH**-tah-starch)
Hespan (Abbreviation: HES) **(Rx)**

How Supplied: *Injection:* 6 g/100 mL-0.9%

Action/Kinetics: Hetastarch is a mixture of synthetic, water-soluble ethoxylated amylopectin molecules with molecular weights ranging from 10,000 to 1,000,000. The colloidal properties of 6% hetastarch are similar to albumin. Its action is similar to dextran, but it produces fewer allergic reactions and does not interfere with blood crossmatching. Hetastarch is not a substitute for whole blood or its fractions. Molecules with a molecular weight less than 50,000 are eliminated quickly by the kidney whereas larger molecules are broken down to smaller ones. **t½:** 17 days for 90% of the dose and 48 days for 10% of the dose.

Uses: Shock (burns, hemorrhages, sepsis, and surgery). Fluid replacement, plasma volume expansion. Adjunct in removal of WBCs (leukopheresis).

Dosage

- **IV infusion only**

Individualized.

Plasma expansion.

500–1,000 mL of 6% solution up to maximum of 1,500 mL (20 mL/kg/day).

For acute hemorrhage.

Rapid rate up to 20 mL/kg/hr. Use slower rates for burns and septic shock.

Leukopheresis.

250–700 mL infused at a constant ratio, usually 1:8 to venous whole blood.

Administration/Storage

1. The solution should not be used if it is turbid deep brown or if a crystalline precipitate forms.
2. The solution should not be frozen; store at room temperature not exceeding 40°C (104°F).
3. Discard partially used bottles.
4. Administer undiluted by IV infusion.

Contraindications: Severe bleeding disorders, severe CHF, or renal failure with oliguria or anuria.

Special Concerns: Use during pregnancy, especially in early pregnancy, only if benefits outweigh risks to the fetus.

Side Effects: *Hematologic:* Prolonged prothrombin, partial thromboplastin, and clotting times; decreased hematocrit. *GI:* Vomiting, enlargement of submaxillary and parotid glands. *Miscellaneous:* Chills, fever, itching, influenza-like syndrome, muscle pain, edema of the lower extremities, ***anaphylaxis,*** circulatory overload, dilution of plasma proteins.

NURSING CONSIDERATIONS

Assessment

1. Note any history of severe bleeding disorders, severe CHF, and/or renal dysfunction.
2. Assess women of childbearing age for pregnancy.
3. Obtain baseline hematologic parameters.

Interventions

1. Monitor I&O. Stop infusion immediately if oliguria, anuria, dyspnea, itching, or flu–like symptoms develop.
2. Check specific gravity of urine (normal: 1.005–1.025). Low values indicate that hetastarch is not being excreted and may require discontinuation of plasma expanders.

3. After administration of 500 mL of hetastarch, obtain a hematocrit. Hematocrit values lower than 30% by volume should be avoided.
4. Note any sudden increase in CVP and/or pulmonary capillary wedge pressure. This may indicate a circulatory overload and CHF.
5. If client has been following a salt-restricted diet, watch closely for evidence of edema (elevated BP, cough, moist rales, cyanosis). Sodium in hetastarch may precipitate pulmonary edema in clients with cardiac disease or kidney dysfunction.
6. Observe client for purpura or other signs of bleeding from orifices or wounds, especially 3–9 hr after drug administration has been completed. Hetastarch may temporarily cause prolonged bleeding times.

Evaluate: Improved circulatory volume (↑ BP, ↑ urine output, ↓ HR).

Hyaluronidase

(hy-al-your-**ON**-ih-days)
Pregnancy Category: C
Wydase **(Rx)**

How Supplied: *Injection:* 150 U/mL; *Powder for injection:* 150 U, 1,500 U

Action/Kinetics: Hyaluronidase, an enzyme that hydrolyzes hyaluronic acid, a constituent of connective tissue, acts to promote the diffusion of injected liquids. The purified enzyme has no effect on BP, respiration, temperature, and kidney function. However, it is antigenic and repeated use may induce the formation of antibodies that neutralize the effect. It will not result in spread of localized infection as long as it is not injected into the infected area. The effects last 24–48 hr.

Uses: Adjunct to promote absorption and dispersion of liquids and drugs, for hypodermoclysis, adjunct in urography to improve resorption of radiopaque agents, administration of local anesthetics. (Hyaluronidase can be added to primary drug solution or injected prior to administration of primary drug solution.)

Dosage

• **SC**

Drug and fluid dispersion.

Adults and older children, usual: 150 units added to the injection solution.

SC urography.

(When IV injection cannot be used.) **With client in prone position:** 75 units **SC** over each scapula, followed by contrast medium in same site.

Hypodermoclysis.

150 units, which facilitates absorption of 1,000 mL fluid (give at a rate no faster than would be used for IV infusion); **pediatric, less than 3 years:** volume of single clysis should be limited to 200 mL; **premature infants, neonates:** volume should not exceed 25 mL/kg/day given at a rate no greater than 2 mL/min.

Administration/Storage

1. Conduct a preliminary skin test for sensitivity by injecting 0.02 mL of the solution intradermally. A positive reaction occurs within 5 min when a wheal with pseudopods appears and persists for 20–30 min and is accompanied by localized itching. The appearance of erythema alone is not a positive reaction.
2. Methods for administering hyaluronidase during clysis therapy:
• Inject hyaluronidase under the skin before clysis is started.
• After the clysis has been started, inject solution of hyaluronidase into tubing close to the needle.
3. Control rate and volume of fluid for the older client so that it will not exceed those used for IV administration.
4. Do not inject hyaluronidase into a malignant area.
5. Check the orders for dosage of hyaluronidase, type and amount of parenteral solution, the rate of flow, and the site of injection.
6. Hyaluronidase is incompatible with heparin and epinephrine.
7. Hyaluronidase solution must be refrigerated. The reconstituted sterile solution maintains potency for 2 weeks if stored below 30°C (86°F).
8. *Treatment of Overdose:* Discontinue and begin supportive treatment

immediately. Epinephrine, corticosteroids, and antihistamines may be required to treat symptoms.
Contraindications: Do not inject into acutely infected or cancerous areas.
Special Concerns: Use with caution during lactation.
Side Effects: Rarely, sensitivity reactions, including urticaria and ***anaphylaxis.***

Symptoms of Overdose: Local edema or urticaria, chills, erythema, dizziness, N&V, tachycardia, hypotension.

NURSING CONSIDERATIONS

Assessment

1. Document indications for therapy, clinical presentation, and onset of symptoms.
2. Describe the pretreatment area. Assess the area receiving clysis for pale color, coldness, hardness, and pain. Reduce the rate of flow and report if evident.
3. Obtain baseline liver and renal function studies and PT/PTT and monitor during parenteral infusion therapy.

Evaluate: Enhanced absorption and dispersion of fluids.

Hydroxypropyl cellulose ophthalmic insert

(hy-**DROX**-ee-proh-pill **SELL**-you-lohs)
Lacrisert **(Rx)**

How Supplied: *Device:* 5 mg
Action/Kinetics: Lacrisert contains 5 mg of hydroxypropyl cellulose in a rod-shaped (1.27-mm-diameter; 3.5-mm-long), water-soluble preparation. It contains no preservatives or other ingredients. This preparation stabilizes and thickens precorneal tear film and prolongs the breakup time for tear film. It also lubricates and protects the eye.
Use: Moderate to severe dry eye syndrome, including keratoconjunctivitis sicca, exposure keratitis, decreased corneal sensitivity, and recurrent corneal lesions. *Investigational:* Ocular lubricant, neuroparalytic keratitis.

Dosage

- **Ocular System**

Dry eye syndrome.

Adults and children: One 5-mg insert daily placed into the inferior cul-de-sac of the eye beneath the base of the tarsus. Some clients may require two inserts daily.
Contraindication: Hypersensitivity to hydroxypropyl cellulose.
Side Effects: Transient blurring of vision, ocular discomfort or irritation, photophobia, hypersensitivity, edema of eyelids, eyelids mat or become sticky, hyperemia. Corneal abrasion may occur if the product is improperly placed in the cul-de-sac. Also, if improperly positioned, the insert will be expelled into the interpalpebral fissure and may cause symptoms of a foreign body.

NURSING CONSIDERATIONS

Client/Family Teaching

1. Instruct client on how to insert and remove Lacrisert. Review the instructions in the package insert and advise to follow the instructions carefully.
2. Avoid rubbing the eyes, thereby preventing a dislodgment of Lacrisert, causing excessive irritation.
3. If Lacrisert is accidentally expelled, client may insert another Lacrisert as needed.
4. Promptly report any S&S of drug side effects. These may include conjunctival hyperemia, exudation, itching, burning, a sensation of the presence of a foreign body, smarting, photophobia, and blurred or cloudy vision or corneal abrasion.
5. Avoid operating a car or other hazardous machinery because the drug may cause transitory blurring of vision.
6. Report for regular ophthalmic examinations as scheduled. Discuss the need to report any adverse reactions to the ophthalmologist.
7. Explain that the medication may retard, stop, or reverse progressive visual deterioration.

Evaluate: Relief of corneal dryness, pain, itching, and sensitivity.

Interferon Beta-1b (r1FN-B)

(in-ter-**FEER**-on **AL**-fah)
Pregnancy Category: C
Betaseron **(Rx)**

How Supplied: *Powder for injection:* 0.3 mg

Action/Kinetics: Interferon beta-1b is made by bacterial fermentation of a strain of *Escherichia coli* that is a genetically engineered plasmid containing the gene for human interferon beta$_{ser17}$. Interferon beta-1b has both antiviral and immunoregulatory effects. The reason for the beneficial effect in MS is not known, although the effects are mediated through combination with specific cell receptors located on the cell membrane. The receptor-drug complex induces the expression of a number of interferon-induced gene products that are thought to be the mediators of the biologic effects of interferon beta-1b. Kinetic information is not available since serum levels are low or not detectable following SC administration to MS clients. Data from healthy volunteers indicate peak serum levels occur within 1–8 hr with a mean serum concentration of 40 IU/mL. Mean terminal half-lives ranged from 8 min to 4.3 hr.

Uses: Treatment of ambulatory clients with relapsing-remitting MS to reduce the frequency of clinical exacerbations. Remitting-relapsing MS is manifested by recurrent attacks of neurologic dysfunction followed by complete or incomplete recovery. *Investigational:* Treatment of AIDS, AIDS-related Kaposi's sarcoma, metastatic renal cell carcinoma, malignant melanoma, cutaneous T-cell lymphoma, and acute non-A/non-B hepatitis.

Dosage

- **SC**

MS clients.

0.25 mg (8 mIU) every other day.

Administration/Storage

1. Effectiveness beyond 2 years of use is not known.
2. To reconstitute, a sterile syringe and needle are required. Inject 1.2 mL of diluent provided (0.54% sodium chloride) into the vial. Swirl gently to dissolve the drug completely (should not be shaken).
3. The reconstituted product should be visually inspected; if it contains particulate matter or is discolored, it should be discarded before use.
4. One mL of the reconstituted solution should be withdrawn from the vial into a sterile syringe fitted with a 27-gauge needle and injected SC. Injection sites include the arms, abdomen, hips, and thighs.
5. Since the reconstituted product contains no preservative, any unused portions should be discarded after one use.
6. Before and after reconstitution with diluent, the drug should be stored at 2°C–8°C (36°F–46°F). The product should be used within 3 hr of reconstitution.

Contraindications: Hypersensitivity to natural or recombinant interferon beta or human albumin. Use during lactation.

Special Concerns: The safety and efficacy for use in chronic progressive MS and in children less than 18 years of age have not been studied. Attempted suicide and suicide have occurred. The drug has the potential to be an abortifacient.

Laboratory Test Interferences: ↑ ALT, total bilirubin, AST, BUN, urine protein. Hypoglycemia or hyperglycemia. Ketosis.

Side Effects: *Body as a whole:* Flu-like symptoms including fever, chills, myalgia, malaise, sweating. Photo-toxicity or photoallergy. Reaction at injection site, headache, pain, asthenia, abdominal pain, weight gain or weight loss, generalized edema, pelvic pain, cyst, necrosis, goiter, abscess, adenoma, ***anaphylaxis,*** ascites, cellulitis, hernia, hydrocephalus, hypothermia, infection, sarcoma, ***sepsis,***

shock. *CV:* Migraine, palpitation, hypertension, tachycardia, peripheral vascular disorder, ***hemorrhage,*** angina, ***arrhythmia,*** atrial fibrillation, cardiomegaly, ***cardiac arrest, cerebral hemorrhage, cerebral ischemia,*** endocarditis, heart failure, hypotension, ***MI,*** pericardial effusion, postural hypotension, ***pulmonary embolus,*** spider angioma, ***subarachnoid hemorrhage,*** syncope, thrombophlebitis, thrombosis, varicose vein, vasospasm, increased venous pressure, ***ventricular extrasystoles or fibrillation.*** *Hematologic:* Lymphocytes below 1,500/mm^3, ANC less than 1,500/mm^3, WBC below 3,000/mm^3, lymphadenopathy, chronic lymphocytic leukemia, hemoglobin less than 9.4 g/dL, petechia, platelets less than 75,000/mm^3, splenomegaly. *Respiratory:* Sinusitis, dyspnea, laryngitis, apnea, asthma, atelectasis, lung carcinoma, hemoptysis, hiccough, hyperventilation, hypoventilation, interstitial pneumonia, lung edema, pleural diffusion, pneumonia, pneumothorax. *GI:* Diarrhea, constipation, vomiting, GI disorder, aphthous stomatitis, cardiospasm, cheilitis, cholecystitis, cholelithiasis, duodenal ulcer, dry mouth, enteritis, esophagitis, fecal impaction, fecal incontinence, flatulence, gastritis, ***GI hemorrhage,*** gingivitis, glossitis, ***hematemesis,*** hepatic neoplasia, hepatitis, hepatomegaly, ileus, increased salivation, intestinal obstruction, melena, nausea, oral leukoplakia, oral moniliasis, pancreatitis, periodontal abscess, proctitis, ***rectal hemorrhage,*** salivary gland enlargement, stomach ulcer, peritonitis, tenesmus. *CNS:* ***Suicide attempts,*** hypertonia, somnolence, speech disorder, ***convulsions,*** hyperkinesia, abnormal gait, acute or chronic brain syndrome, agitation, apathy, aphasia, ataxia, brain edema, ***coma,*** delirium, delusions, dementia, depersonalization, diplopia, dystonia, encephalopathy, euphoria, facial paralysis, foot drop, hallucinations, hemiplegia, hypalgesia, hyperesthesia, incoordination, intracranial hypertension, decreased libido, manic reaction, meningitis, neuralgia, neuropathy, neurosis, nystagmus, oculogyric crisis, ophthalmoplegia, papilledema, paralysis, paranoid reaction, psychosis, decreased reflexes, stupor, subdural hematoma, torticollis, tremor. *Musculoskeletal:* Myasthenia, arthritis, arthrosis, bursitis, leg cramps, muscle atrophy, myopathy, myositis, ptosis, tenosynovitis. *Endocrine:* Cushing's syndrome, diabetes insipidus, hypothyroidism, inappropriate ADH. *Dermatologic:* Sweating, alopecia, contact dermatitis, erythema nodosum, exfoliative dermatitis, furunculosis, hirsutism, leukoderma, lichenoid dermatitis, maculopapular rash, psoriasis, seborrhea, skin benign neoplasm, skin carcinoma, skin hypertrophy, skin necrosis, skin ulcer, urticaria, vesiculobullous rash. *GU:* Dysmenorrhea, menstrual disorder, cystitis, breast pain, menorrhagia, urinary urgency, fibrocystic breast, breast neoplasm, urinary retention, anuria, balanitis, breast engorgement, cervicitis, epididymitis, gynecomastia, hematuria, impotence, kidney calculus or failure, kidney tubular disorder, leukorrhea, nephritis, nocturia, oliguria, polyuria, salpingitis, urethritis, urinary incontinence, enlarged uterine fibroids, uterine neoplasm, ***vaginal hemorrhage.*** *Ophthalmologic:* Blepharitis, blindness, dry eyes, iritis, keratoconjunctivitis, mydriasis, photophobia, retinitis, visual field defect. *Otic:* Ear pain, deafness, otitis externa, otitis media. *Miscellaneous:* Cyanosis, glycosuria, hypoxia, thirst, parosmia, taste loss, taste perversion.

NURSING CONSIDERATIONS

Assessment

1. Document age at onset of diagnosis of MS, frequency of exacerbations, and any other therapies prescribed and the outcome.
2. Note any hypersensitivity to human albumin or interferon beta.
3. Determine if pregnant; drug has abortifacient properties.
4. Obtain baseline hematologic profile and hepatic enzyme levels and monitor throughout therapy (q 3 months).

Client/Family Teaching
1. Explain the appropriate method for drug reconstitution, the proper dose, and administration of drug; provide written guidelines as a reference.
2. Teach client how to self-administer and assess injection technique. Advise on how to dispose of used syringes properly.
3. Do not change dose or administration schedule without provider approval.
4. Advise that flu-like symptoms are common and that acetaminophen may provide some relief.
5. Review the long list of potential drug side effects, stressing those that require immediate medical intervention.
6. Reinforce that any evidence of mental changes, depression, or suicide ideations should be reported immediately.
7. Advise client to practice birth control as drug may harm fetus.
8. Drug may cause photosensitivity reactions. Wear protective clothing, sunscreen, sun glasses, and a hat when exposure is necessary.
9. Avoid alcohol in any form.
10. Advise clients with diabetes to monitor blood sugars closely and to report any overt changes.
11. Identify support groups that may assist family to cope with this chronic disease.

Evaluate: ↓ Frequency and severity of MS exacerbations.

Ketamine hydrochloride

(**KEET**-ah-meen)
Ketalar **(Rx)**

How Supplied: *Injection:* 10 mg/mL, 50 mg/mL, 100 mg/mL

Action/Kinetics: Ketamine is rapid-acting and produces good analgesia. The drug blocks afferent impulses associated with pain perception, depresses spinal cord activity, and affects transmitter systems in the CNS. There is no effect on the pharyngeal-laryngeal reflexes. There is, however, slightly enhanced skeletal muscle tone and cardiovascular and respiratory stimulation. **Onset, IV:** 30 sec following a dose of 2 mg/kg; **onset, IM:** 3–4 min. **Duration, IV:** 5–10 min following a dose of 2 mg/kg; **duration, IM:** 12–25 min following a dose of 10 mg/kg. **t½:** 7–11 min (distribution) and 2–3 hr (elimination). The anesthetic effect is terminated by redistribution to other tissues from the brain and by liver metabolism (the major metabolite is ⅓ as active as ketamine).

Uses: For procedures in which skeletal muscle relaxation is not required. Induction of anesthesia before use of other general anesthetics. As a supplement to nitrous oxide anesthesia. *Investigational:* Adjunct to local anesthesia to produce sedation and analgesia.

Dosage

• **IV, Individualized**

Induction of anesthesia.

Initial: 1–2 mg/kg (of the base) at a rate of 0.5 mg/kg/min.

Maintenance of anesthesia.

0.01–0.05 mg/kg by continuous infusion at a rate of 1–2 mg/min.

Adjunct to local anesthesia.

5–30 mg (of the base) before giving the local anesthetic.

Sedation and analgesia.

0.2–0.75 mg/kg (of the base) given over 2–3 min; **then,** 0.005–0.02 mg/kg (of the base)/min as a continuous IV infusion.

• **IM**

Induction of anesthesia.

Initial: 5–10 mg/kg (of the base). Doses from one-half to the full amount of the induction dose may be used to maintain anesthesia.

Maintenance of anesthesia when ketamine used with diazepam.

0.1–0.5 mg/min ketamine with 2–5 mg diazepam IV as required.

Sedation and analgesia.

2–4 mg/kg (of the base); **then,** 0.005–0.2 mg/kg (of the base)/min by continuous IV infusion.

Administration/Storage
1. The dose should be administered slowly over a 60-sec period to reduce respiratory depression and hypertension.
2. Vials containing 100 mg/mL should always be diluted first with an equal volume of sterile water for injection, NSS, or D5W.
3. A precipitate will form if ketamine is combined with a barbiturate; thus, they should not be mixed in the same syringe.
4. Diazepam and ketamine should not be mixed in the same syringe or infusion flask.
5. Maintenance doses must be determined individually and are dependent, in part, on which additional anesthetic is used.
6. Tonic-clonic movements may occur during anesthesia; if manifested, they are not an indication for additional ketamine.
7. *Treatment of Overdose:* Artificial respiration.

Contraindications: Schizophrenia, acute psychoses, hypertension (or in clients in whom a rise in BP would be dangerous).

Special Concerns: Safe use during pregnancy has not been determined. Use with caution in the chronic alcoholic or if an individual is intoxicated with alcohol.

Side Effects: *Respiratory:* ***Apnea or severe respiratory depression following rapid IV administration, laryngospasm.*** *GI:* N&V, anorexia, increased salivation. *CV:* Increased BP and pulse rate, bradycardia, hypotension, arrhythmias. *Skeletal muscle:* Tonic and clonic movements resembling seizures. *CNS:* Emergence reactions including dream-like states, hallucinations, delirium, vivid imagery, confusion, irrational behavior, excitement. *Ophthalmologic:* Increased intraocular pressure (slight), double vision, nystagmus. *Miscellaneous:* Morbilliform rash, transient erythema.

Symptom of Overdose: ***Respiratory depression.***

Drug Interactions
Barbiturates / ↑ Recovery time from ketamine
Halothane / ↓ Pulse rate, BP, and CO
Muscle relaxants, nondepolarizing / ↑ Neuromuscular effects → respiratory depression
Narcotic analgesics / ↑ Recovery time from ketamine
Thyroid hormones / Tachycardia and hypertension
Tubocurarine / ↑ Neuromuscular effects → respiratory depression

NURSING CONSIDERATIONS
Interventions
1. To prevent dreams that are likely to occur with ketamine, place client in a quiet area after anesthesia. Minimize verbal, tactile, and visual stimulation.
2. If the client is excessively active (emergence delerium) during the recovery phase, anticipate that a low dose of a barbiturate sedative or benzodiazepine may be required. This may also prolong recovery time.
3. Take VS gently. Avoid making noises, bumping bed, and vigorously rousing or stimulating client. Keep side rails up.

Client/Family Teaching
1. Provide printed instructions for postprocedure care. Client frequently experiences amnesia and has difficulty remembering what was previously taught.
2. Do not perform tasks that require mental alertness until drug effects are realized.
3. Avoid alcohol and CNS depressants for at least 24 hr following anesthesia.

Evaluate: Desired anesthetic effect.

Lodoxamide tromethamine
(loh-**DOX**-ah-myd)
Pregnancy Category: B
Alomide **(Rx)**

How Supplied: *Solution:* 0.1%

Action/Kinetics: Lodoxamide is a mast cell stabilizer that inhibits Type I immediate hypersensitivity reac-

tions. It prevents the release of mast cell inflammatory mediators, including slow-reacting substances of anaphylaxis (peptidoleukotrienes), and inhibits eosinophil chemotaxis. The mechanism for the beneficial effect is not known with certainty but may be due to prevention of calcium influx into mast cells upon stimulation by antigens. **Elimination t½:** 8.5 hr. Excreted mainly through the urine.
Uses: To treat ocular disorders such as vernal keratoconjunctivitis, vernal conjunctivitis, and vernal keratitis.

Dosage

- **Ophthalmic Solution**
  Ocular disorders.

Adults and children over 2 years of age: 1–2 gtt in each affected eye 4–6 times daily for up to 3 months.
Contraindication: Use in clients wearing soft contact lenses.
Special Concerns: Use with caution during lactation. The drug is for ophthalmic use only and should not be injected. Safety and efficacy have not been determined for use in children less than 2 years of age.
Side Effects: *Ophthalmologic:* Transient burning, stinging, or discomfort upon instillation. Ocular itching or pruritus, blurred vision, dry eye, tearing, discharge from eyes, hyperemia, crystalline deposits in eye, foreign body sensation, corneal erosion or ulcer, scales on lid or lash, eye pain, ocular edema or swelling, ocular warming sensation, ocular fatigue, chemosis, corneal abrasion, anterior chamber cells, keratopathy, keratitis, blepharitis, allergy, sticky sensation, epitheliopathy. *CNS:* Headache, dizziness, somnolence. *GI:* Nausea, stomach discomfort. *Miscellaneous:* Heat sensation, sneezing, dry nose, rash.

NURSING CONSIDERATIONS

Assessment: Determine onset and describe symptoms. List other agents prescribed and the outcome.
Client/Family Teaching
1. Review the appropriate method and frequency for administration; observe client technique.
2. Stress that soft contact lenses *cannot* be worn during therapy.
3. Advise that some stinging and burning may be evident on instillation, but if symptoms persist after instillation, notify the provider.

Evaluate: Improvement in symptoms of seasonal ocular inflammation.

Nicotine polacrilex (Nicotine Resin Complex)

(**NIK**-oh-teen)
Pregnancy Category: X
Nicorette, Nicorette DS, Nicorette Plus ✦ **(Rx)**

How Supplied: *Gum:* 2 mg, 4 mg
Action/Kinetics: Following chewing, nicotine is released from an ion exchange resin in the gum product, providing blood nicotine levels approximating those produced by smoking cigarettes. The amount of nicotine released depends on the rate and duration of chewing. Following repeated administration q 30 min, nicotine blood levels reach 25–50 ng/mL. If the gum is swallowed, only a minimum amount of nicotine is released. Nicotine is metabolized mainly by the liver, with about 10%–20% excreted unchanged in the urine.
Uses: Adjunct with behavioral modification in smokers wishing to give up the smoking habit. Is considered only as an initial aid, with the ultimate goal being abstention from all forms of nicotine. Most likely to benefit are individuals with the following characteristics:
a. smoke brands of cigarettes containing more than 0.9 mg nicotine;
b. smoke more than 15 cigarettes daily;
c. inhale cigarette smoke deeply and frequently;
d. smoke most frequently during the morning;
e. smoke the first cigarette of the day within 30 min of arising;

f. indicate cigarettes smoked in the morning are the most difficult to give up;
g. smoke even if the individual is ill and confined to bed;
h. find it necessary to smoke in places where smoking is not allowed.
NOTE: Nicotine may be effective in improving the course of difficult-to-treat ulcerative colitis.

Dosage

• **Gum**

Initial: One piece of gum chewed whenever the urge to smoke occurs; **maintenance:** 9–12 pieces of gum daily during the first month, not to exceed 30 pieces daily of the 2-mg strength and 20 pieces daily of the 4-mg strength.

Administration/Storage

1. Nicotine polacrilex is available as a 2-mg (Nicorette) and 4-mg (Nicorette DS) gum. The 4-mg dosage form was introduced since those heavily addicted to smoking had adapted and their symptoms could not be managed by the 2-mg dosage form. Thus, those who smoke more than 25 cigarettes/day should be started on the 4-mg dose.
2. The individual must want to stop smoking and should do so immediately.
3. Each piece of gum should be chewed slowly for about 30 min.
4. Acidic beverages, such as coffee, juices, soft drinks, and wine, interfere with buccal absorption of nicotine from the gum; thus, eating and drinking 15 min before and during chewing of the nicotine gum should be avoided.
5. Clients should be evaluated monthly and if the individual has not smoked for 3 months, the gum should be slowly withdrawn. Nicotine should not be used for longer than 6 months.
6. Suggested procedures for gradual withdrawal of the gum include:
• decreasing the total number of pieces/day by one or more pieces q 4–7 days.
• decreasing the chewing time with each piece from the normal 30 min to 10–15 min for 4–7 days; then gradually decreasing the number of pieces used per day.
• increasing the chewing time for more than 30 min and reducing the number of pieces used per day.
• substituting one or more pieces of sugarless gum for an equal number of pieces of nicotine gum; then, increasing the number of pieces of sugarless gum substituted for nicotine gum q 4–7 days.
• replacing the 4-mg gum with the 2-mg gum and applying any of the first four procedures listed above.
7. *Treatment of Overdose:* Syrup of ipecac if vomiting has not occurred, saline laxative, gastric lavage followed by activated charcoal (if client is unconscious), maintenance of respiration, maintenance of CV function.

Contraindications: Pregnancy, lactation, nonsmokers, serious arrhythmias, angina, vasospastic disease, active temporomandibular joint disease.

Special Concerns: Safety and effectiveness in children and adolescents who smoke have not been determined. Use with caution in hypertension, PUD, oral or pharyngeal inflammation, gastritis, stomatitis, hyperthyroidism, insulin-dependent diabetes, and pheochromocytoma.

Side Effects: *CNS:* Dizziness, irritability, headache. *GI:* N&V, indigestion, GI upset, salivation, eructation. *Other:* Sore mouth or throat, hiccoughs, sore jaw muscles.

Symptoms of Overdose: GI: N&V, diarrhea, salivation, abdominal pain. *CNS:* Headache, dizziness, confusion, weakness, fainting, ***seizures.*** *Respiratory:* Labored breathing, ***respiratory paralysis (cause of death).*** *Other:* Cold sweat, disturbed hearing and vision, hypotension, and rapid, weak pulse.

Drug Interactions

Caffeine / Possibly ↓ blood levels of caffeine due to ↑ rate of breakdown by liver
Catecholamines / ↑ Levels of catecholamines
Cortisol / ↑ Levels of cortisol
Furosemide / Possible ↓ diuretic effect of furosemide

Glutethimide / Possible ↓ absorption of glutethimide
Imipramine / Possibly ↓ blood levels of imipramine due to ↑ rate of breakdown by liver
Pentazocine / Possibly ↓ blood levels of pentazocine due to ↑ rate of breakdown by liver
Theophylline / Possibly ↓ blood levels of theophylline due to ↑ rate of breakdown by liver

NURSING CONSIDERATIONS

Client/Family Teaching

1. Use the gum only as directed. When client has the urge to smoke, chew one piece slowly. When a slight tingling becomes evident, stop chewing until sensation subsides.
2. Advise that too vigorous chewing can increase adverse effects. Provide a printed list of drug (gum) side effects and instruct to report any that are bothersome or of concern.
3. Do not ingest food or liquids 15 min before and during ingestion of the gum as effects may be diminished.
4. Provide the client with names of local support groups that can help with smoking cessation and provide emotional and psychologic support throughout the endeavor.
5. Advise and support participation and enrollment in a formal smoking cessation program.

Evaluate: Evidence of control of nicotine withdrawal symptoms with ↓ number of cigarettes smoked per day or complete smoking cessation.

Nicotine transdermal system

(**NIK**-oh-teen)
Pregnancy Category: D
Habitrol, Nicoderm, Nicotrol, Prostep
(Rx)

How Supplied: *Film, Extended Release:* 5 mg/16 hr, 7 mg/24 hr, 10 mg/16 hr, 11 mg/24 hr, 14 mg/24 hr, 15 mg/16 hr, 21 mg/24 hr, 22 mg/24 hr

Action/Kinetics: Nicotine transdermal system is a multilayered film that provides systemic delivery of varying amounts of nicotine over a 24-hr period after applying to the skin. Nicotine's reinforcing activity is due to two CNS effects. The first is stimulation of the cortex (via the locus ceruleus), producing increased alertness and cognitive performance. The second is a "reward" effect due to an action in the limbic system. At low doses the stimulatory effects predominate, whereas at high doses the reward effects predominate. The nicotine transdermal system produces an initial (first day of use) increase in BP, an increase in HR (3%–7%), and a decrease in SV after 10 days. Nicotine is metabolized in the liver to a large number of metabolites, all of which are less active than nicotine. **t½, following removal of the system from the skin:** 3–4 hr.

Uses: As an aid to stopping smoking for the relief of nicotine withdrawal symptoms. Should be used in conjunction with a comprehensive behavioral smoking cessation program.

Dosage

- **Transdermal System**

HABITROL OR NICODERM

Healthy clients.

Initial: 21 mg/day for the first 6 weeks, followed by 14 mg/day for the next 2 weeks and 7 mg/day for last 2 weeks.

Clients weighing less than 45.5 kg, those who smoke fewer than 10 cigarettes daily, or clients with CV disease. **Initial:** 14 mg/day for the first 6 weeks, followed by 7 mg/day for the next 2 weeks. The entire course of therapy should be from 8 to 12 weeks.

NICOTROL

Initial: 15 mg/day for the first 12 weeks, followed by 10 mg/day for the next 2 weeks and 5 mg/day for the last 2 weeks. The entire course of therapy should be from 14 to 20 weeks.

ProStep
Initial: 22 mg/day for 4–8 weeks followed by 11 mg/day for 2–4 additional weeks. The entire course of therapy should be from 6 to 12 weeks.

Administration/Storage

1. There will be differences in the duration and length of therapy, depending on the product prescribed.
2. The transdermal system should be applied promptly after its removal from the protective pouch to prevent loss of nicotine due to evaporation. Systems should only be used when the pouch is intact.
3. The system should be applied once daily to a nonhairy, clean, and dry site on the trunk or upper, outer arm. After 24 hr, the system should be removed and a new system applied to an alternate skin site when using Habitrol, Nicoderm, or ProStep. Skin sites should not be reused for at least a week. For Nicotrol, a new system should be applied each day upon waking and removed at bedtime.
4. When a used system is removed, it should be folded over and placed in the protective pouch that contained the new system. The used system should be disposed of to ensure access is prevented by children or pets.
5. The goal of therapy with nicotine transdermal systems is complete abstinence. If the client has not stopped smoking by the fourth week of therapy, treatment should be discontinued.
6. The need for adjustment of the dose should be assessed during the first 2 weeks of therapy.
7. Nicotine will continue to be absorbed from the skin for several hours after removal of the system.
8. Use beyond 3 months for Habitrol, Nicoderm, and ProStep and use beyond 5 months for Nicotrol has not been studied.
9. Systems should not be stored above 30°C (86°F) because they are sensitive to heat.
10. *Treatment of Overdose:* Remove the transdermal system immediately. The surface of the skin may be flushed with water and dried; soap should not be used as it may increase the absorption of nicotine. Diazepam or barbiturates may be used to treat seizures and atropine can be given for excessive bronchial secretions or diarrhea. Respiratory support for respiratory failure and fluid support for hypotension and CV collapse. If transdermal systems are ingested PO, activated charcoal should be given to prevent seizures. If the client is unconscious, the charcoal should be administered by an NGT. A saline cathartic or sorbitol added to the first dose of activated charcoal may hasten GI passage of the system. Doses of activated charcoal should be repeated as long as the system remains in the GI tract as nicotine will continue to be released for many hours.

Contraindications: Hypersensitivity or allergy to nicotine or any components of the therapeutic system. Use in children and during labor and delivery. Use in the immediate postmyocardial period, in clients with serious arrhythmias, and in those with severe or worsening angina pectoris. Use with severe renal impairment.

Special Concerns: Pregnant smokers should be encouraged to try to stop smoking using educational and behavioral interventions before using the nicotine transdermal system. The product should only be used during pregnancy if the potential benefit outweighs the potential risk of nicotine to the fetus. The use of nicotine transdermal systems for longer than 3 months has not been studied. Clients with coronary heart disease (history of MI and/or angina pectoris), serious cardiac arrhythmias, or vasospastic diseases (e.g., Buerger's disease, Prinzmetal's variant angina) should be screened carefully before using the transdermal system. Use with caution in clients with hyperthyroidism, pheochromocytoma, or insulin-dependent diabetes (nicotine causes the release of catecholamines). Use with caution in clients with active peptic ulcers, in accelerated hypertension, and during lactation.

Side Effects: *NOTE:* The incidence of side effects is complicated by the fact that clients manifest effects of nicotine withdrawal or by concurrent smoking.

Dermatologic: Erythema, pruritus, or burning at the site of application; cutaneous hypersensitivity, sweating. *Body as a whole:* Allergy, back pain. *GI:* Diarrhea, dyspepsia, dry mouth, abdominal pain, constipation, N&V. *Musculoskeletal:* Arthralgia, myalgia. *CNS:* Abnormal dreams, somnolence, dizziness, impaired concentration, headache, insomnia. *CV:* Tachycardia, hypertension. *Respiratory:* Increased cough, pharyngitis, sinusitis. *GU:* Dysmenorrhea.

Symptoms of Overdose: Pallor, cold sweat, N&V, abdominal pain, salivation, diarrhea, headache, dizziness, disturbed hearing and vision, mental confusion, weakness, tremor. Large overdoses may cause prostration, hypotension, ***respiratory failure, seizures, and death.***

NURSING CONSIDERATIONS

Assessment

1. Determine any evidence of renal or liver dysfunction.
2. Note any history of CAD.
3. List all medications client currently prescribed. Cessation of smoking, with or without nicotine replacement, may alter the response to certain drugs. For example, a decrease in the dosage of acetaminophen, caffeine, imipramine, insulin, oxazepam, pentazocine, propranolol, theophylline, and certain adrenergic blockers (e.g., prazosin, labetalol) may be required. An increase in the dose of adrenergic agonists (e.g., isoproterenol, phenylephrine) may be required.
4. Document any skin disorders as nicotine transdermal systems may be irritating for clients with skin disorders such as atopic or eczematous dermatitis.

Client/Family Teaching

1. Use extreme caution during application and advise all to avoid contact with active systems. If contact does occur, wash the area with water only. The eyes should not be touched.
2. These systems can be a dermal irritant and can cause contact dermatitis. Instruct clients on the proper use of the systems using a return demonstration technique.
3. Any persistent skin irritations such as erythema, edema, or pruritus at the application site as well as any generalized skin reactions such as hives, urticaria, or a generalized rash should be reported and the system should be removed.
4. Advise client to follow the manufacturer's guidelines for proper system application. Review the information sheet that comes with the product as it contains instructions on how to use and dispose of the transdermal systems properly.
5. Stop smoking completely when initiating the nicotine transdermal system. If smoking continues, advise clients that they may experience side effects due to higher nicotine levels in the body.
6. Encourage participation in a formal smoking cessation program. The success or failure of smoking cessation depends on the quality, intensity, and frequency of supportive care. Stress that clients are more likely to stop smoking if they are seen frequently and are active in a formal smoking cessation program.
7. Advise client that nicotine in any form can be toxic and addictive. Review the risks of therapy and stress that the use of nicotine transdermal systems may lead to dependence. To minimize this risk, clients should be encouraged to withdraw use of the transdermal system gradually after 4–8 weeks of use.
8. Review the symptoms of nicotine withdrawal, which include craving, nervousness, restlessness, irritability, mood lability, anxiety, drowsiness, sleep disturbances, impaired con-

centration, increased appetite, headache, myalgia, constipation, fatigue, and weight gain and advise client to report if evident as dosage may require adjustment.
9. Remind client to change sites of application daily and not to reuse this site for 1 week.
10. Client prescribed Nicotrol should remove patch at bedtime and apply upon arising.
11. Keep all products used and unused away from children and pets. Advise that sufficient nicotine is still present in used systems to cause toxicity.
12. If therapy is unsuccessful after 4 weeks, discontinue and identify reasons for failure so that a later attempt may be more successful.
Evaluate: Successful smoking cessation with control of symptoms of nicotine withdrawal.

Ritodrine hydrochloride

(**RYE**-toe-dreen)
Pregnancy Category: B
Yutopar, Yutopar S.R. ✱ **(Rx)**

How Supplied: *Injection:* 10 mg/mL; 15 mg/mL
Action/Kinetics: Stimulates beta-2 receptors of smooth muscle of the uterus, which results in inhibition of uterine contractility. It may also directly inhibit the actin-myosin interaction. The effects of the drug are inhibited by the beta-adrenergic blocking agents. Increased blood levels of insulin, glucose, and free fatty acids and decreased levels of potassium have been observed during IV infusion. **Onset, PO:** 30–60 min; **IV:** 5 min. **Peak plasma concentration, IV:** After a 9-mg infusion over 60 min, 32–50 ng/mL; **PO:** after a dose of 10 mg, 5–15 ng/mL. **Time to peak serum levels:** 20–60 min. **t½, after IV:** 15–17 hr; **after PO:** 12–20 hr. Ninety percent of drug excreted within 24 hr through the urine.
Uses: Preterm labor in selected clients after week 20 of gestation. When indicated, therapy with ritodrine should be initiated as early as possible after diagnosis. However, decision to use ritodrine should include determination of fetal maturity.

Dosage
- **IV, Tablets**
  Preterm labor.

Initial: 0.05–0.1 mg/min (20 gtt/min using microdrip chamber); **then,** depending on response, increase by 0.05 mg/min (10 microdrops/min) q 10 min until desired response occurs. **Effective dose range:** 0.15–0.35 mg/min (30–70 gtt/min). Continue infusion antepartum for a minimum of 12 hr after contractions cease. **PO therapy following initial IV treatment:** 10 mg 30 min before cessation of IV therapy; **then,** for first 24 hr, 10 mg q 2 hr; **maintenance:** 10–20 mg q 4–6 hr, not to exceed 120 mg/day. Dosage is determined by uterine activity and incidence of side effects.
Administration/Storage
1. The drug should be reconstituted with dextrose solution (150 mg in 500 mL). Solutions containing sodium chloride should be avoided, if possible, as their use increases the possibility of pulmonary edema. Final dilution will contain 0.3 mg/mL ritodrine.
2. To minimize hypotension, administer IV dose while the client is in the left lateral position.
3. Use a Y set-up, infusion pump, and microdrip tubing (60 microdrops/mL) for drug administration.
4. Do not use discolored solutions or those containing precipitate. Use diluted solution within 48 hr.
5. PO maintenance therapy is usually initiated 30 min before discontinuing IV therapy.
6. *Treatment of Overdose:* Supportive measures. A beta-adrenergic blocking agent can be used as an antidote. The drug is dialyzable.
Contraindications: Before week 20 of pregnancy (pregnancy category: B) and when continuation of pregnancy is hazardous to mother (e.g., eclampsia, severe preeclampsia, intrauterine fetal death, antepartum hemorrhage,

pulmonary hypertension, chorioamnionitis, and maternal hyperthyroidism, cardiac disease or uncontrolled diabetes mellitus). Also, medical conditions (e.g., uncontrolled hypertension, pheochromocytoma, bronchial asthma, hypovolemia, cardiac arrhythmias due to tachycardia or digitalis toxicity) that would be aggravated by beta-adrenergic agonists.

Laboratory Test Interferences: ↑ Plasma glucose and insulin; ↓ plasma potassium.

Side Effects: All effects are related to the stimulation of beta receptors by the drug. **IV.** *CV:* Increase in maternal and fetal HR, increase in maternal systolic and marked decrease in diastolic BP (widening of pulse pressure), tachycardia, palpitations, ***arrhythmias,*** chest pain, angina, heart murmur, ***myocardial ischemia.*** Sinus bradycardia following drug withdrawal. *GI:* N&V, bloating, ileus, GI upset, diarrhea or constipation. *CNS:* Headache, tremors, malaise, nervousness, jitteriness, restlessness, anxiety, emotional changes, drowsiness, weakness. *Metabolic:* Transient increases in insulin and blood glucose, increases in cyclic AMP and free fatty acids, decrease in potassium, glycosuria, lactic acidosis. *Respiratory:* Dyspnea, hyperventilation. *Other:* Erythema, ***anaphylaxis,*** rash, hemolytic icterus, sweating, chills.

PO. *CV:* Increase in HR of mother, palpitations, ***arrhythmias.*** *Other:* Tremors, nausea, rashes, restlessness. *In the neonate:* Hypoglycemia and ileus are infrequently observed; also hypocalcemia and hypotension in neonates whose mothers also received other beta-receptor agonists.

Symptoms of Overdose: Excessive beta-adrenergic stimulation, including tachycardia (in both the mother and fetus), palpitations, ***cardiac arrhythmias,*** hypotension, dyspnea, tremor, nervousness, N&V.

Drug Interactions

Anesthetics, general / Additive hypotension or cardiac arrhythmias
Atropine / ↑ Systemic hypertension
Beta-adrenergic blocking agents / ↓ Effect of ritodrine
Corticosteroids / ↑ Risk of pulmonary edema
Diazoxide / Additive hypotension or cardiac arrhythmias
Magnesium sulfate / Additive hypotension or cardiac arrhythmias
Meperidine / Additive hypotension or cardiac arrhythmias
Sympathomimetics / Additive effects of sympathomimetics

NURSING CONSIDERATIONS

Assessment

1. Note any evidence or history of preeclampsia, hypertension, or diabetes before initiating drug therapy.
2. Determine that an ultrasound and amniocentesis have been performed to establish fetal maturity. This determines whether ritodrine can be used.
3. Establish gestational age prior to initiating drug therapy. Ritodrine should not be used before week 20 of pregnancy.

Interventions

1. Avoid concomitant administration of beta-adrenergic blocking drugs, such as propranolol, because these drugs inhibit the action of ritodrine.
2. Assess the response to IV therapy with ritodrine by evaluating the strength and frequency of uterine contractions and monitoring the fetal HR. Document and report an increased fetal HR.
3. Monitor and record VS.
• Maintain BP by positioning the client in a left lateral position and evaluating level of hydration.
• Report any increase in SBP, decrease in DBP, and tachycardia.
4. Monitor I&O and auscultate lung sounds to assess fluid status.
5. Prevent circulatory overload. Closely monitor IV flow rate and infused volume during drug administration.
6. Assess for any respiratory dysfunction (i.e., rales, dyspnea, frothy sputum) that may precede pulmo-

nary edema, especially when the client is also receiving corticosteroids.
7. Assess for S&S of electrolyte imbalance. Be particularly alert to hypokalemia, hyperglycemia, and acidosis in clients with diabetes.
8. Assess the postpartum client who has received both ritodrine and general anesthetic for potentiation of hypotensive effects.
9. Neonates of mothers who have received ritodrine should be assessed for hyper- or hypoglycemia, hypocalcemia, hypotension, and ileus. Have emergency medication and equipment available to support the neonate.

Client/Family Teaching
1. Advise to take medication 1 hr before or 2 hr following meals to enhance absorption.
2. Take only as directed at the same time each day.
3. Explain that medication is administered to stop labor and stress the importance of close medical supervision to ensure appropriate dosage.
4. Report any chest pain, tightness, palpitations, dizziness, weakness, tremors, or difficulty breathing immediately.
5. Once IV infusion has been completed, ambulation may be resumed in 3–4 days as long as symptoms do not recur.
6. If contractions resume, membranes rupture, or spotting and/or bleeding occur lie down immediately and notify provider.

Evaluate: Desired inhibition of uterine contractions with suppression of labor.

Sermorelin Acetate

(**sir**-mor-**EL**-in)
Pregnancy Category: C
Geref **(Rx)**

How Supplied: *Powder for injection:* 50 mcg

Action/Kinetics: Sermorelin is the acetate salt of a synthetic amino acid polypeptide that is the amino-terminal segment of naturally occurring human growth hormone (GH). It appears to be equivalent to human growth hormone–releasing hormone. Baseline GH levels are usually low; thus, provocative tests may be of use in assessing the functional ability of the pituitary to secrete GH. Sermorelin increases plasma GH levels by directly stimulating the pituitary gland to release GH.

Use: To evaluate the ability of the somatotroph of the pituitary gland to secrete GH.

Dosage

• **IV**

Dose is individualized for each client based on weight. The drug is given in a single IV dose of 1 mcg/kg in the morning following an overnight fast.

Administration/Storage
1. For clients weighing less than 50 kg, the following procedure should be used:
• The contents of one 50-mcg vial should be reconstituted with a minimum of 0.5 mL of the accompanying sterile diluent.
• Fifteen minutes before and immediately prior to drug administration, venous blood samples are drawn for GH determinations.
• A bolus of 1 mcg/kg IV is given followed by a 3-mL normal saline flush.
• Venous blood samples are drawn for GH determinations 15, 30, 45, and 60 min after drug administration.
2. For clients weighing 50 kg, the following procedure is used:
• The number of ampules of drug is determined based on a dose of 1 mcg/kg.
• The contents of each ampule are reconstituted using a minimum of 0.5 mL of the accompanying sterile diluent.
• The remainder of the procedure is exactly the same as used for clients weighing less than 50 kg.
3. The lyophilized product is to be stored at 2°C–8°C (36°F–46°F).
4. The drug must be used immediately after reconstitution and any unused drug must be discarded.

Contraindications: Hypersensitivity to sermorelin or any of the excipients in the product.
Special Concerns: Use with caution during lactation. Obesity, hyperglycemia, and elevated plasma fatty acids are often associated with subnormal GH responses to sermorelin.
Side Effects: *At injection site:* Pain, redness, or swelling. *GI:* N&V, strange taste in the mouth. *Miscellaneous:* Transient warmth or flushing of the face, headache, paleness, tightness in the chest, antibody formation.

Symptoms of Overdose: Changes in HR and BP in IV doses exceeding 10 mcg/kg.
Drug Interactions: The sermorelin test should not be undertaken in the presence of drugs that directly affect the pituitary secretion of somatotropin. These include insulin, glucocorticoids, products that contain or release somatotropin, cyclooxygenase inhibitors (e.g., aspirin and other nonsteroidal anti-inflammatory agents), clonidine, levodopa, and insulin-induced hypoglycemia. The response to sermorelin may be blunted by atropine and similar drugs, in hypothyroid clients, and in those being treated with antithyroid drugs (e.g., propylthiouracil).

NURSING CONSIDERATIONS

Assessment

1. Determine any history of hyperglycemia, elevated fatty acids, or the presence of obesity.
2. List drugs currently prescribed to ensure none interact unfavorably.
3. A normal response does not preclude GH deficiency because the deficiency is often due to hypothalamic dysfunction in the presence of an intact somatotroph. The sermorelin stimulation test is most easily interpreted when there is a subnormal response to the usual provocative testing and a normal response to sermorelin. When both conventional and sermorelin testing result in subnormal GH responses, the site of the dysfunction cannot be determined with any certainty because some clients with GH deficiency due to hypothalamic dysfunction need multiple sermorelin injections before demonstrating a normal response.

Interventions

1. Monitor VS and I&O.
2. GH therapy should be discontinued 1 week before administering the test.
3. N&V, headaches, warmth or flushing of the face, paleness, pain, or redness or swelling at injection site and chest tightness may be experienced during therapy.

Evaluate: Stimulation of pituitary gland to release GH.

Tacrine Hydrochloride (THA, Tetrahydroaminoacridine)

(**TAH**-krin)
Pregnancy Category: C
Cognex **(Rx)**

How Supplied: *Capsule:* 10 mg, 20 mg, 30 mg, 40 mg
Action/Kinetics: Tacrine is a reversible cholinesterase inhibitor that acts in the CNS. It is believed that during the early stages of Alzheimer's disease, cholinergic neuronal pathways are affected that project from the basal forebrain to the cerebral cortex and hippocampus. Some of the clinical manifestations of dementia are thought to be due to a deficiency of cortical acetylcholine. Tacrine elevates acetylcholine levels in the cerebral cortex by inhibiting cholinesterase and thus the breakdown of acetylcholine. There is no evidence that tacrine alters the progression of dementia, however. Tacrine is rapidly absorbed after PO administration. **Maximal plasma levels:** 1–2 hr. Food will affect the bioavailability of tacrine. Tacrine is extensively metabolized in the liver to several metabolites. The drug undergoes first-pass metabolism, but this can be overcome by increasing the dose. **Elimi-**

nation t½: 2–4 hr. The clearance of tacrine is about 50% higher in females. Also, the mean tacrine levels in smokers are about one-third the levels of nonsmokers.

Use: Treatment of mild to moderate dementia of the Alzheimer's type.

Dosage

• **Tablets**

Alzheimer's disease.

Initial: 10 mg q.i.d. for at least 6 weeks; **then,** after 6 weeks, increase the dose to 20 mg q.i.d. providing there are no significant transaminase elevations and the client tolerates the treatment. Based on the degree of tolerance, the dose may be titrated, at 6-week intervals, to 30 or 40 mg q.i.d.

Administration/Storage

1. The drug should be taken between meals, if possible. If GI upset occurs, the drug can be taken with meals; however, the plasma level will be decreased by 30%–40%.
2. It is important that the initial dose not be increased for 6 weeks as there is the potential for delayed onset of transaminase elevations.
3. *Treatment of Overdose:* General supportive measures. IV atropine sulfate, titrated to effect, may be given in an initial dose of 1–2 mg IV with subsequent doses based on the response.

Contraindications: Hypersensitivity to tacrine or acridine derivatives. Use in clients previously treated with tacrine who developed jaundice due to the drug.

Special Concerns: Tacrine may cause bradycardia that is of importance in clients with sick sinus syndrome. Use with caution in clients at risk for developing ulcers as the drug increases gastric acid secretion. Use with caution in clients with a history of abnormal liver function as indicated by abnormalities in serum ALT, AST, bilirubin, and gamma-glutamyl transpeptidase levels. Use with caution in clients with a history of asthma. There may be worsening of cognitive function following abrupt discontinuation of the drug. There are no studies on the safety and efficacy of tacrine use in children with dementing illness.

Side Effects: *Hepatic:* Increased transaminase levels (most common reason for stopping the drug during treatment). *GI:* N&V diarrhea, dyspepsia, anorexia, abdominal pain, flatulence, constipation, glossitis, gingivitis, dry mouth or throat, stomatitis, increased salivation, dysphagia, esophagitis, gastritis, gastroenteritis, ***GI hemorrhage,*** stomach ulcer, hiatal hernia, hemorrhoids, bloody stools, diverticulitis, fecal impaction, fecal incontinence, ***rectal hemorrhage,*** cholelithiasis, cholecystitis, increased appetite. *Musculoskeletal:* Myalgia, fracture, arthralgia, arthritis, hypertonia, osteoporosis, tendinitis, bursitis, gout, myopathy. *CNS:* ***Precipitation of seizures*** (may also be due to Alzheimer's), dizziness, confusion, ataxia, insomnia, somnolence, tremor, agitation, depression, abnormal thinking, anxiety, hallucinations, hostility, migraine, ***convulsions,*** vertigo, syncope, hyperkinesia, paresthesia, abnormal dreams, dysarthria, aphasia, amnesia, twitching, hypesthesia, delirium, paralysis, bradykinesia, movement disorders, cogwheel rigidity, paresis, neuritis, hemiplegia, Parkinson's disease, neuropathy, extrapyramidal syndrome, decreased or absent reflexes, tardive dyskinesia, dysesthesia, dystonia, encephalitis, ***coma,*** apraxia, oculogyric crisis, akathisia, oral facial dyskinesia, Bell's palsy, nervousness, apathy, increased libido, paranoia, neurosis, ***suicidal episodes,*** psychosis, hysteria. *Respiratory:* Rhinitis, upper respiratory infection, coughing, pharyngitis, sinusitis, bronchitis, pneumonia, dyspnea, epistaxis, chest congestion, asthma, hyperventilation, lower respiratory infection, hemoptysis, lung edema, ***lung cancer, acute epiglottitis.*** *CV:* Hypotension, hypertension, ***heart failure, MI, CVA,*** angina pectoris, transient ischemic attack, phlebitis, venous insufficiency, abdominal aortic aneurysm, atrial fibrillation or flutter, palpitation, tachycardia, bradycardia,

pulmonary embolus, heart arrest, premature atrial contractions, ***AV block,*** bundle branch block. *Dermatologic:* Rash, facial and skin flushing, increased sweating, acne, alopecia, dermatitis, eczema, dry skin, herpes zoster, psoriasis, cellulitis, cyst, furunculosis, herpes simplex, hyperkeratosis, basal cell carcinoma, skin cancer, desquamation, seborrhea, squamous cell carcinoma, skin ulcer, skin necrosis, ***melanoma.*** *GU:* Bladder outflow obstruction, urinary frequency, urinary incontinence, UTI, hematuria, renal stone, kidney infection, glycosuria, dysuria, polyuria, nocturia, pyuria, cystitis, urinary retention, urinary urgency, ***vaginal hemorrhage,*** genital pruritus, breast pain, urinary obstruction, impotence, ***prostate cancer, bladder tumor, renal tumor, renal failure, breast cancer, ovarian carcinoma,*** epididymitis. *Body as a whole:* Headache, fatigue, chest pain, weight decrease, back pain, asthenia, chill, fever, malaise, peripheral edema, facial edema, dehydration, weight increase, cachexia, lipoma, heat exhaustion, sepsis, ***cholinergic crisis, death.*** *Hematologic:* Anemia, lymphadenopathy, leukopenia, thrombocytopenia, hemolysis, pancytopenia. *Ophthalmologic:* Conjunctivitis, cataract, dry eyes, eye pain, visual field defect, diplopia, amblyopia, glaucoma, hordeolum, vision loss, ptosis, blepharitis. *Otic:* Deafness, earache, tinnitus, inner ear infection, otitis media, labyrinthitis, inner ear disturbance. *Miscellaneous:* Purpura, hypercholesterolemia, diabetes mellitus, hypothyroid, hyperthyroid, unusual taste.

Symptoms of Overdose: Cholinergic crisis characterized by severe N&V, sweating, bradycardia, salivation, hypotension, ***collapse, seizures, and increased muscle weakness (may paralyze respiratory muscles leading to death).***

Drug Interactions

Anticholinergic drugs / Tacrine interferes with the action of these drugs

Bethanechol / Tacrine → synergistic effect with bethanechol

Cimetidine / Cimetidine ↑ maximum levels of tacrine

Succinylcholine / Tacrine ↑ muscle relaxation due to succinylcholine

Theophylline / Tacrine ↑ plasma levels of theophylline; ↓ theophylline dose recommended.

NURSING CONSIDERATIONS

Assessment

1. Document onset of symptoms and whether this is a first drug trial for the Alzheimer's client or a rechallenge. If a rechallenge, document serum bilirubin levels during previous treatment.
2. Note any ECG evidence of sick sinus syndrome or any history of ulcer disease, asthma, or liver disease.
3. List drugs currently prescribed to ensure none interact unfavorably. Drug is a cholinesterase inhibitor; notify anesthesia before procedures.
4. Obtain baseline ECG and hematologic and liver profiles. Serum transaminase levels should be monitored weekly for the first 18 weeks and then every 3 months unless dose is increased or the transaminase levels are mildly elevated (in which case weekly monitoring should occur for at least 6 weeks).

Interventions

1. Monitor VS and assess for variations. Drug may cause bradycardia.
2. Assess for symptoms of active or occult GI bleeding; drug may cause a decrease in gastric acid secretion.
3. Observe and record client response carefully as drug is titrated according to client tolerance.

Client/Family Teaching

1. Take between meals unless GI upset is experienced.
2. Explain that clinical manifestations of mild to moderate dementia in Alzheimer's disease are thought to be related to a deficiency of acetylcholine. Tacrine is thought to act to elevate acetylcholine concentrations in the cerebral cortex.

3. Stress that as the disease progresses, tacrine's effect may lessen.
4. Reinforce that drug must be administered as prescribed at regularly spaced intervals. Do not alter dosage without provider approval.
5. Advise to report any new symptoms or any increase in existing symptoms.
6. Smoking may interfere with serum drug levels and should be avoided.
7. During initiation of therapy, N&V and diarrhea may be evident; report if persistent or bothersome.
8. Review delayed-onset side effects that should be reported, e.g., rashes, yellow skin discoloration, and changes in stool color.
9. Do not stop abruptly. Abrupt withdrawal may cause a decline in cognitive function and also contribute to behavioral disturbances.
10. Identify appropriate resources and support groups that may assist the family and caregivers in understanding and coping with this disorder.

Evaluate: Improved level of cognitive functioning in the client with Alzheimer's disease.

Teriparatide acetate

(ter-ih-**PAR**-ah-tyd)
Pregnancy Category: C
Parathar **(Rx)**

How Supplied: *Powder for injection:* 200 U

Action/Kinetics: Teriparatide is a synthetic hormone consisting of the 1–34 fragment of human parathyroid hormone. The drug will initially cause an increased rate of calcium release from bone into blood. The most sensitive indicator for determining the type of hypoparathyroidism is the change in urinary cyclic AMP during the 0–30-min postinfusion period. Clients with hypoparathyroidism will show up to a 10-fold or greater increase over baseline of urinary cyclic AMP in the 0–30-min postinfusion period. Over 90% of these clients will also show a 3-fold or greater increase in urinary phosphate excretion in the 0–60-min postinfusion period. On the other hand, clients with pseudohypoparathyroidism will show less than a 6-fold increase in urinary cyclic AMP excretion in the 0–30-min postinfusion period and less than a 3-fold increase in urinary phosphate excretion in the 0–60-min postinfusion period. **Time to peak excretion of AMP:** During the first 30 min after infusion; **time to peak excretion of phosphate:** during the second 30 min after infusion.

Use: To determine the presence of either hypoparathyroidism or pseudohypoparathyroidism in clients manifesting hypocalcemia.

Dosage

• **IV**

Adults: 5 units/kg infused in 10 mL over 10 min up to a maximum of 200 units. **Pediatric, over 3 years of age:** 3 units/kg, not to exceed 200 units, infused over 10 min.

Administration/Storage

1. The test will distinguish between hypoparathyroidism and pseudohypoparathyroidism but not between these conditions and normal parathyroid function.
2. Clients should be fasting when the drug is administered. To maintain an active urine output during the test, 200 mL water should be ingested per hour for 2 hr before the study as well as during the study.
3. A baseline urine collection should be made during the 60-min period preceding infusion of the drug. Following infusion of the drug, urine should be collected during the 0–30-, 30–60-, and 60–120-min postinfusion periods.
4. Accuracy of the test will be affected by adequate hydration and urine flow, as well as complete collection of urine samples.
5. The reconstituted solution should be used within 4 hr.
6. Have epinephrine 1:1,000 available in the event of an allergic reaction.

Special Concerns: Use with caution during lactation.

Side Effects: *Metabolic:* Hypercalcemia. *GI:* Nausea, diarrhea, abdominal cramps, urge to defecate. *Miscellaneous:* Metallic taste, tingling of extremities, pain at injection site (during or following infusion), ***allergic reactions.***

NURSING CONSIDERATIONS

Assessment

1. Identify indications for testing and any presenting symptoms.
2. Assess urinary output. Document any history of renal dysfunction.
3. Obtain baseline VS and monitor, especially the BP, during the test.

Client/Family Teaching

1. Instruct client to fast for the test.
2. Provide printed guidelines for hydration and preparation for the test.
3. Explain that a metallic taste in the mouth and pain at the injection site may be experienced during drug administration.

Evaluate: Differentiation of hypoparathyroidism (10 times or greater increase of urinary cyclic AMP in 0–30-min postinfusion period) or pseudohypoparathyroidism.

Tiopronin

(tie-oh-**PROH**-nin)
Pregnancy Category: C
Thiola **(Rx)**

How Supplied: *Tablet:* 100 mg
Action/Kinetics: Tiopronin undergoes thiol-disulfide exchange with cystine to form a tiopronin-cystine complex, thus reducing the levels of cystine, which is only sparingly soluble. Reducing cystine levels maintains cystine concentrations below the solubility limit in the urine, thus preventing formation of stones. Up to 48% of the drug will appear in the urine in the first 4 hr following administration and up to 78% by 72 hr.
Uses: Prophylaxis of cystine stone formation. Usually reserved for clients with urinary cystine levels greater than 500 mg/day; those who are resistant to treatment with high fluid intake, alkali and diet modification; and those who show adverse effects to d-penicillamine.

Dosage

- **Tablets**

Prophylaxis of cystine stone formation.

Adults, initial: 800 mg/day in clients with cystine stones; **children,** 15 mg/kg/day. **Maintenance:** Depends on urinary cystine levels and should be based on the dosage required to decrease urinary cystine levels to below its solubility limit (usually <250 mg/L).

Administration/Storage

1. A conservative program including large amounts of fluid and a modest amount of alkali (to maintain urinary pH from 6.5 to 7) in the diet should be tried prior to initiating tiopronin therapy.
2. Maintenance dosage should be given t.i.d. at least 1 hr before or 2 hr after meals.

Contraindications: History of drug-induced agranulocytosis, aplastic anemia, or thrombocytopenia. Lactation.
Special Concerns: Safety and efficacy have not been established in children less than 9 years of age.
Side Effects: *Dermatologic:* Generalized rash—erythematous, maculopapular, morbilliform—accompanied by pruritus. Wrinkling and friability of skin. *Miscellaneous:* Drug fever, lupus erythematosus-like reaction, hypogeusia, vitamin B_6 deficiency.

NURSING CONSIDERATIONS

Assessment

1. Note urinary pH and cystine level prior to initiating therapy.
2. Obtain baseline CBC and liver function studies.

Interventions

1. Monitor and record urinary pH during drug therapy.
2. Measure I&O and promote a high fluid intake (2–3 L/day).
3. Urinary cystine should be measured 1 month after initiation of therapy and every 3 months thereafter.

Client/Family Teaching

1. Take tiopronin only as prescribed on an empty stomach 1 hr before or 2 hr after meals.
2. Drink plenty of fluids (2–3 L/day) during drug therapy. Encourage client to maintain a record of I&O and daily urine pH levels to share with the provider.
3. Provide a printed list and advise the client to report any adverse side effects. Symptoms such as fever, chills, sore throat, or excessive bleeding and bruising may necessitate the discontinuation of drug therapy.
4. Stress the importance of reporting for follow-up lab studies because the dose of drug may need to be adjusted.

Evaluate: ↓ Urinary cystine levels and prevention of cystine stone formation.

APPENDIX ONE

Commonly Used Abbreviations and Symbols

A, aa	of each
ABG	arterial blood gas
a.c.	before meals
ACE	angiotensin-converting enzyme
ACLS	advanced cardiac life support
ACTH	adrenocorticotropic hormone
ad	to, up to
a.d.	right ear
ad lib	as desired, at pleasure
ADA	adenosine deaminase
ADH	antidiuretic hormone
ADL	activities of daily living
AFB	acid fast bacillus
AHF	antihemophilic factor
AIDS	acquired immunodeficiency syndrome
a.l.	left ear
ALT	alanine aminotransferase
A.M., a.m.	morning
AMI	acute myocardial infarction
AML	acute myeloid leukemia
AMP	adenosine monophosphate
ANC	active neutrophil count
ANS	autonomic nervous system
aq	water
aq dest.	distilled water
ARC	AIDS-related complex
ARDS	adult respiratory distress syndrome
ASA	aspirin
ASAP	as soon as possible
AST	aspartate aminotransferase
ATC	around the clock
ATP	adenosine triphosphate
a.u.	each ear, both ears
AV	atrioventricular
AZT	zidovudine
b.i.d.	two times per day
b.i.n.	two times per night
BMR	basal metabolic rate
BP	blood pressure
BPH	benign prostatic hypertrophy
BSA	body surface area
BSE	breast self-exam
BSP	Bromsulphalein

BUN	blood urea nitrogen
C	Centigrade/Celisus
CA	cancer
CABG	coronary artery bypass graft
CAD	coronary artery disease
Caps, caps	capsule(s)
CBC	complete blood count
CD_4	helper T_4 cells
CD_8	suppressor T_8 cells
C&DB	cough and deep breathe
CHF	congestive heart failure
CLL	chronic lymphocytic leukemia
cm	centimeter
CML	chronic myelocytic leukemia
CMV	cytomegalovirus
CN	cranial nerve
CNS	central nervous system
CO	cardiac output
COPD	chronic obstructive pulmonary disease
CPAP	continuous positive airway pressure
CPB	cardiopulmonary bypass
CPR	cardiopulmonary resuscitation
CSF	cerebrospinal fluid
C&S	culture and sensitivity
CT	computerized tomography
CTZ	chemoreceptor trigger zone
CV	cardiovascular
CVA	cerebrovascular accident
CVP	central venous pressure
CXR	chest X ray
d.	day
dATP	deoxy ATP
DBP	diastolic BP
dc	discontinue
DI	diabetes insipidus
DIC	disseminated intravascular coagulation
dil.	dilute
dL	deciliter (one-tenth of a liter)
DNA	deoxyribonucleic acid
dr.	dram (0.0625 ounce)
D5W	5% dextrose in water
EC	enteric-coated
ECB	extracorporeal cardiopulmonary bypass
ECG, EKG	electrocardiogram, electrocardiograph
EDTA	ethylenediaminetetraacetic acid
EENT	eye, ear, nose, and throat
e.g.	for example
elix	elixir
emuls.	emulsion
ESR	erythrocyte sedimentation rate
ET	endotracheal
ext.	extract
F	Fahrenheit, fluoride
FBS	fasting blood sugar
FDA	Food and Drug Administration
FFP	fresh frozen plasma

F/O	follow-up
FSH	follicle-stimulating hormone
g, gm	gram (1,000 mg)
GABA	gamma-aminobutyric acid
GFR	glomerular filtration rate
GI, gi	gastrointestinal
GnRH	gonadotropin-releasing hormone
G6PD	glucose-6-phosphate dehydrogenase
gr	grain
gtt	a drop, drops
GU	genitourinary
h, hr	hour
HA, HAL	hyperalimentation
HCG	human chorionic gonadotropin
HCP	health-care provider
HDL	high density lipoprotein
H&H	hematocrit and hemoglobin
HIV	human immunodeficiency virus
HMG-CoA	3-hydroxy-3-methyl-glutaryl-coenzyme A
HR	heart rate
h.s.	at bedtime
HSV	herpes simplex virus
5-HT	5-hydroxytryptamine
IA	intra-arterial
ICP	intracranial pressure
Ig	immunoglobulin
IM, im	intramuscular
IMV	intermittent mandatory ventilation
IPPB	intermittent positive pressure breathing
ITP	idiopathic thrombocytopenia purpura
IU	international units
IV, iv	intravenous
IVPB	IV piggyback, a secondary IV line
I&O	intake and output
kg	kilogram (2.2 lb)
KVO	keep vein open
L, l	liter (1,000 mL)
Ⓛ	left
LDH	lactic dehydrogenase
LDL	low density lipoprotein
LFT	liver function test
LH	luteinizing hormone
LHRH	luteinizing hormone–releasing hormone
LOC	level of consciousness
LV	left ventricular
M	mix
M^2, m^2	square meter
m., min.	minim
MAO	monoamine oxidase
MAP	mean arterial pressure
max	maximum
mcg	microgram
mCi	millicurie
MDI	metered-dose inhaler
mEq	milliequivalent
mg	milligram

MI	myocardial infarction
MIC	minimum inhibitory concentration
min	minute
mist, mixt	mixture
mL	milliliter
MRI	magnetic resonance imaging
NaCl	sodium chloride
ng	nanogram
NG	nasogastric
NGT	nasogastric tube
NKA	no known allergies
NKDA	no known drug allergies
noct	at night, during the night
non rep	do not repeat
NPO	nothing by mouth
NR	do not refill (e.g., a prescription)
NSAID	nonsteroidal anti-inflammatory drug
NSR	normal sinus rhythm
NSS	normal saline solution
N&V	nausea and vomiting
O_2	oxygen
o.d.	every day
O.D.	right eye
OOB	out of bed
OR	operating room
os	mouth
O.S.	left eye
O_2 sat	oxygen saturation
OTC	over the counter
O.U.	each eye, both eyes
oz.	ounce
PA	pulmonary artery
PABA	para-aminobenzoic acid
PACWP, PAOP	pulmonary artery capillary wedge pressure; pulmonary artery occlusive pressure
PAS	aminosalicylic acid
PBI	protein-bound iodine
p.c.	after meals
PCA	patient-controlled analgesia
PCP	*Pneumocystis carinii* pneumonia
PE	pulmonary embolus
PEEP	positive end expiratory pressure
per	by, through
pH	hydrogen ion concentration
PMH	past medical history
PMS	premenstrual syndrome
PO, po, p.o.	by mouth
PPD	purified protein derivative
PR	by rectum
PRN, p.r.n.	when needed or necessary
PSA	prostatic specific antigen
PT	prothrombin time
PTT	partial thromboplastin time
PUD	peptic ulcer disease
PVC	premature ventricular contraction
PVD	peripheral vascular disease

q.d.	every day
q.h.	every hour
q2h	every two hours
q3h	every three hours
q4h	every four hours
q6h	every six hours
q8h	every eight hours
qhs	every night
q.i.d.	four times per day
q.o.d.	every other day
q.s.	as much as is needed, quantity sufficient
RA	right atrium
RBC	red blood cell
Rept.	let it be repeated
RDA	recommended daily allowance
REM	rapid eye movement
RNA	ribonucleic acid
ROM	range of motion
R/T	related to
RV	right ventricular
Rx	symbol for a prescription
SA	sinoatrial or sustained-action
SAH	subarachnoid hemorrhage
SBE	subacute bacterial endocarditis
SBP	systolic BP
SC, sc, SQ	subcutaneous
SCID	severe combined immunodeficiency disease
SGOT	serum glutamic-oxaloacetic transaminase
SGPT	serum glutamic-pyruvic transaminase
Sig, S.	mark on the label
SIMV	synchronized intermittent mandatory ventilation
SL	sublingual
SLE	systemic lupus erythematosus
SOB	shortness of breath
sol	solution
sp	spirits
SR	sustained-release
ss	one-half
S&S	signs and symptoms
stat	immediately, first dose
STD	sexually transmitted disease
SV	stroke volume
SVT	supraventricular tachycardia
syr	syrup
tab	tablet
TB	tuberculosis
TENS	transcutaneous electric nerve stimulation
t.i.d.	three times per day
t.i.n.	three times per night
T.O.	telephone order
TPN	total parenteral nutrition
TSH	thyroid stimulating hormone
U	unit
μ	micron
μCi	microcurie

µg	microgram
ung	ointment
URTI, URI	upper respiratory infection
USP	U.S. Pharmacopeia
ut dict	as directed
UTI	urinary tract infection
vin	wine
VLDL	very low density lipoprotein
VS	vital signs
V.O.	verbal order
WBC	white blood cell
&	and
>	greater than
<	less than
↑	increased, higher
↓	decreased, lower
-	negative
/	per
%	percent
+	positive
×	times, frequency

APPENDIX TWO

Controlled Substances in the United States and Canada

Controlled Substances Act—United States

The U.S. Federal Controlled Substances Act of 1970 placed drugs controlled by the Act into five categories or schedules based on their potential to cause psychological and/or physical dependence as well as their potential for abuse. The schedules are defined as follows:

Schedule (C-I): Includes substances for which there is a high abuse potential and no current approved medical use (e.g., heroin, marijuana, LSD, other hallucinogens, certain opiates and opium derivatives).

Schedule (C-II): Includes drugs that have a high abuse potential, high ability to produce physical and/or psychological dependence, and for which there is a current approved or acceptable medical use.

Schedule (C-III): Includes drugs for which there is less potential for abuse than drugs in Schedule II and for which there is a current approved medical use. Certain drugs in this category are preparations containing limited quantities of codeine. Also, anabolic steroids are classified in Schedule III.

Schedule (C-IV): Includes drugs for which there is a relatively low abuse potential and for which there is a current approved medical use.

Schedule (C-V): Drugs in this category consist mainly of preparations containing limited amounts of certain narcotic drugs for use as antitussives and antidiarrheals. Federal law provides that limited quantities of these drugs (e.g., codeine) may be bought without a prescription by an individual at least 18 years of age. The product must be purchased from a pharmacist who must keep appropriate records. However, state laws vary, and in many states such products require a prescription.

Controlled Substances—Canada

In Canada, narcotics are governed by the Narcotics Control regulations and are designated by the letter N. Drugs that are considered subject to abuse, which have an approved medical use, and are not narcotics, are designated by the letter C.

Generally prescriptions for Schedule II (high-abuse-potential) drugs cannot be transmitted over the phone and they cannot be refilled. Prescriptions for Schedules III, IV, and V drugs may be refilled up to five times within 6 months. Schedule II drugs are not necessarily "stronger" than drugs in Schedules III, IV, or V; Schedule II drugs are classified as such due to their high abuse potential.

	Drug Schedule	
Drug	*United States*	*Canada*
Alfentanil	II	N
Alprazolam	IV	*
Amobarbital	II	C
Amphetamine	II	Not available
Aprobarbital	III	*
Benzphetamine	III	Not available
Buprenorphine	V	*
Butabarbital	III	C
Butorphanol	*	C
Chloral hydrate	IV	*
Chlordiazepoxide	IV	*
Clonazepam	IV	*
Clorazepate	IV	*
Codeine	II	N
Dextroamphetamine	II	C
Diazepam	IV	*
Diethylpropion	IV	C
Estazolam	IV	*
Ethchlorvynol	IV	*
Fenfluramine	IV	*
Fentanyl	II	N
Flurazepam	IV	*
Glutethimide	III	*
Halazepam	IV	Not available
Hydrocodone	Not available	N
Hydromorphone	II	N
Levomethadyl acetate HC1	II	Not available
Levorphanol	II	N
Lorazepam	IV	*
Mazindol	IV	*
Meperidine	II	N
Mephobarbital	IV	C
Meprobamate	IV	*
Methadone	II	N
Methamphetamine	II	Not available
Metharbital	III	C
Methylphenidate	II	C
Methyprylon	III	*
Midazolam	IV	*
Morphine	II	N
Nalbuphine	*	C
Opium	II	N
Oxazepam	IV	*

Oxycodone	II	N
Oxymorphone	II	N
Paraldehyde	IV	*
Paregoric	III	N
Pemoline	IV	*
Pentazocine	IV	N
Pentobarbital,		
PO, parenteral	II	C
Rectal	III	C
Phendimetrazine	III	Not available
Phenmetrazine	II	Not available
Phenobarbital	IV	C
Phentermine	IV	C
Prazepam	IV	Not available
Propoxyphene	IV	N
Quazepam	IV	Not available
Secobarbital		
PO	II	C
Parenteral	II	*
Rectal	III	*
Sulfentanil	II	N
Talbutal	III	*
Temazepam	IV	*
Triazolam	IV	*
Zolpidem tartrate	IV	*

*Not controlled

APPENDIX THREE

Elements of a Prescription

In order to safely communicate the exact elements desired on a prescription, the following items should be addressed:

A. The prescriber: Name, address, phone number, state license number, and Drug Enforcement Agency (DEA) number (when applicable)
B. The client: Name and address
C. The prescription itself: Name of the medication (generic or trade); quantity to be dispensed (e.g., number of tablets or capsules, 1 vial, 1 tube, volume of liquid); the strength of the medication (e.g., 125-mg tablets, 250 mg/5 mL, 80 mg/1 mL, 10%); and directions for use (e.g., 1 tablet t.i.d.; 2 gtt to each eye q.i.d.; 1 teaspoonful q 8 hr for 10 days; apply a thin film to lesions b.i.d. for 14 days)
D. Other elements: Date prescription is written, signature of the provider, number of refills, and brand product only indication (when applicable).

A typical prescription is depicted as follows:

John Smith, M.D.
1234 N. State Street
Anywhere, PA 12345

Date: Feb. 10, 1995

For: Mary Jones, Age 12
27 East Drive
Anywhere, PA 12345

Rx Amoxicillin 250 mg/5 mL
Disp. 150 mL
Sig: 1 teaspoon PO q 8 hr x 10 days

Refills: 0

Provider signature
State license number

Interpretation of prescription: The above prescription is written by Dr. John Smith for Mary Jones and is for amoxicillin liquid. The concentration desired is 250 mg/5 mL (i.e., 250 mg per teaspoonful). The directions for taking the medication are 1 teaspoon (i.e., 5 mL) by mouth every 8 hr for 10 days. The prescriber wants 150 mL dispensed and there are no refills allowed.

APPENDIX FOUR

Pregnancy Categories: FDA Assigned

A: Adequate and well-controlled studies have failed to demonstrate a risk to the fetus in the first trimester of pregnancy (and there is no evidence of risk in later trimesters).
B: Animal reproduction studies have failed to demonstrate a risk to the fetus and there are no adequate and well-controlled studies in pregnant women.
C: Animal reproduction studies have shown an adverse effect on the fetus and there are no adequate and well-controlled studies in humans, but potential benefits may warrant use of the drug in pregnant women despite potential risks.
D: There is positive evidence of human fetal risk based on adverse reaction data from investigational or marketing experience or studies in humans, but potential benefits may warrant use of the drug in pregnant women despite potential risks.
X: Studies in animals or humans have demonstrated fetal abnormalities and/or there is positive evidence of human fetal risk based on adverse reaction data from investigational or marketing experience and the risks involved in use of the drug in pregnant women clearly outweigh potential benefits.

The use of drugs during pregnancy should be avoided unless the benefits of therapy far outweigh the risk of fetal malformation. This also applies to any OTC drugs, cigarettes, alcohol, excessive caffeine consumption, and street or recreational drugs.

The stages of fetal development include:

1. Days 0–14: Fertilization to implantation
2. Days 18–60: Organogenesis
3. Eight weeks to birth: Organ maturation

APPENDIX FIVE

Commonly Used Laboratory Test Values

Identified normal values will vary depending on the laboratory, quality controls utilized, and methods used for assay. For clarification, check with the laboratory that performed the analysis.

Serum, Plasma, and Blood

Test	Range	Units	SI Range	Units
Acetone, serum	0.3–2.0	mg/dL	51.6–344.0	µmol/L
Acid phosphatase	0.1–5.0	U/L	2.7–10.7	IU/L
Alanine aminotransferase [ALT] (SGPT)	8–20	U/L	8–20	U/L
Albumin, serum	3.5–5.0	g/dL	35–50	g/L
Alcohol (serum levels)				
No significant influence	< 0.05% or 50	mg/dL	10.8	mmol/L
Alcohol influence present	0.05–0.10% or 50–100	mg/dL	10.8–21.6	mmol/L
Reaction time affected	0.10–0.15% or 100–150	mg/dL	21.6–32.5	mmol/L
Indicative of alcohol intoxication	0.15% or 150	mg/dL	32.5	mmol/L
Severe alcohol intoxication	> 0.25% or 250	mg/dL	54.2	mmol/L
Coma	0.30% or 300	mg/dL	65.1	mmol/L

Aldosterone	< 16	ng/dL (fasting)	< 0.45	nmol/L
	4–30	ng/dL (sitting)	0.11–0.84	nmol/L
Alkaline phosphatase	30–120	U/L	0.5–2	μkat/L
Alpha-1-antitrypsin	80–260	mg/dL	0.8–2.6	g/L
Ammonia [NH^+_4]	15–45	μg/dL	11–35	μmol/L
Amylase, serum	60–160	Somogyi U/dL	30–170	U/L
Anion gap	10–17	mEq/L	10–17	mmol/L
Antinuclear antibodies (ANA)	Negative at 1:20 dilution			
Aspartate aminotransferase [AST] (SGOT)	8–33	U/L	8–33	U/L
Bilirubin, total (serum)	0.1–1	mg/dL	2–18	μmol/L
Bilirubin, conjugated (direct)	0.1–0.3	mg/dL	1.7–5.1	μmol/L
Blood urea nitrogen/creatinine ratio	10:1–20:1		Average 15:1	
Calcium, serum	8.8–10.4	mg/dL	2.2–2.58	mmol/L
Calcium, ionized	4.4–5.0	mg/dL	1.1–1.24	mmol/L
Carcinoembryonic antigen (CEA)	<2.5	ng/mL (nonsmoker)	<2.5	μg/L
	<5.0	ng/mL (smoker)	<5.0	μg/L
Ceruloplasmin	18–45	mg/dL	180–450	mg/L
Chloride, serum	95–105	mEq/L	95–105	mmol/L
Cholesterol				
Desirable level	<200	mg/dL	<5.20	mmol/L
Moderate risk	200–240	mg/dL	5.2–6.3	mmol/L
High risk	>240	mg/dL	>6.3	mmol/L
Cold agglutinins	1:8 antibody titer			
Copper	70–140	μg/dL	11–22	μmol/L
Cortisol, serum				
0800 hours	4–19	μg/L	110–520	nmol/L
1600 hours	2–15	μg/L	50–410	nmol/L
2400 hours	5	μg/L	140	nmol/L

Test	Range	Units	SI Range	Units
Creatine kinase (CK)				
Isoenzymes	0–130	U/L	0–2.167	μkat/L
MB fraction	> 5 in MI	%	> 0.05	1
Creatine phosphokinase				
Male	5–35	μg/mL	55–170	U/L
Female	5–25	μg/mL	30–135	U/L
CPK-MB (heart)	0–6%			
Creatinine, serum	0.6–1.2	mg/dL	50–110	μmol/L
Creatinine clearance	75–125	mL/min	1.24–2.08	mL/sec
Erythrocyte count (RBC)				
Male	4.3–5.9	$10^6/mm^3$	4.3–5.9	$10^{12}/L$
Female	3.5–5	$10^6/mm^3$	3.5–5	$10^{12}/L$
Erythrocyte sedimentation rate (ESR)				
Male	0–20	mm/hr	0–20	mm/hr
Female	0–30	mm/hr	0–30	mm/hr
Fibrinogen split products	2–10	μg/mL	Not available	Not available
Free thyroxine index (FTI)	1.1–4.7	mcg/dL		
Gamma-glutamyl transferase (GGT)				
Male	4–23	IU/L	9–69	U/L
Female	3–13	IU/L	4–33	U/L
Gases, arterial blood				
pO_2	75–105	mm Hg	10–14	kPa
pCO_2	35–45	mm Hg	4.7–6	kPa
Glucose, plasma (fasting)	70–110	mg/dL	3.9–6.1	mmol/L
Glucose, postprandial (fasting)	<140	mg/dL/2 hr	<7.77	mmol/L

Test	Conventional values	Conventional units	SI values	SI units
Immunoglobulins (Ig)				
Total	900–2,200	mg/dL	9.0–22.0	g/L
IgG	600–1,900	mg/dL	6.0–19.0	g/L
IgA	60–330	mg/dL	0.6–3.3	g/L
IgM	45–145	mg/dL	0.45–1.45	g/L
IgD	0.5–3.0	mg/dL	0.005–0.03	g/L
IgE	10–506	U/mL	0.1–5.06	U/L
Iron, serum				
Male	80–180	µg/dL	14–32	µmol/L
Female	60–160	µg/dL	11–29	µmol/L
Iron binding capacity	250–460	µg/dL	45–82	µmol/L
Lactic acid				
Arterial	0.5–1.6	mEq/L	0.5–1.6	mmol/L
Venous	0.5–2.2	mEq/L	0.5–2.2	mmol/L
Lactic dehydrogenase (LDH)	70–250	U/L	70–250	U/L
Lead				
Normal	10–20	µg/dL	<0.9	µmol/L
Acceptable	20–40	µg/dL	<1.9	µmol/L
Lipase	14–280	mU/mL	14–280	U/L
	20–180	IU/L		
Lipoproteins				
Low density (LDL)	50–190	mg/dL	1.3–4.9	mmol/L
High density (HDL)				
Male	30–70	mg/dL	0.8–1.8	mmol/L
Female	30–85	mg/dL	0.8–2.2	mmol/L
Leukocyte count (WBC)	4,500–10,000	mm^3	4.5–10	10^9/L
Magnesium, serum	1.8–3	mg/dL	0.8–1.2	mmol/L
	1.6–2.4	mEq/L	0.8–1.2	mmol/L

Test	Range	Units	SI Range	Units
5' Nucleotidase	<17	U/L	<17	U/L
	2–15	IU/L		
Osmolality, plasma	280–300	mOsm/kg	280–300	mmol/kg
Phosphate, serum	2.5–5	mg/dL	0.8–1.6	mmol/L
Potassium, serum	3.5–5	mEq/L	3.5–5	mmol/L
Prostate-specific antigen (PSA)				
Normal	0.4	ng/mL	Not available	Not available
BPH	4–19	ng/mL	Not available	Not available
Prostate CA	10–120	ng/mL	Not available	Not available
Protein				
Total	6–8	g/dL	60–80	g/L
Albumin	3.5–5.0	g/dL	35–50	g/L
Fibrinogen	0.2–0.4	g/dL	2–4	g/L
Globulin	1.5–3.0	g/dL	15–30	g/L
Renin				
Supine	0.2–2.3	ng/mL	0.2–2.3	µg/L
Upright	1.6–4.3	ng/mL	1.6–4.3	µg/L
Reticulocyte count				
Male	0.5–1.5%		$0.005–0.015 \times 10^3$	
Female	0.5–2.5%		$0.005–0.025 \times 10^3$	
Rheumatoid factor	<1:20 titer			
Sodium, serum	135–147	mEq/L	135–147	mmol/L
Thyroid binding globulin (TBG)	12–28	µg/dL	150–360	nmol/L
Thyroid stimulating hormone (TSH)	2–11	µU/mL	2–11	mU/L
Thyroxine (T_4)	5–12	µg/dL	51–142	nmol/L

Thyroxine, free serum	0.8–2.8	ng/dL	10–36	pmol/L
Transferrin	170–370	mg/dL	1.7–3.7	g/L
Triglycerides	< 160	mg/dL	< 1.8	mmol/L
Triiodothyronine (T_3)	0.075–0.2	mg/dL	1.2–3.4	nmol/L
T_3 uptake	25–35%		0.25–0.35	1
T_4	0.8–1.8	ng/dL		
Urea nitrogen	5–20	mg/dL	1.8–7.1	mmol/L
Uric acid				
Male	3.5–7.0	mg/dL	202–416	μmol/L
Female	2.4–6.0	mg/dL	143–357	μmol/L
Zinc protoporphyrin	15–77	μg/dL	0.24–1.23	μmol/L
Zinc, serum	75–150	μg/dL	11.5–23	umol/L

"SI units" is the abbreviation of *Système International d'Unités*. It is a uniform system of reporting numerical values permitting interchangeability of information among nations and between disciplines.

Chernecky, C. C., Krech, R. L., and Berger, B. J. (1993). Laboratory Tests and Diagnostic Procedures. *Philadelphia, PA: W. B. Saunders.*

Jacobs, D. S., Kaster, B. L., Demott, W. R., and Wolfson, W. L. (1988). Laboratory Test Handbook, *2nd ed., St. Louis, MO: Mosby/Lexi-Comp.*

Kee, J. L. (1995). Laboratory and Diagnostic Tests with Nursing Implications, *4th ed., Norwalk, CT: Appleton & Lange.*

Young, D. S. Implementation of SI Units for Clinical Laboratory Data. Annals of Internal Medicine 106:*114–129, 1987. (Courtesy American College of Physicians.)*

ADDITIONAL PHYSIOLOGIC VALUES

HEMATOLOGY

Red blood cell (RBC) count
- Male: 4.3–5.9 × 10^6/mm^3, 4.3–5.9 × 10^{12}/L (SI units)
- Female: 3.5–5 × 10^6/mm^3, 3.5–5.0 × 10^{12}/L (SI units)

RBC indices
- Mean corpuscular hemoglobin (MCH), 27–33 pg (standard and SI)
- Mean corpuscular hemoglobin concentration (MCHC), 33–37 g/dL, 330–370, g/L (SI units)
- Mean corpuscular volume (MCV), 76–100 μm^3, 76–100 fL

Hemoglobin
- Male: 13.5–18 g/dL, 135–180 g/L (SI units)
- Female: 11.5–15.5 g/dL, 115–155 g/L (SI units)
- Glycosylated (HbA_{1c}), < 7.5%

Hematocrit
- Male: 40–52% (0.40–0.52)
- Female: 35–46% (0.35–0.46)

Platelets	130–400 × 10^3/mm^3
White blood cells (leukocytes)	5,000–10,000/mm^3
Neutrophils	50–70%
Segments	50–65%
Bands	0–5%
Basophils	0.25–0.5%
Eosinophils	1–3%
Monocytes	2–6%
Lymphocytes	25–40%
T-lymphocytes	60–80% of lymphocytes
B-lymphocytes	10–20% of lymphocytes
Bleeding time	1–3 min (Duke) 1–5 min (Ivy)
Coagulation time (Lee White)	5–15 min
Prothrombin time	10–15 sec (same as control)
Partial thromboplastin time (PTT)	60–70 sec
Activated partial thromboplastin time (APTT)	30–45 sec
Thrombin time	Within 5 sec of control
INR recommended range	
Standard therapy	2.0–3.0
High-dose therapy	2.5–3.5

BLOOD GASES

Whole blood oxygen, capacity	17–24 vol %
Arterial	
Saturation	96–100% of capacity
pCO_2	35–45 mm Hg
pO_2	75–100 mm Hg
pH	7.38–7.44
Bicarbonate, normal range	24–28 mEq/L
Base excess (BE)	+2 to –2 (±2 mEq/L)
Venous	
Saturation	60–85% capacity
pCO_2	40–54 mm Hg
pO_2	20–50 mm Hg
pH	7.36–7.41

Bicarbonate, normal range	22–28 mEq/L

CEREBROSPINAL FLUID (CSF)

Cell count	0–8/mm^3
Chloride	118–132 mEq/L
Culture	No organisms
Glucose	40–80 mg/dL
Pressure	75–175 cm water
Protein	15–45 mg/dL
Sodium	145–150 mg/dL

URINALYSIS (ROUTINE)

Reference Values (Adult)	
Color	Light straw to dark amber
Appearance	Clear
Odor	Aromatic
Foam	White (small amount)
pH	4.5–8.0 (average is 6)
Specific gravity (SG)	1.005–1.030 (1.015–1.024, normal fluid intake)
Protein	2–8 mg/dL (negative reagent strip test)
Glucose	Negative
Ketones	Negative
Microscopic examination	
RBC	1–2 per low-power field
WBC	3–4
Casts	Occasional hyaline

URINE CHEMISTRY

Aldosterone	2–26 μ/24 hr, 5.6–73 nmol/24 hr (SI units)
Amylase	4–37 U/L/2 hr
Bilirubin and bile	Negative to 0.02 mg/dL
Electrolytes	
Calcium	7.4 mEq/24 hr
Chloride	70–250 mEq/24 hr
Magnesium	15–300 mg/24 hr
Phosphorus, inorganic	0.9–1.3 g/24 hr
Potassium	25–120 mEq/24 hr
Sodium	40–220 mEq/24 hr
Glucose	0
5-Hydroxyindoleacetic acid (HIAA)	2–10 mg/24 hr
Ketones	0
Nitrogenous constituents	
Ammonia	30–50 mEq/24 hr
Creatinine clearance	100–200 mL/min
Creatinine	Males: 20–26 mg/kg/24 hr Females: 14–22 mg/kg/24 hr
Protein	0–5 mg/dL/24 hr
Urea	6–17 g/24 hr
Uric acid	0.25–0.75 g/24 hr
Osmolality	200–1,200 mOsm/L
Porphobilinogen	0.2 mg/24 hr

Steroids	
17-Hydroxycorticosteroids	Males: 5–15 mg/24 hr Females: 3–13 mg/24 hr
17-Ketosteroids	Males: 8–25 mg/24 hr Females: 5–15 mg/24 hr
Urobilinogen	0–4 mg/24 hr
Vanillylmandelic acid (VMA)	1.5–7.5 mg/24 hr

APPENDIX SIX

Nomogram for Estimating Body Surface Area

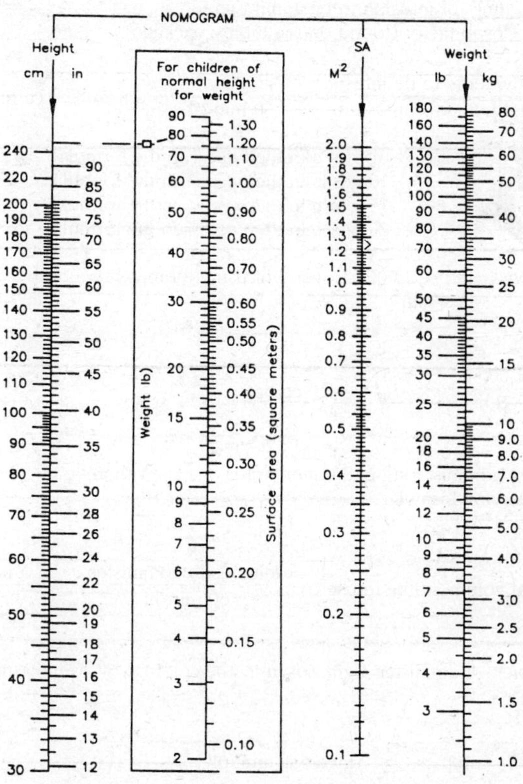

Directions for use: (1) Determine client height. (2) Determine client weight. (3) Draw a straight line to connect the height and weight. Where the line intersects on the SA line is the derived body surface area (M^2).

APPENDIX SEVEN

Easy Formulas for IV Rate Calculation

In order to calculate the continuous drip rate for an IV infusion the following information is necessary:

a. amount of solution to be infused
b. time for infusion to be administered
c. *drop factor (found on the tubing package)

$$\frac{\text{Total volume to be infused}}{\text{Total hours for infusion}} \times \frac{\text{*drop factor}}{\text{60 min/hr}} = \text{gtt/min or cc/hr or mL/hr}$$

*If drop factor is:
60 gtts/min then use 1 in the formula
10 gtts/min then use ⅙ in the formula
15 gtts/min then use ¼ in the formula
20 gtts/min then use ⅓ in the formula

Example: Infuse 1,000 cc over 8 hr using tubing with a drop factor of 10 gtts/min.

$$\frac{\text{1,000 cc}}{\text{8 hr}} \times \frac{1}{6} = \text{20 cc/hr}$$

When administering intermittent infusions, as with antibiotic therapy, use the following formula:

$$\text{Total volume to be infused} \div \frac{\text{minutes to administer}}{\text{60 min/hr}} = \frac{\text{mL}}{\text{hr}}$$

Example: Administer 3 gm Zosyn in 100 cc of D5/W over 45 min

$$100 \div \frac{45}{60} \text{ (invert to multiply)}$$

or

$$100 \times \frac{60}{45} = \text{34 mL/hr}$$

APPENDIX EIGHT

Adult IVPB Medication Administration Guidelines and Riders

Adult IVPB Medication Guidelines

Medication	*Solutions(s)*	*Amount*	*Infuse Over*
Amikin (Amikacin)	D5W; NSS	250–500 mg/ 100 mL	30–60 min
Amphotericin B (Fungizone)	D5W	50 mg/500 mL	6 hr
Ampicillin (Polycillin - N)	NSS	1 g/50 mL	15–30 min
Ancef (Cefazolin Na)	D5W; NSS	1 g/50 mL	40 min
Azactam (Aztreonam)	D5W; NSS	1 g/50 mL	20–30 min
Bactrim (Septra/ Co-Trimoxazole)	D5W	Premixed, usually 5 mL/125 mL sol	60–90 min
Cefotan (Cefotetan disodium)	D5W; NSS	1–2 g/75 mL	30 min
Cipro (Ciprofloxacin)	D5W; NSS	400 mg/200 mL	60 min
Claforan (Cefotaxime)	D5W; NSS	1 g/50 mL	30 min
Cleocin (Clindamycin)	D5W; NSS	300–900 mg/ 100 mL	20–40 min
Decadron (Dexamethasone)	D5W; NSS	40 mg/50 mL	15–30 min
Doxycycline (Vibramycin)	D5W; NSS	100 mg/100 mL	1–2 hr
Erythromycin (Erythrocin)	NSS, RL	500 mg/100 mL	30–60 min
Famotidine (Pepcid)	D5W; NSS	20 mg/50–100 mL	15–30 min
Flagyl (Metronidazole)	Prepackaged	—	60 min
Foscavir (Foscarnet)	D5W	60–90 mg/kg q 8 hr	2 hr
Fortaz (Ceftazidime)	D5W; NSS	1–2 g/100 mL	30 min
Gentamycin (Gentamicin)	D5W; NSS	80 mg/50 mL	30–60 min
Nafcillin (Nafcin)	D5W; NSS	1 g/50–100 mL	30–60 min
Penicillin G	D5W; NSS	5,000,000 U/ 100 mL	40 min
Primaxin (Imipenem-Cilastatin Na)	D5W; NSS	500 mg/100 mL	20–30 min

Medication	*Solutions(s)*	*Amount*	*Infuse Over*
Rocephin (Ceftriaxone Na)	D5W; NSS	1–2 g/100 mL	30 min
Solumedrol (Methylprednisolone)	D5W; NSS	10–250 mg/50 mL	20 min
Tagamet (Cimetidine)	D5W; NSS	300 mg/50 mL	15–20 min
Tetracycline (Achromycin IV)	D5W; NSS	250–500 mg/100 mL	60 min
Tobramycin (Nebcin)	D5W; NSS	80 mg/100 mL	30 min
Vancomycin (Vancocin)	D5W; NSS	1 g/200 mL	60 min
Zantac (Ranitidine HCl)	D5W; NSS	50 mg/100 mL	15–20 min

RIDERS

When ordered for nonemergent IV infusion, the following guidelines may be used for administration:

- Calcium gluconate: 1 ampule Ca gluconate in 100 mL D5W given over 1 hr (each ampule contains approximately 940 mg Ca)

- Magnesium sulfate: 1 g in 100 mL D5W given over 1 hr

- Potassium chloride: 40 mEq in 150 mL D5W given over 4 hr or 60 mEq in 250 mL D5W given over 6 hr. With KCl, a good rule of thumb is not to infuse more than 10 mEq/hr.

- Potassium phosphate: 15 mM phosphate (contains 22 mEq K) in 100 mL D5W given over 2–3 hr

APPENDIX NINE

Drug Preview

Information on the following drugs was received subsequent to the submission of the manuscript. This appendix contains limited information for these drugs; a more complete profile will be included in the next edition of this book.

Abciximab

Pregnancy Category: C
ReoPro **(Rx)**
Classification: Antiplatelet agent

Action/Kinetics: Abciximab is the Fab fragment of the chimeric human-murine monoclonal antibody 7E3. It binds to a glycoprotein receptor on human platelets, thus inhibiting platelet aggregation by preventing the binding of fibrinogen, von Willebrand factor, and other adhesive molecules to receptor sites on activated platelets. **t½, after IV bolus:** 30 min. Platelet function recovers in about 48 hr although the drug remains in the circulation bound to platelets for up to 10 days. Following IV infusion, free drug levels in the plasma decrease rapidly for about 6 hr and then decline at a slower rate.

Uses: Inhibition of platelet aggregation. The drug is used as an adjunct to percutaneous transluminal coronary angioplasty or atherectomy for prophylaxis of acute cardiac ischemic complications in clients at high risk for abrupt closure of the treated coronary vessel. Abciximab is used with aspirin and heparin.

Contraindications: Due to a potential for drug-induced bleeding, abciximab is contraindicated as follows: History of CVA (within 2 years) or CVA with a significant residual neurological deficit; active internal bleeding; within 6 weeks of GI or GU bleeding of clinical significance; bleeding diathesis; within 7 days of administration of oral anticoagulants unless the PT is less than 1.2 times control; thrombocytopenia (less than 100,000 cells/μL); within 6 weeks of major surgery or trauma; intracranial neoplasm; arteriovenous malformation or aneurysm; severe uncontrolled hypertension; presumed or documented history of vasculitis; use of IV dextran before atherectomy or intent to use it during atherectomy; hypersensitivity to murine proteins.

Special Concerns: Benefits versus the risk of increased bleeding should be assessed in clients who weigh less than 75 kg, who are 65 years of age or older, those with a history of GI disease, those receiving thrombolytics, and those receiving heparin. The following conditions are also associated with an increased risk of bleeding in the angioplasty setting and which may be additive to that of abciximab: atherectomy within 12 hr of onset of symptoms for acute MI, atherectomy lasting more than 70 min, and failed atherectomy. Use with caution when abciximab is used with other drugs that affect hemostasis, including thrombolytics, oral anticoagulants, NSAIDs, dipyridamole, and ticlopidine. Use with caution during lactation. Safety and efficacy have not been determined in children.

Side Effects: *CV:* ***Increased bleeding tendencies,*** hypotension, bradycardia, atrial fibrillation or flutter, vascular disorder, pulmonary edema, ***complete AV block,*** supraventricular tachycardia, weak pulse, palpitations, intermittent claudication, pericardial effusion, limb embolism, ***pulmonary embolism, ventricular arrhythmia.*** *GI:*N&V, diarrhea, constipation, ileus. *Hematologic:* Thrombocytopenia, anemia, leukocytosis, hemolytic anemia, petechiae. *CNS:*Hypesthesia, confusion, abnormal thinking, dizziness, ***coma, brain ischemia,*** insomnia. *Respiratory:* Pleural effusion, pleurisy, pneumonia. *Musculoskeletal:* Myopathy, cellulitis, myalgia. *GU:* Urinary tract infection, urinary retention, abnormal renal function. *Miscellaneous:* Pain, peripheral edema, abnormal vision, development of human antichimeric antibody, dysphonia, pruritus.

Dosage

- **IV bolus followed by IV infusion**

Clients undergoing atherectomy with concomitant use of heparin and aspirin.

IV bolus:0.25 mg/kg given 10–60 min before the start of atherectomy. This is followed by **continuous IV infusion:** 10 mcg/min for 12 hr.

NURSING CONSIDERATIONS

Administration/Storage

1. The infusion should be stopped after 12 hr to avoid the effects of prolonged platelet receptor blockade.
2. The continuous infusion of abciximab should be stopped in clients with failed atherectomy as there is no evidence the drug is effective in such situations.
3. Abciximab and heparin should be discontinued if serious bleeding occurs that cannot be controlled by compression.
4. Preparations of abciximab should not be used if they contain visibly opaque particles.
5. If symptoms of an allergic reaction or anaphylaxis occur, the infusion should be stopped immediately and appropriate treatment instituted. Epinephrine, dopamine, theophylline, antihistamines, and corticosteroids should be available for immediate use.
6. The necessary amount (2 mg/mL) of the drug for bolus administration should be withdrawn through a sterile, nonpyrogenic, low-protein-binding 0.2- or 0.22-μm filter into a syringe. The bolus should be given 10–60 min before the procedure.
7. For continuous infusion, withdraw 4.5 mL of abciximab through a sterile, nonpyrogenic, low-protein-binding 0.2- or 0.22-μm filter into a syringe. This should be injected into 250 mL of sterile 0.9% saline or 5% dextrose and infused at a rate of 17 mL/hr (10 mcg/min) for 12 hr using a continuous infusion pump equipped with an in-line sterile, nonpyrogenic, low-protein-binding 0.2- or 0.22-μm filter. Any unused drug should be discarded at the end of the 12-hour infusion.
8. The drug should be given through a separate IV line with no other medication added to the infusion solution. No incompatibilities have been noted with glass bottles or polyvinyl chloride bags or administration sets.
9. Vials should be stored at 2°C–8°C (36°F–46°F) and should not be frozen or shaken.

Assessment

1. Obtain a thorough nursing history.
2. Note any history of CVA, bleeding disorders, recent episodes of bleeding, trauma, or surgery.
3. List other agents prescribed and when last consumed to determine if any enhance the potential for bleeding.
4. Obtain baseline PT, PTT, CBC with differential, VS, and EKG and monitor closely. Check platelet count 2–4 hr after initial bolus and again in 24 hr.

Interventions

1. Anticipate that client undergoing percutaneous transluminal coronary angioplasty (PTCA) and atherectomy will be bolused with abciximab (0.25 mg/kg) 10–60 min before procedure followed by a continous IV infusion of abciximab (10 mcg/min) for 12 hr.

2. Insert lines with saline locks for blood draws.
3. Observe client carefully during abciximab infusion as anaphylaxis may occur at any time.
4. Administer aspirin orally 325 mg 2 hr before procedure and prepare heparin bolus and infusion for administration as prescribed.
5. Observe client carefully for any potential bleeding sites; at all catheter insertion sites, needle puncture sites, GI, GU, and retroperitoneal sites. Remove tape and dressings gently.
6. If serious bleeding develops that cannot be controlled with pressure, stop the infusions of abciximab and heparin.
7. Keep client on complete bedrest while vascular access sheath is in place. Restrain limb in a straight position, and raise HOB no more than 30 degrees. Discontinue heparin infusion at least 4 hr before sheath removal. Monitor distal pulses of involved extremity.
8. Apply pressure for 30 min over femoral artery once sheath is removed. When hemostasis is evident, apply a pressure dressing (sandbag) and check frequently for evidence of bleeding. Monitor any hematoma formation and measure to calculate enlargement. Advise client that bedrest will be enforced for 6–8 hr after abciximab infusion is completed and the sheath has been removed.

Client/Family Teaching

1. Review the indications for therapy, what to expect, how they will be managed clinically, and the anticipated results.
2. Advise client of the risks associated with this therapy, e.g., bleeding from intracranial hemorrhage, which may be lethal, or hematuria or hematemesis, which may require blood and/or platelet transfusions.
3. Explain that this drug may cause the formation of human antichimeric antibody, which may cause allergic or hypersensitivity reactions, thrombocytopenia, or diminshed reponse on readministration.

Evaluate: Prevention of abrupt coronary vessel closure with associated ischemic complications.

Lamotrigine

Pregnancy Category: C
Lamictal **(Rx)**
Classification: Anticonvulsant

See also *Anticonvulsants,* Chapter 36.

Action/Kinetics: Although the mechanism of anticonvulsant action is not known with certainty, lamotrigine may act to inhibit voltage-sensitive sodium channels. This effect stabilizes neuronal membranes and modulates presynaptic transmitter release of excitatory amino acids such as glutamate and aspartate. Lamotrigine is rapidly and completely absorbed after oral use. **Peak plasma levels:** 1.4–4.8 hr following drug administration. The drug is metabolized by the liver with metabolites and unchanged drug excreted mainly through the urine (94%). Lamotrigine induces its own metabolism; also, the drug is eliminated more rapidly in clients who have been taking antiepileptic drugs that induce liver enzymes. However, valproic acid decreases the clearance of lamotrigine.

Uses: As an adjunct in the treatment of partial seizures in adults with epilepsy. *Investigational:* Treat adults with generalized clonic-tonic, absence, atypical absence, and myoclonic seizures. Also, in infants and children with Lennox-Gastaut syndrome.

Contraindication: Use during lactation.

Special Concerns: Safety and efficacy have not been established in children less than 16 years of age, although the drug has been used experimentally in this group. Use with caution in clients with diseases or conditions that could affect metabolism or elimination of the drug, such as in impaired renal, hepatic, or cardiac function.

Side Effects: Side effects listed are those with an incidence of 0.1% or greater. *CNS:* Dizziness, ataxia, somnolence, headache, incoordination, insomnia, tremor, depression, anxiety, irritability, decreased memory, speech disorder, confusion, disturbed concentration, sleep disorder, emotional lability, vertigo, mind racing, amnesia, nervousness, abnormal thinking, abnormal dreams, agitation, akathisia, aphasia, CNS depression, depersonalization, dyskinesia, dysphoria, euphoria, faintness, hallucinations, hostility, hyperkinesia, hypesthesia, myoclonus, panic attack, paranoid reaction, personality disorder, psychosis, stupor. *GI:* N&V, diarrhea, dyspepsia, constipation, tooth disorder, anorexia, dry mouth, abdominal pain, dysphagia, flatulence, gingivitis, gum hyperplasia, increased appetite, increased salivation, abnormal liver function tests, mouth ulceration, stomatitis, thirst. *CV:* Hot flashes, palpitations, flushing, migraine, syncope, tachycardia, vasodilation. *Musculoskeletal:* Arthralgia, joint disorder, myasthenia, dysarthria, muscle spasm, twitching. *Hematologic:* Anemia, ecchymosis, leukocytosis, leukopenia, lymphadenopathy, petechia. *Respiratory:* Rhinitis, pharyngitis, increased cough, dyspnea, epistaxis, hyperventilation. *Dermatologic:* Rash (may be severe enough to require hospitalization), pruritus, alopecia, acne, dry skin, eczema, erythema, hirsutism, maculopapular rash, sweating, urticaria. *Ophthalmologic:* Diplopia, blurred vision, nystagmus, abnormal vision, abnormal accommodation, conjunctivitis, oscillopsia, photophobia. *GU:* Dysmenorrhea, vaginitis, amenorrhea, female lactation, hematuria, polyuria, urinary frequency or incontinence, UTI, vaginal moniliasis. *Body as a whole:* ***Possibility of sudden unexplained death in epilepsy,*** flu syndrome, fever, infection, neck pain, malaise, ***seizure exacerbation,*** chills, halitosis, facial edema, weight gain or loss, peripheral edema, hyperglycemia. *Miscellaneous:* Ear pain, tinnitus, taste perversion.

*Symptoms of Overdose:*Possibility of dizziness, headache, somnolence, coma.

Drug Interactions

Carbamazepine / Lamotrigine concentration is ↓ by about 70%
Phenobarbital / Lamotrigine concentration is ↓ by about 50%
Phenytoin / Lamotrigine concentration is ↓ by 45%–54%
Primidone / Lamotrigine concentration is ↓ by about 40%
Valproic acid / Lamotrigine concentration is ↓ twofold while valproic acid concentration is ↓ by 25%

Dosage

- **Tablets**

Treatment of partial seizures.

Adults and children over 16 years of age who are taking enzyme-inducing antiepileptic drugs, but not valproate: 50 mg once a day for weeks 1 and 2, followed by 100 mg/day in two divided doses for weeks 3 and 4. **Maintenance dose:** 300–500 mg/day given in two divided doses. The dose should be increased by 100 mg/day every week until maintenance levels are reached. **Adults and children over 16 years of age who are taking enzyme-inducing antiepileptic drugs plus valproic acid:** 25 mg every other day for weeks 1 and 2, followed by 25 mg once daily for weeks 3 and 4. **Maintenance dose:** 100–150 mg/day in two divided doses. The dose should be increased by 25–50 mg/day every 1–2 weeks.

NURSING CONSIDERATIONS

See also *Nursing Considerations* for *Anticonvulsant Drugs,* Chapter 36.

Administration/Storage

1. The dosage of lamotrigine should be based on the therapeutic

response since a therapeutic plasma level has not been determined.
2. If a change in seizure control or worsening of side effects is noted in clients receiving lamotrigine in combination with other antiepileptic drugs, a reevaluation of all the drugs in the regimen should be considered.
3. Discontinuing an enzyme-inducing antiepileptic drug should prolong the half-life of lamotrigine whereas discontinuing valproic acid should shorten the half-life of lamotrigine.
4. If it is decided to discontinue lamotrigine therapy, a stepwise reduction of dose over 2 weeks (about 50% per week) is recommended unless safety concerns mandate a more rapid withdrawal.

Assessment
1. Document indications for therapy, onset of symptoms, previous agents used, and the outcome.
2. If client also prescribed other anticonvulsant agents (i.e., valproate, carbamazepine) monitor closely for evidence of adverse effects.
3. Obtain baseline CBC and liver and renal function studies and anticipate reduced dose with liver or renal dysfunction.

Client/Family Teaching
1. Do not stop drug abruptly as this may result in an increase in seizure frequency. Notify provider as drug should be gradually decreased over at least 2 weeks unless safety concerns require rapid withdrawal.
2. Do not perform activities that require mental alertness and/or coordination until drug effects realized as drug may cause dizziness, ataxia, somnolence, headache and blurred vision.
3. Advise that a rash may occur and should be reported immediately so provider can determine if therapy should be interrupted.
4. Photosensitization may occur; wear protective clothing, sunscreen, and sunglasses until tolerance determined.
5. Review drug side effects, stressing those that require immediate reporting, e.g., loss of seizure control, rash.

Evaluate: Control of seizure activity.

Metformin hydrochloride

Pregnancy Category B
Glucophage **(Rx**
Classification: Oral antidiabetic

Action/Kinetics: Metformin is not chemically or pharmacologically related to the oral sulfonylureas. The drug decreases hepatic glucose production, decreases intestinal absorption of glucose, and increases peripheral uptake and utilization of glucose. Metformin does not cause hypoglycemia in either diabetic or nondiabetic clients, and it does not cause hyperinsulinemia. Insulin secretion remains unchanged, while fasting insulin levels and day-long plasma insulin response may decrease. In contrast to sulfonylureas, the body weight of clients treated with metformin remains stable or may decrease somewhat. Food decreases the extent and slightly delays the absorption of metformin. It is negligibly bound to plasma protein; steady state plasma levels (less than 1 mcg/mL) are reached within 24–48 hr. Metformin is excreted unchanged in the urine, and there is no biliary excretion. t½, plasma elimination: 6.2 hr. The plasma and blood half-lives of metformin are prolonged in clients having decreased renal function.

Uses: Alone as an adjunct to diet to lower blood glucose in clients having noninsulin-dependent diabetes mellitus whose blood glucose cannot be managed satisfactorily via diet alone. Also, metformin may be used concomitantly with a sulfonylurea when diet and metformin or a sulfonylurea alone do not result in adequate control of blood glucose.

Contraindications: Renal disease or dysfunction (serum creatinine levels greater than 1.5 mg/dL in males and greater than 1.4 mg/dL in females) or abnormal creatinine clearance due to cardiovascular collapse, acute MI, or septicemia. In clients undergoing radiologic studies using iodinated contrast media, because use of such products may cause alteration of renal function, leading to acute renal failure and lactic acidosis. Acute or chronic metabolic acidosis, including diabetic ketoacidosis, with or without coma. Lactation.

Special Concerns: Cardiovascular collapse, acute CHF, acute MI, and other conditions characterized by hypoxia have been associated with lactic acidosis, which may also be caused by metformin. Use of oral hypoglycemic agents may increase the risk of cardiovascular mortality. Although hypoglycemia does not usually occur with metformin, it may result with deficient caloric intake, strenuous exercise not supplemented by increased intake of calories, or when metformin is taken with sulfonylureas or alcohol. Because of age-related decreases in renal function, use with caution as age increases. Safety and efficacy have not been determined in children.

Side Effects: *Metabolic:* Lactic acidosis (fatal in approximately 50% of cases). *GI:* Diarrhea, N&V, abdominal bloating, flatulence, anorexia, unpleasant or metallic taste. *Hematologic:* Asymptomatic subnormal serum vitamin B_{12} levels.

Symptom of Overdose: Lactic acidosis.

Drug Interactions

Alcohol / Alcohol ↑ the effect of metformin on lactate metabolism

Cimetidine / Cimetidine ↑ (by 60%) peak metformin plasma and whole blood levels

Furosemide / Furosemide ↑ metformin plasma and blood levels; also, metformin ↓ the half-life of furosemide

Iodinated contrast media / ↑ Risk of acute renal failure and lactic acidosis

Nifedipine / Nifedipine ↑ the absorption of metformin, leading to ↑ plasma metformin levels

Dosage

• Tablets

Noninsulin-dependent diabetes mellitus.

Adults, using 500-mg tablet: Starting dose is one 500-mg tablet b.i.d. given with the morning and evening meals. Dosage increases may be made in increments of 500 mg every week, given in divided doses, up to a maximum of 2,500 mg/day. If a 2,500-mg daily dose is required, it may be better tolerated when given in divided doses t.i.d. with meals.

Adults, using 850-mg tablet: Starting dose is 850 mg once daily given with the morning meal. Dosage increases may be made in increments of 850 mg every other week, given in divided doses, up to a maximum of 2,550 mg/day. **Usual maintenance dose:** 850 mg b.i.d. with the morning and evening meals. However, some clients may require 850 mg t.i.d. with meals.

NURSING CONSIDERATIONS

Administration/Storage

1. Dosage must be individualized based on tolerance and effectiveness.

2. Dosage should be given with meals starting at a low dose with gradual escalation. This will reduce GI side effects and allow determination of the minimal dose necessary for adequate control of blood glucose.

3. No transition period is required when transferring clients from standard oral hypoglycemic drugs (other than chlorpropamide) to metformin. When transferring from chlorpropamide, caution should be exercised during the first two weeks because of chlorpropamide's long duration of action.

4. If the maximum dose of metformin for 4 weeks does not provide adequate control of blood glu-

cose, gradual addition of an oral sulfonylurea (data are available for glyburide, chlorpropamide, tolbutamide, and glipizide) may be considered, while maintaining the maximum dose of metformin. The desired control of blood glucose may be attained by adjusting the dose of each drug.
5. If client does not respond to 1–3 months of concomitant metformin and oral sulfonylurea therapy, consideration should be given to initiating insulin therapy and discontinuing the oral agents.
6. The initial and maintenance doses of metformin in geriatric and debilitated clients should be conservative because of the potential for decreased renal function. These clients should not be titrated to the maximum dose.

Assessment

1. Document onset of diabetes, previous therapies utilized, and the outcome.
2. Obtain baseline CBC, BS, and liver and renal function studies; evaluate periodically.
3. Note any evidence of liver or renal failure, because this may precipitate the development of lactic acidosis.
4. Assess for any evidence of metabolic acidosis (i.e., serum lactate levels greater than 5 mmol/L, decreased blood pH or increased anion gap from baseline), because drug is contraindicated.

Interventions

1. Drug may be administered alone or with a sulfonylurea.
2. Do not administer if client is to undergo procedures utilizing iodinated contrast agents.
3. If anemia develops, exclude vitamin B_{12} deficiency, because drug may interfere with B_{12} absorption.
4. If surgery is scheduled, withhold metformin and do not administer until client resumes normal diet.
5. Observe for any sudden changes in a stabilized client that may indicate evidence of ketoacidosis or lactic acidosis; hold drug and report.

Client/Family Teaching

1. Take with food to diminish GI upset.
2. May cause a metallic taste, which will gradually subside.
3. Reinforce that regular exercise, decreased caloric intake, and weight loss are the recommended primary treatment forms to reduce blood glucose levels in Type II diabetes. Stress that medication neither replaces nor excuses compliance with these modalities.
4. Advise that inadequate caloric intake or strenuous exercise without caloric replacement may precipitate hypoglycemia.
5. Stress the importance of regular blood sugar monitoring (fingersticks) at different times during the day and maintaining a written record for provider review.
6. Review the S&S of hypoglycemia (e.g., fatigue, headache, tremors, moist pale skin, etc.) and recommend appropriate actions to correct.
7. Avoid alcohol and any situations that may precipitate dehydration.
8. Advise to consume plenty of fluids and to notify provider when illnesses with fever, vomiting, and diarrhea are persistent and severe.
9. Stop drug and immediately report any of the following symptoms: difficulty breathing, severe weakness or muscle pains, increased sleepiness, or sudden increased abdominal distress.

Evaluate:

• Control of serum glucose levels with prevention of microvascular complications
• Glycosolated hemoglobin within desired range (usually less than 8%)

Nefazodone hydrochloride

Pregnancy Category: C
Serzone **(Rx)**
Classification: Antidepressant

Action/Kinetics: Although the exact antidepressant mechanism is not known, nefazodone inhibits neuronal uptake of serotonin and norepinephrine. The drug antagonizes central 5-HT_2 receptors and alpha-1-adrenergic receptors (which may cause postural hypotension). **Peak plasma levels:** 1 hr. **t½:** 2–4 hr. The drug is extensively metabolized by the liver with less than 1% excreted unchanged in the urine. Nefazodone is an in vitro inhibitor of cytochrome P-450IIIA4 and, as such, may result in drug interactions with other drugs that are metabolized by the same system. Food delays the absorption of nefazodone and decreases the bioavailability by approximately 20%.

Use: Treatment of depression. Use for more than 6–8 weeks has not been studied adequately.

Contraindications: Use with terfenadine or astemizole. Clients hypersensitive to nefazodone or other phenylpiperazine antidepressants. Use in combination with a MAO inhibitor or within 14 days of discontinuing MAO inhibitor therapy.

Special Concerns: Use with caution in clients with a recent history of MI, unstable heart disease in those taking digoxin, and in those with a history of mania. Use with caution during lactation. Safety and efficacy have not been determined in individuals below 18 years of age. There is a possibility of a suicide attempt in depression that may persist until significant remission occurs.

Side Effects: *CNS:* Dizziness, insomnia, agitation, somnolence, lightheadedness, activation of mania or hypomania, confusion, memory impairment, paresthesia, abnormal dreams, decreased concentration, ataxia, incoordination, psychomotor retardation, tremor, hypertonia, decreased libido, vertigo, twitching, depersonalization, hallucinations, ***suicide thoughts/attempt***, apathy, euphoria, hostility, abnormal gait, abnormal thinking, derealization, paranoid reaction, dysarthria, myoclonus, ***neuroleptic malignant syndrome (rare)***. *CV:* Postural hypotension, hypotension, sinus bradycardia, tachycardia, hypertension, syncope, ventricular extrasystoles, angina pectoris, ***CVA (rare)***. *GI:* Nausea, dry mouth, constipation, dyspepsia, diarrhea, increased appetite, vomiting, eructation, periodontal abscess, gingivitis, colitis, gastritis, mouth ulceration, stomatitis, esophagitis, peptic ulcer, rectal hemorrhage. *Dermatologic:* Pruritus, dry skin, acne, alopecia, urticaria, maculopapular rash, vesiculobullous rash, eczema. *Musculoskeletal:* Asthenia, arthralgia, arthritis, tenosynovitis, muscle stiffness, bursitis. *Respiratory:* Pharyngitis, increased cough, dyspnea, bronchitis, asthma, pneumonia, laryngitis, voice alteration, epistaxis, hiccups. *Hematologic:* Ecchymosis, anemia, leukopenia, lymphadenopathy. *Ophthalmologic:* Blurred vision, abnormal vision, visual field defect, dry eye, eye pain, abnormal accommodation, diplopia, conjunctivitis, mydriasis, keratoconjunctivitis, photophobia, night blindness. *Body as a whole:* Headache, infection, flu syndrome, chills, fever, neck rigidity, allergic reaction, malaise, photosensitivity, facial edema, hangover effect, enlarged abdomen, hernia, pelvic pain, halitosis, cellulitis, weight loss, gout, dehydration. *GU:* Urinary frequency, UTI, urinary retention, vaginitis, breast pain, cystitis, urinary urgency, metrorrhagia, amenorrhea, polyuria, vaginal hemorrhage, breast enlargement, menorrhagia, urinary incontinence, abnormal ejaculation, hematuria, nocturia, kidney calculus. *Miscellaneous:* Peripheral edema, thirst, abnormal liver function tests, ear pain, hyperacusis, deafness, taste loss.

Symptoms of Overdose: N&V, somnolence, increased incidence of severity of any of the reported side effects.

Drug Interactions

Alprazolam / ↑ Plasma levels of alprazolam

Astemizole / ↑ Plasma levels of astemizole resulting in QT prolongation and possible serious CV

events, including death due to ventricular tachycardia of the torsades de pointes type
Digoxin / ↑ Plasma levels of digoxin
MAO inhibitors / Serious and possibly fatal reactions including symptoms of hyperthermia, rigidity, myoclonus, autonomic instability with possible rigid fluctuations of VS, and mental status changes that may include extreme agitation progressing to delirium and coma
Propranolol / ↓ Plasma levels of propranolol
Terfenadine / ↑ Plasma levels of terfenadine resulting in QT prolongation and possible serious CV events, including death due to ventricular tachycardia of the torsades de pointes type
Triazolam / ↑ Plasma levels of triazolam
Laboratory Test Interferences: ↑ AST, ALT, LDH. ↓ Hematocrit. Hypercholesterolemia, hypoglycemia.

Dosage

• **Tablets**

Antidepressant.

Adults, initial: 200 mg/day given in two divided doses. Increase dose in increments of 100–200 mg/day at intervals of no less than 1 week. The effective dose range is 300–600 mg/day. The initial dose for elderly or debilitated clients is 100 mg/day given in two divided doses.

NURSING CONSIDERATIONS

Administration/Storage

1. Several weeks may be required for the full beneficial effect to be observed.
2. Although long-term use has not been studied, it is usually recommended that the drug be given for a period of 6 months or longer.
3. At least 14 days should elapse between discontinuation of a MAO inhibitor and initiation of therapy with nefazodone; also, at least 7 days should elapse after stopping nefazodone and before starting an MAO inhibitor.
4. *Treatment of Overdose:*Treatment should be symptomatic and supportive in the cases of hypotension or excessive sedation. Gastric lavage may be used.

Assessment

1. Document indications for therapy, type and onset of symptoms, and any underlying or precipitating factors.
2. List drugs currently prescribed to ensure none interact unfavorably.
3. Determine any history of CAD, recent MI, or conditions requiring digoxin administration.

Client/Family Teaching

1. Take before meals because food may inhibit absorption.
2. Do not perform activities that require mental alertness or coordination until drug effects realized as drug may cause dizziness, somnolence, confusion, incoordination, and decreased concentration and response time.
3. Avoid alcohol and any other CNS depressants. Notify provider before taking any OTC agents or other prescribed agents as many have the potential to interact unfavorably.
4. Advise that it may take several weeks before any effects are realized and not to become discouraged and stop the medication.
5. Stress that therapy must continue with provider supervision once effects are attained in order for client to continue to experience these benefits.
6. Advise client to report any unusual sensations or side effects. Counsel family to observe for any evidence of increased depression or suicidal thoughts/behavior and to report if evident.
7. Use reliable birth control during therapy.

Evaluate

• Reports of symptomatic improvement
• ↓ Symptoms of depression, as evidenced by improved sleeping and eating patterns, ↓ fatigue, and ↑ social involvement and activity

Index

Boldface = generic drug name
italics = therapeutic drug class
Regular type = trade names
CAPITALS = combination drugs

Boldface = generic drug name
italics = therapeutic drug class
Regular type = trade names
CAPITALS = combination drugs

Dicyclomine hydrochloride (Bentyl), **788**
Di-Cyclonex **(Dicyclomine hydrochloride)**, 788
Didanosine (Videx), **219-222**
Dideoxycytidine (Hivid), **236-238**
dideoxyinosine (Videx), **219-222**
Didrex **(Benzphetamine hydrochloride)**, 754
Didronel **(Etidronate disodium)**, 1155
Didronel IV **(Etidronate disodium)**, 1155
Diethylpropion hydrochloride (Tenuate, Tepanil), **756**
Diethylstilbestrol diphosphate (Stilphostrol), **1095-1097**
DIFENOXIN HYDROCHLORIDE WITH ATROPINE SULFATE (Motofen), 984-985
Diflucan **(Fluconazole)**, 161
Diflunisal (Dolobid), **675-677**
Digibind **(Digoxin Immune Fab)**, 1253
Digitaline ✱ **(Digitoxin)**, 484
Digitoxin (Digitaline), **484-485**
Digoxin (Lanoxin), **485-486**
Digoxin Immune Fab (Digibind), **1253-1254**
Dihydrex **(Diphenhydramine hydrochloride)**, 909
Dihydroergotamine mesylate (D.H.E. 45), **827-828**
Dihydroxyaluminum sodium carbonate (Rolaids Antacid), **962**
Dilacor XR **(Diltiazem hydrochloride)**, 426
Dilantin Infatab **(Phenytoin)**, 544
Dilantin Kapseals **(Phenytoin sodium, extended)**, 544
Dilantin Sodium **(Phenytoin sodium, parenteral)**, 544
Dilantin-30 Pediatric **(Phenytoin)**, 544
Dilantin-125 **(Phenytoin)**, 544
Dilatrate-SR **(Isosorbide dinitrate extended-release capsules)**, 386
Dilaudid **(Hydromorphone hydrochloride)**, 714
Dilaudid-HP **(Hydromorphone hydrochloride)**, 714
Dilomine **(Dicyclomine hydrochloride)**, 788
Diltiazem hydrochloride (Cardizem), **426-429**
Dimelor ✱ **(Acetohexamide)**, 1028
Dimenhydrinate (Dramamine), **908-909**
Dimenhydrinate Injection ✱ **(Dimenhydrinate)**, 908
Dimentabs **(Dimenhydrinate)**, 908
Dimercaprol (BAL In Oil), **1255-1256**
Dimetane **(Brompheniramine maleate)**, 905
DIMETANE DECONGESTANT ELIXIR AND TABLETS, 936
Dimetane Extentabs **(Brompheniramine maleate)**, 905
Dimetane-Ten **(Brompheniramine maleate)**, 905
DIMETAPP COLD & ALLERGY CHEWABLE TABLETS, 936
DIMETAPP COLD & FLU CAPLETS, 936
DIMETAPP DM ELIXIR, ELIXIR, EXTENTABS, LIQUIGELS, SINUS CAPLETS, TABLETS, 936
Dinate **(Dimenhydrinate)**, 908
Dinoprostone (Prepidil Gel), **1138-1139**
Diocarpine ✱ **(Pilocarpine hydrochloride)**, 775
Diocto **(Docusate sodium)**, 974
Diocto-K **(Docusate potassium)**, 974
Dioctyl calcium sulfosuccinate (Surfak), **974-975**
Dioctyl potassium sulfosuccinate (Dialose), **974-975**
Dioctyl sodium sulfosuccinate (Colace), **974-975**
Dioeze **(Docusate sodium)**, 974
Diogent ✱ **(Gentamicin sulfate)**, 10
Diomycin ✱ **(Erythromycin base)**, 72
Dionephrine ✱ **(Phenylephrine hydrochloride)**, 816
Diosulf ✱ **(Sulfacetamide sodium)**, 109
Dipalmitoylphosphatidylcholine (Exosurf Neonatal), **921-923**
Dipentum **(Olsalazine sodium)**, 666
Diphen Cough **(Diphenhydramine hydrochloride)**, 909
Diphenacen-10 and -50 **(Diphenhydramine hydrochloride)**, 909
Diphenadryl **(Diphenhydramine hydrochloride)**, 909
Diphenhydramine hydrochloride (Benadryl), **909-910**
DIPHENOXYLATE HYDROCHLORIDE WITH ATROPINE SULFATE (Lomotil), 985
Diphenylan Sodium **(Phenytoin sodium prompt)**, 544
Diphenylhydantoin (Dilantin), **544-550**
Diphenylsulfone (Avlosulfon), **201-202**
Diprolene **(Betamethasone dipropionate)**, 1075

Boldface = generic drug name
italics = therapeutic drug class
Regular type = trade names
CAPITALS = combination drugs

Boldface = generic drug name
italics = therapeutic drug class
Regular type = trade names
CAPITALS = combination drugs

Boldface = generic drug name
italics = therapeutic drug class
Regular type = trade names
CAPITALS = combination drugs